Companion CD

ANATOMY REVIEWS

Changes in Circulation at Birth (Ch. 25)
Conduction System of the Heart (Ch. 25)
Direction of Heart Sounds (Ch. 6)
External and Internal Structures of the Nose (Ch. 6)
External, Middle, and Inner Ear (Ch. 6)
Imaginary Landmarks of the Chest (Ch. 6)
Interior Structures of the Mouth (Ch. 6)
Landmarks of the Pinna (Ch. 6)
Location of Hernias (Ch. 6)
Location of Pulses (Ch. 6)
Location of Retractions (Ch. 23)
Location of Sinuses (Ch. 6)
Location of Sutures and Fontanels (Ch. 8)
Location of Tonsillar Masses (Ch. 23)
Rib Cage (Ch. 6)
Structure of the Eye (Ch. 6)
Structures in the Neck (Ch. 6)
Superficial Lymph Nodes (Ch. 6)

ANIMATIONS

Abdominal Anatomy (Ch. 6)
Adrenal Function (Ch. 29)
Appendicitis (Ch. 24)
Asthma (Ch. 23)
Bag Ventilation (Ch. 23)
Bladder (Ch. 27)
Bone Fractures (Ch. 31)
Brain Lobes (Ch. 28)
Bronchi and Bronchioles (Ch. 23)
Burns in Children (Ch. 30)
Cardiac Tamponade, Infant (Ch. 25)
Catheter Placement, Umbilical Vein (Ch. 25)
Central Venous Access via Femoral Vein (Ch. 22)
Central Venous Access via Jugular Vein (Ch. 22)
Cervical Nerve Examination (Ch. 28)
Cranial Nerves (Ch. 6)
Digestive Tract, Passage of Food (Ch. 24)
Erb's Palsy (Ch. 9)
Foley Catheter Insertion (Ch. 22)
Guillain-Barré Syndrome (Ch. 32)
Heart Sounds (Ch. 25)
Hemophilia A (Ch. 26)
Intubation (Ch. 23)
Intubation in Infant (Ch. 23)
Intubation, Incorrect Placement (Ch. 23)
IV Line Placement (Ch. 22)
Kidney Function (Ch. 27)
Lumbar Puncture, Infant (Ch. 22)
Lung Sounds (Ch. 23)
Organ Systems 3-D Tour (Ch. 6)
PICC Line Placement (Ch. 22)
Platelets and Blood Clotting (Ch. 26)
Respiratory Failure, Infant (Ch. 23)
Seizure, Generalized (Ch. 28)
Shoulder Dystocia (Ch. 9)

Sickle Cell Anemia (Ch. 26)
Spine Structure (Ch. 31)
Structure of the Heart (Ch. 25)
Subaortic Stenosis (Ch. 25)
Subdural Hematoma (Ch. 28)
Ventriculoperitoneal Shunt (Ch. 28)
Volvulus, Pediatric (Ch. 24)

CASE STUDIES

Acne Vulgaris (Ch. 30)
Acute Diarrhea (Gastroenteritis) (Ch. 24)
Acute Epiglottitis (Ch. 23)
Acute Lymphoblastic Leukemia (Ch. 26)
Appendicitis (Ch. 24)
Asthma (Ch. 23)
Attention Deficit/Hyperactivity Disorder (Ch. 17)
Bacterial Conjunctivitis (Ch. 14)
Behaviors Indicative of Future Child Abuse (Ch. 14)
Breast-Feeding (Ch. 8)
Bronchiolitis (Ch. 23)
Burns (Ch. 30)
Chickenpox (Varicella) (Ch. 14)
Child Abuse (Ch. 14)
Cleft Lip and Palate (Ch. 24)
Communicating with Adolescents (Ch. 6)
Cultural Considerations (Ch. 4)
Cystic Fibrosis (Ch. 23)
Dehydration and Diarrhea (Ch. 24)
Developmental Dysplasia of the Hip (Ch. 31)
Diabetes Mellitus (Ch. 29)
Down Syndrome (Ch. 19)
Family Functioning (Ch. 3)
Fractures (Ch. 31)
Health Problems of Infants (Ch. 11)
Health Problems of the Newborn (Ch. 9)
Heavy Metal Poisoning (Ch. 14)
Home Care (Ch. 20)
Hydrocephalus with Myelomeningocele (Ch. 28)
Immunizations (Ch. 10)
Impetigo (Ch. 30)
Infant Growth and Development (Ch. 10)
Ingestion of an Injurious Agent (Ch. 14)
Injury Prevention (Ch. 15)
Meningitis (Ch. 28)
Mononucleosis (Ch. 23)
Osteomyelitis (Ch. 31)
Patent Ductus Arteriosus (Ch. 25)
Pediatric Assessment (Ch. 6)
Pediatric Procedures (Ch. 22)
Poison Ivy (Ch. 30)
Salicylate Ingestion (Ch. 14)
Sickle Cell Anemia (Ch. 26)
Sleep Problems (Ch. 13)
Teen Smoking (Ch. 17)
The Dying Child (Ch. 18)
The Normal Newborn (Ch. 8)
Toilet Training/Toddler Development (Ch. 12)

Tonsillitis (Ch. 23)
Varicella in Spite of Vaccine (Ch. 14)

CRITICAL THINKING EXERCISES

Abdominal Pain (Ch. 24)
Bleeding (Ch. 26)
Bone Marrow Test (Ch. 26)
Cardiac Catheterization (Ch. 25)
Cardiovascular Assessment (Ch. 6)
Central Venous Access Device (Ch. 22)
Circumcision (Ch. 8)
Conjunctivitis (Ch. 14)
Constipation (Ch. 24)
Cystic Fibrosis Inheritance Risks (Ch. 23)
Depression (Ch. 17)
Diagnosis of Down Syndrome in the Neonate (Ch. 18)
Digoxin Administration (Ch. 25)
Discharge Planning (Ch. 21)
Down Syndrome (Ch. 18)
Fetal Alcohol Syndrome/Effects (Ch. 9)
Formula Preparation (Ch. 8)
Fragile X Syndrome (Ch. 18)
Growth Trends During Infancy (Ch. 5)
Guillain-Barré Syndrome (Ch. 32)
Hematemesis (Ch. 24)
HIV Testing in Children (Ch. 26)
Home Care for the Adolescent (Ch. 24)
Hypothyroidism (Ch. 29)
Imitative Play (Ch. 13)
Infant of a Diabetic Mother (Ch. 9)
Infant Safety (Ch. 10)
Ingestion of a Foreign Body (Ch. 23)
Injury Prevention (Ch. 15)
Jaundice (Ch. 9)
Myelomeningocele (Ch. 32)
Neonatal Loss (Ch. 18)
Obesity (Ch. 17)
Osteogenic Sarcoma (Ch. 31)
Patent Ductus Arteriosus (Ch. 9, 25)
Poisoning (Ch. 14)
Seizures (Ch. 28)
Shock (Ch. 25)
The High-Risk Newborn (Ch. 9)
The Interview (Ch. 6)
Turner Syndrome (Ch. 17)

NCLEX REVIEW QUESTIONS

For every chapter

PEDIATRIC ASSESSMENT VIDEO CLIPS

General Assessment (Ch. 6)
Abdomen
Abdomen, Umbilicus
Ankles and Feet, Posterior
Brachial and Femoral Pulses
Breath Sounds, Anterior Chest
Breath Sounds, Posterior Chest
Chest and Abdomen
Chest and Lungs, Posterior
Deep Tendon Reflex, Patellar Tendon

Ear Canal
External Eye
External Genitalia, Female Infant
External Genitalia, Female Neonate
Extraocular Movement
Eye Fixation Using the Cover-Uncover Test
Fine Motor Coordination, Upper Extremities
Genitalia, Supine Position
Head
Head and Neck
Head Circumference
Heart, Anterior Chest
Liver
Lymph Nodes, Head and Neck
Male Genitalia
Mouth, Cranial Nerve X
Muscle Strength, Neck, Shoulders, and Tongue: Cranial Nerves VII, XI, XII
Muscle Strength, Upper Extremities
Oropharynx, Teeth and Tongue
Pedal Pulses
Six Cardinal Fields of Gaze: Cranial Nerves III, IV, and VI
Skin, Back
Thyroid, Posterior Approach
Newborn (Chs. 8 and 9)
Barlow-Ortolani Maneuvers
Buttocks
Cremasteric Reflex
Cry
Male Breasts, Supine Position
Male Genitalia, Circumcision
Moro Reflex
Neck, Posterior
Plantar Grasp
Range-of-Motion, Upper Extremities
Rooting and Sucking Reflexes
Symmetry of Gluteal Folds
Infant (Ch. 10)
Babinski Reflex
Eye Alignment
Eye-Ear Alignment
Head
Motor Development, Head Control
Motor Development, Rolling Over
Motor Development, Sitting
Toddler/Preschooler
Balance Using Hopping (Ch. 13)
Crawling to Standing (Ch. 12)
Fine Motor Skills (Ch. 6)
Motor Development (Ch. 12)
School-Age Child
Balance Using Heel-to-Toe Walking (Ch. 15)
Muscular Development (Ch. 15)
Spine for Alignment (Ch. 31)
Adolescent
Capillary Refill, Upper Extremities (Ch. 25)
Female Breasts, Sitting Position (Ch. 16)

WONG'S

ESSENTIALS *of* PEDIATRIC NURSING

WONG'S

ESSENTIALS *of* PEDIATRIC NURSING

EIGHTH EDITION

Marilyn J. Hockenberry, PhD, RN-CS, PNP, FAAN

Director, Center for Research and Evidence-Based Practice
Nurse Scientist, Texas Children's Hospital;
Director of Nurse Practitioners
Texas Children's Cancer Center;
Professor, Department of Pediatrics
Baylor College of Medicine
Houston, Texas

David Wilson, MS, RNC

Faculty
Langston University School of Nursing;
Staff
Pediatric Emergency Center
Saint Francis Hospital
Tulsa, Oklahoma

with more than 560 illustrations

MOSBY

ELSEVIER

11830 Westline Industrial Drive
St. Louis, Missouri 63146

WONG'S ESSENTIALS OF PEDIATRIC NURSING, ISBN: 978-0-323-05353-2
EIGHTH EDITION

Notice

Knowledge and best practice in this field are constantly changing. As new research and experience broaden
our knowledge, changes in practice, treatment and drug therapy may become necessary or appropriate.
Readers are advised to check the most current information provided (i) on procedures featured or (ii) by the
manufacturer of each product to be administered, to verify the recommended dose or formula, the method
and duration of administration, and contraindications. It is the responsibility of the practitioner, relying
on his or her own experience and knowledge of the patient, to make diagnoses, to determine dosages and
the best treatment for each individual patient, and to take all appropriate safety precautions. To the fullest
extent of the law, neither the Publisher nor the Authors assume any liability for any injury and/or damage to
persons or property arising out of or related to any use of the material contained in this book.

The Publisher

Library of Congress Cataloging-in-Publication Data
Hockenberry, Marilyn J.
Wong's essentials of pediatric nursing. — 8th ed. / Marilyn J. Hockenberry, David Wilson.
  p. ; cm.
Rev. ed. of: Wong's essentials of pediatric nursing. 7th ed. / [edited by] Marilyn J. Hockenberry. c2005.
Includes bibliographical references and index.
ISBN 978-0-323-05353-2 (hardcover : alk. paper)
1. Pediatric nursing. I. Wilson, David, 1950 Aug. 25- II. Wong, Donna L., 1948- III. Wong's essentials of
pediatric nursing. IV. Title. V. Title: Essentials of pediatric nursing.
[DNLM: 1. Pediatric Nursing. WY 159 H685w 2009]
RJ245.W46 2009
618.92'00231—dc22

2008026989

ISBN: 978-0-323-05353-2

Managing Editor: Michele D. Hayden
Publishing Services Manager: Deborah L. Vogel
Senior Project Manager: Deon Lee
Design Direction: Reneé Duenow and Jessica Williams
Chapter Opener Art: © iStockphoto.com

Printed in Canada
Last digit is the print number: 9 8 7 6 5 4 3 2

Chris Humphrey, Photographer

We dedicate this edition of *Wong's Essentials of Pediatric Nursing* to Donna Lee Wong, PhD, RN, PNP, CPN, FAAN, who passed away on May 4, 2008, following complications of leukemia. Donna was the original co-author of this book. Among her numerous publications, she is best known as the author of *Essentials* along with *Wong's Nursing Care of Infants and Children*, *Wong's Clinical Manual of Pediatric Nursing*, and the *Pediatric Quick Reference*. She co-developed the Wong-Baker FACES Pain Rating Scale, a tool used worldwide to assess pain in children and adults and which has been used in extensive research on pain. She was a fellow in the American Academy of Nursing (FAAN) and is listed in *Who's Who in American Nursing* and *The World's Who's Who of Women*. She was awarded many honors including the first recipient of the Audrey Hepburn/Sigma Theta Tau International (Honorary Nursing Society) Award for Contributions to the Health and Welfare of Children, Rutger's University Outstanding Alumni, and the Society of Pediatric Nursing Barbara Larson Humanitarian Award.

For those of us who had the honor of knowing this remarkable individual, she is most remembered for her outstanding generosity and concern for others. Her commitment to pediatric nursing is reflected in her never-ending pursuit of excellence. Her belief that no child should experience pain when interventions were possible led to the development of the concept of "atraumatic care." Donna taught us that nursing is about providing the best care possible and that our patients will be the better for it. She led by example, always looking for ways to improve care for pediatric patients. Donna Wong was an example for all of us who strive for excellence in our nursing profession. We hold her dear to our hearts and will continue to work to carry on her outstanding legacy. She will never be forgotten.

Contributors

CONTRIBUTING EDITOR

Patrick Barrera, BS
Assistant Director
Evidence-Based Clinical Decision Support
Center for Research and Evidence-Based Practice
Texas Children's Hospital
Houston, Texas

CONTRIBUTORS

Debbie Fraser Askin, MN, RNC
Associate Professor
University of Manitoba;
Neonatal Nurse Practitioner
St. Boniface General Hospital
Winnipeg, Manitoba, Canada

Annette L. Baker, MSN, RN, PNP
Pediatric Nurse Practitioner
Cardiovascular Program
Children's Hospital
Boston, Massachusetts

Rose U. Baker, MSN, APRN, BC
Adjunct Faculty
Kent State University
College of Nursing
Kent, Ohio

Faye Blair, MSN, RN
Clinical Specialist
Texas Children's Hospital
Houston, Texas

Christine A. Brosnan, DrPH, RN
Associate Professor
University of Texas Health Science Center at Houston
School of Nursing
Houston, Texas

Terri L. Brown, MSN, RN, CPN
Research Specialist
Center for Research and Evidence-Based Practice
Texas Children's Hospital
Houston, Texas

Rosalind Bryant, APRN, MN, BC, PNP
Pediatric Nurse Practitioner
Texas Children's Cancer Center
Texas Children's Hospital;
Instructor
Department of Pediatrics
Baylor College of Medicine
Houston, Texas

Lisa Creamer, RN, BSN
Case Manager, Child Protection Team
Texas Children's Hospital
Houston, Texas

Martha R. Curry, MS, RN, CPNP
Instructor
Baylor College of Medicine;
Pediatric Nurse Practitioner
Pediatric Rheumatology Department
Texas Children's Hospital
Houston, Texas

Marsha L. Ellett, DNS, RN
Associate Professor
Indiana University School of Nursing
Indianapolis, Indiana

Angela M. Ethier, DSN, RN, CNS, CPN, CT
Research Faculty
Center for Research and Evidence-Based Practice
Texas Children's Hospital
Houston, Texas

Joy Hesselgrave, MSN, RN, CPON
Clinical Specialist
Texas Children's Hospital
Houston, Texas

Mary C. Hooke, PhD(c), APRN-BC, CPON
   Clinical Nurse Specialist
   Hematology-Oncology
   Children's Hospitals and Clinics of Minnesota
   Minneapolis, Minnesota

Eufemia Jacob, PhD, RN
   Assistant Professor
   Department of Pediatrics
   Baylor College of Medicine
   Houston, Texas

Linda M. Kollar, MSN, RN
   Clinical Director
   Division of Adolescent Medicine
   Cincinnati Children's Hospital Medical Center
   Cincinnati, Ohio

Shannon Stone McCord, MS, RN, CPNP, WOCN, CCRN
   Pediatric Nurse Practitioner
   Wound, Ostomy and Continence
   Texas Children's Hospital
   Houston, Texas

Mary A. Mondozzi, MSN, APRN, BC
   Outreach Coordinator, Burn Center Education
   The Paul and Carol David Foundation Burn Institute
   Akron Children's Hospital
   Akron, Ohio

Rebecca A. Monroe, MSN, RN, CPNP, CPON
   Pediatric Nurse Practitioner
   Dallas, Texas

Barbara A. Montagnino, MS, RN, CNS
   Clinical Nurse Specialist
   Progressive Care Unit
   Texas Children's Hospital
   Dallas, Texas

Patricia O'Brien, MSN, RN, CPNP-AC
   Pediatric Nurse Practitioner
   Cardiovascular Program
   Children's Hospital–Boston
   Boston, Massachusetts

Patricia A. Ring, MS, RN, CPNP
   Pediatric Nurse Practitioner
   Pediatric Nephrology Department
   Children's Hospital of Wisconsin
   Milwaukee, Wisconsin

Cheryl C. Rodgers, MSN, RN, CPNP, CPON
   Pediatric Nurse Practitioner
   Texas Children's Hospital;
   Instructor
   Baylor College of Medicine
   Houston, Texas

Jennifer Sanders, RN, BSN
   Nurse Manager
   Texas Children's Hospital
   Houston, Texas

Rebecca J. Schultz, MSN, RN, CPNP
   Instructor
   Baylor College of Medicine;
   Pediatric Nurse Practitioner
   Clinical Coordinator
   Comprehensive Epilepsy Program
   Texas Children's Hospital
   Houston, Texas

Sandra L. Upchurch, PhD, RN
   Chair and Associate Professor
   The University of Texas Health Science Center at Houston
   School of Nursing
   Houston, Texas

Barbara J. Wheeler, MN, RN, IBCLC, RLC
   Neonatal Clinical Nurse Specialist
   Lactation Consultant
   St. Boniface General Hospital
   Winnipeg, Manitoba, Canada

EVIDENCE-BASED PRACTICE BOXES

Terry Jean Brandt, RN, BSN, CPON, CPN
   Education Coordinator
   Inpatient Hematology Oncology Unit
   Texas Children's Cancer Center and Hematology Service
   Texas Children's Hospital
   Houston, Texas

Jessica Hilburn, MT (ASCP), CIC
   Director, Infection Control and Prevention
   Eastern New Mexico Medical Center
   Roswell, New Mexico

Anh Mac, RN, BSN
   Staff Nurse
   Texas Children's Hospital
   Houston, Texas

Theresa E. Reed, RN, BSN
   Clinical Nurse Coordinator
   Nutrition Support Nurses
   Texas Children's Hospital
   Houston, Texas

THE AUTHORS WOULD ALSO LIKE TO ACKNOWLEDGE THE FOLLOWING INDIVIDUALS FOR CONTRIBUTING TO EARLIER EDITIONS

Carol Turnage Carrier, MSN, RN, CNS
Newborn Clinical Nurse Specialist
Texas Children's Hospital;
Clinical Faculty
The University of Texas Health Science Center at Houston
School of Nursing
Houston, Texas

Janet DeJean, RN, CPON
Cancer Center and Hematology Service
Texas Children's Hospital
Houston, Texas

Brandi Horvath, RN, BSN, CPON
Cancer Center and Hematology Service
Texas Children's Hospital
Houston, Texas

Angela C. Morgan, MS, RN, CCRN
Clinical Nurse Specialist, PICU
Texas Children's Hospital
Houston, Texas

Shelly Nalbone, MS, RN, CPNP
Assistant Director
Texas Children's Hospital
Houston, Texas

Curt Roberts, RN
Staff Nurse, PICU
Texas Children's Hospital
Houston, Texas

Danna Salinas, RN, BSN
Staff Nurse, PICU
Texas Children's Hospital
Houston, Texas

INSTRUCTOR'S MANUAL AND OPEN-BOOK QUIZZES

Revised by:
Stephanie C. Butkus, MSN, RN, CPNP, CLC
Assistant Professor
Division of Nursing
Kettering College of Medical Arts
Kettering, Ohio

NCLEX® REVIEW QUESTIONS

Lois S. Marshall, PhD, RN
Nurse Researcher Scholar in Residence
Honor Society of Nursing, Sigma Theta Tau International;
Nurse Education Consultant
LSM Educational Consulting
Miami, Florida

POWERPOINT LECTURE SLIDES

Vivian Gamblian, MSN, RN
Professor of Nursing
Collin County Community College
McKinney, Texas

TEST BANK

Julie White, MSN, RN
Clinical Instructor
Graduate Entry Program
University of Illinois at Chicago
College of Nursing
Maternal/Child Department
Chicago, Illinois

Reviewers

Katherine Dawn Bunting, RD, CSP, LD
Assistant Director, Clinical Nutrition
Food and Nutrition Services
Texas Children's Hospital
Houston, Texas

Kathleen C. Byington, MSN, RN
Pediatric Clinical Nurse Specialist;
Case Manager;
Nurse Practitioner;
Monroe Carell Jr. Children's Hospital at Vanderbilt
Nashville, Tennessee

Miguel F. da Cunha, PhD
Professor
The University of Texas Health Science Center at Houston
School of Nursing
Houston, Texas

Patricia Boyle Egland, MSN, RN, CPNP
Assistant Professor
Pediatric Nursing Department
The Borough of Manhattan Community College
New York, New York

Mary Helen Freter, MS, RN, CPHQ
Assistant Professor
Nursing Department
Tulsa Community College
Tulsa, Oklahoma

Sandra Isburg, MSN, RN
Assistant Professor
Nursing Program
Mount Marty College
Yankton, South Dakota

Mary Knudtson, DNSc, NP
Professor
Family Medicine;
Director
Family Nurse Practitioner Program
University of California
Irvine, California

Marie Kodadek, PhD, RN
Assistant Professor
George Mason University
School of Nursing
Fairfax, Virginia

Debra A. Lewis, MSN, RN, CPN
Instructor;
Senior Level Coordinator
Duquesne University
School of Nursing
Pittsburgh, Pennsylvania

Cynthia G. Sanders, MS, RN, CPNP
Clinical Instructor
Department of Pediatrics
Baylor College of Medicine;
Pediatric Nurse Practitioner
Endocrine Section
Texas Children's Hospital
Houston, Texas

Kerstin I. West-Wilson, MS, RNC, IBCLC
Lactation Consultant
Eastern Oklahoma Perinatal Center
Children's Hospital at Saint Francis
Tulsa, Oklahoma

Linda G. Wofford, RN, CPNP, DNP
Assistant Professor, Nursing
Inman College of Health Science and Nursing
Belmont University
Nashville, Tennessee

Preface

Wong's Essentials of Pediatric Nursing has been a leading book in pediatric nursing since it was first published more than two decades ago. This kind of support places a unique accountability and responsibility on us to earn your future endorsement with each new edition. So, with your encouragement and constructive comments, we offer this extensive revision, the eighth edition of *Wong's Essentials of Pediatric Nursing.*

To accomplish this, Marilyn J. Hockenberry, as Editor-in-Chief, along with David Wilson, Co-Editor, and many expert nurses and multidisciplinary specialists, have revised, rewritten, or authored portions of the text concerning areas that are undergoing rapid and complex change. These areas include community nursing, immunizations, genetics, home care, pain assessment and management, high-risk newborn care, adolescent health issues, end-of-life care, and numerous diseases. We have carefully preserved aspects of the book that have met with universal acceptance—its state-of-the-art research-based information; its strong, integrated focus on the family and community; its logical and user-friendly organization; and its easy-to-read style.

We have tried to meet the increasing demands of faculty and students to teach and to learn in an environment characterized by rapid change, enormous amounts of information, fewer traditional clinical facilities, and less time.

This text encourages students to *think critically.* This edition includes extensively revised nursing care plans that may be individualized according to the patient's needs. The nursing care plans include Nursing Interventions Classification and Nursing Outcomes Classification terminology as well as NANDA Defining Characteristics. The Critical Thinking Exercises ask the nurse to examine the evidence, consider the assumptions, establish priorities, and evaluate alternative perspectives regarding each patient situation. The Critical Thinking Exercises and Ethical Case Studies support our belief that the science of nursing and related health professions is not black and white. In many instances it includes shades of gray, such as in the areas of genetic testing, resuscitation, cultural issues, end-of-life care, and quality of life.

This text also serves as a reference manual for the practicing nurse. The latest recommendations have been included from authoritative organizations such as the American Academy of Pediatrics, the Centers for Disease Control and Prevention, the Institute of Medicine, the Agency for Healthcare Research and Quality, the American Pain Society, the American Nurses Association, and the National Association of Pediatric Nurse Associates and Practitioners. To expand the universe of available information, websites and e-mail addresses have been included for hundreds of organizations and other educational resources.

ORGANIZATION OF THE BOOK

The same general approach to the presentation of content has been preserved from the first edition, although some content has been added, condensed, and rearranged within this framework to improve the flow, minimize duplication, and emphasize health care trends, such as home and community care. The book is divided into two broad parts. The first part of the book, Chapters 1 through 17, follows what is sometimes called the "age and stage" approach, considering infancy, childhood, and adolescence from a developmental context. It emphasizes the importance of the nurse's role in health promotion and maintenance and in considering the family as the focus of care. From a developmental perspective, the care of common health problems is presented, giving readers a sense of the normal problems expected in otherwise healthy children and demonstrating when in the course of childhood these problems are most likely to occur. The remainder of the book, Chapters 18 through 32, presents the more serious health problems of infancy, childhood, and adolescence that are not specific to any particular age-group and that frequently require hospitalization, major medical and nursing intervention, and home care.

UNIT ONE (Chapters 1 through 5) provides a longitudinal view of the child as an individual on a continuum of developmental changes from birth through adolescence and as a member of a family unit maturing within a culture and a community. Chapter 1 includes a discussion of morbidity and mortality in infancy and childhood and examines child health care from a historical perspective. Because unintentional injury is one of the leading causes of death in children, an overview of this topic is included. The nursing process, with emphasis on nursing diagnosis and outcomes and on the importance of developing critical thinking skills, is presented. In this edition, the critical components of evidence-based practice are added and provide the template for exploring the latest pediatric nursing research or practice guidelines throughout the book.

This book is about families with children, and the philosophy of family-centered care is emphasized. This book is also about providing atraumatic care—care that minimizes the psychologic and physical stress that health promotion and illness treatment can inflict. Features such as Family Focus, Community Focus, and Atraumatic Care boxes bring these philosophies to life throughout the text. Finally, the philosophy of delivering nursing care is addressed. We believe strongly that children and families need consistent caregivers. The establishment of the therapeutic relationship with the child and family is explored as the essential foundation for providing quality nursing care.

Chapter 2 provides important information on community-based nursing care, with emphasis on epidemiology as it applies to the detection and identification of causes of morbidity and mortality in pediatrics. A community project presented in this chapter reflects the important components of the nursing process, such as completion of a community needs assessment, planning phase, implementation, and evaluation.

Chapter 3, devoted to the family, further emphasizes the importance of this social group in relation to the health and welfare of children. Family theories establish the tone of the chapter, which includes a variety of parenting situations that reflect contemporary society. Family strengths and vulnerabilities are addressed, and current findings on adoption, divorce, single-parenting, stepfamilies, and dual-earner families have been incorporated.

Chapter 4 provides the opportunity to expand the discussion of social, cultural, and religious influences on child development and health promotion, including socioeconomic factors, customs, and health beliefs and practices. The content more clearly describes the role of the nurse, with emphasis on cultural sensitivity and culturally competent care. Throughout this chapter extensive revisions have been made to the tables detailing cultural and religious factors to make the information more manageable and user friendly. The basic overview of child development in Chapter 5 remains up-to-date and expands on the theoretic approach to personality development and learning. Biologic systems development is not emphasized in this chapter but is discussed more fully in relation to major systems dysfunction in later chapters.

UNIT TWO (Chapters 6 and 7) is concerned with the principles of nursing assessment, including communication and interviewing skills, observation, physical and behavioral assessment, health guidance, and the latest information on preventive care guidelines. Chapter 6 contains guidelines for communicating with children, adolescents, and their families, as well as a detailed description of a health assessment, including discussion of family assessment, nutritional assessment, and a sexual history. Content on communication techniques is outlined to provide a concise format for reference. Chapter 6 continues by providing a comprehensive approach to physical examination and developmental assessment, with updated material on temperature measurement, BMI-for-age guidelines, and the latest CDC clinical growth charts. Chapter 7 is a new chapter in this edition, devoted to critical assessment and management of pain in children. Although the literature on pain assessment and management in children has grown considerably, this knowledge has not been widely applied in practice. Chapter 7 was added to address this concern by presenting detailed assessment and management strategies including discussion of common pain states in children.

UNIT THREE (Chapters 8 and 9) stresses the importance of the neonatal period in relation to child survival during the first few months and the impact on health in later life. In Chapter 8 several areas have been revised to reflect current issues, especially in terms of the educational needs of the family during relatively short postpartum stays and the recognition of newborn problems in the first few weeks of life. An intrauterine growth chart is included that reflects a more homogeneous sample population than previous growth charts. Other current issues that have been updated include proactive measures to prevent infant abduction; hospital-based, baby-friendly breastfeeding initiatives; greater emphasis on choices

for circumcision analgesia; newborn atraumatic care; and newborn screening including universal newborn hearing screening. Newborn skin care guidelines have also been updated, and choices for newborn cord care are discussed. Chapter 9 stresses the nurse's role in caring for the high-risk newborn and the importance of astute observations to the survival of this vulnerable group of infants. Modern advances in neonatal care have mandated extensive revision with a greater sensitivity to the diverse needs of infants, from those with extremely low birth weights, late-preterm infants and those of normal gestational age who have difficulty making an effective transition to extrauterine life. Updates in Chapter 9 include information on near-term infant care, bilirubin monitoring guidelines, preterm infant nutrition, early discharge of the preterm infant, and neonatal exposure to maternal environmental conditions such as alcohol, tobacco, and recreational drugs, as well as exposure to viral infections, including human parvovirus. This chapter also includes updates regarding immunizations required in the neonatal period and detection and management of inborn errors of metabolism.

UNITS FOUR through SIX (Chapters 10 through 17) present the major developmental stages outlined in Unit One, which are expanded to provide a broader concept of these stages and the health problems most often associated with each age-group. Special emphasis is placed on preventive aspects of care. The chapters on health promotion follow a standard approach that is used consistently for each age-group. New information has been added on vitamin intake and food hypersensitivity, as well as complementary and alternative medicine, motor vehicle child safety restraints, and injury prevention in infancy. The influence of nutrition in the preschool-age and school-age child (especially decreasing fat intake) in relation to later chronic diseases such as obesity and hypertension is also discussed. The sections on childhood immunizations and injury prevention have been updated. The potential negative effects of exposure to violence and terrorism are included as well.

The chapters on health problems in these units primarily reflect more typical and age-related concerns. The information on many disorders has been revised to reflect recent changes. Examples include sudden infant death syndrome, lead poisoning, wound healing, attention deficit hyperactivity disorder, contraception, teenage pregnancy, substance abuse, and suicide. The chapters on adolescence include the latest information from the American Medical Association (AMA) Guidelines for Adolescent Preventive Services (GAPS), non-smoking strategies, and current trends in suicide. All psychosocial and physiologic conditions include the latest diagnostic criteria from the *Diagnostic and Statistical Manual of Mental Disorders (DSM-IV-TR)*.

UNIT SEVEN (Chapters 18 through 20) deals with children who have the same developmental needs as growing children but who, because of congenital or acquired physical, cognitive, or sensory impairment, require alternative interventions to facilitate development. Chapter 18 reflects current trends in the care of families and children with chronic illness or disability such as providing home care, normalizing children's lives, focusing on developmental needs, enabling and empowering families, and promoting early intervention. Extensive revisions have been made to reflect increased awareness of the need for quality nursing care at the end of life. This section highlights common fears experienced by the child and family and includes discussion of symptom management and nurses' reactions to caring for dying children.

The content in Chapter 19 on cognitive or sensory impairment includes important updates on the definition and classification of mental retardation. Autism is discussed in this chapter to provide a cohesive overview of cognitive and sensory impairments. Chapter 20 provides an overview of home care in light of the current nursing shortage and its impact on the role of the home health care nurse, care provider, and family. This chapter presents important discussions related to the selection of a home health care agency, the role of the nurse in empowering the family, and case management in home health.

UNIT EIGHT (Chapters 21 and 22) is concerned with the impact of hospitalization on the child and family and presents a comprehensive overview of the stressors imposed by hospitalization and discusses nursing interventions to prevent or eliminate them. New research on short-stay or outpatient admissions addresses preparing children for these experiences. Chapter 21 provides updated information on the effects of illness and hospitalization on children at specific ages and the effects on their development. The increasing role of ambulatory and outpatient settings for surgical procedures is also discussed. Chapter 22 includes numerous new Evidence-Based Practice boxes designed to provide rationales for the interventions discussed in the chapter. A new focus in this chapter is the evidence related to preparation of the child for procedures commonly performed by nurses. Recommendations for practice are based on the evidence and concisely presented in Evidence-Based Practice boxes throughout the chapter.

UNITS NINE through TWELVE (Chapters 23 through 32) consider serious health problems of infants and children primarily from the biologic systems orientation, which has the practical organizational value of permitting health problems and nursing considerations to relate to specific pathophysiologic disturbances. Important revisions include discussions of hepatitis, all blood disorders, respiratory illnesses including acute lung injury and respiratory syncytial virus, tuberculosis, asthma, effects of passive smoking, seizures, chemotherapy, acquired immunodeficiency syndrome, diabetes mellitus, and burns. The information on orthopedic and muscular injuries in childhood as a result of sports participation or other injuries has been extensively revised to reflect current treatment modalities. Chapter 29 includes focused attention on type 2 diabetes and new information on insulin preparations and types of glucose meters.

Extensive **appendixes** are also included and contain information on developmental assessment, growth measurements, pediatric laboratory values, NANDA International–approved nursing diagnoses, and several foreign-language translations of the FACES Pain Rating Scale. An appendix containing Spanish translations of common terms and phrases used in health care and pediatric nursing is included. All of the appendix material reflects the most current versions of forms, charts, and measurements. Additional clinical growth charts can be obtained from the Centers for Disease Control and Prevention website: http://www.cdc.gov/growthcharts.

UNIFYING PRINCIPLES

Several unifying principles have guided the organizational structure of this book since its inception. These principles continue to strengthen the book with each revision in order to produce a text that is consistent in approach throughout each chapter.

The Family as the Unit of Care

The child is an essential member of the family unit. Nursing care is most effective when it is delivered with the belief that *the family is the patient.* This belief permeates the book. When a child is healthy, the child's health is enhanced when the family is a fully functioning, health-promoting system. The family unit can be manifested in a myriad of structures; each has the potential to provide a caring, supportive environment in which the child can grow, mature, and maximize his or her human potential. In addition to the integration of family-centered care into every chapter, an entire chapter is devoted to understanding the family as the core focus in children's lives. Another chapter discusses the social, cultural, and religious influences that impact family beliefs. Separate sections in another chapter deal in depth with family communication and family assessment. The impact of illness and hospitalization, home care, community care, and the death of a child are covered extensively in four additional chapters. The needs of the family are emphasized throughout the text under Nursing Care Management in a separate section on family support. Numerous Family Focus and Family-Centered Care boxes are included to assist nurses in understanding and providing helpful information to families.

An Integrated Approach to Development

Children are not small adults but special individuals with unique minds, bodies, and needs. No book on pediatric nursing is complete without extensive coverage of communication, nutrition, play, safety, dental care, sexuality, sleep, self-esteem, and of course, parenting. Nurses promote the healthy expression of all these dimensions of personhood and need to understand how these functions are expressed by different children at different developmental ages and stages. Effective parenting depends on the parent's knowledge of development, and it is often the nurse's responsibility to provide parents with a developmental awareness of their children's needs. For these reasons, coverage of the many dimensions of childhood is integrated within the growth and development chapters, rather than being presented in separate chapters. For example, safety concerns for a toddler are much different from those for an adolescent. Sleep needs change with age, as do nutritional needs. As a result, the units on each stage of childhood contain complete information on all these functions as they relate to the specific age. In the unit on the school-age child, for instance, information is presented on nutritional needs, age-appropriate play and its significance, safety concerns characteristic of the age-group, appropriate dental care, sleep characteristics, and means of promoting self-esteem—a particularly significant concern for school-age children. The challenges of being the parent of a school-age child are presented, and interventions are suggested that nurses can use to promote healthy parenting. Using the integrated approach, students gain an appreciation for the unique characteristics and needs of children at every age and stage of development.

Focus on Wellness and Illness: Child, Family, and Community

In a pediatric nursing text, a focus on illness is expected. Children become ill, and nurses typically are involved in helping children get well. However, it is not sufficient to prepare nurs-

SpecialFeatures

Much effort has been directed toward making this book easy to teach from and, more important, easy to learn from. In this edition the following features have been included to benefit educators, students, and practitioners.

FAMILY-CENTERED CARE boxes help nurses and students teach parents about the special needs of their infants and children.

EVIDENCE-BASED PRACTICE boxes focus the reader's attention on application of both research and critical thought processes to support and guide the outcomes of nursing care and to provide measurable outcomes that nurses can use to validate their unique role in the health care system.

COMMUNITY FOCUS boxes address issues that expand to the community, such as increasing immunization rates, preventing lead poisoning, or decreasing smoking among teens.

CRITICAL THINKING EXERCISES ask the nurse to examine the evidence, consider the assumptions, establish priorities, and evaluate alternative perspectives regarding each patient situation.

nursing process boxes, new to this edition, streamline the nursing process information on major diseases and conditions for easy identification.

CULTURAL AWARENESS boxes integrate concepts of culturally sensitive care throughout the text. The emphasis is on the clinical application of the information, whether it focuses on toilet training or on male or female circumcision.

ATRAUMATIC CARE boxes emphasize the importance of providing competent care without creating undue physical and psychologic distress. Although many of the boxes provide suggestions for managing pain, atraumatic care also considers approaches to promoting self-esteem and preventing embarrassment.

FYI (For Your Information) segments present information of interest that may increase understanding of a concept or spark an interest in reading about a condition. Unlike the Nursing Alerts, which present essential information, FYIs present information that is optional for the reader and help prioritize what information is most essential for the reader to assimilate.

nursingcareplans include the latest NANDA nursing diagnoses and associated defining characteristics (signs and symptoms), which assist the nurse in the validation of the selected nursing diagnosis. The nursing care plans also include patient outcomes and Nursing Outcomes Classification terminology. Selected nursing interventions and Nursing Interventions Classification terminology are designed to guide the student to individualize the child's and family's care. The inclusion of the classification terminology including NANDA diagnoses, Nursing Interventions Classification, and Nursing Outcomes Classification provides a common language for the nurse to identify the unique needs of children and their families.

FAMILY FOCUS boxes present issues of special significance to families who have a child with a particular disorder. This feature is another method of highlighting the needs or concerns of families that should be addressed when family-centered care is provided.

ETHICAL CASE STUDY boxes have been designed to reflect complex patient care situations that nurses face in clinical practice. The case studies were established using these principles: **E**valuate the issue, **T**reat all involved with respect, **H**ear all sides, **I**nitiate action, and **C**onsider the outcome.

NURSINGALERT features call the reader's attention to considerations that if ignored could lead to a deteriorating or emergency situation. Key assessment data, risk factors, and danger signs are among the kinds of information included.

NURSINGTIP notes present handy information of a nonemergency nature that makes patients more comfortable and the nurse's job easier.

nursingcareguidelines summarize important nursing interventions for a variety of situations and conditions.

emergencytreatment boxes are flagged by colored thumb tabs, enabling the reader to quickly locate interventions for crisis situations.

Numerous pedagogic devices that enhance student learning have been retained from previous editions:

- A functional and attractive **FULL-COLOR DESIGN** visually enhances the organization of each chapter, as well as the special features.

- Many of the **COLOR PHOTOGRAPHS** are new, and anatomic drawings are easy to follow, with color appropriately used to illustrate important aspects, such as saturated and desaturated blood. As an example, the full-color heart illustrations in Chapter 25 clearly depict congenital cardiac defects and associated hemodynamic changes.

- **CHAPTER OUTLINES** with page numbers begin each chapter and allow readers to quickly locate topics of interest.

- The **RELATED TOPICS AND ADDITIONAL RESOURCES** at the beginning of each chapter indicate the chapter or chapters where additional discussion(s) of a given topic can be found. They also highlight additional resources and information included in ancillary products such as the Evolve website, Companion CD, and *Wong's Clinical Manual of Pediatric Nursing.*

- **LEARNING OBJECTIVES** in each chapter provide the reader with a basic guideline for the major points presented in and learned from the chapter.

- **KEY TERMS** are highlighted throughout each chapter to reinforce student learning.

- Hundreds of **TABLES** and **BOXES** highlight key concepts and nursing interventions.

- **KEY POINTS,** located at the end of each chapter, help the reader summarize major concepts, make connections, and synthesize information.

- A detailed, cross-referenced **INDEX** allows readers to quickly access discussions.

ing students to care primarily for sick children. First, health is more than the absence of disease. Being healthy is being whole in mind, body, and spirit. Therefore the majority of the first half of the book is devoted to discussions that promote physical, emotional, psychosocial, mental, and spiritual wellness. Much emphasis is placed on anticipatory guidance of parents to prevent injury or illness in the child. Second, health care is more than ever prevention focused. The objectives set forth in the *Healthy People 2010* report clearly establish a health care agenda in which solutions to medical and social problems lie in preventive strategies. Third, health care is moving from acute care settings to the community, the home, short-stay centers, and clinics. Nurses must be prepared to function in all settings. To be successful, they must understand the pathophysiology, diagnosis, and treatment of health conditions. Competent nursing care flows from this knowledge and is enhanced by an awareness of childhood development, family dynamics, and communication skills.

Nursing Care

Although the information in this text incorporates information from numerous disciplines (medicine, pathophysiology, pharmacology, nutrition, psychology, sociology), its primary purpose is to provide information on the nursing care of children and families. Discussions of all disorders conclude with a section on Nursing Care Management. In addition, 13 care plans are included. Taken together, they cover the nursing care for many childhood diseases, disorders, and conditions. The purposes of the care plans, like every other feature of the book, are to teach and to convey information. They include all current nursing diagnoses approved by NANDA International that have a potential bearing on the health problem. For every diagnosis, defining characteristics, appropriate patient outcomes, and select possible interventions with rationales are presented. The care plans are designed to stimulate critical thinking and encourage the student to individualize outcomes and interventions for the child, rather than to provide an extensive picture of all nursing diagnoses, outcomes, and interventions for every given disease or condition. A new addition to this edition are the Nursing Process boxes, which emphasize the nursing process as a problem-solving method in the provision of individualized patient care.

Culturally Competent Care

Increasing cultural diversity in this country requires nurses caring for children and their families to develop expertise in the care of children from numerous backgrounds. Culturally competent nursing care requires more than acquiring knowledge about ethnic and cultural groups. It encompasses not only awareness of the influence of culture on the child and family, but also the ability to intervene appropriately and effectively. The nurse must learn objective skills to focus on the child's, family's, and community's cultural characteristics. The nurse's self-awareness of unique personal cultural backgrounds must be acknowledged in order to understand how they contribute to cross-cultural communication. The importance of the environment of a cross-cultural care setting must be considered when providing clinical nursing care to culturally diverse families. This edition provides numerous learning experiences that examine cross-cultural communication, cultural assessment, cultural interpretation, and appropriate nursing interventions.

The Critical Role of Research and Evidence-Based Practice

This eighth edition is the product of an extensive review of the literature published since the book was last revised. Many readers and researchers have come to rely on the copious references that reflect significant contributions from a broad audience of professionals. To ensure that information is accurate and current, most citations are less than 5 years old, and almost every chapter has entries dated within 1 year of publication. This book reflects the art and science of pediatric nursing. A central goal in every revision is to base care on research, rather than on tradition. Evidence-based practice produces measurable outcomes that nurses can use to validate their unique role in the health care system. Throughout the book Evidence-Based Practice boxes reflect the importance of the science of nursing care.

CANADIAN CONTENT

The eighth edition of this text includes updated Canadian statistics regarding infant and child health in Chapter 1 and Canadian immunization schedules in Chapter 10. Numerous Canadian resource organizations are also provided throughout the text. These efforts are intended to make the text as valuable as possible to Canadian readers.

TEACHING/LEARNING PACKAGE

For the eighth edition of this text, extensive ancillary products are offered for instructors and students to use in class and clinical settings.

Evolve. Evolve is an innovative website that provides a wealth of continually updated content, resources, and state-of-the-art information on pediatric nursing, including links to related websites, important new content updates, Donna Wong's lectures, and more! Use the web address in the text to access Evolve's wide array of information, including course resources for instructors (Instructor's Manual, Test Bank, Image Collection, PowerPoint slides) and learning resources for students (WebLinks, Interactive Case Studies, NCLEX-style Review Questions, Pediatric Nursing Skills, Assessment Videos, modifiable Nursing Care Plans, and more).

Companion CD. Included with every text, this valuable CD-ROM contains a variety of activities to enhance learning through the use of Critical Thinking Exercises, Case Studies, Anatomy Reviews, Animations, and Assessment Videos. More than 350 NCLEX-style Review Questions are available for students to practice and hone their studying skills.

Instructor's Electronic Resource. This innovative electronic resource for the instructor (available online) contains the following components:

- *Instructor's Manual* contains learning objectives, chapter outlines and accompanying teaching strategies, learning activities, open-book quizzes, and curriculum guides, for courses of various lengths.
- *Electronic Test Bank in ExamView format* contains more than 1000 NCLEX-style test items, including new alternate format questions. An answer key with page references to the text, rationales, and NCLEX-style coding is included.
- *Electronic Image Collection,* containing more than 300 full-color illustrations and photographs from the text, helps in-

structors develop presentations and explain key concepts. All images on the CD can be printed as acetates for overhead projection.

- *PowerPoint Slides,* with lecture outlines for each chapter of the book, assist in presenting materials in the classroom.

AVAILABLE FOR PURCHASE

Clinical Companion. This NEW pocket-sized portable and concise reference for clinical use contains a wealth of information at your fingertips. Brief coverage of more than 130 of the most commonly encountered childhood illnesses and health problems is presented alphabetically for easy reference, and additional sections cover physical assessment, pain assessment and management, diagnostic tests and nursing procedures such as medication administration, specimen collection, and drug calculations.

Study Guide. This comprehensive and challenging study aid presents a variety of questions to enhance learning of key concepts and content from the text. Multiple-choice, matching, and true-false questions are included, as well as Critical Thinking Case Studies. Answers for all questions are included at the back of the study guide.

Virtual Clinical Excursions: CD and Workbook Companion. A CD-ROM and workbook have been developed as a "virtual clinical" experience to expand student opportunities for critical thinking. This package guides the student through a computer-generated virtual clinical environment and helps the user apply textbook content to "virtual patients" in that environment. Case studies are presented that allow students to use this textbook as a reference to assess, diagnose, plan, implement, and evaluate "real" patients using clinical scenarios. The state-of-the-art technologies reflected on this CD-ROM demonstrate *cutting-edge* learning opportunities for students and facilitate knowledge retention of the information found in the textbook. The clinical simulations and workbook represent the next generation of research-based learning tools that promote critical thinking and meaningful learning.

Wong's Clinical Manual of Pediatric Nursing, Seventh Edition. This manual has been extensively revised and contains a wealth of information for use as a reference for students and in the clinical setting. The manual includes more than 45 Nursing Care Plans, patient and family education instructions that can be copied and given to families, detailed descriptions of nursing skills and procedures, and much, much, more!

ACKNOWLEDGMENTS

We are grateful to Donna Wong, whose mentorship and support made us better pediatric nurses. We will miss her greatly. We are also grateful to the many nursing faculty members, practitioners, and students who have offered their comments, recommendations, and suggestions. We are especially grateful to the contributors and the many reviewers who brought constructive criticism, suggestions, and clinical expertise to this edition. This edition could not have been completed without the dedication of these special people.

We are especially thankful to **Patrick Barrera** for his contributions. His commitment to excellence and attention to detail are essential to maintaining the quality of this book. Thanks go to **Kathy McCarthy** and **Gennaro Sambuco** for the beautiful color photography and to the health professionals, children, and parents who generously allowed us to use or take their photographs. Appreciation is also extended to the library staff at Saint Francis Hospital, Tulsa, Oklahoma—**Beth Treaster, Cheryl Stanford,** and **Scott Murray.**

No book is ever a reality without the dedication and perseverance of the editorial staff. Although it is impossible to list every individual at Mosby who has made exceptional efforts to produce this text, we are especially grateful to **Catherine Jackson, Shelly Hayden,** and **Deon Lee** for their support and commitment to excellence.

Finally, we thank our families and our children—for the unselfish love and endless patience that allows us to devote such a large part of our lives to our careers. Our children have given us the opportunity to directly observe the wonders of childhood.

Marilyn J. Hockenberry
David Wilson

Contents

UNIT ONE

CHILDREN, THEIR FAMILIES, AND THE NURSE, 1

1 Perspectives of Pediatric Nursing, 1

Marilyn J. Hockenberry

Health Care for Children, 2
Health Promotion, 2
Nutrition, 2
Dental Care, 3
Immunizations, 3

Childhood Health Problems, 3
Obesity and Type 2 Diabetes, 3
Childhood Injuries, 3
Violence, 6
Substance Abuse, 7
Mental Health Problems, 8

Mortality, 8
Infant Mortality, 8
Childhood Mortality, 9

Morbidity, 10
Childhood Morbidity, 10

The Art of Pediatric Nursing, 10
Philosophy of Care, 10
Family-Centered Care, 10
Atraumatic Care, 11

Role of the Pediatric Nurse, 11
Therapeutic Relationship, 11
Family Advocacy and Caring, 11
Disease Prevention and Health
    Promotion, 12
Health Teaching, 13
Support and Counseling, 13
Coordination and
    Collaboration, 13
Ethical Decision Making, 13
Research, 14

Critical Thinking and the Process of Nursing Children and Families, 14
Critical Thinking, 14
Evidence-Based Practice, 14
Nursing Process, 15
    Assessment, 16
    Nursing Diagnosis, 16
    Planning, 17
    Implementation, 17

Evaluation, 17
Documentation, 17

2 Community-Based Nursing Care of the Child and Family, 20

Christine A. Brosnan and Sandra L. Upchurch

Nursing in the Community, 21

Community Concepts, 21
Community, 21
    Community Health Nursing, 21
    Roles and Functions, 21
Demography, 22
Epidemiology, 22
    Distribution of Disease, Injury, or
        Illness, 22
    Epidemiologic Triangle, 22
    Levels of Prevention, 22
    Screening, 23
Economics, 23

Community Nursing Process, 24
Community Needs Assessment and
    Diagnosis, 24
Community Planning, 25
Community Implementation, 25
Community Evaluation, 25

3 Family Influences on Child Health Promotion, 29

Patrick Barrera

General Concepts, 30
Definition of Family, 30
Family Theories, 30
    Family Systems Theory, 30
    Family Stress Theory, 32
    Developmental Theory, 32
Family Nursing Interventions, 32

Family Structure and Function, 33
Family Structure, 33
    Traditional Nuclear Family, 33
    Nuclear Family, 33
    Blended Family, 33

Extended Family, 33
Single-Parent Family, 33
Binuclear Family, 34
Polygamous Family, 34
Communal Family, 34
Gay/Lesbian Family, 34
Family Strengths and Functioning
    Style, 34

Family Roles and Relationships, 35
Parental Roles, 35
Role Learning, 35
    Family Size and Configuration, 35
    Sibling Interactions, 36
    Ordinal Position, 37
    Multiple Births, 37

Parenting, 38
Motivation for Parenthood, 38
Preparation for Parenthood, 39
Transition to Parenthood, 39
    Parental Factors Affecting
        Transition to Parenthood, 39
Parenting Behaviors, 40
    Parental Styles of Control, 40
Limit Setting and Discipline, 41
    Minimizing Misbehavior, 41
    General Guidelines for
        Implementing Discipline, 41
    Types of Discipline, 41

Special Parenting Situations, *43*
  Parenting the Adopted Child, *43*
    Issues of Origin, *44*
    Adolescence, *44*
    Cross-Racial and International
      Adoption, *44*
  Parenting and Divorce, *45*
    Impact of Divorce on Children, *45*
    Custody and Parenting
      Partnerships, *47*
  Single Parenting, *47*
    Single Fathers, *47*
  Parenting in Reconstituted
    Families, *48*
  Parenting in Dual-Earner
    Families, *48*
    Working Mothers, *48*
  Foster Parenting, *48*
  Accommodating Contemporary
    Parenting Situations, *48*

4   **Social, Cultural, and
    Religious Influences on
    Child Health Promotion, *51***

    Mary C. Hooke

Culture, *52*
  Social Roles, *52*
    Self-Esteem and Culture, *53*
  Subcultural Influences, *53*
    Ethnicity, *53*
    Socioeconomic Class, *54*
    Poverty, *54*
    Homelessness, *54*
    Migrant Farmworker Families, *54*
    Immigrant Children, *55*
    Religion, *55*
    Schools, *55*
    Communities, *55*
    Peer Cultures, *56*

  The Child and Family in North
    America, *56*
    Minority-Group Membership, *56*
  Cultural Shock and Cultural
    Competence, *57*
Cultural and Religious Influences
on Health Care, *58*
  Susceptibility to Health
    Problems, *58*
    Hereditary Factors, *58*
    Socioeconomic Factors, *58*
  Cultural Customs, *59*
    Cultural Relativism, *60*
    Relationships with Health Care
      Providers, *60*
    Food Customs, *61*
  Health Beliefs and Practices, *62*
    Health Beliefs, *62*
    Health Practices, *63*
  Religious Beliefs, *64*
  Importance of Culture and
    Religion to Nurses, *64*

5   **Developmental Influences
    on Child Health
    Promotion, *71***

    Joy Hesselgrave

Growth and Development, *72*
  Foundations of Growth and
    Development, *72*
    Stages of Development, *72*
    Patterns of Growth and
      Development, *72*
    Individual Differences, *74*
  Biologic Growth and Physical
    Development, *74*
    External Proportions, *74*
    Biologic Determinants of Growth
      and Development, *75*
    Skeletal Growth and
      Maturation, *75*
    Neurologic Maturation, *76*
    Lymphoid Tissues, *76*
    Development of Organ
      Systems, *76*
  Physiologic Changes, *76*
    Metabolism, *76*
    Temperature, *77*
    Sleep and Rest, *77*
  Temperament, *77*
    Significance of Temperament, *78*

  Development of Personality
  and Mental Function, *78*
    Theoretic Foundations of
      Personality Development, *78*
      Psychosexual Development
        (Freud), *78*
      Psychosocial Development
        (Erikson), *79*
    Theoretic Foundations of Mental
      Development, *80*
      Cognitive Development
        (Piaget), *80*
      Language Development, *81*
      Moral Development (Kohlberg), *81*
      Spiritual Development (Fowler), *81*
    Development of Self-Concept, *82*
      Body Image, *82*
      Self-Esteem, *82*
  Role of Play in Development, *83*
    Classification of Play, *83*
    Content of Play, *83*
    Social Character of Play, *84*
    Functions of Play, *85*
      Sensorimotor Development, *85*
      Intellectual Development, *85*
      Socialization, *85*
      Creativity, *85*
      Self-Awareness, *85*
      Therapeutic Value, *85*
      Moral Value, *85*
    Toys, *86*
      Toy Safety, *86*
  Selected Factors That Influence
  Development, *86*
    Heredity, *86*
    Neuroendocrine Factors, *86*
    Nutrition, *88*
    Interpersonal Relationships, *88*
    Socioeconomic Level, *89*
    Disease, *89*
    Environmental Hazards, *89*
    Stress in Childhood, *89*
      Coping, *90*
    Influence of the Mass Media, *90*
      Reading Materials, *90*
      Movies, *90*
      Television, *91*
      Video Games, *92*
      Internet, *93*
  Developmental Assessment, *93*
    Denver II, *93*
    Denver II Prescreening
      Developmental
      Questionnaire, *94*

UNIT TWO

ASSESSMENT OF THE CHILD AND FAMILY, 97

6 **Communication and Physical Assessment of the Child, 97**

Marilyn J. Hockenberry

Guidelines for Communication and Interviewing, 98
  Establishing a Setting for Communication, 98
    Appropriate Introduction, 98
    Assurance of Privacy and Confidentiality, 98
  Computer Privacy and Applications in Nursing, 99
  Telephone Triage and Counseling, 99

Communicating with Families, 99
  Communicating with Parents, 99
    Encouraging the Parent to Talk, 100
    Directing the Focus, 100
    Listening and Cultural Awareness, 100
    Using Silence, 101
    Being Empathic, 101
    Providing Anticipatory Guidance, 101
    Avoiding Blocks to Communication, 101
    Communicating with Families Through an Interpreter, 101
  Communicating with Children, 102
    Communication Related to Development of Thought Processes, 102
  Communication Techniques, 105
    Play, 105

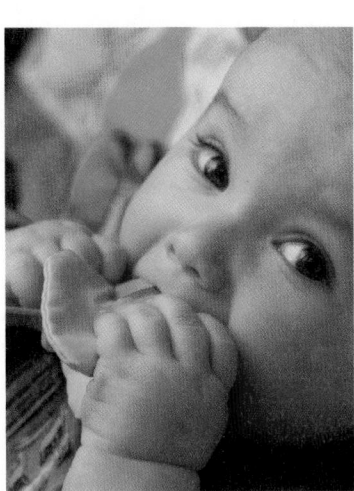

History Taking, 107
  Performing a Health History, 107
    Identifying Information, 107
    Chief Complaint, 107
    Present Illness, 108
    History, 108
    Sexual History, 110
    Family Medical History, 111
    Family Structure, 111
    Psychosocial History, 111
    Review of Systems, 113

Nutritional Assessment, 113
  Dietary Intake, 113
  Clinical Examination, 115
  Evaluation of Nutritional Assessment, 118

General Approaches Toward Examining the Child, 118
  Sequence of the Examination, 118
  Preparation of the Child, 118

Physical Examination, 121
  Growth Measurements, 121
    Growth Charts, 121
    Length, 122
    Height, 122
    Weight, 123
    Skinfold Thickness and Arm Circumference, 124
    Head Circumference, 124
  Physiologic Measurements, 124
    Temperature, 125
    Pulse, 127
    Respiration, 129
    Blood Pressure, 129
  General Appearance, 132
  Skin, 132
    Accessory Structures, 132
  Lymph Nodes, 133
  Head and Neck, 133
  Eyes, 134
    Inspection of External Structures, 134
    Inspection of Internal Structures, 135
    Vision Testing, 135
  Ears, 137
    Inspection of External Structures, 137
    Inspection of Internal Structures, 138
    Auditory Testing, 140
  Nose, 140
    Inspection of External Structures, 140
    Inspection of Internal Structures, 141

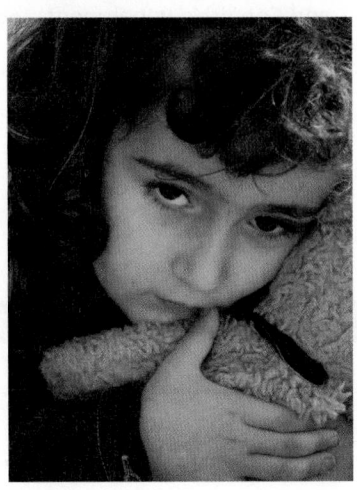

  Mouth and Throat, 141
    Inspection of Internal Structures, 142
  Chest, 143
  Lungs, 144
    Auscultation, 145
  Heart, 145
    Auscultation, 146
  Abdomen, 147
    Inspection, 148
    Auscultation, 149
    Palpation, 149
  Genitalia, 149
    Male Genitalia, 150
    Female Genitalia, 150
  Anus, 151
  Back and Extremities, 151
    Spine, 151
    Extremities, 152
    Joints, 152
    Muscles, 153
  Neurologic Assessment, 153
    Cerebellar Function, 153
    Reflexes, 153
    Cranial Nerves, 153

7 **Pain Assessment and Management in Children, 158**

Eufemia Jacob

Pain Assessment, 159
  Behavioral Measures, 159
  Physiologic Measures, 161
  Self-Report Measures, 162
  Multidimensional Measures, 164

Pain Assessment in Specific
Populations, *165*
  Pain in Neonates, *165*
  Children with Communication
    and Cognitive Impairment, *166*
  Cultural Issues in Pain
    Assessment, *171*
  Children with Chronic Illness
    and Complex Pain, *171*
Pain Management, *171*
  Nonpharmacologic
    Management, *171*

Complementary Pain
  Medicine, *175*
Pharmacologic Management, *175*
  Patient-Controlled Analgesia, *178*
  Epidural Analgesia, *183*
  Transmucosal and Transdermal
    Analgesia, *184*
  Timing of Analgesia, *187*
  Monitoring Side Effects, *188*
  Evaluation of Effectiveness of Pain
    Regimen, *189*

Painful and Invasive
  Procedures, *191*
Postoperative Pain, *191*
Recurrent Headaches
  in Children, *192*
Recurrent Abdominal Pain
  in Children, *192*
Cancer Pain in Children, *193*
Pain and Sedation in End-of-Life
  Care, *194*

UNIT THREE

THE NEWBORN, *197*

**8 Health Promotion of the
    Newborn and Family, *197***

Barbara J. Wheeler

Adjustment to Extrauterine Life, *198*
  Immediate Adjustments, *198*
    Respiratory System, *198*
    Circulatory System, *198*
  Physiologic Status of Other
    Systems, *199*
    Thermoregulation, *199*
    Hematopoietic System, *199*
    Fluid and Electrolyte Balance, *199*
    Gastrointestinal System, *199*
    Renal System, *200*
    Integumentary System, *200*
    Musculoskeletal System, *200*
    Defenses Against Infection, *200*
    Endocrine System, *200*
    Neurologic System, *201*
    Sensory Functions, *201*

Nursing Care of the Newborn
and Family, *201*
  Assessment, *201*
    Initial Assessment: Apgar
      Scoring, *201*
    Clinical Assessment of Gestational
      Age, *203*
    Transitional Assessment: Periods
      of Reactivity, *211*
    Behavioral Assessment, *213*
    Assessment of Attachment
      Behaviors, *215*
    Physical Assessment, *215*
  Maintain a Patent Airway, *215*
  Maintain a Stable Body
    Temperature, *221*
  Protect from Infection and
    Injury, *221*
    Identification, *221*
    Eye Care, *222*
    Vitamin K Administration, *222*

Hepatitis B Vaccine
  Administration, *222*
Newborn Screening for
  Disease, *223*
Universal Newborn Hearing
  Screening, *223*
Bathing, *224*
Care of the Umbilicus, *225*
Circumcision, *225*
Provide Optimal Nutrition, *228*
  Human Milk, *228*
  Breastfeeding, *229*
  Bottle Feeding, *231*
  Commercially Prepared
    Formulas, *232*
  Preparation of Formula, *233*
  Alternate Milk Products, *233*
  Feeding Schedules, *233*
  Feeding Behavior, *234*
Promote Parent-Infant Bonding
  (Attachment), *234*
  Infant Behavior, *234*
  Maternal Attachment, *234*
  Paternal Engrossment, *235*
  Siblings, *236*
  Multiple Births and Subsequent
    Children, *237*
Prepare for Discharge and Home
  Care, *237*

**9 Health Problems
    of Newborns, *243***

Debbie Fraser Askin

Birth Injuries, *244*
  Soft-Tissue Injury, *244*
  Head Trauma, *244*
    Caput Succedaneum, *244*
    Cephalhematoma, *244*
    Subgaleal Hemorrhage, *245*
  Fractures, *246*
  Paralysis, *246*
    Facial Paralysis, *246*

Brachial Palsy, *246*
Phrenic Nerve Paralysis, *247*
Common Problems in the
Newborn, *247*
  Erythema Toxicum
    Neonatorum, *247*
  Candidiasis, *248*
    Oral Candidiasis, *248*
  Herpes, *248*
  Birthmarks, *249*

Nursing Care of the High-Risk
Newborn and Family, *250*
  Identification of High-Risk
    Newborns, *250*
    Classification of High-Risk
      Newborns, *250*
  Care of High-Risk Newborns, *251*
    Systematic Assessment, *251*
    Monitoring Physiologic Data, *252*
    Respiratory Support, *252*
    Thermoregulation, *252*
    Protection from Infection, *254*
    Hydration, *255*
    Nutrition, *255*
    Feeding Resistance, *258*

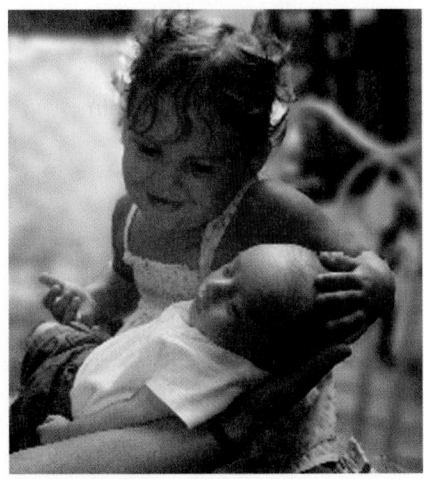

Energy Conservation, *258*
Skin Care, *259*
Administration of
   Medications, *261*
Developmental Outcome, *261*
Family Support and
   Involvement, *264*
Facilitating Parent-Infant
   Relationships, *265*

Discharge Planning and Home
   Care, *268*
   Neonatal Loss, *269*
**High Risk Related to
Dysmaturity,** *271*
   Preterm Infants, *271*
   Postterm Infants, *273*
**High Risk Related to Physiologic
Factors,** *274*
   Hyperbilirubinemia, *274*
   Hemolytic Disease of the
      Newborn, *281*
      Blood Incompatibility, *281*
   Metabolic Complications, *284*
   Respiratory Distress Syndrome, *284*
   Respiratory Complications, *288*
   *Nursing Care Plan: The High-Risk
      Infant with Respiratory Distress
      Syndrome,* *289*
   Cardiovascular Complications, *294*
   Cerebral Complications, *294*
   Neonatal Seizures, *294*
**High Risk Related to Infectious
Processes,** *296*
   Sepsis, *296*
   Necrotizing Enterocolitis, *297*

**High Risk Related to Maternal
Conditions,** *299*
   Infants of Diabetic Mothers, *299*
   Drug-Exposed Infants, *300*
      Alcohol Exposure, *303*
      Cocaine Exposure, *303*
      Methamphetamine Exposure, *304*
      Marijuana Exposure, *304*
   Maternal Infections, *305*
Congenital Anomalies, *308*
   Genetic Etiology of Congenital
      Anomalies, *309*
      Chromosomal Abnormalities, *309*
      Single-Gene Defects, *309*
      Multifactorial Inheritance, *309*
   Defects Caused by Chemical
      Agents, *309*
Inborn Errors of Metabolism, *310*
   Congenital Hypothyroidism, *311*
   Phenylketonuria, *313*
   Galactosemia, *315*
**Genetic Evaluation and
Counseling,** *316*
   Psychologic Aspects of Genetic
      Disease, *317*

UNIT FOUR

INFANCY, *322*

**10 Health Promotion of the
   Infant and Family,** *322*
   David Wilson

**Promoting Optimal Growth
and Development,** *323*
   Biologic Development, *323*
      Proportional Changes, *323*
      Maturation of Systems, *323*
      Fine Motor Development, *325*
      Gross Motor Development, *325*
   Psychosocial Development:
      Developing a Sense of Trust
      (Erikson), *327*
   Cognitive Development:
      Sensorimotor Phase (Piaget), *327*
   Development of Body Image, *330*
   Social Development, *331*
      Attachment, *331*
      Language Development, *332*
      Play, *333*
   Temperament, *334*
      Childrearing Practices Related to
         Temperament, *335*
   Coping with Concerns Related to
      Normal Growth and
      Development, *335*
      Separation and Stranger Fear, *335*
      Alternate Child Care
         Arrangements, *335*

   Limit Setting and Discipline, *341*
   Thumb Sucking and Use of a
      Pacifier, *342*
   Teething, *342*
   Infant Shoes, *343*
**Promoting Optimal Health During
Infancy,** *343*
   Nutrition, *343*
      The First 6 Months, *344*
      The Second 6 Months, *345*
      Selection and Preparation of Solid
         Foods, *345*
      Introduction of Solid Foods, *346*
      Weaning, *347*
   Sleep and Activity, *347*
      Sleep Problems, *347*
   Dental Health, *349*
   Immunizations, *350*
      Schedule for Immunizations, *350*
      Recommendations for Routine
         Immunizations, *351*
      Recommendations for Selected
         Immunizations, *359*
      Reactions, *359*
      Contraindications and
         Precautions, *359*
      Administration, *359*
   Injury Prevention, *365*
      Aspiration of Foreign Objects, *365*

   Suffocation, *368*
   Motor Vehicle Injuries, *369*
   Falls, *370*
   Poisoning, *370*
   Burns, *371*
   Drowning, *372*
   Bodily Damage, *372*
   Nurse's Role in Injury
      Prevention, *372*
**Anticipatory Guidance—Care of
Families,** *374*

11 Health Problems of Infants, 377

David Wilson

Nutritional Disorders, 378
  Vitamin Imbalances, 378
  Complementary and Alternative
    Medicine, 379
  Mineral Imbalances, 379
  Vegetarian Diets, 379
  Nursing Care Management, 380
  Protein-Energy Malnutrition, 381
    Kwashiorkor, 383
    Marasmus, 383
  Food Sensitivity, 384
    Cow's Milk Allergy, 386
    Lactose Intolerance, 387

Feeding Difficulties, 395
  Regurgitation and "Spitting
    Up," 395
  Paroxysmal Abdominal Pain
    (Colic), 395
  Growth Failure (Failure to
    Thrive), 396
Positional Plagiocephaly, 400
Disorders of Unknown Etiology, 401
  Sudden Infant Death
    Syndrome, 401
  Apnea and Apparent Life-
    Threatening Event, 404

UNIT FIVE

EARLY CHILDHOOD, 409

12 Health Promotion of the Toddler and Family, 409

David Wilson

Promoting Optimal Growth and
Development, 410
  Biologic Development, 410
    Proportional Changes, 410
    Sensory Changes, 410
    Maturation of Systems, 410
    Gross and Fine Motor
      Development, 411
  Psychosocial Development, 411
    Developing a Sense of Autonomy
      (Erikson), 411
  Cognitive Development:
    Sensorimotor and Preoperational
    Phase (Piaget), 412
  Spiritual Development, 413
  Development of Body Image, 414
  Development of Gender
    Identity, 415
  Social Development, 415
    Language, 415
    Personal-Social Behavior, 416
    Play, 416
  Coping with Concerns Related
    to Normal Growth
    and Development, 417
    Toilet Training, 417
    Sibling Rivalry, 420
    Temper Tantrums, 421
    Negativism, 421
    Regression, 422
Promoting Optimal Health During
Toddlerhood, 422
  Nutrition, 422
    Nutritional Counseling, 422
    Dietary Guidelines, 423

Sleep and Activity, 424
Dental Health, 424
  Regular Dental Examinations, 424
  Removal of Plaque, 424
  Fluoride, 425
  Low-Cariogenic Diet, 426
Injury Prevention, 426
  Motor Vehicle Injuries, 428
  Drowning, 431
  Burns, 431
  Poisoning, 432
  Falls, 433
  Aspiration and Suffocation, 433
  Bodily Damage, 433
  Terrorism and Violence, 434
Anticipatory Guidance—Care
  of Families, 434

13 Health Promotion of the Preschooler and Family, 437

Rebecca A. Monroe

Promoting Optimal Growth and
Development, 438
  Biologic Development, 438
    Gross and Fine Motor Skills, 438
  Psychosocial Development, 438
    Developing a Sense of Initiative
      (Erikson), 438
  Cognitive Development, 439
    Preoperational Phase (Piaget), 439
  Moral Development, 439
    Preconventional or Premoral Level
      (Kohlberg), 439
  Spiritual Development, 439
  Development of Body Image, 440
  Development of Sexuality, 440
  Social Development, 440
    Language, 440
    Personal-Social Behavior, 440
    Play, 441
  Coping with Concerns Related
    to Normal Growth
    and Development, 442
    Preschool and Kindergarten
      Experience, 442
    Sex Education, 443
    Fears, 446
    Stress, 446
    Aggression, 447
    Speech Problems, 447
Promoting Optimal Health During
the Preschool Years, 447
  Nutrition, 447
  Sleep and Activity, 448
    Sleep Problems, 449

Dental Health, *450*
Injury Prevention, *450*
Anticipatory Guidance—Care
   of Families, *450*

14 Health Problems of Toddlers and Preschoolers, *452*

David Wilson, Lisa Creamer, and Faye Blair

Infectious Disorders, *453*
   Communicable Diseases, *453*
   Conjunctivitis, *464*
   Stomatitis, *465*
Intestinal Parasitic Diseases, *466*
   **General Nursing Care
      Management, *466***
   Giardiasis, *466*
   Enterobiasis (Pinworms), *468*
Ingestion of Injurious Agents, *469*
   **Principles of Emergency
      Treatment, *470***
      Assessment, *473*
      Gastric Decontamination, *473*
      Prevention of Recurrence, *474*

Heavy Metal Poisoning, *475*
Lead Poisoning, *475*
   Causes of Lead Poisoning, *476*
   Screening for Lead Poisoning, *478*
Child Maltreatment, *480*
   Child Neglect, *480*
      Types of Neglect, *480*
   Emotional Abuse, *480*
   Physical Abuse, *480*
      Shaken Baby Syndrome, *481*
      Munchausen Syndrome
         by Proxy, *481*
      Factors Predisposing to Physical
         Abuse, *481*
   Sexual Abuse, *482*
      Characteristics of Abusers
         and Victims, *482*
      Initiation and Perpetuation
         of Sexual Abuse, *482*
   **Nursing Care of the Maltreated
      Child, *483***
      Caregiver-Child Interaction, *485*
      History and Interview, *485*
      Physical Assessment, *486*
   *Nursing Care Plan: The Child Who
      Is Maltreated, 489*

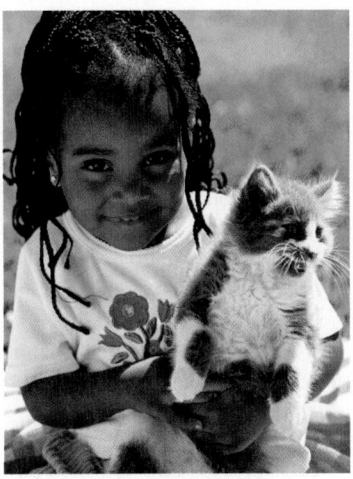

UNIT SIX

MIDDLE CHILDHOOD AND ADOLESCENCE, *492*

15 Health Promotion of the School-Age Child and Family, *492*

Cheryl C. Rodgers

**Promoting Optimal Growth and
Development, *493***
   Biologic Development, *493*
      Proportional Changes, *493*
      Maturation of Systems, *493*
      Prepubescence, *494*
   **Psychosocial Development:
      Developing a Sense of Industry
      (Erikson), *494***
   **Cognitive Development
      (Piaget), *495***
   **Moral Development
      (Kohlberg), *495***
   Spiritual Development, *496*
   Social Development, *497*
      Social Relationships and
         Cooperation, *497*
      Relationships with Families, *498*
      Play, *498*
   Developing a Self-Concept, *499*
      Developing a Body Image, *500*
   **Coping with Concerns Related to
      Normal Growth and
      Development, *500***

School Experience, *500*
Latchkey Children, *500*
Limit Setting and Discipline, *501*
Dishonest Behavior, *501*
Stress and Fear, *504*
**Promoting Optimal Health During
the School Years, *504***
   Nutrition, *504*
   Sleep and Rest, *505*
   Exercise and Activity, *505*
      Sports, *505*
      Acquisition of Skills, *506*
   Dental Health, *506*
      Dental Problems, *506*
   Sex Education, *507*
      Nurse's Role in Sex Education, *507*
   School Health, *508*
   Injury Prevention, *508*
   **Anticipatory Guidance—Care
      of Families, *509***

16 Health Promotion of the Adolescent and Family, *513*

Linda M. Kollar

**Promoting Optimal Growth and
Development, *514***

Biologic Development, *514*
   **Hormonal Changes of
      Puberty, *514***
   Sexual Maturation, *515*
   Physical Growth, *515*
   Physiologic Changes, *518*
**Psychosocial Development:
   Developing a Sense of Identity
   (Erikson), *518***
**Cognitive Development
   (Piaget), *519***

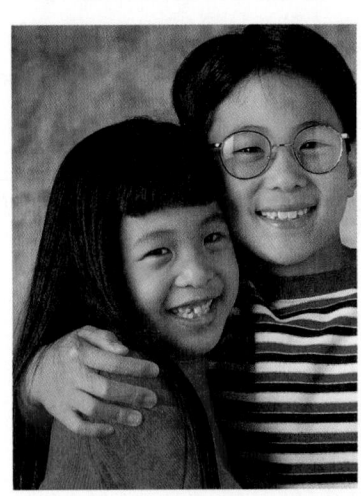

Moral Development
(Kohlberg), 519
Spiritual Development, 520
Social Development, 520
Relationships with Parents, 520
Relationships with Peers, 520
Interests and Activities, 521
Adolescent Sexuality, 522
Development of Self-Concept and
Body Image, 523
Responses to Puberty, 524
**Promoting Optimal Health During
Adolescence, 524**
Immunizations, 526
Nutrition, 526
Eating Habits and Behavior, 527
Sleep and Rest, 528
Exercise and Activity, 528
Dental Health, 528
Personal Care, 528
Vision, 528
Hearing, 529
Posture, 529
Body Art, 529
Tanning, 529
Stress Reduction, 529
Sexuality Education
and Guidance, 530
Injury Prevention, 531
Motor Vehicle–Related
Injuries, 532
Firearms, 532
Sports Injuries, 532
Anticipatory Guidance—Care
of Families, 532

17 **Health Problems of School-
Age Children and
Adolescents, 536**

Linda M. Kollar and David Wilson

Problems Related to Elimination, 537
Enuresis, 537
Encopresis, 538
**Health Problems Related to Sports
Participation, 538**
Overuse Syndromes, 538
Stress Fractures, 539
Nurse's Role in Sports for Children
and Adolescents, 539
Altered Growth and Maturation, 540
Sex Chromosome Disorders, 540
Turner Syndrome, 540
Klinefelter Syndrome, 540

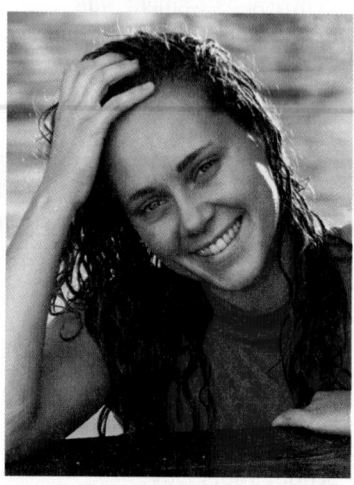

Disorders Related to the
Reproductive System, 541
Amenorrhea, 541
Dysmenorrhea, 541
Vaginitis, 542
Disorders of the Male
Reproductive System, 542
Gynecomastia, 543
**Health Problems Related to
Sexuality, 543**
Adolescent Pregnancy, 543
Contraception, 544
Sexually Transmitted Diseases, 547
Pelvic Inflammatory Disease, 547
Sexual Assault (Rape), 549
Rape Trauma Syndrome, 550
Eating Disorders, 551
Obesity, 551
Anorexia Nervosa and Bulimia
Nervosa, 556
**Disorders with Behavioral
Components, 559**
Attention Deficit Hyperactivity
Disorder and Learning
Disability, 559
Posttraumatic Stress Disorder, 562
School Phobia, 562
Recurrent Abdominal Pain, 562
Conversion Reaction, 563
Childhood Depression, 563
Childhood Schizophrenia, 564
**Serious Health Problems of Later
Childhood and Adolescence, 564**
Substance Abuse, 564
Motivation, 564
Types of Drugs Abused, 565
Suicide, 568
Methods, 569
Motivation, 570

UNIT SEVEN

THE CHILD AND FAMILY WITH SPECIAL NEEDS, 574

18 **Chronic Illness, Disability,
or End-of-Life Care for the
Child and Family, 574**

Angela M. Ethier

**Perspectives on the Care of Children
with Special Needs, 575**
Scope of the Problem, 575
Trends in Care, 575
Developmental Focus, 575
Family-Centered Care, 576
Family–Health Care Provider
Communication, 576
Establishing Therapeutic
Relationships, 576

The Role of Culture in Family-
Centered Care, 577
Shared Decision Making, 577
Normalization, 577
Managed Care, 578
**The Family of the Child with Special
Needs, 578**
Impact of the Child's Chronic
Illness or Disability, 578
Parents, 579
Siblings, 580
Coping with Ongoing Stress and
Periodic Crises, 581
Concurrent Stresses Within the
Family, 581

Coping Mechanisms, 581
Parental Empowerment, 581
**Assisting Family Members in
Managing Their Feelings, 581**
Shock and Denial, 582
Adjustment, 582
Reintegration and
Acknowledgment, 582
Establishing a Support System, 583
The Child with Special Needs, 583
Developmental Aspects, 583
Coping Mechanisms, 584
Hopefulness, 584
Health Education and
Self-Care, 584

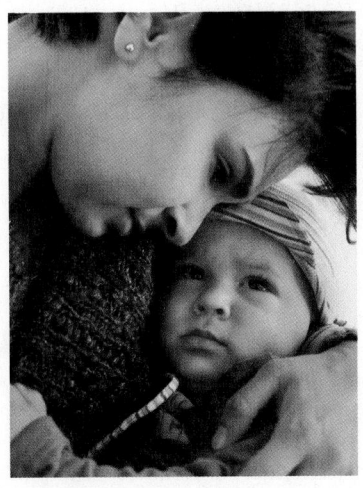

Responses to Parental
Behavior, *585*
Type of Illness or Disability, *585*
**Nursing Care of the Family and Child
with Special Needs, *585***
Assessment, *585*
Provide Support at the Time of
Diagnosis, *586*
Support Family's Coping
Methods, *587*
Parents, *587*
Parent-to-Parent Support, *589*
Advocate for Empowerment, *589*
The Child, *589*
Siblings, *590*
Educate About the Disorder and
General Health Care, *590*
Activities of Daily Living, *590*
Safe Transportation, *591*
Primary Health Care, *591*
Promote Normal
Development, *591*
Early Childhood, *591*
School Age, *593*
Adolescence, *594*
Establish Realistic Future
Goals, *594*
**Perspectives on the Care of Children
at the End of Life, *595***
Principles of Palliative Care, *595*

Decision Making at the End of
Life, *595*
Ethical Considerations in End-of-
Life Decision Making, *595*
Physician–Health Care Team
Decision Making, *596*
Parental Decision Making, *597*
The Dying Child, *597*
Treatment Options for Terminally Ill
Children, *599*
**Nursing Care of the Child and Family
at the End of Life, *600***
*Nursing Care Plan: The Child Who
Is Terminally Ill or Dying, 600*
Fear of Pain and Suffering, *600*
Pain and Symptom
Management, *602*
Parents' and Siblings' Need for
Education and Support, *603*
Fear of Dying Alone or of Not
Being Present When the Child
Dies, *603*
Fear of Actual Death, *603*
Home Deaths, *603*
Hospital Deaths, *604*
Organ or Tissue Donation and
Autopsy, *605*
Grief and Mourning, *605*
Parental Grief, *606*
Sibling Grief, *606*
Nurses' Reactions to Caring for
Dying Children, *607*

**19 Impact of Cognitive or
Sensory Impairment on the
Child and Family, *610***
Rosalind Bryant

Cognitive Impairment, *611*
General Concepts, *611*
Nursing Care of Children
with Impaired Cognitive
Function, *612*
*Nursing Care Plan: The Child
with Impaired Cognitive
Function, 614*
Down Syndrome, *619*
Fragile X Syndrome, *622*

Sensory Impairment, *623*
Hearing Impairment, *623*
Visual Impairment, *628*
Deaf-Blind Children, *633*
Retinoblastoma, *633*
Autism Spectrum Disorders, *635*

**20 Family-Centered Home
Care, *641***
Marilyn J. Hockenberry

General Concepts of Home Care, *642*
Home Care Trends, *642*
Effective Home Care, *643*
Discharge Planning and Selection
of a Home Care Agency, *644*
Care Coordination (Case
Management), *646*
Role of the Nurse, Training, and
Standards of Care, *647*

Family-Centered Home Care, *648*
Diversity in Home Care, *648*
Parent-Professional
Collaboration, *649*
The Nursing Process, *650*
Promotion of Optimum
Development, Self-Care, and
Education, *651*
Safety Issues in the Home, *653*
Family-to-Family Support, *654*

UNIT EIGHT

IMPACT OF HOSPITALIZATION ON THE CHILD AND FAMILY, *658*

**21 Family-Centered Care of
the Child During Illness and
Hospitalization, *658***
Jennifer Sanders

**Stressors of Hospitalization and
Children's Reactions, *659***

Separation Anxiety, *659*
Early Childhood, *661*
Later Childhood and
Adolescence, *661*
Loss of Control, *661*
Infants, *661*
Toddlers, *662*

Preschoolers, *662*
School-Age Children, *662*
Adolescents, *662*
Effects of Hospitalization on the
Child, *663*
Individual Risk Factors, *663*
Beneficial Effects of
Hospitalization, *664*

22 Pediatric Variations of Nursing Interventions, 686
Terri L. Brown

General Concepts Related to Pediatric Procedures, 687
Informed Consent, 687
    Requirements for Obtaining
        Informed Consent, 687
    Eligibility for Giving Informed
        Consent, 689
Preparation for Diagnostic and
    Therapeutic Procedures, 689
    Psychologic Preparation, 689
    Performance of the Procedure, 693
    Postprocedural Support, 694
    Use of Play in Procedures, 694
Surgical Procedures, 694
    Preoperative Care, 694
    Postoperative Care, 697
Compliance, 698
    Compliance Strategies, 699

General Hygiene and Care, 700
Maintaining Healthy Skin, 700
Bathing, 701
Oral Hygiene, 701
Hair Care, 702
Feeding the Sick Child, 702
Controlling Elevated
    Temperatures, 702
    Fever, 703
    Hyperthermia, 704
Family Teaching and Home
    Care, 704

Safety, 705
Environmental Factors, 705
    Toy Safety, 705
    Preventing Falls, 706
Infection Control, 706
Transporting Infants and
    Children, 708

Restraining Methods and
    Therapeutic Holding, 708
    Jacket Restraint, 709
    Mummy Restraint or Swaddle, 709
    Arm and Leg Restraints, 709
    Elbow Restraint, 710
Positioning for Procedures, 710
    Femoral Venipuncture, 710
    Extremity Venipuncture, 710
    Lumbar Puncture, 710
    Bone Marrow Aspiration
        or Biopsy, 711

Collection of Specimens, 711
Urine Specimens, 711
    Clean-Catch Specimens, 712
    Twenty-Four-Hour Collection, 712
    Bladder Catheterization and Other
        Techniques, 713
Stool Specimens, 715
Blood Specimens, 715
Respiratory Secretion
    Specimens, 717

Administration of Medication, 717
Determination of Drug
    Dosage, 717
    Checking Dosage, 718
    Identification, 718
Oral Administration, 718
    Preparation, 718
    Administration, 719
Intramuscular Administration, 719
    Selecting the Syringe and
        Needle, 719
    Determining the Site, 720
    Administration, 720
Subcutaneous and Intradermal
    Administration, 723
Intravenous Administration, 725
    Peripheral Intermittent Infusion
        Device, 725
    Central Venous Access Device, 725
Nasogastric, Orogastric, or
    Gastrostomy Administration, 730
Rectal Administration, 730
Optic, Otic, and Nasal
    Administration, 730
Family Teaching and Home
    Care, 731

Maintaining Fluid Balance, 732
Measurement of Intake and
    Output, 732
    Special Needs When the Child Is
        NPO, 732
Parenteral Fluid Therapy, 733
    Site and Equipment, 733
    Safety Catheters and Needleless
        Systems, 734
    Infusion Pumps, 735
    Securement of a Peripheral
        Intravenous Line, 735

Stressors and Reactions of the Family of the Child Who Is Hospitalized, 664
Parental Reactions, 664
Sibling Reactions, 664
Altered Family Roles, 664

Nursing Care of the Child Who Is Hospitalized, 664
Preparation for
    Hospitalization, 664
    Admission Assessment, 665
    Preparing Child for Admission, 665
Nursing Interventions, 668
    Preventing or Minimizing
        Separation, 668
    Minimizing Loss of Control, 670
    Preventing or Minimizing Fear of
        Bodily Injury, 672
    Providing Developmentally
        Appropriate Activities, 672
    Providing Opportunities for Play
        and Expressive Activities, 673
    Maximizing Potential Benefits of
        Hospitalization, 675

Nursing Care of the Family, 676
Supporting Family Members, 676
Providing Information, 677
Encouraging Parent
    Participation, 677
Preparing for Discharge and Home
    Care, 678

Care of the Child and Family in Special Hospital Situations, 679
Ambulatory or Outpatient
    Setting, 679
Isolation, 680
Emergency Admission, 680
Intensive Care Unit, 681

Removal of a Peripheral
Intravenous Line, *737*
Complications, *738*
**Procedures for Maintaining
Respiratory Function, *738***
Inhalation Therapy, *738*
Oxygen Therapy, *738*
Monitoring Oxygen Therapy, *739*
Aerosol Therapy, *740*
Bronchial (Postural) Drainage, *741*
Chest Physical Therapy, *741*

Artificial Ventilation, *741*
Artificial Airways, *741*
Tracheostomy, *741*
**Procedures Related to Alternative
Feeding Techniques, *745***
Gavage Feeding, *745*
Gastrostomy Feeding, *746*
Nasoduodenal and Nasojejunal
Tubes, *749*

Total Parenteral Nutrition, *749*
Family Teaching and Home
Care, *750*
**Procedures Related to
Elimination, *750***
Enema, *750*
Ostomies, *750*
Family Teaching and Home
Care, *751*

UNIT NINE

THE CHILD WITH PROBLEMS RELATED TO THE TRANSFER OF OXYGEN AND NUTRIENTS, *754*

23 **The Child with Respiratory
Dysfunction, *754***
David Wilson

Respiratory Infection, *755*
*Nursing Care Plan: The Child with
Acute Respiratory Tract
Infection, 759*
**Upper Respiratory Tract
Infections, *759***
Nasopharyngitis, *759*
Pharyngitis, *762*
Tonsillitis, *763*
Influenza, *764*
Otitis Media, *765*
Infectious Mononucleosis, *768*
Croup Syndromes, *769*
Acute Epiglottitis, *769*
Acute Laryngitis, *770*
Acute
Laryngotracheobronchitis, *770*
Acute Spasmodic Laryngitis, *771*
Bacterial Tracheitis, *772*
Infections of the Lower Airways, *772*
Bronchitis, *773*
Respiratory Syncytial Virus and
Bronchiolitis, *773*
Pneumonias, *774*
Viral Pneumonia, *775*
Primary Atypical Pneumonia, *775*
Severe Acute Respiratory
Syndrome, *775*
Avian Influenza Virus, *775*
Bacterial Pneumonia, *776*
**Other Infections of the Respiratory
Tract, *777***
Pertussis (Whooping Cough), *777*
Tuberculosis, *777*

**Pulmonary Dysfunction Caused by
Noninfectious Irritants, *780***
Foreign Body Aspiration, *780*
Aspiration Pneumonia, *781*
Acute Respiratory Distress
Syndrome/Acute Lung Injury, *781*
Smoke Inhalation Injury, *782*
Environmental Tobacco Smoke
Exposure, *783*
**Long-Term Respiratory
Dysfunction, *783***
Asthma, *783*
*Nursing Care Plan: The Child with
Asthma, 792*
Cystic Fibrosis, *795*
Obstructive Sleep-Disordered
Breathing, *803*
Respiratory Emergency, *803*
Respiratory Failure, *803*
Cardiopulmonary
Resuscitation, *804*
Resuscitation Procedure, *805*
Airway Obstruction, *809*
Infants, *809*
Children, *809*

24 **The Child with
Gastrointestinal
Dysfunction, *813***
Marsha L. Ellett

Gastrointestinal Dysfunction, *814*
Dehydration, *814*
Water Balance in Infants, *814*
Types of Dehydration, *815*

Disorders of Motility, *817*
Diarrhea, *817*
Constipation, *823*
Newborn Period, *824*
Infancy, *824*
Childhood, *824*
Hirschsprung Disease, *825*
Vomiting, *826*
Gastroesophageal Reflux, *827*
**Functional Abdominal Pain
Disorders, *829***
Inflammatory Disorders, *829*
Acute Appendicitis, *829*
*Nursing Care Plan: The Child with
Appendicitis, 831*
Meckel Diverticulum, *831*
Inflammatory Bowel Disease, *833*
Peptic Ulcer Disease, *836*
Hepatic Disorders, *838*
Acute Hepatitis, *838*
Cirrhosis, *841*
Biliary Atresia, *842*

Structural Defects, 843
    Cleft Lip or Cleft Palate, 843
    Esophageal Atresia with
        Tracheoesophageal Fistula, 846
    Hernias, 849
Obstructive Disorders, 849
    Hypertrophic Pyloric Stenosis, 849
    Intussusception, 852

Malrotation and Volvulus, 853
Anorectal Malformations, 854
Malabsorption Syndromes, 855
    Celiac Disease, 855
    Short-Bowel Syndrome, 856

UNIT TEN

THE CHILD WITH PROBLEMS RELATED TO THE PRODUCTION AND CIRCULATION OF BLOOD, 861

25 The Child with
Cardiovascular
Dysfunction, 861

Patricia O'Brien and
Annette L. Baker

Cardiovascular Dysfunction, 862
    History and Physical
        Examination, 862
Congenital Heart Disease, 865
    Circulatory Changes at Birth, 866
    Altered Hemodynamics, 866
    Classification of Defects, 866
        Defects with Increased Pulmonary
            Blood Flow, 867
        Obstructive Defects, 867
        Defects with Decreased Pulmonary
            Blood Flow, 867
        Mixed Defects, 870
Clinical Consequences of Congenital
Heart Disease, 876
    Congestive Heart Failure, 876
    Nursing Care Plan: The Child with
        Congestive Heart Failure
        (CHF), 880
    Hypoxemia, 884
Nursing Care of the Family and Child
with Congenital Heart Disease, 886
    Help Family Adjust to the
        Disorder, 886
    Educate Family About the
        Disorder, 887
    Help Families Manage the Illness
        at Home, 887
    Prepare Child and Family for
        Invasive Procedures, 888

Provide Postoperative Care, 889
    Observe Vital Signs, 889
    Maintain Respiratory Status, 890
    Monitor Fluids, 890
    Provide Rest and Progressive
        Activity, 890
    Provide Comfort and Emotional
        Support, 891
Plan for Discharge and Home
Care, 891

Acquired Cardiovascular
Disorders, 891
    Bacterial (Infective)
        Endocarditis, 891
    Rheumatic Fever, 893
    Hyperlipidemia
        (Hypercholesterolemia), 894
    Cardiac Dysrhythmias, 896
    Pulmonary Artery
        Hypertension, 897
    Cardiomyopathy, 898
Heart Transplantation, 899
Vascular Dysfunction, 899
    Systemic Hypertension, 899
    Kawasaki Disease (Mucocutaneous
        Lymph Node Syndrome), 901
    Shock, 902
    Anaphylaxis, 904
    Septic Shock, 906
    Toxic Shock Syndrome, 907

26 The Child with Hematologic
or Immunologic
Dysfunction, 911

Rosalind Bryant

Hematologic and Immunologic
Dysfunction, 912
Red Blood Cell Disorders, 912
    Anemia, 912
        Classification, 912
        Consequences of Anemia, 912
    Iron Deficiency Anemia, 915
    Sickle Cell Anemia, 916
    β-Thalassemia (Cooley
        Anemia), 923
    Aplastic Anemia, 924
Defects in Hemostasis, 925
    Hemophilia, 925

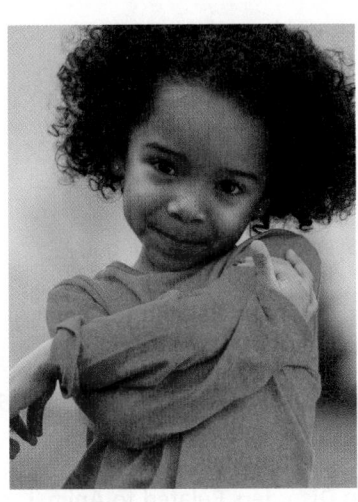

Idiopathic Thrombocytopenic
Purpura, 927
Disseminated Intravascular
Coagulation, 929
Epistaxis (Nosebleeding), 929

Neoplastic Disorders, 930
Leukemias, 930
Prognosis, 931
Late Effects of Treatment, 932
*Nursing Care Plan: The Child with
Cancer,* 932
Lymphomas, 937
Hodgkin Disease, 937
Non-Hodgkin Lymphoma, 939

Immunologic Deficiency
Disorders, 939
Human Immunodeficiency Virus
Infection and Acquired
Immunodeficiency
Syndrome, 939
Severe Combined
Immunodeficiency Disease, 943
Wiskott-Aldrich Syndrome, 943

**Technologic Management of
Hematologic and Immunologic
Disorders,** 943
Blood Transfusion Therapy, 943
Hematopoietic Stem Cell
Transplantation, 945
Apheresis, 946

UNIT ELEVEN

THE CHILD WITH A DISTURBANCE OF REGULATORY MECHANISMS, 949

**27 The Child with
Genitourinary
Dysfunction,** 949

*Barbara A. Montagnino
and Patricia A. Ring*

Genitourinary Dysfunction, 950
**Genitourinary Tract Disorders and
Defects,** 950
Urinary Tract Infection, 950
Obstructive Uropathy, 956
External Defects, 957
Psychologic Problems Related to
Genital Surgery, 957

Glomerular Disease, 958
Nephrotic Syndrome, 958
Acute Glomerulonephritis, 961

Miscellaneous Renal Disorders, 962
Hemolytic Uremic Syndrome, 962
Wilms Tumor, 963

Renal Failure, 965
Acute Renal Failure, 965
*Nursing Care Plan: The Child with
Acute Renal Dysfunction,* 967
Chronic Renal Failure, 967

**Technologic Management of Renal
Failure,** 970
Dialysis, 970
Transplantation, 971

**28 The Child with Cerebral
Dysfunction,** 974

Marilyn J. Hockenberry

Cerebral Dysfunction, 975
General Aspects, 975

Increased Intracranial Pressure, 975
Altered States of
Consciousness, 976
Levels of Consciousness, 976
Coma Assessment, 976
Neurologic Examination, 977
Vital Signs, 977
Skin, 977
Eyes, 977
Motor Function, 978
Posturing, 979
Reflexes, 979
Special Diagnostic Procedures, 979

**Nursing Care of the Unconscious
Child,** 981
Respiratory Management, 982
Intracranial Pressure
Monitoring, 982
Nursing Activities, 983
Suctioning, 984
Nutrition and Hydration, 984
Altered Pituitary Secretion, 984
Medications, 984
Thermoregulation, 984
Elimination, 984
Hygienic Care, 985
Positioning and Exercise, 985
Stimulation, 985
Regaining Consciousness, 985
Family Support, 985

Cerebral Trauma, 986
Head Injury, 986
Near-Drowning, 993

Nervous System Tumors, 995
Brain Tumors, 995
Neuroblastoma, 997

Intracranial Infections, 998
Bacterial Meningitis, 998
Nonbacterial (Aseptic)
Meningitis, 1002
Encephalitis, 1002
Rabies, 1003
Reye Syndrome, 1004

Seizure Disorders, 1005
Epilepsy, 1005
*Nursing Care Plan: The Child with
Seizure Disorder,* 1011
Febrile Seizures, 1016

Cerebral Malformations, 1016
Cranial Deformities, 1016
Hydrocephalus, 1017

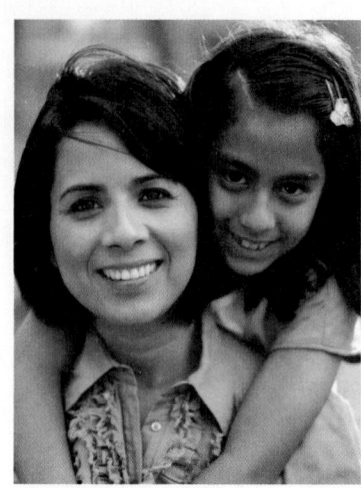

29 The Child with Endocrine Dysfunction, *1023*

Marilyn J. Hockenberry

Disorders of Pituitary Function, *1024*
Hypopituitarism, *1024*
Pituitary Hyperfunction, *1029*
Precocious Puberty, *1029*
Diabetes Insipidus, *1030*
Syndrome of Inappropriate
  Antidiuretic Hormone, *1031*

Disorders of Thyroid Function, *1032*
Juvenile Hypothyroidism, *1032*
Goiter, *1033*
Lymphocytic Thyroiditis, *1033*
Hyperthyroidism, *1034*

Disorders of Parathyroid Function, *1035*
Hypoparathyroidism, *1035*
Hyperparathyroidism, *1036*

Disorders of Adrenal Function, *1037*
Acute Adrenocortical
  Insufficiency, *1037*
Chronic Adrenocortical
  Insufficiency (Addison
  Disease), *1038*
Cushing Syndrome, *1039*
Congenital Adrenal
  Hyperplasia, *1040*
Pheochromocytoma, *1042*

Disorders of Pancreatic Hormone Secretion: Diabetes Mellitus, *1042*
Nursing Care Plan: The Child with Diabetes Mellitus, 1052

30 The Child with Integumentary Dysfunction, *1060*

Shannon Stone McCord, Rose U. Baker, and Mary A. Mondozzi

Integumentary Dysfunction, *1061*
Skin Lesions, *1061*
  Skin of Younger Children, *1061*
Wounds, *1062*
  Epidermal Injuries, *1062*
  Injury to Deeper Tissues, *1062*
  Process of Wound Healing, *1062*
  Factors That Influence
    Healing, *1065*
General Therapeutic
  Management, *1065*
  Dressings, *1067*
  Topical Therapy, *1067*
  Systemic Therapy, *1067*
Nursing Care Management, *1067*
  Wound Care, *1068*
  Relief of Symptoms, *1068*
  Topical Therapy, *1068*

Home Care and Family
  Support, *1069*

Infections of the Skin, *1069*
Bacterial Infections, *1069*
Viral Infections, *1071*
Dermatophytoses (Fungal
  Infections), *1071*
Systemic Mycotic (Fungal)
  Infections, *1072*

Skin Disorders Related to Chemical or Physical Contacts, *1074*
Contact Dermatitis, *1074*
Poison Ivy, Oak, and Sumac, *1075*
Drug Reactions, *1076*
Foreign Bodies, *1076*

Skin Disorders Related to Animal Contacts, *1076*
Arthropod Bites and Stings, *1076*
Scabies, *1079*
Pediculosis Capitis, *1079*
Rickettsial Diseases, *1082*
Lyme Disease, *1082*
Mammal Bites and Scratches, *1083*
Pet and Wild Animal Bites, *1083*
Human Bites, *1083*
Cat Scratch Disease, *1083*

Miscellaneous Skin Disorders, *1084*

Skin Disorders Associated with Specific Age-Groups, *1084*
Diaper Dermatitis, *1084*
Atopic Dermatitis (Eczema), *1086*
Seborrheic Dermatitis, *1089*
Acne, *1089*

Thermal Injury, *1091*
Burns, *1091*
Sunburn, *1103*
Cold Injury, *1103*

UNIT TWELVE

THE CHILD WITH A PROBLEM THAT INTERFERES WITH PHYSICAL MOBILITY, *1106*

31 The Child with Musculoskeletal or Articular Dysfunction, *1106*

David Wilson, Martha R. Curry, and Marilyn J. Hockenberry

The Immobilized Child, *1107*
Immobilization, *1107*
  Physiologic Effects of
    Immobilization, *1107*
  Psychologic Effects of
    Immobilization, *1108*
  Effect on Families, *1109*

Traumatic Injury, *1110*
Soft-Tissue Injury, *1110*
  Contusions, *1110*

Dislocations, *1111*
Sprains, *1111*
Strains, *1112*
Fractures, *1112*
  Epiphyseal (or Physeal)
    Injuries, *1112*
  Types of Fractures, *1112*
  Bone Healing and
    Remodeling, *1113*
The Child in a Cast, *1115*
  The Cast, *1115*
The Child in Traction, *1117*
  Purposes of Traction, *1117*
  Types of Traction (General), *1118*
  Upper Extremity Traction, *1118*
  Lower Extremity Traction, *1118*
  Cervical Traction, *1119*

Distraction, *1121*
  External Fixation, *1121*
Amputation, *1121*

Congenital Defects, *1122*
Developmental Dysplasia of the
  Hip, *1122*
Congenital Clubfoot, *1125*
Metatarsus Adductus (Varus), *1126*
Skeletal Limb Deficiency, *1127*
Osteogenesis Imperfecta, *1127*

Acquired Defects, *1128*
Legg-Calvé-Perthes Disease, *1128*
Slipped Capital Femoral
  Epiphysis, *1130*
Kyphosis and Lordosis, *1130*
Idiopathic Scoliosis, *1130*

Infections of Bones and Joints, *1134*
  Osteomyelitis, *1134*
  Septic Arthritis, *1135*
  Skeletal Tuberculosis, *1135*

Bone and Soft-Tissue Tumors, *1136*
  General Concepts: Bone
    Tumors, *1136*
  Osteosarcoma, *1136*
  Ewing Sarcoma (Primitive
    Neuroectodermal Tumor), *1137*
  Rhabdomyosarcoma, *1138*

Disorders of Joints, *1139*
  Juvenile Idiopathic Arthritis
    (Juvenile Rheumatoid
    Arthritis), *1139*
  Systemic Lupus
    Erythematosus, *1142*

32 **The Child with
    Neuromuscular or Muscular
    Dysfunction,** *1145*
    David Wilson

Congenital Neuromuscular or
Muscular Disorders, *1146*
  Cerebral Palsy, *1146*

*Nursing Care Plan: The Child with
    Cerebral Palsy, 1151*
Spina Bifida
    (Myelomeningocele), *1154*
  Latex Allergy, *1159*
Spinal Muscular Atrophy, Type 1
    (Werdnig-Hoffmann
    Disease), *1161*
Spinal Muscular Atrophy, Type 3
    (Kugelberg-Welander
    Disease), *1162*
Muscular Dystrophies, *1162*
Duchenne (Pseudohypertrophic)
    Muscular Dystrophy, *1162*

Acquired Neuromuscular
Disorders, *1165*
  Guillain-Barré Syndrome
    (Infectious Polyneuritis), *1165*
  Tetanus, *1167*
  Botulism, *1168*
    Infant Botulism, *1169*
  Spinal Cord Injuries, *1170*

Appendixes
  A Developmental/Sensory
     Assessment, *1174*
  B Growth Measurements, *1180*
  C Common Laboratory
     Tests, *1192*
  D NANDA International–
     Approved Nursing Diagnoses
     2007-2008, *1201*
  E Translations of Wong-Baker
     FACES Pain Rating Scale, *1202*
  F Spanish-English
     Translations, *1204*
  G Dietary Reference
     Intakes, *1206*

1

Perspectives of Pediatric Nursing

MARILYN J. HOCKENBERRY

CHAPTER OUTLINE

HEALTH CARE FOR CHILDREN, 2
Health Promotion, 2
Nutrition, 2
Dental Care, 3
Immunizations, 3
CHILDHOOD HEALTH PROBLEMS, 3
Obesity and Type 2 Diabetes, 3
Childhood Injuries, 3
Violence, 6
Substance Abuse, 7
Mental Health Problems, 8
MORTALITY, 8
Infant Mortality, 8
Childhood Mortality, 9
MORBIDITY, 10
Childhood Morbidity, 10

THE ART OF PEDIATRIC NURSING, 10
Philosophy of Care, 10
Family-Centered Care, 10
Atraumatic Care, 11
ROLE OF THE PEDIATRIC NURSE, 11
Therapeutic Relationship, 11
Family Advocacy and Caring, 11
Disease Prevention and Health
   Promotion, 12
Health Teaching, 13
Support and Counseling, 13
Coordination and Collaboration, 13
Ethical Decision Making, 13
Research, 14

**CRITICAL THINKING AND THE PROCESS
OF NURSING CHILDREN AND
FAMILIES, 14**
Critical Thinking, 14
Evidence-Based Practice, 14
Nursing Process, 15
   Assessment, 16
   Nursing Diagnosis, 16
   Planning, 17
   Implementation, 17
   Evaluation, 17
   Documentation, 17

LEARNING OBJECTIVES

On completion of this chapter the reader will be able to:
- Define the terms *mortality* and *morbidity*.
- Identify two ways that knowledge of mortality and morbidity can improve child health.
- List three major causes of death during infancy, early childhood, later childhood, and adolescence.
- List two major causes of illness during childhood.
- Describe five broad functions of the pediatric nurse in promoting the health of children.
- Define *critical thinking*.
- Identify the five steps of the nursing process.
- Define *nursing diagnosis*.
- Define *evidence-based practice*.

RELATED TOPICS and ADDITIONAL RESOURCES

IN TEXT

Care Coordination (Case Management),
  Ch. 20
Classification of High-Risk Newborns, *Ch. 9*
Cultural and Religious Influences on Health
  Care, *Ch. 4*
Immunizations, *Ch. 10*

Injury Prevention: Infant, *Ch. 10*; Toddler,
  Ch. 12; Preschooler *Ch. 13*; School-Age
  Child, *Ch. 15*; Adolescent, *Ch. 16*
Preschool and Kindergarten Experience,
  Ch. 13
Scope of the Problem (Chronic Illness or
  Disability), *Ch. 18*
Suicide, *Ch. 17*

   COMPANION CD

NCLEX Review Questions

evolve

evolve.elsevier.com/Wong/essentials/

NCLEX Review Questions
WebLinks

HEALTH CARE FOR CHILDREN

The major goal for pediatric nursing is to improve the quality of health care for children. There are 73 million children 0 to 18 years of age in the United States, comprising 25% of the population (Dougherty, Meikle, Owens, and others, 2005). The health of children living in the United States has improved in numerous areas, including vaccination coverage, adolescent birth rates, and child mortality. Although child mortality rates have declined dramatically, millions of families have no child health insurance, resulting in lack of access to care and health promotion services. And although most American children are healthy, disparities related to race, ethnicity, socioeconomic status, and geography prevail. Patterns of child health are shaped by medical progress and societal trends (Dougherty, Meikle, Owens, and others, 2005; Wise, 2004, 2005). The *Healthy People 2010* Leading Health Indicators (Box 1-1) provide a framework for identifying essential components for child health promotion programs designed to prevent future health problems in our nation's children.

The National Children's Study is the largest long-term study of children's health and development conducted in the United States. The study is designed to follow 100,000 children and their families from birth to age 21 to understand the link between children's environments and their physical and emotional health and development (American Academy of Pediatrics, 2004). It is hoped that a study of this magnitude will provide innovative interventions for families, children, and health care providers to eradicate unhealthy diets, dental caries, and childhood obesity, and bring a significant reduction in violence, injury, substance abuse, and mental health disorders among the nation's children. This study supports the *Healthy People 2010* primary goals to increase the quality and years of healthy life and eliminate health disparities related to race, ethnicity, and socioeconomic status (US Department of Health and Human Services, 2007).

HEALTH PROMOTION

Many of tomorrow's leading causes of death, disease, and disability (cardiovascular disease, cancer, chronic lung diseases, depression, violence, substance abuse, injuries, nutritional deficiencies, human immunodeficiency virus/acquired immunodeficiency syndrome [HIV/AIDS]) can be significantly reduced in children and adolescents by preventing six categories of behavior (World Health Organization [WHO], 2007):

1. Tobacco use
2. Behavior that results in injury and violence
3. Alcohol and substance use
4. Dietary and hygienic practices that cause disease
5. Sedentary lifestyle
6. Sexual behavior that causes unintended pregnancy and disease

Child health promotion provides opportunities to reduce differences in current health status among members of different groups and ensure equal opportunities and resources to enable all children to achieve their fullest health potential.

NUTRITION

Nutrition is an essential component for healthy growth and development, and its promotion begins at birth. Human milk is the preferred form of nutrition for all infants. **Breastfeeding** provides the infant with micronutrients, immunologic properties, and several enzymes that enhance digestion and absorption of these nutrients. Many working mothers tend to wean their infants early to avoid the hassle of breast pumping during the workday. However, over the past several years, there has been resurgence in breastfeeding due to the education of mothers and fathers regarding its benefits.

Young children tend to establish eating habits during the first 2 to 3 years of life, and the nurse is instrumental in guiding parents in the selection of nutritious foods. During child-

---

BOX 1-1

Healthy People 2010

GOALS
Increase quality and length of healthy life
Eliminate health disparities

LEADING HEALTH INDICATORS
Physical activity
Overweight and obesity
Tobacco use
Substance abuse
Responsible sexual behavior
Mental health
Injury and violence
Environmental quality
Immunization
Access to health care

From US Department of Health and Human Service: Healthy people 2010: *understanding and improving health*, ed 2, Washington, DC, 2000, US Government Printing Office.

hood, the eating preferences and attitudes related to food habits are established by family influences and culture. During adolescence, parental influence diminishes as the adolescent make food choices related to peer acceptability and sociability; these choices may be detrimental to the chronically ill child with diabetes, hypertension, or heart or renal disease.

Unhealthy diets are common among lower income families, often because of the lack of nutritious fresh fruits and vegetables and adequate milk and protein intake. In addition, the lifestyles of homeless and migrant children place these populations at risk for inadequate food, causing nutrient deficiencies, developmental and growth delays, depression, hunger, and behavior problems.

DENTAL CARE

The *Healthy People 2010* project reports that nearly one in five children between the ages of 2 and 4 years, particularly Latino children, has visible cavities (Edelstein, 2005). **Dental caries** is the single most common chronic disease of childhood (Heuer, 2007). The most common form of early dental disease is early childhood caries, which may begin at the first birthday and progress to pain and infection within the first 2 years of life (Edelstein, 2005). Preschoolers of low-income families are twice as likely to develop tooth decay and only half as likely to visit the dentist as other children (Edelstein, 2005). Since this is a preventable disease, nursing plays an essential role in promoting early tooth care by instructing the children and parents on practicing dental hygiene beginning with the first tooth eruption; drinking fluoridated water, including bottled water; and instituting early dental preventive care.

IMMUNIZATIONS

The two public health interventions that have had the greatest impact on world health are clean drinking water and vaccines. Differences in **immunizations rates** exist among children of different races and ethnicities, family incomes, states, types of vaccinations, and adolescents and younger children (Dougherty, Meikle, Owens, and others, 2005). A child's immunization record should be reviewed at each clinic visit, and parents should be instructed to keep immunizations current, reinforcing the *Healthy People 2010* goal of vaccinating 90% of 2-year-olds (US Department of Health and Human Services, 2007).

CHILDHOOD HEALTH PROBLEMS

The health of the nation's children continues to improve in many areas, such as lower pregnancy rates for adolescents and expanded vaccine coverage. However, changes in modern society, including disruptive influences on the family, the explosion of technology, and the proliferation of information systems, are influencing the emergence of significant medical problems that affect the health of children (Lichter, 2005). Recent concern has focused on groups of children who have increased morbidity: homeless and immigrant children, children living in poverty, low-birth-weight (LBW) children, children with chronic illnesses, foreign-born adopted children, and children in daycare centers. A number of factors place these groups at risk for poor health. A major cause is barriers to health care, especially for the homeless, the poverty stricken, and those with chronic health problems. Other factors include improved survival of children with chronic health problems, particularly infants of very low birth weight (VLBW).

In addition to disease and injury, children face behavior, social (family), and educational problems that are referred to as the **new morbidity** or **pediatric social illness**. These problems (e.g., poverty, violence, aggression, noncompliance, school failure, and adjustment to divorce or bereavement) interfere with children's social and academic development. **Mental health issues** also affect our children and adolescents. One out of five has mental health problems, and one out of 10 has serious emotional problems that affect daily functioning (Coury, 2006). Examples of increasing pediatric problems include obesity, type 2 diabetes, injuries, violence, substance abuse, and emotional and mental health problems during adolescence.

OBESITY AND TYPE 2 DIABETES

Childhood obesity is the most common nutritional problem among American children and is increasing in epidemic proportions, along with type 2 diabetes (Yensel, Preud'Homme, and Curry, 2004). **Obesity** in children and adolescents is defined as a body mass index at or greater than the 95th percentile for youth of the same age and gender (Dietz, 2005; Covington, Cybulski, Davis, and others, 2001). The National Health and Nutrition Examination Survey reported that the prevalence of overweight children doubled and the prevalence of overweight adolescents tripled between 1980 and 2000 (Dietz, 2005).

Advancements in entertainment and technology such as television, computers, and video games have contributed to the growing childhood obesity problem in the United States. Approximately 63% of 8- to 18-years-olds have a television in their bedrooms and watch television an average of 4 hours a day (Robinson and Sargent, 2005). Minority populations, especially African-American and Hispanic children from families of low socioeconomic status, watch more than 4 hours of television daily, exacerbating the effects of sedentary activity with intake of high-caloric, fatty foods (Fitzgibbon and Stolley, 2004).

Lack of outside physical activity because of unsafe environments and inconvenient facilities for physical activities, combined with easy assess to video games and television within the home, tend to promote obesity among low-income minority children. Overweight youth, especially of Hispanic, African-American, and Native American descent, have increased risk for developing diabetes, insulin resistance, hypertension, and heart disease (Jackson, 2001; Yensel, Preud'Homme, and Curry, 2004) (Fig. 1-1). A major nursing health prevention focus, consistent with the *Healthy People 2010* primary goals, is the reduction of overweight children, ages 6 to 19 years, from the current 20% in all ethnic groups, to less than 6% (Duderstadt, 2004; US Department of Health and Human Services, 2007).

CHILDHOOD INJURIES

Injuries are the most common cause of death and disability to children in the United States (Schnitzer, 2006) (Table 1-1). **Unintentional injuries** among children ages 19 and under have dropped to 39%, and the violent death rate has dropped 36% in the same age bracket; however, the trend has now plateaued (Rivara, 2005). Despite the decrease in injuries to children, motor vehicle (MV)–related accidents continue as the most common cause of death in children older than 1 year of age. As children grow older, the percentage of deaths from injuries increases. The most common types of unintentional

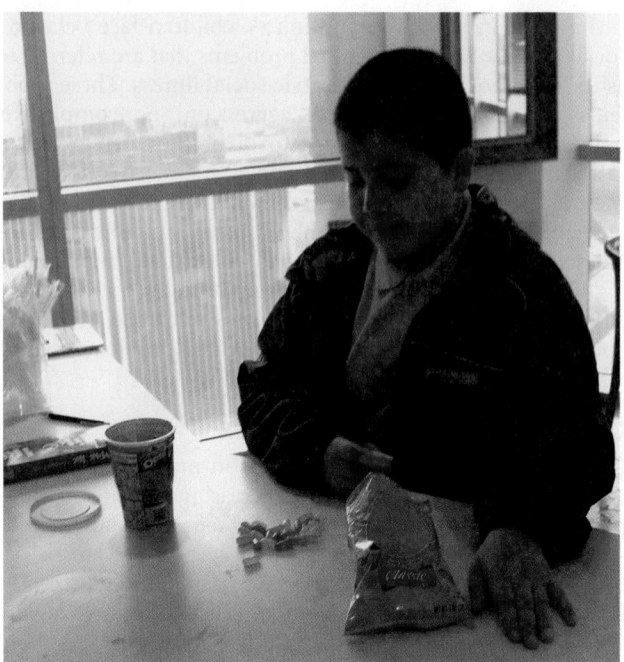

FIG. 1-1 ■ The American culture's intake of high-caloric fatty foods contributes to obesity in children.

injuries, in addition to MV accidents, include drowning, burns, and firearm accidents. Many childhood injury fatalities could be avoided. For example, the majority of bicycling deaths are from head injuries. Although helmets reduce the risk of head injury by 85%, few children wear them (National Safety Council, 2000).

The type of injury and the circumstances surrounding it are closely related to normal growth and developmental behavior (Box 1-2). As children develop, their innate curiosity impels them to investigate activities and to mimic the behavior of others. This is essential to acquire competency as an adult, but it predisposes children to numerous hazards.

The child's **developmental stage** partially determines the types of injuries that are most likely to occur at a specific age and helps provide clues to preventive measures. For example, small infants are helpless in any environment. When they begin to roll over or propel themselves, they can fall from unprotected surfaces. The crawling infant, who has a natural tendency to place objects in the mouth, is at risk for aspiration or poisoning. The mobile toddler, with the instinct to explore and investigate and the ability to run and climb, may experience falls, burns, and collisions with objects. As children grow older, their absorption with play makes them oblivious to environmental hazards such as street traffic or water. The need

TABLE 1-1

Mortality from Leading Types of Unintentional Injuries, United States, 1997 (Rate Per 100,000 Population in Each Age-Group)

	AGE (years)			
TYPE OF ACCIDENT	<1	1-4	5-14	15-24
MALES				
All causes	818.0	39.8	24.0	124.4
Unintentional injuries (all types)	22.3	15.2	10.6	52.3
Motor vehicle	4.4 (2)	5.3 (1)	5.8 (1)	38.3 (1)
Drowning	1.8 (4)	3.9 (2)	1.6 (2)	3.2 (2)
Fires and burns	1.5 (5)	2.5 (3)	0.8 (3)	—
Firearms	—	0.5 (4)	0.5 (4)	—
Ingestion of food/object	2.5 (3)	0.5 (5)	—	—
Falls	—	—	—	1.2 (5)
Mechanical suffocation	9.1 (1)	0.6 (4)	0.4 (5)	—
Poisoning	—	—	—	2.8 (3)
All other unintentional injuries	3.1	2.3	1.4	5.3
Accidents as a percent of all deaths	2.7%	38.2%	44.3%	42.0%
FEMALES				
All causes	662.9	31.8	17.4	46.0
Unintentional injuries (all types)	18.1	10.9	6.7	20.0
Motor vehicle	4.4 (2)	4.7 (1)	4.3 (1)	17.1 (1)
Drowning	1.4 (4)	2.0 (2)	0.6 (3)	0.4 (3)
Fires and burns	1.2 (5)	2.0 (2)	0.7 (2)	—
Firearms	—	—	0.1 (4)	0.1 (5)
Ingestion of food/object	1.5 (3)	0.4 (4)	—	—
Falls	—	—	—	0.2 (4)
Mechanical suffocation	6.9 (1)	0.3 (5)	0.1 (4)	—
Poisoning	—	—	—	0.8 (2)
All other unintentional injuries	2.7	1.5	0.9	1.5
Accidents as a percent of all deaths	2.7%	34.2%	38.2%	43.4%

Modified from National Safety Council: *Injury facts*, Itaska, Ill, 2000, The Council. Data from National Center for Health Statistics.

to conform and gain acceptance compels older children and adolescents to accept challenges and dares. Although the rate of injuries is high in children less than 9 years of age, most fatal injuries occur in later childhood and adolescence.

The pattern of deaths caused by unintentional injuries, especially from MVs, drowning, and burns, is remarkably consistent in most Western societies. However, the United States far exceeds other countries in the number of **violent deaths.** The leading causes of death from injuries for each age-group according to sex are presented in Table 1-1. Although the incidence of violence is increasing in the United States, it is important to note that accidents continue to account for more than three times as many teen deaths as any other cause (Heron, 2007). Fortunately, prevention strategies

such as the use of car restraints, bicycle helmets, and smoke detectors have resulted in a significant decrease in fatalities for children. Currently, all states have enacted legislation requiring young children to be properly restrained in MVs. Despite safety efforts, the overwhelming cause of death in children is MV-related fatalities, including occupant, pedestrian, bicycle, and motorcycle deaths. In fact, MV-related accidents now account for more than half of all injury deaths (National Center for Injury Prevention and Control, 2001). The majority of deaths from injuries occur in males. Even though the percentage of infants dying from MV injuries is small compared with the total number of deaths in that age-group, children under 1 year of age still have a high death rate from MV accidents, primarily from a failure to use proper restraints (Fig. 1-2).

Pedestrian injuries in children account for significant numbers of MV-related deaths. Most pedestrian injuries occur at midblock, at intersections, in driveways, and in parking lots. Driveway injuries typically involve small children and large vehicles backing up. Parents may not be alert to the dangers leading to such injuries and consequently fail to protect their children.

Bicycle injuries are another important cause of childhood deaths. Children ages 5 to 9 years are at greatest risk of bicycling fatalities. The majority of bicycling deaths are from head injuries. Helmets reduce the risk of head injury by 85%, but few children wear helmets (National Safety Council, 2000). Community-wide bicycle helmet campaigns and mandatory-use laws have resulted in significant increases in helmet use. Still, issues such as stylishness, comfort, and social acceptability remain important factors in compliance. Nurses can educate children and families about pedestrian and bicycle safety. In particular, school nurses can promote helmet wearing and encourage peer leaders to act as role models.

Drowning and **burns** are among the top five leading causes of deaths for males and females throughout childhood (Fig. 1-3). In addition, improper use of firearms is a major cause of death among males (Fig. 1-4). During infancy, more males succumb to death from aspiration or suffocation than do females (Fig. 1-5). More than half of all **poisonings** re-

---

BOX 1-2
Childhood Injuries: Risk Factors

Sex—Preponderance of males; difference mainly the result of behavioral characteristics, especially aggression

Temperament—Children with difficult temperament profile, especially persistence, high activity level, and negative reactions to new situations

Stress—Predisposes children to increased risk taking and self-destructive behavior; general lack of self-protection

Alcohol and drug use—Associated with higher incidence of motor vehicle injuries, drownings, homicides, and suicides

History of previous injury—Associated with increased likelihood of another injury, especially if initial injury required hospitalization

Developmental characteristics
- Mismatch between child's developmental level and skill required for activity (e.g., all-terrain vehicles)
- Natural curiosity to explore environment
- Desire to assert self and challenge rules
- In older child, desire for peer approval and acceptance

Cognitive characteristics (age specific)
Infancy—Sensorimotor: explores environment through taste and touch
Young child
- Object permanence—actively searches for attractive object
- Cause and effect—unaware of consequential dangers
- Transductive reasoning—may fail to learn from experiences (e.g., perceives falling from a step as a different type of danger from climbing a tree)
- Magical and egocentric thinking—cannot comprehend danger to self or others; cannot take place of others to realize danger
School-age child—Transitional cognitive processes: unable to fully comprehend causal relationships; attempts dangerous acts without detailed planning regarding consequences
Adolescent—Formal operations: preoccupied with abstract thinking and loses sight of reality; may lead to feeling of invulnerability

Anatomic characteristics (especially in young children)
- Large head—predisposes to cranial injury
- Large spleen and liver with wide costal arch—predisposes to direct trauma to these organs
- Small and light body—may be thrown easily, especially inside a moving vehicle

Other factors—Poverty, family stress (e.g., maternal illness, recent environmental change), substandard alternative child care, young maternal age, low maternal education, multiple siblings

FIG. 1-2 ■ Motor vehicle injuries are the leading cause of death in children older than 1 year of age. The majority of fatalities involve occupants who are unrestrained.

FIG. 1-3 ■ **A,** Drowning is one of the leading causes of death. Children left unattended are unsafe even in shallow water. **B,** Burns are among the top three leading cause of death from injury in children ages 1 to 14 years.

FIG. 1-4 ■ Improper use of firearms is the fourth leading cause of death from injury in children 5 to 14 years of age.

FIG. 1-5 ■ Mechanical suffocation is the leading cause of death from injury in infants.

ported in 1999 occurred in children under 6 years of age (National Center for Injury Prevention and Control, 2001) (Fig. 1-6). By ages 4 to 5 years, unintentional poisonings are uncommon. Another increase occurs in the 15- to 24-year age-group, where poisoning is the third leading cause of death in males and second in females. Poisoning in this age-group is typically intentional and usually represents death from suicide (especially among females) or drug abuse.

VIOLENCE

Each day, 10 children in the United States are murdered by gunfire, equivalent to approximately one child every 2½ hours (Groves, 2005). Strikingly higher homicide rates are found among minority populations, especially African-American children. Violence permeates American households through television programs, commercials, video games, and movies that tend to desensitize the child toward violence. By the time preschoolers graduate from high school, they will have viewed more than 200,000 violent acts on television (Groves, 2005). Violence also permeates the schools with the availability of guns and illicit drugs and the presence of gangs, exemplified by one of the deadliest school shootings in U.S. history at Columbine High School in Colorado in 1999 (Fisher and

Kettl, 2003). Although declines from peak levels in 1993 have been observed in serious violent crimes with children as victims or as offenders (ages 12 to 17) (Federal Interagency Forum on Child and Family Statistics, 2007), assessment of high-risk behaviors in our youth must continue to be a major focus of health promotion.

The causes of increased violence against children and self-inflicted violence are not fully understood. In young children the increase in homicide may represent a more accurate identification of child abuse. In all cases the problem of child homicide is extremely complex and involves numerous social, economic, and other influences. Prevention lies in better understanding of the social and psychologic factors that lead to

COMMUNITY FOCUS

Violence in Children

Community violence has reached epidemic proportions in the United States. Recently, political leaders have recognized violence as a public health emergency and a preventable problem (Groves, 2005). The serious problem of community violence affects the lives of many children and expands throughout the family, schools, and the workplace. Nurses working with children, adolescents, and families have a critical role in reducing violence through early identification and symptom recognition of the mental-emotional stress that can result from these experiences.

During the past decade the incidence of violent crimes has dramatically increased, making the United States the most violent country in the industrialized world. The multifaceted origins of the problem of violence include developmental factors, gang involvement, access to firearms, drugs, the media, poverty, and family conflict. Often, the silent and underrecognized victims are the children who witness acts of community violence. Studies suggest that chronic exposure to violence has a negative effect on a child's cognitive, social, psychologic, and moral development. Also, multiple exposures to episodes of violence do not inoculate children against the negative effects; continued exposure can result in lasting symptoms of stress. Children living with chronic violence may exhibit behaviors such as difficulty concentrating in school, memory impairment, aggressive play, uncaring behaviors, and constricted activities and thinking for fear of reliving the traumatic event (Groves, 2005).

The growing national concern about the increasing prevalence of violent crimes has prompted nurses to actively participate in ensuring that children grow up in safe environments. Pediatric nurses are positioned to assess children and adolescents for signs of exposure to violence and well-known risk factors, as well as to provide nonviolent problem-solving strategies, counseling, and referrals. These activities will affect community practice and expand the nurse's role in the future health environment. Suggestions for professional resources include the following.

Brady Center to Prevent Gun Violence
1225 Eye St. NW, Suite 1100
Washington, DC 20005
(202) 289-7319
http://www.bradycenter.org

National Domestic Violence Hotline
PO Box 161810
Austin, TX 78716
(800) 799-SAFE
http://www.ndvh.org

National Organization for Victim Assistance
Courthouse Square
510 King St., Suite 424
Alexandria, VA 22314
(703) 535-NOVA or (800) TRY-NOVA
http://www.trynova.org

National School Safety Center
141 Duesenberg Drive, Suite 11
Westlake Village, CA 91362
(805) 373-9977
http://www.schoolsafety.us

Parent Teacher Association—National Headquarters
541 North Fairbanks Court, Suite 1300
Chicago, IL 60611-3396
(312) 670-6782 or (800) 307-4PTA (4782)
http://www.pta.org

Targeted Outreach Program
Boys and Girls Club of America
National Headquarters
1275 Peachtree St. NE
Atlanta, GA 30309
(404) 487-5700
http://www.bgca.org

the high rates of homicide and suicide. Nurses need to be especially aware of young people who are depressed, repeatedly in trouble with the criminal justice system, or associated with groups known to be violent. Prevention requires identification of these young people and therapeutic intervention by qualified professionals.

Pediatric nurses can assess children and adolescents for risk factors related to violence. Families that own firearms must be educated about their safe use and storage. The presence of a gun in a household increases the risk of suicide by about fivefold and the risk of homicide by about threefold. Legislative efforts may focus on preventing specific groups, such as felons and children, from having access to firearms. Technologic changes such as childproof safety devices and loading indicators could improve the safety of firearms (see Community Focus Box).

SUBSTANCE ABUSE

Risk-taking behaviors, particularly in males, tends to begin in the first decade of life and continue into adolescence with drinking alcohol while driving, speeding, carrying a weapon, or using illicit drugs. Alcohol and illicit drug use occurs most

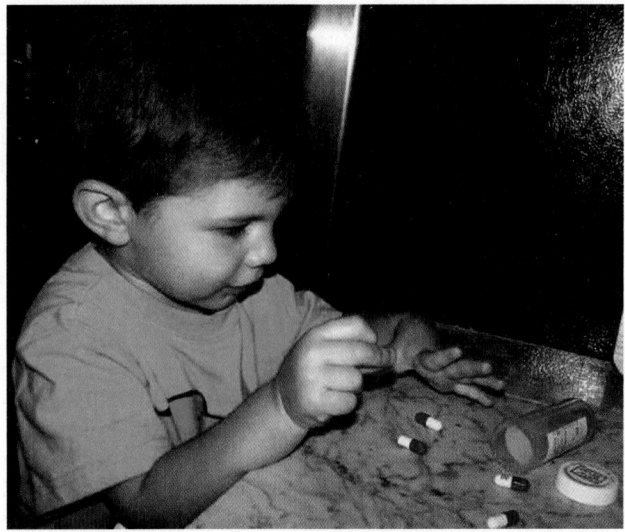

FIG. 1-6 ■ Poisoning causes a considerable number of injuries in children under 4 years of age. Prescription drugs should never be left where young children can reach them.

commonly between ages 12 and 17 years and is associated with violence and injury (Jackson, 2001). About 10.9 million youths between the ages of 12 and 20 (primarily males) report drinking alcohol, with nearly 19.2% reported as being binge drinkers and 6.1% as being heavy drinkers (Substance Abuse and Mental Health Services Administration, 2004). Sixty-six percent of youths who drank alcohol heavily and 52% of youths from 12 to 17 years of age who smoked cigarettes daily were also users of illicit drugs (Substance Abuse and Mental Health Services Administration, 2004). An estimated 2.6 million new marijuana users emerged in 2002, with 69% under age 18 years. Use of marijuana, the most commonly used illicit drug, declined slightly from 20.6% in 2002 to 19.6% in 2003 (National Center for Health Statistics, 2007). During the same period, decreases were also seen in use of lysergic acid diethylamide (LSD) (1.3% to 0.6%), 3,4-methylenedioxymethamphetamine (MDMA, or ecstasy) (2.2% to 1.3%), and methamphetamine (0.9% to 0.7%) (National Center for Health Statistics, 2007). The slight decline in American youth's illicit drug use is attributed to education regarding the adverse effects of illicit drugs, parental disapproval, decreased availability of drugs, and consistent participation in church and organized activities such as scouts and sports.

MENTAL HEALTH PROBLEMS

Mental health problems affect one out of five school-age children in the United States. Children and adolescents with mental health problems are more likely to drop out of school than those with other disabilities (Kelleher, 2005). One of the most common mental health problems is **attention deficit hyperactivity disorder** (ADHD) (Kelleher, 2005). ADHD is characterized by inattentiveness, impulsivity, and at times hyperactivity occurring in children as early as 3 years of age (Medd, 2003). ADHD affects every aspect of the child's life, but is most obvious in the classroom. Family education, counseling, medication, proper classroom placement, environmental manipulation, and behavior therapy are important management strategies for these children.

Suicide is defined as a self-chosen death and is the third leading cause of death in children ages 10 to 19 (Doucette, 2005). The American Association of Suicidology (2007) estimates that in a typical high school classroom, three students (one boy and two girls) have likely made a suicide attempt in the last year. Suicide is a preventable occurrence, placing a heavy burden on the nurse's ability to identify the at-risk child or adolescent who may display mental health and emotional problems. There is a need to more completely integrate a system of care for children and adolescents that will provide integrated medical and mental health services that promote health (Coury, 2006).

MORTALITY

Figures describing rates of occurrence for events such as death in children are referred to as **vital statistics. Mortality statistics** describe the incidence or number of individuals who have died over a specific period. They are usually presented as rates per 100,000. Mortality rates are calculated from a sample of death certificates. In the United States the National Center for Health Statistics, under the Department of Health and Human Services, Public Health Service, is responsible for the collection, analysis, and dissemination of data on the health of the American people (Federal Interagency Forum on Child and Family Statistics, 2007).

The tabulation of race for live births (the denominator of infant mortality rates) has changed from race of child to race of mother. Formerly, to determine the child's race in mixed parentage in which one parent was Caucasian, the child was assigned the race of the other parent. In general, this change in assignment of race from child to mother has resulted in more Caucasian births and fewer non-Caucasian births. However, infant deaths are recorded by the decedent's race, resulting in a lower infant mortality rate for Caucasians than non-Caucasians. As a result of these changes in the early 1990s, figures for births, deaths, and infant mortality rates by race are not comparable to statistics reported before these changes were made.

INFANT MORTALITY

The **infant mortality rate** is the number of deaths during the first year of life per 1000 live births. It may be further divided into **neonatal mortality** (<28 days of life) and **postneonatal mortality** (28 days to 11 months). In the United States infant mortality has decreased dramatically. At the beginning of the twentieth century the rate was approximately 200 infant

---

TABLE 1-2

Infant Mortality Rate (IMR) for Countries of >2,500,000 Population with IMR Equal to or Less Than the U.S. Rate for 2004 (Rate Per 1000 Live Births)

COUNTRY	IMR 2004
Singapore	—
Hong Kong	2.7
Japan	2.8
Finland	3.3
Sweden	3.1
Norway	3.2
Czech Republic	3.7
Spain	3.5
France	—
Germany	4.1
Italy	4.1
Austria	4.4
Denmark	4.4
Switzerland	4.2
Portugal	3.8
Belgium	4.7
Greece	—
Israel	4.6
Canada	—
Australia	4.4
Korea	4.6
Netherlands	4.4
United Kingdom	—
Ireland	4.9
New Zealand	5.6
Cuba	5.8
United States	6.8

From Martin JA, Kung HC, Mathews TJ, and others: Annual summary of vital statistics: 2006, *Pediatrics* 121(4):788-801, 2008.
—, Data are not available.

deaths per 1000 live births. In 2004 the infant mortality rate was 6.78 deaths per 1000 live births (Martin, Kung, Mathews, and others, 2008).

From a worldwide perspective, however, the United States lags behind other nations in reducing infant mortality. In 2004 the United States ranked last among 27 nations that have a population of at least 2.5 million and had infant mortality rates equal to or lower than that of the United States in 2000. Hong Kong, Singapore, and Japan have the three lowest rates, with the United States ranked last behind Cuba and Croatia (Martin, Kung, Mathews, and others, 2008) (Table 1-2).

Birth weight is considered the major determinant of neonatal death in technologically developed countries. There is a relationship between LBW and infant morbidity and mortality (Martin, Kochanek, Strobino, and others, 2005). The lower the birth weight, the higher the mortality. The relatively high incidence of LBW (<2500 g [5.5 pounds]) in the United States is considered a key factor in its higher neonatal mortality rate when compared with other countries. Access to and the use of high-quality prenatal care is a promising preventive strategy to decrease early delivery and infant mortality. Other factors that increase the risk of infant mortality include African-American race, male gender, short or long gestation, maternal age, and lower level of maternal education (Martin, Kochanek, Strobino, and others, 2005).

As Table 1-3 demonstrates, many of the leading causes of death during infancy continue to occur during the perinatal period. The first four causes—congenital anomalies, disorders relating to short gestation and unspecified LBW, sudden infant death syndrome (SIDS), and newborn affected by maternal complications of pregnancy—accounted for about half (49%) of all deaths of infants under 1 year of age (Heron, 2007). LBW is a major indicator of infant health and a significant predictor of infant mortality (Martin, Kung, Mathews, and others, 2008). Many birth defects are associated with LBW, and reducing the incidence of LBW will prevent congenital anomalies. Infant mortality resulting from HIV infection decreased significantly during the 1990s. In 2003 HIV/AIDS accounted for less than 0.2% of all infant deaths (Hoyert, Heron, Murphy, and others, 2006).

When infant death rates are categorized according to race, a disturbing difference is seen. Infant mortality for Caucasians is considerably lower than for all other races in the United States, with African Americans having twice the rate of Caucasians. Although the infant mortality of all racial groups increased slightly between 2001 and 2002, the gap has remained constant, with the infant mortality rate expressed as a ratio of African-American to Caucasian deaths being relatively unchanged for the past decade (Martin, Kochanek, Strobino, and others, 2005). The LBW rate is also much higher for African-American infants than for any other group. One encouraging note is that the gap in mortality rates between Caucasian and non-Caucasian races other than African Americans has narrowed in recent years. Infant mortality rates for Hispanics and Asian–Pacific Islanders have decreased dramatically during the past 2 decades (Martin, Kochanek, Strobino, and others, 2005).

CHILDHOOD MORTALITY

Death rates for children older than 1 year of age have always been lower than those for infants (see Table 1-2). Children ages 5 to 14 years have the lowest rate of death. However, a sharp rise occurs during later adolescence, primarily from injuries, homicide, and suicide (Table 1-4). In 2005 these causes were responsible for approximately 75% of deaths in teenagers and young adults 15 to 19 years old (Martin, Kung, Mathews, and others, 2008). The trend in racial differences that occurs in infant mortality is also apparent in childhood deaths for all ages and for both sexes. Caucasians have fewer deaths for all ages, and male deaths outnumber female deaths.

After 1 year of age, the cause of death changes dramatically, with unintentional injuries (accidents) being the leading cause from the youngest ages to the adolescent years. **Violent deaths** have been steadily increasing among young people ages 10 through 25 years, especially African Americans and males. Homicide is the second leading cause of death in the 15- to 19-year age-group (see Table 1-4). Children 12 years of age and older tend to be killed by nonfamily members (acquaintances and gangs, typically of the same race) and most frequently by firearms. In 2004 African-American adolescent males were twice as likely to die as a result of a firearm injury as an MV injury (Federal Interagency Forum on Child and

TABLE 1-3

Infant Mortality Rate and Percentage of Total Deaths for 10 Leading Causes of Infant Death in 2004 (Rate Per 1000 Live Births)

RANK	CAUSE OF DEATH (BASED ON 10TH REVISION, INTERNATIONAL CLASSIFICATION OF DISEASES)	PERCENT	RATE
	All races, all causes	100.00%	679.4
1	Congenital anomalies	20.1	136.7
2	Disorders relating to short gestation and unspecified low birth weight	16.6	112.9
3	Sudden infant death syndrome	8.0	54.6
4	Newborn affected by maternal complications of pregnancy	6.1	41.7
5	Accidents (unintentional injuries)	3.8	25.6
6	Newborn affected by complications of placenta, cord, and membranes	3.7	25.3
7	Respiratory distress of newborn	3.1	21.3
8	Bacterial sepsis of newborn	3.0	20.1
9	Neonatal hemorrhage	2.2	15.0
10	Diseases of circulatory system	2.1	14.4

Modified from Heron M: Deaths: leading causes for 2004, *Natl Vital Stat Rep* 56(5):1-96, 2007.

TABLE 1-4

Five Leading Causes of Death in Children in the United States: Selected Age Intervals, 2005 (Rate Per 100,000 Population)

RANK	AGES 1-4 YEARS		AGES 5-9 YEARS		AGES 10-14 YEARS		AGES 15-19 YEARS	
	CAUSE	RATE	CAUSE	RATE	CAUSE	RATE	CAUSE	RATE
	All causes	29.3	All causes	14.5	All causes	18.0	All causes	65.0
1	Accidents	10.1	Accidents	5.5	Accidents	6.4	Accidents	31.2
2	Congenital anomalies	3.2	Cancer	2.5	Cancer	2.4	Homicide	9.7
3	Cancer	2.3	Congenital anomalies	1.0	Suicide	1.3	Suicide	7.5
4	Homicide	2.2	Homicide	0.6	Homicide	1.0	Cancer	3.5
5	Heart disease	0.9	Heart disease	0.5	Congenital anomalies	0.9	Heart disease	1.8

Modified from Martin JA, Kung HC, Mathews TJ, and others: Annual summary of vital statistics—2006, *Pediatrics* 121(4):788-801, 2008.

Family Statistics, 2007). Suicide, a form of self-violence, is the third leading cause of death among children and adolescents 10 to 19 years of age.

MORBIDITY

Measurements of the prevalence of a specific illness in the population at a particular time are known as **morbidity statistics.** Morbidity statistics are generally presented as rates per 1000 population. Unlike mortality, morbidity is difficult to define and may denote acute illness, chronic disease, or disability. Source of data also influences the statistics. Common sources include reasons for visits to physicians; diagnoses for hospital admission; or household interviews such as the National Health Interview Survey, Child Health Supplement. Unlike death rates, which are updated annually, morbidity statistics are revised less frequently and do not necessarily represent the general population.

CHILDHOOD MORBIDITY

Acute illness is defined as an illness with symptoms severe enough to limit activity or require medical attention. Respiratory illness accounts for approximately 50% of all acute conditions, 11% are caused by infections and parasitic disease, and 15% are caused by injuries. The chief illness of childhood is the common cold.

The types of diseases that children contract during childhood vary according to age. For example, upper respiratory tract infections and diarrhea decrease in frequency with age, whereas other disorders, such as acne and headaches, increase. Children who have had a particular type of problem are more likely to have that problem again. Morbidity is not distributed randomly in children. Children from poor families do not fare as well on health indicators as children from nonpoor families (Federal Interagency Forum on Child and Family Statistics, 2007). This finding suggests the need for heightened efforts to improve access to health care for low-income children.

Recent concern has focused on groups of children who have increased morbidity: homeless children, children living in poverty, LBW children, children with chronic illnesses, foreign-born adopted children, and children in daycare centers. A number of factors place these groups at risk for poor health. A major cause is barriers to health care, especially for the homeless, the poverty stricken, and those with chronic health problems. Other factors include improved survival of children with chronic health problems, particularly infants of VLBW.

THE ART OF PEDIATRIC NURSING
PHILOSOPHY OF CARE

Nursing of infants, children, and adolescents is consistent with the **definition of nursing** as "the diagnosis and treatment of human responses to actual or potential health problems." This definition incorporates the four essential features of contemporary nursing practice (American Nurses Association, 2003):

1. Attention to the full range of human experiences and responses to health and illness without restriction to a problem-focused orientation
2. Integration of objective data with knowledge gained from an understanding of the patient or group's subjective experience
3. Application of scientific knowledge to the processes of diagnosis and treatment
4. Provision of a caring relationship that facilitates health and healing

FAMILY-CENTERED CARE

The philosophy of **family-centered care** recognizes the family as the constant in a child's life. Service systems and personnel must support, respect, encourage, and enhance the strength and competence of the family by developing a partnership with parents (Newton, 2000). Nurses support families in their natural caregiving and decision-making roles by building on their unique strengths and acknowledging their expertise in caring for their child both within and outside the hospital setting (Newton, 2000). The needs of all family members, not just the child's, are considered (Box 1-3). The philosophy acknowledges diversity among family structures and backgrounds; family goals, dreams, strategies, and actions; and family support, service, and information needs.

Two basic concepts in family-centered care are enabling and empowerment. Professionals **enable** families by creating opportunities and means for all family members to display their current abilities and competencies and to acquire new ones to meet the needs of the child and family. **Empowerment** describes the interaction of professionals with families in such a way that families maintain or acquire a sense of control over their family lives and acknowledge positive changes that result from helping behaviors that foster their own strengths, abilities, and actions.

Although caring for the family is strongly emphasized throughout this text, it is highlighted in features such as Cultural Awareness, Family Focus (see p. 17), and Family-Centered Care boxes.

ATRAUMATIC CARE

Although tremendous advances have been made in pediatric care, much of what is done to children to cure illness and prolong life is traumatic, painful, upsetting, and frightening. Unfortunately, attempts to minimize the trauma of medical interventions have not kept pace with technologic advances. With knowledge of the stressors imposed on ill children and their families and armed with interventions that are safe and effective in eliminating or reducing the stressors, health professionals must direct their attention to providing atraumatic care.

Atraumatic care is the provision of therapeutic care in settings, by personnel, and through the use of interventions that eliminate or minimize the psychologic and physical distress experienced by children and their families in the health care system. **Therapeutic care** encompasses the prevention, diagnosis, treatment, or palliation of chronic or acute conditions. *Setting* refers to the place in which that care is given—the home, the hospital, or any other health care setting. **Personnel** includes anyone directly involved in providing therapeutic care. **Interventions** range from psychologic approaches, such as preparing children for procedures, to physical interventions, such as providing space for a parent to room in with a child. **Psychologic distress** may include anxiety, fear, anger, disappointment, sadness, shame, or guilt. **Physical distress** may range from sleeplessness and immobilization to disturbing sensory stimuli such as pain, temperature extremes, loud noises, bright lights, or darkness. Thus atraumatic care is con-

cerned with the who, what, when, where, why, and how of any procedure performed on a child for the purpose of preventing or minimizing psychologic and physical stress (Wong, 1989).

The overriding goal in providing atraumatic care is: **first, do no harm.** Three principles provide the framework for achieving this goal: (1) prevent or minimize the child's separation from the family, (2) promote a sense of control, and (3) prevent or minimize bodily injury and pain. Examples of providing atraumatic care include fostering the parent-child relationship during hospitalization, preparing the child before any unfamiliar treatment or procedure, controlling pain, allowing the child privacy, providing play activities for expression of fear and aggression, providing choices to children, and respecting cultural differences.

ROLE OF THE PEDIATRIC NURSE

Pediatric nurses are involved in every aspect of a child's and family's growth and development. Nursing functions vary according to regional job structures, individual education and experience, and personal career goals. Just as patients (children and their families) have unique backgrounds, each nurse brings an individual set of variables that affects the nurse-patient relationship. No matter where pediatric nurses practice, their primary concern is the welfare of the child and family.

THERAPEUTIC RELATIONSHIP

The establishment of a therapeutic relationship is the essential foundation for providing high-quality nursing care. Pediatric nurses need to have meaningful relationships with children and their families and yet remain separate enough to distinguish their own feelings and needs. In a **therapeutic relationship,** caring, well-defined boundaries separate the nurse from the child and family. These boundaries are positive and professional and promote the family's control over the child's health care. Effective family advocacy demands that these boundaries be established and promote therapeutic relationships (Jacobson, 2002). Both the nurse and the family are empowered, and open communication is maintained. In a **nontherapeutic relationship** these boundaries are blurred, and many of the nurse's actions may serve personal needs, such as a need to feel wanted and involved, rather than the family's needs.

Exploring whether relationships with patients are therapeutic or nontherapeutic helps nurses identify problem areas early in their interactions with children and families (see Nursing Care Guidelines box). Although questions for exploring types of involvement label certain actions negative or positive, no one action makes a relationship therapeutic or nontherapeutic. For example, a nurse may spend additional time with the family but still recognize his or her own needs and maintain professional separateness. An important clue to nontherapeutic relationships is the staff's concerns about their peer's actions with the family.

FAMILY ADVOCACY AND CARING

Although nurses are responsible to themselves, the profession, and the institution of employment, their primary responsibility is to the consumer of nursing services—the child and family. The nurse must work with family members, identify their goals and needs, and plan interventions that best address the defined problems. As an advocate, the nurse assists the child and family in making informed choices and acting in the

nursingcareguidelines

Exploring Your Relationships with Children and Families

To foster therapeutic relationships with children and families, you must first become aware of your caregiving style, including how effectively you take care of yourself. The following questions should help you understand the therapeutic quality of your professional relationships.

NEGATIVE ACTIONS

Are you overinvolved with children and their families?
- Do you work overtime to care for the family?
- Do you spend off-duty time with children's families, either in or out of the hospital?
- Do you call frequently (either the hospital or home) to see how the family is doing?
- Do you show favoritism toward certain patients?
- Do you buy clothes, toys, food, or other items for the child and family?
- Do you compete with other staff members for the affection of certain patients and families?
- Do other staff members comment to you about your closeness to the family?
- Do you attempt to influence families' decisions rather than facilitate their informed decision making?

Are you underinvolved with children and families?
- Do you restrict parent or visitor access to children, using excuses such as the unit is too busy?
- Do you focus on the technical aspects of care and lose sight of the person who is the patient?

Are you overinvolved with children and underinvolved with their parents?
- Do you become critical when parents do not visit their children?
- Do you compete with parents for their children's affection?

POSITIVE ACTIONS

Do you strive to empower families?
- Do you explore families' strengths and needs in an effort to increase family involvement?
- Have you developed teaching skills to instruct families rather than doing everything for them?
- Do you work with families to find ways to decrease their dependence on health care providers?
- Can you separate families' needs from your own needs?

Do you strive to empower yourself?
- Are you aware of your emotional responses to different people and situations?
- Do you seek to understand how your own family experiences influence reactions to patients and families, especially as they affect tendencies toward overinvolvement or underinvolvement?
- Do you have a calming influence, not one that will amplify emotionality?
- Have you developed interpersonal skills in addition to technical skills?
- Have you learned about ethnic and religious family patterns?
- Do you communicate directly with persons with whom you are upset or take issue?
- Are you able to "step back" and withdraw emotionally, if not physically, when emotional overload occurs, yet remain committed?
- Do you take care of yourself and your needs?
- Do you periodically interview family members to determine their current issues (e.g., feelings, attitudes, responses, wishes), communicate these findings to peers, and update records?
- Do you avoid relying on initial interview data, assumptions, or gossip regarding families?
- Do you ask questions if families are not participating in care?
- Do you assess families for feelings of anxiety, fear, intimidation, worry about making a mistake, a perceived lack of competence to care for their child, or fear of health care professionals overstepping their boundaries into family territory, or vice versa?
- Do you explore these issues with family members and provide encouragement and support to enable families to help themselves?
- Do you keep communication channels open among self, family, physicians, and other care providers?
- Do you resolve conflicts and misunderstandings directly with those who are involved?
- Do you clarify information for families or seek the appropriate person to do so?

Do you recognize that from time to time a therapeutic relationship can change to a social relationship or an intimate friendship?
- Are you able to acknowledge the fact when it occurs and understand why it happened?
- Can you ensure that there is someone else who is more objective who can take your place in the therapeutic relationship?

For information on one hospital's guidelines for establishing therapeutic relationships between nurses and children and families, contact Jane H. Barnsteiner, PhD, RN, FAAN, Director of Nursing Practice and Research, Children's Hospital of Philadelphia, 34th and Civic Center Blvd., Philadelphia, PA 19104-4399, (215) 898-4142; e-mail: barnstnr@nursing.upenn.edu.

child's best interest. Advocacy involves ensuring that families are aware of all available health services, informed adequately of treatments and procedures, involved in the child's care, and encouraged to change or support existing health care practices. The United Nations' Declaration of the Rights of the Child (Box 1-4) provides guidelines for nursing practice to ensure that every child receives optimum care. The nurse uses this knowledge to adapt care for the child's optimum physical and emotional well-being.

As nurses care for children and families, they must demonstrate **caring,** compassion, and empathy for others. Aspects of caring embody the concept of atraumatic care and the development of a therapeutic relationship with patients. Parents perceive caring as a sign of quality in nursing care, which is often focused on the nontechnical needs of the child and fam-

ily. Parents describe "personable" care as actions by the nurse that include acknowledging the parent's presence, listening, making the parent feel comfortable in the hospital environment, involving the parent and child in the nursing care, showing interest in and concern for their welfare, showing affection and sensitivity to the parent and child, communicating with them, and individualizing the nursing care. Parents perceive personable nursing care as being integral to establishing a positive relationship.

DISEASE PREVENTION AND HEALTH PROMOTION

Every nurse involved with child care must practice preventive health care. Regardless of the identified problem, the nurse's role is to plan care that fosters every aspect of growth and development. Based on a thorough assessment process, problems related to nutrition, immunizations, safety, dental care, development, socialization, discipline, or schooling often become obvious. Once the problem is identified, the nurse acts to intervene directly or to refer the family to other health care providers or agencies.

The best approach to prevention is **education** and **anticipatory guidance.** In this text each chapter on health promotion includes sections on anticipatory guidance. An appreciation of the hazards or conflicts of each developmental period enables the nurse to guide parents regarding childrearing practices aimed at preventing potential problems. One of the most significant examples is safety. Because each age-group is at risk for special types of injuries, preventive teaching can significantly reduce injuries, lowering permanent disability and mortality rates.

Prevention also involves less obvious aspects of child care. Besides preventing physical disease or injury, the nurse also promotes mental health. For example, it is not sufficient to administer immunizations without regard to the psychologic trauma associated with the procedure. Optimum health care involves providing care with a humane approach; the nurse and all other health care professionals must ensure that **humane care** is provided.

HEALTH TEACHING

Health teaching is inseparable from family advocacy and prevention. Health teaching may be a direct goal of the nurse, such as during parenting classes, or may be indirect, such as helping parents and children understand a diagnosis or medical treatment, encouraging children to ask questions about their bodies, referring families to health-related professional or lay groups, supplying patients with appropriate literature, and providing anticipatory guidance.

Health teaching is one area in which nurses often need preparation and practice with competent role models, since it involves transmitting information at the child's and family's level of understanding and desire for information. As an effective educator, the nurse focuses on providing the appropriate health teaching with generous feedback and evaluation to promote learning.

SUPPORT AND COUNSELING

Attention to emotional needs requires support and, sometimes, counseling. The role of child advocate or health teacher is supportive by virtue of the individualized approach. The nurse can offer support by listening, touching, and being physically present. Touching and physical presence are most helpful with children because they facilitate nonverbal communication.

Counseling involves a mutual exchange of ideas and opinions that provides the basis for mutual problem solving. It involves support, teaching, techniques to foster the expression of feelings or thoughts, and approaches to help the family cope with stress. Optimally, counseling not only helps resolve a crisis or problem but also enables the family to attain a higher level of functioning, greater self-esteem, and closer relationships. Although counseling is often the role of nurses in specialized areas, counseling techniques are discussed in various sections of this text to help students and nurses cope with immediate crises and refer families for additional professional assistance.

COORDINATION AND COLLABORATION

The nurse, as a member of the health care team, collaborates and coordinates nursing services with the activities of other professionals. Working in isolation does not serve the child's best interests. The concept of holistic care can be realized only through a unified, interdisciplinary approach. Being aware of individual contributions and limitations to the child's care, the nurse must collaborate with other specialists to provide high-quality health services. Failure to recognize limitations can be nontherapeutic at best and destructive at worst. For example, the nurse who feels competent in counseling but who is really inadequate in this area may not only prevent the child from dealing with a crisis but may also impede future success with a qualified professional.

Even nurses who practice in isolated geographic areas widely separated from other health professionals cannot be considered independent. Every nurse works interdependently with the child and family, collaborating on assessing needs and planning interventions so that the final care plan is one that truly meets the child's needs. Unfortunately, this aspect of collaboration and coordination frequently is lacking in health care planning. Numerous disciplines often work together to formulate a comprehensive approach without consulting patients regarding their ideas or preferences. The nurse is in a vital position to include patients in their care, either directly or indirectly, by communicating their thoughts to the health care team.

ETHICAL DECISION MAKING

Ethical dilemmas arise when competing moral considerations underlie various alternatives. Parents, nurses, physicians, and other health care team members may reach different but morally defensible decisions by assigning different weights to competing moral values. These competing moral values may include **autonomy,** the patient's right to be self-governing; **nonmaleficence,** the obligation to minimize or prevent harm; **beneficence,** the obligation to promote the patient's well-being; and **justice,** the concept of fairness. Nurses must determine the most beneficial or least harmful action within the framework of societal mores, professional practice standards, the law, institutional rules, the family's value system and religious traditions, and the nurse's personal values. Nurses are important role models for demonstrating how to create an environment of mutual respect and understanding for patients and their families. Respect for the

BOX 1-5

American Nurses Association Standard 12: Ethics

The registered nurse integrates ethical provisions in all areas of practice.

MEASUREMENT CRITERIA

The registered nurse:

1. Uses the Code of Ethics for Nurses with Interpretive Statements to guide practice.
2. Delivers care in a manner that preserves and protects patient autonomy, dignity, and rights.
3. Maintains patient confidentiality within legal and regulatory parameters.
4. Serves as a patient advocate, assisting patients in developing skills for self-advocacy.
5. Maintains a therapeutic and professional patient-nurse relationship with appropriate professional role boundaries.
6. Demonstrates a commitment to practicing self-care, managing stress, and connecting with self and others.
7. Contributes to resolving ethical issues of patients, colleagues, or systems as evidenced in such activities as participating on ethics committees.
8. Reports illegal, incompetent, or impaired practices.

The advanced practice registered nurse:

1. Informs the patient of the risks, benefits, and outcomes of health care regimens.
2. Participates in interdisciplinary teams that address ethical risks, benefits, and outcomes.

The registered nurse in a nursing role specialty:

1. Participates on multidisciplinary and interdisciplinary teams that address ethical risks, benefits, and outcomes.
2. Informs administrators or others of the risks, benefits, and outcomes of programs and decisions that affect health care delivery.

Reprinted with permission from American Nurses Association: *Nursing: scope and standards of practice,* Silver Spring, Md, 2004, Nursesbooks.org.

individuals they care for is the affirmation that other persons matter in the same way as the nurses themselves (Milton, 2005).

Nurses must prepare themselves systematically for collaborative ethical decision making. This can be accomplished through formal course work, continuing education, contemporary literature, and work to establish an environment conducive to ethical discourse. Moreover, nurses must be educated on the mechanisms for dispute resolution, case review by ethics committees, procedural safeguards, state statutes, and case law (Woods, 2005).

The nurse also uses the professional code of ethics for guidance and as a means for professional self-regulation. The Code of Ethics for Nurses by the American Nurses Association focuses on the nurse's accountability and responsibility to the patient and emphasizes the nursing role as an independent professional, one that upholds its own legal liability (Box 1-5).

Nurses may face ethical issues regarding patient care, such as the use of lifesaving measures for VLBW newborns or the terminally ill child's right to refuse treatment. They may struggle with questions regarding truthfulness, balancing their rights and responsibilities in caring for children with AIDS, whistle-blowing, or allocating resources. Throughout the text such dilemmas are addressed in boxes titled Ethical Case Studies. Conflicting ethical arguments are presented to help nurses clarify their value judgments when confronted with sensitive issues.

RESEARCH

Practicing nurses should contribute to research because they are the individuals observing human responses to health and illness. The current emphasis on measurable outcomes to determine the efficacy of interventions (often in relation to the cost) demands that nurses know whether clinical interventions result in positive outcomes for their patients. This demand has influenced the current trend toward **evidence-based practice** (EBP), which implies questioning why something is effective and whether a better approach exists. The concept of EBP also involves analyzing and translating published clinical research into the everyday practice of nursing. When nurses base their clinical practice on science and research and document their clinical outcomes, they will be able to validate their contributions to health, wellness, and cure, not only to their patients, third-party payers, and institutions but also to the nursing profession. Evaluation is essential to the nursing process, and research is one of the best ways to accomplish this.

CRITICAL THINKING AND THE PROCESS OF NURSING CHILDREN AND FAMILIES

CRITICAL THINKING

A systematic thought process is essential to a profession. It assists the professional in meeting the patient's needs. **Critical thinking** is purposeful, goal-directed thinking that assists individuals in making judgments based on evidence rather than guesswork (Alfaro-LeFevre, 2005). It is based on the scientific method of inquiry, which is also the roots of the nursing process. Critical thinking and the nursing process are considered crucial to professional nursing in that they constitute a holistic approach to problem solving.

Critical thinking is a complex developmental process based on rational and deliberate thought. Becoming a critical thinker provides a common denominator for knowledge that exemplifies disciplined and self-directed thinking. The knowledge is acquired, assessed, and organized by thinking through the clinical situation and developing an outcome focused on optimum patient care. The cognitive skills used in high-quality thinking include intellectual discipline, self-evaluation, creativity, persistence, risk taking, and intuition (Ignatavicius, 2001). Critical thinking transforms the way in which individuals view themselves, understand the world, and make decisions. In recognition of the importance of this skill, Critical Thinking Exercises are included in this text. These exercises present a nursing practice situation that challenges the student to use the skills of critical thinking to come to the best conclusion. The student is led by a series of questions that explore the evidence, assumptions underlying the problem, nursing priorities, and support for nursing interventions that allow the nurse make a rational and deliberate response based on self-directed thinking. The benefit of these thinking exercises is that they may enhance nursing performance in clinical judgment.

EVIDENCE-BASED PRACTICE

EBP is the collection, interpretation, and integration of valid, important, and applicable patient-reported, nurse-observed, and research-derived information (Simpson, 2004). Evidence-

TABLE 1-5
The Nursing Process and Evidence-Based Practice

NURSING PROCESS	ACTIONS	EVIDENCE-BASED PRACTICE	ACTIONS
Assessment	Collects patient data	Ask the question	Clearly identifies specific patient problems and needs
Diagnosis	Analyzes assessment data and determines diagnosis	Search for evidence	Collects information relevant to patient's identified problems and needs
Planning	Develops care plan	Analyze evidence	Critically appraises published literature
Implementation	Initiates interventions identified in care plan	Apply evidence to practice	Integrates evidence with clinical expertise and patient's unique needs
Evaluation	Evaluates patient's progress toward attainment of outcomes	Evaluate effectiveness	Evaluates effectiveness of integration of evidence

based nursing practice combines knowledge with clinical experience and intuition. It provides a rational approach to decision making that facilitates best practice (Newhouse, Dearholt, Poe, and others, 2005). EBP is an important tool that complements the nursing process by using critical thinking skills to make decisions based on existing knowledge. The traditional nursing process approach to patient care can be used to conceptualize the essential components of EBP nursing (Table 1-5). During the assessment and diagnostic phases of the nursing process, the nurse establishes important clinical questions and completes a critical review of existing knowledge. EBP also begins with identification of the problem. The nurse asks clinical questions in a concise, organized way that allows for clear answers. Once the specific questions are identified, extensive searching for the best information to answer the question begins. The nurse evaluates clinically relevant research, analyzes findings from the history and physical examinations, and reviews the specific pathophysiology of the defined problem. The third step in the nursing process is to develop a care plan. In evidence-based nursing practice, the care plan is established on completion of a critical appraisal of what is known and not known about the defined problem. Next, in the traditional nursing process, the nurse implements the care plan. By integrating evidence with clinical expertise, the nurse focuses care on the patient's unique needs. A template for organizing the evidence is found in Box 1-6. The final step in EBP is consistent with the final phase of the nursing process: to evaluate the effectiveness of the care plan.

Searching for evidence in this modern era of technology can be overwhelming. Appropriate **resources** must be available for nurses to implement EBP. Resources include online search engines and journal access to the most recent information. In many institutions computer terminals are available on patient care units, with the Internet and online journals easily accessible. Another important resource for the implementation of EBP is **time.** The nursing shortage and ongoing changes that many institutions face have compounded the issue of nursing time allocation for patient care, education, and training. In some institutions nurses are given paid time away from performing patient care to participate in activities that promote EBP. This requires an organizational environment that values EBP and its potential impact on patient care. As knowledge is generated regarding the significant impact of EBP on patient care outcomes, it is hoped that the organizational culture will change to support

BOX 1-6
Evidence-Based Practice Template

ASK THE QUESTION

SEARCH FOR EVIDENCE
Search Strategies:

Databases Used:

CRITICALLY ANALYZE THE EVIDENCE

APPLY THE EVIDENCE: NURSING IMPLICATIONS

REFERENCES

the staff nurse's participation in EBP. As the amount of available evidence increases, so does our need to critically evaluate the evidence.

NURSING PROCESS
The nursing process is a method of problem identification and problem solving that describes what the nurse actually does (Alfaro-LeFevre, 2005). The five-step model that is accepted as the nursing process is assessment, diagnosis (problem identification), planning (with outcome development), implementation, and evaluation. The second step of the nursing process, nursing diagnosis, is the naming of the child's or family's problem in standardized nursing language. In the American Nurses Association (2003) Standards of Practice, the nursing diagnosis phase of the nursing process is separated into two steps: nursing diagnosis and outcome identification. Throughout this text Nursing Process boxes provide organization for the nursing care, following the template in Box 1-7.

BOX 1-7
Nursing Process

Assessment—Assess for signs and symptoms. Observe for subjective and objective data.
Diagnosis (problem identification)—After a thorough assessment, establish a nursing diagnosis. Validate nursing diagnosis with defining characteristics.
Planning—Establish expected patient outcomes.
Implementation—Develop and implement nursing intervention strategies.
Evaluation—Establish method for continual assessment of care and evaluation of outcomes based on specific guidelines.

Assessment

Assessment is a continuous process that operates at all phases of problem solving and is the foundation for decision making. Assessment involves multiple nursing skills and consists of the purposeful collection, classification, and analysis of data from a variety of sources. To provide an accurate and comprehensive assessment, the nurse must consider information about the patient's biophysical, psychologic, sociocultural, and spiritual background.

Nursing Diagnosis

The second stage of the nursing process is problem identification and nursing diagnosis. At this point the nurse must interpret and make decisions about the data gathered. The nurse organizes or clusters these data into categories to identify significant areas and makes one of the following decisions:

- **No dysfunctional health problems are evident;** no interventions are indicated.
- **Risk for dysfunctional health problems exists;** interventions are needed to facilitate health promotion.
- **Actual dysfunctional health problems are evident;** interventions are needed to facilitate health promotion.

The nursing diagnosis is the naming of the cue clusters that are obtained during the assessment phase. According to NANDA International (formerly the North American Nursing Diagnosis Association), the currently accepted definition of the term **nursing diagnosis** is that it is a clinical judgment about individual, family, or community responses to actual and potential health problems and life processes. Box 1-8 reviews the classification systems for nursing diagnoses. Nursing diagnoses provide the basis for selecting nursing interventions to achieve outcomes for which the nurse is accountable (Johnson, Bulechek, Dochterman, and others, 2001). The Nursing Interventions Classification (NIC) consists of a standardized list of more than 400 examples of care provided by nurses in clinical practice. The Nursing Outcomes Classification (NOC) is a comprehensive, standardized system of patient outcomes that can be used to evaluate the results of specific nursing interventions. Examples of NIC and NOC concepts are listed in each Nursing Care Plan (NCP) in this text to provide an understanding of the standardized language and its interrelatedness within the individualized NCP.

Not all children have actual health problems; some have a potential health problem, which is a risk state that requires

---

BOX 1-8
Classification Systems for Nursing Diagnoses

HUMAN RESPONSE PATTERNS
Exchanging—Mutual giving and receiving
Communicating—Sending messages
Relating—Establishing bonds
Valuing—Assigning relative worth
Choosing—Selecting alternatives
Moving—Activity
Perceiving—Receiving information
Knowing—The meaning associated with information
Feeling—The subjective awareness of sensation or affect

FUNCTIONAL HEALTH PATTERNS
Health perception–health management pattern—Perceptions related to general health management and preventive practices
Nutritional-metabolic pattern—Intake of food and fluids related to metabolic requirements
Elimination pattern—Regularity and control of excretory functions, bowel, bladder, skin, and wastes
Activity-exercise pattern—Activity patterns that require energy expenditure and provide for rest
Sleep-rest pattern—Effectiveness of sleep and rest periods
Cognitive-perceptual pattern—Adequacy of language, cognitive skills, and perception related to required or desired activities; includes pain perception
Self-perception–self-concept pattern—Beliefs and evaluation of self-worth
Role-relationship pattern—Family and social roles, especially parent-child relationships
Sexuality and reproductive pattern—Problems or potential problems with sexuality or reproduction
Coping–stress tolerance pattern—Stress tolerance level and coping patterns, including support systems
Value-belief pattern—Values, goals, or beliefs that influence health-related decisions and actions

TAXONOMY II DOMAINS
Domain 1—Health Promotion
Domain 2—Nutrition
Domain 3—Elimination
Domain 4—Activity/Rest
Domain 5—Perception/Cognition
Domain 6—Self-Perception
Domain 7—Role Relationships
Domain 8—Sexuality
Domain 9—Coping/Stress Tolerance
Domain 10—Life Principles
Domain 11—Safety/Protection
Domain 12—Comfort
Domain 13—Growth/Development

Adapted from North American Nursing Diagnosis Association: *Nursing diagnoses: definitions and classifications, 2005-2006,* Philadelphia, 2005, The Association.

---

nursing intervention to prevent the development of an actual problem. Potential health problems may be indicated by the presence of **risk factors,** or signs, that predispose a child and family to a dysfunctional health pattern and are limited to individuals at greater risk than the population as a whole. Nursing intervention is directed toward reducing risk factors. To differentiate actual from potential health problems, the

FAMILY FOCUS

Using Defining Characteristics to Select an Appropriate Nursing Diagnosis

An 18-month-old only child is admitted with respiratory distress and a presumptive diagnosis of epiglottitis. Initial nursing actions focus on the child's physiologic status. As the condition stabilizes, family assessment data are gathered. The child's immunizations are current, he is clean and well nourished, and his developmental age is appropriate. The parents are both present at admission. The mother is distraught about the sudden onset of respiratory distress. She states that earlier her child had only a "runny nose" and she thought it was just a cold. When the child suddenly began to have difficulty breathing, she felt helpless and unable to relieve her child's discomfort. She states: "Nothing I did made him any better. If I had known this could happen, I would have brought him to the hospital sooner. I feel like a bad mother." In the hospital, after explanations by the nurses, the mother understands that epiglottitis is a sudden illness that typically follows symptoms of a cold. She is cooperative and asks what she can do to make her child more comfortable. She implements all the suggestions of the health care team. The father supports both the child and mother, although he assumes a more passive, "listening" role.

Three nursing diagnoses that relate to family and parent situations may be relevant. The first step is to review the diagnoses and the defining characteristics and decide which one is most appropriate:

1. **Parenting, Impaired**—Inability of the primary caretaker to create, maintain, or regain an environment that nurtures the child's growth and development
   Selected defining characteristics:
   Insecure (or lack of) attachment to infant
   Poor or inappropriate caretaking skills

2. **Conflict, Parental Role**—Parent experience of role confusion and conflict in response to crisis
   Selected defining characteristics:
   Parent expressing concerns about changes in parental role
   A demonstrated disruption in care or caretaking routines
   Parent expressing concerns or feelings of inadequacy to provide for the child's physical and emotional needs during hospitalization or in home
   Parent verbalizing or demonstrating feelings of guilt, anger, fear, anxiety, or frustration about effect of child's illness on family process

3. **Family Processes, Interrupted**—A change in family relationships or functioning.
   Selected defining characteristics:
   Expressions of conflict within the family
   Changes in communication patterns among family members

Of these three diagnoses, the most relevant one is *Conflict, Parental Role*. The parents demonstrate attachment behavior to their child and are attentive to his needs. They appear to have appropriate parenting skills and are able to communicate effectively with each other. Neither parent expressed any conflict within the family. The sudden onset of this child's illness has interrupted the mother's usual role and caused her to feel inadequate, anxious, and guilty. However, the mother is able to adapt to this crisis. She demonstrates an ability to cope by learning and implementing new comforting skills for her child. The defining characteristics of the other two diagnoses require maladaptive characteristics that are clearly not demonstrated by these parents.

---

word *risk* is included in the nursing diagnosis statement (e.g., Risk for Infection).

Signs and symptoms refer to a cluster of cues and defining characteristics that are derived from patient assessment and indicate actual health problems. When a defining characteristic is essential for the diagnosis to be made, it is considered critical. These critical defining characteristics help differentiate between diagnostic categories. For example, in deciding between the diagnostic categories related to family function and coping, the defining characteristics are critical in choosing the most appropriate nursing diagnosis (see Family Focus box).

Planning

Once the nursing diagnoses have been identified, the nurse develops a care plan and establishes outcomes or goals. The **outcome** is the projected or expected change in a patient's health status, clinical condition, or behavior that occurs after nursing interventions have been instituted. The ultimate goal of nursing care is to convert the nursing diagnoses into a desired health state. The care plan must be established before specific nursing interventions are developed and implemented.

Implementation

The implementation phase begins when the nurse puts the selected intervention into action and accumulates feedback data regarding its effects (or the patient's response to the intervention). The feedback returns in the form of observation and communication and provides a database on which to evaluate the outcome of the nursing intervention. It is imperative that continuous assessment of the patient's status occur throughout all phases of the nursing process, thus making the process a dynamic rather than static problem-solving method. Throughout the implementation stage, the patient's physical safety and psychologic comfort in terms of atraumatic care are the main concerns.

Evaluation

Evaluation is the last step in the decision-making process. The nurse gathers, sorts, and analyzes data to determine whether (1) the established outcome has been met, (2) the nursing interventions were appropriate, (3) the plan requires modification, or (4) other alternatives should be considered. The evaluation phase either completes the nursing process (outcome is met) or serves as the basis for the selection of other alternatives for intervention in solving the specific problem.

Documentation

Although documentation is not one of the five steps of the nursing process, it is essential for evaluation. The nurse can assess, diagnose and identify problems, plan, and implement without documentation; however, evaluation is best performed with written evidence of progress toward outcomes. The patient's medical record should include evidence of those elements listed in the Nursing Care Guidelines box.

Currently attention in health care is also focused on patient outcomes. The patient's care is evaluated not only at discharge but thereafter as well to ensure that the outcomes are met and there is adequate care for assisting the patient in resolving existing or potential health problems.

One federal agency that has developed clinical guidelines is the Agency for Healthcare Research and Quality.*

---

*540 Gaither Road, Suite 2000, Rockville, MD 20850; (301) 427-1364; info@ahrq.gov; http://www.ahrq.gov.

KEY POINTS

■ *Healthy People 2010* broadened the health care objectives achieved in the 1990s and focuses on prevention as the method of achieving its goals.
■ Although the infant mortality rate in the United States has declined over the past few decades, the United States lags significantly behind most other major countries, such as Canada.

■ LBW, which is closely related to early gestational age, is considered the leading cause of neonatal death in the United States.
■ Injuries are the leading cause of death in children over age 1 year, with the majority being MV injuries.
■ Childhood morbidity encompasses acute illness, chronic disease, and disability.
■ Eighty percent of childhood illnesses are attributable to infections, with respiratory tract infections occurring two or three times more often than all other illnesses combined.
■ The *new morbidity* refers to behavioral, social, and educational problems that can significantly alter a child's health.
■ Developmental stage and environment are important determinants in the prevalence of injuries at a given age and thus help to direct preventive measures.
■ The philosophy of family-centered care recognizes that the family is the constant in a child's life and that service systems and personnel must support, respect, and enhance the family's strength and competence.
■ Atraumatic care is the provision of therapeutic care in settings, by personnel, and through the use of interventions that eliminate or minimize the psychologic and physical distress experienced by children and their families in the health care system.
■ The pediatric nurse's roles include a therapeutic relationship, family advocacy, disease prevention and health promotion, health teaching, support and counseling, coordination and collaboration, ethical decision making, and research.
■ EBP is the collection, interpretation, and integration of valid, important, and applicable patient-reported, nurse-observed, and research-derived information.
■ The process of nursing children and families includes accurate and comprehensive assessment, analysis and synthesis of assessment data to arrive at a nursing diagnosis, planning of care, implementation of the plan, and evaluation of interventions.

REFERENCES

Alfaro-LeFevre R: *Applying nursing process: a tool for critical thinking,* ed 6, Philadelphia, 2005, Lippincott.

American Academy of Pediatrics: *The National Children's Study,* retrieved Dec 1, 2004, from http://www.aap.org/family/natlchstudy.htm.

American Association of Suicidology: *About AAS,* retrieved Feb 2, 2007, from http://www.suicidology.org.

American Nurses Association: *Nursing: scope and standards of practice,* Washington, DC, 2003, The Association.

Coury DL: Over the rainbow: advancing child health in the new millennium, *Ambul Pediatr* 6(3):134-137, 2006.

Covington CY, Cybulski MJ, Davis TL, and others: Kids on the move: preventing obesity among urban children, *Am J Nurs* 101(3):73-77, 79, 81-82, 2001.

Dietz WH: Overweight: an epidemic. In Cosby AG, Greenberg RE, Southward LH, and others, editors: *About children: an authoritative resource on the state of childhood today,* Elk Grove Village, Ill, 2005, American Academy of Pediatrics.

Doucette A: Youth suicide. In Cosby AG, Greenberg RE, Southward LH, and others, editors: *About children: an authoritative resource on the state of childhood today,* Elk Grove Village, Ill, 2005, American Academy of Pediatrics.

Dougherty D, Meikle SF, Owens P, and others: Children's health care in the First National Healthcare Quality Report and National Healthcare Disparities Report, *Med Care* 43(3 Suppl): I58-I63, 2005.

Duderstadt KG: Advocacy for reducing childhood obesity, *J Pediatr Health Care* 18:103-105, 2004.

Edelstein BL: Tooth decay: the best of times, the worst of times. In Cosby AG, Greenberg RE, Southward LH, and others, editors: *About children: an authoritative resource on the state of childhood today,* Elk Grove Village, Ill, 2005, American Academy of Pediatrics.

Federal Interagency Forum on Child and Family Statistics: *America's children: key national indicators of well-being,* Washington, DC, 2007, US Government Printing Office.

Fisher K, Kettl P: Teachers' perceptions of school violence, *J Pediatr Health Care* 17:79-83, 2003.

Fitzgibbon ML, Stolley MR: Environmental changes may be needed for prevention of overweight in minority children, *Pediatr Ann* 33:45-49, 2004.

Groves BM: Violence in the lives of children. In Cosby AG, Greenberg RE, Southward LH, and others, editors: *About children: an authoritative resource on the state of childhood today,* Elk Grove Village, Ill, 2005, American Academy of Pediatrics.

Heron M: Deaths: leading causes for 2004, *Natl Vital Stat Rep* 56(5):1-96, 2007.

Heuer S: Family-centered care, *J Spec Pediatr Nurs* 12(1):61-65, 2007.

Hoyert DL, Heron M, Murphy SL, and others: *Deaths: final data for 2003,* 2006, National Center for Health Statistics, retrieved Jan 20, 2006, from http://www.cdc.gov/nchs/products/pubs/pubd/hestats/finaldeaths03/finaldeaths03.htm.

Ignatavicius D: Critical thinking skills for at the bedside success, *Nurs Manage* 32(1):37-39, 2001.

Jackson PL: *Healthy people 2010:* the pediatric nursing challenge for the next decade, *Pediatr Nurs* 27:498-502, 2001.

Jacobson GA: Maintaining professional boundaries: preparing nursing students for the challenge, *J Nurs Educ* 41(6):279-281, 2002.

Johnson M, Bulechek G, Dochterman J, and others: *Nursing diagnosis, outcomes and interventions,* St Louis, 2001, Mosby.

Kelleher K: Mental health. In Cosby AG, Greenberg RE, Southward LH, and others, editors: *About children: an authoritative resource on the state of childhood today,* Elk Grove Village, Ill, 2005, American Academy of Pediatrics.

Lichter DT: Families: diversity and change. In Cosby AG, Greenberg RE, Southward LH, and others, editors: *About children: an authoritative resource on the state of childhood today,* Elk Grove Village, Ill, 2005, American Academy of Pediatrics.

Martin JA, Kochanek KD, Strobino DM, and others: Annual summary of vital statistics: 2003, *Pediatrics* 115(3):619-634, 2005.

Martin JA, Kung HC, Mathews TJ, and others: Annual summary of vital statistics: 2006, *Pediatrics* 121(4):788-801, 2008.

Medd SE: Children with ADHD need our advocacy, *J Pediatr Health Care* 17:102-104, 2003.

Milton CL: The ethics of respect in nursing, *Nurs Sci Q* 18(1):20-23, 2005.

National Center for Health Statistics: *About* Healthy People 2010, retrieved Feb 2, 2007, from http://www.cdc.gov/nchs/about/otheract/hpdata2010/abouthp.htm.

National Center for Injury Prevention and Control: *Injury fact book 2001-2002,* Atlanta, 2001, Centers for Disease Control and Prevention.

National Safety Council: *Injury facts,* Itaska, Ill, 2000, The Council.

Newhouse R, Dearholt S, Poe S, and others: Evidence-based practice: a practical approach to implementation, *JONA* 35(1):35-40, 2005.

Newton MS: Family-centered care: current realities in parent participation, *Pediatr Nurs* 26(2):164-168, 2000.

Rivara FP: Impact of injury. In Cosby AG, Greenberg RE, Southward LH, and others, editors: *About children: an authoritative resource on the state of childhood today,* Elk Grove Village, Ill, 2005, American Academy of Pediatrics.

Robinson TN, Sargent JD: Children and media. In Cosby AG, Greenberg RE, Southward LH, and others, editors: *About children: an authoritative resource on the state of childhood today,* Elk Grove Village, Ill, 2005, American Academy of Pediatrics.

Schnitzer PG: Prevention of unintentional childhood injuries, *Am Fam Physician* 74(11):1864-1869, 2006.

Simpson R: Evidence-based nursing offers certainty in the uncertain world of healthcare, *Nurs Manage* 35(10):10-12, 2004.

Substance Abuse and Mental Health Services Administration, Office of Applied Studies: *2003 National survey on drug use and health: results,* 2004, retrieved Feb 2, 2007, from http://www.drugabusestatistics.samhsa.gov/NHSDA/2k3NSDUH/2k3results.htm.

US Department of Health and Human Services: *Healthy people 2010,* 2007, retrieved Jan 8, 2008, from http://www.healthypeople.gov/default.htm.

Wise PH: Medical progress and inequalities in child health. In Cosby AG, Greenberg RE, Southward LH, and others, editors: *About children: an authoritative resource on the state of childhood today,* Elk Grove Village, Ill, 2005, American Academy of Pediatrics.

Wise PH: The transformation of child health in the United States, *Health Affairs* 23(5):9-25, 2004.

Wong D: Principles of atraumatic care. In Feeg V, editor: *Pediatric nursing: forum on the future: looking toward the 21st century,* Pitman, NJ, 1989, Anthony J Jannetti.

Woods M: Nursing ethics education: are we really delivering the good(s)? *Nurs Ethics* 12(1):5-18, 2005.

World Health Organization: *School health and youth health promotion,* 2007, retrieved Jan 26, 2007, from http://www.who.int/school_youth_health/en.

Yensel CS, Preud'Homme D, Curry DM: Childhood obesity and insulin-resistant syndrome, *J Pediatr Nurs* 19:238-246, 2004.

2

Community-Based Nursing Care of the Child and Family

CHRISTINE A. BROSNAN AND SANDRA L. UPCHURCH

CHAPTER OUTLINE

NURSING IN THE COMMUNITY, 21
COMMUNITY CONCEPTS, 21
Community, 21
  Community Health Nursing, 21
  Roles and Functions, 21
Demography, 22

Epidemiology, 22
  Distribution of Disease, Injury,
    or Illness, 22
  Epidemiologic Triangle, 22
  Levels of Prevention, 22
  Screening, 23
Economics, 23

COMMUNITY NURSING PROCESS, 24
Community Needs Assessment and
  Diagnosis, 24
Community Planning, 25
Community Implementation, 25
Community Evaluation, 25

LEARNING OBJECTIVES

On completion of this chapter the reader will be able to:
- Define a community.
- Describe community health nursing.

- Identify the roles and functions of the community health nurse.
- Discuss selected aspects of the epidemiologic process.

- Explain the purpose of an economic evaluation.
- Discuss the components of the community nursing process.

RELATED TOPICS and ADDITIONAL RESOURCES

 IN TEXT
Family-Centered Home Care, *Ch. 20*
Health Care for Children, *Ch. 1*
Immunizations, *Ch. 1*
Nursing Process, *Ch. 1*

 COMPANION CD
NCLEX Review Questions

evolve
evolve.elsevier.com/Wong/essentials/
NCLEX Review Questions
WebLinks

NURSING IN THE COMMUNITY

The health of children and their families is greatly influenced by their community, and nurses can make a significant contribution by working with the community to promote children's heath. Nurses working with pediatric populations in the community need an understanding of the concepts and processes critical to address pediatric concerns from a community health perspective. Healthy communities provide not only excellent medical care, but also a nurturing, safe place for children to live and grow. Healthy communities and cities address concerns through collaboration between and among citizens, health care providers, businesses, and governmental and private agencies (Flynn and Ivanov, 2004).

This chapter discusses community health nursing as it relates to children. First, it identifies and defines the concepts and principles that serve as the basis of community health nursing. Then it describes the community health nursing process, step by step. It includes a box that demonstrates use of the process to address a very real child health concern: obesity.

COMMUNITY CONCEPTS
COMMUNITY

There are several ways to define a community. A community is a group of individuals with shared characteristics or interests who interact with each other (Allender and Spradley, 2005). A community is a system that includes children and families, the physical environment, educational facilities, safety and transportation resources, political and governmental agencies, health and social services, communication resources, economic resources, and recreational facilities. The community is also the client of the community health nurse (Anderson, 2008). Community health initiatives are directed at either the general health of the community as a whole or at specific populations within the community that have unique needs. In this context, **populations** can be described as groups of people who live in a community and have characteristics in common, for example, school-age children. **Target populations** or **subpopulations** are more narrowly defined groups (e.g., nonimmunized preschoolers, obese middle school children) toward whom nurses direct activities to improve the health status of individuals in the group. Common values often guide behaviors of populations and subpopulations in relation to health promotion and disease prevention (McEwen and Nies, 2007; Williams, 2004).

Community-oriented care involves a collaboration of individuals and groups, including health care providers, advocates, government, managed care organizations, businesses, children, and families, within a specific community. The goal of the collaborative effort is to provide services that promote the child health initiatives of *Healthy People 2010.** Community care is "without walls" in that the services of the health care system are frequently redesigned to meet the changing needs of the community. Those involved in community care partner with the community to identify, plan, intervene, and evaluate activities that improve the community's health (Anderson and McFarlane, 2008).

Community Health Nursing

Community health nursing focuses on promoting and maintaining the health of individuals, families, and groups in a community setting. Community health nursing is a synthesis

*http://www.healthypeople.gov.

of nursing and public health. It is population focused and involves collaboration with other disciplines to assess, plan, and implement care that emphasizes personal responsibility for health and self-care by community members (Allender and Spradley, 2005; Williams, 2004). Community health nursing, at its best, empowers communities by enabling its members to gain the knowledge and skills needed to fulfill their own needs.

Although community health concepts can be used to address health concerns in any setting, traditional community health settings include the following: home health agencies, schools, physician offices, ambulatory health clinics, emergency departments, triage call centers, insurance agencies, health departments, international relief agencies, health education agencies, juvenile detention facilities, camps, daycare centers, foster care facilities, hospice centers, and rehabilitation agencies. The American Nurses Association (1986) has established nine standards for community health nursing to guide practice across settings. They include the following categories: theory, data collection, diagnosis, planning, intervention, evaluation, quality assurance and professional development, interdisciplinary collaboration, and research. The revised scope and standards of public health nursing (American Nurses Association, 2007) describe the major components and measurement criteria for each standard.

Roles and Functions

The roles and functions of the community health nurse continue to evolve. In the future, more pediatric nurses will be working in community settings. The Health Resources and Services Administration (2004) reported that 14.9% of the total registered nurse work force was employed in a community or public health setting and 11.5% in ambulatory care. Only 56.2% of registered nurses were employed in hospital settings. An example of the role evolution is the need for competent public health/community health nurses to work during times of natural disasters, public health threats, and terrorism attacks (Gebbie and Turnock, 2006) (Box 2-1).

Traditionally, the roles of community health nurses included caregiver, advocate, case manager, case finder, counselor, educator, epidemiologist, group process leader, health planner, and manager. For example, the nurse employed in a pediatric outpatient clinic will function in a number of roles to provide care to a child with type 2 diabetes. The nurse provides case management by coordinating care between the disciplines, counseling by supporting the child and family through developmental crisis, and case finding by identifying risk factors in the child's siblings.

The Institute of Medicine (1988) developed a list of core functions to guide the work of public health professionals, including nurses. The core functions are directed to population-wide services and to personal and home services for people at risk. The population-wide service is based on assessment of health status monitoring and disease **surveillance, policy development,** and **assurance** that policies are translated into service. The Council on Linkages Between Academia and Public Health Practice (2001), a group of university educators and public health professionals, further delineated the core functions and developed a list of skills to improve the ability of all public health workers, including nurses, to implement them. The eight categories of skills include analytic/assessment, policy development/program plan-

---

BOX 2-1

Evolving Role of the Pediatric Nurse: Natural and Man-Made Disasters

Communities are affected by disasters, either natural disasters like hurricanes and wildfires or man-made disasters like terrorist attacks. During disasters, communities may not have the resources to respond and recover on their own. Pediatric nurses in all settings need to know **disaster management stages,** which include:

Prevention—Identification of disaster risks; education about what actions to take.

Preparedness and planning
- For individuals and families—Training in first aid, an emergency disaster kit, a predetermined place to meet, and a communication plan.
- For communities and agencies—Determination of the lines of authority and communication; coordination of personnel, supplies, and equipment; evacuation; rescue; and care of the dead.

Response—Begins after the disaster; plans are implemented, which may include shelter in place for individuals, evacuation, or search and rescue. Calmness and patience are essential characteristics for all individuals involved.

An important question for nurses to consider: Will nurses care for patients in the community during the disaster, or will they stay with their own family? (See Internet Resources.)

Modified from Mendias EP, Grimes DE: Preventing and managing community emergencies: disasters and infectious diseases. In Anderson ET, McFarlane J: *Community as partner: theory and practice in nursing,* Philadelphia, 2008, Lippincott Williams & Wilkins; and Summerlin EB: Natural and man-made disasters. In Nies MA, McEwen M: *Community/public health nursing: promoting the health of populations,* Philadelphia, 2007, Saunders.

ning, communication, cultural competency, community dimensions of practice, basic public health sciences, financial planning and management, and leadership and systems thinking. Thus the pediatric nurse employed in a managed care environment may be asked to develop a creative approach to teaching children from different cultures who have asthma about peak flow meters during emergency department visits. Included in the request may be a mechanism to evaluate the cost of the approach and the occurrence of repeated emergency department visits.

NURSING ALERT

Nurses must be able to communicate and work with professionals from other disciplines. This includes being able to understand the terms used by demographers, epidemiologists, and economists.

DEMOGRAPHY

Demography is the study of population characteristics. **Demographic characteristics** include age, gender, race or ethnicity, socioeconomic status, and education. Individuals, families, and communities may have demographic characteristics that affect their health risks (Cashaw, 2008). **Risk** is an increased probability of developing a disease, injury, or illness. Age is one of the most important risk factors for disease prevention and certain health conditions. For example, infants are most likely to die as a result of congenital malformations, children and adolescents as a result of accidents, and middle-aged adults as a result of cancer (National Center for Health Statistics, 2006). Gender also plays an important role. Males are at much greater risk of hemophilia A and B than females.

Race or ethnicity has long been associated with increased risk for disease and disability, but it is now thought that, aside from genetic predisposition, there is a complicated relationship between minority status and socioeconomic status that increases the risk for disease and disability (Smith, 2000). Low socioeconomic status predisposes children to a variety of problems. Poor children are more likely to be obese and to have untreated dental problems. They are more likely to have no regular site for medical care and to be treated in emergency departments (National Center for Health Statistics, 2006).

EPIDEMIOLOGY

Epidemiology is that science of population health applied to the detection of morbidity and mortality in a population. The epidemiologic process identifies the distribution and causes of disease or injury across a population (Cashaw, 2008). It also serves as an important component in developing health programs. For example, *Healthy People 2010* incorporated the process to develop a set of health objectives for the United States. Health professionals in community, state, and national health care organizations use the objectives as a guide to develop programs that have the greatest impact on the health of children.

Distribution of Disease, Injury, or Illness

Morbidity rates are used to measure disease and injury and, along with **natality and mortality rates,** present an objective picture of the health status of a community. There are two types of morbidity rates: incidence and prevalence. **Incidence** measures the occurrence of *new* events in a population during a time period. **Prevalence** measures *existing* events in a population during a time period (Hennekens and Buring, 1987). For example, the incidence of type 1 diabetes in a community is estimated by counting the new cases of type 1 diabetes in a population and dividing that figure by the population at risk. The prevalence of type 1 diabetes is estimated by counting the existing cases of type 1 diabetes in a population and dividing that figure by the population at risk. Both incidence and prevalence are usually given as rates per 1000, 10,000, or 100,000 population, depending on their frequency. Box 2-2 presents frequently used mortality and morbidity rates.

Epidemiologic Triangle

Three factors form the epidemiologic triangle, and their interrelationship alters the risk of acquiring a disease or condition (McKeown and Hilfinger, 2004). These factors are agent, host, and environment (Fig. 2-1).

An **agent** is responsible for causing a disease and may be an infectious agent such as *Mycobacterium tuberculosis*, a chemical agent such as lead in paint, or a physical agent such as fire. **Host** factors are those that are specific to an individual or group. These may be genetic factors that cannot be controlled, or they can be lifestyle factors (e.g., food selections or exercise patterns). **Environmental factors** provide a setting for the host and include the climatic conditions in which the host lives and factors related to the home, neighborhood, and school.

Levels of Prevention

Community health programs are based on three classic levels of prevention (Leavell and Clark, 1965). **Primary prevention** focuses on health promotion and prevention of disease or

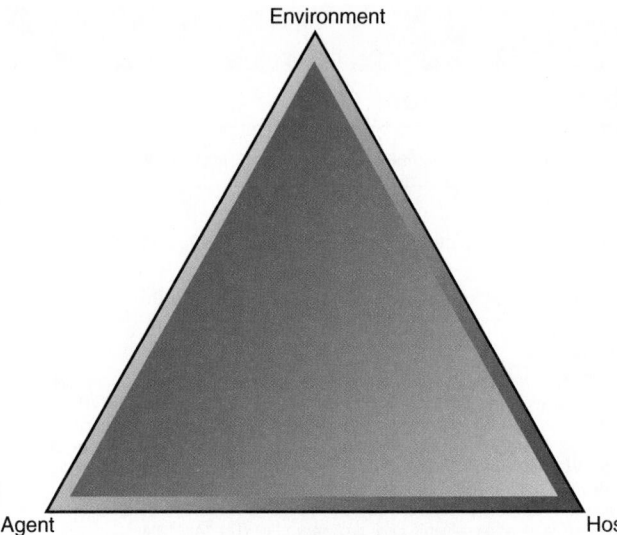

FIG. 2-1 ■ The epidemiologic triangle.

BOX 2-2
Frequently Used Mortality and Morbidity Rates

CRUDE BIRTH RATE

$$\frac{\text{Number of births in a population}}{\text{Total population}} \text{ within a time period} \times 1000$$

CRUDE DEATH RATE

$$\frac{\text{Number of deaths in a population}}{\text{Total population}} \text{ within a time period} \times 1000$$

CAUSE-SPECIFIC DEATH RATE

$$\frac{\text{Number of deaths in a population due to a certain disease}}{\text{Total population}}$$
$$\text{within a time period} \times 1000$$

AGE-SPECIFIC DEATH RATE

$$\frac{\text{Number of deaths in a population in a certain age-group}}{\text{Total population in that age-group}}$$
$$\text{within a time period} \times 1000$$

INCIDENCE OF DISEASE

$$\frac{\text{Number of new events in a population}}{\text{Total at-risk population}}$$
$$\text{within a time period} \times 1000$$

PREVALENCE OF DISEASE

$$\frac{\text{Number of existing events in a population}}{\text{Total at-risk population}}$$
$$\text{within a time period} \times 1000$$

---

injury. Examples of primary prevention activities include well-child care clinics, immunization programs, safety programs (bike helmets, car seats, seat belts, childproof containers), nutrition programs, environmental efforts (clean air programs), sanitation measures (chlorinated water, garbage removal, sewage treatment), and community parenting classes. **Secondary prevention** focuses on screening and early diagnosis of disease. Examples of secondary interventions include tuberculosis and lead screening programs and mental health counseling for stressful events such as separation, divorce, death, or community natural disasters (e.g., earthquakes, floods, hurricanes). **Tertiary prevention** focuses on optimizing function for children with a disability or chronic disease. Tertiary interventions include rehabilitation and disease management programs for asthma, sickle cell disease, cancer, and anorexia and special education programs for children.

Screening

Community health nurses are frequently involved in **screening,** a secondary prevention activity. The purpose of screening is to detect and treat disease early in the period of pathogenesis to prevent the spread and progression of the disease (Wilson and Jungner, 1968). However, screening is not appropriate for every condition. Although screening may bring benefit, there is a certain amount of risk associated with any intervention. It is essential to determine the evidence for a proposed screening program before beginning the program so that the benefits of screening exceed the risks and cost. For example, acanthosis nigricans (AN) is a thickening and darkening of the skin that is commonly found on the neck and is associated with insulin resistance (Centers for Disease Control and Prevention, 2007). Some school health officials have recommended screening for AN as a way to identify early type 2 diabetes in children, but others have argued that screening may not be effective. Because of this controversy, AN is a good example of the need to determine the evidence before establishing a screening program (see Evidence-Based Practice box).

ECONOMICS

A basic understanding of the **economics** of health care is essential because it enables the nurse to participate in decision making about the worth of children's health programs. Economists theorize that individuals and societies view health as a basic utility, that is, something that is perceived as valuable (Gold, Patrick, Torrance, and others, 1996). Other basic utilities are food, shelter, and clothing. People are willing to trade resources, such as money and time, for a program or intervention that will improve their health. Economists measure the amount of resources individuals and communities are willing to pay for good health. They also examine how different groups prioritize health care needs and allocate health care dollars. Methods for defining and estimating cost have been well described, as has the need for a standardized approach to the measurement of cost and effects (Drummond, Sculpher, Torrance, and others, 2005; Brosnan and Swint, 2001).

Economic evaluation provides objective information to establish the value of a program to the community. An example is an evaluation of a school-based hepatitis B vaccination program by Wilson (2000). He concluded that the percentage of vaccinated sixth graders increased from 8% without the program to 82% with the program. The higher vaccination rate potentially saved money that might have eventually been spent to treat these children for hepatitis, cirrhosis, or cancer. The program resulted in potential cost savings of $24 million when compared with the no-program alternative.

EVIDENCE-BASED PRACTICE

Acanthosis Nigricans and the Risk of Type 2 Diabetes in Children

ASK THE QUESTION   How effective is acanthosis nigricans (AN) screening in detecting insulin resistance in a school-aged population?

SEARCH FOR EVIDENCE

Search Strategies   Keywords *acanthosis nigricans* and *screening* were used to find articles published in English between 1996 and 2007. Studies were limited to children 0 to 18 years of age.

Databases Used   PubMed, CINAHL, Cochrane Database of Systematic Reviews, Centers for Disease Control and Prevention (CDC)

CRITICALLY ANALYZE THE EVIDENCE

Six correlational studies were reviewed (evidence level 6). Four of the studies screened community or school populations, and two studies screened clinic populations.

The prevalence of AN ranged from 5% in a general pediatric population (Drobac, Brickman, Smith, and others, 2004) to 73% in a sample of overweight children (Kobaissi, Weigensberg, Ball, and others, 2004). Obesity was found to be a more effective predictor of insulin resistance than AN (Kobaissi, Weigensberg, Ball, and others; Mukhtar, Cleverley, Voorhees, and others, 2001; Nguyen, Keil, Russell, and others, 2001).

The CDC discourages community and school screening for AN because there is insufficient evidence that it predicts diabetes development (CDC, 2007).

APPLY THE EVIDENCE: NURSING IMPLICATIONS

AN screening should not be adopted as part of a community or schoolwide screening program. Further research is needed to determine the most predictive indicator of diabetes development.

References

Bent KN, Shuster GF 3rd, Hurley JS, and others: Acanthosis nigricans as an early clinical proxy marker of increased risk of type II diabetes, *Public Health Nurs* 15(6):415-421, 1988.

Centers for Disease Control and Prevention: *CDC statement on screening children for acanthosis nigricans in schools and communities,* 2007, retrieved Jan 4, 2008, from http://www.cdc.gov/diabetes/news/docs/an.htm.

Drobac S, Brickman W, Smith T, and others: Evaluation of a type 2 diabetes screening protocol in an urban pediatric clinic, *Pediatrics* 114(1):141-148, 2004.

Hirschler V, Aranda C, Oneto A, and others: Is acanthosis nigricans a marker of insulin resistance in obese children? *Diabetes Care* 25(12):2353, 2002.

Kobaissi HA, Weigensberg MJ, Ball GD, and others: Relation between acanthosis nigricans and insulin sensitivity in overweight Hispanic children at risk for type 2 diabetes, *Diabetes Care* 27(6):1412-1416, 2004.

Mukhtar Q, Cleverley G, Voorhees RE, and others: Prevalence of acanthosis nigricans and its association with hyperinsulinemia in New Mexico adolescents, *J Adolesc Health* 28(5):372-376, 2001.

Nguyen TT, Keil MF, Russell DL, and others: Relation of acanthosis nigricans to hyperinsulinemia and insulin sensitivity in overweight African American and white children, *J Pediatr* 138(4):474-480, 2001.

COMMUNITY NURSING PROCESS

In community nursing the focus of the nursing process shifts from the individual child and family to the community or target population (Box 2-3). The stages of the process (assessment, diagnosis, planning, implementation, and evaluation) are similar whether the client is one child or a population of children; only the type of interventions and indicators of wellness and illness differ (Anderson, 2008). **Assessment** is focused on collecting subjective and objective information about the target population to **diagnose** problems based on community needs. **Planning** involves the development of community-centered goals. During the **implementation** stage, the nurse works with the community to implement a program that enables members to reach their goals. Finally, the nurse **evaluates** whether the goals were met. Community nursing is collaborative, and the nurse is one member of a community team that includes other health professionals, educators, politicians, religious leaders, members of public and voluntary organizations, and consumers. The nurse's role depends on the scope of the project, the target population, and the expertise of team members.

Students may be introduced to community collaboration through service learning. The community partnership model is an example of a model that enables nursing students to become part of a collaborative team and to directly contribute to a community's well-being. In this model the missions of nursing education, research, and practice are linked through three pro-

BOX 2-3

The Community Nursing Process

Assessment and diagnosis—The nurse collects subjective and objective information about a community and develops a diagnosis based on community needs and problems.

Planning—The nurse develops community-centered goals to address the identified needs and problems.

Implementation—The nurse implements a program that enables community members to reach their goals.

Evaluation—The nurse conducts a systematic evaluation to determine whether goals and program objectives were met.

cesses: evidence-based practice, service learning, and scholarly teaching (Brosnan, Upchurch, Meininger, and others, 2005).

COMMUNITY NEEDS ASSESSMENT AND DIAGNOSIS

The assessment phase of the community nursing process is called a **community needs assessment.** Assessment involves the collection of subjective and objective information about a community. **Subjective information** indicates what community members say are their most important needs and can be determined in a number of ways. One way is to distribute questionnaires to a sample of people living in the community. Another way is to interview community members directly, phoning or meeting with individuals (such as community leaders) who represent the group or who have a special role in the group.

Objective information is data that the nurse collects either by direct observation or through written sources. A windshield tour is one method of direct observation. Nurses drive through a neighborhood and take notes about the environment, including the appearance of houses, the presence of sidewalks and gutters, the number of public areas, and so on. Objective information about the community's health status can also be obtained from such sources as the Chamber of Commerce, Census Bureau, libraries, state health departments, and the Internet sites of voluntary health organizations or government agencies. Information about service agencies can be found in resource directories, including the local telephone book, community resource directories compiled by such organizations as the United Way, and population-specific books provided by public and voluntary agencies.

One way to organize an assessment is to use a guide that lists community systems that need to be examined. This process is similar to using a physical assessment guide to examine the different body systems in an individual patient. Anderson and McFarlane (2008) described eight community systems that the nurse should examine: health and social services, communication, recreation, physical environment, education, safety and transportation, politics and government, and economics. During the assessment the nurse studies how well each component in the community functions and interacts to meet the health needs of children, identifies the strengths of the community, and determines whether any barriers disrupt the components and prevent access to care for children and their families.

After the assessment is completed, the community nurse collaborates with team members to analyze the results of surveys and questionnaires, determine whether the needs described by community members can be met by existing community agencies, and identify individuals at highest risk. During the analysis the demographic characteristics, the morbidity rates, and the mortality rates in the community are compared with a standard. Comparisons can be made on the basis of time or place. In time comparisons the nurse contrasts the rates in the current year with the rates during an earlier period. In comparisons of place the nurse contrasts the rates in the community with those of a standard population. Standard rates may come from another community or from city, state, or national rates. For example, the rate of tuberculosis in a group of preschool children in the community in 2002 could be compared with the rate of tuberculosis in preschool children in the state in 2002.

A **community health diagnosis** is the reflection of health status, risks, or needs as determined by a causative agent. The format of a community diagnosis is similar to that of an individual nursing diagnosis, with a problem (need) and etiology related to that problem (causative agent). An example of a community nursing diagnosis is "Child abuse related to a violent environment" (Visiting Nurse Association, 1986).

> **NURSING TIP**
>
> All communities have strengths and limitations. The community health nurse draws on the strengths of a community to solve problems.

COMMUNITY PLANNING

The nurse collaborates with community members in developing a plan that addresses the needs and problems of the target population. To maximize the use of community resources, problems should first be prioritized on the basis of their severity, the felt needs of the community, and the ability of the community nurse to bring about change. After prioritizing the problems, the nurse works with community members to develop at least one goal for each problem the members will address. **Goals** are outcomes that give direction to interventions and provide a measure of the change the interventions produced. Community interventions frequently take the form of **health programs** for improving the health status of the target population. Community health programs are based on the three levels of prevention: primary, secondary, and tertiary. For example, a goal for preventing bicycle injuries is, "Within 1 year all students in the first grade will wear bicycle helmets." The nurse and community members then plan a program that includes a health education program about bicycle safety for students and their parents (primary prevention).

The planning group considers the resources that are already available in the community and resources that will be needed for implementing a health program, including personnel, supplies and equipment, office space, phones, and computers. Decisions are made about the timeline of the program, the budget, and strategies that can be used to obtain funding. The nurse may also contact health professionals who have implemented successful programs in other communities; they can provide valuable, time-saving tips and suggestions. Program descriptions are found through professional contacts, online resources, and reviews of the literature. An example of a community assessment and planning project is presented in Box 2-4.

COMMUNITY IMPLEMENTATION

During program implementation, the nurse and community members carry out the intervention. Whether the program is simple or complex, oversight is needed to ensure that everyone involved is communicating with one another, following the guidelines of the plan, keeping within the timeline, and documenting daily activities and expenses. The documentation will prove invaluable during the evaluation phase of the process.

COMMUNITY EVALUATION

Evaluation identifies whether the goals and program objectives were met. There are various models of program evaluation. The structure, process, and outcomes (evaluation) method is commonly used by health care organizations. Donabedian (1980) described this approach as:

Structure—Where and by whom is the care delivered in a program?
Process—Was the care delivered using operational standards and within the financial guidelines of the program?
Outcomes—What was the impact on health status? Was there any improvement?

Structure focuses on the qualifications of personnel; the adequacy of buildings, offices, supplies, and equipment; and the characteristics of the target population. Process focuses on

BOX 2-4

An Example of Community Assessment and Planning

Sabine is an elementary school with 500 prekindergarten to sixth-grade children. The school nurse has been asked to conduct an assessment of the school community and to develop a care plan. The schoolchildren and their families are the target population.

COMMUNITY NEEDS ASSESSMENT AND DIAGNOSIS

The school nurse formed a team of community members that included parents of students who attend Sabine Elementary School, faculty and staff, health care professionals, local religious leaders, and politicians. The group met at regularly scheduled intervals. Their first task was to complete the community assessment. Team members mailed questionnaires to a random sample of families who had children attending Sabine. They held focus groups with community members to obtain subjective information about the needs of the school community. Team members obtained objective data from the local health department, school records, and the U.S. Census Bureau. The nurse also conducted a windshield tour of the neighborhood surrounding the school. The following information was collected:

People—Sabine is located in an ethnically diverse area composed of 30% Hispanics, 30% African Americans, 30% non-Hispanic Caucasians, and 10% Asians. The ethnicity of students in the school is representative of the surrounding area. Sabine is located in a large southwestern city.

Safety and transportation—School bus service was rated very good to excellent by a majority of those surveyed. Transportation records indicated that the last school bus accident occurred 1 year ago. There were no fatalities, but a number of children were injured. Other accidents occurred 2 years and 10 years prior to the most recent accident.

Economics—Although 94% of families had at least one fully employed member, 25% of the families lived below the poverty level. The number below poverty level had not changed in 10 years.

Education—Sixty percent of the adult population had a high school diploma, and 10% of this group had completed at least 1 year of college. School attendance at Sabine was higher than overall state attendance rates.

Communication—Ninety-five percent of homes had telephones, compared with 85% 10 years ago. An estimated 10% of the target population did not speak English, and Spanish was the primary language spoken in this group.

Recreation—Few places were available for small children to play. The focus groups recommended more parks and playgrounds.

Politics and government—The school system was strongly centralized and headed by a school superintendent. The city had a mayor and city council.

Social—Of those families living below the poverty level, 60% received some type of welfare assistance, including food stamps. The school lunch program served 95% of the children attending the school.

Health—The childhood immunization rate for all diseases among children in the community who were between 19 and 35 months of age was 90%, which compared favorably with the national level of 82% in 2005 (National Center for Health Statistics, 2006). The immunization rate for children attending Sabine Elementary School was 100%. Vision and hearing screening programs at Sabine resulted in the referral of 5% of the students for vision problems and 2% of the students for hearing problems. Review of student records indicated that all those children referred received diagnostic follow-up and treatment when indicated. Heights and weights were obtained on all students annually, and the body mass index (BMI) was determined for each student. BMI is calculated by dividing the weight in kilograms by the square of the height in meters (Flegal, Carroll, Kuzmarski, and others, 1998). Results indicated that 30% of students were above the 95th percentile for age and sex, compared with 19% nationally (National Center for Health Statistics, 2006). In focus groups, students and teachers noted that school breakfasts and lunches were high in carbohydrates and fats. They also observed that decreased recess time resulted in decreased student activity during school hours.

On the basis of these assessments, the following community diagnoses were made:

1. Increase in injuries related to school bus accidents.
2. Increase in obesity among students compared with the national standard related to high intake of calories and sedentary lifestyle.

PLANNING

Team members agreed that the number of school bus accidents should be closely monitored over the next 5 years. However, there was a consensus that increased obesity among students was the priority problem, and the team developed the following two goals:

1. Within 2 years the percentage of students with BMIs above the 95th percentile for age and sex will be 20%.
2. Within 5 years that percentage will be 10%.

Team members reviewed the literature for examples of communities that had experienced similar problems, contacted school and health department officials in other areas of the country, examined the results of successful programs, and planned a health program that addressed the unique needs of the target population. The program was titled "Sabine Excels in Health." Program activities were:

- Each September the nurse will address the school's parent association about the program and will discuss the importance of a healthy diet and exercise for all family members.
- Every month teachers will set aside 1 hour to talk with their students about healthy food choices and about the importance of limiting television viewing time.
- Within 6 months school administrators and community members will petition the city to provide a neighborhood park.
- Within 1 year the school dietitian will assess the nutritional value of the current school meals and, if indicated, revise the meal plan to ensure a healthy diet.
- Within 1 year the school will develop a plan to allow a minimum of 30 minutes of unrestricted play during the school day.

Team members determined the resources needed to implement the program, including personnel, supplies, and equipment. They estimated the total cost of setting up the program and maintaining it for 5 years and applied for funding to the school district and to the city and state health departments.

IMPLEMENTATION AND EVALUATION

The school nurse and other team members assumed responsibility for the timely implementation and evaluation of the Sabine Excels in Health program.

the interaction of patients and providers. Process indicators include the number of people who attended a health education program, the number of pamphlets distributed, and the efficiency of the program. Outcome focuses on whether program objectives and community goals were met. Program evaluation should be ongoing so that performance improvement initiatives are monitored and so that an improvement in the way health care is delivered will affect the health status of the target population.

KEY POINTS

- Caring for children within a community requires a multidisciplinary approach.
- Healthy communities provide children with high-quality medical care and a nurturing, safe place to live and grow.
- Community health nursing focuses on promoting and maintaining the health of individuals, families, and groups in the community setting.
- Individual families and communities may have demographic characteristics that affect their risk for disease or injury.
- Epidemiology is the science of population health applied to the detection of morbidity and mortality in a population.
- Community health programs are based on three levels of intervention: primary, secondary, and tertiary.
- Economic evaluations provide objective information to establish the value of a program to society.
- A community needs assessment involves collection of subjective and objective information about the community.
- A community health diagnosis is a problem with a defined cause related to a community problem.
- Program planning and implementation in the community require collaboration between the nurse and community members who are in positions to promote change.
- Evaluation of effective community programs includes consideration of the structure, process, and outcomes related to the program.

REFERENCES

Allender JA, Spradley BW: Opportunities and challenges of community health nursing. In Allender JA, Spradley BW: *Community health nursing: promoting and protecting the public's health,* Philadelphia, 2005, Lippincott Williams & Wilkins.

American Nurses Association: *Public health nursing scope and standards,* Washington, DC, 2007, The Association.

American Nurses Association: *Standards of community health nursing practice,* Kansas City, Mo, 1986, The Association.

Anderson ET: A model to guide practice. In Anderson ET, McFarlane J: *Community as partner: theory and practice in nursing,* Philadelphia, 2008, Lippincott Williams & Wilkins.

Anderson ET, McFarlane J: Community assessment. In Anderson ET, McFarlane J: *Community as partner: theory and practice in nursing,* Philadelphia, 2008, Lippincott Williams & Wilkins.

Brosnan CA, Swint JM: Cost analysis: concepts and application, *Public Health Nurs* 18(1):13-18, 2001.

Brosnan CA, Upchurch SL, Meininger JC, and others: Student nurses participate in public health research and practice through a school-based screening program, *Public Health Nurs* 22(3):260-266, 2005.

Cashaw SA: Epidemiology, demography and community health. In Anderson ET, McFarlane J, editors: *Community as partner,* Philadelphia, 2008, Lippincott Williams & Wilkins.

Centers for Disease Control and Prevention: *CDC statement on screening children for acanthosis nigricans in schools and communities,* 2007, retrieved Jan 4, 2008, from http://www.cdc.gov/diabetes/news/docs/an.htm.

Council on Linkages Between Academia and Public Health Practice: *Core competencies for public health professionals,* 2001, retrieved Jan 4, 2008, from http://www.phf.org/competencies.htm.

Donabedian A: *The definition of quality and approaches to its assessment,* Ann Arbor, Mich, 1980, Health Administration Press.

Drummond MF, Sculpher MJ, Torrance GW, and others: *Methods for the economic evaluation of health care programmes,* ed 3, New York, 2005, Oxford University Press.

Flegal KM, Carroll MD, Kuzmarski RJ, and others: Overweight and obesity in the United States: prevalence and trends, *Int J Obes Relat Metab Disord* 22(1):39-47, 1998.

Flynn BC, Ivanov LL: Health promotion through healthy communities and cities. In Stanhope M, Lancaster J: *Community and public health nursing,* St Louis, 2004, Mosby.

Gebbie KM, Turnock BJ: The public health workforce, 2006. new challenges, *Health Affairs* 25(4):923-933, 2006.

Gold MR, Patrick DL, Torrance GW, and others: Identifying and valuing outcomes. In Gold MR, Siegel JE, Russell LB, and others, editors: *Cost-effectiveness in health and medicine,* New York, 1996, Oxford University Press.

Health Resources and Services Administration: *The registered nurse population,* Rockville, Md, 2004, US Department of Health and Human Services.

Hennekens CH, Buring JE: *Epidemiology in medicine,* Boston, 1987, Little, Brown.

Institute of Medicine: *The future of public health,* Washington, DC, 1988, National Academy Press.

Leavell HR, Clark EG: *Preventive medicine for the doctor in his community: an epidemiologic approach,* New York, 1965, McGraw-Hill.

McEwen M, Nies MA: Health: a community view. In Nies MA, McEwen M: *Community/public health: promoting the health of populations,* Philadelphia, 2007, Saunders.

McKeown RE, Hilfinger DK: Epidemiology. In Stanhope M, Lancaster J: *Community and public health nursing,* St Louis, 2004, Mosby.

National Center for Health Statistics: *Health, United States, 2006: with chartbook on trends in the health of Americans,* DHS Pub No 2006-1232, Hyattsville, Md, 2006, US Department of Health and Human Services, retrieved Jan 4, 2008, from http://www.cdc.gov/nchs/data/hus/hus06.pdf.

Smith GD: Learning to live with complexity: ethnicity, socioeconomic position, and health in Britain and the United States, *Am J Public Health* 90:1694-1698, 2000.

Visiting Nurse Association of Omaha: *Client management information system for community health nursing agencies,* Rockville, Md, 1986, US Department of Health and Human Services.

Williams CA: Community-oriented populations-focused practice: the foundation of specialization in public health practice. In Stanhope M, Lancaster J: *Community and public health nursing,* St Louis, 2004, Mosby.

Wilson JMG, Jungner G: Principles and practice of screening for disease, *Public Health Papers,* no. 34, Geneva, 1968, World Health Organization.

Wilson T: Economic evaluation of a metropolitan-wide, school-based hepatitis B vaccination program, *Public Health Nurs* 17(3):222-227, 2000.

INTERNET RESOURCES

Children Now: http://www.childrennow.org

Healthy People 2010: http://www.healthypeople. gov

Kids Count Data, Annie E. Casey Foundation: http:// www.aecf.org/MajorInitiatives/KIDSCOUNT.aspx

National Center for Health Statistics: http://www. cdc.gov/nchs

National Institute of Environmental Health Sciences: http://www. niehs.nih.gov

National Safety Council: http://www.nsc.org

Office of Disease Prevention and Health Promotion: http://www.odphp.osophs.dhhs.gov

Safe Kids Worldwide: http://www.safekids.org

U.S. Census Bureau (U.S. and state census information): http://www. census.gov

U.S. Department of Education: http://www.ed.gov

U.S. Department of Health and Human Services: http://www.os.dhhs.gov

World Health Organization: http://www.who.int

Family Influences on Child Health Promotion

PATRICK BARRERA

CHAPTER OUTLINE

GENERAL CONCEPTS, 30
Definition of Family, 30
Family Theories, 30
  Family Systems Theory, 30
  Family Stress Theory, 32
  Developmental Theory, 32
Family Nursing Interventions, 32
**FAMILY STRUCTURE AND
FUNCTION, 33**
Family Structure, 33
  Traditional Nuclear Family, 33
  Nuclear Family, 33
  Blended Family, 33
  Extended Family, 33
  Single-Parent Family, 33
  Binuclear Family, 34
  Polygamous Family, 34
  Communal Family, 34
  Gay/Lesbian Family, 34
Family Strengths and Functioning
  Style, 34

**FAMILY ROLES AND
RELATIONSHIPS, 35**
Parental Roles, 35
Role Learning, 35
  Family Size and Configuration, 35
  Sibling Interactions, 36
  Ordinal Position, 37
  Multiple Births, 37
PARENTING, 38
Motivation for Parenthood, 38
Preparation for Parenthood, 39
Transition to Parenthood, 39
  Parental Factors Affecting Transition to
    Parenthood, 39
Parenting Behaviors, 40
  Parental Styles of Control, 40
Limit Setting and Discipline, 41
  Minimizing Misbehavior, 41
  General Guidelines for Implementing
    Discipline, 41
  Types of Discipline, 41

SPECIAL PARENTING SITUATIONS, 43
Parenting the Adopted Child, 43
  Issues of Origin, 44
  Adolescence, 44
  Cross-Racial and International
    Adoption, 44
Parenting and Divorce, 45
  Impact of Divorce on Children, 45
  Custody and Parenting Partnerships, 47
Single Parenting, 47
  Single Fathers, 47
Parenting in Reconstituted Families, 48
Parenting in Dual-Earner Families, 48
  Working Mothers, 48
Foster Parenting, 48
**Accommodating Contemporary Parenting
  Situations, 48**

LEARNING OBJECTIVES

**On completion of this chapter the
reader will be able to:**
- Discuss definitions of family.
- Describe three major family theories.
- Identify different family structures found
  in the United States.

- Discuss the effect of family size and
  configuration on personality development.
- Discuss the role transition experienced by
  new parents.
- Explain various parenting behaviors such
  as parenting styles, disciplinary patterns,
  and communication skills.

- Demonstrate an understanding of special
  parenting situations such as adoption,
  divorce, single parenting, parenting in
  reconstituted families, and dual-earner
  families.

RELATED TOPICS and ADDITIONAL RESOURCES

 IN TEXT

Adolescent Pregnancy, *Ch. 17*
Alternate Child Care Arrangements, *Ch. 10*
Communicating with Families, *Ch. 6*
Growth and Development, *Ch. 5*
History Taking and Physical Examination,
   Ch. 6

Impact of the Child's Chronic Illness or
   Disability, *Ch. 18*
Preschool and Kindergarten Experience,
   Ch. 13
Promote Parent-Infant Bonding
   (Attachment), *Ch. 8*
Sibling Rivalry, *Ch. 12*

 COMPANION CD

Case Study—Family Functioning
NCLEX Review Questions

evolve

evolve.elsevier.com/Wong/essentials/

NCLEX Review Questions
WebLinks

GENERAL CONCEPTS

DEFINITION OF FAMILY

The term **family** has been defined in many different ways according to the individual's own frame of reference, value judgment, or discipline. There is no universal definition of family; a family is what an individual considers it to be. Biology describes the family as fulfilling the biologic function of perpetuation of the species. Psychology emphasizes the interpersonal aspects of the family and its responsibility for personality development. Economics views the family as a productive unit providing for material needs. Sociology depicts the family as a social unit interacting with the larger society, creating the context within which cultural values and identity are formed. Others define family in terms of the relationships of the persons who make up the family unit. The most common type of relationships are **consanguineous** (blood relationships), **affinal** (marital relationships), and **family of origin** (family unit a person is born into).

Earlier definitions of family emphasized that family members were related by legal ties or genetic relationships and lived in the same household with specific roles. Later definitions have been broadened to reflect both structural and functional changes. A family can be defined as an institution where individuals, related through biology or enduring commitments, and representing similar or different generations and genders, participate in roles involving mutual socialization, nurturance, and emotional commitment (Lerner, Sparks, and McCubbin, 1999).

Considerable controversy has been generated about the newer concepts of family, such as communal families, single-parent families, and homosexual families. To accommodate these and other varieties of family styles, the descriptive term **household** is frequently used.

> **NURSINGALERT**
>
> The nurse's knowledge and the sensitivity with which he or she assesses a household will determine the types of interventions that are appropriate to support family members.

Nursing of infants and children is intimately involved with care of the child *and* the family. Family structure and dynamics can have an enduring influence on a child, affecting the child's health and well-being (American Academy of Pediatrics, 2003). Consequently, nurses must be aware of the functions of the family, various types of family structures, and

theories that provide a foundation for understanding the changes within a family and for directing family-oriented interventions.

FAMILY THEORIES

A **family theory** can be used to describe families and how the family unit responds to events both within and outside the family. Each family theory makes assumptions about the family and has inherent strengths and limitations. Most nurses use a combination of theories in their work with children and families. Commonly used theories are family systems theory, family stress theory, and developmental theory (Table 3-1).

Family Systems Theory

Family systems theory is derived from general systems theory, a science of "wholeness" that is characterized by interaction among the components of the system and between the system and the environment. **General systems theory** expanded scientific thought from a simplistic view of direct cause and effect (A causes B) to a more complex and interrelated theory (A influences B, but B also affects A). In family systems theory, the family is viewed as a system that continually interacts with its members and the environment. The emphasis is on the interaction between the members; a change in one family member creates a change in other members, which in turn results in a new change in the original member. Consequently, a problem or dysfunction does not lie in any one member but rather in the type of interactions used by the family. Because the interactions, not the individual members, are viewed as the source of the problem, the family becomes the patient and the focus of care. Examples of the application of family systems theory to clinical problems are nonorganic failure to thrive and child abuse. According to family systems theory, the problem does not rest solely with the parent or child but with the type of interactions between the parent and child and the factors that affect their relationship.

The family is viewed as a whole that is different from the sum of the individual members. For example, in a household of parents and one child, there are not only three individuals, but four interactive units. These units include three dyads (the marital relationship, the mother-child relationship, and the father-child relationship) and a triangle (the mother-father-child relationship). The family system functions within a larger system composed of the extended family, the subculture, the culture, and society. This ecologic model of family

TABLE 3-1

Summary of Family Theories and Applications

ASSUMPTIONS	STRENGTHS	LIMITATIONS	APPLICATIONS
FAMILY SYSTEMS THEORY A change in any one part of a family system affects all other parts of the family system (circular causality). Family systems are characterized by periods of rapid growth and change and periods of relative stability. Both too little change and too much change are dysfunctional for the family system; therefore a balance between morphogenesis (change) and morphostasis (no change) is necessary. Family systems can initiate change, as well as react to it.	Applicable for family in normal everyday life, as well as for family dysfunction and pathology Useful for families of varying structure and various stages of life cycle	More difficult to determine cause-and-effect relationships because of circular causality	Mate selection, courtship processes, family communication, boundary maintenance, power and control within family, parent-child relationships, adolescent pregnancy and parenthood
FAMILY STRESS THEORY Stress is an inevitable part of family life, and any event, even if positive, can be stressful for family. Family encounters both normative expected stressors and unexpected situational stressors over life cycle. Stress has a cumulative effect on family. Families cope with and respond to stressors with a wide range of responses and effectiveness.	Potential to explain and predict family behavior in response to stressors and to develop effective interventions to promote family adaptation Focuses on positive contribution of resources, coping, and social support to adaptive outcomes Can be used by many disciplines in health field	Relationships between all variables in framework not yet adequately described Not yet known if certain combinations of resources and coping strategies are applicable to all stressful events	Transition to parenthood and other normative transitions, single-parent families, families experiencing work-related stressors (dual-earner family, unemployment), acute or chronic childhood illness or disability, infertility, death of a child, divorce, teenage pregnancy and parenthood
DEVELOPMENTAL THEORY Families develop and change over time in similar and consistent ways. Family and its members must perform certain time-specific tasks set by themselves and by persons in the broader society. Family role performance at one stage of family life cycle influences family's behavioral options at next stage. Family tends to be in stage of disequilibrium when entering a new life-cycle stage and strives toward homeostasis within stages.	Provides a dynamic, rather than static, view of family Addresses both changes within family and changes in family as a social system over its life history Anticipates potential stressors that normally accompany transitions to various stages and when problems may peak because of lack of resources	Traditional model more easily applied to two-parent families with children Use of age of oldest child and marital duration as marker of stage transition sometimes problematic (e.g., in stepfamilies, single-parent families)	Anticipatory guidance, educational strategies, and developing or strengthening family resources for management of transition to parenthood; family adjustment to children entering school, becoming adolescents, leaving home; management of "empty nest" years and retirement

systems theory places the family dyads in the center of a circle surrounded by the extended family, the subculture, and the culture, with the larger society at the periphery. The concept of **nonsummativity**—"the whole is greater than the sum of its parts"—implies that the nurse must consider relationships between family members as well as the family's relationship to its environment. To effect positive change in a family, it is necessary to work with and through the various systems that affect family life.

Another concept, **adaptability,** views the family as a highly adaptable unit. When problems exist within the family, change occurs by altering the interaction or feedback messages that perpetuate disruptive behavior. **Feedback** refers to processes in the family that help identify strengths and needs and determine how well goals are accomplished. Positive feedback initiates change; negative feedback resists change. When the family system is disrupted, change can occur at any point in the sys-

tem. Although family systems theorists pursue the family history to understand current family interaction and problem patterns, the emphasis is on what is occurring *now* and how to change that pattern. This focus allows for sometimes rapid and dramatic changes.

A major factor that influences a family's adaptability is its **boundary,** an imaginary line that exists between the family and its environment. Families have varying degrees of openness and closure in these boundaries. For example, one family has the capacity to reach out for help, whereas another considers help threatening. Knowledge of boundaries is critical when teaching or counseling families. Families with open boundaries may demonstrate a greater receptivity to interventions, whereas families demonstrating closed boundaries often require increased sensitivity and skill on the part of the nurse to gain their trust and acceptance. The nurse who uses family systems theory should assess the family's ability to accept new ideas, information, resources, and opportunities and to plan strategies.

Family Stress Theory

Family stress theory explains how families react to stressful events and suggests factors that promote adaptation to stress. Families encounter **stressors** (events that cause stress and have the potential to effect a change in the family social system), including those that are predictable (e.g., parenthood) and those that are unpredictable (e.g., illness, unemployment). These stressors are cumulative, involving simultaneous demands from work, family, and community life. Too many stressful events occurring within a relatively short period (usually 1 year) can overwhelm the family's ability to cope and place it at risk for breakdown or physical and emotional health problems among its members. When the family experiences too many stressors for it to cope adequately, a state of crisis ensues. For adaptation to occur, a change in family structure or interaction is necessary.

The **resiliency model of family stress, adjustment, and adaptation** emphasizes that the stressful situation is not necessarily pathologic or detrimental to the family but demonstrates that the family needs to make fundamental structural or systemic changes to adapt to the situation (McCubbin and McCubbin, 1994). For example, bringing a child with special needs to a treatment facility for therapy might be considered a crisis for a family without a car or money for public transportation, but may be defined as only a minor inconvenience by another family with adequate resources.

Developmental Theory

Developmental theory is an outgrowth of several theories of development. Foremost among the developers is Duvall (1977), who described eight developmental tasks of the family throughout its life span (Box 3-1). The family is described as a small group, a semiclosed system of personalities that interacts with the larger cultural social system. As an interrelated system, changes do not occur in one part without a series of changes in other parts.

Developmental theory addresses family change over time using Duvall's family life cycle stages, based on the predictable changes in the structure, function, and roles of the family, with the age of the oldest child as the marker for stage transition. The arrival of the first child marks the transition from stage I to stage II. As the first child grows and develops, the family enters subsequent stages. In every stage the family faces certain developmental tasks. At the same time, each member of the family must achieve individual developmental tasks as part of each family life cycle stage.

Developmental theory can be applied to nursing practice. For example, the nurse can assess how well new parents are accomplishing the individual and family developmental tasks associated with transition to parenthood. New applications should emerge as more is learned about developmental stages for nonnuclear and nontraditional families.

FAMILY NURSING INTERVENTIONS

In working with children, the nurse must include family members in their care plan. To discover family dynamics, strengths, and weaknesses, a thorough family assessment is necessary (see Chapter 6). When working with families, the nurse's choice of interventions depends on the theoretic fam-

---

BOX 3-1

Duvall's Developmental Stages of the Family

STAGE I—MARRIAGE AND AN INDEPENDENT HOME: THE JOINING OF FAMILIES
Reestablish couple identity.
Realign relationships with extended family.
Make decisions regarding parenthood.

STAGE II—FAMILIES WITH INFANTS
Integrate infants into the family unit.
Accommodate to new parenting and grandparenting roles.
Maintain marital bond.

STAGE III—FAMILIES WITH PRESCHOOLERS
Socialize children.
Parents and children adjust to separation.

STAGE IV—FAMILIES WITH SCHOOLCHILDREN
Children develop peer relations.
Parents adjust to their children's peer and school influences.

STAGE V—FAMILIES WITH TEENAGERS
Adolescents develop increasing autonomy.
Parents refocus on midlife marital and career issues.
Parents begin a shift toward concern for the older generation.

STAGE VI—FAMILIES AS LAUNCHING CENTERS
Parents and young adults establish independent identities.
Parents renegotiate marital relationship.

STAGE VII—MIDDLE-AGED FAMILIES
Reinvest in couple identity with concurrent development of independent interests.
Realign relationships to include in-laws and grandchildren.
Deal with disabilities and death of older generation.

STAGE VIII—AGING FAMILIES
Shift from work role to leisure and semiretirement or full retirement.
Maintain couple and individual functioning while adapting to the aging process.
Prepare for own death and dealing with the loss of spouse and/or siblings and other peers.

Modified from Wright LM, Leahey M: *Nurses and families: a guide to family assessment and intervention*, Philadelphia, 1984, Davis.

---

ily model that is used (Box 3-2). For example, in family systems theory, the focus is on the interaction of family members within the larger environment. In this case, using group dynamics to involve all members in the intervention process and being a skillful communicator are essential. Systems theory also presents excellent opportunities for anticipatory guidance. Because each family member reacts to every stress experienced by that system, nurses can intervene to help the family prepare for and cope with changes. Each stress point represents an opportunity for change and learning because families are more open to interventions at this time (Brazelton, 1995). In the family stress theory, crisis intervention strategies are employed to help family members cope with the challenging event. In the developmental theory, the nurse provides anticipatory guidance to prepare members for transition to the next family stage.

Family Nursing Interventions

- Behavior modification
- Case management and coordination
- Collaborative strategies
- Contracting
- Counseling, including support, cognitive reappraisal, and reframing
- Empowering families through active participation
- Environmental modification
- Family advocacy
- Family crisis intervention
- Networking, including use of self-help groups and social support
- Providing information and technical expertise
- Role modeling
- Role supplementation
- Teaching strategies, including stress management, lifestyle modifications, and anticipatory guidance

From Friedman MM, Bowden VR, Jones EG: *Family nursing: research theory and practice*, ed 5, Upper Saddle River, NJ, 2003, Pearson Education.

FIG. 3-1 ■ Children benefit from interaction with grandparents, who sometimes assume the parenting role.

FAMILY STRUCTURE AND FUNCTION

FAMILY STRUCTURE

The **family structure,** or **family composition,** consists of individuals, each with a socially recognized status and position, who interact with one another on a regular, recurring basis in socially sanctioned ways. When members are gained or lost through events such as marriage, divorce, birth, death, abandonment, or incarceration, the family composition is altered and roles must be redefined or redistributed.

Traditionally, the family structure was either a nuclear or extended family. In recent years, family composition has assumed new configurations, with the single-parent family and blended family becoming prominent forms. The predominant structural pattern in any society depends on the mobility of families as they pursue economic goals and as relationships change. It is not uncommon for children to belong to several different family groups during their lifetime.

Nurses must be able to meet the needs of children from many diverse family structures and home situations. The particular family structure a child participates in affects the direction of nursing care. The U.S. Census Bureau uses four definitions for families: the traditional nuclear family, the nuclear family, the blended family or household, and the extended family or household.

Traditional Nuclear Family

A traditional nuclear family consists of a married couple and their biologic children. Children in this type of family live with both biologic parents and, if siblings are present, only full brothers and sisters (i.e., siblings who share the same two biologic parents). No other persons are present in the household (i.e., no steprelatives, foster or adopted children, half-siblings, other relatives, or nonrelatives).

Nuclear Family

The nuclear family is composed of two parents and their children. The parent-child relationship may be biologic, step, adoptive, or foster. Sibling ties may be biologic, step, half, or adoptive. The parents are not necessarily married. No other relatives or nonrelatives are present in the household.

Blended Family

A blended family or household, also called a *reconstituted family,* includes at least one stepparent, stepsibling, or half-sibling. A stepparent is the spouse of a child's biologic parent but is not the child's biologic parent. Stepsiblings do not share a common biologic parent; the biologic parent of one child is the stepparent of the other. Half-siblings share only one biologic parent. Nurses may have opportunities to interact with blended families in the community.

Extended Family

An extended family or household includes at least one parent, one or more children, and one or more members (related or unrelated) other than a parent or sibling. Parent-child and sibling relationships may be biologic, step, adoptive, or foster.

In many nations and among many ethnic and cultural groups, households with extended families are common. Within the extended family, grandparents often find themselves rearing their grandchildren (Fig. 3-1). In extended families, young parents are often considered too young or too inexperienced to make decisions independently. Often, the older relative holds the authority and makes decisions in consultation with the young parents. Sharing residence with relatives is also beneficial because this arrangement assists with the management of scarce resources and provides child care for working families. A resource for extended families is the Grandparent Information Center.*

Single-Parent Family

In the United States an estimated 21.7 million children lived in **single-parent families** in 2005 (Annie E Casey Foundation, 2007). The contemporary single-parent family has emerged partially as a consequence of the women's rights movement and also as a result of more women (and men) establishing separate households because of divorce, death, desertion, or illegitimacy. In addition, a more liberal attitude in the courts has made it possible for single people, both male

---

*For information, contact the local AARP representative or office; http://www.aarp.org/families/grandparents.

and female, to adopt children. Although mothers usually head single-parent families, it is becoming more common for fathers to be awarded custody of dependent children in divorce settlements. With the increased psychologic and financial independence of women and the increased acceptability of illegitimacy in society, more unmarried women are deliberately choosing mother-child families. Frequently, these mothers and children are absorbed into the extended family. The challenges of single-parent families are discussed on p. 47.

Binuclear Family

The term **binuclear family** is used to describe the situation that allows parents to continue the parenting role while terminating the spousal unit. The degree of cooperation between households and the time the child spends with each can vary. In **joint custody,** the court assigns divorcing parents equal rights and responsibilities concerning the minor child or children. These alternate family forms are efforts on the part of those concerned to view divorce as a process of reorganization and redefinition of a family rather than as a family dissolution. Joint custody and co-parenting are discussed further on p. 47.

Polygamous Family

Although it is not legally sanctioned in the United States, the conjugal unit is sometimes extended by the addition of spouses in polygamous matings. **Polygamy** refers to either wives (**polygyny**) or, rarely, husbands (**polyandry**). Many societies practice polygyny that is further designated as **sororal,** in which the wives are sisters, or **nonsororal,** in which the wives are unrelated. Sororal polygyny is widespread throughout the world. Most often, mothers and their children share a husband and father, with each mother and her children living in the same or separate household.

Communal Family

The **communal family** emerged from disenchantment with most contemporary life choices. Although communal families may have divergent beliefs, practices, and organization, the basic impetus for formation has been dissatisfaction with the nuclear family structure, social systems, and goals of the larger community. Relatively uncommon today, communal groups share common ownership of property. In cooperatives, there is private ownership of property, but certain goods and services are shared and exchanged without monetary consideration. There is strong reliance on group members and material interdependence. Both provide collective security for nonproductive members, share homemaking and childrearing functions, and help overcome the problem of interpersonal isolation or loneliness.

Gay/Lesbian Family

A **same-sex, homosexual,** or **gay/lesbian family** is one in which there is a legal or common-law tie between two persons of the same sex who have children. With the social stigma attached to being gay or lesbian, it is difficult to state the number of children of gay or lesbian parents; estimates range from 1 million to 14 million (Ariel and McPherson, 2000; Pawelski, Perrin, Foy, and others, 2006). Although some children in gay/lesbian households are biologic from a former marriage or relationship, there are other circumstances where children may be present. They may be foster or adoptive parents, lesbian mothers may conceive through artificial fertilization, or a gay male couple may become parents through use of a surrogate mother.

Disclosure of parental homosexuality ("coming out") to children can be a concern for families. There are a number of factors to consider before disclosing this information to children. Parents should be comfortable with their own sexual preference and should discuss this with the children as they become old enough to understand relationships. Discussions should be planned and take place in a quiet setting where interruptions are unlikely. Children should be assured that the parent's relationship with them will not change as a result of the discussion (Lynch and Murray, 2000).

There are a growing number of families with same-sex parents in the United States, with an estimated one fourth of all same-sex couples raising children (Pawelski, Perrin, Foy, and others, 2006). The gay/lesbian family environment can be as healthy as any other. Nurses need to be nonjudgmental and to learn to accept differences rather than demonstrate a homophobic prejudice that can have a detrimental effect on the nurse-child-family relationship. Moreover, the more knowledge of the child's family constellation and lifestyle that nurses have, the more help they can provide to the parents and the child.

FAMILY STRENGTHS AND FUNCTIONING STYLE

Family function refers to the interactions of family members, especially the quality of those relationships and interactions. Researchers are interested in family characteristics that help families function effectively. Knowledge of these factors guides the nurse throughout the nursing process, and helps the nurse

---

BOX 3-3

Qualities of Strong Families

- A belief and sense of **commitment** toward promoting the well-being and growth of individual family members, as well as the family unit
- **Appreciation** for the small and large things that individual family members do well and **encouragement** to do better
- Concentrated effort to spend **time** and do things together, no matter how formal or informal the activity or event
- A sense of **purpose** that permeates the reasons and basis for "going on" in both bad and good times
- A sense of **congruence** among family members regarding the value and importance of assigning time and energy to meet needs
- The ability to **communicate** with one another in a way that emphasizes positive interactions
- A clear set of **family rules, values,** and **beliefs** that establishes expectations about acceptable and desired behavior
- A varied repertoire of **coping strategies** that promote positive functioning in dealing with both normative and nonnormative life events
- The ability to engage in **problem-solving** activities designed to evaluate options for meeting needs and procuring resources
- The ability to be **positive** and see the positive in almost all aspects of their lives, including the ability to see crisis and problems as an opportunity to learn and grow
- **Flexibility** and **adaptability** in the roles necessary to procure resources to meet needs
- A **balance** between the use of internal and external family resources for coping and adapting to life events and planning for the future

From Dunst C, Trivette C, Deal A: *Enabling and empowering families: principles and guidelines for practice,* Cambridge, Mass, 1988, Brookline Books.

to predict ways in which families may cope and respond to a stressful event, to provide individualized support that builds on family strengths and unique functioning style, and to assist family members in obtaining resources.

Family strengths and unique functioning styles (Box 3-3) are significant resources that nurses can use to meet family needs. Building on qualities that make a family work well and strengthening family resources make the family unit even stronger. All families have strengths as well as vulnerabilities.

FAMILY ROLES AND RELATIONSHIPS

Each individual has a position, or status, in the family structure and plays culturally and socially defined roles in interactions within the family. Each family also has its own traditions and values and sets its own standards for interaction within and outside the group. Each determines the experiences the children should have, those they are to be shielded from, and how each of these experiences meets the needs of family members. When family ties are strong, social control is highly effective, and most members conform to their roles willingly and with commitment. Conflicts arise when people do not fulfill their roles in ways that meet other family members' expectations, either because they are unaware of the expectations or because they choose not to meet them.

PARENTAL ROLES

In all family groups the socially recognized status of father and mother exists with socially sanctioned roles that prescribe appropriate sexual behavior and childrearing responsibilities. The guides for behavior in these roles serve to control sexual conflict in society and provide for prolonged care of children. The degree to which parents are committed and the way they play their roles are influenced by a number of variables and by the parents' unique socialization experience.

Parental role definitions are changing as a result of the changing economy and increased opportunities for women. Women are achieving equality with men in education, more of them have entered the work force, and the number of women who choose to have fewer children or none at all is increasing. As the role of the woman has changed, the complementary role of the man has also changed. Many fathers are taking a more active role in childrearing and household tasks. As the redefinition of sex roles continues in American families, there may be role conflicts in many families because of a cultural lag of the persisting traditional role definitions.

ROLE LEARNING

Roles are learned through the socialization process. During all stages of development children learn and practice, through interaction with others and in their play, a set of social roles and the characteristics of other roles. They behave in patterned and more or less predictable ways because they learn roles that define mutual expectations in typical social relationships. Although role definitions are changing, the basic determinants of parenting remain the same. Several determinants of parenting infants and young children are parental personality and mental well-being, systems of support, and child characteristics. These determinants have been used as consistent measurements to determine a person's success in fulfilling the parental role.

Parents, peers, authority figures, and other socializing agents who use positive and negative sanctions to ensure con-

formity to their norms transmit role conceptions. Role behaviors positively reinforced by rewards such as love, affection, friendship, and honors are strengthened. Negative reinforcement takes the form of ridicule, withdrawal of love, expressions of disapproval, or banishment.

In some cultures the role behavior expected of children conflicts with desirable adult behavior. For example, in the United States, children are expected to be submissive in childhood but dominant as adults. This conflict of expectations is known as **role discontinuity.** Other cultures value the same behaviors, such as courage and aggression, in both children and adults; this provides **role continuity.**

One responsibility of the family is to develop culturally appropriate role behavior in children. Children learn to perform in expected ways consistent with their position in the family and culture. The observed behavior of each child is a single manifestation—a combination of social influences and individual psychologic processes. In this way the uniting of the child's intrapersonal system (the self) with the interpersonal system (the family) is simultaneously understood as the child's conduct.

Role structuring initially takes place within the family unit, in which the children fulfill a set of roles and respond to the roles of their parents and other family members. The roles of the children are shaped primarily by the parents, who apply direct or indirect pressures to induce or force children into the desired patterns of behavior or direct their efforts toward modification of the role responses of the child on a mutually acceptable basis. Parents have their own techniques and determine the course that the process of socialization follows.

Children respond to life situations according to behaviors learned in reciprocal transactions. As they acquire important role-taking skills, their relationships with others change. For instance, when a teenager is also the mother but lives in a household with the grandmother, the teenager may be viewed more as an adolescent than as a mother. Children become proficient at understanding others as they acquire the ability to discriminate their own perspectives from those of others. Children who get along well with others and attain status in the peer group have well-developed role-taking skills.

Family Size and Configuration

Parenting practices differ between small and large families. In small families, more emphasis is placed on the individual development of the children. Parenting is intensive rather than extensive, and there is constant pressure to measure up to family expectations. Children's development and achievement are measured against those of other children in the neighborhood and social class. In small families, there is more democratic participation by the children than in larger families. Adolescents in small families identify more strongly with their parents and rely more on their parents for advice. They have well-developed, autonomous inner controls as contrasted with adolescents from larger families, who rely more on adult authority.

Children in a large family are able to adjust to a variety of changes and crises. There is more emphasis on the group and less on the individual (Fig. 3-2). Cooperation is essential, often because of economic necessity. The large number of people sharing a limited amount of space requires a greater degree of organization, administration, and authoritarian control. A dominant family member (a parent or older child)

FIG. 3-2 ■ Family structure promotes strong relationships among its members.

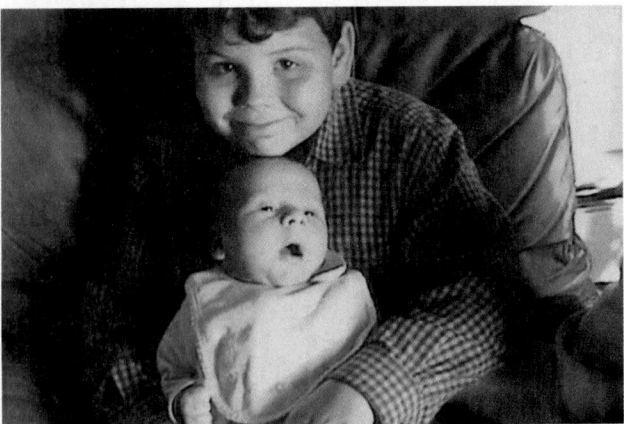

FIG. 3-3 ■ Older school-age children often enjoy taking responsibility for the care of a younger sibling.

wields control. The number of children reduces the intimate, one-to-one contact between the parent and any individual child. Consequently, children turn to each other for what they cannot get from their parents. The reduced parent-child contact encourages individual children to adopt specialized roles to gain recognition in the family.

Older siblings in large families often administer discipline. Siblings are usually attuned to what constitutes misbehavior. Sibling disapproval or ostracism is frequently a more meaningful disciplinary measure than parental interventions. In situations such as death or illness of a parent, an older sibling often assumes responsibility for the family at considerable personal sacrifice. Large families generate a sense of security in the children that is fostered by sibling support and cooperation. However, adolescents from a large family are more peer oriented than family oriented.

Sibling Interactions

Spacing of Children. Age differences between siblings affect the childhood environment, but to a lesser extent than does the sex of the sibling. The arrival of a sibling is difficult for toddlers and preschool children, especially between the ages of 2 and 3 years old. At this age, they are still very attached to their parents and do not understand the concept of sharing. An older child is able to understand the situation and is less likely to see the newcomer as a threat, although the child does feel the loss of the only-child status. In general, the narrower the spacing between siblings, the more the children influence one another, especially in emotional characteristics. The wider the spacing, the greater the influence of the parents.

Traditionally, sibling relationships were viewed from a Freudian perspective that emphasized the concept of sibling rivalry. Recently, researchers have viewed siblings through developmental or ecologic frameworks that focus on interactions within family systems (Friedman, Bowden, and Jones, 2003). The results of these broader perspectives provide a picture of rich and varied sibling interactions (Fig. 3-3).

Sibling Functions. The sibling relationship's most unique feature is its duration. The longest relationship one will share with another human being is the sibling relationship, which lasts through a lifetime (often 50 to 80 years), compared with the child-parent relationship of approximately 30 to 50 years. Siblings spend long periods together and get to know each other at their best and worst.

Siblings exert power, exchange services, and express feelings in reciprocal ways that are often not revealed in the presence of the parents. They see themselves in their brother or sister, experience life vicariously through their sibling's behavior, and begin to expand on their own possibilities. Siblings can also be touchstones for what the other would *not* like to be, and they use each other as yardsticks for comparison. They provide a sounding board for each other and offer a safe forum for experimenting with new behaviors and roles. Brothers and sisters provide each other with tangible services (e.g., lending money, clothing, toys, or sports equipment; teaching a skill), help each other with childhood problems, provide support in dealing with parents or others outside the family, and provide introductions to new friendship groups. Children learn to negotiate and bargain, and sometimes to manipulate, from their siblings. Their interactions with each other provide opportunities for conflict and conflict resolution. They protect one another from parental-executive abuse of power and can form a coalition to deal with the issues of authority, power, and emotional support. Negotiating with parents is stronger when siblings act together rather than singly.

Siblings interpret the outside world for each other and perform educative functions for the parents. A related function is **pioneering,** in which one sibling initiates a process, thereby giving the others permission to follow. These patterns include breaking explicit family rules, taking new pathways (such as leaving the family), or adopting different moral or political codes and lifestyles.

Tattling can be an important lever in sibling interactions. On the other hand, there is often a conspiracy of silence among siblings, leaving the parents feeling isolated and excluded. A willingness to maintain each other's privacy often serves as a powerful bond of loyalty that distinguishes the relationship between siblings from that between friends.

More Active Sibling Relationships. Sibling relationships vary among cultures. Some factors may be giving the sibling relationship greater significance in American families than in the past. Shrinking family size, longer life spans, divorce and remarriage, geographic mobility, maternal employment, alternative sources of child care, competitive pressures, stress, and parental insufficiency may be propelling siblings into greater contact and emotional interdependence than ever before. Siblings often join forces to confront the trauma of divorce, and they frequently rely on each other for support when parents remarry. The large number of working mothers means that young siblings today have significant amounts of time when a personally committed adult does not monitor their relationship. Often an older sibling is required to babysit, resulting in children spending more and more time together unsupervised. In a worried, mobile, small-family, high-stress, fast-paced, parent-absent society, children often turn to a brother or sister to meet their needs for contact, constancy, and permanency.

Ordinal Position

Researchers have observed that the birth position of children affects their personalities. Parents treat children differently, and sibling interactions are different, depending on the child's position within the family. Power is unequally distributed among siblings. Older siblings attempt to dominate younger ones. Therefore younger siblings develop interpersonal skills, the ability to negotiate, and an ability to accept unfavorable outcomes to a greater extent than older siblings. Later-born children are obliged to interact with other siblings from birth and seem to be more outgoing and make friends more easily than firstborns. Children vary tremendously, and generalizations do not always apply to the individual. General characteristics of children in the various ordinal positions are presented in Box 3-4.

The Only Child. Being the only child in a family has traditionally been considered a disadvantage. Only children have been described as selfish, spoiled, dependent, and lonely. However, they do not demonstrate more evidence of maladjustment or self-centeredness than other children and tend to strongly resemble firstborn children in respects such as higher educational goals. Only children perform better on cognitive tests, are more mature, are more socially sensitive, and demonstrate superiority in language facility compared with other children.

Only children also enjoy the advantage of having parents who can devote more time to them, talk to them, and stimulate them in intellectual activities. However, parents also exert greater pressure for mature behavior at an early age and for achievement. Relative isolation from peers contributes to intellectual pursuits and encourages a rich fantasy life, independence, and originality.

Multiple Births

A deviation in early development that occurs with variable frequency is multiple births. Twins are not uncommon in the population, but triplets are rare and quadruplets or quintuplets are extremely unusual. In any of these situations, the offspring can be of the like or unlike sex (i.e., derived from a single ovum; from multiple ova; or from a combination of the two, which can involve one or more cell divisions). The cause of twinning is unknown, but the increase in the number of larger multiples (quintuplets, sextuplets) during recent years has been associated with fertility treatments such as ovulation-inducing drugs or in vitro fertilization. Because women in their thirties are almost 2.5 times as likely as women in their

BOX 3-4

Influence of Ordinal Position on Children

FIRSTBORN CHILDREN
Are more achievement oriented
Are more dominant
Receive more physical punishment
Are allowed to show more aggression to siblings
Have stronger consciences; are more self-disciplined and inner directed
Are more socially anxious
Are prone to feelings of guilt
Identify more with parents than with peers
Are more conservative
Are subject to greater parental expectations
Begin to speak earlier in life
Demonstrate higher intellectual achievement
Plan better and experience fewer frustrations
Are likely to be most wanted

MIDDLE CHILDREN
Have more demands made on them for household help
Are praised less often
Receive less of the parents' time
Learn to compromise and be adaptable
Are less stimulated toward achievement
Are more difficult to characterize because of a variety of positions in the family

YOUNGEST CHILDREN
Are less dependent than firstborn children
Are less tense, more affectionate, and more good natured
Tend to identify more with peer group than with parents
Are more flexible in their thinking
Are popular with classmates
Have fewer demands placed on them for household help

ONLY CHILDREN
Have many of the same characteristics as firstborn children
Are more mature and cultivated
Experience greater parental pressure for mature behavior and achievement
Demonstrate superiority in language facility
Rarely develop into stereotype of spoiled, selfish child
Often enjoy a rich fantasy life as a result of isolation

twenties to have higher-order plural births, the rise in the multiple-birth ratio has been associated with increased childbearing among older women and the expanded use of fertility drugs (Hamilton, Minino, Martin, and others, 2007).

Twins are of two distinct types: **identical,** or **monozygotic (MZ),** and **fraternal** (Fig. 3-4), or **dizygotic (DZ)** (Box 3-5). In 2004 in the United States the overall rate of twin birth was 32.2 per 1000 births, a record high (Hamilton, Minino, Martin, and others, 2007); one third are MZ twins, and two thirds are DZ twins.

A special kind of sibling relationship is observed in twins, although getting along with each other and quarreling are not much different from these behaviors in any other two siblings, especially if they are different-sex fraternal twins. Twins tend to work out a relationship that is reasonably satisfactory to both and demonstrate early independence from parental at-

BOX 3-5

Characteristics of Twins

MONOZYGOTIC (MZ) OR IDENTICAL TWINS	DIZYGOTIC (DZ) OR FRATERNAL TWINS
Result of one fertilized ovum that became separated early in development	Result of fertilization of two ova
Alike physically and genetically	Differ physically and genetically
Same sex	May be same or opposite sex
Frequency:	Frequency:
Occurs uniformly in all populations	Varies among races (highest—blacks, lowest—Asians, intermediate—whites)
Unaffected by maternal age	More common with advancing maternal age (maximum at age 35-39, then decreases rapidly)
Tendency unaffected by heredity	Marked familial tendency
	Expressed only in the female
	Fathers appear to transmit disposition toward double ovulation to daughters
Similar behavior	Dissimilar behavior; more sibling rivalry

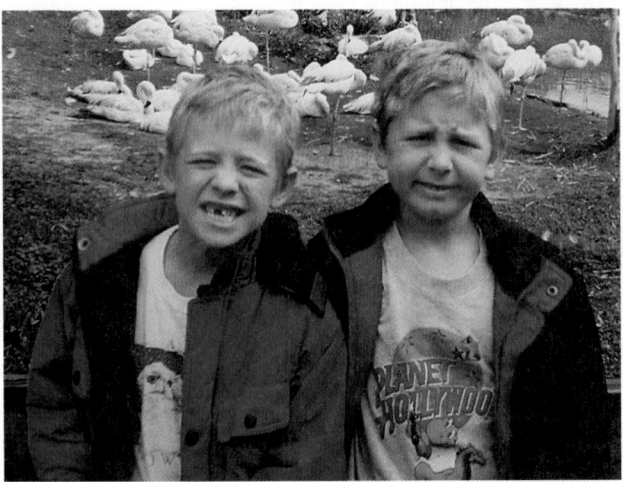

FIG. 3-4 ■ Fraternal twins.

tention. They develop a remarkable capacity for cooperative play and considerable loyalty and generosity toward each other. It is not uncommon for them to evolve a private language between themselves that may interfere with the development of the family language.

In a twinship, one member of the pair, to a greater or lesser extent, is more dominant, outgoing, and assertive than the other, often to the consternation of their parents. However, the seemingly more passive twin is able to accomplish as much and get his or her way as frequently as the more assertive twin.

Researchers have also observed a difference in behavior between identical and fraternal twins. There is near-unison in the actions of identical twins (although they alternate in assuming the leadership), but fraternal twins, even of the same sex, do not display this quality. Sibling rivalry can be pronounced in fraternal twins, especially in different-sex twins.

Identical twins also differ in their response to the tendency of some parents to treat twins exactly alike. The present philosophy is to determine the degree to which the children demonstrate an inclination toward togetherness. Some twins thrive best when they are constantly in each other's company; others prefer more individuality and separateness. The conservative approach is to allow the children to follow their natural inclinations. Early years of togetherness are often the basis of the children's security, and separating them too early may produce unnecessary stresses. Fostering individual differences as they become evident could ease the process of separation when it becomes advisable.

Parental Adjustment. The entrance of any new member into a household creates stress, but with multiple births two or more new members must be incorporated into the family at the same time. The problems are obvious. Two infants must be provided with physical care, including feeding, diapering, and all of the purchasing and preparation that accompanies the care of any infant. Scheduling becomes crucial, and advancement in development brings new problems and adjustments (e.g., space and sleeping arrangements, selection of a stroller and other equipment). Care must be observed in selecting toys. As play becomes a serious business, some toys that would be safe and appropriate for a single child become weapons when two infants share a playpen. It is a good idea to select different toys for each child as they grow older and encourage sharing.

It is especially important for parents to maintain relationships with each other and other family members. It is doubly important for parents to arrange time together as often as possible. The National Organization of Mothers of Twins Clubs, Inc.,* has local chapters throughout the United States to offer information and support to parents of twins and is highly recommended as a resource for all new parents of twins. *Twins Magazine*† is a place to seek and give advice about parenting multiples.

PARENTING

MOTIVATION FOR PARENTHOOD

A dominant characteristic in all societies is that adults are expected to become parents and to be gratified by the experience. Pressures of tradition, sentiment regarding the state of parenthood, and religious beliefs influence decision making

---

*NOMOTC Executive Office, PO Box 700860, Plymouth, MI 48170-0955; http://www.nomotc.org.
†http://www.twinsmagazine.com.

because conformity to social-role expectations is a strong influence in family planning.

Factors that influence family size are social class, religion, race, financial stability, type of conjugal-role relationships, and the social-psychologic aspects of sexual relations. In the case of divorce and remarriage, an individual may decide to have more children with the new spouse.

PREPARATION FOR PARENTHOOD

The basic goals of parenting are to promote the physical survival and health of children, to foster the skills and abilities necessary to be a self-sustaining adult, and to foster behavioral capabilities for optimizing cultural values and beliefs. However, new parents often approach parenthood with limited experience and knowledge. Parents learn by trial and error, committing the same mistakes committed by countless other parents, but they somehow manage to accomplish the task, becoming more skilled with each additional child. Tradition, rather than rational planning, furnishes the chief norms for childrearing. Experience in having been nurtured as a child is an essential component of successful parenting.

Their own parents are probably the only persons whom parents observe intimately in the parental role. This results in a **generational continuity**—parents rear their own children in much the same way as they themselves were reared. Other essential skills that parents need to feel comfortable in the parenting role include a basic understanding of childhood growth and development, bathing, feeding, use of play, and interpersonal communication skills.

TRANSITION TO PARENTHOOD

Although experts disagree as to whether the birth of the first child should be labeled a crisis, the early weeks of an infant's life call for parents to make drastic adjustments. Even though the parents have anticipated and prepared for the child's arrival, the birth presents the challenge of providing total care 24 hours a day for a new member of the family. A crisis may occur if the event is perceived as disturbing old habits and relationships and eliciting new responses. The birth requires role changes or significantly modifies former relationships. In addition to the roles of husband and wife, the couple must assume the roles of father and mother.

The advent of a new family member requires that the family cope with greater financial responsibilities, a possible loss of income, changes in sleeping habits, and less time for the parents to spend with each other (especially if it is a firstborn) and with other children. If these events are perceived as aversive, it can disrupt the couple's bond and reduce the couple's intimacy and affection.

Parental Factors Affecting Transition to Parenthood

No amount of preparation can fully prepare prospective parents for the constant and immediate needs of an infant. The importance of early parent-infant interactions is addressed in the discussion of the neonate, especially the attachment process (see Chapter 8). Factors affecting parenting are the age of the parents, the quality of the parental relationship, the amount of previous experience with childrearing, parental support systems, and the effects of stress on parental behavior.

Parental Age. From a physiologic health perspective, the most satisfactory ages for childbearing are the years between

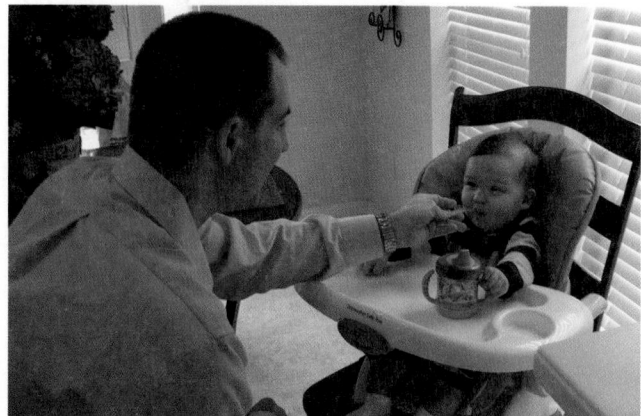

FIG. 3-5 ■ Fathers who assume care of their children may feel more comfortable and successful in their parenting role.

18 and 35. During this time, parents are considered to be in optimum health, with a predicted life span that allows sufficient time and vigor to raise a family. However, the age at which parents begin their families has changed over the past few decades in the United States, with a substantial increase in the birth rate for women 30 to 44 years of age and a decline for women ages 20 to 29 years.

Father Involvement. Current practices that encourage early father-infant interaction indicate that fathers are as intrigued with their newborns as mothers are (see discussion on paternal engrossment under Promote Parent-Infant Bonding [Attachment], Chapter 8). Even fathers who have little initial contact with their newborn become involved with them over the next few months (Fig. 3-5), although the type of interaction is different from that of the mother. For example, mothers are more likely to hold, soothe, care for, or play quietly with their infants, whereas fathers are more boisterous and engage in more physically stimulating activities. However, fathers are more than just playmates. They are often successful at soothing a distressed infant. A secure attachment to the father can help offset the consequences of an insecure attachment to the mother.

Parenting Education. First-time parents who have prepared themselves to be parents experience less stress adjusting to the birth of new baby than those who have not. Programs designed to take place near the time of birth or soon after can be more helpful in easing transitional stress than programs that take place earlier.

Many parents are looking for ways to be a better parent. Nurses can offer a number of suggestions: being an active listener, having an active role in education, keeping up with technology, keeping up with regular visits to the child's health care provider and vaccinations, ensuring safety in and out of the home, spending quality time with the child, and focusing on improving overall family communication (Fig. 3-6).

Other factors influencing the transition to the parental role include the following:

- Parents with previous experience, such as another child, appear to be more relaxed, have less conflict in disciplinary relationships, and are more aware of normal growth and development.
- The amount of stress experienced by one or both parents may interfere with their ability to exhibit patience and understanding and to cope with their children's behavior.

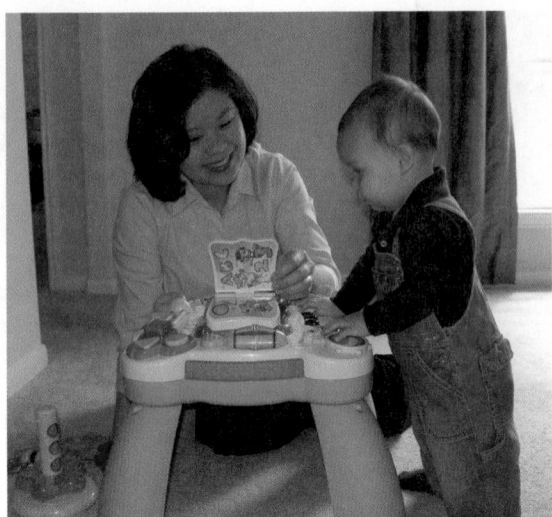

FIG. 3-6 ■ Quality time spent with a child is essential to a family's health and well-being.

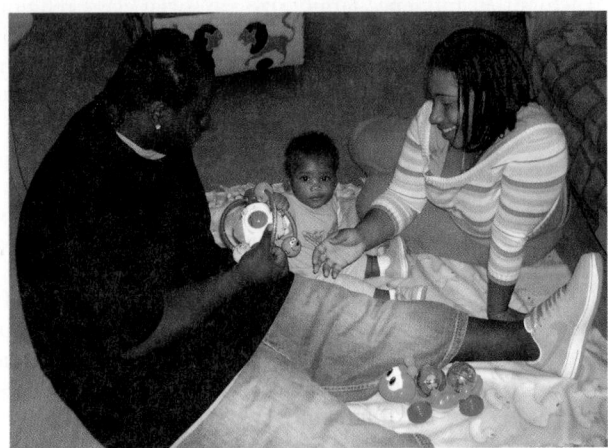

FIG. 3-7 ■ Learning new roles together as a mother and father can enhance parenting relationships.

■ Special characteristics of the infant, such as being temperamentally difficult, can cause the parents to lose confidence and doubt their abilities. Infants with special care needs (such as those associated with a disability) can be a significant source of added stress.

■ Stressed marital relationships can have a negative effect on parental transition because marital tension can alter caregiving routines and interfere with enjoyment of the infant. Conversely, parents' support and encouragement of one another serve as positive influences on establishing a satisfying parental role.

Support Systems. Successful adaptation to the stress of transition to parenthood involves at least two types of family resources (McCubbin and McCubbin, 1994). **Internal resources** such as adaptability and integration are the first type of resource. Changing from an orderly, predictable life to a relatively disordered, unpredictable one is a universal adaptation that families must make. Rigid schedules are impossible to maintain, and former activities must be curtailed or abandoned. **Adaptation** is reflected in learning to be patient, becoming better organized, and becoming more flexible. **Integration** refers to the couple's attempt to continue some activities they engaged in before they became parents. In this way couples are able to maintain a sense of continuity and appreciate the importance of the husband-wife relationship.

The second resource for coping with stress is the use of ***coping strategies*** that strengthen the organization and functioning of the family. These include the use of social support systems and community resources and the adoption of a future orientation. Interpersonal supports that provide information, advice, and caretaking can be derived from friends, relatives, and neighbors. Relationships with family, friends, and community are essential. For parents, positive, supportive work relationships are important. Equally important is time spent with friends. Arranging for time away from the child or children is also beneficial. One parent can assume care of the family to allow the other parent some time to himself or herself. Adoption of a future orientation provides reassurance to parents that things will get better, that they will cope, and that it is realistic to plan for the time when they will be able to engage in self-fulfilling activities.

It is also reassuring to know that others experience ambivalent feelings toward parenthood and share the same difficulties and frustrations. Exchanging ideas and experiences with other parents and each other provides an opportunity to voice concerns and to learn new ways to cope with multiple childrearing problems (Fig. 3-7).

PARENTING BEHAVIORS
Parental Styles of Control
Parenting styles can be described as authoritarian, permissive, or authoritative. **Authoritarian** or **dictatorial** parents try to control their children's behavior and attitudes through unquestioned mandates. They establish rules and regulations or standards of conduct that they expect to be followed rigidly and unquestioningly. They value and reward absolute obedience, mute acceptance of their word, and unfailing respect for the family's principles and beliefs. They forcefully punish any behavior that is contrary to parental standards. Parental authority is exercised with little explanation and little involvement of the child in decision making. The message is: "Do it because I say so."

Punishment need not be corporal but may be stern withdrawal of love and approval. Careful training often results in rigidly conforming behavior in the children, who tend to be sensitive, shy, self-conscious, retiring, and submissive. They are more apt to be courteous, loyal, honest, and dependable but docile. These behaviors are more typically observed when close supervision and affection accompany parental authority. If not, this style of parenting may be associated with both defiant and antisocial behavior.

Permissive or **laissez-faire** parents exert little or no control over their children's actions. They avoid imposing their own standards of conduct and allow their children to regulate their own activity as much as possible. These parents consider themselves to be resources for the children, not role models. If rules do exist, the parents explain the underlying reason, elicit the children's opinions, and consult them in decision-making processes. They employ lax, inconsistent discipline; do not set sensible limits; and do not prevent the children from upsetting the home routine. These parents rarely punish the children. Consequently, the children control the parents and are often disobedient, disrespectful, and generally defiant of authority.

Authoritative or **democratic** parents combine practices from both of the previously described parenting styles. They direct their children's behavior and attitudes by emphasizing the reason for rules and negatively reinforcing deviations. They respect the individuality of each child and allow the child to voice objections to family standards or regulations. Parental control is firm and consistent but tempered with encouragement, understanding, and security. Control is focused on the issue, not on withdrawal of love or the fear of punishment. These parents foster "inner-directedness," a conscience that regulates behavior based on feelings of guilt or shame for wrongdoing, not on fear of being caught or punished. Parents' realistic standards and reasonable expectations produce children with high self-esteem who are self-reliant, assertive, inquisitive, content, and highly interactive with other children.

There are differing philosophies in regard to parenting. Childrearing is a culturally bound phenomenon, and children are socialized to behave in ways that are important to their family. In the authoritative style, authority is shared and children are included in discussions, fostering an independent and assertive style of participation in family life. When working with individual families, nurses should give these differing styles equal respect.

LIMIT SETTING AND DISCIPLINE

In its broadest sense, **discipline** means *to teach* or refers to a set of rules governing conduct. In a narrower sense, it refers to the action taken to enforce the rules after noncompliance. **Limit setting** refers to establishing the rules or guidelines for behavior. For example, parents can place limits on the amount of time children spend watching television or chatting online. The clearer the limits that are set and the more consistently they are enforced, the less need there is for disciplinary action.

Nurses can help parents establish realistic and concrete "rules." Limit setting and discipline are positive, necessary components of childrearing and serve several useful functions as they help children:

- Test their limits of control
- Achieve in areas appropriate for mastery at their level
- Channel undesirable feelings into constructive activity
- Protect themselves from danger
- Learn socially acceptable behavior

Children want and need limits. Unrestricted freedom is a threat to their security and safety. Through testing the limits imposed on them, children learn the extent to which they can manipulate their environment and gain reassurance from knowing that others are there to protect them from potential harm.

Minimizing Misbehavior

The reasons for misbehavior may include attention, power, defiance, and a display of inadequacy (e.g., the child misses classes because of a fear that he or she is unable to do the work). Children may also misbehave because the rules are not clear or consistently applied. Acting out behavior, such as a temper tantrum, may represent uncontrolled frustration, anger, depression, or pain. The best approach is to structure in-

FAMILY-CENTERED CARE

Minimizing Misbehavior

- Set realistic goals for acceptable behavior and expected achievements.
- Structure opportunities for small successes to lessen feelings of inadequacy.
- Praise children for desirable behavior with attention and verbal approval.
- Structure the environment to prevent unnecessary difficulties (e.g., place fragile objects in inaccessible area).
- Set clear and reasonable rules; expect the same behavior regardless of the circumstances; if exceptions are made, clarify that the change is for one time only.
- Teach desirable behavior through own example, such as using a quiet, calm voice rather than screaming.
- Review expected behavior before special or unusual events, such as visiting a relative or having dinner in a restaurant.
- Phrase requests for appropriate behavior positively, such as "Put the book down," rather than "Don't touch the book."
- Call attention to unacceptable behavior as soon as it begins; use distraction to change the behavior or offer alternatives to annoying actions, such as a quiet toy for one that is excessively noisy.
- Give advance notice or "friendly reminders," such as "When the TV program is over, it is time for dinner" or "I'll give you to the count of three and then we have to go."
- Be attentive to situations that increase the likelihood of misbehaving, such as overexcitement or fatigue, or decreased personal tolerance to minor infractions.
- Offer sympathetic explanations for not granting a request, such as "I am sorry I can't read you a story now, but I have to finish dinner. Then we can spend time together."
- Keep any promises made to children.
- Avoid outright conflicts; temper discussions with statements such as "Let's talk about it and see what we can decide together" or "I have to think about it first."
- Provide children with opportunities for power and control.

teractions with children so that unacceptable behavior is prevented or minimized (see Family-Centered Care box).

General Guidelines for Implementing Discipline

Regardless of the type of discipline used, certain principles are essential to ensure the efficacy of the approach (see Family-Centered Care box). Many strategies, such as behavior modification, can only be implemented effectively when principles of consistency and timing are followed. A pattern of intermittent or occasional enforcement of limits actually prolongs the undesired behavior because children learn that if they are persistent, the behavior is permitted eventually. Delaying punishment weakens its intent, and practices such as telling the child, "Wait until your father comes home," are not only ineffectual, but also convey negative messages about the other parent.*

Types of Discipline

To deal with misbehavior, parents need to implement appropriate disciplinary action. Many approaches are available. **Reasoning** involves explaining why an act is wrong and is usu-

*For parenting of kindergarten through sixth grade children, see http://child parenting.about.com and http://www.kidshealth.org.

Implementing Discipline

Consistency—Implement disciplinary action exactly as agreed on and for each infraction.

Timing—Initiate discipline as soon as child misbehaves; if delays are necessary, such as to avoid embarrassment, verbally disapprove of the behavior and state that disciplinary action will be implemented.

Commitment—Follow through with the details of the discipline, such as timing of minutes; avoid distractions that may interfere with the plan, such as telephone calls.

Unity—Make certain that all caregivers agree on the plan and are familiar with the details to prevent confusion and alliances between child and one parent.

Flexibility—Choose disciplinary strategies that are appropriate to child's age and temperament and the severity of the misbehavior.

Planning—Plan disciplinary strategies in advance and prepare child if feasible (e.g., explain use of time-out); for unexpected misbehavior, try to discipline when you are calm.

Behavior orientation—Always disapprove of the behavior, not the child, with such statements as "That was a wrong thing to do. I am unhappy when I see behavior like that."

Privacy—Administer discipline in private, especially with older children, who may feel ashamed in front of others.

Termination—After the discipline is administered, consider child as having a "clean slate," and avoid bringing up the incident or lecturing.

ally appropriate for older children, especially when moral issues are involved. However, young children cannot be expected to "see the other side" because of their egocentrism. Children in the preoperative stage of cognitive development (toddlers and preschoolers) have a limited ability to distinguish between their point of view and those of others. Sometimes children use "reasoning" as a way of gaining attention. For example, they may misbehave thinking the parents will give them a lengthy explanation of the wrongdoing and knowing that negative attention is better than no attention. When children use this technique, parents should end the explanation by stating, "This is the rule, and this is how I expect you to behave. I won't explain it any further."

Unfortunately, reasoning is often combined with **scolding,** which sometimes takes the form of shame or criticism. For example, the parent may state, "You are a bad boy for hitting your brother." Children take such remarks seriously and personally, believing that they *are* bad.

NURSINGALERT

When reprimanding children, focus only on the misbehavior, not on the child. Use of "I" messages rather than "you" messages expresses personal feelings without accusation or ridicule. For example, an "I" message attacks the behavior—"I am upset when Johnny is punched; I don't like to see him hurt"—not the child.

Positive and negative reinforcement is the basis of **behavior modification** theory—behavior that is rewarded will be repeated; behavior that is not rewarded will be extinguished. Using **rewards** is a positive approach. By encouraging children to behave in specified ways, the parents can decrease the ten-

dency to misbehave. With young children, using paper stars is an effective method. For older children, the "token system" is appropriate, especially if a certain number of stars or tokens yields a special reward, such as a trip to the movies or a new book. In planning a reward system, the parents must explain expected behaviors to the child and establish rewards that are reinforcing. A chart should be used to record the stars or tokens, and an earned reward should be given promptly. Verbal approval should always accompany extrinsic rewards.

Consistently **ignoring** behavior will eventually extinguish or minimize the act. Although this approach sounds simple, it is often difficult to implement consistently. Parents frequently "give in" and resort to previous patterns of discipline. Consequently, the behavior is actually reinforced because the child learns that persistence gains parental attention. For ignoring to be effective, parents should (1) understand the process, (2) record the undesired behavior before using ignoring to determine whether a problem exists and to compare results after ignoring is begun, (3) determine whether parental attention acts as a reinforcer, and (4) be aware of "response burst." Response burst is a phenomenon that occurs when the undesired behavior increases after ignoring is initiated because the child is "testing" the parents to see if they are serious about the plan.

The strategy of **consequences** involves allowing children to experience the results of their misbehavior. It includes three types:

Natural—Those that occur without any intervention, such as being late and missing dinner

Logical—Those that are directly related to the rule, such as not being allowed to play with another toy until the used ones are put away

Unrelated—Those that are imposed deliberately, such as no playing until homework is completed or the use of time-out

Natural or logical consequences are preferred and effective if they are meaningful to children. For example, the natural consequence of living in a messy room may do little to encourage cleaning up, but allowing no friends over until the room is neat can be motivating! Withdrawing privileges is often an unrelated consequence. After the child experiences the consequence, the parent should refrain from any comment, because the usual tendency is for the child to try to place blame for imposing the rule.

Time-out is actually a refinement of the common practice of "sending the child to his or her room" and is a type of unrelated consequence. It is based on the premise of removing the reinforcer (i.e., the satisfaction or attention the child is receiving from the activity). When placed in an unstimulating and isolated place, children become bored and consequently agree to behave in order to reenter the family group (Fig. 3-8). Time-out avoids many of the problems of other disciplinary approaches. No physical punishment is involved; no reasoning or scolding is given; and the parent does not need to be present for all of the time-out, thus facilitating his or her ability to consistently apply this type of discipline. Time-out offers both the child and the parent a "cooling off" time. To be effective, however, time-out must be planned in advance (see Family-Centered Care box).

Corporal or **physical punishment** most often takes the form of spanking. Based on the principles of aversive therapy,

FIG. 3-8 ■ Time-out is an excellent disciplinary strategy for young children.

inflicting pain through spanking causes a dramatic short-term decrease in the behavior. However, there are serious flaws in this approach: (1) it teaches children that violence is acceptable; (2) it may physically harm the child if it is the result of parental rage; and (3) children become "accustomed" to spanking, requiring more severe corporal punishment each time. Spanking can result in severe physical and psychologic injury, and it interferes with effective parent-child interaction. In addition, when the parent is not around, the misbehavior is likely to occur, since children have not learned to behave well for their own sake. Parental use of corporal punishment may also interfere with the child's development of moral reasoning.

SPECIAL PARENTING SITUATIONS

Parenting is a demanding task under the most ideal circumstances, but when parents and children are faced with situations that deviate from what is considered the norm, the potential for family disruption is increased. Situations that are encountered frequently are divorce, single parenthood, blended families, adoption, and dual-career families. In addition, as cultural diversity increases in our communities, many immigrants are making the transition to parenthood and a new country, culture, and language simultaneously. Other situations that create unique parenting challenges are parental alcoholism, homelessness, and incarceration. Although these topics are not addressed here, the reader may wish to investigate them further.

PARENTING THE ADOPTED CHILD

Adoption establishes a legal relationship between a child and parents who are not related by birth, but who have the same rights and obligations that exist between children and their biologic parents. In the past the biologic mother alone made the decision to relinquish the rights to her child. In recent years the courts have acknowledged the legal rights of the biologic father regarding this decision. Concerned child advocates have questioned whether decisions that honor the father's rights are in the best interests of the child. As the rights of the child have become recognized, older children have successfully dissolved their legal bond with their biologic parents to pursue adoption by adults of their choice. Furthermore, there is a growing interest and demand within the gay and lesbian community to adopt.

Unlike biologic parents, who prepare for their child's birth with prenatal classes and the support of friends and relatives, adoptive parents have few sources of support and preparation for the new addition to their family. Nurses can provide the information, support, and reassurance needed to reduce parental anxiety regarding the adoptive process and refer adoptive parents to state parental support groups. Such sources can be contacted through a state or county welfare office.

Most problems faced by adoptive parents are not different from those encountered by natural parents, but the desire to be a good parent is often intensified in adoptive parents. Adoptive parents have been portrayed as more apprehensive, insecure, and in need of more assistance than biologic parents. However, some adoptive parents may actually need less assistance than biologic parents. This situation may be related to the adoptive parents' completely voluntary decision to become parents, the relatively long time they have to prepare for parenting, and the maturity associated with adopting.

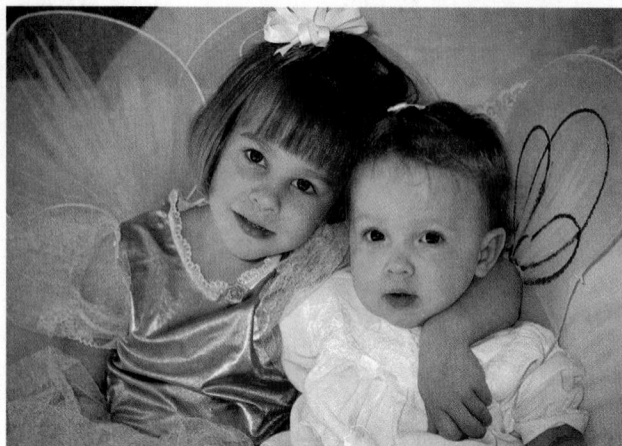

FIG. 3-9 ▪ An older sister lovingly embraces her adopted sister.

Parenting the Adopted Child

Twelve-month-old Justin was adopted at birth. His parents tell you that they wonder when they should tell Justin that he is adopted. As the nurse, what counseling and advice should you give Justin's parents?

QUESTIONS
1. Evidence—Is there sufficient information to draw any conclusions about this situation?
2. Assumptions—Describe some underlying assumptions about the following:
   a. The best time to tell children that they are adopted
   b. The manner in which parents should tell their child about adoption
   c. Children's reactions to being told they are adopted
3. What implications for nursing care can be drawn at this time?
4. Does the evidence support your conclusion?
5. Are there alternative perspectives to consider?

The sooner infants enter their adoptive home, the better the chances of parent-infant attachment. However, the more caregivers the infant has had before adoption, the greater the risk for attachment problems. The infant must break the bond with the previous caregiver and form a new bond with the adoptive parents. Difficulties in forming an attachment depend on the amount of time the infant has spent with earlier caregivers (e.g., the birth mother, nurse, adoption agency personnel).

Siblings, adopted or biologic, who are old enough to understand should be included in decisions regarding the commitment to adopt, with reassurance that they are not being replaced. Ways that the siblings can interact with the adopted child should be stressed (Fig. 3-9).

Issues of Origin

The task of telling children that they are adopted can be a cause of deep concern and anxiety. There are no clear-cut guidelines for parents to follow in determining when and at what age children are ready for the information. Parents are naturally reluctant to present the children with such potentially unsettling news. However, it is important that parents not withhold the adoption from the child, since it is an essential component of the child's identity (see Critical Thinking Exercise).

The timing arises naturally, as parents become aware of the child's readiness. Most authorities believe that children should be informed at an age young enough so that, as they grow older, they do not remember a time when they did not know they were adopted. The time is highly individual, but must be right for both the parents and the child. It may be when children ask where babies come from, at which time children can also be told the facts of their adoption. If they are told in a way that conveys the idea that they were active participants in the selection process, they will be less likely to feel that they were abandoned victims in a helpless situation. For example, parents can tell children that their personal qualities drew the parents to them. It is wise for parents who have not previously discussed adoption to tell children that they are adopted before the children enter school to avoid third parties inadvertently telling the children before the parents have had the opportunity to do so. Complete honesty between parents and children strengthens the relationship.

Parents should anticipate behavior changes after the disclosure, especially in older children. Children who are struggling with the revelation that they are adopted may benefit from individual and family counseling. Children may use the fact of their adoption as a weapon to manipulate and threaten parents. Statements such as "My real mother would not treat me like this" or "You don't love me as much because I'm adopted" hurt parents and increase their feelings of insecurity. Such statements may also cause parents to become overpermissive. Adopted children need the same undemanding love, combined with firm discipline and limit setting, as any other child.

Adolescence

Adolescence may be an especially trying time for parents of adopted children. The normal confrontations of adolescents and parents assume more painful aspects in adoptive families. Adolescents may use their adoption to defy parental authority or as a justification for aberrant behavior. As they attempt to master the task of identity formation, the feeling of abandonment by their biologic parents comes into awareness and may be intensified. Gender differences in reacting to adoption may surface.

Adopted children fantasize about their biologic parents and may feel the need to discover their parents' identity to define themselves and their own identity. It is important for parents to keep the lines of communication open and to reassure their child that they understand the need to search for their identity. In some states, birth certificates are made legally available to adopted children when they come of age. It is important for parents to be honest with questioning adolescents and to tell them of this possibility (the parents themselves are unable to obtain the birth certificate; it is the children's responsibility if they desire it).

Cross-Racial and International Adoption

Adoption of children from racial backgrounds different from that of the family is commonplace. In addition to the problems faced by adopted children in general, children of a cross-racial adoption must deal with physical and sometimes cultural differences. It is advised that parents who adopt such children do everything to preserve the adopted children's racial heritage.

> **NURSINGALERT**
>
> As a health care provider, it is important not to ask the wrong questions, such as "Is she yours, or is she adopted?" "What do you know about the 'real' mother?" "Do they have the same father?" or "How much did it cost to adopt him?"

Although the children are full-fledged members of an adopting family and citizens of the adopted country, if they have a strikingly different appearance from other family members or exhibit distinct racial or ethnic characteristics, challenges may be encountered outside the family. Bigotry may appear among relatives and friends. Strangers may make thoughtless comments and talk about the children as though they were not members of the family. It is vital that family members declare to others that this is their child and a cherished member of the family.

In international adoptions the medical information the parents receive may be incomplete or sketchy; weight, height, and head circumference are often the only objective information present in the child's medical record. Many internationally adopted children were born preterm, and common health problems such as infant diarrhea and malnutrition delay growth and development. Some children have serious or multiple health problems that can be very stressful for the parents.

PARENTING AND DIVORCE

Since the mid-1960s, a marked change in the stability of families has been reflected in increased rates of divorce, single parenthood, and remarriage. In 2005 the divorce rate for the United States was 3.8 per 1000 total population (Munson and Sutton, 2006). The divorce rate has changed little since 1987. In the previous decade, the rate increased yearly, with a peak in 1979. Although almost half of all divorcing couples are childless, it is estimated that more than 1 million children experience divorce each year.

The process of divorce begins with a period of marital conflict of varying length and intensity, followed by a separation, the actual legal divorce, and the reestablishment of different living arrangements (Box 3-6). Because a function of parenthood is to provide for the security and emotional welfare of children, disruption of the family structure often engenders strong feelings of guilt in the divorcing parents.

During a divorce, parents' coping abilities may be compromised. The parents may be preoccupied with their own feelings, needs, and life changes and unable to be available and supportive to their children. Newly employed parents, usually mothers, are likely to leave children with new caregivers, in strange settings, or alone after school. The parent may also spend more time away from home, searching for or establishing new relationships. Sometimes, however, the adult feels frightened and alone and begins to depend on the child as a substitute for the absent parent. This dependence places an enormous burden on the child.

Common characteristics in the custodial household after separation and divorce include disorder, coercive types of control, inflammable tempers in both parents and children,

---

> **BOX 3-6**
> **Stages of the Divorce Process**
>
> **ACUTE PHASE**
> The married couple makes the decision to separate.
> This phase includes the legal steps of filing for dissolution of the marriage and, usually, the departure of the father from the home.
> This phase lasts from several months to more than a year and is accompanied by familial stress and a chaotic atmosphere.
>
> **TRANSITIONAL PHASE**
> The adults and children assume unfamiliar roles and relationships within a new family structure.
> This phase is often accompanied by a change of residence, a reduced standard of living and altered lifestyle, a larger share of the economic responsibility being shouldered by the mother, and radically altered parent-child relationships.
>
> **STABILIZING PHASE**
> The postdivorce family reestablishes a stable, functioning family unit. Remarriage frequently occurs, with concomitant changes in all areas of family life.

Modified from Wallerstein JS: Children of divorce: stress and developmental tasks. In Garmezy N, Rutter M, editors: *Stress, coping, and development in children,* New York, 1983, McGraw-Hill.

reduced parental competence, a greater sense of parental helplessness, poorly enforced discipline, and diminished regularity in enforcing household routines. Noncustodial parents are seldom prepared for the role of visitor, may assume the role of recreational and "fun" parent, and may not have a residence suitable for children's visits. They may also be concerned about maintaining the arrangement over the years to follow.

Impact of Divorce on Children

Numerous studies indicate that divorce has a profound effect on children. Many youngsters suffer for years from psychologic and social difficulties associated with continuing or new stresses in the postdivorce family. Even when a divorce is amicable and open, children recall parental separation with the same emotions felt by victims of a natural disaster: loss, grief, and vulnerability to forces beyond their control.

The impact of divorce on children depends on several factors, including the age and sex of the children, the outcome of the divorce, and the quality of the parent-child relationship and parental care during the years following the divorce. Family characteristics are more crucial to the child's well-being than specific child characteristics, such as age or sex. High levels of ongoing family conflict are related to problems of social development, emotional stability, and cognitive skills for the child.

Complications associated with divorce include efforts on the part of one parent to subvert the child's loyalties to the other, abandonment to other caregivers, and adjustment to a stepparent. A major problem occurs when children are "caught in the middle" between the divorced parents. They become the message bearer between the parents, are often quizzed about the activities of the other parent, and have to listen to one parent criticize the other. A nurse may be able to intercede by helping the child get out of the middle by stating "I messages" based on the formula of "I feel … (state the feeling) when you … (state the source). I would like it if you …." This approach

BOX 3-7
Feelings and Behaviors of Children Related to Divorce

INFANCY
Effects of reduced mothering or lack of mothering
Increased irritability
Disturbance in eating, sleeping, and elimination
Interference with attachment process

EARLY PRESCHOOL CHILDREN (AGES 2 TO 3 YEARS)
Frightened and confused
Blame themselves for the divorce
Fear of abandonment
Increased irritability, whining, tantrums
Regressive behaviors (e.g., thumb sucking, loss of elimination control)
Separation anxiety

LATER PRESCHOOL CHILDREN (AGES 3 TO 5 YEARS)
Fear of abandonment
Blame themselves for the divorce; decreased self-esteem
Bewilderment regarding all human relationships
Become more aggressive in relationships with others (e.g., siblings, peers)
Engage in fantasy to seek understanding of the divorce

EARLY SCHOOL-AGE CHILDREN (AGES 5 TO 6 YEARS)
Depression and immature behavior
Loss of appetite and sleep disorders
May be able to verbalize some feelings and understand some divorce-related changes
Increased anxiety and aggression
Feelings of abandonment by departing parent

MIDDLE SCHOOL-AGE CHILDREN (AGES 6 TO 8 YEARS)
Panic reactions
Feelings of deprivation—loss of parent, attention, money, and secure future
Profound sadness, depression, fear, and insecurity
Feelings of abandonment and rejection

Fear regarding the future
Difficulty expressing anger at parents
Intense desire for reconciliation of parents
Impaired capacity to play and enjoy outside activities
Decline in school performance
Altered peer relationships—become bossy, irritable, demanding, and manipulative
Frequent crying, loss of appetite, sleep disorders
Disturbed routine, forgetfulness

LATER SCHOOL-AGE CHILDREN (AGES 9 TO 12 YEARS)
More realistic understanding of divorce
Intense anger directed at one or both parents
Divided loyalties
Ability to express feelings of anger
Ashamed of parental behavior
Desire for revenge; may wish to punish the parent they hold responsible
Feelings of loneliness, rejection, and abandonment
Altered peer relationships
Decline in school performance
May develop somatic complaints
May engage in aberrant behavior such as lying, stealing
Temper tantrums
Dictatorial attitude

ADOLESCENTS (AGES 12 TO 18 YEARS)
Able to disengage themselves from parental conflict
Feelings of a profound sense of loss—of family, childhood
Feelings of anxiety
Worry about themselves, parents, siblings
Expression of anger, sadness, shame, embarrassment
May withdraw from family and friends
Disturbed concept of sexuality
May engage in acting-out behaviors

empowers the child to feel in control. An example of an "I message" is: "I do not feel comfortable when you ask me questions about mom; maybe you could ask her yourself."

Feelings of children toward divorce vary with age (Box 3-7). Some children feel a sense of shame and embarrassment concerning the family situation. Some feelings cause children to see themselves as different, inferior, or unworthy of love, especially if they feel responsible for the family dissolution. Although the social stigma attached to divorce no longer produces the emotions it did in the past, such feelings may still exist in small towns or in some cultural groups and can reinforce children's negative self-image. The lasting effects of divorce depend on the children's and the parents' adjustment to the transition from an intact family to a single-parent family and, often, to a reconstituted family.

Although most studies have concentrated on the negative effects of divorce on youngsters, some positive outcomes of divorce have been reported. A successful postdivorce family, either a single-parent or a reconstituted family, can improve the quality of life for both adults and children. If conflict is resolved, a better relationship with one or both parents may result, and some children may have less contact with a dis-

turbed parent. Greater stability in the home setting and the removal of arguing parents can be a positive outcome for the child's long term well-being.

Age- and Sex-Related Responses to Divorce. Previously, it was believed that divorce had a greater impact on younger children, but recent observations indicate that divorce constitutes a major disruption for children of all ages. The feelings and behaviors of children may be different for various ages and gender, but all children suffer stress second only to the stress produced by the death of a parent. Although considerable research has looked at sex differences in children's adjustments to divorce, the findings are not conclusive.

Telling the Children. Parents are understandably hesitant to tell children about their decision to divorce. Most parents neglect to discuss either the divorce or its inevitable changes with their preschool child. Without preparation, even children who remain in the family home are confused by the parental separation. Frequently, children are already experiencing vague, uneasy feelings that are more difficult to cope with than being told the truth about the situation. If possible, the initial disclosure should include both parents and siblings, followed by individual discussions with each child. Sufficient time should be set aside for these discussions, and they should take place during a period of calm, not after an argument. Parents who physically hold or touch their children provide them with a feeling of warmth and reassurance. The discussions should include the reason for the divorce (if age appropriate) and reassurance that the divorce is not the fault of the children.

Parents should not fear crying in front of the children, because their crying gives the children permission to cry also. Children need to ventilate their feelings. Children may feel guilt, a sense of failure, or that they are being punished for misbehavior. They normally feel anger and resentment and should be allowed to communicate these feelings without punishment. They also have feelings of terror and abandonment. They need consistency and order in their lives. They want to know where they will live, who will take care of them, if they will be with their siblings, and if there will be enough money to live on. Children fear that if their parents stopped loving each other, they could stop loving them. Their need for love and reassurance is tremendous at this time. Children may also wonder what will happen on special days such as birthdays and holidays, whether both parents will come to school events, and whether the child will still have the same friends.

Custody and Parenting Partnerships

In the past, when parents separated, the mother was given custody of the children with visitation agreements for the father. Now both parents and the courts are seeking alternatives. Current belief is that neither fathers nor mothers should be awarded custody automatically. Custody should be awarded to the parent who is best able to provide for the children's welfare. In some cases, children experience severe stress when living or spending time with a parent. Many fathers have demonstrated both their competence and their commitment to care for their children.

Often overlooked are the changes that may occur in the children's relationships with other relatives, especially grandparents. Grandparents on the noncustodial side are often kept from their grandchildren, whereas those on the custodial side may be overwhelmed by their adult child's return to the household with grandchildren.

Two other types of custody arrangements are divided custody and joint custody. **Divided, or split, custody** means that each parent is awarded custody of one or more of the children, thereby separating siblings. For example, sons might live with the father and daughters with the mother.

Joint custody takes one of two forms. In **joint physical custody,** the parents alternate the physical care and control of the children on an equitable basis while maintaining shared parenting responsibilities legally. This custody arrangement works well for families who live close to each other and whose occupations permit an active role in the care and rearing of the children. In **joint legal custody,** the children reside with one parent but both parents are the children's legal guardians, and both participate in childrearing.

Co-parenting offers substantial benefits for the family: children can be close to both parents, and life with each parent can be more normal (as opposed to having a disciplinarian mother and a recreational father). To be successful, parents in these arrangements must place high value on the commitment to provide normal parenting and to separate their marital conflicts from their parenting roles. No matter what type

of custody arrangement is awarded, the primary consideration is the welfare of the children.

SINGLE PARENTING

An individual may acquire single-parent status as a result of divorce, separation, death of a spouse, or birth or adoption of a child. Although divorce rates have stabilized, the number of single-parent households continues to rise. In 2005, 32% of children younger than 18 years of age lived in single-parent families, and the majority of single parents are women (US Census Bureau, 2003; Annie E Casey Foundation, 2007). It is estimated that at least half of the children born during the 1990s will spend part of their life in a family headed by a divorced, separated, widowed, or never-married mother. Although some women are single parents by choice, most of these women never planned on being single parents, and many feel pressure to marry or remarry.

Managing shortages of money, time, and energy are major concerns for single parents. Studies repeatedly confirm the financial difficulties of single-parent families, particularly in the case of single mothers. In 2004 only one third of mother-headed households received any child support or alimony (Annie E Casey Foundation, 2007). In fact, the stigma of poverty may be more keenly felt than the discrimination associated with being a single parent. These families are often forced by their financial status to live in communities with inadequate housing and personal safety concerns. Single parents often feel guilty about the time spent away from their children. Divorced mothers, from marriages in which the father assumed the role of breadwinner and the mother the household maintenance and parenting roles, have considerable difficulty adjusting to their new role of breadwinner. Many single parents have trouble arranging for adequate child care, particularly care for a sick child.

Being a teenage parent adds to the financial burden of being a single parent and can have long-term consequences for the mother and child. Poverty is a well-known predictor of adverse effects on a child's health and well-being. Approximately 78% of children born to a teenage mother who did not marry or graduate high school live in poverty. In contrast, only 9% of children born to women over 20 who marry and finish high school live in poverty (Annie E Casey Foundation, 2007).

Social supports and community resources needed by single-parent families include health care services that are open on evenings and weekends; high-quality child care; respite child care to relieve parental exhaustion and prevent burnout; and parent enhancement centers for advancing education and job skills, providing recreational activities, and offering parenting education. Single parents need social contacts separate from their children for their own emotional growth and that of their children. Parents Without Partners, Inc.,* is an organization designed to meet the needs of single parents.

Single Fathers

Fathers who have custody of their children have many of the same problems as divorced mothers. They feel overburdened by the responsibility, depressed, and concerned about their ability to cope with the emotional needs of the children, espe-

*1650 South Dixie Hwy., Suite 510, Boca Raton, FL 33432; (800) 637-7974; http://parentswithoutpartners.org.

cially girls. Some fathers lack home-making skills. They find it difficult at first to coordinate household tasks, school visits, and other activities associated with managing a household alone. Fathers often demand more assistance with household tasks and more independence from their children than custodial mothers do, and they are likely to make use of alternative caregiving and support systems.

PARENTING IN RECONSTITUTED FAMILIES

In the United States, many of the children living in homes where parents have divorced will experience another major change in their lives such as the addition of a stepparent or new siblings. The entry of a stepparent into a ready-made family requires adjustments for all family members. Some obstacles to the role adjustments and family problem solving include disruption of previous lifestyles and interaction patterns, complexity in the formation of new ones, and lack of social supports. Despite these problems, most children from divorced families want to live in a two-parent home.

Cooperative parenting relationships can allow more time for each set of parents to be alone to establish their own relationship with the children. Under ideal circumstances, power conflicts between the two households can be reduced, and tension and anxiety can be lessened for all family members. In addition, the children's self-esteem can be increased, and there is a greater likelihood of continued contact with grandparents. Flexibility, mutual support, and open communication are critical in successful relationships in stepfamilies and stepparenting situations. Unfortunately, stepfamilies usually do not seek help to prevent problems. Typically, information and counseling are sought only when problems have surfaced and can no longer be ignored. A preventive rather than remedial approach is needed.

PARENTING IN DUAL-EARNER FAMILIES

No change in family lifestyle has had more impact than the large numbers of women entering the workplace. As women moved away from the traditional homemaker role, the numbers of dual-earner families increased dramatically. This trend is unlikely to diminish significantly. As a result, the family is subjected to considerable stress as members attempt to meet the challenge of the often competing demands of occupational needs and those regarded as necessary for a rich family life.

Role definitions are frequently altered to arrange an equitable division of time and labor, as well as to resolve conflict, especially conflict related to the traditional norms of the culture. Overload is a common source of stress in a dual-earner family, and social activities are significantly curtailed. Time demands and scheduling are major problems for all individuals who work. When the individuals are parents, the demands can be even more intense. Dual-earner couples may increase the strain on themselves to avoid creating stress for their children. Although there is no evidence to indicate that the dual-earner lifestyle is stressful to children, the stress experienced by the parents may affect the children indirectly.

Working Mothers

Working mothers have become the norm in the United States. Child care is critical to the working mother's sense of well-being. The quality of child care is a persistent concern for all working parents (see Evidence-Based Practice box).

Determinants of child care quality are based on health and safety requirements, responsive and warm interaction between staff and children, developmentally appropriate activities, trained staff, limited group size, age-appropriate caregivers, adequate staff-to-child ratios, and adequate indoor and outdoor space. Nurses play an important role in helping families to find suitable sources of child care and to prepare children for this experience (see Alternate Child Care Arrangements, Chapter 10).

FOSTER PARENTING

The term **foster care** is defined as placement in an approved living situation away from the family of origin. The living situation may be an approved foster home, possibly with other children, or a preadoptive home. Each state provides a standard for the role of foster parent and a process by which to become one. These "parents" contract with the state to provide a home for children for a limited duration. Most states require about 27 hours of training before being on contract and at least 12 hours of continuing education a year. Foster parents may be required to attend a foster parent support group that is often separate from a state agency. Each state has guidelines regarding the relative health of the prospective foster parents and their families, background checks regarding legal issues for the adults, personal interviews, and a safety inspection of the residence and surroundings.

Foster homes include both kinship and nonrelative placements. Since the 1980s, the proportion of children in out-of-home care placed with relatives has increased rapidly and been accompanied by a decrease in the number of foster families. As with their nonfoster counterparts, much of the child's adjustment depends on the family's stability and available resources. Even though foster homes are designed to provide short-term care, it is not unusual for children to stay for many years.

Nurses should be aware that nearly 700,000 children will spend time living in foster care in a given year, many of them facing developmental concerns (Annie E Casey Foundation, 2007; American Academy of Pediatrics, 2000). Children in foster care tend to have a higher than normal incidence of acute and chronic health problems and may experience feelings of isolation or confusion (Annie E Casey Foundation, 2007). Foster children are often at risk because of their previous caretaking environment. Nurses should strive to implement strategies that will improve the health care for this group of children. In particular, assessment and case management skills are required to involve other disciplines to meet their needs.

ACCOMMODATING CONTEMPORARY PARENTING SITUATIONS

During recent years, both the private and government sectors have identified specific problems of contemporary families. Many of these issues involve working parents. One significant stressor for the working single parent or for dual-earner families is when a child becomes ill. The frequency of childhood illness, exclusion practices of most licensed child care programs, and employer's limited sick-leave policies are other contributing factors. Most authorities agree that a familiar face and place are important components of sick-child care, and some argue that the only place for an ill child is at home with a parent or other relative.

EVIDENCE-BASED PRACTICE

Daycare for Preschool Children

ASK THE QUESTION   Does daycare have an effect on preschool education, health, and welfare?

SEARCH FOR EVIDENCE

Search Strategies   Randomized controlled trials of daycare for preschool children were identified using electronic databases, hand searches of relevant literature, and contact with authors.

Databases Used   MEDLINE, EMBASE, Cochrane Controlled Trials Register, Social Science Citation Index, PsycLIT, Eric, and BIRD (French)

CRITICALLY ANALYZE THE EVIDENCE

Seven randomized control trials and one quasi-randomized study were identified after examining 920 abstracts and 19 books (Zortich, Roberts, and Oakley, 2005). All of the eight studies were conducted in the United States. In these eight studies, a total of 2203 children were randomized to daycare or a control group. All subjects were less than 4 years old at enrollment. Daycare ranged from 2 hr/wk for 8 months to 7 hr/day, 5 day/wk, for 7 years. All studies examined cognitive development, six studies examined school performance, four studies evaluated behavior, and one study assessed children's health.

- Brooks-Gunn, McCarton, Casey, and others (1994)—Two-year follow-up study of 985 preterm subjects of varying socioeconomic background. Outcomes: Developmental quotient and intelligence quotient (IQ), behavior, health status, health care usage, weight gain, maternal employment, public assistance, health insurance, and mother-child interactions.
- Campbell, Breitmayer, and Ramey (1994)—Follow up of 12 to 15 years. Age at enrollment was 6 weeks; 111 children of disadvantaged families. Outcomes: IQ, school achievement, mother-child interaction, maternal employment and education, child's psychologic well-being.
- Deutsch (1966)—Thirteen-year follow up, high attrition led to unbalanced groups. Subjects were 4 years old at enrollment; 504 children from disadvantaged families. Outcomes: School competence, developed abilities, child's attitude, and impact on family.
- Garber (1988)—Quasi-randomized study, 7-year follow up. Age 3 years at enrollment, 40 children from disadvantaged background and low maternal IQ. Outcomes: Developmental quotient, IQ, school achievement.
- Gray and Klaus (1970)—Twelve-year study, subjects 3 years at enrollment, 65 subjects from varying social backgrounds. Outcomes: IQ, achievement and language, follow up of school competence, developed abilities, child's attitude, and impact on family.
- Palmer and Siegel (1977)—Nine-year follow up, boys only, 2 years old at enrollment, 310 subjects of mixed socioeconomic status. Outcomes: IQ, language, developmental outcomes, school competence, developed abilities, child's attitude, and impact on family.
- Schweinhart, Barnes, and Wiekart (1993)—Twenty-four–year follow up, 3 years old at enrollment, 128 disadvantaged children.

Outcomes: IQ, special education placement, grade retention, social development, parental satisfaction, delinquent behavior, employment, self-confidence, relationship with parents.
- Wasik, Ramey, Bryant, and others (1990)—Six-month follow up, 6 weeks old at enrollment, 65 children from disadvantaged families. Outcomes: Developmental index, IQ, home environment, childrearing attitudes; home-based group performed worse than control.

APPLY THE EVIDENCE: NURSING IMPLICATIONS

- Studies revealed out-of-home daycare has beneficial effects for children, enhancing cognitive development and preventing later school failures.
- Observational studies have reported that daycare can negatively affect child development. The studies reviewed show that preschool education has a beneficial effect on a child's behavior.
- Center-based daycare increases maternal employment and education, which could lead to improved socioeconomic status.
- Mother-child interaction can be improved by daycare, with studies showing improved communication between mother and child when compared with children who receive no daycare.
- Evidence suggests that out-of-home daycare can have a positive effect on social outcomes for children and their families.

References

Brooks-Gunn J, McCarton CM, Casey PH, and others: Early intervention in low-birth-weight premature infants: results through age 5 years from the Infant Health and Development Program, *JAMA* 272(16):1257-1262, 1994.

Campbell FA, Breitmayer B, Ramey CT: Effects of early intervention on intellectual and academic achievement: a follow-up study of children from low-income families, *Child Devel* 65:684-698, 1994.

Deutsch M: Facilitating development in pre-school child: social and psychological perspectives. In Hechinger FM, editor: *Pre-school education today*, vol 73-97, Garden City, NJ, 1966, Doubleday.

Garber HL: *The Milwaukee project: preventing mental retardation in children at risk*, Washington, DC, 1988, American Association on Mental Retardation.

Gray SW, Klaus RA: The early training project: a seventh year report, *Child Devel* 41:909-924, 1970.

Palmer FH, Siegel RJ: Minimal intervention at ages 2 and 3 and subsequent intellectual changes. In Day MC, Parker RK, editors: *The pre-school in action: exploring early childhood programs*, ed 2, Boston, 1977, Allyn & Bacon.

Schweinhart LJ, Barnes HV, Wiekart DP: *Significant benefits: the High/Scope Perry Preschool Study through age 27*, Ypsilanti, Mich, 1993, High/Scope Press.

Wasik BH, Ramey CT, Bryant DM, and others: A longitudinal study of two early intervention strategies: Project CARE, *Child Devel* 61:1682-1696, 1990.

Zortich B, Roberts I, and Oakley A: Day care for pre-school children, *Cochrane Database Syst Rev* (2):CD000564, 2000. In *The Cochrane Library*, issue 3, 2005.

Some employers have become more family focused and provide time off for parents to be with sick children. Increasing numbers are becoming more generous in the amount of time they allow parents (fathers as well as mothers) to remain at home after the birth or adoption of a child. Flexible work schedules and family-oriented legislation can ease the burden of managing family and work responsibilities. The passage of the Family and Medical Leave Act (FMLA) in 1993 set the stage for a greater focus on the issues of contemporary families. FMLA allows eligible employees to take up to 12 weeks of unpaid leave each year to care for newborn or newly adopted children, parents, or spouses who have serious health conditions, or to recover from their own serious health condition.

KEY POINTS

- Because there is no agreement about the definition of family, a family is what an individual considers it to be.
- Three theories that have significant relevance and application to pediatric nursing are family systems theory, family stress theory, and developmental theory.
- Although the traditional family structure was nuclear or extended, in recent years other forms, such as the single-parent family, have emerged.
- Family size and position within the family structure have a strong impact on a child's development.
- Interpersonal skills and a basic understanding of childhood growth and development are two essential areas of focus for parents.
- Parental control tends to be predominantly one of three types: authoritarian, permissive, or authoritative.
- Three areas of special concern to adoptive families include the initial attachment process, the task of telling the children they are adopted, and identity formation during adolescence.
- Marital factors within the home significantly influence a child's development. The impact of divorce on a child depends on the child's age, the outcome, and the quality of the parent-child relationship and parental care following the divorce.
- Single parenting and stepparenting create adjustment difficulties and add stress to the already demanding parental role. Significant numbers of children will live in a single-parent or reconstituted family at some point.

answers to CRITICAL THINKING EXERCISE

PARENTING THE ADOPTED CHILD

1. Yes. Although there is no one best time to tell children they are adopted, most authorities believe that children should be informed before they enter school to avoid learning about it from third parties.

In addition, authorities agree that children should be told at an age young enough so that, as they grow older, they do not remember a time when they did not know they were adopted.

2. a. The best time is highly individualized and based on the child's readiness. For some children, this may be when they ask about where babies come from. Children have a more difficult adjustment if disclosure occurs when they are older, and waiting until adolescence is too late.
   b. Parents should be completely honest with the child and provide information about the adoption in a matter-of-fact way with complete honesty. Sharing the story of adoption is an important parental responsibility and can be handled much like a parent shares birth experiences with a biologic child.
   c. Parents should anticipate that children may act out after being told that they are adopted. Some children use the fact of their adoption as a weapon to manipulate and threaten their parents. Allowing children to express their feelings and emotions after they have been told about their adoption is very important.

3. Because Justin's parents have requested guidance, it is appropriate for you, as the nurse, to provide information about how and when they should tell Justin he is adopted. However, the nurse's first priority is to be certain that Justin's parents are comfortable with this information, and that they feel free to ask any further questions and to obtain additional information. Because Justin is only 12 months old, his parents have time to think about how they will present this information to Justin and to prepare for the disclosure. They also have time to discuss how they will react to the feelings, emotions, and behaviors that Justin may demonstrate after he learns he is adopted.

4. Yes, at the present time, most authorities agree that children should be told about the fact that they are adopted, and that disclosure of this information should occur before the school-age years.

5. The nurse might ask Justin's parents if they would like additional materials such as books and pamphlets. The nurse could also refer Justin's parents to community resources on adoption if they request additional information.

REFERENCES

American Academy of Pediatrics: Family pediatrics: report of the Task Force on the Family, *Pediatrics* 111(6):1541-1571, 2003.

American Academy of Pediatrics, Committee on Early Childhood, Adoption, and Dependent Care: Development issues for young children in foster care (RE0012), *Pediatrics* 106(5):1145-1150, 2000.

Annie E Casey Foundation: *2007 Kids count data book: state profiles of child well-being*, Baltimore, 2007, The Foundation.

Ariel J, McPherson DW: Therapy with lesbian and gay parents and their children, *J Marriage Fam Ther* 26(4):421-432, 2000.

Brazelton TB: Working with families: opportunities for early intervention, *Pediatr Clin North Am* 42(1):1-10, 1995.

Duvall ER: *Family development*, ed 5, Philadelphia, 1977, Lippincott.

Friedman MM, Bowden VR, Jones EG: *Family nursing: research theory and practice*, ed 5, Upper Saddle River, NJ, 2003, Prentice Hall.

Hamilton BE, Minino AM, Martin JA, and others: Annual summary of vital statistics: 2005, *Pediatrics* 119(2):345-360, 2007.

Lerner RM, Sparks EE, McCubbin LD: *Family diversity and family policy: strengthening families for America's children*, Boston, 1999, Kluwer Academic Publishers.

Lynch JM, Murray K: For the love of the children: the coming out process for lesbian and gay parents and stepparents, *J Homosex* 39(1):1-24, 2000.

McCubbin MA, McCubbin HI: Families coping with illness: the resiliency model of family stress, adjustment, and adaptation. In Danielson CB, Bissel BH, Winstead-Fry P, editors: *Families, health, and illness*, St Louis, 1994, Mosby.

Munson ML, Sutton PD: Births, marriages, divorces, and deaths: provisional data for 2005, *Natl Vital Stat Rep* 54(20):1-7, 2006.

Pawelski JG, Perrin EC, Foy JM, and others: The effects of marriage, civil union, and domestic partnership laws on the health and well-being of children, *Pediatrics* 118(1):349-364, 2006.

US Census Bureau: *Two married parents the norm*, Washington, DC, 2003, Department of Commerce News, retrieved Jan 8, 2008, from http://www.census.gov/Press-Release/www/2003/cb03-97.html.

4

Social, Cultural, and Religious Influences on Child Health Promotion

MARY C. HOOKE

CHAPTER OUTLINE

CULTURE, 52
Social Roles, 52
 Self-Esteem and Culture, 53
Subcultural Influences, 53
 Ethnicity, 53
 Socioeconomic Class, 54
 Poverty, 54
 Homelessness, 54
 Migrant Farmworker Families, 54
 Immigrant Children, 55
 Religion, 55
 Schools, 55

Communities, 55
 Peer Cultures, 56
The Child and Family in North
 America, 56
 Minority-Group Membership, 56
Cultural Shock and Cultural
 Competence, 57
CULTURAL AND RELIGIOUS INFLUENCES
ON HEALTH CARE, 58
Susceptibility to Health Problems, 58
 Hereditary Factors, 58
 Socioeconomic Factors, 58

Cultural Customs, 59
 Cultural Relativism, 60
 Relationships with Health Care
  Providers, 60
 Food Customs, 61
Health Beliefs and Practices, 62
 Health Beliefs, 62
 Health Practices, 63
Religious Beliefs, 64
Importance of Culture and Religion
 to Nurses, 64

LEARNING OBJECTIVES

On completion of this chapter the reader will be able to:

- Define culture, cultural competence, ethnocentrism, and cultural relativism.
- Describe the subcultural influences on child development in the areas of socioeconomic class, poverty, religion, and schools.

- Discuss the population shifts in number of minority children in the United States.
- Identify four common diseases or disorders that affect certain ethnic or cultural groups.

- Identify areas of potential conflict of values and customs for a nurse interacting with a family from a different cultural or ethnic group.
- Describe three religious groups whose beliefs significantly affect their health practices.

RELATED TOPICS and ADDITIONAL RESOURCES

 IN TEXT

Communicating with Families Through an
 Interpreter, *Ch. 6*
Family Assessment Interview, *Ch. 6*
Family Influences on Child Health
 Promotion, *Ch. 3*
Listening and Cultural Awareness, *Ch. 6*
Lactose Intolerance, *Ch. 11*

Nutritional Assessment, *Ch. 6*
Sickle Cell Anemia, *Ch. 26*
Skin, *Ch. 6*
Spiritual Development: General, *Ch. 5*;
 Toddler, *Ch. 12*; Preschooler, *Ch. 13*;
 School-Age Child, *Ch. 15*; Adolescent,
 Ch. 16
Vegetarian Diets, *Ch. 11*

 COMPANION CD

Case Study—Cultural Considerations
NCLEX Review Questions

evolve

evolve.elsevier.com/Wong/essentials/

NCLEX Review Questions
Skill—Providing Culturally Sensitive Care
WebLinks

CULTURE

The future of any society depends on its children; therefore society must provide for their care, nurturing, and socialization. Culture plays a critical role in the parenting behaviors that facilitate children's development (Meléndez, 2005). The customs and values of the culture help to organize a society's childrearing system and are transmitted from one generation to the next through the medium of the family. A holistic view of any child requires that nurses develop some understanding of the ways that culture contributes to the development of social and emotional relationships and influences childrearing practices and attitudes toward health.

As the ethnic, racial, and cultural diversity in the composition of the U.S. population increases, it is imperative that nurses become competent in transcultural nursing knowledge (Muñoz and Luckmann, 2005). This orientation to transcultural nursing includes an awareness of the nurse's own culture. The nurse who is becoming culturally competent learns about other cultures, becomes able to assess the perspectives of others, and shares his or her own culture with others (Dunn, 2002).

Culture is a pattern of learned beliefs, values, and practices that are shared within a group; it includes practices; customs; views on roles and relationships, including parenting; and communication patterns and language (Betancourt, 2004). Culture differs from both race and ethnicity. **Race** is defined as a division of humans possessing traits that are transmissible by descent and that are sufficient to characterize it as a distinct human type. One classification of race, based on skin color, is Caucasian (white), Negroid (African American), and Mongoloid (yellow). **Ethnicity** is the affiliation of a set of persons who share a unique cultural, social, and linguistic heritage (Fig. 4-1). **Socialization** is the process by which society imparts its competencies, values, and expectations to children (Trawick-Smith, 2006).

Culture is a complex whole in which each part is interrelated. It provides the lens through which all facets of human behavior can be interpreted (Spector, 2004). Culture is not a surface veneer that covers a basic outlook shared by all human beings; rather, it is an ingrained orientation to life that serves as a frame of reference for individual perception and judgment. People from one culture differ from those in other cultures in the ways they think, solve problems, and perceive and structure the world. Culture is, essentially, the way of life of a group of people that incorporates experiences of the past, influences thought and action in the present, and transmits these traditions to future group members. Adaptation is necessary, however, for the culture to survive in an ever-changing world. Consciously and unconsciously, the members abandon, modify, or assume new patterns to meet the needs of the group.

The cultural setting in which children are raised can influence many aspects of their life, from the food they eat to the way they behave in a social setting. To be acceptable members of the culture, children must learn how the culture expects them to behave toward others in the group. In turn, they learn how they can expect others to behave toward them.

Cultures and subcultures contribute to the uniqueness of child members in such a subtle way and at such an early age that children grow up to think that their beliefs, attitudes, values, and practices are the "correct" or "normal" ones. By age 5, children can identify persons who belong to their own race or cultural background. During later primary years, children are able to identify people from different cultures (Trawick-

FIG. 4-1 ■ Ethnicity is an individual's association with shared cultural, social, and linguistic heritage.

Smith, 2006). A set of values learned in childhood is likely to characterize children's attitudes and behavior for life, guiding their long-range strivings and monitoring their short-range, impulsive inclinations. Thus every ongoing society socializes each succeeding generation to its cultural heritage.

The manner and sequence of the growth and development phenomenon are universal and fundamental features of all children; however, the variations in behavioral responses that children display to similar events are believed to be determined by their culture. Children acquire the skills, knowledge, beliefs, and values important to their own family and culture. The pace of acquisition of cognitive and motor skills can differ by cultural background as well as the child's social and emotional development (Trawick-Smith, 2006).

Cultures may also differ in whether status in the group is based on age or on skill. Even children's play and their types of games are culturally determined. In some cultures children play in groups composed of members of the same sex; in others, they play in mixed-sex groups. In some cultures team games predominate; in others, most play is limited to individual games.

Standards and norms vary from culture to culture and from location to location; a practice that is accepted in one area may meet with disapproval or create tension in another. The extent to which cultures tolerate divergence from the established norm varies among cultures and subcultural groups. Although conformity provides a degree of security, it is often a deterrent to change.

SOCIAL ROLES

Much of children's self-concept is derived from their ideas about their social roles. **Roles** are cultural creations; therefore the culture prescribes patterns of behavior for persons in a variety of social positions. All persons who hold similar social positions have an obligation to behave in a particular manner. A role prohibits some behaviors and allows others. Because it delineates and clarifies roles, the culture is a significant influence on the development of children's self-concept (i.e., attitudes and beliefs they have about themselves).

A social group consists of a system of roles carried out in both primary and secondary groups. A **primary group** is characterized by intimate, continued, face-to-face contact; mutual support of members; and the ability to order or constrain a considerable proportion of individual members' behavior. Two such groups are the family and the peer group, both of which exert a great deal of influence on the child.

Secondary groups are groups that have limited, intermittent contact and in which there is generally less concern for members' behavior. These groups offer little in terms of support or pressure toward conformity except in rigidly limited areas. Examples of secondary groups are professional associations and church organizations (also considered in relation to subgroups). The childrearing orientation in a secondary-group environment, such as urban communities, differs considerably from that of a primary-group community. An urban community is dynamic and rapidly changing; therefore many of the traditional behaviors and values do not meet its needs. Consequently, parents are often uncertain about what to teach their children. They may wish to rear their children with values consistent with their own, but the differences in experience between the generations are too great. As a result, they often grant their children autonomy in some areas of decision making early in the developmental process, and other secondary groups assume a greater influence. The children are exposed to an assortment of social groups with diverse sets of values and expectations. None of the groups is highly dominant in its influence; therefore the children are exposed to an eclectic set of values, some in agreement and some in conflict with the others. From these they must ultimately select those that they determine to be best for them and adopt them to form a consistent set of roles and behaviors to be incorporated into the self-concept.

Self-Esteem and Culture

A child's sense of self-esteem is influenced by his or her culture (Trawick-Smith, 2006). Some cultures are more collective in thought and action. A child from a collective culture will hold an inclusive view of self. Self-evaluation is related to the accomplishments or competencies of the entire family or community. School experiences that focus on personal achievement may promote positive self-esteem in some children but not in others, who are more dependent on the success of a whole family or peer group. A child's sense of control may not come from individual self-reliance but rather from a feeling of worth in his or her family or community (Trawick-Smith, 2006).

Families and culture also influence the criteria children use to evaluate their own abilities. Additionally, cultures vary in whether they instill an internal locus of control (a belief in the ability to regulate one's own life). Effects on self-esteem are minimal if these beliefs are directed by parents and are in accordance with cultural customs (Trawick-Smith, 2006). What is damaging to emotional health is helplessness that stems from prejudice. Ethnic pride is a factor that has helped maintain positive self-image and protect against the damage that prejudice can cause (Trawick-Smith, 2006).

SUBCULTURAL INFLUENCES

Except in rare situations, children grow and develop in a blend of cultures and subcultures. In a large, complex society such as that of the United States, different groups have their own set

FIG. 4-2 ■ Teenagers from different cultural backgrounds interact within the larger culture.

of standards, values, and expectations within the collective ways of the large culture. Although many cultural differences are related to geographic boundaries, subcultures are not always restricted by location.

Children's membership in a cultural subgroup is, for the most part, involuntary. They are born into a family with a specific ethnic or racial heritage, socioeconomic level, and religious beliefs. Although in the complex North American society there are countless subcultures and considerable variation in the way of life, those subcultures that seem to exert the greatest influence on childrearing are ethnicity, social class, and occupational role. In addition, schools and peer-group subcultures are strong influences in the socialization of the child (Fig. 4-2).

Ethnicity

Ethnicity is the classification of or affiliation with any of the basic groups or divisions of humans or any heterogeneous population differentiated by customs, characteristics, language, or similar distinguishing factors. Ethnic differences extend to many areas and include such manifestations as family structure, language, food preferences, moral codes, and expression of emotion. Some standards of behavior result from the cultural heritage of the specific ethnic group. The term *ethnic* has aroused strong negative feelings and is often rejected by the general population (Spector, 2004).

To establish their place in the group, children learn how to adhere to a mode of behavior that is in accordance with standards distinctive to the group and learn how they can expect others to behave toward them. They take their cues by observing and imitating those to whom they are exposed. For example, children of a racial minority form a perception of their role as a group member by observing the manner in which role models within the subgroup respond to treatment by people outside the subgroup. When they see group members display an attitude of inferiority, they assume this to be the appropriate behavior and incorporate these perceptions into their own self-concept.

In the United States the cross-cultural lines are becoming blurred as subcultures are assimilated and blend into the larger culture. It is particularly difficult for persons to attempt to maintain an identity with a subculture while living and conforming to the requirements of the dominant culture. Universal customs and language used in commercial and educational systems are different from those of the minority culture. Consequently, children reared in this environment are confused about roles and values, and they usually adopt those of the more influential or higher status culture. Youths, in particular, are influenced by the locally dominant group.

Ethnocentrism is the concept that one's own culture proves the right and natural way to do things while all other ways are unnatural and inferior (Galanti, 2004). **Ethnic stereotyping** or labeling stems from ethnocentric views of people. Ethnocentrism implies that all other groups are inferior and that their ways are not in the best interests of the group. It is a common attitude among a dominant ethnic group and strongly influences the ability of one person to objectively evaluate the beliefs and behaviors of others. This inherent viewpoint of individuals tends to bias their interpretation and understanding of the behavior of others. The culturally competent nurse should be empathetic and aware of his or her own views and that they may differ from another's based on culture or ethnicity. The nurse should be willing to ask questions that will provide a better understanding of patient or family views when appropriate.

Socioeconomic Class

It is important to recognize that family relationships may be stronger among some ethnic or cultural groups than others. However, the influence of socioeconomic class cannot be overlooked. Socioeconomic class relates to the family's economic and education levels. Strong family relationships exist among those of lower socioeconomic class who have few resources and must rely on the support of a family network to meet physical and emotional needs. Middle- and upper-class people often have resources that reach beyond the extended family. They are able to access physical and emotional support in the community (Giger and Davidhizar, 2004).

The term **socioeconomic class** should not be confused with cultural or ethnic diversity. Children of a specific race are not necessarily of low socioeconomic status. Additionally, children of poverty do not automatically have developmental delays (Trawick-Smith, 2006).

Poverty

A subcultural influence closely related to, but different from, social class is the condition known as poverty. It is a relative concept and is usually associated with the general standards of a population. The term **poverty** implies both visible and invisible impoverishment. It is a condition in which families live without adequate resources (Trawick-Smith, 2006). **Visible poverty** refers to lack of money or material resources, which includes insufficient clothing, poor sanitation, and deteriorating housing. **Invisible poverty** refers to social and cultural de-

privation, such as limited employment opportunities, inferior educational opportunities, lack of or inferior medical services and health care facilities, and an absence of public services.

An **absolute standard** of poverty attempts to delimit some basic set of resources needed for adequate existence. **Relative poverty** reflects the median income and median standard of living in a society or country and is the term used in referring to childhood poverty in the United States (Scruggs and Allan, 2006); that is, what appears to be substandard living conditions in one area may be a standard or norm in another.

The number of children living in poverty has continued to increase during the twenty-first century. The child poverty rate in the United States is among the highest in the developed world (American Academy of Pediatrics, 2005). In 2006, 18% of children were living in poverty, a 6% increase since the year 2000. In 2005, nearly 29 million U.S. children lived in low-income families. **Low income** is defined as having a family income (for a family of four) that is less than twice the federal poverty threshold with at least one parent working 50 or more weeks during the year. The majority of these children, or nearly 15 million, had at least one parent who worked regularly but were living on the economic edge and struggling to make ends meet (Annie E Casey Foundation, 2006). Poverty is a strong predictor of child health and is closely associated with poorer physical, developmental, and mental health outcomes (American Academy of Pediatrics, 2005).

Homelessness

One of the most pressing problems in the United States is the growing number of homeless families. **Homeless individuals** are those who lack resources and community ties necessary to provide for their own adequate shelter. Homeless children have increased in numbers as poverty has become feminized, minorities have become poorer, and low-income housing has become less accessible. Estimates on the number of homeless children in the United States are at 1.6 million children each year, with the number growing (American Academy of Pediatrics, 2005). The majority of children are younger than 5 years of age and predominantly from minority groups.

Most homelessness is a direct result of increasing numbers of people in poverty combined with a lack of decent, affordable housing. Government housing subsidies have decreased, whereas the number of working poor has increased (Tropello, 2000). Other reasons include job layoffs, low income, parental mental illness, domestic conflict, and unexpected family or economic crises. Many families move into homelessness gradually after family members and friends are no longer willing to provide housing. Another group of homeless children are the "runaway" and "throwaway" adolescents. Many runaways are victims of physical and sexual abuse and leave home because of long-term family or school problems.

Migrant Farmworker Families

One of the most disadvantaged groups is migrant farm workers and their children. Indications suggest that in the United States there are between 3 million and 5 million migrant and seasonal workers and their dependents, whose average yearly income is well below the poverty level. In addition, most of these families have no health insurance.

The low position of these families on the economic scale and their rootless, mobile existence subject them to inadequate sanitation, substandard housing, social isolation, and lack of educational and medical facilities (American Academy of Pediatrics, 2005). This lifestyle is especially deleterious to the children. Schooling and health care are inadequate. Children are likely to live in a number of localities and attend a variety of schools over the course of a year, with no continuity in either education or health care. Because both parents work in the fields, children receive little adult supervision; therefore injury rates are high, and meals are erratic.

Immigrant Children

The 2000 U.S. Census informed us that there are a growing number of immigrants who currently are living in the United States (US Census Bureau, 2001). In 2005 it is estimated that 21% of children (15.7 million) lived in immigrant families; the children were either born outside the United States or had at least one foreign-born parent (Annie E Casey Foundation, 2007). These children and families face unique stressors, including depression, grief, and anxiety related to migration and acculturation, separation from extended family and supports, language barriers, disparities in socioeconomic status compared with their country of origin, and possibly traumatic events that necessitated their immigration (American Academy of Pediatrics, 2005). Current laws restrict health benefits under government programs for immigrants who lawfully entered the United States after 1996; they must wait for 5 years to become eligible for comprehensive health benefits (American Academy of Pediatrics, 2005). Immigrant issues continue to require the attention of policymakers and child advocates.

Religion

An influential factor shaping the culture of the United States is the Judeo-Christian faith. Many immigrants came to the United States for religious freedom and established a religious and moral atmosphere that persists today. However, there are individual differences that are part of the general culture.

The religious orientation of the family dictates a code of morality and influences the family's attitudes toward education, male and female role identity, and beliefs regarding their ultimate destiny (Fig. 4-3). Religion may also be a factor in determining the school the children attend, the companions with whom they associate, and often their mate selection. In a few instances, such as in the Mennonite and Amish communities, religion is the basis for a common way of life that determines where children are reared and their lifestyle. (See also Religious Beliefs, p. 64.)

Schools

Next to the family, schools exert the major force in providing continuity between generations by conveying a vast amount of culture from the older members to the young. In this way children are prepared to carry out the traditional social roles they are expected to assume as adults in society. School rules and regulations regarding attendance, authority relationships, and the system of sanctions and rewards based on achievement transmit to the child the behavioral expectations of the adult world of employment and relationships. School is often the only institution in which children systematically learn about the negative consequences of behaviors that deviate from social expectations. Teachers are expected to stimulate and guide the intellectual development of children and their

FIG. 4-3 ■ Soon after an infant is born, many families have special religious ceremonies.

sense of esthetics and to foster their capacity for creative problem solving. Through education, individuals in the lower classes are offered the opportunity and the capacity to move up in the social strata.

Traditionally, the socialization process of school began when the child entered kindergarten or first grade. Today, with more than 65% of mothers of preschool children working outside the home, this socialization process begins much earlier for a significant number of children in a variety of child care settings (Annie E Casey Foundation, 2006).

Children of some cultural groups fare less well in school. They come from under-represented groups, including African-American, Mexican-American, Puerto Rican, and Native American children (Trawick-Smith, 2006). These cultural variations can be attributed to high rates of poverty, different cognitive styles, ineffective schools, and parents' views of schools as oppressive to cultural and traditional values (Trawick-Smith, 2006).

Communities

Surveys of more than 1 million young persons in the United States in grades 6 through 12 have shown that those who experience a higher number of specific assets in their lives are more likely to make healthy choices and avoid high-risk behaviors. These assets offer a framework for positive child and adolescent development. The child's or adolescent's community is made up of the family, school, neighborhood, youth organization, and other members. They all contribute to the young person's experience within any culture (Search-Institute, 2007).

Four categories of external assets that youth receive from the community include (Search-Institute, 2007):

1. **Support**—Young people need to feel support, care, and love from their families, neighbors, and others. They also need organizations and institutions that offer positive, supportive environments.
2. **Empowerment**—Young people need to feel valued by their community and be able to contribute to others. They need to feel safe and secure.

3. **Boundaries and expectations**—Young people need to know what is expected of them and what actions and behaviors are within the community boundaries and what are outside of them.
4. **Constructive use of time**—Young people need opportunities for growth through constructive, enriching opportunities and quality time at home.

Internal assets must also be nurtured in the community's young members. These internal qualities guide choices and create a sense of centeredness, purpose, and focus. The four categories of internal assets include (Search-Institute, 2007):

1. **Commitment to learning**—Young people need to develop a commitment to education and life-long learning
2. **Positive values**—Youth need to have a strong sense of values that direct their choices.
3. **Social competencies**—Young people need competencies that help them make positive choices and build relationships.
4. **Positive identity**—Young people need a sense of their own power, purpose, worth, and promise.

Peer Cultures

Peer groups also have an impact on the socialization of children. Peer relationships become increasingly important and influential as children proceed through school. In school, children have what can be regarded as a culture of their own. It is most apparent in the school and in the unsupervised play group. The play group presents this culture in a much purer form than does the school, in which culture is partly produced by adults.

During their lives children are exposed to value systems such as those of the family, ethnic group, and social class. In peer-group interaction they are confronted with a variety of these sets of values. The values imposed by the peer group are especially compelling because children must accept and conform to them to be accepted as members of the group. When the peer values are not too different from those of family and teachers, the mild conflict created by these small differences serves to separate children from the adults in their lives and to strengthen the feeling of belonging to the peer group. The relationships in a peer group change over time, and leadership may shift (Trawick-Smith, 2006).

The kind of socialization provided by the peer group depends on the special subculture that develops from the background, interests, and capabilities of its members. Some groups support school achievement, others focus on athletic prowess, and still others are decidedly antithetic to educative goals. Scholastic achievement is strongly related to the value system of the peer groups. Many conflicts between teachers and students and between parents and students can be attributed to fear of rejection by peers. A conflict between what is expected from parents regarding academic achievement and what is expected from the peer culture is especially pronounced in high school.

Although it has neither the traditional authority of the parents nor the legal authority of the schools for teaching information, the peer group manages to convey a substantial amount of information to its members. Peer relationships also provide an important social context for the development of body image among both adolescent girls and boys. Although other subcultural forces such as the family and media influence the development of body image, adolescents' perception of what is a desirable appearance is created by norms and expectations that are modeled and reinforced within the peer group (Jones and Crawford, 2006). It is through peer relationships that children learn ways to deal with dominance and hostility and to relate with persons in positions of leadership and authority. The peer subculture relieves boredom and provides recognition that individual members do not receive from teachers and other authority figures.

THE CHILD AND FAMILY IN NORTH AMERICA

The frontier background of the North American culture has contributed to the overall orientation to life and childrearing. There has always been a basic optimistic view of the world, a belief that things can be better and that the children can and will be better off than the parents. This hopeful outlook and a general future orientation, together with the possibility of upward social mobility, have created a pervasive overall attitude of optimism. Increasing development of self-confidence and autonomy in children is fostered and encouraged. Children in North America are generally permitted a greater degree of freedom than in more tradition-oriented cultures, where individuals remain in one class for life.

Family life in North America is characterized by increasing geographic and economic mobility. There is less reliance on tradition, families are fragmented, and there is limited opportunity to transmit and acquire the traditional and accepted customs of a culture. Consequently, young adults rely to a greater extent on professed experts, peers, and mass media for acquisition of acceptable patterns of behavior, including childrearing practices. Conflicting information can be a source of confusion and frustration as parents attempt to determine the comparatively stable, essential components of the culture and transmit these to their children.

Children in North America grow up with a number of adults who differ from one another but who all provide input as role models, teachers, and standards for behavior. Most children live in some form of nuclear family located in sharply differentiated neighborhoods determined by income and ethnic status within a highly technical, largely urban society. Class differences in childrearing persist, but they are becoming less divergent as a result of the increased homogeneity of the culture.

Minority-Group Membership

The United States has more racial, ethnic, and religious minority groups than any other country as a result of high immigration rates and high birth rates among these groups. Ethnic minority groups are becoming increasingly important because it is anticipated that these groups will produce children at a faster rate than will the majority Caucasian population. Consequently, the minority population is increasing, whereas the majority Caucasian population is decreasing. When people from different cultures interact, this is termed **cultural diversity** (Purnell and Paulanka, 2003).

The 2000 U.S. Census found that there are more than 280 million people in the United States, with 6.8 million reporting more than two races. African Americans alone or in combination with another race comprise more than 35 million, and Hispanics or Latinos of any race comprise more than 35 million. The Hispanic population increased 58%, or 13 million people, from 1990 to 2000 (US Census Bureau, 2001). (See Cultural Awareness box.)

CULTURAL AWARENESS

Overview of Race and Hispanic Origin in Census 2000

The federal government defines race and Hispanic origin as two separate and distinct concepts. In the 2000 U.S. Census, responders were first asked if they are of Spanish/Hispanic/Latino origin. The second question asked respondents to report the race or races they considered themselves to be. The definitions of racial groups included the following (US Census Bureau, 2001):

- **Caucasians** are people having "origins in any of the original peoples of Europe, the Middle East, or North Africa."
- **African Americans,** sometimes referred to as **blacks,** are defined as "people having origins in any of the Black racial groups of Africa."
- An **Asian** is any person with "origins in any of the original peoples of the Far East, Southeast Asia, or the Indian subcontinent."
- **Native Hawaiians** and **Other Pacific Islanders** are "people having origins in any of the original peoples of Hawaii, Guam, Samoa, or other Pacific Islands."
- **Native Americans** (referred to as **American Indians)** and **Alaska Natives** are defined as "people having origins in any of the original peoples of North and South America (including Central America), and who maintain tribal affiliation or community attachment."

NURSINGALERT
Because American cultures and subcultures can be so diverse, it is essential that nurses be aware of and knowledgeable about the predominant groups in their work community and apply the knowledge in their practice.

NURSINGALERT
Generalizations made about an ethnic group may not apply to certain groups and individuals.

When minority groups immigrate to another country, a certain degree of cultural and ethnic blending occurs through the involuntary process of **acculturation,** those gradual changes produced in a culture by the influence of another culture that cause one or both cultures to be more similar to the other. This process is involuntary; the minority group member is forced to learn the new culture to survive (Spector, 2004). However, the changes occur to various degrees in different families and groups. Many groups continue to identify with their traditional heritage while adapting to the ill-defined concept of the "American way." Acculturation may be referred to as **assimilation,** which is the process of developing a new cultural identity (Spector, 2004).

Evidence indicates that changes in attitudes are slowly taking place in some groups and in some places. An attitude of **cultural relativism** provides for understanding behaviors in their cultural context and sees other ways of doing things as different but equally valid (Galanti, 2004). With growing awareness, interest, and understanding by increasing numbers of the majority group, which have accompanied the recent emergence of racial and ethnic pride, minority-group children are becoming more secure and confident in their racial or ethnic identity. Individuals vary in their reactions to membership in a minority group, and much of this variation can be attrib-

CRITICAL THINKING EXERCISE

Reducing Cultural Shock
A woman from the Middle East is visiting her child who is hospitalized for a serious illness. Her husband left for home a short time ago to wash and change clothes. She speaks little English. You need to obtain consent from her for an emergency procedure. She is hesitant and refuses to sign the consent form. What should you do?

QUESTIONS
1. Evidence—Is there sufficient information to draw any conclusions about this woman's actions?
2. Assumptions—Describe some underlying assumptions about each of the following:
   a. Arab culture
   b. Need for interpreter
   c. Approval for emergency procedures
   d. Documentation of the need for the emergency procedure
3. What priorities for nursing care should be established at this time?
4. Does the evidence support your nursing intervention(s)?
5. What alternative perspectives might you have?

uted to familial factors. As with all children, the most important influences on development of a positive self-image are warm, understanding parents who take an active interest in fostering their children's growth. Parents who accept their children and react positively and constructively rather than in a negative and demeaning manner will help their children develop feelings of self-worth, self-esteem, and self-acceptance. The more adequate children feel, the more positive will be their attitudes toward both majority and minority children, the greater their ability to withstand prejudice and intolerance, and the less their need for counteraggressive behavior.

CULTURAL SHOCK AND CULTURAL COMPETENCE
The term **cultural shock** describes the "feelings of helplessness and discomfort and a state of disorientation experienced by an outsider attempting to comprehend or effectively adapt to a different cultural group because of differences in cultural practices, values, and beliefs" (Leininger, 1978). This state occurs with both patients and health care providers who move from one cultural setting to another. It can happen to persons who immigrate to a new country (such as Asian refugees) or to those from a subcultural group who must adjust to the ways of an unfamiliar subgroup (such as children entering the school subculture or consumers entering the hospital subculture). Cultural shock is characterized by the inability to respond to or function in a new or strange situation (see Critical Thinking Exercise).

Numerous factors influence reactions to a new environment. Language barriers, including dialects and jargon (such as medical language) specific to a subcultural group, inhibit effective communication. Habits and customs (such as different role behaviors or etiquette) and differences in attitudes and beliefs are puzzling to the stranger in the new environment. The outsider experiences intense feelings of isolation, loneliness, and nonrelatedness.

Nurses are challenged to overcome cultural shock and develop the dynamics of **cultural sensitivity,** an awareness of cultural similarities and differences. In doing so, the nurse is helped to practice **culturally competent care**. This requires changing the way people think about, understand, and interact within the world around them. Cultural competence is an ongoing process that is interactive and without end (Dunn, 2002). Six elements included in the process of developing cultural competence are (Dunn, 2002):

1. Working on changing one's world view through examining one's own values and behaviors and striving to reject racism and institutions that support it
2. Becoming familiar with core cultural issues by recognizing these issues and exploring them with patients
3. Becoming knowledgeable about the cultural groups we work with while learning about each individual patient's unique history
4. Becoming familiar with core cultural issues related to health and illness and communicating in a way that encourages patients to explain what an illness means to them
5. Developing a relationship of trust with the patient and creating a welcoming atmosphere in the health care setting
6. Negotiating for mutually acceptable and understandable interventions of care

NURSING ALERT

Cultural knowledge helps us understand the behavior of our patients and families so that we do not consider it pathologic. This knowledge does not allow us to make assumptions about their behavior clinically. A **cultural assessment** is a strategy to elicit the patient's and family's understanding of their illness and to individualize the patient's care plan. Cultural competence is nursing competence (Dreher and MacNaugton, 2002).

CULTURAL AND RELIGIOUS INFLUENCES ON HEALTH CARE

SUSCEPTIBILITY TO HEALTH PROBLEMS

Some groups of people are more susceptible than others to certain illnesses. An innate susceptibility is acquired through generations of evolutionary changes that take place within constrained or segregated populations. The proximity to disease, environmental factors, and general physical status are significant factors associated with health problems.

Hereditary Factors

Advances in science have found that many diseases have a genetic basis. The access to screening for these diseases will challenge genetic testing and counseling and can present complex moral dilemmas for the individual patient and family and for society.

A number of conditions show ethnic or racial differences based on genetics. For example, Tay-Sachs disease, characterized by early neurologic deterioration and mental retardation, affects primarily Ashkenazi Jewish families, particularly those of Northeastern European origin, whereas Sephardic Jewish families appear to be no more at risk for the disease than are other populations. The incidence of cystic fibrosis is highest in Caucasians and almost nonexistent in Asians, and the rare affected African Americans are usually in areas where there is apt to be mixed ancestry. A classic disorder of African Americans is sickle cell disease (see Chapter 26); however, the incidence of cardiovascular disease, pneumonia, and diabetes is also high among African Americans. Native Americans are at risk for type 2 diabetes and lactose intolerance. Racial and

ethnic differences are further considered in relation to diseases and defects as they are discussed throughout the book.

Common food items and drugs may cause health problems in certain ethnic groups. For example, persons of Mediterranean, African, Near Eastern, and Asian origin frequently have glucose-6-phosphate dehydrogenase deficiency. They may develop acute hemolytic anemia after they ingest fava (horse or broad) beans or certain drugs such as aspirin preparations, sulfonamides, or primaquine. Other groups, especially Southern Europeans, Jews, Arabs, African Americans, Asians, and Native Americans, have a deficiency of lactase, the enzyme needed to metabolize lactose. Ingestion of lactose can cause abdominal distention, flatus, and diarrhea (Purnell and Paulanka, 2003). Unknowing but well-meaning health care workers may be responsible for these symptoms in their clients when they prescribe foods or food supplements containing lactose as sources of nutrients.

Physical Characteristics. Among racial groups there are observable differences in physical appearance. The most obvious are skin and hair coloring and texture. Skin color is determined by the amount of melanin pigment present in the skin. Persons from countries located near the equator have darkly pigmented skin, which serves to protect the skin from the year-round exposure to the sun's rays; persons from northern countries have very light skin, which provides for maximum exposure to the sun's rays (necessary for vitamin D metabolism) during the short daylight hours. There can be wide variations in skin color between these two extremes as a result of geographic origin or intermixing of persons with dark and light skin color. In patients with dark pigmentation, the detection of skin color changes (e.g., vasomotor alterations, cyanosis, jaundice) can be difficult and requires modification of assessment techniques.

Variations in the newborn are often related to racial or ethnic origin. For example, newborn infants of Asian and African-American parents are smaller than infants of Caucasian parentage, and bluish pigmented areas (mongolian spots) on the sacral region are a common observation in Asian, African-American, Native American, and Mexican-American infants. It is important that health care providers be familiar with these birthmarks. They should be documented at newborn examinations and subsequent visits so they are not suddenly interpreted as bruises (Garwick and Auger, 2000).

Evaluation of stature and body build reveals some racial tendencies. "Typical" growth descriptions are often based on observations of middle-class Caucasian children from the United States. Children from Asian countries are commonly smaller, falling below the 10th percentile on weight and height charts used for children in the United States, whereas African and African-American children are more advanced in physical growth (Trawick-Smith, 2006). This difference in stature can lead to misinterpretation of health status and capabilities.

Socioeconomic Factors

The most overwhelming adverse influence on health is socioeconomic status. A higher percentage of lower-class individuals are suffering from some health problem at any one time than are those in any other group. The sum of all aspects of their situation contributes to and compounds health problems; this includes crowded living conditions and poor sanitation, which facilitate transfer of disease (e.g., tuberculosis). There is a higher incidence of lead poisoning in children from families from the lower socioeconomic classes because there is more ready access to lead in the environment, especially lead-based paint in old housing (Centers for Disease Control and Prevention, 2007).

In the lower classes, children are less likely to be immunized against preventable diseases than are children in the upper and middle classes. Lack of funds or inaccessibility of health services inhibits treatment for any but severe illness or injury. Sometimes health care is inadequate because of lack of information. In some areas a disorder is so commonplace that it is looked on as unavoidable; it is not recognized as something that requires (or is amenable to) treatment. The parents may not have information regarding causes, treatment, outcome of the illness, or preventive measures. The nurse can use the limited opportunities when the family does come into contact with the health care system to inquire about immunizations, screen for vision problems, provide nutritional information, and offer additional prevention and health promotion resources.

Poverty. A high correlation between poverty and the prevalence of illness has long been observed. Impoverished families suffer from poor nutrition; without medical insurance, they have little if any preventive health care, inadequate health maintenance, and limited access to medical treatment. One of the most significant health problems related to poverty is a high infant mortality rate. Although the infant mortality rate in the United States is at an all-time low, our nation's infant survival rate remains lower than that of most industrialized nations (Annie E Casey Foundation, 2006).

Poor families are denied access to many health institutions for emergency or other hospital care. Frequently they must travel long distances to service centers that are willing to assume their care. In an emergency they must find money for taxi fare, borrow an automobile, or seek other means of transportation. They must find care for dependents, such as other infants and small children, or have them accompany them when taking the ill child for care. Families tend to delay preventive care indefinitely unless health services are relatively accessible. They are more likely to consult folk practitioners or other persons within their community. Day-to-day needs of food, clothing, and lodging take precedence over health care as long as the ailing person feels able to perform activities of daily living.

Poor nutrition accounts for many health problems in the lower classes. Lack of funds and knowledge results in a diet that may be seriously deficient in essential food substances, especially protein, vitamins, and iron. This inadequate diet often leads to nutritional deficiency disorders and growth retardation in children. In many the total intake is insufficient to support normal growth. Unstructured eating patterns and irregularly scheduled mealtimes can also contribute to erratic food intake and a proportionately larger consumption of nonnourishing snacks, which can result in excessive weight gain.

Because of deficient preventive care, dental problems are more prevalent. Lack of standard immunizations, together with reduced resistance from poor nutrition, renders the exposed children in poor segments of the population vulnerable to communicable diseases. Poor sanitation and crowded living conditions also contribute to the higher incidence and perpetuation of illness. In general, poor people become ill more frequently and remain ill for longer periods than do persons in the general population.

Homelessness. Research indicates that families are the fastest-growing subgroup of the homeless population (American Academy of Pediatrics, 2005). Homeless children experience all of the health problems associated with poverty, as well as other types of disorders. A majority of these children experience poor health. They not have a regular source of health care, and the focus of their care is not preventive. Their care is fragmented, crisis oriented, and often sought in emergency departments. Children who are homeless experience a higher incidence of trauma-related injuries, developmental delays, sinusitis, anemia, asthma, bowel dysfunction, eczema, and visual and neurologic deficits (American Academy of Pediatrics, 2005). Additionally, homeless adolescent youth are at risk for violence and victimization, substance abuse, pregnancy, and sexually transmitted diseases (American Academy of Pediatrics, 2005).

Migrant Farmworker Families. Migrants generally suffer more illness, both acute and chronic, than the general population. They live in an environment of poverty, unstable and overcrowded housing, poor sanitation, unreliable transportation, and social isolation. Children of migrant farmworkers have a higher risk of respiratory and ear infections, gastroenteritis, intestinal parasites, skin infections, dental problems, lead and pesticide exposure, tuberculosis, short stature, undiagnosed congenital abnormalities, delayed development, and injuries (American Academy of Pediatrics, 2005).

When medical care is provided to migrant families, follow-up care is usually impossible because of their transient lifestyle. Compliance with medical therapies is primarily related to accessibility and availability. For example, medications provided by health workers are more likely to be taken than those that must be obtained at a pharmacy. In addition, medications are often discontinued after self-perceived recovery.

Immigrant Families. Children who have immigrated may have diseases such as malaria or hepatitis A that are more common in their country but rarely diagnosed in the United States. Immigrants have a higher rate of tuberculosis infections than U.S.-born persons. Immigrant children may not have been screened at birth for congenital diseases such as hemoglobinopathies and inborn errors of metabolism. Immunizations may not have been adequate as well (American Academy of Pediatrics, 2005).

CULTURAL CUSTOMS

Nurses must be aware of the need to consider cultural differences in patients when providing health care. An understanding of the various beliefs regarding the causation of illness and disease, as well as traditional health practices, is essential to successful intervention. The more nurses know about the values, beliefs, and customs of other ethnic groups, the better able they are to meet the needs of these families and to gain their cooperation and compliance.

NURSINGTIP

Cultural resources that include a brief description of the culture and views on health, illness, diet, and other matters are available on the Internet; some institutions develop their own quick references. A newer approach to cultural competence focuses on educating providers to be aware of certain cross-cutting cultural and social issues and health beliefs that are present in all cultures (Betancourt, Green, Carrillo, and others, 2003).

Cultural Relativism

Although clinical characteristics of a disease or condition are essentially the same across cultures, how a child or family interprets or experiences it varies. Culture as an influence is one obvious explanation for variance. **Cultural relativism** is the concept that any behavior must be judged first in the context of the culture in which it occurs (Purnell and Paulanka, 2003). Nurses must first relate to the family's perceptions and interpretations of experiences from the family's background and cultural belief system before they can effectively intervene.

Some cultures, for example, may view a chronic illness or disability as affecting only particular aspects of a child's life, and the child as a whole is viewed as normal. In contrast, Chinese families frequently describe the illness as having global effects on many aspects of the child's present and future life (Martinson, Armstrong, and Qiao, 1997). These contrasting views may result in a difference in goals and expectations that parents have for their children.

In some cultures the child's gender may influence a family's perception of the implications of an illness or disability. For example, in the Arabic and Asian cultures the male child is held in higher esteem than the female child. This also holds true for some families of Jewish, Italian, Greek, and Indian origin. The male child may receive better health care and more food because this is the child who will take care of his parents in their old age (Galanti, 2004).

Perceptions of disease or signs and symptoms of illness are also influenced by culture. Some cultures, for example, see diarrhea as a cleansing of the body that is essential for health maintenance and illness prevention or cure. Furthermore, signs or symptoms resulting from diarrhea and ensuing dehydration, such as malaise, fever, anorexia, and irritability, may be viewed as separate illness entities.

Nurses can often recognize a family's health-related cultural perceptions and interpretations through discussion and observation. Implications of these perceptions should be explored and considered when planning culturally appropriate interventions.

Relationships with Health Care Providers

Communication in the health care setting can be challenging when both parties speak the same language. It becomes even more complex when the patient and health care provider speak different languages. The same word can have different meaning in different cultures. Patients may say yes to a question they do not understand when they mean no. Communication styles can differ by style and demeanor, use of silence, use of eye contact, gestures, and body language (Galanti, 2004).

In relation to time, some cultures are oriented toward the clock, whereas others are more focused on activities. Conflicts can arise during an interaction involving these two orientations. For example, African Americans tend to be flexible in their time orientation; an African-American family may be late for or miss appointments because other issues take precedence, and the family may not communicate this to the health agency. The Japanese, on the other hand, consider time to be valuable and to be used wisely.

Family roles differ by culture as well. Decision making may involve the extended family. Authority figures in a family may be a mother or father or grandparent. Kinship structure is also determined by culture. Many cultures are unilateral in that

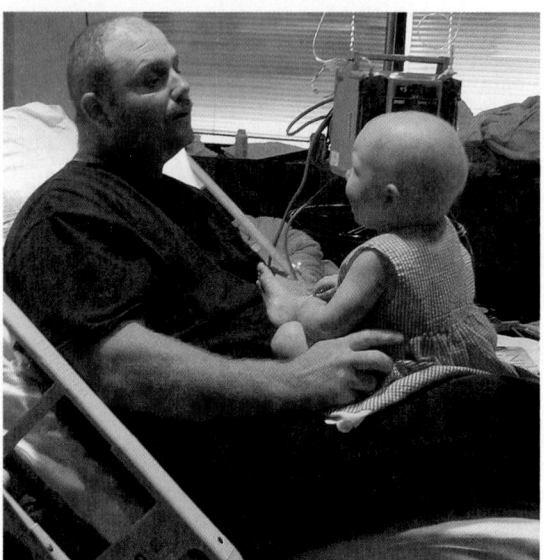

FIG. 4-4 ■ A father with his hospitalized child. (Courtesy E. Jacob, Texas Children's Hospital, Houston.)

they trace their descent from either a male or a female ancestor (Galanti, 2004) (Fig. 4-4).

> **NURSINGALERT**
>
> In working with families, it is essential for nurses to identify key members. Failure to include these significant individuals in teaching can seriously hinder adherence to the care plan.

Nurses should inform themselves of any specific attitudes regarding the manner of approach to a child in a given culture. A primary social premise for Navajo Indians is that no person has the right to speak for another. They may allow a child to decide whether to take a medicine or not, whereas in other cultures this view might be viewed as irresponsible (Purnell and Paulanka, 2003). Some ethnic groups, such as the Amish, consider a child's admission to the hospital a family affair, with all members gathering to support and console the child and parents. In others, such as the Samoan family, the family is willing to relinquish the care of the child to the hospital authority without interference. Their visits with the child are short, although intense, but this behavior may be misinterpreted by the hospital staff as indifference or abandonment.

Nurses who are members of a majority culture may encounter tension and distrust in a child from a minority culture as a result of the child's learned perception or relationships with other persons in the majority group. Based on these biases, minority children may suspect that nurses have hostile feelings toward them and fear ill treatment. When such children are hospitalized, this feeling compounds the feelings of loneliness, helplessness, and retribution that accompany frightening experiences and separation from families. The reverse situation may be encountered by a nurse from a minority culture attempting to meet the needs of a child who has been conditioned to view the nurse's cultural or ethnic group as inferior.

Communication. Communication may be a source of distress and misunderstanding between persons from different ethnic groups, especially if the languages are different.

Lack of interpreter services and linguistically appropriate health education materials are associated with patient dissatisfaction, poor understanding and adherence, and lower-quality health care (Betancourt, Green, Carrillo, and others, 2003). The Office of Minority Health of the U.S. Department of Health and Human Services has established national standards on culturally and linguistically appropriate services in health care. Health care organizations must ensure the competence of language assistance provided to persons with limited English proficiency (LEP) by interpreters and bilingual staff. Family and friends should not be used for interpretation services except on request by the patient (Shaw-Taylor, 2002).

Some persons with poor or limited language comprehension may simply smile and nod in agreement if they do not understand the questions or directives. It is vital that the family fully understand all implications of a child's care and management before they sign permits for special procedures or assume responsibility for the child's care. It is not uncommon for a Vietnamese or a Japanese family to indicate "yes" when in fact they mean "no" in order to avoid social disharmony. They tend to use indirectness rather than confrontation and may become evasive when direct questioning makes them uncomfortable.

NURSINGTIP

Helpful communication tools include the following:
- Have a series of audio and audiovisual recordings in several languages designed to greet and familiarize the family with the hospital.
- If an interpreter is not available on site, the Language Line, a national telephonic interpreter service for all languages, can be accessed by institutions as a back-up system.
- Have legal consent forms and explanations of common diagnostic tests available in several languages.
- Keep cards with common greetings, phrases, and names of body parts in the family's language with the patient's chart (e.g., miseries [pain] and locked bowels [constipation] in African Americans; and caida de la mollera [fallen fontanel from dehydration], susto [fright], dolor, duele, or lele [pain], and la diarrhea [diarrhea] in Hispanics).

Nonverbal communication is a practiced art in many Native American tribes, and the members are highly sensitive to body language. They emphasize periods of silence to formulate thoughts in preparation for speech and often remain silent after listening to statements by others to properly assimilate what has been said. Interruption, interjection, or haste to arrive at abrupt conclusions is perceived as immature behavior.

The level of comfort with body space or distance from others varies among cultures. For example, Hispanics tend to get closer, and Asians prefer a greater distance.

Eye contact is viewed differently in cultures. Although Anglos are advised to look people straight in the eye, it is not uncommon for persons in some ethnic groups to avoid eye contact and become uncomfortable when conversing with health workers. A Vietnamese patient may not look directly into the nurse's eyes as a sign of respect. Some Native Americans will make eye contact during the initial greeting, but continued, unwavering eye contact is considered insulting and disrespectful. Asians may consider eye contact a sign of hostility or impoliteness.

Gestures also may have different meanings. For example, some Asians consider finger or foot pointing disrespectful. Native Americans consider vigorous handshaking a sign of aggression, whereas to Anglos the gesture is a sign of good will.

Families may be reluctant to question or otherwise initiate contact with health professionals. In the Asian cultures, for example, it is considered a sign of disrespect to question those who are viewed as persons of authority. A Japanese family may wait silently rather than ask or question. They believe that the health professionals know best and will meet their needs without being asked. It is also important to avoid criticism. Criticism can cause Asians to "lose face," to feel ashamed, which is highly undesirable.

Language and bureaucracy have been considered the biggest barriers to the use of health care services by many families (Betancourt, Green, Carrillo, and others, 2003). Long intake processes and wait times are also barriers for minority patients. Often families may have poor language comprehension, so it is necessary to speak slowly and carefully, not loudly, when conversing with them. Many persons are able to read and write English better than they can speak or understand it. Also, the dominant language usually takes over in anxiety-provoking situations, even in those who are able to communicate satisfactorily under ordinary circumstances.

Terms of address and use of first and last names vary among cultures and can create confusion. For example, in Asian cultures the family name is given first in respect for the family and the given name follows. Therefore all siblings in a family have the same first name. Ethiopians have a complex system whereby women retain their last names after marriage and the paternal grandfather's name becomes the child's last name.

The expression of emotion also varies ethnically. In some cultures (e.g., Hispanic or Jewish) emotions are expressed openly and members are accustomed to sharing their sorrows and joys with family and friends. Conversely, Nordic and Asian groups are more restrained.

Health care providers generally ask questions and use handouts, booklets, and—particularly with children—dolls and pictures as communication aids. This is uncommon in some cultures. For example, Native American healers ask few questions and do not use forms. Nurses need to consider both verbal and nonverbal communication techniques to interact effectively with children and their families from different cultures (see Nursing Care Guidelines box).

Food Customs

Food customs and symbolism are an integral part of various cultural, ethnic, and religious groups. Although in a large country such as the United States most persons have adopted the eclectic food habits that have evolved over countless generations, many ethnic and geographic food traditions and preferences are retained. Special holidays, ceremonies, and life experiences such as births, birthdays, weddings, and death are often marked by special food items or feasts. In many cultures specific food practices are followed during pregnancy in the belief that certain foods damage the developing fetus.

The distinctive food customs of ethnic groups are a product of their native environment, determined by availability. Fish is a staple food of persons living near the ocean, such as people from Japan, Polynesia, Southern Europe, and Scandinavia. Fruit and vegetable preferences are directly related to the climate in which they grow naturally or can be cultivated. The types of grain that are ethnically associated are also those

nursingcareguidelines

Culturally Sensitive Interactions
NONVERBAL STRATEGIES

Invite family members to choose where they would like to sit or stand, allowing them to select a comfortable distance.

Observe interactions with others to determine which body gestures (e.g., shaking hands) are acceptable and appropriate. Ask when in doubt.

Avoid appearing rushed.

Be an active listener.

Observe for cues regarding appropriate eye contact.

Learn appropriate use of pauses or interruptions for different cultures.

Ask for clarification if nonverbal meaning is unclear.

VERBAL STRATEGIES

Learn proper terms of address.

Use a positive tone of voice to convey interest.

Speak slowly and carefully, not loudly, when families have poor language comprehension.

Encourage questions.

Learn basic words and sentences of family's language, if possible.

Avoid professional terms.

When asking questions, tell family why the questions are being asked, the way in which the information they provide will be used, and how it might benefit their child.

Repeat important information more than once.

Always give the reason or purpose for a treatment or prescription.

Use information written in family's language.

Obtain the services of an interpreter whenever there is uncertainty regarding full comprehension in a medical encounter (see Chapter 6).

Learn from families and representatives of their culture methods of communicating information without creating discomfort.

Address intergenerational needs (e.g., family's need to consult with others).

Be sincere, open, and honest and, when appropriate, share personal experiences, beliefs, and practices to establish rapport and trust.

FIG. 4-5 ■ Food customs outside the home can differ significantly from traditional cultural practices.

that grow best in the native lands. Even in the continental United States there are regional favorites, such as rice, hominy grits, and okra in the Southern states. In some cultures food is highly spiced; in others, foods tend to be bland.

Children may have a number of restrictions related to food items. Some have a physiologic origin, such as lack of dairy foods in the diets of some persons of African or Asian ancestry in whom a hereditary lactase deficiency prevents digestion of foods containing lactose. Others have religious restrictions, such as kosher foods and food preparation of the Orthodox Jewish faith, avoidance of pork in the diet of persons of Islamic faith, and the vegetarian diet of Seventh-Day Adventists (see Vegetarian Diets, Chapter 11).

Children in a strange environment, such as the hospital, feel much more comfortable when they are served familiar foods (Fig. 4-5). Hospital food often tastes strange and bland. The family may be concerned that their child is not receiving foods appropriate to their culture and beliefs. When possible, it is advisable to provide children ethnic foods or allow families to bring favorite foods. Concern for differences in food habits and patterns projects an attitude of respect for the family's ethnic or religious heritage.

HEALTH BELIEFS AND PRACTICES
Health Beliefs

Beliefs related to the cause of illness and the maintenance of health are an integral part of the cultural heritage of families. Often inseparable from religious beliefs, they influence the way that families cope with health problems and the way that they respond to health care providers. Predominant among most cultures are beliefs related to natural forces, supernatural forces, and imbalance between forces.

Natural Forces. The most common natural forces held responsible for ill health if the body is not adequately protected include cold air entering the body, impurities in the air, or other natural sources. For example, a Chinese mother may overdress her infant in an effort to keep cold wind from entering the child's body. The Chinese believe that cold weather, rain, and wind are responsible for "cold" conditions. In the African-American culture, natural phenomena such as phases of the moon, seasons of the year, and planet positions are believed to affect the body and its processes; therefore health maintenance is strongly associated with the ability to read "the signs." Most Native Americans consider health to be a state of harmony with nature and the universe.

Supernatural Forces. High on the list of causes of illness are forces beyond comprehension and logical explanation. Evil influences such as voodoo, witchcraft, or evil spirits are viewed in some cultures as causes of adverse health, especially those illnesses that cannot be explained by other means.

A health belief that is common among people from Central America, the Middle East, the Mediterranean, some Asian, and some African societies is the concept of the **evil eye** (Galanti, 2004). The general belief is that one person inflicts evil on another and causes the victim to fall ill. The motive is usually envy. Each culture that believes compliment can cause the evil eye also has ways to neutralize them. This is part of the concept of health as a state of balance, and illness as a state of imbalance (see Imbalance of Forces). Infants and small children, because of immature development of their internal strength-weakness states, are especially vulnerable to the gaze of the evil eye. Consequently, the evil eye concept serves to rationalize an inexplicable onset of illness in children who display such symptoms as restlessness, crying, diarrhea, vomiting, and fever.

Although seldom expressed to health care providers, the belief that a witch can cast a spell over others at the request of someone who wishes them ill is found in Caribbean, African, and Australian aboriginal cultures. The victim is often tortured in effigy by pins driven into a doll at the location where the intended victim is to be hurt. "Voodoo deaths" have occurred from the victim's belief in the curse and may result from dehydration as the victim gives up the will to live and refuses to drink (Chidester, 2001).

Imbalance of Forces. The concept of balance or equilibrium is widespread throughout the world. One of the most common imbalances supported by the Hispanic, Filipino, Chinese, and Arab cultures is that which exists between "hot" and "cold." This belief is reputedly derived from the Hippocratic theory of humoral pathology, which states that illness is caused by an imbalance of the four humors: phlegm, blood, black bile, and yellow bile. "Hot" and "cold" describe certain properties and conditions completely unrelated to temperature. Diseases, areas of the body, foods, and illnesses are classified as either "hot" or "cold." In Chinese health belief, the forces are termed **yin (cold)** and **yang (hot).** To maintain health, these "hot" and "cold" forces must be kept in balance.

Illness is treated by restoring normal balance through the application of appropriate "hot" or "cold" remedies. A "cold" condition such as a respiratory disease is believed to be caused by exposure to cold weather, rain, or cold wind entering the body; it is treated by administering "hot" foods, herbs, or drugs. Menstruation is considered to be a "hot" condition; therefore women are cautioned against ingesting "hot" foods, which might increase menstrual flow or produce cramping. Ingesting too much of either "hot" or "cold" foods can also be interpreted as a cause of illness.

Health care workers who are aware of this belief are better able to understand why some persons refuse to eat certain foods. It is possible to help families devise a diet that contains the necessary balance of basic food groups prescribed by the medical subculture while conforming to the beliefs of the ethnic subculture.

The hot-cold food classification may have adverse effects. For example, newborn infants are often started on evaporated milk formulas. Evaporated milk is considered to be a "hot" food, whereas whole milk is viewed as a "cold" food. Infants tend to develop rashes, which are believed to be caused by "hot" foods; in such cases, parents may decide to switch to whole milk. However, parents fear that it is dangerous to change too rapidly, so they often feed the child some type of neutralizing substance, which may create additional health problems. Such a problem might be averted if the family's preference is determined before discharge from the hospital, with a formula prescribed that is agreeable to both the family and the practitioner.

Health Practices

There are numerous similarities among cultures regarding prevention and treatment of illness. All cultures have some types of home remedies that they apply before seeking help from other persons. Within the ethnic community, folk healers who are endowed with the ability to "cure" maladies are sought for special situations and when home remedies are unsuccessful. There is the ***curandero*** (male) or ***curandera*** (female) of the Mexican-American community whose healing powers are believed to be a gift from God. The Asian consults an herbalist, knowledgeable in medicines, or an ethnic practitioner practiced in Asian therapies, including **acupuncture** (insertion of needles), **acupressure** (application of pressure), and **moxibustion** (application of heat). Native Americans consult a variety of healers with specific skills and knowledge. Specialized medicine persons diagnose illness, provide nonsacred treatments (usually by way of massage and herbs), and care for souls. Other specialists perform services or affect cures through spiritual means. Native Hawaiians consult ***kahunas*** and practice ***ho'oponopono*** to heal family imbalance or disputes.

The folk healers are powerful persons in their community. They "speak the language" of the family who seeks help and often combine their rituals and potions with prayer and entreaties to God. They also are able to create an atmosphere conducive to successful management. Furthermore, they exhibit a sincere interest in the family and their problem.

Some folk remedies are compatible with the medical regimen and can be used to reinforce the treatment plan. For example, most of the foods contraindicated for persons with peptic ulcers are "hot" foods and would be avoided because of their belief systems. Also, aspirin (a "hot" medication) is an appropriate therapy for "cold" diseases such as the common cold and arthritis. It is not uncommon to discover that a folk prescription has a scientific basis. However, numerous health remedies or preventive practices have no scientific basis, such as the use of garlic or ***asafetida*** (a bad-smelling gum resin obtained from various Asiatic plants that looks like a dried sponge), which is worn around the neck to prevent contagious diseases. Also, the wearing of copper or silver bracelets to protect the wearer as he or she grows has no scientific basis. Practices that do no harm should be respected. Overcoming the effect of the evil eye usually requires specialized rituals conducted by the appropriate practitioner. For example, the Chicano *curandera* ascertains that the condition is truly the result of the evil eye by performing an assessment ritual and then, with a confirmed diagnosis, performs a curative ritual. Sometimes the faith in the folk practitioner results in a delay in obtaining needed medical treatment, although the practitioner will usually suggest medical care if his or her ministrations are unsuccessful.

Health practices of different cultures may also present problems in assessment and interpretation. For example, certain cultural practices or remedies can be misdiagnosed as evidence of child abuse by uninformed professionals (Box 4-1). It is important to explain why these and other familiar remedies may now be considered harmful. Health care providers need to be aware of the practices so they do not misinterpret symptoms such as red welts from coining. Families need to understand how such practices can place them in jeopardy with child protective services (Galanti, 2004). Cultural health remedies that are detrimental to health include eating clay, excessive amounts of salt, or compounds that contain lead or mercury. A careful history can reveal these remedies, but it may require the collaboration of a folk healer to convince a user to stop the practice.

Faith healing and religious rituals are closely allied with many folk-healing practices. Wearing of amulets, medals, and other religious relics believed by the culture to protect the individual and facilitate healing is a common practice. It is important for health workers to recognize the value of this practice and keep the items where the family has placed them

---

BOX 4-1

Cultural Practices Possibly Considered Abusive by the Dominant Culture

Coining—An Asian practice that may produce weltlike lesions on the child's back when a coin, held on edge, is repeatedly rubbed lengthwise on the oiled skin to rid the body of a disease (Galanti, 2004).

Cupping—A practice in many parts of the world (Asia, Latin American, parts of Europe) of placing a container (e.g., tumbler, bottle, jar) containing steam against the skin surface to "draw out the poison" or other evil element. When the heated air within the container cools, a vacuum is created that produces a bruiselike blemish on the skin directly beneath the mouth of the container (Galanti, 2004).

Burning—A practice of some Southeast Asian groups whereby small areas of skin are burned to treat enuresis and temper tantrums.

Female genital mutilation (female circumcision)—Removal of or injury to any part of the female genital organ; practiced in some parts of Africa (Galanti, 2004).

Forced kneeling—A discipline measure of some Caribbean groups in which a child is forced to kneel for a long time.

Topical garlic application—A practice of Yemenite Jews in which crushed garlic cloves or garlic–petroleum jelly plaster is applied to the wrists to treat infectious disease. The practice can result in blisters or garlic burns.

Traditional remedies that contain lead—**Greta** and **azarcon** (Mexico; used for digestive problems), **paylooah** (Southeast Asia; used for rash or fever), and **surma** (India; used as a cosmetic to improve eyesight).

BOX 4-2

BELIEF Framework for Integrating Culture and Spirituality into the Nursing Assessment

Belief system—A spiritual belief system is the tenet regarding a higher power that gives structure and form to everyday lives.

Ethics or values—Ethical or personal belief systems that guide the family's everyday life. The family may not follow a formal religion but still follow core values.

Lifestyle—Diet, nutrition, use of caffeine and alcohol, prayer and meditation, clothing, and medicinal practices all are examples where culture, religion, and spirituality may be closely connected.

Involvement in a spiritual community—The community can provide the family the benefits of identity, socialization, and support, while keeping children and adolescents involved in safe and healthy social activities.

Education—Religious education affects the cultural, moral, and ethical development of children. The children's belief system influences their coping mechanisms, especially during chronic illness.

Future events—Knowledge of the patient and family's belief system allows the nurse to provide individualized and sensitive anticipatory guidance for future health events.

From McEvoy M: Culture and spirituality as an integrated concept in pediatric care, *MCN* 28(1):39-43, 2003.

---

or nearby. It offers comfort and support and rarely impedes medical and nursing care. If an item must be removed during a procedure, it should be replaced, if possible, when the procedure is completed. The reason for its temporary removal is explained to the family, and they are reassured that their wishes will be respected.

Nurses can be most effective by operating from a multicultural perspective. Adopting a multicultural perspective means using appropriate aspects of each culture's orientation to health to develop culturally acceptable health care interventions.

NURSINGALERT

Avoid directly criticizing traditional health cultural beliefs and practices as wrong or harmful or implying that biomedical measures are uniformly correct and effective and the only way to prevent illness or treat sickness. Such criticisms usually result in rejection of both biomedical health care practitioners and their health teaching. When folk practices do not interfere with the patient's welfare, they need not be discouraged. Often a compromise can be reached that accomplishes the nurse's goal while maintaining the dignity and self-esteem of the child and family.

RELIGIOUS BELIEFS

Religious and spiritual dimensions are among the most important influences in many people's lives. The term **spirituality** relates to an individual's personal beliefs, transcendent experiences, and principles; **religion** refers to an organized system of beliefs or a place of worship. The pediatric nurse who learns how the patient and family view their traditions, values, and beliefs can understand how these dimensions may affect the patient's health (McEvoy, 2003). Three areas to explore for information about the family's culture, religion, or

spirituality are beliefs and values, daily practices, and community involvement. An assessment tool can be easily used for integrating culture and spirituality into the nursing assessment (Box 4-2).

Religion affects the way people interpret and respond to illness (Spector, 2004). Among many groups, illness, injury, or death is believed to be sent by God as a punishment for sin. Some may believe that health workers will be unable to help a person whom God is punishing and may express a fatalistic attitude toward treatment, stating it is "the will of God." Others view it as a test of strength, like the testing of Job in the Bible, and strive to remain faithful and overcome the conflicts.

Religious affiliation has implications for many health-related functions and procedures. It is comforting for the family of an ill child to have this need recognized and respected. Nurses need to determine whether there are any special considerations, including dietary restrictions, related to spiritual practices that are important to the family. Family members are asked whether they want a clergy member present and whether they prefer hospital staff to call or prefer to do this on their own.

It is also important to determine the wishes of the family regarding baptism, rites or practices related to death, and other religious rituals (such as circumcision, communion, or use of amulets or icons). Religion, which offers families understanding and spiritual support, is a valuable asset to health care. Characteristics of selected religions with beliefs that affect health care are outlined in Table 4-1.

IMPORTANCE OF CULTURE AND RELIGION TO NURSES

A general agreement exists among nurses to raise the cultural competence of professional nursing practice. To begin to understand and deal effectively with families in a multicultural community, nurses need to recognize barriers to transcultural communication and work to remove these barriers (Muñoz

TABLE 4-1

Religious Beliefs That May Affect Nursing Care

BIRTH AND DEATH	DIET AND FOOD PRACTICES	MEDICAL CARE
BUDDHIST		
Birth: No baptism Infant presentation **Death:** Last rite chanting is often practiced at bedside soon after death; the deceased's family or Buddhist priest should be contacted. **Organ donation/transplantation:** Organ donation is a matter of individual conscience.	Restrictions on some food combinations; extremes must be avoided. Some sects are strictly vegetarian. Discourage use of alcohol and drugs.	Illness is believed to be a trial to aid development of soul; illness results from Karmic causes. Surgery is permitted, but extremes must be avoided. Cleanliness is of great importance. Family, community, and Buddhist priest are supportive visitors.
CHURCH OF CHRIST, SCIENTIST (CHRISTIAN SCIENCE)		
Birth: No baptism **Death:** No last rites; autopsy is not permitted except in cases of sudden death; individuals can choose burial or cremation. **Organ donation/transplantation:** Church takes no specific position on transplantation as distinct from other medical or surgical procedures. Individuals decide on organ donation.	Abstain from alcohol and some forms of tea and coffee.	Oppose human intervention with drugs or other therapies; however, accept legally required immunizations. Accept physical and moral healing. Family, friends, and members of spiritual community may visit.
CHURCH OF JESUS CHRIST OF LATTER DAY SAINTS (MORMON)		
Birth: No baptism Infant is blessed by church official at first opportunity after birth (in church). Baptism by immersion at 8 years. **Death:** Believe that it is proper to bury the dead in the ground; cremation is discouraged. **Organ donation/transplantation:** Individuals can choose whether to will organs to be used in transplants.	Prohibit tea (except herbal), coffee, and alcohol. Some individuals avoid chocolate and other products that contain caffeine. Fasting for 24 hours each month.	Devout adherents believe in divine healing. Medical therapy is not prohibited. Spiritual items: a "garment" (type of underwear) that is considered sacred; person may not want to remove it. Family, friends, and church members are supportive visitors.
HINDU		
Birth: No baptism **Death:** Certain prescribed rites are followed after death; priest may tie thread around neck or wrist to signify blessing; family will wash the body; are particular about who touches their dead; bodies are to be cremated. **Organ donation/transplantation:** No religious laws prohibiting donation; individual decision.	Many dietary restrictions. Eating meat is forbidden.	With an amputation, loss of a limb is believed to represent sins committed in previous life. Accept most modern medical practices; some belief in faith healing. Spiritual item: Person may wear a thread around wrist or body; do not remove it. Family, community members, and priest are supportive visitors.
ISLAM (MUSLIM/MOSLEM)		
Birth: At birth, the first words said to the infant in his or her right ear are *Allah-o-Akbar* (Allah is great), and the remainder of the Call for Prayer is recited. An *Aqeeqa* (party) to celebrate the birth of the child is arranged by the parents. Male children are circumcised. **Death:** At the time of death, specific rituals (e.g., bathing, wrapping the body in cloth) must be done by same-sex Muslim. Before moving and handling the body, it is preferable to contact someone from the person's mosque or the local Islamic Society to perform these rituals. **Organ donation/transplantation:** Individual decides on organ donation/transplantation.	Prohibit all pork products and alcohol. Fasting is practiced during the ninth month of the Islamic year (Ramadan).	Believers are encouraged in the Qu'ran to seek treatment. It is taught that only Allah cures; however, Muslims are taught not to refuse treatment in the belief that Allah will take care of them because he also chooses at times to work through the efforts of humans. Other practices: Right hand is used for eating; left hand is for hygiene. Family and friends are supportive visitors.

Data from Galanti G: *Caring for patients from different cultures,* ed 3, Philadelphia, 2004, University of Pennsylvania Press; Lipson JG, Dibble SL, Minarik PA: *Culture and clinical care: a pocket guide,* San Francisco, 2005, UCSF Nursing Press; Purnell LD, Paulanka BJ: *Transcultural health care: a culturally competent approach,* Philadelphia, 2003, Davis; Spector RE: *Cultural diversity in health and illness,* ed 6, Upper Saddle River, NJ, 2004, Pearson Prentice Hall.

Continued

TABLE 4-1		
Religious Beliefs That May Affect Nursing Care—cont'd		
BIRTH AND DEATH	DIET AND FOOD PRACTICES	MEDICAL CARE
JEHOVAH'S WITNESSES **Birth:** No baptism **Death:** No official last rites are practiced when death occurs. **Organ donation/transplantation:** Organ donation is forbidden.	No tobacco; moderate alcohol permissible.	Blood or blood products are not allowed; volume expanders are permissible if not derived from blood.
JUDAISM (ORTHODOX AND CONSERVATIVE) **Birth:** No baptism Ritual circumcision of male infants on eighth day; performed by mohel (ritual circumciser familiar with Jewish law and aseptic technique). **Death:** According to tradition, during last moments of life, relatives and close friends remain with the deceased. Amputated limbs or surgically removed tissues should be made available to family for burial. Cremation not allowed. **Organ donation/transplantation:** Organ transplantation/donation is complex issue; sometimes they are practiced.	Numerous dietary kosher laws exist; followers are allowed only meat from animals that are vegetable eaters and are ritually slaughtered; predatory fowl, shellfish, and pork are prohibited. Milk products served first can be followed by meat in a few minutes, but milk may not be consumed for several hours after eating meat. Fasting is part of Yom Kippur observance. Matzo replaces leavened bread during Passover week.	May resist surgical procedures during Sabbath, which extends from sundown Friday until sundown Saturday. Illness is grounds for violating dietary laws. Spiritual items: Men may wear prayer shawl, yarmulka (cap) while praying. Family, friends, and rabbi are supportive visitors.
ROMAN CATHOLIC **Birth:** Infant baptism; especially urgent if poor prognosis, when it may be performed by anyone **Death:** Sacrament of the Sick is performed if prognosis is poor while patient is alive. **Organ donation/transplantation:** Transplantation of organs is viewed by Catholics as ethically and morally acceptable to Vatican; organ donation is viewed as an act of charity.	Abstaining from meat is practiced on Ash Wednesday, Good Friday, and Fridays during Lent (as a rule).	Encourage anointing of the sick. Spiritual items: Rosary beads, crucifix Traditional church teaching does not approve of contraceptives or abortion.

Data from Galanti G: *Caring for patients from different cultures,* ed 3, Philadelphia, 2004, University of Pennsylvania Press; Lipson JG, Dibble SL, Minarik PA: *Culture and clinical care: a pocket guide,* San Francisco, 2005, UCSF Nursing Press; Purnell LD, Paulanka BJ: *Transcultural health care: a culturally competent approach,* Philadelphia, 2003, Davis; Spector RE: *Cultural diversity in health and illness,* ed 6, Upper Saddle River, NJ, 2004, Pearson Prentice Hall.

BOX 4-3
Exploring Your Cultural Competence: ASKED Model of Cultural Competence

Awareness—Am I aware of my personal biases and prejudices toward cultural groups different from mine?

Skill—Do I have the skill to conduct a cultural assessment and perform a culturally based physical assessment in a sensitive manner?

Knowledge—Do I have knowledge of the patient's world view and the field of biocultural ecology?

Encounters—How many face-to-face encounters have I had with patients from diverse cultural backgrounds?

Desire—What is my genuine desire to "want to be" culturally competent?

Data from Campinha-Bacote J: Many faces: addressing diversity in health care, *Online J Issues Nurs* 8:1, 2003; retrieved May 5, 2007, from http://www.nursingworld.org/ojin/topic20/tpc20_2.htm.

and Luckmann, 2005). Nurses, too, are a product of their own cultural background. They also need to recognize that they are part of the "nursing culture." Nurses function within the framework of a professional culture with its own values and traditions and, as such, become socialized into their professional culture in their educational program and later in their work environments and professional associations.

Frequently, nurses and other health care workers are not aware of their own cultural values and how those values influence their thoughts and actions. A model for self-examination on cultural competence is the *ASKED* model (Box 4-3). Recognizing that a behavior may be characteristic of a culture rather than an "abnormal" behavior places nurses at an advantage in their relationships with families. When nurses respect a family's cultural differences, they are better able to determine whether the behavior is distinctive to the individual or a characteristic of the culture.

Cultural standards and values, family structure and function, and experience with health care influence a family's feelings and attitudes toward health, their children, and health care delivery systems. It is often difficult for nurses to be nonjudgmental and objective in working with families whose behaviors and attitudes differ from or conflict with their own. The nurse needs to understand how one's own cultural background influences the way care is delivered (American Nurses Association, 1991). Relying on one's own values and experiences for guidance can result in frustration and disappointment. It is one thing to know what is needed to deal with a health problem; it is often quite another to implement a fruitful course of action unless nurses work within the cultural and socioeconomic framework of the family.

It is beneficial to adapt ethnic practices to the family's health needs rather than to attempt to change longstanding beliefs. To aid their efforts to understand and respect the cultural beliefs of families, nurses need to develop knowledge on how cultural groups understand life processes, define health and illness, and view the causes of illness. Nurses should combine their cross-cultural knowledge with excellent communication skills to learn from the individual patient and family about issues important to their care (Betancourt, Green, Carrillo, and others, 2003).

Some broad characteristics of selected cultures are outlined in Table 4-2. Tables 4-1 and 4-2 are presented as beginning frameworks for practicing transcultural nursing. Nurses must assess the cultural and religious practices of families to identify how these practices are similar to and different from those of their own cultural and religious backgrounds.

> **NURSINGALERT**
>
> These generalizations are presented to help nurses learn the unique beliefs and practices of various groups and are not meant to be used as stereotypes of any group. A stereotype is an end point. The nurse does not attempt to learn where the individual fits the statement. A generalization provides a beginning point from which the nurse can inquire further to obtain more information and individualize the patient's care (Galanti, 2004).

TABLE 4-2

Broad Cultural Characteristics Related to Health Care of Children and Families

HEALTH BELIEFS	HEALTH PRACTICES	FAMILY RELATIONSHIPS	COMMUNICATION
AFRICAN			
Illness classified as: **Natural**—affected by forces of nature without adequate protection (e.g., cold air, pollution, food and water) **Unnatural**—God's punishment for improper behavior May see illness as the "will of God"	Self-care and folk medicine prevalent Folk therapies usually religious in origin Folk therapies often not shared with the medical provider Prayer as common means for prevention and treatment	Strong kinship bonds in extended family; members come to aid of others in crisis Less likely to view illness as a burden Place strong emphasis on work and ambition Elders cared for and respected	Alert to any evidence of discrimination Place importance on nonverbal behavior Affection shown by touching and hugging Silence may indicate lack of trust Initial eye contact to show respect; maintaining eye contact can be viewed as aggressive Best to use direct but caring approach
CHINESE			
A healthy body viewed as gift from parents and ancestors and must be cared for Health seen as one of the results of balance between the forces of **yin** (cold) and **yang** (hot)—energy forces that rule the world Illness caused by imbalance Blood believed to be source of life and is not regenerated **Chi** is innate energy	Goal of therapy—to restore balance of yin and yang Acupuncturist needles applied to appropriate meridians identified in terms of yin and yang Acupressure and **tai chi** replacing acupuncture in some areas **Moxibustion**—application of heat to skin over specific meridians Wide use of medicinal herbs procured and applied in prescribed ways Meals may or may not be planned to balance hot and cold	Extended family pattern common Strong concept of loyalty of young to old Respect for elders taught at early age—acceptance without questioning or talking back Children's behavior a reflection on family Family and individual honor and "face" important Self-reliance and self-esteem highly valued; self-expression repressed	Open expression of emotions unacceptable Often smile when they do not comprehend Eye contact avoided as sign of respect

Data from Galanti G: *Caring for patients from different cultures*, ed 3, Philadelphia, 2004, University of Pennsylvania Press; Lipson JG, Dibble SL, Minarik PA: *Culture and clinical care: a pocket guide*, San Francisco, 2005, UCSF Nursing Press; Purnell LD, Paulanka BJ: *Transcultural health care: a culturally competent approach*, Philadelphia, 2003, Davis; Spector RE: *Cultural diversity in health and illness*, ed 6, Upper Saddle River, NJ, 2004, Pearson Prentice Hall.

Continued

TABLE 4-2

Broad Cultural Characteristics Related to Health Care of Children and Families—cont'd

HEALTH BELIEFS	HEALTH PRACTICES	FAMILY RELATIONSHIPS	COMMUNICATION
HAITIAN			
Illness seen as a punishment **Natural** cause (*maladi bone die*—disease of the Lord) caused by environmental factors, movement of blood within the body, changes between hot and cold, and bone displacement **Supernatural** (*loa*—spirits' anger) Good health seen as the maintenance of equilibrium Prayer and good spiritual habits important	Health a personal responsibility Foods have properties of "hot"/"cold" and "light"/"heavy" and must be in harmony with one's life cycle and bodily states Natural illnesses treated by home and folk remedies first May use religious medallions, rosary beads, or figure of saint to pray with	Maintenance of family reputation paramount Lineal authority supreme; children in a subordinate position in family hierarchy Children valued for parental security in old age and expected to contribute to family welfare at an early age	Recent immigrants and older persons may speak only Haitian Creole Often smile and nod in agreement when do not understand Quiet and gentle communication style and lack of assertiveness lead health care providers to falsely believe they comprehend health teaching and are compliant May not ask questions if health care provider is busy or rushed
JAPANESE			
Shinto religious influence Human inherently good Evil caused by outside spirits Illness caused by contact with polluting agents (e.g., blood, corpses, skin diseases) Health achieved through harmony and balance between self and society Disease caused by disharmony with society and not caring for body	Energy restored by means of acupuncture, acupressure, massage, and moxibustion along affected meridians *Kampō* medicine—use of natural herbs Believe in removal of diseased parts Trend is to use both Western and Asian healing methods Care for disabled viewed as family's responsibility Take pride in child's good health Seek preventive care, medical care for illness	Close intergenerational relationships Generational categories: *Issei*—first generation to live in United States *Nisei*—second generation *Sansei*—third generation *Yonsei*—fourth generation Family tends to keep problems to self Value self-control and self-sufficiency Concept of *haji* (shame) imposes strong control; unacceptable behavior of children reflects on family	Make significant use of nonverbal communication with subtle gestures and facial expression Tend to suppress emotions Will often wait silently
MEXICAN-AMERICAN			
Health controlled by environment, fate, and will of God Certain illnesses considered "hot" and "cold" states and are treated with food that complements those states Disease based on imbalance between individual and environment	Seek help from *curandero* or *curandera*, especially in rural areas *Curandero(a)* receives position by birth, apprenticeship, or a "calling" via dream or vision Treatments involve use of herbs, rituals, and religious artifacts Practice for severe illness—make promises, visit shrines, offer medals and candles, offer prayers Adhere to "hot" and "cold" food prescriptions and prohibitions for prevention and treatment of illness	Strong kinship—extended families include **compadres** (godparents) established by ritual kinship Children valued highly and desired, taken everywhere with family Elderly treated with respect	Spanish speaking or bilingual May have a strong preference for native language and revert to it in times of stress May shake hands or engage in introductory embrace Interpret prolonged eye contact as disrespectful Relaxed concept of time—may be late to appointments
NATIVE AMERICAN			
Believe health is state of harmony with nature and universe Respect bodies through proper management Depend on individual belief in traditional culture Traditional health beliefs holistic and wellness oriented	Distinction made between indigenous health problem requiring native healer or practice and Western disease requiring other medical care Health practices include self-sufficiency and harmonious living Participation in religious ceremonies and prayer promotes health	Cultures vary in kinship structure Extended family structure—usually includes relatives from both sides of family Elder members assume leadership roles	Use anecdotes or metaphors to discuss a situation Long pauses indicate careful consideration Nonverbal communication Respect indicated by avoiding eye contact Individuals usually speak for themselves

Data from Galanti G: *Caring for patients from different cultures*, ed 3, Philadelphia, 2004, University of Pennsylvania Press; Lipson JG, Dibble SL, Minarik PA: *Culture and clinical care: a pocket guide*, San Francisco, 2005, UCSF Nursing Press; Purnell LD, Paulanka BJ: *Transcultural health care: a culturally competent approach*, Philadelphia, 2003, Davis; Spector RE: *Cultural diversity in health and illness*, ed 6, Upper Saddle River, NJ, 2004, Pearson Prentice Hall.

TABLE 4-2			
Broad Cultural Characteristics Related to Health Care of Children and Families—cont'd			
HEALTH BELIEFS	HEALTH PRACTICES	FAMILY RELATIONSHIPS	COMMUNICATION
PUERTO RICAN			
Subscribe to the "hot-cold" theory of causation of illness Believe some illness caused by evil forces Destiny (*Si Dios quiere*—if God wants) is in control of health	Infrequent use of health care system Seek folk healers (*espiritistas*)—use of herbs, rituals Treatment classified as "hot" or "cold" Many varieties of herbal teas used to treat illness and promote healing	Family usually large and home centered—the core of existence Father has authority in family Great respect for elders Children valued—seen as a gift from God Children taught to obey and respect parents	Spanish speaking or bilingual Strong sense of family privacy—may view questions regarding family as impudent
VIETNAMESE			
Good health considered to be balance between yin and yang Concept of health based on harmony and balance Rituals used to prevent illness	Family uses all means possible before using outside agencies for health care Regard health as family responsibility; outside aid sought when resources run out Use herbal medicine, spiritual practices, and acupuncture May consider head sacred and feet profane; avoid touching head after feet May use cupping, coin rubbing, or pinching skin May inhale aromatic oils, take herbal teas, or wear strings tied on body	Family is revered institution Multigenerational families Family is chief social network Children highly valued Individual needs and interests subordinate to those of a family group Father is main decision maker Women taught submission to men Parents expect respect and obedience from children	May hesitate to ask questions Questioning authority is sign of disrespect; asking questions considered impolite May avoid eye contact with health professionals as a sign of respect

KEY POINTS

- Culture is the sum total of mores, traditions, and beliefs about how people function and encompasses other products of human works and thoughts specific to members of an intergenerational group, community, or population.
- Nurses have a responsibility to continually develop cultural competence. This includes understanding and respecting the influence of culture, race, and ethnicity on the development of social and emotional relationships, childrearing practices, and attitudes toward health.
- A child's self-concept evolves from ideas about his or her social roles.
- Important subcultural influences on children include ethnicity, socioeconomic class, poverty, homelessness, immigration, religion, schools, community, and peers.
- A trend that has significantly influenced the American family is increasing geographic and economic mobility.
- Membership in a minority group presents special challenges for children, although changes in societal attitudes are slowly taking place.

- A child's physical characteristics and susceptibility to health problems can be related to ethnic and cultural variations of hereditary and socioeconomic forces.
- Groups of children suffering from greater physical and mental health problems are those living in poverty, those who are homeless, those who live in migrant farm families, and those who are recent immigrants to the United States.
- Because verbal and nonverbal communication is an important cultural consideration, nurses need to acknowledge and respect their patient's practices for productive interaction to occur.
- Cultural beliefs related to cause of illness and maintenance of health may focus on natural forces, supernatural forces, or imbalance of forces.
- In planning and implementing patient care, nurses need to strive to adapt ethnic practices to the family's health needs rather than attempt to change longstanding beliefs.
- No cultural group is homogeneous; every racial and ethnic group contains great diversity.

??? answers to
CRITICAL THINKING EXERCISE

REDUCING CULTURAL SHOCK

1. Yes. An understanding of the Arab culture provides insight into the woman's hesitancy to make decisions in her husband's absence.

2. a. Typically in the Arab culture men make the decisions and women are expected to support these decisions.

   b. The need for an interpreter is evident to make certain the mother understands the seriousness of the situation.

   c. Knowledge of the procedures for obtaining approval for emergency procedures without informed consent will facilitate obtaining the best care for the child.

   d. Appropriate documentation of how approval was obtained without parental consent is essential.

3. The first priority is to make certain the child is receiving the best care possible and that the necessary procedure is performed as soon as possible. The next priority is to use an interpreter to ensure the mother understands that the situation is an emergency.

4. Yes. The health status of the child is most important at this time.

5. Attempts to reach the father by phone should continue, and continued support of the mother during this stressful time is important.

REFERENCES

American Academy of Pediatrics: Committee on Community Health Services: providing care for immigrant, homeless, and migrant children, *Pediatrics* 115(4):1095-1100, 2005.

American Nurses Association: *Position statement: cultural diversity in nursing practice,* 1991, retrieved April 15, 2007, from http://nursingworld.org/readroom/position/ethics/etcldv.htm.

Annie E Casey Foundation: One out of five U.S. children is living in an immigrant family, *Data Snapshot,* no. 4, March 2007, retrieved April 15, 2007, from http://www.kidscount.org/sld/snapshot_immigrant.pdf.

Annie E Casey Foundation: *2006 Kids count data book; state profiles of child well-being,* 2006, retrieved April 20, 2007, from http://www.aecf.org/upload/PublicationFiles/DA36221056.pdf.

Betancourt JR: Cultural competence—marginal or mainstream movement, *N Engl J Med* 351(10):953-954, 2004.

Betancourt JR, Green AR, Carrillo JE, and others: Defining cultural competence: a practical framework for addressing racial/ethnic disparities in health and healthcare, *Pub Health Rep* 118:292-302, 2003.

Centers for Disease Control and Prevention: *Childhood lead poisoning prevention program,* 2007, retrieved April 22, 2007, from http://www.cdc.gov/nceh/publications/factsheets/ChildhoodLeadPoisoningPreventionProgram.pdf.

Chidester D: *Patterns of transcendence: religion, death, and dying,* ed 2, Belmont, Calif, 2001, Wadsworth.

Dreher M, MacNaughton N: Cultural competence in nursing: foundation or fallacy? *Nurs Outlook* 50:181-186, 2002.

Dunn AM: Culture competence and the primary care provider, *J Pediatr Health Care* 16:105-111, 2002.

Galanti G: *Caring for patients from different cultures,* ed 3, Philadelphia, 2004, University of Pennsylvania Press.

Garwick A, Auger S: What do providers need to know about American Indian culture? Recommendations from urban Indian family caregivers, *Fam Systems Health* 18:177-189, 2000.

Giger JN, Davidhizar RE: *Transcultural nursing: assessment and intervention,* ed 4, St Louis, 2004, Mosby.

Jones DC, Crawford JK: The peer appearance culture during adolescence: gender and body mass variations, *J Youth Adolesc* 2:257-269, 2006.

Leininger M: *Transcultural nursing,* New York, 1978, John Wiley & Sons.

Martinson IM, Armstrong V, Qiao J: The experience of the family of children with chronic illness at home in China, *Pediatr Nurs* 23(4):371-375, 1997.

McEvoy M: Culture and spirituality as an integrated concept in pediatric care, *MCN* 28(1):39-43, 2003.

Meléndez L: Parental beliefs and practices around early self-regulation: the impact of culture and immigration, *Infants Young Child* 18(2):136-146, 2005.

Muñoz C, Luckmann J: *Transcultural communication in nursing,* ed 2, Clifton Park, NY, 2005, Thomson Delmar Learning.

Purnell LD, Paulanka BJ: *Transcultural health care: a culturally competent approach,* ed 2, Philadelphia, 2003, Davis.

Scruggs L, Allan JP: The material consequences of welfare states: benefit generosity and absolute poverty in 16 OECD countries, *Comp Pol Studies* 39:880-904, 2006.

Search-Institute: *Developmental asset categories 2007,* retrieved May 2, 2007, from http://www.search-institute/org/assets/assetcategories.html.

Shaw-Taylor Y: Culturally and linguistically appropriate health care for racial or ethnic minorities: analysis of the US Office of Minority Health's recommended standards, *Health Policy* 62:211-221, 2002.

Spector RE: *Cultural diversity in health and illness,* ed 6, Upper Saddle River, NJ, 2004, Prentice-Hall.

Trawick-Smith J: *Early childhood development: a multicultural perspective,* ed 4, Upper Saddle River, NJ, 2006, Pearson Education.

Tropello PD: The many faces of homelessness. In Kelley ML, Fitzsimons VM, editors: *Understanding cultural diversity,* Sudbury, Mass, 2000, Jones & Bartlett.

US Census Bureau: *Overview of race and Hispanic origin: Census 2000 brief,* 2001, retrieved May 5, 2007, from http://www.census.gov/prod/2001pubs/c2kbr01-1.pdf.

Developmental Influences on Child Health Promotion

JOY HESSELGRAVE

CHAPTER OUTLINE

GROWTH AND DEVELOPMENT, 72
Foundations of Growth and
  Development, 72
  Stages of Development, 72
  Patterns of Growth and Development, 72
  Individual Differences, 74
Biologic Growth and Physical
  Development, 74
  External Proportions, 74
  Biologic Determinants of Growth and
    Development, 75
  Skeletal Growth and Maturation, 75
  Neurologic Maturation, 76
  Lymphoid Tissues, 76
  Development of Organ Systems, 76
Physiologic Changes, 76
  Metabolism, 76
  Temperature, 77
  Sleep and Rest, 77
Temperament, 77
  Significance of Temperament, 78
**DEVELOPMENT OF PERSONALITY
AND MENTAL FUNCTION, 78**
Theoretic Foundations of Personality
  Development, 78
  Psychosexual Development (Freud), 78
  Psychosocial Development (Erikson), 79

Theoretic Foundations of Mental
  Development, 80
  Cognitive Development (Piaget), 80
  Language Development, 81
  Moral Development (Kohlberg), 81
  Spiritual Development (Fowler), 81
Development of Self-Concept, 82
  Body Image, 82
  Self-Esteem, 82
ROLE OF PLAY IN DEVELOPMENT, 83
Classification of Play, 83
Content of Play, 83
Social Character of Play, 84
Functions of Play, 85
  Sensorimotor Development, 85
  Intellectual Development, 85
  Socialization, 85
  Creativity, 85
  Self-Awareness, 85
  Therapeutic Value, 85
  Moral Value, 85
Toys, 86
  Toy Safety, 86

**SELECTED FACTORS THAT INFLUENCE
DEVELOPMENT, 86**
Heredity, 86
Neuroendocrine Factors, 86
Nutrition, 88
Interpersonal Relationships, 88
Socioeconomic Level, 89
Disease, 89
Environmental Hazards, 89
Stress in Childhood, 89
  Coping, 90
Influence of the Mass Media, 90
  Reading Materials, 90
  Movies, 90
  Television, 91
  Video Games, 92
  Internet, 93
DEVELOPMENTAL ASSESSMENT, 93
Denver II, 93
Denver II Prescreening Developmental
  Questionnaire, 94

LEARNING OBJECTIVES

On completion of this chapter the
reader will be able to:
- Describe major trends in growth and
  development.
- Explain the alterations in the major body
  systems that take place during the
  process of growth and development.

- Discuss the development and
  relationships of personality, cognition,
  language, morality, spirituality, and self-
  concept.
- Describe the role of play in the growth
  and development of children.

- Demonstrate an understanding of the role
  of innate and environmental factors in
  the physical and emotional development
  of children.

RELATED TOPICS and ADDITIONAL RESOURCES

IN TEXT

Growth Failure (Failure to Thrive), *Ch. 11*
Health Promotion of the Adolescent and
    Family, *Ch. 16*
Health Promotion of the Infant and Family,
    Ch. 10
Health Promotion of the Preschooler and
    Family, *Ch. 13*

Health Promotion of the School-Age Child
    and Family, *Ch. 15*
Health Promotion of the Toddler and Family,
    Ch. 12
Providing Opportunities for Play and
    Expressive Activities, *Ch. 21*
Use of Play in Procedures, *Ch. 22*

COMPANION CD

Critical Thinking Exercise—Growth Trends
    During Infancy
NCLEX Review Questions

evolve

evolve.elsevier.com/Wong/essentials/

NCLEX Review Questions
WebLinks

GROWTH AND DEVELOPMENT

FOUNDATIONS OF GROWTH AND DEVELOPMENT

Growth and development, usually referred to as a unit, express the sum of the numerous changes that take place during the lifetime of an individual. The entire course is a dynamic process that encompasses several interrelated dimensions:

> **Growth**—an increase in number and size of cells as they divide and synthesize new proteins; results in increased size and weight of the whole or any of its parts
>
> **Development**—a gradual change and expansion; advancement from lower to more advanced stages of complexity; the emerging and expanding of the individual's capacities through growth, maturation, and learning
>
> **Maturation**—an increase in competence and adaptability; aging; usually used to describe a qualitative change; a change in the complexity of a structure that makes it possible for that structure to begin functioning; to function at a higher level
>
> **Differentiation**—processes by which early cells and structures are systematically modified and altered to achieve specific and characteristic physical and chemical properties; sometimes used to describe the trend of mass to specific; development from simple to more complex activities and functions

All these processes are interrelated, simultaneous, and ongoing; none occurs apart from the others. The processes depend on a sequence of endocrine, genetic, constitutional, environmental, and nutritional influences (Seidel, Ball, Dains, and others, 2007). The child's body becomes larger and more complex; the personality simultaneously expands in scope and complexity. Very simply, growth can be viewed as a **quantitative** change, and development as a **qualitative** change.

Stages of Development

Most authorities in the field of child development conveniently categorize child growth and behavior into approximate age stages or in terms that describe the features of an age-group. The age ranges of these stages are admittedly arbitrary and, because they do not take into account individual differences, cannot be applied to all children with any degree of precision. However, categorization affords a convenient means to describe the characteristics associated with the majority of children at periods when distinctive developmental changes appear and specific developmental tasks must be accomplished. (A **developmental task** is a set of skills and competencies peculiar to each developmental stage that children must accomplish or master to deal effectively with their environment.) It is also significant for nurses to know that there

are characteristic health problems peculiar to each major phase of development. The sequence of descriptive age periods and subperiods that are used here and elaborated in subsequent chapters is listed in Box 5-1.

Patterns of Growth and Development

There are definite and predictable patterns in growth and development that are continuous, orderly, and progressive. These patterns, or trends, are universal and basic to all human beings, but each human being accomplishes these in a manner and time unique to that individual.

Directional Trends. Growth and development proceed in regular, related directions or gradients and reflect the physical development and maturation of neuromuscular functions (Fig. 5-1). The first pattern is the **cephalocaudal,** or **head-to-tail,** direction. The head end of the organism develops first and is large and complex, whereas the lower end is small and simple and takes shape at a later period. The physical evidence of this trend is most apparent during the period before birth, but it also applies to postnatal behavior development. Infants achieve structural control of the head before they have control of the trunk and extremities, hold their back erect before they stand, use their eyes before their hands, and gain control of their hands before they have control of their feet.

Second, the **proximodistal,** or **near-to-far,** trend applies to the midline-to-peripheral concept. A conspicuous illustration is the early embryonic development of limb buds, which is followed by rudimentary fingers and toes. In the infant, shoulder control precedes mastery of the hands, the whole hand is used as a unit before the fingers can be manipulated, and the central nervous system develops more rapidly than the peripheral nervous system.

These trends or patterns are bilateral and appear symmetric—each side develops in the same direction and at the same rate as the other. For some of the neurologic functions, this symmetry is only external because of unilateral differentiation of function at an early stage of postnatal development. For example, by the age of approximately 5 years the child has demonstrated a decided preference for the use of one hand over the other, although previously either one had been used.

The third trend, **differentiation,** describes development from simple operations to more complex activities and functions. From broad, global patterns of behavior, more specific, refined patterns emerge. All areas of development (physical, mental, social, and emotional) proceed in this direction.

BOX 5-1

Developmental Age Periods

PRENATAL PERIOD—CONCEPTION TO BIRTH
Germinal—Conception to approximately 2 weeks
Embryonic—2 to 8 weeks
Fetal—8 to 40 weeks (birth)
A rapid growth rate and total dependency make this one of the most crucial periods in the developmental process. The relationship between maternal health and certain manifestations in the newborn emphasizes the importance of adequate prenatal care to the health and well-being of the infant.

INFANCY PERIOD—BIRTH TO 12 MONTHS
Neonatal—Birth to 27 or 28 days
Infancy—1 to approximately 12 months
The infancy period is one of rapid motor, cognitive, and social development. Through mutuality with the caregiver (parent), the infant establishes a basic trust in the world and the foundation for future interpersonal relationships. The critical first month of life, although part of the infancy period, is often differentiated from the remainder because of the major physical adjustments to extrauterine existence and the psychologic adjustment of the parent.

EARLY CHILDHOOD—1 TO 6 YEARS
Toddler—1 to 3 years
Preschool—3 to 6 years
This period, which extends from the time children attain upright locomotion until they enter school, is characterized by intense activity and discovery. It is a time of marked physical and personality development. Motor development advances steadily. Children at this age acquire language and wider social relationships, learn role standards, gain self-control and mastery, develop increasing awareness of dependence and independence, and begin to develop a self-concept.

MIDDLE CHILDHOOD—6 TO 11 OR 12 YEARS
Frequently referred to as the *school age*, this period of development is one in which the child is directed away from the family group and centered around the wider world of peer relationships. There is steady advancement in physical, mental, and social development, with emphasis on developing skill competencies. Social cooperation and early moral development take on more importance with relevance for later life stages. This is a critical period in the development of a self-concept.

LATER CHILDHOOD—11 TO 19 YEARS
Prepubertal—10 to 13 years
Adolescence—13 to approximately 18 years
The tumultuous period of rapid maturation and change known as adolescence is considered to be a transitional period that begins at the onset of puberty and extends to the point of entry into the adult world—usually high school graduation. Biologic and personality maturation are accompanied by physical and emotional turmoil, and there is redefining of the self-concept. In the late adolescent period the young person begins to internalize all previously learned values and to focus on an individual, rather than a group, identity.

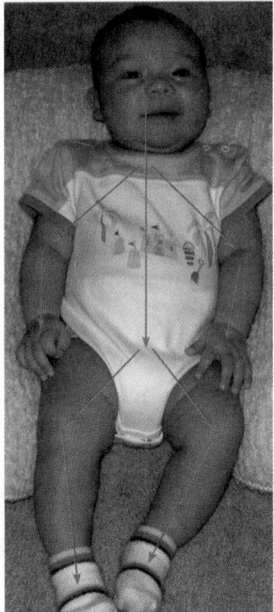

FIG. 5-1 ■ Directional trends in growth.

ment; gross, random muscle movements take place before fine muscle control.

Sequential Trends. In all dimensions of growth and development there is a definite, predictable sequence, with each child normally passing through every stage. Children crawl before they creep, creep before they stand, and stand before they walk. Later facets of the personality are built on the early foundation of trust. The child babbles, then forms words and, finally, sentences; writing emerges from scribbling.

Developmental Pace. Although development has a fixed, precise order, it does not progress at the same rate or pace. There are periods of accelerated growth and periods of decelerated growth in both total body growth and the growth of subsystems. Not all areas of development occur at the same pace. When a spurt occurs in one area such as gross motor, minimal advances may take place in language, fine motor, or social skills. Once the gross motor skill has been achieved, then development focus will shift to another area. The rapid growth before and after birth gradually levels off throughout early childhood. Growth is relatively slow during middle childhood, markedly increases at the beginning of adolescence, and levels off in early adulthood. Each child grows at his or her own pace. Distinct differences are observed between children as they reach developmental milestones.

FYI

Research suggests that normal growth, particularly height in infants, may occur in brief (possibly even 24-hour) bursts that punctuate long periods in which no measurable growth takes place. The researchers noted sex differences, with girls growing in length during the week they gained weight and boys growing in the week following a significant weight gain. Sex-specific growth hormone pulse patterns may coordinate body composition, weight gain, and linear growth (Lampl, Johnson, and Frongillo, 2001; Lampl, Thompson, Frongillo, 2005). Further, findings indicate a stuttering or saltatory pattern of growth that follows no regular cycle and can occur after "quiet" periods that last as long as 4 weeks. Mothers reported that their children were usually fussy and voraciously hungry a day or two before the growth spurt.

Through the process of development and differentiation, early embryonal cells with vague, undifferentiated functions progress to an immensely complex organism composed of highly specialized and diversified cells, tissues, and organs. Generalized development precedes specific or specialized develop-

Critical Thinking Exercise—Growth Trends During Infancy

Sensitive Periods. There are limited times during the process of growth when the organism will interact with a particular environment in a specific manner. Periods termed **critical, sensitive, vulnerable,** and **optimal** are those times in the lifetime of an organism when it is more susceptible to positive or negative influences.

The quality of interactions during these sensitive periods determines whether the effects on the organism will be beneficial or harmful. For example, physiologic maturation of the central nervous system is influenced by adequacy and timing of contributions from the environment such as stimulation and nutrition. The first 3 months of prenatal life are sensitive periods for physical growth of the fetus.

Psychologic development also appears to have sensitive periods, when an environmental event has maximal influence on the developing personality. For example, primary socialization occurs during the first year when the infant makes the initial social attachments and establishes a basic trust in the world. A warm relationship with a parent figure is fundamental to a healthy personality. The same concept might be applied to readiness for learning skills such as toilet training or reading. In these instances there appears to be an opportune time when the skill is best learned.

Individual Differences

Each child grows in his or her own unique and personal way. Great individual variation exists in the age at which developmental milestones are reached. The sequence is predictable; the exact timing is not. Rates of growth vary, and measurements are defined in terms of ranges to allow for individual differences. Some children are fast growers, others are moderate, and some are slower to reach maturity. Periods of fast growth, such as the pubescent growth spurt, may begin earlier or later in some children than in others. Children may grow fast or slowly during the spurt and may finish sooner or later than other children. Gender is an influential factor because girls seem to be more advanced in physiologic growth at all ages.

BIOLOGIC GROWTH AND PHYSICAL DEVELOPMENT

As children grow, their external dimensions change. These changes are accompanied by corresponding alterations in structure and function of internal organs and tissues that reflect the gradual acquisition of physiologic competence. Each part has its own rate of growth, which may be directly related to alterations in the size of the child (e.g., the heart rate). Skeletal muscle growth approximates whole body growth; brain, lymphoid, adrenal, and reproductive tissues follow distinct and individual patterns (Fig. 5-2). When growth deficiency has a secondary cause, such as severe illness or acute malnutrition, recovery from the illness or the establishment of an adequate diet will produce a dramatic acceleration of the growth rate that usually continues until the child's individual growth pattern is resumed.

External Proportions

Variations in the growth rate of different tissues and organ systems produce significant changes in body proportions during childhood. The cephalocaudal trend of development is most evident in total body growth as indicated by these changes. During fetal development the head is the fastest-growing body part, and at 2 months of gestation the head

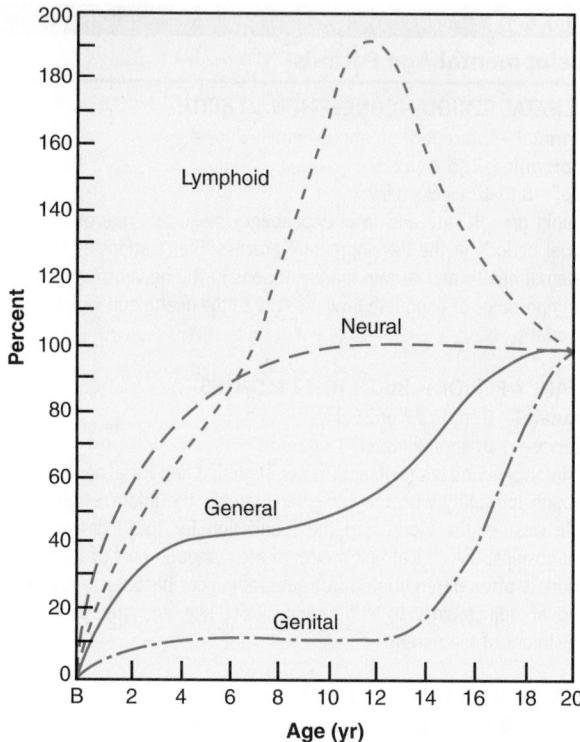

FIG. 5-2 ■ Growth rates for the body as a whole and three types of tissues. *Lymphoid:* thymus, lymph nodes, and intestinal lymph masses. *Neural:* brain, dura, spinal cord, optic apparatus, and head dimensions. *General:* body as a whole; external dimension; and respiratory, digestive, renal, circulatory, and musculoskeletal systems. (From Jackson JA, Patterson DG, and Harris RE: *The measurement of man,* Minneapolis, 1930, University of Minnesota Press.)

FIG. 5-3 ■ Changes in body proportions occur dramatically during childhood.

constitutes 50% of total body length. During infancy growth of the trunk predominates; the legs are the most rapidly growing part during childhood; in adolescence, the trunk once again elongates. In the newborn infant the lower limbs are one third the total body length but only 15% of the total body weight; in the adult the lower limbs constitute one half of the total body height and 30% or more of the total body weight. As growth proceeds, the midpoint in head-to-toe measurements gradually descends from a level even with the umbilicus at birth to the level of the symphysis pubis at maturity.

TABLE 5-1

General Trends in Height and Weight Gain During Childhood

AGE-GROUP	WEIGHT*	HEIGHT*
Infants		
Birth–6 months	Weekly gain—140-200 g (5-7 ounces) Birth weight doubles by end of first 4-7 months†	Monthly gain—2.5 cm (1 inch)
6-12 months	Weight gain—85-140 g (3-5 ounces) Birth weight triples by end of first year	Monthly gain—1.25 cm (0.5 inch) Birth length increases by approximately 50% by end of first year
Toddlers	Birth weight quadruples by age 2.5	Height at age 2 is approximately 50% of eventual adult height Gain during second year—about 12 cm (4.7 inches) Gain during third year—about 6-8 cm (2.4-3.1 inches)
Preschoolers	Yearly gain—2-3 kg (4.5-6.5 pounds)	Birth length doubles by age 4 Yearly gain—5-7.5 cm (2-3 inches)
School-age children	Yearly gain—2-3 kg (4.5-6.5 pounds)	Yearly gain after age 7—5 cm (2 inches) Birth length triples by about age 13
Pubertal growth spurt		
Females—10-14 years	Weight gain—7-25 kg (15.5-55 pounds) Mean—17.5 kg (38.5 pounds)	Height gain—5-25 cm (2-10 inches); approximately 95% of mature height achieved by onset of menarche or skeletal age of 13 Mean—20.5 cm (8 inches)
Males—11-16 years	Weight gain—7-30 kg (15.5-66 pounds) Mean—23.7 kg (52.2 pounds)	Height gain—10-30 cm (4-12 inches); approximately 95% of mature height achieved by skeletal age of 15 years Mean—27.5 cm (11 inches)

*Yearly height and weight gains for each age-group represent averaged estimates from a variety of sources.
†Jung FE, Czajka-Narins DM: Birth weight doubling and tripling times: an updated look at the effects of birth weight, sex, race, and type of feeding, *Am J Clin Nutr* 42:182-189, 1985.

Biologic Determinants of Growth and Development

The most prominent feature of childhood and adolescence is physical growth (Fig. 5-3). Throughout development various tissues in the body undergo changes in growth, composition, and structure. In some tissues the changes are continuous (e.g., bone growth and dentition); in others, significant alterations occur at specific stages (e.g., appearance of secondary sex characteristics). When these measurements are compared with standardized norms, a child's developmental progress can be determined with a high degree of confidence (Table 5-1). Growth in children with Down syndrome differs from that in other children. They have slower growth velocity between 6 months and 3 years and then again in adolescence. Puberty occurs earlier, and they achieve shorter stature. This population of patients are frequent users of the health care system, often with multiple providers, and benefit from the use of the Down syndrome growth chart to monitor their growth (Cronk, Crocker, Pueschel, and others, 1988; Myrelid, Gustafsson, Ollars, and others, 2002).

Linear growth, or **height,** occurs almost entirely as a result of skeletal growth and is considered a stable measurement of general growth. Growth in height is not uniform throughout life but ceases when maturation of the skeleton is complete. The maximum rate of growth in length occurs before birth, but the newborn continues to grow at a rapid, though slower, rate.

NURSING TIP

Double the child's height at the age of 2 years to estimate how tall he or she may be as an adult.

At birth, **weight** is more variable than height and is, to a greater extent, a reflection of the intrauterine environment. The average newborn weighs from 3175 to 3400 g (7 to 7.5 pounds). In general, the birth weight doubles by 4 to 7 months of age and triples by the end of the first year. By the age of 2 to 2½ years the birth weight usually quadruples. After this point the "normal" rate of weight gain, just as the growth in height, assumes a steady annual increase of approximately 2 to 2.75 kg (4.4 to 6 pounds) per year until the adolescent growth spurt.

Both **bone age** determinants and state of **dentition** are used as indicators of development. Because both are discussed elsewhere, neither is elaborated here (see next section for bone age; see also Chapters 10 and 12 for dentition).

Skeletal Growth and Maturation

The most accurate measure of general development is **skeletal** or **bone age,** the radiologic determination of osseous maturation. Skeletal age appears to correlate more closely with other measures of physiologic maturity (such as onset of menarche) than with chronologic age or height. Bone age is determined by comparing the mineralization of ossification centers and advancing bony form to age-related standards.

Bone formation begins during the second month of fetal life when calcium salts are deposited in the intercellular substance (matrix) to form calcified cartilage first and then true bone. Bone formation exhibits some differences. In small bones the bone continues to form in the center and cartilage continues to be laid down on the surfaces. In long bones the ossification begins in the **diaphysis** (the long central portion of the bone) and continues in the **epiphysis** (the end portions of the bone). Between the diaphysis and the epiphysis, an **epiphyseal cartilage plate** (or **growth plate**) unites with the diaphysis by columns of spongy tissue, the **metaphysis.** Active growth in length takes place in the epiphyseal growth plate. Interference with this growth site by trauma or infection can result in deformity.

The first centers of ossification appear in the 2-month-old embryo, and at birth the number is approximately 400, about half the number at maturity. New centers appear at regular intervals during the growth period and provide the basis for assessment of bone age. Postnatally the earliest centers to appear (at 5 to 6 months of age) are those of the capitate and hamate bones in the wrist. Therefore radiographs of the hand and wrist provide the most useful areas for screening to determine skeletal age, especially before age 6 years. These centers appear earlier in girls than in boys.

Nurses must understand that the growing bones of children possess many unique characteristics. Bone fractures occurring at the growth plate may be difficult to discover and may significantly affect subsequent growth and development (Urbanski and Hanlon, 1996). Factors that may influence skeletal muscle injury rates and types in children and adolescents include (Kaczander, 1997; Caine, DiFiori, and Maffulli; 2006):

■ Less protective sports equipment for children
■ Less emphasis on conditioning, especially flexibility
■ In adolescents, fractures that are more common than ligamentous ruptures because of the rapid growth rate of the physeal (segment of tubular bone that is concerned mainly with growth) zone of hypertrophy

Neurologic Maturation

In contrast to other body tissues, which grow rapidly after birth, the nervous system grows proportionately more rapidly before birth. Two periods of rapid brain cell growth occur during fetal life: a dramatic increase in the number of neurons between 15 and 20 weeks of gestation and another increase at 30 weeks, which extends to 1 year of age. The rapid growth of infancy continues during early childhood and then slows to a more gradual rate during later childhood and adolescence.

Postnatal growth consists of increasing the amount of cytoplasm around the nuclei of existing cells, increasing the number and intricacy of communications with other cells, and advancing their peripheral axons to keep pace with expanding body dimensions. This allows for increasingly complex movement and behavior. Neurophysiologic changes also provide the foundation for language, learning, and behavior development. Neurologic or electroencephalographic development is sometimes used as an indicator of maturational age in the early weeks of life.

Lymphoid Tissues

Lymphoid tissues contained in the lymph nodes, thymus, spleen, tonsils, adenoids, and blood lymphocytes follow a growth pattern unlike that of other body tissues. These tissues are small in relation to total body size, but they are well developed at birth. They increase rapidly to reach adult dimensions by 6 years of age and continue to grow. At about age 10 to 12 years they reach a maximum development that is approximately twice their adult size. This is followed by a rapid decline to stable adult dimensions by the end of adolescence.

Development of Organ Systems

All tissues and organ systems undergo changes during development. Some are striking; others are subtle. Many have implications for assessment and care. Because the major importance of these changes relates to their dysfunction, the

TABLE 5-2
Dietary Reference Intake for Calories and Protein Throughout Adolescence*

AGE (years)	ENERGY ALLOWANCE (kcal/kg)	PROTEIN (g/day)
INFANTS		
0-0.5	108	9.1
0.5-1	98	11
CHILDREN		
1-3	102	13
4-8	90	19
MALES		
9-13	55	34
14-18	45	52
FEMALES		
9-13	47	34
14-18	40	46

Data from Otten JJ, Hellwig JP, Meyers LD, editors: *Dietary reference intakes: the essential guide to nutrient requirements,* Washington, DC, 2006, National Academies Press.
*According to the American Academy of Pediatrics, energy and protein needs during adolescence should be based on height rather than weight.

developmental characteristics of various systems and organs are discussed throughout the book as they relate to these areas. Physical characteristics and physiologic changes that vary with age are included in age-group descriptions.

PHYSIOLOGIC CHANGES

Physiologic changes that take place in all organs and systems are discussed as they relate to dysfunction. Other changes such as pulse and respiratory rates and blood pressure are an integral part of physical assessment (see Chapter 6). In addition, there are changes in basic functions, including metabolism, temperature, and patterns of sleep and rest.

Metabolism

The rate of metabolism when the body is at rest (**basal metabolic rate,** or **BMR**) demonstrates a distinctive change throughout childhood. Highest in the newborn infant, the BMR closely relates to the proportion of surface area to body mass, which changes as the body increases in size. In both sexes the proportion decreases progressively to maturity. The BMR is slightly higher in boys at all ages and further increases during pubescence over that in girls.

The rate of metabolism determines the caloric requirements of the child. The basal energy requirement of infants is about 108 kcal/kg of body weight and decreases to 40 to 45 kcal/kg at maturity (Table 5-2). Water requirements throughout life remain at approximately 1.5 ml/calorie of energy expended. Children's energy needs vary considerably at different ages and with changing circumstances. The energy requirement to build tissue steadily decreases with age, following the general growth curve; however, energy needs vary with the individual child and may be considerably higher. For short periods (e.g., during strenuous exercise) and more prolonged periods (e.g., illness), the needs can be very high.

Temperature

Body temperature, reflecting metabolism, decreases over the course of development (see inside back cover). Thermoregulation is one of the most important adaptation responses of the infant during the transition from intrauterine to extrauterine life. In the healthy neonate hypothermia can result in several negative metabolic consequences such as hypoglycemia, elevated bilirubin levels, and metabolic acidosis. Skin-to-skin care, also referred to as kangaroo care, is an effective way to prevent neonatal hypothermia in infants. Unclothed, diapered infants are placed on the parent's bare chest after birth, promoting thermoregulation and attachment (Galligan, 2006). After the unstable regulatory ability in the neonatal period, heat production steadily declines as the infant grows into childhood. Individual differences of 0.5° to 1° F are normal, and occasionally a child normally displays an unusually high or low temperature. Beginning at approximately 12 years of age, girls display a temperature that remains relatively stable, whereas the temperature in boys continues to fall for a few more years. Females maintain a temperature slightly above that of males throughout life.

Even with improved temperature regulation, infants and young children are highly susceptible to temperature fluctuations. Body temperature responds to changes in environmental temperature and is increased with active exercise, crying, and emotional stress. Infections can cause a higher and more rapid temperature increase in infants and young children than in older children. In relation to body weight, an infant produces more heat per unit than adolescents. Consequently, during active play or when heavily clothed, an infant or small child is likely to become overheated.

Sleep and Rest

Sleep, a protective function in all organisms, allows for repair and recovery of tissues after activity. As in most aspects of development, there is wide variation among individual children in the amount and distribution of sleep at various ages. As children mature, there is a change in the total time they spend in sleep and the amount of time they spend in deep sleep.

Newborn infants sleep much of the time that is not occupied with feeding and other aspects of their care. As infants grow older, the total time spent in sleep gradually decreases, they remain awake for longer periods, and they sleep longer at night. For example, the length of a sleep cycle increases from approximately 50 to 60 minutes in the newborn infant to approximately 90 minutes in adolescence (Anders, Sadeh, and Appareddy, 2005). During the latter part of the first year, most children sleep through the night and take one or two naps during the day. By the time they are 12 to 18 months old, most children have eliminated the second nap. After age 3 years the child has usually given up daytime naps, except in cultures in which an afternoon nap or siesta is customary. Sleep time declines slightly from ages 4 to 10 and then increases somewhat during the pubertal growth spurt.

The quality of sleep changes as children mature. As children develop through adolescence, their need for sleep does not decline, but their opportunity for sleep may be affected by social, activity, and academic schedules. The time spent in deep, restful sleep increases from 50% in infancy to 80% in the older child.

TEMPERAMENT

Temperament is defined as "the manner of thinking, behaving, or reacting characteristic of an individual" (Chess and Thomas, 1999) and refers to the way in which a person deals with life. From the time of birth, children exhibit marked individual differences in the way they respond to their environment and the way others, particularly the parents, respond to them and their needs. A genetic basis has been suggested for some differences in temperament. Nine characteristics of temperament have been identified through interviews with parents (Box 5-2). Temperament refers to behavioral tendencies, not to discrete behavioral acts. There are no implications of good or bad. Most children can be placed into one of three common categories based on their overall pattern of temperamental attributes:

The easy child—Easy-going children are even tempered, are regular and predictable in their habits, and have a positive approach to new stimuli. They are open and adaptable to change and display a mild to moderately intense mood that is typically positive. Approximately 40% of children fall into this category.

The difficult child—Difficult children are highly active, irritable, and irregular in their habits. Negative withdrawal responses are typical, and they require a more structured environment. These children adapt slowly to new routines, people, or situations. Mood expressions are usually intense and primarily

---

BOX 5-2

Attributes of Temperament

Activity—Level of physical motion during activity such as sleep, eating, play, dressing, and bathing

Rhythmicity—Regularity in the timing of physiologic functions such as hunger, sleep, and elimination

Approach-withdrawal—Nature of initial responses to a new stimulus such as people, situations, places, foods, toys, and procedures (**Approach** responses are positive and are displayed by activity or expression; **withdrawal** responses are negative expressions or behaviors.)

Adaptability—Ease or difficulty with which the child adapts or adjusts to new or altered situations

Threshold of responsiveness (sensory threshold)—Amount of stimulation, such as sounds or light, required to evoke a response in the child

Intensity of reaction—Energy level of the child's reactions, regardless of quality or direction

Mood—Amount of pleasant, happy, friendly behavior compared with unpleasant, unhappy, crying, unfriendly behavior exhibited by the child in various situations

Distractibility—Ease with which a child's attention or direction of behavior can be diverted by external stimuli

Attention span and persistence—Length of time a child pursues a given activity (**attention**) and the continuation of an activity in spite of obstacles (**persistence**)

BOX 5-3

Activities to Promote Mastery Motivation

- Encourage unobtrusive assistance during play.
- Share pleasure with infant in accomplishments.
- Don't give immediate assistance during tasks.
- Don't interrupt infant during tasks.
- Let infant initiate activities.
- Limit controlling feedback during play.
- Provide audio and visually responsive toys.
- Provide early kinesthetic stimulation (picking up, rocking).

From Morrow JD, Camp BW: Mastery motivation and temperament of 7-month-old infants, *Pediatr Nurs* 22(3):211-217, 1996.

negative. They exhibit frequent periods of crying, and frustration often produces violent tantrums. This group represents about 10% of children.

The slow-to-warm-up child—Slow-to-warm-up children typically react negatively and with mild intensity to new stimuli and, unless pressured, adapt slowly with repeated contact. They respond with only mild but passive resistance to novelty or changes in routine. They are inactive and moody but show only moderate irregularity in functions. Fifteen percent of children demonstrate this temperament pattern.

Thirty-five percent of children either have some, but not all, of the characteristics of one of the categories or are inconsistent in their behavioral responses. Many normal children demonstrate this wide range of behavioral patterns.

Significance of Temperament

Observations indicate that children who display the difficult or slow-to-warm-up patterns of behavior are more vulnerable to the development of behavior problems in early and middle childhood. Any child can develop behavior problems if there is dissonance between the child's temperament and the environment. Demands for change and adaptation that are in conflict with the child's capacities can become excessively stressful. However, authorities emphasize that it is not the temperament patterns of children that place them at risk; it is the **degree of fit** between children and their environment, specifically their parents, that determines the degree of vulnerability. The potential for optimum development exists when environmental expectations and demands fit with the individual's style of behavior and the parents' ability to navigate this period (Chess and Thomas, 1999) (see Growth Failure [Failure to Thrive], Chapter 11).

Early identification of temperament provides a useful tool for caregivers in anticipating probable areas of difficulty or risk associated with development. For example, "difficult" children may be prone to colic in infancy, active children require more vigilance to prevent injury, and school entry requires different approaches for children with different temperaments.

Research indicates that irritable and unadaptable infants can raise doubts in mothers about their competence (Beck, 1996). Additional research indicates that a child's temperament can affect parent-child interactions and can influence the parents' self-esteem, marital harmony, mood, and overall satisfaction as parents (Carey, 1998). Studies on the relationship between temperament and the ability to perform a task

successfully (mastery motivation) have found that infants with high mastery are more cooperative and less difficult (Morrow and Camp, 1996). Principles that can be used by nurses in direct patient care and in providing anticipatory guidance are listed in Box 5-3.

DEVELOPMENT OF PERSONALITY AND MENTAL FUNCTION

Personality and cognitive skills develop in much the same manner as biologic growth—new accomplishments build on previously mastered skills. Many aspects depend on physical growth and maturation. This is not a comprehensive account of the multiple facets of personality and behavior development. Many aspects are integrated with the child's emotional and social development in later discussion of various age-groups. Table 5-3 summarizes some of the developmental theories.

THEORETIC FOUNDATIONS OF PERSONALITY DEVELOPMENT

Psychosexual Development (Freud)

According to Freud, all human behavior is energized by psychodynamic forces, and this psychic energy is divided among three components of personality: the id, the ego, and the superego. The **id**, the **unconscious mind**, is the inborn component that is driven by instincts. The id obeys the pleasure principle of immediate gratification of needs, regardless of whether the object or action can actually do so. The **ego**, the **conscious mind**, serves the reality principle. It functions as the conscious or controlling self that is able to find realistic means for gratifying the instincts while blocking the irrational thinking of the id. The **superego**, the **conscience**, functions as the moral arbitrator and represents the ideal. It is the mechanism that prevents individuals from expressing undesirable instincts that might threaten the social order.

Freud considered the sexual instincts to be significant in the development of the personality. However, he used the term **psychosexual** to describe any **sensual pleasure**. During childhood certain regions of the body assume a prominent psychologic significance as the source of new pleasures and new conflicts gradually shifts from one part of the body to another at particular stages of development:

Oral stage (birth to 1 year)—During infancy the major source of pleasure seeking is centered on oral activities such as sucking, biting, chewing, and vocalizing. Children may prefer one of these over the others, and the preferred method of oral gratification can provide some indication of the personality they develop.

Anal stage (1 to 3 years)—Interest during the second year of life centers in the anal region as sphincter muscles develop and children are able to withhold or expel fecal material at will. At this stage the climate surrounding toilet training can have lasting effects on children's personalities.

Phallic stage (3 to 6 years)—During the phallic stage the genitalia become an interesting and sensitive area of the body. Children recognize differences between the sexes and become curious about the dissimilarities. This is the period around which the controversial issues of the Oedipus and Electra complexes, penis envy, and castration anxiety are centered.

Latency period (6 to 12 years)—During the latency period children elaborate on previously acquired traits and skills. Physical and psychic energy are channeled into acquisition of knowledge and vigorous play.

TABLE 5-3

Summary of Personality, Cognitive, and Moral Development Theories

PSYCHOSEXUAL (FREUD)	PSYCHOSOCIAL (ERIKSON)	COGNITIVE (PIAGET)	MORAL JUDGMENT (KOHLBERG)	SPIRITUAL (FOWLER)
I. INFANCY—BIRTH–1 YEAR				
Oral	Trust vs mistrust	Sensorimotor (birth–2 years)		Undifferentiated
II. TODDLERHOOD—1-3 YEARS				
Anal	Autonomy vs shame and doubt	Preoperational thought, pre-conceptual phase (transductive reasoning [e.g., specific to specific]) (2-4 years)	Preconventional (premoral) level Punishment and obedience orientation	Intuitive-projective
III. EARLY CHILDHOOD—3-6 YEARS				
Phallic	Initiative vs guilt	Preoperational thought, intuitive phase (transductive reasoning) (4-7 years)	Preconventional (premoral) level Naive instrumental orientation	Mythical-literal
IV. MIDDLE CHILDHOOD—6-12 YEARS				
Latency	Industry vs inferiority	Concrete operations (inductive reasoning and beginning logic) (7-11 years)	Conventional level Good-boy, nice-girl orientation Law-and-order orientation	Synthetic-convention
V. ADOLESCENCE—12-18 YEARS				
Genital	Identity vs role confusion	Formal operations (deductive and abstract reasoning) (11-15 years)	Postconventional or principled level Social-contract orientation	Individuating-reflexive

Genital stage (age 12 and older)—The last significant stage begins at puberty with maturation of the reproductive system and production of sex hormones. The genital organs become the major source of sexual tensions and pleasures, but energies are also invested in forming friendships and preparing for marriage.

Psychosocial Development (Erikson)

The most widely accepted theory of personality development is that advanced by Erikson (1963). Although built on Freudian theory, it is known as **psychosocial** development and emphasizes a healthy personality as opposed to a pathologic approach. Erikson also uses the biologic concepts of critical periods and epigenesis, describing key conflicts or core problems that the individual strives to master during critical periods in personality development. Successful completion or mastery of each of these core conflicts is built on the satisfactory completion or mastery of the previous stage.

Each psychosocial stage has two components—the favorable and the unfavorable aspects of the core conflict—and progress to the next stage depend on resolution of this conflict. No core conflict is ever mastered completely but remains a recurrent problem throughout life. No life situation is ever secure. Each new situation presents the conflict in a new form. For example, when children who have satisfactorily achieved a sense of trust encounter a new experience (e.g., hospitalization), they must again develop a sense of trust in those responsible for their care in order to master the situation. Erikson's life-span approach to personality development consists of eight stages; however, only the first five relating to childhood are included here:

Trust vs mistrust (birth to 1 year)—The first and most important attribute to develop for a healthy personality is basic **trust.** Establishment of basic trust dominates the first year of life and describes all of the child's satisfying experiences at this age. Corresponding to Freud's oral stage, it is a time of "getting" and "taking in" through all the senses. It exists only in relation to something or someone; therefore consistent, loving care by a mothering person is essential for development of trust. **Mistrust** develops when trust-promoting experiences are deficient or lacking or when basic needs are inconsistently or inadequately met. Although shreds of mistrust are sprinkled throughout the personality, from a basic trust in parents stems trust in the world, other people, and oneself. The result is **faith** and **optimism.**

Autonomy vs shame and doubt (1 to 3 years)—Corresponding to Freud's anal stage, the problem of **autonomy** can be symbolized by the holding on and letting go of the sphincter muscles. The development of autonomy during the toddler period is centered on children's increasing ability to control their bodies, themselves, and their environment. They want to do things for themselves, using their newly acquired motor skills of walking, climbing, and manipulating and their mental powers of selecting and decision making. Much of their learning is acquired by imitating the activities and behavior of others. Negative feelings of **doubt** and **shame** arise when children are made to feel small and self-conscious, when their choices are disastrous, when others shame them, or when they are forced to be dependent in areas in which they are capable of assuming control. The favorable outcomes are **self-control** and **willpower.**

Initiative vs guilt (3 to 6 years)—The stage of **initiative** corresponds to Freud's phallic stage and is characterized by vigorous, intrusive behavior; enterprise; and a strong imagination. Children explore the physical world with all their senses and powers (Fig. 5-4). They develop a conscience. No longer guided only by outsiders, they have an inner voice that warns

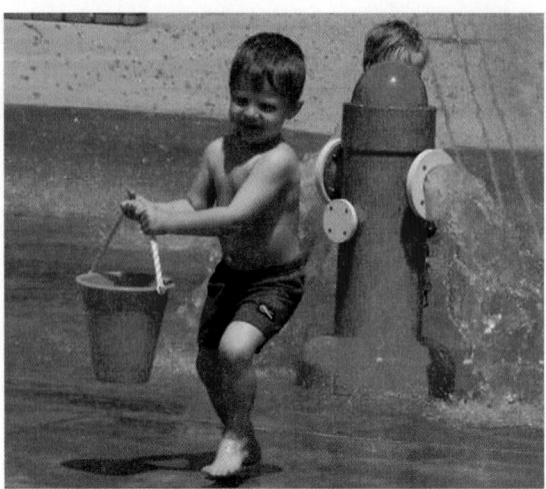

FIG. 5-4 ■ The stage of initiative is characterized by physical activity and imagination while children explore the physical world around them.

and threatens. Children sometimes undertake goals or activities that are in conflict with those of parents or others, and being made to feel that their activities or imaginings are bad produces a sense of **guilt.** Children must learn to retain a sense of initiative without impinging on the rights and privileges of others. The lasting outcomes are **direction** and **purpose.**

Industry vs inferiority (6 to 12 years)—The stage of **industry** is the latency period of Freud. Having achieved the more crucial stages in personality development, children are ready to be workers and producers. They want to engage in tasks and activities that they can carry through to completion; they need and want real achievement. Children learn to compete and cooperate with others, and they learn the rules. It is a decisive period in their social relationships with others. Feelings of **inadequacy** and **inferiority** may develop if too much is expected of them or if they believe that they cannot measure up to the standards set for them by others. The ego quality developed from a sense of industry is **competence.**

Identity vs role confusion (12 to 18 years)—Corresponding to Freud's genital period, the development of **identity** is characterized by rapid and marked physical changes. Previous trust in their bodies is shaken, and children become overly preoccupied with the way they appear in the eyes of others as compared with their own self-concept. Adolescents struggle to fit the roles they have played and those they hope to play with the current roles and fashions adopted by their peers, to integrate their concepts and values with those of society, and to come to a decision regarding an occupation. Inability to solve the core conflict results in **role confusion.** The outcome of successful mastery is **devotion** and **fidelity** to others and to values and ideologies.

THEORETIC FOUNDATIONS OF MENTAL DEVELOPMENT

The term **cognition** refers to the process by which developing individuals become acquainted with the world and the objects it contains. Children are born with inherited potentials for intellectual growth, but they must develop that potential through interaction with the environment. By assimilating information through the senses, processing it, and acting on it, they come to understand relationships between objects and between themselves and their world. With cognitive development, children acquire the ability to reason abstractly,

to think in a logical manner, and to organize intellectual functions or performances into higher-order structures. Language, morals, and spiritual development emerge as cognitive abilities advance.

Cognitive Development (Piaget)

Cognitive development consists of age-related changes that occur in mental activities. The best-known theory regarding children's thinking, and a more comprehensive developmental theory than those already described, was developed by the Swiss psychologist Jean Piaget (1969). According to Piaget, intelligence enables individuals to make adaptations to the environment that increase the probability of survival, and through their behavior individuals establish and maintain equilibrium with the environment.

Piaget (1969) proposed three stages of reasoning: (1) intuitive, (2) concrete operational, and (3) formal operational. When they enter the stage of concrete logical thought at about age 7 years, children are able to make logical inferences, classify, and deal with quantitative relationships about concrete things. Not until adolescence are they able to reason abstractly with any degree of competence. Each stage is derived from and builds on the accomplishments of the previous stage in a continuous, orderly process. The course of intellectual development is both maturational and invariant and is divided into the following stages (ages are approximate):

Sensorimotor (birth to 2 years)—The sensorimotor stage of intellectual development consists of six substages (see pp. 327 and 412) that are governed by sensations in which simple learning takes place. Children progress from reflex activity through simple repetitive behaviors to imitative behavior. They develop a sense of cause and effect as they direct behavior toward objects. Problem solving is primarily by trial and error. They display a high level of curiosity, experimentation, and enjoyment of novelty and begin to develop a sense of self as they are able to differentiate themselves from their environment. They become aware that objects have **permanence**—that an object exists even though it is no longer visible. Toward the end of the sensorimotor period, children begin to use language and representational thought.

Preoperational (2 to 7 years)—The predominant characteristic of the preoperational stage of intellectual development is **egocentrism,** which in this sense does not mean selfishness or self-centeredness, but the inability to put oneself in the place of another. Children interpret objects and events not in terms of general properties, but in terms of their relationships or their use to them. They are unable to see things from any perspective other than their own; they cannot see another's point of view, nor can they see any reason to do so (see Cognitive Development, Chapter 13).

Preoperational thinking is concrete and tangible. Children cannot reason beyond the observable, and they lack the ability to make deductions or generalizations. Thought is dominated by what they see, hear, or otherwise experience. However, they are increasingly able to use language and symbols to represent objects in their environment. Through imaginative play, questioning, and other interactions, they begin to elaborate concepts and to make simple associations between ideas. In the latter stage of this period their reasoning is **intuitive** (e.g., the stars have to go to bed just as they do), and they are only beginning to deal with problems of weight, length, size, and time. Reasoning is also **transductive**—because two events occur together, they cause each other, or knowledge of one characteristic is transferred to another (e.g., all women with big bellies have babies).

Concrete operations (7 to 11 years)—At this age thought becomes increasingly logical and coherent. Children are able to classify, sort, order, and otherwise organize facts about the world to use in problem solving. They develop a new concept of permanence—**conservation** (see Cognitive Development [Piaget], Chapter 16); that is, they realize that physical factors such as volume, weight, and number remain the same even though outward appearances are changed. They are able to deal with a number of different aspects of a situation simultaneously. They do not have the capacity to deal in abstraction; they solve problems in a concrete, systematic fashion based on what they can perceive. Reasoning is **inductive**. Through progressive changes in thought processes and relationships with others, thought becomes less self-centered. They can consider points of view other than their own. Thinking has become socialized.

Formal operations (11 to 15 years)—Formal operational thought is characterized by adaptability and flexibility. Adolescents can think in abstract terms, use abstract symbols, and draw logical conclusions from a set of observations. For example, they can solve the following question: If *A* is larger than *B,* and *B* is larger than *C,* which symbol is the largest? (The answer is *A.*) They can make hypotheses and test them; they can consider abstract, theoretic, and philosophic matters. Although they may confuse the ideal with the practical, most contradictions in the world can be dealt with and resolved.

Language Development

Children are born with the mechanism and capacity to develop speech and language skills. However, they do not speak spontaneously. The environment must provide a means for them to acquire these skills. Speech requires intact physiologic structure and function (including respiratory, auditory, and cerebral) plus intelligence, a need to communicate, and stimulation.

The rate of speech development varies from child to child and is directly related to neurologic competence and cognitive development. Gesture precedes speech, and in this way a small child communicates satisfactorily. As speech develops, gesture recedes but never disappears entirely. Research suggests that infants can learn sign language before vocal language and that it may enhance the development of vocal language (Thompson, Cotner-Bichelman, McKerchar, and others, 2007). At all stages of language development, children's comprehension vocabulary (what they understand) is greater than their expressed vocabulary (what they can say), and this development reflects a continuing process of modification that involves both the acquisition of new words and the expanding and refining of word meanings previously learned. By the time they begin to walk, children are able to attach a name to objects and persons.

The first parts of speech used are nouns, sometimes verbs (e.g., "go"), and combination words (such as "bye-bye"). Responses are usually structurally incomplete during the toddler period, although the meaning is clear. Next they begin to use adjectives and adverbs to qualify nouns, followed by adverbs to qualify nouns and verbs. Later, pronouns and gender words are added (such as "he" and "she"). By the time children enter school, they are able to use simple, structurally complete sentences that average five to seven words.

Moral Development (Kohlberg)

Children also acquire moral reasoning in a developmental sequence. Moral development, as described by Kohlberg (1968), is based on cognitive developmental theory and consists of the following three major levels, each of which has two stages:

Preconventional level—The preconventional level of moral development parallels the preoperational level of cognitive development and intuitive thought. Culturally oriented to the labels of good/bad and right/wrong, children integrate these in terms of the physical or pleasurable consequences of their actions. At first children determine the goodness or badness of an action in terms of its consequences. They avoid punishment and obey without question those who have the power to determine and enforce the rules and labels. They have no concept of the basic moral order that supports these consequences. Later, children determine that the right behavior consists of that which satisfies their own needs (and sometimes the needs of others). Although elements of fairness, give and take, and equal sharing are evident, they are interpreted in a practical, concrete manner without loyalty, gratitude, or justice.

Conventional level—At the conventional stage children are concerned with conformity and loyalty. They value the maintenance of family, group, or national expectations regardless of consequences. Behavior that meets with approval and pleases or helps others is considered good. One earns approval by being "nice." Obeying the rules, doing one's duty, showing respect for authority, and maintaining the social order are the correct behaviors. This level is correlated with the stage of concrete operations in cognitive development.

Postconventional, autonomous, or principled level—At the postconventional level the individual has reached the cognitive stage of formal operations. Correct behavior tends to be defined in terms of general individual rights and standards that have been examined and agreed on by the entire society. Although procedural rules for reaching consensus become important, with emphasis on the legal point of view, there is also emphasis on the possibility for changing law in terms of societal needs and rational considerations.

The most advanced level of moral development is one in which self-chosen ethical principles guide decisions of conscience. These are abstract and ethical but universal principles of justice and human rights with respect for the dignity of persons as individuals. It is believed that few persons reach this stage of moral reasoning.

Spiritual Development (Fowler)

Spiritual beliefs are closely related to the moral and ethical portion of the child's self-concept and, as such, must be considered as part of the child's basic needs assessment. Children need to have meaning, purpose, and hope in their lives. Also, the need for confession and forgiveness is present, even in very young children. Extending beyond religion (an organized set of beliefs and practices), spirituality affects the whole person: mind, body, and spirit. Fowler (1981) has identified seven stages in the development of faith, four of which are closely associated with and parallel cognitive and psychosocial development in childhood:

Stage 0: Undifferentiated—This stage of development encompasses the period of infancy during which children have no concept of right or wrong, no beliefs, and no convictions to guide their behavior. However, the beginnings of a faith are established with the development of basic trust through their relationships with the primary caregiver.

Stage 1: Intuitive-projective—Toddlerhood is primarily a time of imitating the behavior of others. Children imitate the religious gestures and behaviors of others without comprehending any meaning or significance to the activities. During the preschool years children assimilate some of the values and beliefs of their parents. Parental attitudes toward moral codes and religious beliefs convey to children what they consider to be good and bad. Children still imitate behavior at this age and follow parental beliefs as part of their daily lives rather than through an understanding of their basic concepts.

Stage 2: Mythical-literal—Through the school-age years, spiritual development parallels cognitive development and is closely related to children's experiences and social interaction. Most have a strong interest in religion during the school-age years. They accept the existence of a deity, and petitions to an omnipotent being are important and expected to be answered; good behavior is rewarded, and bad behavior is punished. Their developing conscience bothers them when they disobey. They have a reverence for thoughts and matters and are able to articulate their faith. They may even question its validity.

Stage 3: Synthetic-convention—As children approach adolescence, however, they become increasingly aware of spiritual disappointments. They recognize that prayers are not always answered (at least on their own terms) and may begin to abandon or modify some religious practices. They begin to reason, to question some of the established parental religious standards, and to drop or modify some religious practices.

Stage 4: Individuating-reflexive—Adolescents become more skeptical and begin to compare the religious standards of their parents with those of others. They attempt to determine which to adopt and incorporate into their own set of values. They also begin to compare religious standards with the scientific viewpoint. It is a time of searching rather than reaching. Adolescents are uncertain about many religious ideas but will not achieve profound insights until late adolescence or early adulthood.

DEVELOPMENT OF SELF-CONCEPT

Self-concept is how an individual describes himself or herself. The term **self-concept** includes all the notions, beliefs, and convictions that constitute an individual's self-knowledge and that influence that individual's relationships with others. It is not present at birth but develops gradually as a result of unique experiences within the self, with significant others, and with the realities of the world. However, an individual's self-concept may or may not reflect reality.

In infancy the self-concept is primarily an awareness of one's independent existence learned in part as a result of social contacts and experiences with others. The process becomes more active during toddlerhood as children explore the limits of their capacities and the nature of their impact on others. School-age children are more aware of differences among people, are more sensitive to social pressures, and become more preoccupied with issues of self-criticism and self-evaluation. During early adolescence children focus more on physical and emotional changes taking place and on peer acceptance. Self-concept is crystallized during later adolescence as young people organize their self-concept around a set of values, goals, and competencies acquired throughout childhood.

Body Image

A vital component of self-concept, **body image** refers to the subjective concepts and attitudes that individuals have toward their own bodies. It consists of the physiologic (the perception of one's physical characteristics), psychologic (values and attitudes toward the body, abilities, and ideals), and social nature of one's image of self (the self in relation to others). All three

of the components interrelate with one another. Body image is a complex phenomenon that evolves and changes during the process of growth and development. Any actual or perceived deviation from the "norm" (no matter how this is interpreted) is cause for concern. The extent to which a characteristic, defect, or disease affects children's body image is influenced by the attitudes and behavior of those around them.

The significant others in their lives exert the most important and meaningful impact on children's body image. Labels that are attached to them (such as "skinny," "pretty," or "fat") or body parts (such as "ugly mole," "bug eyes," or "yucky skin") are incorporated into the body image. Because they lack the understanding of deviations from the physical standard or norm, children notice prominent differences in others and unwittingly make rude or cruel remarks about such minor deviations as large or widely spaced front teeth, large or small eyes, moles, or extreme variations in height.

Infants receive input about their bodies through self-exploration and sensory stimulation from others. As they begin to manipulate their environment, they become aware of their bodies as separate from others. Toddlers learn to identify the various parts of their bodies and are able to use symbols to represent objects. Preschoolers become aware of the wholeness of their bodies and discover the genitalia. Exploration of the genitalia and the discovery of differences between the sexes become important. There is only a vague concept of internal organs and function (Stuart and Laraia, 2000).

School-age children begin to learn about internal body structure and function and become aware of differences in body size and configuration. They are highly influenced by the cultural norms of society and current fads. Children whose bodies deviate from the norm are often criticized or ridiculed. Adolescence is the age when children become most concerned about the physical self. The unfamiliar body changes, and the new physical self must be integrated into the self-concept. Adolescents face conflicts over what they see and what they visualize as the ideal body structure. Body image formation during adolescence is a crucial element in the shaping of identity, the psychosocial crisis of adolescence.

Self-Esteem

Self-esteem is the value that an individual places on oneself and refers to an overall evaluation of oneself (Willoughby, King, and Polatajko, 1996). Self-esteem is described as the affective component of the self, whereas self-concept is the cognitive component; however, the two terms are almost indistinguishable and are often used interchangeably.

The term **self-esteem** refers to a personal, subjective judgment of one's worthiness derived from and influenced by the social groups in the immediate environment and individuals' perceptions of how they are valued by others. Self-esteem changes with development. Highly egocentric toddlers are unaware of any difference between competence and social approval. On the other hand, preschool and early school-age children are increasingly aware of the discrepancy between their competencies and the abilities of more advanced children. Being accepted by adults and peers outside the family group becomes more important to them. Positive feedback enhances their self-esteem; they are vulnerable to feelings of worthlessness and are anxious about failure.

As children's competencies increase and they develop meaningful relationships, their self-esteem rises. Their self-esteem is again at risk during early adolescence when they are defining an identity and sense of self in the context of their peer group. Unless children are continually made to feel incompetent and of little worth, a decrease in self-esteem during vulnerable times is only temporary. Children assess the following aspects of themselves in forming an overall evaluation of their self-esteem (Sieving and Zirbel-Donisch, 1990):

Competence—How adequate are my cognitive, physical, and social skills?

Sense of control—How well can I complete tasks needed to produce desired actions? Is someone or something specific vs luck or chance responsible for my successes and failures?

Moral worth—How closely do my actions and behaviors meet moral standards that have been set?

Worthiness of love and acceptance—How worthy am I of love and acceptance from parents, other significant adults, siblings, and peers?

Factors that influence the formation of a child's self-esteem include (1) the child's temperament and personality, (2) abilities and opportunities available to accomplish age-appropriate developmental tasks, (3) how significant others interact with the child, and (4) social roles assumed and the expectations of these roles (see also Psychosocial History, Chapter 6).

ROLE OF PLAY IN DEVELOPMENT

Through the universal medium of play, children learn what no one can teach them. They learn about their world and how to deal with this environment of objects, time, space, structure, and people. They learn about themselves operating within that environment—what they can do, how to relate to things and situations, and how to adapt themselves to the demands society makes on them. Play is the *work* of the child. In play, children continually practice the complicated, stressful processes of living, communicating, and achieving satisfactory relationships with other people.

CLASSIFICATION OF PLAY

From a developmental point of view, patterns of children's play can be categorized according to content and social character. In both there is an additive effect; each builds on past accomplishments, and some element of each is maintained throughout life. At each stage in development the new predominates.

CONTENT OF PLAY

The content of play involves primarily the physical aspects of play, although social relationships cannot be ignored. The content of play follows the directional trend of the simple to the complex:

Social-affective play—Play begins with social-affective play, wherein infants take pleasure in relationships with people. As adults talk, touch, nuzzle, and in various ways elicit a response from an infant, the infant soon learns to provoke parental emotions and responses with such behaviors as smiling, cooing, or initiating games and activities. The type and intensity of the adult behavior with children vary among cultures.

Sense-pleasure play—Sense-pleasure play is a nonsocial stimulating experience that originates from without. Objects in the environment—light and color, tastes and odors, textures and consistencies—attract children's attention, stimulate their

FIG. 5-5 ■ Children derive pleasure from handling raw materials.

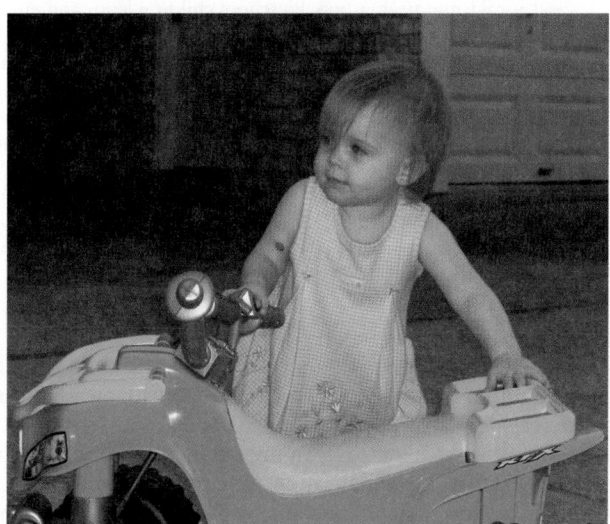

FIG. 5-6 ■ After infants develop new skills to grasp and manipulate, they begin to conquer new abilities such as getting on a play motorcycle.

senses, and give pleasure. Pleasurable experiences are derived from handling raw materials (water, sand, food), from body motion (swinging, bouncing, rocking), and from other uses of senses and abilities (smelling, humming) (Fig. 5-5).

Skill play—After infants have developed the ability to grasp and manipulate, they persistently demonstrate and exercise their newly acquired abilities through skill play, repeating an action over and over again. The element of sense-pleasure play is often evident in the practicing of a new ability, but all too frequently the determination to conquer the elusive skill produces pain and frustration (e.g., learning to get into a play car) (Fig. 5-6).

Unoccupied behavior—In unoccupied behavior children are not playful but focusing their attention momentarily on anything that strikes their interest. Children daydream, fiddle with clothes or other objects, or walk aimlessly. This role differs from that of onlookers, who actively observe the activity of others.

Dramatic, or pretend, play—One of the vital elements in children's process of identification is dramatic play, also known as symbolic or pretend play. It begins in late infancy (11 to 13 months) and is the predominant form of play in the preschool child. After children begin to invest situations and people with meanings and to attribute affective significance to the world, they can pretend and fantasize almost anything. By acting out events of daily life, children learn and practice the roles and identities modeled by the members of their family and society. Children's toys, replicas of the tools of society, provide a medium for learning about adult roles and activities that may be puzzling and frustrating to them. Interacting with the world is one way children get to know it. The simple, imitative, dramatic play of the toddler, such as using the telephone, driving a car, or rocking a doll, evolves into more complex, sustained dramas of the preschooler, which extend beyond common domestic matters to the wider aspects of the world and the society, such as playing police officer, storekeeper, teacher, or nurse. Older children work out elaborate themes, act out stories, and compose plays.

Games—Children in all cultures engage in games alone and with others. Solitary activity involving games begins as very small children participate in repetitive activities and progress to more complicated games that challenge their independent skills such as puzzles, solitaire, and computer or video games. Very young children participate in simple, **imitative games** such as pat-a-cake and peek-a-boo. Preschool children learn and enjoy **formal games,** beginning with ritualistic, self-sustaining games such as ring-around-a-rosy and London Bridge. With the exception of some simple board games, preschool children do not engage in **competitive games.** Preschoolers hate to lose and will try to cheat, want to change rules, or demand exceptions and opportunities to change their moves. School-age children and adolescents enjoy competitive games, including cards, checkers, and chess, and physically active games such as baseball.

SOCIAL CHARACTER OF PLAY

The play interactions of infancy are between the child and an adult. Children continue to enjoy the company of an adult but are increasingly able to play alone. As age advances, interaction with age-mates increases in importance and becomes an essential part of the socialization process. Through interaction, highly egocentric infants, unable to tolerate delay or interference, ultimately acquire concern for others and the ability to delay gratification or even to reject gratification at the expense of another. A pair of toddlers will engage in considerable combat because their personal needs cannot tolerate delay or compromise. By the time they reach age 5 or 6 years, children are able to arrive at a compromise or make use of arbitration, usually after they have attempted but failed to gain their own way. Through continued interaction with peers and the growth of conceptual abilities and social skills, children are able to increase participation with others in the following types of play:

Onlooker play—During onlooker play, children watch what other children are doing but make no attempt to enter into the play activity. There is an active interest in observing the interaction of others but no movement toward participating. Watching an older sibling bounce a ball is a common example of the onlooker role.

Solitary play—During solitary play, children play alone with toys different from those used by other children in the same area. They enjoy the presence of other children but make no effort to get close to or speak to them. Their interest is centered on their own activity, which they pursue with no reference to the activities of the others.

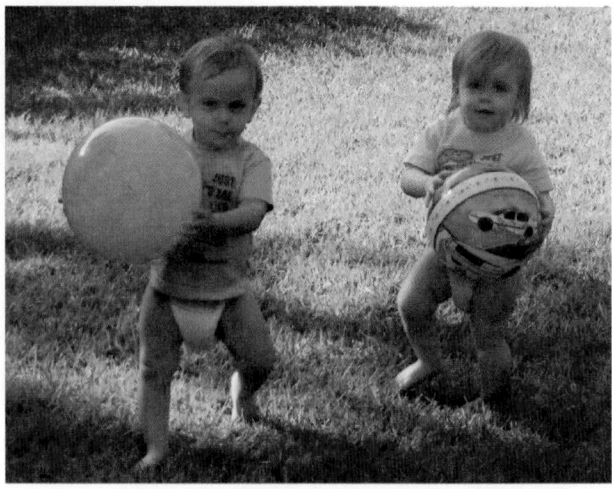

FIG. 5-7 ■ Parallel play.

FIG. 5-8 ■ Associative play.

Parallel play—During parallel activities children play independently but among other children. They play with toys like those the children around them are using, but as each child sees fit, neither influencing nor being influenced by the other children. Each plays beside, but not with, other children (Fig. 5-7). There is no group association. Parallel play is the characteristic play of toddlers, but it may also occur in other groups of any age. Individuals who are involved in a creative craft with each person separately working on an individual project are engaged in parallel play.

Associative play—In associative play, children play together and are engaged in a similar or even identical activity, but there is no organization, division of labor, leadership assignment, or mutual goal. Children borrow and lend play materials, follow each other with wagons and tricycles, and sometimes attempt to control who may or may not play in the group. Each child acts according to his or her own wishes; there is no group goal (Fig. 5-8). For example, two children play with dolls, borrowing articles of clothing from each other and engaging in similar conversation, but neither directs the other's actions or establishes rules regarding the limits of the play session. There is a great deal of behavioral contagion: when one child initiates an activity, the entire group follows the example.

FIG. 5-9 ■ Cooperative play.

Cooperative play—Cooperative play is organized, and children play in a group *with* other children (Fig. 5-9). They discuss and plan activities for the purposes of accomplishing an end—to make something, to attain a competitive goal, to dramatize situations of adult or group life, or to play formal games. The group is loosely formed, but there is a marked sense of belonging or not belonging. The goal and its attainment require organization of activities, division of labor, and role playing. The leader-follower relationship is definitely established, and the activity is controlled by one or two members who assign roles and direct the activity of the others. The activity is organized to allow one child to supplement another's function to complete the goal.

FUNCTIONS OF PLAY
Sensorimotor Development

Sensorimotor activity is a major component of play at all ages and is the predominant form of play in infancy. Active play is essential for muscle development and serves a useful purpose as a release for surplus energy. Through sensorimotor play, children explore the nature of the physical world. Infants gain impressions of themselves and their world through tactile, auditory, visual, and kinesthetic stimulation. Toddlers and preschoolers revel in body movement and exploration of objects in space. With increasing maturity, sensorimotor play becomes more differentiated and involved. Whereas very young children run for the sheer joy of body movement, older children incorporate or modify the motions into increasingly complex and coordinated activities such as races, games, roller skating, and bicycle riding.

Intellectual Development

Through exploration and manipulation children learn colors, shapes, sizes, textures, and the significance of objects. They learn the significance of numbers and how to use them; they learn to associate words with objects; and they develop an understanding of abstract concepts and spatial relationships, such as *up, down, under,* and *over.* Activities such as puzzles and games help them develop problem-solving skills. Books, stories, films, and collections expand knowledge and provide enjoyment as well. Play provides a means to practice and expand language skills. Through play, children continually rehearse past experiences to assimilate them into new perceptions and

relationships. Play helps children comprehend the world in which they live and distinguish between fantasy and reality.

Socialization

From very early infancy children show interest and pleasure in the company of others. Their initial social contact is with the mothering person, but through play with other children they learn to establish social relationships and solve the problems associated with these relationships. They learn to give and take, which is more readily learned from critical peers than from the more tolerant adults. They learn the sex role that society expects them to fulfill, as well as approved patterns of behavior and deportment. Closely associated with socialization is development of moral values and ethics. Children learn right from wrong, the standards of the society, and to assume responsibility for their actions.

Creativity

In no other situation is there more opportunity to be creative than in play. Children can experiment and try out their ideas in play through every medium at their disposal, including raw materials, fantasy, and exploration. Creativity is stifled by pressure toward conformity; therefore striving for peer approval may inhibit creative endeavors in the school-age or adolescent child. Creativity is primarily a product of solitary activity, yet creative thinking is often enhanced in group settings where listening to others' ideas stimulates further exploration of one's own ideas. After children feel the satisfaction of creating something new and different, they transfer this creative interest to situations outside the world of play.

Self-Awareness

Beginning with active explorations of their bodies and awareness of themselves as separate from the mother, the process of developing a self-identity is facilitated through play activities. Children learn who they are and their place in the world. They become increasingly able to regulate their own behavior, to learn what their abilities are, and to compare their abilities with those of others. Through play, children are able to test their abilities, to assume and try out various roles, and to learn the effect their behavior has on others. They learn the sex role that society expects them to fulfill, as well as approved patterns of behavior and deportment.

Therapeutic Value

Play is therapeutic at any age (Fig. 5-10). In play, children can express emotions and release unacceptable impulses in a socially acceptable fashion. Children are able to experiment and test fearful situations and can assume and vicariously master the roles and positions that they are unable to perform in the world of reality. Children reveal much about themselves in play. Through play, children are able to communicate to the alert observer the needs, fears, and desires that they are unable to express with their limited language skills. Throughout their play, children need the acceptance of adults and their presence to help them control aggression and to channel their destructive tendencies.

Moral Value

Although children learn at home and at school those behaviors considered right and wrong in the culture, the interaction with peers during play contributes significantly to their moral

FIG. 5-10 ■ Play is therapeutic at any age and provides a means for release of tension and stress.

training. Nowhere is the enforcement of moral standards as rigid as in the play situation. If they are to be acceptable members of the group, children must adhere to the accepted codes of behavior of the culture (e.g., fairness, honesty, self-control, consideration for others). Children soon learn that their peers are less tolerant of violations than are adults and that to maintain a place in the play group, they must conform to the standards of the group.

TOYS

The type of toys chosen by or provided for children can support and enhance the child's development in the areas just described. Although no scientific evidence shows that any toy is necessary for optimal learning, toys offer an opportunity to bring the child and parent together. Research has indicated that a positive parent-child interaction can enhance early childhood brain development (American Academy of Pediatric, 2003). Toys that are small replicas of the culture and its tools help children assimilate into their culture. Toys that require pushing, pulling, rolling, and manipulating teach them about physical properties of the items and help develop muscles and coordination. Rules and the basic elements of cooperation and organization are learned through board games.

Because they can be used in a variety of ways, raw materials with which children can exercise their own creativity and imaginations are sometimes superior to ready-made items. For example, building blocks can be used to construct a variety of structures, to count, and to learn shapes and sizes.

Toy Safety

Selection of toys and play equipment is a joint effort between parents and children, but evaluation of their safety is the responsibility of the adult. Government agencies do not inspect and police all toys on the market. Therefore adults

who purchase, supervise purchases, or allow children to use play equipment need to evaluate such equipment for its safety and age appropriateness. This includes toys that are gifts or those that are purchased by the children themselves (see Family-Centered Care box). A choke tube tester, about the same diameter as a child's windpipe, can be used to determine whether a toy is small enough to be a choking hazard. Parents should also be alert to notices of toys determined to be defective and recalled by the manufacturers. Parents and health workers can obtain information on a variety of recalled products and can report potentially dangerous toys and child products to the U.S. Consumer Product Safety Commission (CPSC)* or, in Canada, the Canadian Toy Testing Council.†

SELECTED FACTORS THAT INFLUENCE DEVELOPMENT

HEREDITY

Inherited characteristics have a profound influence on development. The sex of the child, determined by random selection at the time of conception, directs both the pattern of growth and the behavior of others toward the child. In all cultures, attitudes and expectations are shaped by the sex of the child. Sex and other hereditary determinants strongly affect the end result of growth and the rate of progress toward it. There is a high correlation between parent and child with regard to traits such as height, weight, and rate of growth. Most physical characteristics, including shape and form of features, body build, and physical peculiarities, are inherited and can influence the way in which children grow and interact with their environment. Many dimensions of personality, such as temperament, activity level, responsiveness, and a tendency toward shyness, are believed to be inherited.

Differences in health and vigor of children may be attributed to hereditary traits. An inherited physical or mental disorder will alter or modify a child's physical or emotional growth and interactions. The extent to which disabling conditions interfere with the child's growth and well-being is considered in relation to numerous disabilities throughout the remainder of the book.

NEUROENDOCRINE FACTORS

The hypothalamic-pituitary axis produces a number of releasing and inhibitory hormones that influence growth. There is evidence, based on observations of denervated skeletal muscles, that the peripheral nervous system may influence growth, since muscles deprived of nerve supply degenerate. Many of these effects are not sufficiently explained by disuse or diminished blood supply.

Probably all hormones affect growth in some fashion. Three hormones—growth hormone, thyroid hormone, and androgens—when given to persons deficient in these hormones, stimulate protein anabolism and thereby produce retention of elements essential for building protoplasm and bony tissue. It appears that each of the hormones that has a significant influence on growth manifests its major effect at a different period of growth (see Chapter 29).

---

*CPSC hotline: (800) 638-2772; http://www.cpsc.gov (assistance is also available in Spanish).
†1973 Baseline Road, Ottawa ON K2C 0C7, Canada; (613) 228-3155; fax: (613) 228-3242; http://www.toy-testing.org.

FAMILY-CENTERED CARE

Toy Safety*

SELECTION

Select toys that suit the skills, abilities, and interests of children.

Select toys that are safe for the specific child; look for a label that indicates the intended age-group. Toys that are safe for one age may not be safe for another.

For infants, toddlers, and all children who still mouth objects, avoid toys with small parts that may pose a fatal choking or aspiration hazard. Toys in this category are usually labeled, "Not recommended for children under 3 years."

For infants avoid toys with strings or cords that are 7 inches or longer because they may cause strangulation.

For all children younger than 8 years avoid electric toys with heating elements.

For children younger than 5 years avoid arrows or darts.

Check for safety labels such as "flame retardant" or "flame resistant."

Select toys durable enough to survive rough play; look for sturdy construction such as tightly secured eyes, nose, or any small parts.

Select toys light enough that they will not cause harm if one falls on a child.

Look for toys with smooth, rounded edges. Avoid toys with sharp edges that can cut or that have sharp points. Points on the inside of the toy can puncture the skin if the toy is broken.

Avoid toys with any shooting or throwing objects that can injure eyes. This includes toys with which other missiles such as sticks or pebbles might be used as substitutes for the intended projectiles.

Arrows and darts used by children should have blunt tips and be manufactured from resilient materials; make certain the tips are securely attached.

Make certain that materials in toys are nontoxic by checking where the toy is manufactured, looking for recalls on toys, and checking the news.

Avoid toys that make loud noises that might damage a child's hearing. Even some squeaking toys are too loud when held close to the ear.

If selecting caps for cap guns, look for the label required by federal law to be on boxes or packages of caps, which states: "Warning—Do not fire closer than 1 foot to the ear. Do not use indoors."

If selecting a toy gun, be certain that the barrel or the entire gun is brightly colored to avoid being mistaken for a real gun.

BB guns or pellet rifles should not be given to children under the age of 16.

Electric toys should be labeled UL, which means they have met the safety standards of the Underwriters Laboratories.

Check toy instructions for clarity. They should be clear to an adult and, when appropriate, to the child.

SUPERVISION

Maintain a safe play environment.

Remove and discard plastic wrappings on toys immediately; they could suffocate a child.

Remove large toys, bumper pads, and boxes from playpens; an adventuresome child can use such items as a means of climbing or falling out.

Set ground rules for play.

Supervise young children closely during play.

Teach children how to use toys properly and safely.

Instruct older children to keep their toys away from younger brothers, sisters, and friends.

Keep children who are playing with riding toys away from stairs, hills, traffic, and swimming pools.

Establish and enforce rules regarding protective gear.

- Insist that children wear helmets when using bicycles, skateboards, or in-line skates.
- Insist that children wear gloves and wrist, elbow, and knee pads when using skateboards or in-line skates.

Instruct children on electrical safety.

- Teach children the proper way to unplug an electric toy—pull on the plug, not the cord.
- Teach children to beware of electrical appliances and even electrically operated playthings; often children are unfamiliar with the hazards of electricity in association with water.

Teach children the safe use of utensils that under certain circumstances can cause injury—scissors, knives, needles, heating elements, loops, long string, or cord.

MAINTENANCE

Inspect old and new toys regularly for breakage, loose parts, and other potential hazards.

Look for jagged or sharp edges or broken parts that might constitute a choking hazard.

Check movable parts to make certain they are attached securely to the toys; sometimes pieces that are safe when attached to the toy become a danger when detached.

Examine all outdoor toys regularly for rust and weak or sharp parts that could become a danger to a child.

Check electrical cords and plugs for cracked or fraying parts.

Maintain toys in good repair, without signs of possible hazards such as sharp edges, splinters, weak seams, or rust.

Make repairs immediately, or discard out of reach of children.

Sand sharp wooden toys or splintered surfaces so they are smooth.

Use only paint labeled "nontoxic" to repaint toys, toy boxes, or children's furniture.

STORAGE

Provide a safe place for children to store toys, and teach them how to store toys safely to prevent accidental injury from stepping, tripping, or falling on a toy.

Select a toy chest or toy box that is ventilated, is free of self-locking devices that could trap a child inside, and has a lid designed not to pinch a child's fingers or fall on a child's head.

To avoid entrapment and suffocation, containers other than toy chests used for storage purposes should be fitted with spring-loaded support devices if they have a hinged lid.

Playthings meant for older children and adults should be safely stowed away on high shelves, in locked closets, or in other areas unavailable to younger children.

*Another helpful resource is *Toy safety: guidelines for parents* from American Academy of Pediatrics, Division of Publications, 141 Northwest Point Blvd., Elk Grove Village, IL 60007-1098; http://www.aap.org.

COMMUNITY FOCUS

Healthy Food Choices

Current research indicates that new lower-fat recipes in school lunch programs are well accepted by children (Matvienko, 2007). However, less-healthy foods are still more readily available than more-healthy foods in our nation's schools (Delva, O'Malley, Johnston, 2007).

NUTRITION

Nutrition is probably the single most important influence on growth. Dietary factors regulate growth at all stages of development, and their effects are exerted in numerous and complex ways. During the rapid prenatal growth period, poor nutrition may influence development from the time of implantation of the ovum until birth. During infancy and childhood the demand for calories is relatively great, as evidenced by the rapid increase in both height and weight. At this time protein and caloric requirements are higher than at almost any period of postnatal development. As the growth rate slows, with its concomitant decrease in metabolism, there is a corresponding reduction in caloric and protein requirements (see Table 5-2).

Growth is uneven during the periods of childhood between infancy and adolescence, when there are plateaus and small growth spurts. The child's appetite fluctuates in response to these variations until the turbulent growth spurt of adolescence, when adequate nutrition is extremely important but may be subjected to numerous emotional influences. Adequate nutrition is closely related to good health throughout life, and an overall improvement in nourishment is evidenced by the gradual increase in size and early maturation of children in this century (see Community Focus box).

INTERPERSONAL RELATIONSHIPS

Relationships with significant others play a critical role in development, particularly in emotional, intellectual, and personality development. Not only do the quality and quantity of contacts with other persons exert an influence on the growing child, but the widening range of contacts is essential to learning and developing a healthy personality.

The mothering person is unquestionably the single most influential person during early infancy. This person is the one who meets the infant's basic needs of food, warmth, comfort, and love. He or she provides stimulation for the child's senses and facilitates his or her expanding capacities. Through this person the child learns to trust the world and feel secure to venture in increasingly wider relationships.

It is generally the parents who are most influential in helping the child to assume sex-role identification. Parents define and reinforce acceptable sex-role behavior and provide sex-appropriate role models for the child. In the absence of a sex-role model in the family setting, the child may adopt some characteristics of the opposite-sex parent or sibling. Frequently the child identifies with a teacher or other significant person of the same sex.

Siblings are children's first peers, and the way in which they learn to relate to each other affects later interactions with

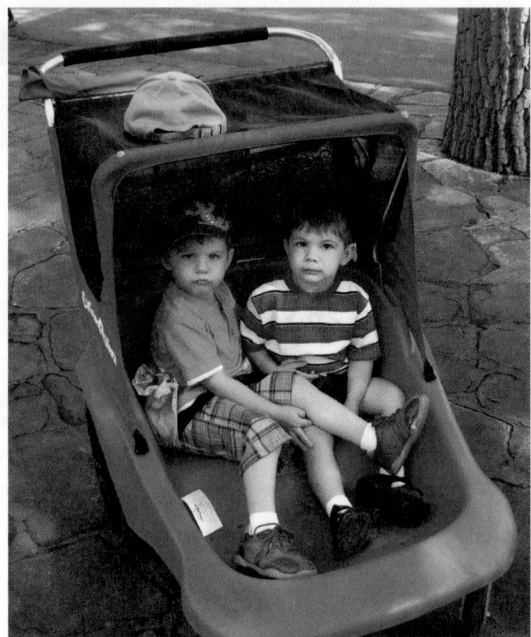

FIG. 5-11 ■ Peers become increasingly important as children develop friendships outside the family group.

peers outside the family group. The sphere of persons from whom children seek approval widens to include other members of their family, their peers, and, to a lesser extent, other authority figures (e.g., teachers). The increasing importance of the peer group in determining the behavior of school-age children and adolescents is well documented (Fig. 5-11).

When children fail to have high-quality interpersonal relationships with mothering persons, they experience **emotional deprivation.** The most prominent feature of emotional deprivation, particularly during the first year, is developmental delays. Much of the information regarding the adverse effects of interpersonal influences on development has been acquired through retrospective studies of gross deprivation and trauma. The most notable instances involved homeless infants who were placed in institutions for care. Those infants who did not receive consistent mothering care failed to gain weight even with an adequate diet; were pale, listless, and immobile; and were unresponsive to stimuli such as smiling or cooing that usually elicit a response from the normal infant. If emotional deprivation continues for a sufficient length of time, the child may not survive infancy.

Although the most remarkable examples of emotional deprivation were first recognized among infants in institutions, the term **masked deprivation** has been used to describe children reared in homes in which there is a distorted parent-child relationship or otherwise disordered home environment. Infants do not thrive if the caregiving person is hostile, fearful of handling them, or indifferent to them and their needs. Such children exhibit poor growth even though they are apparently free of physical disease. Growth delays in these children are believed to be caused by a psychologically induced endocrine imbalance that interferes with growth. These same infants and children display "catch-up" growth in a changed environment (see Growth Failure [Failure to Thrive], Chapter 11).

SOCIOECONOMIC LEVEL

Evidence indicates that the socioeconomic level of children's families has a significant impact on growth and development. At all ages, children from upper- and middle-class families are taller than comparative children of families in the lower socioeconomic strata. The cause of these differences is less definite, although the poorer health and nutrition of lower socioeconomic levels are probably significant factors. Nutritious food sources (especially proteins) are scarce, and other factors (e.g., larger family size and irregularity in eating, sleeping, and exercise) may play a role.

Families from lower socioeconomic groups may lack the knowledge or resources needed to provide the safe, stimulating, and enriched environment that fosters optimum development for children. They may be unable to move from unsafe neighborhoods where drug traffic and drive-by shootings are the norm. The effects on the emotional development of children living under these conditions have been compared with those experienced by children living in war zones.

DISEASE

Altered growth and development are one of the clinical manifestations in a number of hereditary disorders. Growth impairment is particularly marked in skeletal disorders, such as the various forms of dwarfism and at least one of the chromosomal anomalies (Turner syndrome). Many of the disorders of metabolism, such as vitamin D–resistant rickets, the mucopolysaccharidoses, and the numerous endocrine disorders, interfere with the normal growth pattern. In other disorders the tendency is toward the upper percentile of height (e.g., Klinefelter and Marfan syndromes).

Many chronic illnesses that are associated with varying degrees of growth failure are congenital cardiac anomalies and respiratory disorders such as cystic fibrosis. Any disorder characterized by the inability to digest and absorb body nutrients will have an adverse effect on growth and development.

ENVIRONMENTAL HAZARDS

Hazards in the environment are a source of concern to health care providers and others interested in health and safety. Physical injuries are the most prevalent consequences of environmental dangers, and these are discussed extensively throughout the book in relation to age, specific hazards, and selected physical disabilities.

Children are at a high risk for harm resulting from the chemical residues of modern life present in the environment. The hazards of these chemical residues relate to their potential carcinogenicity, enzymatic effects, and accumulation (Baum and Shannon, 1995) (see Community Focus box). The harmful agents most often associated with health risks are chemicals and radiation. Water, air, and food contamination from a variety of sources are well documented. Significant causes of exposure are substances in the immediate environment such as lead and asbestos, chemicals secreted in breast milk (especially prescribed drugs and nicotine), and contamination within well-insulated homes (especially from disinfectants or burning of substances that produce toxic fumes). Passive inhalation of tobacco smoke by infants and children is a hazard at all stages of development. The harmful effects of large doses of radiation are unquestioned, although the effects of low-dose or short-term radiation are debatable, as are the safe vs harmful dosage levels.

COMMUNITY FOCUS

Sun Protection Basics

Skin cancer is increasing in children, accounting for about 4% of pediatric malignancies. Each Global Solar UV Index level has associated precautions, including sunglasses, sunscreens, sun protective clothing, and sun avoidance.

- Children's sunglasses must absorb at least 99% of ultraviolet radiation (UV). Choose sunglasses with the label "Blocks 99% of UV rays," "UV absorption up to 400 nm," "Special purpose," or "Meets American National Standards Institute (ANSI) requirements."
- Allow children to choose their sunglasses. A child who wears prescription glasses should also wear prescription sunglasses.
- Avoid sun exposure between 10 AM and 2 PM. High altitude, sand, concrete, snow, and water increase UV exposure.
- Wear wide-brim hats and sun protective clothing.
- Apply an adequate layer of sunscreen, preferably waterproof or water resistant, and reapply at regular intervals.

From Maguire-Eisen M, Rothman K, Demierre M: The ABC's of sun protection, *Dermatol Nurs* 17(6):419-433, 2005.

STRESS IN CHILDHOOD

Defined from both a physiologic and an emotional point of view, essentially **stress** is "an imbalance between environmental demands and a person's coping resources that . . . disrupts the equilibrium of the person" (Masten, Garmezy, Tellegen, and others, 1988).

Although all children experience stress, some youngsters appear to be more vulnerable than others. Children's age, temperament, life situation, and state of health affect their vulnerability, reactions, and ability to handle stress. Also, the responses to a stressor can be behavioral, psychologic, or physiologic. It is impossible and undesirable to protect children from stress, but providing them with interpersonal security helps them develop coping strategies for dealing with stress. The concept of an **emotional bank,** in which deposits and withdrawals can be made, can help parents and caregivers maintain a proper perspective regarding the effects of stress and coping. Children with a good, positive balance in the account can tolerate significant withdrawal experiences. For children with a low balance, even a minor withdrawal may bankrupt the account, causing it to be overdrawn.

Parents and other caregivers can try to recognize signs of stress to help children deal with stressors before they become overwhelming. Signs of stress take many forms but are typically the same ones seen in children who are abused (see Chapter 14) or depressed (see Chapter 17). If a number of stressors are imposed on children at the same time, the children are more vulnerable. When a succession of stressors produces an excessive stress load, children may experience a serious change in health or behavior.

It is important that parents and persons working with children understand the nature of childhood stress and ways it can be recognized or anticipated. Caregivers must *listen* to children so they are aware of children's fears and concerns and must let them know that they are important and that what they say matters. Physical contact is comforting and reassuring to children. Simply holding, touching, or hugging children is both relaxing and comforting and facilitates communication. Spending unhurried time with children, taking family outings or vacations, and exposing children to positive influences help build children's strength and security. Supportive interpersonal relationships are essential to the psychologic well-being of children.

Coping

Coping refers to a special class of individual reactions to stressors—specifically, a reaction to a stressor that resolves, reduces, or replaces the affective state classified as stressful. **Coping strategies** are the specific ways in which children cope with stressors, as distinguished from **coping styles,** which are relatively unchanging personality characteristics or outcomes of coping (Wachs, 2006). Research indicates that, as children age, they tend toward a more internal locus of control and use more vigilant modes of coping (LaMontagne, Hepworth, Johnson, and others, 1996). Children, like adults, respond to everyday stress by trying to change the circumstances or trying to adjust to circumstances the way they are. Any strategy that provides relaxation is effective in reducing stress, and most children have their own natural methods such as withdrawal, physical activity, reading, listening to music, working on a project, or taking a nap. Some turn to parents to solve their problems, or they may develop socially unacceptable strategies, such as cheating, stealing, or lying.

Children can be taught stress-reduction techniques to use in coping. First, they must be helped to recognize signs of tension in themselves and then taught any of a variety of appropriate strategies—special exercises, relaxation and breathing, mental imagery, and numerous other simple activities. Also, parents and other caregivers can anticipate possible stress-provoking events and prepare children for coping by role playing a scenario or "talking it through" beforehand. Probably the most useful tool that children can learn is how to solve problems. When children can view any new situation as a problem to be solved and an opportunity to learn, they are not vulnerable to the control of others. It provides them with a sense of mastery over their own lives and reinforces the fact that they have within themselves the ability and information to handle whatever comes their way. Problem-solving skill gives them the confidence to know where and how to seek help when they need it.

INFLUENCE OF THE MASS MEDIA

Media can have an enormous influence on the developing child. There is no doubt that the media provide children with a means for extending their knowledge about the world in which they live and have helped narrow the differences between classes. However, there is growing concern regarding the enormous influence the media can have on the developing child because of the large number of hours spent watching television. The images of risky behavior presented by the media may serve to establish or reinforce teenagers' perceptions of their social environment. Children may identify closely with people or characters portrayed in reading materials, movies, video games, and television programs and commercials.

Today, children tend to select media and sports figures as their ideal role models, whereas in the past the majority of children chose their parents or parent surrogates as the people they most wanted to be like (Duck, 1990). This trend can be viewed as a grave concern or a magnificent opportunity to promote positive role models.

Reading Materials

Books, newspapers, and magazines are the oldest form of mass media. They contribute to children's competence in almost every respect and also provide enjoyment. Recognition of the impact that reading matter used in the schools has on the value system and socialization processes has prompted reevaluation of the content of textbooks in terms of the biased presentation of male and female role models, the sugar-coated view of life situations, and the biased history of minority groups.

Fairy tales, for generations the mainstay of young children's literature, for a time were condemned for being sexist; violent; and riddled with unfavorable stereotypes, such as the wicked stepmother, dwarfs, and physical unattractiveness associated with evil. They are now believed to provide an excellent medium for explaining puzzling and important topics such as death, stepparents, and inner feelings and turmoil. Although they do not provide solutions, fairy tales confront children with emotional predicaments and offer suggestions for dealing with them.

Comic books and other pulp reading material have been popular in every generation, usually at the expense of literature provided by schools, libraries, and parents. Many children have nothing else to read. The easy reading, quick action, and adventure in brief episodes seem to fulfill a need for children who are striving to understand both aggression in others and their own impulses. Reading ability, intelligence, and school adjustment apparently have no relationship to the number and type of comic books read. Most comic books appear to be relatively harmless to the majority of children and may be beneficial. Comic books seem to have only a minor influence on acquisition of beliefs, values, and behaviors. The popularity of this medium has prompted some educators to encourage translations of literature into comic book form to stimulate students' interest in the classics.

Movies

Movies that are not closely bound to reality and often portray an assortment of socially approved behaviors may contribute to children's value systems and provide opportunities for desirable social learning. On the other hand, children, especially adolescents, flock to the "macho" movies and those whose heroes resort to violent resolution of problems, such as karate and wild automobile chases. The carryover of these influences into daily life and relationships may account in part for the increase in violent behavior of young persons.

Another concern is the plethora of "slasher" and R-rated movies available to children and teenagers in theaters and through cable television and videocassettes. The content of movies has changed markedly during the past few decades, with violence and mutilation being major themes. To children who are unable to distinguish between reality and fantasy, these films play on their deepest fears and result in bedtime fears, nightmares, and a fearful view of the world.

Young children can be frightened by some of the movies considered safe for family viewing. For example, *Bambi* can frighten young children, and the villainous witches in *Snow White* and the *Wizard of Oz* are terrifying figures. Also, certain classic children's movies, such as *Snow White* and *Cinderella,* depict stepmothers as evil, destructive persons; such portrayals can have a deleterious effect on children-stepmother relationships or can be confusing to children who have developed a positive relationship with a stepmother.

Movie rating categories are available on the Motion Picture Association of America website.*

Television

The medium with the most impact on children in North America today is television, which has become one of the most significant socializing agents in the lives of young children. The content of programs and commercials provides multiple sources for acquiring information, modeling behaviors, and observing value orientations. Besides producing a leveling effect on class differences in general information and vocabulary, television exposes children to a wider variety of topics and events than they encounter in day-to-day life. Television always has time to talk to children and is a form of access to the adult world.

> **FYI**
>
> Researchers have reported that the television is on for more than 6 hours per day in more than half of American homes and that children watch an average of more than 21 hours of television per week; with other media like video games, screen time may increase to as much as 35 to 55 hours a week (Gentile, Oberg, Sherwood, and others, 2004).

Television viewing has a direct impact on child development and behavior. Several studies have found that violence on television and the mass media in general can have a negative influence on the development of unhealthy behaviors and violence in children (Earles, Alexander, Johnson, and others, 2002; Monsen, 2002; Brown and Witherspoon, 2002). Several factors encourage the learning or performing of television-influenced behaviors (Box 5-4).

Most researchers have concluded that protracted television viewing can have detrimental effects on children. For example, in one study, television viewing was implicated as contributing to irregular sleep schedules in children under 3 years of age (Thompson and Christakis, 2005). Recognizing the negative effects of television viewing, the American Academy of Pediatrics has recommended that children older than age 2 watch less than 2 hours of high-quality television a day and that children younger than 2 years watch no television (American Academy of Pediatrics, 2001a; Certain and Kahn, 2002). However, this warning has not been heeded, with approximately 40% of infants already watching by 3 months of age and the number increasing to 90% by 24 months. Parents reported the three primary reasons they allowed their infants to watch television was because they thought it was educational for them, they thought it was entertaining, and they needed time to get other things done. Parents did watch television with their infants more than half the time (Zimmerman, Christakis, and Meltzoff, 2007).

The passive activity associated with television viewing is frequently accompanied by eating—in many cases, high-calorie snacks. Furthermore, children may expend tremendous mental energy processing the audiovisual messages from television, which may be exhausting and make them less likely to engage in physical activity later. Andersen, Crespo, Bartlett,

*http://www.mpaa.org.

> ■ **BOX 5-4**
>
> ### Factors That Encourage Learning or Performing Television-Influenced Behaviors
>
> **Age**—Younger children focus on behaviors rather than on motives or consequences. They view alternatives in a concrete manner, and they are unable to differentiate between central and peripheral plot information.
>
> **Identification with characters or situations**—Children often imitate behaviors of persons and situations similar to those in their own lives.
>
> **Reward and punishment syndrome**—Children imitate behaviors they see rewarded or not punished when it is expected. They are less likely to repeat an act they see punished; their attention is immediately attracted when they see an act committed that they know should be punished but is not.
>
> **Opportunity to reproduce behaviors**—Children imitate behaviors when given the right environment or when violence seems an accepted solution. When children see a situation on television, they use this information when they encounter a similar situation that requires a solution.
>
> **Motivation to reproduce behaviors**—Children imitate behavior when given the appropriate incentives: expectation of reward or lack of punishment. Some children have self-control; others do not.

and others (1998) found that the incidence of body fat increased in direct proportion to the amount of hours of television watched by children in the United States; as the number of hours of television viewing increased, children were less likely to participate in vigorous physical activities.

In a study to identify children at risk for heart disease, researchers found that more than half of the children with high cholesterol levels watched at least 2 hours of television each day. Using a family history of heart disease or high cholesterol as the screening indicator for cholesterol testing in children, researchers identified three out of four children with high cholesterol levels. When these families were also questioned about the time their children spent watching television, investigators were able to identify 90% of the children with high cholesterol levels by using 2 or more viewing hours as the risk factor (Goldsmith, 1990).

Television programs and commercials, like movies, contain many implicit and explicit messages that promote alcohol consumption, smoking, violence, and promiscuous or unsafe sexual activity. An area of increasing concern is media violence, especially in programs featuring heavy metal rock groups, whose lyrics and videos sensationalize violent sex, suicide, and satanism. There is now clear evidence documenting a relationship between television viewing and the use of alcohol or tobacco, violence and aggressive behavior, the use of guns to commit violent acts, and early sexual activity (American Academy of Pediatrics, 2001a; Strasburger and Donnerstein, 1999).

Parents can help children evaluate television violence by pointing out the subtleties children miss, such as the aggressor's motives and intentions and the unpleasant consequences the perpetrators suffer as a result of their aggressive acts. Often the consequence is separated from the act by a commercial, and therefore children cannot make the correlation. Parents need to point out that conflicts can be resolved without resorting to violent behavior. They can also stress the purpose of the programs—primarily entertainment—and explain why they like or dislike something on television (e.g., "This show is trying to tell you that crime does not pay and that if one does wrong, one will go to jail"). Explanations and discussions can take place between shows (with the volume turned down), and young children can learn from both older children and adults. These discussions can be effective when begun early and carried out consistently.

It is especially important to identify at-risk children and control their viewing. House rules that specify the type and amount of television help children understand limits, and video-recorded selections of appropriate programs can be substituted for less desirable offerings. Parents need to carefully monitor cable and other pay-television programming because these popular options present more uncensored programming. Locked boxes, V-chips, and blocking devices are available for cable receivers to prevent children from viewing programs when unsupervised. Vessey, Yim-Chiplis, MacKenzie, and others (1998) suggest that parental role modeling may have a more positive influence on the child's behavior than television programming. They further recommend that parents watch television with children and help children understand the difference between their life and habits and those of persons represented on television.

Television is the medium by which most children learn of a natural disaster or act of terrorism. Research on the effects of September 11, 2001, and the Oklahoma City bombing suggests that posttraumatic stress reactions increase with increased exposure to media coverage. Reading, rather than watching the event on television, may lead to better retention of the experience (Pfefferbaum, Seale, Brandt, and others, 2003). After September 11, 2001, 85% of children in one study reported concerns for their safety and security (Phillips, Prince, and Schiebelhut, 2004). More than half of the children in this study coped by volunteering their time or donating materials for relief teams. In addition, parents should limit the exposure to media coverage of traumatic events, talk to their child about the event, and maintain routines as much as possible.

On the positive side, television has been shown to be a positive influence on children's abilities to deal with a variety of social issues such as divorce, the arrival of a new baby, discrimination, honesty, and helpfulness. Children who view educational programming (such as "Mister Rogers' Neighborhood" and "Sesame Street") for a long period become more affectionate, considerate, cooperative, and helpful toward their playmates. A systematic review of preschoolers and television found that educational viewing can increase their knowledge, affect their racial attitudes, and increase their imaginative be-

havior (Thakkar, Garrison, and Christakis, 2006). The ways that minority and ethnic characters are portrayed on television can have an impact on the way the majority culture views minority persons and on the self-image of minority children.

Parents need to supervise the amount and type of television programs their children watch and to teach their children how to watch television (Box 5-5 and Family-Centered Care box).

NURSING TIP
During an assessment, consider that parents may not be aware of how much time their children spend watching television. Parents may also not understand the child's inability to distinguish between the "fantasy" of television and life events (Vessey, Yim-Chiplis, and MacKenzie, 1998).

Nurses and parents can be powerful forces in influencing the media. They can watch closely for an increase in violence and other undesirable programming and complain to sponsors and television stations if they believe it is not appropriate. Good programming can be both educational and entertaining.

Video Games

With the popularity of home gaming systems, children are spending increased hours playing video games. Unfortunately, many of the video games available are violent, portraying vir-

---

FAMILY-CENTERED CARE

Television Viewing

Provide a positive role model by developing television substitutes such as reading, athletics, physical conditioning, and hobbies.
Construct a time chart of child's activities (homework, television viewing, scheduled outside activities, playing with a friend).
Discuss with child what you both believe to be a balanced set of activities.
At the beginning of each week, select appropriate programs from television schedules.
Allow child to select programs from this approved list.
Limit child's viewing to 2 hours or less per day.
Rule out television at specific times (e.g., before breakfast or on school nights).
Leave the television off at mealtimes.
Make a list of alternative activities (e.g., riding a bicycle, reading a book, or working on a hobby).
Require that child choose to do something from this list before watching television.
Watch programs with child.
Discuss program and commercial content with child:
- Distinguish between the real and the unreal.
- Correlate consequences with actions.
- Point out subtle messages.
- Explore alternatives to aggressive conflict resolution.
- Stress purpose of program (e.g., entertainment, education).
- Explain likes and dislikes.
Turn the television off after the selected program is over.
Remove televisions from children's bedrooms.
Monitor cable and pay television selections; use a lockbox if necessary.
Limit use of television as a safe distraction to potentially stressful times (e.g., keeping the children occupied while the parent gets organized after a difficult day).

BOX 5-5

Five Important Ideas to Teach Children and Adolescents About Television

1. You are smarter than what you see on your television.
2. Television world is not real.
3. Television teaches that some people are more important than others.
4. Television keeps showing the same things over and over again.
5. Somebody is always trying to make money with television.

Modified from Davis J: Five important ideas to teach your children about TV, *Media Values* 59/60:10-14, 1992.

tual crimes and violence against others, particularly women. Video games allow the player to be the aggressor, making an ideal environment for a child to learn violent behavior (American Academy of Pediatrics, 2001b). Although video games come with violence and age ratings, many parents are not aware of or choose to ignore the rating appropriate for their child. The American Academy of Pediatrics (2001b) recommends that health care providers encourage parents to adhere to the game ratings and limit the amount of time spent playing games and watching television to less than 2 hours a day combined. Video games have two ratings criteria. The front cover has the rating symbol for age appropriateness, and the back cover has a descriptor indicating the elements of the game. The ratings can be found on the Entertainment Software Rating Board website.*

Internet

The use of computers in both the classroom and household has affected childhood learning and development. Schools offer a wide variety of computer programs that enable children of all ages to broaden their world views. Computers offer the advantage of interactive learning and improved hand-eye coordination. Parents have a wide variety of computer software choices for learning and gaming.

Although computer technology has enhanced many forms of learning and recreation, there are potential dangers to children. The Internet and e-mail have made correspondence and information available to children from around the world in minutes. Social networking sites (e.g., MySpace, FaceBook) provide opportunities for children and adolescents to express themselves through blogs, music, pictures, and videos. Although the site owner can accept new friends, many experts are concerned that on-line friendships do not have the same depth as in-person relationships and that security filters are inadequate to protect vulnerable teenagers. Some activities such as "cybersex" and "kiddie porn," as well as some "chat rooms," may expose children to individuals who may attempt to take advantage of the child's naïveté for illicit purposes. Government officials are working to curb illegal activities on the Internet that involve children, yet at the same time maintain freedom of speech. Filtered Internet service providers are available that may serve to protect children from objectionable sites. Nurses must be involved in encouraging parents to be knowledgeable of their children's Internet activities while providing appropriate learning activities unique to computers. One helpful strategy is to locate the computer in a public area of the home such as the kitchen or family room to enable parents to easily monitor its use.

DEVELOPMENTAL ASSESSMENT

One of the most essential components of a complete health appraisal is assessment of developmental function. **Screening** procedures are designed to identify quickly and reliably those children whose developmental level is below normal for their age and who therefore require further investigation. They also provide a means of recording objective measurements of present developmental function for future reference. Since the passage of Public Law 99-457, the Education of the Handicapped Act Amendments of 1986, much greater emphasis is placed on developmental assessment of children with disabili-

ties, and nurses can play a vital role in providing this service. It is estimated that 16% of children are affected by developmental disabilities, but fewer than 30% of these children are identified before kindergarten (Wagner, Jenkins, and Smith, 2006). All the procedures discussed in this section can be administered in a variety of settings: home, school, daycare center, hospital, practitioner's office, or clinic.

DENVER II

The most widely used developmental screening tests for young children are the series of tests developed by William Frankenburg and his colleagues (1994a). The oldest and best known—the **Denver Developmental Screening Test (DDST)** and its revision, the **DDST-R**—have been revised, restandardized, and renamed the **Denver II.** Before administering the Denver II, the examiner should be trained by, and receive certification from, a master instructor who has been trained by the Denver faculty.* The Denver II differs from the DDST in items, test form, interpretation, and referral (see Appendix A). The previous total of 105 items has been increased to 125, including an increase from 21 DDST to 39 Denver II language items. Previous items that were difficult to administer or interpret have been either modified or eliminated. Many items that were previously tested by parental report now require observation by the examiner.

Each item was evaluated to determine whether significant differences exist on the basis of sex, ethnic group, maternal education, and place of residence. Items for which clinically significant differences exist were replaced or, if retained, are discussed in the technical manual. When evaluating children delayed on one of these items, the examiner can look up norms for the subpopulations to consider whether the delay may be caused by sociocultural or environmental differences.

The items on the test form are arranged in the same format as the DDST-R. The norms for the distribution bars were updated with the new standardization data but retain the 25th, 50th, 75th, and 90th percentile divisions. The test form contains a place to rate the child's behavioral characteristics (compliance, interest in surroundings, fearfulness, and attention span).

To determine relative areas of advancement and delay, enough items should be administered to establish the basal and ceiling levels in each sector. By scoring appropriate items as "pass," "fail," "refusal," or "no opportunity" and relating such scores to the child's age, the examiner can interpret each item as described in Box 5-6. To identify "cautions," all items intersected by the age line are administered. To screen solely for developmental delays, only the items located totally to the *left* of the child's age line are administered. Criteria for referral are based on the availability of resources in the community.

Research on the Denver II's validity and accuracy continues. One study found that it identified most children with even subtle developmental problems. However, almost half the children without developmental problems received suspect scores, resulting in a high rate of overreferrals (Glascoe, Byrne, Ashford, and others, 1992). To minimize overreferrals, a decision for referral depends not only on the results of the Denver II, but also on the practitioner's clinical judgment af-

---

*http://www.esrb.org/ratings.

*Forms and complete instructions are available from Denver Developmental Materials, PO Box 371075, Denver, CO 80237-5075; (800) 419-4729; http://www.denverii.com. The DDST and DDST-R are no longer available.

BOX 5-6
Denver II Scoring

INTERPRETATION OF DENVER II SCORES
Advanced—Passed an item completely to the right of the age line (passed by less than 25% of children).

OK—Passed, failed, or refused an item intersected by the age line between the 25th and 75th percentiles.

Caution—Failed or refused items intersected by the age line on or between the 75th and 90th percentiles.

Delay—Failed an item completely to the left of the age line. Refusals to the left of the age line may also be considered delays, since the reason for the refusal may be inability to perform the task.

INTERPRETATION OF TEST
Normal—No delays and a maximum of one caution

Suspect—One or more delays or two or more cautions

Untestable—Refusals on one or more items completely to the left of the age line or on more than one item intersected by the age line in the 75th to 90th percentile area

RECOMMENDATIONS FOR REFERRAL FOR SUSPECT AND UNTESTABLE RESULTS
Rescreen in 1 to 2 weeks to rule out temporary factors.

If rescreen is suspect or untestable, use clinical judgment based on the following: number of cautions and delays; which items are cautions and delays; rate of past development; clinical examination and history; and availability of referral resources.

ter considering the child's developmental history; general health status; social, cultural, and emotional environment; and the availability of local resources for diagnosis and treatment (Frankenburg, 1994a, 1994b).

Although it is not the purpose of this discussion to detail the instruction manual, some points concerning preparation, administration, and interpretation of the Denver II are important to stress. Before beginning the screening, ask whether the child was born preterm and correctly calculate the adjusted age. Up to 24 months of age, allowances are made for preterm infants by subtracting the number of weeks of missed gestation from their present age and testing them at the adjusted age. For example, a 16-week-old infant who was born 4 weeks early is tested at a 12-week adjusted age level.

Explain to the parents and child, if appropriate, that the screenings are *not* intelligence tests but rather are a method of showing what the child can do at a particular age. Emphasize that the child is *not* expected to perform each item on the test. Tell the parent before the screening begins that the results of the child's performance will be explained after all the items have been concluded. It is the nurse's responsibility to properly inform parents of any testing or screening procedure before its administration so that they are fully aware of its purpose and intent.

Prepare toddlers and preschoolers for the procedure by presenting it as a game. Frequently, the Denver II is an excellent way to begin a health appraisal because it is nonthreatening, requires no painful or unfamiliar procedures, and capitalizes on the child's natural activity of play. Because children are easily distracted, perform each item quickly and present only one toy from the kit at a time. After that toy's purpose is concluded, such as building a tower of blocks or identifying

its color, replace the toy in the bag and take out another one. Temporary factors that may interfere with the child's performance include fatigue, illness, fear, hospitalization, separation from the parent, or general unwillingness to perform the activities. In addition, undiagnosed mental retardation, hearing loss, vision loss, or neurologic impairment or a familial pattern of slow development greatly influences the child's performance.

After completion of the Denver II, ask the parent whether the child's performance was typical of behavior at other times. If the parent replies affirmatively and the child's cooperation was satisfactory, explain the results, emphasizing all successful items first, then those items the child failed but was not expected to pass, and finally those items that represent delays. If the parent replies that the child's performance was not typical of usual behavior, it is best to defer any scoring or discussion of results, especially if the refusals yield a suspect score. In this situation reschedule testing for a time when the child is more likely to cooperate.

In explaining a normal score, focus on how well the child performed and reinforce the parents' efforts in satisfactorily stimulating their child. In addition to assessing the child's present developmental level, the Denver II can be used to guide parents toward those activities that are appropriate, although not necessarily expected, for the child's age. By testing for items to the right of the age line (ones the child is not expected to perform), the examiner can identify children with advanced development, who may be gifted.

In explaining delays, carefully note the parent's response, especially casual acceptance such as "He'll catch up" or questions such as "Does this mean my child is retarded?" Be aware of personal anxieties during these situations and refrain from giving glib reassurances such as "I'm sure he will do better next time." Rather, respond honestly to parents' questions, yet with appropriate flexibility and concern, stressing the need for further developmental testing.

DENVER II PRESCREENING DEVELOPMENTAL QUESTIONNAIRE

The Prescreening Developmental Questionnaire (PDQ II) is a further revision of the PDQ and the R-PDQ. This version uses the norms (90th and 75th percentiles) from the Denver II. The PDQ II is a parent-answered prescreen consisting of 91 questions from the Denver II, although only a subset of questions is asked for each age-group. The form may need to be read to parents and caregivers who are less educated.

Four different forms are available and are selected based on age: orange (0 to 9 months), purple (9 to 24 months), cream (2 to 4 years), and white (4 to 6 years). The caregiver answers questions until (1) three "nos" are circled (they do not have to be consecutive) or (2) all the questions on both sides of the form have been answered. Scoring is based on the number of delays or cautions (see Box 5-6). Children who have no delays or cautions are considered to be developing normally. If a child has one delay or two cautions, the caregiver is provided with age-appropriate developmental activities to pursue with the child, and a rescreen with the PDQ II is done 1 month later. If on rescreening the child has one or more delays, the Denver II is administered as soon as possible. If a child has two or more delays or three or more cautions on the first screening with the PDQ II, the Denver II is administered as soon as possible.

Several additional parent report developmental screening tools meet the standards for screening test accuracy. Some of the most common include the Ages and Stages Questionnaires (ASQ), Parents' Evaluation of Developmental Status (PEDS), Child Development Inventory, and the Pediatric Symptom Checklist. Although it is beyond the scope of this chapter to describe each screening tool, using a tool can aid the nurse in providing anticipatory guidance and appropriate referral (Wagner, Jenkins, and Smith, 2006).

KEY POINTS

- Growth describes a change in quantity and occurs when cells divide and synthesize new proteins.
- Maturation, a qualitative change, describes the aging process or an increase in competence and adaptability.
- Differentiation refers to a biologic description of the processes by which early cells and structures are modified and altered to achieve specific and characteristic physical and chemical properties.
- Development involves change from a lower to a more advanced stage of complexity.
- The five major developmental periods are prenatal, infancy, early childhood, middle childhood, and later childhood (pubescence and adolescence).
- Growth and development proceed in predictable patterns of direction, sequence, and pace.

- The directional trends in growth and development are cephalocaudal, proximodistal, and mass to specific.
- Physical development includes increase in height and weight and changes in body proportion, dentition, and some body tissues.
- The three broad classifications of child temperament are the easy child, the difficult child, and the slow-to-warm-up child.
- The developmental theories most widely used in explaining child growth and development are Freud's psychosexual stages, Erikson's stages of psychosocial development, Piaget's stages of cognitive development, Kohlberg's stages of moral development, and Fowler's stages of spiritual development.
- To develop a positive self-concept, children need recognition for their achievements and the approval of others.
- Through play, children learn about their world and how to relate to objects, people, and situations.
- Play provides a means of development in the areas of sensorimotor and intellectual progress, socialization, creativity, self-awareness, and moral behavior; it serves as a means for release of tension and expression of emotions.
- Growth and development are affected by a variety of conditions and circumstances, including heredity, physiologic function, gender, disease, physical environment, nutrition, and interpersonal relationships.
- Children's vulnerability and reaction to stress depend to a large extent on their age, coping behaviors, and support systems.
- The mass media can be influential in children's learning and behavior.
- Developmental screening tools are valuable in identifying infants and children who are at risk for developmental delays.

REFERENCES

American Academy of Pediatrics, Committee on Early Childhood, Adoption, and Dependent Care: Selecting appropriate toys for young children: the pediatrician's role, *Pediatrics* 111(4):911-913, 2003.

American Academy of Pediatrics, Committee on Public Education: Children, adolescents, and television, *Pediatrics* 107(2):423-426, 2001a.

American Academy of Pediatrics, Committee on Public Education: Media violence, *Pediatrics* 108(5):1222-1226, 2001b.

Anders TF, Sadeh A, Appareddy V: Normal sleep in neonates and children. In Sheldon S, Ferber R, Kryger M, editors: *Principles and practice of sleep medicine in the child*, Philadelphia, 2005, Saunders.

Andersen RE, Crespo CJ, Bartlett SJ, and others: Relationship of physical activity and television watching with body weight and level of fatness among children, *JAMA* 279(12):938-943, 1998.

Baum C, Shannon M: Environmental toxins: cutting the risks, *Contemp Pediatr* 12(7):20-43, 1995.

Beck CT: A meta-analysis of the relationship between postpartum depression and infant temperament, *Nurs Res* 45(4):225-230, 1996.

Brown JD, Witherspoon EM: The mass media and American adolescents' health, *J Adolesc Health* 31(6S):153-170, 2002.

Caine D, DiFiori J, Maffulli N: Physeal injuries in children's and youth sports: reasons for concern? *Br J Sports Med* 40(9):749-760, 2006.

Carey WB: Teaching parents about infant temperament, *Pediatrics* 102(5 Suppl E):1311-1316, 1998.

Certain LK, Kahn RS: Prevalence, correlates, and trajectory of television viewing among infants and toddlers, *Pediatrics* 109(4):634-642, 2002.

Chess S, Thomas A: *Goodness of fit: clinical applications from infancy through adult life*, London, 1999, Routledge.

Cronk C, Crocker AC, Pueschel SM, and others: Growth charts for children with Down syndrome: 1 month to 18 years of age, *Pediatrics* 81(1):102-110, 1988.

Delva J, O'Malley PM, Johnston LD: Availability of more-healthy and less-healthy food choices in American schools: a national study of grade, racial/ethnic, and socioeconomic differences, *Am J Prev Med* 33(4 Suppl):S226-S239, 2007.

Duck J: Children's ideals: the role of real-life versus media figures, *Aust J Psychol* 42:19-29, 1990.

Earles KA, Alexander R, Johnson M, and others: Media influences on children and adolescents: violence and sex, *J Natl Med Assoc* 94(9):797-801, 2002.

Erikson EH: *Childhood and society*, ed 2, New York, 1963, Norton.

Fowler J: *Stages of faith: the psychology of human development and the quest for meaning*, New York, 1981, HarperCollins.

Frankenburg WK: Preventing developmental delays: is developmental screening sufficient? I. Developmental screening and the Denver II, *Pediatrics* 93(4):586-589, 1994a.

Frankenburg WK: Preventing developmental delays: is developmental screening sufficient? II. Partners in health care, *Pediatrics* 93(4):589-593, 1994b.

Galligan M: Proposed guidelines for skin to skin treatment of neonatal hypothermia, *MCN* 31(5):298-304, 2006.

Gentile D, Oberg C, Sherwood N, and others: Well-child visits in the video age: pediatricians and the American Academy of Pediatrics guidelines for children's media use, *Pediatrics* 114(5):1235-1241, 2004.

Glascoe FP, Byrne KE, Ashford LG, and others: Accuracy of the Denver-II in developmental screening, *Pediatrics* 89(6 Pt 2):1221-1225, 1992.

Goldsmith M: Youngsters dialing up cholesterol levels? *JAMA* 264(23):2976, 1990.

Kaczander BI: Pediatric sports medicine: a unique perspective, *Podiatr Manage* 16(2):53-60, 1997.

Kohlberg L: Moral development. In Sills DL, editor: *International encyclopedia of the social sciences*, New York, 1968, Macmillan.

LaMontagne LL, Hepworth JT, Johnson BD, and others: Children's preoperative coping and its effects on postoperative anxiety and return to normal activity, *Nurs Res* 45(3):141-147, 1996.

Lampl M, Thompson A, Frongillo EA: Sex differences in the relationships among weight gain, subcutaneous skinfold tissue and salutatory length growth spurts in infancy, *Pediatr Res* 58(6):1238-1242, 2005.

Lampl M, Johnson ML, Frongillo EA: Mixed distribution analysis identifies saltation and stasis growth, *Ann Hum Biol* 28(4):403-411, 2001.

Masten AS, Garmezy N, Tellegen A, and others: Competence and stress in school children: moderating effects of individual and family qualities, *J Child Psychol Psychiatry* 29:747-764, 1988.

Matvienko O: Impact of a nutrition education curriculum on snack choices of children ages six and seven years, *J Nutr Educ Behav* 39(5):281-285, 2007.

Monsen RB: Children and the media, *J Pediatr Nurs* 17(4):309-310, 2002.

Morrow JD, Camp BW: Mastery motivation and temperament of 7-month-old infants, *Pediatr Nurs* 22(3):211-217, 1996.

Myrelid A, Gustafsson J, Ollars B, and others: Growth charts for Down's syndrome from birth to 18 years of age, *Arch Dis Child* 87(2):97-103, 2002.

Pfefferbaum B, Seale T, Brandt E, and others: Media exposure in children 100 miles from a terrorist bombing, *Ann Clin Psychiatry* 15(1):1-8, 2003.

Phillips D, Prince S, Schiebelhut L: Elementary school children's responses 3 months after the September 11 terrorist attacks: a study in Washington, DC, *Am J Orthopsych* 75(4):509-528, 2004.

Piaget J: *The theory of stages in cognitive development*, New York, 1969, McGraw-Hill.

Seidel HM, Ball JW, Dains JE, and others: *Mosby's guide to physical examination*, ed 6, St Louis, 2007, Mosby.

Sieving RE, Zirbel-Donisch ST: Development and enhancement of self-esteem in children, *J Pediatr Health Care* 4(6):290-296, 1990.

Strasburger VC, Donnerstein E: Children, adolescents, and the media: issues and solution, *Pediatrics* 103(1):129-139, 1999.

Stuart GW, Laraia MT: *Principles and practice of psychiatric nursing*, ed 7, St Louis, 2000, Mosby.

Thakkar R, Garrison M, Christakis D: A systematic review for the effects of television viewing by infants and preschoolers, *Pediatrics* 118(5):2025-2031, 2006.

Thompson DA, Christakis DA: The association between television viewing and irregular sleep schedules among children less than 3 years of age, *Pediatrics* 116(4):851-856, 2005.

Thompson R, Cotner-Bichelman N, McKerchar P, and others: Enhancing early communication through infant sign training, *J Appl Behav Anal* 40(1):15-23, 2007.

Urbanski LF, Hanlon DP: Pediatric orthopedics, *Top Emerg Med* 18(2):73-90, 1996.

Vessey JA, Yim-Chiplis PK, MacKenzie NR: Effects of television viewing on children's development, *Pediatr Nurs* 23(5):483-486, 1998.

Wachs T: Contributions of temperament to buffering and sensitization processes in children's development, *Ann NY Acad Sci* 1094:28-30, 2006.

Wagner J, Jenkins B, Smith J: Nurses' utilization of parent questionnaires for developmental screening, *Pediatr Nurs* 32(5): 409-412, 2006.

Willoughby C, King G, Polatajko H: A therapist's guide to children's self-esteem, *Am J Occup Ther* 50(2):124-132, 1996.

Zimmerman F, Christakis D, Meltzoff A: Television and DVD/video viewing in children younger than 2 years, *Arch Pediatr Adolesc Med* 161:473-479, 2007.

6

Communication and Physical Assessment of the Child

MARILYN J. HOCKENBERRY

CHAPTER OUTLINE

GUIDELINES FOR COMMUNICATION AND INTERVIEWING, 98
Establishing a Setting for Communication, 98
 Appropriate Introduction, 98
 Assurance of Privacy and Confidentiality, 98
Computer Privacy and Applications in Nursing, 99
Telephone Triage and Counseling, 99
COMMUNICATING WITH FAMILIES, 99
Communicating with Parents, 99
 Encouraging the Parent to Talk, 100
 Directing the Focus, 100
 Listening and Cultural Awareness, 100
 Using Silence, 101
 Being Empathic, 101
 Providing Anticipatory Guidance, 101
 Avoiding Blocks to Communication, 101
 Communicating with Families Through an Interpreter, 101
Communicating with Children, 102
 Communication Related to Development of Thought Processes, 102
Communication Techniques, 105
 Play, 105
HISTORY TAKING, 107
Performing a Health History, 107
 Identifying Information, 107
 Chief Complaint, 107
 Present Illness, 108
 History, 108
 Sexual History, 110
 Family Medical History, 111

Family Structure, 111
Psychosocial History, 111
Review of Systems, 113
NUTRITIONAL ASSESSMENT, 113
Dietary Intake, 113
Clinical Examination, 115
Evaluation of Nutritional Assessment, 118
GENERAL APPROACHES TOWARD EXAMINING THE CHILD, 118
Sequence of the Examination, 118
Preparation of the Child, 118
PHYSICAL EXAMINATION, 121
Growth Measurements, 121
 Growth Charts, 121
 Length, 122
 Height, 122
 Weight, 123
 Skinfold Thickness and Arm Circumference, 124
 Head Circumference, 124
Physiologic Measurements, 124
 Temperature, 125
 Pulse, 127
 Respiration, 129
 Blood Pressure, 129
General Appearance, 132
Skin, 132
 Accessory Structures, 132
Lymph Nodes, 133
Head and Neck, 133
Eyes, 134
 Inspection of External Structures, 134
 Inspection of Internal Structures, 135
 Vision Testing, 135

Ears, 137
 Inspection of External Structures, 137
 Inspection of Internal Structures, 138
 Auditory Testing, 140
Nose, 140
 Inspection of External Structures, 140
 Inspection of Internal Structures, 141
Mouth and Throat, 141
 Inspection of Internal Structures, 142
Chest, 143
Lungs, 144
 Auscultation, 145
Heart, 145
 Auscultation, 146
Abdomen, 147
 Inspection, 148
 Auscultation, 149
 Palpation, 149
Genitalia, 149
 Male Genitalia, 150
 Female Genitalia, 150
Anus, 151
Back and Extremities, 151
 Spine, 151
 Extremities, 152
 Joints, 152
 Muscles, 153
Neurologic Assessment, 153
 Cerebellar Function, 153
 Reflexes, 153
 Cranial Nerves, 153

LEARNING OBJECTIVES

On completion of this chapter the reader will be able to:
- Identify communication strategies for interviewing parents.
- Formulate guidelines for using an interpreter.
- Identify communication strategies for communicating with children of different age-groups.

- Describe four communication techniques that are useful with children.
- State the components of a complete health history.
- List three areas that are evaluated as part of nutritional assessment.
- Prepare a child for a physical examination based on his or her developmental needs.

- Perform a comprehensive physical examination in a sequence appropriate to the child's age.
- Recognize expected normal findings for children at various ages.
- Record the physical examination according to the head-to-toe format.

RELATED TOPICS and ADDITIONAL RESOURCES

 IN TEXT

Altered States of Consciousness, *Ch. 28*
Assessment of Cardiac Function, *Ch. 25*
Biologic Development (Adolescents), *Ch. 16*
Dental Problems, *Ch. 15*
Family Structure and Function, *Ch. 3*
Hearing Impairment; Visual Impairment, *Ch. 19*
Idiopathic Scoliosis, *Ch. 31*
Immunizations, *Ch. 10*
Neurologic Examination, *Ch. 28*
Pain Assessment, *Ch. 7*
Physical Assessment (Newborn), *Ch. 8*
Preparation for Diagnostic and Therapeutic Procedures, *Ch. 22*
Sex Education: Preschooler, *Ch. 13;* School-Age Child, *Ch. 15;* Adolescent, *Ch. 16*
Sexually Transmitted Diseases, *Ch. 17*

Skin Lesions, *Ch. 30*
Social, Cultural, and Religious Influences on Child Health Promotion, *Ch. 4*
Systemic Hypertension, *Ch. 25*
Use of Play in Procedures, *Ch. 22*

 COMPANION CD

Anatomy Reviews—Superficial Lymph Nodes; Location of Sinuses; Structures in the Neck; Structures of the Eye; Landmarks of the Pinna; External, Middle, and Inner Ear; External and Internal Structures of the Nose; Interior Structures of the Mouth; Rib Cage; Imaginary Landmarks of the Chest; Percussion Sounds in the Thorax; Location of Pulses; Direction of Heart Sounds; Location of Hernias

Animations—Abdominal Anatomy; Cranial Nerves; Organ Systems 3-D Tour
Case Studies—Communicating with Adolescents; Pediatric Assessment
Critical Thinking Exercises—The Interview; Cardiovascular Assessment
NCLEX Review Questions
Pediatric Assessment Video Clips

evolve
evolve.elsevier.com/Wong/essentials/

NCLEX Review Questions
Pediatric Assessment Video Clips
Skills—Communicating with Children; Measuring Physical Growth; Measuring Body Temperature
WebLinks

GUIDELINES FOR COMMUNICATION AND INTERVIEWING

The most widely used method of communicating with parents on a professional basis is the interview process. Unlike social conversation, **interviewing** is a specific form of goal-directed communication. As nurses converse with children and adults, they focus on the individuals to determine the kind of persons they are, their usual mode of handling problems, whether help is needed, and the way they react to counseling. Developing interviewing skills requires time and practice, but following some guiding principles can facilitate this process. An organized approach is most effective when using interviewing skills in patient teaching.

ESTABLISHING A SETTING FOR COMMUNICATION
Appropriate Introduction

Introduce yourself to, and ask the name of, each family member who is present. Address parents or other adults by their appropriate titles, such as "Mr." and "Mrs.," unless they specify a preferred name. Record the preferred name on the medical record. Using formal address or their preferred names, rather than using first names or "mother" or "father," conveys respect and regard for the parents or other caregivers (Seidel, Ball, Dains, and others, 2003).

At the beginning of the visit, include children in the interaction by asking them their name, age, and other information. Nurses often direct all questions to adults, even when children are old enough to speak for themselves. This serves to terminate one extremely valuable source of information: the patient. When the child is included, follow the general rules for communicating with children given in the Nursing Care Guidelines box on p. 103.

Assurance of Privacy and Confidentiality

The place where the interview is conducted is almost as important as the interview itself. The physical environment should allow for as much privacy as possible, with distractions, such as interruptions, noise, or other visible activity, kept to a minimum. At times it is necessary to turn off a television or radio. The environment should also have some play provision for young children to keep them occupied during the parent-nurse interview (Fig. 6-1). Parents who are constantly interrupted by their children are unable to concentrate

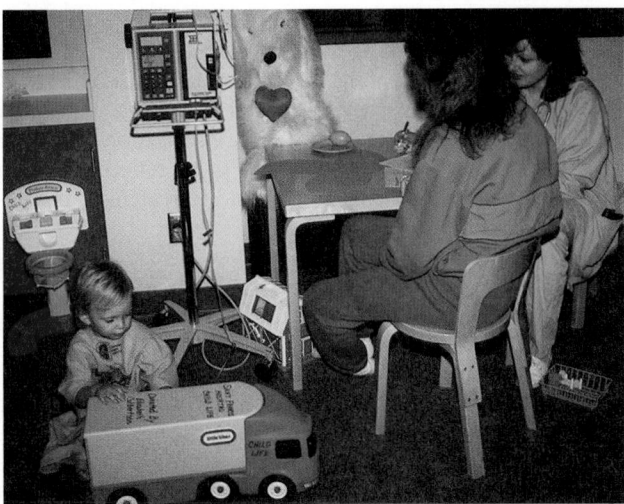

FIG. 6-1 ■ Child plays while nurse interviews parent.

fully and tend to give brief answers to finish the interview as quickly as possible.

Confidentiality is another essential component of the initial phase of the interview. Since the interview is usually shared with other members of the health team care or the teacher (in the case of students), be certain to inform the family of the limits regarding confidentiality. If confidentiality is a concern in a particular situation, such as when talking to a parent suspected of child abuse or a teenager contemplating suicide, deal with this directly and inform the person that in such instances confidentiality cannot be ensured. However, the nurse judiciously protects information of a confidential nature (Sullivan, 1997).

> **NURSINGALERT**
>
> In 2003 the Health Insurance Portability and Accountability Act (HIPAA) was implemented to ensure patient privacy and limit access to sensitive health information. Nurses and students should become familiar with their institution's policy regarding HIPAA compliance.*

COMPUTER PRIVACY AND APPLICATIONS IN NURSING

The use of computer technology to store and retrieve health information has become widespread. The privacy and security of this health information has generated a growing concern throughout the health care community. Any person accessing confidential health information is charged with managing safeguards for disclosure, since violations might incur civil damages.

In 1994 a committee of the Institute of Medicine recommended a national code of fair health information practices. It suggested that health data organizations establish data protection units to develop privacy policies and security practices for manual and automated data processing systems. Technologic safeguards, such as encryption and managerial security procedures, can be applied to computer hardware across a network to ensure protection of individual patient privacy.

*For more information, visit http://www.hhs.gov/ocr/hipaa.

Many institutions use computer and information applications in nursing (**nursing informatics**), such as electronic medical records, to record care and access information. Two important health care applications are record transmission, including facsimile (fax), electronic mail (e-mail), and telemedicine. The telemedicine application is capable of two-way video conferencing, transmission of radiographs, and clinical consultation between remote sites and centralized resources.*

TELEPHONE TRIAGE AND COUNSELING

Nurses are increasingly responsible for assessment of children's symptoms and clinical judgment for further medical care (**triage**) via telephone report. Most often, health problems are assessed and prioritized according to urgency, and treatment is judiciously provided via telephone services. Successful outcomes are based on the consistency and accuracy of the information provided, and parents are empowered to participate in their child's medical care. Telephone triage care management has increased access to high-quality health care services, and patient satisfaction has significantly improved. Unnecessary emergency department and clinic visits have decreased, saving medical costs and time (with less absence from work) for families in need of health care. The most common telephone triage call is for a fever. Approximately 37% of the triage calls related to fever require emergency care, and nearly 50% benefit from home management (Deadrick and Boggess, 1996).

> **NURSINGALERT**
>
> Legal issues can emerge from errors in telephone triage care management. Always advise the parent that the child should be seen if there is any doubt as to the seriousness of the illness.

A well-designed telephone triage program is essential for safe, prompt, and consistent-quality health care (Rutenberg, 2000). Telephone triage is more than "just a phone call," since a child's life is a high price to pay for poorly managed or incompetent telephone assessment skills. Typically, guidelines for telephone triage include asking screening questions; determining when to immediately refer to emergency medical services (dial 911); and determining when to refer to same-day appointments, appointments in 24 to 72 hours, appointments in 4 days or more, or home care (Box 6-1).

COMMUNICATING WITH FAMILIES

COMMUNICATING WITH PARENTS

Although the parent and child are separate and distinct individuals, the nurse's relationship with the child is frequently mediated by the parent, particularly in the case of younger children. For the most part, information about the child is acquired by direct observation or is communicated to the nurse by the parents. Usually it can be assumed that because of the close contact with the child, the parent gives reliable information. Making an assessment of the child requires input from the child (verbal and nonverbal), information from the parent, and the nurse's own observations of the child and interpretation of the relationship between the child and the parent. Counseling and guidance must be directed to the care-

*Resources: Nicoll LH: *Nurses' guide to the Internet,* ed 3, Philadelphia, 2001, Lippincott. Also available is a bimonthly publication, *CIN: Computers, Informatics, Nursing.* To order, call (800) 638-3030; fax (301) 714-2300; e-mail: CustomerService@LWW.com; http://www.cinjournal.com.

BOX 6-1

Telephone Triage Guidelines

Date and time
Background
  ■ Name, age, sex
  ■ Chronic illness
  ■ Allergies, current medications, treatments, or recent immunizations
Chief complaint
General symptoms
  ■ Severity
  ■ Duration
  ■ Other symptoms
  ■ Pain
Systems review
Steps taken
  ■ Advised to call emergency medical services (911)
  ■ Advised to see practitioner
  ■ Advice given for home care
  ■ Call back if symptoms worsen or fail to improve

RESOURCES FOR TELEPHONE TRIAGE PROTOCOLS

Brown J: *Pediatric telephone medicine: principles, triage and advice,* ed 3, Philadelphia, 1998, Lippincott.

Murphy KA: *Pediatric triage guidelines,* St Louis, 1997, Mosby.

Schmitt BD: *Pediatric telephone protocols,* Elk Grove Village, Ill, 1998, American Academy of Pediatrics.

Simonsen SM: *Telephone assessment: guidelines for practice,* ed 2, St Louis, 2001, Mosby.

giver of infants and small children; when children are old enough to be active participants in their own health maintenance, the parent becomes a collaborator in health care.

Encouraging the Parent to Talk

Interviewing parents not only offers the opportunity to determine the child's health and developmental status, but also offers information about factors that influence the child's life. Whatever the parent sees as a problem should be a concern of the nurse. These problems are not always easy to identify. Nurses need to be alert for clues and signals by which a parent communicates worries and anxieties. Careful phrasing with broad, open-ended questions such as "What is Jimmy eating now?" provides more information than several single-answer questions, such as "Is Jimmy eating what the rest of the family eats?"

Sometimes the parent will take the lead without prompting. At other times it may be necessary to direct another question on the basis of an observation, such as "Connie seems unhappy today" or "How do you feel when David cries?" If the parent appears to be tired or distraught, consider asking, "What do you do to relax?" or "What help do you have with the children?" A comment such as "You handle the baby very well. What kinds of experience have you had with babies?" to new parents who appear comfortable with their first child gives positive reinforcement and provides an opening for any questions they might have regarding the infant's care. Often all that is required to keep parents talking is a nod or saying "yes" or "uh-huh."

When attempting to elicit feelings and covert problem areas, avoid closed-ended questions that begin with "Does . . .,"

"Did . . .," or "Is . . .," which usually require only a single response. In addition, asking questions such as "Does your son have any problems at school?" subtly implies a lack of parental skills and evokes defensiveness. Instead, say, "What . . .," "How . . .," "Tell me about . . ." and encourage elaboration with "You were saying . . ." or "You say that . . .," or by reflecting back a key word. Open-ended questions are nonthreatening and encourage description.

Directing the Focus

The ability to direct the focus of the interview while allowing for maximum freedom of expression is one of the most difficult goals in effective communication. One approach is the use of open-ended or broad questions, followed by guiding statements. For example, if the parent proceeds to list the other children by name, say, "Tell me their ages, too." If the parent continues to describe each child in depth, which is not the purpose of the interview, redirect the focus by stating, "Let's talk about the other children later. You were beginning to tell me about Paul's activities at school." This approach conveys interest in the other children but focuses the assessment on the patient.

If a parent suggests that a problem exists with one of the other children, reintroduce this subject at the end of the interview to assess the need for further family follow-up. Saying to the parent, "Before, you mentioned that your older son is having trouble in school. Tell me what you see as the problem," reintroduces this subject but only in terms of the possible problem.

Listening and Cultural Awareness

Listening is the most important component of effective communication. When listening is truly aimed at understanding the client, it is an active process that requires concentration and attention to all aspects of the conversation—verbal, nonverbal, and abstract. Major blocks to listening are environmental distraction and premature judgment.

The nurse's attitudes and feelings are easily injected into an interview. Often nurses' perceptions of a parent's behavior are influenced by their own perceptions, prejudices, and assumptions, which may include racial, religious, and cultural stereotypes. What may be interpreted as passive hostility or a lack of interest in a parent may be shyness or an expression of anxiety. For example, in Western cultures eye contact and directness are signs of paying attention. However, in many non-Western cultures, including that of Native Americans, directness, such as looking someone in the eye, is considered rude. Children are taught to avert their gaze and to look down when being addressed by an adult, especially one with authority (Seidel, Ball, Dains, and others, 2003). Therefore judgments about "listening," as well as verbal interactions, need to be made with an appreciation of cultural differences (see Nursing Care Guidelines box, p. 62, and Chapter 3).

Although it is necessary to make some preliminary judgments, listen with as much objectivity as possible by clarifying meanings and attempting to see the situation from the parent's point of view. Effective interviewers consciously control their reactions, responses, and the techniques they use.

Minimum verbal activity with active listening facilitates parent involvement. It is tempting to spend time explaining, describing, and interpreting health information when the opportunity presents itself. However, it is possible to provide effective health education by timing the information properly and presenting only as much as is necessary at the moment.

Careful listening facilitates the use of clues, verbal leads, or signals from the interviewee to move the interview along. Frequent references to an area of concern, repetition of certain key words, or a special emphasis on something or someone serves as cues to the interviewer for the direction of inquiry. Concerns and anxieties are often mentioned in a casual, off-hand manner. Even though they are casual, they are important and deserve careful scrutiny to identify problem areas. For example, a parent who is concerned about a child's habit of bed-wetting may casually mention that the child's bed was "wet this morning."

Listening is also helpful in assessing reliability. For example, the answers elicited at the beginning of the interview may differ from those at the end, when the parent feels more confident in revealing problems. It is important to identify any discrepancies and reintroduce those topics for further investigation.

Using Silence

Silence as a response is often one of the most difficult interviewing techniques to learn. It requires a sense of confidence and comfort on the part of the interviewer to allow the interviewee space in which to think without interruptions. Silence permits the interviewee to sort out thoughts and feelings and search for responses to questions. Silence can also be a cue for the interviewer to go more slowly, reexamine the approach, and not push too hard (Seidel, Ball, Dains, and others, 2003).

Sometimes it is necessary to break the silence and reopen communication. Do this in a way that encourages the person to continue talking about what is considered important. Breaking a silence by introducing a new topic or by prolonged talking essentially terminates the interviewee's opportunity to use the silence. Suggestions for breaking the silence include statements such as "Is there anything else you wish to say?" "I see you find it difficult to continue; how may I help?" or "I don't know what this silence means. Perhaps there is something you would like to put into words but find difficult to say."

Being Empathic

Empathy is the capacity to understand what another person is experiencing from within that person's frame of reference; it is often described as the ability to put oneself in another's shoes. The essence of empathic interaction is accurate understanding of another's feelings (Price and Archbold, 1997; White, 1997; Reynolds, Scott, and Jessiman, 1999). Empathy differs from **sympathy,** which is *having* feelings or emotions in common with another person, rather than *understanding* those feelings. Sympathy is not therapeutic in the helping relationship because it leads to overinvolvement emotionally and potentially to professional burnout (Yegdich, 1999).

Providing Anticipatory Guidance

The ideal way to handle a situation is to deal with it *before* it becomes a problem. The best preventive measure is anticipatory guidance. Traditionally, **anticipatory guidance** has focused on providing families information on normal growth and development, as well as nurturing childrearing practices. For example, one of the most significant areas in pediatrics is

injury prevention. Beginning prenatally, parents need specific instructions on home safety. Because of the child's maturing developmental skills, home safety changes must be implemented early to minimize risks to the child.

Many normal developmental changes can disturb unprepared parents, such as a toddler's diminished appetite, negativism, altered sleeping patterns, and anxiety toward strangers. Such topics are discussed in the chapters on health promotion to provide the nurse with information for counseling parents.

However, anticipatory guidance should extend beyond giving information to empowering families to use the information as a means of building competence in their parenting abilities. To achieve this level of anticipatory guidance (Desselle and Pearlmutter, 1997), the nurse should:

- Base interventions on needs identified by the family, not by the professional
- View the family as competent or as having the ability to be competent
- Provide opportunities for the family to achieve competence

> **NURSINGTIP**
>
> Often parents need early guidance with their children (Desselle and Pearlmutter, 1997), and anticipatory guidance builds competence in their parenting skills.

Avoiding Blocks to Communication

A number of blocks to communication can adversely affect the quality of the helping relationship. Many of these blocks are initiated by the interviewer, such as giving unrestricted advice or forming prejudged conclusions. Another type of block occurs primarily with the interviewees and concerns **information overload.** When individuals are presented with too much information or information that is overwhelming, they will often demonstrate signs of increasing anxiety or decreasing attention. Such signals should alert the interviewer to give less information or to clarify what has been said. Some of the more common blocks to communication, including signs of information overload, are listed in Box 6-2.

Communication blocks can be corrected by careful analysis of the interview process. One of the best methods for improving interviewing skills is audiotape or videotape feedback. With supervision and guidance, the interviewer can recognize the blocks and consciously avoid them.

Communicating with Families Through an Interpreter

Sometimes communication is impossible because two people speak different languages. In this case it is necessary to obtain information through a third party, the interpreter. When an interpreter is used, the same interviewing guidelines apply. Specific guidelines for using an adult interpreter are presented in the Nursing Care Guidelines box.

Communicating with families through an interpreter requires sensitivity to cultural, legal, and ethical considerations. For example, in some cultures using a child as an interpreter is considered an insult to an adult because children are expected to show respect by not questioning their elders. In some cultures class differences between the interpreter and the family may cause the family to feel intimidated and less inclined to offer information. Therefore it is important to

BOX 6-2
Blocks to Communication

COMMUNICATION BARRIERS (NURSE)
Socializing
Giving unrestricted and sometimes unasked for advice
Offering premature or inappropriate reassurance
Giving overready encouragement
Defending a situation or opinion
Using stereotyped comments or clichés
Limiting expression of emotion by asking directed, closed-ended
    questions
Interrupting and finishing the person's sentence
Talking more than the interviewee
Forming prejudged conclusions
Deliberately changing the focus

SIGNS OF INFORMATION OVERLOAD (PATIENT)
Long periods of silence
Wide eyes and fixed facial expression
Constant fidgeting or attempting to move away
Nervous habits (e.g., tapping, playing with hair)
Sudden disruptions (e.g., asking to go to the bathroom)
Looking around
Yawning, eyes drooping
Frequently looking at a watch or clock
Attempting to change topic of discussion

nursingcareguidelines

Using an Interpreter
- Explain to interpreter the reason for the interview and the type of questions that will be asked.
- Clarify whether a detailed or brief answer is required and whether the translated response can be general or literal.
- Introduce interpreter to family and allow some time before the interview for them to become acquainted.
- Communicate directly with family members when asking questions to reinforce interest in them and to observe nonverbal expressions, but do not ignore interpreter.
- Pose questions to elicit only one answer at a time, such as "Do you have pain?" rather than "Do you have any pain, tiredness, or loss of appetite?"
- Refrain from interrupting family member and interpreter while they are conversing.
- Avoid commenting to interpreter about family members, since they may understand some English.
- Be aware that some medical words, such as *allergy*, may have no similar word in another language; avoid medical jargon whenever possible.
- Be aware that cultural differences may exist regarding views on sex, marriage, or pregnancy.
- Allow time after the interview for interpreter to share something that he or she thought could not be said earlier; ask about the interpreter's impression of nonverbal clues to communication and family members' reliability or ease in revealing information.
- Arrange for family to speak with same interpreter on subsequent visits whenever possible.

choose the translator carefully and provide time for the interpreter and family to establish rapport.

Issues of legal and ethical concerns may also arise. For example, in obtaining informed consent through an interpreter, it is important that the family be fully informed of all aspects of the particular procedure to which they are consenting. Issues of confidentiality may arise when family members related to another patient are asked to interpret for the family, thus revealing sensitive information that may be shared with other families on the unit. With increased sensitivity toward patient rights and confidentiality, many institutions now require consent forms to be produced in the patient's primary language.

When no one else is available to translate, children within the family are often asked to assume this role. In this situation it is important to stress *literal* translation of parent responses. To ensure correct translations, it may be necessary to interrupt the parent and ask the child to translate every few sentences. When using children as interpreters, ask questions directed at specific answers and assess the interpreted translation in terms of nonverbal expressions of communication. It should be noted that some institutions prohibit or discourage the use of children as interpreter; check institutional policy for compliance.

NURSINGALERT
When using translated materials, such as a health history form, be certain the informant is literate in the foreign language.

COMMUNICATING WITH CHILDREN

Although the greatest amount of verbal communication is usually carried out with the parent, do not exclude the child during the interview. Pay attention to infants and younger children through play or by occasionally directing questions or remarks to them. Include older children as active participants.

In communication with children of all ages, the nonverbal components of the communication process convey the most significant messages. It is difficult to disguise feelings, attitudes, and anxiety when relating to children. They are alert to surroundings and attach meaning to every gesture and move that is made; this is particularly true of very young children.

Active attempts to make friends with children before they have had an opportunity to evaluate an unfamiliar person tend to increase their anxiety. It is helpful to continue to talk to the child and parent but go about activities that do not involve the child directly, thus allowing the child to observe from a safe position. If the child has a special toy or doll, "talk" to the doll first. Ask simple questions such as "Does your teddy bear have a name?" to ease the child into conversation. Other guidelines for communicating with children are presented in the Nursing Care Guidelines box. Specific guidelines for preparing children for procedures, a common nursing function, are discussed in Chapter 22.

Communication Related to Development of Thought Processes

The normal development of language and thought offers a frame of reference for communicating with children. Thought processes progress from sensorimotor to perceptual to concrete and finally to abstract, formal operations. The early social communicative development of children has been divided

nursingcareguidelines

Communicating with Children

- Allow children time to feel comfortable.
- Avoid sudden or rapid advances, broad smiles, extended eye contact, or other gestures that may be seen as threatening.
- Talk to the parent if child is initially shy.
- Communicate through transition objects such as dolls, puppets, and stuffed animals before questioning a young child directly.
- Give older children the opportunity to talk without the parents present.
- Assume a position that is at eye level with child (Fig. 6-2).
- Speak in a quiet, unhurried, and confident voice.
- Speak clearly, be specific, and use simple words and short sentences.
- State directions and suggestions positively.
- Offer a choice only when one exists.
- Be honest with children.
- Allow them to express their concerns and fears.
- Use a variety of communication techniques.

FIG. 6-2 ■ Nurse assumes position at child's level.

into three stages: (1) **perlocutionary stage**—unintentional communication behavior; (2) **illocutionary stage**—true intent in communication efforts; and (3) **locutionary stage**—intentional communication behaviors and use of symbols (Hoge and Parette, 1995). An understanding of the typical characteristics of these stages provides the nurse with a framework to facilitate social communication (Box 6-3).

Infancy. Because they are unable to use words, infants primarily use and understand nonverbal communication. Infants communicate their needs and feelings through nonverbal behaviors and vocalizations that can be interpreted by someone who is around them for a sufficient time. Infants smile and coo when content and cry when distressed. Crying is provoked by unpleasant stimuli from inside or outside, such as hunger, pain, body restraint, or loneliness. Adults interpret this to mean that an infant needs something and consequently try to alleviate the discomfort and reduce tension. Crying (or the desire to cry) persists as a part of everyone's communication repertoire.

Infants respond to adults' nonverbal behaviors. They become quiet when they are cuddled, are patted, or receive other forms of gentle physical contact. They derive comfort from the sound of a voice, even though they do not understand the words that are spoken. Until infants reach the age at which they experience stranger anxiety, they readily respond to any firm, gentle handling and quiet, calm speech. Loud, harsh sounds and sudden movements are frightening.

Older infants' attention is centered on themselves and their parents; therefore any stranger is a potential threat until proved otherwise. Holding out the hands and asking the child to "come" is seldom successful, especially if the infant is with the parent. If infants must be handled, simply pick them up firmly without gestures. Observe the position in which the parent holds the infant. Most infants learn to prefer a particular position and manner of handling. In general, infants are more at ease upright than horizontal. Also, hold infants so they can see their parents. Until they develop the understand-

BOX 6-3

Characteristics of Communicative Development in Young Children

PERLOCUTIONARY STAGE (0 TO 8-9 MONTHS)
Child is reflexive to stimuli.
Child shows increasing purpose in action.

EMERGING ILLOCUTIONARY STAGE (8-9 TO 12-15 MONTHS)
Child communicates intentionally with signals and gestures.

CONVENTIONAL ILLOCUTIONARY–EMERGING LOCUTIONARY STAGE (12-15 TO 18-24 MONTHS)
Child communicates intentionally with gestures, vocalizations, and verbalizations.

Modified from Hoge DR, Parette HP: Facilitating communicative development in young children with disabilities, *Transdisc J* 5(2):113-130, 1995.

ing that an object (in this case the parent) removed from sight can still be present, they have no way of knowing the object is still there.

Early Childhood. Children younger than 5 years of age are egocentric. They see things only in relation to themselves and from their point of view. Therefore, focus communication on them. Tell them what they can do or how they will feel. Experiences of others are of no interest to them. It is futile to use another child's experience in an attempt to gain the cooperation of small children. Allow them to touch and examine articles that will come in contact with them. A stethoscope bell will feel cold; palpating a neck might tickle. Although they have not yet acquired sufficient language skills to express their feelings and wants, toddlers are able to communicate effectively with their hands to transmit ideas without words. They push an unwanted object away, pull another person to show them something, point, and cover the mouth that is saying something they do not wish to hear.

FIG. 6-3 ■ A young child may take the expression "a little stick in the arm" literally.

Everything is direct and concrete to small children. They are unable to work with abstractions and interpret words literally. Analogies escape them because they are unable to separate fact from fantasy. For example, they attach literal meaning to such common phrases as "two-faced," "sticky fingers," or "coughing your head off." Children who are told they will get "a little stick in the arm" may not be able to envision an injection (Fig. 6-3). Therefore, avoid using a phrase that might be misinterpreted by a small child (see Nursing Care Guidelines box, Chapter 22, p. 693).

Young children assign human attributes to inanimate objects. Consequently they fear that objects may jump, bite, cut, or pinch all by themselves. Children do not know that these devices are unable to perform without human direction. To minimize their fear, keep unfamiliar equipment out of view until it is needed.

School-Age Years. Younger school-age children rely less on what they see and more on what they know when faced with new problems. They want explanations and reasons for everything but require no verification beyond that. They are interested in the functional aspect of all procedures, objects, and activities. They want to know why an object exists, why it is used, how it works, and the intent and purpose of its user. They need to know what is going to take place and why it is being done to them specifically. For example, to explain a procedure such as taking blood pressure, show the child how squeezing the bulb pushes air into the cuff and makes the "silver" in the tube go up. Let the child operate the bulb. An explanation for the procedure might be as simple as, "I want to see how far the silver goes up when the cuff squeezes your arm." Consequently, the child becomes an enthusiastic participant.

School-age children have a heightened concern about body integrity. Because of the special importance they place on their body, they are sensitive to anything that constitutes a threat or suggestion of injury to it. This concern extends to their possessions, so that they may appear to overreact to loss or threatened loss of treasured objects. Helping children voice their concerns enables the nurse to provide reassurance and to implement activities that reduce their anxiety. For example, if a shy child dislikes being the center of attention, ignore that particular child by talking and relating to other children in the family or group. When children feel more comfortable, they will usually interject personal ideas, feelings, and interpretations of events.

Older children have an adequate and satisfactory use of language. They still require relatively simple explanations, but their ability to think concretely can facilitate communication and explanation. Commonly, they have sufficient experience with health and health care workers to understand what is transpiring and what is generally expected of them.

Adolescence. As children move into adolescence, they fluctuate between child and adult thinking and behavior. They are riding a current that is moving them rapidly toward a maturity that may be beyond their coping ability. Therefore, when tensions rise, they may seek the security of the more familiar and comfortable expectations of childhood. Anticipating these shifts in identity allows the nurse to adjust the course of interaction to meet the needs of the moment. No single approach can be relied on consistently, and encountering cooperation, hostility, anger, bravado, and a variety of other behaviors and attitudes can be expected. It is as much a mistake to regard the adolescent as an adult with an adult's wisdom and control as it is to assume that the teenager has the concerns and expectations of a child.

Frequently adolescents are more willing to discuss their concerns with an adult outside the family, and they often welcome the opportunity to interact with a nurse outside the presence of their parents. They are accepting of anyone who displays a genuine interest in them. However, adolescents are quick to reject persons who attempt to impose their values on them, whose interest is feigned, or who appear to have little respect for who they are and what they think or say.

Interviewing the adolescent presents some special issues. The first may be whether to talk with the adolescent alone or with the adolescent and parents together. Of course, if the parent is not there, the only question is whether to suggest to the teenager that the parents be interviewed at another time. If the parents and teenager are together, talking with the adolescent first has the advantage of immediately identifying with the young person, thus fostering the interpersonal relationship. However, talking with the parents initially may provide insight into the family relationship. In either case, give both parties an opportunity to be included in the interview. If time constraints are important, such as during history taking, clarify these at the onset to avoid appearing to "take sides" by talking more with one person than with the other.

Confidentiality is of great importance when interviewing adolescents. Explain to parents and teenagers the limits of confidentiality, specifically that young persons' disclosures will not be shared unless they indicate a need for intervention, as in the case of suicidal behavior.

Another dilemma in interviewing adolescents is that two views of a problem frequently exist—the teenager's and the parents'. Clarification of the problem is a major task. However, providing both parties an opportunity to discuss their perceptions in an open and unbiased atmosphere can, by itself, be therapeutic. Demonstrating positive communication skills

nursingcareguidelines

Communicating with Adolescents

BUILD A FOUNDATION
Spend time together.
Encourage expression of ideas and feelings.
Respect their views.
Tolerate differences.
Praise good points.
Respect their privacy.
Set a good example.

COMMUNICATE EFFECTIVELY
Give undivided attention.
Listen, listen, listen.
Be courteous, calm, and open minded.
Try not to overreact. If you do, take a break.
Avoid judging or criticizing.
Avoid the "third degree" of continuous questioning.
Choose important issues when taking a stand.
After taking a stand:
- Think through all options.
- Make expectations clear.

can help families communicate more effectively (see Nursing Care Guidelines box).

NURSINGALERT

Studies have indicated that family communication patterns significantly influence self-esteem in deaf children. Adolescents whose parents use total communication (speech, finger spelling, and sign language) had higher self-esteem scores than those with parents who used speech only (Desselle and Pearlmutter, 1997).

COMMUNICATION TECHNIQUES

In addition to such conventional interviewing methods as reflection and open-ended questions, a number of techniques encourage family members to express their thoughts and feelings in a less directive and confrontational manner. Several approaches are **projective**—they present nonspecific material that enables individuals to externalize or project inner aspects of themselves to others.

A variety of verbal techniques can be used to encourage communication. Some of these techniques can be used to pose questions or explore concerns in a less threatening manner. Others can be presented as "word games," which are often well received by children. However, for many children and adults, talking about feelings is difficult, and verbal communication may be more stressful than supportive. In such instances several nonverbal techniques can be used to encourage communication.

Both verbal and nonverbal techniques are described in Box 6-4. Because of the importance of play in communicating with children, play is discussed more extensively below. Any of the verbal or nonverbal techniques can give rise to strong feelings that surface unexpectedly. Be prepared to handle them or to recognize when issues go beyond your ability to deal with them. At that point, consider an appropriate referral.

Play

Play is a universal language of children. It is one of the most important forms of communication and can be an effective technique in relating to them. Clues about physical, intellectual, and social developmental progress can often be gleaned from the form and complexity of a child's play behaviors. Play requires minimum equipment or none at all. Therapeutic play is often used to reduce the trauma of illness and hospitalization (see Chapter 21) and to prepare children for therapeutic procedures (see Chapter 22).

Because their ability to perceive precedes their ability to transmit, infants respond to activities that register on their senses. Patting, stroking, and other skin play conveys messages. Repetitive actions, such as stretching infants' arms out to the side while they are lying on their back and then folding the arms across the chest or raising and revolving the legs in a bicycling motion, will elicit pleasurable sounds. Colorful items to catch the eye or interesting sounds, such as a ticking clock, chimes, bells, or singing, can be used to attract children's attention.

Older infants respond to simple games. The old game of peek-a-boo is an excellent means of initiating communication with infants while maintaining a "safe," nonthreatening distance. After this intermittent eye contact, the nurse is no longer viewed as a stranger but as a friend. This can be followed by touch games. Clapping an infant's hands together for pat-a-cake or wiggling the toes for "this little piggy" delights an infant or small child. Talking to a foot or other part of the child's body is another effective tactic. Much of the nursing assessment can be carried out with the use of games and simple play equipment while the infant remains in the safety of the parent's arms or lap.

The nurse can capitalize on the natural curiosity of small children by playing games such as "Which hand do you take?" and "Guess what I have in my hand" or by manipulating items such as a flashlight or stethoscope. Finger games are useful. More elaborate materials, such as puppets and replicas of familiar or unfamiliar items, serve as excellent means of communicating with small children. The variety and extent are limited only by the nurse's imagination.

Through play, children reveal their perceptions of interpersonal relationships with their family, friends, or hospital personnel. Children may also reveal the wide scope of knowledge they have acquired from listening to others around them. For example, through needle play, children may disclose how carefully they have watched each procedure by precisely duplicating the technical skills. They may also reveal how well they remember those who performed procedures. One child who painstakingly reenacted every detail of a tedious medical procedure also played the role of the physician who had repeatedly shouted at her to be still for the long ordeal. Her anger at him was most evident during the play session and revealed the cause for her abrupt withdrawal and passive hostility toward the medical and nursing staff after the test.

Play sessions serve not only as assessment tools for determining children's awareness and perception of their illness, but also as methods of intervention and evaluation. In the previous example, when the child revealed anger toward the physician, the nurse acted the part of the patient but this time did not accept the physician's harsh commands to stay still. Instead, the nurse said to the physician all the things the child had wished she could say.

BOX 6-4

Creative Communication Techniques with Children

VERBAL TECHNIQUES

"I" Messages

Relate a feeling about a behavior in terms of "I."

Describe effect behavior had on the person.

Avoid use of "you."

"You" messages are judgmental and provoke defensiveness.

Example—"You" message: "You are being uncooperative about doing your treatments."

Example—"I" message: "I am concerned about how the treatments are going because I want to see you get better."

Third-Person Technique

Express a feeling in terms of a third person ("he," "she," "they"). This is less threatening than directly asking children how they feel because it gives them an opportunity to agree or disagree without being defensive.

Example—"Sometimes when a person is sick a lot, he feels angry and sad because he cannot do what others can." Either wait silently for a response or encourage a reply with a statement such as "Did you ever feel that way?"

Approach allows children three choices: (1) to agree and, one hopes, express how they feel; (2) to disagree; or (3) to remain silent, which means they probably have such feelings but are unable to express them at this time.

Facilitative Response

Listen carefully and reflect back to patients the feelings and content of their statements.

Responses are empathic and nonjudgmental and legitimize the person's feelings.

Formula for facilitative responses: "You feel _____ because ___ _____."

Example—If child states, "I hate coming to the hospital and getting needles," a facilitative response is, "You feel unhappy because of all the things that are done to you."

Storytelling

Use the language of children to probe into areas of their thinking while bypassing conscious inhibitions or fears.

The simplest technique is asking children to relate a story about an event, such as "being in the hospital."

Other approaches:

- Show children a picture of a particular event, such as a child in a hospital with other people in the room, and ask them to describe the scene.
- Cut out comic strips, remove words, and have child add statements for scenes.

Mutual Storytelling

Reveal child's thinking and attempt to change child's perceptions or fears by retelling a somewhat different story (more therapeutic approach than storytelling).

Begin by asking child to tell a story about something, then tell another story that is similar to child's tale but with differences that help child in problem areas.

Example—Child's story is about going to the hospital and never seeing his or her parents again. Nurse's story is also about a child (using different names but similar circumstances) in a hospital whose parents visit every day, but in the evening after work, until the child is better and goes home with them.

Bibliotherapy

Use books in a therapeutic and supportive process.

Provide children with an opportunity to explore an event that is similar to their own but sufficiently different to allow them to distance themselves from it and remain in control.

General guidelines for using bibliotherapy are:

1. Assess child's emotional and cognitive development in terms of readiness to understand the book's message.
2. Be familiar with the book's content (intended message or purpose) and the age for which it is written.
3. Read the book to the child if child is unable to read.
4. Explore the meaning of the book with the child by having child:
   - Retell the story
   - Read a special section with the nurse or parent
   - Draw a picture related to the story and discuss the drawing
   - Talk about the characters
   - Summarize the moral or meaning of the story

Dreams

Dreams often reveal unconscious and repressed thoughts and feelings.

Ask child to talk about a dream or nightmare.

Explore with child what meaning the dream could have.

"What If" Questions

Encourage child to explore potential situations and to consider different problem-solving options.

Example—"What if you got sick and had to go the hospital?" Children's responses reveal what they know already and what they are curious about, providing an opportunity for them to learn coping skills, especially in potentially dangerous situations.

Three Wishes

Ask, "If you could have any three things in the world, what would they be?"

If child answers, "That all my wishes come true," ask child for specific wishes.

Rating Game

Use some type of rating scale (numbers, sad to happy faces) to have child rate an event or feeling.

Example—Instead of asking youngsters how they feel, ask how their day has been "on a scale of 1 to 10, with 10 being the best."

Word Association Game

State key words and ask children to say the first word they think of when they hear the word.

Start with neutral words and then introduce more anxiety-producing words, such as "illness," "needles," "hospitals," and "operation."

Select key words that relate to some relevant event in the child's life.

Sentence Completion

Present a partial statement and have the child complete it. Some sample statements are:

- The thing I like best (least) about school is _____.
- The best (worst) age to be is _____.
- The most (least) fun thing I ever did was _____.
- The thing I like most (least) about my parents is _____.
- The one thing I would change about my family is _____.
- If I could be anything I wanted, I would be _____.
- The thing I like most (least) about myself is _____.

BOX 6-4

Creative Communication Techniques with Children—cont'd

VERBAL TECHNIQUES—cont'd

Pros and Cons

Select a topic, such as "being in the hospital," and have child list "five good things and five bad things" about it.

This is an exceptionally valuable technique when applied to relationships, such as things family members like and dislike about each other.

NONVERBAL TECHNIQUES

Writing

Writing is an alternative communication approach for older children and adults.

Specific suggestions include:

- Keep a journal or diary.
- Write down feelings or thoughts that are difficult to express.
- Write "letters" that are never mailed (a variation is making up a "pen pal" to write to).

Keep an account of child's progress from both a physical and an emotional viewpoint.

Drawing

Drawing is one of the most valuable forms of communication—both nonverbal (from looking at the drawing) and verbal (from child's story of the picture).

Children's drawings tell a great deal about them because they are projections of their inner selves.

Spontaneous drawing involves giving child a variety of art supplies and providing the opportunity to draw.

Directed drawing involves a more specific direction, such as "draw a person" or the "three themes" approach (state three things about child and ask child to choose one and draw a picture).

Guidelines for Evaluating Drawings

Use spontaneous drawings and evaluate more than one drawing whenever possible.

Interpret drawings in light of other available information about child and family, including the child's age and stage of development.

Interpret drawings as a whole rather than focusing on specific details of the drawing.

Consider individual elements of the drawing that may be significant:

Sex of figure drawn first—Usually relates to child's perception of own sex role.

Size of individual figures—Expresses importance, power, or authority.

Order in which figures are drawn—Expresses priority in terms of importance.

Child's position in relation to other family members—Expresses feelings of status or alliance.

Exclusion of a member—May denote feeling of not belonging or desire to eliminate.

Accentuated parts—Usually express concern for areas of special importance (e.g., large hands may be a sign of aggression).

Absence of or rudimentary arms and hands—Suggest timidity, passivity, or intellectual immaturity; tiny, unstable feet may express insecurity, and hidden hands may mean guilt feelings.

Placement of drawing on the page and type of stroke—Free use of paper and firm, continuous strokes express security, whereas drawings restricted to a small area and lightly drawn in broken or wavering lines may be a sign of insecurity.

Erasures, shading, or cross-hatching—Expresses ambivalence, concern, or anxiety with a particular area.

Magic

Use simple magic tricks to help establish rapport with child, encourage compliance with health interventions, and provide effective distraction during painful procedures.

Although the "magician" talks, no verbal response from child is required.

Play

Play is the universal language and "work" of children.

It tells a great deal about children because they project their inner selves through the activity.

Spontaneous play involves giving child a variety of play materials and providing the opportunity to play.

Directed play involves a more specific direction, such as providing medical equipment or a dollhouse for focused reasons, such as exploring child's fear of injections or exploring family relationships.

HISTORY TAKING

PERFORMING A HEALTH HISTORY

The format used for history taking may be (1) **direct,** where the nurse asks for information via direct interview with the informant; or (2) **indirect,** where the informant supplies the information by completing some type of questionnaire. The direct method is superior to the indirect approach or a combination of both. However, in view of time constraints, the direct approach is not always practical. If the direct approach cannot be used, review parents' written responses and question them regarding any unusual answers. The categories listed in Box 6-5 encompass children's current and past health status and information about their psychosocial environment.

Identifying Information

Much of the identifying information may already be available from other recorded sources. However, if the parent and youngster seem anxious, use this opportunity to ask about such information to help them feel more comfortable.

Informant. One of the important elements of identifying information is the **informant,** the person(s) who furnish the information. Record (1) who the person is (child, parent, or other), (2) an impression of reliability and willingness to communicate, and (3) any special circumstances such as the use of an interpreter or conflicting answers by more than one person.

Chief Complaint

The chief complaint is the specific reason for the child's visit to the clinic, office, or hospital. It may be viewed as the theme, with the present illness viewed as the description of the problem. The chief complaint is elicited by asking open-ended, neutral questions such as "What seems to be the matter?" "How may I help you?" or "Why did you come here today?" Avoid labeling-type questions such as "How are you sick?" or "What is the problem?"; it is possible that the reason for the visit is not an illness or problem.

Occasionally, it is difficult to isolate one symptom or problem as the chief complaint because the parent may identify

---

BOX 6-5

Outline of a Pediatric Health History

Identifying information

1. Name	6. Sex
2. Address	7. Religion
3. Telephone	8. Date of interview
4. Birth date and place	9. Informant
5. Race/ethnic group	

Chief complaint (CC)—To establish the major specific reason for the child's and parents' seeking professional health attention

Present illness (PI)—To obtain all details related to the chief complaint

Past history (PH)—To elicit a profile of the child's previous illnesses, injuries, or operations

1. Birth history (pregnancy, labor and delivery, perinatal history)	3. Allergies
	4. Current medications
	5. Immunizations
2. Previous illnesses, injuries, or operations	6. Growth and development
	7. Habits

Review of systems (ROS)—To elicit information concerning any potential health problem

1. General	10. Chest
2. Integument	11. Respiratory
3. Head	12. Cardiovascular
4. Eyes	13. Gastrointestinal
5. Ears	14. Genitourinary
6. Nose	15. Gynecologic
7. Mouth	16. Musculoskeletal
8. Throat	17. Neurologic
9. Neck	18. Endocrine

Family medical history—To identify genetic traits or diseases that have familial tendencies and to assess exposure to a communicable disease in a family member and family habits that may affect the child's health, such as smoking and chemical use

Psychosocial history—To elicit information about the child's self-concept

Sexual history—To elicit information concerning the child's sexual concerns or activities and any pertinent data regarding adults' sexual activity that influences the child

Family history—To develop an understanding of the child as an individual and as a member of a family and a community

1. Family composition
2. Home and community environment
3. Occupation and education of family members
4. Cultural and religious traditions
5. Family function and relationships

Nutritional assessment—To elicit information on the adequacy of the child's nutritional intake and needs

1. Dietary intake
2. Clinical examination

---

nursingcareguidelines

Analyzing the Symptom: Pain

TYPE

Be as specific as possible. With young children, asking the parents how they know the child is in pain may help describe its type, location, and severity. For example, a parent may state, "My child must have a severe earache because she pulls at her ears, rolls her head on the floor, and screams. Nothing seems to help." Help older children describe the "hurt" by asking them if it is sharp, throbbing, dull, or stabbing. Record whatever words they use in quotes.

LOCATION

Be specific. "Stomach pains" is too general a description. Children can better localize the pain if they are asked to "point with one finger to where it hurts" or to "point to where Mommy or Daddy would put a Band-Aid." Determine if the pain radiates by asking, "Does the pain stay there or move? Show me with your finger where the pain goes."

SEVERITY

Severity is best determined by finding out how it affects the child's usual behavior. Pain that prevents a child from playing, interacting with others, sleeping, and eating is most often severe. Assess pain intensity using a rating scale, such as a numeric or FACES scale (see Chapter 7).

DURATION

Include the duration, onset, and frequency. Describe this in terms of activity and behavior, such as "pain reported to last all night, child refused to sleep and cried intermittently."

INFLUENCING FACTORS

Include anything that causes a change in the type, location, severity, or duration of the pain: (1) precipitating events (those that cause or increase the pain), (2) relieving events (those that lessen the pain, such as medications), (3) temporal events (times when the pain is relieved or increased), (4) positional events (standing, sitting, lying down), and (5) associated events (meals, stress, coughing).

---

many. In this situation be as specific as possible when asking questions. For example, asking informants to state which *one* problem or symptom prompted them to seek help now may help them focus on the most immediate concern.

Present Illness

The history of the present illness* is a narrative of the chief complaint from its earliest onset through its progression to the present. Its four major components are (1) the details of

onset, (2) a complete **interval** history, (3) the **present** status, and (4) the reason for seeking help **now.** The focus of the present illness is on all factors relevant to the main problem, even if they have disappeared or changed during the onset, interval, and present.

Analyzing a Symptom. Because pain is often the most characteristic symptom denoting the onset of a physical problem, it is used as an example for analysis of a symptom. Assessment includes (1) type, (2) location, (3) severity, (4) duration, and (5) influencing factors (see Nursing Care Guidelines box; see also Pain Assessment, Chapter 7).

History

The history contains information relating to all previous aspects of the child's health status and concentrates on several areas that are ordinarily passed over in the history of an adult, such as birth history, detailed feeding history, immunizations, and growth and development. Since a great deal of information is included in this section, use a combination of open-ended and fact-finding questions. For example, begin interviewing for each section with an open-ended statement such as "Tell me about your child's birth" to provide the informants

---

*The term *illness* is used in its broadest sense to denote any problem of a physical, emotional, or psychosocial nature. It is actually a history of the chief complaint.

with the opportunity to relate what they think is most important. Ask fact-finding questions related to specific details whenever necessary to focus the interview on certain topics.

Birth History. The birth history includes all data concerning (1) the mother's health during pregnancy, (2) the labor and delivery, and (3) the infant's condition immediately after birth. Since prenatal influences have significant effects on a child's physical and emotional development, a thorough investigation of the birth history is essential. Because parents may question what relevance pregnancy and birth have on the child's present condition, particularly if the child is past infancy, explain why such questions are included. An appropriate statement may be, "I will be asking you some questions about your pregnancy and ____'s [refer to child by name] birth. Your answers will give me a more complete picture of his [or her] overall health."

Because emotional factors also affect the outcome of pregnancy and the subsequent parent-child relationship, investigate (1) concurrent crises during pregnancy and (2) prenatal attitudes toward the fetus. It is best to approach the topic of parental acceptance of pregnancy through indirect questioning. Asking parents if the pregnancy was planned is a leading statement because they may respond affirmatively for fear of criticism if the pregnancy was unexpected. Rather, encourage parents to disclose their true reactions by referring to specific facts relating to the pregnancy, such as the spacing between offspring, an extended or short interval between marriage and conception, or the concurrent experience of pregnancy and adolescence. The parent can choose to explore such statements with further explanations or, for the moment, may not be able to reveal such feelings. If the parent remains silent, return to this topic later in the interview.

Dietary History. Because parental concerns are common and nursing interventions are important in ensuring optimum nutrition, the dietary history is discussed in detail later in this chapter under Nutritional Assessment.

Previous Illnesses, Injuries, and Operations. When inquiring about past illnesses, begin with a general statement such as "What other illnesses has your child had?" Since parents are most likely to recall serious health problems, ask specifically about colds; earaches; and childhood diseases such as measles, rubella (German measles), chickenpox, mumps, pertussis (whooping cough), diphtheria, tuberculosis, scarlet fever, strep throat, tonsillitis, or allergic manifestations.

In addition to illnesses, ask about injuries that required medical intervention, operations, and any other reason for hospitalization, including the dates of each incident. It is important to focus on injuries such as accidental falls, poisoning, choking, or burns, since these may be potential areas for parental guidance.

Allergies. Ask about commonly known allergic disorders such as hay fever and asthma; unusual reactions to drugs, food, or latex products; and reactions to other contact agents such as poisonous plants, animals, household products, or fabrics. If asked appropriate questions, most people can give reliable information about drug reactions (see Nursing Care Guidelines box).

NURSINGALERT

Information about allergic reactions to drugs or other products is essential. Failure to document a serious reaction places the child at risk if the agent is given.

---

nursingcareguidelines

Taking an Allergy History

- Has your child ever taken any drugs or tablets that have disagreed with him or her or caused an allergy? If yes, can you remember the name(s) of these drugs?
- Can you describe the reaction?
- Was the drug taken by mouth (as a tablet or syrup), or was it an injection?
- How soon after starting the drug did the reaction happen?
- How long ago did this happen?
- Did anyone tell you it was an allergic reaction, or did you decide for yourself?
- Has your child ever taken this drug, or a similar one, again? If yes, did your child experience the same problems?
- Have you told the doctors or nurses about your child's reaction or allergy?

Modified from Cantrill JA, Cottrell WN: Accuracy of drug allergy documentation, *Am J Health Syst Pharm* 54:1627-1629, 1997.

Current Medications. Inquire about current drug regimens, including vitamins, antipyretics (especially aspirin), antibiotics, antihistamines, decongestants, or antitussives. List all medications, including name, dose, schedule, duration, and reason for administration. Often parents are unaware of the drug's actual name. Whenever possible, ask parents to bring the containers with them to the next visit, or ask for the name of the pharmacy and call for a list of all the child's recent prescription medications. However, this list will not include over-the-counter medications, which are important to know.

Immunizations. A record of all immunizations is essential. Since many parents are unaware of the exact name and date of each immunization, the most reliable source of information is a hospital, clinic, or private practitioner's record. All immunizations and "boosters" are listed, stating (1) the name of the specific disease, (2) the number of injections, (3) the dosage (sometimes lesser amounts are given if a reaction is anticipated), (4) the ages when administered, and (5) the occurrence of any reaction following the immunization.

NURSINGALERT

Inquire about previous administration of any horse or other foreign serum, recent administration of gamma globulin or blood transfusion, and anaphylactic reactions to neomycin or chicken eggs.

Growth and Development. The most important previous growth patterns to record are:

- Approximate weight at 6 months, 1 year, 2 years, and 5 years of age
- Approximate length at ages 1 and 4 years
- Dentition, including age of onset, number of teeth, and symptoms during teething

Developmental milestones include:

- Age of holding up head steadily
- Age of sitting alone without support
- Age of walking without assistance
- Age of saying first words with meaning

BOX 6-6
Habits to Explore During a Health Interview

- Behavior patterns such as nail biting, thumb sucking, pica (habitual ingestion of nonfood substances), rituals ("security" blanket or toy), and unusual movements (head banging, rocking, overt masturbation, walking on toes)
- Activities of daily living, such as hour of sleep and arising, duration of nighttime sleep and naps, type and duration of exercise, regularity of stools and urination, age of toilet training, and daytime or nighttime bed-wetting
- Unusual disposition; response to frustration
- Use or abuse of alcohol, drugs, coffee, or tobacco

- Present grade in school
- Scholastic grades
- Interactions with other children, peers, and adults

Use specific and detailed questions when inquiring about each developmental milestone. For example, "sitting up" can mean many different activities, such as sitting propped up, sitting in someone's lap, sitting with support, sitting up alone but in a hyperflexed position for assisted balance, or sitting up unsupported with the back slightly rounded. A clue to misunderstanding of the requested activity may be an unusually early age of achievement (see Developmental Assessment, p. 93).

Habits. Habits are an important area to explore (Box 6-6). Parents frequently express concerns during this part of the history. Encourage their input by saying, "Please tell me any concerns you have about your child's habits, activities, or development." Investigate further any concerns that are expressed.

One of the most common concerns relates to sleep. Many children develop a normal sleep pattern, and all that is required during the assessment is a general overview of nighttime sleep and nap schedules. However, a number of children also develop sleep problems (see Sleep Problems, Chapters 10 and 13). When sleep problems occur, a more detailed sleep history is required to guide appropriate interventions.*

Habits related to use of chemicals apply primarily to older children and adolescents. If a youngster admits to smoking, drinking, or drug use, ask about the quantity and frequency. Questions such as "Have you ever had a drinking or drug problem?" or "When was the last time you had a drink or took drugs?" may yield more reliable data than questions such as "How much do you drink?" or "How often do you drink or take drugs?" Clarify that "drinking" includes all types of alcohol, such as beer and wine. When quantities such as a "glass" of wine or a "can" of beer are given, ask about the size of the container.

If older children deny use of chemical substances, inquire about past experimentation. Asking, "You mean you never tried to smoke or drink?" implies that the nurse expects some such activity, and the youngster may be more inclined to answer truthfully. Be aware of the confidential nature of such questioning, the adverse effect that the parents' presence may

BOX 6-7
Anticipatory Guidance—Sexuality

AGES 12 TO 14 YEARS
Have adolescent identify supportive adult to discuss sexuality issues and concerns with.
Discuss advantages of delaying sexual activity.
Discuss making responsible decisions regarding normal sexual feelings.
Discuss role of gender, peer pressure, and the media in sexual decision making.
Discuss contraceptive options (advantages and disadvantages).
Provide education regarding sexually transmitted diseases (STDs) and human immunodeficiency virus (HIV) infection; clarify risks and discuss condoms.
Discuss abuse prevention: avoiding dangerous situations, role of drugs and alcohol, and use of self-defense.
Have adolescent clarify values, needs, and ability to be assertive.
If adolescent is sexually active, discuss limiting partners, use of condoms, and contraceptive options.
Have confidential interview with adolescent (including a sexual history).
Discuss the evolution of sexual identity and expression.
Discuss breast examination or testicular examination.

AGES 15 TO 18 YEARS
Support delaying sexual activity.
Discuss alternatives to intercourse.
Discuss "When are you ready for sex?"
Clarify values; encourage responsible decision making.
Discuss consequences of unprotected sex: early pregnancy, STDs, including HIV infection.
Discuss negotiating with partner and barriers to safer sex.
If adolescent is sexually active, discuss limiting partners, use of condoms, and contraceptive options.
Emphasize that sex should be safe and pleasurable for both partners.
Have confidential interview with adolescent.
Discuss concerns about sexual expression and identity.

Modified from Wright K: Anticipatory guidance: developing a healthy sexuality, *Pediatr Ann* 26(2 Suppl):S142-S144, C3, 1997.

have on the adolescent's willingness to answer, and the fact that self-reporting may not be an accurate account of chemical abuse.

Sexual History

The sexual history is an essential component of adolescents' health assessment. The history uncovers areas of concern related to sexual activity; alerts the nurse to circumstances that may indicate screening for sexually transmitted diseases or testing for pregnancy; and provides information related to the need for sexual counseling, such as safe sex practices. Guidelines for anticipatory guidance topics for parents and adolescents are found in Box 6-7.

One approach to initiating a conversation about sexual concerns is to begin with a history of peer interactions. Open-ended statements such as "Tell me about your social life" or "Who are your closest friends?" generally lead into a discussion of dating and sexual issues. To probe further, include questions about the adolescent's attitudes on such topics as sex education, "going steady," "living together," and premarital sex. Phrase questions to reflect concern rather than judgment or criticism of sexual practices.

*A sleep history and a sleep chart for the family to record the child's daily sleep and wake activities is available in Wilson D, Hockenberry M: *Wong's clinical manual of pediatric nursing*, ed 7, St Louis, 2008, Mosby.

In any conversation regarding sexual history, be aware of the language that is used in either eliciting or conveying sexual information. For example, avoid asking if the adolescent is "sexually active," because this term is broadly defined. "Are you having sex with anyone?" is probably the most direct and best understood question. Since same-sex experimentation may occur, refer to all sexual contacts in nongender terms, such as "anyone" or "partners," rather than "girlfriends" or "boyfriends."

A detailed account of sexual partners is needed if the patient has a history of, displays any symptoms of, or asks for treatment of a sexually transmitted disease. A difficult but necessary part of the interview is to determine the sites of possible infection. Since sexual diseases can be contracted in any of the body orifices, inform the adolescent that a sexually transmitted disease can be acquired without visible signs of disease at nongenital sites.

Family Medical History

The family medical history is used primarily for the purpose of discovering the potential existence of hereditary or familial diseases in the parents and child. In general, it is confined to first-degree relatives (parents, siblings, grandparents, and immediate aunts and uncles). Information for each family member includes age, marital status, state of health if living, cause of death if deceased, and any evidence of the following conditions: heart disease, hypertension, cancer, diabetes mellitus, obesity, congenital anomalies, allergy, asthma, seizures, tuberculosis, sickle cell disease, mental retardation, mental disorders such as depression or psychosis, emotional problems, syphilis, or rheumatic fever. Confirm the accuracy of the reported disorders by inquiring about the symptoms, course, treatment, and sequelae of each diagnosis.

Geographic Location. One of the important areas to explore when assessing the family health history is geographic location, including the birthplace and travel to different areas in or outside of the country, for identification of possible exposure to endemic diseases. Although the primary interest focuses on the child's temporary residence in various localities, also inquire about close family members' travel, especially during tours of military service or business trips. Children are especially susceptible to parasitic infestation in areas of poor sanitary conditions and to vector-borne diseases, such as those from mosquitoes or ticks in warm and humid or heavily wooded regions.

Family Structure

Assessment of the family, both its structure and function, is an important component of the history-taking process. Because the quality of the functional relationship between the child and family members is a major factor in emotional and physical health, family assessment is discussed separately and in greater detail apart from the more traditional health history.

Family assessment is the collection of data about the composition of the family and the relationships among its members. In its broadest sense, **family** refers to all those individuals who are considered by the family member to be significant to the nuclear unit, including relatives, friends, and social groups such as the school and church. Although family assessment is not family therapy, it can and frequently is therapeutic. Involving family members in discussing family characteristics

nursingcareguidelines

Initiating a Comprehensive Family Assessment

Perform a comprehensive assessment on:
- Children receiving comprehensive well-child care
- Children experiencing major stressful life events (e.g., chronic illness, disability, parental divorce, death of a family member)
- Children requiring extensive home care
- Children with developmental delays
- Children with repeated accidental injuries and those with suspected child abuse
- Children with behavioral or physical problems that could be caused by family dysfunction

Modified from Cantrill JA, Cottrell WN: Accuracy of drug allergy documentation, *Am J Health Syst Pharm* 54:1627-1629, 1997.

and activities can provide insight into family dynamics and relationships.

Because of the time involved in performing an in-depth family assessment as presented here, be selective in deciding when knowledge of family function may facilitate nursing care (see Nursing Care Guidelines box). During brief contacts with families, a full assessment is not appropriate, and screening with one or two questions from each category may reflect the health of the family system or the need for additional assessment.

Family structure refers to the composition of the family—who lives in the home and those social, cultural, religious, and economic characteristics that influence the child's and family's overall psychobiologic health (see also Chapters 3 and 4). Since the information elicited in this part of the history is often the most personal and confidential, include it toward the end of the interview when rapport is well established.

The most common method of eliciting information on the family structure is to interview family members. The principal areas of concern (Box 6-8) are (1) family composition, (2) home and community environment, (3) occupation and education of family members, and (4) cultural and religious traditions.

NURSINGALERT

In assessing family composition, it is sometimes difficult to ascertain the status of the adult relationships. If the parent fails to mention the other parent, ask, "Where is the child's father [or mother]?" Avoid saying "husband" or "wife" because this assumes that only marital relationships exist.

Psychosocial History

The traditional medical history includes a personal and social section that concentrates on children's personal status, such as school adjustment and any unusual habits, and the family and home environment. Since several personal aspects are covered under development and habits, only those issues related to children's ability to cope and their self-concept are presented here.

Through observation, obtain a general idea of how children handle themselves in terms of confidence in dealing with others, answering questions, and coping with new situations.

BOX 6-8

Family Assessment Interview

GENERAL GUIDELINES

Schedule the interview with the family at a time that is most convenient for all parties; include as many family members as possible; clearly state the purpose of the interview.

Begin the interview by asking each person's name and their relationship to one another.

Restate the purpose of the interview and the objective.

Keep the initial conversation general to put members at ease and to learn the "big picture" of the family.

Identify major concerns and reflect these back to the family to be certain that all parties receive the same message.

Terminate the interview with a summary of what was discussed and a plan for additional sessions if needed.

STRUCTURAL ASSESSMENT AREAS

Family Composition

Immediate members of the household (names, ages, and relationships)

Significant extended family members

Previous marriages, separations, death of spouses, or divorces

Home and Community Environment

Type of dwelling, number of rooms, occupants

Sleeping arrangements

Number of floors, accessibility of stairs and elevators

Adequacy of utilities

Safety features (fire escape, smoke and carbon monoxide detectors, guardrails on windows, use of car restraint)

Environmental hazards (e.g., chipped paint, poor sanitation, pollution, heavy street traffic)

Availability and location of health care facilities, schools, play areas

Relationship with neighbors

Recent crises or changes in home

Child's reaction and adjustment to recent stresses

Occupation and Education of Family Members

Types of employment

Work schedules

Work satisfaction

Exposure to environmental or industrial hazards

Sources of income and adequacy

Effect of illness on financial status

Highest degree or grade level attained

Cultural and Religious Traditions

Religious beliefs and practices

Cultural and ethnic beliefs and practices

Language spoken in home

Assessment questions include:

- Does the family identify with a particular religious or ethnic group? Are both parents from that group?
- How is religious or ethnic background part of family life?
- What special religious or cultural traditions are practiced in the home (e.g., food choices and preparation)?
- Where were family members born, and how long have they lived in this country?
- What language does the family speak most frequently?
- Do they speak and understand English?
- What do they believe causes health or illness?
- What religious or ethnic beliefs influence the family's perception of illness and its treatment?

- What methods are used to prevent or treat illness?
- How does the family know when a health problem needs medical attention?
- Whom does the family contact when a member is ill?
- Does the family rely on cultural or religious healers or remedies? If so, ask them to describe the type of healer or remedy.
- Whom does the family go to for support (clergy, medical healer, relatives)?
- Does the family experience discrimination because of their race, beliefs, or practices? Ask them to describe.

FUNCTIONAL ASSESSMENT AREAS

Family Interactions and Roles

Interactions refer to ways family members relate to each other.

Chief concern is the amount of intimacy and closeness among the members, especially spouses.

Roles refer to behaviors of people as they assume a different status or position.

Observations include:

- Family members' responses to each other (cordial, hostile, cool, loving, patient, short tempered)
- Obvious roles of leadership vs submission
- Support and attention shown to various members

Assessment questions include:

- What activities does the family perform together?
- Whom do family members talk to when something is bothering them?
- What are members' household chores?
- Who usually oversees what is happening with the children, such as at school or health care?
- How easy or difficult is it for the family to change or accept new responsibilities for household tasks?

Power, Decision Making, and Problem Solving

Power refers to individual member's control over others in family; it is manifested through family decision making and problem solving.

Chief concern is clarity of boundaries of power between parents and children.

One method of assessment involves offering a hypothetical conflict or problem, such as a child failing school, and asking family how they would handle this situation.

Assessment questions include:

- Who usually makes the decisions in the family?
- If one parent makes a decision, can the child appeal to the other parent to change it?
- What input do children have in making decisions or discussing rules?
- Who makes and enforces the rules?
- What happens when a rule is broken?

Communication

Communication is concerned with clarity and directness of communication patterns.

Further assessment includes periodically asking family members if they understood what was just said and to repeat the message.

Observations include:

- Who speaks to whom
- If one person speaks for another or interrupts
- If members appear uninterested when certain individuals speak
- If there is agreement between verbal and nonverbal messages

Family Assessment Interview—cont'd

FUNCTIONAL ASSESSMENT AREAS—cont'd
Communication—cont'd
Assessment questions include:

- How often do family members wait until others are through talking before "having their say"?
- Do parents or older siblings tend to lecture and preach?
- Do parents tend to "talk down" to the children?

Expression of Feelings and Individuality
Expressions are concerned with personal space and freedom to grow with limits and structure needed for guidance.
Observing patterns of communication offers clues to how freely feelings are expressed.

Assessment questions include:

- Is it OK for family members to get angry or sad?
- Who gets angry most of the time? What do they do?
- If someone is upset, how do other family members try to comfort this person?
- Who comforts specific family members?
- When someone wants to do something, such as try out for a new sport or get a job, what is the family's response (offer assistance, discouragement, or no advice)?

Observe the parent-child relationship for the types of messages sent to children about their coping skills and self-worth. Do the parents treat the child with respect, focusing on strengths, or is the interaction one of constant reprimands, with emphasis on weaknesses and faults? Do the parents help the child learn new coping strategies or support the ones the child uses?

Messages about body image are also conveyed through the parent-child interaction. Do the parents label the child and body parts, such as "bad boy," "skinny legs," or "ugly scar"? Do the parents handle the child gently, using soothing touch to calm an anxious child, or do they treat the child roughly, using slaps or restraint to force compliance? If the child touches certain parts of the body, such as the genitalia, do the parents make comments that suggest a negative connotation?

With older children many of the communication strategies discussed earlier in the chapter are useful in eliciting more definitive information about their coping and self-concept. Children can write down five things they like and dislike about themselves. The nurse can use sentence completion statements, such as "The thing I like best (or worst) about myself is _____," "If I could change one thing about myself, it would be _____," or "When I am scared, I _____."

Review of Systems

The review of systems is a specific review of each body system, following an order similar to that of the physical examination (see Nursing Care Guidelines box). Often the history of the present illness provides a complete review of the system involved in the chief complaint. Since asking questions about other body systems may appear unrelated and irrelevant to the parents or child, precede the questioning with an explanation of why the data are needed (similar to the explanation concerning the relevance of the birth history) and reassure the parents that the child's main problem has not been forgotten.

Begin the review of a specific system with a broad statement such as "How has your child's general health been?" or "Has your child had any problems with his eyes?" If the parent states that the child has had problems with some body function, pursue this with an encouraging statement such as "Tell me more about that." If the parent denies any problems, query

for specific symptoms (e.g., "No headaches, bumping into objects, or squinting?"). If the parent reconfirms the absence of such symptoms, record positive statements in the history, such as "Mother denies headaches, bumping into objects, or squinting." In this way, anyone who reviews the health history is aware of exactly what symptoms were investigated.

NUTRITIONAL ASSESSMENT

DIETARY INTAKE

Food consumption patterns of children have changed over the past 30 years (Nicklas, Demory-Luce, Yang, and others, 2004). The prevalence of overweight and obesity among children and adolescents has significantly increased (Hedley, Ogden, Johnson, and others, 2004). Knowledge of the child's dietary intake is an essential component of a nutritional assessment. However, it is also one of the most difficult factors to assess. Individuals' recall of food consumption, especially amounts eaten, is frequently unreliable. The food intake history of children and adolescents is prone to reporting error, mostly in the form of underreporting (Livingstone, Robson, and Wallace, 2004). People from different cultures may have difficulty adequately describing the types of food they eat. Despite these obstacles, a dietary evaluation is an important component of the child's assessment.

The **dietary reference intakes** (DRIs) are a set of four nutrient-based reference values that provide quantitative estimates of nutrient intake for use in assessing and planning dietary intake (American Academy of Pediatrics, 2004; Murphy and Poos, 2002). The specific DRIs include:

Estimated average requirement (EAR)—Nutrient intake estimated to meet the requirement of half the healthy individuals (50%) for a specific age and gender group. Used to examine the possibility of inadequacy.
Recommended dietary allowance (RDA)—Average daily dietary intake sufficient to meet the nutrient requirement of nearly all (97% to 98%) of healthy individuals for a specific age and gender group. Dietary intake at or above this level usually has a low probability of inadequacy.
Adequate intake (AI)—Recommended intake level based on estimates of nutrient intake by healthy groups of individuals. Dietary intake at or above this level usually has a low probability of inadequacy.

nursingcareguidelines

Review of Systems

General—Overall state of health, fatigue, recent or unexplained weight gain or loss (period of time for either), contributing factors (change of diet, illness, altered appetite), exercise tolerance, fevers (time of day), chills, night sweats (unrelated to climatic conditions), frequent infections, general ability to carry out activities of daily living

Integument—Pruritus, pigment or other color changes, acne, eruptions, rashes (location), tendency for bruising, petechiae, excessive dryness, general texture, disorders or deformities of nails, hair growth or loss, hair color change (for adolescent, use of hair dyes or other potentially toxic substances, such as hair straighteners)

Head—Headaches, dizziness, injury (specific details)

Eyes—Visual problems (behaviors indicative of blurred vision, such as bumping into objects, clumsiness, sitting close to television, holding a book close to face, writing with head near desk, squinting, rubbing the eyes, bending head in an awkward position), cross-eyes (strabismus), eye infections, edema of lids, excessive tearing, use of glasses or contact lenses, date of last optic examination

Ears—Earaches, discharge, evidence of hearing loss (ask about behaviors, such as need to repeat requests, loud speech, inattentive behavior), results of any previous auditory testing

Nose—Nosebleeds (epistaxis), constant or frequent runny or stuffy nose, nasal obstruction (difficulty breathing), alteration or loss of sense of smell

Mouth—Mouth breathing, gum bleeding, toothaches, toothbrushing, use of fluoride, difficulty with teething (symptoms), last visit to dentist (especially if temporary dentition is complete), response to dentist

Throat—Sore throats, difficulty swallowing, choking (especially when chewing food—may be from poor chewing habits), hoarseness or other voice irregularities

Neck—Pain, limitation of movement, stiffness, difficulty holding head straight (torticollis), thyroid enlargement, enlarged nodes or other masses

Chest—Breast enlargement, discharge, masses, enlarged axillary nodes (for adolescent girl, ask about breast self-examination)

Respiratory—Chronic cough, frequent colds (number per year), wheezing, shortness of breath at rest or on exertion, difficulty breathing, sputum production, infections (pneumonia, tuberculosis), date of last chest x-ray examination, and skin reaction from tuberculin testing

Cardiovascular—Cyanosis or fatigue on exertion, history of heart murmur or rheumatic fever, anemia, date of last blood count, blood type, recent transfusion

Gastrointestinal (questions in regard to appetite, food tolerance, and elimination habits are asked elsewhere)—Nausea, vomiting (not associated with eating, may be indicative of brain tumor or increased intracranial pressure), jaundice or yellowing skin or sclera, belching, flatulence, recent change in bowel habits (blood in stools, change of color, diarrhea, or constipation)

Genitourinary—Pain on urination, frequency, hesitancy, urgency, hematuria, nocturia, polyuria, unpleasant odor to urine, force of stream, discharge, change in size of scrotum, date of last urinalysis (for adolescent, sexually transmitted disease, type of treatment; for male adolescent, ask about testicular self-examination)

Gynecologic—Menarche, date of last menstrual period, regularity or problems with menstruation, vaginal discharge, pruritus, date and result of last Papanicolaou (Pap) smear (include obstetric history, as discussed under birth history, when applicable); if sexually active, type of contraception, sexually transmitted disease and type of treatment

Musculoskeletal—Weakness, clumsiness, lack of coordination, unusual movements, back or joint stiffness, muscle pains or cramps, abnormal gait, deformity, fractures, serious sprains, activity level

Neurologic—Seizures, tremors, dizziness, loss of memory, general affect, fears, nightmares, speech problems, any unusual habits

Endocrine—Intolerance to weather changes, excessive thirst or urination, excessive sweating, salty taste to skin, signs of early puberty

---

Tolerable upper intake level (UL)—Highest average daily nutrient intake level likely to pose no risk of adverse health effects. As intake increases above the UL, risk of adverse effects increases. Dietary intake above this level usually places an individual at risk of adverse effects from excessive nutrient intake.

MyPyramid for Kids describes dietary intake in children (see Fig. 11-1). Specific questions used to conduct a nutritional assessment are also included in Box 6-9. Every nutritional assessment should begin with a **dietary history.** The exact questions used to elicit a dietary history vary with the child's age. In general, the younger the child, the more specific and detailed the history should be.

The overview elicited from the dietary history can be helpful in evaluating food frequency records. The history is also concerned with financial and cultural factors that influence food selection and preparation (see Cultural Awareness box).

The most common and probably easiest method of assessing daily intake is the **24-hour recall.** The child or parent recalls every item eaten in the past 24 hours and the approximate amounts. The 24-hour recall is most beneficial when it represents a typical day's intake. Some of the difficulties with a daily recall are the family's inability to remember exactly what was eaten and inaccurate estimation of portion size. To increase accuracy of reporting portion sizes, the use of food models and additional questioning are recommended. In general, this method is most useful in providing *qualitative* information about the child's diet.

To improve the reliability of the daily recall, the family can complete a **food diary** by recording every food and liquid consumed for a certain number of days. A 3-day record consisting of 2 weekdays and 1 weekend day is representative for most people. Providing specific charts to record intake can improve compliance. The family should record items immediately after eating.

A **food frequency questionnaire** or record provides information about the number of times in a day, week, or month a child consumes items from the different food groups. In general, it provides a qualitative overview but has the advantage of avoiding recall based on a "typical" day. It can be especially useful when verifying a food history or diary.

BOX 6-9

Nutrition Assessment

DIETARY HISTORY

What are the family's usual mealtimes?

Do family members eat together or at separate times?

Who does the family grocery shopping and meal preparation?

How much money is spent to buy food each week?

How are most foods prepared—baked, broiled, fried, other?

How often does the family or your child eat out?
- What kinds of restaurants do you go to?
- What kinds of food does your child typically eat at restaurants?

Does your child eat breakfast regularly?

Where does your child eat lunch?

What are your child's favorite foods, beverages, and snacks?
- What are the average amounts eaten per day?
- What foods are artificially sweetened?
- What are your child's snacking habits?
- When are sweet foods usually eaten?
- What are your child's toothbrushing habits?

What special cultural practices are followed? What ethnic foods are eaten?

What foods and beverages does your child dislike?

How would you describe your child's usual appetite (hearty eater, picky eater)?

What are your child's feeding habits (breast, bottle, cup, spoon, eats by self, needs assistance, any special devices)?

Does your child take vitamins or other supplements? Do they contain iron or fluoride?

Does your child have any known or suspected food allergies? Is your child on a special diet?

Has your child lost or gained weight recently?

Are there any feeding problems (excessive fussiness, spitting up, colic, difficulty sucking or swallowing)? Are there any dental problems or appliances, such as braces, that affect eating?

What types of exercise does your child do regularly?

Is there a family history of cancer, diabetes, heart disease, high blood pressure, or obesity?

ADDITIONAL QUESTIONS FOR INFANTS

What was the infant's birth weight? When did it double? Triple?

Was the infant preterm?

Are you breastfeeding or have you breast-fed your infant? For how long?

If you use a formula, what is the brand?
- How long has the infant been taking it?
- How many ounces does the infant drink a day?

Are you giving the infant cow's milk (whole, low fat, skim)?
- When did you start?
- How many ounces does the infant drink a day?

Do you give your infant extra fluids (water, juice)?

If the infant takes a bottle to bed at nap or nighttime, what is in the bottle?

At what age did the child start on cereal, vegetables, meat or other protein sources, fruit or juice, finger food, table food?

Do you make your own baby food or use commercial foods, such as infant cereal?

Does the infant take a vitamin or mineral supplement? If so, what type?

Has the infant had an allergic reaction to any food(s)? If so, list the foods and describe the reaction.

Does the infant spit up frequently; have unusually loose stools; or have hard, dry stools? If so, how often?

How often do you feed your infant?

How would you describe your infant's appetite?

Modified from Murphy SP, Poos MI: Dietary reference intakes: summary of applications in dietary assessment, *Pub Health Nutr* 5(6A):843-849, 2002.

 CULTURAL AWARENESS

Food Practices

Because cultural practices are prevalent in food preparation, consider carefully the kinds of questions that are asked and the judgments made during counseling. For example, some cultures, such as Hispanic, African American, and Native American, include many vegetables, legumes, and starches in their diet that together provide sufficient essential amino acids, even though the actual amount of meat or dairy protein is low. (See Food Customs, Chapter 4.)

CLINICAL EXAMINATION

A significant amount of information regarding nutritional deficiencies is elicited from a clinical examination, especially from assessing the skin, hair, teeth, gums, lips, tongue, and eyes. Hair, skin, and mouth are vulnerable because of the rapid turnover of epithelial and mucosal tissue. Table 6-1 summarizes clinical signs of possible nutritional deficiency or excess. Few are diagnostic for a specific nutrient, and if suspicious signs are found, they must be confirmed with dietary

and biochemical data. Generally, the clinical examination does not reveal children *at risk* for a deficiency or excess.

Anthropometry, an essential parameter of nutritional status, is the measurement of height, weight, head circumference, proportions, skinfold thickness, and arm circumference in young children. Height and head circumference reflect past nutrition, whereas weight, skinfold thickness, and arm circumference reflect present nutritional status, especially of protein and fat reserves. Skinfold thickness is a measurement of the body's fat content because approximately half the body's total fat stores are directly beneath the skin. The upper arm muscle circumference is correlated with measurements of total muscle mass. Since muscle serves as the body's major protein reserve, this measurement is considered an index of the body's protein stores. Ideally, growth measurements are recorded over time, and comparisons are made regarding the *velocity* of growth based on previous and present values. Numerous **biochemical tests** are available for assessing nutritional status and include analysis of plasma; blood cells; urine; and tissues from liver, bone, hair, and fingernails. Many of these tests are complicated and are not performed routinely. Common laboratory procedures for nutritional status include measurement of hemoglobin, hematocrit, transferrin, albu-

TABLE 6-1		

Clinical Assessment of Nutritional Status

EVIDENCE OF ADEQUATE NUTRITION	EVIDENCE OF DEFICIENT OR EXCESS NUTRITION	DEFICIENCY OR EXCESS*
GENERAL GROWTH		
Between 5th and 95th percentiles for height, weight, and head circumference	Below 5th or above 95th percentile for growth	Protein, calories, fats, and other essential nutrients, especially vitamin A, pyridoxine, niacin, calcium, iodine, manganese, zinc
Steady gain with expected growth spurts during infancy and adolescence	Absence of or delayed growth spurts; poor weight gain	
Sexual development appropriate for age	Delayed sexual development	Excess vitamins A, D
SKIN		
Smooth, slightly dry to touch	Hardening and scaling	Vitamin A
Elastic and firm	Seborrheic dermatitis	Excess niacin
Absence of lesions	Dry, rough, petechiae	Riboflavin
Color appropriate to genetic background	Delayed wound healing	Vitamin C
	Scaly dermatitis on exposed surfaces	Riboflavin, vitamin C, zinc
	Wrinkled, flabby	Niacin
	Crusted lesions around orifices, especially nares	Protein, calories, zinc
	Pruritus	Excess vitamin A, riboflavin, niacin
	Poor turgor	Water, sodium
	Edema	Protein, thiamine
		Excess sodium
	Yellow tinge (jaundice)	Vitamin B$_{12}$
		Excess vitamin A, niacin
	Depigmentation	Protein, calories
	Pallor (anemia)	Pyridoxine, folic acid, vitamins B$_{12}$, C, E (in preterm infants), iron
		Excess vitamin C, zinc
	Paresthesia	Excess riboflavin
HAIR		
Lustrous, silky, strong, elastic	Stringy, friable, dull, dry, thin	Protein, calories
	Alopecia	Protein, calories, zinc
	Depigmentation	Protein, calories, copper
	Raised areas around hair follicles	Vitamin C
HEAD		
Even molding, occipital prominence, symmetric facial features	Softening of cranial bones, prominence of frontal bones, skull flat and depressed toward middle	Vitamin D
Fused sutures after 18 months	Delayed fusion of sutures	Vitamin D
	Hard, tender lumps in occiput	Excess vitamin A
	Headache	Excess thiamine
NECK		
Thyroid not visible, palpable in midline	Thyroid enlarged, may be grossly visible	Iodine
EYES		
Clear, bright	Hardening and scaling of cornea and conjunctiva	Vitamin A
Good night vision	Night blindness	Vitamin A
Conjunctiva—Pink, glossy	Burning, itching, photophobia, cataracts, corneal vascularization	Riboflavin
EARS		
Tympanic membrane—Pliable	Calcified (hearing loss)	Excess vitamin D
NOSE		
Smooth, intact nasal angle	Irritation and cracks at nasal angle	Riboflavin
Excess vitamin A		

*Nutrients listed are deficient unless specified as excess.

TABLE 6-1

Clinical Assessment of Nutritional Status—cont'd

EVIDENCE OF ADEQUATE NUTRITION	EVIDENCE OF DEFICIENT OR EXCESS NUTRITION	DEFICIENCY OR EXCESS*
MOUTH		
Lips—Smooth, moist, darker color than skin	Fissures and inflammation at corners	Riboflavin Excess vitamin A
Gums—Firm, coral pink, stippled	Spongy, friable, swollen, bluish red or black, bleed easily	Vitamin C
Mucous membranes—Bright pink, smooth, moist	Stomatitis	Niacin
Tongue—Rough texture, no lesions, taste sensation	Glossitis Diminished taste sensation	Niacin, riboflavin, folic acid Zinc
Teeth—Uniform white color, smooth, intact	Brown mottling, pits, fissures Defective enamel Caries	Excess fluoride Vitamins A, C, D, calcium, phosphorus Excess carbohydrates
CHEST		
In infants, shape almost circular	Depressed lower portion of rib cage	Vitamin D
In children, lateral diameter increased in proportion to anteroposterior diameter	Sharp protrusion of sternum	Vitamin D
Smooth costochondral junctions	Enlarged costochondral junctions	Vitamins C, D
Breast development—Normal for age	Delayed development	See under General Growth; especially zinc
CARDIOVASCULAR SYSTEM		
Pulse and blood pressure (BP) within normal limits	Palpitations	Thiamine
	Rapid pulse	Potassium Excess thiamine
	Arrhythmias	Magnesium, potassium Excess niacin, potassium
	Increased BP	Excess sodium
	Decreased BP	Thiamine Excess niacin
ABDOMEN		
In young children, cylindric and prominent	Distended, flabby, poor musculature	Protein, calories
	Prominent, large	Excess calories
In older children, flat	Potbelly, constipation	Vitamin D
Normal bowel habits	Diarrhea	Niacin Excess vitamin C
	Constipation	Excess calcium, potassium
MUSCULOSKELETAL SYSTEM		
Muscles—Firm, well-developed, equal strength bilaterally	Flabby, weak, generalized wasting Weakness, pain, cramps	Protein, calories Thiamine, sodium, chloride, potassium, phosphorus, magnesium Excess thiamine
	Muscle twitching, tremors	Magnesium
	Muscular paralysis	Excess potassium
Spine—Cervical and lumbar curves (double S curve)	Kyphosis, lordosis, scoliosis	Vitamin D
Extremities—Symmetric; legs straight with minimum bowing	Bowing of extremities, knock-knees	Vitamin D, calcium, phosphorus
	Epiphyseal enlargement	Vitamins A, D
	Bleeding into joints and muscles, joint swelling, pain	Vitamin C
Joints—Flexible, full range of motion, no pain or stiffness	Thickening of cortex of long bones with pain and fragility, hard tender lumps in extremities	Excess vitamin A
	Osteoporosis of long bones	Calcium Excess vitamin D

Continued

TABLE 6-1

Clinical Assessment of Nutritional Status—cont'd

EVIDENCE OF ADEQUATE NUTRITION	EVIDENCE OF DEFICIENT OR EXCESS NUTRITION	DEFICIENCY OR EXCESS*
NEUROLOGIC SYSTEM		
Behavior—Alert, responsive, emotionally stable	Listless, irritable, lethargic, apathetic (sometimes apprehensive, anxious, drowsy, mentally slow, confused)	Thiamine, niacin, pyridoxine, vitamin C, potassium, magnesium, iron, protein, calories
		Excess vitamins A, D, thiamine, folic acid, calcium
Absence of tetany, convulsions	Masklike facial expression, blurred speech, involuntary laughing	Excess manganese
	Convulsions	Thiamine, pyridoxine, vitamin D, calcium, magnesium
		Excess phosphorus (in relation to calcium)
Intact peripheral nervous system	Peripheral nervous system toxicity (unsteady gait, numb feet and hands, fine motor clumsiness)	Excess pyridoxine
Intact reflexes	Diminished or absent tendon reflexes	Thiamine, vitamin E

*Nutrients listed are deficient unless specified as excess.

min, creatinine, and nitrogen. Laboratory values for these tests and more specific nutrient measurements are given in Appendix C.

EVALUATION OF NUTRITIONAL ASSESSMENT

After collecting the data needed for a thorough nutritional assessment, evaluate the findings to plan appropriate counseling. From the data, assess whether the child is (1) malnourished, (2) at risk for becoming malnourished, or (3) well nourished with adequate reserves.

Analyze the daily food diary for the variety and amounts of foods suggested in MyPyramid (see Fig. 11-1). For example, if the list includes no vegetables, inquire about this rather than assuming that the child dislikes vegetables, since it could be that none were served that day. Also, evaluate the information in terms of the family's ethnic practices and financial resources. Encouraging increased protein intake with additional meat may be unfeasible for families on a limited budget or in conflict with food practices that use meat sparingly, such as in Asian meal preparation.

GENERAL APPROACHES TOWARD EXAMINING THE CHILD

SEQUENCE OF THE EXAMINATION

Ordinarily, the sequence for examining patients follows a head-to-toe direction. The main function of such a systematic approach is to provide a general guideline for assessment of each body area to avoid omitting segments of the examination. The standard recording of data also facilitates exchange of information among different professionals. The typical organization of a physical examination is indicated in the chapter outline. In examining children, this orderly sequence is frequently altered to accommodate the child's developmental needs, although the examination is recorded following the head-to-toe model. Using developmental and chronologic age as the main criteria for assessing each body system accomplishes several goals:

- Minimizes stress and anxiety associated with assessment of various body parts
- Fosters a trusting nurse-child-parent relationship
- Allows for maximum preparation of the child

- Preserves the essential security of the parent-child relationship, especially with young children
- Maximizes the accuracy and reliability of assessment findings

PREPARATION OF THE CHILD

Although the physical examination consists of painless procedures, to a child the use of a tight arm cuff, probes in the ears and mouth, pressure on the abdomen, and a cold piece of metal to listen to the chest can be stressful. Therefore the same considerations discussed in Chapter 22 for preparing children for procedures are followed here. In addition to that discussion, general guidelines related to the examining process are presented in the Nursing Care Guidelines box.

The physical examination should be as pleasant as possible, as well as educational. For example, the nurse can use a detailed drawing or anatomically correct doll to help preschoolers and older children learn about their bodies (Vessey, 1995). The paper-doll technique is a useful approach to teaching children about the body part that is being examined (Fig. 6-4). At the conclusion of the visit, the child can bring home the paper doll as a memento of the experience.

Table 6-2 summarizes guidelines for positioning, preparing, and examining children at various ages. Because no child fits precisely into one age category, it may be necessary to vary the approach after a preliminary assessment of the child's developmental achievements and needs. Even with the best approach, many toddlers are uncooperative and inconsolable for much of the physical examination. However, some seem intrigued by the new surroundings and unusual equipment and respond more like preschoolers than toddlers. Likewise, some early preschoolers may require more of the "security measures" employed with younger children, such as continued parent-child contact, and less of the preparatory measures used with preschoolers, such as playing with the equipment before and during the actual examination (Fig. 6-5).

Although the variations in the general approaches are numerous, some common ones are elaborated on here. For example, the suggested sequence may change considerably when the child is in pain or when obvious physical defects are present. In either situation, examine the affected area last to

nursingcareguidelines

Performing Pediatric Physical Examination

Perform examination in appropriate, nonthreatening area.
- Have room well lit and decorated with neutral colors.
- Have room temperature comfortably warm.
- Place all strange and potentially frightening equipment out of sight.
- Have some toys, dolls, stuffed animals, and games available for child.
- If possible, have rooms decorated and equipped for different-age children.
- Provide privacy, especially for school-age children and adolescents.

Provide time for play and becoming acquainted.

Observe behaviors that signal child's readiness to cooperate:
- Talking to the nurse
- Making eye contact
- Accepting the offered equipment
- Allowing physical touching
- Choosing to sit on examining table rather than parent's lap

If signs of readiness are not observed, use the following techniques:
- Talk to parent while essentially "ignoring" child; gradually focus on child or a favorite object, such as a doll.
- Make complimentary remarks about child, such as appearance, dress, or a favorite object.
- Tell a funny story or play a simple magic trick.
- Have a nonthreatening "friend" available, such as a hand puppet to "talk" to child for the nurse (see Fig. 6-25, *A*).

If child refuses to cooperate, use the following techniques:
- Assess reason for uncooperative behavior; consider that a child who is unduly afraid may have had a traumatic experience.
- Try to involve child and parent in process.
- Avoid prolonged explanations about examining procedure.
- Use a firm, direct approach regarding expected behavior.
- Perform examination as quickly as possible.
- Have attendant gently restrain child.
- Minimize any disruptions or stimulation.
- Limit number of people in room.
- Use isolated room.
- Use quiet, calm, confident voice.

Begin examination in a nonthreatening manner for young children or children who are fearful:
- Use activities that can be presented as games, such as test for cranial nerves (see Table 6-12) or parts of developmental screening tests (p. 93).
- Use approaches such as Simon Says to encourage child to make a face, squeeze a hand, stand on one foot, and so on.
- Use paper-doll technique:
  1. Lay child supine on an examining table or floor that is covered with a large sheet of paper.
  2. Trace around child's body outline.
  3. Use body outline to demonstrate what will be examined, such as drawing a heart and listening with stethoscope before performing activity on child.

If several children in the family will be examined, begin with most cooperative child to model desired behavior.

Involve child in examination process:
- Provide choices, such as sitting on table or in parent's lap.
- Allow child to handle or hold equipment.
- Encourage child to use equipment on a doll, family member, or examiner.
- Explain each step of the procedure in simple language.

Examine child in a comfortable and secure position:
- Sitting in parent's lap
- Sitting upright if in respiratory distress

Proceed to examine the body in an organized sequence (usually head to toe) with the following exceptions:
- Alter sequence to accommodate needs of different-age children (see Table 6-2).
- Examine painful areas last.
- In emergency situation, examine vital functions (airway, breathing, and circulation) and injured area first.

Reassure child throughout examination, especially about bodily concerns that arise during puberty.

Discuss findings with family at end of examination.

Praise child for cooperation during examination; give reward such as a small toy or sticker.

FIG. 6-4 ■ Using paper-doll technique to prepare child for physical examination.

FIG. 6-5 ■ Preparing children for physical examination.

TABLE 6-2

Age-Specific Approaches to Physical Examination During Childhood

POSITION	SEQUENCE	PREPARATION
INFANT		
Before able to sit alone—Supine or prone, preferably in parent's lap; before 4-6 months, can place on examining table **After able to sit alone**—Sitting in parent's lap whenever possible; if on table, place with parent in full view	If quiet, auscultate heart, lungs, abdomen. Record heart and respiratory rates. Palpate and percuss same areas. Proceed in usual head-to-toe direction. Perform traumatic procedures last (eyes, ears, mouth [while crying]). Elicit reflexes as body part is examined. Elicit Moro reflex last.	Completely undress if room temperature permits. Leave diaper on male infant. Gain cooperation with distraction, bright objects, rattles, talking. Smile at infant; use soft, gentle voice. Pacify with bottle of sugar water or feeding. Enlist parent's aid for restraining to examine ears, mouth. Avoid abrupt, jerky movements.
TODDLER		
Sitting or standing on or by parent Prone or supine in parent's lap	Inspect body area through play: "count fingers," "tickle toes." Use minimum physical contact initially. Introduce equipment slowly. Auscultate, percuss, palpate whenever quiet. Perform traumatic procedures last (same as for infant).	Have parent remove outer clothing. Remove underwear as body part is examined. Allow to inspect equipment; demonstrating use of equipment is usually ineffective. If uncooperative, perform procedures quickly. Use restraint when appropriate; request parent's assistance. Talk about examination if cooperative; use short phrases. Praise for cooperative behavior.
PRESCHOOL CHILD		
Prefer standing or sitting Usually cooperative prone or supine Prefer parent's closeness	If cooperative, proceed in head-to-toe direction. If uncooperative, proceed as with toddler.	Request self-undressing. Allow to wear underpants if shy. Offer equipment for inspection; briefly demonstrate use. Make up story about procedure (e.g., "I'm seeing how strong your muscles are" [blood pressure]). Use paper-doll technique. Give choices when possible. Expect cooperation; use positive statements (e.g., "Open your mouth").
SCHOOL-AGE CHILD		
Prefer sitting Cooperative in most positions Younger child prefers parent's presence Older child may prefer privacy	Proceed in head-to-toe direction. May examine genitalia last in older child.	Respect need for privacy. Request self-undressing. Allow to wear underpants. Give gown to wear. Explain purpose of equipment and significance of procedure, such as otoscope to see eardrum, which is necessary for hearing. Teach about body function and care.
ADOLESCENT		
Same as for school-age child Offer option of parent's presence	Same as older school-age child. May examine genitalia last.	Allow to undress in private. Give gown. Expose only area to be examined. Respect need for privacy. Explain findings during examination: "Your muscles are firm and strong." Matter-of-factly comment about sexual development: "Your breasts are developing as they should be." Emphasize normalcy of development. Examine genitalia as any other body part; may leave to end.

Clinical Preventive Services for Normal-Risk Children

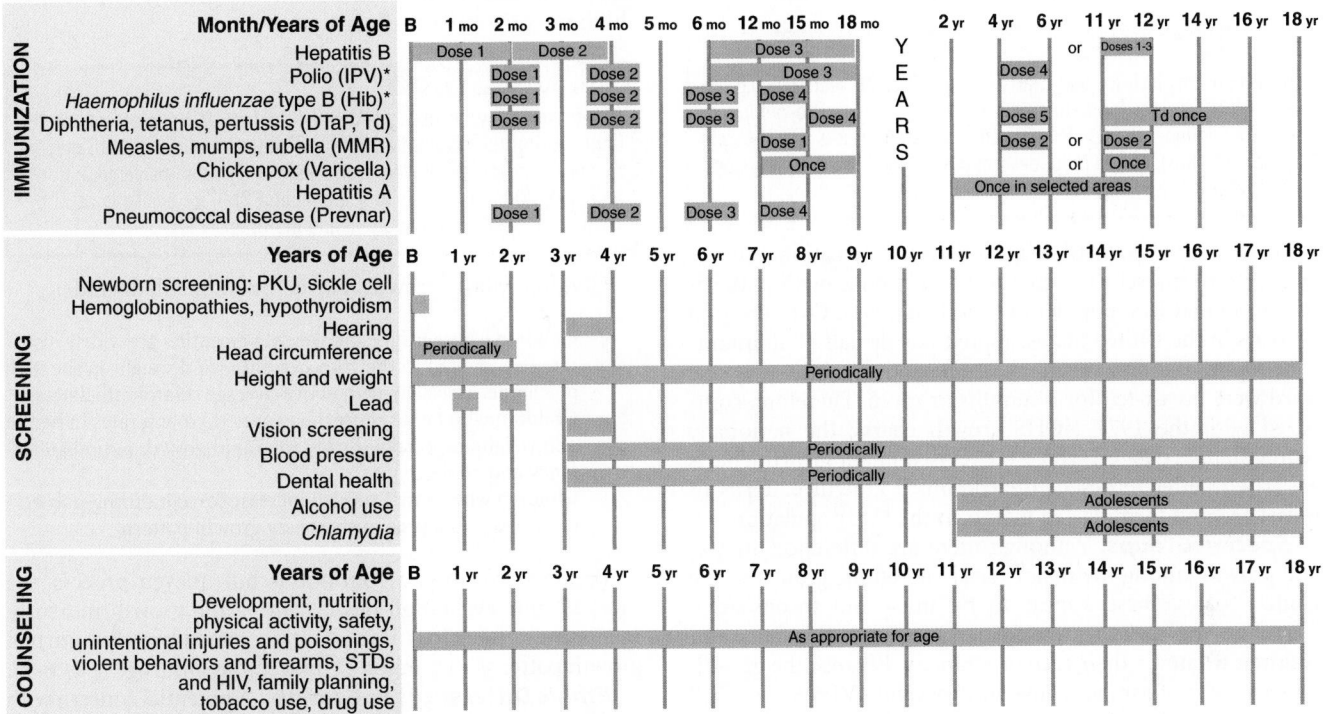

Recommended by most U.S. authorities

*Schedules may vary according to vaccine type.

FIG. 6-6 ■ Child preventive care time line. The information on immunizations is based on recommendations issued by Advisory Committee on Immunization Practices, American Academy of Pediatrics, and American Academy of Family Physicians. *B,* Birth; *HIV,* human immunodeficiency virus; *PKU,* phenylketonuria; *STDs,* sexually transmitted diseases. (From US Department of Health and Human Services: *Child health guide: put prevention into practice,* Washington, DC, Jan 2003 [rev], The Department.)

minimize distress early in the examination and to focus on normal, healthy, functioning body parts.

PHYSICAL EXAMINATION

Although the approach to and sequence of the physical examination differ according to the child's age, the following discussion outlines the traditional model for physical assessment. The focus includes all pediatric age-groups, but the reader is referred to Chapter 8 for a detailed discussion of a newborn assessment. Because the physical examination is a vital part of preventive pediatric care, a schedule for periodic health visits is given in Fig. 6-6.

GROWTH MEASUREMENTS

Measurement of physical growth in children is a key element in evaluating their health status. Physical growth parameters include weight, height (length), skinfold thickness, arm circumference, and head circumference. Values for these growth parameters are plotted on percentile charts, and the child's measurements in percentiles are compared with those of the general population.

Growth Charts

The most commonly used growth charts in the United States are from the National Center for Health Statistics (NCHS) (Kuczmarski RJ, Ogden CL, Grummer-Strawn, LM, and oth-

ers, 2000). The growth charts have been revised to include the body mass index–for-age (BMI-for-age) charts, 3rd and 97th smoothed percentiles for all charts, and the 85th percentile for the weight-for-stature and BMI-for-age charts (see Appendix B). The data were collected from five national surveys between 1963 and 1994. The revised charts have eliminated the disjunctions between the curves for infants and other children and have been extended for children and adolescents to 20 years.

The weight-for-age percentile distributions are now continuous between the infant and the older child charts at 24 to 36 months. The length-for-age to stature-for-age and weight-for-length to weight-for-stature curves are parallel in the overlapping ages of 24 to 36 months. The revised weight-for-stature charts provide a smoother transition from the weight-for-length charts for preschool-age children.

The most prominent change to the complement of growth charts for older children and adolescents is the addition of the BMI-for-age growth curves. The BMI-for-age charts were developed with national survey data (1963 to 1994), excluding data from the 1988 to 1994 National Health and Nutrition Examination Surveys III (NHANES III) for children older than 6 years because an increase in body weight and BMI occurred between NHANES III and previous national surveys. Without this exclusion, the 85th and 95th percentile curves would have been higher, and fewer children and adolescents would have been classified as at risk of or overweight. Therefore the BMI-for-age growth curves do not represent the current population of children older than 6 years of age.

Breast- and Formula-Fed Infants. The national survey data better represent the combined size and growth patterns of the general U.S. population (1971 to 1994). Over the past 30 years in the United States, approximately half of all infants were reported to have been breast-fed, and approximately one third were breast-fed for 3 months or more. Therefore, compared with the 1977 NCHS growth charts, the nationally representative data on which the revised infant growth charts are based better represent the combined growth patterns of breast-fed and formula-fed infants in the U.S. population.

Special Groups. Although there are differences in size and growth among the major racial and ethnic groups in the United States, these appear to be small and inconsistent. Therefore the revised growth charts include all infants and children whatever their race or ethnicity. Because the growth patterns of preterm, very low–birth-weight (VLBW) (<1500 g [3.3 pounds]) infants are considerably different from those of higher birth-weight, full-term infants and specialized growth charts exist to track the growth of VLBW infants, data for VLBW infants were excluded from the revised charts.

Version of the Growth Charts. Three different versions of the charts are available.* The first set contains all nine smoothed percentile lines (3rd, 5th, 10th, 25th, 50th, 75th, 90th, 95th, 97th), and the second and third sets contain seven smoothed percentile lines. The second set contains the 5th and 95th percentile lines, and the third set contains the 3rd and 97th percentile lines at the extreme ends of the distribution. In addition, the charts for weight-for-stature and BMI-for-age contain the 85th percentile. In all the growth charts, age is truncated to the nearest full month, for example, 1 month (1.0 to 1.9 months), 11 months (11.0 to 11.9 months), 23 months (23.0 to 23.9 months).

The three sets of charts are provided to meet the needs of various users. Set 1 shows all the major percentile curves but may have limitations when the curves are close together, especially at the youngest ages. Most users in the United States may wish to use the format shown in set 2 for the majority of routine clinical applications (see Appendix B). Pediatric endocrinologists and others dealing with special populations, such as children with failure to thrive, may wish to use the format in set 3.

Nurses are often responsible for measuring growth in children, so it is essential that they understand the revised growth charts. Several important differences exist between the 1977 and the revised charts with significant implications for classifying children as underweight or overweight. Nurses need to become familiar with determining BMI, which only requires information about the child's weight and height.† With the

---

*http://www.cdc.gov/growthcharts.
†BMI = [Weight in pounds ÷ (Height in inches × Height in inches)] × 703.
NOTE: Formula is BMI calculation for adults, used in some pediatric settings; for child and adolescent BMI table and plotting, see Appendix B.

increasing number of overweight children in the United States, the BMI charts will become a critical component of children's physical assessment.

Children whose growth may be questionable include:

- Children whose height and weight percentiles are widely disparate (e.g., height in the 10th percentile and weight in the 90th percentile, especially with above-average skinfold thickness)
- Children who fail to show the expected growth rates in height and weight, especially during the rapid growth periods of infancy and adolescence
- Children who show a sudden increase (except during puberty) or decrease in a previously steady growth pattern

Because growth is a continuous but uneven process, the most reliable evaluation lies in comparing growth measurements over time. It is important to remember that normal growth patterns vary among children the same age (Fig. 6-7).

Ethnic Differences in Growth. A potential concern with the U.S. growth charts is their accuracy in evaluating the growth of children from different ethnic and socioeconomic backgrounds. Research findings indicate that these growth charts can serve as a reference guide for all racial or ethnic groups if used from the perspective that different groups of children have varying normal distributions on the growth curves. The NCHS charts are accurate for U.S. African-American children because this group was included in the sample population. Special growth charts for Chinese children are given in Appendix B.

Length

The term **length** refers to measurements taken when children are supine (also referred to as **recumbent length**). Until children are 24 months old (or 36 months if using the chart for birth to 36 months), measure recumbent length. Because of the normally flexed position during infancy, fully extend the body by (1) holding the head in midline, (2) grasping the knees together gently, and (3) pushing down on the knees until the legs are fully extended and flat against the table. If using a measuring board, place the head firmly at the top of the board and the heels of the feet firmly against the footboard.

If such a measuring device is not available, measure length by placing the child on a paper-covered surface, marking the end points of the top of the head and the heels of the feet, and measuring between these two points (Fig. 6-8). For accurate measurement, hold the writing utensil at a right angle to the table when marking the cephalic point; position the feet with the toes pointing directly to the ceiling when marking the heel point. Regardless of the method used, have someone assist in holding the child's head in midline while you extend the legs and take the measurements.

Height

The term **height** (or **stature**) refers to the measurement taken when children are standing upright. Measure height by having the child, with shoes removed, stand as tall and straight as

FIG. 6-7 ■ These children of identical age (8 years) are markedly different in size. Child on left, of Asian descent, is at 5th percentile for height and weight. Child on right is above 95th percentile for height and weight. However, both children demonstrate normal growth patterns.

FIG. 6-8 ■ Measurement of head, chest, and abdominal circumference and crown-to-heel (recumbent) length.

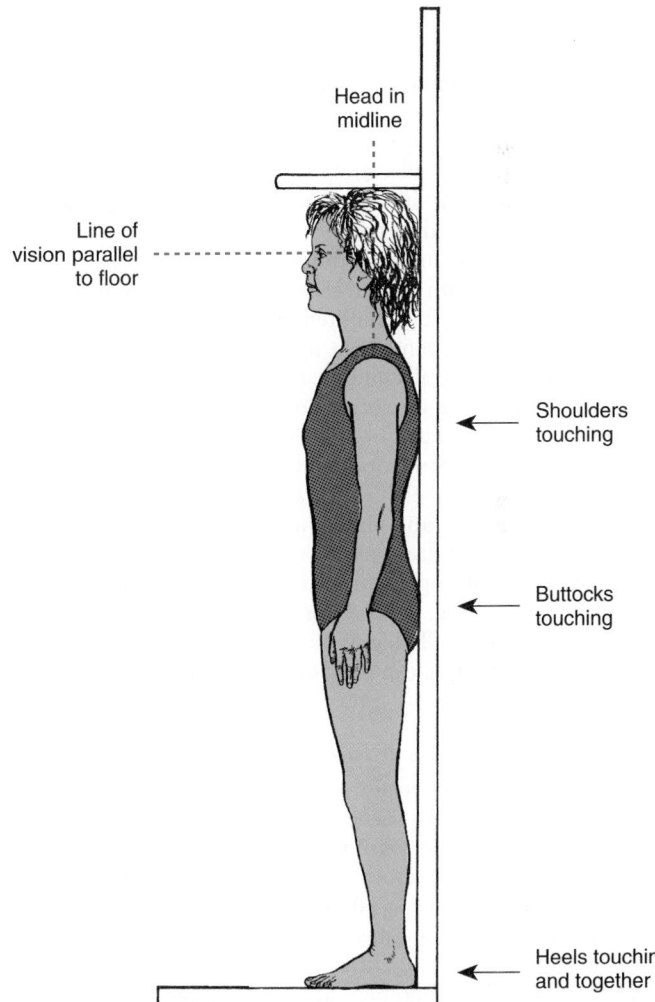

FIG. 6-9 ■ Measurement of height. (Redrawn from *Human growth and growth disorders: an update*, San Francisco, 1989, Genentech.)

possible, with the head in midline and the line of vision parallel to the ceiling and floor. Be certain the child's back is to the wall or other vertical flat surface, with the heels, buttocks, and back of the shoulders touching the wall and the medial malleoli touching if possible (Fig. 6-9). Check for and correct bending of the knees, slumping of the shoulders, or raising of the heels.

> **NURSINGTIP**
>
> Normally, height is less if measured in the afternoon than in the morning. To minimize this variation, apply modest upward pressure under the jaw or the mastoid processes behind the ears.

For the most accurate measurement, use a wall-mounted unit (**stadiometer;** see Fig. 6-9). The movable measuring rod of platform scales is accurate only if it maintains a parallel position to the floor and rests securely on the topmost part of the head. To improvise a flat surface for measuring length, attach a paper or metal tape or yardstick to the wall, position the child adjacent to the tape, and place a three-dimensional object, such as a thick book or box, on top of the head. Rest the side of the object firmly against the wall to form a right angle. Measure length or stature to the nearest 1 mm or ⅛ inch.

Weight

Weight is measured with an appropriately sized beam balance scale, which measures weight to the nearest 10 g (0.35 ounce) for infants and 100 g (0.22 pound) for children. Before the child is weighed, balance the scale by setting it at 0 and noting

if the balance registers exactly in the middle of the mark. If the end of the balance beam rises to the top or bottom of the mark, more or less weight, respectively, is needed. Some scales are designed to allow for self-correction, but others need to be recalibrated by the manufacturer. Scales vary in their accu-

FIG. 6-10 ■ **A**, Infant on scale. **B**, Toddler on scale. Note presence of nurse to prevent falls. (**B**, Courtesy Paul Vincent Kuntz, Texas Children's Hospital, Houston.)

racy; infant scales tend to be more accurate than adult platform scales, and newer scales tend to be more accurate than older ones, especially at the upper levels of weight measurement. When precise measurements are needed, two nurses should take the weight independently; if there is a discrepancy, a third reading should be taken.

Take measurements in a comfortably warm room. When the birth to 36-month growth charts are used, children should be weighed nude. Older children are usually weighed while wearing their underpants or a light gown. However, always respect the privacy of all children. If the child must be weighed wearing some article of clothing or some type of special device, such as a prosthesis or an armboard for an intravenous device, note this when recording the weight. Children who are measured for recumbent length are usually weighed on an infant platform scale and placed in a lying or sitting position. When weighing children, place your hand lightly above the body of the infant to prevent the child from accidentally falling off the scale (Fig. 6-10, *A*) or stand close to the toddler, ready to prevent a fall (Fig. 6-10, *B*). For maximum asepsis, cover the scale with a clean sheet of paper between each child's measurement.

Skinfold Thickness and Arm Circumference

Measures of relative weight and stature cannot distinguish between adipose (fat) tissue and muscle. One convenient measure of body fat is **skinfold thickness,** which is increasingly recommended as a routine measurement. Skinfold thickness is measured with special calipers, such as the Lange calipers. The most common sites for measuring skinfold thickness are the triceps (most practical for routine clinical use), subscapula, suprailiac, abdomen, and upper thigh. For greatest reliability the exact procedure for measurement must be followed and the average of at least two measurements of one site recorded.

Arm circumference is an indirect measure of muscle mass. Measurement of arm circumference follows the same procedure for skinfold thickness except the midpoint is measured with a paper or steel tape. Place the tape vertically, along the posterior aspect of the upper arm to the acromial process and to the olecranon process; half the measured length is the midpoint. Percentiles for triceps skinfold and arm circumference

in children are listed in Appendix B and may be used as reference data. However, the percentiles are not standards or norms, since values between the 5th and 95th percentiles are not ranges of normal.

Head Circumference

Measure head circumference in children up to 36 months of age and in any child whose head size is questionable. Measure the head at its greatest circumference, usually slightly above the eyebrows and pinna of the ears and around the occipital prominence at the back of the skull (see Fig. 6-8). Because head shape can affect the location of the maximum circumference, more than one measurement at points above the eyebrows may be needed to obtain the most accurate measure. Use a paper or metal tape, since a cloth tape can stretch and give a falsely small measurement. For greatest accuracy, use devices with tenths of a centimeter, since the percentile charts have only 0.5-cm increments.

Plot the head size on the appropriate growth chart under head circumference. Generally, head and chest circumferences are equal at about 1 to 2 years of age. During childhood, chest circumference exceeds head size by about 5 to 7 cm (2 to 2.75 inches). (For newborns see Physical Assessment, Chapter 8.)

PHYSIOLOGIC MEASUREMENTS

Physiologic measurements, key elements in evaluating physical status of vital functions, include temperature, pulse, respiration, and blood pressure. Compare each physiologic recording with normal values for that age-group (see inside back cover). In addition, compare the values taken on preceding health visits with present recordings. For example, a falsely elevated blood pressure reading may not indicate hypertension if previous recent readings have been within normal limits. The isolated recording may indicate some stressful event in the child's life.

As in most procedures carried out with children, older children and adolescents are treated much the same as adults. However, special consideration must be given to preschool children (see Atraumatic Care box).

For best results in taking vital signs of infants, count respirations first (before the infant is disturbed), take the pulse next, and measure temperature last. If vital signs cannot be

ATRAUMATIC CARE

Reducing Young Children's Fears

Young children, especially preschoolers, fear intrusive procedures because of their poorly defined body boundaries. Therefore avoid invasive procedures, such as measuring rectal temperature, whenever possible. Also, avoid using the word "take" when measuring vital signs, since young children interpret words literally and may think that their temperature or other function will be taken away. Instead, say, "I want to know how warm you are."

BOX 6-10

Fever in Infants and Children

Temperature depends on the time of day, age, and physical activity. In general evaluation is recommended for the following:

Infants ≤3 months of age: ≥100.4° F (38° C)
Infants 3 to 36 months of age: ≥102° F (38.9° C)
Children of any age: ≥104° F (40° C)

BOX 6-11

Recommended Temperature Screening Routes in Infants and Children

BIRTH TO 2 YEARS
Axillary
Rectal—if definitive temperature reading is needed for infants over 1 month of age

2 TO 5 YEARS
Axillary
Tympanic
Oral—when child can hold thermometer under tongue
Rectal—if definitive temperature reading is needed

OVER 5 YEARS
Oral
Axillary
Tympanic

BOX 6-12

Alternative Temperature Measurement Sites for the Ill Child

SKIN
Probe is placed on the skin to determine heat output in response to changes in the patient's skin temperature.
Skin temperature sensors are most often used for neonates and infants placed in radiant heat warmers or isolettes (using servocontrol feature of the apparatus). In turn, the heater unit warms to a set point to maintain the infant's temperature within a specified range.
ThermoSpot is an example of a device allowing continuous thermal monitoring in neonates.

URINARY BLADDER
A thermistor or thermocouple is placed within the indwelling bladder catheter. The catheter tip immersed in the bladder provides a continuous temperature read-out on the bedside monitor.
This is not a true measure of core temperature but responds better than rectal and skin temperatures to core body changes.
Because of thermistor sizes, this method is unusable with neonates and small infants.

PULMONARY ARTERY
A catheter is placed into the heart to obtain a reading in the pulmonary artery.
It is used in critical care settings or operating rooms only in patients requiring aggressive monitoring.
Catheter is not available in sizes for neonates or small infants.

ESOPHAGEAL SITE
Probe is inserted into the lower third of the esophagus at the level of the heart.
This is used in critical care settings or operating rooms.
Several companies have esophageal stethoscopes with temperature probe monitors for patients in the operating room that show a continuous temperature reading.

NASOPHARYNGEAL SITE
Probe is inserted into the nasopharynx, posterior to the soft palate, and provides an estimate of hypothalamic temperature.
This is used in critical care settings or operating rooms.

Data from Kumar PR, Nisarga R, Gowda B: Temperature monitoring in newborns using ThermoSpot, *Indian J Pediatr* 71(9):795-796, 2004; Martin SA, Kline AM: Can there be a standard for temperature measurement in the pediatric intensive care unit? *AACN Clin Issues* 15(2):254-266, 2004; and Maxton FJC, Justin L, Gilles D: Estimating core temperature in infants and children after cardiac surgery: a comparison of six methods, *J Adv Nurs* 45(2):214-222, 2004.

---

taken without disturbing the child, record the child's behavior (e.g., crying) along with the measurement.

Temperature

Temperature is the measure of heat content within an individual's body. The **core temperature** most closely reflects the temperature of the blood flow through the carotid arteries to the hypothalamus. Core temperature is relatively constant despite wide fluctuations in the external environment. When a child's temperature is altered, receptors in the skin, spinal cord, and brain respond in an attempt to achieve normothermia, a normal temperature state. In pediatrics, there is a lack of consensus regarding what temperature constitutes normothermia for every child. For rectal temperatures in children, a value of 37° to 37.5° C (98.6° to 99.5° F) is an acceptable range, where heat loss and heat production are balanced. For neonates, a core body temperature between 36.5° and 37.6° C

(97.7° and 99.7° F) is a desirable range. In the neonate, temperature measurements are obtained for monitoring adequacy of thermoregulation, not fever; therefore temperature measurements in each infant should be carefully considered in the context of the *purpose* and the environment. Temperature definitions of fever based on age are found in Box 6-10.

Temperature in healthy children can be measured at several body sites via oral, rectal, axillary, ear canal, tympanic membrane, temporal artery, or skin route (Box 6-11). For the ill child other sites for temperature measurement that have been investigated include the urinary bladder, pulmonary artery, and esophageal and nasopharyngeal sites (Martin and Kline, 2004) (Box 6-12). One of the most important influences on the accuracy of temperature is improper temperature-taking

TABLE 6-3

Temperature Measurement Locations for Infants and Children

TEMPERATURE SITE

ORAL

Place tip under tongue in right or left posterior sublingual pocket, not in front of tongue. Have child keep mouth closed, without biting on thermometer.

Pacifier thermometers measure intraoral or supralingual temperature and are available but lack support in the literature.

Several factors affect mouth temperature: eating and mastication, hot or cold beverages, open-mouth breathing, ambient temperature.

AXILLARY

Place tip under arm in center of axilla and keep close to skin, not clothing. Hold child's arm firmly against side. Temperature may be affected by poor peripheral perfusion (results in lower value), clothing or swaddling, use of radiant warmer, or amount of brown fat in cold-stressed neonate (results in higher value).

Advantage: avoids intrusive procedure and eliminates risk of rectal perforation.

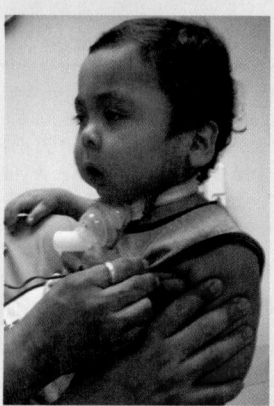

EAR BASED (AURAL)

Insert small infrared probe deeply into canal to allow sensor to obtain measurement. Size of probe (most are 8 mm) may influence accuracy of result. In young children this may be a problem because of small diameter of canal. Proper placement of ear is controversial related to whether the pinna should be pulled in manner similar to that used during otoscopy (see p. 140).

RECTAL

Place well-lubricated tip at maximum 2.5 cm (1 inch) into rectum for children and 1.5 cm (0.6 inch) for infants; securely hold thermometer close to anus.

Child may be placed in side-lying, supine, or prone position (i.e., supine with knees flexed toward abdomen); cover penis, since procedure may stimulate urination. A small child may be placed prone across parent's lap.

TEMPORAL ARTERY

An infrared sensor probe scans across forehead, capturing heat from arterial blood flow. Temporal artery is only artery close enough to skin's surface to provide access for accurate temperature measurement.

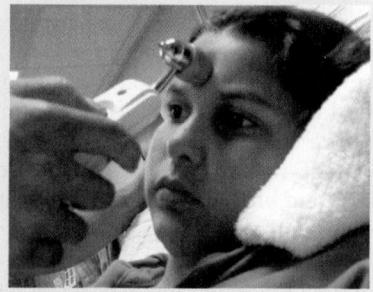

Data from Martin SA, Kline AM: Can there be a standard for temperature measurement in the pediatric intensive care unit? *AACN Clin Issues* 15(2):254-266, 2004; and Falzon A, Grech V, Caruana B, and others: How reliable is axillary temperature measurement? *Acta Paediatr* 92(3):309-313, 2003. Oral, axillary, rectal, and temporal artery images courtesy Paul Vincent Kuntz, Texas Children's Hospital, Houston.

technique. Detailed discussion of temperature-taking methods and visual examples of proper techniques are shown in Table 6-3. For a critical review of the evidence on temperature taking methods, see the Evidence-Based Practice box.

NURSINGALERT

Glass mercury thermometers used in many studies as the "gold standard" are no longer recommended for use (Goldman and Shannon, 2001).

The most frequently used temperature measurement devices in infants and children are as follows (Healthcare Product Comparison System, 2004a, 2004b):

Electronic intermittent thermometers—Measure the patient's temperature at oral, rectal, and axillary sites and are used as primary diagnostic indicators
Infrared thermometers—Measure the patient's temperature by collecting emitted thermal radiation from a particular site (e.g., ear canal)
Electronic continuous thermometers—Measure the patient's temperature during the administration of general anesthesia, treatment of hypothermia or hyperthermia, and other situations that require continuous monitoring

A detailed description of these devices is found in Box 6-13.

NURSINGALERT

The belief that core temperature can be estimated by adding 1° C to the temperature taken in the axilla is incorrect. Do not add a degree to the finding obtained by taking a temperature by the axillary route (Craig, Lancaster, Williamson, and others, 2000).

Pulse

A satisfactory pulse can be taken radially in children older than 2 years of age. However, in infants and young children, the **apical impulse** (heard through a stethoscope held to the chest at the apex of the heart) is more reliable (see Fig. 6-32 for location of pulses). Count the pulse for 1 full minute in infants and young children because of possible irregularities in rhythm. However, when frequent apical rates are needed, use shorter counting times (e.g., 15- or 30-second intervals). For greater accuracy, measure the apical rate while the child is asleep; record the child's behavior along with the rate. Pulses may be graded according to the criteria in Table 6-4. Compare radial and femoral pulses at least once during infancy to detect the presence of circulatory impairment, such as coarcta-

---

BOX 6-13

Types of Thermometers Used to Measure Temperature in Infants and Children

ELECTRONIC THERMOMETER
Temperature is sensed with an electronic component called thermistor mounted at the tip of a plastic and stainless steel probe, which is connected to an electronic recorder. A disposable plastic cover is used for infection control.
Temperature measurement appears on digital display within 60 seconds.
Probe can be placed in mouth, axilla, or rectum.

INFRARED THERMOMETER
Thermal radiation is measured from axilla, ear canal, or tympanic membrane.
Temperature measurement appears on digital display in approximately 1 second.
Three types are available for ear-based use: tympanic, ear canal, and arterial heat balance via the ear canal (AHBE).
Often these devices are all inappropriately referred to as *tympanic thermometers*.
Temperatures measured in this way reflect arterial (bloodstream) temperature.

EAR-BASED TEMPERATURE SENSOR
Although this is frequently used in pediatric settings (especially ambulatory clinics), debate still continues on the reliability of ear-based thermometry in screening febrile children.
Most models use "offsets" for internal calculations that transform ear temperature into supposedly equivalent oral or rectal temperatures.

EAR SENSOR (LIGHTOUCH LTX)
This measures the infrared heat energy radiating from canal opening, scans canal for highest temperature reading, and then calculates arterial temperature (correlates highly with core or internal body temperature).
It is available in two sizes; smaller size of LightTouch Pedi-Q is for infants and toddlers.

AXILLARY SENSOR (LIGHTOUCH LTN)
This measures the infrared heat energy radiating from the axilla.
It can be used on wet skin; in incubators; or under radiant heaters, warming pads, or other heat sources.

DIGITAL THERMOMETER
A probe is connected to a microprocessor chip, which translates signals into degrees and sends temperature measurement to digital display.
It is used like an oral electronic thermometer and can be used for measuring oral, rectal, and axillary temperature.
It is more accurate and easier to read, but somewhat more expensive, than plastic strip thermometer.

LIQUID CRYSTAL SKIN CONTACT THERMOMETER (CHEMICAL DOT THERMOMETER)
This single-use, disposable, flexible thermometer has a specific chemical mixture in each circle that changes color to measure temperature increments of $2/10$ of a degree.
There are two types:
1. Kept in mouth (1 minute), axilla (3 minutes), or rectum (3 minutes); color change is read 10 to 15 seconds after removing thermometer
2. Wearable, continuous-use thermometer, which is placed under axilla; may be read within 2 to 3 minutes after placement and continuously thereafter; discard and replace every 48 hours

EVIDENCE-BASED PRACTICE

Temperature Measurement in Pediatrics

ASK THE QUESTION   In infants and children, what is the most accurate method for measuring temperature?

SEARCH FOR EVIDENCE

Search Strategies   Searched the literature to obtain clinical research studies related to this issue. Selection criteria included English, publications within past 10 years, research-based articles (level 3 or lower), infant and child populations, comparisons to gold standard: rectal thermometry.

Databases Used   PubMed, Cochrane Collaboration, MD Consult, Joanna Briggs Institute, National Guideline Clearinghouse (AHRQ), TRIP Database Plus, PedsCCM, BestBETs

CRITICALLY ANALYZE THE EVIDENCE

Rectal temperature—Rectal measurement remains the clinical gold standard for the precise diagnosis of fever in infants and children (Greenes and Fleisher, 2004; Riddell and Eppich, 2003; University of Michigan, 2003). However, this procedure is more invasive and is contraindicated for infants less than 1 month old, children with recent rectal surgery, children with diarrhea or anorectal lesions, and children receiving chemotherapy (cancer treatment usually affects mucosa and causes neutropenia). Findings are affected by depth of insertion and presence of stool. Rectal temperatures are slow to change in relation to changing core temperature. Many parents are uncomfortable with this method, and children may resent it. It has capacity to spread contaminants found in stool.

Oral temperature (OT)—OT indicates rapid changes in core body temperature, but accuracy may be an issue when compared with rectal site (Jensen, Jensen, Madsen, and others, 2000). OTs are considered the standard for temperature measurement (Gilbert, Barton, and Counsell, 2002), but are contraindicated in children who have an altered level of consciousness, are receiving oxygen, are mouth breathing, are experiencing mucositis, had recent oral surgery or trauma, and are under 5 years of age (Carroll, 2000; Holtzclaw, 1998; El-Radhi and Barry, 2006). Limitations of OTs include the effect of ambient room temperature and recent oral intake (Carroll, 2000; Holtzclaw, 1998; Martin and Kline, 2004). Even patients with no obvious mouth breathing were found to have OTs in the normal range despite the presence of clinical fever (Tandberg and Sklar, 1983). O'Brien, Rogers, Holden, and others (2000) found OT-predictive thermometers to read significantly lower than other core temperature measurements and miss one out of seven fevers.

Axillary temperature—This is inconsistent and insensitive in infants and children over 1 month old (Jean-Mary, Dicanzio, Shaw, and others, 2002; Falzon, Grech, Caruana, and others, 2003). Despite its low sensitivity and specificity in detecting fever, the axillary site is recommended by the American Academy of Pediatrics (2001) as a screening test for fever in infants 1 month of age.

Ear (aural) temperature—This is not a precise measurement of body temperature. Meta-analysis of 101 studies comparing tympanic membrane temperatures with rectal temperatures in children concluded that the tympanic method demonstrated a wide range of variability, limiting its application in a pediatric setting (Craig, Lancaster, Taylor, and others, 2002). Diagnosis of fever without a focus should not be made based on tympanic thermometry, since it is not an accurate measure of core temperature (Craig, Lancaster, Taylor, and others, 2002; Riddell and Eppich, 2003).

Temporal artery temperature (TAT)—TAT was not predictable for fever in children under 3 months but could be used as a screening tool for detecting fever less than 38° C (100.4° F) in children 3 to 24 months old (Schuh, Komar, Stephens, and others, 2004). Temporal temperature can be used as a rapid assessment screening tool to identify rectal fever over 39° C (102.2° F) in children 3 to 24 months old, but is unreliable as a screening tool for infants under 3 months (Siberry, Diener-West, Schappell, and others, 2002). These published studies examining the accuracy and precision of TATs in infants and children are limited by small sample sizes. Previous samples included subjects primarily under the age of 36 months, although

one abstract was found of a study that examined 75 TATs in children 6 to 12 years old (Pidwell, Heavrin, Santen, and others, 2000). Settings that have been used to study TATs in pediatric patients include the emergency center (Greenes & Fleisher, 2001; Pidwell, Heavrin, Santen, and others, 2000; Schuh, Komar, Stephens, and others, 2004; Siberry, Diener-West, Schappell, and others, 2002), physician's office (Callanan, 2003), pediatric intensive care unit (Hebbar, Fortenberry, Rogers, and others, 2005), and operating room (Al-Mukhaizeem, Allen, Komar, and others, 2004).

APPLY THE EVIDENCE: NURSING IMPLICATIONS

No single site used for temperature assessment provides unequivocal estimates of core body temperature. Studies show that the axillary and tympanic measures demonstrate poor agreement when these modes are compared with more accurate core temperature methods. The differences are more evident as temperature increases, regardless of age. When an accurate method for obtaining a correct reflection of core temperature is needed, the rectal temperature is recommended in younger children and the oral route in older children. For infants less than 1 month of age, the American Academy of Pediatrics (2001) recommends axillary temperatures.

References

Al-Mukhaizeem F, Allen U, Komar L, and others: Comparison of temporal artery, rectal and esophageal core temperatures in children: results of a pilot study, *Paediatr Child Health* 9(7):461-465, 2004.

American Academy of Pediatrics, Committee on Environmental Health: Technical report: mercury in the environment: implications for pediatricians, *Pediatrics* 108(1):197-205, 2001.

Callanan D: Detecting fever in young infants: reliability of perceived, pacifier, and temporal artery temperatures in infants younger than 3 months of age, *Pediatr Emerg Care* 19(4):240-243, 2003.

Carroll M: An evaluation of temperature measurement, *Nurs Stand* 14(44):39-43, 2000.

Craig JV, Lancaster GA, Taylor S, and others: Infrared ear thermometry compared with rectal thermometry in children: a systemic review, *Lancet* 360:603-609, 2002.

El-Radhi AS, Barry W: Thermometry in paediatric practice, *Arch Dis Child* 91(4):351-356, 2006.

Falzon A, Grech V, Caruana B, and others: How reliable is axillary temperature measurement? *Acta Paediatr* 92(3):309-313, 2003.

Gilbert M, Barton AJ, Counsell CM: Comparison of oral and tympanic temperatures in adult surgical patients, *Appl Nurs Res* 15(1):42-47, 2002.

Greenes DS, Fleisher GR: When body temperature changes, does rectal temperature lag? *J Pediatr* 144(6):824-826, 2004.

Greenes DS, Fleisher GR: Accuracy of a noninvasive temporal artery thermometer for use in infants, *Arch Pediatr Adolesc Med* 155(3):376-381, 2001.

Hebbar K, Fortenberry JD, Rogers K, and others: Comparison of temporal artery thermometer to standard temperature measurement in pediatric intensive care unit patients, *Pediatr Crit Care Med* 6(5):557-561, 2005.

Holtzclaw BJ: New trends in thermometry for the patient in the ICU, *Crit Care Nurs Q* 21(3):12-25, 1998.

Jean-Mary MB, Dicanzio J, Shaw J, and others: Limited accuracy and reliability of infrared axillary and aural thermometers in a pediatric outpatient population, *J Pediatr* 141(5):671-676, 2002.

Jensen BN, Jensen FS, Madsen SN, and others: Accuracy of digital tympanic, oral, axillary, and rectal thermometers compared with standard rectal mercury thermometers, *Eur J Surg* 166(11):848-851, 2000.

Martin SA, Kline AM: Can there be a standard for temperature measurement in the pediatric intensive care unit? *AACN Clin Issues* 15(2):254-266, 2004.

EVIDENCE-BASED PRACTICE

Temperature Measurement in Pediatrics—cont'd

O'Brien DL, Rogers IR, Holden W, and others: The accuracy of oral predictive and infrared emission detection tympanic thermometers in an emergency department setting, *Acad Emerg Med* 7(9):1061-1064, 2000.

Pidwell WB, Heavrin BS, Santen SA, and others: Accuracy of temporal artery thermometer (abstract), *Ann Emerg Med* 36(4):S5, 2000.

Riddell A, Eppich W: *Should tympanic temperature measurement be trusted?* BestBETs, 2003, retrieved April 2005 from http://www.bestbets.org/cgi-bin/bets.pl?record500340.

Schuh S, Komar L, Stephens D, and others: Comparison of the temporal artery and rectal thermometry in children in the emergency department, *Pediatr Emerg Care* 20(11):736-741, 2004.

Siberry GK, Diener-West M, Schappell E, and others: Comparison of temple temperatures with rectal temperatures in children under 2 years of age, *Clin Pediatr* 41(6):405-414, 2002.

Tandberg D, Sklar D: Effect of tachypnea on the estimation of body temperature by an oral thermometer, *N Engl J Med* 308(16):945-946, 1983.

University of Michigan: *Rectal temperature is still the gold standard for determining the presence or absence of fever*, Evidence-Based Pediatrics Web Site, 2003, retrieved April 2005 from http://www.med.umich.edu/pediatrics/ebm/cats/fever.htm.

TABLE 6-4

Grading of Pulses

GRADE	DESCRIPTION
0	Not palpable
+1	Difficult to palpate, thready, weak, easily obliterated with pressure
+2	Difficult to palpate, may be obliterated with pressure
+3	Easy to palpate, not easily obliterated with pressure (normal)
+4	Strong, bounding, not obliterated with pressure

TABLE 6-5

Normative Dinamap Blood Pressure Values (Systolic/Diastolic; Mean Arterial Pressure in Parentheses)

AGE-GROUP	MEAN	90TH PERCENTILE	95TH PERCENTILE
Newborn (1-3 days)	65/41 (50)	75/49 (59)	78/52 (62)
1 month–2 years	95/58 (72)	106/68 (83)	110/71 (86)
2-5 years	101/57 (74)	112/66 (82)	115/68 (85)

From Park M, Menard S: Normative oscillometric blood pressure values in the first 5 years in an office setting, *Am J Dis Child* 143(7):860-864, 1989.

tion of the aorta. (See inside back cover for normal rates for pediatric age-groups.)

Respiration

Count the respiratory rate in children in the same manner as for the adult patient. However, in infants observe abdominal movements, since respirations are primarily diaphragmatic. Because the movements are irregular, count them for 1 full minute for accuracy (see also p. 144). (See inside back cover for normal respiratory rates in children.)

Blood Pressure

Blood pressure (BP) measurement by noninvasive methods is part of a routine vital sign determination. BP should be measured annually in children 3 years of age through adolescence and in children with symptoms of hypertension, children in emergency departments and intensive care units, and high-risk infants (National High Blood Pressure Education Program Working Group, 2004). Ambulatory BP monitoring in children and adolescents is a valuable method for assessing and managing suspected hypertension (Bald, 2002).

Measurement Devices. BP can also be measured using electronic devices that employ oscillometric or Doppler techniques. In **oscillometry,** pressure changes are transmitted through the arterial wall to the pressure cuff, and the oscillations are detected by a pressure-sensitive indicator. Oscillometers have digital read-outs for systolic, diastolic, and **mean arterial pressures (MAP)** and for pulse. The MAP is not the same as the mean BP (arithmetic average of systolic and diastolic pressures). Rather, it is a value somewhat lower than the arithmetic mean. BP readings using oscillometry, such as Dinamap, are generally higher (10 mm Hg higher) than measurements using auscultation (Park, Menard, and Yuan, 2001)

(Table 6-5). Differences between Dinamap and auscultatory readings prevent the interchange of the readings by the two methods. The oscillometric BP monitoring method is a reliable screening tool used in a variety of age-groups (Mattu, Heran, and Wright, 2004a, 2004b).

Doppler ultrasound translates changes in ultrasound frequency caused by blood movement within the artery to audible sound by means of a transducer in the cuff. This technique is useful for systolic pressure measurement but is unreliable for diastolic pressure measurement. Oscillometric and Doppler instruments are useful in measuring BP in infants and have largely replaced the flush method, which reflects only the mean BP, and the auscultatory method.

Selection of Cuff. No matter what type of noninvasive technique is used, the most important factor in accurately measuring BP is the use of an appropriately sized cuff (**cuff size** refers only to the inner inflatable bladder, not the cloth covering). A technique to establish an appropriate cuff size is to choose a cuff having a bladder width that is approximately 40% of the arm circumference midway between the olecranon and the acromion. This will usually be a cuff bladder that covers 80% to 100% of the circumference of the arm (Fig. 6-11) (Beevers, Lip, and O'Brien, 2001; National Institutes of Health, 1996). Researchers have found that selection of a cuff with a bladder width equal to 40% of the upper arm circumference most accurately reflects directly measured radial arterial pressure (Clark, Kieh-Lai, Sarnaik, and others, 2002) (Table 6-6).

Using limb circumference for selecting cuff width more accurately reflects direct arterial BP than using limb length, since this method takes into account variations in arm thick-

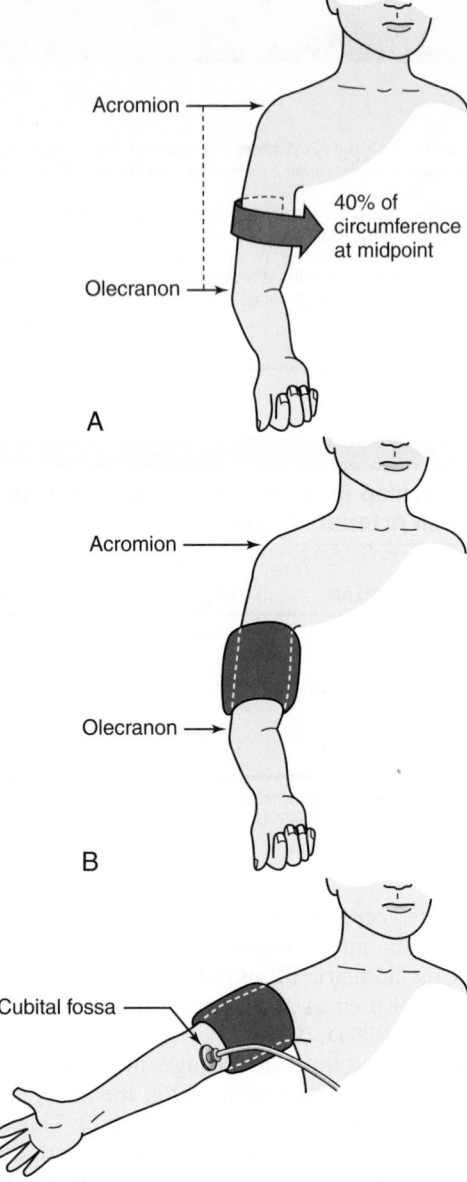

FIG. 6-11 ■ Determination of proper cuff size. **A,** Cuff bladder width should be approximately 40% of circumference of arm measured at a point midway between olecranon and acromion. **B,** Cuff bladder length should cover 80% to 100% of circumference of arm. **C,** Blood pressure should be measured with cubital fossa at heart level. Arm should be supported. Stethoscope bell is placed over brachial artery pulse, proximal and medial to cubital fossa and below bottom edge of cuff. (From National Institutes of Health, National Heart, Lung, and Blood Institute: *Update on the Task Force Report [1987] on high blood pressure in children and adolescents: a working group report from the National High Blood Pressure Education Program*, NIH Pub No 96-3790, Bethesda, Md, Sept 1996, The Institutes.)

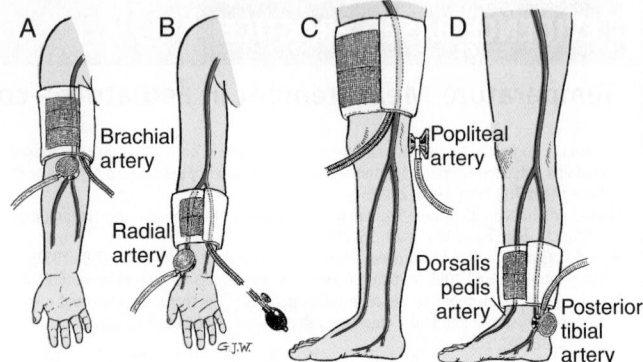

FIG. 6-12 ■ Sites for measuring blood pressure. **A,** Upper arm. **B,** Lower arm or forearm. **C,** Thigh. **D,** Calf or ankle.

TABLE 6-6
Recommended Dimensions for Blood Pressure Cuff Bladders

AGE RANGE	WIDTH (cm)	LENGTH (cm)	MAXIMUM ARM CIRCUMFERENCE (cm)*
Newborn	4	8	10
Infant	6	12	15
Child	9	18	22
Small adult	10	24	26
Adult	13	30	34
Large adult	16	38	44
Thigh	20	42	52

From National High Blood Pressure Education Program Working Group on High Blood Pressure in Children and Adolescents: The fourth report on the diagnosis, evaluation, and treatment of high blood pressure in children and adolescents, *Pediatrics* 114(2 Suppl 4th Rep):555-576, 2004.

*Calculated so that largest arm would still allow bladder to encircle arm by at least 80%.

TABLE 6-7
Differences in Oscillometric Systolic Blood Pressure Between Arm and Lower Extremity Sites in Normal Children

AGE-GROUP (years)	SYSTOLIC BLOOD PRESSURE × (mean ± SD)	
	ARM-THIGH	ARM-CALF
4-8	−7.1 ± 6.8	−9.3 ± 7.4
9-16	−2.4 ± 7.7	−5.0 ± 26.9

From Park M, Lee D, Johnson GA: Oscillometric blood pressures in the arm, thigh, and calf in healthy children and those with aortic coarctation, *Pediatrics* 91(4):761-765, 1993.

ness and the amount of pressure required to compress the artery (Gillman and Cook, 1995). For measurement sites other than the upper arms, the limb circumference guidelines can be used, although the shape of the limb (e.g., conical shape of the thigh) may prevent appropriate placement of the cuff and inaccurately reflect intraarterial BP.

Cuffs that are either too narrow or too wide affect the accuracy of BP measurements. If the cuff size is too small, the reading on the device is falsely high. If the cuff size is too large, the reading is falsely low (Clark, Kieh-Lai, Sarnaik, and others, 2002).

When another site is used, BP measurements using noninvasive techniques may differ. Generally, systolic pressure in the lower extremities (thigh or calf) is greater than pressure in the upper extremities, and systolic BP in the calf is higher than that in the thigh (Fig. 6-12). These differences are listed in Table 6-7 and apply to oscillometric measurements taken on the right extremities with the child supine and the cuff size based on the circumference method (Park, Lee, and Johnson, 1993).

> **NURSINGALERT**
>
> When taking BP, use an appropriately sized cuff. When the correct size is not available, use an oversized cuff rather than an undersized one or use another site that more appropriately fits the cuff size. Do not choose a cuff based on the name of the cuff (e.g., an "infant" cuff may be too small for some infants).

> **NURSINGALERT**
>
> Compare BP in the upper and lower extremities at least once to detect abnormalities, such as coarctation of the aorta, in which the lower extremity pressure is less than the upper extremity pressure.

Measurement and Interpretation. Measuring and interpreting BP in infants and children requires additional attention to correct procedure because (1) limb sizes vary and cuff selection must accommodate the circumference; (2) excessive pressure on the antecubital fossa affects the Korotkoff sounds; (3) children easily become anxious, which can elevate BP; and (4) BP values change with age and growth. In children and adolescents the normal range of BP is determined by body size and age. BP standards that are based on gender, age, and height provide a more precise classification of BP according to body size. This approach avoids misclassifying children who are very tall or very short. The revised BP tables now include the 50th, 90th, 95th, and 99th percentiles (with standard deviations) by gender, age, and height (see inside back cover).

To use the tables in a clinical setting, the height percentile is determined by using the newly revised Centers for Disease Control and Prevention growth charts.* The child's measured systolic BP and diastolic BP are compared with the numbers provided in the table (boys or girls) according to the child's age and height percentile. The child is normotensive if the BP is below the 90th percentile. If the BP is at or above the 90th percentile, the BP measurement should be repeated at that visit to verify an elevated BP. BP measurements between the 90th and 95th percentiles indicate prehypertension and warrant reassessment and consideration of other risk factors. In addition, if an adolescent's BP is more than 120/80 mm Hg, the patient should be considered prehypertensive even if this value is below the 90th percentile. This BP level typically occurs for systolic BP at 12 years old and for diastolic BP at 16 years old. If the child's BP (systolic or diastolic) is at or above the 95th percentile, the child may be hypertensive, and the measurement must be repeated on at least two occasions to confirm diagnosis (National High Blood Pressure Education Program Working Group, 2004). (See Nursing Care Guidelines box.)

Orthostatic Hypotension. Orthostatic hypotension (OH), also called postural hypotension or orthostatic intolerance, is often manifested as syncope (fainting), vertigo (dizzi-

> ## nursingcareguidelines
>
> ### Using the Blood Pressure Tables
>
> 1. Use the standard height charts to determine the height percentile.
> 2. Measure and record the child's systolic blood pressure (SBP) and diastolic blood pressure (DBP).
> 3. Use the correct gender table for SBP and DBP.
> 4. Find the child's age on the left side of the table. Follow the age row horizontally across the table to the intersection of the line for the height percentile (vertical column).
> 5. There, find the 50th, 90th, 95th, and 99th percentiles for SBP in the left columns and for DBP in the right columns.
>   - BP less than 90th percentile is normal.
>   - BP between the 90th and 95th percentile is prehypertension. In adolescents, BP of 120/80 mm Hg or greater is prehypertension, even if this figure is less than the 90th percentile.
>   - BP over than 95th percentile may be hypertension.
> 6. If the BP is over the 90th percentile, the BP should be repeated twice at the same office visit, and an average SBP and DBP should be used.
> 7. If the BP is over the 95th percentile, BP should be staged. If stage 1 (95th to 99th percentile plus 5 mm Hg), BP measurements should be repeated on two more occasions. If hypertension is confirmed, evaluation should proceed. If BP is stage 2 (>99th percentile plus 5 mm Hg), prompt referral should be made for evaluation and therapy. If the patient is symptomatic, immediate referral and treatment are indicated.

From National High Blood Pressure Education Program Working Group on High Blood Pressure in Children and Adolescents: The fourth report on the diagnosis, evaluation, and treatment of high blood pressure in children and adolescents, *Pediatrics* 114(2 Suppl 4th Rep):555-576, 2004.

ness), or lightheadedness and is caused by decreased blood flow to the brain (**cerebral hypoperfusion**). Normally blood flow to the brain is maintained at a constant level by a number of compensating mechanisms that regulate systemic BP. When one assumes a sitting or standing position from a supine or recumbent position, peripheral capillary vasoconstriction occurs, and blood that was pooling in the lower vasculature is returned to the heart for redistribution to the head and remainder of the body. When this mechanism fails or is slow to respond, the person may experience vertigo or syncope. One of the most common causes of OH is hypovolemia, which may be induced by medications such as diuretics, vasodilator medications, and prolonged immobility or bed rest. Other causes of OH include dehydration, diarrhea, emesis, fluid loss from sweating and exertion, alcohol intake, dysrhythmias, diabetes mellitus, sepsis, and hemorrhage.

BP measurements taken with the child supine then standing (at least 2 minutes in each position) may demonstrate variability and assist in the diagnosis of OH. The child with a sustained drop in systolic pressure of more than 20 mm Hg or in diastolic pressure of more than 10 mm Hg after standing for 2 minutes without an increase in heart rate of more than 15 beats/min most likely has an autonomic deficit. Nonneurogenic causes of OH have a compensatory increase in pulse of more than 15 beats/min as well as a drop in BP, as noted previously. For the child or adolescent who is seen with vertigo, lightheadedness, nausea, syncope, diaphoresis, and pallor, it is important to monitor BP and heart rate to determine the original cause. BP is an important diagnostic measurement in children and adolescents and must be a part of the routine monitoring of vital signs.

NURSINGALERT

Published norms for BP, such as those on the inside back cover, are valid only if the same method of measurement (auscultation and cuff size determination) is used in clinical practice.

GENERAL APPEARANCE

The child's general appearance is a cumulative, subjective impression of the child's physical appearance, state of nutrition, behavior, personality, interactions with parents and nurse (also siblings if present), posture, development, and speech. Although general appearance is recorded at the beginning of the physical examination, it encompasses all the observations of the child during the interview and physical assessment.

Note the **facies,** the child's facial expression and appearance. For example, the facies may give clues to children who are in pain; have difficulty breathing; feel frightened, discontented, or unhappy; are mentally deficient; or are acutely ill.

Observe the **posture, position,** and types of **body movement.** The child with hearing or vision loss may characteristically tilt the head in an awkward position to hear or see better. The child in pain may favor a body part. The child with low self-esteem or a feeling of rejection may assume a slumped, careless, and apathetic pose. Likewise, a child with confidence, a feeling of self-worth, and a sense of security usually demonstrates a tall, straight, well-balanced posture. While observing such body language, do not interpret too freely but rather record objectively.

Note the child's **hygiene** in terms of cleanliness; unusual body odor; the condition of the hair, neck, nails, teeth, and feet; and the condition of the clothing. Such observations are excellent clues to possible instances of neglect, inadequate financial resources, housing difficulties (e.g., no running water), or lack of knowledge concerning children's needs.

Behavior includes the child's personality, activity level, reaction to stress, requests, frustration, interactions with others (primarily the parent and nurse), degree of alertness, and response to stimuli. Some mental questions that serve as reminders for observing behavior include: What is the child's overall personality? Does the child have a long attention span, or is he or she easily distracted? Can the child follow two or three commands in succession without the need for repetition? What is the youngster's response to delayed gratification or frustration? Is eye contact used during conversation? What is the child's reaction to the nurse and family members? Is the child quick or slow to grasp explanations?

Development can be assessed by carefully observing the child, but verify your impressions with screening tests. Various tests for assessing development, speech, vision, and hearing are discussed later in this chapter and in Chapter 19.

Under general appearance, record an overall estimate of the child's speech development, motor skills, coordination, and recent area of achievement. For example, the following statement may apply to an 18-month-old child: "Motor development advanced for age; climbs, runs, jumps (most recent motor skill), manipulates small objects with ease; excellent coordination and balance; beginning to name many objects; uses two-word phrases; and enjoys 'talking' to self and others."

SKIN

Skin is assessed for color, texture, temperature, moisture, and turgor. Examination of the skin and its accessory organs primarily involves inspection and palpation. Touch allows the nurse to assess the texture, turgor, and temperature of the skin (Turnbull, 2000). The normal **color** in light-skinned children varies from a milky white and rose to a deeply hued pink. Dark-skinned children, such as those of Native American, Hispanic, or African descent, have inherited various brown, red, yellow, olive green, and bluish tones in their skin. Asian persons have skin that is normally of a yellow tone. Several variations in skin color can occur, some of which warrant further investigation. The types of color change and their appearance in children with light or dark skin are summarized in Table 6-8.

Normally the skin **texture** of young children is smooth, slightly dry, and not oily or clammy. Evaluate skin **temperature** by symmetrically feeling each part of the body and comparing upper areas with lower ones. Note any difference in temperature.

Determine **tissue turgor,** or elasticity in the skin, by grasping the skin on the abdomen between the thumb and index finger, pulling it taut, and quickly releasing it. Elastic tissue immediately assumes its normal position without residual marks or creases. In children with poor skin turgor, the skin remains suspended or tented for a few seconds before slowly falling back on the abdomen. Skin turgor is one of the best estimates of adequate hydration and nutrition.

Accessory Structures

Inspection of the accessory structures of the skin may be performed while the skin is being examined or when the scalp and extremities are being assessed.

Inspect the **hair** for color, texture, quality, distribution, and elasticity. Children's scalp hair is usually lustrous, silky, strong, and elastic. Genetic factors affect the appearance of hair. For example, the hair of African-American children is usually curlier and coarser than that of Caucasian children. Hair that is stringy, dull, brittle, dry, friable, and depigmented may suggest poor nutrition. Record any bald or thinning spots. Loss of hair in infants may indicate lying in the same position and may be a clue for counseling parents concerning the child's stimulation needs.

Inspect the hair and scalp for general cleanliness. Persons in various ethnic groups condition their hair with oils or lubricants that, if not thoroughly washed from the scalp, clog the sebaceous glands, causing scalp infections. Also examine the area for lesions; scaliness; evidence of infestation, such as lice or ticks; and signs of trauma, such as ecchymosis, masses, or scars.

In children who are approaching puberty, look for growth of secondary hair as a sign of normally progressing pubertal changes. Note precocious or delayed appearance of hair growth because, although not always suggestive of hormonal dysfunction, it may be of great concern to the early- or late-maturing adolescent.

Inspect the **nails** for color, shape, texture, and quality. Normally the nails are pink, convex, smooth, and hard but flexible (not brittle). The edges, which are usually white, should extend over the fingers. Dark-skinned individuals may have more deeply pigmented nail beds. Short, ragged nails are typical of habitual biting. Uncut, dirty nails are a sign of poor hygiene.

TABLE 6-8
Differences in Color Changes of Racial Groups

DESCRIPTION	APPEARANCE IN LIGHT SKIN	APPEARANCE IN DARK SKIN
Cyanosis—Bluish tone through skin; reflects reduced (deoxygenated) hemoglobin	Bluish tinge, especially in palpebral conjunctiva (lower eyelid), nail beds, earlobes, lips, oral membranes, soles, and palms	Ashen gray lips and tongue
Pallor—Paleness; may be sign of anemia, chronic disease, edema, or shock	Loss of rosy glow in skin, especially face	Ashen gray appearance in black skin; More yellowish brown color in brown skin
Erythema—Redness; may be result of increased blood flow from climatic conditions, local inflammation, infection, skin irritation, allergy, or other dermatoses, or may be caused by increased numbers of red blood cells as compensatory response to chronic hypoxia	Redness easily seen anywhere on body	Much more difficult to assess; rely on palpation for warmth or edema
Ecchymosis—Large, diffuse areas, usually black and blue, caused by hemorrhage of blood into skin; typically result of injuries	Purplish to yellow-green areas; may be seen anywhere on skin	Very difficult to see unless in mouth or conjunctiva
Petechiae—Same as ecchymosis except for size: small, distinct, pinpoint hemorrhages 2 mm in size; can denote some type of blood disorder, such as leukemia	Purplish pinpoints most easily seen on buttocks, abdomen, and inner surfaces of arms or legs	Usually invisible except in oral mucosa, conjunctiva of eyelids, and conjunctiva covering eyeball
Jaundice—Yellow staining of skin usually caused by bile pigments	Yellow staining seen in sclerae of eyes, skin, fingernails, soles, palms, and oral mucosa	Most reliably assessed in sclerae, hard palate, palms, and soles

FIG. 6-13 ■ Examples of flexion creases on palm. A, Normal. B, Transpalmar crease.

The palm normally shows three flexion creases (Fig 6-13, A). In some situations such as Down syndrome, the two distal horizontal creases are fused to form a single horizontal crease (the single palmar crease, or transpalmar crease) (Fig. 6-13, B). If grossly abnormal lines or folds are observed, sketch a picture to describe them and refer the finding to a specialist for further investigation.

LYMPH NODES
Lymph nodes are usually assessed when the part of the body in which they are located is examined. The body's lymphatic drainage system is extensive; the usual sites for palpating accessible lymph nodes are shown in Fig. 6-14.

Palpate nodes using the distal portion of the fingers and gently but firmly pressing in a circular motion along the regions where nodes are normally present. During assessment of the nodes in the head and neck, tilt the child's head upward slightly but without tensing the sternocleidomastoid or trapezius muscles. This position facilitates palpation of the submental, submandibular, tonsillar, and cervical nodes. Palpate the axillary nodes with the child's arms relaxed at the sides but slightly abducted. Assess the inguinal nodes with the child in the supine position. Note size, mobility, temperature, and tenderness, as well as reports by the parents regarding any visible change of enlarged nodes. In children, small, nontender, movable nodes are usually normal. Tender, enlarged, warm lymph nodes generally indicate infection or inflammation close to their location. Report such findings for further investigation.

HEAD AND NECK
Observe the head for general shape and symmetry. A flattening of one part of the head, such as the occiput, may indicate that the child continually lies in this position. Marked asymmetry is usually abnormal and may indicate premature closure of the sutures (craniosynostosis).

NURSINGALERT
Significant head lag after 6 months of age strongly indicates cerebral injury and is referred for further evaluation.

Note head control in infants and head posture in older children. Most infants by 4 months of age should be able to hold the head erect and in midline when in a vertical position.

Evaluate range of motion by asking the older child to look in each direction (to either side, up, and down) or by manually putting the younger child through each position. Limited range of motion may indicate wryneck, or torticollis, in which the child holds the head to one side with the chin pointing toward the opposite side a result of injury to the sternocleidomastoid muscle.

NURSINGALERT
Hyperextension of the head (opisthotonos) with pain on flexion is a serious indication of meningeal irritation and is referred for immediate medical evaluation.

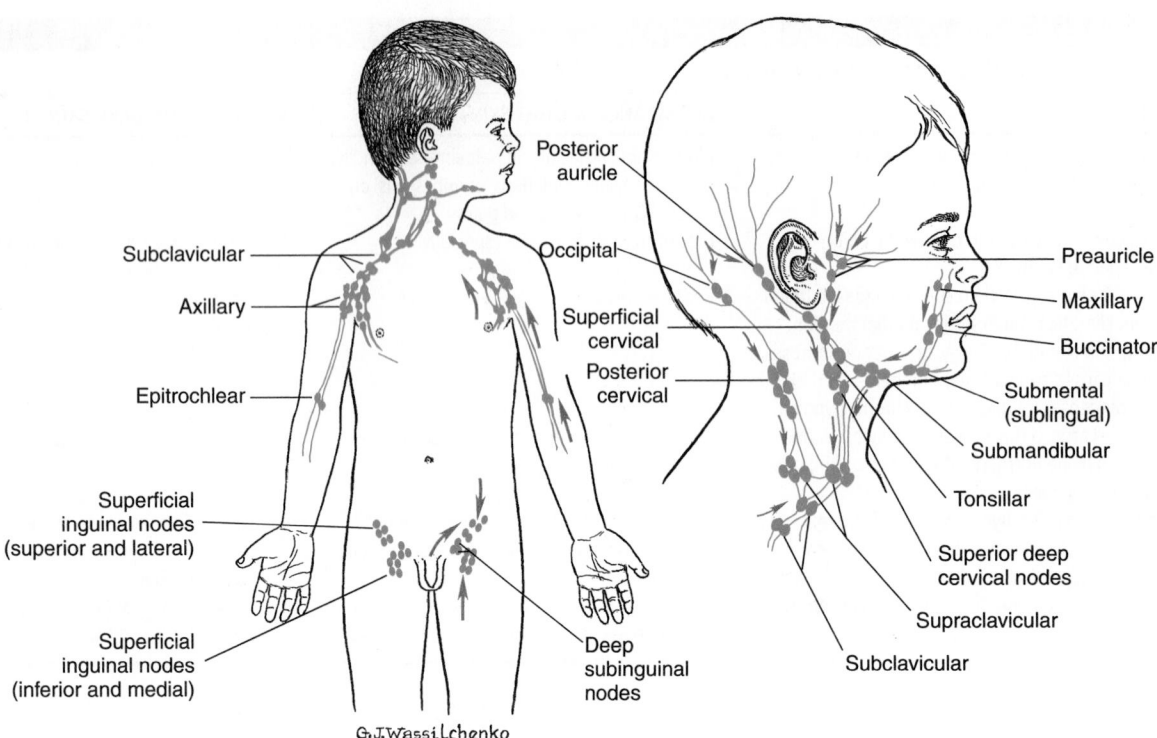

FIG. 6-14 ■ Location of superficial lymph nodes. *Arrows* indicate directional flow of lymph.

Palpate the **skull** for patent sutures, fontanels, fractures, and swellings. Normally the posterior fontanel closes by the second month of life, and the anterior fontanel fuses between 12 and 18 months of age. Early or late closure is noted, since either may be a sign of a pathologic condition. (For a more detailed discussion of the cranial bones, see Chapter 8.)

While examining the head, observe the **face** for symmetry, movement, and general appearance. Ask the child to "make a face" to assess symmetric movement and disclose any degree of paralysis. Note any unusual facial proportion, such as an unusually high or low forehead; wide- or close-set eyes; or a small, receding chin.

In addition to assessment of the head and neck for movement, inspect the neck for size and palpate its associated structures. The neck is normally short, with skinfolds between the head and shoulders during infancy; however, it lengthens during the next 3 to 4 years.

> **NURSINGALERT**
>
> If any masses are detected in the neck, report them for further investigation. Large masses can block the airway.

EYES

Inspection of External Structures

Inspect the **lids** for proper placement on the eye. When the eye is open, the upper lid should fall near the upper iris. When the eyes are closed, the lids should completely cover the cornea and sclera (Fig. 6-15).

Determine the general slant of the **palpebral fissures** or lids by drawing an imaginary line through the two points of the medial canthus and across the outer orbit of the eyes and

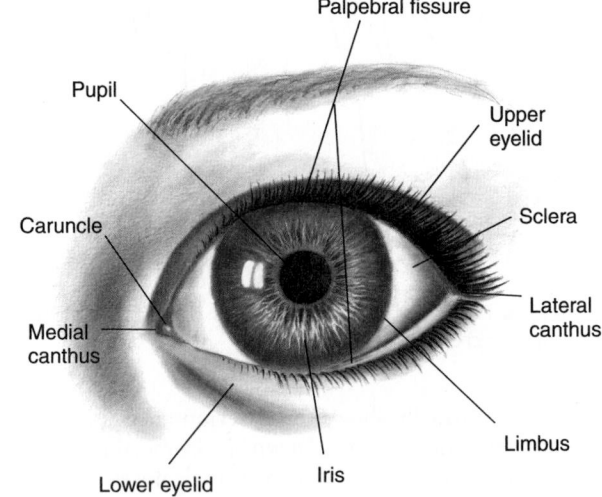

FIG. 6-15 ■ External structures of eye.

aligning each eye on the line. Usually the palpebral fissures lie horizontally. However, in Asians the slant is normally upward.

Also inspect the inside lining of the lids, the **palpebral conjunctiva.** To examine the lower conjunctival sac, pull the lid down while the patient looks up. To evert the upper lid, hold the upper lashes and gently pull *down* and *forward* as the child looks down. Normally the conjunctiva appears pink and glossy. Vertical yellow striations along the edge are the **meibomian,** or **sebaceous, glands** near the hair follicle. Located in the inner or medial canthus and situated on the inner edge of the upper and lower lids is a tiny opening, the **lacrimal punc-**

tum. Note any excessive tearing, discharge, or inflammation of the lacrimal apparatus.

The **bulbar conjunctiva,** which covers the eye up to the limbus, or junction of the cornea and sclera, should be transparent. The **sclera,** or white covering of the eyeball, should be clear. Tiny black marks in the sclera of heavily pigmented individuals are normal.

The **cornea,** or covering of the iris and pupil, should be clear and transparent. Record opacities because they can be signs of scarring or ulceration, which can interfere with vision. The best way to test for opacities is to illuminate the eyeball by shining a light at an angle (obliquely) toward the cornea.

Compare the **pupils** for size, shape, and movement. They should be round, clear, and equal. Test their **reaction to light** by quickly shining a light toward the eye and removing it. As the light approaches, the pupils should constrict; as the light fades, the pupils should dilate. Test the pupil for any response of **accommodation** by having the child look at a bright, shiny object at a distance and quickly moving the object toward the face. The pupils should constrict as the object is brought near the eye. Normal findings on examination of the pupils may be recorded as *PERRLA,* which stands for "*P*upils *E*qual, *R*ound, *R*eact to *L*ight, and *A*ccommodation."

Inspect the **iris** and pupil for color, size, shape, and clarity. Permanent eye color is usually established by 6 to 12 months of age. While inspecting the iris and pupil, look for the lens. Normally the lens is not visible through the pupil.

Inspection of Internal Structures

The ophthalmoscope permits visualization of the interior of the eyeball with a system of lenses and a high-intensity light. The lenses permit clear visualization of eye structures at different distances from the nurse's eye and correct visual acuity differences in the examiner and child. Use of the ophthalmoscope requires practice to know which lens setting produces the clearest image.

The ophthalmic and otic heads are usually interchangeable on one "body" or handle, which encloses the power source, either disposable or rechargeable batteries. The nurse should practice changing the heads, which snap on and are secured with a quarter turn, and replacing the batteries and light bulbs. Nurses who are not directly involved in physical assessment are often responsible for ensuring that the equipment functions properly.

Preparing the Child. The nurse can prepare the child for the ophthalmoscopic examination by showing the child the instrument, demonstrating the light source and how it shines in the eye, and explaining the reason for darkening the room. For infants and young children who do not respond to such explanations, it is best to use distraction to encourage them to keep their eyes open. Forcibly parting the lids results in an uncooperative, watery eyed child and a frustrated nurse. Usually, with some practice, the nurse can elicit a red reflex almost instantly while approaching the child and may also gain a momentary inspection of the blood vessels, macula, or optic disc.

Funduscopic Examination. Fig. 6-16 shows the structures of the back of the eyeball, or the **fundus.** The fundus is immediately apparent as the **red reflex.** The intensity of the color increases in darkly pigmented individuals.

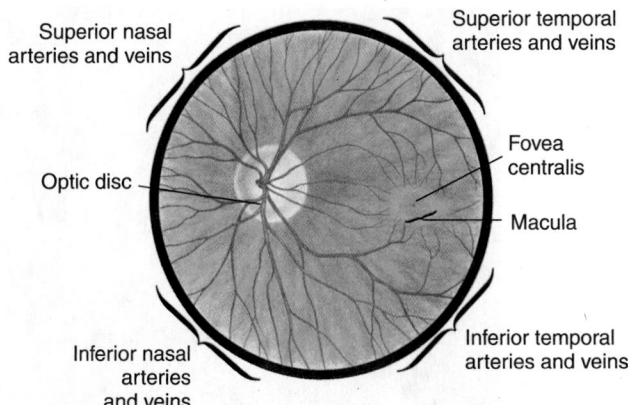

FIG. 6-16 ■ Structures of fundus. (From Seidel HM, Ball JW, Dains JE, and others: *Mosby's guide to physical examination,* ed 4, St Louis, 1999, Mosby.)

NURSINGALERT

A brilliant, uniform red reflex is an important sign because it rules out many serious defects of the cornea, aqueous chamber, lens, and vitreous chamber. Any dark shadows or opacities are recorded because they indicate some abnormality in any of these structures.

As the ophthalmoscope is brought closer to the eye, the most conspicuous feature of the fundus is the **optic disc,** the area where the blood vessels and optic nerve fibers enter and exit from the eye. The color of the disc is creamy pink; it is lighter in color than the surrounding fundus. Normally it is round or vertically oval.

After the optic disc is located, the area is inspected for **blood vessels.** The central retinal artery and vein appear in the depths of the disc and emanate outward with visible branching. The **veins** are darker and about one fourth larger than the **arteries.** Normally the branches of the arteries and veins cross each other.

Other structures that may be seen are the **macula,** the area of the fundus with the greatest concentration of visual receptors, and, in the center of the macula, a minute glistening spot of reflected light called the **fovea centralis;** this is the area of most perfect vision.

Vision Testing

Several tests are available for assessing vision. This discussion focuses on four areas: (1) ocular alignment, (2) visual acuity, (3) peripheral vision, and (4) color vision. Vision screening should be performed at the earliest possible age and at regular intervals (American Academy of Pediatrics, 2003a; Wall, Marsh-Tootle, Evans, and others, 2002). Behavioral and physical signs of visual impairment are discussed in Chapter 19.

Ocular Alignment. Normally, by the age of 3 to 4 months, children are able to fixate on one visual field with both eyes simultaneously (binocularity). One of the most important tests for binocularity is alignment of the eyes to detect nonbinocular vision, or **strabismus** (Halle, 2002). In strabismus, or cross-eye, one eye deviates from the point of fixation. If the misalignment is constant, the weak eye becomes "lazy," and the brain eventually suppresses the image produced by that eye. If strabismus is not detected and cor-

FIG. 6-17 ■ **A,** Corneal light reflex test demonstrating orthophoric eyes. **B,** Pseudostrabismus. Inner epicanthal folds cause eyes to appear misaligned; however, corneal light reflexes fall perfectly symmetrically.

FIG. 6-18 ■ Alternate cover test to detect amblyopia in patient with strabismus. **A,** Eye is occluded, and child is fixating on light source. **B,** If eye does not move when uncovered, eyes are aligned.

rected by ages 4 to 6 years, blindness from disuse, known as **amblyopia,** may result.

Tests commonly used to detect misalignment are the corneal light reflex and the cover tests. To perform the **corneal light reflex test,** or **Hirschberg test,** shine a flashlight or the light of the ophthalmoscope directly into the patient's eyes from a distance of about 40.5 cm (16 inches). If the eyes are **orthophoric,** or normal, the light falls symmetrically within each pupil (Fig. 6-17, *A*). If the light falls off center in one eye, the eyes are misaligned. **Epicanthal folds,** excess folds of skin that extend from the roof of the nose to the inner termination of the eyebrow and that partially or completely overlap the inner canthus of the eye, may give a false impression of misalignment **(pseudostrabismus)** (Fig. 6-17, *B*). Epicanthal folds are often found in Asian children.

In the **cover test,** one eye is covered, and the movement of the *uncovered* eye is observed while the child looks at a near (33 cm [13 inches]) or distant (6 m [20 feet]) object. If the uncovered eye does not move, it is aligned. If the uncovered eye moves, a misalignment is present because, when the stronger eye is temporarily covered, the misaligned eye attempts to fixate on the object.

In the **alternate cover test,** occlusion shifts back and forth from one eye to the other, and movement of the eye that was *covered* is observed as soon as the occluder is removed while

the child focuses on a point in front of him or her (Fig. 6-18). If normal alignment is present, shifting the cover from one eye to the other will not cause the eye to move. If misalignment is present, eye movement will occur when the cover is moved. This test takes more practice than the other cover test because the occluder must be moved back and forth quickly and accurately to see the eye move. Because deviations can occur at different ranges, it is important to perform the cover tests at both close and far distances.

> **NURSINGALERT**
>
> The cover test is usually easier to perform if the examiner uses his or her own hand rather than a card-type occluder (see Fig. 6-18). Attractive occluders fashioned like an ice cream cone or happy-face lollipop cut from cardboard are also well received by young children.

Photoscreening is a technique used to screen for amblyopia, refractive disorders, and media opacities (American Academy of Pediatrics, 2003a; Berry, Simons, Siatkowski, and others, 2001). Using a camera, the nurse obtains images of the pupillary reflexes (reflections) and red reflexes (Bruckner test) (American Academy of Pediatrics, 2003a). Photoscreening offers an effective way to screen infants, preverbal children, and those with developmental delays who are difficult to screen.

Visual Acuity Testing in Children Beyond Infancy. The most common test for measuring visual acuity is the **Snellen letter chart,** which consists of lines of letters of decreasing size (see Appendix B). During testing, the American Academy of Pediatrics (2003a) now recommends that children stand 10 feet from the chart with their heels at the 10-foot line. When screening for visual acuity in children, the nurse tests the child's right eye first by covering the left. Children who wear glasses should be screened with them on. Tell the child to keep both eyes open during the examination. If the child fails to read the current line, move up the chart to the next larger line. Continue up the chart until a line is found that the child can pass. Then begin moving down the chart again until the child fails to read the line. To pass each line, the child must correctly identify four of six symbols on the line. Repeat the procedure, covering the right eye.

For children unable to read letters and numbers, the **tumbling E** or **HOTV** test is useful (Coats and Jenkins, 1997). The tumbling E test uses the capital letter E pointing in four different directions. The child is asked to point in the direction the E is facing. The HOTV test consists of a wall chart composed of the letters H, O, T, and V. The child is given a board containing a large H, O, T, and V. The examiner points to a letter on the wall chart, and the child matches the correct letter on the board held in his or her hand. The tumbling E and HOTV are excellent tests for preschool-age children.

When a child is unable to perform the tumbling E or HOTV test, the LEA symbol or Allen card test may be used. The **Allen card test** uses common figures to test the child's vision. It is important to assess whether the child is able to identify the pictures before actual vision testing. The examiner walks backward slowly, flipping through the cards and presenting different pictures to the child. The examiner continues to move backward as the child correctly calls out the figures. When the child begins to miss the figure on the cards, the examiner moves forward to confirm that the child is able to identify the figures at that point. All Allen card figures are 20/30 in size. The farthest distance at which the child is able to accurately identify the pictures becomes the numerator, and 30 becomes the denominator. For example, if the child is able to identify the pictures accurately at 15 feet, the visual acuity is recorded as 15/30. This is equivalent to 20/40 or 10/20 visual acuity.

Visual Acuity Testing in Infants and Difficult-to-Test Children. In newborns, vision is tested mainly by checking for **light perception** by shining a light into the eyes and noting responses such as pupillary constriction, blinking, following the light to midline, increased alertness, or refusal to open the eyes after exposure to the light. Although the simple maneuver of checking light perception and eliciting the pupillary light reflex indicates that the anterior half of the visual apparatus is intact, it does not confirm that the infant can see. In other words, this test does not assess whether the brain receives the visual message and interprets the signals.

Another test of visual acuity is the infant's ability to fix on and follow a target. Although any brightly colored or patterned object can be used, the human face is excellent. Hold the infant upright while moving your face slowly from side to side.

> **NURSING ALERT**
>
> If visual fixation and following are not present by 3 to 4 months of age, further ophthalmologic evaluation is needed.

Other signs that may indicate visual loss or other serious eye problems include fixed pupils, strabismus, constant nystagmus, the setting-sun sign, and slow lateral movements. Unfortunately, it is difficult to test each eye separately; the presence of such signs in one eye could indicate unilateral blindness.

Special tests are available for testing infants and other difficult-to-test children to assess acuity or confirm blindness. For example, in **visually evoked potentials,** the eyes are stimulated with a bright light or pattern, and electrical activity to the visual cortex is recorded through scalp electrodes. Acuity is assessed by using progressively smaller patterns.

Peripheral Vision. In children who are old enough to cooperate, estimate **peripheral vision,** or the visual field of each eye, by having the children fixate on a specific point directly in front of them as an object, such as a finger or a pencil, is moved from beyond the field of vision into the range of peripheral vision. Check each eye separately and for each quadrant of vision. As soon as children see the object, have them say "stop." At that point measure the angle from the anteroposterior axis of the eye (straight line of vision) to the peripheral axis (point at which the object is first seen). Normally children see about 50 degrees upward, 70 degrees downward, 60 degrees nasalward, and 90 degrees temporally. Limitations in peripheral vision may indicate blindness from damage to structures within the eye or to any of the visual pathways.

Color Vision. Another important test is for color vision. It is estimated that 8% to 10% of Caucasian males and less than half that percentage of African-American males inherit the X-linked disorder known as **color vision deficit** (also known as **color blindness,** a less acceptable term). From 0.5% to 1% of Caucasian females are affected. Although the severity of impaired perception of color varies considerably, the two most common types are **protanomaly,** in which the child confuses gray with pink or pale blue with green, and **deuteranomaly,** in which the child confuses gray with pale purple or green. In most of these individuals the color vision deficit causes no major problems. However, some individuals with more severe deficits may be unable to distinguish amber or red traffic lights, fail to see a red brake light on the rear of a car, have difficulty distinguishing green traffic lights from certain types of incandescent street lamps, and have a poor sense of color coordination of clothing. For school-age children the greatest difficulty lies in performance of academic skills that use color as a visual aid. Adolescents may be ineligible for certain vocational opportunities, such as electronics, photography, printing, interior decorating, pharmaceuticals, textiles, police work, and several types of military service.

The tests available for color vision include the **Ishihara test** and the **Hardy-Rand-Rittler test.** Each consists of a series of cards (pseudoisochromatic) on which is printed a color field composed of spots of a certain "confusion" color. Against the field is a number or symbol similarly printed in dots but of a color likely to be confused with the field color by the person with a color vision deficit. As a result, the figure or letter is invisible to an affected individual but is clearly seen by a person with normal vision.

EARS

Inspection of External Structures

The entire external earlobe is called the **pinna,** or **auricle;** one is located on each side of the head. Measure the **height** alignment of the pinna by drawing an imaginary line from the

FIG. 6-19 ■ Ear alignment.

ATRAUMATIC CARE

Reducing Distress from Otoscopy in Young Children

Make examining the ear a game by explaining that you are looking for a "big elephant" in the ear. This kind of make-believe is an absorbing distraction and usually elicits cooperation. After examining the ear, clarify that "looking for elephants" was only pretend and thank the child for letting you look in his or her ear. Another great distraction technique is asking the child to put a finger on the opposite ear to keep the light from getting out.

Anatomy Review—External, Middle, and Inner Ear

outer orbit of the eye to the occiput, or most prominent protuberance of the skull. The top of the pinna should meet or cross this line. Low-set ears are commonly associated with renal anomalies or mental retardation. Measure the **angle** of the pinna by drawing a perpendicular line from the imaginary horizontal line and aligning the pinna next to this mark. Normally the pinna lies within a 10-degree angle of the vertical line (Fig. 6-19). If it falls outside this area, record the deviation and look for other anomalies.

Normally the pinna extends slightly outward from the skull. Except in newborn infants, ears that are flat against the head or protruding away from the scalp may indicate problems. Flattened ears in an infant may suggest a frequent side-lying position and, just as with isolated areas of hair loss, may be a clue to investigating parents' understanding of the child's stimulation needs.

Inspect the **skin** surface around the ear for small openings, extra tags of skin, or sinuses. If a sinus is found, note this because it may represent a fistula that drains into some area of the neck or ear. Cutaneous tags represent no pathologic process but may cause parents concern in terms of the child's appearance.

Also assess the ear for **hygiene.** An otoscope is not necessary for looking into the external canal to note the presence of **cerumen,** a waxy substance produced by the ceruminous glands in the outer portion of the canal. Cerumen is usually yellow-brown and soft. If an otoscope is used and any discharge is seen, its color and odor are noted. Avoid transmitting potentially infectious material to the other ear or to another child through hand washing and using disposable specula or sterilizing reusable specula between each examination.

Inspection of Internal Structures

The head of the otoscope permits visualization of the tympanic membrane by use of a bright light, a magnifying glass, and a speculum. Some otoscopes have an attachment for a pneumonic device to insert air into the canal to determine membrane compliance (movement). The speculum, which is inserted into the external canal, comes in a variety of sizes to accommodate different canal widths. The largest speculum that fits comfortably into the ear is used to achieve the greatest

area of visualization. The lens, or magnifying glass, is movable, allowing the examiner to insert an object, such as a curette, into the ear canal through the speculum while still viewing the structures through the lens.

Positioning the Child. Before beginning the otoscopic examination, position the child properly and restrain if necessary. Older children usually cooperate and do not need restraint. However, prepare them for the procedure by allowing them to play with the instrument, demonstrating how it works, and stressing the importance of remaining still. A helpful suggestion is to let them observe you examining the parent's ear. Restraint is needed for younger children because the ear examination upsets them (see Atraumatic Care box).

As you insert the speculum into the meatus, move it around the outer rim to accustom the child to the feel of something entering the ear. If examining a painful ear, touch a nonpainful part of the affected ear, then examine the unaffected ear, and finally return to the painful ear. By this time the child is usually less fearful of anything causing discomfort to the ear and will cooperate more.

For their protection and safety, infants and toddlers must be restrained for the otoscopic examination. There are two general positions of restraint. In one the child is seated sideways in the parent's lap with one arm hugging the parent and the other arm at the side. The ear to be examined is toward the nurse. With one arm the parent holds the child's head firmly against his or her chest, and with the other arm hugs the child, thereby securing the child's free arm (Fig. 6-20, *A*). The ear is examined using the same procedure for holding the otoscope as described later.

The other position involves placing the child on the side, back, or abdomen with the arms at the side and the head turned so that the ear to be examined points toward the ceiling. Lean over the child, use the upper part of the body to restrain the arms and upper trunk movements, and use the examining hand to stabilize the head. This position is practical for young infants or for older children who need minimum restraint, but it may not be feasible for other children who protest vigorously. For safety enlist the parent's or an assistant's help in immobilizing the head by firmly placing one hand above the ear and the other on the child's side, abdomen, or back (Fig. 6-20, *B*).

With cooperative children, examine the ear with the child in a side-lying, sitting, or standing position. One disadvantage to standing is that the child may "walk away" as the otoscope enters the canal. If the child is standing or sitting, tilt the head

FIG. 6-20 ■ Position for restraining child (**A**) and infant (**B**) during otoscopic examination.

FIG. 6-21 ■ Positioning head by tilting it toward opposite shoulder for full view of tympanic membrane.

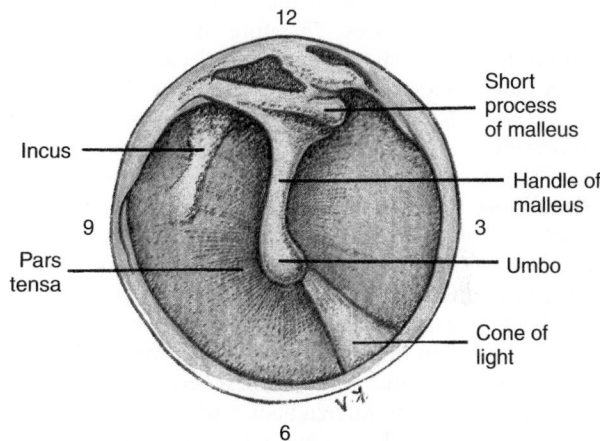

FIG. 6-22 ■ Landmarks of tympanic membrane with "clock" superimposed. (Modified from Potter PA, Perry AG: *Basic nursing: theory and practice,* ed 2, St Louis, 1991, Mosby.)

slightly toward the child's opposite shoulder to achieve a better view of the drum (Fig. 6-21).

With the thumb and forefinger of the free (usually nondominant) hand, grasp the auricle. For the two positions of restraint, hold the otoscope upside down at the junction of its head and handle with the thumb and index finger. Place the other fingers against the skull to allow the otoscope to move with the child in case of sudden movement. In examining a cooperative child, hold the handle with the otic head upright or upside down. Use the dominant hand to examine both ears or reverse hands for each ear, whichever is more comfortable.

Before using the otoscope, visualize the external ear and the tympanic membrane as being superimposed on a clock (Fig. 6-22). The numbers become important geographic landmarks. Introduce the speculum into the meatus between the 3 and 9 o'clock positions in a *downward* and *forward* position.

Because the canal is curved, the speculum does not permit a panoramic view of the tympanic membrane unless the canal is straightened. In infants the canal curves upward. Therefore pull the pinna *down* and *back* to the 6 to 9 o'clock range to straighten the canal (Fig. 6-23, *A*).

With older children, usually those older than 3 years of age, the canal curves downward and forward. Therefore pull the pinna *up* and *back* toward a 10 o'clock position (Fig. 6-23, *B*). If you have difficulty visualizing the membrane, try repositioning the head, introducing the speculum at a different angle, and pulling the pinna in a slightly different direction. Do not insert the speculum past the cartilaginous (outermost) portion of the canal, usually a distance of 0.60 to 1.25 cm (0.23 to 0.5 inch) in older children. Insertion of the speculum into the posterior or bony portion of the canal causes pain.

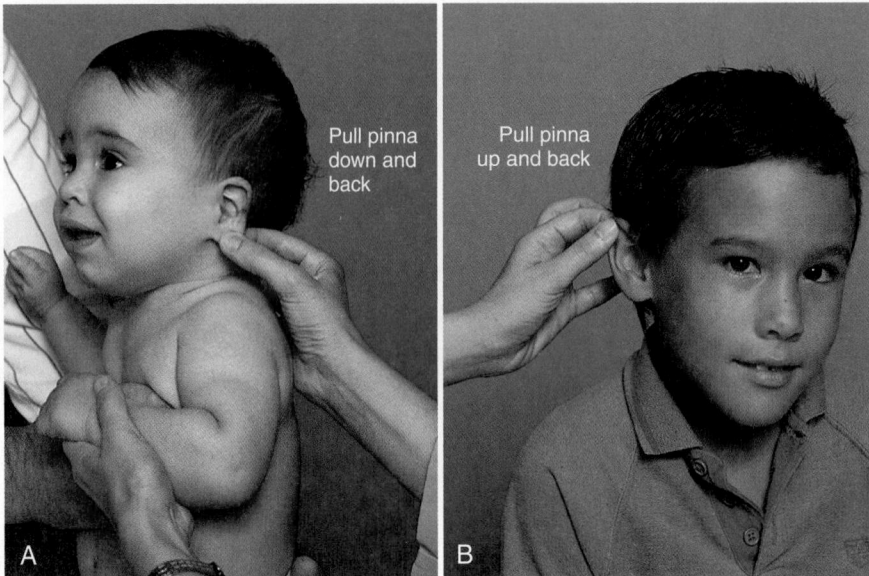

FIG. 6-23 ■ Positioning for visualizing eardrum in infant (**A**) and in child older than 3 years of age (**B**).

In neonates and young infants the walls of the canal are pliable and floppy because of the underdeveloped cartilaginous and bony structures. Therefore the very small 2-mm speculum usually needs to be inserted deeper into the canal than in older children. Great care must be exercised not to damage the walls or drum. For this reason, only an experienced examiner should insert an otoscope into the ears of very young infants.

Otoscopic Examination. As you introduce the speculum into the external canal, inspect the walls of the canal, the color of the tympanic membrane, the light reflex, and the usual landmarks of the bony prominences of the middle ear. The **walls** of the external auditory canal are pink, although they are more pigmented in dark-skinned children. Minute hairs are evident in the outermost portion, where cerumen is produced. Note signs of irritation, foreign bodies, or infection.

Foreign bodies in the ear are not uncommon in children and range from erasers to beans. Symptoms may include pain, discharge, and affected hearing. Soft objects, such as paper or insects, can be removed with forceps. Small, hard objects, such as pebbles, can be removed with a suction tip, a hook, or irrigation. However, irrigation is contraindicated if the object is vegetative matter, such as beans or pasta, which swells when in contact with fluid.

> **NURSINGALERT**
> If there is any doubt about the type of object in the ear and the appropriate method to remove it, refer the child to the appropriate practitioner.

The **tympanic membrane** is a translucent, light pearly pink or gray. Note marked erythema (which may indicate suppurative otitis media), a dull nontransparent grayish color (sometimes suggestive of serous otitis media), or ashen gray areas (signs of scarring from a previous perforation). A black area usually suggests a perforation of the membrane that has not healed.

The characteristic tenseness and slope of the tympanic membrane cause the light of the otoscope to reflect at about the 5 or 7 o'clock position. The **light reflex** is a fairly well-defined, cone-shaped reflection, which normally points away from the face.

The **bony landmarks** of the drum are formed by the **umbo,** or tip of the malleus. It appears as a small, round, opaque, concave spot near the center of the drum. The **manubrium** (long process or handle) of the malleus appears to be a whitish line extending from the umbo upward to the margin of the membrane. At the upper end of the long process near the 1 o'clock position (in the right ear) is a sharp, knoblike protuberance, representing the short process of the malleus. Note the absence of the light reflex or loss or abnormal prominence of any of these landmarks.

Auditory Testing

Several types of hearing tests are available and recommended for screening in infants and children (American Academy of Pediatrics, 2003b) (Table 6-9). The nurse must operate under a high index of suspicion for those children who may have conditions associated with hearing loss and who may have developed behaviors that indicate auditory impairment (Cunningham and Cox, 2003). Types of hearing loss, causes, clinical manifestations, and appropriate treatment are discussed in Chapter 19.

NOSE
Inspection of External Structures

The nose is located in the middle of the face just below the eyes and above the lips. Compare its placement and alignment by drawing an imaginary vertical line from the center point between the eyes down to the notch of the upper lip. The nose should lie exactly vertical to this line, with each side exactly symmetric. Note its location, any deviation to one side, and asymmetry in overall size and in diameter of the nares (nostrils). The **bridge** of the nose is sometimes flat in Asian and African-American children. Observe the **alae nasi** for any sign of flaring, which indicates respiratory difficulty. Always report any flaring of the alae nasi. Fig. 6-24 illustrates

TABLE 6-9

Audiologic Tests for Infants and Children

AGE	AUDITORY TEST AND AVERAGE TIME	TYPE OF MEASUREMENT	PROCEDURE
All ages	Evoked otoacoustic emissions, 10-minute test	Physiologic test specifically measuring cochlear (outer hair cell) response to presentation of stimulus	Small probe containing sensitive microphone is placed in ear canal for stimulus delivery and response detection.
Birth–9 months	Auditory brainstem response, 15-minute test	Electrophysiologic measurement of activity in auditory nerve and brainstem pathways	Placement of electrodes on child's head detects auditory stimuli presented through earphones one ear at a time.
9 months–2½ years	Conditioned oriented responses or visual reinforced audiometry, 30-minute test	Behavioral tests measuring child's responses to speech and frequency-specific stimuli presented through speakers	Both techniques condition child to associate speech or frequency-specific sound with reinforcement stimulus, such as lighted toy.
2½–4 years	Play audiometry, 30-minute test	Behavioral test measuring auditory thresholds in response to speech and frequency-specific stimuli presented through earphones and/or bone vibrator	Child is conditioned to put peg in peg board or drop block in a box when stimulus tone is heard.
4 years–adolescence	Conventional audiometry, 30-minute test	Behavioral test measuring auditory thresholds in response to speech and frequency-specific stimuli presented through earphone and/or bone vibrator	Patient is instructed to raise hand when stimulus is heard.

Modified with permission from Bachmann KR, Arvedson JC: Early identification and intervention for children who are hearing impaired, *Pediatr Rev* 19:155-165, 1998.

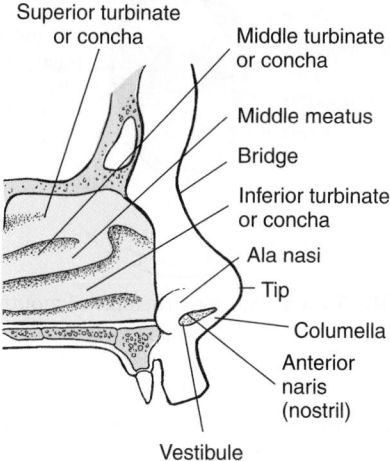

FIG. 6-24 ■ External landmarks and internal structures of nose.

Superior turbinate or concha
Middle turbinate or concha
Middle meatus
Bridge
Inferior turbinate or concha
Ala nasi
Tip
Columella
Anterior naris (nostril)
Vestibule

spaces or channels between the turbinates are called the **meatus** and correspond to each of the three turbinates. Normally the front end of the inferior and middle turbinate and the middle meatus are seen. They should be the same color as the lining of the vestibule.

Inspect the **septum,** which should divide the vestibules equally. Note any deviation, especially if it causes an occlusion of one side of the nose. A perforation may be evident within the septum. If this is suspected, shine the light of the otoscope into one naris and look for admittance of light to the other. Because olfaction is an important function of the nose, testing for smell may be done at this point or as part of cranial nerve assessment (see Table 6-12).

MOUTH AND THROAT

With a cooperative child, almost the entire examination of the mouth and throat can be accomplished without the use of a tongue blade. Ask the child to open the mouth wide; to move the tongue in different directions for full visualization; and to say "ahh," which depresses the tongue for full view of the back of the mouth (tonsils, uvula, and oropharynx) (Fig. 6-25, *A*). For a closer look at the buccal mucosa, or lining of the cheeks, ask children to use their fingers to move the outer lip and cheek to one side (see Atraumatic Care box).

Infants and toddlers usually resist attempts to keep the mouth open. Because inspecting the mouth is upsetting, leave it for the end of the physical examination (along with examination of the ears) or do it during episodes of crying. However, the use of a tongue blade (preferably flavored) to depress the tongue is necessary. Place the tongue blade along the *side* of the tongue, not in the center back area where the gag reflex is elicited. Fig 6-25, *B*, illustrates proper positioning of the child for the oral examination.

The major structure of the exterior of the mouth is the **lips.** The lips should be moist, soft, smooth, and pink, or a

the landmarks used in describing the external structures of the nose.

Inspection of Internal Structures

Inspect the **anterior vestibule** of the nose by pushing the tip upward, tilting the head backward, and illuminating the cavity with a flashlight or otoscope without the attached ear speculum. Note the **color** of the **mucosal lining,** which is normally redder than the oral membranes, as well as any swelling, discharge, dryness, or bleeding. There should be no discharge from the nose.

On looking deeper into the nose, inspect the **turbinates,** or **concha,** plates of bone that jut into the nasal cavity and are enveloped by mucous membrane. The turbinates greatly increase the surface area of the nasal cavity as air is inhaled. The

FIG. 6-25 ■ **A,** Encouraging child to cooperate. **B,** Positioning child for examination of mouth.

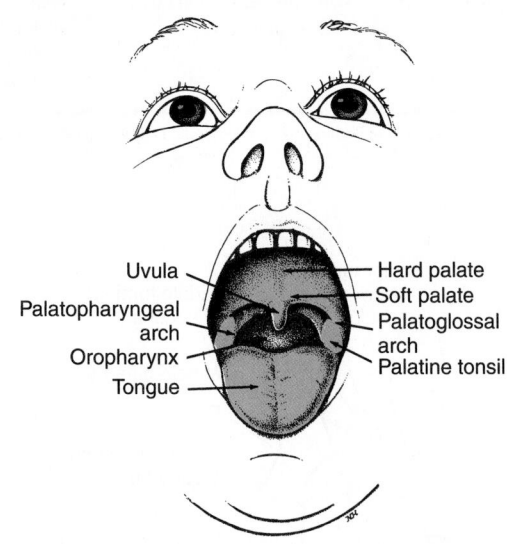

FIG. 6-26 ■ Interior structures of mouth.

ATRAUMATIC CARE

Encouraging Opening the Mouth for Examination

- Perform the examination in front of a mirror.
- Let child first examine someone else's mouth, such as the parent, the nurse, or a puppet (see Fig. 6-25, *A*), and then examine child's mouth.
- Instruct child to tilt the head back slightly, breathe deeply through the mouth, and hold the breath; this action lowers the tongue to the floor of the mouth without the use of a tongue blade.
- Lightly brushing the palate with a cotton swab also may open the mouth for assessment.

deeper hue than the surrounding skin. The lips should be symmetric when relaxed or tensed. Assess symmetry when the child talks or cries.

Inspection of Internal Structures

The major structures that are visible within the oral cavity and oropharynx are the mucosal lining of the lips and cheeks, gums (or gingiva), teeth, tongue, palate, uvula, tonsils, and posterior oropharynx (Fig. 6-26). Inspect all areas lined with **mucous membranes** (inside the lips and cheeks, gingiva, underside of the tongue, palate, and back of the pharynx) for color, any areas of white patches or ulceration, bleeding, sensitivity, and moisture. The membranes should be bright pink, smooth, glistening, uniform, and moist.

Inspect the **teeth** for number in each dental arch, for hygiene, and for occlusion or bite (see also Teething, Chapter 10). Discoloration of tooth enamel with obvious plaque (whitish coating on the surface of the teeth) is a sign of poor dental hygiene and indicates a need for counseling. Brown spots in the crevices of the crown of the tooth or between the teeth may be caries (cavities). Chalky white to yellow or brown areas on the enamel may indicate fluorosis (excessive fluoride ingestion). Teeth that appear greenish black may be stained temporarily from ingestion of supplemental iron.

Examine the **gums (gingiva)** surrounding the teeth. The color is normally coral pink, and the surface texture is stippled, similar to the appearance of an orange peel. In dark-skinned children the gums are more deeply colored, and a brownish area is often observed along the gum line.

Inspect the **tongue** for papillae, small projections that contain several taste buds and give the tongue its characteristic rough appearance. Note the size and mobility of the tongue. Normally the tip of the tongue should extend to the lips or beyond.

The roof of the mouth consists of the **hard palate,** which is located near the front of the oral cavity, and the **soft palate,** which is located toward the back of the pharynx and has a small midline protrusion called the **uvula.** Carefully inspect the palates to ensure they are intact. The arch of the palate should be dome shaped. A narrow, flat roof or a high, arched palate affects the placement of the tongue and can cause feeding and speech problems. Test movement of the uvula by eliciting a gag reflex. It should move upward to close off the nasopharynx from the oropharynx.

Examine the oropharynx and note the size and color of the **palatine tonsils.** They are normally the same color as the surrounding mucosa; glandular, rather than smooth in appear-

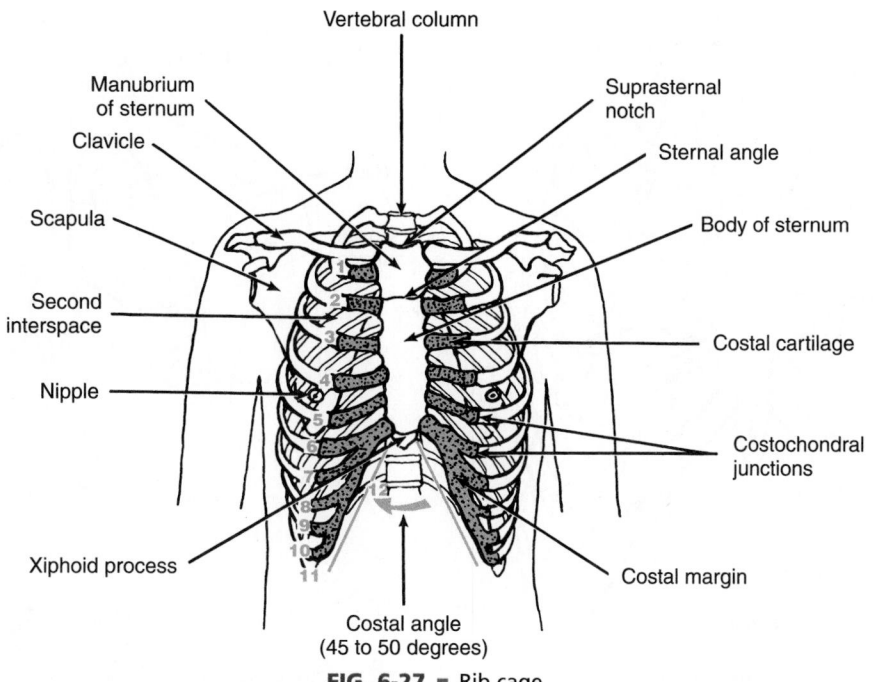

FIG. 6-27 ▪ Rib cage.

ance; and barely visible over the edge of the palatoglossal arches. The size of the tonsils varies considerably during childhood. However, report any swelling, redness, or white areas on the tonsils.

CHEST

Inspect the **chest** for size, shape, symmetry, movement, breast development, and the bony landmarks formed by the ribs and sternum. The **rib cage** consists of 12 ribs on each side and the sternum, or breast bone, located in the midline of the trunk (Fig. 6-27). The **sternum** is composed of three main parts. The **manubrium,** the uppermost portion, can be felt at the base of the neck at the **suprasternal notch.** The largest segment of the sternum is the **body,** which forms the **sternal angle (angle of Louis)** as it articulates with the manubrium. At the end of the body is a small, movable process called the **xiphoid.** The angle of the costal margin as it attaches to the sternum is called the **costal angle** and is normally about 45 to 50 degrees. These bony structures are important landmarks in the location of ribs and **intercostal spaces (ICSs),** which are the spaces between the ribs. They are numbered according to the rib directly *above* the space. For example, the space immediately below the second rib is the second ICS.

The **thoracic cavity** is also divided into segments by drawing imaginary lines on the chest and back. Fig. 6-28 illustrates the anterior, lateral, and posterior divisions.

Measure the **size** of the chest by placing the measuring tape around the rib cage at the nipple line (see Fig. 6-8). For greatest accuracy, take two measurements—one during inspiration and the other during expiration—and record the average. Chest size is important mainly in relation to head circumference, which is discussed on p. 124. Always report marked disproportions because most are caused by abnormal head growth, although some may be a result of altered chest shape, such as **barrel chest** (chest is round) or **pigeon chest** (sternum protrudes outward).

FIG. 6-28 ▪ Imaginary landmarks of chest. **A,** Anterior. **B,** Right lateral. **C,** Posterior.

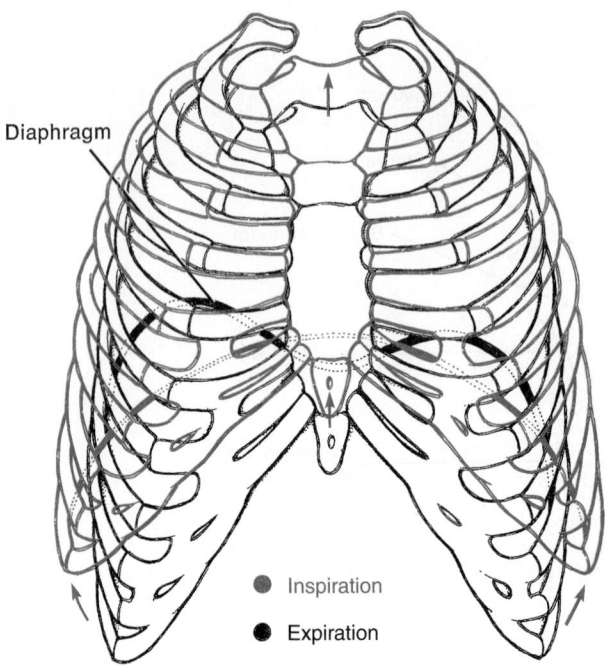

FIG. 6-29 ■ Movement of chest during respiration.

Inspiration

Expiration

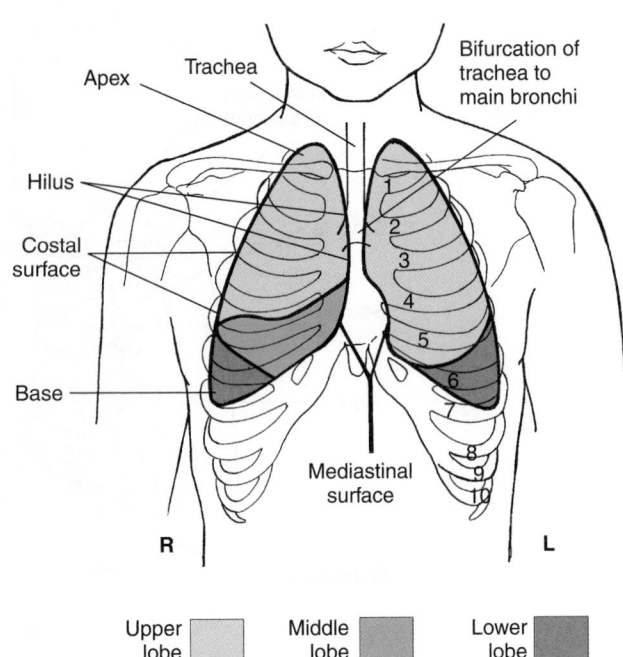

FIG. 6-30 ■ Location of lobes of lungs within thoracic cavity.

Upper lobe   Middle lobe   Lower lobe

During infancy the chest's **shape** is almost circular, with the anteroposterior (front-to-back) diameter equaling the transverse, or lateral (side-to-side), diameter. As the child grows, the chest normally increases in the transverse direction, causing the anteroposterior diameter to be less than the lateral diameter. Note the **angle** made by the lower costal margin and the sternum, and palpate the junction of the ribs with the costal cartilage (costochondral junction) and sternum, which should be fairly smooth.

Movement of the chest wall should be symmetric bilaterally and coordinated with breathing. During inspiration the chest rises and expands, the diaphragm descends, and the costal angle increases. During expiration the chest falls and decreases in size, the diaphragm rises, and the costal angle narrows (Fig. 6-29). In children younger than 6 or 7 years of age, respiratory movement is principally abdominal or diaphragmatic. In older children, particularly girls, respirations are chiefly thoracic. In either type the chest and abdomen should rise and fall together. Always report any asymmetry of movement.

While inspecting the skin surface of the chest, observe the position of the **nipples** and any evidence of **breast development.** Normally the nipples are located slightly lateral to the midclavicular line between the fourth and fifth ribs. Note symmetry of nipple placement and normal configuration of a darker pigmented areola surrounding a flat nipple in the prepubertal child.

Pubertal breast development usually begins in girls between 10 and 14 years of age (see Chapter 16). Record early (precocious) or delayed breast development, as well as evidence of any other secondary sexual characteristics. In males **breast enlargement (gynecomastia)** may be caused by hormonal or systemic disorders, but more commonly it is a result of adipose tissue from obesity or a transitory body change during early puberty. In either situation investigate the child's feelings regarding breast enlargement.

In adolescent girls who have achieved sexual maturity, palpate the breasts for evidence of any masses or hard nodules. Use this opportunity to discuss the importance of routine breast self-examination. Emphasize that most palpable masses are benign to decrease any fear or concern that results when a mass is felt.

LUNGS

The lungs are situated inside the thoracic cavity, with one lung on each side of the sternum. Each lung is divided into an **apex,** which is slightly pointed and rises above the first rib; a **base,** which is wide and concave and rides on the dome-shaped diaphragm; and a **body,** which is divided into lobes. The right lung has three lobes: the upper, middle, and lower. The left lung has only two lobes, the upper and lower, because of the space occupied by the heart (Fig. 6-30).

Inspection of the lungs primarily involves observation of respiratory movements, which are discussed previously. Evaluate respirations for **rate** (number per minute), **rhythm** (regular, irregular, or periodic), **depth** (deep or shallow), and **quality** (effortless, automatic, difficult, or labored). Note the character of **breath sounds,** such as noisy, grunting, snoring, or heavy.

Evaluate respiratory movements by placing each hand flat against the back or chest with the thumbs in midline along the lower costal margin of the lungs. The child should be sitting during this procedure and, if cooperative, should take several deep breaths. During respiration your hands will move with the chest wall. Assess the amount and speed of respiratory excursion and note any asymmetry of movement.

Experienced examiners may percuss the lungs. The anterior lung is percussed from apex to base, usually with the child in the supine or sitting position. Each side of the chest is percussed in sequence to compare the sounds. When the posterior lung is percussed, the procedure and sequence are the same, although the child should be sitting. Resonance is heard

BOX 6-14
Classification of Normal Breath Sounds

VESICULAR BREATH SOUNDS
Heard over entire surface of lungs, with exception of upper intrascapular area and area beneath manubrium.
Inspiration is louder, longer, and higher pitched than expiration.
Sound is soft, swishing noise.

BRONCHOVESICULAR BREATH SOUNDS
Heard over manubrium and in upper intrascapular regions where trachea and bronchi bifurcate.
Inspiration is louder and higher pitched than in vesicular breathing.

BRONCHIAL BREATH SOUNDS
Heard only over trachea near suprasternal notch.
Inspiratory phase is short, and expiratory phase is long.

nursingcareguidelines

Effective Auscultation
- Make certain child is relaxed and not crying, talking, or laughing. Record if child is crying.
- Check that room is comfortable and quiet.
- Warm stethoscope before placing it against skin.
- Apply firm pressure on chest piece but not enough to prevent vibrations and transmission of sound.
- Avoid placing stethoscope over hair or clothing, moving it against skin, breathing on tubing, or sliding fingers over chest piece, which may cause sounds that falsely resemble pathologic findings.
- Use a symmetric and orderly approach to compare sounds.

ATRAUMATIC CARE

Encouraging Deep Breaths
- Ask child to "blow out" the light on an otoscope or pocket flashlight; discreetly turn off the light on the last try so that the child feels successful.
- Place a cotton ball in child's palm; ask child to blow the ball into the air and have parent catch it.
- Place a small tissue on the top of a pencil and ask child to blow the tissue off.
- Have child blow a pinwheel, a party horn, or bubbles.

BOX 6-15
Various Patterns of Respiration

Tachypnea—Increased rate
Bradypnea—Decreased rate
Dyspnea—Distress during breathing
Apnea—Cessation of breathing
Hyperpnea—Increased depth
Hypoventilation—Decreased depth (shallow) and irregular rhythm
Hyperventilation—Increased rate and depth
Kussmaul respiration—Hyperventilation, gasping and labored respiration; usually seen in diabetic coma or other states of respiratory acidosis
Cheyne-Stokes respiration—Gradually increasing rate and depth with periods of apnea
Biot respiration—Periods of hyperpnea alternating with apnea (similar to Cheyne-Stokes except that depth remains constant)
Seesaw (paradoxic) respirations—Chest falls on inspiration and rises on expiration
Agonal—Last gasping breaths before death

over all the lobes of the lungs that are not adjacent to other organs. Any deviation from the expected sound is recorded and reported.

Auscultation

Auscultation involves using the stethoscope to evaluate breath sounds (see Nursing Care Guidelines box). Breath sounds are best heard if the child inspires deeply (see Atraumatic Care box). In the lungs breath sounds are classified as vesicular, bronchovesicular, or bronchial (Box 6-14).

Absent or **diminished breath sounds** are always an abnormal finding warranting investigation. Fluid, air, or solid masses in the pleural space all interfere with the conduction of breath sounds. Diminished breath sounds in certain segments of the lung can alert the nurse to pulmonary areas that may benefit from chest physiotherapy. Increased breath sounds after pulmonary therapy indicate improved passage of air through the respiratory tract. Terms used to describe various respiration patterns are found in Box 6-15.

Various pulmonary abnormalities produce **adventitious sounds** that are not normally heard over the chest. These sounds occur in addition to normal or abnormal breath sounds. They are classified into two main groups: **crackles,** which result from the passage of air through fluid or moisture, and **wheezes,** which are produced as air passes through narrowed passageways, regardless of the cause, such as exudate, inflammation,

spasm, or tumor. Considerable practice with an experienced tutor is necessary to differentiate the various types of lung sounds. Often it is best to describe the type of sound heard in the lungs rather than trying to label it. Always report any abnormal sounds for further medical evaluation.

HEART

The heart is situated in the thoracic cavity between the lungs in the mediastinum and above the diaphragm (Fig. 6-31). About two thirds of the heart lies within the left side of the rib cage, with the other third on the right side as it crosses the sternum. The heart is positioned in the thorax like a trapezoid:

Vertically along the right sternal border (RSB) from the second to the fifth rib
Horizontally (long side) from the lower right sternum to the fifth rib at the left midclavicular line (LMCL)
Diagonally from the left sternal border (LSB) at the second rib to the LMCL at the fifth rib
Horizontally (short side) from the RSB and LSB at the second ICS—base of the heart

Inspection is best done with the child sitting in a semi-Fowler position. Look at the anterior chest wall from an angle, comparing both sides of the rib cage with each other. Nor-

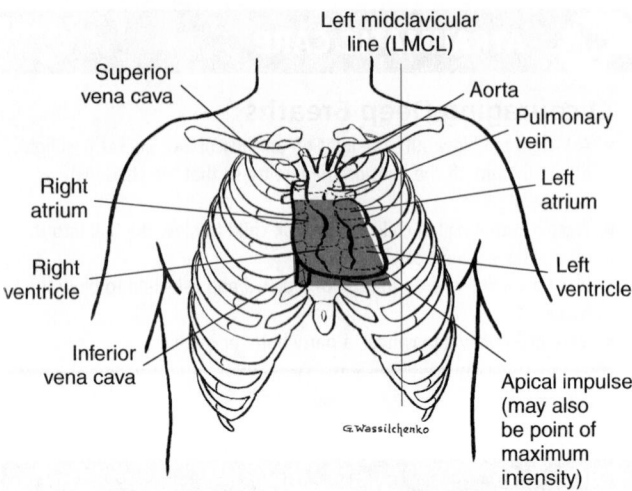

FIG. 6-31 ■ Position of heart within thorax.

FIG. 6-32 ■ Location of pulses.

mally they should be symmetric. In children with thin chest walls, a pulsation may be visible. Because comprehensive evaluation of cardiac function is not limited to the heart, also consider other findings such as the presence of all pulses (especially the femoral pulses) (Fig. 6-32), distended neck veins, clubbing of the fingers, peripheral cyanosis, edema, blood pressure, and respiratory status.

Use palpation to determine the location of the **apical impulse (AI),** the most lateral cardiac impulse that may correspond to the apex. The AI is found:

■ Just lateral to the LMCL and fourth ICS in children over 7 years of age
■ At the LMCL and fifth ICS in children less than 7 years of age

Although the AI gives a general idea of the size of the heart (with enlargement, the apex is lower and more lateral), its normal location is variable, making it an unreliable indicator of heart size.

The **point of maximum intensity (PMI),** as the name implies, is the area of most intense pulsation. Usually the PMI is located at the same site as the AI, but it can occur elsewhere. For this reason, the two terms should not be used synonymously.

Assess **capillary refill time,** an important test for peripheral circulation, by pressing the skin lightly on a central site, such as the forehead, or a peripheral site, such as the top of the hand, to produce a slight blanching. The time it takes for the blanched area to return to its original color is the **capillary refill time.**

NURSINGALERT

Capillary refill should be brisk—less than 2 seconds; prolonged refill may be associated with poor systemic perfusion or a cool ambient temperature.

Auscultation

Origin of Heart Sounds. The heart sounds are produced by the opening and closing of the valves and the vibration of blood against the walls of the heart and vessels. Normally two sounds—S_1 and S_2—are heard, which correspond, respectively, to the familiar "lub dub" often used to describe the

sounds. S_1 is caused by closure of the **tricuspid** and **mitral valves** (sometimes called the **atrioventricular valves**). S_2 is the result of closure of the **pulmonic** and **aortic valves** (sometimes called **semilunar valves**). Normally the split of the two sounds in S_2 is distinguishable and widens during inspiration. **Physiologic splitting** is a significant normal finding.

NURSINGALERT

Fixed splitting, in which the split in S_2 does not change during inspiration, is an important diagnostic sign of atrial septal defect.

Two other heart sounds—S_3 and S_4—may be produced. S_3 is normally heard in some children; S_4 is rarely heard as a normal heart sound; it usually indicates the need for further cardiac evaluation.

Differentiating Normal Heart Sounds. Fig. 6-33 illustrates the approximate anatomic position of the valves within the heart chambers. Note that the anatomic location of valves does not correspond to the area where the sounds are heard best. The auscultatory sites are located in the direction of the blood flow through the valves.

Normally S_1 is louder at the apex of the heart in the mitral and tricuspid area, and S_2 is louder near the base of the heart in the pulmonic and aortic area (Table 6-10). Listen to each sound by inching down the chest. The following areas should also be auscultated for sounds, such as murmurs, which may radiate to these sites: sternoclavicular area above the clavicles and manubrium, area along the sternal border, area along the left midaxillary line, and area below the scapulae.

TABLE 6-10		
Sequence of Auscultating Heart Sounds*		
AUSCULTATORY SITE	CHEST LOCATION	CHARACTERISTICS OF HEART SOUNDS
Aortic area	Second right intercostal space close to sternum	S_2 heard louder than S_1; aortic closure heard loudest
Pulmonic area	Second left intercostal space close to sternum	Splitting of S_2 heard best, normally widens on inspiration; pulmonic closure heard best
Erb point	Second and third left intercostal spaces close to sternum	Frequent site of innocent murmurs and those of aortic or pulmonic origin
Tricuspid area	Fifth right and left intercostal spaces close to sternum	S_1 heard as louder sound preceding S_2 (S_1 synchronous with carotid pulse)
Mitral or apical area	Fifth intercostal space, left midclavicular line (third to fourth intercostal space and lateral to left midclavicular line in infants)	S_1 heard loudest; splitting of S_1 may be audible because mitral closure is louder than tricuspid closure
		S_3 heard best at beginning of expiration with child in recumbent or left side-lying position; occurs immediately after S_2; sounds like word S_1 S_2 S_3: "Ken-tuc-ky"
		S_4 heard best during expiration with child in recumbent position (left side-lying position decreases sound); occurs immediately before S_1; sounds like word S_4 S_1 S_2: "Ten-nes-see"

*Use both diaphragm and bell chest pieces when auscultating heart sounds. Bell chest piece is necessary for low-pitched sounds of murmurs, S_3, and S_4.

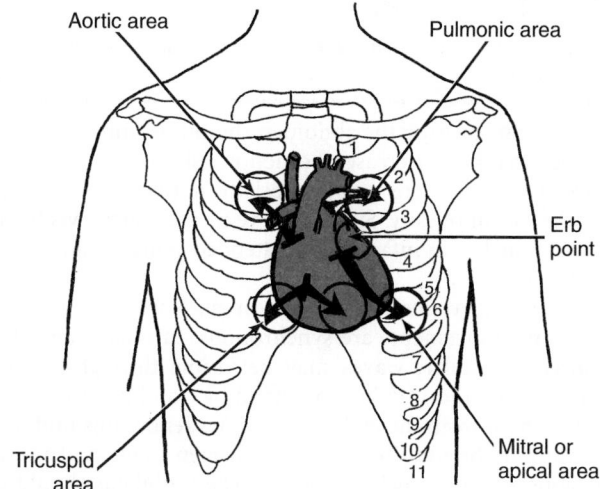

FIG. 6-33 ■ Direction of heart sounds for anatomic valve sites and areas *(circled)* for auscultation.

NURSINGTIP

To distinguish between S_1 and S_2 heart sounds, simultaneously palpate the carotid pulse with the index and middle fingers and listen to the heart sounds; S_1 is synchronous with the carotid pulse.

Auscultate the heart with the child in at least two positions: sitting and reclining. If adventitious sounds are detected, further evaluate them with the child standing, sitting and leaning forward, and lying on the left side. For example, atrial sounds such as S_4 are heard best with the person in a recumbent position and usually fade if the person sits or stands.

Evaluate heart sounds for (1) **quality** (they should be clear and distinct, not muffled, diffuse, or distant); (2) **intensity,** especially in relation to the location or auscultatory site (they should not be weak or pounding); (3) **rate** (they should have the same rate as the radial pulse); and (4) **rhythm** (they should be regular and even). A particular arrhythmia that oc-

curs normally in many children is **sinus arrhythmia,** in which the heart rate increases with inspiration and decreases with expiration. Differentiate this rhythm from a truly abnormal arrhythmia by having children hold their breath. In sinus arrhythmia, cessation of breathing causes the heart rate to remain steady.

Heart Murmurs. Another important category of the heart sounds is **murmurs,** which are produced by vibrations within the heart chambers or in the major arteries from the back-and-forth flow of blood. (For a more detailed discussion, see Assessment of Cardiac Function, Chapter 25.) Murmurs are classified as:

Innocent—No anatomic or physiologic abnormality exists.
Functional—No automatic cardiac defect exists, but a physiologic abnormality such as anemia is present.
Organic—A cardiac defect with or without a physiologic abnormality exists.

The description and classification of murmurs are skills that require considerable practice and training. In general, recognize murmurs as distinct swishing sounds that occur in addition to the normal heart sounds and record the (1) **location,** or the area of the heart in which the murmur is heard best; (2) **time** of the occurrence of the murmur within the S_1, S_2 cycle; (3) **intensity** (evaluate in relationship to the child's position); and (4) **loudness.** The usual subjective method of grading the loudness or intensity of a murmur is listed in Table 6-11.

ABDOMEN

Examination of the abdomen involves inspection, followed by auscultation and then palpation. Perform palpation last because it may distort the normal abdominal sounds. Knowledge of the anatomic placement of the abdominal organs is essential to differentiate normal, expected findings from abnormal ones (Fig. 6-34).

For descriptive purposes, the abdominal cavity is divided into four quadrants by drawing a vertical line midway from the sternum to the symphysis pubis and a horizontal line

Anatomy Review—Direction of Heart Sounds

Animation—Abdominal Anatomy

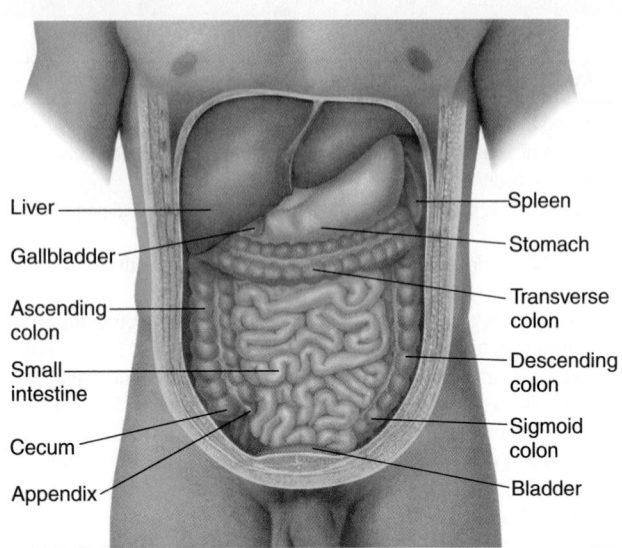

FIG. 6-34 ■ Location of structures in abdomen. (From Seidel HM, Ball JW, Dains JE, and others: *Mosby's guide to physical examination*, ed 5, St Louis, 2003, Mosby.)

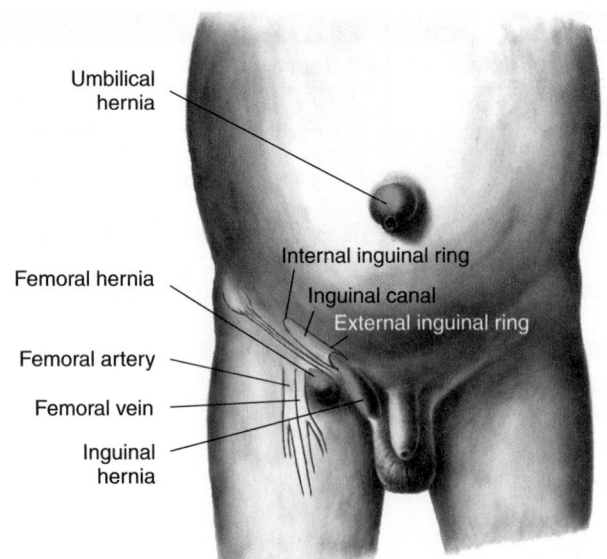

FIG. 6-35 ■ Location of hernias.

TABLE 6-11
Grading of the Intensity of Heart Murmurs

GRADE	DESCRIPTION
I	Very faint; often not heard if child sits up
II	Usually readily heard; slightly louder than grade I; audible in all positions
III	Loud, but not accompanied by a thrill
IV	Loud, accompanied by a thrill
V	Loud enough to be heard with a stethoscope barely touching the chest; accompanied by a thrill
VI	Loud enough to be heard with the stethoscope not touching the chest; often heard with the human ear close to the chest; accompanied by a thrill

across the abdomen through the umbilicus. The sections are named:

- Left upper quadrant
- Left lower quadrant
- Right upper quadrant
- Right lower quadrant

Inspection

Inspect the **contour** of the abdomen with the child erect and supine. Normally the abdomen of infants and young children is cylindric and, in the erect position, fairly prominent because of the physiologic lordosis of the spine. In the supine position the abdomen appears flat. A midline protrusion from the xiphoid to the umbilicus or symphysis pubis is usually **diastasis recti,** or failure of the rectus abdominis muscles to join in utero. In a healthy child a midline protrusion is usually a variation of normal muscular development.

A tense, boardlike abdomen is a serious sign of paralytic ileus and intestinal obstruction.

The **skin** covering the abdomen should be uniformly taut, without wrinkles or creases. Sometimes silvery, whitish striae ("stretch marks") are seen, especially if the skin has been stretched as in obesity. Superficial veins are usually visible in light-skinned, thin infants, but distended veins are an abnormal finding.

Observe **movement** of the abdomen. Normally chest and abdominal movements are synchronous. In infants and thin children **peristaltic waves** may be visible through the abdominal wall; they are best observed by standing at eye level to and across from the abdomen. Always report this finding.

Examine the **umbilicus** for size, hygiene, and evidence of any abnormalities, such as hernias. The umbilicus should be flat or only slightly protruding. If a herniation is present, palpate the sac for abdominal contents and estimate the approximate size of the opening. **Umbilical hernias** are common in infants, especially in African-American children.

Hernias may exist elsewhere on the abdominal wall (Fig. 6-35). An **inguinal hernia** is a protrusion of peritoneum through the abdominal wall in the inguinal canal. It occurs mostly in males, is frequently bilateral, and may be visible as a mass in the scrotum. To locate a hernia, slide the little finger into the external inguinal ring at the base of the scrotum and ask the child to cough. If a hernia is present, it will hit the tip of the finger.

NURSINGTIP

If the child is too young to cough, have the child blow up a balloon or laugh to raise the intraabdominal pressure sufficiently to demonstrate the presence of an inguinal hernia.

A **femoral hernia,** which occurs more frequently in girls, is felt or seen as a small mass on the anterior surface of the thigh just below the inguinal ligament in the femoral canal

Promoting Relaxation During Abdominal Palpation

Position child comfortably, such as in a semireclining position in the parent's lap, with knees flexed.

Warm the hands before touching the skin.

Use distraction, such as telling stories or talking to child.

Teach child to use deep breathing and to concentrate on an object.

Give infant a bottle or pacifier.

Begin with light, superficial palpation and gradually progress to deeper palpation.

Palpate any tender or painful areas last.

Have child hold the parent's hand and squeeze it if palpation is uncomfortable.

Use the nonpalpating hand to comfort child, such as placing the free hand on the child's shoulder while palpating the abdomen.

To minimize sensation of tickling during palpation:

- Have children "help" with palpation by placing a hand over the palpating hand.
- Have them place a hand on the abdomen with the fingers spread wide apart, and palpate between their fingers.

FIG. 6-36 ■ Palpating femoral pulses.

(a potential space medial to the femoral artery). Feel for a hernia by placing the index finger of your right hand on the child's right femoral pulse (left hand for left pulse) and the middle finger flat against the skin toward the midline. The ring finger lies over the femoral canal, where the herniation occurs. Palpation of hernias in the pelvic region is often part of the genital examination.

Auscultation

The most important finding to listen for is **peristalsis,** or **bowel sounds,** which sound like short metallic clicks and gurgles. Their frequency per minute should be recorded (e.g., 5 sounds/min). Bowel sounds may be stimulated by stroking the abdominal surface with a fingernail. Report absence of bowel sounds or hyperperistalsis, since either usually denotes an abdominal disorder.

Palpation

Two types of palpation are performed: superficial and deep. For **superficial palpation,** lightly place your hand against the skin and feel each quadrant, noting any areas of tenderness, muscle tone, and superficial lesions such as cysts. Because superficial palpation is often perceived as tickling, several techniques can be used to minimize this sensation and relax the child (see Atraumatic Care box). Admonishing the child to stop laughing only draws attention to the sensation and decreases cooperation.

Deep palpation is used for palpating organs and large blood vessels and for detecting masses and tenderness that were not discovered during superficial palpation. Palpation usually begins in the lower quadrants and proceeds upward to avoid missing the edge of an enlarged liver or spleen. Except for palpating the liver, successful identification of other organs, such as the spleen, kidney, and part of the colon, requires considerable practice with tutored supervision. Report any

questionable mass. The lower edge of the liver is sometimes felt in infants and young children as a superficial mass 1 to 2 cm (0.4 to 0.8 inch) below the right costal margin (the distance is sometimes measured in fingerbreadths). Normally, the liver descends during inspiration as the diaphragm moves downward. Do not mistake this downward displacement as a sign of liver enlargement.

> **NURSING ALERT**
>
> If the liver is palpable 3 cm (1.2 inch) below the right costal margin or the spleen is palpable more than 2 cm (0.8 inch) below the left costal margin, these organs are enlarged—a finding that is always reported for further medical investigation.

Palpate the **femoral pulses** by placing the tips of two or three fingers (index, middle, or ring) along the inguinal ligament about midway between the iliac crest and symphysis pubis. Feel both pulses simultaneously to make certain that they are equal and strong (Fig. 6-36).

> **NURSING ALERT**
>
> Absence of femoral pulses is a significant sign of coarctation of the aorta and is referred for medical evaluation.

GENITALIA

Examination of genitalia conveniently follows assessment of the abdomen while the child is still supine. In adolescents inspection of the genitalia may be left to the end of the examination. The best approach is to examine the genitalia matter-of-factly, placing no more emphasis on this part of the assessment than on any other segment. It helps to relieve children's and parents' anxiety by telling them the results of the findings; for example, the nurse might say, "Everything looks fine here."

If it is necessary to ask questions, such as about discharge or difficulty urinating, respect the child's privacy by covering the lower abdomen with the gown or underpants. To prevent embarrassing interruptions, keep the door or curtain closed and post a "do not disturb" sign. Have a drape ready to cover the genitalia if someone enters the room.

In examining the genitalia, wear gloves when touching body substances. It might be helpful for the adolescent to know that wearing gloves also prevents skin-to-skin contact.

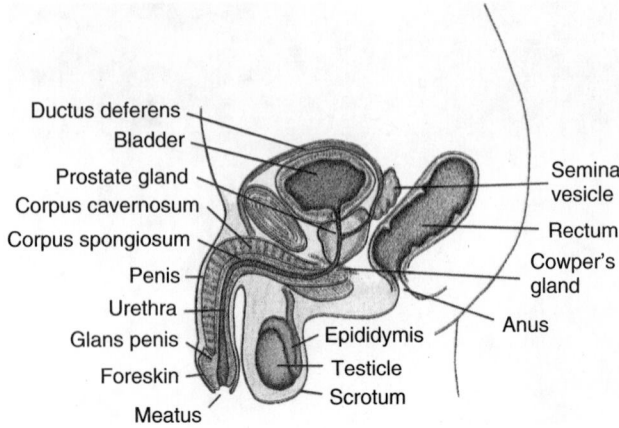

FIG. 6-37 ■ Major structures of genitalia in uncircumcised post-pubertal male. (From Potter PA, Perry AG: *Basic nursing: theory and practice,* ed 4, St Louis, 1999, Mosby.)

FIG. 6-38 ■ **A,** Preventing cremasteric reflex by having child sit in "tailor" position. **B,** Blocking inguinal canal during palpation of scrotum for descended testes.

The genital examination is an excellent time for eliciting questions or concern about body function or sexual activity. Also use this opportunity to increase or reinforce the child's knowledge of reproductive anatomy by naming each body part and explaining its function. This part of the health assessment is an opportune time to teach testicular self-examination to boys.*

Male Genitalia

Note the external appearance of the glans and shaft of the penis, the prepuce, the urethral meatus, and the scrotum (Fig. 6-37). The **penis** is generally small in infants and young boys until puberty, when it begins to increase in both length and width. In an obese child the penis often looks abnormally small because of the folds of skin partially covering it at the base. Be familiar with normal pubertal growth of the external male genitalia to compare the findings with the expected sequence of maturation (see Chapter 16).

Examine the **glans** (head of the penis) and **shaft** (portion between the perineum and prepuce) for signs of swelling, skin lesions, inflammation, or other irregularities. Any of these signs may indicate underlying disorders, especially sexually transmitted diseases.

The **urethral meatus** is carefully inspected for location and evidence of discharge. Normally it is centered at the tip of the glans.

Hair distribution is also noted. Normally, before puberty, no pubic hair is present. Soft, downy hair at the base of the penis is an early sign of pubertal maturation. In older adolescents hair distribution is diamond-shaped from the umbilicus to the anus.

The location and size of the **scrotum** are noted. The scrota hang freely from the perineum behind the penis, and the left scrotum normally hangs lower than the right. In infants the scrota appear large in relation to the rest of the genitalia. The skin of the scrotum is loose and highly rugated (wrinkled). During early adolescence the skin normally becomes redder and coarser. In dark-skinned children the scrota are usually more deeply pigmented.

Palpation of the scrotum includes identification of the testes, epididymis, and, if present, inguinal hernias. The two **testes** are felt as small, ovoid bodies about 1.5 to 2 cm (0.6 to 0.8 inch) long—one in each scrotal sac. They do not enlarge until puberty, when they approximately double in size.

When palpating for the presence of the testes, avoid stimulating the **cremasteric reflex,** which is stimulated by cold, touch, emotional excitement, or exercise. This reflex pulls the testes higher into the pelvic cavity. Several measures are useful in preventing the cremasteric reflex during palpation of the scrotum. First, warm the hands. Second, if the child is old enough, examine him in a tailor or "Indian" position, which stretches the muscle, preventing its contraction (Fig. 6-38, *A*). Third, block the normal pathway of ascent of the testes by placing the thumb and index finger over the upper part of the scrotal sac along the inguinal canal (Fig. 6-38, *B*). If there is any question concerning the existence of two testes, place the index and middle fingers in a scissors fashion to separate the right and left scrota. If, after using these techniques, you have not palpated the testes, feel along the inguinal canal and perineum to locate masses that may be undescended testes. Although undescended testes may descend at any time during childhood and are checked at each visit, failure to palpate testes is reported.

Female Genitalia

The examination of female genitalia is limited to inspection and palpation of external structures. If a vaginal examination is required, an appropriate referral is made unless the nurse is qualified to perform the procedure. A convenient position for examination of the genitalia involves placing the young child

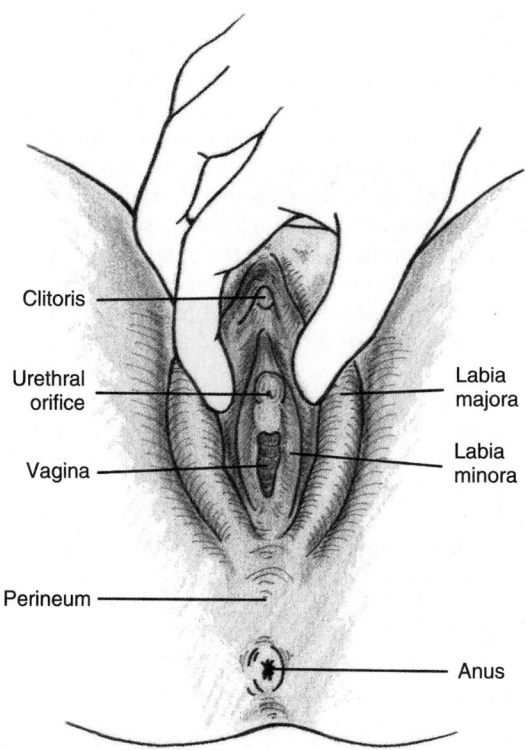

FIG. 6-39 ■ External structures of genitalia in postpubertal female. Labia are spread to reveal deeper structures. (From Potter PA, Perry AG: *Basic nursing: theory and practice,* ed 4, St Louis, 1999, Mosby.)

supine on the examining table or in a semireclining position on the parent's lap with the feet supported on your knees as you sit facing the child. Divert the child's attention from the examination by instructing her to try to keep the soles of her feet pressed against each other. Separate the labia majora with the thumb and index finger and retract outward to expose the labia minora, urethral meatus, and vaginal orifice.

Examine the female genitalia for size and location of the structures of the **vulva,** or **pudendum** (Fig. 6-39). The **mons pubis** is a pad of adipose tissue over the symphysis pubis. At puberty the mons is covered with hair, which extends along the labia. The usual pattern of female **hair distribution** is an inverted triangle. The appearance of soft, downy hair along the labia majora is an early sign of sexual maturation. Note the size and location of the **clitoris,** a small, erectile organ located at the anterior end of the labia minora. It is covered by a small flap of skin, the **prepuce.**

The **labia majora** are two thick folds of skin running posteriorly from the mons to the posterior commissure of the vagina. Internal to the labia majora are two folds of skin called the **labia minora.** Although the labia minora are usually prominent in the newborn, they gradually atrophy, which makes them almost invisible until their enlargement during puberty. The inner surface of the labia should be pink and moist. Note the size of the labia and any evidence of fusion, which may suggest male scrota. Normally no masses are palpable within the labia.

The **urethral meatus** is located posterior to the clitoris and is surrounded by the Skene glands and ducts. Although not a prominent structure, the meatus appears as a small V-shaped slit. Note its location, especially if it opens from the clitoris or inside the vagina. Gently palpate the glands, which are common sites of cysts and sexually transmitted lesions.

The **vaginal orifice** is located posterior to the urethral meatus. Its appearance varies depending on individual anatomy and sexual activity. Ordinarily, examination of the vagina is limited to inspection. In virgins a thin crescent-shaped or circular membrane, called the **hymen,** may cover part of the vaginal opening. In some instances it completely occludes the orifice. After rupture, small rounded pieces of tissue called **caruncles** remain. Although an imperforate hymen denotes lack of penile intercourse, a perforate one does not necessarily indicate sexual activity (see also Sexual Abuse, Chapter 14).

> **NURSING ALERT**
>
> In girls who have been circumcised, the genitalia will appear different. Do not show surprise or disgust, but note the appearance and discuss the procedure with the young woman.

Surrounding the vaginal opening are **Bartholin glands,** which secrete a clear, mucoid fluid into the vagina for lubrication during intercourse. Palpate the ducts for cysts. Also note the discharge from the vagina, which is usually clear or white.

ANUS

After examination of the genitalia, the anal area is easily examined, although the child should be placed on the abdomen. Note the general firmness of the **buttocks** and symmetry of the **gluteal folds.** Assess the tone of the anal sphincter by eliciting the **anal reflex.** Gently scratching the anal area results in an obvious quick contraction of the external anal sphincter.

BACK AND EXTREMITIES
Spine

The general **curvature** of the spine is noted. Normally the back of a newborn is rounded or C shaped from the thoracic and pelvic curves. The development of the cervical and lumbar curves approximates development of various motor skills, such as cervical curvature with head control, and gives the older child the typical double S curve.

Marked curvatures in posture are abnormal. **Scoliosis,** lateral curvature of the spine, is an important childhood problem, especially in girls. Although scoliosis may be identified by observing and palpating the spine and noting a sideways displacement, more objective tests include:

- With the child standing erect, clothed only in underpants (and bra if older girl), observe from behind, noting asymmetry of the shoulders and hips.
- With the child bending forward so that the back is parallel to the floor, observe from the side, noting asymmetry or prominence of the rib cage.

A slight limp, a crooked hemline, or complaints of a sore back are other signs and symptoms of scoliosis.

Inspect the **back,** especially along the spine, for any tufts of hair, dimples, or discoloration. **Mobility** of the vertebral column is easily assessed in most children because of their propensity for constant motion during the examination. However, mobility can be tested by asking the child to sit up from a prone position or to do a modified sit-up exercise.

Movement of the cervical spine is an important diagnostic sign of neurologic problems, such as meningitis. Normally movement of the head in all directions is effortless.

Extremities

Inspect each extremity for symmetry of length and size; refer any deviation for orthopedic evaluation. Count the fingers and toes to be certain of the normal number. This is so often taken for granted that an extra digit (**polydactyly**) or fusion of digits (**syndactyly**) may go unnoticed.

Inspect the arms and legs for **temperature** and **color,** which should be equal in each extremity, although the feet may normally be colder than the hands.

Assess the **shape** of bones. Several variations of bone shape may be observed in children. Although many of them cause parents concern, most are benign and require no treatment. **Bowleg,** or **genu varum,** is lateral bowing of the tibia. It is clinically present when the child stands with the medial malleoli (rounded prominence on either side of the ankle) opposite each other and the space between the knees is greater than approximately 5 cm (2 inches) (Fig. 6-40). Toddlers are usually bowlegged after beginning to walk until all their lower back and leg muscles are well developed. Unilateral or asymmetric bowlegs that are present beyond the age of 2 to 3 years, particularly in African-American children, may represent pathologic conditions requiring further investigation.

Knock-knee, or **genu valgum,** appears as the opposite of bowleg, in that the knees are close together but the feet are spread apart. It is determined clinically by using the same method as for genu varum but by measuring the distance between the malleoli, which normally should be less than 7.5 cm (3 inches) (Fig. 6-41). Knock-knee is normally present in children from about 2 to 7 years of age. Knock-knee that is excessive, asymmetric, accompanied by short stature, or evident in a child nearing puberty requires further evaluation.

Next inspect the **feet.** Infants' and toddlers' feet appear flat because the foot is normally wide and the arch is covered by a fat pad. Development of the arch occurs naturally from the action of walking. Normally, at birth the feet are held in a valgus (outward) or varus (inward) position. To determine whether a foot deformity at birth is a result of intrauterine position or development, scratch the outer, then inner, side of the sole. If the foot position is self-correctable, it will assume a right angle to the leg. As the child begins to walk, the feet turn outward less than 30 degrees and inward less than 10 degrees.

Toddlers have a "toddling" or broad-based gait, which facilitates walking by lowering the center of gravity. As the child reaches preschool age, the legs are brought closer together. By school age the walking posture is much more graceful and balanced.

The most common gait problem in young children is **pigeon toe,** or **toeing in,** which usually results from torsional deformities, such as internal tibial torsion (abnormal rotation or bowing of the tibia). Tests for tibial torsion include measuring the thigh-foot angle, which requires considerable practice for accuracy.

Elicit the **plantar** or **grasp reflex** by exerting firm but gentle pressure with the tip of the thumb against the lateral sole of the foot from the heel upward to the little toe and then across to the big toe. The normal response in children who are walking is flexion of the toes. **Babinski sign,** dorsiflexion of the big toe and fanning of the other toes, is normal during infancy but abnormal after about 1 year of age or when locomotion begins (see Fig. 10-6).

Joints

Evaluate the joints for **range of motion.** Normally this requires no specific testing if the nurse has observed the child's movements during the examination. However, the hips should be routinely investigated in infants for congenital dislocation. Report any evidence of joint immobility or hyperflexibility.

FIG. 6-40 ■ Bowleg.

FIG. 6-41 ■ Knock-knee.

Palpate the joints for heat, tenderness, and swelling. These signs, as well as redness over the joint, warrant further investigation.

Muscles

Note symmetry and quality of muscle development, tone, and strength. Observe **development** by looking at the shape and contour of the body in both a relaxed and a tensed state. Estimate **tone** by grasping the muscle and feeling its firmness when it is relaxed and contracted. A common site for testing tone is the biceps muscle of the arm. Children are usually willing to "make a muscle" by clenching their fist.

Estimate **strength** by having the child use an extremity to push or pull against resistance, as in the following examples:

Arm strength—Child holds the arms outstretched in front of the body and tries to raise the arms while downward pressure is applied.
Hand strength—Child shakes hands with nurse and squeezes one or two fingers of the nurse's hand.
Leg strength—Child sits on a table or chair with the legs dangling and tries to raise the legs while downward pressure is applied.

Note symmetry of strength in the extremities, hands, and fingers, and report evidence of paresis, or weakness.

NEUROLOGIC ASSESSMENT

The assessment of the nervous system is the broadest and most diverse part of the examination process, since every human function, both physical and emotional, is controlled by neurologic impulses. Much of the neurologic examination has already been discussed, such as assessment of behavior, sensory testing, and motor function. The following focuses on a general appraisal of cerebellar function, deep tendon reflexes, and the cranial nerves.

Cerebellar Function

The cerebellum controls balance and coordination. Much of the assessment of cerebellar function is included in observing the child's posture, body movements, gait, and development of fine and gross motor skills. Tests such as balancing on one foot and the heel-to-toe walk assess **balance.** Test **coordination** by asking the child to reach for a toy, button clothes, tie shoes, or draw a straight line on a piece of paper (provided the child is old enough to do these activities). Coordination can also be tested by any sequence of rapid, successive movements, such as quickly touching each finger with the thumb of the same hand.

Several tests for cerebellar function can be performed as games (Box 6-16). When a Romberg test is done, stay beside the child if there is a possibility that the child may fall. School-age children should be able to perform these tests, although in the finger-to-nose test preschoolers normally can only bring the finger within 5 to 7.5 cm (2 to 3 inches) of the nose. Difficulty in performing these exercises indicates poor sense of position (especially with the eyes closed) and incoordination (especially with the eyes opened).

Reflexes

Testing reflexes is an important part of the neurologic examination. Persistence of primitive reflexes (see Chapter 8), loss of reflexes, or hyperactivity of deep tendon reflexes is usually a result of a cerebral insult.

Elicit reflexes by using the rubber head of the reflex hammer, flat of the finger, or side of the hand. If the child is easily frightened by equipment, use your hand or finger. Although testing reflexes is a simple procedure, the child may inhibit the reflex by unconsciously tensing the muscle. To avoid tensing, distract younger children with toys or talk to them. Older children can concentrate on the exercise of grasping their two hands in front of them and trying to pull them apart. This diverts their attention from the testing and causes involuntary relaxation of the muscles.

Deep tendon reflexes are stretch reflexes of a muscle. The most common deep tendon reflex is the **knee jerk,** or **patellar reflex** (sometimes called the **quadriceps reflex**). The reflexes normally elicited are described in Figs. 6-42 to 6-45. Report any diminished or hyperreflexive response for further evaluation.

Cranial Nerves

Assessment of the cranial nerves is an important area of neurologic assessment (Table 6-12). With young children, present the tests as games to foster trust and security at the beginning of the examination. Or include the cranial nerve test when each system is examined, such as tongue movement and strength, gag reflex, swallowing, cardinal positions of gaze (Fig. 6-46), and position of the uvula during examination of the mouth.

FIG. 6-42 ■ Testing for triceps reflex. Child is placed supine, with forearm resting over chest, and triceps tendon is struck. Alternate procedure: child's arm is abducted, with upper arm supported and forearm allowed to hang freely. Triceps tendon is struck. Normal response is partial extension of forearm.

BOX 6-16

Tests for Cerebellar Function

Finger-to-nose test—With child's arm extended, ask child to touch the nose with the index finger with eyes open and then closed.
Heel-to-shin test—Have child stand and run the heel of one foot down the shin or anterior aspect of the tibia of the other leg, both with eyes opened and then closed.
Romberg test—Have child stand with eyes closed and heels together; falling or leaning to one side is abnormal and is called **Romberg sign.**

FIG. 6-43 ■ Testing for biceps reflex. Child's arm is held by placing partially flexed elbow in examiner's hand with thumb over antecubital space. Examiner's thumbnail is struck with hammer. Normal response is partial flexion of forearm.

FIG. 6-44 ■ Testing for patellar, or knee jerk, reflex, using distraction. Child sits on edge of examining table (or on parent's lap) with lower legs flexed at knee and dangling freely. Patellar tendon is tapped just below kneecap. Normal response is partial extension of lower leg.

FIG. 6-45 ■ Testing for Achilles reflex. Child should be in same position as for knee jerk reflex. Foot is supported lightly in examiner's hand, and Achilles tendon is struck. Normal response is plantar flexion of foot (foot pointing downward).

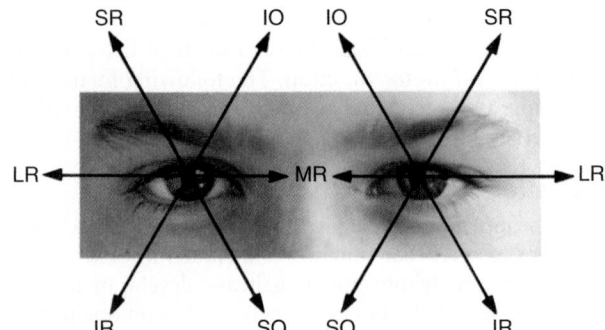

FIG. 6-46 ■ Testing cardinal positions of gaze. Muscles responsible for movement: *SR,* Superior rectus; *IR,* inferior rectus; *MR,* medial rectus; *IO,* inferior oblique; *SO,* superior oblique; *LR,* lateral rectus.

TABLE 6-12

Assessment of Cranial Nerves

DESCRIPTION AND FUNCTION	TESTS
I—OLFACTORY NERVE Olfactory mucosa of nasal cavity Smell	With eyes closed, have child identify odors such as coffee, alcohol from a swab, or other smells; test each nostril separately.
II—OPTIC NERVE Rods and cones of retina, optic nerve Vision	Check for perception of light, visual acuity, peripheral vision, color vision, and normal optic disc.

III—OCULOMOTOR NERVE
Extraocular muscles of eye:
    Superior rectus (SR)—moves eyeball up and in
    Inferior rectus (IR)—moves eyeball down and in
    Medial rectus (MR)—moves eyeball nasally
    Inferior oblique (IO)—moves eyeball up and out
Pupil constriction and accommodation
Eyelid closing
	Have child follow an object (toy) or light in 6 cardinal positions of gaze (see Fig. 6-46).
	
	Perform *PERRLA* (*P*upils *E*qual, *R*ound, *R*eact to *L*ight, and *A*ccommodation).
	Check for proper placement of lid.

IV—TROCHLEAR NERVE Superior oblique muscle (SO)—moves eye down and out	Have child look down and in (see Fig. 6-46).
V—TRIGEMINAL NERVE Muscles of mastication Sensory—face, scalp, nasal and buccal mucosa	Have child bite down hard and open jaw; test symmetry and strength. With child's eyes closed, see if child can detect light touch in mandibular and maxillary regions. Test corneal and blink reflex by touching cornea lightly (approach from side so that child does not blink before cornea is touched).
VI—ABDUCENS NERVE Lateral rectus (LR) muscle—moves eye temporally	Have child look toward temporal side (see Fig. 6-46).
VII—FACIAL NERVE Muscles for facial expression Anterior ⅔ of tongue (sensory)	Have child smile, make funny face, or show teeth to see symmetry of expression. Have child identify sweet or salty solution; place each taste on anterior section and sides of protruding tongue; if child retracts tongue, solution will dissolve toward posterior part of tongue.
VIII—AUDITORY, ACOUSTIC, OR VESTIBULOCOCHLEAR NERVE Internal ear Hearing and balance	Test hearing; note any loss of equilibrium or presence of vertigo.
IX—GLOSSOPHARYNGEAL NERVE Pharynx, tongue Posterior ⅓ of tongue Sensory	Stimulate posterior pharynx with a tongue blade; child should gag. Test sense of sour or bitter taste on posterior segment of tongue.
X—VAGUS NERVE Muscles of larynx, pharynx, some organs of gastrointestinal system, sensory fibers of root of tongue, heart, and lung	Note hoarseness of voice, gag reflex, and ability to swallow. Check that uvula is in midline; when stimulated with tongue blade, it should deviate upward and to stimulated side.
XI—ACCESSORY NERVE Sternocleidomastoid and trapezius muscles of shoulder	Have child shrug shoulders while applying mild pressure; with examiner's hands placed on shoulders, have child turn head against opposing pressure on either side; note symmetry and strength.
XII—HYPOGLOSSAL NERVE Muscles of tongue	Have child move tongue in all directions; have child protrude tongue as far as possible; note any midline deviation. Test strength by placing tongue blade on one side of tongue and having child move it away.

KEY POINTS

- To effectively establish a setting for communication, nurses must make an appropriate introduction, and ensure privacy and confidentiality.
- When communicating with parents, nurses need to encourage parental involvement, listen carefully, use silence, and be empathic.
- Communication with children must reflect their developmental stage.
- Nonverbal communication with children may take the form of writing, drawing, and play.
- The objectives of performing a health history are to identify pertinent information, determine the chief complaint, analyze the present illness, secure the patient's health history, review biologic systems, and record a family medical history and child psychosocial and sexual history.
- Family assessment is the collection of data about family composition and relationships among its members; it also focuses on home and community environment, parents' occupation and education, and cultural and religious traditions.
- Nutritional assessment is performed by determination of dietary intake, clinical examination, and biochemical analysis.
- Growth measurements during the physical examination focus on length or height, weight, skinfold thickness, and arm and head circumference. Assessment of growth is measured against standard growth charts to determine a child's status in comparison with other children of the same age.
- Measurements of temperature, pulse, respiration, and blood pressure constitute the physiologic approach to assessment.

- The general appearance of a child is a cumulative, subjective impression of physical appearance, state of nutrition, behavior, personality, interactions with parents and nurse, posture, development, and speech.
- Assessment of the skin, which primarily involves inspection and palpation, focuses on color, texture, temperature, moisture, and turgor. The nurse needs to be aware of both physiologic and ethnic factors that may affect these areas.
- In assessment of the lymph nodes, the nurse examines, by palpation, the part of the body in which the glands are located.
- The head is inspected for shape, symmetry, mobility, and muscle control.
- Examination of the eyes includes placement and alignment, inspection of external and internal structures, and vision testing.
- The ear examination encompasses placement and alignment, external and internal structures, and auditory testing.
- The lungs are examined by inspection, palpation, percussion, and auscultation.
- Auscultation is the most important procedure for examining the heart.
- Abdominal assessment follows an orderly sequence of inspection, auscultation, and palpation, since palpation may distort normal abdominal sounds.
- Examination of the genitalia may provoke anxiety in the child, and the nurse must avoid any transference of anxiety.
- Neurologic assessment addresses behavior; motor, sensory, and cerebellar function; reflexes; and cranial nerves.

REFERENCES

American Academy of Pediatrics: *Pediatric nutrition handbook,* ed 5, Elk Grove Village, Ill, 2004, The Academy.

American Academy of Pediatrics, Committee on Practice and Ambulatory Medicine, Section on Ophthalmology: Eye examination in infants, children, and young adults by pediatricians, *Pediatrics* 111(4):902-907, 2003a.

American Academy of Pediatrics, Committee on Practice and Ambulatory Medicine, Section on Otolaryngology and Bronchoesophagology: Hearing assessment in infants and children: recommendations beyond neonatal screening, *Pediatrics* 111(2):436-440, 2003b.

Bald M: Ambulatory blood pressure monitoring in children and adolescents, *Minerva Pediatr* 54(1):13-24, 2002.

Beevers G, Lip GYH, O'Brien E: ABC of hypertension blood pressure measurement, part I, Sphygmomanometry: factors common to all techniques, *BMJ* 322(7292):981-985, 2001.

Berry BE, Simons BD, Siatkowski RM, and others: Preschool vision screening using the MTI-Photoscreener, *Pediatr Nurs* 27(1):27-34, 2001.

Clark JA, Kieh-Lai MW, Sarnaik A, and others: Discrepancies between direct and indirect blood pressure measurements using various recommendations for arm cuff selection, *Pediatrics* 110(5):920-923, 2002.

Coats DK, Jenkins RH: Vision assessment of the pediatric patient: refinements, *Am Acad Ophthalmol* 1(1):1-12, 1997.

Craig JV, Lancaster GA, Williamson PR, and others: Temperature measured at the axilla compared with rectum in children and young people: systematic review, *BMJ* 320(7243):1174-1178, 2000.

Cunningham M, Cox EO: Hearing assessment in infants and children: recommendations beyond neonatal screening, *Pediatrics* 111(2):436-440, 2003.

Deadrick D, Boggess P: *Pediatrics on telephone line,* paper presented at the First Annual National Conference for Advanced Practice Nurses, New Brunswick, NJ, Nov 6-8, 1996, Rutgers University.

Desselle DD, Pearlmutter L: Navigating two cultures: deaf children, self-esteem, and parents' communication patterns, *Soc Work Educ* 19(1):23-30, 1997.

Gillman MW, Cook NR: Blood pressure measurement in childhood epidemiological studies, *Circulation* 92(4):1049-1057, 1995.

Goldman LR, Shannon MW: Technical report: mercury in the environment: implications for pediatricians, *Pediatrics* 108(1):197-205, 2001.

Halle C: Achieve new vision screening objectives, *Nurse Pract* 27(3):15-35, 2002.

Healthcare Product Comparison System: *Thermometers, electronic, infrared,* Plymouth Meeting, Penn, July 2004a, ECRI.

Healthcare Product Comparison System: *Thermometers, electronic, thermistor/thermocouple, patient,* Plymouth Meeting, Penn, July 2004b, ECRI.

Hedley AA, Ogden CL, Johnson CL, and others: Prevalence of overweight and obesity among US children, adolescents, and adults, 1999-2002, *JAMA* 291(23):2847-2850, 2004.

Hoge DR, Parette HP: Facilitating communicative development in young children with disabilities, *Transdisc J* 5(2):113-130, 1995.

Kuczmarski RJ, Ogden CL, Grummer-Strawn LM, and others: CDC growth charts: United States, *Adv Data* 314:1-27, 2000.

Livingstone MBE, Robson PJ, Wallace MW: Issues in dietary intake assessment of children and adolescents, *Br J Nutr* 92(Suppl 2):S213-S222, 2004.

Martin SA, Kline AM: Can there be a standard for temperature measurement in the pediatric intensive care unit? *AACN Clin Issues* 15(2):254-266, 2004.

Mattu GS, Heran BS, Wright JM: Comparison of the automated non-invasive oscillometric blood pressure monitor (BpTRU™) with the auscultatory mercury sphygmomanometer in a paediatric population, *Blood Pressure Monit* 9(1):39-45, 2004a.

Mattu GS, Heran BS, Wright JM: Overall accuracy of the BpTRU™—an automated electronic blood pressure device, *Blood Press Monit* 9(1):47-52, 2004b.

Murphy SP, Poos MI: Dietary reference intakes: summary of applications in dietary assessment, *Public Health Nutr* 5(6A):843-849, 2002.

National High Blood Pressure Education Program Working Group on High Blood Pressure in Children and Adolescents: The fourth report on the diagnosis, evaluation, and treatment of high blood pressure in children and adolescents, *Pediatrics* 114(2 Suppl 4th Rep):555-576, 2004.

National Institutes of Health, National Heart, Lung, and Blood Institute: *Update on the Task Force Report (1987) on high blood pressure in children and adolescents: a working group report from the National High Blood Pressure Education Program,* NIH Pub No 96-3790, Bethesda, Md, Sept 1996, The Institutes.

Nicklas TA, Demory-Luce D, Yang SJ, and others: Children's food consumption patterns have changed over 2 decades (1973-1994): the Bogalusa heart study, *J Am Diet Assoc* 104(7):1127-1140, 2004.

Park M, Lee D, Johnson GA: Oscillometric blood pressures in the arm, thigh, and calf in healthy children and those with aortic coarctation, *Pediatrics* 91(4):761-765, 1993.

Park MK, Menard SW, Yuan C: Comparison of auscultatory and oscillometric blood pressures, *Arch Pediatr Adolesc Med* 155(1):50-53, 2001.

Price V, Archbold J: What's it all about, empathy? *Nurs Educ Today* 17(2):106-110, 1997.

Reynolds WH, Scott B, Jessiman WC: Empathy has not been measured in clients' terms or effectively taught: a review of the literature, *J Adv Nurs* 30(5):1177-1185, 1999.

Roche AF, Guo S: The new growth charts, *Pediatr Basics* 94:2-13, 2001.

Rutenberg CD: Telephone triage, *Am J Nurs* 100(3):77-78, 80-81, 2000.

Seidel HM, Ball JW, Dains JE, and others: *Mosby's guide to physical examination,* ed 5, St Louis, 2003, Mosby.

Sullivan GH: Protecting patient's privacy, *RN* 60(6):55-56, 58-59, 1997.

Turnbull R: Skin assessment in children: a methodical approach, *Nurs Times* 96(41):33-34, 2000.

Vessey JA: Developmental approaches to examining young children, *Pediatr Nurs* 21(1):53-56, 1995.

Wall TC, Marsh-Tootle W, Evans HH, and others: Compliance with vision-screening guidelines among a national sample of pediatricians, *Ambul Pediatr* 2(6):449-455, 2002.

White SJ: Empathy: a literature review and concept analysis, *J Clin Nurs* 6(4):253-257, 1997.

Yegdich T: On the phenomenology of empathy in nursing: empathy or sympathy? *J Adv Nurs* 30(1):83-93, 1999.

Pain Assessment and Management in Children

EUFEMIA JACOB

CHAPTER OUTLINE

PAIN ASSESSMENT, 159
Behavioral Measures, 159
Physiologic Measures, 161
Self-Report Measures, 162
Multidimensional Measures, 164
**PAIN ASSESSMENT IN SPECIFIC
POPULATIONS, 165**
Pain in Neonates, 165
Children with Communication and
    Cognitive Impairment, 166
Cultural Issues in Pain Assessment, 171

Children with Chronic Illness and
    Complex Pain, 171
PAIN MANAGEMENT, 171
Nonpharmacologic Management, 171
Complementary Pain Medicine, 175
Pharmacologic Management, 175
    Patient-Controlled Analgesia, 178
    Epidural Analgesia, 183
    Transmucosal and Transdermal
        Analgesia, 184
    Timing of Analgesia, 187

Monitoring Side Effects, 188
Evaluation of Effectiveness of Pain
    Regimen, 189
Painful and Invasive Procedures, 191
Postoperative Pain, 191
Recurrent Headaches in Children, 192
Recurrent Abdominal Pain
    in Children, 192
Cancer Pain in Children, 193
Pain and Sedation in End-of-Life
    Care, 194

LEARNING OBJECTIVES

On completion of this chapter the
reader will be able to:
- Identify measures to assess pain in
  children.

- List various types of pain assessment
  tools for use with children.
- Outline essential pain management
  strategies to reduce pain in children.

- Review common types of pain
  experienced by children.
- Discuss evidence to support specific pain
  management strategies.

RELATED TOPICS and ADDITIONAL RESOURCES

 IN TEXT

Communication and Physical and
    Developmental Assessment of the Child,
    Ch. 6
Compliance, *Ch. 22*
Cultural and Religious Influences on Health
    Care, *Ch. 4*
Family-Centered Care, *Ch. 21*

Family-Centered Home Care, *Ch. 20*
Impact of Chronic Illness or Disability on the
    Child and Family, *Ch. 18*
Nursing Diagnosis, *Ch. 1*
Physical and Developmental Assessment of
    the Child, *Ch. 6*
Preparation for Diagnostic and Therapeutic
    Procedures, *Ch. 22*

 COMPANION CD

NCLEX Review Questions

evolve

evolve.elsevier.com/Wong/essentials/

NCLEX Review Questions
Skills—Calculating Safe Dosages for
    Children; Managing Pain
Nursing Care Plan—The Child in Pain
WebLinks

PAIN ASSESSMENT

Although the ability to measure pain in children has improved dramatically in recent years, assessment of pain in children continues to be complex and challenging. Children's ability to describe pain changes as they grow older and as they cognitively and linguistically mature (Box 7-1). Three types of measures—behavioral, physiologic, and self-report—have been developed to measure children's pain, and their applicability depends on the child's cognitive and linguistic ability.

BEHAVIORAL MEASURES

Distress behaviors, such as vocalization, facial expression, and body movement, have been associated with pain (Figs. 7-1 and 7-2). These behaviors are helpful in evaluating pain in

---

BOX 7-1

Developmental Characteristics of Children's Responses to Pain

YOUNG INFANT

Generalized body response of rigidity or thrashing, possibly with local reflex withdrawal of stimulated area

Loud crying

Facial expression of pain (brows lowered and drawn together, eyes tightly closed, mouth open and squarish)

No association demonstrated between approaching stimulus and subsequent pain

OLDER INFANT

Localized body response with deliberate withdrawal of stimulated area

Loud crying

Facial expression of pain or anger

Physical resistance, especially pushing the stimulus away after it is applied

YOUNG CHILD

Loud crying, screaming

Verbal expressions such as "Ow," "Ouch," "It hurts"

Thrashing of arms and legs

Attempts to push stimulus away before it is applied

Lack of cooperation; need for physical restraint

Requests termination of procedure

Clinging to parent, nurse, or other significant person

Requesting emotional support, such as hugs or other forms of physical comfort

May become restless and irritable with continuing pain

Behaviors occurring in anticipation of actual painful procedure

SCHOOL-AGE CHILD

May see all behaviors of young child, especially during actual painful procedure, but less in anticipatory period

Stalling behavior, such as "Wait a minute" or "I'm not ready"

Muscular rigidity, such as clenched fists, white knuckles, gritted teeth, contracted limbs, body stiffness, closed eyes, wrinkled forehead

ADOLESCENT

Less vocal protest

Less motor activity

More verbal expressions, such as "It hurts" or "You're hurting me"

Increased muscle tension and body control

Data from Craig KD, McMahon RJ, Morison JD, and others: Developmental changes in infant pain expression during immunization injections, *Soc Sci Med* 19(12):1331-1337, 1984; and Katz ER, Kellerman J, Siegel SE: Behavioral distress in children with cancer undergoing medical procedures: developmental considerations, *J Consult Clin Psychol* 48(3):356-365, 1980.

---

infants and children with limited communication skills. However, discriminating between pain behaviors and reactions from other sources of distress, such as hunger, anxiety, or other types of discomfort, is not always easy. These factors decrease the specificity and sensitivity of behavioral measures (Table 7-1).

Behavioral assessment is useful for measuring pain in infants and preverbal children who do not have the language skills to communicate that they are in pain, or in children with mental clouding and confusion that limit their ability to communicate meaningfully (McGrath, 1998). Behavior provides important information that cannot be obtained from self-report. Behavioral assessment may provide a more complete picture of the total pain experience when administered in conjunction with a subjective self-report measure. However, behavioral pain scales may be more time consuming than self-reports. These measures depend on a trained observer to watch and record children's behaviors such as vocalization, facial expression, and body movements that suggest discomfort.

Behavioral measures are most reliable when measuring short, sharp procedural pain, such as during injections or lumbar punctures. They are less reliable when measuring longer-lasting pain. In older children pain scores on behavioral measures do not always correlate with the children's own reports of pain intensity. The four most commonly used behav-

FIG. 7-1 ■ Full, robust crying of preterm infant after heel stick. (Courtesy Halbouty Premature Nursery, Texas Children's Hospital, Houston; photo by Paul Vincent Kuntz.)

FIG. 7-2 ■ The face of pain after heel stick. Note eye squeeze, brow bulge, nasolabial furrow, and widespread mouth. (Courtesy Halbouty Premature Nursery, Texas Children's Hospital, Houston; photo by Paul Vincent Kuntz.)

TABLE 7-1

Selected Behavioral Pain Assessment Scales for Young Children

AGES OF USE	RELIABILITY AND VALIDITY	VARIABLES	SCORING RANGE
OBJECTIVE PAIN SCORE (OPS) (HANNALLAH, BROADMAN, BELMAN, AND OTHERS, 1987)			
4 months–18 years	Concurrent validity with linear analog pain scale, Spearman's r—0.721 with scores 6 and 0.419 with scores <6 Interrater agreement, coefficient alpha—0.986 for one rater and 0.983 for the other Concurrent validity with CHEOPS, Pearson correlation coefficient—0.88 and 0.94	Blood pressure (0-2) Crying (0-2) Moving (0-2) Agitation (0-2) Verbal evaluation/body language (0-2)	0 = no pain; 10 = worst pain
CHILDREN'S HOSPITAL OF EASTERN ONTARIO PAIN SCALE (CHEOPS) (MCGRATH, JOHNSON, GOODMAN, AND OTHERS, 1985)			
1-5 years	Interrater reliability—90%-99.5% Internal correlation—significant correlations between pairs of items Concurrent validity between CHEOPS and visual analog scale (VAS)—0.91; between individual and total scores of CHEOPS and VAS—0.50-0.86 Construct validity with preanalgesia and postanalgesia scores—9.9-6.3	Cry (1-3) Facial (0-2) Child verbal (0-2) Torso (1-2) Touch (1-2) Legs (1-2)	4 = no pain; 13 = worst pain
NURSES ASSESSMENT OF PAIN INVENTORY (NAPI) (STEVENS, 1990)			
Newborn–16 years	Not tested by original author; later tested by Joyce, Schade, Keck, and others (1994) Interrater agreement—weighted kappa 0.37-0.80 Discriminant validity—statistically significant differences between preanalgesia and postanalgesia scores (p <.0001) Reliability—Cronbach alpha: 0.35-0.69	Body movement (0-2) Facial (0-3) Touching (0-2)	0 = no pain; 7 = worst pain
BEHAVIORAL PAIN SCORE (BPS) (ROBIEUX, KUMAR, RADHAKRISHNAN, AND OTHERS, 1991)			
3-36 months	Original article describes limited details of reliability and validity testing	Facial expression (0-2) Cry (0-3) Movements (0-3)	0 = no pain; 8 = worst pain
MODIFIED BEHAVIORAL PAIN SCALE (MBPS) (TADDIO, NULMAN, KOREN, AND OTHERS, 1995)			
4-6 months	Concurrent validity between MBPS and VAS scores—correlation coefficient 0.68 (p <.001) and 0.74 (p <.001) Construct validity using prevaccination and postvaccination scores with EMLA vs placebo—significantly lower scores with EMLA (p <.01) Internal consistency of items—significant correlations between items Interrater agreement ICC—0.95, p <.001 Test-retest reliability—0.95, p <.001	Facial expression (0-3) Cry (0-4) Movements (0, 2, 3)	0 = no pain; 10 = worst pain
RILEY INFANT PAIN SCALE (RIPS) (SCHADE, JOYCE, GERKENSMEYER, AND OTHERS, 1996)			
<36 months; children with cerebral palsy	Interrater agreement using intraclass correlation coefficient—0.53-0.83, p <.0001 Discriminant validity using Mann-Whitney U test with preanalgesia and postanalgesia scores—statistically significant (p <.001) Sensitivity—0.31-0.23 Specificity—0.86-0.90 Interrater reliability using 2-way cross tabulations and kappa statistics (r[87] = 0.94; p <.001) and kappa values above 0.50 for each category	0: Neutral face/smiling, calm, sleeping quietly, no cry, consolable, moves easily 1: Frowning/grimace, restless body movements, restless sleep, whimpering, winces with touch 2: Clenched teeth, moderate agitation, sleeps intermittently, difficult to console, cries with touch 3: Full cry expression, thrashing/flailing, sleeping prolonged periods interrupted by jerking or no sleep, screaming/high-pitched cry, inconsolable, screams when touched/moved	0 = no pain; 3 = worst pain

TABLE 7-1			
Selected Behavioral Pain Assessment Scales for Young Children—cont'd			
AGES OF USE	RELIABILITY AND VALIDITY	VARIABLES	SCORING RANGE
FLACC POSTOPERATIVE PAIN TOOL (MERKEL, VOEPEL-LEWIS, SHAYEVITZ, AND OTHERS, 1997)			
2 months–7 years	Validity using analysis of variance for repeated measures to compare FLACC scores before and after analgesia; preanalgesia FLACC scores significantly higher than postanalgesia scores at 10, 30, and 60 minutes ($p < .001$ for each time) Correlation coefficients used to compare FLACC pain scores and OPS pain scores; significant positive correlation between FLACC and OPS scores ($r = 0.80; p < .001$); positive correlation also found between FLACC scores and nurses' global ratings of pain ($r[47] = 0.41; p < .005$)	Face (0-2) Legs (0-2) Activity (0-2) Cry (0-2) Consolability (0-2)	0 = no pain; 10 = worst pain

FLACC Scale*

	0	1	2
Face	No particular expression or smile	Occasional grimace or frown, withdrawn, disinterested	Frequent to constant frown, clenched jaw, quivering chin
Legs	Normal position or relaxed	Uneasy, restless, tense	Kicking, or legs drawn up
Activity	Lying quietly, normal position, moves easily	Squirming, shifting back and forth, tense	Arched, rigid, or jerking
Cry	No cry (awake or asleep)	Moans or whimpers, occasional complaint	Crying steadily, screams or sobs, frequent complaints
Consolability	Content, relaxed	Reassured by occasional touching, hugging, or talking to; distractible	Difficult to console or comfort

*From Merkel SI, Voepel-Lewis T, Shayevitz JR, and others: The FLACC: a behavioral scale for scoring postoperative pain in young children, *Pediatr Nurs* 23(3):293-297, 1997. Used with permission of Jannetti Publications, Inc., and the University of Michigan Health System. Can be reproduced for clinical and research use.

ioral pain measures are the FLACC, CHEOPS, TPPPS, and PPPRS (see Table 7-1).

The **FLACC Pain Assessment Tool** is an interval scale that includes five categories of behavior: *F*acial expression, *L*eg movement, *A*ctivity, *C*ry, and *C*onsolability (Manworren and Hynan, 2003). It measures pain by quantifying pain behaviors with scores ranging from 0 (no pain behaviors) to 10 (most possible pain behaviors). The FLACC observational pain tool has been revised and validated to include behaviors specific to those with cognitive impairment (Malviya, Voepel-Lewis, Burke, and others, 2006). The revised FLACC includes an open-ended descriptor under each category to allow parents or caregivers to record individual pain behaviors. In 52 children (4 to 19 years) with cognitive impairment, interrater reliability was supported with intraclass correlation coefficients 0.76 to 0.90. Construct validity was demonstrated by the decrease in FLACC scores following analgesic administration (Malviya, Voepel-Lewis, Burke, and others, 2006).

The **Children's Hospital of Eastern Ontario Pain Scale (CHEOPS)** was developed in collaboration with experienced recovery room nurses who were queried as to what behaviors they most frequently observed to determine whether a child is in pain (McGrath, Johnson, Goodman, and others, 1985). Six categories of behaviors are identified: cry, facial, verbal, torso, touch, and legs. Scoring was devised as: 0 = behavior that is the antithesis of pain, 1 = behavior that is not indicative of pain and is not the antithesis of pain, 2 = behavior

indicating mild or moderate pain, and 3 = behavior indicating severe pain. The range of the total score is 4 to 13.

The **Toddler-Preschooler Postoperative Pain Scale (TPPPS)** is an observational scale developed for measuring postoperative pain in children ages 1 to 5 years (Tarbell, Cohen, and Marsh, 1992). It consists of seven items divided among three pain behavior categories: (1) vocal pain expression (verbal pain complaints—cry, scream, groan, moan, grunt), (2) facial pain expression (open mouth, lips pulled back at corners, squint, closed eyes, furrowed forehead, brow bulge), and (3) bodily pain expression (restless behavior).

The **Parent's Postoperative Pain Rating Scale (PPPRS)** is a scale that parents may use to rate their children's pain by noting changes in the frequency of a number of behaviors (Chambers, Reid, McGrath, and others, 1996).

PHYSIOLOGIC MEASURES

Physiologic measures are not able to distinguish between physical responses to pain and other forms of stress to the body (Sweet and McGrath, 1998). Profound physiologic changes often accompany the experience of pain. Physiologic parameters such as heart rate, respiratory rate, blood pressure, palmar sweating, cortisone levels, transcutaneous oxygen, vagal tone, and endorphin concentrations reflect a generalized and complex response to stress. They are not localized responses to pain, but they provide useful information about the general distress levels of children who are experiencing pain. Like behavioral scales, physiologic measures may be useful for infants and children who are not able to communicate verbally. The physiologic parameters provide indirect estimates of pain, and the presence and strength of pain can only be inferred from the changes in these parameters. Most of the studies on the physiologic parameters involved predominantly infants.

SELF-REPORT MEASURES

Although children who are 4 and 5 years old are able to use self-report measures (Table 7-2), their ability to use them may be influenced by the cognitive characteristics of the preoperational stage (Stanford, Chambers, and Craig, 2006). The child's thinking tends to be egocentric, concrete, and perceptually dominated. Simple, concrete anchor words, such as "no

TABLE 7-2
Pain Rating Scales for Children

PAIN SCALE, DESCRIPTION	INSTRUCTIONS	RECOMMENDED AGE, COMMENTS
FACES PAIN RATING SCALE* (WONG AND BAKER, 1988) Consists of 6 cartoon faces ranging from smiling face for "no pain" to tearful face for "worst pain"	*Original instructions:* Explain to child that each face is for a person who feels happy because there is no pain (hurt) or sad because there is some or a lot of pain. FACE 0 is very happy because there is no hurt. FACE 1 hurts just a little bit. FACE 2 hurts a little more. FACE 3 hurts even more. FACE 4 hurts a whole lot, but FACE 5 hurts as much as you can imagine, although you don't have to be crying to feel this bad. Ask child to choose face that best describes own pain. Record number under chosen face on pain assessment record. *Brief word instructions:* Point to each face using the words to describe the pain intensity. Ask child to choose face that best describes own pain, and record appropriate number.	For children as young as 3 years. Using original instructions without affect words, such as happy or sad, or brief words resulted in same range of pain rating, probably reflecting child's rating of pain intensity. For coding purposes, numbers 0, 2, 4, 6, 8, 10 can be substituted for 0-5 system to accommodate 0-10 system. FACES provides three scales in one: facial expressions, numbers, and words. Research supports cultural sensitivity of FACES for Caucasian, African-American, Hispanic, Thai, Chinese, and Japanese children.

0	1 or 2	2 or 4	3 or 6	4 or 8	5 or 10
No hurt	Hurts little bit	Hurts little more	Hurts even more	Hurts whole lot	Hurts worst

OUCHER (BEYER, DENYES, AND VILLARRUEL, 1992) Consists of 6 photographs of Caucasian child's face representing "no hurt" to "biggest hurt you could ever have"; also includes vertical scale with numbers from 0 to 100; scales for African-American and Hispanic children have been developed (Villarruel and Denyes, 1991)	*Numeric scale:* Point to each section of scale to explain variations in pain intensity: "0 means no hurt." "This means little hurts" (pointing to lower part of scale, 1-29). "This means middle hurts" (pointing to middle part of scale, 30-69). "This means big hurts" (pointing to upper part of scale, 70-99). "100 means the biggest hurt you could ever have." Score is actual number stated by child. *Photographic scale:* Point to each photograph and explain variations in pain intensity using following language: 1st picture from the bottom is "no hurt," 2nd is "a little hurt," 3rd is "a little more hurt," 4th is "even more hurt than that," 5th is "pretty much or a lot of hurt," and 6th is "biggest hurt you could ever have." Score pictures from 0 to 5, with bottom picture scored as 0. *General:* Have child practice using Oucher by recalling and rating previous pain experiences (e.g., falling off bike). Child points to number or photograph that describes pain intensity associated with experience. Obtain current pain score from child by asking, "How much hurt do you have right now?"	Children 3-13 years Use numeric scale if child can count to 100 by ones and identify the larger of any 2 numbers, or by tens (Jordan-Marsh, Yoder, Hall, and others, 1994). Determine whether child has cognitive ability to use photographic scale; child should be able to rate 6 geometric shapes from largest to smallest. Determine which ethnic version of Oucher to use. Allow child to select version of Oucher, or use version that most closely matches physical characteristics of child. Note: Ethnically similar scale may not be preferred by child when given choice of ethnically neutral cartoon scale (Luffy and Grove, 2003).

*Wong-Baker FACES Pain Rating Scale reference manual describing development and research of the scale is available from City of Hope Pain and Palliative Care Resource Center, 1500 East Duarte Road, Duarte, CA 91010, (626) 359-8111, ext. 3829; fax (626) 301-8941.

TABLE 7-2

Pain Rating Scales for Children—cont'd

PAIN SCALE, DESCRIPTION	INSTRUCTIONS	RECOMMENDED AGE, COMMENTS
POKER CHIP TOOL (HESTER, FOSTER, JORDAN-MARSH, AND OTHERS, 1998)		
Uses 4 red poker chips placed horizontally in front of child	Say to child: "I want to talk with you about the hurt you may be having right now." Align chips horizontally in front of child on bedside table, clipboard, or other firm surface. Tell child, "These are pieces of hurt." Beginning at chip nearest child's left side and ending at one nearest right side, point to chips and say, "This (1st chip) is a little bit of hurt and this (4th chip) is the most hurt you could ever have." For a young child or for any child who may not fully comprehend the instructions, clarify by saying, "That means this (1) is just a little hurt, this (2) is a little more hurt, this (3) is more yet, and this (4) is the most hurt you could ever have." Do not give children an option for 0 hurt. Research with Poker Chip Tool has verified that children without pain will so indicate by responses such as, "I don't have any." Ask child, "How many pieces of hurt do you have right now?" After initial use of Poker Chip Tool, some children internalize the concept "pieces of hurt." If child gives response such as "I have 1 right now," before you ask or before you lay out poker chips, record number of chips on Pain Flow Sheet. Clarify child's answer by statements such as "Oh, you have a little hurt? Tell me about the hurt."	Children as young as 4 years Determine whether child has cognitive ability to use numbers by identifying larger of any 2 numbers.
WORD-GRAPHIC RATING SCALE† (TESLER, SAVEDRA, HOLZEMER, AND OTHERS, 1991)		
Uses descriptive words (may vary in other scales) to denote varying intensities of pain	Explain to child, "This is a line with words to describe how much pain you may have. This side of the line means no pain, and over here the line means worst possible pain." (Point with your finger where "no pain" is, and run your finger along the line to "worst possible pain.") "If you have no pain, you would mark like this." (Show example.) "If you have some pain, you would mark somewhere along the line, depending on how much pain you have." (Show example.) "The more pain you have, the closer to worst pain you would mark. The worst pain possible is marked like this." (Show example.) "Show me how much pain you have right now by marking with a straight, up-and-down line anywhere along the line." With millimeter rule, measure from the "no pain" end to mark and record this measurement as pain score.	Children 4-17 years

No pain	Little pain	Medium pain	Large pain	Worst possible pain

NUMERIC SCALE		
Uses straight line with end points identified as "no pain" and "worst pain" and sometimes "medium pain" in the middle; divisions along line marked in units from 0-10 (high number may vary)	Explain to child that at one end of line is 0, which means that person feels no pain (hurt). At other end is usually 5 or 10, which means the person feels worst pain imaginable. The numbers 1-5 or 1-10 are for very little pain to a whole lot of pain. Ask child to choose number that best describes own pain.	Children as young as 5 years, as long as they can count and have some concept of numbers and their values in relation to other numbers Scale may be used horizontally or vertically Number coding should be same as other scales used in facility

No pain   Worst pain

0 1 2 3 4 5 6 7 8 9 10

†Instructions for Word-Graphic Rating Scale from Acute Pain Management Guideline Panel: *Acute pain management in infants, children, and adolescents: operative and medical procedures; quick reference guide for clinicians,* ACHPR Pub No 92-0020, Rockville, Md, 1992, Agency for Healthcare Research and Quality, US Department of Health and Human Services. Word-Graphic Rating Scale is part of the Adolescent Pediatric Pain Tool and is available from Pediatric Pain Study, University of California, School of Nursing, Department of Family Health Care Nursing, San Francisco, CA 94143-0606.

Continued

TABLE 7-2		
Pain Rating Scales for Children—cont'd		
PAIN SCALE, DESCRIPTION	INSTRUCTIONS	RECOMMENDED AGE, COMMENTS
VISUAL ANALOG SCALE (VAS) (CLINE, HERMAN, SHAW, AND OTHERS, 1992)		
Vertical or horizontal line that is drawn to certain length, such as 10 cm (4 inches), and anchored by items that represent extremes of the subjective phenomenon, such as pain, that is measured	Ask child to place mark on line that best describes amount of own pain. With centimeter ruler, measure from "no pain" end to the mark, and record this measurement as the pain score. 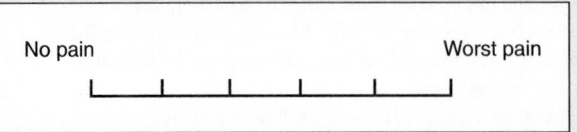	Children as young as 4½ years; preferably 7 years Vertical or horizontal scale may be used Research shows that children ages 3-18 years prefer VAS less than other scales (Luffy and Grove, 2003; Wong and Baker, 1988)
COLOR TOOL (ELAND AND BANNER, 1999)		
Uses markers for child to construct own scale that is used with body outline	Present 8 markers to child in random order. Ask child, "Of these colors, which color is like _____?" (the event identified by child as having hurt the most). Place the marker (representing severe pain) away from other markers. Ask child, "Which color is like a hurt, but not quite as much as _____?" (the event identified by child as having hurt the most). Place this marker with the marker chosen to represent severe pain. Ask child, "Which color is like something that hurts just a little?" Place the marker with the other colors. Ask child, "Which color is like no hurt at all?" Show the 4 marker choices to the child in order from worst to no-hurt color. Ask child to show on body outlines where he or she hurts, using markers chosen. After child has colored hurts, ask if they are current hurts or hurts from the past. Ask if child knows why the area hurts if it is not clear why it does.	Children as young as 4 years, provided they know their colors, are not color blind, and are able to construct the scale if in pain

hurt" to "biggest hurt," are more appropriate than "least pain sensation to worst intense pain imaginable."

The ability to discriminate degrees of pain in facial expressions appears to be reasonably established by 3 years of age (Stanford, Chambers, and Craig, 2006). **Faces pain scales** that were developed for young children may be a measure of pain intensity, pain affect, or both, particularly when the faces are anchored by a smiling face on one end and a face with tears on the other end (Chambers, Giesbrecht, Craig, and others, 1999; Chambers, Hardial, Craig, and others, 2005). Although clinicians may think that the smiling face anchor confounds the emotion of "feeling happy" with being "pain free," there is no evidence to support this notion. Researchers looked at the effects of the smiling face (e.g., the Wong-Baker [WB] FACES Pain Scale) vs the neutral anchor faces (e.g., Bieri Faces Pain Scale–Revised) on measurement of pain. Chambers, Hardial, Craig, and others (2005) demonstrated a high correlation between the two forms of faces scales, with r = 0.91 between the Bieri Faces (neutral anchor) and WB-FACES Pain Scale (smiling anchor). These data suggest that children are able to use either scale for communicating the amount of pain they experience.

MULTIDIMENSIONAL MEASURES

Several cognitive skills, such as measurement, classification, and seriation (the ability to accurately place in ascending or descending order), become explicit between approximately 7 and 10 years of age. Older children are able to use the 0 to 10 numeric rating scale that is currently used by adolescents and adults. However, the use of the 0 to 10 numeric rating scale is only an assessment of pain intensity, which may not change in some pain states (Jacob, Miaskowski, Savedra, and others, 2003a). Other dimensions such as pain quality, pain location, and spatial distribution of pain may change without a change in pain intensity.

Two multidimensional assessment tools have been well validated in children 8 years and older that assess not only pain intensity, but also pain location and pain quality. Modeled after the McGill Pain Questionnaire (Melzack, 1975), the **Adolescent Pediatric Pain Tool (APPT)** is a multidimensional pain instrument for children and adolescents that is used to assess three dimensions of pain: location, intensity, and quality (Fig. 7-3). The APPT is a one-page, two-sided instrument with a front and back body outline on one side (Savedra, Holzemer, Tesler, and others, 1993, 1989). On the back side is a 100 mm word-graphic rating scale (Tesler, Savedra, Holzemer, and others, 1991) and a pain descriptor list (Wilkie, Holzemer, Tesler, and others, 1990). Each of the three components of the APPT is scored separately. The body outline is scored by placing a clear plastic template overlay with 43 body areas on the body outline diagram. An estimate of the pervasiveness of the pain is made by counting the number of body areas marked. A ruler

Right   Left   Left   Right

Hips

FIG. 7-3 ■ Adolescent Pediatric Pain Tool: body outlines for pain assessment. Instructions: "Color in the areas on these drawings to show where you have pain. Make the marks as big or as small as the place where the pain is." Tool has been completed by a child with sickle cell disease. (From Savedra MC, Tesler MD, Holzemer WL, Ward JA, School of Nursing, University of California–San Francisco; copyright 1989, 1992.)

BOX 7-2

Manifestations of Acute Pain in the Neonate

PHYSIOLOGIC RESPONSES

Vital signs—Observe for variations.
- Increased heart rate or blood pressure
- Rapid, shallow respirations

Oxygenation
- Decreased transcutaneous oxygen saturation ($tcPo_2$)
- Decreased arterial oxygen saturation (Sao_2)

Skin—Observe color and character.
- Pallor or flushing
- Diaphoresis
- Palmar sweating

Laboratory evidence of metabolic or endocrine changes
- Hyperglycemia
- Lowered pH
- Elevated corticosteroids

Other observations
- Increased muscle tone
- Dilated pupils
- Decreased vagal nerve tone
- Increased intracranial pressure

BEHAVIORAL RESPONSES

Vocalizations—Observe quality, timing, and duration.
- Crying or whimpering
- Groaning

Facial expression—Observe characteristics, timing, orientation of eyes and mouth.
- Grimaces
- Brow furrowed
- Chin quivering
- Eyes tightly closed
- Mouth open and squarish

Body movements and posture—Observe type, quality, and amount of movement or lack of movement; relationship to other factors.
- Limb withdrawal
- Thrashing
- Rigidity or flaccidity
- Fist clenching

Changes in state—Observe sleep, appetite, activity level.
- Changes in sleep-wake cycles, feeding behavior, or activity level
- Fussiness, irritability
- Listlessness

or micrometer preprinted on the APPT is used to score the word-graphic rating scale. The number of millimeters from the left side of the scale to the point marked by the child is measured; and the numeric value provides an overall evaluation of the amount of pain the child is experiencing. The total number of words on the descriptor list is counted, and scores range from 0 to 56. The clinician then counts the number of words selected in each of three categories—evaluative, sensory, and affective—and calculates a percentage score for each one (Savedra, Holzemer, Tesler, and others, 1993).

The **Pediatric Pain Questionnaire (PPQ)** is a multidimensional pain instrument to assess patient and parental perceptions of the pain experience in a manner appropriate for the cognitive-developmental level of children and adolescents. The PPQ represents an attempt to assess the complexities of pediatric chronic, recurrent pain and targeted chronic musculoskeletal pain in children with juvenile rheumatoid arthritis. It consists of eight questions: (1) the pain history, (2) pain language, (3) the colors children associate with pain, (4) the emotions they experience, (5) their worst pain experiences, (6) the ways they cope with pain, (7) the positive aspects of pain, and (8) the location of their current pain. The PPQ includes three components: (1) visual analog scales; (2) color-coded rating scales; and (3) verbal descriptors to provide information about the sensory, affective, and evaluative dimensions of chronic pain (Varni, Thompson, and Hanson, 1987). It also has information about the child's and family's pain history, symptoms, pain relief interventions, and socioenvironmental situations that may influence pain. The child, parent, and physician complete the form separately.

PAIN ASSESSMENT IN SPECIFIC POPULATIONS

PAIN IN NEONATES

Assessment of pain in the preverbal child is difficult, especially in the neonate, since the most reliable indicator of pain, self-report, is not possible. Evaluation must be based on physiologic changes and behavioral observations (Box 7-2). Although behaviors such as vocalizations, facial expressions, and body movements are common to all infants, they vary with different situations. Crying associated with pain is more intense and sustained (see Fig. 7-1). Facial expression is the most consistent and specific characteristic; scales are available to systematically evaluate facial features, such as eye squeeze, brow bulge, open mouth, and taut tongue (Hadjistavropoulos, Craig, Grunau, and others, 1997). Most infants respond with increased body movements, but the infant may be experiencing pain even when lying quietly with eyes closed. The preterm infant's response to pain may be behaviorally blunted or absent; however, there is ample evidence that such infants are neurologically capable of feeling pain. In addition, infants in awake or alert states demonstrate a more robust reaction to painful stimuli than infants in sleep states. Also, an infant receiving a muscle-paralyzing agent such as vecuronium will be incapable of a behavioral or visible pain response.

Although regular use of pain assessment tools can assist caregivers in determining whether the infant is in pain, caregivers must consider the infant's maturity, behavioral state, energy resources available to respond, and risk factors for pain. In infants with diminished ability to respond robustly to pain, it is imperative to presume that pain exists in all situations that are usually considered painful for adults and children, even in the absence of behavioral or physiologic signs (Sweet and McGrath, 1998).

Several pain assessment tools have been developed for the assessment of pain in the neonate (Table 7-3). One pain assessment tool used by nurses who work with preterm and full-term infants in the neonatal intensive care setting is called **CRIES,** which is an acronym for the tool's physiologic and behavioral indicators of pain: *C*rying, *R*equiring increased oxygen, *I*ncreased vital signs, *E*xpression, and *S*leeplessness. Each indicator is scored from 0 to 2—similar to the Apgar score for neonates. The total possible pain score, representing the worst pain, is 10. A pain score greater than 4 should be considered significant. This tool has been tested for reliability and validity for postoperative pain in infants between the ages of 32 weeks of gestation up to 20 weeks postterm (60 weeks) (Sweet and McGrath, 1998).

The **Premature Infant Pain Profile (PIPP)** is unique because it has been developed specifically for preterm infants (Sweet and McGrath, 1998). The category "gestational age at time of observation" gives a higher pain score to infants with lower gestational age. Infants who are asleep 15 seconds before the painful procedure also receive additional points for their blunted behavioral responses to painful stimuli.

The **Neonatal Pain, Agitation, and Sedation Scale (NPASS)** was originally developed to measure pain or sedation in preterm infants after surgery. It measures five criteria (see Table 7-3) in two dimensions (pain and sedation) and may be used in neonates as young as 23 weeks of gestation up to infants 100 days old. Extra points are added in the pain scale dimension for preterm infants based on gestational age (Sweet and McGrath, 1998).

CHILDREN WITH COMMUNICATION AND COGNITIVE IMPAIRMENT

The assessment of pain in children with communication and cognitive impairment can be challenging. Children who have significant difficulties in communicating with others about

their pain include those with significant neurologic impairments (e.g., cerebral palsy), mental retardation, metabolic disorders, autism, severe brain injury, and communication barriers (e.g., critically ill children who are on ventilators or heavily sedated or have neuromuscular disorders, loss of hearing, or loss of vision). These children are at greater risk than other children for undertreatment of pain because they have medical problems that may cause pain during numerous painful procedures. Their behaviors include moaning, inconsistent patterns of play and sleep, changes in facial expression, and other physical problems that may mask expression of pain and be difficult to interpret (Hadden and von Baeyer, 2002). These children often experience spasticity, contractures, and orthopedic surgical treatment that may be painful.

The mother or primary caregiver is an important source of information during assessment (Breau, MacLaren, McGrath, and others, 2003). Up to 60% of parents of children with severe cognitive impairment reported that their child experienced pain or severe discomfort that was not being effectively managed (Lenton, Stallard, Lewis, and others; 2001; Stallard, Williams, Velleman, and others, 2002a). The most frequently reported pain behaviors are crying; being less active; seeking comfort; moaning; not cooperating; being irritable; being stiff, spastic, tense, or rigid; sleeping less; being difficult to satisfy or pacify; flinching or moving body part away; and being agitated or fidgety (Hadden and von Baeyer, 2002). Parents also reported pain during some daily living activities such as assisted stretching and walking, independent standing, toileting, putting on splints, occupational therapy, range of motion, and physical therapy.

Stallard, Williams, Lenton, and others (2001) asked the parents of cognitively impaired and noncommunicative children to assess the presence, severity, and duration of their pain during a 2-week observation period. Parents reported that 84% experienced pain on 5 or more separate days, with 32% experiencing pain on 12 or more days. Of the 74 episodes that lasted longer than 30 minutes, 33.8% occurred at night. Most pain episodes were judged to last longer than 10 minutes, with 48% of the children having episodes lasting longer than 10 minutes on 5 or more days. Although the experience of pain was common among this group of children, none was receiving treatment for relief or management of pain.

The **Non-communicating Children's Pain Checklist** is a pain measurement tool specifically designed for children with cognitive impairments (Breau, McGrath, Camfield, and others, 2002). The scale discriminates between periods of pain and calm and can predict behavior during subsequent episodes of pain (Fig. 7-4). The scale consists of six subscales (vocal, social, facial, activity, body and limbs, physiologic), which are scored based on the number of times the items are observed over a 10-minute period (0 = not at all; 1 = just a little; 2 = fairly often; 3 = very often).

Another tool, the **Pain Indicator for Communicatively Impaired Children (PICIC),** distinguishes between pain and nonpain in communicatively impaired children with life-threatening illness (Stallard, Williams, Velleman, and others, 2002a, 2002b). The PICIC has six core pain cues: (1) crying with or without tears; (2) screaming, yelling, groaning, or moaning; (3) screwed up or distressed looking face; (4) body appearing stiff or tense; (5) difficulty in comforting

Text continued on p. 171

TABLE 7-3

Pain Assessment Scales for Infants

AGES OF USE	RELIABILITY AND VALIDITY	VARIABLES	SCORING RANGE
POSTOPERATIVE PAIN SCORE (POPS) (BARRIER, ATTIA, MAYER, AND OTHERS, 1987)			
1-7 months	Not tested by original authors Later tested by Joyce, Schade, Keck, and others (1994) High interrater agreement (reliability); discriminant validity ($p <.0001$); reliability with high Cronbach alpha—0.79-0.88	Sleep (0-2) Flexion fingers/toes (0-2) Facial expression (0-2) Sucking (0-2) Quality of cry (0-2) Tone (0-2) Spontaneous motor activity (0-2) Consolability (0-2) Spontaneous excitability (0-2) Sociability (0-2)	0 = worst pain; 20 = no pain
NEONATAL INFANT PAIN SCALE (NIPS) (LAWRENCE, ALCOCK, MCGRATH, AND OTHERS, 1993)			
Average gestational age 33.5 weeks	Interrater reliability—0.92 and 0.97 Construct validity using analysis of variance between before, during, and after procedure scores—$F = 18.97$, df = 2.42, $p <.001$ Concurrent validity between NIPS and visual analog scale (VAS) using Pearson correlations—0.53-0.84 Internal consistency using Cronbach alpha—0.95, 0.87, and 0.88 for before, during, and after procedure scores	Facial expression (0-1) Arms (0-1) Cry (0-2) Legs (0-1) Breathing patterns (0-1) State of arousal (0-1)	0 = no pain; 7 = worst pain
PAIN ASSESSMENT TOOL (PAT) (HODGKINSON, BEAR, THORN, AND OTHERS, 1994)			
27 weeks of gestational age–full term	No reliability or validity discussed by original authors	Posture/tone (1-2) Respirations (1-2) Sleep pattern (0-2) Heart rate (1-2) Expression (1-2) Saturations (0-2) Color (0-2) Blood pressure (0-2) Cry (0-2) Nurse's perception (0-2)	4 = no pain; 20 = worst pain
PAIN RATING SCALE (PRS) (JOYCE, SCHADE, KECK, AND OTHERS, 1994)			
1-36 months	Interrater agreement—$r = 0.65$-0.84, $p <.0001$ Discriminant validity—statistically significant t-tests ($p <0.0001$)	0: Smiling, sleeping, no change when moved/touched 1: Takes small amount orally, restless, moving, cries 2: Not drinking/eating, short periods of cries, distracted with rocking or pacifier 3: Change in behavior, irritable, arms/legs shake/jerk, facial grimace 4: Flailing, high-pitched wailing, parents request pain medication, unable to distract 5: Sleeping prolonged periods interrupted by jerking, continuous crying, rapid and shallow respirations	0 = no pain; 5 = worst pain

Continued

TABLE 7-3

Pain Assessment Scales for Infants—cont'd

AGES OF USE	RELIABILITY AND VALIDITY	VARIABLES	SCORING RANGE
CRIES (KRECHEL AND BILDNER, 1995)			
32-60 weeks of gestational age	Concurrent validity between CRIES and POPS—0.73 (p <.0001, n = 1382); Spearman correlation between subjective report and POPS and CRIES—0.49 (p <.0001, n >1300) Discriminant validity using before and after analgesia scores—Wilcoxon sign rank test: mean decline of 3.0 units (p <.0001, n = 74) Interrater reliability using Spearman correlation coefficient—r = .72 (p <.0001, n = 680)	Crying (0-2) Requires increased oxygen (0-2) Increased vital signs (0-2) Expression (0-2) Sleepless (0-2)	0 = no pain; 10 = worst pain
PREMATURE INFANT PAIN PROFILE (PIPP) (STEVENS, JOHNSTON, PETRYSHEN, AND OTHERS, 1996)			
28-40 weeks of gestational age	Internal consistency using Cronbach alpha—0.75-0.59; standardized item alpha for 6 items—0.71 Construct validity using handling vs painful situations—statistically significant differences (paired t = 12.24, 2-tailed p <.0001, and Mann-Whitney U = 765.5, p <.00001) and using real vs sham heel stick procedures with infants ages 28-30 weeks of gestational age (t = 2.4, 2-tailed p <.02, and Mann-Whitney U = 132, p <.016) and with full-term boys undergoing circumcision with topical anesthetic vs placebo (t = 2.6, 2-tailed p <.02, or nonparametric equivalent Mann-Whitney U test, U = 145.7, 2-tailed p <.02)	Gestational age (0-3) Eye squeeze (0-3) Behavioral state (0-3) Nasolabial furrow (0-3) Heart rate (0-3) Oxygen saturation (0-3) Brow bulge (0-3)	0 = no pain; 21 = worst pain
SCALE FOR USE IN NEWBORNS (SUN) (BLAUER, GERSTMANN, 1998)			
0-28 days	No reliability; face validity, content validity, construct validity using extreme groups	Central nervous system state (0-4) Movement (0-4) Breathing (0-4) Tone (0-4) Heart rate (0-4) Face (0-4) Mean blood pressure (0-4)	0 = no pain; 28 = worst pain Average baseline score 10-14 Score of 2 represents normal or baseline value
NEONATAL PAIN, AGITATION, AND SEDATION SCALE (NPASS) (PUCHALSKI AND HUMMEL, 2002)			
Birth (23 weeks of gestational age) and full-term newborns up to 100 days	Interrater reliability using ICC—0.95 CI for preintervention and postintervention pain scale; 0.95 CI for preintervention and postintervention sedation scale Internal consistency (Cronbach alpha): Preintervention pain scale—0.75 and 0.71 raters 1 and 2 Postintervention pain scale—0.25 and 0.27 raters 1 and 2 Preintervention sedation scale—0.88 and 0.81 raters 1 and 2 Postintervention sedation scale—0.86 and 0.89 raters 1 and 2	Cry/irritability (0-2) Behavior/state (0-2) Facial expression (0-2) Extremities/tone (0-2) Vital signs—heart rate, respiratory rate, blood pressure, Sao₂ (0-2)	Pain score—0 = no pain; 10 = intense pain Sedation score—0 = no sedation; 10 = deep sedation

CRIES Neonatal Postoperative Scale*

	0	1	2
Crying	No	High pitched	Inconsolable
Requires oxygen for saturation >95%	No	<30%	>30%
Increased vital signs	Heart rate and blood pressure preoperative state	Heart rate and blood pressure increase <20% of preoperative state	Heart rate and blood pressure increase >20% of preoperative state
Expression	None	Grimace	Grimace/grunt
Sleepless	No	Wakes at frequent intervals	Constantly awake

*Neonatal pain assessment tool developed at the University of Missouri–Columbia (Krechel SW, Bildner J: CRIES: a new neonatal postoperative pain measurement score: initial testing of validity and reliability, *Pediatr Anaesth* 5:53-61, 1995). Copyright S Krechel, MD, and J Bildner, RNC, CNS, 1995. Used with permission.

Non-communicating Children's Pain Checklist — Postoperative Version (NCCPC-PV)

NAME:_____   UNIT/FILE #: _____   DATE:_____ (dd/mm/yy)

OBSERVER:_____   START TIME:_____ AM/PM   STOP TIME:_____AM/PM

How often has this child shown these behaviours in the last 10 minutes? Please circle a number for each behaviour. If an item does not apply to this child (for example, this child cannot reach with his/her hands), then indicate "not applicable" for that item.

| 0 = NOT AT ALL | 1 = JUST A LITTLE | 2 = FAIRLY OFTEN | 3 = VERY OFTEN | NA = NOT APPLICABLE |

I. Vocal

1. Moaning, whining, whimpering (fairly soft)	0	1	2	3	NA
2. Crying (moderately loud)	0	1	2	3	NA
3. Screaming/yelling (very loud)	0	1	2	3	NA
4. A specific sound or word for pain (e.g., a word, cry, or type of laugh)	0	1	2	3	NA

II. Social

5. Not cooperating, cranky, irritable, unhappy	0	1	2	3	NA
6. Less interaction with others, withdrawn	0	1	2	3	NA
7. Seeking comfort or physical closeness	0	1	2	3	NA
8. Being difficult to distract, not able to satisfy or pacify	0	1	2	3	NA

III. Facial

9. A furrowed brow	0	1	2	3	NA
10. A change in eyes, including: squinching of eyes, eyes opened wide, eyes frowning	0	1	2	3	NA
11. Turning down of mouth, not smiling	0	1	2	3	NA
12. Lips puckering up, tight, pouting, or quivering	0	1	2	3	NA
13. Clenching or grinding teeth, chewing, or thrusting tongue out	0	1	2	3	NA

IV. Activity

14. Not moving, less active, quiet	0	1	2	3	NA
15. Jumping around, agitated, fidgety	0	1	2	3	NA

V. Body and Limbs

16. Floppy	0	1	2	3	NA
17. Stiff, spastic, tense, rigid	0	1	2	3	NA
18. Gesturing to or touching part of the body that hurts	0	1	2	3	NA
19. Protecting, favoring, or guarding part of the body that hurts	0	1	2	3	NA
20. Flinching or moving the body part away, being sensitive to touch	0	1	2	3	NA
21. Moving the body in a specific way to show pain (e.g., head back, arms down, curls up, etc.)	0	1	2	3	NA

VI. Physiological

22. Shivering	0	1	2	3	NA
23. Change in color, pallor	0	1	2	3	NA
24. Sweating, perspiring	0	1	2	3	NA
25. Tears	0	1	2	3	NA
26. Sharp intake of breath, gasping	0	1	2	3	NA
27. Breath holding	0	1	2	3	NA

SCORE SUMMARY

Category	I	II	III	IV	V	VI	TOTAL
Score							

FIG. 7-4 ■ Non-communicating Children's Pain Checklist. (Reprinted with permission from Breau L, McGrath P, Finley A, and others: Psychometric properties of the Non-communicating Children's Pain Checklist revised, *Pain* 99[1-2]:349-357, 2002.)

Continued

USING THE NCCPC-PV

The NCCPC-PV was designed to be used for children, aged 3 to 18 years, who are unable to speak because of cognitive (mental/intellectual) impairments or disabilities. It can be used *whether or not* a child has physical impairments or disabilities. Descriptions of the types of children used to validate the NCCPC-PV can be found in: Breau, L.M., Finley, G.A., McGrath, P.J. & Camfield, C.S. (2002). Validation of the Non-communicating Children's Pain Checklist — Postoperative Version. *Anesthesiology, 96* (3), 528-535. The NCCPC-PV was designed to be used without training by parents and caregivers (carers), or by other adults who are not familiar with a specific child (do not know them well).

The NCCPC-PV may be freely copied for clinical use or use in research funded by not-for-profit agencies. For-profit agencies should contact Lynn Breau: Pediatric Pain Research, IWK Health Centre, 5850 University Avenue, Halifax, Nova Scotia, Canada, B3J 3G9 (lbreau@ns.sympatico.ca).

The NCCPC-PV was intended for use for pain after surgery or due to other procedures conducted in hospital. If short- or long-term pain is suspected for a child at home or in a long-term residential setting, the **Non-communicating Children's Pain Checklist — Revised** may be used. It can be obtained by contacting Lynn Breau. Information regarding the NCCPC-R can be found in: Breau, L.M., McGrath, P.J., Camfield, C.S. & Finley, G.A. (2002). Psychometric Properties of the Non-communicating Children's Pain Checklist—Revised. *Pain, 99,* 349-357.

ADMINISTRATION

To complete the NCCPC-R, base your observations on the child's behavior over **10 minutes**. *It is not necessary to watch the child continuously for this period*. However, it is recommended that the observer be in the child's presence for the majority of this time (e.g., be in the same room with the child). Although shorter observation periods may be used, the cut-off scores described below may not apply.

At the end of the observation time, indicate how frequently (how often) each item was seen or heard. This should not be based on the child's typical behavior or in relation to what he or she usually does. A guide for deciding the frequency of items is below:

> 0 = Not present at all during the observation period. (Note: If the item is not present because the child is not capable of performing that act, it should be scored as "NA").
> 1 = Seen or heard rarely (hardly at all), but is present.
> 2 = Seen or heard a number of times, but not continuous (not all the time).
> 3 = Seen or heard often, almost continuous (almost all the time); anyone would easily notice this if they saw the child for a few moments during the observation time.
> NA = Not applicable. This child is not capable of performing this action.

SCORING

1. Add up the scores for each subscale and enter below that subscale number in the Score Summary at the bottom of the sheet. Items marked "NA" are scored as "0" (zero).
2. Add up all subscale scores for Total Score.
3. Check whether the child's score is greater than the cut-off score.

CUT-OFF SCORE

Based on the scores of 24 children aged 3 to 18 (Breau, Finley, McGrath & Camfield, 2002), a **Total Score of 11 or more** indicates a child has **moderate to severe pain**. Based on unpublished data from this same sample, a *Total score of 6-10* indicates a child has **mild pain**. When parents and caregivers completed the NCCPC-PV in hospital for the study group, this was accurate 88% of the time. When other observers completed the NCCPC-PV, this was accurate 75% of the time. A Total Score of 10 or less indicates less than moderate/severe pain. This was correct in the study group for parents and caregivers 81% of the time, and for other observers 63% of the time.

USE OF CUT-OFF SCORES

As with all observational tools, caution should be taken in using cut-off scores, because they may not be 100% accurate. They should not be used as the only basis for deciding whether a child should be treated for pain. In some cases children may have lower scores when pain is present. For more detailed instructions for use of the NCCPC-PV in such situations, please refer to the full manual, available from Lynn Breau: Pediatric Pain Research, IWK Health Centre, 5850 University Avenue, Halifax, Nova Scotia, Canada, B3J 3G9 (lbreau@ns.sympatico.ca).

FIG. 7-4, cont'd ■ Non-communicating Children's Pain Checklist. (Reprinted with permission from Breau L, McGrath P, Finley A, and others: Psychometric properties of the Non-communicating Children's Pain Checklist revised, *Pain* 99[1-2]:349-357, 2002.)

or consoling; and (6) flinching or moving away if touched. The items are rated using a 4-point Likert scale (1 = not at all, 2 = a little, 3 = often, 4 = all the time).

CULTURAL ISSUES IN PAIN ASSESSMENT

A major challenge in the assessment and management of pain in children is the **cultural appropriateness** of pain assessment tools that have been validated only in Caucasian and English-speaking children. Observational scales and interview questionnaires for pain may not be as reliable for pain assessment as self-report scales in Hispanic children. In Chinese children who learned to read Chinese characters vertically downward and from right to left, the use of vertically oriented visual analog scales resulted in less error than horizontally oriented scales. Cultural background may therefore influence the reliability of pain assessment tools developed in a single cultural context (Bernstein and Pachter, 2003).

The **Oucher Pain Scale** (see Table 7-2), originally developed and validated as a self-report of pain intensity for Caucasian children 3 to 12 years old, now features culturally specific photographs with pictures of children who more closely match the physical characteristics of African-American and Hispanic children (Beyer and Knott, 1998). The Oucher Faces Pain Scale consists of six photographs on the right side and a 0 to 100 scale marked off in tens on the left side. The photographs show the face of one child with the pictures arranged to show increasing levels of discomfort. Each version has been tested primarily with children in the ethnic group (Caucasian, African American, Hispanic) depicted in the photographs. It has been used by children ages 3 to 12 years old. Children use the Oucher by selecting a photograph or number that most closely represents the level of pain intensity they are experiencing (Beyer and Knott, 1998). These tools address cultural issues in accuracy of pain assessment and were designed to promote cultural sensitivity and self-esteem for minority, non-Caucasian children.

CHILDREN WITH CHRONIC ILLNESS AND COMPLEX PAIN

Questionnaires and pain assessment scales do not always provide the most meaningful means of assessing pain in children, particularly for those with complex pain. Some children cannot relate to a face or a number that describes their pain and may not be able to isolate pain from other symptoms they are experiencing. In children with cancer, experiencing multiple symptoms makes it difficult to isolate the pain symptom from other symptoms. Rating the pain does not always accurately convey to others how they really feel (Woodgate and Yanofsky, 2004).

In children with chronic illness, particularly those with complex pain, the most important aspect during assessment is to develop a trusting relationship with the child and the family, so that a deeper understanding of the pain experience may be obtained. The pain experience may be complicated by pain processes that occur in the central nervous system (such as hyperalgesia, central sensitization, windup), by other symptoms (such as fatigue, nausea, vomiting, diarrhea, constipation) that accompany medical treatments, and by complications (such as infections, unexpected development of fistulas, typhlitis) from disease or treatments (Turner, 2005). The pain experience may interfere with the child's ability to eat, sleep, and perform daily activities and routines (Miaskowski and Lee, 1999; Morin, Gibson, and Wade, 1998).

Other important components of assessment include the onset of pain; pain duration or pattern; the effectiveness of the current treatment; factors that aggravate or relieve the pain; other symptoms and complications concurrently felt; and interference with the child's mood, function, and interactions with family (Turner, 2005). In addition to asking the child or parent when the pain started and how long the pain lasts, the nurse can assess variations and rhythms by asking if the pain is better or worse at certain times during the day or night. If the child has had pain for a while, the child or parent may know which medications and doses are helpful. They may also have found some nonpharmacologic methods that have helped. The nurse may ask the child or parent if there are activities, positions, and other events that may increase the pain. Pain may be accompanied by other symptoms such as nausea and poor appetite.

Other factors warranting careful assessment that may pose barriers to effective management include family issues and relationships, fears and concerns about addiction (see Community Focus box, p. 189), the clinician's and family's lack of knowledge about pain, inappropriate use of pain medications, ineffective management of adverse effects from medications, and the use of different pain interventions (Turner, 2005).

PAIN MANAGEMENT

Unrelieved pain may lead to potential long-term physiologic, psychosocial, and behavioral consequences (Goldschneider and Anand, 2003; Weisman, Bernstein, and Schechter, 1998). Management of pain should be a priority for all clinicians.

NONPHARMACOLOGIC MANAGEMENT

Pain is often associated with fear, anxiety, and stress (Kain, Mayes, Caldwell-Andrews, and others, 2006). A number of **nonpharmacologic techniques** (see Nursing Care Guidelines box), such as distraction, relaxation, guided imagery, and cutaneous stimulation, provide coping strategies that may help reduce pain perception, make pain more tolerable, decrease anxiety, and enhance the effectiveness of analgesics or reduce the dosage required (Rusy and Weisman, 2000). In addition, these techniques decrease the perceived threat of pain, provide a sense of control, enhance comfort, and promote rest and sleep (Greco and Berde, 2005). Although there is a paucity of research on the effectiveness of many of these interventions, the strategies are safe, noninvasive, and inexpensive, and most are independent nursing functions. Environmental and psychologic factors may exert a powerful influence on children's pain perceptions and may be modified by using psychosocial strategies, education, parental support, and cognitive-behavioral interventions. For children undergoing repeated painful procedures, cognitive-behavioral interventions are effective for decreasing anxiety and distress (McGrath and Hillier, 2003).

If the child cannot identify a familiar coping technique, the nurse can describe several strategies and let the child select the most appealing one. Experimentation with several strategies that are suitable to the child's age, pain intensity, and abilities is often necessary to determine the most effective approach. Parents should be involved in the selection process; they may be familiar with the child's usual coping skills and can help identify potentially successful strategies. Involving parents also encourages their participation in learning the skill with the child and acting as coach. If the parent cannot assist the

nursingcareguidelines

Nonpharmacologic Strategies for Pain Management

GENERAL STRATEGIES

Use nonpharmacologic interventions to supplement, not replace, pharmacologic interventions, and use for mild pain and pain that is reasonably well controlled with analgesics.

Form a trusting relationship with child and family.

Express concern regarding their reports of pain and intervene appropriately.

Take an active role in seeking effective pain management strategies.

Use general guidelines to prepare child for procedure.

Prepare child before potentially painful procedures, but avoid "planting" the idea of pain.

- For example, instead of saying, "This is going to (or may) hurt," say, "Sometimes this feels like pushing, sticking, or pinching, and sometimes it doesn't bother people. Tell me what it feels like to you."
- Use "nonpain" descriptors when possible (e.g., "It feels like heat" rather than "It's a burning pain"). This allows for variation in sensory perception, avoids suggesting pain, and gives the child control in describing reactions.
- Avoid evaluative statements or descriptions (e.g., "This is a terrible procedure" or "It really will hurt a lot").

Stay with child during a painful procedure.

- Allow parents to stay with child if child and parent desire; encourage parent to talk softly to child and to remain near child's head.
- Involve parents in learning specific nonpharmacologic strategies and in assisting child with their use.

Educate child about the pain, especially when explanation may lessen anxiety (e.g., that pain may occur after surgery and does not indicate something is wrong); reassure the child that he or she is not responsible for the pain.

For long-term pain control, give child a doll, which represents "the patient," and allow child to do everything to the doll that is done to the child; pain control can be emphasized through the doll by stating, "Dolly feels better after the medicine."

Teach procedures to child and family for later use.

SPECIFIC STRATEGIES

Distraction

Involve parent and child in identifying strong distracters.

Involve child in play; use radio, tape recorder, CD player, or computer game; have child sing or use rhythmic breathing.

Have child take a deep breath and blow it out until told to stop.

Have child blow bubbles to "blow the hurt away."

Have child concentrate on yelling or saying "ouch," with instructions to "yell as loud or soft as you feel it hurt; that way I know what's happening."

Have child look through kaleidoscope (type with glitter suspended in fluid-filled tube) and encourage him or her to concentrate by asking, "Do you see the different designs?"

Use humor, such as watching cartoons, telling jokes or funny stories, or acting silly with child.

Have child read, play games, or visit with friends.

Relaxation

With an infant or young child:

- Hold in a comfortable, well-supported position, such as vertically against the chest and shoulder.
- Rock in a wide, rhythmic arc in a rocking chair or sway back and forth, rather than bouncing child.
- Repeat one or two words softly, such as "Mommy's here."

With a slightly older child:

- Ask child to take a deep breath and "go limp as a rag doll" while exhaling slowly; then ask child to yawn (demonstrate if needed).
- Help child assume a comfortable position (e.g., pillow under neck and knees).
- Begin progressive relaxation: starting with the toes, systematically instruct child to let each body part "go limp" or "feel heavy"; if child has difficulty relaxing, instruct child to tense or tighten each body part and then relax it.
- Allow child to keep eyes open, since children may respond better if eyes are open rather than closed during relaxation.

Guided Imagery

Have child identify some highly pleasurable real or imaginary experience.

Have child describe details of the event, including as many senses as possible (e.g., "feel the cool breezes," "see the beautiful colors," "hear the pleasant music").

Have child write down or tape record script.

Encourage child to concentrate only on the pleasurable event during the painful time; enhance the image by recalling specific details through reading the script or playing the tape.

Combine with relaxation and rhythmic breathing.

Positive Self-Talk

Teach child positive statements to say when in pain (e.g., "I will be feeling better soon," "When I go home, I will feel better, and we will eat ice cream").

Thought Stopping

Identify positive facts about the painful event (e.g., "It does not last long").

Identify reassuring information (e.g., "If I think about something else, it does not hurt as much").

Condense positive and reassuring facts into a set of brief statements and have child memorize them (e.g., "Short procedure, good veins, little hurt, nice nurse, go home").

Have child repeat the memorized statements whenever thinking about or experiencing the painful event.

Behavioral Contracting

Informal—May be used with children as young as 4 or 5 years of age:

- Use stars, tokens, or cartoon character stickers as rewards.
- Give a child who is uncooperative or procrastinating during a procedure a limited time (measured by a visible timer) to complete the procedure.
- Proceed as needed if child is unable to comply.
- Reinforce cooperation with a reward if the procedure is accomplished within specified time.

Formal—Use written contract, which includes:

- Realistic (seems possible) goal or desired behavior
- Measurable behavior (e.g., agreeing not to hit anyone during procedures)
- Date and signature of all persons involved in any of the agreements
- Identified rewards or consequences that are reinforcing
- Goals that can be evaluated
- Commitment and compromise requirements for both parties (e.g., while timer is used, nurse will not nag or prod child to complete procedure)

child, other appropriate persons may include a grandparent, older sibling, nurse, or child life specialist (McGrath and Hillier, 2003).

Children should learn to use a specific strategy before pain occurs or before it becomes severe. Children are responsive to pain-controlling strategies that involve their imaginations and senses of play (Gerik, 2005). To reduce the child's effort, instructions for a strategy, such as distraction or relaxation, can be audiotaped and played during a period of comfort. However, even after they have learned an intervention, children often need help using it during a painful procedure. The intervention can also be used after the procedure. This gives the child a chance to recover, feel mastery, and cope more effectively (McGrath and Hillier, 2003).

Virtual reality has been identified as a potentially effective tool for pain distraction (Gold, Kim, Kant, and others, 2006). The participant's attention is drawn away from the "real world" and into the "virtual world" with the incorporation of visual, auditory, and tactile stimuli.

Several studies have documented the effectiveness of nonpharmacologic analgesia, such as containment, positioning, nonnutritive sucking (Fig. 7-5), and kangaroo holding during painful procedures in neonates. **Containment** is achieved through positioning and blanket rolls (Cole and Jorgensen, 1997). It provides a "nest" that enhances the infant's feelings of security and decreases stress. Comforting measures and **swaddling** have been demonstrated to reduce crying and heart rate after procedures such as heel punctures and injections. In infants between 27 and 34 weeks of gestational age, those infants who were swaddled after a routine heel stick procedure were able to calm crying immediately, decrease heart rate, and return to a sleep state; in comparison, infants who were not swaddled took a minimum of 10 minutes to return to baseline physiologic and behavioral levels (Fearon, Kisilevsky, Hains, and others, 1997). **Proper positioning** with the infant held in a midline orientation, hand to mouth activity, and proper flexion can promote self-soothing behaviors. **Facilitated tucking,** which is holding the infant's extremities

FIG. 7-5 ■ Sucking following oral sucrose can enhance analgesia before a heel stick in a preterm infant.

flexed and contained close to the trunk, during heel lance procedures has been demonstrated to decrease heart rate, decrease crying time, and promote stability in the sleep-wake cycles after the lance.

Nonnutritive sucking (pacifier) attenuates behavioral, physiologic, and hormonal responses to pain from procedures, such as heel punctures, venipuncture, and immunization injections. The administration of concentrated sucrose with and without nonnutritive sucking has been demonstrated to have calming and pain-relieving effects for invasive procedures in neonates (see Evidence-Based Practice box). The amount of time crying was decreased with the oral administration of 2 ml of a 12% to 24% sucrose solution, 2 minutes before a heel lance or venipuncture (Stevens, Yamada, and Ohlsson, 2005).

Kangaroo care is skin-to-skin holding of infants dressed only in diapers against their mother's or father's chest (Gray, Watt, and Blass, 2000; Johnston, Stevens, Pinelli, and others, 2003). Infants who spent 1 to 3 hours in kangaroo care showed increased frequency in quiet sleep, longer duration of quiet

EVIDENCE-BASED PRACTICE

Reduction of Minor Procedural Pain in Infants
Carol Turnage Carrier

ASK THE QUESTION	In newborns and infants, does sucrose provide adequate analgesia during minor painful procedures? Are the effects age dependent?

SEARCH FOR EVIDENCE

Search Strategies	Search selection criteria included English publications within past 10 years, research-based articles (level 3 or lower) on neonates or infants undergoing venipuncture or immunizations.
Databases Used	PubMed, Cochrane Collaboration, MD Consult, Joanna Briggs Institute, National Guideline Clearinghouse (AHQR), TRIP Database Plus, PedsCCM, BestBETs

CRITICALLY ANALYZE THE EVIDENCE
Venipuncture Versus Heel Lance for Blood Sampling. Four randomized controlled trials reviewed by the Cochrane Collaboration (Shah and Ohlsson, 2004) compared the efficacy and painfulness of blood sampling by venipuncture or heel lance in full-term neonates. The researchers

concluded that venipuncture performed by skilled phlebotomists results in less pain than heel stick for blood sampling. Decreased pain scores, cry duration, and mother's rating of infant's pain demonstrated venipuncture as the preferred method of blood collection.

Continued

EVIDENCE-BASED PRACTICE

Reduction of Minor Procedural Pain in Infants—cont'd

Glucose vs EMLA Cream for Venipuncture in Neonates

- In a randomized control, double-blind study (Gradin, Lenclen, Gajdos, and others, 2002) of 201 newborn infants, 99 received EMLA (lidocaine and prilocaine) and oral placebo and 102 were given 30% oral glucose and placebo on the skin. The 30% glucose group had significantly lower PIPP scores and duration of crying than EMLA group. Significantly fewer patients in the glucose group were scored on the PIPP as having pain or a score above 6 (19.3% compared with 41.7%). Glucose compared with EMLA for venipuncture pain.
- In a randomized control, double-blind study, Lindh, Wiklund, Blomquist, and others (2003) compared the pain response of 90 infants divided equally into EMLA plus 1 ml water by mouth as control placebo with treatment group given occlusive dressing plus 1 ml oral glucose (300 mg/ml). The combination of EMLA and oral glucose significantly reduced pain response associated with diphtheria-pertussis-tetanus immunizations in 3-month-old infants.

Sucrose for Minor Painful Procedures (Heel Lance and Venipuncture)

- One hundred fifty full-term newborns were randomly assigned to one of six treatment groups: (1) no treatment, (2) 2 ml sterile water placebo, (3) 2 ml 30% glucose, (4) 2 ml 30% sucrose, (5) 2 ml 30% sucrose with pacifier, and (6) pacifier alone. Results: The pacifier alone was more effective than sweet solutions, sweet solutions and pacifier were significantly more effective than the placebo, and sucrose and glucose were equally effective in lowering pain scores (Carbajal, Chauvet, Couderc, and others, 1999).
- Acharya, Annamali, Taub, and others (2004) studied 28 infants (mean gestation at birth of 30.5 weeks and postnatal age of 27.2 days) who received either 2 ml of a placebo of sterile water or 25% sucrose slowly over 2 minutes into the mouth by syringe 4 minutes before two routine venipunctures. Results: Behavioral state and difficulty and duration of venipuncture were not significantly different between the two liquids. Heart rate, crying times, and neonatal facial coding system scores were significantly lower in the treatment group.
- Abad, Diaz-Gomez, Domenech, and others (2001) compared oral sucrose with EMLA in a prospective randomized trial of 51 full-term newborn infants less than 4 days old receiving venipuncture. The 2 ml of 24% sucrose solution alone was the most effective analgesic compared with placebo (spring water), EMLA, or EMLA combined with 2 ml sucrose. The combination of EMLA and sucrose did not enhance the analgesic effects.
- In the Stevens, Yamada, and Ohlsson (2005) review, 21 randomized control trials met criteria for review, 11 with full-term infants and 9 with preterm infants, with 1 study including both populations (1616 infants; maximum postnatal age of 28 days after reaching 40 weeks corrected age). Heel lance was the most common procedure observed as the painful stimulus; three studies used venipuncture. Sucrose in a wide variety of dosages delivered by syringe or pacifier was found to decrease crying time, heart rate, facial action, and composite pain scores during venipuncture and heel lance. These reviewers recommend the use of sucrose in a range of 0.012 to 0.12 g (0.05 to 0.5 ml) of a 24% solution 2 minutes before a single heel lance or venipuncture for safe and effective pain relief. They also recommend concomitant use of other methods of pain relief, since some studies included use of pacifier, rocking, kangaroo care, or holding along with sucrose intervention.

Sucrose Compared with Glucose for Analgesia for Minor Pain (Heel Stick)

- Guala, Pastore, Liverani, and others (2001) evaluated the effects of three glucose solutions (5%, 33%, and 50%) compared with two sucrose solutions (33% and 50%) and a control (water). Twenty healthy newborn infants in each group received 1 ml of the placebo, glucose, or sucrose solution on the tongue right before heel stick. The main outcome, heart rate changes, did not reach significance in any group, although the rates were lower in the glucose group.

APPLY THE EVIDENCE: NURSING IMPLICATIONS
Sucrose
- Sucrose is effective in reducing pain response in infants 6 months and less undergoing minor acute painful procedures.
- Adverse effects such as hyperglycemia, aspiration, or necrotizing enterocolitis have not been reported with sucrose administered without additives.
- The most effective dose has been 24% solution given at least 2 minutes before a procedure.
- Doses of 50% to 75% have been effective for relieving pain during immunizations in infants up to 6 months of age, suggesting that higher concentrations may be required for older infants.
- Effective dose volumes range from 0.05 to 2 ml, with lower volumes used for low-birth-weight infants and larger volumes used for older infants.
- The analgesic effect of sucrose in combination with sucking a bottle or pacifier appears to be enhanced.
- Administration can be by labeled oral syringe, dipped pacifier, or bottle, depending on the infant's ability and age.
- The advantages of minimum wait time, low cost, and decreased risk of adverse effects were significant.

Glucose
- Glucose, 1 ml 30% given by syringe, is more effective than EMLA for venipuncture pain.
- Comparisons between sucrose and glucose have been inconclusive.

Topical Anesthetics
- EMLA is not as effective as either sucrose or glucose for venipuncture pain and takes 60 minutes for application before a procedure.

References

Abad F, Diaz-Gomez NM, Domenech E, and others: Oral sucrose compares favorably with lidocaine-prilocaine cream for pain relief during venepuncture in neonates, *Acta Paediatr* 90:160-165, 2001.
Acharya AB, Annamali S, Taub NA, and others: Oral sucrose analgesia for preterm infant venepuncture, *Arch Dis Child Fetal Neonatal Educ* 89:F17-F18, 2004.
Carbajal R, Chauvet X, Couderc S, and others: Randomised trial of analgesic effects of sucrose, glucose, and pacifiers in term neonates, *BMJ* 319(7222):1393-1397, 1999.
Gradin M, Lenclen R, Gajdos V, and others: Crossover trial of analgesic efficacy of glucose and pacifier in very preterm neonates during subcutaneous injections, *Pediatrics* 110(6):1053-1057, 2002.
Guala A, Pastore G, Liverani ME, and others: Glucose or sucrose as an analgesic for newborns: a randomized controlled blind trial, *Minerva Pediatrica* 53:271-274, 2001.
Lindh V, Wiklund U, Blomquist HK, and others: EMLA cream and oral glucose for immunization pain in 3-month old infants, *Pain* 104(1-2):381-388, 2003.
Shah V, Ohlsson A: Venepuncture versus heel lance for blood sampling in term neonates, *Cochrane Database Syst Rev* (4):CD001452.pub2; DOI: 10.1002/14651858.CD001452.pub2, 2004.
Stevens B, Yamada J, Ohlsson A: *Sucrose for analgesia in newborn infants undergoing painful procedures* (review), 2005. In Cochrane Neonatal Collaboration, retrieved March 6, 2007, from http://www.thecochranelibrary.com.

sleep, and decreased crying in the neonatal intensive care unit. They also cried less at the age of 6 months when compared with neonates who did not receive skin-to-skin contact. Significant differences were found in pain responses during heel lancing between infants who were kangaroo held and those who were not. In the study by Gray, Watt, and Blass (2000), heart rate increased by 8 to 10 beats/min in the kangaroo care group vs an increase by 36 to 38 beats/min in the control group of neonates who were swaddled in bassinets. Grimacing was 64% less, and crying was 82% less frequent.

In another study, infant responses to pain during heel lance procedures were compared using kangaroo holding (Fig. 7-6), with the neonate held upright at a 60-degree angle between the mother's breasts for maximal skin-to-skin contact (Johnston, Stevens, Pinelli, and others, 2003). A blanket was placed over the neonate's back, and the mother's clothes were wrapped around the neonate for 30 minutes before the lancing procedure, during, and at least 30 minutes after the heel stick. Another group remained in the isolette in a prone position, swaddled with a blanket and the heel accessible, for 30 minutes before the heel lancing procedure. Pain scores were significantly lower in kangaroo-held infants.

COMPLEMENTARY PAIN MEDICINE

Many terms are used to describe approaches to health care that are outside the realm of conventional medicine as practiced in the United States. **Complementary and alternative medicine (CAM),** as defined by the National Center for Complementary and Alternative Medicine, is a group of diverse medical and health care systems, practices, and products that are not currently considered part of conventional medicine (Myers, Stuber, Bonamer-Rheingans, and others, 2005). Although some scientific evidence exists regarding the efficacy of some CAM therapies, questions are yet to be answered through well-designed scientific studies, such as whether these therapies are safe and whether they work for the diseases or medical conditions for which they are used.

CAM therapies may be grouped into five classes:

1. **Biologically based**—foods, special diets, herbal or plant preparations, vitamins, other supplements
2. **Manipulative treatments**—chiropractic, osteopathy, massage
3. **Energy based**—Reiki, bioelectric or magnetic treatments, pulsed fields, alternating and direct currents
4. **Mind-body techniques**—mental healing, expressive treatments, spiritual healing, hypnosis, relaxation
5. **Alternative medical systems**—homeopathy; naturopathy; ayurvedic; and traditional Chinese medicine, including acupuncture and moxibustion

Current estimates of pediatric CAM use range from 10% to 15%, derived from children sampled at health care facilities, with chronic conditions, and/or from countries other than the United States. For the U.S. population, pediatric CAM use was estimated to be 31% to 84% (Myers, Stuber, Bonamer-Rheingans, and others, 2005; Rusy and Weisman, 2000). Those who used CAM were found in each age-group, and the mean age was 10.3 years. The majority used unconventional therapy for chronic, as opposed to life-threatening, medical conditions. The therapies that are increasingly used include herbal medicine, massage, megavitamins, self-help groups, folk remedies, energy healing, and homeopathy (Myers, Stuber, Bonamer-Rheingans, and others, 2005; Rusy and Weisman, 2000).

FIG. 7-6 ■ Mother using kangaroo hold with her newborn infant. Note placement of the infant directly on the mother's skin.

PHARMACOLOGIC MANAGEMENT

Nonopioids, including acetaminophen (Tylenol, Paracetamol) and nonsteroidal antiinflammatory drugs (NSAIDs), are suitable for mild to moderate pain (Table 7-4); **opioids** are needed for moderate to severe pain (Table 7-5). A combination of the two analgesics acts on the pain system on two levels: nonopioids primarily act at the peripheral nervous system and opioids primarily act at the central nervous system. The combination of NSAIDs and opioids provides increased analgesia without increased side effects. Several combinations, such as acetaminophen with codeine, may have increasing doses of the opioid but a constant dose of the nonopioid (Table 7-6). Before increasing the opioid, it may be preferable to increase the nonopioid component, for example, adding one regular-strength acetaminophen tablet (325 mg) to acetaminophen 300 mg with codeine 15 mg (Tylenol No. 2) before advancing to acetaminophen 300 mg with codeine 30 mg (Tylenol No. 3) or codeine 60 mg (Tylenol No. 4). However, if this approach is not successful, pain management will require a stronger opioid (see Table 7-5).

Oxycodone is available without a nonopioid in an immediate release and controlled release preparation (OxyContin). The oxycodone dose can be safely increased without the risk of toxicity from excessive acetaminophen use. Actions of various opioids differ. Morphine is considered the gold standard for the management of severe pain. When morphine is not a suitable opioid, drugs such as hydromorphone (Dilaudid) and fentanyl (Sublimaze) are effective substitutes. Although fentanyl is used as an anesthetic in the operating room, it is classified as an analgesic. It can be safely administered by nurses by the intravenous (IV), intramuscular (IM), transmucosal, and transdermal routes (Algren, Gursoy, Johnson, and others, 1998; Golianu, Krane, Galloway, and others, 2000).

TABLE 7-4

Nonsteroidal Antiinflammatory Drugs (NSAIDs) Approved for Children*

DRUG	DOSAGE	COMMENTS
Acetaminophen (Tylenol)	10-15 mg/kg/dose q 4-6 hr not to exceed 5 doses in 24 hr or 75 mg/kg/day, PO	Available in numerous preparations; nonprescription Higher dosage range may provide increased analgesia
Choline magnesium trisalicylate (Trilisate)	Children <37 kg (81.5 pounds)—50 mg/kg/day divided into 2 doses Children >37 kg (81.5 pounds)—2250 mg/day divided into 2 doses	Available in suspension, 500 mg/5 ml; prescription
Ibuprofen (children's Motrin, children's Advil)	Children <6 months—5-10 mg/kg/dose q 6-8 hr; maximum: 40 mg/kg/day	Available in numerous preparations Available in suspension (100 mg/5 ml) and drops (100 mg/2.5 ml); nonprescription
Naproxen (Naprosyn)	Children >2 years—10 mg/kg/day divided into 2 doses	Available in suspension (125 mg/5 ml) and several different dosages for tablets; nonprescription
Tolmetin (Tolectin)	Children >2 years—20 g/kg/day divided into 3-4 doses	Available in 200-mg, 400-mg, and 600-mg tablets; prescription

Data from: *Drug facts and comparisons*, Philadelphia, 2008, Lippincott Williams & Wilkins.

NOTE: Newer formulations of NSAIDs selectively inhibit one of the enzymes of cyclooxygenase (COX-2, which is responsible for pain transmission) but do not inhibit the other (COX-1). Inhibition of COX-1 decreases prostaglandin production, which is necessary for normal organ function. For example, prostaglandins help maintain gastric mucosal blood flow and barrier protection, regulate blood flow to the liver and kidneys, and facilitate platelet aggregation and clot formation. Theoretically, the COX-2 NSAIDs provide similar analgesic and antiinflammatory benefits with fewer gastric and platelet side effects than the nonselective agents. COX-2 NSAIDs are approved for use in patients older than 18 years of age.

*All NSAIDs in this table (except acetaminophen) have significant antiinflammatory, antipyretic, and analgesic actions. Acetaminophen has a weak antiinflammatory action, and its classification as an NSAID is controversial. Patients respond differently to various NSAIDs; therefore changing from one drug to another may be necessary for maximum benefit.

Acetylsalicylic acid (aspirin) is also an NSAID but is not recommended for children because of its possible association with Reye syndrome. The NSAIDs in this table have no known association with Reye syndrome. However, caution should be exercised in prescribing any salicylate-containing drug (e.g., choline magnesium trisalicylate) for children with known or suspected viral infection. Side effects of ibuprofen, naproxen, and tolmetin include nausea, vomiting, diarrhea, constipation, gastric ulceration, bleeding nephritis, and fluid retention.

Acetaminophen and choline magnesium trisalicylate are well tolerated in the gastrointestinal tract and do not interfere with platelet function. NSAIDs (except acetaminophen) should not be given to patients with allergic reactions to salicylates. All the NSAIDs should be used cautiously in patients with renal impairment.

TABLE 7-5

Dosage of Selected Opioids for Children

DRUG	APPROPRIATE EQUIANALGESIC	APPROXIMATE EQUIANALGESIC PARENTERAL DOSE	RECOMMENDED STARTING DOSAGE (CHILDREN <50 kg [110 pounds] BODY WEIGHT)* ORAL	PARENTERAL*
Morphine	30 mg q 3-4 hr	10 mg q 3-4 hr	0.2-0.4 mg/kg q 3-4 hr 0.3-0.6 mg/kg time released q 12 hr	0.1-0.2 mg/kg IM q 3-4 hr 0.02-0.1 mg/kg IV bolus q 2 hr 0.015 mg/kg q 8 min PCA 0.01-0.02 mg/kg/hr IV infusion (neonates) 0.01-0.06 mg/kg/hr IV infusion (child)
Fentanyl (Sublimaze) (oral mucosal form [Actiq])†	Not available	0.1 mg IV	5-15 mcg/kg; maximum dose: 400 mcg	0.5-1.5 mcg/kg IV bolus q 30 min 1-2 mcg/hr IV infusion
Codeine‡	200 mg q 3-4 hr	130 mg q 3-4 hr	1 mg/kg q 3-4 hr	Not recommended
Hydromorphone§ (Dilaudid)	7.5 mg q 3-4 hr	1.5 mg q 3-4 hr	0.04-0.1 mg/kg q 3-4 hr	0.02-0.1 mg/kg q 3-4 hr 0.005-0.2 mg/kg IV bolus q 2 hr
Hydrocodone and acetaminophen (Lorcet, Lortab, Vicodin)	30 mg q 3-4 hr	Not available	0.2 mg/kg q 3-4 hr	Not available
Levorphanol (Levo-Dromoran)	4 mg q 6-8 hr	2 mg q 6-8 hr	0.04 mg/kg q 6-8 hr	0.02 mg/kg q 6-8 hr
Methadone (Dolophine)	20 mg q 6-8 hr	10 mg q 6-8 hr	0.2 mg/kg q 6-8 hr	0.1 mg/kg q 6-8 hr
Oxycodone (Roxicodone, OxyContin; also in Percocet, Percodan, Tylox)	20 mg q 3-4 hr	Not available	2 mg/kg q 3-4 hr¶	Not available

Data from Acute Pain Management Guideline Panel: *Acute pain management: operative or medical procedures and trauma: clinical practice guideline*, AHCPR Pub No 92-0032, Rockville, Md, 1992, Agency for Health Care Policy and Research, Public Health Service, US Department of Health and Human Services; and Berde C, Albin A, Glazer J, and others: American Academy of Pediatrics report of the Subcommittee on Disease-Related Pain in Childhood Cancer, *Pediatrics* 86(5 pt 2):818-825, 1990. Codeine dosages from McCaffery M, Pasero C: *Pain: a clinical manual*, ed 2, St Louis, 1999, Mosby.

IM, Intramuscular; *IV*, intravenous; *PCA*, patient-controlled analgesia; *q*, every.

NOTE: Published tables vary in suggested doses that are equianalgesic to morphine. Clinical response is criterion that must be applied for each patient; titration to clinical response is necessary. Because there is not complete cross-tolerance among these drugs, it is usually necessary to use a lower than equianalgesic dose when changing drugs and to retitrate to response.

CAUTION: Recommended doses do not apply to patients with renal or hepatic insufficiency or other conditions affecting drug metabolism and kinetics.

*CAUTION: Doses listed for patients with body weight <50 kg (110 pounds) cannot be used as initial starting doses in infants <6 months of age. For nonventilated infants <6 months, the initial opioid dose should be about ¼ to ⅓ of the dose recommended for older infants and children. For example, morphine could be used at a dose of 0.03 mg/kg instead of the traditional 0.1 mg/kg.

†Actiq is indicated only for management of breakthrough cancer pain in patients with malignancies who are already receiving and are tolerant to opioid therapy, but it can be used for preoperative or preprocedural sedation and analgesia.

‡CAUTION: Codeine doses above 65 mg often are not appropriate because of diminishing incremental analgesia with increasing doses but continually increasing constipation and other side effects.

§For morphine, hydromorphone, and oxymorphone, rectal administration is an alternate route for patients unable to take oral medications, but equianalgesic doses may differ from oral and parenteral doses because of pharmacokinetic differences.

¶CAUTION: Doses of aspirin and acetaminophen in combination with opioid or nonsteroidal antiinflammatory drug preparations must also be adjusted to patient's body weight. Daily dose of acetaminophen should not exceed 75 mg/kg, or 4000 mg.

TABLE 7-6
Coanalgesic Adjuvant Drugs

DRUG	DOSAGE	INDICATIONS	COMMENTS
ANTIDEPRESSANTS			
Amitriptyline	0.2-0.5 mg/kg PO hs Titrate upward by 0.25 mg/kg q 5-7 days prn Available in 10- and 25-mg tablets Usual starting dose—10-25 mg	Continuous neuropathic pain with burning, aching, dysthesia with insomnia	Provides analgesia by blocking reuptake of serotonin and norepinephrine, possibly slowing transmission of pain signals Helps with pain related to insomnia and depression (use nortriptyline if patient is oversedated)
Nortriptyline	0.2-1.0 mg/kg PO AM or bid Titrate up by 0.5 mg q 5-7 days Maximum—25 mg/dose	Neuropathic pain as above without insomnia	Analgesic effects seen earlier than antidepressant effects Side effects include dry mouth, constipation, urinary retention
ANTICONVULSANTS			
Gabapentin	5 mg/kg PO hs Increase to bid on day 2, tid on day 3 Maximum—300 mg/day	Neuropathic pain	Mechanism of action unknown Side effects include sedation, ataxia, nystagmus, dizziness
Carbamazepine	*<6 years:* 2.5-5 mg/kg PO bid initially Increase 20 mg/kg/24 hr, divide bid every week prn Maximum—100 mg bid *6-12 years:* 5 mg/kg PO bid initially Increase 10 mg/kg/24 hr, divide bid every week prn to usual maximum—100 mg bid *>12 years:* 200 mg PO bid initially Increase 200 mg/24 hr, divide bid every week prn to maximum—1.6-2.4 g/24 hr	Sharp, lancinating neuropathic pain Peripheral neuropathies Phantom limb pain	Similar analgesic effect to amitriptyline Monitor blood levels for toxicity only Side effects include decreased blood counts, ataxia, gastrointestinal irritation
ANXIOLYTICS			
Lorazepam	0.03-0.1 mg/kg q 4-6 hr PO or IV Maximum—2 mg/dose	Muscle spasm Anxiety	May increase sedation in combination with opioids Can cause depression with prolonged use
Diazepam	0.1-0.3 mg/kg q 4-6 hr PO or IV Maximum—10 mg/dose		
CORTICOSTEROIDS			
Dexamethasone	Dose dependent on clinical situation; higher bolus doses in cord compression, then lower daily dose Try to wean to NSAIDs if pain allows Cerebral edema—1-2 mg/kg load then 1-1.5 mg/kg/day divided q 6 hr Maximum—4 mg/dose Antiinflammatory—0.08-0.3 mg/kg/day divided q 6-12 hr	Pain from increased intracranial pressure Bony metastasis Spinal or nerve compression	Side effects include edema, gastrointestinal irritation, increased weight, acne Use gastroprotectants such as H_2-blockers (ranitidine) or proton pump inhibitors such as omeprazole for long-term administration of steroids or NSAIDs in end-stage cancer with bony pain
OTHERS			
Clonidine	2-4 mcg/kg PO q 4-6 hr May also use a 100 mcg transdermal patch q 7 days for patients >40 kg (88 pounds)	Neuropathic pain Lancinating, sharp, electrical, shooting pain Phantom limb pain	α_2-Adenoreceptor agonist modulates ascending pain sensations Routes of administration: oral, transdermal, and spinal Management of withdrawal symptoms Monitor for orthostatic hypertension, decreased heart rate Sedation common

bid, Twice a day; *hs*, at bedtime; *IV*, intravenous; *NSAIDs*, nonsteroidal antiinflammatory drugs; *PO*, by mouth; *prn*, as needed; *q*, every; *tid*, three times a day.

Continued

TABLE 7-6

Coanalgesic Adjuvant Drugs—cont'd

DRUG	DOSAGE	INDICATIONS	COMMENTS
OTHERS—cont'd			
Mexiletine	2-3 mg/kg/dose PO tid, may titrate 0.5 mg/kg q 2-3 wk prn Maximum—300 mg/dose		Similar to lidocaine, longer acting Stabilizes sodium conduction in nerve cells, reduces neuronal firing Can enhance action of opioids, antidepressants, anticonvulsants Side effects include dizziness, ataxia, nausea, vomiting May measure blood levels for toxicity

bid, Twice a day; *hs,* at bedtime; *IV,* intravenous; *NSAIDs,* nonsteroidal antiinflammatory drugs; *PO,* by mouth; *prn,* as needed; *q,* every; *tid,* three times a day.

Several drugs, known as **coanalgesics** or **adjuvant analgesics,** may be used alone or with opioids to control pain symptoms and opioid side effects. Drugs frequently used to relieve anxiety, cause sedation, and provide amnesia are diazepam (Valium) and midazolam (Versed); however, these drugs are not analgesics and should be used to enhance the effects of analgesics, not as a substitute for analgesics. Other adjuvants include tricyclic antidepressants (e.g., amitriptyline, imipramine) and antiepileptics (e.g., gabapentin, carbamazepine, clonazepam) for neuropathic pain (see Table 7-6), stool softeners and laxatives for constipation, antiemetics for nausea and vomiting, diphenhydramine for itching, steroids for inflammation and bone pain, and dextroamphetamine and caffeine for possible increased analgesia and decreased sedation (Table 7-7) (Greco and Berde, 2005).

The use of **placebos** to determine whether the patient is having pain is unjustified and unethical; a positive response to a placebo, such as a saline injection, is common in patients who have a documented organic basis for pain. Therefore the deceptive use of placebos does not provide useful information about the presence or severity of pain. The use of placebos can cause side effects similar to those of opioids, can destroy the patient's trust in the health care staff, and raises serious ethical and legal questions. The American Society for Pain Management Nursing has issued a position statement against the use of placebos to treat pain (McCaffery and Pasero, 1999).

NURSING ALERT

The optimum dosage of an analgesic is one that controls pain without causing severe side effects. This usually requires titration, the gradual adjustment of drug dosage (usually by increasing the dose) until optimum pain relief without excessive sedation is achieved. Dosage recommendations are only safe initial dosages (see Tables 7-6 and 7-7), not optimum dosages.

Children (except infants younger than about 3 to 6 months) metabolize drugs more rapidly than adults; younger children may require higher doses of opioids to achieve the same analgesic effect. Therefore the therapeutic effect and duration of analgesia vary. Children's dosages are usually calculated according to body weight, except in children with a weight greater than 50 kg (110 pounds), where the weight formula may exceed the average adult dosage. In this case the adult dosage is used.

A reasonable starting dose of opioid for infants under 6 months who are not mechanically ventilated is one fourth to one third of the recommended starting dose for older children. The infant is monitored closely for signs of pain relief and respiratory depression. The dose is titrated to effect. Because tolerance can develop rapidly, large doses may be needed for continued severe pain (Greco and Berde, 2005). If pain relief is inadequate, the initial dose is increased (usually by 25% to 50% if pain is moderate, or by 50% to 100% if pain is severe) to provide greater analgesic effectiveness. Decreasing the interval between doses may also provide more continuous pain relief. A major difference between opioids and nonopioids is that nonopioids have a **ceiling effect,** which means that doses higher than the recommended dose will not produce greater pain relief. Opioids do not have a ceiling effect other than that imposed by side effects; therefore larger dosages can be safely given for increasing severity of pain.

Parenteral and oral dosages of opioids are not the same. Because of the **first-pass effect,** an oral opioid is rapidly absorbed from the gastrointestinal tract and is partially metabolized in the liver before reaching the central circulation. Therefore oral dosages must be larger to compensate for the partial loss of analgesic potency to achieve **equianalgesia** (equal analgesic effect). Conversion factors (Table 7-8) for selected opioids must be used when a change is made from IV (preferred) or IM to oral administration. Immediate conversion from IM or IV to the suggested equianalgesic oral dose may result in a substantial error. For example, the dose may be significantly more or less than what the child requires. Small changes ensure small errors. Several routes of analgesic administration can be used (Box 7-3); the most effective and least traumatic should be selected.

Patient-Controlled Analgesia

A significant advance in the administration of IV, epidural, or subcutaneous analgesics is the use of patient-controlled analgesia (PCA). As the name implies, the patient controls the amount and frequency of the analgesic, which is typically delivered through a special infusion device. Children who are physically able to "push a button" (i.e., 5 to 6 years of age) and who can understand the concept of pushing a button to obtain pain relief can use PCA (Maxwell and Yaster, 2000). Although it is controversial, parents and nurses have used the IV PCA system for the child. Nurses can efficiently use the infusion device on a

Text continued on p. 183

TABLE 7-7

Management of Opioid Side Effects

SIDE EFFECT	ADJUVANT DRUGS	NONPHARMACOLOGIC TECHNIQUES
Constipation	**Senna and docusate sodium** *Tablet:* 2-6 years—Start with ½ tablet once a day; maximum: 1 tablet bid 6-12 years—Start with 1 tablet once a day; maximum: 2 tablets bid >12 years—Start with 2 tablets once a day; maximum: 4 tablets bid *Liquid:* 1 month–1 year: 1.25-5 ml hs 1-5 years—2.5-5 ml hs 5-15 years—5-10 ml hs >15 years—10-25 ml hs **Casanthranol and docusate sodium** *Liquid*—5-15 ml hs *Capsules*—1 cap PO hs **Bisacodyl**—PO or PR 3-12 years—5 mg/dose/day >12 years—10-15 mg/dose/day **Lactulose** 7.5 ml/day after breakfast Adult—15-30 ml/day PO **Mineral oil**—1-2 tsp/day PO **Magnesium citrate** <6 years—2-4 ml/kg PO once 6-12 years—100-150 ml PO once >12 years—150-300 ml PO once **Milk of Magnesia** <2 years—0.5 ml/kg PO once 2-5 years—5-15 ml/day PO once 6-12 years—15-30 ml PO once >12 years—30-60 ml PO once	Increase water intake Prune juice, bran cereal, vegetables Exercise
Sedation	**Caffeine**—single dose of 1-1.5 mg PO **Dextroamphetamine**—2.5-5 mg PO in AM and early afternoon **Methylphenidate**—2.5-5 mg PO in AM and early afternoon Consider opioid switch if sedation is persistent	Caffeinated drinks (e.g., Mountain Dew, cola drinks)
Nausea, vomiting	**Promethazine**—0.5 mg/kg q 4-6 hr; maximum: 25 mg/dose **Ondansetron**—0.1-0.15 mg/kg IV or PO q 4 hr; maximum: 8 mg/dose **Granisetron**—10-40 mcg/kg q 2-4 hr; maximum: 1 mg/dose **Droperidol**—0.05-0.06 mg/kg IV q 4-6 hr; can be very sedating	Imagery, relaxation Deep, slow breathing
Pruritus	**Diphenhydramine**—1 mg/kg IV or PO q 4-6 hr prn; maximum: 25 mg/dose **Hydroxyzine**—0.6 mg/kg PO q 6 hr; maximum: 50 mg/dose **Naloxone**—0.5 mcg/kg q 2 min until pruritus improves (diluted in solution of 0.1 mg naloxone per 10 ml saline) **Butorphanol**—0.3-0.5 mg/kg IV (use cautiously in opioid-tolerant children; may cause withdrawal symptoms); maximum: 2 mg/dose because mixed agonist-antagonist	Oatmeal baths, good hygiene Exclude other causes of itching Change opioids
Respiratory depression: mild to moderate	Hold dose of opioid Reduce subsequent doses by 25%	Arouse gently, give oxygen, encourage to deep breathe
Respiratory depression: severe	**Naloxone** *During disease pain management:* 0.5 mcg/kg in 2 min increments until breathing improves (American Pain Society, 1999; McCaffery and Pasero, 1999) Reduce opioid dose if possible Consider opioid switch *During sedation for procedures:* 5-10 mcg/kg until breathing improves (Yaster, Krance, Kaplan, and others, 1997) Reduce opioid dose if possible Consider opioid switch	Oxygen, bag and mask if indicated

bid, Twice a day; *hs*, at bedtime; *IV*, intravenous; *PO*, by mouth; *PR*, by rectum; *prn*, as needed; *q*, every; *tid*, three times a day.

Continued

TABLE 7-7

Management of Opioid Side Effects—cont'd

SIDE EFFECT	ADJUVANT DRUGS	NONPHARMACOLOGIC TECHNIQUES
Dysphoria, confusion, hallucinations	Evaluate medications; eliminate adjuvant medications with central nervous system effects as symptoms allow Consider opioid switch if possible **Haloperidol** (Haldol)—0.05-0.15 mg/kg/day divided in 2-3 doses; maximum: 2-4 mg/day	Rule out other physiologic causes
Urinary retention	Evaluate medications; eliminate adjuvant medications with anticholinergic effects (e.g., antihistamines, tricyclic antidepressants) Occurs with spinal analgesia more frequently than with systemic opioid use **Oxybutynin** 1 year—1 mg tid 1-2 years—2 mg tid 2-3 years—3 mg tid 4-5 years—4 mg tid >5 years—5 mg tid	Rule out other physiologic causes In/out or indwelling urinary catheter

bid, Twice a day; *hs*, at bedtime; *IV*, intravenous; *PO*, by mouth; *PR*, by rectum; *prn*, as needed; *q*, every; *tid*, three times a day.

TABLE 7-8

Equianalgesia of Selected Analgesics

DRUG*	EQUAL TO ORAL MORPHINE (mg)	EQUAL TO IM OR IV MORPHINE (mg)
Hydromorphone (Dilaudid) 1 mg	4	1.3
Codeine 30 mg	4.5	1.5
Meperidine (Demerol) 50 mg	4.8	1.6
Codeine 30 mg, acetaminophen 300 mg (Tylenol No. 3)	7.2	2.4
Oxycodone 5 mg, acetaminophen 325 mg (Percocet)	7.2	2.4
Oxycodone 5 mg, aspirin 325 mg (Percodan)	7.2	2.4
Hydrocodone 5 mg, acetaminophen 500 mg (Vicodin, Lortab)	9	3
Oxycodone 5 mg, acetaminophen 500 mg (Tylox)	9	3
Methadone (Dolophine) 10 mg	15	7.5
Acetaminophen 325 mg (Tylenol)	2.7	0.9
Aspirin 325 mg	2.7	0.9
Acetaminophen 500 mg (Tylenol Extra Strength)	4	1.3
Codeine 60 mg, +acetaminophen 300 mg (Tylenol No. 4)	11.7	3.9
Fentanyl transdermal patch (Duragesic) (based on 25 mcg/hr patch applied q 3 days = 50 mg oral morphine q 24 hr or divided into 6 doses = 8.3 mg) or use:	8.3	2.77

RECOMMENDED INITIAL DURAGESIC DOSE BASED ON DAILY ORAL MORPHINE DOSE†

ORAL 24-HOUR MORPHINE (mg/day)	DURAGESIC DOSE (mg/hr)
45-134	25
135-224	50
225-314	75
315-404	100
405-494	125
495-584	150
585-674	175
675-764	200
765-854	225
855-944	250
945-1034	275
1035-1124	300

Courtesy Betty R. Ferrell, PhD, FAAN, 1999. Used with permission.

IM, Intramuscular; *IV*, intravenous; *q*, every.

NOTE: When converting to oral oxycodone from oral morphine, an appropriate conservative estimate is 15-20 mg oxycodone per 30 mg morphine; however, when converting to oral morphine from oral oxycodone, an appropriate conservative estimate is 30 mg morphine per 30 mg oxycodone (McCaffery M, Pasero C: *Pain: a clinical manual*, ed 2, St Louis, 1999, Mosby).

*Oral medication with exception of fentanyl.

†Data from Duragesic package insert, Janssen Pharmaceutical Products, Titusville, NJ, 2001.

BOX 7-3

Routes and Methods of Analgesic Drug Administration

ORAL

Oral route preferred because of convenience, cost, and relatively steady blood levels

Higher dosages of oral form of opioids required for equivalent parenteral analgesia

Peak drug effect after 1 to 2 hours for most analgesics

Delay in onset a disadvantage when rapid control of severe pain or of fluctuating pain is desired

SUBLINGUAL, BUCCAL, OR TRANSMUCOSAL

Tablet or liquid placed between cheek and gum (buccal) or under tongue (sublingual)

Highly desirable because more rapid onset than oral route

- Produced less first-pass effect through liver than oral route, which normally reduces analgesia from oral opioids (unless sublingual or buccal form is swallowed, which occurs often in children)

Few drugs commercially available in this form

Many drugs able to be compounded into sublingual troche or lozenge*

Actiq—Oral transmucosal fentanyl citrate in hard confection base on a plastic holder; indicated only for management of breakthrough cancer pain in patients with malignancies who are already receiving and are tolerant to opioid therapy, but can be used for preoperative or preprocedural sedation and analgesia

INTRAVENOUS (IV) (BOLUS)

Preferred for rapid control of severe pain

Provides most rapid onset of effect, usually in about 5 minutes

Advantage for acute pain, procedural pain, and breakthrough pain

Needs to be repeated hourly for continuous pain control

Preferable for drugs with short half-life (morphine, fentanyl, hydromorphone) to avoid toxic accumulation of drug

IV (CONTINUOUS)

Preferred over bolus and intramuscular injection for maintaining control of pain

Provides steady blood levels

Easy to titrate dosage

SUBCUTANEOUS (SC) (CONTINUOUS)

Used when oral and IV routes not available

Provides equivalent blood levels to continuous IV infusion

Suggested initial bolus dose to equal 2-hour IV dose; total 24-hour dose usually requires concentrated opioid solution to minimize infused volume; use smallest gauge needle that accommodates infusion rate

PATIENT-CONTROLLED ANALGESIA (PCA)

Generally refers to self-administration of drugs, regardless of route

Typically uses programmable infusion pump (IV, epidural, SC) that permits self-administration of boluses of medication at preset dose and time interval (lockout interval is time between doses)

PCA bolus administration often combined with initial bolus and continuous (basal or background) infusion of opioid

Optimum lockout interval not known but must be at least as long as time needed for onset of drug

- Should effectively control pain during movement or procedures
- Longer lockout provides larger dose

FAMILY-CONTROLLED ANALGESIA

One family member (usually a parent) or other caregiver designated as child's primary pain manager with responsibility for pressing PCA button

Guidelines for selecting a primary pain manager for family-controlled analgesia:

- Spends a significant amount of time with the patient
- Is willing to assume responsibility of being primary pain manager
- Is willing to accept and respect patient's reports of pain (if able to provide) as best indicator of how much pain the patient is experiencing; knows how to use and interpret a pain rating scale
- Understands the purpose and goals of patient's pain management plan
- Understands concept of maintaining a steady analgesic blood level
- Recognizes signs of pain and side effects and adverse reactions to opioid

NURSE-ACTIVATED ANALGESIA

Child's primary nurse designated as primary pain manager and is only person who presses PCA button during that nurse's shift

Guidelines for selecting primary pain manager for family-controlled analgesia also applicable to nurse-activated analgesia

May be used in addition to a basal rate to treat breakthrough pain with bolus doses; patients assessed every 30 minutes for the need for a bolus dose

May be used without a basal rate as a means of maintaining analgesia with around-the-clock bolus doses

INTRAMUSCULAR

NOTE: Not recommended for pain control; not current standard of care

Painful administration (hated by children)

Tissue and nerve damage possible with some drugs

Wide fluctuation in absorption of drug from muscle

Faster absorption from deltoid than from gluteal sites

Shorter duration and more expensive than oral drugs

Time consuming for staff and unnecessary delay for child

INTRANASAL

Available commercially as butorphanol (Stadol NS); approved for those older than 18 years of age

Should not be used in patient receiving morphinelike drugs because butorphanol is partial antagonist that will reduce analgesia and may cause withdrawal

INTRADERMAL

Used primarily for skin anesthesia (e.g., before lumbar puncture, bone marrow aspiration, arterial puncture, skin biopsy)

Local anesthetics (e.g., lidocaine) cause stinging, burning sensation

Duration of stinging dependent on type of "caine" used

To avoid stinging sensation associated with lidocaine:

- Buffer the solution by adding 1 part sodium bicarbonate (1 mEq/ml) to 9 or 10 parts 1% or 2% lidocaine with or without epinephrine (see Evidence-Based Practice box, p. 187)

Normal saline with preservative, benzyl alcohol, anesthetizes venipuncture site

Use same dose as for buffered lidocaine (see Evidence-Based Practice box, p. 187)

Data primarily from American Pain Society: *Principles of analgesic use in the treatment of acute pain and chronic cancer pain*, ed 4, Skokie, Ill, 1999, The Society; and McCaffery M, Pasero C: *Pain: a clinical manual*, ed 2, St Louis, 1999, Mosby.

*For further information about compounding drugs in troche or suppository form, contact Professional Compounding Centers of America (PCCA), 9901 S. Wilcrest Drive, Houston, TX 77009; (800) 331-2498; http://www.pccarx.com.

Continued

█ BOX 7-3

Routes and Methods of Analgesic Drug Administration—cont'd

TOPICAL OR TRANSDERMAL

EMLA (eutectic mixture of local anesthetics [lidocaine and prilocaine]) cream and anesthetic disk or LMX4 (4% lidocaine cream)

- Eliminates or reduces pain from most procedures involving skin puncture
- Must be placed on intact skin over puncture site and covered by occlusive dressing or applied as anesthetic disc for 1 hour or more before procedure (see Evidence-Based Practice box, p. 185)

LAT (lidocaine-adrenaline-tetracaine) or tetracaine-phenylephrine (tetraphen)

- Provides skin anesthesia about 15 minutes after application on nonintact skin
- Gel (preferable) or liquid placed on wounds for suturing
- Adrenaline not for use on end arterioles (fingers, toes, tip of nose, penis, earlobes) because of vasoconstriction

Numby Stuff

- Uses iontophoresis to transport lidocaine 2% and epinephrine 1:100,000 (Iontocaine) into the skin
- Current delivered by small battery-powered device that has an electrode with Iontocaine and a ground electrode
- Produces local dermal anesthesia in about 10 minutes to a depth of approximately 10 mm at maximum setting
- May be frightening to young children when they see the device and feel the current
- Observe child during iontophoresis and remove all metal, such as jewelry, from application site to prevent burns

Transdermal fentanyl (Duragesic)

- Available as patch for continuous pain control
- Safety and efficacy not established in children younger than 12 years of age
- Not appropriate for initial relief of acute pain because of long interval to peak effect (12 to 24 hours); for rapid onset of pain relief, give an immediate-release opioid
- Orders for "rescue doses" of an immediate-release opioid recommended for breakthrough pain, a flare of severe pain that breaks through the medication being administered at regular intervals for persistent pain
- Has duration of up to 72 hours for prolonged pain relief
- If respiratory depression occurs, possible need for several doses of naloxone

Vapocoolant

- Use of prescription spray coolant, such as fluorimethane (Spray and Stretch) or ethyl chloride (Pain Ease); applied to the skin for 10 to 15 seconds immediately before the needle puncture; anesthesia lasts about 15 seconds

- Cold disliked by some children; may be less uncomfortable to spray coolant on a cotton ball and then apply this to the skin
- Application of ice to the skin for 30 seconds found to be ineffective

RECTAL

Alternative to oral or parenteral routes

Variable absorption rate

Generally disliked by children

Many drugs able to be compounded into rectal suppositories*

REGIONAL NERVE BLOCK

Use of long-acting local anesthetic (bupivacaine or ropivacaine) injected into nerves to block pain at site

Provides prolonged analgesia postoperatively, such as after inguinal herniorrhaphy

May be used to provide local anesthesia for surgery, such as dorsal penile nerve block for circumcision or for reduction of fractures

INHALATION

Use of anesthetics, such as nitrous oxide, to produce partial or complete analgesia for painful procedures

Side effects (e.g., headache) possible from occupational exposure to high levels of nitrous oxide

EPIDURAL OR INTRATHECAL

Involves catheter placed into epidural, caudal, or intrathecal space for continuous infusion or single or intermittent administration of opioid with or without a long-acting local anesthetic (e.g., bupivacaine, ropivacaine)

Analgesia primarily from drug's direct effect on opioid receptors in spinal cord

Respiratory depression rare but may have slow and delayed onset; can be prevented by checking level of sedation and respiratory rate and depth hourly for initial 24 hours and decreasing dose when excessive sedation is detected

Nausea, itching, and urinary retention common dose-related side effects from the epidural opioid

Mild hypotension, urinary retention, and temporary motor or sensory deficits common unwanted effects of epidural local anesthetic

Catheter for urinary retention inserted during surgery to decrease trauma to child; if inserted when child is awake, anesthetize urethra with lidocaine

---

Data primarily from American Pain Society: *Principles of analgesic use in the treatment of acute pain and chronic cancer pain*, ed 4, Skokie, Ill, 1999, The Society; and McCaffery M, Pasero C: *Pain: a clinical manual*, ed 2, St Louis, 1999, Mosby.

*For further information about compounding drugs in troche or suppository form, contact Professional Compounding Centers of America (PCCA), 9901 S. Wilcrest Drive, Houston, TX 77009; (800) 331-2498; http://www.pccarx.com.

child of any age to administer analgesics to avoid signing for and preparing opioid injections every time one is needed (Fig. 7-7). When PCA is used as "nurse- or parent-controlled" analgesia, the concept of patient control is negated, and the inherent safety of PCA needs to be monitored. Research has reported safe and effective analgesia in children when the PCA was controlled by patient, parent, or nurse (Algren, Gursoy, Johnson, and others, 1998; Maxwell and Yaster, 2000).

PCA infusion devices typically allow for three methods or modes of drug administration to be used alone or in combination:

- **Patient-administered boluses** that can only be infused according to the preset amount and **lockout interval** (time between doses). More frequent attempts at self-administration usually mean the patient may need the dose and time adjusted for better pain control.
- **Nurse-administered boluses** that are typically used to give an initial loading dose to increase blood levels rapidly and to relieve **breakthrough pain** (pain not relieved with the usual programmed dose).
- **Continuous basal rate infusion** that delivers a constant amount of analgesic and prevents pain from returning during those times, such as sleep, when the patient cannot control the infusion.

FIG. 7-7 ■ Nurse programming a patient-controlled analgesia pump to administer analgesia.

As with any type of analgesic management plan, continued assessment of the child's pain relief is essential for the greatest benefit from PCA. Typical uses of PCA are for controlling pain from surgery, sickle cell crisis, trauma, and cancer. Morphine is the drug of choice for PCA and is usually prepared in a concentration of 1 mg/ml (Table 7-9). Other options are hydromorphone (0.2 mg/ml) and fentanyl (0.01 mg/ml). Hydromorphone is often used when patients are not able to tolerate side effects such as pruritus and nausea from the morphine PCA (Algren, Gursoy, Johnson, and others, 1998; Maxwell and Yaster, 2000).

Some physicians may still prescribe meperidine. However, meperidine is the least potent and shortest-acting of the synthetic opioids and the least effective in providing analgesia for severe pain. More important, it may increase the risk of seizures when administered chronically because of the excitatory effects on the nervous system of its metabolite, normeperidine. Some authors (Nadvi, Sarnaik, and Ravindranath, 1999) have argued that the incidence of meperidine-associated seizures is extremely small (0.4% of patients; 0.06% of admissions) and the risk of seizures should not dissuade clinicians from using this drug. However, the American Pain Society recommends that meperidine be reserved for brief treatment courses for patients who have reported and demonstrated its effectiveness, or who have allergies or uncorrectable intolerances to other opioids. Meperidine should not be used for longer than 48 hours or in doses greater than 600 mg/24 hr (Max, Byas-Smith, Gracely, and others, 1995).

Epidural Analgesia

Epidural analgesia may also be used to manage pain in selected cases. Although an epidural catheter may be inserted at any vertebral level, it is usually placed into the epidural space of the spinal column at the lumbar or caudal level (Fig. 7-8). The thoracic level is usually reserved for older children or adolescents who have had an upper abdominal or thoracic procedure, such as a lung transplant. An opioid (usually fentanyl, hydromorphone, or preservative-free morphine, which is often combined with a long-acting local anesthetic such as bupivacaine or ropivacaine) is instilled via single or intermittent bolus, continuous infusion, or patient-controlled epidural analgesia. Analgesia results from the drug's effect on opiate receptors in the dorsal horn of the spinal cord, rather than the brain. As a result, respiratory depression is rare, but if it occurs, it develops slowly, typically 6 to 8 hours after administration (Golianu, Krane, Galloway, and others, 2000). Properly securing the epidural catheter with an occlusive dressing decreases the possibility of soiling or inadvertently displacing the catheter (Fig. 7-9). Careful monitoring of sedation level and respiratory status is critical to prevent opioid-induced respiratory depression. Assessment of pain and the skin con-

TABLE 7-9

Suggested Intravenous Patient-Controlled Analgesia Opioid Infusion Orders

DRUG	BASAL RATE (mcg/kg/hr)	BOLUS RATE (mcg/kg/dose)	LOCKOUT PERIOD (min)	MAXIMUM DOSE/HR (mg/kg)
Morphine	10-30	10-30	6-10	0.1-0.15
Hydromorphone	3-5	6-10	0.015-0.02	3-5
Fentanyl	0.5-1.0	0.5-1.0	6-10	0.002-0.004

From Yaster M, Krance EJ, Kaplan RF, and others: *Pediatric pain management and sedation handbook*, St Louis, 1997, Mosby.

FIG. 7-8 ■ Epidural analgesia catheter placement.

FIG. 7-9 ■ Dressing covering site of epidural catheter.

FIG. 7-10 ■ LMX is an effective analgesic before intravenous insertion or blood draw.

dition around the catheter site are important aspects of nursing care (Golianu, Krane, Galloway, and others, 2000).

Transmucosal and Transdermal Analgesia

Fentanyl is also available as a transdermal patch (Duragesic). Although contraindicated for acute pain management, it may be used for older children and adolescents who have cancer pain or sickle cell pain or for patients who are opioid tolerant.

One of the most significant improvements in the ability to provide atraumatic care to children is the **anesthetic cream** LMX (a 4% liposomal lidocaine cream) or EMLA (an eutectic mixture of local anesthetics) (Abdelkefi, Abdennebi, Mellouli, and others, 2004; Choi, Irwin, Hui, and others, 2003; Egekvist and Bjerring, 2000; Gad, Olsen, Lysgaard, and others, 2005; Rogers and Ostrow, 2004; Santiago, Abad, Fernandez, and others, 2000; Uziel, Berkovitch, Gazarian, and others, 2003). The eutectic mixture (lidocaine 2.5% and prilocaine 2.5%), whose melting point is lower than that of the two anesthetics alone, permits effective concentrations of the drug to penetrate intact skin (see Evidence-Based Practice box and Fig. 7-10).

In some situations there is not ample time for topical preparations like LMX or EMLA to take effect, and **refriger-**

ant sprays such as ethyl chloride and fluorimethane can be used (Reis and Holubkov, 1997). When sprayed on the skin, these sprays vaporize, rapidly cool the area, and provide superficial anesthesia. Hospital formularies may have other products with lidocaine, prilocaine, or amethocaine topical preparations that require less time for application.

A randomized controlled trial compared the efficacy and safety of amethocaine gel (which is applied for 30 minutes) and EMLA cream (which is applied for 60 minutes) before a port-a-cath puncture. Children rated the pain following the puncture using the FACES rating scale (coded 0 to 5). Both groups had low pain scores, less than or equal to 2, and it did not make a significant difference whether the amethocaine or the EMLA cream was used. The researchers concluded that the amethocaine was clinically equivalent to EMLA, but the amethocaine gel required less time for anesthesia (Bishai, Taddio, Bar-Oz, and others, 1999). Another transdermal option is Numby Stuff, which uses **iontophoresis** (mild electrical current) to actively push the drug into the skin. This preparation of Iontocaine (lidocaine hydrochloride 2% with epinephrine 1:100,000 topical solution) provides dermal anesthesia to a depth of 10 mm in approximately 10 minutes (Squire, Kirchhoff, and Hissong, 2000). It can be used for IV placement, insertion of percutaneous central catheters lines, lumbar punctures, implantable port needle insertion, and pulsed dye laser therapy. It is important to provide explanations and let the child become familiar with the equipment. Some children may find the tingling sensation uncomfortable or frightening while the drug is administered (Squire, Kirchhoff, and Hissong, 2000).

The LidoSite Topical System is another method to help reduce needlestick pain associated with procedures such as IV cannulation, venipuncture, or laser ablation of superficial skin lesions for patients age 5 years and older. The LidoSite system delivers numbing medication to the proce-

EVIDENCE-BASED PRACTICE

EMLA Versus LMX for Pain Reduction During Peripheral Intravenous Access in Children

ASK THE QUESTION   In children is EMLA (lidocaine and prilocaine) a better anesthetic cream than LMX (lidocaine) in reducing pain from peripheral intravenous (PIV) access?

SEARCH FOR EVIDENCE

Search Strategies   Search selection criteria included English publications within past 5 years, research-based articles (level 3 or lower) on children undergoing PIV access.

Databases Used   PubMed, Cochrane Collaboration, MD Consult, Joanna Briggs Institute, National Guideline Clearinghouse (AHQR), TRIP Database Plus, PedsCCM, BestBETs

CRITICALLY ANALYZE THE EVIDENCE

Three studies were found that evaluated the two anesthetics for PIV access. All three were randomized control trials (level 1). All three studies found that a 30-minute application of LMX is as effective as a 60-minute application of EMLA for producing topical anesthesia for PIV access in children. None of the studies found PIV access difficulty was influenced by EMLA or LMX.

- The two local anesthetics (EMLA vs LMX) were compared in a group of 120 children 5 to 17 years of age scheduled for venipuncture in two sites. No differences were found in patients' perception of pain or parental and nurse observation scores (Eichenfield, Funk, Fallon-Friedlander, and others, 2002).
- EMLA and LMX were compared in a group of 30 healthy children 7 to 13 years of age. Self-report measures showed no difference in reported pain when examining the two anesthetics (Kleiber, Sorenson, Whiteside, and others, 2002).
- EMLA and LMX were compared in 60 children, 8 to 17 years of age, randomized to either LMX or EMLA. No differences were found between the groups. LMX caused less blanching (Koh, Harrison, Myers, and others, 2004).

APPLY THE EVIDENCE: NURSING IMPLICATIONS

LMX offers several advantages: rapid onset of action, lower cost, and lack of risk of methemoglobinemia in children of all ages. Apply LMX for 30 minutes before establishing PIV access.

Nursing implications include the following:
- Age—More than 34 weeks of gestation
- Time of onset—30 minutes
- Duration—1 hour
- Removal—No greater than 2 hours after application
- Multiple sites—Yes
- Use with abraded skin—No
- Impact on PIV access difficulty—None
- Do not use within 2 hours before vesicants
- Maximum area/dose—For children weighing less than 20 kg (44 pounds), apply to area less than 100 cm^2
- Cover with occlusive dressing

References

Eichenfield LF, Funk A, Fallon-Friedlander S, and others: A clinical study to evaluate the efficacy of Ela-Max as compared with eutectic mixture of local anesthetics cream for pain reduction of venipuncture in children, *Pediatrics* 109(6):1092-1099, 2002.

Kleiber C, Sorenson M, Whiteside K, and others: Topical anesthetics for intravenous insertion in children: a randomized equivalency study, *Pediatrics* 110:758-761, 2002.

Koh JL, Harrison D, Myers R, and others: A randomized, double-blind comparison study of EMLA and ELA-Max for topical anesthesia in children undergoing intravenous insertion, *Pediatr Anesth* 14:977-982, 2004.

dure site quickly and effectively after a 10-minute application (Fig. 7-11 and Evidence-Based Practice box). The system consists of a single-use, prefilled LidoSite patch, filled with lidocaine hydrochloride 10% and epinephrine 0.1%, and the LidoSite controller, an easy-to-use preprogrammed device that activates the patch. It provides pain reduction equivalent to a lidocaine (Xylocaine) injection without the needlestick. Through iontophoresis, a mild current from the controller activates the patch to accelerate delivery of lidocaine—the anesthetic medication—to the injection site. Epinephrine contained in the LidoSite patch helps focus the anesthetic effect directly under the patch and extends the duration of the effect for an hour.

The **intradermal route** is sometimes used to inject a local anesthetic, typically lidocaine, into the skin to reduce the pain from a lumbar puncture, bone marrow aspiration, or venous or arterial access. One problem with the use of lidocaine is the stinging and burning that initially occur. However, the used of buffered lidocaine with sodium bicarbonate (see Evidence-Based Practice box) reduces the stinging sensation (Wong and Pasero, 1997a, 1997b). Warming the lidocaine to 37° C (98.6° F) may accomplish the same effect.

FIG. 7-11 ■ The LidoSite system delivers analgesia quickly to the intravenous site.

Lidocaine Iontophoresis for Pain Reduction During Peripheral Intravenous Access in Children

Joy Hesselgrave

ASK THE QUESTION In children is lidocaine iontophoresis an effective anesthetic for peripheral intravenous (PIV) access pain relief?

SEARCH FOR EVIDENCE

Search Strategies Search selection criteria included English publications within past 5 years, research-based articles (level 3 or lower) on children undergoing PIV access.

Databases Used PubMed, Cochrane Collaboration, MD Consult, Joanna Briggs Institute, National Guideline Clearinghouse (AHQR), TRIP Database Plus, PedsCCM, BestBETs

CRITICALLY ANALYZE THE EVIDENCE

Five studies were found that evaluated the effectiveness of iontophoresis as a topical anesthetic in pediatric patients for PIV access. Four were randomized control trials (level 1) and one was level 6 evidence. All the studies found that a 10-minute application of lidocaine and epinephrine using iontophoresis was effective in providing pain relief for procedures. None of the studies found intravenous placement difficulty was influenced by iontophoresis. Common side effects included blanching or erythema at the application site that resolved within 24 hours. Other side effects included tingling and discomfort during the iontophoresis process. There is a low risk of electrical burn from the iontophoresis unit; no burns were reported in these clinical trials.

- A study of 272 children, ages 12 to 17 years, evaluated effectiveness of 10-minute iontophoresis with lidocaine vs a saline placebo before venipuncture or PIV access. Results indicated that the iontophoresis with lidocaine was an effective anesthetic for venipuncture after 10 minutes (Zempsky and Parkinson, 2004).
- Iontophoresis was also evaluated in 12 subjects, ages 5 to 15 years, using three different applications on various anatomic sites. Plasma concentrations of lidocaine were serially evaluated and found to be below 10 ng/ml at all time points. The researchers did dermal assessment over several time points and concluded that percutaneous lidocaine administration using iontophoresis is safe and well tolerated (Kearns, Heacook, Daly, and others, 2003).
- Twenty-six children ages 7 to 16 were enrolled in a study that compared PIV access using EMLA and iontophoresis. The PIV access procedures were 1 week apart. There was no difference in pain scores between the two methods by subject, parent, and observer rating (Galinkin, Rose, Harris, and others, 2002).
- Thirty-eight patients, ages 12 to 84 months, were included in this study to determine the safety, tolerability, and efficacy of iontophoresis for dermal anesthesia before venous access in an emergency department. They used a maximum of 30 mA over 20 minutes for the procedure. Lidocaine levels and pain scores by nurses and parents suggest that iontophoresis is safe and well tolerated in this younger population (Schultz, Strout, Jordan, and others, 2002).
- Forty-nine patients, ages 7 and older, received either lidocaine by iontophoresis or placebo before nonemergent PIV insertion. Based on pain scores, lidocaine iontophoresis was more effective than placebo for peripheral IV insertion (Kim, Kini, Troshynski, and others, 1999).

APPLY THE EVIDENCE: NURSING IMPLICATIONS

- Apply iontophoresis unit to one site for 10 minutes before venipuncture. Once removed, the anesthetic continues to be effective for 75 minutes and increases to a depth of 6 to 10 mm. Children accept this better than injected anesthetic.
- Lidocaine hydrochloride with epinephrine offers several advantages: rapid onset of action, prolonged duration of anesthesia, and comparable cost to topical lidocaine.
- Disadvantages include sensations from the electrical impulses that can cause discomfort, the ability to anesthetize only one site at a time, and the rare risk of electrical burn. It is currently approved only for children 5 years of age and older.

Several iontophoresis units are available, but LidoSite and Numby Stuff are most commonly used in pediatrics.

Characteristic	LidoSite	Numby Stuff
Age	Approved for 5 years	No lower age identified by manufacturer, except not recommended for neonates
Time of onset	Controller preset to deliver over 10 minutes	Set to deliver 40 mA/min over 10-20 minutes based on adjustable current level (2.0, 3.0, and 4.0 mA)
Duration	75 minutes	20 minutes with lidocaine alone and 90 minutes with lidocaine and epinephrine
Depth of penetration	6.4 mm after 10 minutes	10 mm
Multiple sites	No, one site at a time; second patch may be applied to different site after 30 minutes	No, one site at a time
Contraindications	Pacemakers or other electrical support systems, do not use within 2 hours before vesicants, allergy to lidocaine or epinephrine, abraded skin or new scar tissue	Pacemakers or other electrical support systems, do not use within 2 hours before vesicants, allergy to lidocaine or epinephrine, abraded shin or new scar tissue
Maximum area and dose	Prefilled lidocaine and epinephrine patch	Various sizes of electrodes that require nurse to fill with medication
Impact on PIV access difficulty	None reported	None reported

References

Galinkin JL, Rose JB, Harris K, and others: Lidocaine iontophoresis versus eutectic mixture of local anesthetics (EMLA) for IV placement in children, *Anesth Analg* 94(6):1484-1488, 2002.

Kearns GL, Heacook J, Daly SJ, and others: Percutaneous lidocaine administration via a new iontophoresis system in children: tolerability and absence of systemic bioavailability, *Pediatrics* 112(3 Pt 1):578-582, 2003.

Kim MK, Kini NM, Troshynski TJ, and others: A randomized clinical trial of dermal anesthesia by iontophoresis for peripheral intravenous catheter placement in children, *Ann Emerg Med* 33(4):395-399, 1999.

Schultz AA, Strout TD, Jordan P, and others: Safety, tolerability, and efficacy of iontophoresis with lidocaine for dermal anesthesia in ED pediatric patients, *J Emerg Nurs* 28(4):289-296, 2002.

Zempsky WT, Parkinson TM: Lidocaine iontophoresis for topical anesthesia before dermatologic procedures in children: a randomized controlled trial, *Pediatr Dermatol* 20(4):364-368, 2004.

EVIDENCE-BASED PRACTICE

Buffered Lidocaine for Pain Reduction During Peripheral Intravenous Access in Children
Angela C. Morgan

ASK THE QUESTION   In children is buffered lidocaine an appropriate anesthetic for reducing pain during peripheral intravenous (PIV) access?

SEARCH FOR EVIDENCE

Search Strategies   Search criteria included English publications within the past 5 years, research-based articles (level 3 or lower) on children undergoing PIV access. Two of the articles reviewed were more than 5 years old but were included based on the limited literature in this area.

Databases Used   PubMed, Cochrane Collaboration, MD Consult, Joanna Briggs Institute, National Guideline Clearinghouse (AHQR), TRIP Database, PedsCCM, Best BETs

CRITICALLY ANALYZE THE EVIDENCE

A review of the literature revealed 10 studies evaluating buffered lidocaine given before PIV access from 1991 through 1999 (Murphy, 2000). Four of the studies were specific to pediatrics. Findings from the pediatric studies support buffered lidocaine as a pain reduction measure in children before PIV access.

- A randomized trial consisting of 69 subjects ranging from 4 to 17 years of age (61% female) evaluated buffered lidocaine vs LMX (liposomal lidocaine cream) before PIV access. Results showed both interventions decreased pain and no significant differences in pain levels between the buffered lidocaine and LMX groups. The LMX group stated that the pain came with the removal of the occlusive dressing from the site (Luhmann, Hurt, Shootman, and others, 2004).
- Fein, Boardman, Stevenson, and others (1998) evaluated buffered lidocaine vs no pain control measures in a group of 99 children requiring PIV access in the emergency department (ED). PIV access without buffered lidocaine was significantly more painful than PIV access with buffered lidocaine.
- Sacchetti and Carraccio (1996) evaluated subcutaneous lidocaine vs no pain control measures in 110 children under 2 years of age before PIV access in the ED. No significant differences in pain levels were found in the groups. A weakness to this trial was that it was not blinded or randomized.
- A randomized clinical trial of 59 children requiring PIV access in the ED evaluated the use and nonuse of subcutaneous lidocaine before PIV access. PIV access without lidocaine was significantly more painful than PIV access with lidocaine regardless of catheter size. Trial weaknesses included a small sample size with wide confidence levels and no randomization (Klein, Shugerman, Leigh-Taylor, and others, 1995).

APPLY THE EVIDENCE: NURSING IMPLICATIONS
Buffered Lidocaine
- Age—More than 2 years
- Time of onset—Immediate
- Duration—1 hour
- Multiple sites—Yes
- Use with abraded skin—No
- Impact on PIV access difficulty—Possibility of some vasoconstriction
- Do not use within 2 hours before vesicants
- Dose—0.1 to 0.5 ml buffered 1% lidocaine, to a maximum of 0.45 ml/kg/dose; can repeat dose after 2 hours
- Consideration—An "extra stick" and ineffective buffered lidocaine administration may result in pain during both local administration and PIV access. Expertise in administering buffered lidocaine is an important factor related to its effectiveness.

References

Fein JA, Boardman CR, Stevenson S, and others: Saline with benzyl alcohol as intradermal anesthesia for intravenous line placement in children, *Pediatr Emerg Care* 14(2):119-122, 1998.
Klein EJ, Shugerman RP, Leigh-Taylor K, and others: Buffered lidocaine: analgesia for intravenous line placement in children, *Pediatrics* 95(5):709-712, 1995.
Luhmann J, Hurt S, Shootman M, and others: A comparison of buffered lidocaine versus ELA-Max before peripheral intravenous catheter insertions in children, *Pediatrics* 113(3 Pt 1):217-220, 2004.
Murphy R: *Prior injection of local anaesthetic and the pain and success of intravenous cannulation,* 2000, retrieved March 2005 from http://www.bestbets.org.
Sacchetti AD, Carraccio C: Subcutaneous lidocaine does not affect the success rate of intravenous access in children less than 24 months of age, *Acad Emerg Med* 3(11):1016-1019, 1996.

Timing of Analgesia

The right timing for administering analgesics depends on the type of pain. For **continuous pain control,** such as for postoperative or cancer pain, a preventive schedule of medication **around the clock (ATC)** is effective. The ATC schedule avoids the low concentrations of medications in plasma that permit breakthrough pain. If analgesics are administered only when pain returns (a typical use of the prn, or "as needed," order), pain relief may take several hours. This may require higher doses, leading to a cycle of undermedication of pain alternating with periods of overmedication and drug toxicity. This cycle of erratic pain control also promotes **"clock watching,"** which may be erroneously equated with addiction. Nurses can effectively use prn orders by giving the drug at regular intervals, since "as needed" should be interpreted as "as needed to prevent pain," not "as little as possible."

Preventive pain control is best provided through continuous IV infusion rather than intermittent boluses. If intermittent boluses are given, the intervals between doses should not exceed the drug's expected duration of effectiveness. For extended pain control with fewer administration times, drugs that provide longer duration of action (e.g., some NSAIDs, time-released morphine or oxycodone, methadone, levorphanol) can be used.

Continuous analgesia is not always appropriate, since not all pain is continuous. Frequently, temporary pain control or conscious sedation is needed to provide analgesia before a scheduled procedure. When pain can be predicted, the drug's **peak effect** should be timed to coincide with the painful event. For example, with opioids the peak effect is approximately a half hour for the IV route; with nonopioids the peak effect occurs about 2 hours after oral administration. For

---

BOX 7-4
Side Effects of Opioids

GENERAL
Constipation (possibly severe)
Respiratory depression
Sedation
Nausea and vomiting
Agitation, euphoria
Mental clouding
Hallucinations
Orthostatic hypotension
Pruritus
Urticaria
Sweating
Miosis (may be sign of toxicity)
Anaphylaxis (rare)

SIGNS OF TOLERANCE
Decreasing pain relief
Decreasing duration of pain relief

**SIGNS OF WITHDRAWAL SYNDROME IN PATIENTS
WITH PHYSICAL DEPENDENCE**
Initial Signs of Withdrawal
Lacrimation
Rhinorrhea
Yawning
Sweating

Later Signs of Withdrawal
Restlessness
Irritability
Tremors
Anorexia
Dilated pupils
Gooseflesh
Nausea, vomiting

---

nursingcareguidelines

Managing Opioid-Induced Respiratory Depression

IF RESPIRATIONS ARE DEPRESSED
Assess sedation level.
Reduce infusion by 25% when possible.
Stimulate patient (shake shoulder gently, call by name, ask to breathe).

IF PATIENT CANNOT BE AROUSED OR IS APNEIC
Administer naloxone (Narcan).
- For children weighing less than 40 kg (88 pounds), dilute 0.1 mg naloxone in 10 ml sterile saline to make 10 mcg/ml solution and give 0.5 mcg/kg.
- For children weighing more than 40 kg (88 pounds), dilute 0.4-mg ampule in 10 ml sterile saline and give 0.5 ml.
Administer bolus by slow intravenous push every 2 minutes until effect is obtained.
Closely monitor patient. Naloxone's duration of antagonist action may be shorter than that of opioid, requiring repeated doses of naloxone.
NOTE: Respiratory depression caused by benzodiazepines (e.g., diazepam [Valium] or midazolam [Versed]) can be reversed with flumazenil (Romazicon). Pediatric dosing experience suggests 0.01 mg/kg (0.1 ml/kg); if no (or inadequate) response after 1 to 2 minutes, administer same dose and repeat as needed at 60-second intervals for maximum dose of 1 mg (10 ml) (Yaster, Krance, Kaplan, and others, 1997).

---

rapid onset and peak of action, opioids that quickly penetrate the blood-brain barrier (e.g., IV fentanyl) provide excellent pain control.

Monitoring Side Effects

Both NSAIDs and opioids have side effects, although the major concern is with those from opioids (Box 7-4). **Respiratory depression** is the most serious complication and is most likely to occur in sedated patients. The respiratory rate may decrease gradually, or respirations may cease abruptly. Lower limits of normal are not established for children, but any significant change from a previous rate calls for increased vigilance. A slower respiratory rate does not necessarily reflect decreased arterial oxygenation; an increased depth of ventilation may compensate for the altered rate. If respiratory depression or arrest occurs, the nurse must be prepared to intervene quickly (see Nursing Care Guidelines box).

Although respiratory depression is the most feared side effect, **constipation** is a common, and sometimes serious, side effect of opioids, which decrease peristalsis and increase anal sphincter tone. Prevention with stool softeners and laxatives is more effective than treatment once constipation occurs. Di-

etary treatment, such as increased fiber, is usually not sufficient to promote regular bowel evacuation. However, dietary measures, such as increased fluid and fruit intake, and physical activity are encouraged. **Pruritus** from epidural or IV infusion can be treated with low doses of IV naloxone, nalbuphine, or diphenhydramine. **Nausea, vomiting,** and **sedation** usually subside after two days of opioid administration; however, oral or rectal antiemetics may be necessary.

Both tolerance and physical dependence can occur with prolonged use of opioids (see Community Focus box). **Physical dependence** is a normal, natural, physiologic state of neuroadaptation. When opioids are abruptly discontinued without weaning, **withdrawal symptoms** occur. Symptoms of withdrawal occur at 24 hours after abrupt discontinuation and reach a peak within 72 hours. Symptoms of withdrawal include signs of neurologic excitability (irritability, tremors, seizures, increased motor tone, insomnia), gastrointestinal dysfunction (nausea, vomiting, diarrhea, abdominal cramps), and autonomic dysfunction (sweating, fever, chills, tachypnea, nasal congestion, rhinitis). Withdrawal symptoms can be anticipated and prevented by weaning patients from opioids that were administered for more than 5 to 10 days. Adherence to a weaning protocol to prevent or minimize withdrawal symptoms from opioids will be required. A weaning flow sheet (Fig. 7-12) may be used to assess the efficacy of opioid weaning in neonates (Franck and Vilardi, 1995; Franck, Vilardi, Durand, and others, 1998).

Tolerance occurs when the dose of an opioid needs to be increased to achieve the same analgesic effects that was previously achieved at a lower dose (see Community Focus box).

COMMUNITY FOCUS

Fear of Opioid Addiction

One of the reasons for the unfounded but prevalent fear of addiction from opioids used to relieve pain is a misunderstanding of the differences between physical dependence, tolerance, and addiction. Health care professionals and the community often confuse addiction with the physiologic effects of opioids, when in reality these three states are unrelated. The American Society of Addiction Medicine defines these terms as follows:

Physical dependence on an opioid is a physiologic state in which abrupt cessation of the opioid, or administration of an opioid antagonist, results in withdrawal syndrome. Physical dependence on opioids is an expected occurrence in all individuals in the presence of continuous use of opioids for therapeutic or nontherapeutic purposes. It does not, in and of itself, imply addiction.

Tolerance is a form of neuroadaptation to the effects of chronically administered opioids (or other medications) that is indicated by the need for increasing or more frequent doses of the medication to achieve the initial effects of the drug. A person may develop tolerance both to the analgesic effects of opioids and to some of the unwanted side effects, such as respiratory depression, sedation, or nausea. Tolerance is variable in occurrence, but it does not, in and of itself, imply addiction.

Addiction in the context of pain treatment with opioids is characterized by a persistent pattern of dysfunctional opioid use that may involve any or all of the following:

- Adverse consequences associated with the use of opioids
- Loss of control over the use of opioids
- Preoccupation with obtaining opioids, despite the presence of adequate analgesia

Unfortunately, individuals who have severe, unrelieved pain may become intensely focused on finding relief. Sometimes behaviors such as "clock watching" make patients appear to others to be preoccupied with obtaining opioids. However, this preoccupation focuses on finding relief of pain, not on using opioids for reasons other than pain control. This phenomenon has been termed **pseudoaddiction** and must not be confused with real addiction.

Nurses must educate older children, parents, and health professionals about the extremely low risk of real addiction (less than 1%) from the use of opioids to treat pain. Infants, young children, and comatose or terminally ill children simply cannot become addicted because they are incapable of a consistent pattern of drug-seeking behavior, such as stealing, drug dealing, prostitution, or use of family income, to obtain opioids for nonanalgesic reasons.

Data from American Society of Addiction Medicine: *Public policy statement on definitions related to the use of opioids for pain treatment*, Feb 2001, retrieved May 7, 2007 from http://www.asam.org/Pain.html.

Tolerance may develop after 10 to 21 days of morphine administration. Treatment of tolerance involves increasing the dose or decreasing the duration between doses. Treatment of physical dependence involves gradually reducing the dose over several days to prevent withdrawal symptoms. The following are guidelines for treating physical dependence from morphine (Max, Byas-Smith, Gracely, and others, 1995):

- Gradually reduce dose (similar to tapering of steroids).
- Give one half of previous daily dose every 6 hours for first 2 days.
- Then reduce dose by 25% every 2 days. Continue this schedule until total daily dose of 0.6 mg/kg/day of morphine (or

equivalent) is reached. After 2 days on this dose, discontinue opioid.
- A switch to oral methadone may also be done, using one fourth of equianalgesic dose as initial weaning dose and proceeding as described above.

Parents and older children may fear addiction when opioids are prescribed. The nurse should address these concerns with assurance that any such risk is extremely low. It may be helpful to ask the question, "If you did not have this pain, would you want to take this medicine?" The answer is invariably no, which reinforces the solely therapeutic nature of the drug. It is also important to avoid making statements to the family such as "We don't want you to get used to this medicine," or "By now you shouldn't need this medicine," which may reinforce the fear of becoming addicted. Whereas both physical dependence and tolerance are physiologic states, **addiction** or **psychologic dependence** is a psychologic state and implies a "cause-effect" mode of thinking, such as "I need the drug because it makes me feel better." Infants and children do not have the cognitive ability to make the cause-effect association and therefore cannot become addicted. The use of opioid analgesics early in life has not been demonstrated to increase the risk for addiction later in life. Nurses need to explain to parents the differences among physical dependence, tolerance, and addiction and allow parents to express concerns about the use and duration of use of opioids. Infants and children, when treated appropriately with opioids, may be at risk for physical tolerance and physical dependence, but not psychologic dependence or addiction (Turner, 2005; Greco and Berde, 2005).

Evaluation of Effectiveness of Pain Regimen

The effectiveness of analgesics can be enhanced by a supportive attitude toward the child. By reinforcing the cause and effect of the medication and analgesia, the nurse can condition the child to expect pain relief, provided the regimen is likely to be effective. A pain relief scale or periodic ratings of pain intensity should be used for evaluation of effectiveness of pain regimens.

The response to therapy should be evaluated 15 to 30 minutes after each dose, and titration should continue to the highest achievable amount of relief (Max, Byas-Smith, Gracely, and others, 1995). In a retrospective study that examined the pain experience of children with sickle cell disease, evidence of pain relief from medications was documented for less than half (44.8%) of the patients in the emergency department (ED) (Jacob and Mueller, 2006). Even though The Joint Commission required documentation of pain assessments with vital signs, evidence of pain relief was not documented in 41.4% of the episodes. Titration methods in the ED or during the course of hospitalization, if used, were not reflected in the amount of medications received by the children (Jacob, Miaskowski, Savedra, and others, 2003a; 2003b).

Several harmful effects occur with unrelieved pain, particularly when pain is prolonged. A number of **physiologic stress responses** in the body are triggered during pain, and they lead to negative consequences that involve multiple systems. Unrelieved pain may prolong the stress response and adversely affect an infant's or child's recovery, whether it is from trauma, surgery, or disease. In a landmark study by Anand and Hickey (1992), 30 neonates received deep intraop-

Children's Hospital Oakland Opioid Weaning Flowsheet and Guidelines for Use of the Form
Analgesia/sedation orders (drug/dose/frequency)

		Time:		
Date				
Drug				
Administration time				
Dose ↑ or ↓ or freq change				
Choose one: Crying/agitated 25%-50% of interval Crying/agitated >50% of interval	2 3			
Choose one: Sleeps ≤25% of interval Sleeps 26%-75% of interval Sleeps >75% of interval	3 2 1			
Choose one: Hyperactive Moro Markedly hyperactive Moro	2 3			
Choose one: Mild tremors, disturbed Moderate/severe tremors, disturbed	1 2			
Increased muscle tone	2			
Temperature 37.2°-38.4°C	1			
Temperature >38.4°C	2			
Respiratory rate >60 (extubated)	2			
Suction >twice/interval (intubated)	2			
Sweating	1			
Frequent yawning (>3-4/interval)	1			
Sneezing (>3-4/interval)	1			
Nasal stuffiness	1			
Emesis	2			
Projectile vomiting	3			
Loose stools	2			
Watery stools	3			
TOTAL SCORE				
ADJUSTED SCORE				
INITIALS OF PERSON SCORING				

Directions: Score every 2-4 hours per guideline
Score greater than 8-12 may indicate withdrawal

Guidelines for use of the flow sheet

Use of form
Use the flowsheet for all infants who have received continuous or around-the-clock opioid medication for 3 days or more, or more than 3 doses per day for more than 5 days. This patient population will most often include postoperative patients, agitated intubated infants, and all post-ECMO patients.

Instructions
1. Write drug, dose, and frequency of analgesics and sedatives ordered
2. Enter date, name of drug (abbreviated MS=morphine sulfate or FENT=fentanyl), and administration time of drugs given in the appropriate boxes; indicate if dose frequency given is an increase or decrease from the ordered dose
3. Scoring must be performed every 4 hours during weaning of opioids, every 2 hours if score is 8 or greater. The score for each item indicates the presence of the sign during the previous 2-4 hours (depending on the scoring interval). Every 4-hour scoring should continue until the patient is off all opioids for 48-72 hours. Place a "0" in the column after the sign if it is not seen during the scoring period.

Central nervous system
Crying behavior: Score 2 points if patient exhibits crying or cry behavior for a duration of ≤50% of the scoring interval. Score 3 points if cumulative crying behavior totals >50% of the scoring interval.
NOTE: Crying behavior is accompanied by the facial expressions associated with crying, but without audible sounds because of endotracheal intubation.
Sleeping: Score 3 points if patient sleeps for ≤25% of the scoring interval. Score 2 points if patient sleeps for 26%-75% of the scoring interval. Score 1 point if patient sleeps for >75% of the scoring interval.
Moro (startle) reflex: Score 2 points if patient has some arm and/or leg extension when touched or when disturbed by loud noises. Score 3 points if patient has marked arm and/or leg extension that is accompanied by crying behavior, hyperalert state, or continued arm and/or leg tremors after being startled.
Tremors—disturbed: Score 1 point if patient has mild tremors when disturbed. Score 2 points if patient has moderate to severe tremors when disturbed. NOTE: Tremors are alternating movements that are rhythmic, of equal rate and amplitude, and can usually be stopped by flexion of the limb.
Increased muscle tone: Score 2 points if patient exhibits fisting or tight flexion of extremities that are difficult to extend.

Metabolic
Temperature: Score 1 point if patient's temperature is 37.2°-38.4°C. Score 2 points if patient's temperature is >38.4°C.
Respiratory rate: Score 1 point if patient's spontaneous respiratory rate is >60/minute. Score 2 points if patient's spontaneous respiratory rate is >60/minute and accompanied by retractions.
Suction: Score 2 points if patient is suctioned more than twice during a 4-hour period.
Sweating: Score 1 point if patient exhibits any type of sweating, including beads of sweat, or if skin is moist to touch.
Yawning: Score 1 point if patient yawns >3-4 times in succession or yawns 1-2 times often during a 4-hour period.
Sneezing: Score 1 point if patient sneezes >3-4 times in succession or sneezes 1-2 times during a 4-hour period.
Nasal stuffiness: Score 1 point for nasal stuffiness.

Gastrointestinal
Emesis of formula/stomach contents: Score 2 points if patient has 1 or more episodes of emesis during a 4-hour period.
Projectile vomiting: Score 3 points if patient has 1 or more episodes of projectile vomiting.
Loose stools: Score 2 points if patient has loose stools characterized by a water ring around some solid stool. The stools will often be frequent. NOTE: Do not score for "breast milk" stools: frequent, small, seedy, yellow stools.
Watery stools: Score 3 points if patient has stools that consist of only liquid. The stools will often be frequent.

Total score: Add up all the scores in the column and place the total score in this box. Clinical signs that appear continuously, such as respiratory rate >60 or regular poor feeding, should be included in the total score.
Adjusted score: The adjusted score is used when a sign is detected that is expected to occur independently of withdrawal, due to a preexisting condition (high respiratory rate in infant with bronchopulmonary dysplasia). The decision to adjust the score should be made after discussion with the healthcare team during rounds, and the rationale should be recorded in a problem-oriented note. Circle the signs to be excluded and deduct the points from the total score to obtain the adjusted score.
Initials of person scoring: The person scoring should write his/her initials in this space.

FIG. 7-12 ■ Weaning flow sheet to monitor opioid weaning in neonates.

erative anesthesia with high doses of the opioid sufentanil, followed postoperatively by an infusion of opioids for 24 hours, and 15 neonates received lighter anesthesia with halothane and morphine followed postoperatively by intermittent morphine and diazepam. The 15 neonates who received the lighter anesthesia and intermittent postoperative opioids had more severe hyperglycemia and lactic acidemia, and four postoperative deaths occurred in the group. The 30 neonates who received deep anesthesia had a lower incidence of complications (sepsis, metabolic acidosis, disseminated intravascular coagulation) and no deaths.

Poorly controlled acute pain can predispose patients to **chronic pain syndromes.** A guiding principle in pain management is that prevention of pain is always better than treatment (Benjamin, Swinson, and Nagel, 2000). Pain that is established and severe is often more difficult to control. When pain is unrelieved, sensory input from injured tissues reaches spinal cord neurons and may enhance subsequent responses. Long-lasting changes in cells within spinal cord pain pathways may occur after a brief painful stimulus and may lead to the development of chronic pain conditions. Basbaum (1999a, 1999b) reported a series of studies that emphasize a distinct neurochemistry of acute and persistent pain and concluded that persistent pain is not merely a prolonged acute pain symptom of some other disease. Underlying physiologic mechanisms lead to the persistence of pain (Marx, 2004; Woolf and Salter, 2000).

In a study of nursing practice related to pain assessment and management in different pediatric specialty units (Jacob and Puntillo, 2000), complaints of pain were noted, but specific pain scores or notations about responses to analgesics after administration were seldom documented. Pain scores were not available before and after analgesics, and it was therefore not possible to conclude whether analgesics were effective. Nurses therefore need to evaluate and monitor pain in a timely fashion after administration of analgesics; titrate dosage to effect; or make recommendations for an alternate analgesic, for addition of another analgesic, or for a combination of analgesics, adjuvants, and nonpharmacologic strategies.

PAINFUL AND INVASIVE PROCEDURES

Several painful and invasive procedures require the administration of anesthetics and analgesics. For circumcision pain, caudal or penile blocks are employed before the procedure. Parents are then instructed how to apply lidocaine gels for the first 24 to 36 hours after the circumcision. For open wounds, bupivacaine may be instilled with or without epinephrine onto the dressing applied to skin to minimize pain for up to 48 hours after the procedure. For graft donor sites, analgesia is maintained by using a foam dressing soaked with bupivacaine (0.25%, 2 mg/kg; 0.8 ml/kg) applied to the donor surface. A continuous infusion of 0.25% bupivacaine at 1 to 3 ml/hr via a standard 18-gauge epidural catheter is then curled on the outer or inner surface of the foam (Cousins and Power, 2003). Wound perfusion of bupivacaine is useful for iliac crest bone graft donor sites (used for alveolar bone grafting in some techniques of cleft palate repair). A standard 18-gauge epidural catheter is also used with a very low infusion rate (1 to 3 ml/hr) of bupivacaine. For minor and some intermediate procedures, the local anesthetic infiltration with bupivacaine is commonly used. Some examples of these procedures include surface wounds and tunneling procedures in the anesthetized child requiring inguinal surgery; insertion of ventriculoperitoneal shunts, central venous lines, or central venous catheter-reservoir systems; and similar procedures.

Nitrous oxide, which is taken up rapidly and eliminated by the lungs, is highly insoluble in the blood and is delivered quickly to the brain to produce an analgesic effect equivalent to that of IV morphine. After approximately 2 minutes of inhalation, maximum pain relief can be achieved. The child breathes via face mask, nasal mask, or mouthpiece. It is not suitable for children younger than 3 years old and works best for children older than 5 years of age. Nitrous oxide inhalations are used frequently for a wide variety of procedures that require potent analgesia for a short time, such as suture insertion or removal, dressing removal or changes (including burns), drain or catheter removal, venipuncture or cannulation, lumbar puncture, physical therapy, and biopsies (skin, muscle, renal, or bone marrow). However, in children with pneumothorax, bowel obstruction, abnormal airway, recent head injury (especially with an intracranial air pocket), chronic respiratory disease with air trapping or bullous changes in the lung, and some types of uncorrected congenital heart disease (such as pulmonary hypertension), the use of nitrous oxide is contraindicated. Nitrous oxide may lead to expansion of air pockets in confined spaces (chest, cranial cavities, bowel lumens) and create an increased pressure and tension effect. Tension pneumothorax, ischemia or shift of intracranial contents, and bowel distention with risk of perforation could oc-

cur. In addition, because nitrous oxide produces a degree of sedation and potentiates the sedative effects of other central nervous system depressants, caution is required when concurrently giving opioids, benzodiazepines, antihistamines, and similar drugs. Inspired concentrations of up to 50% nitrous oxide used for less than 30 minutes do not affect airway reflexes. Only trained personnel may administer nitrous oxide and monitor the child (Cousins and Power, 2003).

POSTOPERATIVE PAIN

Surgery and traumatic injuries (e.g., fractures, dislocations, strains, sprains, lacerations, burns) generate a **catabolic state** as a result of increased secretion of catabolic hormones. Consequently, alterations in blood flow, coagulation, fibrinolysis, substrate metabolism, and water and electrolyte balance can occur and increase the demands on the cardiovascular and respiratory systems (Cousins and Power, 2003). The major endocrine and metabolic changes are elicited during the first 48 hours after surgery or trauma. Local anesthetics and opioid neural blockade may effectively modify the responses to surgical injury and mitigate the physiologic response.

Pain associated with surgery to the chest (e.g., repair of congenital heart defects, chest trauma) or abdominal regions (e.g., appendectomy, cholecystectomy, splenectomy) may result in pulmonary complications. Pain leads to decreased muscle movement in the thorax and abdominal area and leads to decreased tidal volume, vital capacity, functional residual capacity, and alveolar ventilation. The patient is unable to cough and clear secretions, and the risk for complications such as pneumonia and atelectasis is high. Severe postoperative pain also results in sympathetic overactivity, which leads to increases in heart rate, peripheral resistance, blood pressure, and cardiac output. The patient eventually experiences an increase in cardiac demand and myocardial oxygen consumption and a decrease in oxygen delivery to the tissues.

The basis for good postoperative pain control in children is preemptive analgesia. **Preemptive analgesia** involves administration of medications (e.g., local and regional anesthetics, analgesics) before the child experience the pain or before surgery is performed so that the sensory activation and changes in the pain pathways of the peripheral and central nervous system can be controlled. Preemptive analgesia has been demonstrated to lower postoperative pain, lower analgesic requirement, lower hospital stay, lower complications after surgery, and minimize the risks for peripheral and central nervous system sensitization that can lead to persistent pain (Cousins and Power, 2003).

A combination of medications (**multimodal** or **balanced analgesia**) is used for postoperative pain and may include NSAIDs, local anesthetics, nonopioids, and opioid analgesics to achieve optimum relief and minimize side effects. Opioids (see Table 7-5) administered ATC during the first 48 hours or administered via PCA (see Table 7-9) are commonly prescribed postoperatively. The duration of use is frequently limited to days, since the cause of pain usually resolves. The combination of the IV NSAID ketorolac and morphine using a PCA device is frequently prescribed after thoracic surgery. Morphine delivered by PCA leads to a lower total dosage of opioid analgesia when compared with the administration of intermittent doses of analgesic as required. After bowel surgery, a mixture of local anesthetics (bupivacaine) and a low-dose opioid (fentanyl) delivered by epidural route improves the rate of recovery and minimizes the gastrointestinal effects (e.g., bowel stasis, nausea, vomiting). Once bowel function has been restored, oral opioids such as immediate release and controlled release preparations are preferred in older children. Controlled release opioids facilitate ATC dosing and improve sleep. They are also associated with lower incidence of nausea, sedation, and breakthrough pain.

RECURRENT HEADACHES IN CHILDREN

Recurrent headaches in children can be caused by several factors, including tension, dental braces, and imbalance or weakness of eye muscles causing deviation in alignment and refractive errors. Headaches may be the sequelae to accidents, sinusitis and other cranial infection or inflammation, increased intracranial pressure, epileptic attacks, drugs, obstructive sleep apnea, and rarely hypertension. Other causes may include arteriovenous malformations, disturbances in cerebrospinal fluid flow or absorption, intracranial hemorrhages, ocular and dental diseases, bacterial infections, and brain tumors. Severe pain is the most disturbing symptom in migraine. Tension-type headache is usually mild or moderate, often producing a pressing feeling in the temples, like a "tight band around the head." Continuous, daily, or near-daily headache with no specific cause occurs in a small subgroup of children. In epilepsy, headaches commonly occur before, during, or after a seizure attack.

Treatment of recurrent headaches requires an understanding of the antecedents and consequences of headache pain. A **headache diary** can allow the child to record the time of onset, activities before the onset, any worries or concerns as far back as 24 hours before the onset, severity and duration of pain, pain medications taken, and activity pattern during headache episodes. The headache diary allows ongoing monitoring of headache activity, indicates the effects of interventions, and guides treatment planning.

There are two main approaches to prevention of headache using behavioral approaches:

■ Teaching patients self-control skills to prevent headache (e.g., biofeedback techniques and relaxation training)
■ Modifying behavior patterns that increase the risk of headache occurrence or reinforce headache activity (e.g., cognitive-behavioral stress management techniques)

Biofeedback is a technology-based form of relaxation therapy and can be useful in assessing and reinforcing learning of relaxation skills such as progressive muscle relaxation, deep breathing, and imagery. Children as young as 7 years of age have been taught these skills and with 2 to 3 weeks of practice are able to decrease the time needed to achieve relaxation.

To modify behavior patterns that increase the risk of headache occurrence or reinforce headache activity, the nurse instructs parents to avoid giving excessive attention to their child's headache and to respond matter-of-factly to pain behavior and requests for special attention (Holden, Deichmann, and Levy, 1999). Parents are taught to assess whether school or social performance demands are being avoided because of headache. Parents are taught to focus attention on **adaptive coping** such as the use of relaxation techniques and maintenance of normal activity patterns. When using cognitive-behavioral stress management techniques, the parents identify negative thoughts and situations that may be associated with

increased risk for headache. The child is then taught to activate positive thoughts and engage in adaptive behavior appropriate to the situation.

RECURRENT ABDOMINAL PAIN IN CHILDREN

Recurrent abdominal pain (RAP) or functional abdominal pain is defined as pain that occurs at least once per month for 3 consecutive months, accompanied by pain-free periods, and is severe enough that it interferes with a child's normal activities. Management of RAP is highly individualized to reflect the causes of the pain and the psychosocial needs of the child and family. A clear understanding of the child's characteristics (anxiety, physical health, temperament, coping skills, experience, learned response, depression), child's disability (school attendance, activities with family, social interactions, pain behaviors), environmental factors (family attitudes and behavioral patterns, school environment, community, friendships), and the pain stimulus (disease, injury, stress) is important in planning management strategies (Collins and Weisman, 2003).

Before any workup of the pain, the nurse informs the family that RAP is common in children and only 10% of children with RAP have an identifiable organic cause for their pain symptom. Medical workup is dictated by the child's symptoms and signs in combination with knowledge about common organic causes of RAP. If an organic cause is found, it will be treated appropriately. Even if no organic cause is found, the nurse needs to communicate to the child and family a belief that the pain is real. Usually the abdominal pain goes away, but even if problems are identified, they may not be the actual cause and pain may persist, may be replaced by another symptom, or may go away on its own. The management plan includes regular follow-up at a 3- to 4-month intervals, a list of symptoms that call for earlier contact, and biobehavioral pain management techniques. The goal is to minimize the impact the pain has on the child's activities and the family's life (Collins and Weisman, 2003).

Case reports have demonstrated the effectiveness of implementing a time-out procedure, token systems, and positive reinforcement based on operant theory treatment modalities. Stress management and cognitive-behavioral strategies have also been reported to be successful. Parent training in how to avoid positive reinforcement of sick behaviors and focus on rewarding healthy behaviors is important. Over the course of several sessions, parents are educated about RAP, how to distinguish between sick and well behaviors, a reward system for well behaviors, and the importance of reinforcing relaxation and stressing coping skills taught to children for pain management. Treatment may consist of a varying number of sessions over 1 to 6 months and may include various components such as monitoring of symptoms, limited parent attention, relaxation training, increased dietary fiber, and requirements of school attendance. Response rates are 25% without abdominal pain and 56% to 75% improvements in symptoms (Collins and Weisman, 2003).

The use of cognitive-behavioral therapy has been documented to reduce or eliminate pain in children with RAP and highlights the involvement of parents in supporting their child's self-management behavior. No negative side effects of symptom substitution occurred with the interventions. The combination of self-regulation and cognitive-behavioral interventions along with fiber intervention is more effective for treating RAP than using fiber alone (Weydert, Ball, and Davis, 2003).

Famotidine is an H_2-receptor antagonist that may be given twice daily (0.5 mg/kg/dose). It was demonstrated to improve pain in 68% of children and decreased the peptic index score. The **peptic index score** is a composite score for nausea, vomiting, appetite, epigastric pain, weight loss, and nocturnal awakening. Pizotifen is a serotonin antagonist that was tested in 14 children given at 5 ml (0.25 mg) twice daily for 1 month. Patients who received pizotifen had fewer days of abdominal pain, a lower index of severity, and a lower index of misery when compared with those receiving a placebo. The only side effects noted were slight drowsiness and slight weight gain. Pizotifen is available worldwide but not approved for use in the United States (Symon and Russell, 1995).

CANCER PAIN IN CHILDREN

Pain in children with cancer was reported to be the most prevalent symptom (84.4%) and was rated to be moderate to severe (86.6%) and highly distressing (52.8%) (Collins, Byrnes, Dunkel, and others, 2000). Pain may be related to an operation; mucositis; a phantom limb; infection; chemotherapy; and procedures such as bone marrow aspiration, needle puncture, or lumbar puncture. Tumor-related pain frequently occurs when the child relapses or when tumors become resistant to treatment. Intractable pain may occur in patients with solid tumors that metastasize to the central or peripheral nervous system. In young adult survivors of childhood cancer, chronic pain conditions may develop, including complex regional pain syndrome of the lower extremity, phantom limb pain, avascular necrosis, mechanical pain related to bone that failed to unite after tumor resection, and postherpetic neuralgia.

Other treatment-related pain includes (1) abdominal pain after allogeneic bone marrow transplantation, which may be associated with acute graft-versus-host disease; (2) abdominal pain associated with typhlitis (infection of the cecum), which occurs when the patient is immunocompromised; (3) phantom sensations and phantom limb pain after an amputation; (4) peripheral neuropathy after administration of vincristine; and (5) medullary bone pain, which may be associated with administration of granulocyte colony–stimulating factor (Collins and Weisman, 2003).

Almost 40% of all pain episodes in children with cancer may be attributed to procedures (Ljungman, Gordh, Sorensen, and others, 2001, 2000, 1999; Ljungman, Kreuger, Andreasson, and others, 2000). Survivors of childhood cancer describe vivid memories of their experience with repeated painful procedures during treatment. These procedures include needle puncture for IM chemotherapy (L-asparaginase), IV lines, port access and blood draws, lumbar puncture, bone marrow aspiration and biopsy, removal of central venous catheters, and other invasive diagnostic procedures. Fear and anxiety related to these procedures may be minimized with parent and child preparation. The preparation starts with obtaining information from the parent about the child's coping styles, explaining the procedure, and enlisting their support. Topical analgesics (e.g., cold sprays, EMLA, amethocaine gels), as discussed previously, have been effective in providing analgesia before needle procedures.

Lumbar puncture for administration of chemotherapy (e.g., cytarabine, methotrexate) and collection of cerebrospinal fluid may lead to a leak at the puncture site and low intra-

cranial pressure (Collins and Weisman, 2003). Some children may experience postdural puncture headache, which may be treated by administering nonopioid analgesics and placing the patient in the supine position for 1 hour after the procedure. The pain related to bone marrow aspiration is due to the insertion of a large needle into the posterior iliac space and the unpleasant sensation experienced at the time of marrow aspiration. Cognitive-behavioral therapy (e.g., guided imagery, relaxation, music therapy, hypnosis), conscious sedation, and general anesthesia have been proven effective in decreasing pain and distress during the procedure.

If the patient is neutropenic (absolute neutrophil count $<500/mm^3$), the antipyretic action of acetaminophen may mask a fever. In patients with thrombocytopenia (platelet count $<50,000/mm^3$), who may be at risk for bleeding, NSAIDs are contraindicated. Morphine is the most widely used opioid for moderate to severe pain and may be administered via the oral (including sustained release formulations such as MS Contin and Kadian), IV, subcutaneous, epidural, and intrathecal routes. When dose-limiting side effects of morphine develop, hydromorphone has been reported to be effective in several studies of children with cancer (Drake, Longworth, and Collins, 2004). In children and adolescents with mucositis after bone marrow transplantation, hydromorphone was well tolerated and had a potency ratio of approximately 6:1 relative to morphine (Drake, Longworth, and Collins, 2004).

The most common clinical syndrome of neuropathic pain is painful **peripheral neuropathy** caused by chemotherapeutic agents, particularly vincristine and cisplatin, and rarely cytarabine (Collins and Weisman, 2003). Withdrawal of the chemotherapy may resolve the neuropathy over weeks to months, or it may persist even after withdrawal. Neuropathic pain is associated with at least one of the following: (1) pain that is described as electric or shocklike, stabbing, or burning; (2) signs of neurologic involvement (e.g., paralysis, neuralgia, pain hypersensitivity) other than those associated with the progression of the tumor; and (3) the location of the solid organ cancer consistent with neurologic damage that could give rise to neuropathic pain. Dying children with cancer who experience neuropathic pain have higher baseline requirements of morphine and require rapid increases of morphine than dying children without neuropathic pain (Dougherty and DeBaun, 2003). Children with neuropathic pain often require massive opioid infusion (>3 mg/kg/hr of IV morphine dose equivalent, or approximately 100-fold greater than standard starting infusion rates). An epidural or subarachnoid infusion may be initiated if the patient experiences dose-limiting side effects of opioids or if pain was resistant to opioids.

Tricyclic antidepressants (amitriptyline, desipramine) and anticonvulsants (gabapentin, carbamazepine) have demonstrated effectiveness in neuropathic cancer pain. Randomized controlled trials showed that 60% to 70% of patients with neuropathic pain achieve relief with tricyclic antidepressants (Sindrup, Otto, Finnerup, and others, 2005). The tricyclic antidepressants have many actions that could be involved in their pain-relieving effect and have been considered the mainstay of therapy for neuropathic pain (Sindrup, Otto, Finnerup, and others, 2005).

Klepstad, Borchgrevink, Hval, and others (2001) reported the pain experience of a 12-year-old girl with severe neuropathic pain caused by a cervical spinal tumor. Two weeks after resection of the tumor, the child experienced increased pain in her neck, which was superficial and distributed in the dermatomes below the cervical medullary lesion. Pain was provoked by touch and did not decrease in intensity despite a subcutaneous infusion of morphine at 160 mg/24 hr. The child screamed from increased pain when her parents or siblings tried to comfort her with bodily contact. Pain was relieved after administration of 7.5 to 10 mg IV ketamine. Ketamine is an N-methyl-D-aspartate (NMDA) antagonist, which has undesirable side effects (e.g., sedation, nausea, dissociative reactions, muteness, dizziness, and visual distortions) and short duration of action (Sang, 2000). After administration of ketamine, the child was able to tolerate touch without pain paroxysms. A continuous IV infusion was eventually initiated for convenience, and benzodiazepines were added to avoid the psychomimetic effects associated with ketamine.

Although ketamine is frequently used to ensure analgesia and sedation during painful procedures in children, the long-term use of ketamine for the treatment of neuropathic pain in children has not been systematically studied and is not of clinical benefit for all patients (Klepstad, Borchgrevink, Hval, and others, 2001). In randomized studies of patients with chronic neuropathic pain, only some patients had a beneficial response to ketamine (Haines and Gaines, 1999; Max, Byas-Smith, Gracely, and others, 1995; Mitchell, 2001).

PAIN AND SEDATION IN END-OF-LIFE CARE

Many patients require doses of opioids that make them sedated but arousable as their disease progresses (e.g., cancer, human immunodeficiency virus, cystic fibrosis, neurodegenerative disease) at the end of life. Comfort can be achieved with a combination of opioids and adjuvant analgesics in most situations. Parents need reassurance that the opioids are treating pain but not causing the child's death and the child's advancing disease is the cause of death.

A small group of patients have intolerable side effects or inadequate analgesia despite extremely aggressive use of medications to relieve pain and side effects. Continuous sedation may be a means of relieving suffering when there is no feasible or acceptable means of providing analgesia that preserves alertness. A continuing high-dose infusion of opioids along with sedation is prescribed to reduce the possibility that a child might experience unrelieved pain but be too sedated to report it. Sedation in these situations is widely regarded as providing comfort, not euthanasia. Clinicians and ethicists have a range of views regarding assisted suicide and euthanasia, but they all agree that no child or parent should choose death because of inadequate efforts to relieve pain and suffering (Berde and Collins, 2003).

KEY POINTS

■ Although the ability to measure pain in children has improved dramatically in recent years, assessment of pain in children continues to be complex and challenging.

■ Behavioral assessment is useful for measuring pain in infants and preverbal children who do not have the language skills to communicate that they are in pain, or when mental clouding and confusion limit a child's ability to communicate.

■ Physiologic measures are not able to distinguish between physical responses to pain and other forms of stress to the body.

■ The number of pain measures that are available for use in infants and young children has increased dramatically and adds a layer of complexity to the assessment of pain in children.

■ Important components of assessment include the onset of pain; pain duration or pattern; effectiveness of the current treatment; factors that aggravate or relieve the pain; other symptoms and complications concurrently felt; and interference with the child's mood, function, and interactions with family.

■ The administration of sucrose with and without nonnutritive sucking has been demonstrated to have calming and pain-relieving effects for invasive procedures in neonates.

■ One of the most significant improvements in the ability to provide atraumatic care to children is the anesthetic creams LMX and EMLA.

■ Nonopioids, including acetaminophen (Tylenol, Paracetamol) and NSAIDs, are suitable for mild to moderate pain; opioids are needed for moderate to severe pain.

■ Several drugs, known as coanalgesics or adjuvant analgesics, may be used alone or with opioids to control pain symptoms and opioid side effects.

■ A significant advance in the administration of IV, epidural, or subcutaneous analgesics is the use of PCA.

■ Although respiratory depression is the most feared side effect, constipation is a common, and sometimes serious, side effect of opioids, which decrease peristalsis and increase anal sphincter tone.

■ Several harmful effects occur with unrelieved pain, particularly when pain is prolonged.

■ Surgery and traumatic injuries (fractures, dislocations, strains, sprains, lacerations, burns) generate a catabolic state as a result of increased secretion of catabolic hormones and lead to alterations in blood flow, coagulation, fibrinolysis, substrate metabolism, and water and electrolyte balance, and increase the demands on the cardiovascular and respiratory systems.

■ Treatment of recurrent headaches requires an understanding of the antecedents and consequences of headache pain.

■ RAP or functional abdominal pain is defined as pain that occurs at least once per month for 3 consecutive months, accompanied by pain-free periods, and is severe enough that it interferes with a child's normal activities.

■ Injections from immunizations, IM antibiotics in the ED or physician's office, and blood draws are common sources of pain in children.

■ For nonpainful procedures such as radiologic imaging studies several medications are used to sedate, minimize anxiety, and induce amnesia.

■ Several painful and invasive procedures require the administration of anesthetics and analgesics.

REFERENCES

Abdelkefi A, Abdennebi YB, Mellouli F, and others: Effectiveness of fixed 50% nitrous oxide oxygen mixture and EMLA cream for insertion of central venous catheters in children, *Pediatr Blood Cancer* 43(7):777-779, 2004.

Algren JT, Gursoy F, Johnson TD, and others: The effect of nitrous oxide diffusion on laryngeal mask airway cuff inflation in children, *Paediatr Anaesth* 8(1):31-36, 1998.

Anand KJ, Hickey PR: Halothane-morphine compared with high-dose sufentanil for anesthesia and postoperative analgesia in neonatal cardiac surgery, *N Engl J Med* 326(1):1-9, 1992.

American Pain Society: *Principles of analgesic use in the treatment of acute pain and chronic cancer pain,* ed 4, Glenview, Ill, 1999, The Society.

Barrier G, Attia J, Mayer MN, and others: Measurement of postoperative pain and narcotic administration in infants using a new clinical scoring system, *Anesthesiology* 67(3A):A532, 1987.

Basbaum AI: Distinct neurochemical features of acute and persistent pain, *Proc Natl Acad Sci USA* 96(14):7739-7743, 1999a.

Basbaum AI: Spinal mechanisms of acute and persistent pain, *Reg Anesth Pain Med* 24(1):59-67, 1999b.

Benjamin L, Swinson G, Nagel R: Sickle cell anemia day hospital: an approach for the management of uncomplicated painful crises, *Blood* 95:1130-1137, 2000.

Berde C, Collins J: Cancer pain and palliative care in children. In Melzack R, Wall P, editors: *Handbook of pain management,* St Louis, 2003, Churchill Livingstone.

Bernstein B, Pachter L: Cultural considerations in children's pain. In Schechter N, Berde C, Yaster M, editors: *Pain in infants, children, and adolescents,* Philadelphia, 2003, Lippincott Williams & Wilkins.

Beyer JE, Denyes MJ, Villarruel AM: The creation, validation and continuing development of the Oucher: a measure of pain intensity in children, *J Pediatr Nurs* 7(5):335-346, 1992; retrieved May 3, 2007, from http://www.oucher.org.

Beyer JE, Knott CB: Construct validity estimation for the African-American and Hispanic versions of the Oucher scale, *J Pediatr Nurs* 13(1):20-31, 1998.

Bishai R, Taddio A, Bar-Oz B, and others: Relative efficacy of amethocaine gel and lidocaine-prilocaine cream for port-a-cath puncture in children, *Pediatrics* 104(3):e31, 1999.

Blauer T, Gerstmann D: A simultaneous comparison of three neonatal pain scales during common NICU procedures, *Clin J Pain* 14(1):39-47, 1998.

Breau LM, MacLaren J, McGrath PJ, and others: Caregivers' beliefs regarding pain in children with cognitive impairment: relation between pain sensation and reaction increases with severity of impairment, *Clin J Pain* 19(6):335-344, 2003.

Breau LM, McGrath PJ, Camfield CS, and others: Psychometric properties of the Non-communicating Children's Pain Checklist–Revised, *Pain* 99:349-357, 2002.

Chambers CT, Giesbrecht K, Craig KD, and others: A comparison of faces scales for the measurement of pediatric pain: children's and parents' ratings, *Pain* 83:25-35, 1999.

Chambers CT, Hardial J, Craig KD, and others: Faces scales for the measurement of postoperative pain intensity in children following minor surgery, *Clin J Pain* 21(3):277-285, 2005.

Chambers CT, Reid GJ, McGrath PJ, and others: Development and preliminary validation of a postoperative pain measure for parents, *Pain* 68:307-313, 1996.

Choi WY, Irwin MG, Hui TW, and others: EMLA cream versus dorsal penile nerve block for postcircumcision analgesia in children, *Anesth Analg* 96(2):396-399, 2003.

Cline ME, Herman J, Shaw ER, and others: Standardization of the visual analogue scale, *Nurs Res* 41(6):378-380, 1992.

Cole J, Jorgensen K: Medical, developmental, and pharmacologic intervention: the essence of collaboration, *Neonatal Netw* 16:56-58, 1997.

Collins JJ, Byrnes ME, Dunkel IJ, and others: The measurement of symptoms in children with cancer, *J Pain Symptom Manage* 19(5):363-377, 2000.

Collins J, Weisman S: Management of pain in childhood cancer. In Schechter N, Berde C, Yaster M, editors: *Pain in infants, children, and adolescents,* Philadelphia, 2003, Lippincott Williams & Wilkins.

Cousins M, Power I: Acute and postoperative pain. In Melzack R, Wall P, editors: *Handbook of pain management,* St Louis, 2003, Churchill Livingstone.

Dougherty M, DeBaun MR: Rapid increase of morphine and benzodiazepine usage in the last 3 days of life in children with cancer is related to neuropathic pain, *J Pediatr* 142(4):373-376, 2003.

Drake R, Longworth J, Collins JJ: Opioid rotation in children with cancer, *J Palliat Med* 7(3):419-422, 2004.

Egekvist H, Bjerring P: Effect of EMLA cream on skin thickness and subcutaneous venous diameter: a randomized, placebo-controlled study in children, *Acta Dermatol Venereol* 80(5):340-343, 2000.

Eland JA, Banner W: Analgesia, sedation, and neuromuscular blockage in pediatric critical care. In Hazinski ME, editor: *Manual of pediatric critical care,* St Louis, 1999, Mosby.

Fearon I, Kisilevsky BS, Hains SM, and others: Swaddling after heel lance: age-specific effects on behavioral recovery in preterm infants, *Develop Behav Pediatr* 18:222-232, 1997.

Franck L, Vilardi J: Assessment and management of opioid withdrawal in ill neonates, *Neonatal Netw* 14(2):39-48, 1995.

Franck LS, Vilardi J, Durand D, and others: Opioid withdrawal in neonates after continuous infusions of morphine or fentanyl during extracorporeal membrane oxygenation, *Am J Crit Care* 7(5):364-369, 1998.

Gad LN, Olsen KS, Lysgaard AB, and others: Optimized use of EMLA cream in children—secondary publication: a randomized, prospective, controlled comparison of two application regimes, *Ugeskr Laeger* 167(4):404-407, 2005.

Gerik SM: Pain management in children: developmental considerations and mind-body therapies, *South Med J* 98(3):295-302, 2005.

Gold JI, Kim SH, Kant AJ, and others: Effectiveness of virtual reality for pediatric pain distraction during i.v. placement, *Cyberpsychol Behav* 9(2):207-212, 2006.

Goldschneider K, Anand K: Long-term consequences of pain in neonates. In Schechter N, Berde C, Yaster M, editors: *Pain in infants, children, and adolescents,* Philadelphia, 2003, Lippincott Williams & Wilkins.

Gray L, Watt L, Blass E: Skin-to-skin contact is analgesic in healthy newborns, *Pediatrics* 105(1):110-111, 2000.

Greco C, Berde C: Pain management for the hospitalized pediatric patient, *Pediatr Clin North Am* 52(4):995-1027, 2005.

Hadden KL, von Baeyer CL: Pain in children with cerebral palsy: common triggers and expressive behaviors, *Pain* 99(1-2):281-288, 2002.

Hadjistavropoulos HD, Craig KD, Grunau RE, and others: Judging pain in infants: behavioural, contextual, and developmental determinants, *Pain* 73(3):319-324, 1997.

Haines DR, Gaines SP: N of 1 randomised controlled trials of oral ketamine in patients with chronic pain, *Pain* 83(2):283-287, 1999.

Hannallah RS, Broadman LM, Belman AB, and others: Comparison of caudal and ilioinguinal/iliohypogastric nerve blocks for control of postorchiopexy pain in pediatric ambulatory surgery, *Anesthesiology* 66:832-834, 1987.

Hester NO, Foster RL, Jordan-Marsh M, and others: Putting pain measurement into clinical practice. In Finley GA, McGrath PJ, editors: *Measurement of pain in infants and children,* vol 10, Seattle, 1998, IASP Press.

Hodgkinson K, Bear M, Thorn J, and others: Measuring pain in neonates: evaluating an instrument and developing a common language, *Aust J Adv Nurs* 12(1):17-22, 1994.

Holden E, Deichmann M, Levy J: Empirically supported treatments in pediatric psychology: recurrent pediatric headache, *J Pediatr Psychol* 24:91-100, 1999.

Jacob E, Miaskowski C, Savedra M, and others: Changes in intensity, location, and quality of vaso-occlusive pain in children with sickle cell disease, *Pain* 102(1-2):187-193, 2003a.

Jacob E, Miaskowski C, Savedra M, and others: Management of vaso-occlusive pain in hospitalized children with sickle cell disease, *J Pediatr Hematol Oncol* 25(4):307-311, 2003b.

Jacob E, Mueller BU: Pain experience of children with sickle cell disease who had prolonged hospitalizations for acute painful episodes, *Pain Med* 2006 (Online Early Articles). DOI: 10.1111/j.1526-4637.2006.00252.x.

Jacob E, Puntillo KA: Variability of analgesic practices for hospitalized children on different pediatric specialty units, *J Pain Symptom Manage* 20(1):59-67, 2000.

Johnston CC, Stevens B, Pinelli J, and others: Kangaroo care is effective in diminishing pain response in preterm neonates, *Arch Pediatr Adolesc Med* 157(11):1084-1088, 2003.

Jordan-Marsh M, Yoder L, Hall D, and others: Alternate Oucher form testing: gender ethnicity, and age variations, *Res Nurs Health* 17:111-118, 1994.

Joyce BA, Schade JG, Keck JF, and others: Reliability and validity of preverbal pain assessment tools, *Issues Comp Pediatr Nurs* 17:121-135, 1994.

Kain ZN, Mayes LC, Caldwell-Andrews AA, and others: Preoperative anxiety, postoperative pain, and behavioral recovery in young children undergoing surgery, *Pediatrics* 118(2):651-658, 2006.

Klepstad P, Borchgrevink P, Hval B, and others: Long-term treatment with ketamine in a 12-year-old girl with severe neuropathic pain caused by a cervical spinal tumor, *J Pediatr Hematol Oncol* 23(9):616-619, 2001.

Krechel SW, Bildner J: CRIES: a new neonatal post-operative pain measurement score: initial testing of validity and reliability, *Pediatr Anaesth* 5:53-61, 1995.

Lawrence J, Alcock D, McGrath P, and others: The development of a tool to assess neonatal pain, *Neonatal Netw* 12(6):59-66, 1993.

Lenton S, Stallard P, Lewis M, and others: Prevalence and morbidity associated with non-malignant, life-threatening conditions in childhood, *Child Care Health Devel* 27(5):389-398, 2001.

Ljungman G, Gordh T, Sorensen S, and others: Lumbar puncture in pediatric oncology: conscious sedation vs. general anesthesia, *Med Pediatr Oncol* 36(3):372-379, 2001.

Ljungman G, Gordh T, Sorensen S, and others: Pain variations during cancer treatment in children: a descriptive survey, *Pediatr Hematol Oncol* 17(3):211-221, 2000.

Ljungman G, Gordh T, Sorensen S, and others: Pain in paediatric oncology: interviews with children, adolescents and their parents, *Acta Paediatr* 88(6):623-630, 1999.

Ljungman G, Kreuger A, Andreasson S, and others: Midazolam nasal spray reduces procedural anxiety in children, *Pediatrics* 105(1 Pt 1):73-78, 2000.

Luffy R, Grove SK: Examining the validity, reliability, and preference of three pediatric pain measurement tools in African-American children, *Pediatr Nurs* 29(1):54-60, 2003.

Malviya S, Voepel-Lewis T, Burke C, and others: The revised FLACC observational pain tool: improved reliability and validity for pain assessment in children with cognitive impairment, *Paediatr Anaesth* 16(3):258-265, 2006.

Manworren R, Hynan L: Clinical validation of FLACC: Preverbal Patient Pain Scale, *Pediatr Nurs* 29(2):140-146, 2003.

Marx J: Pain research: prolonging the agony, *Science* 305(5682):326-329, 2004.

Max MB, Byas-Smith MG, Gracely RH, and others: Intravenous infusion of the NMDA antagonist, ketamine, in chronic posttraumatic pain with allodynia: a double-blind comparison to alfentanil and placebo, *Clin Neuropharmacol* 18(4):360-368, 1995.

Maxwell L, Yaster M: Perioperative management issues in pediatric patients, *Anesthesiol Clin North Am* 18(3):601-632, 2000.

McCaffery M, Pasero C: *Pain clinical manual*, St Louis, 1999, Mosby.

McGrath P: Behavioral measures of pain. In Finley G, McGrath P, editors: *Measurement of pain in infants and children*, Seattle, 1998, IASP Press.

McGrath P, Hillier L, editors: *Modifying the psychologic factors that intensify children's pain and prolong disability*, Philadelphia, 2003, Lippincott Williams & Wilkins.

McGrath PJ, Johnson G, Goodman JT, and others: The CHEOPS: a behavioral scale to measure postoperative pain in children. In Fields H, Dubner R, Cervero F, editors: *Advances in pain research and therapy*, New York, 1985, Raven Press.

Melzack R: The McGill pain questionnaire: major properties and scoring methods, *Pain* 1:277-299, 1975.

Merkel SI, Voepel-Lewis T, Shayevitz JR, and others: The FLACC: a behavioral scale for scoring postoperative pain in young children, *Pediatr Nurs* 23(3):293-297, 1997.

Miaskowski C, Lee K: Pain, fatigue, and sleep disturbances in oncology outpatients receiving radiation therapy for bone metastasis: a pilot study, *J Pain Symptom Manage* 17(5):320-332, 1999.

Mitchell AC: An unusual case of chronic neuropathic pain responds to an optimum frequency of intravenous ketamine infusions, *J Pain Symptom Manage* 21(5):443-446, 2001.

Morin C, Gibson D, Wade J: Self-reported sleep and mood disturbance in chronic pain patients, *Clin J Pain* 14(4):311-314, 1998.

Myers C, Stuber ML, Bonamer-Rheingans JI, and others: Complementary therapies and childhood cancer, *Cancer Control* 12(3):172-180, 2005.

Nadvi SZ, Sarnaik S, Ravindranath Y: Low frequency of meperidine-associated seizures in sickle cell disease, *Clin Pediatr (Phila)* 38(8):459-462, 1999.

Puchalski M, Hummel P: The reality of neonatal pain, *Adv Neonatal Care* 2(5):233-244, 2002.

Reis E, Holubkov R: Vapocoolant spray is equally effective as EMLA cream in reducing immunization pain in school-aged children, *Pediatrics* 100(6):E5, 1997.

Robieux I, Kumar R, Radhakrishnan S, and others: Assessing pain and analgesia with a lidocaine-prilocaine emulsion in infants and toddlers during venipuncture, *J Pediatr* 118(6):971-973, 1991.

Rogers TL, Ostrow CL: The use of EMLA cream to decrease venipuncture pain in children, *J Pediatr Nurs* 19(1):33-39, 2004.

Rusy L, Weisman S: Complementary therapies for acute pediatric pain management, *Pediatr Clin North Am* 47(3):589-599, 2000.

Sang CN: NMDA-receptor antagonists in neuropathic pain: experimental methods to clinical trials, *J Pain Symptom Manage* 19(1 Suppl):S21-S25, 2000.

Santiago A, Abad P, Fernandez C, and others: Premedication with EMLA cream for ambulatory surgery in children, *Ambul Surg* 8(3):157, 2000.

Savedra MC, Holzemer WL, Tesler MD, and others: Assessment of postoperation pain in children and adolescents using the adolescent pediatric pain tool, *Nurs Res* 42(1):5-9, 1993.

Savedra MC, Tesler MD, Holzemer WL, and others: Pain location: validity and reliability of body outline markings by hospitalized children and adolescents, *Res Nurs Health* 12:307-314, 1989.

Schade JG, Joyce BA, Gerkensmeyer J, and others: Comparison of three preverbal scales for postoperative pain assessment in a diverse pediatric sample, *J Pain Symptom Manage* 12(6):348-359, 1996.

Sindrup SH, Otto M, Finnerup NB, and others: Antidepressants in the treatment of neuropathic pain, *Basic Clin Pharmacol Toxicol* 96(6):399-409, 2005.

Squire SJ, Kirchhoff KT, Hissong K: Comparing two methods of topical anesthesia used before intravenous cannulation in pediatric patients, *J Pediatr Health Care* 14(2):68-72, 2000.

Stallard P, Williams L, Lenton S, and others: Pain in cognitively impaired, non-communicating children, *Arch Dis Child* 85(6):460-462, 2001.

Stallard P, Williams L, Velleman R, and others: The development and evaluation of the pain indicator for communicatively impaired children (PICIC), *Pain* 98(1-2):145-149, 2002a.

Stallard P, Williams L, Velleman R, and others. Intervening factors in caregivers' assessments of pain in non-communicating children, *Devel Med Child Neurol* 44(3):213-214, 2002b.

Stanford EA, Chambers CT, Craig KD: The role of developmental factors in predicting young children's use of a self-report scale for pain, *Pain* 120(1-2):16-23, 2006.

Stevens B: Development and testing of a pediatric pain management sheet, *Pediatr Nurs* 16(6):543-548, 1990.

Stevens B, Johnston C, Petryshen P, and others: Premature Infant Pain Profile: development and initial validation, *Clin J Pain* 12:13-22, 1996.

Stevens B, Yamada J, Ohlsson A: *Sucrose for analgesia in newborn infants undergoing painful procedures* (review), 2005. In Cochrane Neonatal Collaboration, retrieved May 4, 2007, from http://www.thecochranelibrary.com.

Sweet S, McGrath P: Physiological measures of pain. In Finley G, McGrath P, editors: *Measurement of pain in infants and children*, Seattle, 1998, IASP Press.

Symon DN, Russell G: Double blind placebo controlled trial of pizotifen syrup in the treatment of abdominal migraine, *Arch Dis Child* 72(1):48-50, 1995.

Taddio A, Nulman I, Koren BS, and others: A revised measure of acute pain in infants, *J Pain Symptom Manage* 10(6):456-463, 1995.

Tarbell SE, Cohen IT, Marsh JL: The Toddler-Preschooler Postoperative Pain Scale: an observational scale for measuring postoperative pain in children aged 1-5: preliminary report, *Pain* 50(3):273-280, 1992.

Tesler MD, Savedra MC, Holzemer WL, and others: The word-graphic rating scale as a measure of children's and adolescents' pain intensity, *Res Nurs Health* 14:361-371, 1991.

Turner HN: Complex pain consultations in the pediatric intensive care unit, *AACN Clin Issues* 16(3):388-395, 2005.

Uziel Y, Berkovitch M, Gazarian M, and others: Evaluation of eutectic lidocaine/prilocaine cream (EMLA) for steroid joint injection in children with juvenile rheumatoid arthritis: a double blind, randomized, placebo controlled trial, *J Rheumatol* 30(3):594-596, 2003.

Varni JW, Thompson KL, Hanson V: The Varni/Thompson Pediatric Pain Questionnaire, part I, Chronic musculoskeletal pain in juvenile rheumatoid arthritis, *Pain* 28:27-38, 1987.

Villarruel AM, Denyes MJ: Pain assessment in children: theoretical and empirical validity, *Adv Nurs Sci* 14(2):32-41, 1991.

Weisman S, Bernstein B, Schechter N: Consequences of inadequate analgesia during painful procedures in children, *Arch Pediatr Adolesc Med* 152:147-149, 1998.

Weydert J, Ball T, Davis M: Systematic review of treatments for recurrent abdominal pain, *Pediatrics* 111(1):1-3, 2003.

Wilkie DJ, Holzemer WL, Tesler MD, and others: Measuring pain quality: validity and reliability of children's and adolescents' pain language, *Pain* 41(2):151-159, 1990.

Wong DL, Baker CM: Pain in children: comparison of assessment scales, *Pediatr Nurs* 14(1):9-17, 1988.

Wong D, Pasero CL: Reducing the pain of lidocaine, *Am J Nurs* 97(1):17-18, 1997a.

Wong D, Pasero CL: Using local anesthetics to control procedural pain, *Am J Nurs* 97(1):17, 1997b.

Woodgate R, Yanofsky R: A different perspective to approaching cancer symptoms in children, *J Pain Symptom Manage* 26(3):800-817, 2004.

Woolf CJ, Salter MW: Neuronal plasticity: increasing the gain in pain, *Science* 288(5472):1765-1769, 2000.

Yaster M, Krance EJ, Kaplan RF, and others: *Pediatric pain management and sedation handbook*, St Louis, 1997, Mosby.

Health Promotion of the Newborn and Family

BARBARA J. WHEELER

CHAPTER OUTLINE

ADJUSTMENT TO EXTRAUTERINE LIFE, 198
Immediate Adjustments, 198
  Respiratory System, 198
  Circulatory System, 198
Physiologic Status of Other Systems, 199
  Thermoregulation, 199
  Hematopoietic System, 199
  Fluid and Electrolyte Balance, 199
  Gastrointestinal System, 199
  Renal System, 200
  Integumentary System, 200
  Musculoskeletal System, 200
  Defenses Against Infection, 200
  Endocrine System, 200
  Neurologic System, 201
  Sensory Functions, 201
NURSING CARE OF THE NEWBORN AND FAMILY, 201
Assessment, 201
  Initial Assessment: Apgar Scoring, 201
  Clinical Assessment of Gestational Age, 203

Transitional Assessment: Periods of Reactivity, 211
  Behavioral Assessment, 213
  Assessment of Attachment Behaviors, 215
  Physical Assessment, 215
Maintain a Patent Airway, 215
Maintain a Stable Body Temperature, 221
Protect from Infection and Injury, 221
  Identification, 221
  Eye Care, 222
  Vitamin K Administration, 222
  Hepatitis B Vaccine Administration, 222
  Newborn Screening for Disease, 223
  Universal Newborn Hearing Screening, 223
  Bathing, 224
  Care of the Umbilicus, 225
  Circumcision, 225
Provide Optimal Nutrition, 228
  Human Milk, 228
  Breastfeeding, 229

Bottle Feeding, 231
  Commercially Prepared Formulas, 232
  Preparation of Formula, 233
  Alternate Milk Products, 233
  Feeding Schedules, 233
  Feeding Behavior, 234
Promote Parent-Infant Bonding (Attachment), 234
  Infant Behavior, 234
  Maternal Attachment, 234
  Paternal Engrossment, 235
  Siblings, 236
  Multiple Births and Subsequent Children, 237
Prepare for Discharge and Home Care, 237

LEARNING OBJECTIVES

On completion of this chapter the reader will be able to:

- Identify the principal cardiorespiratory changes that occur during transition to extrauterine life.
- Identify the immature physiologic functioning of each body system and its significance to nursing care of the newborn.

- Perform an initial and transitional assessment of the newborn, including the Apgar score and gestational age assessment.
- Perform a newborn physical assessment based on recognition of expected normal findings.

- Outline a nursing plan of care for the well newborn.
- Assess and promote parent-infant attachment behaviors.

RELATED TOPICS and ADDITIONAL RESOURCES

 IN TEXT

Administration of Medication, *Ch. 22*
Birth Injuries, *Ch. 9*
Common Problems in the Newborn, *Ch. 9*
Congenital Heart Disease, *Ch. 25*
Diaper Dermatitis, *Ch. 30*
Fluoride, *Ch. 12*
Health Problems of Newborns, *Ch. 9*
Motor Vehicle Injuries, *Ch. 10*
Multiple Births, *Ch. 3*
Nutrition, *Ch. 10*
Physical Examination, *Ch. 6*
Sibling Rivalry, *Ch. 12*

 COMPANION CD

Anatomy Review—Location of Sutures and
    Fontanels
Case Studies—Breastfeeding; The Normal
    Newborn
Critical Thinking Exercises—Circumcision;
    Formula Preparation
NCLEX Review Questions
Pediatric Assessment Video Clips

evolve
evolve.elsevier.com/Wong/essentials/

NCLEX Review Questions
Pediatric Assessment Video Clips
WebLinks

 **WONG'S CLINICAL MANUAL
OF PEDIATRIC NURSING, 7th Ed**

Patient and Family Education: Suctioning
    the Nose and Mouth, *p. 566*
Guidelines for Automobile Seat Safety,
    p. 237

ADJUSTMENT TO EXTRAUTERINE LIFE

The most profound physiologic change required of the neonate is transition from fetal or placental circulation to independent respiration. The loss of the placental connection means the loss of complete metabolic support, especially the supply of oxygen and the removal of carbon dioxide. The normal stresses of labor and delivery produce alterations of placental gas exchange patterns, acid-base balance in the blood, and cardiovascular activity in the infant. Factors that interfere with this normal transition or that increase fetal **asphyxia** (a condition of hypoxemia, hypercapnia, and acidosis) will affect the fetus's adjustment to extrauterine life.

IMMEDIATE ADJUSTMENTS
Respiratory System

The most critical and immediate physiologic change required of the newborn is the onset of breathing. The stimuli that help initiate the first breath are primarily chemical and thermal. **Chemical factors** in the blood (low oxygen, high carbon dioxide, and low pH) initiate impulses that excite the respiratory center in the medulla. The primary **thermal stimulus** is the sudden chilling of the infant who leaves a warm environment and enters a relatively cooler atmosphere. This abrupt change in temperature excites sensory impulses in the skin that are transmitted to the respiratory center.

Tactile stimulation may assist in initiating respiration. Descent through the birth canal and normal handling during delivery help stimulate respiration in uncompromised infants. Acceptable methods of tactile stimulation include slapping or flicking the soles of the feet or gently rubbing the newborn's back, trunk, or extremities (American Academy of Pediatrics, 2006a). Slapping the newborn's buttocks or back is a harmful technique and should not be done. Prolonged tactile stimulation, beyond one or two slaps or flicks to the soles of the feet or rubbing the back once or twice, can waste precious time in the event of respiratory difficulty and can cause additional damage in infants who have become hypoxemic before or during the birth process.

The initial entry of air into the lungs is opposed by the surface tension of the fluid that filled the fetal lungs and the alveoli. Some lung fluid may also be removed during the nor-

mal forces of labor and delivery. As the chest emerges from the birth canal, fluid is squeezed from the lungs through the nose and mouth. After complete delivery of the chest, brisk recoil of the thorax occurs, and air enters the upper airway to replace the lost fluid. Remaining lung fluid is absorbed by the pulmonary capillaries and lymphatic vessels.

In the alveoli the surface tension of the fluid is reduced by **surfactant,** a substance produced by the alveolar epithelium that coats the alveolar surface. The effect of surfactant in facilitating breathing is discussed in relation to respiratory distress syndrome (see Chapter 9).

Circulatory System

As important as the initiation of respiration are the circulatory changes that allow blood to flow through the lungs. These changes, which occur more gradually, are the result of pressure changes in the lungs, heart, and major vessels. The transition from fetal to postnatal circulation involves the functional closure of the **fetal shunts:** the foramen ovale, the ductus arteriosus, and eventually the ductus venosus. (For a review of fetal circulation, see Chapter 25.) Increased blood flow dilates the pulmonary vessels, pulmonary vascular resistance decreases, and systemic resistance increases, thus maintaining blood pressure. As the pulmonary vessels receive blood, the pressure in the right atrium, right ventricle, and pulmonary arteries decreases. Left atrial pressure increases above right atrial pressure, with subsequent foramen ovale closure. With the increase in pulmonary blood flow and dramatic reduction of pulmonary vascular resistance, the ductus arteriosus begins to close.

The most important factors controlling ductal closure are the increased oxygen concentration of the blood and the fall in endogenous prostaglandins. The foramen ovale closes functionally at or soon after birth. The ductus arteriosus is closed functionally by the fourth day. Anatomic closure takes considerably longer. Failure of the ductus arteriosus or foramen ovale to close results in persistence of fetal shunting of blood away from the lungs (see Chapter 25).

Because of the reversible flow of blood through the ductus during the early neonatal period, a functional murmur occasionally may be heard. In conditions such as crying or straining, the increased pressure shunts unoxygenated blood from the right side of the heart across the ductal opening, causing **transient cyanosis.**

PHYSIOLOGIC STATUS OF OTHER SYSTEMS
Thermoregulation

Next to establishing respiration, heat regulation is most critical to the newborn's survival. Although the newborn's capacity for heat production is adequate, three factors predispose the newborn to excessive heat loss:

- The newborn's large surface area facilitates heat loss to the environment, although this is partially compensated for by the newborn's usual position of flexion, which decreases the amount of surface area exposed to the environment.
- The newborn's thin layer of subcutaneous fat provides poor insulation for conservation of heat.
- The newborn's mechanism for producing heat is different from that of the adult, who can increase heat production through shivering. The chilled neonate cannot shiver but produces heat through **nonshivering thermogenesis (NST),** which involves increased metabolism and oxygen consumption.

The principal thermogenic sources are the heart, liver, and brain. An additional source unique to the newborn is known as **brown adipose tissue,** or **brown fat.** Brown fat, which owes its name to its larger content of mitochondrial cytochromes, has a greater capacity for heat production through intensified metabolic activity than does ordinary adipose tissue. Heat generated in brown fat is distributed to other parts of the body by the blood, which is warmed as it flows through the layers of this tissue. Superficial deposits of brown fat are located between the scapulae, around the neck, in the axillae, and behind the sternum. Deeper layers surround the kidneys, trachea, esophagus, some major arteries, and adrenals. The location of brown fat may explain why the nape of the neck often feels warmer than the rest of the infant's body.

Because of these factors predisposing infants to loss of body heat, it is essential that newly born infants are quickly dried and either provided with warm, dry blankets, or placed skin-to-skin with their mothers after delivery.

Although newborns' ability to conserve heat is usually a matter of concern, they also can have difficulty dissipating heat in an overheated environment, which increases the risk of hyperthermia.

Hematopoietic System

The **blood volume** of the newborn depends on the amount of placental transfer of blood. The blood volume of the full-term infant is about 80 to 85 ml/kg of body weight. Immediately after birth the total blood volume averages 300 ml, but depending on how long cord clamping is delayed, as much as 100 ml can be added to the blood volume. Blood values for the newborn are listed in Appendix C.

Fluid and Electrolyte Balance

Changes occur in the **total body water volume,** extracellular fluid volume, and intracellular fluid volume during the transition from fetal to postnatal life. At birth the total weight of the infant is 73% fluid, compared with 58% in the adult. The infant has a proportionately higher ratio of extracellular fluid than the adult and consequently has a higher level of total body sodium and chloride and a lower level of potassium, magnesium, and phosphate.

An important aspect of fluid balance is its relationship to other systems. In addition to the rate of fluid exchange being seven times greater in the infant than in the adult, the infant's **rate of metabolism** is twice as great in relation to body weight. As a result, twice as much acid is formed, leading to more rapid development of acidosis. In addition, the immature kidneys cannot sufficiently concentrate urine to conserve body water. These three factors make the infant more prone to dehydration, acidosis, and possible overhydration or water intoxication.

Gastrointestinal System

The ability of the newborn to digest, absorb, and metabolize foodstuff is adequate but limited in certain functions. Enzymes are adequate to handle the proteins and simple carbohydrates (monosaccharides and disaccharides), but deficient production of pancreatic amylase impairs use of complex carbohydrates (polysaccharides). Deficiency of pancreatic lipase limits absorption of fats, especially with ingestion of foods with high saturated fatty acid content such as cow's milk. Human milk, despite its high fat content, is easily digested because it contains enzymes such as lipase, which assist in digestion.

The liver is the most immature of the gastrointestinal organs. The activity of the enzyme **glucuronyl transferase** is reduced, which affects the conjugation of bilirubin with glucuronic acid and contributes to the physiologic jaundice of the newborn. The liver is also deficient in forming plasma proteins. The decreased plasma protein concentration probably plays a role in the edema usually seen at birth. Prothrombin and other coagulation factors are also low. The liver stores less glycogen at birth than later in life. Consequently, the newborn is prone to hypoglycemia, which may be prevented by early and effective feeding, especially breastfeeding.

Some **salivary glands** are functioning at birth, but the majority do not begin to secrete saliva until about age 2 to 3 months, when drooling is frequent. Stomach capacity is limited to about 90 ml; thus the infant requires frequent small feedings. The colon also has a small volume; the newborn may have a bowel movement after each feeding. Newborns who breastfeed usually have more frequent feedings and more frequent stools than infants who receive formula.

The infant's **intestine** is longer in relation to body size than that of the adult. Therefore there are a larger number of secretory glands and a larger surface area for absorption as compared with the adult's intestine. Infants have rapid peristaltic waves and simultaneous nonperistaltic waves along the entire esophagus, which propel nutrients forward. The relative immaturity of the peristaltic waves, combined with decreased lower esophageal sphincter (LES) pressure, inappropriate relaxation of the LES, and delayed gastric emptying, make regurgitation a common occurrence. Progressive changes in the stooling pattern indicate a properly functioning gastrointestinal tract (Box 8-1).

The neonatal gastrointestinal mucosa may perform an important function as a barrier to foreign antigens. Both immune and nonimmune factors may play a vital role in decreasing the absorption of antigens capable of causing serious neonatal illness; however, the functional capacity of this system may be immature or altered. Feeding the infant human milk may increase the effectiveness of this defense mechanism.

Change in Stooling Patterns of Newborns

MECONIUM
Infant's first stool; composed of amniotic fluid and its constituents, intestinal secretions, shed mucosal cells, and possibly blood (ingested maternal blood or minor bleeding of alimentary tract vessels).
Passage of meconium should occur within the first 24 to 48 hours, although it may be delayed up to 7 days in very low–birth-weight infants.

TRANSITIONAL STOOLS
Usually appear by third day after initiation of feeding; greenish brown to yellowish brown, thin, and less sticky than meconium; may contain some milk curds.

MILK STOOL
Usually appears by fourth day.
In **breast-fed infants** stools are yellow to golden, are pasty in consistency, and have an odor similar to that of sour milk.
In **formula-fed infants** stools are pale yellow to light brown, are firmer in consistency, and have a more offensive odor.

Renal System

All structural components are present in the renal system, but there is a functional deficiency in the kidney's ability to concentrate urine and to cope with conditions of fluid and electrolyte stress such as dehydration or a concentrated solute load.

Total volume of urine per 24 hours is about 200 to 300 ml by the end of the first week. However, the bladder voluntarily empties when stretched by a volume of 15 ml, resulting in as many as 20 voidings per day. The first voiding should occur within 24 hours. The urine is colorless and odorless and has a specific gravity of about 1.020.

Integumentary System

At birth all the structures within the skin are present, but many of the functions of the integument are immature. The outer two layers of the skin, the epidermis and dermis, are loosely bound to each other and very thin. **Rete pegs,** which later in life anchor the epidermis to the dermis, are not developed. Slight friction across the epidermis, such as from rapid removal of adhesive tape, can cause separation of these layers and blister formation. The transitional zone between the cornified and living layers of the epidermis is effective in preventing fluid from reaching the skin surface.

The **sebaceous glands** are very active late in fetal life and in early infancy because of the high levels of maternal androgens. They are most densely located on the scalp, face, and genitalia and produce the greasy vernix caseosa that covers the infant at birth. Plugging of the sebaceous glands causes **milia.**

The **eccrine glands,** which produce sweat in response to heat or emotional stimuli, are functional at birth, and palmar sweating on crying reaches levels equivalent to those of anxious adults by 3 weeks of age. The eccrine glands produce sweat in response to higher temperatures than those required in adults, and the retention of sweat may result in miliaria. The **apocrine glands** remain small and nonfunctional until puberty.

The growth phases of **hair follicles** usually occur simultaneously at birth. During the first few months the synchrony between hair loss and regrowth is disrupted, and there may be overgrowth of hair or temporary alopecia. Boys' hair grows faster than girls' hair, and in both sexes scalp hair growth is slower at the crown.

Because the amount of **melanin** is low at birth, newborns are lighter skinned than they will be as children. Consequently, they are more susceptible to the harmful effects of the sun.

Musculoskeletal System

At birth the **skeletal system** contains larger amounts of cartilage than of ossified bone, although the process of ossification is fairly rapid during the first year. The nose, for example, is predominantly cartilage at birth and may be temporarily flattened or asymmetric because of the force of delivery. The six skull bones are relatively soft and are separated only by membranous seams. The sinuses are incompletely formed in the newborn.

Unlike the skeletal system, the **muscular system** is almost completely formed at birth. Growth in size of muscular tissue is caused by hypertrophy, rather than hyperplasia, of cells.

Defenses Against Infection

The infant is born with several defenses against infection. The first line of defense is the **skin** and **mucous membranes,** which protect the body from invading organisms. The mature neonatal intestinal mucosal (gut) barrier may also play a vital role as an important defense mechanism against antigens. The second line of defense is the macrophage system, which produces several types of cells capable of attacking a pathogen. The **neutrophils** and **monocytes** are phagocytes, which means they can engulf, ingest, and destroy foreign agents. **Eosinophils** also probably have a phagocytic property, since they increase in number in the presence of foreign protein. The **lymphocytes** (T cells and B cells) are capable of being converted to other cell types, such as monocytes and antibodies. Although the phagocytic properties of the blood are present in the infant, the inflammatory response of the tissues to localize an infection is immature.

The third line of defense is the formation of specific **antibodies** to an antigen. Exposure to various foreign agents is necessary for antibody production to occur. Infants are generally not capable of producing their own immunoglobulin (Ig) until the beginning of the second month of life, but they receive considerable passive immunity in the form of IgG from the maternal circulation and from human milk (see p. 228). They are protected against most major childhood diseases, including diphtheria, measles, poliomyelitis, and rubella, for about 3 months, provided the mother has developed antibodies to these illnesses.

Endocrine System

Ordinarily the endocrine system of the newborn is adequately developed, but its functions are immature. For example, the posterior lobe of the pituitary gland produces limited quantities of **antidiuretic hormone,** or **vasopressin,** which inhibits diuresis. This renders the young infant highly susceptible to dehydration.

The effect of maternal **sex hormones** is particularly evident in the newborn. The labia are hypertrophied, and the breasts of both genders may be engorged and secrete milk (witch's milk) from the first few days of life to as long as 2 months of age. Female newborns may have **pseudomen-**

struation (more often seen as a milky secretion than actual blood) from a sudden drop in progesterone and estrogen levels.

Neurologic System

At birth the nervous system is incompletely integrated but sufficiently developed to sustain extrauterine life. Most neurologic functions are **primitive reflexes.** The **autonomic nervous system** is crucial during transition because it stimulates initial respirations, helps maintain acid-base balance, and partially regulates temperature control.

Myelination of the nervous system follows cephalocaudal-proximodistal (head-to-toe–center-to-periphery) laws of development and is closely related to observed mastery of fine and gross motor skills. **Myelin** is necessary for rapid and efficient transmission of some, but not all, nerve impulses along the neural pathway. The tracts that develop myelin earliest are the sensory, cerebellar, and extrapyramidal tracts. This accounts for the acute senses of taste, smell, and hearing in the newborn, as well as the perception of pain. All **cranial nerves** are present and myelinated except for the optic and olfactory nerves.

Sensory Functions

The newborn's sensory functions are remarkably well developed and have a significant effect on growth and development, including the attachment process.

Vision. At birth the eye is structurally incomplete. The **fovea centralis** is not yet completely differentiated from the macula. The **ciliary muscles** are also immature, limiting the eyes' ability to accommodate and focus on an object for any length of time. The infant can track and follow objects. The **pupils** react to light, the blink reflex is responsive to minimal stimulus, and the corneal reflex is activated by a light touch. **Tear glands** usually do not begin to function until 2 to 4 weeks of age.

The newborn has the ability to focus momentarily on a bright or moving object that is within 20 cm (8 inches) and in the midline of the visual field. In fact, the infant's ability to fixate on coordinated movement is greater during the first hour of life than during the succeeding several days. **Visual acuity** is reported to be between 20/100 and 20/400, depending on the vision measurement techniques.

The infant also demonstrates visual preferences: medium colors (yellow, green, pink) over bright (red, orange, blue) or dim colors; black-and-white contrasting patterns, especially geometric shapes and checkerboards; large objects with medium complexity rather than small, complex objects; and reflecting objects over dull ones.

Hearing. After the amniotic fluid has drained from the ears, the infant probably has **auditory acuity** similar to that of an adult. The neonate reacts to a loud sound of about 90 decibels with a startle reflex. The newborn's response to sounds of low frequency vs those of high frequency differs; the former, such as the sound of a heartbeat, metronome, or lullaby, tends to decrease an infant's motor activity and crying, whereas the latter elicits an alerting reaction. There is also an early sensitivity to the sound of human voices, although not specifically speech sounds. For example, infants younger than 3 days of age can discriminate the mother's voice from that of other women. As early as age 5 days, newborns can differentiate between stories repeated to them during the last trimester of pregnancy by their mother and the same stories recited after birth by a different woman.

The internal and middle **ear** is large at birth, but the external canal is small. The mastoid process and the bony part of the external canal have not yet developed. Consequently the tympanic membrane and facial nerve are very close to the surface and can be easily damaged.

Smell. Newborns react to strong odors such as alcohol or vinegar by turning their heads away. Breast-fed infants are able to smell breast milk and will cry for their mothers when they smell leaking milk. Infants are also able to differentiate the breast milk of their mother from the breast milk of other women by smell. Maternal odors are believed to influence the attachment process and successful breastfeeding. Unnecessary routine washing of the breast may interfere with establishment of early breastfeeding.

Taste. The newborn has the ability to distinguish between tastes. Various types of solutions elicit differing gustofacial reflexes. A tasteless solution elicits no facial expression; a sweet solution elicits an eager suck and a look of satisfaction; a sour solution causes the usual puckering of the lips; and a bitter liquid produces an angry, upset expression. Newborns demonstrate preferential taste for glucose water to sterile water. During early childhood the taste buds are distributed mostly on the tip of the tongue.

Touch. At birth the infant is able to perceive tactile sensation in any part of the body, although the face (especially the mouth), hands, and soles of the feet seem to be most sensitive. There is increasing documentation that touch and motion are essential to normal growth and development. Gentle patting of the back or rubbing of the abdomen usually elicits a calming response from the infant. In turn, painful stimuli, such as a pinprick, will elicit an upset response.

NURSING CARE OF THE NEWBORN AND FAMILY

ASSESSMENT

The newborn requires thorough, skilled observation to ensure a satisfactory adjustment to extrauterine life. Physical assessment following delivery can be divided into four phases:

1. The initial assessment, which includes the Apgar scoring system
2. Transitional assessment during the periods of reactivity
3. Assessment of gestational age
4. Systematic physical examination.

In addition, the nurse must be aware of behaviors that signal successful reciprocal attachment between the infant and parents. Awareness of the expected normal findings during each assessment process helps the nurse recognize any deviation that may prevent the infant from progressing uneventfully through the early postnatal period. With shorter hospitalizations, the accomplishment of thorough newborn assessment and parent teaching has become a challenge.

Initial Assessment: Apgar Scoring

The most frequently used method to assess the newborn's immediate adjustment to extrauterine life is the **Apgar** scoring system (Papile, 2001). The score is based on observation of heart rate, respiratory effort, muscle tone, reflex irritability, and color (Table 8-1). Each item is given a score of 0, 1, or 2. Evaluations of all five categories are made at 1 and 5 minutes

TABLE 8-1

Infant Evaluation at Birth—Apgar Scoring System

SIGN	0	1	2
Heart rate	Absent	Slow, <100 beats/min	>100 beats/min
Respiratory effort	Absent	Irregular, slow, weak cry	Good, strong cry
Muscle tone	Limp	Some flexion of extremities	Well flexed
Reflex irritability	No response	Grimace	Cry, sneeze
Color	Blue, pale	Body pink, extremities blue	Completely pink

ESTIMATION OF GESTATIONAL AGE BY MATURITY RATING

NEUROMUSCULAR MATURITY

PHYSICAL MATURITY

Skin	sticky friable transparent	gelatinous red, translucent	smooth pink, visible veins	superficial peeling &/or rash, few veins	cracking pale areas rare veins	parchment deep cracking no vessels	leathery cracked wrinkled
Lanugo	none	sparse	abundant	thinning	bald areas	mostly bald	
Plantar Surface	heel-toe 40-50 mm: -1 <40 mm: -2	>50 mm no crease	faint red marks	anterior transverse crease only	creases ant. 2/3	creases over entire sole	
Breast	imperceptible	barely perceptible	flat areola no bud	stippled areola 1-2 mm bud	raised areola 3-4 mm bud	full areola 5-10 mm bud	
Eye/Ear	lids fused loosely: -1 tightly: -2	lids open pinna flat stays folded	slightly curved pinna; soft; slow recoil	well-curved pinna; soft but ready recoil	formed & firm instant recoil	thick cartilage ear stiff	
Genitals (male)	scrotum flat, smooth	scrotum empty faint rugae	testes in upper canal rare rugae	testes descending few rugae	testes down good rugae	testes pendulous deep rugae	
Genitals (female)	clitoris prominent labia flat	prominent clitoris small labia minora	prominent clitoris enlarging minora	majora & minora equally prominent	majora large minora small	majora cover clitoris & minora	

MATURITY RATING

score	weeks
-10	20
-5	22
0	24
5	26
10	28
15	30
20	32
25	34
30	36
35	38
40	40
45	42
50	44

A

FIG. 8-1 ■ A, New Ballard Scale for newborn maturity rating. Expanded scale includes extremely preterm infants and has been refined to improve accuracy in more mature infants. (**A,** From Ballard JL, Khoury JC, Wedig K, and others: New Ballard Score, expanded to include extremely premature infants, *J Pediatr* 119(3): 418, 1991.)   *Continued*

FIG. 8-1, cont'd ■ **B,** Intrauterine growth: birth weight percentiles based on live single births at gestational ages 20 to 44 weeks. (**B,** Data from Alexander GR, Himes JH, Kaufman RB, and others: A United States national reference for fetal growth, *Obstet Gynecol* 87(2):163-168, 1996.)

after birth and repeated until the infant's condition stabilizes. Total scores of 0 to 3 represent severe distress, scores of 4 to 6 signify moderate difficulty, and scores of 7 to 10 indicate absence of difficulty in adjusting to extrauterine life. The Apgar score is affected by the degree of physiologic immaturity, infection, congenital malformations, maternal sedation or analgesia, and neuromuscular disorders.

The Apgar score reflects the general condition of the infant at 1 and 5 minutes based on the five parameters described previously. The Apgar score is not a tool, however, that stands on its own to either interpret past events or predict future events linked to the infant's eventual neurologic or physical status. Considerable discussion and controversy have centered on Apgar scoring because of its misuse as an indicator for the presence or absence of perinatal asphyxia in the medicolegal field (American Academy of Pediatrics and American College of Obstetricians and Gynecologists, 2006). In addition, the Apgar score is not used to determine the newborn's need for resuscitation at birth.

Clinical Assessment of Gestational Age

Assessment of gestational age is an important criterion because perinatal morbidity and mortality are related to gestational age and birth weight. A frequently used method of determining gestational age is the **New Ballard Scale (NBS)** by Ballard, Khoury, Wedig, and others (1991) (Fig. 8-1, *A*). This scale, an abbreviated version of the **Dubowitz scale,** assesses six external physical and six neuromuscular signs. Each sign

has a number score, and the cumulative score correlates with a maturity rating of 20 to 44 weeks of gestation.

The NBS includes −1 and −2 scores that reflect signs of extremely preterm infants, such as fused eyelids; imperceptible breast tissue; sticky, friable, transparent skin; no lanugo; and square-window (flexion of wrist) angle of greater than 90 degrees (see Fig. 8-1, *A,* and the description of the tests in Box 8-2). The examination of infants with a gestational age of 26 weeks or less should be performed at a postnatal age of less than 12 hours. For infants with a gestational age of at least 26 weeks, the examination can be performed up to 96 hours after birth. To ensure accuracy, it is recommended that the initial examination be performed within the first 48 hours of life. Neuromuscular adjustments after birth in extremely immature neonates require that a follow-up examination be performed to further validate neuromuscular criteria. The NBS scale overestimates gestational age by 2 to 4 days in infants younger than 37 weeks of gestation, especially at gestational ages of 32 to 37 weeks (Ballard, Khoury, Wedig, and others, 1991). In a blinded Spanish study, Marín, Martín, Lliteras, and others (2006) compared estimations of gestational age using NBS vs ultrasonography or mother's last menstrual period. Researchers found general agreement between NBS and ultrasonography or last menstrual period; however, they noted that NBS tends to overestimate gestational age in very preterm newborns and in infants whose mothers had received prenatal corticosteroid therapy.

Weight Related to Gestational Age. The weight of the infant at birth also correlates with the incidence of perina-

---

BOX 8-2

Tests Used in Assessing Gestational Age

Posture—With infant quiet and in a supine position, observe degree of flexion in arms and legs. Muscle tone and degree of flexion increase with maturity.
*Full flexion of the arms and legs—4.**

Square window—With thumb supporting back of arm below wrist, apply gentle pressure with index and third fingers on dorsum of hand without rotating infant's wrist. Measure angle between base of thumb and forearm.
Full flexion (hand lies flat on ventral surface of forearm)—4.

Arm recoil—With infant supine, fully flex both forearms on upper arms, hold for 5 seconds; pull down on hands to fully extend and rapidly release arms. Observe rapidity and intensity of recoil to a state of flexion.
A brisk return to full flexion—4.

Popliteal angle—With infant supine and pelvis flat on a firm surface, flex lower leg on thigh and then flex thigh on abdomen. While holding knee with thumb and index finger, extend lower leg with index finger of other hand. Measure degree of angle behind knee (popliteal angle).
An angle of less than 90 degrees—5.

Scarf sign—With infant supine, support head in midline with one hand; use other hand to pull infant's arm across the shoulder so that infant's hand touches shoulder. Determine location of elbow in relation to midline.
Elbow does not reach midline—4.

Heel to ear—With infant supine and pelvis flat on a firm surface, pull foot as far as possible up toward ear on same side. Measure distance of foot from ear and degree of knee flexion (same as popliteal angle).
Knees flexed with a popliteal angle of less than 90 degrees—4.

*Numeric ratings correspond with Fig. 8-1, *A*, on p. 202.

FIG. 8-2 ■ Three infants, same gestational age, weight 600, 1400, and 2750 g, respectively, from left to right. (From Korones SB: *High-risk newborn infants: the basis for intensive nursing care*, ed 4, St Louis, 1986, Mosby.)

tal morbidity and mortality. However, birth weight alone is a poor indicator of gestational age and fetal maturity. Maturity implies **functional capacity**—the degree to which the neonate's organ systems are able to adapt to the requirements of extrauterine life. Therefore gestational age is more closely related to fetal maturity than is birth weight. Because heredity influences a newborn's size, noting the size of other family members is part of the assessment process.

Intrauterine growth curves are used to classify infants according to birth weight and gestational age. The primary intrauterine growth charts that provide national reference data include the work of Alexander, Himes, Kaufman, and others (1996), which is representative of more than 3.1 million live births in the United States, and Thomas, Peabody, Turnier, and others (2000). Arbuckle, Wilkins, and Sherman (1993), and Kramer, Platt, Wen, and others (2001), have produced intrauterine growth charts using large numbers of infants representative of the Canadian population. Thomas and others (2000) concluded that intrauterine growth measured by head circumference, birth weight, and length varies according to race and gender. These researchers also found that altitude did not seem to significantly affect birth weight, as has been suggested by other authors. It is recommended that the reader access and use the most current intrauterine growth chart specific to the referent population being evaluated.

Classification of infants at birth by both **birth weight** and **gestational age** provides a more satisfactory method for predicting mortality risks and providing guidelines for management of the neonate than estimating gestational age or birth weight alone. The infant's birth weight, length, and head circumference are plotted on standardized graphs that identify normal values for gestational age (for birth weight see Fig. 8-1, *B*). The infant whose weight is **appropriate for gestational age (AGA)** (between 10th and 90th percentiles) can be presumed to have grown at a normal rate regardless of the time of birth—preterm, term, or postterm. The infant who is **large for gestational age (LGA)** (above 90th percentile) can be presumed to have grown at an accelerated rate during fetal life; the **small-for-gestational-age (SGA)** infant (below 10th percentile) can be assumed to have intrauterine growth restriction or delay.

When gestational age is determined according to a standardized gestational age scale such as the NBS, the newborn will fall into one of the following nine possible categories for birth weight and gestational age: AGA—term, preterm, postterm; SGA—term, preterm, postterm; LGA—term, preterm, postterm. Fig. 8-2 illustrates the disparity between birth weights of three preterm infants of the same gestational age, 32 weeks. Birth weight and gestational age both influence morbidity and mortality; the lower the birth weight and gestational age, the higher the morbidity and mortality.

General Measurements. Several important measurements of the newborn have significance when compared with each other and when recorded over time on a graph. For the full-term infant, average **head circumference** is between 33 and 35.5 cm (13 and 14 inches). Head circumference may be somewhat less immediately after birth because of the molding process that occurs during a vaginal delivery. Usually by the second or third day the skull is normal in size and contour.

Chest circumference is 30.5 to 33 cm (12 to 13 inches). Head circumference is usually about 2 to 3 cm (about 1 inch) greater than chest circumference. Because of the molding of the head during delivery, these measurements may initially appear equal.

Head circumference may also be compared with crown-to-rump length, or sitting height. **Crown-to-rump** measure-

FIG. 8-3 ■ Measurement of infant length.

FIG. 8-4 ■ Mother taking axillary temperature with digital thermometer.

ments are usually 31 to 35 cm (12.2 to 13.8 inches) and are approximately equal to head circumference. The relationship of the head and crown-to-rump measurements is more reliable than that of the head and chest. Neonatal head circumference and crown-to-rump length may provide a more accurate means for identifying infants at risk; head circumference has been shown to be equal to or up to 1 cm more than crown-to-rump length in 62% of the infants examined and determined to be normocephalic.

Abdominal circumference need not be routinely measured in the newborn, but should be done in the event of abdominal distention to determine changes in girth over time (Conner, 2003). Abdominal circumference is measured just above the level of the umbilicus, since the umbilical cord is still attached, making measurements across the umbilicus too variable in newborns. Measuring the abdominal circumference below the umbilical region is unsuitable because bladder status may affect the reading.

Head-to-heel length is also measured. Because of the usual flexed position of the infant, it is important to extend the leg completely when measuring total body length. The average length of the newborn is 48 to 53 cm (19 to 21 inches) (Fig. 8-3).

Measure **body weight** soon after birth because weight loss occurs fairly rapidly. Normally the neonate loses about 10% of the birth weight by 3 to 4 days of age because of loss of extracellular fluid and meconium, as well as limited food intake, especially in breast-fed infants. The birth weight is usually regained by the tenth to fourteenth day of life. Most newborns weigh 2700 to 4000 g (6 to 9 pounds), the average weight being about 3400 g (7.5 pounds). Accurate birth weights and lengths are important because they provide a baseline for assessment of future growth.

Another category of measurements is vital signs. **Axillary temperatures** are taken because insertion of a thermometer into the rectum can potentially cause perforation of the mucosa if performed incorrectly (see Table 6-3 and Fig. 8-4). Core body temperature varies according to the periods of reactivity but is usually 36.5° to 37.6° C (97.7° to 99.7° F). Skin temperature is slightly lower than core body temperature. Therefore axillary temperature may be less than rectal temperature, although the difference is small (as little as 0.2° F) between axillary and rectal sites. Because brown adipose tissue

is located in the axillary pocket, axillary readings may be elevated whenever NST occurs. However, axillary readings may be normal in cold-stressed infants when NST is not triggered or is overwhelmed.

The single best method for determining the newborn infant's temperature in any given situation remains elusive when considering the available studies. Controversy exists regarding the accuracy of tympanic membrane sensors. Bliss-Holtz (1993) compared axillary and tympanic membrane temperatures in neonates and found that tympanic membrane temperature measurements were helpful in determining the infant's thermal state. However, other studies have found tympanic membrane temperatures to have high variability according to neonatal environment (bassinet or open crib, radiant warmer, and incubator) (Hicks, 1996; Leick-Rude and Bloom, 1998) and limited usefulness in critically ill neonates (Weiss, Poeltler, and Gocka, 1993; Wilshaw, Beckstrand, Waid, and others, 1999). One study concluded that tympanic membrane temperatures were unacceptable for detecting fever in children under 6 years of age (Lanham, Walker, Klocke, and others, 1999). A meta-analysis of 101 studies comparing tympanic membrane temperatures with rectal temperatures in children concluded that the tympanic method demonstrated a wide range of variability, limiting its application in a pediatric setting (Craig, Lancaster, Taylor, and others, 2002). The Canadian Paediatric Society (CPS) (2007) outlines concerns regarding safety and accuracy of tympanic temperature measurement in newborns because of the size of a newborn's external ear canal relative to the size of the thermometer probe. To ensure accuracy, the probe, which may be up to 8 mm (0.3 inch) in diameter, must be deeply inserted into the ear canal to allow orientation of the sensor near or against the tympanic membrane. At birth, the average diameter of the canal is just 4 mm (0.16 inch); at 2 years of age it is just 5 mm (0.2 inch). The CPS concurs with earlier writers Bliss-Holtz (1993) and Yetman, Coody, West, and others (1993) in their conclusion that infrared tympanic membrane technology has yet to meet clinical needs for use in newborn infants.

Infrared axillary and digital thermometers are used in many neonatal units because they give rapid readings and are easy to clean; studies demonstrate their usefulness in well, full-term newborns (Sganga, Wallace, Kiehl, and others, 2000), whereas accuracy with critically ill neonates is less predictable (Seguin and Terry, 1999; Wilshaw, Beckstrand, Waid, and others, 1999). Bailey and Rose (2001) concluded that tympanic membrane temperatures (vs axillary) in healthy preterm infants were reliable, were cost effective, and decreased the amount of handling required for monitoring. Skin temperature readings have also been found to vary with probe site placement; bed type; environmental temperature; and the use of blankets, clothing, and nesting devices (Leick-Rude and Bloom, 1998). Jones, Kleber, Eckert, and others (2003) compared rectal temperatures of infants under 2 months of age with calibrated digital thermometers and mercury glass thermometers; the study of 120 infants found that the digital thermometers measured a higher temperature (mean average of 0.7° F; range 0° to 1.6° F) than the mercury glass thermometers. The researchers concluded that the error in measurement was attributable to the digital thermometer used. Advantages of digital thermometers in neonatal care include relatively easy readability by parents and caretakers in the home, improvement of discharge planning effectiveness, and decreased risk of breakage and associated complications compared with glass thermometers.

Temporal artery thermometers (TATs) are available for use in the general pediatric population, and parents often report ease of use and less discomfort with such methods. Greenes and Fleisher (2001) concluded that the TAT had limited sensitivity in infants for detecting rectal fever, yet the TAT was more accurate than the tympanic thermometer. Siberry, Diener-West, Schappell, and others (2002) compared the infrared TAT (using an infrared device) with the rectal temperature measurement (digital thermometer) and found poor predictability for fever in children 0 to 3 months old. The authors concluded that the TAT could be used as a rapid assessment screening tool to identify rectal fever in children 3 to 24 months old, but TAT was unreliable as a screening tool for infants under 3 months. Schuh, Komar, Stephens, and others (2004) compared rectal temperatures with TAT measurements in an emergency department population of children under 24 months and concluded that the TAT was not reliable for detecting rectal fever in children under 3 months but could be used as a screening tool for detecting fever of at least 38.3° C (100.9° F) in children 3 to 24 months.

In most studies regarding newborn temperature, the glass mercury thermometer is the gold standard against which other methods are compared. There is no universal agreement on placement times for glass thermometers, although 3 minutes for rectal temperature and 5 minutes for axillary temperature are considered to be adequate. The American Academy of Pediatrics (2001) has, however, issued a statement

FIG. 8-5 ■ Measurement of blood pressure using oscillometry.

recommending that mercury thermometers no longer be used in clinics and homes to decrease mercury exposure hazard.

Nurses must be cognizant of the many variables involved (site—axillary, rectal, tympanic, skin; skin blood flow at site of measurement; environment—radiant warmer, open crib, incubator, clothing, or nesting; purpose—fever, possible sepsis, in which case the temperature may be lower than normal in newborns, and thermoregulation in the transition phase; instrument—electronic, digital, infrared) and able to make clear clinical decisions based on accurate and objective data. Further research is needed to perfect thermometers that accurately reflect the infant's core temperature in order to effectively plan nursing care and maintain a stable temperature.

Pulse and **respirations** also vary according to the periods of reactivity and the infant's behaviors but are usually in the range of 120 to 140 beats/min and 30 to 60 breaths/min, respectively. Both are counted for a full 60 seconds to detect irregularities in rate or rhythm. The heart rate is taken apically with a stethoscope, and the femoral arteries are palpated for equality of strength or fullness.

Measurement of **blood pressure** (BP) provides baseline data and may indicate cardiovascular problems. BP is most easily and accurately assessed using oscillometry (Dinamap), when the newborn is in a quiet or sleep state, using an appropriate cuff width–to-arm ratio of 0.45 to 0.70 (approximately half to three quarters) (Nuntnarumit, Yand, and Bada-Ellzey, 1999). Oscillometry is less reliable when mean arterial pressure is below 40 mm Hg (Chia, Ang, Wong, and others, 1990) (Fig. 8-5). The average oscillometric systolic/diastolic pressure is 65/41 mm Hg at 1 to 3 days of age. Compare BP in the upper and lower extremities, which should be equal.

A suggested schedule for monitoring heart rate, respiratory rate, and temperature is on admission to the nursery, once every 30 minutes until the newborn has been stable for 2 hours (American Academy of Pediatrics and American College of Obstetricians and Gynecologists, 2007), then once every 8 hours until discharge. However, this schedule may vary according to institutional policy. Any change in the infant, such as color, breathing, muscle tone, or behavior, necessitates more frequent monitoring.

General Appearance. Before each body system is assessed, it is important to describe the general **posture** and behavior of the newborn. The overall appearance yields valuable clues to the infant's physical status.

In the full-term neonate the posture is one of complete **flexion** as a result of in utero position. Most infants are born in a vertex presentation with the head flexed and the chin resting on the upper chest, the arms flexed with the hands clenched, the legs flexed at the knees and hips, and the feet dorsiflexed. The vertebral column is also flexed. It is important to recognize any deviation from this characteristic fetal position.

The infant's **behavior** is carefully noted, especially the degree of alertness, drowsiness, and irritability; the latter two factors may reflect common signs of neurologic problems. Some questions to mentally ask when assessing behavior include:

- Is the infant awakened easily by a loud noise?
- Is the infant comforted by rocking, sucking, or cuddling?
- Do there seem to be periods of deep and light sleep?
- When awake, does the infant seem satisfied after a feeding?
- What stimuli elicit responses from the infant?
- When disturbed, how much does the infant protest?

Skin. The **texture** of the newborn's skin is velvety smooth and puffy, especially about the eyes, the legs, the dorsal aspect of the hands and the feet, and the scrotum or labia. Skin **color** depends on racial and familial background and varies greatly among newborns. In general, the Caucasian infant is usually pink to red. The African-American newborn may appear a pinkish or yellowish brown. Infants of Hispanic descent may have an olive tint or a slight yellow cast to the skin. Infants of Asian descent may be a rosy or yellowish tan. The color of Native American newborns depends on the tribe and can vary from a light pink to a dark, reddish brown. By the second or third day the skin turns to its more natural tone and is drier and flakier. Several other color changes that may be noted on the skin are described later in this chapter (see Table 8-4).

At birth the skin may be partially covered with a grayish white, cheeselike substance called **vernix caseosa,** a mixture of sebum and desquamating cells. It will be absorbed by 24 to 28 hours. A fine, downy hair called **lanugo** may be present on the skin, especially on the forehead, cheeks, shoulders, and back.

Head. General observation of the **contour** of the head is important, since **molding** occurs in almost all vaginal deliveries. In a vertex delivery the head is usually flattened at the forehead, with the apex rising and forming a point at the end of the parietal bones and the posterior skull or occiput dropping abruptly. The usual, more oval contour of the head is apparent by 1 to 2 days after birth. The change in shape occurs because the bones of the cranium are not fused, allowing for overlapping of the edges of these bones to accommodate to the size of the birth canal during delivery. Such molding usually does not occur in infants born by elective cesarean section.

Six bones—the frontal, occipital, two parietals, and two temporals—make up the cranium. Between the junction of these bones are bands of connective tissue called **sutures.** At the junction of the sutures are wider spaces of unossified membranous tissue called **fontanels.** The two most prominent fontanels in infants are the **anterior fontanel,** formed by the junction of the sagittal, coronal, and frontal sutures, and the **posterior fontanel,** formed by the junction of the sagittal and lambdoid sutures (Fig. 8-6, *A*).

The skull is palpated for all patent sutures and fontanels, noting size, shape, molding, or abnormal closure. The sutures feel like cracks between the skull bones, and the fontanels feel like wider **soft spots** at the junction of the sutures. These are palpated by using the tip of the index finger and running it along the ends of the bones (see Fig. 8-6, *B*).

The anterior fontanel is diamond shaped and measures anywhere from barely palpable to 4 to 5 cm (about 2 inches) at its widest point (from bone to bone, rather than from suture to suture). The posterior fontanel is easily located by following the sagittal suture toward the occiput. The posterior fontanel is triangular, usually measuring between 0.5 and 1 cm (less than ½ inch) at its widest part. The fontanels should feel flat, firm, and well demarcated against the bony edges of the skull. Frequently pulsations are visible at the anterior fontanel. Coughing, crying, or lying down may temporarily cause the fontanels to bulge and become more taut.

Palpate the skull for any unusual masses or prominences, particularly those resulting from birth trauma, such as caput succedaneum or cephalhematoma (see Chapter 9). Because of the pliability of the skull, exerting pressure at the margin of the parietal and occipital bones along the lambdoid suture may produce a snapping sensation similar to the indentation of a Ping-Pong ball. This phenomenon, known as **physiologic craniotabes,** may be found normally, especially in newborns of breech birth, but also may indicate hydrocephalus, congenital syphilis, or rickets.

Assess the degree of **head control.** Although **head lag** is normal in the newborn, the degree of ability to control the head in certain positions should be recognized. If the supine infant is pulled from the arms into a semi-Fowler position, marked head lag and hyperextension are noted (Fig. 8-7, *A*). However, as the infant is brought forward into a sitting position, the infant will attempt to control the head in an upright position. As the head falls forward onto the chest, many infants will attempt to right it into the erect position. Also, if the infant is held in ventral suspension (i.e., held prone above and parallel to the examining surface), the infant will hold the head in a straight line with the spinal column (see Fig. 8-7, *B*). When lying on the abdomen, the newborn has the ability to lift the head slightly, turning it from side to side. Marked head lag is seen in neonates with Down syndrome, prematurity, hypoxia, and neuromuscular compromise.

Frontal suture

Anterior fontanel

Frontal bone

Coronal
suture

Sagittal
suture

Parietal
bone

Posterior fontanel

Lambdoid
suture

Occipital
bone

A

B

FIG. 8-6 ■ A, Location of sutures and fontanels. **B,** Palpating anterior fontanel.

FIG. 8-7 ■ Head control in infant. **A,** Inability to hold head erect when pulled to sitting position. **B,** Ability to hold head erect when placed in ventral suspension.

Eyes. Because newborns tend to have their eyes tightly closed, it is best to begin the examination of the eyes by observing the lids for edema, which is normally present for the first 2 days after delivery. The eyes are observed for symmetry. **Tears** may be present at birth, but purulent discharge from the eyes shortly after birth is abnormal. To visualize the surface structures of the eye, the infant is held supine, and the head is gently lowered. The eyes will usually open, similar to the mechanism of a doll's eyes. The **sclera** should be white and clear.

The cornea is examined for the presence of any opacities or haziness. The **corneal reflex** is normally present at birth but may not be elicited unless neurologic or eye damage is suspected. The pupil will usually respond to light by constricting.

The pupils are normally malaligned. A searching **nystagmus** is common. **Strabismus** is a normal finding because of the lack of binocularity. The color of the iris is noted. Most light-skinned newborns have slate gray or dark blue eyes, whereas dark-skinned infants have brown eyes.

A funduscopic examination is difficult to perform because of the infant's tendency to keep the eyes tightly closed. However, a **red reflex** should be elicited (see Chapter 6).

NURSINGTIP

To elicit a red reflex, place the infant in a dark room. In an alert state many newborns will open the eyes in a supported sitting position.

Ears. The ears are examined for position, structure, and auditory function. The top of the pinna should lie in a horizontal plane to the outer canthus of the eye (see Fig. 6-19). The pinna is often flattened against the side of the head from pressure in utero. An otoscopic examination ordinarily may not be performed because the **canals** are filled with vernix caseosa and amniotic fluid, making visualization of the **tympanic membrane** difficult.

Auditory ability is tested by a number of objective hearing tests (see p. 140). Making a loud noise close to the infant's head may or may not elicit a response; the lack of a response, however, is not a definite indication of hearing loss. The **startle reflex** (see Table 8-2) may be observed when there is a sudden loud noise near the infant or the bassinet is accidentally bumped, but this often depends on the infant's state at the time.

Nose. The nose is usually flattened after birth, and bruises are common. Patency of the **nasal canals** can be assessed by holding a hand over the infant's mouth and one canal and noting the passage of air through the unobstructed opening. If nasal patency is questionable, it is reported, because most newborns are obligatory nose breathers. Sneezing and thin white mucus are common up to several hours after birth.

Mouth and Throat. An external defect of the mouth such as cleft lip is readily apparent; however, the internal structures require careful inspection. The **palate** is normally highly arched and somewhat narrow. Rarely teeth may be present. A common finding is **Epstein pearls,** small, white, epithelial cysts along both sides of the midline of the hard palate. They are insignificant and disappear in several weeks.

The **frenulum** of the upper lip is a band of thick, pink tissue that lies under the inner surface of the upper lip and extends to the maxillary alveolar ridge. It is particularly evident when the infant yawns or smiles. It disappears as the maxilla grows.

The **lingual frenulum** attaches the underside of the tongue to the lower palate midway between the ventral surface of the tongue and the tip. In some cases a tight lingual frenulum, formerly referred to as tongue-tie, may restrict adequate sucking. Further evaluation may be required to ascertain adequate sucking, particularly in breast-fed infants. The treatment for a tight lingual frenulum advocated by the American Academy of Pediatrics is **frenotomy,** a safe and effective surgical procedure that improves comfort, effectiveness, and ease of breastfeeding for mother and infant (Barclay, 2002; Ballard, Auer, and Khoury, 2002; Coryllos, Genna, and Salloum, 2004).

Elicit the **sucking reflex** by placing a nipple or nonlatex gloved finger in the infant's mouth. The infant should exhibit a strong, vigorous suck. The **rooting reflex** is elicited by stroking the cheek and noting the infant's response of turning toward the stimulated side and sucking.

The **uvula** can be inspected while the infant is crying and the chin is depressed. However, it may be retracted upward and backward during crying. Tonsillar tissue is generally not seen in the newborn. **Natal teeth,** teeth present at birth, as opposed to **neonatal teeth,** which erupt during the first month of life, are seen infrequently and erupt chiefly at the position of the lower incisors. Teeth are reported because they are frequently found with developmental abnormalities and syndromes, including cleft lip and palate. Most natal teeth are loosely attached. However, current thinking suggests preserving them until they exfoliate naturally (McDonald and Avery,

2004), unless the tooth is attached loosely or breastfeeding is impaired by the neonate biting the breast.

Neck. Because the newborn's neck is short and covered with folds of tissue, adequate assessment of the neck requires allowing the head to fall gently backward in hyperextension while the back is supported in a slightly raised position. Observe for range of motion, shape, and any abnormal masses, and palpate each clavicle for possible fractures.

Chest. The **shape** of the newborn's chest is almost circular because the anteroposterior and lateral diameters are equal. The ribs are flexible, and slight **intercostal retractions** are normally seen on inspiration. The xiphoid process is commonly visible as a small protrusion at the end of the sternum. The sternum is generally raised and slightly curved.

Inspect the **breasts** for size; shape; and nipple formation, location, and number. Breast enlargement appears in many newborns of either gender by the second or third day and is caused by maternal hormones. Occasionally a milky substance, sometimes called **witch's milk,** is secreted by the infant's breasts by the end of the first week. **Supernumerary nipples** may be found on the chest, on the abdomen, or in the axilla.

Lungs. The normal **respirations** of the newborn are irregular and abdominal, and the rate is between 30 and 60 breaths/min. Pauses in respiration of less than 20 seconds' duration are considered normal. After the initial forceful breaths required to initiate respiration, subsequent breaths should be nonlabored and fairly regular in rhythm. **Periodic breathing** is commonly seen in full-term newborns and consists of rapid nonlabored respirations followed by pauses of less than 20 seconds; periodic breathing may be more prominent during sleep and is not accompanied by status changes such as cyanosis or bradycardia. Occasional irregularities occur in relation to crying, sleeping, stooling, and feeding.

Perform auscultation when the infant is quiet. Bronchial breath sounds should be equal bilaterally. Any differences in auscultatory findings between symmetric sites is reported. **Crackles** soon after birth indicate the presence of fluid, which represents the normal transition of the lungs to extrauterine life. However, wheezes, persistence of medium or coarse crackles after the first few hours of life, and stridor should be reported for further investigation.

Heart. **Heart rate** is auscultated and may range from 100 to 180 beats/min shortly after birth and, when the infant's condition has stabilized, from 120 to 140 beats/min. The **point of maximum impulse** (PMI) may be palpated and is usually found at the fourth to fifth intercostal space, medial to the left midclavicular line. The PMI gives some indication of the location of the heart, which may be displaced in conditions such as congenital diaphragmatic hernia or pneumothorax. **Dextrocardia,** an anomaly wherein the heart is on the right side of the body, is reported, because the abdominal organs may also be reversed, with associated circulatory abnormalities.

NURSING TIP

Because auscultation of neonatal breath sounds and heart tones is often difficult for the untrained ear, practice auscultating one parameter at a time. Close your eyes and mentally block out the extraneous sounds heard, such as room noise or neonatal movement; offer the newborn a pacifier or a nonlatex gloved finger. Auscultation of a murmur and decreased air movement in specific lung fields requires patience and practice; it may require auscultating the heart tones or breath sounds for 1 to 3 minutes each.

Auscultation of the specific components of the **heart sounds** is difficult because of the rapid rate and effective transmission of respiratory sounds. However, the **first** (S1) and **second** (S2) sounds should be clear and well defined; the second sound is somewhat higher in pitch and sharper than the first. A **murmur** is frequently heard in the newborn, especially over the base of the heart or at the left sternal border at the third or fourth interspace. Ordinarily a murmur is not associated with specific cardiac defects, but frequently represents the incomplete functional closure of fetal shunts. (See Chapter 6 for other characteristics of murmurs.) However, always record and report any murmur or other unusual sounds.

Abdomen. The normal **contour** of the abdomen is cylindric and usually prominent with few visible veins. Bowel sounds are heard within the first 15 to 20 minutes after birth. Visible peristaltic waves may be observed in some newborns. Diastasis recti is a gap in the rectus muscles; this usually benign condition is visible as a raised and palpable bulge at midline, especially in the crying infant.

Inspect the **umbilical cord** to determine the presence of two arteries, which look like papular structures, and one vein, which has a larger lumen than the arteries and a thinner vessel wall. At birth the cord appears bluish white and moist. After clamping, it begins to dry and appears a dull, yellowish brown. It progressively shrivels in size and turns greenish black.

If the umbilical cord appears unusually large in diameter at the base, inspect for the presence of a hematoma or small omphalocele. If the cord is clamped over an existing omphalocele, part of the intestine will be clamped, causing tissue necrosis. One practical rule of thumb is to cut the cord distally 4 to 5 inches from a questionable enlargement until further examination is carried out by a practitioner. The extra length can later be cut once no pathologic condition has been identified.

NURSINGALERT

A cord that is draining and erythematous at the base should be investigated by the primary practitioner. The cord undergoes a process of dry gangrene decay, which has an odor; therefore odor alone may not be a reliable index of suspicion for omphalitis.

Palpate after inspecting the abdomen. The **liver** is normally palpable 1 to 3 cm (about 0.5 to 1 inch) below the right costal margin. The tip of the **spleen** can sometimes be felt, but a palpable spleen more than 1 cm below the left costal margin suggests enlargement and warrants further investigation. Although both **kidneys** should be palpated, this maneuver requires considerable practice. When felt, the lower half of the right kidney and the tip of the left kidney are 1 to 2 cm above the umbilicus.

During examination of the lower abdomen, it is particularly important to palpate for **femoral pulses,** which should be strong and equal bilaterally.

Female Genitalia. Normally, the **labia minora, labia majora,** and **clitoris** are edematous, especially after a breech delivery. However, the labia and clitoris must be carefully inspected to identify any evidence of ambiguous genitalia or other abnormalities. Normally, in a female, the urethral opening is located behind and below the clitoris.

A **hymenal tag** is occasionally visible from the posterior opening of the vagina. It is composed of tissue from the hymen and the labia minora. It usually disappears in several weeks. Generally, the vaginal vault is not inspected.

Vaginal discharge may be noted during the first week of life. This **pseudomenstruation** is a manifestation of the abrupt decrease of maternal hormones and usually disappears by 2 to 4 weeks. Fecal discharge from the vaginal opening indicates a rectovaginal fistula and is always reported. Vernix caseosa may be present in large amounts between the labia.

Male Genitalia. The **penis** is inspected for the urethral opening, which is located at the tip. However, the opening may be totally covered by the **prepuce,** or foreskin, which covers the glans penis. A tight prepuce is a common finding in the newborn. It should not be forcefully retracted; locating the urinary meatus is usually possible without retracting the foreskin. **Smegma,** a white cheesy substance, is commonly found around the glans penis, under the foreskin. Small, white, firm lesions called **epithelial pearls** may be seen at the tip of the prepuce. An erection is common in the newborn.

The **scrotum** may be large, edematous, and pendulous in the full-term neonate, especially in the infant born in breech position. It is more deeply pigmented in dark-skinned races. A noncommunicating **hydrocele** commonly occurs unilaterally and disappears within a few months. Always palpate the scrotum for the presence of **testes** (see Chapter 6). In small newborns, particularly preterm infants, the undescended testes may be palpable within the inguinal canal. Absence of the testes may also be a sign of ambiguous genitalia, especially when accompanied by a small scrotum and penis. **Inguinal hernias** may or may not be manifested immediately after birth. A hernia is more easily detected when the infant is crying. Palpable **lymph nodes** are most commonly found in the inguinal area.

Back and Rectum. Inspect the **spine** with the infant prone. The shape of the spine is gently rounded, with none of the characteristic S-shaped curves seen later in life. Any abnormal openings, masses, dimples, or soft areas are noted. A protruding sac anywhere along the spine, but most commonly in the sacral area, indicates some type of **spina bifida.** A small sinus, which may or may not be communicating with the spine, is a **pilonidal sinus.** It is frequently covered with a tuft of hair. Although it may have no pathologic significance, a pilonidal cyst may indicate the existence of spina bifida occulta or be a portal of entry into the spinal column. With the infant still prone, note symmetry of the gluteal folds. Report any evidence of asymmetry; tests for developmental dysplasia of the hip are performed by trained (or skilled) examiners (see Chapter 31).

The presence of an anal orifice and passage of meconium from the anal orifice during the first 24 to 48 hours of life indicates **anal patency.** If an imperforate anus is suspected, report this to the primary practitioner for further evaluation.

NURSINGALERT

The presence of meconium or stool in the rectal area is not an indication of rectal patency; a fistula may exist wherein stool is evacuated via the vagina, scrotum, or raphe. Therefore it is imperative that anal patency be checked with a small rubber catheter should any doubt regarding patency exist.

Extremities. Examine the extremities for symmetry, range of motion, and reflexes. Count the fingers and toes, and note supernumerary digits (**polydactyly**) or fusion of digits (**syndactyly**). A partial syndactyly between the second and third toes is a common variation seen in otherwise normal infants. The nail beds should be pink, although slight blueness is evident in acrocyanosis.

The palms of the hands should have the usual creases (see Fig. 6-13). The full-term newborn usually has creases covering the entire sole of the foot. The soles of the feet are flat with prominent fat pads.

Observe **range of motion** of the extremities throughout the entire examination. The absence of arm movement signals a potential birth injury paralysis such as Klumpke or Erb-Duchenne palsy. An asymmetric or partial Moro reflex should alert the practitioner to further evaluate upper extremity mobility. Examine the lower extremities for limb length, symmetry, and hip abduction and flexion. The newborn will demonstrate full range of motion in the elbow, hip, shoulder, and knee joints. Movements should be symmetric, smooth, and unrestricted.

Also assess **muscle tone.** By attempting to extend a flexed extremity, determine if tone is equal bilaterally. Extension of any extremity is usually met with resistance, and when released, the extremity returns to its previous flexed position. **Hypotonia** suggests some degree of hypoxia or neurologic disorder and is common in an infant with Down syndrome. **Asymmetry** of muscle tone may indicate a degree of paralysis from brain damage or nerve damage. Failure to move the lower limbs suggests a spinal cord lesion or injury. Sustained rhythmic tremors, twitches, and myoclonic jerks characterize neonatal seizures or may indicate **neonatal abstinence syndrome.** (See Neonatal Seizures and Drug-Exposed Infants, Chapter 9.) Sudden asynchronous jerking movements, quivering, or momentary tremors are usually normal.

Two reflexes are elicited. The first is the **grasp reflex.** Touching the palms of the hands or soles of the feet near the base of the digits causes flexion or grasping (Fig. 8-8, *A*). The other is the **Babinski reflex.** Stroking the outer sole of the foot upward from the heel across the ball of the foot causes the big toe to dorsiflex and the other toes to hyperextend (see Fig. 8-8, *B*).

Neurologic System. Assessing neurologic status is a critical part of the physical examination of the newborn. Much of the neurologic testing takes place during evaluation of body systems, such as eliciting localized reflexes and observing posture, muscle tone, head control, and movement. However, several important mass (total body) reflexes also need to be elicited. Test these at the end of the examination, since they may disturb the infant and interfere with auscultation. These reflexes, as well as several local reflexes, are described in Table 8-2. Record and report the absence, asymmetry, persistence, or weakness of a reflex.

Transitional Assessment: Periods of Reactivity

The newborn exhibits behavioral and physiologic characteristics that may at first appear to be signs of stress. However, during the initial 24 hours, changes in heart rate, respiration, motor activity, color, mucus production, and bowel activity occur in an orderly, predictable sequence that is normal and indicates lack of stress.

For 6 to 8 hours after birth, the newborn is in the **first period of reactivity.** During the first 30 minutes the infant is very alert, cries vigorously, may suck his or her fingers or fist, and appears very interested in the environment. At this time the newborn's eyes are usually open, making this an excellent opportunity for mother, father, and child to see each other. Because the newborn has a vigorous suck, this is also an opportune time to begin breastfeeding. The infant will usually grasp the nipple quickly, satisfying both mother and infant. This is particularly important to point out to parents, because after this initially highly active state the infant may be sleepy and uninterested in sucking. Physiologically, the respiratory rate during this period is as high as 80 breaths/min, crackles may be heard, heart rate reaches 180 beats/min, bowel sounds are active, mucus secretions are increased, and temperature may decrease. Maintaining appropriate temperature for the newborn is best accomplished by practicing skin-to-skin care whereby only a diaper is worn, to allow majority of skin surface

FIG. 8-8 ■ **A,** Plantar or grasp reflex. **B,** Babinski reflex. *1,* Direction of stroke. *2,* Dorsiflexion of big toe. *3,* Fanning of toes. (**A,** From Zitelli BJ, Davis HW: *Atlas of pediatric physical diagnosis,* ed 4, St Louis 2002, Mosby.)

TABLE 8-2	

Assessment of Reflexes in the Newborn

REFLEXES	EXPECTED BEHAVIORAL RESPONSES
LOCALIZED	
Eyes	
Blinking or corneal	Infant blinks at sudden appearance of a bright light or at approach of an object toward cornea; persists throughout life.
Pupillary	Pupil constricts when a bright light shines toward it; persists throughout life.
Doll's eye	As head is moved slowly to right or left, eyes lag behind and do not immediately adjust to new position of head; disappears as fixation develops; if persists, indicates neurologic damage.
Nose	
Sneeze	Sneezing is a spontaneous response of nasal passages to irritation or obstruction; persists throughout life.
Glabellar	Tapping briskly on glabella (bridge of nose) causes eyes to close tightly.
Mouth and Throat	
Sucking	Infant begins strong sucking movements of circumoral area in response to stimulation; persists throughout infancy, even without stimulation, such as during sleep.
Gag	Stimulation of posterior pharynx by food, suction, or passage of a tube causes infant to gag; persists throughout life.
Rooting	Touching or stroking the cheek along side of mouth causes infant to turn head toward that side and begin to suck; should disappear at about age 3-4 months, but may persist for up to 12 months.
Extrusion	When tongue is touched or depressed, infant responds by forcing it outward; disappears by age 4 months.
Yawn	Yawning is a spontaneous response to decreased oxygen by increasing amount of inspired air; persists throughout life.
Cough	Irritation of mucous membranes of larynx or tracheobronchial tree causes coughing; persists throughout life; usually present after first day of birth.
EXTREMITIES	
Grasp	Touching palms of hands or soles of feet near base of digits causes flexion of fingers and toes (see Fig. 8-8, *A*); palmar grasp lessens after age 3 months, to be replaced by voluntary movement; plantar grasp lessens by 8 months of age.
Babinski	Stroking outer sole of foot upward from heel and across ball of foot causes toes to hyperextend and hallux to dorsiflex (see Fig. 8-8, *B*); disappears after age 1 year.
Ankle clonus	Briskly dorsiflexing foot while supporting knee in partially flexed position results in 1-2 oscillating movements ("beats"); eventually no beats should be felt.
MASS	
Moro	Sudden jarring or change in equilibrium causes sudden extension and abduction of extremities and fanning of fingers, with index finger and thumb forming a C shape, followed by flexion and adduction of extremities; legs may weakly flex; infant may cry (Fig. 8-9); disappears after age 3-4 months, usually strongest during first 2 months.
Startle	A sudden loud noise causes abduction of the arms with flexion of elbows; hands remain clenched; disappears by age 4 months.
Perez	While infant is prone on a firm surface, thumb is pressed along spine from sacrum to neck; infant responds by crying, flexing extremities, and elevating pelvis and head; lordosis of the spine, as well as defecation and urination, may occur; disappears by age 4-6 months.
Tonic neck	When infant's head is turned to one side, arm and leg extend on that side, and opposite arm and leg flex (Fig. 8-10); disappears by age 3-4 months, to be replaced by symmetric positioning of both sides of body.
Trunk incurvation (Galant)	Stroking infant's back alongside spine causes hips to move toward stimulated side; disappears by age 4 weeks.
Dance or step	If infant is held so that sole of foot touches a hard surface, there is a reciprocal flexion and extension of the leg, simulating walking; disappears after age 3-4 weeks, to be replaced by deliberate movement.
Crawl	When placed on abdomen, infant makes crawling movements with arms and legs (Fig. 8-11); disappears at about age 6 weeks.
Placing	When infant is held upright under arms and dorsal side of foot is briskly placed against hard object, such as table, leg lifts as if foot is stepping on table; age of disappearance varies.

to be in contact with mother's skin. A light blanket may be used to cover mother and newborn. Research has shown mother's skin temperature will increase to ensure the newborn does not become hypothermic (Kimura and Matsuoka, 2007).

After this initial stage of alertness and activity, the infant enters the **second stage** of the first reactive period, which generally lasts 2 to 4 hours. Heart and respiratory rates decrease, temperature continues to fall, mucus production decreases,

and urine or stool is usually not passed. The infant is in a state of sleep and relative calm. Any attempt at stimulation usually elicits minimal response. Because of the continued decline in body temperature, undressing or bathing is avoided during this time.

The **second period of reactivity** begins when the infant awakes from this deep sleep; it lasts about 2 to 5 hours and provides another excellent opportunity for child and parents

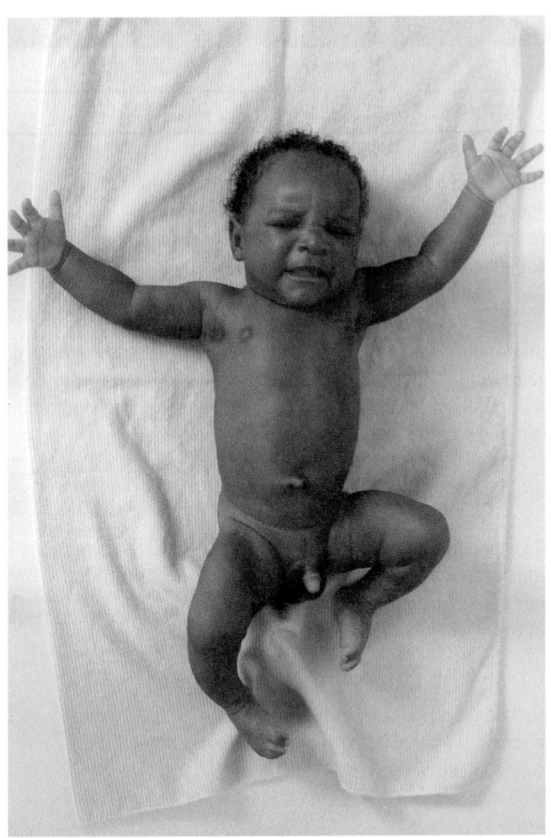

FIG. 8-9 ■ Moro reflex. (Photo by Paul Vincent Kuntz, Texas Children's Hospital, Houston.)

FIG. 8-10 ■ Tonic neck reflex. (Photo by Paul Vincent Kuntz, Texas Children's Hospital, Houston.)

to interact. The infant is again alert and responsive, heart and respiratory rates increase, the gag reflex is active, gastric and respiratory secretions are increased, and passage of meconium frequently occurs. This period is usually over when the amount of respiratory mucus has decreased. After this stage is a period of stabilization of physiologic systems and a vacillating pattern of sleep and activity.

Behavioral Assessment

Another important area of assessment is observation of behavior. Infants' behavior helps shape their environment, and their ability to react to various stimuli affects how others relate to them. The principal areas of behavior for newborns are sleep, wakefulness, and activity, such as crying.

One method of systematically assessing the infant's behavior is the use of the **Brazelton Neonatal Behavioral Assessment Scale (BNBAS)** (Brazelton and Nugent, 1996). The BNBAS is an interactive examination that assesses the infant's response to 28 items organized according to the clusters in Box 8-3. It is generally used as a research or diagnostic tool and requires special training.

In addition to its use as an initial and ongoing tool to assess neurologic and behavioral responses, the scale can be used in assessment of initial parent-child relationships, as a preventive instrument that identifies a caregiver who may benefit from a role model, and as a guide to help parents focus on their infant's individuality and develop a deeper attachment to their child. Studies have demonstrated that showing parents the unique characteristics of their infant causes a more positive

FIG. 8-11 ■ Crawl reflex. (Photo by Paul Vincent Kuntz, Texas Children's Hospital, Houston.)

BOX 8-3

Clusters of Neonatal Behaviors in Brazelton Neonatal Behavioral Assessment Scale

Habituation—Ability to respond to and then inhibit response to discrete stimulus (light, rattle, bell, pinprick) while asleep

Orientation—Quality of alert states and ability to attend to visual and auditory stimuli while alert

Motor performance—Quality of movement and tone

Range of state—Measure of general arousal level or arousability of infant

Regulation of state—How infant responds when aroused

Autonomic stability—Signs of stress (tremors, startles, skin color) related to homeostatic (self-regulating) adjustment of the nervous system

Reflexes—Assessment of several neonatal reflexes

TABLE 8-3
States of Sleep and Activity

STATE/BEHAVIOR	IMPLICATIONS FOR PARENTING
DEEP SLEEP (QUIET) Closed eyes Regular breathing No movement except for occasional sudden bodily twitch No eye movement	Continue usual house noises because external stimuli do not arouse infant. Leave infant alone if sudden loud noise awakens infant and child cries. Do not attempt to feed.
LIGHT SLEEP (ACTIVE) Closed eyes Irregular breathing Slight muscular twitching of body Rapid eye movement (REM) under closed eyelids May smile	External stimuli that did not arouse infant during deep sleep may minimally arouse child. Periodic groaning or crying is usual; do not interpret as an indication of pain or discomfort.
DROWSY Eyes may be open Irregular breathing Active body movement variable, with occasional mild startles	Most stimuli arouse infant but may return to sleep state. Pick infant up during this time rather than leaving in crib. Provide mild stimulus to awaken. Infant may enjoy nonnutritive sucking.
QUIET ALERT Eyes wide open and bright Responds to environment by active body movement and staring at close-range objects Minimal body activity Regular breathing Focuses attention on stimuli	Satisfy infant's needs such as hunger or nonnutritive sucking. Place infant in area of home where activity is continuous. Place toys in crib or playpen. Place objects within 17.5-20 cm (7-8 inches) of infant's view. Intervene to console.
ACTIVE ALERT May begin with whimpering and slight body movement Eyes open Irregular breathing	Remove intense internal or external stimuli because infant has increased sensitivity to stimuli.
CRYING Progresses to strong, angry crying and uncoordinated thrashing of extremities Eyes open or tightly closed Grimaces Irregular breathing	Comforting measures that were effective during alert state are usually ineffective. Rock and swaddle to decrease crying. Intervene to reduce fatigue, hunger, or discomfort.

Portions adapted from Blackburn S, Loper DL: *Maternal, fetal, and neonatal physiology: a clinical perspective*, Philadelphia, 1992, Saunders.

perception of the infant to develop, with increased interaction between infant and parent.

Patterns of Sleep and Activity. Newborns begin life with a systematic schedule of sleep and wakefulness that is initially evident during the periods of reactivity. After this initial period, it is not unusual for the infant to sleep almost constantly for the next 2 to 3 days to recover from the exhausting birth process.

Infants have six distinct sleep-wake states, which represent a particular form of neural control (Table 8-3). As maturity increases, each state becomes more precisely defined according to the behaviors observed. **State** is defined as a "group of characteristics that regularly occur together" (Blackburn, 2003) and includes body activity, eye and facial movements, respiratory pattern, and response to internal and external stimuli. The six sleep-wake states are quiet (deep) sleep, active (light) sleep, drowsy, quiet alert, active alert, and crying. Infants respond to internal and external environmental factors

by controlling sensory input and regulating the sleep-wake states; the ability to make smooth transitions between states is called **state modulation.** The ability to regulate sleep-wake states is essential in the neurobehavioral development of the infant. The more immature the infant, the less able he or she is able to cope with external and internal factors that affect the sleep-wake patterns.

Recognition and knowledge of sleep-wake states is important in the planning of nursing care. It is also important for nurses to help parents and caregivers understand the significance of the infant's behavioral responses to daily caregiving and how these states can be altered. A classic example is the newborn who feeds vigorously in the active alert state but poorly once he or she progresses to the crying state. The neurologic assessment of a newborn in the active alert state will differ significantly from the deep sleep state.

Newborns typically spend as much as 16 to 18 hours sleeping and do not necessarily follow a pattern of light-dark diur-

---

nursingcareguidelines

Assessing Attachment Behavior

- When the infant is brought to the parents, do they reach out for the child and call the child by name?
- Do the parents speak about the child in terms of identification— whom the infant looks like; what appears special about their child compared with other infants?
- When parents are holding the infant, what kind of body contact is there? Do they feel at ease in changing the infant's position; are fingertips or whole hands used; are there parts of the body they avoid touching or parts of the body they investigate and scrutinize?
- When the infant is awake, what kinds of stimulation do the parents provide? Do they talk to the infant, to each other, or to no one? How do they look at the infant—direct visual contact, avoidance of eye contact, or looking at other people or objects?
- How comfortable do the parents appear in terms of caring for the infant? Do they express any concern regarding their ability or disgust for certain activities, such as changing diapers?
- What type of affection do they demonstrate to the newborn, such as smiling, stroking, kissing, or rocking?
- If the infant is fussy, what kinds of comforting techniques do the parents use, such as rocking, swaddling, talking, or stroking?

nursingcareguidelines

Physical Examination of the Newborn

1. Provide a normothermic and nonstimulating examination area.
2. Check that equipment and supplies are working properly and are accessible.
3. Undress only body area examined to prevent heat loss.
4. Proceed in an orderly sequence (usually head to toe) with the following exceptions:
   - Observe infant's attitude and position of flexion first to avoid disturbing him or her.
   - Perform all procedures that require quiet next, such as auscultating the lungs, heart, and abdomen.
   - Perform disturbing procedures, such as testing reflexes, last.
   - Measure head, chest, and length at same time to compare results.
5. Proceed quickly to avoid stressing infant.
6. Comfort infant during and after the examination.
   - Talk softly.
   - Hold infant's hands against chest.
   - Swaddle and hold.
   - Offer pacifier or nonlatex gloved finger to suck.
   - Use containment and positioning to maximize developmental state regulation.

---

nal rhythm. With increasing age, sleep-wake states will change, with increasing amounts of time spent in awake alert states and decreasing amounts of sleep time. Approximately 50% of total sleep time is spent in irregular or rapid eye movement sleep.

Cry. The newborn should begin extrauterine life with a strong, lusty cry. The sounds produced by crying can be described as hunger, anger, pain, and "bid for attention" cries. Discomfort (pain) sounds initially consist of gasps and cries in which the consonant *H* is clearly distinguishable. The duration of crying is as variable in each infant as the duration of sleep patterns. Newborns may cry as little as 5 minutes or as much as 2 hours or more per day. Feeding usually terminates the state of crying when hunger is the cause. Swaddling or wrapping an infant snugly in a blanket promotes sleep and maintains body temperature. Rocking the infant reduces crying and induces quiet alertness or sleep. Variations in the initial cry can indicate abnormalities. A weak, groaning cry or grunting during expiration usually indicates respiratory disturbance. Absent, weak, or constant crying requires further investigation for possible drug withdrawal or a neurologic problem.

Assessment of Attachment Behaviors

One of the most important areas of assessment is careful observation of behaviors that are thought to indicate the formation of emotional bonds between the newborn and family, especially the mother. Such behaviors include the **en face position;** undressing and touching the infant; smiling, kissing, and talking to the infant; and holding, rocking, and cradling the child close to the body (see Nursing Care Guidelines box). Because assessment is closely related to interventions that promote attachment (e.g., encouraging these behaviors in parents), assessing attachment behaviors is further discussed on pp. 234-235.

Physical Assessment

An essential aspect of the care of the newborn is a thorough physical assessment that includes estimation of gestational age and physical examination to identify normal characteristics and existing abnormalities. These initial and ongoing assessments are critical to establishing baseline data for planning, implementing, and evaluating care and are a nursing priority in caring for the newborn. The discussion of physical examination focuses on normal findings and variations from the norm that require little or no intervention. The reader is encouraged to review Chapter 6 for further discussion of examination techniques. General guidelines for conducting a physical examination are presented in the Nursing Care Guidelines box. Table 8-4 summarizes physical examination of the newborn.

The nursing care of the newborn is discussed on the following pages. The nursing process in the care of the newborn is outlined in the Nursing Process box.

MAINTAIN A PATENT AIRWAY

Establishing a patent airway is a primary objective in the delivery room and is the responsibility of the attending nurses and practitioners. However, maintaining a patent airway continues to be a priority goal in the nursery, with attention to proper positioning of the infant to facilitate drainage of secretions, especially after feeding. The American Academy of Pediatrics (2000a) recommends the supine position during sleep for healthy newborns. This recommendation is based on the possible association between sleeping prone and sudden infant death syndrome (see Chapter 11). Since the initial recommendation in 1992 that all infants be placed in the supine position to sleep, there has been no evidence of an increased number of complications, such as choking or vomiting, when infants are placed in this position (Malloy, 2002). There has,

Text continued on p. 221

nursingprocess | The Healthy Newborn and Family

ASSESSMENT
Assess the newborn according to the guidelines on pp. 215-220.

DIAGNOSIS (PROBLEM IDENTIFICATION)
After a thorough assessment, several nursing diagnoses for the healthy newborn include:
- Readiness for Enhanced Parenting
- Risk for Injury
- Effective Breastfeeding
- Risk for Imbalanced Body Temperature
- Readiness for Enhanced Nutrition
- Ineffective Breathing Pattern
- Risk for Infection

PLANNING
Numerous goals for the healthy newborn are discussed on pp. 215-239. Expected patient outcomes include:
- Newborn airway will remain patent.
- Effective breathing pattern will be established.
- Thermoregulation will be maintained.
- Parent-infant attachment behaviors will be exhibited.
- Breastfeeding or bottle feeding will be established.
- Infant will exhibit no evidence of infection; immune status will be maintained.
- Newborn will remain free of injury.
- Family will demonstrate ability to care for infant's basic needs.

IMPLEMENTATION
Intervention strategies for the healthy newborn and family are discussed on pp. 215-239.

EVALUATION
The effectiveness of nursing interventions for the newborn and family is determined by continual assessment and evaluation of care based on the following guidelines:
- Observe infant's color and respiratory pattern.
- Monitor axillary temperature regularly; observe for signs of temperature instability such as respiratory distress.
- Observe for any evidence of infection, especially at the umbilicus or site of circumcision; check identification bands; verify administration of prophylactic eye treatment, vitamin K injection, hepatitis B vaccine, and hearing and newborn screening tests.
- Monitor infant's feeding ability and oral intake.
- Monitor daily weight.
- Observe interactions between infant and family members; interview family regarding their feelings about the newborn.
- Observe parents' ability to provide care for infant; interview parents regarding any concerns about infant's care at home.
- Observe parents' correct use of car safety seat restraint on discharge.

TABLE 8-4
Physical Assessment of the Newborn

USUAL FINDINGS	COMMON VARIATIONS OR MINOR ABNORMALITIES	POTENTIAL SIGNS OF DISTRESS OR MAJOR ABNORMALITIES
GENERAL MEASUREMENTS		
Head circumference—33-33.5 cm (13-14 inches); about 2-3 cm (1 inch) larger than chest circumference	Molding after birth altering head circumference Head and chest circumferences equal for first 1-2 days after birth	Head circumference <10th or >90th percentile
Chest circumference—30.5-33 cm (12-13 inches)		
Crown-to-rump length—31-35 cm (12.2-13.8 inches); approximately equal to head circumference		
Head-to-heel length—48-53 cm (19-21 inches)		
Birth weight—2700-4000 g (6-9 pounds)	Loss of 10% of birth weight in first week; regained in 10-14 days, depending on feeding method	Birth weight <10th or >90th percentile
VITAL SIGNS		
Axillary temperature—36.5°-37.6° C (97.9°-99.7° F)	Crying slightly increasing body temperature Radiant warmer falsely increasing axillary temperature	Hypothermia Hyperthermia
Apical heart rate—120-140 beats/min	Crying increasing heart rate; sleep decreasing heart rate During first period of reactivity (6-8 hours), rate reaching 180 beats/min	**Bradycardia**—Resting rate <80-100 beats/min **Tachycardia**—Rate >160-180 beats/min Irregular rhythm

TABLE 8-4

Physical Assessment of the Newborn—cont'd

USUAL FINDINGS	COMMON VARIATIONS OR MINOR ABNORMALITIES	POTENTIAL SIGNS OF DISTRESS OR MAJOR ABNORMALITIES
VITAL SIGNS—cont'd		
Respirations—30-60 breaths/min	Crying increasing respiratory rate; sleep decreasing respiratory rate During first period of reactivity (6-8 hours), rate reaching 80 breaths/min	**Tachypnea**—Rate >60 breaths/min **Apnea**—Breathing stops for 20 seconds
Oscillometric blood pressure—65/41 mm Hg in arm and calf (age 1-2 days; mean 50 mm Hg)	Crying and activity increasing blood pressure (BP)	Oscillometric systolic pressure in calf 6-9 mm Hg less than in upper extremity (possible sign of coarctation of aorta)
GENERAL APPEARANCE		
Posture—Flexion of head and extremities, which rest on chest and abdomen	**Frank breech**—Extended legs, abducted and fully rotated thighs, flattened occiput, extended neck	Limp posture, extension of extremities
SKIN		
At birth, bright red, puffy, smooth Second to third day, pink, flaky, dry Vernix caseosa Lanugo Edema around eyes, face, legs, dorsa of hands, feet, and scrotum or labia **Acrocyanosis**—Cyanosis of hands and feet **Cutis marmorata**—Transient mottling when infant is exposed to decreased temperature	Neonatal jaundice after first 24 hours Ecchymoses or petechiae caused by birth trauma **Milia**—Distended sebaceous glands that appear as tiny white papules on cheeks, chin, and nose **Miliaria or sudamina**—Distended sweat (eccrine) glands that appear as minute vesicles, especially on face **Erythema toxicum**—Pink papular rash with vesicles superimposed on thorax, back, buttocks, and abdomen; may appear in 24-48 hours and resolve after several days **Harlequin color change**—Clearly outlined color change as infant lies on side; lower half of body becomes pink, and upper half is pale **Mongolian spots**—Irregular areas of deep blue pigmentation, usually in sacral and gluteal regions; seen predominantly in newborns of African, Native American, Asian, or Hispanic descent **Telangiectatic nevi ("stork bites")**—Flat, deep pink localized areas usually seen on back of neck	Progressive jaundice, especially in first 24 hours Generalized cyanosis Pallor Mottling Grayness Plethora Hemorrhage, ecchymoses, or petechiae that persist **Sclerema**—Hard and stiff skin Poor skin turgor Rashes, pustules, or blisters **Café-au-lait spots**—Light brown spots **Nevus flammeus**—Port-wine stain
HEAD		
Anterior fontanel—Diamond shaped; size varying from barely palpable to 4-5 cm (1.5-2 inches) (see Fig. 8-6) **Posterior fontanel**—Triangular, 0.5-1 cm (<0.5 inch) Fontanels flat, soft, and firm Widest part of fontanel measured from bone to bone, not suture to suture	Molding after vaginal delivery Third sagittal (parietal) fontanel Bulging fontanel because of crying or coughing **Caput succedaneum**—Edema of soft scalp tissue **Cephalhematoma** (uncomplicated)—Hematoma between periosteum and skull bone	Fused sutures Bulging or depressed fontanels when quiet Widened sutures and fontanels **Craniotabes**—Snapping sensation along lambdoid suture that resembles indentation of Ping-Pong ball

Continued

TABLE 8-4

Physical Assessment of the Newborn—cont'd

USUAL FINDINGS	COMMON VARIATIONS OR MINOR ABNORMALITIES	POTENTIAL SIGNS OF DISTRESS OR MAJOR ABNORMALITIES
EYES		
Lids usually edematous	Epicanthal folds in Asian infants	Pink color of iris
Color—Slate gray, dark blue, brown	Searching nystagmus or strabismus	Purulent discharge
Absence of tears	**Subconjunctival (scleral) hemorrhages**—	Upward slant in non-Asians
Presence of red reflex	Ruptured capillaries, usually at limbus	Hypertelorism (3 cm)
Corneal reflex in response to touch		Hypotelorism
Pupillary reflex in response to light		Congenital cataracts
Blink reflex in response to light or touch		Constricted or dilated fixed pupil
Rudimentary fixation on objects and ability to follow to midline		Absence of red reflex
		Absence of pupillary or corneal reflex
		Inability to follow object or bright light to midline
		Yellow sclera
EARS		
Position—Top of pinna on horizontal line with outer canthus of eye	Inability to visualize tympanic membrane because of filled aural canals	Low placement of ears
Startle reflex elicited by a loud, sudden noise	Pinna flat against head	Absence of startle reflex in response to loud noise
Pinna flexible, cartilage present	Irregular shape or size	Minor abnormalities may be signs of various syndromes, especially renal
	Pits or skin tags	
NOSE		
Nasal patency	Flattened and bruised	Nonpatent canals
Nasal discharge—Thin white mucus		Thick, bloody nasal discharge
Sneezing		Flaring of nares (alae nasi)
		Copious nasal secretions or stuffiness (may be minor)
MOUTH AND THROAT		
Intact, high-arched palate	**Natal teeth**—Teeth present at birth; benign but may be associated with congenital defects	Cleft lip
Uvula in midline	**Epstein pearls**—Small, white epithelial cysts along midline of hard palate	Cleft palate
Frenulum of tongue		Large, protruding tongue or posterior displacement of tongue
Frenum of upper lip		Profuse salivation or drooling
Sucking reflex—Strong and coordinated		**Candidiasis (thrush)**—White, adherent patches on tongue, palate, and buccal surfaces
Rooting reflex		Inability to pass nasogastric tube
Gag reflex		Hoarse, high-pitched, weak, absent, or other abnormal cry
Extrusion reflex		
Absent or minimal salivation		
Vigorous cry		
NECK		
Short, thick, usually surrounded by skinfolds	**Torticollis (wry neck)**—Head held to one side with chin pointing to opposite side	Excessive skinfolds
Tonic neck reflex		Resistance to flexion
		Absence of tonic neck reflex
		Fractured clavicle; crepitus
CHEST		
Anteroposterior and lateral diameters equal	Funnel chest (pectus excavatum)	Depressed sternum
Slight sternal retractions evident during inspiration	Pigeon chest (pectus carinatum)	Marked retractions of chest and intercostal spaces during respiration
Xiphoid process evident	Supernumerary nipples	Asymmetric chest expansion
Breast enlargement	Secretion of milky substance from breasts ("witch's milk")	Redness and firmness around nipples
		Wide-spaced nipples

TABLE 8-4

Physical Assessment of the Newborn—cont'd

USUAL FINDINGS	COMMON VARIATIONS OR MINOR ABNORMALITIES	POTENTIAL SIGNS OF DISTRESS OR MAJOR ABNORMALITIES
LUNGS Respirations chiefly abdominal Cough reflex absent at birth, present by 1-2 days Bilateral equal bronchial breath sounds	Irregular rate and depth of respirations, periodic breathing Crackles shortly after birth	Inspiratory stridor Expiratory grunt Retractions Persistent irregular breathing Periodic breathing with repeated apneic spells Seesaw respirations (paradoxic) Unequal breath sounds Persistent fine, medium, or coarse crackles Wheezing Diminished breath sounds Peristaltic bowel sounds on one side, with diminished breath sounds on same side
HEART **Apex**—Fourth to fifth intercostal space, lateral to left sternal border S_2 slightly sharper and higher in pitch than S_1	**Sinus arrhythmia**—Heart rate increasing with inspiration and decreasing with expiration Transient cyanosis on crying or straining	**Dextrocardia**—Heart on right side Displacement of apex, muffled Cardiomegaly Abdominal shunts Murmur Thrill Persistent central cyanosis Hyperactive precordium
ABDOMEN Cylindric **Liver**—Palpable 2-3 cm below right costal margin **Spleen**—Tip palpable at end of first week of age **Kidneys**—Palpable 1-2 cm above umbilicus **Umbilical cord**—Bluish white at birth with two arteries and one vein **Femoral pulses**—Equal bilaterally	Umbilical hernia **Diastasis recti**—Midline gap between recti muscles **Wharton jelly**—unusually thick umbilical cord	Abdominal distention Localized bulging Distended veins Absent bowel sounds Enlarged liver and spleen Ascites Visible peristaltic waves Scaphoid or concave abdomen Moist umbilical cord Presence of only one artery in cord Urine, stool, or pus leaking from cord or cord insertion site Periumbilical erythema Palpable bladder distention following scanty voiding Absent femoral pulses Cord bleeding or hematoma **Omphalocele or gastroschisis**—Protrusion of abdominal contents through abdominal wall or cord
FEMALE GENITALIA Labia and clitoris usually edematous Urethral meatus behind clitoris Vernix caseosa between labia Urination within 24 hours	**Pseudomenstruation**—Blood-tinged or mucoid discharge Hymenal tag	Enlarged clitoris with urethral meatus at tip Fused labia Absence of vaginal opening Meconium from vaginal opening No urination within 24 hours Masses in labia Ambiguous genitalia Bladder exstrophy

Continued

TABLE 8-4

Physical Assessment of the Newborn—cont'd

USUAL FINDINGS	COMMON VARIATIONS OR MINOR ABNORMALITIES	POTENTIAL SIGNS OF DISTRESS OR MAJOR ABNORMALITIES
MALE GENITALIA		
Urethral opening at tip of glans penis	Urethral opening covered by prepuce	**Hypospadias**—Urethral opening on ventral surface of penis
Testes palpable in each scrotum	Inability to retract foreskin	**Epispadias**—Urethral opening on dorsal surface of penis
Scrotum usually large, edematous, pendulous, and covered with rugae; usually deeply pigmented in dark-skinned ethnic groups	**Epithelial pearls**—Small, firm, white lesions at tip of prepuce	**Chordee**—Ventral curvature of penis
Smegma	Erection or priapism	Testes not palpable in scrotum or inguinal canal
Urination within 24 hours	Testes palpable in inguinal canal	No urination within 24 hours
	Scrotum small	Inguinal hernia
		Hypoplastic scrotum
		Hydrocele—Fluid in scrotum
		Masses in scrotum
		Meconium from scrotum
		Discoloration of testes
		Ambiguous genitalia
		Bladder exstrophy
BACK AND RECTUM		
Spine intact; no openings, masses, or prominent curves	Green liquid stools in infant under phototherapy	Anal fissures or fistulas
Trunk incurvation reflex	Delayed passage of meconium in very low–birth-weight neonates	Imperforate anus
Anal reflex		Absence of anal reflex
Patent anal opening		No meconium within 36-48 hours
Passage of meconium within 48 hours		Pilonidal cyst or sinus
		Tuft of hair along spine
		Spina bifida (any degree)
EXTREMITIES		
Ten fingers and toes	Partial syndactyly between second and third toes	**Polydactyly**—Extra digits
Full range of motion	Second toe overlapping third toe	**Syndactyly**—Fused or webbed digits
Nail beds pink, with transient cyanosis immediately after birth	Wide gap between first (hallux) and second toes	**Phocomelia**—Hands or feet attached close to trunk
Creases on anterior two thirds of sole	Deep crease on plantar surface of foot between first and second toes	**Hemimelia**—Absence of distal part of extremity
Sole usually flat	Asymmetric length of toes	Hyperflexibility of joints
Symmetry of extremities	Dorsiflexion and shortness of hallux	Persistent cyanosis of nail beds
Equal muscle tone bilaterally, especially resistance to opposing flexion		Yellowing of nail beds
Equal bilateral brachial pulses		Sole covered with creases
		Transverse palmar (simian) crease
		Fractures
		Decreased or absent range of motion
		Dislocated or subluxated hip
		Limitation in hip abduction
		Unequal gluteal or leg folds
		Unequal knee height (Allis or Galeazzi sign)
		Audible clunk on abduction of hip (Ortolani sign)
		Asymmetry of extremities
		Unequal muscle tone or range of motion
NEUROMUSCULAR SYSTEM		
Extremities usually in some degree of flexion	Quivering or momentary tremors	**Hypotonia**—Floppy, poor head control, extremities limp
Extension of an extremity followed by previous position of flexion		**Hypertonia**—Jittery, arms and hands tightly flexed, legs stiffly extended, startles easily
Head lag while sitting, but momentary ability to hold head erect		Asymmetric posturing (except tonic neck reflex)
Ability to turn head from side to side when prone		**Opisthotonic posturing**—Arched back
Ability to hold head in horizontal line with back when held prone		Signs of paralysis
		Tremors, twitches, and myoclonic jerks
		Marked head lag in all positions

however, been an increase in the number of infants with cranial asymmetry, particularly unilateral flattening of the occiput (American Academy of Pediatrics, 2003c). Health care professionals must educate parents on prevention of deformational plagiocephaly by encouraging alternate positions when the infant is awake.

A bulb syringe is kept near the infant and is used if suctioning is required. If more forceful removal of secretions is required, mechanical suction is used. The use of the proper-size catheter and correct suctioning technique is essential to prevent mucosal damage and edema. Gentle suctioning is necessary to prevent reflex bradycardia, laryngospasm, and cardiac arrhythmias from vagal stimulation. Oropharyngeal suctioning is performed for 5 seconds, with sufficient time between suctioning to allow the infant to recuperate and reoxygenate.

> **NURSINGALERT**
>
> To avoid aspiration of amniotic fluid or mucus, clear the pharynx first, then the nasal passages using a bulb syringe: remember, *mouth* before *nose.* Vital signs are closely monitored, and any indication of respiratory distress is immediately reported.

> **NURSINGALERT**
>
> The cardinal signs of respiratory distress in the newborn include tachypnea, nasal flaring, grunting, intercostal retractions, and cyanosis.

MAINTAIN A STABLE BODY TEMPERATURE

Conserving the newborn's body heat is an essential nursing goal. At birth a major cause of heat loss is **evaporation,** the loss of heat through moisture. The amniotic fluid that bathes the infant's skin favors evaporation, especially when combined with the cool atmosphere of the delivery room. Heat loss through evaporation is minimized by rapidly drying the skin and hair with a warmed towel and placing the infant in a heated environment or skin-to-skin contact with the mother.

Another major cause of heat loss is **radiation,** the loss of heat to cooler solid objects in the environment that are not in direct contact with the infant. Loss of heat through radiation increases as these solid objects become colder and closer to the infant. The temperature of ambient or surrounding air in the incubator essentially has no effect on loss of heat through radiation. This is a critical point to remember when attempting to maintain a constant temperature for the infant, because even though the temperature of the ambient air is optimal, the infant can become hypothermic.

An example of radiant heat loss is the placement of the incubator close to a cold window, drafty doorway, or air-conditioning unit. The cold from any of these sources will cool the walls of the incubator and, subsequently, the body of the neonate. To prevent this, the infant is placed as far away as possible from exterior walls, windows, and ventilating units. If heat loss continues to be a problem, a radiant warmer may be placed over the infant or infant and mother.

The use of radiant heating devices such as heat lamps or phototherapy lights with an incubator may cause overheating of the infant because infants cannot effectively dissipate radiant heat through the Plexiglas wall of the incubator. For this same reason, an incubator should not be exposed to direct sunlight.

Heat loss can also occur through conduction and convection. **Conduction** involves loss of heat from the body because of direct contact of skin with a cooler solid object. This can be minimized by placing the infant on a padded, covered surface and providing insulation through clothes and blankets rather than by placing the infant directly on a hard table. Placing the newborn close to the mother, such as in her arms or on her abdomen immediately after delivery, is physically beneficial in terms of conserving heat, as well as fostering maternal attachment.

Convection is similar to conduction, except that heat loss is aided by surrounding air currents. For example, placing the infant in the direct flow of air from a fan or air-conditioner vent will cause rapid heat loss through convection. Transporting the neonate in a crib with solid sides reduces airflow around the infant.

PROTECT FROM INFECTION AND INJURY

The most important practice for preventing cross-infection is thorough hand washing of all individuals involved in the infant's care. Other procedures to prevent infection include eye care, umbilical care, bathing, and care of the circumcision. Artificial and long fingernails are discouraged for those working in neonatal care because the former have been implicated in the transmission of *Pseudomonas* organisms (Moolenaar, Crutcher, San Joaquin, and others, 2000) and *Klebsiella pneumoniae* (Gupta, Della-Latta, Todd, and others, 2004). Vitamin K is administered to protect against hemorrhage. In addition, several safety measures are practiced, particularly in terms of proper identification, and screening tests are used to detect various disorders.

Identification

Proper identification of the newborn is absolutely essential. The nurse must verify that identifying bands are securely fastened and verify the information (name, gender, mother's admission number, date, and time of birth) against the birth records and the child's actual gender. This identification process should take place optimally in the delivery room. Some institutions use methods of infant identification such as a color photograph kept in the medical record, storage of blood for DNA genotyping, or electronic surveillance systems for infant security. Footprinting or fingerprinting alone is *not* currently recommended for newborn identification (American Academy of Pediatrics and American College of Obstetricians and Gynecologists, 2007); however, the National Center for Missing and Exploited Children (NCMEC) does recommend the use of footprints as a form of identification in addition to a cord blood sample, which is stored until the day after discharge. Electronic tags that give off a radio frequency may also be used to prevent newborn abductions. A tag is placed on the newborn and removed at the time of discharge by hospital personnel.

A proactive hospital emergency plan should be implemented to prevent infant abduction and to respond promptly and effectively in the event one happens. A mock newborn abduction drill is an effective method that can be used to evaluate staff competence and response to the incident (Shogan, 2002). *All* hospital personnel should be educated regarding newborn abduction, preventive aspects, and methods to identify the potential risk of such an occurrence.

The nurse needs to discuss safety issues with the mother the first time the infant is brought to her. The NCMEC* has reported that 55% of infant abductions occur in the mother's room (Rabun, 2000). A written copy of the safety instructions should also be given to the parent. Parents are instructed to look at identification badges of nurses and hospital personnel who come to take infants and not to relinquish their infants to anyone without proper identification. Mothers are also advised not to leave the infant alone in the crib while they shower or use the bathroom; rather, they should ask to have the infant observed by a health care worker if a family member is not present in the room. Parents and staff are encouraged to use a password system when the newborn is taken from the room as a routine security measure (Carroll, 2000). The nurse should document in the chart that these instructions were given and that appropriate identification band checks are routinely made throughout each shift. Nursing staff are also educated regarding the "typical" abductor profile and to be constantly aware of visitors with unusual behavior.

The typical profile of an abductor is a female between the ages of 15 and 44 who is often overweight and has low self-esteem; she may be emotionally disturbed because of the loss of her own child or inability to conceive and may have a strained relationship with her husband or partner. The typical abductor may also be seen visiting the newborn nursery or neonatal intensive care unit area before the abduction and may ask questions about the care of or the health of a specific newborn. The abductor may familiarize herself with the hospital routine and may also impersonate a health care worker. Parents are made aware of the fact that infant safety measures must be implemented in the home as well. Measures to prevent and decrease infant abduction after discharge to the home include avoiding the publication of birth announcements in the local newspaper and avoiding using yard decorations to announce a newborn's arrival (Shogan, 2002).

Eye Care

Prophylactic eye treatment against **ophthalmia neonatorum,** infectious conjunctivitis of the newborn, includes the use of (1) silver nitrate (1%) solution, (2) erythromycin (0.5%) ophthalmic ointment or drops, or (3) tetracycline (1%) ophthalmic ointment or drops (preferably in single-dose ampules or tubes) (see Nursing Care Guidelines box). *Chlamydia trachomatis* is the major cause of ophthalmia neonatorum in the United States. Silver nitrate is effective against gonococcal conjunctivitis.

Topical antibiotics such as tetracycline and erythromycin, silver nitrate, and a 2.5% povidone-iodine solution (currently unavailable in commercial form in the United States) have not proved to be effective in the treatment of chlamydial conjunctivitis.

A 14-day course of oral erythromycin or an oral sulfonamide may be given for chlamydial conjunctivitis (American Academy of Pediatrics and American College of Obstetricians and Gynecologists, 2007). Administration of oral erythromycin in infants younger than 6 weeks old has been associated with infantile hypertrophic pyloric stenosis; therefore parents

nursingcareguidelines

Ophthalmia Neonatorum Prophylaxis
1. Clean the eyelids with sterile cotton and sterile water if needed.
2. Separate lids and apply 2 drops or a 1- to 2-cm (½-inch) ribbon of ointment in each conjunctival sac.
3. Massage lids gently to ensure spread of the medication.
4. Wipe excess medication from eye with sterile cotton 1 minute after application.
5. Do not rinse eyes.

should be informed of the potential risks and signs of the illness (American Academy of Pediatrics, 2006b). Herpes simplex virus may also cause neonatal conjunctivitis; treatment in such cases involves the use of topical and systemic antiviral medications.

Because studies on maternal attachment emphasize that in the first hour of life a newborn has a greater ability to focus on coordinated movement than at any other time during the next several days and because eye contact is very important in the development of maternal-infant bonding, the routine administration of silver nitrate or topical ophthalmic antibiotics can be postponed for up to 1 hour in the United States and up to 2 hours in Canada. However, a checklist should be used to ensure that the drug is given.

NURSINGTIP

A chemical conjunctivitis may occur within 24 hours of instillation of ophthalmic prophylaxis. The clinical features include mild lid edema and a sterile, nonpurulent eye discharge (Fuloria and Kreiter, 2002). Purulent eye discharge should be reported to the primary practitioner for further investigation.

Vitamin K Administration

Shortly after birth, vitamin K is administered as a single intramuscular dose of 0.5 to 1 mg to prevent hemorrhagic disease of the newborn, also called **vitamin K deficiency bleeding (VKDB).** Normally, vitamin K is synthesized by the intestinal flora. However, because the infant's intestine is sterile at birth and because breast milk contains low levels of vitamin K, the supply is inadequate for at least the first 3 or 4 days. The major function of vitamin K is to catalyze the synthesis of prothrombin in the liver, which is needed for blood clotting. The vastus lateralis muscle is the traditionally recommended injection site, but the ventrogluteal (not dorsogluteal) muscle can be used.

Several countries have noted a resurgence in later onset of VKDB after practicing orally administered prophylaxis (American Academy of Pediatrics, 2003a). Current recommendations are that vitamin K be given to all newborns as a single intramuscular dose of 0.5 to 1.0 mg (American Academy of Pediatrics, 2003a). Additional study is needed on the efficacy, safety, and bioavailability of oral preparations and on the most effective dosing regimens to prevent VKDB.

Hepatitis B Vaccine Administration

To decrease the incidence of hepatitis B virus in children and its serious consequences, cirrhosis and liver cancer, in adulthood, the first of three doses of hepatitis B vaccine is recommended soon after birth and before hospital discharge for all newborns in the United States; this first dose may also be given at the practitioner's discretion at the first well-newborn visit if the mother is hepatitis B surface antigen (HBsAg) negative. The injection is given in the vastus lateralis muscle, since this site is associated with a better immune response than is the dorsogluteal area (a muscle typically not used in infants in the United States) (see also Immunizations, Chapter 10). Giving the infant concentrated oral sucrose can reduce the pain of the injection (Stevens, Yamada, and Ohlsson, 2004).

Preterm infants who weigh less than 2000 g (4.4 pounds) and are born to HBsAg-negative women may be vaccinated at a chronologic age of 1 month if medically stable or at hospital discharge, if discharged before the infant reaches 1 month chronologic age (American Academy of Pediatrics, 2007). Infants born to HBsAg-positive mothers should be immunized within 12 hours after birth with hepatitis B vaccine and hepatitis B immune globulin (HBIG) at separate sites, regardless of gestational age or birth weight; the birth dose in such infants should not be counted in the series of three hepatitis B vaccines, and the full three-dose series should be administered starting at age 1 month (American Academy of Pediatrics, 2006b). An infant who weighs less than 2000 g and whose mother's HBsAg status is unknown should receive the hepatitis B vaccine within 12 hours of birth; maternal status should be determined readily and, if unavailable, the infant should receive the dose of HBIG as soon as possible but within 7 days of birth. In Canada, hepatitis B vaccine is given to the newborn only if the mother is HBsAg positive at birth (see Immunizations, Chapter 10).

Newborn Screening for Disease

A number of genetic disorders can be detected in the newborn period. There is no national policy for such detection in the United States; therefore the extent of neonatal screening is determined by state laws and voluntary guidelines. Most states require screening for phenylketonuria (PKU), congenital hypothyroidism, galactosemia, and hemoglobin defects such as sickle cell disease (see Chapters 9 and 26); screening for congenital hearing loss is recommended at the same time as disease screening. Because concern has been voiced regarding the inconsistency among states in screening for genetic disorders based on cost, population demographics, resource availability, and political environment, the Task Force on Newborn Screening was formed by the American Academy of Pediatrics and other federal health care agencies to address this issue. A number of resolutions and policies have been developed to better address the issue of newborn screening (see American Academy of Pediatrics, 2000b).

The advent of tandem mass spectrometry has expanded newborn screening to include detection of disorders of fatty acid oxidation, amino acids, and organic acids. This technology uses a minimum amount of blood and can identify more than 20 different disorders in 2 minutes (Bryant, Horns, Longo, and others, 2004). Tandem mass spectrometry has improved sensitivity and specificity for the detection of such conditions as PKU and has a lower rate of false-positive results than other standardized testing methods.

The nurse's responsibility is to educate parents regarding the importance of screening and to collect appropriate specimens at the recommended time (after 24 hours of age). With early newborn discharge before 24 hours, adequate screening for PKU requires a follow-up test within 2 weeks (American Academy of Pediatrics and American College of Obstetricians and Gynecologists, 2007). Accurate screening depends on high-quality blood spots on approved filter paper forms. The blood should completely saturate the filter paper spot on one side only. The paper should not be handled, placed on wet surfaces, or contaminated with any substance. (See Atraumatic Care box.)

The American Academy of Pediatrics and American College of Obstetricians and Gynecologists (2007) also recommend routine prenatal and perinatal human immunodeficiency virus (HIV) counseling and testing for all pregnant women and their newborns. Benefits of early identification of HIV-infected infants are early antiretroviral therapy and aggressive nutritional supplementation; appropriate changes in their immunization schedule; monitoring and evaluation of immunologic, neurologic, and neuropsychologic functions for possible changes caused by antiretroviral therapy; initiation of interventions for special educational needs; evaluation for the need of other therapies, such as immunoglobulin for the prevention of bacterial infections; tuberculosis screening and treatment; and management of communicable disease exposures. In addition, vertical transmission of HIV from mother to newborn may be reduced to 2% with a cesarean section before the rupture of membranes and onset of labor (American Academy of Pediatrics and American College of Obstetricians and Gynecologists, 2007). As a result of virologic diagnostic techniques such as HIV culture, polymerase chain reaction, and immune complex–dissociated p24 antigen, diagnosis of HIV infection can be made in 30% to 50% of infants at birth and in 100% of infants by 4 to 6 months of age. For information on additional diseases that may be screened in the newborn period, see *Newborn Screening Fact Sheets* (Kaye and American Association of Pediatrics Committee on Genetics, 2006).

Universal Newborn Hearing Screening

Approximately 1 to 6 per 1000 newborns may have significant hearing loss, which may go undetected until later in life. Such deficits may lead to subsequent speech and language delays, which could be treated with early detection. The Joint Committee on Infant Hearing, American Academy of Pediatrics (2000c), recommends that all birthing hospitals establish programs to screen *all* newborn infants before discharge for hearing loss by automated auditory brainstem response or transient evoked otoacoustic emissions. Newborns who fail the initial screening require documentation and referral for further testing by 1 month of age; newborns who do not receive initial screening before discharge should also be tested by 1 month. It is estimated that screening by high-risk factors alone fails to identify approximately 50% of all newborns with a congenital hearing loss. Guidelines for screening infants and older children for hearing loss have been published by the American Academy of Pediatrics (2003b).

Because approximately 50% of all causes of childhood hearing loss are attributed to genetic causes, molecular genetic tests on blood in all newborns has been proposed to detect infants with late-onset or prelingual hearing loss; in such infants hearing loss may not be detected by standard screening in early infancy and would not otherwise be identified until later in life (Morton and Nance, 2006).

ATRAUMATIC CARE

Heel Punctures

Repeated heel lancing is often necessary to obtain sufficient blood for a number of newborn blood tests, including newborn screening. It has been anecdotally observed that newborns appear to withdraw the heel when touched for subsequent heel punctures. Taddio, Shah, Gilbert-MacLeod, and others (2002) found that infants of diabetic mothers exposed to multiple heel punctures in the first 24 to 36 hours of life learned to anticipate pain and exhibited more intense pain responses. The use of automated lancet devices such as Tenderfoot* has been found to cause less pain and require fewer punctures than manual lance blades (Blain-Lewis, 1992; Paes, Janes, Vegh, and others, 1993). Additional studies have shown that venipuncture performed by an experienced phlebotomist elicited fewer pain responses (as measured by the Premature Infant Pain Profile [PIPP]) from full-term newborns than did heel punctures (Shah and Ohlsson, 2001). Furthermore, the need for additional skin punctures was reduced with venipuncture. Although maternal anxiety was initially higher in the venipuncture group, mothers who observed the venipuncture reported observing less pain response than mothers who observed heel punctures.

Oral sucrose and nonnutritive sucking have proved effective in decreasing the pain associated with heel punctures in preterm and full-term infants during the first week of life (Stevens, Yamada, and Ohlsson, 2004; Gibbins, Stevens, Hodnett, and others, 2002; Harrison, Johnston, and Loughnan, 2003); however, the exact dose range that proves effective varies among several studies (Stevens, Yamada, and Ohlsson, 2004). In one study, infants experiencing venipuncture were either given oral sucrose (30%) and a skin placebo or the eutectic mixture of local anesthetic (EMLA). Pain scores were measured with the PIPP, and infants receiving the oral sucrose solution exhibited fewer pain symptoms than those in the EMLA group (Gradin, Eriksson, Holmqvist, and others, 2002). Giving newborns 2 ml of oral sucrose solution (25% and 50%) significantly reduced crying time and heart rate after 3 minutes in comparison with controls (sterile water) during heel stick sampling for serum bilirubin concentrations (Haouari, Wood, Griffith, and others, 1995). Newborns given 2 ml of concentrated oral sucrose solution showed a significant reduction in crying time and heart rate in comparison with controls (given sterile water) during heel stick sampling and other painful stimuli (Stevens, Yamada, and Ohlsson, 2004).

Evidence indicates that as little as 2 ml of a 24% oral sucrose solution is effective in decreasing pain in full-term and preterm infants. In addition, the best analgesic effect is achieved when sucrose is administered 2 minutes before the painful procedure with a pacifier or syringe. In one study protocol where oral sucrose was effective, 0.5 ml of 24% oral sucrose solution was administered 2 minutes before the heel puncture,

during, and 5 minutes after the heel puncture (Gibbins, Stevens, Hodnett, and others, 2002). Eriksson and Finnstrom (2004) found that repeated administration of a 30% sucrose solution before heel lance in healthy full-term infants did not decrease the pain-relieving effect of the sucrose solution; the study's aim was to determine whether multiple oral sucrose administrations would cause tolerance to sucrose. Monitoring for adverse effects must accompany each administration (Noerr, 2001).

The mother's holding the infant in skin-to-skin contact has also been shown to significantly reduce the child's distress during the procedure (Blass and Watt, 1999; Gray, Watt, and Blass, 2000; Johnston, Stevens, Pinelli, and others, 2003). Breastfeeding during heel puncture in full-term newborns has been shown to be effective in decreasing pain scores when compared with placebo or a 30% oral sucrose solution (Carbajal, Veerapen, Couderc, and others, 2003).

The application of the topical anesthetic EMLA to reduce the pain of heel lance has produced mixed results in full-term and preterm infants (Fitzgerald, Millard, and McIntosh, 1989; Taddio, Ohlsson, Einarson, and others, 1998; Stevens, Johnston, Taddio, and others, 1999). Grunau, Linhares, Holsti, and others (2004) noted that placing preterm infants in a prone (vs supine) position for heel stick did not decrease the pain response and that additional pain-relieving measures for this population are necessary.

Music was found to decrease the pain response to heel stick in a small group of preterm infants (Butt and Kisilevsky, 2000). A study comparing the effects of swaddling and containment on preterm infants undergoing heel stick failed to demonstrate significant differences between the two interventions (Huang, Tung, Kuo, and others, 2004).

These studies provide evidence of a number of effective ways to decrease the pain associated with heel puncture in full-term and preterm newborns. It is essential that nurses use *all* available resources to advocate for the prevention and management of neonatal pain during such procedures. Because the overall goal is to decrease the effect of painful interventions such as heel stick on infants, a combination of pharmacologic and nonpharmacologic interventions is recommended. (See also Atraumatic Care box, pp. 226-227.)

A number of commercially available oral sucrose solutions now exist, including Ora-Sweet† (54% solution), which can be diluted 1:1 to produce a 27% solution, and Sweet-Ease,‡ 24% sucrose solution. When these are not available, the pharmacy may mix an oral sucrose solution to ensure a clean product. An approximate 25% sucrose solution is made by mixing 1 teaspoon of granulated (table) sugar with 4 teaspoons of sterile water; however, this method is the least desirable to prevent contamination of the solution and subsequent problems.

*International Technidyne, Inc., Edison, NJ.
†Paddock Laboratories, Minneapolis.
‡Children's Medical Ventures, Norwell, Massachusetts.

Bathing

Bath time is an opportunity for the nurse to accomplish much more than general hygiene. It is an excellent time for observing the infant's behavior, state of arousal, alertness, and muscular activity. Bathing is usually performed after the vital signs have stabilized, especially the temperature.

With the possibility of transmission of viruses such as hepatitis B virus and HIV via maternal blood and blood-stained amniotic fluid, the traditional timing of the newborn's bath has been questioned. The newborn must be considered a potential contamination source until proved otherwise. As part of **standard precautions,** nurses should wear gloves when handling the newborn until blood and amniotic fluid are removed by bathing.

Studies indicate that healthy full-term newborns with a stable body temperature can be bathed as early as 1 hour of age without experiencing problems, provided that effective thermoregulation measures are taken after the bath (Penny-MacGillivray, 1996; Behring, Vezeau, and Fink, 2003; Varda and Behnke, 2000; Medves and O'Brien, 2004). Nurses are cautioned, however, to avoid instituting routine newborn bathing according to a rigid schedule; nursing interventions such as bathing should instead be based on individualized assessment and family interaction needs.

The bath time provides an opportunity for the nurse to involve the parents in the care of their child, to teach correct hygiene procedures, and to learn about their infant's individual characteristics (Fig. 8-12). The appropriate types of bath-

FIG. 8-12 ■ Bath time is an excellent opportunity for parents to learn about their newborn.

ing supplies and the need for safety in terms of water temperature and supervision of the infant at all times during the bath are stressed.

Parents are encouraged to examine their infant closely during bathing. Frequently, normal variations such as Epstein pearls, mongolian spots, or "stork bites" cause parents much worry because they are unaware of the significance of such findings. Minor birth injuries may appear as major defects to them. Explaining how these occurred and when they will disappear reassures parents of their infant's normalcy. Common variations are discussed further in Chapter 9.

One of the most important considerations in skin cleansing is preservation of the skin's **acid mantle,** which is formed from the uppermost horny layer of the epidermis; sweat; superficial fat; metabolic products; and external substances such as amniotic fluid, microorganisms, and chemicals. The infant's skin surface has a pH of about 5 soon after birth, and the bacteriostatic effects of this pH are significant. Consequently, only plain warm water or soap with appropriate pH should be used for the bath. Alkaline soaps, oils, powder, and lotions are not used because they alter the acid mantle, thus providing a medium for bacterial growth. Talcum powder has the added risk of aspiration if it is applied too close to the infant's face. A safer alternative is a cornstarch-based powder (see also Diaper Dermatitis, Chapter 30).

Parents should be involved in a discussion regarding the newborn's bath at home. It is recommended that for the first 2 weeks the infant be bathed no more than two or three times per week with a plain warm sponge bath. This practice will help maintain the integrity of the newborn's skin and allow time for the umbilical cord to completely dry. Routine daily soap bathing for newborns is no longer recommended (Association of Women's Health, Obstetric and Neonatal Nursing, 2007; Darmstadt and Dinulos, 2000).

Care of the Umbilicus

Because the umbilical stump is an excellent medium for bacterial growth, various methods of cord care are practiced to prevent infection. Common methods include the use of an antimicrobial agent such as bacitracin or triple dye, although some experts advocate the use of alcohol alone, soap and water,

sterile water, povidone-iodine, or no treatment (natural healing). The use of antiseptic agents has been shown to prolong cord drying and separation (Zupan, Garner, and Omari, 2004). Studies regarding bacterial growth and colonization according to the cleansing method used have produced varied results (Janssen, Selwood, Dobson, and others, 2003; Golombek, Brill, and Salice, 2002; Dore, Buchan, Coulas, and others, 1998). A Cochrane Review of 21 studies found no significant difference between cords treated with antiseptics compared with dry cord care or placebo; there were no reported systemic infections or deaths, and a trend toward reduced colonization was found in cords treated with antiseptics (Zupan, Garner, and Omari, 2004). Recommendations for cord care by the Association of Women's Health, Obstetric and Neonatal Nursing (2007) include cleaning the cord initially with sterile water or a neutral pH cleanser, then subsequently cleaning the cord with water. A one-time application of triple dye has been shown to be superior to alcohol, povidone-iodine, or topical antibiotics in reducing colonization or infection; the use of alcohol is associated with prolonged cord drying and separation (McConnell, Lee, Couillard, and others, 2004).

Nurses working in neonatal care must carefully evaluate the available studies and compare the risks and benefits regarding the method of cord care within their own population of newborns and families. Regardless of the method used, nurses must include cord care teaching in the discharge planning because it has been demonstrated to be a concern for parents following discharge to the home.

The diaper is folded in front below the cord to avoid irritation and wetness on the site. The area is kept free of urine and stool and cleansed daily with the cleanser of choice. Parents are instructed regarding stump deterioration and proper umbilical care. The stump deteriorates through the process of dry gangrene. Cord separation time is influenced by a number of factors, including type of cord care, type of delivery, and other perinatal events. The average cord separation time is 10 to 14 days.

It takes a few more weeks for the cord base to heal completely after cord separation. During this time, care consists of keeping the base clean and dry and observing for any signs of infection.

> **NURSINGALERT**
>
> With early hospital discharge, newborns may be discharged before it is safe to remove the cord clamp. Teach the parent how to safely remove the clamp once the newborn is at least 24 hours old and no oozing from the cord is noted.

Circumcision

Circumcision, the surgical removal of the foreskin on the glans penis, may be done in the hospital or in an outpatient clinic, although it is not a common practice in most countries. In the United States, however, circumcision rates have increased significantly over time: 61.1% of boys born in the United States from 1997 to 2000 were circumcised, compared with 48.3% of boys born from 1988 to 1991 (Nelson, Dunn, Wan, and others, 2005). Despite the frequency of the procedure in the United States, there is still much controversy regarding the benefits and risks (Box 8-4). The American Academy of Pediatrics (1999) issued a circumcision policy statement stating that the medical benefits of male newborn circumcision are not sufficiently significant to recommend it as a rou-

Critical Thinking Exercise—Circumcision

BOX 8-4

Risks and Benefits of Neonatal Circumcision

RISKS

Complications:
- Hemorrhage
- Infection
- Dehiscence (separation of approximated edges of skin)
- Meatitis (from loss of protective foreskin)
- Adhesions
- Concealed penis
- Urethral fistula
- Meatal stenosis

Pain in unanesthetized infants (long-term consequences unknown, but short-term stresses include increased heart rate, behavior changes, prolonged crying, increased cortisol levels, and decreased blood oxygenation)

BENEFITS

Prevention of penile cancer and posthitis (inflammation of prepuce)

Decreased incidence of balanitis (inflammation of glans), urinary tract infections in male infants, and some sexually transmitted diseases later in life (herpes, syphilis, gonorrhea)

Decreased incidence of human immunodeficiency virus (HIV) infection, human papillomavirus (HPV), and cervical cancer (in female partner)

Prevention of complications associated with later circumcision

Preservation of male's body image that is consistent with peers (only in countries or cultures where procedure is common)

 ATRAUMATIC CARE

Guidelines for Pain Management During Neonatal Circumcision*

PHARMACOLOGIC INTERVENTIONS

Use of Topical Anesthetic

One hour before the procedure, administer acetaminophen.

Place a thick layer (1 g) of EMLA† (lidocaine-prilocaine) cream around the penis where the prepuce (foreskin) attaches to the glans. Avoid placing cream on the tip of the penis where EMLA may come in contact with urethral opening. LMX4 (4% lidocaine cream) has also been proved effective and safe for term newborn circumcision (Lehr, Cepeda, Frattarelli, and others, 2005). Apply a small dollop of topical cream to a small area (1 cm²) before large application to ensure infant does not have an allergic reaction to the anesthetic.

Cover the penis with a "finger cot" that is cut from a vinyl or latex glove or a piece of plastic wrap, and secure bottom of covering with tape. Avoid using Tegaderm or large amounts of tape on the skin because removing the adhesive causes pain and can irritate or remove the fragile skin.

If the infant urinates during the time EMLA is applied (1 hour) and a significant amount of EMLA is removed, reapply the cream and covering. The total application of EMLA should not exceed a surface area of 10 cm² (1.25 3 1.25 inches).

Remove cream with clean cloth or tissue. Blanching of skin is an expected reaction to EMLA's application under an occlusive dressing; erythema and some edema may occur also.

Two minutes before starting the procedure, give the infant a concentrated sucrose solution (24%). Use this solution to coat the pacifier (recoat several times before and during the procedure) or administer 2 ml to the tongue.

Following procedure, apply petrolatum or A&D ointment on a 4×4 dressing before diapering infant to prevent the wound from adhering to the dressing or diaper. Topical anesthetic alone is not recommended for pain management of circumcision.

Administer acetaminophen as ordered by the practitioner 4 hours after the initial dose; give additional doses as needed but not to exceed five doses in 24 hours or a maximum dosage of 75 mg/kg/day.

Data from Broadman LM, Hannallah RS, Belman AB, and others: Post-circumcision analgesia: a prospective evaluation of subcutaneous ring block of the penis, *Anesthesiology* 67:339-402, 1987; Howard CR, Howard FM, Weitzman ML: Acetaminophen analgesia in neonatal circumcision: the effect on pain, *Pediatrics* 93(4):641-646, 1994; Lander J, Brady-Fryer B, Metcalfe JB, and others: Comparison of ring block, dorsal penile nerve block, and topical anesthesia for neonatal circumcision, *JAMA* 278:2157-2162, 1997; Mintz MR, Grillo R: Dorsal penile nerve block for circumcision, *Clin Pediatr* 28:590-591, 1989; Serour F, Mandelberg A, Mori J: Slow injection of local anesthetic will decrease pain during dorsal penile nerve block, *Acta Anaesthesiol Scand* 42:926-928, 1998; Spencer DM, Miller KA, O'Quinn M, and others: Dorsal penile nerve block in neonatal circumcision: chloroprocaine versus lidocaine, *Am J Perinatol* 9(3):214-218, 1992; Stang H, Snellman LW, Condon LM, and others: Beyond dorsal penile nerve block: a more humane circumcision, *Pediatrics* 100(2):e3, 1997, retrieved from http://www.pediatrics.org/cgi/content/full/100/2/e3; Stevens B, Taddio A, Ohlsson A, and others: The efficacy of sucrose for relieving procedural pain in neonates—a systematic review and meta-analysis, *Acta Paediatr* 86:837-842, 1997; Taddio A, Stevens B, Craig K, and others: Efficacy and safety of lidocaine-prilocaine cream (EMLA) for pain during circumcision, *N Engl J Med* 336(17):1197-1201, 1997; Taddio A: Pain management for neonatal circumcision, *Paediatr Drugs* 3(2):101-111, 2001; Taddio A, Ohlsson K, Ohlsson A: Lidocaine-prilocaine cream for analgesia during circumcision in newborn boys, *Cochrane Syst Rev* (1):CD000496, 2003; Geyer J, Ellsbury D, Kleiber C, and others: An evidence-based multidisciplinary protocol for neonatal circumcision pain management, *J Obstet Gynecol Neonatal Nurs* 31(4):403-410, 2002; Taddio A, Pollock N, Gilbert-MacLeod C, and others: Combined analgesia and local anesthesia to minimize pain during circumcision, *Arch Pediatr Adolesc Med* 154(6):620-623, 2000; Kraft NL: A pictorial and video guide to circumcision without pain, *Adv Neonatal Care* 3(2):50-64, 2003; and Lehr VT, Cepeda E, Frattarelli DA, and others: Lidocaine 4% cream compared with lidocaine 2.5% and prilocaine 2.5% or dorsal penile block for circumcision, *Am J Perinatol* 22(5):231-237, 2005.

*There is sufficient evidence and support for use of a combination of pharmacologic and nonpharmacologic interventions to holistically manage neonatal circumcision pain. Combined analgesia, nonpharmacologic interventions (such as swaddling), and local anesthesia may be used during the procedure to provide holistic pain management (Taddio A, Pollock N, Gilbert-MacLeod C, and others: Combined analgesia and local anesthesia to minimize pain during circumcision, *Arch Pediatr Adolesc Med* 154(6):620-623, 2000; Anand KJS and International Evidence-Based Group for Neonatal Pain: Consensus statement for the prevention and management of pain in the newborn, *Arch Pediatr Adolesc Med* 155(2):173-180, 2001; Geyer J, Ellsbury D, Kleiber C, and others: An evidence-based multidisciplinary protocol for neonatal circumcision pain management, *J Obstet Gynecol Neonatal Nurs* 31(4):403-410, 2002; Razmus I, Dalton M, Wilson D: Pain management for newborn circumcision, *Pediatr Nurs* 20(5):414-417, 427, 2004).

†NOTE: In March, 1999, the Food and Drug Administration (FDA) approved the use of EMLA in infants age 37 weeks of gestation. Although the package insert lists under "warnings" that patients taking drugs associated with drug-induced methemoglobinemia, such as acetaminophen, are at greater risk for developing methemoglobinemia, there have been no reported cases of this complication occurring in children taking acetaminophen and using EMLA. In fact, there is no evidence that acetaminophen is a methemoglobin-inducing drug in humans (Prescott LF: *Paracetamol (acetaminophen): a critical bibliographic review*, Bristol, 1996, Taylor & Francis). The only reported cases of methemoglobinemia from acetaminophen have been in cats and dogs (Hjelle JJ, Grauer GF: Acetaminophen-induced toxicosis in dogs and cats, *J Am Vet Med Assoc* 188(7):742-749, 1986).

tine procedure; this policy was reaffirmed in 2005 (American Academy of Pediatrics, 2005a). The Academy's statement emphasizes parental autonomy to determine what is in the best interest of their male newborn. The policy encourages the physician to ensure that parents have been given accurate and unbiased information about the risks, benefits, and alternatives before making an informed choice and that they understand that circumcision is an elective procedure. In addition to examining the medical benefits of male newborn circumcision, the American Academy of Pediatrics recommends that procedural analgesia be provided if parents decide to have their male infant circumcised.

Nurses are in a unique position to help educate parents regarding the care of their newborns, and they must take responsibility for ensuring that each parent has accurate and unbiased information with which to make an informed decision regarding the appropriateness of the circumcision procedure for their newborn. Parents need to know the options for pain control, especially the choice of topical or injected anesthesia, and their option of observing the procedure. Nurses should also be proactive in advocating for circumcision analgesia.

The nurse should also use every nonpharmacologic intervention that can reduce the pain of this operative procedure (see Atraumatic Care box). Despite adequate scientific evidence that newborns feel and respond to pain, circumcisions are still being performed in the United States with either insufficient analgesia or no analgesia at all. Nurses can use the American Academy of Pediatrics' policy statement to advocate more effectively for the use of optimal pain relief for circumcision.

Four types of anesthesia and analgesia are used in newborns undergoing circumcision: ring block, dorsal penile nerve block (DPNB), topical anesthetic such as EMLA (prilocaine-lidocaine) or LMX4 (4% lidocaine), and concentrated oral sucrose. Oral acetaminophen and comfort measures such as music, sucking on a pacifier, and soothing voices have not proved to be effective in reducing the pain of circumcision when used alone (Williamson, 1997); however, these may be used in addition to analgesia and anesthesia to decrease procedural pain.

The Cochrane group exploring pain relief for neonatal circumcision (Brady-Fryer, Wiebe, and Lander, 2007) found

ATRAUMATIC CARE

Guidelines for Pain Management During Neonatal Circumcision—cont'd
PHARMACOLOGIC INTERVENTIONS—cont'd
Use of Dorsal Penile Nerve Block or Ring Block
One hour before procedure administer acetaminophen.
One hour before procedure, apply EMLA. For the dorsal penile nerve block (DPNB) apply EMLA to the prepuce as described previously and at the penile base. For the ring block apply EMLA to the prepuce as described previously and to the shaft of the penis. A topical anesthetic should be used in conjunction with the DPNB or ring block to avoid the pain of injecting the anesthetic.
Use a 30-gauge needle to administer the lidocaine.‡ For the DPNB, 0.4 ml of the lidocaine is infiltrated at the 10:30 o'clock and 1:30 o'clock positions in Buck's fascia at the penile base. For the ring block, 0.4 ml of lidocaine is infiltrated subcutaneously on each side of the shaft of the penis below the prepuce. Using buffered lidocaine (with sodium bicarbonate) and warming the solution may further decrease pain. (Lidocaine with epinephrine is not used in neonates.)
For maximum anesthesia, wait 5 minutes after the injection of lidocaine. An alternative anesthetic is chloroprocaine, which is as effective as lidocaine after 3 minutes.
During the circumcision, administer sucrose as described previously.
Apply A&D ointment or petrolatum as described previously.

Acetaminophen
Administer acetaminophen as ordered by the practitioner (10 to 15 mg/kg) every 4 to 6 hours for 24 hours not to exceed five doses in 24 hours or a maximum dosage of 75 mg/kg/day.

Oral Sucrose
Administer 2 ml of a concentrated solution (12% to 25%) of oral sucrose 2 minutes before the procedure.
Allow infant to suck on pacifier dipped in oral sucrose during procedure.

NONPHARMACOLOGIC INTERVENTIONS (TO ACCOMPANY PRECEDING PHARMACOLOGIC INTERVENTIONS)
If Circumstraint board is used, pad with blankets or other thick, soft material such as "lamb's wool." A more comfortable, padded, and physiologic restraint that places the infant semireclining can also decrease distress (Stang, Snellman, Condon, and others, 1997).§
Provide the parents, caregiver, or another staff member with the option of holding the infant during the procedure or of being present during the circumcision.
Swaddle the upper body and legs during the procedure to provide warmth and containment and to reduce movement (see Fig. 8-13).
If the patient is not swaddled and is unclothed, use a radiant warmer to prevent hypothermia. Shield infant's eyes from overhead lights as needed.
Prewarm any topical solutions to be used in sterile preparation of the surgical site by placing in a warm blanket or towel.
Play infant relaxation music¶ before, during, and after procedure; allow parents or other caregiver the option of providing the music of choice.
After the procedure, remove restraints and swaddle. Immediately have the parent, other caregiver, or nursing staff hold the infant. Continue to have the infant suck on pacifier or offer feeding.
Recommend use of combination analgesia; oral sucrose, acetaminophen, and topical anesthetic; or oral sucrose, acetaminophen, topical anesthetic, and DPNB or ring block, in addition to nonpharmacologic comfort measures such as containment.

‡NOTE: In one study, the use of buffered lidocaine, which normally reduces the stinging sensation of lidocaine, did not provide effective anesthesia for DPNB (Stang, Snellman, Condon, and others, 1997). The study on slow injection of the anesthetics lidocaine and bupivacaine compared 40 vs 80 seconds in patients ages 15-53 years (Serour F, Mandelberg A, Mori J: Slow injection of local anesthetic will decrease pain during dorsal penile nerve block, *Acta Anaesthesiol Scand* 42:926-928, 1998).
§For information on the Stang Circ Chair, contact Pedicraft, 4134 Augustine Road, Jacksonville, FL 32247; (800) 223-7649; http://www.pedicraft.com.
¶Suggested infant relaxation music: *Heartbeat Lullabies* by Terry Woodford. Available from Baby-Go-To-Sleep Center, Audio Therapy Innovations, Inc., PO Box 550, Colorado Springs, CO 80901; (800) 537-7748; http://www.babygotosleep.com.

FIG. 8-13 ■ Proper positioning of infant in Circumstraint. (Photo by Paul Vincent Kuntz, Texas Children's Hospital, Houston.)

that DPNB was the most effective intervention for decreasing pain of circumcision. Studies exploring the use of several strategies concurrently, such as that conducted by Razmus, Dalton, and Wilson (2004), which included groups receiving both sucrose and ring block compared with ring block alone, have the most potential to clarify optimum strategies.

Circumcision should not be performed immediately after delivery because of the neonate's unstabilized physiologic status and increased susceptibility to stress. Preoperative nursing care usually includes allowing the infant nothing by mouth before the procedure to prevent aspiration of vomitus (about 2 hours); however, the necessity of this practice has been questioned (Kraft, 2003). Additional measures include checking for a signed consent form and adequately restraining the infant, usually on a special board (Fig. 8-13) or physiologic circumcision restraint chair. All of the equipment used for the procedure, such as gloves, instruments, dressings, and draping towels, must be sterile.

The procedure involves freeing the foreskin from the glans penis by using a scalpel, Gomco or Mogen clamp (see Cultural Awareness box), or Plastibell. In the **Gomco technique** the foreskin is clamped, cut with a scalpel, and removed; the clamp crushes the nerve endings and blood vessels, promoting hemostasis. In the **Plastibell procedure** the foreskin is removed using a plastic ring and a string tied around the foreskin like a tourniquet. The excess foreskin is trimmed. In about 5 to 8 days the plastic ring separates and falls off.

After the procedure is completed, the infant is released from the restraints and comforted. If the parents were not present during the procedure, they are informed of the infant's status and reunited with their son.

Care of the circumcised penis depends on the type of procedure performed. If a clamp (Gomco or Mogen) was used, a petrolatum gauze dressing may be applied loosely to prevent adherence to the diaper. If the Plastibell was applied, no special dressing is required. Because the area is tender, the diaper is applied loosely to prevent friction against the penis. The penis is evaluated for excessive bleeding in the first few hours after the procedure, and the first void is recorded.

Normally, on the second day a yellowish white exudate forms as part of the granulation process. This is not a sign of infection and is not forcibly removed. As healing progresses, the exudate disappears. Parents are educated to report any evidence of bleeding, unusual swelling, or absence of voiding to the practitioner.

PROVIDE OPTIMAL NUTRITION

Selection of a feeding method is one of the major decisions faced by parents. In general, there are three acceptable choices: human milk, commercially prepared whole cow's milk formula, and modified evaporated cow's milk. There are significant nutritional, economic, and psychologic advantages and differences among these methods. Nurses should be at the forefront in providing the parent(s) with accurate and unbiased information needed to make a conscientious informed decision regarding the feeding method.

Human Milk

Human milk is the best option for infant nutrition up to 1 year of age. Breast milk consists of a number of micronutrients that are called **bioavailable,** meaning these nutrients are available in quantities and qualities that make them easily digestible by the newborn's intestine and absorbed for energy and growth. Breast milk offers a variety of immunologic properties that are found exclusively in human milk. Human milk has been shown to be effective in protecting the newborn against respiratory tract infections, gastrointestinal infections caused by enterococci, otitis media, numerous allergies, type 2 diabetes, and atopy.

The fat content of human milk is composed of lipids, triglycerides, and cholesterol; cholesterol is an essential element for brain growth. The function of these lipids is to allow optimal intestinal absorption of essential fatty acids and polyunsaturated fatty acids (PUFAs). Furthermore, lipids contribute approximately 50% of the total calories in human milk (Lawrence and Lawrence, 2005). Although the overall fat content in human milk is higher than in cow's milk, it is used more efficiently by the infant.

The primary source of carbohydrate in human milk is lactose, which is present in higher concentrations (6.8 g/dl) than in cow's milk–based formula (4.9 g/dl). The carbohydrates not only serve as a large portion of total calories in human milk, but they also have protective functions; the oligosaccharides in human milk stimulate the growth of *Lactobacillus bifidus* and prevent bacteria from adhering to epithelial surfaces. Additional carbohydrates found in human milk include glucose, galactose, and glucosamine.

Human milk also contains two proteins, whey (lactalbumin) and casein (curd), in a ratio of approximately 60:40 (vs 80:20 in most cow's milk–based formula). This ratio in human milk makes it more digestible and produces the soft stools seen in breast-fed infants. Thus human milk has a laxative effect, and constipation is uncommon. The whey protein, lactoferrin, in human milk has iron-binding characteristics with bacteriostatic capabilities, particularly against gram-positive and gram-negative aerobes, anaerobes, and yeasts (Lawrence and Lawrence, 2005).

Lysozyme is found in large quantities in human milk and has bacteriostatic functions against gram-positive bacteria and Enterobacteriaceae. Human milk also contains numerous other host defense factors such as macrophages, granulocytes, and T and B lymphocytes. Casein in human milk greatly enhances the absorption of iron, thus preventing iron-dependent bacteria from proliferating in the gastrointestinal tract (Biancuzzo, 2003). Secretory IgA is found in high levels in colostrum, but levels gradually decline over the first 14 days of life. Secretory IgA prevents bacteria and viruses from invading the intestinal mucosa in breast-fed newborns, thus protecting from infection (Hanson and Korotkova, 2002). The whey protein is also believed to play an important role in preventing the development of certain allergies.

Several digestive enzymes also present in human milk include amylases, lipases, proteases, and ribonucleases, which enhance the digestion and absorption of various nutrients. The amounts of lipid- and water-soluble vitamins, electrolytes, minerals, and trace elements in human milk are sufficient for growth, development, and energy needs during the first 6 months of life. The one possible exception is vitamin D, which is found in varying amounts depending on the mother's intake of vitamin D–fortified food and exposure to ultraviolet light. Therefore, to prevent vitamin-D–deficiency rickets, the American Academy of Pediatrics (2003d) now recommends that infants who are exclusively breast-fed or who are ingesting less than 500 ml/day of vitamin D–fortified formula be supplemented with 200 IU vitamin D (oral) per day.

Additional beneficial components of human milk include prostaglandins; epidermal growth factor; desoxyhexanoic acid

(DHA); arachidonic acid (AA); taurine; cystine; carnitine; cytokine; interleukins; and natural hormones such as thyroid-releasing hormone, gonadotropin-releasing hormone, and prolactin. Studies have demonstrated that breastfeeding is associated with a decrease in the incidence of type 2 diabetes (Kue Young, Chateau, and Zhang, 2002; Young, Martens, Taback, and others, 2002), a decrease in the incidence of hospital admissions for respiratory tract illnesses in generally healthy infants (Bachrach, Schwarz, and Bachrach, 2003), and higher intelligence scores compared with cow's milk–based formula–fed infants (Anderson, Johnston, and Remley, 1999). Some studies have demonstrated that breastfeeding has an analgesic effect on newborns during painful procedures such as heel puncture (Carbajal, Veerapen, Couderc, and others, 2003; Gray, Miller, Phillips, and others, 2002; Shah, Aliwalas, and Shah, 2006).

Breastfeeding

Human milk is the preferred form of nutrition for all infants. *Healthy People 2010* has a goal to increase breastfeeding rates in the United States to 75% in early postpartum and to 50% for mothers who continue to breastfeed for at least 6 months (US Department of Health and Human Services, 2000). A survey by Ross Products (Ryan, Zhou, and Gaston, 2004) indicates that 70.1% of women breastfeed in early postpartum, and 33.2% continued to breastfeed for 6 months. Some have voiced concern that early discharge of new mothers from hospitals, more aggressive marketing of infant formulas to the public, and more employed mothers contributed to the decline of breastfeeding in the 1990s. In addition, some hospital practices intended to provide optimal maternal-newborn health may instead undermine breastfeeding. Early separation of mother and newborn, delays in initiating breastfeeding, provision of formula in the hospital and in discharge packs, conflicting information by health care workers, and formula coupons given at discharge have been implicated in the decline of breastfeeding after discharge. Rooming-in has correlated positively with successful breastfeeding, whereas the use of a pacifier has sometimes been associated with earlier weaning from breast to bottle.

A survey of breastfeeding mothers indicated that the determining factors for changing to bottle feeding included the mother's perception of the father's attitude toward breastfeeding and the mother's uncertainty regarding the amount of milk the infant would receive (Arora, McJunkin, Wehrer, and others, 2000). These findings have important implications for involving fathers in education and discussion regarding breastfeeding before and during the pregnancy. Fathers may express concerns of feeling left out during the newborn period if they have little involvement other than diapering and holding the infant. Encouraging fathers regarding their positive role in supporting the mother in breastfeeding may enhance the mother-infant interaction and decrease her sense of helplessness and isolation.

The American Academy of Pediatrics (2005b) has reaffirmed its position exclusively recommending breastfeeding until at least 1 year of age as the best form of infant nutrition. The Academy also supports programs that enable women to continue breastfeeding after returning to work. In its support of breastfeeding practices, the Academy further discourages the advertisement of infant formula to breastfeeding mothers

BOX 8-5

Ten Steps to Successful Breastfeeding

Every facility providing maternity services and care for newborn infants should:

1. Have a written breastfeeding policy that is routinely communicated to all health care staff.
2. Train all health care staff in skills necessary to implement this policy.
3. Inform all pregnant women about the benefits and management of breastfeeding.
4. Help mothers initiate breastfeeding within a half hour of birth.
5. Show mothers how to breastfeed and how to maintain lactation, even if they should be separated from their infants.
6. Give newborn infants no food or drink other than breast milk, unless medically indicated.
7. Practice rooming-in—allowing mothers and infants to remain together—24 hours a day.
8. Encourage breastfeeding on demand.
9. Give no artificial teats or pacifiers (also called *dummies* or *soothers*) to breastfeeding infants.
10. Foster the establishment of breastfeeding support groups, and refer mothers to them on discharge from the hospital or clinic.

Data from Kyenkya-Isabirye M: UNICEF launches the Baby-Friendly Hospital Initiative, *MCN* 17(4):177-179, 1992; Wright A, Rice S, Wells S: Changing hospital practices to increase the duration of breastfeeding, *Pediatrics* 97(5):669-676, 1996.

FIG. 8-14 ■ Simultaneous breastfeeding of twins.

and distribution of formula discharge packs without the advice of a health care provider.

The Baby-Friendly Hospital Initiative (BFHI) is a joint effort of the World Health Organization and the United Nations Children's Fund to encourage, promote, and support breastfeeding as the model for optimum infant nutrition. Ten research-supported practices were developed by BFHI as a guideline for maternity facilities worldwide to promote breastfeeding (Wright, Rice, and Wells, 1996; Kyenkya-Isabirye, 1992) (Box 8-5). Research indicates that Baby-Friendly designated hospitals in the United States have higher rates for breastfeeding initiation and exclusivity than hospitals that are not Baby-Friendly designates (Merewood, Mehta, Chamberlain, and others, 2005).

In addition to the physiologic qualities of human milk, the most outstanding psychologic benefit of breastfeeding is the close maternal-child relationship. The infant is nestled close to the mother's skin, can hear the rhythm of her heartbeat, can feel the warmth of her body, and has a sense of peaceful security. The mother has a close feeling of union with her child and feels a sense of accomplishment and satisfaction as the infant sucks milk from her.

Human milk is the most economical form of feeding. It is always available, ready to serve at room temperature, and free of contamination. Although human milk is not sterile, healthy full-term infants can tolerate varying amounts of nonpathogenic and pathogenic organisms. The protection against infection can provide additional cost savings in terms of fewer medical visits and less time lost from work for the employed mother.

Breast-fed infants, especially beyond 2 to 3 months of age, tend to grow at a satisfactory but slower rate than bottle-fed infants.

Contraindications to breastfeeding include (Lawrence and Lawrence, 2005; American Academy of Pediatrics, 2005b):

- Maternal chemotherapy-antimetabolites and certain antineoplastic drugs
- Active tuberculosis not under treatment in mother
- HIV in mother
- Galactosemia in infant
- Maternal herpes simplex lesion on a breast
- Cytomegalovirus (CMV)—primary risk for preterm infants receiving CMV-infected donor milk, not for infected mother's infant (who already has CMV)
- Maternal substance abuse (e.g., cocaine, methamphetamine, and marijuana) (NOTE: Maternal methadone treatment for substance abuse is *not* a contraindication to breastfeeding.)
- Human T-cell leukemia virus types I and II
- Mothers who are receiving diagnostic or radioactive isotopes or who have had exposure to radioactive materials (for as long as there is radioactivity in milk)

Mastitis is usually not a contraindication if the discomfort is tolerable.

A small number of medications are contraindicated for breastfeeding mothers. Consult a reference text such as Hale (2006). Some herbal products are presented as safe and effective alternatives to prescription or over-the-counter medications; certain herbal agents, called **galactogogues,** are reported to increase breast milk production. There is insufficient data to confirm or deny the assertion of increased milk production using galactogogues, and mothers are cautioned to seek advice from a practitioner to ensure that the herbal preparations will not harm the breastfeeding infant (Conover and Buehler, 2004).

Breastfeeding can be done with twins and other multiples. If both twins are full term, they can begin feeding immediately after birth (Fig. 8-14); late preterm (near-term) infants should be evaluated individually but may be put to breast if stable. Simultaneous feeding promotes the rapid production of milk needed for both infants and makes the milk that would normally be lost in the letdown reflex available to one of the twins. When only one infant is hungry, the mother should feed singly. She should also alternate breasts when feeding each infant and avoid favoring one breast for one

FIG. 8-15 ■ The tongue is under the areola, with the tip of the nipple at the back of the wide-open mouth.

infant. The suckling patterns of infants vary, and each infant needs the visual stimulation and exercise that alternating breasts provides.

A concern many mothers have is the perceived inconvenience of loss of freedom and independence. Being committed to feeding the infant every 2 to 3 hours can be overwhelming, especially to women with multiple responsibilities. Many women resume their careers shortly after their pregnancy and prefer to bottle-feed. Combining breastfeeding and employment is possible, and suggestions for the mother are discussed in Chapter 10. Although breastfeeding is the preferred form of infant feeding, mothers' decisions regarding their preferences must be supported and respected.

Successful breastfeeding probably depends more on the mother's desire to breastfeed, satisfaction with breastfeeding, and available support systems than on any other factors. Mothers need support, encouragement, and assistance during their postpartum hospital stay and at home to enhance their opportunities for success and satisfaction.

Three main criteria have been proposed as essential in promoting positive breastfeeding: absence of a rigid feeding schedule, correct positioning of the infant at the breast to achieve latch-on, and correct suckling technique. Correct suckling for breastfeeding is defined as a wide-open mouth, tongue under the areola, and expression of milk by effective alveolar compression (Fig. 8-15).

The following interventions promote breastfeeding:

- Frequent and early breastfeeding, especially during the first hour of life; immediate skin-to-skin contact; rooming-in; and feeding on demand
- Direct modeling of the importance of breastfeeding by health care providers, such as implementing demand nursing with no formula supplementation and decreased emphasis on infant formula products
- Increased information and support to mothers following discharge, especially phone follow-up
- Early breast pumping every 2 to 3 hours for 10 to 15 minutes bilaterally if the newborn is unable to nurse immediately (increases oxytocin production and thus milk production)

Nurses play a significant role in the breastfeeding decision and must make themselves available to families for guidance and support. Several excellent books and organizations, such as LaLeche League International,* are available as resources for professionals and breastfeeding mothers.

NURSINGALERT

Do not use microwaves to defrost frozen human milk. High-temperature microwaving (72° to 98° C [162° to 208° F]) significantly destroys the antiinfective factors and vitamin C content (Quan, Yang, Rubinstein, and others, 1992). The safety of low-temperature microwaving (20° to 53° C [68° to 127° F]) remains questionable. One of the best ways to thaw frozen human milk is to place it under a warm flow of tap water. Another option is to let the frozen milk thaw overnight in the refrigerator to maintain high levels of secretory IgA (Biancuzzo, 2003). Test the temperature of the milk before feeding.

Bottle Feeding

Bottle feeding generally refers to the use of bottles for feeding commercial or evaporated milk formula rather than using the breast, although human milk may be expressed and fed with a bottle when necessary. Bottle feeding is an acceptable method of feeding. Nurses should not assume that new parents automatically know how to bottle feed their infant. Parents who choose bottle feeding also need support and assistance in meeting their infant's needs.

Providing newborns with nutrition is only one aspect of the feeding. Holding them close to the body while rocking or cuddling them helps to ensure the emotional component of feeding. Like breast-fed infants, bottle-fed infants need to be held on alternate sides of the lap to expose them to different stimuli. The feeding should not be hurried. Even though they may suck vigorously for the first 5 minutes and seem to be satisfied, they should be allowed to continue sucking. Infants need at least 2 hours of sucking a day. If there are six feedings per day, then about 20 minutes of sucking at each feeding provides for oral gratification.

NURSINGTIP

A recent study suggests bottles with a soft nipple system and a collapsible liner may promote more natural posture and a more stable breathing pattern than other bottle systems (Brown, 2007).

Propping the bottle is discouraged for the following reasons:

- It denies the infant the important component of close human contact.
- The infant may aspirate formula into the trachea and lungs while sleeping.
- It may facilitate the development of middle ear infections. If the infant lies flat and sucks, milk that has pooled in the pharynx becomes a suitable medium for bacterial growth. Bacteria then enters the eustachian tube, which leads to the middle ear, causing acute otitis media.
- It encourages continuous pooling of formula in the mouth, which can lead to nursing caries when the teeth erupt (see Chapter 12).

---

*PO Box 4079, Schaumburg, IL 60168-4079; (847) 519-7730; http://www. lalecheleague.org. In Canada: PO Box 700, Winchester, Ontario, KOC 2KO; (800) 665-4324; http://www.lllc.ca.

Commercially Prepared Formulas

The analysis of human and whole cow's milk indicates that the latter is unsuitable for infant nutrition. Whole cow's milk has a high protein content and low fat and lipid content, and there is evidence that it may cause intestinal bleeding and lead to iron deficiency anemia in infants. Questions have also been raised regarding the unmodified protein content of whole cow's milk, which may trigger an undesired immune response and thus increase the incidence of allergies in children at an early age.

Commercially prepared formulas are cow's milk based and have been modified to resemble the nutritional content of human milk. These formulas are altered from cow's milk by removing butterfat, decreasing the protein content, and adding vegetable oil and carbohydrate. Some cow's milk–based formulas have demineralized whey added to yield a whey/casein ratio of 60:40. The standard cow's milk–based formulas, regardless of the commercial brand, have essentially the same compositions of vitamins, minerals, protein, carbohydrates, and essential amino acids, with minor variations such as the source of carbohydrate; nucleotides to enhance immune function; and long-chain polyunsaturated fatty acids (LCPUFAs), DHA and arachidonic acid (AA), which are thought to improve brain function (Georgieff, 2001). DHA and AA are both found in large quantities in human milk but until recently were not present in most infant formulas. Studies in full-term infants receiving supplements with DHA and AA have produced mixed results regarding brain function and visual acuity. Many studies report a variety of sources for LCPUFAs, including egg yolk lipid, phospholipids, and triglyceride. The evidence for supplementation of formula for preterm infants with LCPUFAs, however, has been more convincing, producing some transient improvement in visual acuity and general development (American Academy of Pediatrics, 2004b). There do not appear to be any adverse effects associated with LCPUFA supplementation in preterm infants with respect to the incidence of bronchopulmonary disease, necrotizing enterocolitis, or other conditions of prematurity (American Academy of Pediatrics, 2004b). The Food and Drug Administration (FDA) regulates the manufacture of infant formula in the United States to ensure product safety. Standard cow's milk–based formulas are sold as low iron and iron fortified; however, only the iron-fortified formulas meet the requirements of infants (American Academy of Pediatrics, 2004b).

There are four main categories of commercially prepared infant formulas: (1) **cow's milk–based formulas,** available in 20 kcal/fl oz as liquid (ready to feed), as powder (requires reconstitution with water), or as a concentrated liquid (requires dilution with water); (2) **soy-based formulas,** available commercially in ready-to-feed 20 kcal/fl oz powder and concentrated liquid forms, commonly used for children who are lactose or cow's milk protein intolerant; (3) **casein- or whey-hydrolysate formulas,** commercially available in ready-to-feed and powder forms and used primarily for children who cannot tolerate or digest cow's milk– or soy-based formulas; and (4) **amino acid formulas.**

The American Academy of Pediatrics (2004b) recommends the use of soy protein–based formulas for infants with galactosemia, hereditary lactase deficiency, documented IgE allergies caused by cow's milk, and documented evidence of lactose intolerance. Soy protein–based formulas, however, have not been proved to be effective in preventing colic or allergy in healthy or high-risk infants (American Academy of Pediatrics, 2004b). Soy-based formulas, however, are not hypoallergenic, and a small percentage of the population may also be allergic to soy. Some researchers have speculated that exclusive use of soy formula in infants may adversely affect their endocrine, reproductive, and immune systems. This concern is related to isoflavones in soy and possible alteration in sexual maturity, immune response, and thyroid function (Greim, 2004; Chen and Rogan, 2004). Others report no long-term untoward effects from the ingestion of isoflavones in soy formula (Merritt and Jenks, 2004; Giampietro, Bruno, Furcolo, and others, 2004).

The casein- or whey-hydrolysate formulas are considered to be less antigenic than either cow's milk–based or soy-based formulas. The protein hydrolysate formulas (casein and whey) are derived from cow's milk–based formulas by a process of heat, filtration, and enzyme treatment designed to break the peptide chains into more digestible and hypoallergenic proteins. The hydrolysate formulas have the disadvantage of tasting bad; however, these may be made more palatable by adding a hypoallergenic flavoring such as Vari-Flavor. To reduce the incidence of cow's milk allergy and atopic dermatitis in infants at high risk for these conditions, use of hydrolyzed formula must be combined with strict avoidance of solid food during the first 4 to 6 months of life (Host and Halken, 2004).

Neocate and EleCare are extensively hydrolyzed amino acid formulas, designed for infants who are sensitive to cow's milk–based, soy-based, and partially hydrolyzed casein- and whey-based formulas. Both products are available in powder form. A wide variety of formulas are manufactured for infants and children with special needs; it is not within the scope of this text to discuss each one, but a formula company representative can provide product books that describe the purpose and content of each formula.

Follow-up formulas are marketed as a transitional formula for infants older than 6 months who are also eating solid foods. These generally contain a higher percentage of calories from protein and carbohydrate sources, a higher amount of iron and vitamins, and a lower amount of fat than standard cow's milk–based formulas. Many nutrition experts and the

Academy of Pediatrics (2004b), however, dispute the necessity of follow-up formulas if the infant is receiving an adequate amount of solid foods containing sufficient iron, vitamins, and minerals.

Preparation of Formula

Persons preparing infant formula wash their hands well and then wash all of the equipment used to prepare the formula with soap and water. Sterilizing bottles and nipples 5 minutes in boiling water may be required in certain situations where a hot-water dishwasher is not available. It is generally recommended that the tap water used to reconstitute powdered infant formula or to dilute concentrated liquid be brought to a rolling boil for 1 minute, then allowed to cool before use (American Academy of Pediatrics, 2004b). Using warm or hot tap water or placing the prepared formula bottle in the microwave is not adequate for preventing bacterial growth. Following the manufacturer's instructions for preparing the formula is essential to ensure the infant receives adequate calories and fluid for adequate growth. Parents are cautioned not to alter the reconstitution or dilution of infant formula except under the specific directions of the primary practitioner. Powdered formula and concentrated formula are prepared and bottled immediately before each feeding. Warming the formula is optional, although many parents prefer to warm it before feeding. Any milk remaining in the bottle after the feeding is discarded because it is an excellent medium for bacterial growth. Opened cans of ready-to-feed or concentrated formula are covered and refrigerated immediately until the next feeding. Bottled water should not be considered sterile unless otherwise indicated; bottled water without fluoride should be avoided for mixing infant formula (Morin, 2007). Because of incidents involving contamination of powdered formula with *Enterobacter sakazakii* and subsequent infant death in a neonatal unit, it is now recommended that hospital formula preparation for newborns follow separate guidelines; these are discussed in Chapter 9.

Laws governing the labeling of infant formulas require that the directions for preparation and use of the formula include pictures and symbols for nonreading individuals. In addition, manufacturers are translating the directions into foreign languages, such as Spanish and Vietnamese, to prevent misunderstanding and errors in formula preparation.

NURSING ALERT
Stress to families that the proportions must not be altered—neither diluted with extra water to extend the amount of formula, nor concentrated to provide more calories.

Alternate Milk Products

In the United States few infants are fed **evaporated milk formula,** and its use is not recommended by the American Academy of Pediatrics (2004b). However, it has many advantages over whole milk. It is readily available in cans; needs no refrigeration if unopened; is less expensive than commercial formula; provides a softer, more digestible curd; and contains more lactalbumin and a higher calcium/phosphorus ratio. Disadvantages of evaporated milk for infant nutrition include low iron and vitamin C concentrations, excessive sodium and phosphorus, decreased vitamin A and D (except in fortified forms), and poorly digested fat. A common rule for preparing evaporated milk formula is diluting the 13-ounce can of milk with 19½ ounces of water and adding 3 tablespoons of sugar or commercially processed corn syrup.

Evaporated milk must not be confused with condensed milk, which is a form of evaporated milk with 45% more sugar. Because of its high carbohydrate concentration and disproportionately low fat and protein content, condensed milk is not used for infant feeding. Likewise, skim and low-fat milk must not be used for infant milk because they are deficient in caloric concentration, significantly increase the renal solute load and water demands, and deprive the body of essential fatty acids.

Goat's milk is a poor source of iron and folic acid. It has an excessively high renal solute load as a result of its high protein content, making it unsuitable for infant nutrition (Hendriksz and Walter, 2004). Some parents believe that goat's milk is less allergenic than other available milk sources and may feed it to their infant to reduce allergic milk reactions. However, infants allergic to cow's milk have experienced anaphylaxis with their first exposure to goat's milk (Pessler and Nejat, 2004). Raw, unpasteurized milk from any animal source is unacceptable for infant nutrition.

Feeding Schedules

Ideally, feeding schedules should be determined by the infant's hunger. **Demand feedings** involve feeding infants when they signal readiness. **Scheduled feedings** are arranged at predetermined intervals. Some hospital routinely feed infants every 3 to 4 hours. Although this may be satisfactory for bottle-fed infants, it hinders the breastfeeding process. Breastfed infants tend to be hungry every 2 to 3 hours because of the easy digestibility of the milk; therefore they should be fed on demand.

Supplemental feedings should *not* be offered to breast-fed infants before lactation is well established, since they may satiate the infant and may cause nipple preference (see Evidence-Based Practice box, p. 301). Supplemental water is not needed in breast-fed infants, even in hot climates (American Academy of Pediatrics, 2005b). Satiated infants suck less vigorously at the breast, and milk production depends on the breast being emptied at each feeding. If milk is allowed to accumulate in the ducts, causing breast engorgement, ischemia results, suppressing the activity of the acini, or milk-secreting cells. Consequently, milk production is reduced. In addition, the process of sucking from a bottle is different from breast nipple compression. The relatively inflexible rubber nipple prevents the tongue from its usual rhythmic action. Infants learn to put the tongue against the nipple holes to slow down the more rapid flow of fluid. When infants use these same tongue movements during breastfeeding, they may push the human nipple out of the mouth and may not grasp the areola properly.

Usually by 3 weeks of age lactation is well established. Bottle-fed infants retain about 2 to 3 ounces of formula at each feeding and are fed approximately six times a day. The quantity of formula consumed is based on the caloric need of 108 kcal/kg/day; therefore a newborn who weighs 3 kg requires 324 kcal/day. Because commercial formula has 20 kcal/oz, approximately 16 ounces (480 ml) will provide the daily caloric requirement. Breast-fed infants may feed as frequently as 10 to 12 times a day.

Feeding Behavior

Five behavioral stages occur during successful feeding. Recognizing these steps can assist nurses in identifying potential feeding problems caused by improper feeding techniques. **Prefeeding behavior,** such as crying or fussing, demonstrates the infant's level of arousal and degree of hunger. To encourage the infant to grasp the breast properly, it is preferable to begin feeding during the quiet alert state, before the infant becomes upset. **Approach behavior** is indicated by sucking movements or the rooting reflex. **Attachment behavior** includes activities that occur from the time the infant receives the nipple and sucks (sometimes more pronounced during initial attempts at breastfeeding). **Consummatory behavior** consists of coordinated sucking and swallowing. Persistent gagging might indicate unsuccessful consummatory behavior. **Satiety behavior** is observed when infants let the parent know that they are satisfied, usually by falling asleep.

PROMOTE PARENT-INFANT BONDING (ATTACHMENT)

The process of parenting is based on a relationship between parent and infant. As more is learned of the complexity of neonates and of their potential for influencing and shaping their environments, particularly their interaction with significant others, it is apparent that promoting positive parent-child relationships necessitates an understanding of behavioral steps in attachment, variables that enhance or hinder this process, and methods of teaching parents to develop a stronger relationship with their children, especially by recognizing potential problems. (See also Assessment of Attachment Behaviors, p. 215.)

Infant Behavior

Nurses must appreciate the individuality and uniqueness of each infant. According to the individual temperament, the infant will change and shape the environment, which will influence future development. (See Patterns of Sleep and Activity, p. 214.) An infant who sleeps 20 hours a day will be exposed to fewer stimuli than one who sleeps 16 hours a day. In turn, each infant will likely elicit a different response from parents. The infant who is quiet, undemanding, and passive may receive much less attention than one who is responsive, alert, and active. Behavioral characteristics such as irritability and consolability can influence the ease of transition to parenthood and the parents' perception of the infant.

Nurses can positively influence the attachment of parent and child. The first step is recognizing individual differences and explaining to parents that such characteristics are normal. For example, some people believe that infants sleep throughout the day, except for feedings. For some newborns this may be true, but for many it is not. Understanding that the infant's wakefulness is part of a biologic rhythm and not a reflection of inadequate parenting can be crucial in promoting healthy parent-child relationships. Another aspect of helping parents concerns supplying guidelines on how to enhance the infant's development during awake periods. Placing the child in a crib to stare at the same mobile every day is not exciting, but carrying the infant into each room as one does daily chores can be fascinating. A few suggestions can make life more stimulating for the infant and gratifying for the parents (Box 8-6).

Maternal Attachment

Research has suggested that there is a **maternal sensitive period** immediately and for a short time after birth when parents have a unique ability to attach to their infants (Klaus, Kennell, and Klaus, 1995). Mothers demonstrate a predictable and orderly pattern of behavior during the development of the attachment process. When mothers are presented with their nude infants, they begin to examine the infant with their fingertips, concentrating on touching the extremities, and then proceed to massage and encompass the trunk with their entire hands. Assuming the **en face position,** in which the mother's and infant's eyes meet in visual contact in the same vertical plane, is significant in the formation of affectional ties (Fig. 8-16). Although similar patterns of touching have been observed, additional studies demonstrate different patterns for mothers, as well as the same pattern for nonmaternal persons, such as male and female nurses. Consequently, nurses must exercise caution in interpreting behaviors such as touching.

Several studies have attempted to substantiate the long-term benefits of providing parents with opportunities to optimally bond with their infant during the initial postpartum period. Although there has been some evidence that increased parent-child contact encourages prolonged breastfeeding and may minimize the risks of parenting disorders, conclusions

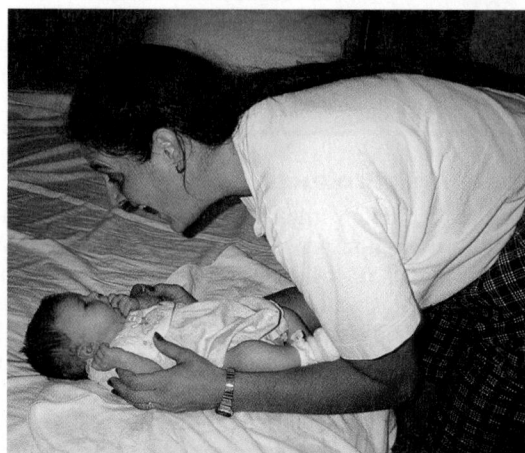

FIG. 8-16 ■ En face position between parent and infant can be significant in attachment process.

BOX 8-6

How to Make the Infant's World More Exciting*

- Infants prefer animated and auditory objects.
- Infants enjoy novelty and quickly tire of seeing same objects; mobiles should be changed frequently.
- Infants prefer to look at medium-intensity colors and contrasting colors, such as black and white.
- Infants like geometric shapes and checkerboards; they prefer patterns over straight lines.
- Contrasting lights and reflective surfaces such as mirrors are especially interesting.
- But most of all, nothing is as fascinating as the human face and voice!

*Objects should be placed about 20 cm (8 inches) away from infant.

about the long-term effects of such early intervention on parenting and child development must be viewed cautiously. In addition, some authorities claim that the emphasis on bonding has been unjustified and may lead to guilt and fear in parents who did not have early contact with their infant. There is concern that the literal interpretation of "sensitive" or "critical" might imply that without early contact, optimum bonding cannot occur or, conversely, that early contact alone is sufficient to ensure competent parenting. Examples of cases where a strong maternal-infant attachment develops in less than ideal situations include adoption and the birth of a child with a congenital defect (Billings, 1995).

The nurse should stress to parents that, although early bonding is valuable, it does not represent an "all or none" phenomenon. Throughout the child's life there will be multiple opportunities for development of parent-child attachment. Bonding is a complex process that develops gradually and is influenced by numerous factors, only one of which is the type of initial contact between the newborn and parent.

In a concept analysis of parent-infant attachment, Goulet, Bell, St-Cyr, and others (1998) describe attributes of parent-infant attachment as **proximity, reciprocity,** and **commitment.** Within these attributes are further dimensions, which include contact, emotional state, individualization, complementarity, sensitivity, centrality, and parent role exploration. The researchers describe the parent-infant attachment process as one that is complex and therefore cannot be evaluated simply by the observations of attitudes and behaviors of parents toward their infants (Goulet, Bell, St-Cyr, and others, 1998). Further research into the reciprocal relationships between infant and parent and the situational factors that influence such relationships are recommended.

One component of successful maternal attachment is the concept of **reciprocity** (Brazelton, 1974). As the mother responds to the infant, the infant must respond to the mother by some signal, such as sucking, cooing, eye contact, grasping, or molding (conforming to other's body during close physical contact). The first step is **initiation,** in which interaction between infant and parent begins. Next is **orientation,** which establishes the partners' expectations of each other during the interaction. Following orientation is **acceleration** of the attention cycle to a peak of excitement. The infant reaches out and coos, both arms jerk forward, the head moves backward, the eyes dilate, and the face brightens. After a short time, **deceleration** of the excitement and **turning away** occur, in which the infant's eyes shift away from the parent's and the child grasps his or her shirt. During this cycle of nonattention, repeated verbal or visual attempts to reinitiate the infant's attention are ineffective. This deceleration and turning away probably prevents the infant from being overwhelmed by excessive stimuli. In a good interaction both partners have synchronized their attention-nonattention cycles. Parents or other caregivers who do not allow the infant to turn away and who continually attempt to maintain visual contact encourage the infant to turn off the attention cycle and thus prolong the nonattention phase.

Although this description of reciprocal interacting behavior is usually observed in the infant by 2 to 3 weeks of age, nurses can use this information to teach parents how to interact with their infant. Recognizing the attention vs nonattention cycles and understanding that the latter is not a rejection of the parent helps parents develop competence in parenting.

Paternal Engrossment

Fathers also show specific attachment behaviors to the newborn. This process of **paternal engrossment,** forming a sense of absorption, preoccupation, and interest in the infant, includes (1) visual awareness of the newborn, especially focusing on the beauty of the child; (2) tactile awareness, often expressed in a desire to hold the infant; (3) awareness of distinct characteristics with emphasis on those features of the infant that resemble the father; (4) perception of the infant as perfect; (5) development of a strong feeling of attraction to the child that leads to intense focusing of attention on the infant; (6) experiencing a feeling of extreme elation; and (7) feeling a sense of deep self-esteem and satisfaction. These responses are greatest during the early contacts with the infant and are intensified by the neonate's normal reflex activity, especially the grasp reflex and visual alertness. In addition to behavioral reactions, fathers also demonstrate physiologic responses such as increased heart rate and BP during interactions with their newborns.

The process of engrossment has significant implications for nurses. It is imperative to recognize the importance of early father-infant contact in releasing these behaviors. Fathers need to be encouraged to express their positive feelings, especially if such emotions are contrary to any popular belief that fathers should remain stoic. If this is not clarified, fathers may feel confused and attempt to suppress the natural sensations of absorption, preoccupation, and interest in order to conform with societal expectations.

Mothers also need to be aware of the responses of the father toward the newborn, especially because one of the consequences of paternal preoccupation with the infant is less overt attention toward the mother. If both parents are able to share their feelings, each can appreciate the process of attachment toward their child and will avoid the unfortunate conflict of being insensitive and unaware of the other's needs. In addition, a father who is encouraged to form a relationship with his newborn is less likely to feel excluded and abandoned after the family returns home and the mother directs her attention toward caring for the infant.

Ideally, the process of engrossment should be discussed with parents before the delivery, such as in prenatal classes, to reinforce the father's awareness of his natural feelings toward the expected child. Focusing on the future experience of seeing, touching, and holding one's newborn may also help expectant fathers become more comfortable in accepting their paternal feelings. This in turn can assist them in being more supportive toward the mother, especially as the labor and delivery draw near.

At the infant's birth, the nurse can play a vital role in helping the father express engrossment by assessing the neonate in front of the couple; pointing out normal characteristics; encouraging identification through consistent referral to the child by name; encouraging the father to cuddle, hold, talk to, or feed the infant; and demonstrating whenever necessary the soothing powers of caressing, stroking, and rocking the child (Fig. 8-17). Fathers are encouraged to be with the mother during labor and delivery, to spend time alone with the mother and newborn after delivery, and to room-in with the mother and infant. Many birthing centers have adopted a family-centered focus, including sleeping accommodations that more closely resemble the home environment for the new mother and father.

FIG. 8-17 ■ A desire to hold the infant and participate in caregiving activities is an indication of paternal engrossment.

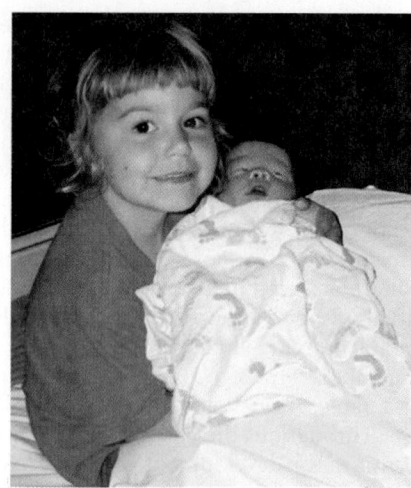

FIG. 8-18 ■ Sibling visitation shortly after birth can facilitate the attachment process.

Fathers, like mothers, may demonstrate attachment not only after the infant's birth but during fetal life as well. Paternal attachment may proceed at a different pace than maternal attachment. Paternal preoccupation with events of labor and delivery and the spouse's health may detract from paternal attachment (Anderson, 1996). Research has noted that, although fathers spend similar amounts of time in interaction with their newborns as do mothers, the nature of their interaction is different. Mothers and infants focus on face-to-face exchange and mutual gazing, co-vocalization, and affectionate touch. Fathers' time with their infants includes quick peaks of high positive emotionality, including joint laughter and open exuberance. Interactions with fathers tend to center on physical games or games with an object focus, rather than on face-to-face signals (Feldman, 2007).

The nurse observes for the same indications of affection from the father as those expected in the mother, such as making visual contact in the en face position and embracing the infant close to the body. When present, such behaviors are reinforced. If such responses are not obvious, the nurse needs to assess the father's feelings regarding this birth, cultural beliefs that may affect his expression of emotions, and other factors that influence his perception of the infant and the mother in order to facilitate a positive attachment during this critical period.

Siblings

Although the attachment process has been discussed almost exclusively in terms of the parents and infants, it is essential that nurses be aware of other family members, such as siblings and members of the extended family, who need preparation for the acceptance of this new child. Young children in particular need sensitive preparation for the birth to minimize sibling jealousy.

In support of **family-centered care,** there is an increasing trend to allow siblings to visit the mother on the postpartum unit and to hold the newborn (Fig. 8-18). Another trend has been the presence of siblings at childbirth. Unlike sibling visitation, the evidence supporting this practice has been controversial, yet the nature of truly providing family-centered care encompasses siblings, grandparents, and other significant persons who comprise the extended family unit (Tomlinson, Bryan, and Esau, 1996). The American Academy of Pediatrics and American College of Obstetricians and Gynecologists (2007) support the presence of siblings at childbirth and visitation of the newborn and mother; basic guidelines for infection control and adult supervision are also recommended.

Children exhibit different degrees of involvement in the birth process. Some reported benefits include children's increased knowledge of the birth process, less regressive behavior after the birth, and more mothering and caregiving behavior toward the infant. Some practitioners add facilitated family bonding and assimilation of the newborn into the family as positive outcomes. Parents whose children attended the birth have echoed these same benefits and have expressed their desire to repeat the experience should another pregnancy occur. Despite these positive findings, opponents believe that allowing children to observe a delivery could lead to emotional difficulties, although there is no research to support this contention. As research mounts, birthing centers that allow siblings at the birth are developing more definitive guidelines, such as an age requirement of at least 4 to 5 years, the presence of a supportive person for the sibling only, and an adequate sequence of preparation in which parents explore all options for preparing their other children.

From observations during sibling visitation, there is evidence that sibling attachment occurs. However, the en face position is assumed much less often among the newborn and siblings than between mother and newborn, and when this position is used, it is brief. Siblings focus more on the head or face than on touching or talking to the infant. The siblings' verbalizations are focused less on attracting the infant's attention and more on addressing the mother about the newborn. Children who have established a prenatal relationship with the fetus have demonstrated more attachment behaviors, supporting the suggestion of encouraging prenatal acquaintance. Additional research is needed to establish theories on sibling bonding as have been constructed for parental bonding.

Multiple Births and Subsequent Children

A component of attachment that has special meaning for families with multiple births, **monotropy** refers to the principle that a person can become optimally attached to only one individual at a time. If a parent can form only one attachment at a time, how can all the siblings of a multiple birth receive optimum emotional care? Research on bonding and multiple births is still lacking despite the recent increase in multiple births, and even less is known about paternal engrossment and sibling attachment. In regard to maternal-twin bonding, the conclusions of different authors vary. Some report that mothers bond equally to each twin at the time of birth, even if one twin is ill. Others suggest that mothers of twins may take months or years to form individual attachments to each child, or even longer if the twins are identical.

Nurses can be instrumental in promoting bonding of multiple births. The most important principle is to assist the parents in recognizing the individuality of the children, especially in monozygotic (identical) twins. The mother should visit with each newborn, including a sick infant, as much as possible after birth. Rooming-in and breastfeeding are encouraged. Any characteristics that are unique to each child are emphasized, and each infant is called by name, rather than referring to "the twins." Asking the family questions such as "How do you tell Sally and Amy apart?" and "In what ways are Sally and Amy different and similar?" helps point out their individual characteristics. Behaviors on the BNBAS can be used to illustrate these differences and to stress effective strategies for dealing with multiple personalities at the same time. Cobedding (bed sharing) of twins or other multiples may also be encouraged in the hospital and home, with the goal of maintaining the bond between siblings that was formed in utero (Fig. 8-19). Much research is focused on exploring the safety and benefits of the practice of cobedding (Hayward, Campbell-Yeo, Price, and others, 2007) (see also Sudden Infant Death Syndrome, Chapter 11); however, the cobedding of infant siblings differs from forms of cobedding that involve older siblings or adults. Other strategies for promoting individualism are discussed under Multiple Births in Chapter 3.

Another area of attachment that has received minimal attention is maternal bonding of multiparous mothers. Research suggests that there are several additional tasks to "taking on" a second child. These include:

- Promoting acceptance and approval of the second child
- Grieving and resolving the loss of an exclusive dyadic relationship with the first child
- Planning and coordinating family life to include a second child
- Reformulating a relationship with the first child
- Identifying with the second child by comparing this child with the first child in terms of physical and psychologic characteristics
- Assessing one's affective capabilities in providing sufficient emotional support and nurturance simultaneously to two children

Employed mothers who have a second child report fewer concerns than with the first child regarding general aspects of separation from their child and the effect of separation on the child, but they have similar concerns regarding separation due to employment. It appears that, although experience may decrease some concerns, it may not minimize others.

FIG. 8-19 ■ Newborn twins are placed in same bed during newborn transition period.

PREPARE FOR DISCHARGE AND HOME CARE

With short postpartum hospital stay, as well as a trend toward **mother-infant care,** also called **dyad** or **couplet care,** discharge planning, referral, and home visits have become increasingly important components of comprehensive newborn care. First-time, as well as experienced, parents benefit from guidance and assistance with the infant's care, such as breastfeeding or bottle feeding, and with the family's integration of a new member, particularly sibling adjustment.

To assess and meet these needs, teaching must begin early, ideally *before the birth.* Not only is the postpartum stay sometimes very short (12 to 24 hours), but also mothers are in the **taking-in phase,** where they demonstrate passive and dependent behaviors. On the first postpartum day, as a result of fatigue and excitement, mothers may not be able to absorb large amounts of information. This time may need to be spent highlighting essential aspects of care, such as infant safety and feeding. Parents may also be given a list of mother and infant care topics as part of the nursing admission history to choose issues they wish to review. Teaching before discharge should focus on newborn feeding patterns, monitoring diapers for voiding and stooling, jaundice, and infant crying.

The American Academy of Pediatrics (2004a) has established guidelines for postpartum discharge before 48 hours of age (see Family-Centered Care box). The Academy emphasizes that the primary care physician rather than an insurance company should make the determination of appropriate discharge time.

Despite concerns expressed regarding early discharge and newborn rehospitalizations for dehydration, jaundice, breastfeeding failure, and other issues, studies in various parts of the United States and Canada continue to be reassuring. They show that rehospitalizations, emergency department visits, and infant morbidities have not significantly increased since early postpartum discharge was implemented (Gries, Phyall, and Barfield, 2000; Danielsen, Castles, Damberg, and others, 2000; Martens, Derksen, and Gupta, 2004). The American Academy of Pediatrics (2004a) recommends that newborns discharged early receive follow-up care within 48 hours either in the primary practitioner's office or in the home.

Although many mothers and newborns may be safely discharged within 12 to 24 hours without detriment to their health, others require a longer stay. Follow-up home care within days (or even hours after discharge when minor problems are anticipated) appears to be the emerging trend in an

FAMILY-CENTERED CARE

Early Newborn Discharge Criteria

■ It was a singleton birth between 38 and 42 weeks of gestation.
■ Baby was delivered by uncomplicated vaginal delivery.
■ Birth weight is appropriate for gestational age.
■ Physical examination was normal.
■ Vital signs are normal and stable as measured in an open crib with adequate clothing.
■ Infant has urinated and passed at least one stool.
■ Infant has completed at least two successful feedings.
■ Clinical significance of jaundice, if present, has been determined and appropriate management or follow-up plans put in place.
■ Appropriate maternal and infant blood tests have been performed.
■ Appropriate neonatal immunizations have been administered.
■ Newborn hearing screening has been completed per hospital protocol and state regulations.
■ Family, environmental, and social risk factors have been assessed.
■ Documentation is in place that mother has received usual infant care training and has demonstrated competency.
■ Support persons are available to assist mother and her infant after discharge.
■ Continuing medical care is planned, including that infants discharged sooner than 48 hours be examined within 48 hours of discharge from hospital.

Data from American Academy of Pediatrics, Committee on Fetus and Newborn: Hospital stay for healthy terms newborns, *Pediatrics* 113(5):1434-1436, 2004.

COMMUNITY FOCUS

Early Newborn Discharge Checklist

Feeding—Adequate latch-on demonstrated for breastfeeding newborn; successfully feeding 2 to 3 ounces of formula every 3 to 4 hours with minimum spitting up and no vomiting; wet diapers indicating adequate hydration and intake
Elimination—Voiding every 4 to 6 hours or more often; one stool passed in first 24 to 28 hours
Circumcision—Evidence of voiding; nonbleeding circumcision (does not require pressure); no excess edema at site
Color—Pink centrally and buccal mucosa moist; no evidence of jaundice in first 24 hours
Cord—No signs or symptoms of infection; if used, drying agent applied per institution protocol (see Care of the Umbilicus, p. 225)
Newborn screening—Completed phenylketonuria and other screenings per state law
Vital signs—Stable heart rate, respiratory rate, and temperature for at least 8 to 12 hours; no apnea
Activity—Wakeful periods before feedings; moves all extremities
Home visit or primary practitioner visit—Follow-up appointment within 48 hours after discharge

COMMUNITY FOCUS

Newborn Home Care After Early Discharge*

Wet diapers—Six to 10 per day
Breastfeeding—Successful latch-on and feeding every 1.5 to 3 hours daily; audible swallowing
Formula feeding—Successfully taking at least 1 to 2 ounces every 3 to 4 hours; voiding as above
Circumcision—Wash with warm water only; yellow exudate forming, with no bleeding; Plastibell intact for 48 hours
Stools—At least one every 48 to 72 hours (bottle feeding), or two or three per day (breastfeeding)
Color—Pink to ruddy when crying; pink centrally when at rest or asleep
Activity—Has four or five wakeful periods per day and alerts to environmental sounds and voices
Jaundice—Physiologic jaundice (i.e., jaundice not appearing in the first 24 hours); feeding, voiding, and stooling as noted above or practitioner notification for suspicion of pathologic jaundice (appears within 24 hours of birth; hemolysis and ABO/Rh problem suspected), decreased activity, poor feeding, or dark orange skin color persisting on the fifth day in light-skinned newborn; obtain transcutaneous bilirubin before discharge and identify risk with an hour-specific nomogram (see Hyperbilirubinemia, Chapter 9)
Cord—Kept above diaper line; drying, no drainage; periumbilical area nonerythematous
Vital signs—Heart rate 120 to 140 beats/min at rest; respiratory rate 30 to 55 breaths/min at rest without evidence of sternal retractions, grunting, or nasal flaring; temperature 36.3° to 37° C (97.3° to 98.6° F) axillary
Position of sleep—Back

*Any deviation from the above or suspicion of poor newborn adaptation should be reported to the practitioner at once.

family unit. The ultimate safety and success of early newborn discharge from hospital are contingent on using clear discharge criteria and having a high-quality early follow-up program (Radmacher, Massey, and Adamkin, 2002).

With family structures changing, it is essential that nurses identify the primary caregiver, which may not always be the mother but may be a father, grandparent, or baby-sitter. Depending on the family composition, the mother's primary support system in the care of the newborn may not always be the traditional husband or male companion.

Nurses should not assume that terminology associated with mother-infant care is understood. Words relating to the anatomy (e.g., *meconium, labia, edema,* and *genitalia*) and to breastfeeding (e.g., *areola, colostrum,* and *let-down reflex*) may be unfamiliar to mothers. Mothers with other children do not necessarily understand more words, and younger, less educated moms may be at particular risk for not understanding teaching.

An essential area of discharge counseling is the safe transportation of the newborn home from the hospital. Ideally this information should also be provided *before* delivery to allow parents an opportunity to purchase a suitable infant car safety seat. When purchasing a car safety seat, parents should consider cost and convenience. The convertible-type seats are more expensive initially but cost less than two separate systems

effort to curtail hospital costs and provide adequate maternal-newborn care with minimal complications. (See Community Focus boxes.)

Despite the changing spectrum of well-newborn health care, the nurse's role continues to be that of providing ongoing assessments of each mother-newborn dyad to ensure a safe transition to home and a successful adaptation into the (infant-only model and infant-toddler convertible model). Convenience is a major factor, since a cumbersome restraint may be used less often or used improperly. Before buying a car safety seat, it is best to try out different models. For example, some types are too large for subcompact cars. Asking friends about the advantages and disadvantages of their restraints is helpful, but borrowing their car seat or purchasing a used one can be dangerous. Parents should use only a restraint that has directions for use and a certification label stating that it complies with federal motor vehicle safety standards (both should be on the seat). They should not use a restraint that has been involved in a crash. Some service clubs and hospitals have loan programs for restraints. Information about approved models and other aspects of car safety seat restraints is available from several organizations and sources.*

Parents are cautioned against placing an infant in the front seat of a car with a passenger-side air bag. Infants weighing less than 9 kg (20 pounds) or younger than 1 year should always be placed in a rear-facing child safety seat in the back seat of the car (American Academy of Pediatrics, 2002).

NURSING ALERT

In a car seat, padding is never placed underneath or behind the infant because it creates slackness in the harness, leading to the possibility of the child's ejection from the seat in the event of a crash. In vehicles with front passenger-side air bags, the rear-facing safety seat must be placed in the back seat to avoid injury to the infant from the released air bag forcing the safety seat against the vehicle seat or passenger door.

Although federal safety standards do not specify the *minimum* weight of an infant and the appropriate type of restraint, newborns weighing 2 kg (4.4 pounds) receive relatively good support in convertible seats with a seat back–to-crotch strap height of 14 cm (5.7 inches) or less. Rolled blankets or towels may be needed between the crotch and legs to prevent slouching and can be placed along the sides to minimize lateral movements. Placing the infant in a safety seat at a 45-degree angle will prevent slumping and airway obstruction (American Academy of Pediatrics, 2002). Seats with shields (large padded surfaces in front of the child) and armrests (found on some other models) are unacceptable because of their proximity to the infant's face and neck. (For a discussion of appropriate car restraints for preterm infants, see p. 268, and for infants, see Motor Vehicle Injuries in Chapters 10 and 12.)

In the United States and Canada all states and provinces have mandated the use of child restraints. Therefore hospitals and birthing centers should have policies regarding the safe discharge of a newborn in a car safety seat and provisions for parents to learn to use the device correctly. In addition, hospital personnel should ensure that infants born before 37 weeks of gestation have a period of observation in the selected car seat to monitor for possible apnea, bradycardia, and oxygen desaturation (American Academy of Pediatrics, 2002). Parents are more likely to use a restraint correctly and consistently if the proper use of one is demonstrated and its necessity is stressed. Infants and children continue to be hurt and killed because car seat restraints are not installed properly.

KEY POINTS

- Transition from fetal or placental circulation to independent respiration is the most important physiologic change required of the newborn.
- Chemical and thermal factors help initiate the neonate's first respiration.
- Circulatory changes in the neonate result from shifts in pressure in the heart and major vessels and from functional closures of the fetal shunts.
- The newborn's large surface area, thin layer of subcutaneous fat, and unique mechanism for producing heat predispose the newborn to excessive heat loss.
- The infant's high rate of metabolism is closely correlated with the rate of fluid exchange, which is seven times greater in the infant than in the adult.
- The skin and mucous membranes, the macrophage system, and antibodies are the first, second, and third lines, respectively, of defense against infection.
- The Apgar score, the initial assessment of the newborn, focuses on heart rate, respiratory effort, muscle tone, reflex irritability, and color.
- Physical assessment of the newborn includes clinical assessment of gestational age, general measurements, general appearance, head-to-toe assessment, and parent-infant attachment or bonding.
- Neurologic assessment focuses on localized reflexes and posture, muscle tone, head control, and movement and is best accomplished during the general physical examination.
- Behavioral assessment of newborns with the BNBAS examines responses to seven categories: habituation, orientation, motor performance, range of state, regulation of state, autonomic stability, and reflexes.
- Physical care for the newborn includes maintaining a patent airway, maintaining a stable body temperature, protecting from infection and injury, and providing optimal nutrition.
- Although the attachment, or bonding, process primarily affects infants and parents, siblings also play an important role.
- An essential aspect of discharge teaching is ensuring the newborn's safe transportation home in a federally approved, backward-facing car safety seat.

---

*American Academy of Pediatrics, 141 Northwest Point Blvd., Elk Grove Village, IL 60007; (847) 434-4000; http://www.aap.org; and local division of traffic safety or National Highway Traffic Safety Administration Auto Safety Hotline, (888) 327-4236. For children with special needs, contact the Easter Seals, (800) 221-6827, and ask about Special KARS (Kids Are Riding Safe).

REFERENCES

Abubakar I, Iliyasu Z, Kabir M, and others: Knowledge, attitude and practice of female genital cutting among antenatal patients in Aminu Kano Teaching Hospital, *Nigerian J Med* 13(3):254-258, 2004.

Alexander GR, Himes JH, Kaufman RB, and others: A United States national reference for fetal growth, *Obstet Gynecol* 87(2):163-168, 1996.

American Academy of Pediatrics, Committee on Infectious Diseases: Recommended immunization schedules for children and adolescents—United States, 2007, *Pediatrics* 119(1):207-208, 2007.

American Academy of Pediatrics: *Neonatal resuscitation textbook*, ed 5, Dallas, 2006a, American Heart Association.

American Academy of Pediatrics, Committee on Infectious Diseases: *Red book: 2006 report of the Committee on Infectious Diseases*, ed 27, Elk Grove Village, Ill, 2006b, The Academy.

American Academy of Pediatrics: AAP publications retired and reaffirmed, *Pediatrics* 116(3):796, 2005a.

American Academy of Pediatrics, Section on Breastfeeding: Breastfeeding and the use of human milk (policy statement), *Pediatrics* 115(2):496-506, 2005b.

American Academy of Pediatrics, Committee on Fetus and Newborn: Hospital stay for healthy term newborns, *Pediatrics* 113(5):1434-1436, 2004a.

American Academy of Pediatrics, Committee on Nutrition: *Pediatric nutrition handbook*, ed 5, Elk Grove Village, Ill, 2004b, The Academy.

American Academy of Pediatrics: Controversies concerning vitamin K and the newborn (policy statement), *Pediatrics* 112(1):191-192, 2003a.

American Academy of Pediatrics: Hearing assessments in infants and children: recommendations beyond neonatal screening, *Pediatrics* 111(2):436-440, 2003b.

American Academy of Pediatrics: Prevention and management of positional skull deformities in infants (clinical report), *Pediatrics* 112(1):199-202, 2003c.

American Academy of Pediatrics: Prevention of rickets and vitamin D deficiency: new guidelines for vitamin D intake (clinical report), *Pediatrics* 111(4):908-910, 2003d.

American Academy of Pediatrics, Committee on Injury and Poison Prevention: Selecting and using the most appropriate car safety seats for growing children: guidelines for counseling parents, *Pediatrics* 109(3):550-553, 2002.

American Academy of Pediatrics, Committee on Environmental Health: Mercury in the environment: implications for pediatricians (technical report), *Pediatrics* 108(1):197-205, 2001.

American Academy of Pediatrics, Task Force on Infant Sleep Position and Sudden Infant Death Syndrome: Changing concepts of sudden infant death syndrome: implications for infant sleeping environment and sleep position, *Pediatrics* 105(3):650-656, 2000a.

American Academy of Pediatrics: Serving the family from birth to the medical home: newborn screening: a blueprint for the future, *Pediatrics* 106(2 pt 2 Suppl):389-427, 2000b.

American Academy of Pediatrics, Joint Committee on Infant Hearing: Year 2000 Position Statement: principle and guidelines for early hearing detection and intervention, *Pediatrics* 106(4):798-824, 2000c.

American Academy of Pediatrics, Task Force on Circumcision: Circumcision policy statement, *Pediatrics* 103(3):686-693, 1999.

American Academy of Pediatrics, Committee on Bioethics: Female genital mutilation, *Pediatrics* 102(1):153-156, 1998.

American Academy of Pediatrics, Committee on Fetus and Newborn, and American College of Obstetricians and Gynecologists, Committee on Obstetric Practice: The Apgar score, *Pediatrics* 117(4):1444-1447, 2006.

American Academy of Pediatrics and American College of Obstetricians and Gynecologists: *Guidelines for perinatal care*, ed 6, Elk Grove Village, Ill, 2007, The Academy.

Anderson AM: The father-infant relationship: becoming connected, *J Soc Pediatr Nurs* 1(2):83-92, 1996.

Anderson JW, Johnstone BM, Remley DT: Breastfeeding and cognitive development: a meta-analysis, *Am J Clin Nutr* 70(4):525-535, 1999.

Arbuckle T, Wilkins R, Sherman G: Birth weight percentiles by gestational age in Canada, *Obstet Gynecol* 81(1):39-48, 1993.

Arora S, McJunkin C, Wehrer J, and others: Major factors influencing breastfeeding rates: mother's perception of father's attitude and milk supply, *Pediatrics* 106(5):e67, 2000.

Association of Women's Health, Obstetric and Neonatal Nursing: *Evidence-based clinical practice guideline: neonatal skin care*, Washington, DC, 2007, The Association.

Bachrach VR, Schwarz E, Bachrach LR: Breastfeeding and the risk of hospitalization for respiratory disease in infancy, *Arch Pediatr Adolesc Med* 157(3):237-243, 2003.

Bailey J, Rose P: Axillary and tympanic temperature recording in the preterm neonate: a comparative study, *J Adv Nurs* 34(4):465-474, 2001.

Ballard JL, Auer CE, Khoury JC: Ankyloglossia: assessment, incidence, and effect of frenuloplasty on the breastfeeding dyad, *Pediatrics* 110(5):e63, 1001, 2002.

Ballard JL, Khoury JC, Wedig K, and others: New Ballard Score, expanded to include extremely premature infants, *J Pediatr* 119(3):417-423, 1991.

Barclay L: Frenuloplasty corrects ankyloglossia disrupting breastfeeding, *Pediatrics* 110:63, 2002.

Behring A, Vezeau TM, Fink R: Timing of the newborn first bath: a replication, *Neonat Netw* 22(1):39-46, 2003.

Biancuzzo M: *Breastfeeding the newborn: clinical strategies for nurses*, ed 2, St Louis, 2003, Mosby.

Billings JR: Bonding theory—tying mothers in knots? A critical review of the application of a theory to nursing, *J Clin Nurs* 4(4):207-211, 1995.

Blackburn ST: *Maternal, fetal, and neonatal physiology: a clinical perspective*, St Louis, 2003, Saunders.

Blain-Lewis N: Comparative studies of bruising and healing after heelstick, *Neonat Intensive Care* 5(5):18-21, 1992.

Blass EM, Watt LB: Suckling- and sucrose-induced analgesia in human newborns, *Pain* 83(3):611-623, 1999.

Bliss-Holtz J: Methods of newborn infant temperature monitoring: a research review, *Issues Compr Pediatr Nurs* 18(4):287-298, 1993.

Brady-Fryer B, Wiebe N, Lander JA: Pain relief for neonatal circumcision, *Cochrane Database Syst Rev* 18(4):CD004217, 2007.

Brazelton TB: Mother-infant reciprocity. In Klaus M, Leger T, Trause MA, editors: *Maternal attachment and mothering disorders*, New Brunswick, NJ, 1974, Johnson & Johnson Baby Products.

Brazelton TB, Nugent JK: *Neonatal behavioural assessment scale*, London, 1996, MacKeith Press.

Brown R: Can bottle-feeding really mimic breastfeeding? *J Hum Lactation* 23(1):118-119, 2007.

Bryant KG, Horns KM, Longo N, and others: A primer on newborn screening, *Adv Neonat Care* 4(5):306-317, 2004.

Butt ML, Kisilevsky BS: Music modulates behaviour of premature infants following heel lance, *Can J Nurs Res* 31(4):17-39, 2000.

Canadian Paediatric Society, Community Paediatrics Committee: *Temperature measurement in paediatrics*, 2007, retrieved May 22, 2007, from http://www.cps.ca/english/statements/cp/cp00-01.htm.

Carbajal R, Veerapen S, Couderc S, and others: Analgesic effect of breast feeding in term neonates: randomized controlled trial, *BMJ* 326 (7379):13, 2003.

Carroll V: Infant abduction: lowering the risk, *AWHONN Lifelines* 3(6):25-27, 2000.

Chen A, Rogan W: Isoflavones in soy infant formula: a review of evidence for endocrine and other activity in infants, *Ann Rev Nutr* 24:33-54, 2004.

Chia F, Ang AT, Wong TW, and others: Reliability of the Dinamap noninvasive monitor in the measurement of blood pressure of ill Asian newborns, *Clin Pediatr* 29(5):262-267, 1990.

Cohen HA, Drucker MM, Vainer S, and others: Postcircumcision urinary tract infection, *Clin Pediatr* 31(6):322-324, 1992.

Conner GK: Abdominal assessment. In Tappero EP, Honeyfield ME: *Physical assessment of the newborn: a comprehensive approach to the art of physical examination*, ed 3, Petaluma, Calif, 2003, NICU Ink.

Conover E, Buehler BA: Use of herbal agents by breastfeeding women may affect infants, *Pediatr Ann* 33(4):235-240, 2004.

Coryllos A, Genna C, Salloum A: Congenital tongue-tie and its impact on breastfeeding. In American Academy of Pediatrics, Section on Breastfeeding: *Breastfeeding: best for baby and mother*, Elk Grove Village, Ill, 2004, The Academy.

Craig JV, Lancaster GA, Taylor S, and others: Infrared ear thermometry compared with rectal thermometry in children: a systematic review, *Lancet* 360(9333):603-609, 2002.

Danielson B, Castles AG, Damberg CL, and others: Newborn discharge timing and readmissions: California, 1992-1995, *Pediatrics* 106(1):31-39, 2000.

Darmstadt GL, Dinulos JG: Neonatal skin care, *Pediatr Clin North Am* 47(4):757-782, 2000.

Dore S, Buchan D, Coulas S, and others: Alcohol versus natural drying for newborn cord care, *J Obstet Gynecol Neonat Nurs* 27(6):621-627, 1998.

Eriksson M, Finnstrom O: Can daily repeated doses of orally administered glucose induce tolerance when given for neonatal pain relief? *Acta Paediatr* 93(2):246-249, 2004.

Fein SB, Falci CD: Infant formula preparation, handling, and related practices in the United States, *J Am Diet Assoc* 99(10):1234-1239, 1999.

Feldman R: Parent-infant synchrony and the construction of shared timing: physiological precursors, developmental outcomes, and risk conditions, *J Child Psychol Psychiatry* 48(3):329-354, 2007.

Female genital mutilation, *AAP News* 10(2):3, 1994.

Fitzgerald M, Millard C, McIntosh N: Cutaneous hypersensitivity following peripheral tissue damage in newborn infants and its reversal with topical anaesthesia, *Pain* 39:31-36, 1989.

Fuloria M, Kreiter S: The newborn examination, part I, Emergencies and common abnormalities involving the skin, head, neck, chest, and respiratory and cardiovascular systems, *Am Fam Physician* 65(1):61-68, 2002.

Georgieff MK: Taking a rational approach to the choice of formula, *Contemp Pediatr* 18(8):112-130, 2001.

Giampietro PG, Bruno G, Furcolo G, and others: Soy protein formulas in children: no hormonal effects in long-term feeding, *J Pediatr Endocrinol Metab* 17(2):191-196, 2004.

Gibbins S, Stevens B, Hodnett E, and others: Efficacy and safety of sucrose for procedural pain relief in preterm and term neonates, *Nurs Res* 51(6):375-382, 2002.

Golombek SG, Brill PE, Salice AL: Randomized trial of alcohol versus triple dye for umbilical cord care, *Clin Pediatr* 41(6):419-423, 2002.

Goulet C, Bell L, St-Cyr D, and others: A concept analysis of parent-infant attachment, *J Adv Nurs* 28(5):1071-1081, 1998.

Gradin M, Eriksson M, Holmqvist G, and others: Pain reduction at venipuncture in newborns: oral glucose compared with local anesthetic cream, *Pediatrics* 110(6):1053-1057, 2002.

Gray L, Miller LW, Phillips BL, and others: Breastfeeding is analgesic in healthy newborns, *Pediatrics* 109(4):590-593, 2002.

Gray L, Watt L, Blass EM: Skin-to-skin contact is analgesic in healthy newborns, *Pediatrics* 105(1):110-111, 2000; retrieved July 20, 2007, from http://www.pediatrics.org/cgi/content/full/105/1/e14.

Greenes DS, Fleisher GR: Accuracy of a noninvasive temporal artery thermometer for use in infants, *Arch Pediatr Adolesc Med* 155(3):376-381, 2001.

Greim HA: The endocrine and reproductive system: adverse effects of hormonally active substances? *Pediatrics* 113(4):1070-1075, 2004.

Gries DM, Phyall G, Barfield WD: Evaluation of early discharge program for infants after childbirth in a military population, *Mil Med* 165(8):616-621, 2000.

Grunau RE, Linhares MB, Holsti L, and others: Does prone or supine position influence pain responses in preterm infants at 32 weeks gestational age? *Clin J Pain* 20(2):76-82, 2004.

Gupta A, Della-Latta P, Todd B, and others: Outbreak of extended-spectrum beta-lactamase-producing *Klebsiella pneumoniae* in a neonatal intensive care unit linked to artificial nails, *Infect Control Hosp Epidemiol* 25(3):210-215, 2004.

Hale T: *Medications and mothers' milk,* Amarillo, Tex, 2006, Pharmasoft.

Hanson LA, Korotkova M: The role of breastfeeding in prevention of neonatal infection, *Semin Neonatol* 7(4):275-281, 2002.

Haouari N, Wood C, Griffith G, and others: The analgesic effect of sucrose in full-term infants: a randomised controlled trial, *BMJ* 310(6993):1498-1500, 1995.

Harrison D, Johnston L, Loughnan P: Oral sucrose for procedural pain in sick hospitalized infants: a randomized-controlled trial, *J Paediatr Child Health* 39(8):591-597, 2003.

Hayward K, Campbell-Yeo M, Price S, and others: Co-bedding twins: how pilot study findings guided improvements in planning a larger multicenter trial, *Nurs Res* 56(2):137-143, 2007.

Hendriksz CJ, Walter JH: Feeding infants with undiluted goat's milk can mimic tyrosinaemia type 1, *Acta Paediatr* 93(4):552-553, 2004.

Hicks MA: A comparison of the tympanic and axillary temperatures of the preterm and term infant, *J Perinatol* 16(4):261-267, 1996.

Host A, Halken S: Hypoallergenic formulas—when, to whom and how long: after more than 15 years we know the right indication! *Allergy* 59(Suppl 78):45-52, 2004.

Huang CM, Tung WS, Kuo LL, and others: Comparison of pain responses of premature infants to the heelstick between containment and swaddling, *J Nurs Res* 12(1):31-40, 2004.

Janssen PA, Selwood BL, Dobson SR, and others: To dye or not to dye: a randomized, clinical trial of a triple dye/alcohol regime versus dry cord care, *Pediatrics* 111(1):15-20, 2003.

Johnston CC, Stevens B, Pinelli J, and others: Kangaroo care is effective in diminishing pain response in preterm neonates, *Arch Pediatr Adolesc Med* 157(11):1084-1088, 2003.

Jones HL, Kleber CB, Eckert GJ, and others: Comparison of rectal temperature measured by digital vs. mercury glass thermometer in infants under 2 months old, *Clin Pediatr* 42(4):357-359, 2003.

Kaye CI, and American Association of Pediatrics Committee on Genetics: Newborn screening fact sheets, *Pediatrics* 118(3):e934-e963, 2006.

Kimura C, Matsuoka M: Changes in breast skin temperature during the course of breastfeeding, *J Hum Lact* 23(1):60-69, 2007.

Klaus MH, Kennell JH, Klaus PH: *Bonding: building the foundations of secure attachment and independence,* Menlo Park, Calif, 1995, Addison-Wesley.

Kraft NL: A pictorial and video guide to circumcision without pain, *Adv Neonatal Care* 3(2):50-64, 2003.

Kramer MS, Platt RW, Wen SW, and others: A new and improved population-based Canadian reference for birth weight for gestational age, *Pediatrics* 108(2):e35, 462, 2001.

Kue Young T, Chateau D, Zhang M: Type 2 diabetes mellitus in children: prenatal and early infancy risk factors among native Canadians, *Arch Pediatr Adolesc Med* 156(7):651-655, 2002.

Kyenkya-Isabirye M: UNICEF launches the Baby-Friendly Hospital Initiative, *MCN* 17(4):177-179, 1992.

Lanham DM, Walker B, Klocke E, and others: Accuracy of tympanic temperature readings in children under 6 years of age, *Pediatr Nurs* 25(1):39-42, 1999.

Lawrence RA, Lawrence RM: *Breastfeeding: a guide for the medical profession,* ed 6, St Louis, 2005, Mosby.

Lehr VT, Cepeda E, Frattarelli DA, and others: Lidocaine 4% cream compared with lidocaine 2.5% and prilocaine 2.5% or dorsal penile block for circumcision, *Am J Perinatol* 22(5):231-237, 2005.

Leick-Rude MK, Bloom LF: A comparison of temperature-taking methods in neonates, *Neonat Netw* 17(5):21-37, 1998.

Malloy MH: Trends in postneonatal aspiration deaths and reclassification of sudden infant death syndrome: impact of the "Back to Sleep" program, *Pediatrics* 109(4):661-665, 2002.

Marín Gabriel MA, Martín Moreiras J, Lliteras Fleixas G, and others: Assessment of the new Ballard score to estimate gestational age, *An Pediatr (Barc.)* 64(2):140-145, 2006.

Martens PJ, Derksen S, Gupta S: Predictors of hospital readmission of Manitoba newborns within 6 weeks postbirth discharge: a population-based study, *Pediatrics* 114(3):708-713, 2004.

McCleary PH: Female genital mutilation and childbirth: a case report, *Birth* 21(4):221-223, 1994.

McConnell TP, Lee CW, Couillard M, and others: Trends in umbilical cord care: scientific evidence for practice, *Newborn Infant Nurs Rev* 4(4):211-222, 2004.

McDonald RE, Avery DR: *Dentistry for the child and adolescent,* ed 8, St Louis, 2004, Mosby.

Medves M, O'Brien B: The effect of bather and location of first bath on maintaining thermal stability in newborns, *J Obstet Gynecol Neonat Nurs* 33(2):175-182, 2004.

Merewood A, Mehta SD, Chamberlain LB, and others: Breastfeeding rates in US Baby-Friendly hospitals: results of a national survey, *Pediatrics* 116(3):628-634, 2005.

Merritt RJ, Jenks BH: Safety of soy-based formulas containing isoflavones: the clinical evidence, *J Nutr* 134(5):1220S-1224S, 2004.

Moolenaar RL, Crutcher JM, San Joaquin VH, and others: A prolonged outbreak of *Pseudomonas aeruginosa* in a neonatal intensive care unit: did staff fingernails play a role in disease transmission? *Infect Control Hosp Epidemiol* 21(2):80-85, 2000.

Morin KH.: Infant nutrition: what about water softeners and bottled water for babies? *MCN* 32(1):57, 2007.

Morrone A, Hercogova J, Lotti T: Stop female genital mutilation: appeal to the international dermatologic community, *Int J Dermatol* 41(5):253-263, 2002.

Morton CC, Nance WE: Newborn hearing screening—a silent revolution, *N Engl J Med* 354(20):2151-2164, 2006.

Nelson CP, Dunn R, Wan J, and others: The increased incidence of newborn circumcision: data from the nationwide inpatient sample, *J Urology* 173(30):978-981, 2005.

Noerr B: Sucrose for neonatal procedural pain, *Neonat Netw* 20(7):63-67, 2001.

Nuntnarumit P, Yang W, Bada-Ellzey HS: Blood pressure measurements in the newborn, *Clin Perinatol* 26(4):981-996, 1999.

Paes B, Janes M, Vegh P, and others: A comparative study of heel-stick devices for infant blood collection, *Am J Dis Child* 147(3):346-348, 1993.

Papile LA: The Apgar score in the 21st century, *N Engl J Med* 344(7):519-520, 2001.

Penny-MacGillivray T: A newborn's first bath: when? *J Obstet Gynecol Neonat Nurs* 25(6):481-487, 1996.

Pessler F, Nejat M: Anaphylactic reactions to goat's milk in a cow's milk allergic infant, *Pediatr Allergy Immunol* 15(2):183-185, 2004.

Quan R, Yang C, Rubinstein S, and others: Effects of microwave radiation on anti-infective factors in human milk, *Pediatrics* 89(4 Pt 1):667-669, 1992.

Rabun J: *For healthcare professionals: guidelines on prevention of and response to infant abductions,* ed 6, Alexandria, Va, 2000, National Center for Missing and Exploited Children.

Radmacher P, Massey C, Adamkin D: Hidden morbidity with "successful" early discharge, *J Perinatol* 22:15-20, 2002.

Razmus I, Dalton M, Wilson D: Pain management for newborn circumcision, *Pediatr Nurs* 20(5):414-417, 427, 2004.

Ryan AS, Zhou W, Gaston MH: Regional and sociodemographic variation of breastfeeding in the United States, 2002, *Clin Pediatr* 43(9):815-824, 2004.

Schuh S, Komar L, Stephens D, and others: Comparison of the temporal artery and rectal thermometry in children in the emergency department, *Pediatr Emerg Care* 20(11):736-741, 2004.

Seguin J, Terry K: Neonatal infrared axillary thermometry, *Clin Pediatr* 38(1):35-40, 1999.

Sganga A, Wallace R, Kiehl E, and others: A comparison of four methods of normal newborn temperature measurement, *MCN* 25(2):76-79, 2000.

Shah PS, Aliwalas LI, Shah V: Breastfeeding or breast milk for procedural pain in neonates, *Cochrane Database Syst Rev* (3):CD004950, 2006.

Shah V, Ohlsson A: Venepuncture versus heel lance for blood sampling in term neonates, *Cochrane Database Syst Rev* (2):CD001452, 2001.

Shogan MG: Emergency management plan for newborn abduction, *J Obstet Gynecol Neonat Nurs* 31(3):340-346, 2002.

Siberry GK, Diener-West M, Schappell E, and others: Comparison of temple temperatures with rectal temperatures in children under 2 years of age, *Clin Pediatr* 41(6):405-414, 2002.

Sigman-Grant M, Bush G, Anantheswaran R: Microwave heating of infant formula: a dilemma resolved, *Pediatrics* 90(3):412-415, 1992.

Stang HJ, Snellman LW, Condon LM, and others: Beyond dorsal penile nerve block: a more humane circumcision, *Pediatrics* 100(2):e3, 1997.

Stevens B, Johnston C, Taddio A, and others: Management of pain from heel lance with lidocaine-prilocaine (EMLA) cream: is it safe and efficacious in preterm infants? *J Dev Behav Pediatr* 20(4):216-221, 1999.

Stevens B, Yamada J, Ohlsson A: Sucrose for analgesia in newborn infants undergoing painful procedures, *Cochrane Database Syst Rev* (3): CD001069, 2004.

Taddio A, Ohlsson A, Einarson TR, and others: A systematic review of lidocaine-prilocaine cream (EMLA) in the treatment of acute pain in neonates, *Pediatrics* 101(2):e1, 1998; retrieved May 18, 2007, from http://www.pediatrics.org/cgi/content/full/101/2/e1.

Taddio A, Shah V, Gilbert-MacLeod C, and others: Conditioning and hyperalgesia in newborns exposed to repeated heel lances, *JAMA* 288(7):857-861, 2002.

Thomas P, Peabody J, Turnier V, and others: A new look at intrauterine growth and the impact of race, altitude, and gender, *Pediatrics* 106(2):e21, 2000.

Tomlinson PS, Bryan AA, Esau AL: Family centered intrapartum care: revisiting an old concept, *J Obstet Gynecol Neonat Nurs* 25(4):331-337, 1996.

Trochtenberg DS: Neonatal circumcision, *N Engl J Med* 323(17):1206, 1990 (letter to the editor).

US Department of Health and Human Services: *Healthy people 2010: understanding and improving health*, Washington, DC, 2000, The Department, retrieved June 15, 2007, from http://www.health.gov/healthypeople.

Varda KE, Behnke RS: The effect of timing the initial bath on newborn's temperature, *J Obstet Gynecol Neonat Nurs* 29(1):27-32, 2000.

Weiss ME, Poeltler D, Gocka I: Infrared tympanic thermometry for neonatal temperature assessment, *J Obstetric Gynecol Neonat Nurs* 23(9):798-803, 1993.

WHO Study Group on Female Genital Mutilation and Obstetric Outcome: Female genital mutilation and obstetric outcome: WHO collaborative prospective study in six African countries, *Lancet* 367(9525):1835-1841, 2006.

Williamson ML: Circumcision anesthesia: a study of nursing implications for dorsal penile nerve block, *Pediatr Nurs* 23(10):59-63, 1997.

Wilshaw R, Beckstrand R, Waid D, and others: A comparison of the use of tympanic, axillary, and rectal thermometers in infants, *J Pediatr Nurs* 14(2):88-93, 1999.

Wright A, Rice S, Wells S: Changing hospital practices to increase the duration of breast-feeding, *Pediatrics* 97(5):669-676, 1996.

Yetman RJ, Coody DK, West MS, and others: Comparison of temperature measurements by an aural infrared thermometer with measurements by traditional rectal and axillary techniques, *J Pediatr* 122(5):769-773, 1993.

Young TK, Martens PJ, Taback SP, and others: Type 2 diabetes mellitus in children: prenatal and early infancy risk factors among native Canadians, *Arch Pediatr Adolesc Med* 156(7):651-655, 2002.

Zupan J, Garner P, Omari AA: Topical umbilical cord care at birth, *Cochrane Database Syst Rev* (3):CD001057, 2004.

9

Health Problems of Newborns

DEBBIE FRASER ASKIN

CHAPTER OUTLINE

BIRTH INJURIES, 244
Soft-Tissue Injury, 244
Head Trauma, 244
  Caput Succedaneum, 244
  Cephalhematoma, 244
  Subgaleal Hemorrhage, 245
Fractures, 246
Paralysis, 246
  Facial Paralysis, 246
  Brachial Palsy, 246
  Phrenic Nerve Paralysis, 247
COMMON PROBLEMS IN THE NEWBORN, 247
Erythema Toxicum Neonatorum, 247
Candidiasis, 248
Herpes, 248
Birthmarks, 249
NURSING CARE OF THE HIGH-RISK NEWBORN AND FAMILY, 250
Identification of High-Risk Newborns, 250
Care of High-Risk Newborns, 251
  Systematic Assessment, 251
  Monitoring Physiologic Data, 252
  Respiratory Support, 252
  Thermoregulation, 252
  Protection from Infection, 254
  Hydration, 255
  Nutrition, 255

Feeding Resistance, 258
Energy Conservation, 258
Skin Care, 259
Administration of Medications, 261
Developmental Outcome, 261
Family Support and Involvement, 264
Facilitating Parent-Infant Relationships, 265
Discharge Planning and Home Care, 268
Neonatal Loss, 269
HIGH RISK RELATED TO DYSMATURITY, 271
Preterm Infants, 271
Postterm Infants, 273
HIGH RISK RELATED TO PHYSIOLOGIC FACTORS, 274
Hyperbilirubinemia, 274
Hemolytic Disease of the Newborn, 281
  Blood Incompatibility, 281
Metabolic Complications, 284
Respiratory Distress Syndrome, 284
Respiratory Complications, 288
Nursing Care Plan: The High-Risk Infant with Respiratory Distress Syndrome, 289
Cardiovascular Complications, 294
Cerebral Complications, 294
Neonatal Seizures, 294

HIGH RISK RELATED TO INFECTIOUS PROCESSES, 296
Sepsis, 296
Necrotizing Enterocolitis, 297
HIGH RISK RELATED TO MATERNAL CONDITIONS, 299
Infants of Diabetic Mothers, 299
Drug-Exposed Infants, 300
  Alcohol Exposure, 303
  Cocaine Exposure, 303
  Methamphetamine Exposure, 304
  Marijuana Exposure, 304
Maternal Infections, 305
CONGENITAL ANOMALIES, 308
Genetic Etiology of Congenital Anomalies, 309
  Chromosomal Abnormalities, 309
  Single-Gene Defects, 309
  Multifactorial Inheritance, 309
Defects Caused by Chemical Agents, 309
INBORN ERRORS OF METABOLISM, 310
Congenital Hypothyroidism, 311
Phenylketonuria, 313
Galactosemia, 315
GENETIC EVALUATION AND COUNSELING, 316
Psychologic Aspects of Genetic Disease, 317

LEARNING OBJECTIVES

On completion of this chapter the reader will be able to:
- Recognize common deviations from normal characteristics in the newborn.
- Perform a systematic assessment of a high-risk newborn.
- Outline a general care plan for a high-risk infant.

- Recognize physiologic factors that compromise the preterm infant's health status.
- Discuss the role of the nurse in facilitating positive parent-infant relationships.
- Contrast physical characteristics of preterm and full-term infants.
- Discuss the basis for screening newborns for health problems.

- Discuss the rationale for performing newborn screening and genetic counseling when a newborn has a hereditary condition.
- Modify a general care plan to meet the needs of an infant with specific high-risk health needs.

RELATED TOPICS and ADDITIONAL RESOURCES

 IN TEXT

Administration of Medication, *Ch. 22*
Assessment (Newborn), *Ch. 8*
Cognitive Impairment, *Ch. 19*
Collection of Specimens, *Ch. 22*
Congenital Adrenal Hyperplasia, *Ch. 29*
Diaper Dermatitis, *Ch. 30*
Family-Centered Home Care, *Ch. 20*
Impact of Chronic Illness or Disability on the
    Child, *Ch. 18*
Infant Mortality, *Ch. 1*
Infection Control, *Ch. 22*
Pain Assessment, *Ch. 7*
Pain Management, *Ch. 7*
Pain in Neonates, *Ch. 7*
Preparing for Discharge and Home Care,
    Ch. 21

Procedures for Maintaining Respiratory
    Function, *Ch. 22*
Procedures Related to Alternative Feeding
    Techniques, *Ch. 22*
Promote Parent-Infant Bonding
    (Attachment), *Ch. 8*

 COMPANION CD

Animations—Shoulder Dystocia; Erb's Palsy
Case Study—Health Problems of the
    Newborn
Critical Thinking Exercises—Jaundice; The
    High-Risk Newborn; Infant of a Diabetic
    Mother; Patent Ductus Arteriosus; Fetal
    Alcohol Syndrome/Effects
NCLEX Review Questions

 EVOLVE WEBSITE

http://evolve.elsevier.com/Wong/essentials/
Critical Thinking Case Study—
    Hyperbilirubinemia
Nursing Care Plans—The Newborn with
    Jaundice; The High-Risk Infant with
    Respiratory Distress Syndrome
NCLEX Review Questions
WebLinks

**WONG'S CLINICAL MANUAL
OF PEDIATRIC NURSING, 7th Ed**

Nursing Care Plans—The Newborn with
    Jaundice, *p. 409;* The Infant with
    Bronchopulmonary Dysplasia, *p. 411*
Patient and Family Education—Measuring
    Your Child's Temperature, *p. 508*

BIRTH INJURIES

Several factors predispose an infant to birth injuries (Mangurten, 2006; Paige and Moe, 2006). Maternal factors include uterine dysfunction that leads to prolonged or precipitous labor, preterm or postterm labor, and cephalopelvic disproportion. Injury may result from dystocia caused by fetal macrosomia, multifetal gestation, abnormal or difficult presentation (not caused by maternal uterine or pelvic conditions), and congenital anomalies. Intrapartum events that can result in scalp injury include the use of intrapartum monitoring of fetal heart rate and collection of fetal scalp blood for acid-base assessment. Obstetric birth techniques can cause injury. Forceps birth, vacuum extraction, version and extraction, and cesarean birth are potential contributory factors. Often more than one factor is present, and multiple predisposing factors may be related to a single maternal condition.

SOFT-TISSUE INJURY

Various types of soft-tissue injury may be sustained during the process of birth, primarily in the form of bruises or abrasions secondary to dystocia. Soft-tissue injury usually occurs when there is some degree of disproportion between the presenting part and the maternal pelvis (**cephalopelvic disproportion**). The use of forceps to facilitate a difficult vertex delivery may produce bruising or abrasion on the sides of the neonate's face. Petechiae or ecchymoses may be observed on the presenting part after a breech or brow delivery. After a difficult or precipitous delivery, the sudden release of pressure on the head can produce scleral hemorrhages or generalized petechiae over the face and head. Petechiae and ecchymoses may also appear on the head, neck, and face of an infant born with a nuchal cord, giving the infant's face a cyanotic appearance. A well-defined circle of petechiae and ecchymoses or abrasions may also be seen on the occipital region of the newborn's head when a vacuum suction cup is applied during delivery. Rarely, lacerations occur during cesarean section.

These traumatic lesions generally fade spontaneously within a few days, without treatment. However, petechiae may be a manifestation of an underlying bleeding disorder or a systemic illness such as an infection and should be further evaluated as to their origin. Nursing care is primarily directed toward assessing the injury and providing an explanation and reassurance to the parents.

HEAD TRAUMA

Trauma to the head and scalp that occurs during the birth process is usually benign but occasionally results in more serious injury. The injuries that produce serious trauma, such as intracranial hemorrhage and subdural hematoma, are discussed in relation to neurologic disorders in the newborn (see Table 9-9). Skull fractures are discussed in association with other fractures sustained during the birth process. The three most common types of extracranial hemorrhagic injury are caput succedaneum, subgaleal hemorrhage, and cephalhematoma.

Caput Succedaneum

The most commonly observed scalp lesion is **caput succedaneum,** a vaguely outlined area of edematous tissue situated over the portion of the scalp that presents in a vertex delivery (Fig. 9-1, *A*). The swelling consists of serum or blood, or both, accumulated in the tissues *above* the bone, and it often extends beyond the bone margins. The swelling may be associated with overlying petechiae or ecchymoses. No specific treatment is needed, and the swelling subsides within a few days.

Cephalhematoma

Infrequently, a cephalhematoma is formed when blood vessels rupture during labor or delivery to produce bleeding into the area between the bone and its periosteum. The injury occurs most often with primiparous delivery and is often associated with forceps delivery and vacuum extraction. Unlike caput

FIG. 9-1 ■ **A,** Caput succedaneum. **B,** Cephalhematoma. **C,** Subgaleal hemorrhage. (**A** and **B,** From Seidel HM, Ball JM, Davis JE, and others: *Mosby's guide to physical examination,* ed 6, St Louis, 2006, Mosby.)

succedaneum, the boundaries of the cephalhematoma are sharply demarcated and do not extend beyond the limits of the bone (suture lines) (see Fig. 9-1, *B*). The cephalhematoma may involve one or both parietal bones. The occipital bones are less commonly affected, and the frontal bones are rarely affected. The swelling is usually minimal or absent at birth and increases in size on the second or third day. Blood loss is usually not significant.

No treatment is indicated for uncomplicated cephalhematoma. Most lesions are absorbed within 2 weeks to 3 months. Lesions that result in severe blood loss to the area or that involve an underlying fracture require further evaluation. Hyperbilirubinemia may result during resolution of the hematoma. A local infection can develop and is suspected when a sudden increase in swelling occurs. Parents should be counseled that, in some cases, a small area of calcification may develop and persist.

Subgaleal Hemorrhage

Subgaleal hemorrhage is bleeding into the subgaleal compartment (see Fig. 9-1, *C*). The **subgaleal compartment** is a potential space that contains loosely arranged connective tissue; it is located beneath the galea aponeurosis, the tendinous sheath that connects the frontal and occipital muscles and forms the inner surface of the scalp. The injury occurs as a result of forces that compress and then drag the head through

the pelvic outlet (Paige and Moe, 2006). There have been reports of concern regarding the increased use of the vacuum extractor at birth and an association with cases of subgaleal hemorrhage, neonatal morbidity, and deaths (Boo, Foong, Mahdy, and others, 2005; Uchil and Arulkumaran, 2003); however, the rates of such outcomes have reportedly declined (Putta and Spencer, 2000). The bleeding extends beyond bone, often posteriorly into the neck, and continues after birth, with the potential for serious complications such as anemia or hypovolemic shock.

Early detection of the hemorrhage is vital; serial head circumference measurements and inspection of the back of the neck for increasing edema and a firm mass are essential. A boggy fluctuant mass over the scalp that crosses the suture line and moves as the baby is repositioned is an early sign of subgaleal hemorrhage (Doumouchtsis and Arulkumaran, 2006). Other signs include pallor, tachycardia, and increasing head circumference (Putta and Spencer, 2000). An early sign of subgaleal hemorrhage is a forward and lateral positioning of the newborn's ears because the hematoma extends posteriorly. Computed tomography or magnetic resonance imaging is useful in confirming the diagnosis. Replacement of lost blood and clotting factors is required in acute cases of hemorrhage. Monitoring the infant for changes in level of consciousness and a decrease in the hematocrit are also key to early recognition and management. An increase in serum bilirubin levels may be seen as a result of the degradation of red blood cells within the hematoma.

Nursing Care Management

Nursing care is directed toward assessment and observation of the common scalp injuries and vigilance in observing for possible associated complications such as infection or, rarely, acute blood loss and hypovolemia. Because these visible injuries resolve spontaneously, parents need reassurance of their usual benign nature.

FRACTURES

The **clavicle,** or **collarbone,** is the bone most frequently fractured during the birth process. It is often associated with shoulder dystocia or a difficult vertex or breech delivery of infants who are large for gestational age. **Crepitus** (the coarse crackling sensation produced by the rubbing together of fractured bone fragments) may be felt or heard on examination. A palpable, spongy mass, representing localized edema and hematoma, may also be a sign of a fractured clavicle. The infant may be reluctant to move the arm on the affected side, and the Moro reflex may be asymmetric. Radiographs usually reveal a complete fracture with overriding of the fragments.

Fractures of **long bones,** such as the femur or the humerus, are sometimes difficult to detect by radiographic examination. Although osteogenesis imperfecta is a rare finding, a newborn infant with a fracture should be assessed for other evidence of this congenital disorder.

Fractures of the neonatal **skull** are uncommon. The bones, which are less mineralized and more compressible than bones in older infants and children, are separated by membranous seams that allow sufficient alteration in the head contour so that it adjusts to the birth canal during delivery. Skull fractures usually follow a prolonged, difficult delivery or forceps extraction. Most fractures are linear, but some may be visible as depressed indentations that compress or decompress like a Ping-Pong ball. Management of depressed skull fractures is controversial; many resolve without intervention. Nonsurgical elevation of the indentation using a hand breast pump or vacuum extractor has been reported (Mangurten, 2006). Surgery may be required in the presence of bone fragments or signs of increased intracranial pressure (Uhing, 2004). A similar finding in neonates is **craniotabes,** which is usually benign or may be associated with prematurity or hydrocephalus (Johnson, 2003). In this condition the cranial bone(s) move freely on palpation and may easily compress.

> **NURSING ALERT**
>
> The newborn with a fractured clavicle may have no symptoms, but suspect a fracture if an infant has limited use of the affected arm, malpositioning of the arm, asymmetric Moro reflex, or focal swelling or tenderness, or if he or she cries in pain when the arm is moved. Eliciting the scarf sign (extending arm across chest toward opposite shoulder) for assessment of gestational age is contraindicated if a fractured clavicle is suspected.

> **NURSING ALERT**
>
> Any newborn who is large for gestational age or weighs more than 3855 g (8.5 pounds) and is delivered vaginally should be evaluated for a fractured clavicle.

Nursing Care Management

Often, no intervention is needed other than maintaining proper body alignment, careful dressing and undressing of the infant, and handling and carrying that support the affected bone. For example, if the infant has a fractured clavicle, it is important to support the upper and lower back rather than pull the infant up from under the arms. Placing the infant in a side-lying position with the affected side down is also avoided. Linear skull fractures usually require no treatment. A Ping-Pong ball–type skull fracture may require decompression by surgical intervention. The infant is carefully observed for signs of neurologic complications. The parents of infants with a fracture of any bone should be involved in caring for the infant during hospitalization as part of discharge planning for care at home.

PARALYSIS
Facial Paralysis

Pressure on the facial nerve (cranial nerve VII) during delivery may result in injury to that nerve. The primary clinical manifestations are loss of movement on the affected side, such as an inability to completely close the eye, drooping of the corner of the mouth, and absence of wrinkling of the forehead and nasolabial fold (Fig. 9-2). The paralysis is most noticeable when the infant cries. The mouth is drawn to the unaffected side, the wrinkles are deeper on the normal side, and the eye on the involved side remains open.

No medical intervention is necessary. The paralysis usually disappears spontaneously in a few days but may take as long as several months.

Brachial Palsy

Plexus injury results from forces that alter the normal position and relationship of the arm, shoulder, and neck. **Erb palsy (Erb-Duchenne paralysis)** is caused by damage to the upper plexus and usually results from stretching or pulling away of the shoulder from the head, as might occur with shoulder dystocia or with a difficult vertex or breech delivery. Other

A   B

FIG. 9-2 ■ A, Paralysis of right side of face 15 minutes after forceps delivery. Absence of movement on affected side is especially noticeable when infant cries. **B,** The same infant 24 hours later.

identified risk factors include an infant with birth weight of over 4000 g (8.8 pounds), a second stage of labor of less than 15 minutes, maternal body mass index greater than 29, and a vacuum-assisted extraction (Hudic, Fatusic, Sinanovic, and others, 2006). The less common lower plexus palsy, or **Klumpke palsy,** results from severe stretching of the upper extremity while the trunk is relatively less mobile.

The clinical manifestations of Erb palsy are related to the paralysis of the affected extremity and muscles. The arm hangs limp alongside the body while the shoulder and arm are adducted and internally rotated. The elbow is extended, and the forearm is pronated, with the wrist and fingers flexed; a grasp reflex may be present because finger and wrist movement remain normal (Tappero, 2003) (Fig. 9-3). In lower plexus palsy the muscles of the hand are paralyzed, with consequent wrist drop and relaxed fingers. In a third and more severe form of brachial palsy, the entire arm is paralyzed and hangs limp and motionless at the side. The Moro reflex is absent on the affected side for all forms of brachial palsy.

Treatment of the affected arm is aimed at preventing contractures of the paralyzed muscles and maintaining correct placement of the humeral head within the glenoid fossa of the scapula. Complete recovery from stretched nerves usually takes 3 to 6 months. Full recovery is expected in 88% to 92% of infants (Paige and Moe, 2006). However, avulsion of the nerves (complete disconnection of the ganglia from the spinal cord that involves both anterior and posterior roots) results in permanent damage. For those injuries that do not improve spontaneously by 3 months, surgical intervention may be needed to relieve pressure on the nerves or to repair the nerves with grafting (Joyner, Soto, and Adam, 2006). In some cases injection of botulinum toxin A into the pectoralis major muscle may be effective in reducing muscle contractures after birth-related brachial plexus injuries (Price, Ditaranto, Yaylali, and others, 2007).

Phrenic Nerve Paralysis

Phrenic nerve paralysis results in diaphragmatic paralysis as demonstrated by ultrasonography, which shows paradoxic chest movement and an elevated diaphragm. Initially, radiography may not demonstrate an elevated diaphragm if the neonate is receiving positive pressure ventilation (Volpe, 2001). The injury sometimes occurs in conjunction with brachial palsy. Respiratory distress is the most common and important sign of injury. Because injury to the phrenic nerve is usually unilateral, the lung on the affected side does not expand, and respiratory efforts are ineffectual. Breathing is primarily thoracic, and cyanosis, tachypnea, or complete respiratory failure may be seen. Pneumonia and atelectasis on the affected side may also occur.

Nursing Care Management

Nursing care of the infant with facial nerve paralysis involves aiding the infant in sucking and helping the mother with feeding techniques. Because part of the mouth cannot close tightly around the nipple, the use of a soft rubber nipple with a large hole may be helpful. The infant may require gavage feeding to prevent aspiration. Breastfeeding is not contraindicated, but the mother will need additional assistance in helping the infant grasp and compress the areolar area.

If the lid of the eye on the affected side does not close completely, artificial tears can be instilled daily to prevent drying of the conjunctiva, sclera, and cornea. The lid is often taped shut to prevent accidental injury. If eye care is needed at home, the parents are taught the procedure for administering eye drops before the infant is discharged from the nursery (see Chapter 22).

Nursing care of the newborn with brachial palsy is concerned primarily with proper positioning of the affected arm. The affected arm should be gently immobilized on the upper abdomen; passive range-of-motion exercises of the shoulder, wrist, elbow, and fingers are initiated at 7 to 10 days of age (Joyner, Soto, and Adam, 2006). Wrist flexion contractures may be prevented with the use of supportive splints. In dressing the infant, preference is given to the affected arm. Undressing begins with the unaffected arm, and redressing begins with the affected arm to prevent unnecessary manipulation and stress on the paralyzed muscles. Parents are taught to use the "football" position when holding the infant and to avoid picking the child up from under the axillae or by pulling on the arms.

The infant with phrenic nerve paralysis requires the same nursing care as any infant with respiratory distress.

The family's emotional needs are also an important part of nursing care; the family will need reassurance regarding the neonate's progress toward an optimal outcome.

Follow-up is also essential because of the extended length of recovery. Parents may wish to contact the Brachial Plexus Palsy Foundation* and visit the website for further information.

COMMON PROBLEMS IN THE NEWBORN

ERYTHEMA TOXICUM NEONATORUM

Erythema toxicum neonatorum, also known as **flea-bite dermatitis** or **newborn rash,** is a benign, self-limiting eruption of unknown cause that usually appears within the first 2 days of life. The lesions are firm, 1- to 3-mm, pale yellow or white papules or pustules on an erythematous base; they resemble flea bites. The rash appears most commonly on the face, proximal extremities, trunk, and buttocks, but it may be located anywhere on the body except the palms and soles. The rash is more obvious during crying episodes. There are no systemic manifestations, and successive crops of lesions heal

FIG. 9-3 ■ Left-sided brachial plexus (Erb) palsy. Note extended, internally rotated arm and pronated wrist on affected side.

*210 Spring Haven Circle, Royersford, PA 19468; http://www.brachialplexus palsyfoundation.org.

without pigmentation changes. The rash usually lasts about 5 to 7 days. The etiology is unknown. However, a smear of the pustule will show numerous eosinophils and a relative absence of neutrophils. When the diagnosis is questionable, bacterial, fungal, or viral cultures should be obtained. Although no treatment is necessary, parents are usually concerned about the rash and need to be reassured of its benign and transient nature.

CANDIDIASIS

Candidiasis, also known as **moniliasis,** is not uncommon in the newborn. *Candida albicans,* the usual organism responsible, may cause disease in any organ system. It is a yeastlike fungus (it produces yeast cells and spores) that can be acquired from a maternal vaginal infection during delivery; from person-to-person transmission (especially from poor hand-washing technique); or from contaminated hands, bottles, nipples, or other articles. Mucocutaneous, cutaneous, and disseminated candidal infections are all observed in this age-group. Candidiasis is usually a benign disorder in the neonate, often confined to the oral and diaper regions. **Diaper dermatitis** caused by *Candida* organisms manifests as a moist, erythematous eruption with small white or yellow pebbly pustules. Small areas of skin erosion may also be seen.

Oral Candidiasis

Oral candidiasis (**thrush**) is characterized by white, adherent patches on the tongue, palate, and inner aspects of the cheeks (Fig. 9-4). It is often difficult to distinguish from coagulated milk. The infant may refuse to suck because of pain in the mouth.

This condition tends to be acute in the newborn and chronic in infants and young children. Thrush appears when the oral flora is altered as a result of antibiotic therapy or poor hand washing by the infant's caregiver. Although the disorder is usually self-limiting, spontaneous resolution may take as long as 2 months, during which time lesions may spread to the larynx, trachea, bronchi, and lungs and along the gastrointestinal tract. The disease is treated with good hygiene, application of a fungicide, and correction of any underlying disturbance. The source of infection should be treated to prevent reinfection.

FIG. 9-4 ■ Oral candidiasis (thrush). (From *Variations and minor departures in infants,* Evansville, Ind, 1978, Mead Johnson & Co.)

Topical application of 1 ml nystatin (Mycostatin) over the surfaces of the oral cavity four times a day, or every 6 hours, is usually sufficient to prevent spread of the disease or prolongation of its course. Several other drugs may be used, including amphotericin B (Fungizone), clotrimazole (Lotrimin, Mycelex), fluconazole (Diflucan), or miconazole (Monistat, Micatin) given intravenously, orally, or topically. To prevent relapse, therapy should be continued for at least 2 days after the lesions disappear (Lawrence and Lawrence, 2005). Gentian violet solution may be used in addition to one of the antifungal drugs in chronic cases of oral thrush; however, the former does not treat gastrointestinal *Candida* infection and may be irritating to the oral mucosa.

> **NURSINGALERT**
>
> Oral candidiasis can be distinguished from coagulated milk when attempts to remove the patches with a tongue blade are unsuccessful. The primary caregiver may also report that the infant does not nurse well or bottle feed as previously.

Nursing Care Management

Nursing care is directed toward preventing spread of the infection and correctly applying the prescribed topical medication. For candidiasis in the diaper area, the caregiver is taught to keep the diaper area clean and to apply the medication to affected areas as prescribed (see also Diaper Dermatitis, Chapter 30). Infants with candidal diaper dermatitis can introduce the yeast into the mouth from contaminated hands. Placing clothes over the diaper can prevent this cycle of self-infection.

In cases of oral thrush, nystatin is administered after feedings. The medication is distributed over the surface of the oral mucosa and tongue with an applicator or syringe; the remainder of the dose is deposited in the mouth to be swallowed by the infant to treat any gastrointestinal lesions.

In addition to good hygienic care, other measures to control thrush include rinsing the infant's mouth with plain water after each feeding before applying the medication and boiling reusable nipples and bottles for at least 20 minutes after a thorough washing (spores are heat resistant). If used, pacifiers should be boiled for at least 20 minutes once daily. If the mother is breastfeeding it is recommended that simultaneous treatment of the infant and mother occur if either is infected (Lawrence and Lawrence, 2005).

HERPES

Neonatal herpes is one of the most serious viral infections in the newborn, with a mortality rate of up to 60% in infants with disseminated disease. Approximately 86% to 90% of herpes simplex transmission occurs during passage through the birth canal (Parker and Montrowl, 2004). The risk of infection during vaginal birth in the presence of genital herpes is estimated to be as high as 57% with active primary infection at term (Brown, Wald, Morrow, and others, 2003). However, in up to 80% of cases of neonatal herpes simplex virus (HSV) infection, the mother has no history or symptoms of infection at the time of birth, but serologic testing reveals evidence of the herpesvirus (Kimberlin, 2005).

Neonatal herpes manifests in one of three ways: (1) with skin, eye, and mouth involvement; (2) as localized central nervous system (CNS) disease; or (3) as disseminated disease involving multiple organs. In skin and eye disease a rash appears as vesicles or pustules on an erythematous base. Clusters of lesions are common. The lesions ulcerate and crust over rapidly. Most infants with neonatal herpes eventually develop this characteristic rash, but up to 20% of neonates with disseminated disease do not develop a skin rash (Kimberlin, 2007). Ophthalmologic clinical findings include chorioretinitis and microphthalmia; neurologic involvement such as microcephaly and encephalomalacia may also develop (Kimberlin, 2007). Disseminated infections may involve virtually every organ system, but the liver, adrenal glands, and lungs are most commonly affected. In HSV meningitis infants develop multiple lesions of cortical hemorrhagic necrosis. It can occur alone or with oral, eye, or skin lesions. The presenting symptoms, which may occur in the second to fourth week of life, include lethargy, poor feeding, irritability, and local or generalized seizures.

Nursing Care Management

Neonates with herpesvirus or suspected infection (as a result of exposure) should be carefully evaluated for clinical manifestations. The absence of skin lesions in the neonate exposed to maternal herpesvirus does not indicate absence of disease. Contact precautions (in addition to standard precautions) should be instituted according to American Academy of Pediatrics and American College of Obstetricians and Gynecologists guidelines or hospital protocol. It is recommended that swabs of the mouth, nasopharynx, conjunctivae, rectum, and any skin vesicles be obtained from the exposed neonate; in addition, urine, stool, blood, and CSF specimens should be obtained for culture. Antiviral therapy with acyclovir is initiated if the cultures are positive or if there is strong suspicion of herpesvirus infection (American Academy of Pediatrics, 2006a).

BIRTHMARKS

Discolorations of the skin are common findings in the newborn infant (see discussion on skin assessment of the newborn, Chapter 8). Most, such as mongolian spots or telangiectatic nevi, involve no therapy other than reassurance to parents of the benign nature of these discolorations. However, some can be a manifestation of a disease that suggests further examination of the child and other family members (e.g., the multiple light brown **café-au-lait spots** that often characterize the autosomal dominant hereditary disorder neurofibromatosis and are common findings in Albright syndrome).

Darker or more extensive lesions demand further scrutiny, and excision of the lesion is recommended when feasible. Such lesions include the reddish brown solitary nodule that appears on the face or upper arm and usually represents a spindle and epithelioid cell nevus (**juvenile melanoma**); a **giant pigmented nevus** (or **bathing trunk nevus**), a dark brown to black, irregular plaque that is at risk of transformation to malignant melanoma; and the dark brown or black macules that become more numerous with age (**junctional** or **compound nevi**).

Vascular birthmarks may be divided into the following categories: vascular malformations, capillary hemangiomas, and mixed hemangiomas. **Vascular stains (malformations)** are permanent lesions that are present at birth and are initially flat and erythematous. Any vascular structure, capillary, vein, artery, or lymphatic may be involved. The two most common vascular stains are the **transient macular stain** (stork bite, salmon patch, or angel kiss) and the **port-wine stain,** or **nevus flammeus.** The port-wine lesions are pink, red, or, rarely, purple stains of the skin that thicken, darken, and proportionately enlarge as the child grows (Fig. 9-5, *A*). The macular stain is most often located on the eyelids, glabella, or nape of the neck and usually fades by 1 year of age (Conlon and Drolet, 2004).

Port-wine stains may also be associated with structural malformations, such as glaucoma or leptomeningeal angiomatosis (tumor of blood or lymph vessels in the pia-arachnoid) (**Sturge-Weber syndrome**) or bony or muscular overgrowth (**Klippel-Trenaunay-Weber syndrome**). Children with port-wine stains on the eyelids, forehead, or cheeks should be monitored for these syndromes with periodic ophthalmologic examination, neurologic imaging, and measurement of extremities.

The treatment of choice for port-wine stains is the use of the flashlamp-pumped pulsed dye laser. A series of treatments is usually needed. The treatments can significantly lighten or completely clear the lesions with almost no scarring or pigment change.

Capillary hemangiomas, sometimes referred to as **strawberry hemangiomas,** are benign cutaneous tumors that involve only capillaries. These hemangiomas are bright red, rubbery nodules with a rough surface and a well-defined margin (see Fig. 9-5, *B*). Strawberry hemangiomas may not be apparent at birth but may appear within a few weeks and

FIG. 9-5 ■ A, Port-wine stain. **B,** Strawberry hemangioma. (From Zitelli BJ, Davis HW: *Atlas of pediatric physical diagnosis,* ed 5, St Louis, 2007, Mosby.)

enlarge considerably during the first year of life and then begin to involute spontaneously. It may take 5 to 12 years for complete resolution. As many as 50% of patients may be left with residual findings such as telangiectasia, redundant fatty tissue, or skin atrophy (Alster and Railan, 2006). **Cavernous venous hemangiomas** involve deeper vessels in the dermis and have a bluish red color and poorly defined margins. These latter forms may be associated with the trapping of platelets (**Kasabach-Merritt syndrome**) and subsequent thrombocytopenia (Witt, 2003; Conlon and Drolet, 2004).

Although most hemangiomas require no treatment because of their high rate of spontaneous involution, some vision and airway obstruction may necessitate therapy. The pulsed dye laser can effectively reduce some hemangiomas; systemic prednisone administered for 2 to 3 weeks or longer may also deter further growth. Subcutaneous injections of interferon alfa-2a or interferon alfa-2b may be required if prednisone therapy and the pulsed dye laser fail to control a problematic hemangioma; however, associated side effects may outweigh the benefits of therapy in some cases (Dohil, Baugh, and Eichenfield, 2000).

Nursing Care Management

Birthmarks, especially those on the face, are upsetting to parents. Families need an explanation of the type of lesion, its significance, and possible treatment.* They can benefit from seeing photographs of other infants before and after treatment for port-wine stains or after the passage of time for hemangiomas. Pictures taken to follow the involution process may further help parents gain confidence that progress is taking place.

If laser therapy is performed, the lesion will have a purplish black appearance for 7 to 10 days, after which the blackness fades and gives way to redness with an eventual lightening of the treated area. During the treatment phase parents are cautioned to avoid any trauma to the lesion or picking at the scab. The child's fingernails are trimmed as an added precaution. Washing the area gently with water and dabbing it dry is adequate, although in some cases a topical antibiotic ointment may be used. No salicylates should be taken during the treatment phase because they decrease the effects of the therapy. The child should be kept out of the sun for several weeks and then protected with a sunscreen of at least SPF 25. Complications associated with laser treatment include redness and bruising and, less commonly, hyperpigmentation, hypopigmentation, and atrophic scarring (Alster and Railan, 2006).

NURSING CARE OF THE HIGH-RISK NEWBORN AND FAMILY

IDENTIFICATION OF HIGH-RISK NEWBORNS

The **high-risk neonate** can be defined as a newborn, regardless of gestational age or birth weight, who has a greater-than-average chance of morbidity or mortality because of conditions or circumstances associated with birth and the adjustment to extrauterine existence. The high-risk period encompasses human growth and development from the time of **viability** (the gestational age at which survival outside the uterus is believed to be possible, or as early as 23 weeks of gestation) up to 28 days following birth; thus it includes threats to life and health that occur during the prenatal, perinatal, and postnatal periods.

Classification of High-Risk Newborns

High-risk infants are most often classified according to birth weight, gestational age, and predominant pathophysiologic problems. The more common problems related to physiologic status are closely associated with the state of maturity of the infant and usually involve chemical disturbances (e.g., hypoglycemia, hypocalcemia) or consequences of immature organs and systems (e.g., hyperbilirubinemia, respiratory distress, hypothermia). Because high-risk factors are common to sev-

---

BOX 9-1
Classification of High-Risk Infants

CLASSIFICATION ACCORDING TO SIZE

Low-birth-weight (LBW) infant—An infant whose birth weight is less than 2500 g (5.5 pounds), regardless of gestational age

Very low–birth-weight (VLBW) infant—An infant whose birth weight is less than 1500 g (3.3 pounds)

Extremely low–birth-weight (ELBW) infant—An infant whose birthweight is less than 1000 g (2.2 pounds)

Appropriate-for-gestational-age (AGA) infant—An infant whose weight falls between the 10th and 90th percentiles on intrauterine growth curves

Small-for-date (SFD) or small-for-gestational-age (SGA) infant—An infant whose rate of intrauterine growth was slowed and whose birth weight falls below the 10th percentile on intrauterine growth curves (see also Fig. 8-1, *B*)

Intrauterine growth restriction (IUGR)—Found in infants whose intrauterine growth is restricted (sometimes used as a more descriptive term for the SGA infant)

Symmetric IUGR—Growth restriction in which the weight, length, and head circumference are all affected

Asymmetric IUGR—Growth restriction in which the head circumference remains within normal parameters while the birth weight falls below the 10th percentile

Large-for-gestational-age (LGA) infant—An infant whose birth weight falls above the 90th percentile on intrauterine growth charts

CLASSIFICATION ACCORDING TO GESTATIONAL AGE

Preterm (premature) infant—An infant born before completion of 37 weeks of gestation, regardless of birth weight

Full-term infant—An infant born between the beginning of the 38 weeks and the completion of the 42 weeks of gestation, regardless of birth weight

Postterm (postmature) infant—An infant born after 42 weeks of gestational age, regardless of birth weight

Near-term (late-preterm) infant—An infant born between 34⁶/₇ and 36⁶/₇ weeks of gestation, regardless of birth weight*

CLASSIFICATION ACCORDING TO MORTALITY

Live birth—Birth in which the neonate manifests any heartbeat, breathes, or displays voluntary movement, regardless of gestational age

Fetal death—Death of the fetus after 20 weeks of gestation and before delivery, with absence of any signs of life after birth

Neonatal death—Death that occurs in the first 27 days of life; early neonatal death occurs in the first week of life; late neonatal death occurs at 7 to 27 days

Perinatal mortality—Total number of fetal and early neonatal deaths per 1000 live births

---

*Information is available from Vascular Birthmarks Foundation, http://www. birthmark.org.

*NOTE: Definitions on near-term (late preterm) vary among experts, but Engle (2006) suggests the above (which corresponds to 239th day to 259th day from first day of last menstrual period).

eral specialty areas—particularly obstetrics, pediatrics, and neonatology—specific terminology is needed to describe the developmental status of the newborn (Box 9-1).

Formerly, weight at birth was considered to reflect a reasonably accurate estimation of gestational age; that is, if an infant's birth weight exceeded 2500 g (5.5 pounds), the infant was considered to be mature. However, accumulated data have shown that intrauterine growth rates are not the same for all infants and that other factors (e.g., heredity, placental insufficiency, maternal disease) influence intrauterine growth and

birth weight. From these data a more definitive and meaningful classification system that encompasses birth weight, gestational age, and neonatal outcome has been developed. (See Fig. 8-2 for size comparison of newborn infants.)

CARE OF HIGH-RISK NEWBORNS
Systematic Assessment

A thorough systematic physical assessment is an essential component in the care of the high-risk infant (see Nursing Care Guidelines box). Subtle changes in feeding behavior, ac-

nursingcareguidelines

Physical Assessment

GENERAL ASSESSMENT
Using electronic scale, weigh daily, or more often if indicated.
Measure length and head circumference periodically.
Describe general body shape and size, posture at rest, ease of breathing, presence and location of edema.
Describe any apparent deformities.
Describe any signs of distress—poor color, hypotonia, lethargy, apnea.

RESPIRATORY ASSESSMENT
Describe shape of chest (barrel, concave), symmetry, presence of incisions, chest tubes, or other deviations.
Describe use of accessory muscles—nasal flaring or substernal, intercostal, or suprasternal retractions.
Determine respiratory rate and regularity.
Auscultate and describe breath sounds—crackles, wheezing, wet or diminished sounds, grunting, diminished air movement, stridor, equality of breath sounds.
Describe cry if not intubated.
Describe ambient oxygen and method of delivery; if intubated, describe size and position of tube, type of ventilator, and settings.
Determine oxygen saturation by pulse oximetry and partial pressure of oxygen, and describe carbon dioxide by transcutaneous carbon dioxide (tcPco$_2$).

CARDIOVASCULAR ASSESSMENT
Determine heart rate and rhythm.
Describe heart sounds, including any murmurs.
Determine the point of maximum impulse (PMI), the point at which the heartbeat sounds and palpates loudest (a change in the PMI may indicate a mediastinal shift).
Describe infant's color (may be of cardiac, respiratory, or hematopoietic origin)—cyanosis, pallor, plethora, jaundice, mottling.
Assess color of mucous membranes, lips.
Determine blood pressure as indicated. Indicate extremity used and cuff size.
Describe peripheral pulses, capillary refill, peripheral perfusion (mottling).
Describe monitors, their parameters, and whether alarms are in "on" position.

GASTROINTESTINAL ASSESSMENT
Determine presence of abdominal distention—increase in circumference, shiny skin, evidence of abdominal wall erythema, visible peristalsis, visible loops of bowel, status of umbilicus.
Determine any signs of regurgitation, and time related to feeding; describe character and amount of residual if gavage fed; if nasogastric tube is in place, describe type of suction, drainage (color, consistency, pH, guaiac).

Describe amount, color, consistency, and odor of any emesis.
Palpate liver margin (1 to 3 cm below right costal margin).
Describe amount, color, and consistency of stools; check for occult blood or reducing substances if ordered or indicated by appearance of stool.
Describe bowel sounds—presence or absence (must be present if feeding).

GENITOURINARY ASSESSMENT
Describe any abnormalities of genitalia.
Describe amount (as determined by weight), color, pH, labstick findings, and specific gravity of urine (to screen for adequacy of hydration).
Check weight (the most accurate measure for assessment of hydration).

NEUROLOGIC-MUSCULOSKELETAL ASSESSMENT
Describe infant's movements—random, purposeful, jittery, twitching, spontaneous, elicited; describe level of activity with stimulation; evaluate based on gestational age.
Describe infant's position or attitude—flexed, extended.
Describe reflexes observed—Moro, sucking, Babinski, plantar, and other expected reflexes.
Determine level of response and consolability.
Determine changes in head circumference (if indicated), size and tension of fontanels, suture lines.
Determine pupillary responses in infant over 32 weeks of gestation.
Check hip alignment (only experienced practitioner should perform).

TEMPERATURE
Determine axillary temperature.
Determine relationship to environmental temperature.

SKIN ASSESSMENT
Describe any discoloration, reddened area, signs of irritation, blisters, abrasions, or denuded areas, especially where monitoring equipment, infusions, or other apparatus come in contact with skin; also check and note any skin preparation used (e.g., povidone-iodine).
Determine texture and turgor of skin—dry, smooth, flaky, peeling, etc.
Describe any rash, skin lesion, or birthmarks.
Determine whether intravenous infusion catheter or needle is in place, and observe for signs of infiltration.
Describe parenteral infusion lines—location, type (arterial, venous, peripheral, umbilical, central, peripheral central venous); type of infusion (medication, saline, dextrose, electrolyte, lipids, total parenteral nutrition); type of infusion pump and rate of flow; type of catheter; and appearance of insertion site.

tivity, color, oxygen saturation (Sao_2), or vital signs often indicate an underlying problem. The low-birth-weight (LBW) preterm infant, especially the very low–birth-weight (VLBW) or extremely low–birth-weight (ELBW) infant, is ill equipped to withstand prolonged physiologic stress and may die within minutes of exhibiting abnormal symptoms if the underlying pathologic process is not corrected. The alert nurse is aware of subtle changes and reacts promptly to implement interventions that promote optimum functioning in the high-risk neonate. Changes in the infant's status are noted through ongoing observations of the infant's adaptation to the extrauterine environment.

Observational assessments of the high-risk infant are made according to the infant's acuity; the critically ill infant requires close observation and assessment of respiratory function, including continuous pulse oximetry, electrolytes, and evaluation of blood gases. Accurate documentation of the infant's status is an integral component of nursing care. With the aid of continuous, sophisticated cardiopulmonary monitoring, nursing assessments and daily care may be coordinated to allow for minimal handling of the infant (especially the VLBW or ELBW infant) to decrease the effects of environmental stress.

Monitoring Physiologic Data

Most neonates under intensive observation are placed in a controlled thermal environment and monitored for heart rate, respiratory activity, and temperature. The monitoring devices are equipped with an alarm system that indicates when the vital signs are above or below preset limits. However, it is essential to check the apical heart rate and compare it with the monitor reading.

Blood pressure (BP) is monitored routinely in the sick neonate by either internal or external means. Direct recording with arterial catheters is often used but carries the risks inherent in any procedure in which a catheter is introduced into an artery. Normal BP ranges for healthy preterm infants are listed in Table 9-1. Infants who have birth asphyxia, have low Apgar scores, or are mechanically ventilated may have lower mean BPs. In the neonatal intensive care unit (NICU), frequent laboratory examinations and their interpretation are integral parts of the ongoing assessment of infants' progress. Accurate intake and output records are kept on all acutely ill infants. An accurate output can be obtained by collecting urine in a plastic urine collection bag specifically made for preterm infants (see Urine Specimens, Chapter 22) or by weighing the diapers, which is the simplest and least traumatic means of measuring urinary output. The preweighed wet diaper is weighed on a gram scale, and the gram weight of the urine is converted directly to milliliters (e.g., 25 g = 25 ml).

One study has shown that urine obtained from cloth diapers or disposable diapers containing absorbent gelling material yields inaccurate results for urine specific gravity, pH, and protein. Urine samples obtained from cotton balls of 100% cotton that were strategically placed in the diaper proved to be the most accurate (Kirkpatrick, Alexander, and Cain, 1997).

Blood examinations are a necessary part of the ongoing assessment and monitoring of the high-risk newborn's progress. The tests most often performed are blood glucose, bilirubin, calcium, hematocrit, serum electrolytes, and blood gases. Samples may be obtained from the heel; by venipuncture; by arte-

TABLE 9-1		
Blood Pressure Ranges in Different Weight Groups of Healthy Preterm Infants*		
BIRTH WEIGHT (g)	SYSTOLIC (mm Hg)	DIASTOLIC (mm Hg)
501-750	50-62	26-36
751-1000	48-59	23-36
1001-1250	49-61	26-35
1251-1500	46-56	23-33
1501-1750	46-58	23-33
1751-2000	48-61	24-35

Modified from Hegyi T, Carbone MT, Anwar M, and others: Blood pressure ranges in premature infants, part I, The first hours of life, *J Pediatr* 124(4):630, 1994.
*Defined as infants without a history of maternal hypertension, Apgar scores of <3 at 1 minute and <6 at 5 minutes, pneumothorax, hematocrit 32%, serum pH 7.1, use of dopamine, infusion of erythrocytes or colloid, mechanical ventilation, or cardiopulmonary resuscitation.

rial puncture; or by an indwelling catheter in an umbilical vein, an umbilical artery, or a peripheral artery (see Atraumatic Care box, p. 224, and Collection of Specimens, Chapter 22).

When numerous blood samples must be drawn, it is important to maintain an accurate record of the amount of blood being removed, especially in ELBW and VLBW infants, who can ill afford to have their blood supply depleted during the acute phase of their illness. There is an increased emphasis on drawing as little blood as possible from high-risk neonates to minimize the depletion of blood volume and avoid blood transfusions and associated complications. To obtain frequent samples for monitoring arterial blood gas levels without repeated arterial punctures, pulse oximetry, which measures the saturation or percentage of oxygen in the hemoglobin, is typically used. Although used less frequently than pulse oximetry, transcutaneous carbon dioxide ($tcPco_2$) is monitored in some situations. The nurse notes changes in oxygenation (or other aspects being monitored) associated with handling and adjusts the infant's care accordingly. The frequency of vital signs is determined by the infant's acuity level (seriousness of condition) and response to handling.

The nursing process in the care of the high-risk newborn and family is described in the Nursing Process box.

Respiratory Support

The primary objective in the care of high-risk infants is to establish and maintain respiration. Many infants require supplemental oxygen and assisted ventilation. All infants require appropriate positioning to maximize oxygenation and ventilation. Oxygen therapy is provided on the basis of the infant's requirements and illness (see Respiratory Distress Syndrome, p. 284).

Thermoregulation

After or concurrent with the establishment of respiration, the most crucial need of the LBW infant is application of external warmth. Prevention of heat loss in the distressed infant is absolutely essential for survival, and maintaining a neutral thermal environment is a challenging aspect of neonatal intensive nursing care. Heat production is a complicated process that involves the cardiovascular, neurologic, and metabolic systems, and the immature neonate has all of the problems related to heat production that are faced by the full-term infant (see

nursingprocess | The High-Risk Newborn and Family

ASSESSMENT

At birth the newborn is given a rapid, yet thorough, assessment to determine any apparent problems and identify those that demand immediate attention. This examination is primarily concerned with evaluation of cardiopulmonary and neurologic functions. The assessment includes assignment of an Apgar score (see Chapter 8) and evaluation for any obvious congenital anomalies or evidence of neonatal distress. A systematic assessment (see p. 251) is carried out once the high-risk newborn is stable. (See also Clinical Assessment of Gestational Age, Chapter 8.)

DIAGNOSIS (PROBLEM IDENTIFICATION)

Many nursing diagnoses may be evident after a careful assessment of the infant at risk. Some apply to all infants; others vary according to the needs and characteristics of individual infants and their families. Because a number of health problems accompany the high-risk infant, the nurse is also alert to other conditions and complications discussed later in this chapter and elsewhere in the book. The nursing diagnoses that represent general guides for nursing intervention are:

- Ineffective Breathing Pattern related to pulmonary and neuromuscular immaturity
- Ineffective Thermoregulation related to immature temperature control and decreased subcutaneous fat
- Risk for Infection (risk factors include deficient immunologic defenses, exposure to environmental pathogens, required invasive procedures)
- Imbalanced Nutrition: Less Than Body Requirements related to inability to ingest nutrients
- Risk for Impaired Skin Integrity (risk factors include immature skin structure, physical immobility, decreased fluid intake, and invasive procedures)
- Risk for Imbalanced Fluid Volume (risk factors include immature skin structure; extra fluid losses via skin, lungs, and urine; decreased ability to take in required amount of fluid to sustain hydration)
- Delayed Growth and Development related to preterm birth, immature physiologic capabilities at birth, neonatal intensive care unit environment, separation from parents, effects of concomitant illnesses
- Interrupted Family Processes related to preterm birth, situational crisis, interruption of parent-infant interaction
- Anticipatory Grieving related to unexpected birth of high-risk infant, knowledge deficit regarding infant's prognosis and eventual outcome

PLANNING

The nursing care plan for the high-risk infant depends to a large extent on the diagnosis of the health problem(s) that place the infant at risk. However, the following expected outcomes are appropriate for many high-risk infants and their families:

- Infant will exhibit adequate oxygenation.
- Infant will maintain stable body temperature.
- Infant will exhibit no evidence of nosocomial infection.
- Infant will receive adequate hydration and nutrition.
- Infant will maintain skin integrity.
- Infant will receive appropriate developmental support and care.
- Parents will experience positive parent-infant interactions.
- Parents will exhibit positive caretaking abilities with high-risk infant.
- Family will receive appropriate support, including preparation for home care or for infant's death.

IMPLEMENTATION

Intervention strategies for the high-risk infant and family are discussed on pp. 251-270.

EVALUATION

The effectiveness of nursing interventions is determined by continual reassessment and evaluation of care based on the following observational guidelines:

- Take vital signs and perform respiratory assessments at time intervals based on infant's condition and needs; observe infant's respiratory efforts and response to therapy; check functioning of equipment; review laboratory test results.
- Measure body temperature at specified intervals.
- Observe infant's behavior and appearance for evidence of sepsis.
- Assess for hydration; assess and measure fluid intake; observe infant during feeding; measure amount of human milk, formula, or parenteral intake; weigh daily.
- Observe infant's skin for signs of irritation, excoriation, and breakdown.
- Observe infant's response to developmental care.
- Observe parental interaction with infant; interview family regarding their feelings, concerns, and readiness for home care.
- Assess family and observe their behaviors during and after the death of their infant.

Thermoregulation, Chapter 8). However, LBW infants are placed at further disadvantage by a number of additional problems. They have an even smaller muscle mass and fewer deposits of brown fat for producing heat, lack insulating subcutaneous fat, and have poor reflex control of skin capillaries.

To delay or prevent the effects of cold stress, at-risk newborns are placed in a heated environment immediately after birth, where they remain until they are able to maintain **thermal stability**—the capacity to balance heat production and conservation with heat dissipation. Because overheating produces an increase in oxygen and calorie consumption, the infant is also jeopardized in a hyperthermic environment. A **neutral thermal environment** is one that permits the infant to maintain a normal core temperature with minimum oxygen consumption and calorie expenditure. Studies indicate that optimum thermoneutrality cannot be predicted for every

high-risk infant's needs. In healthy term infants it is recommended that axillary temperatures be maintained at 36.5° to 37.5° C (97.7° to 99.5° F), whereas in preterm infants axillary temperatures of 36.3° and 36.9° C (97.3° and 98.4° F) are considered appropriate (Blake and Murray, 2006). Other guidelines for VLBW infants suggest that a skin temperature of 36° to 36.3° C (96.8° to 97.3° F) may be appropriate for some infants providing the infant is medically stable and growing appropriately (Kenner, 2003). The lower temperature range in preterm infants reflects the increased risk of apnea of prematurity and thermal stress in these infants.

VLBW and ELBW infants, with thin skin and almost no subcutaneous fat, can control body heat loss or gain only within a limited range of environmental temperatures. In these infants heat loss from radiation, evaporation, and transepidermal water loss is three to five times greater than in larger in-

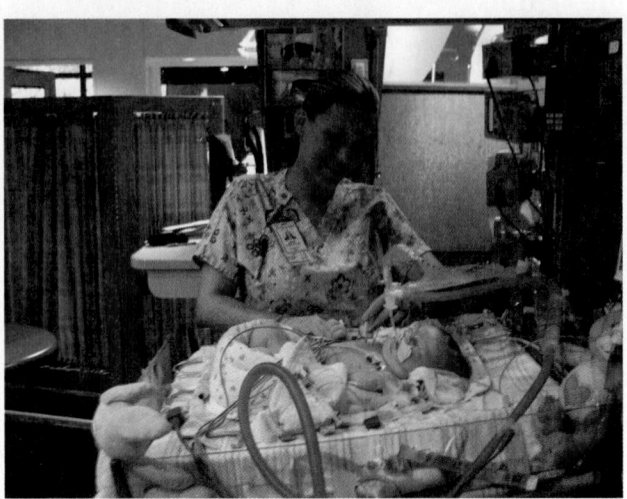

FIG. 9-6 ■ Nurse caring for infant in a radiant warmer. (Photo courtesy E. Jacobs, Texas Children's Hospital, Houston.)

FIG. 9-7 ■ Infant under plastic wrap, which produces a draft-free environment. (Photo courtesy E. Jacobs, Texas Children's Hospital, Houston.)

fants, and a decrease in body temperature is associated with an increase in mortality. Further research is needed to define a neutral thermal environment for the ELBW infant.

The consequences of cold stress that produce additional hazards to the neonate are (1) hypoxia, (2) metabolic acidosis, and (3) hypoglycemia. Increased metabolism in response to chilling creates a compensatory increase in oxygen and calorie consumption. If available oxygen is not increased to accommodate this need, arterial oxygen tension is decreased. This is further complicated by a smaller lung volume in relation to the metabolic rate, which creates diminished oxygen in the blood and concurrent pulmonary disorders. A small advantage is gained by the presence of fetal hemoglobin because its increased capacity to carry oxygen allows the infant to exist for longer periods in conditions of lowered oxygen tension.

The three primary methods for maintaining a neutral thermal environment are the use of an incubator, a radiant warming panel (Fig. 9-6), and an open bassinet with cotton blankets. The dressed infant under blankets can maintain a certain temperature within a wider range of environmental temperatures; however, the close observations required with a high-risk infant are best accomplished if the infant remains partially unclothed. The incubator should always be prewarmed before placing an infant in it. The use of **double-walled incubators** significantly improves the infant's ability to maintain a desirable temperature and reduce energy expenditure related to heat regulation. Inside or outside the incubator, head coverings are effective in preventing heat loss. A fabric-insulated or wool cap is more effective than one fashioned from stockinette. The use of a heated gel mattress with radiant heat has been shown to significantly decrease the incidence of radiation heat loss and preserve an adequate neutral thermal environment for the VLBW neonate (L'Herault, Petroff, and Jeffrey, 2001).

An effective means for maintaining the desired range of temperature in the infant is the use of a **manually adjusted** or **automatically controlled (servo-controlled) incubator.** The latter mechanism, when set at the upper and lower limits of the desired circulating air temperature range, adjusts auto-

matically in response to signals from a thermal sensor attached to the abdominal skin. If the infant's temperature drops, the warming device is triggered to increase heat output. The servo control is usually set to a desired skin temperature between 36° and 36.5° C (96.8° and 97.7° F) (Blake and Murray, 2006).

A high-humidity atmosphere contributes to body temperature maintenance by reducing **evaporative heat loss.** A number of "microenvironments" may be used with the VLBW and ELBW infant to minimize evaporative and **insensible water losses.** These include items such as food-grade plastic bags or plastic wrap, humidified reservoirs for incubators, and humidified plastic heat shields covered with plastic wrap (Fig. 9-7). When such environments are used, special care must be taken to avoid bacterial contamination of the warm and humid environment by organisms such as *Pseudomonas* and *Serratia*, which have an affinity for moist environments; postnatally acquired pneumonia from such organisms may be fatal, particularly in VLBW infants. A systematic review of practices to decrease hypothermia at birth in LBW infants found that plastic wraps or bags kept preterm infants warmer, leading to higher temperatures on admission to neonatal units and less hypothermia (McCall, Alderdice, Halliday, and others, 2005). This practice is now recommended in the Neonatal Resuscitation Program guidelines published by the American Heart Association (2005).

Skin-to-skin (kangaroo) contact between the stable preterm infant and parent is also a viable option for interaction because of the maintenance of appropriate body temperature by the infant. Other benefits of skin-to-skin contact are discussed later in this chapter.

Protection from Infection

Protection from infection is an integral part of all newborn care, but preterm and sick neonates are particularly susceptible. The protective environment of a regularly cleaned and changed incubator provides effective isolation from airborne infective agents. However, thorough, meticulous, and frequent hand washing is the foundation of a preventive program. This includes *all* persons who come in contact with infants and their equipment. After handling another infant or equipment, no one ever touches an infant without first washing hands.

Personnel with infectious disorders are either barred from the unit until they are no longer infectious or are required to wear suitable shields, such as masks or gloves, to reduce the likelihood of contamination. An annual influenza vaccination is recommended for NICU personnel. **Standard precautions** as a method of infection control are instituted in all nursery areas to protect the infants and staff (see Chapter 22). The benefit of "gowning" by visitors and hospital staff to control infection is not supported by research. Sibling visitation in the NICU has not been shown to increase nosocomial infections (Polak, Ringler, and Daugherty, 2004).

The sources of infection rise in direct relationship to the number of persons and pieces of equipment coming in contact with the infants. Equipment used in the care of infants is cleaned on a regular basis in accordance with the manufacturer's recommendations or institutional protocol; this includes cleaning of cribs, mattresses, incubators, radiant warmers, cardiorespiratory monitors, pulse oximeters, and vital sign–monitoring equipment after usage with one infant and before usage with another. Because organisms thrive best in water, plumbing fixtures and humidifying equipment are particularly hazardous. Disposable equipment used for water-related therapies, such as nebulizers and plastic tubing, is changed regularly.

Hydration

High-risk infants often receive supplemental parenteral fluids to supply additional calories, electrolytes, or water. Adequate hydration is particularly important in preterm infants because their extracellular water content is higher (70% in full-term infants and up to 90% in preterm infants), their body surface is larger, and the capacity for osmotic diuresis is limited in preterm infants' underdeveloped kidneys. Therefore these infants are highly vulnerable to fluid depletion.

Parenteral fluids may be given to the high-risk neonate via several routes depending on the nature of the illness, the duration and type of fluid therapy, and unit preference. Common routes of fluid infusion include peripheral, peripherally inserted central venous (or percutaneous central venous), surgically inserted central venous, and umbilical venous catheters. The preferred sites for peripheral intravenous (IV) infusions in neonates are the peripheral veins on the dorsal surfaces of the hands or feet. Alternative sites are scalp veins and antecubital veins. Special precautions and frequent observations must accompany the use of peripheral lines (Beauman and Swanson, 2006). In many neonatal centers the percutaneous central venous catheter is used for parenteral therapy and medication administration because of less expense and decreased neonatal trauma.

In most facilities NICU nurses insert peripheral IV catheters and maintain the infusions. IVs must always be delivered by continuous infusion pumps that deliver minute volumes at a preset flow rate. The catheter is secured to the skin with a minimum amount of tape (see Skin Care, p. 259), with care taken not to cause undue pressure from the catheter hub and tubing. Because all infants, especially those who are ELBW and VLBW, are highly vulnerable to any fluid shifts, infusion rates are carefully regulated and checked hourly to prevent tissue damage from extravasation, fluid overload, or dehydration. Pulmonary edema, congestive heart failure, patent duc-

tus arteriosus, and intraventricular hemorrhage may occur with fluid overload. Dehydration may cause electrolyte disturbances with potentially serious CNS effects.

Infants who are ELBW, tachypneic, receiving phototherapy, or in a radiant warmer have increased insensible water losses that require appropriate fluid adjustments. Nurses must monitor fluid status by daily (or more frequent) weights and accurate intake and output of all fluids, including medications and blood products. Urine-specific gravity and dipstick measurements are monitored per unit protocol, and serum electrolytes are obtained as warranted by the infant's condition. ELBW infants often require more frequent monitoring of these parameters because of their inordinate transepidermal fluid loss, immature renal function, and propensity to dehydration or overhydration. Intolerance of even dextrose 5% is not uncommon in the ELBW infant, with subsequent glycosuria and osmotic diuresis. Alterations in behavior, alertness, or activity level in these infants receiving IV fluids may signal an electrolyte imbalance, hypoglycemia, or hyperglycemia. The nurse is also observant for tremors or seizures in the VLBW or ELBW infant, since these may be a sign of hyponatremia or hypernatremia.

> **NURSING ALERT**
>
> Nurses should be constantly alert for signs of IV infiltration (e.g., erythema, edema, color change of tissue, blanching at site) and for signs of overhydration (weight gain of more than 30 g [1 ounce] in 24 hours, periorbital edema, tachypnea, and crackles on lung auscultation).

A common problem observed in infants who have an umbilical artery catheter in place is vasoconstriction of peripheral vessels, which can seriously impair circulation. The response is triggered by arterial vasospasm caused by the presence of the catheter, the infusion of fluids, or injection of medication. Blanching of the buttocks, genitalia, or legs or feet is an indication of vasospasm. The problem is recognized promptly and reported to the practitioner. The nurse must also observe for signs of thrombi in infants with umbilical venous or arterial lines. The precipitation of microthrombi in the vascular bed with the use of such catheters is commonly manifested by a sudden bluish discoloration seen in the toes, called **catheter toes.** The problem is promptly reported to the practitioner because failure to alleviate the existing pathologic condition may result in the loss of toes or even a foot or leg.

> **NURSING ALERT**
>
> Circulatory effects are observed first in the toes but may extend to include the legs and buttocks. The toes first flush and then turn a mulberry color; if the condition is not corrected, there may be serious complications involving the loss of a limb. The infant with an umbilical venous or arterial catheter should also be observed closely for catheter dislodging and subsequent bleeding or hemorrhage; urinary output, renal function, and gastrointestinal function are also evaluated in these infants. Although the intent of such catheters is to effectively deliver IV fluids (and sometimes medications) and to obtain arterial blood gas samples, they are not without inherent complications.

Nutrition

Optimum nutrition is critical in the management of LBW and preterm infants, but there are difficulties in providing for their nutritional needs. The various mechanisms for ingestion and digestion of foods are not fully developed; the more immature the infant, the greater the problem. In addition, the nutritional requirements for this group of infants are not known with certainty. It is known that all preterm infants are at risk because of poor nutritional stores and several physical and developmental characteristics.

An infant's nutritional needs for rapid growth and daily maintenance must be met in the presence of several anatomic and physiologic disabilities. Although some sucking and swallowing activities are demonstrated before birth and in preterm infants, coordination of these mechanisms does not occur until approximately 32 to 34 weeks of gestation, and they are not fully synchronized until 36 to 37 weeks. Initial sucking is not accompanied by swallowing, and esophageal contractions are uncoordinated. Consequently, infants are highly prone to aspiration and its attendant dangers. As infants mature, the suck-swallow pattern develops but is slow and ineffectual, and these reflexes may also become easily exhausted.

The amount and method of feeding are determined by the infant's size and condition. Nutrition can be provided by either the parenteral or enteral route or by a combination of the two. Infants who are ELBW, VLBW, or critically ill often obtain the majority of their nutrients by the parenteral route because of their inability to digest and absorb enteral nutrition. Illness factors resulting in hypoxia and major organ immaturity further preclude the use of enteral feeding until the infant's condition has stabilized; necrotizing enterocolitis (NEC) has previously been associated with enteral feedings in acutely ill or distressed infants (see Necrotizing Enterocolitis, p. 297). Total parenteral nutritional support of acutely ill infants may be accomplished successfully with commercially available IV solutions specifically designed to meet the infant's nutritional needs, including protein, amino acids, trace minerals, vitamins, carbohydrates (dextrose), and fat (lipid emulsion).

Studies have shown that there are benefits to the early introduction of small amounts of enteral feedings in metabolically stable preterm infants. These **minimal enteral (trophic gastrointestinal priming) feedings** have been shown to stimulate the infant's gastrointestinal tract, preventing mucosal atrophy and subsequent enteral feeding difficulties. Minimal enteral feedings with as little as 0.1 to 4 ml/kg breast milk or preterm formula may be given by gavage as early as the second or third postnatal day. These minimal enteral feedings have been shown to simulate the infant's gastrointestinal tract, preventing mucosal atrophy and subsequent enteral feeding difficulties. Parenteral hydration and nutrition are continued until the infant is able to tolerate an amount of enteral feeding sufficient to sustain growth. An increased incidence of NEC in those VLBW infants receiving minimal enteral nutrition has not been substantiated (Reynolds and Thureen, 2007). In fact, minimal enteral feedings have been proved to increase mineral absorption, increase serum calcium and alkaline phosphatase activity, and substantially decrease the incidence of bilious gastric residuals and feeding intolerance in preterm infants (Schanler, Shulman, Lau, and others, 1999). Minimal enteral feedings have been recommended as the standard of care for feeding VLBW infants (Kliegman, 2003).

Although the timing of the first feeding has been a matter of controversy, most authorities now believe that early feeding (provided that the infant is medically stable) reduces the incidence of complicating factors, such as hypoglycemia and dehydration, and the degree of hyperbilirubinemia. The feeding regimen used varies in different units. The initial enteral feeding is usually not attempted until infants have adapted to extrauterine existence as evidenced by adequate oxygenation; gastrointestinal motility, including passage of meconium; and stable cardiopulmonary status.

Breastfeeding. There is now sufficient evidence indicating that human milk is the best source of nutrition for term and preterm infants. Studies indicate that preterm infants as young as 32 weeks are able to breastfeed if they have adequate sucking and swallowing reflexes and there are no other contraindications, such as respiratory complications or concurrent illness (McCain, 2003). Mothers who wish to breastfeed their preterm infants are encouraged to pump their breasts until their infants are sufficiently stable to tolerate breastfeeding. Appropriate guidelines for the storage of **expressed mother's milk** should be followed to decrease the risk of milk contamination and destruction of its beneficial properties.

Preterm infants may be able to successfully breastfeed earlier than previously believed (32 to 36 weeks); in addition, preterm infants who are breast-fed rather than bottle-fed demonstrate fewer incidences of oxygen desaturation; absence of bradycardia; warmer skin temperature; and better coordination of breathing, sucking, and swallowing (Gardner, Snell, and Lawrence, 2006). The preterm infant should be carefully evaluated for readiness to breastfeed, including assessment of behavioral state, ability to maintain body temperature outside an artificial heat source, respiratory status, and readiness to suckle at the mother's breast. The latter may be accomplished with nonnutritive suckling at the breast during skin-to-skin (kangaroo) contact so that the mother and newborn may become accustomed to each other (Gardner, Snell, and Lawrence, 2006). Nasal cannula oxygen may also be provided during preterm breastfeeding on the basis of the infant's assessed requirements.

Time, patience, and dedication on the part of the mother and the nursing staff are needed to help infants with breastfeeding. The process is begun slowly—beginning with one feeding daily and gradually increasing the feedings as the infant tolerates them. Supplementary bottle feeding is inefficient because the infant expends energy and calories to feed twice. Supplementing by gavage feeding or using a training nipple is more energy and calorie efficient. Breastfeeding the preterm infant often requires additional guidance by a lactation consultant; continued support and encouragement by the nursing staff and family members are essential. In addition, postdischarge breastfeeding often requires further guidance, counseling, and support by nursing staff (McCain, 2003).

For those infants who cannot be breast-fed but who also cannot survive except on human milk, banked **donor milk** is important. Because of the antiinfective and growth-promoting properties of human milk, as well as its superior nutrition, donor milk is used in many NICUs for preterm or sick infants when the mother's own milk is not available (American Academy of Pediatrics, 2005a). Donor milk is also used therapeutically for medical purposes, such as in transplant recipients who are immunocompromised. Unprocessed human milk from unscreened donors is not recommended because of the risk of transmission of infectious agents (American Academy of Pediatrics, 2005a).

The Human Milk Banking Association of North America* has established guidelines for the operation of donor human

---

*http://www.hmbana.org.

milk banks. Donor milk banks collect, screen, process (pasteurize), and distribute milk donated by breastfeeding mothers who are feeding their own infants and pumping a few extra ounces each day for the milk bank.

Nipple Feeding. Vigorous infants can be fed from a nipple with little difficulty, whereas compromised preterm infants will require alternative methods. The amount to be fed is determined largely by the infant's weight gain and tolerance of previous feeding and is increased by small increments until a satisfactory caloric intake is ensured.

The rate of increase that is well tolerated varies from one infant to another, and determining this rate is often a nursing responsibility. Preterm infants require more time and patience to feed compared with full-term infants, and the oropharyngeal mechanism may be stressed by an attempt to feed too rapidly. It is important not to tire the infants or overtax their capacity to retain the feedings. When infants require a prolonged time (arbitrarily, more than 30 minutes) to complete a feeding, gavage feeding may be considered for the next time.

A developmental approach to feeding considers the individual infant's readiness rather than initiating feedings based on weight and age or a predetermined time schedule. **Feeding readiness** is determined by each infant's medical status, energy level, ability to sustain a brief quiet alert state, gag reflex (demonstrated with a gavage tube insertion), spontaneous rooting and sucking behaviors, and functional sucking reflex (McCain, 2003). The preterm infant may experience difficulty coordinating sucking, swallowing, and breathing, with resultant apnea, bradycardia, and decreased oxygen saturation. The infant's ability to suck on a pacifier does not indicate complete readiness for nipple feeding or ability to coordinate the above-mentioned activities without some degree of stress; a gradual introduction of nippling in preterm infants is based on careful evaluation of their ability to maintain adequate cardiopulmonary functions while feeding. When infants are unable to tolerate bottle feedings, intermittent feedings by gavage are instituted until they gain enough strength and coordination to use the nipple.

NURSING ALERT

Poor feeding behaviors such as apnea, bradycardia, cyanosis, pallor, and decreased oxygen saturation in any infant who has previously fed well may indicate an underlying illness.

The nipple used should be relatively firm and stable. Although a high-flow, pliable nipple requires less energy to use, it may provide a flow rate that is too rapid for some preterm infants to manage without risk of aspiration. A firmer nipple facilitates a more "cupped" tongue configuration and allows for a more controlled, manageable flow rate.

The infant is positioned in the feeder's arms or placed semiupright in the lap (Fig. 9-8) and is held with the back curved slightly to simulate the position assumed naturally by most full-term newborns. The use of gentle cheek and jaw support for preterm infants has been shown to facilitate feedings. Stroking the infant's lips, cheeks, and tongue before feeding helps promote oral sensitivity. Inward and upward support to the infant's cheeks and a slightly upward lift to the chin are provided by the fingers to assist nipple compression during feeding.

Bottle feedings are continued if infants are able to tolerate the feedings and take the required amount. Some preterm

FIG. 9-8 ■ Nipple feeding the preterm infant. **A,** Infant is first brought to a quiet alert state in preparation for feeding. **B,** After readiness is demonstrated, infant is nipple fed. (Courtesy Jeff Barnes, Education and Eastern Oklahoma Perinatal Center, St. Francis Hospital, Tulsa.)

infants respond more slowly than full-term infants; therefore the feeding interval and the amount of the feeding are individualized. Preterm infants are often slow feeders and require patience, frequent rest periods, and burping (or bubbling).

Gavage Feeding. Gavage feeding is a safe means of meeting the nutritional requirements of infants who are unable to feed orally. These infants are usually too weak to suck effectively, are unable to coordinate swallowing, and lack a gag reflex. Gavage feedings may be provided by continuous drip regulated via infusion pump or by intermittent bolus feedings. Studies have demonstrated an overall decrease in total milk fat concentration delivery when continuous gavage infusions are administered, which suggests that intermittent or bolus gavage of expressed mother's milk be administered when possible (Premji, Paes, Jacobson, and others, 2002). Intermittent gavage feeding is used as an energy-conserving technique for infants learning to nipple feed who become excessively tired, listless, or cyanotic.

A size 3.5, 5, 6, or 8 French feeding tube is used to instill the feeding, and the usual methods for determining correct placement are used (see Chapter 22 for technique). Although the more relaxed lower esophageal sphincter makes passage of the tube easier, there may be changes in heart rate and BP in response to vagal stimulation. For intermittent feeding it is preferable to insert the tube through the mouth rather than the nares. Nasal insertion obstructs nose breathing and may irritate the delicate nasal mucosa. Passage through the mouth also provides an opportunity to observe the sucking response. However, because of less stimulation of the gag reflex, nasal tube gavage may be used in certain situations, such as when continuous or frequent feedings (every 2 hours) are required or in older preterm infants who need supplementation after nipple feeding but who fight, gag, and vomit with oral tube management. When an indwelling tube is required, consideration should be given to using a product made of Silastic rather than polyvinyl chloride (PVC), since PVC becomes stiff when exposed to body fluids.

The stomach is aspirated, the contents measured, and the aspirate returned as part of the feeding. However, this practice may vary depending on circumstances and individual unit protocol. The amount of aspirate depends on the time since the previous feeding or concurrent illness. Some advocate deducting the amount aspirated to avoid overdistending the stomach.

The milk or formula is allowed to flow by gravity, and the length of time varies. This procedure is not used as a timesaving method for the nurse. Complications of indwelling tubes include aspiration, obstructed nares, mucous plugs, purulent rhinitis, epistaxis, infection, and possible stomach perforation.

> **NURSINGALERT**
>
> Contamination of powdered infant formula in hospitals by *Enterobacter sakazakii* has been associated with serious neonatal infections, NEC, and death (Forsythe, 2005). When possible, alternatives to powdered formula should be chosen; otherwise such formula should be carefully mixed in a designated preparation room using aseptic technique, and continuous infusion of powdered formula should not exceed 4 hours (Centers for Disease Control and Prevention, 2002a).

The nurse must observe preterm infants closely for behaviors that indicate readiness for oral feedings. These include:

- A strong, vigorous suck
- Coordination of sucking and swallowing
- A gag reflex
- Sucking on the gavage tube, hands, or a pacifier
- Rooting and wakefulness before and sleeping after feedings

When these behaviors are noted, infants can be challenged with nipple feedings that are introduced slowly.

The infant may be held during gavage feedings by the caregiver or parent. Oxygen may be supplied via nasal cannula to facilitate handling. It is not recommended that the infant be removed from a primary source of oxygen for feedings, since doing so decreases oxygen availability. **Nonnutritive sucking (NNS)** on a pacifier may help bring the infant to a quiet alert state in preparation for feeding. Proposed benefits of NNS include improved weight gain, improved milk intake, more

stable heart rate and oxygen saturation, earlier age at full oral feeds, and improved behavioral state. A systematic review of NNS found that infants receiving NNS were discharged significantly earlier than non-NNS infants and also experienced a more rapid transition from tube to bottle feedings and better bottle-feeding performance. Support for the other benefits of NNS were less consistent (Pinelli and Symington, 2005).

> **NURSINGALERT**
>
> An increase in gastric residuals, abdominal distention, bilious vomiting, temperature instability, apneic episodes, and bradycardia may be indicative of early NEC and should be reported to the practitioner.

Feeding Resistance

Any feeding technique that bypasses the mouth precludes the opportunity for the child to practice sucking and swallowing, or to experience normal hunger and satiation cycles. Infants may demonstrate aversion to oral feedings by such behaviors as averting the head to the presentation of the nipple, extruding the nipple by tongue thrust, gagging, or even vomiting.

Other observations include disinterest in or active resistance to oral play, diminished spontaneity and motivation, and shallow interpersonal relationships, probably related to the absence of some early incorporative patterns of normal oral experiences. The longer the period of nonoral feeding, the more severe the feeding problems, especially if this period occurs during a time when the infant progresses from reflexive to learned and voluntary feeding actions. Infancy is the period during which the mouth is the primary instrument for reception of stimulation and pleasure.

Infants identified as being at risk for feeding resistance should be provided with regular oral stimulation such as stroking the oral area from cheeks to lips, touching the tongue, placing some of the feeding on the lips and tongue, and associating feeding with pleasurable activities (holding, talking, making eye contact) based on the child's developmental level. Those who exhibit feeding aversion should begin a stimulation program to overcome resistance and acquire the ability to take nourishment by the oral route. Because management requires long-term commitment, successful implementation of a plan for oral stimulation depends on maximum parental involvement and promotion of primary nursing (see Family Focus box).

Energy Conservation

One of the major goals of care for the high-risk infant is conservation of energy. Much of the care described in this section is directed toward this end (e.g., disturbing the infant as little

> ## FAMILY FOCUS
>
> ### Feeding Resistance
>
> Our son was in the NICU for several months. Now at 6 years of age he is normal in every way except one—he refuses almost all food. He lives on a diet of mashed bananas, mashed potatoes, fruit juice, milk, and a daily multivitamin-mineral pill. Getting him to eat has been a 6-year battle that we have lost. Now I know that simple oral stimulation techniques could have prevented or lessened this problem. Please tell nurses the importance of these interventions when any infant is NPO for a prolonged time.
>
> *—A mother and a nurse*

as possible, maintaining a neutral thermal environment, gavage feeding as appropriate, promoting oxygenation, judiciously implementing any caregiving activities that increase oxygen intake and caloric consumption). The infant who is not required to expend excess energy to breathe, eat, or alter body temperature can use this energy for growth and development. Diminishing environmental noise levels and shading the infant from bright lights also promote rest (see Developmental Outcome, p. 261).

Early in hospitalization, the prone position is best for most preterm infants and results in improved oxygenation, better-tolerated feedings, and more organized sleep-rest patterns. Infants exhibit less physical activity and energy expenditure when placed in the prone position (Fig. 9-9). Prolonged supine positioning for preterm infants is not desirable, since they appear to lose their sense of equilibrium when supine and use vital energy in attempts to recover balance by postural changes. In addition, prolonged supine positioning is associated with long-term problems such as decreased flexion of the limbs, pelvis, and trunk; widely abducted hips (frog-leg position); retracted and abducted shoulders; ankle and foot eversion; increased neck extension; and increased trunk extension with neck and back arching (Holditch-Davis, Blackburn, and VandenBerg, 2003). The American Academy of Pediatrics (2005b) continues to affirm its position that *healthy* infants be placed to sleep in a supine position.* When medically stable, preterm infants should also be placed in a supine position to sleep unless conditions such as gastroesophageal reflux or upper airway anomalies make this impractical (see also Sudden Infant Death Syndrome, Chapter 11). Prone positioning for play should be provided in the nursery and encouraged after discharge.

Skin Care

The skin of preterm infants is characteristically immature relative to that of full-term infants. In most preterm infants the skin barrier properties resemble those of the term infant

---

*Information is available from the National Institute of Child Health and Human Development's SIDS: "Back to Sleep" Campaign, http://www.nichd.nih.gov/sids.

by 2 to 4 weeks' postnatal age, regardless of gestational age at birth. Because of its increased sensitivity and fragility, no alkaline-based soap that might destroy the skin's **acid mantle** is used. The increased permeability of the skin facilitates absorption of ingredients. All skin products (e.g., alcohol or povidone-iodine) should be used with caution; the skin is rinsed with water afterward because these substances may cause severe irritation and chemical burns in VLBW and ELBW infants.

The skin is easily excoriated and denuded; therefore care must be taken to avoid damage to the delicate structure. The total skin is thinner than that of full-term infants and lacks **rete pegs,** appendages that anchor the epidermis to the dermis. Therefore there is less cohesion between the thinner skin layers. The use of adhesive tape or bandages may excoriate the skin or adhere to the skin surface so well that the epidermis can be separated from the dermis and pulled away with the tape. The use of pectin barriers and hydrocolloid adhesives may be useful, since these products mold well to skin contours and adhere in moist conditions. Recommendations for protecting the integrity of the skin of preterm infants include using minimal adhesive tape, backing the tape with cotton, and delaying adhesive and pectin barrier removal until adherence is reduced (Lund and Kuller, 2003). Emollients such as Eucerin or Aquaphor have been used to promote skin integrity and prevent dry, cracking, and peeling skin in infants at risk for skin breakdown; however, the use of such agents should be weighed against the increased risk for coagulase-negative infections in preterm infants (Edwards, Conner, Soll, and others, 2004).

It is unsafe to use scissors to remove dressings or tape from the extremities of very small and immature infants, since it is easy to snip off tiny extremities or nick loosely attached skin. Solvents used to remove tape are avoided because they tend to dry and burn the delicate skin. Guidelines for skin care are listed in the Nursing Care Guidelines box.

During skin assessment of preterm infants, nurses are alert to the subtle signs that indicate **zinc deficiency,** a problem sometimes seen in infants who have inadequate intake or abnormal losses of zinc. Breakdown usually occurs in the areas around the mouth, buttocks, fingers, and toes. In preterm and

FIG. 9-9 ■ **A,** Preterm infant slowly transitioned to prone position on prone roll. **B,** Preterm infant positioned on prone roll. (Courtesy Halbouty Premature Nursery, Texas Children's Hospital, Houston; photos by Paul Vincent Kuntz.)

nursingcareguidelines

Neonatal Skin Care

GENERAL SKIN CARE
Assessment
Assess skin every day or more often as needed for redness, dryness, flaking, scaling, rashes, lesions, excoriation, or breakdown.

Identify risk factors for skin injury: gestational age <30 weeks, adhesive use, high-frequency ventilation, ECMO, hypotension requiring vasopressors.

Use a valid assessment tool to provide reliable and objective measurement of skin condition.

Evaluate and report abnormal skin findings and analyze for possible causes.

Intervene according to interpretation of findings or physician order.

Bathing
Initial Bath
Assess for stable temperature a minimum of 2 to 4 hours before first bath.

Use cleansing agents with neutral pH or minimal dyes or perfume, in water.

Use universal precautions; wear gloves.

Do not completely remove vernix; allow vernix to wear off with normal care and handling.

Bathe preterm infant younger than 32 weeks in warm water only for the first week.

Routine
Decrease frequency of baths to every second or third day by daily cleansing of eye, oral, and diaper areas and pressure points.

Use cleanser or soaps no more than two or three times a week.

Avoid rubbing skin during bathing or drying.

Immerse stable infants fully (except head) in an appropriate-size tub.

Use swaddled immersion bathing technique: slow unwrapping after gently lowering into water for sensitive, but stable, infants needing assistance with motor system reactivity.

Emollients
Apply sparingly to dry, flaking, fissured areas as needed.

Chose petrolatum-based products that are free of preservatives, dyes, and perfumes.

Observe neonates <750 g receiving emollient therapy for increased risk of coagulase-negative *Staphylococcus* infections.

Consider dispensing emollients from hospital pharmacy, unit dose, or patient-specific container.

Adhesives
Decrease use as much as possible.

Use semipermeable dressings to secure intravenous lines (IVs), NG/OG tubes, silicone catheters, and central lines.

Use hydrogel or limb electrodes.

Consider pectin barriers beneath adhesives to protect skin.

Secure pulse oximeter probe or electrodes with elasticized dressing material (carefully avoid restricting blood flow).

Do not use adhesive remover, solvents, or bonding agents.

Avoid removing adhesives for at least 24 hours after application.

Adhesive removal can be facilitated using water, mineral oil, or petrolatum.

Remove adhesives or skin barriers slowly, supporting the skin underneath with one hand and gently peeling away the product from the skin with the other hand.*

Antiseptic Agents
Apply before invasive procedures.

Consider the potential for skin breakdown or irritation with disinfectant.

No specific disinfectant is recommended over another for all neonates; remove completely with water or saline after use.

Avoid use of isopropyl alcohol for skin prep or removal of other disinfectants.

Transepidermal Water Loss (TEWL)
Minimize TEWL and heat loss in small preterm infants at less than 30 weeks of gestation by:
- Measuring ambient humidity during first weeks of life
- Apply occlusive polyethylene body bag immediately at delivery and remove after infant is stabilized in the NICU.
- Consider increasing humidity to 70% to 90% by using a humidified incubator for first 7 days; decrease to 50% until 28 days of age.
- Use supplemental conductive heat and reduce radiant heat source.
- Apply semipermeable transparent dressings to skin surfaces on infant's chest, abdomen and back.

SKIN BREAKDOWN
Prevention
Decrease pressure from externally applied forces using water, air, or gel mattresses; sheepskin; or cotton bedding.

Provide adequate nutrition, including protein, fat, and zinc.

Apply transparent adhesive dressings to protect arms, elbows, and knees from friction injury.

Use tracheostomy and gastrostomy dressings (Hydrasorb or Lyofoam) for drainage and relief of pressure from trach or gastrostomy tube.

Use emollient in the diaper area (groin and thighs) to reduce urine irritation.

Treating Skin Breakdown
Irrigate wound every 4 to 8 hours with warm half-strength normal saline using a 20-ml or larger syringe and 20-gauge Teflon catheter.

Culture wound and treat if signs of infection are present (excessive redness, swelling, pain on touch, heat, or resistance to healing).

Use transparent adhesive dressing for uninfected wounds.

Apply hydrogel with or without antibacterial or antifungal ointments (as ordered) for infected wounds (may need to moisten before removal).

Use hydrocolloid for deep, uninfected wounds (leave in place for 5 to 7 days) or as an ostomy barrier and to improve appliance adhesion; warm barrier in hand for several minutes to soften before applying to skin.

Avoid use of antiseptic solutions for wound cleansing (use for intact skin only).

Data from Kuller JM: Skin breakdown: risk factors, prevention, and treatment, *NINR* 1(1):33-42, 2001; Lund CH, Kuller J, Raines DA, and others: *Neonatal skin care: evidence-based clinical practice guideline,* ed 2, Washington, DC, 2007, AWHONN; Johnson FE, Maikler VE: Nurses' adoption of the AWHONN/NANN Neonatal Skin Care Project, *NINR* 1(1):59-67, 2001; Lund CH, Kuller J, Lott JW: Neonatal skin care: clinical outcomes of the AWHONN/NANN evidence-based clinical practice guideline, *J Obstet Gynecol Neonatal Nurs* 30(1):41-51, 2001; Taquino LT: Promoting wound healing in the neonatal setting: process versus protocol, *J Perinat Neonatal Nurs* 14(1):108-118, 2000; Lund C, Lane A, Raines DA: Neonatal skin care: the scientific basis for practice, *J Obstet Gynecol Neonatal Nurs* 28(3):241-254, 1999; Malloy MB, Perez-Woods R: Neonatal skin care: prevention of skin breakdown, *Pediatr Nurs* 17(1):41-48, 1991.

*CAUTION: Scissors are not to be used for tape or dressing removal because of hazard of cutting skin or amputating tiny digits.

nursingcareguidelines

Neonatal Skin Care—cont'd

SKIN BREAKDOWN—cont'd
Treating Diaper Dermatitis
Maintain clean, dry skin; use absorbent diapers and change often.
If mild irritation occurs, use petrolatum barrier.
For developing dermatitis, apply a generous quantity of zinc-oxide barrier.
For severe dermatitis, identify cause and treat (frequent stooling from spina bifida, severe opiate withdrawal, or malabsorption syndrome).
Treat *Candida albicans* with antifungal ointment or cream.
Avoid powders and antibiotic ointments. (See Cord and Circumcision Care, Chapter 8.)

OTHER SKIN CARE CONCERNS
Use of Substances on Skin
Evaluate all substances that come in contact with infant's skin.
Before using any topical agent, analyze components of preparation and:
  ■ Use sparingly and only when necessary.
  ■ Confine use to smallest possible area.
  ■ Whenever possible and appropriate, wash off with water.
  ■ Monitor infant carefully for signs of toxicity and systemic effects.

Use of Thermal Devices
Avoid heat lamps because of increased potential for burns. If needed, measure actual temperature of exposed skin every 15 minutes.
When using heating pads:
  ■ Change infant's position every 15 minutes initially and then every 1 to 2 hours.
  ■ Preset temperature of heating pads to less than 40° C (104° F).

When using preheated transcutaneous electrodes:
  ■ Avoid use on infants.
  ■ Set at lowest possible temperature.
  ■ Use pulse oximetry rather than transcutaneous monitoring whenever possible.
When prewarming heels before phlebotomy, avoid temperatures over 40° C.
Provide warm ambient humidity, directed away from infant; use aerosolized sterile water and maintain ambient temperature so as to not exceed 40° C.
Document use of all heating devices.

Use of Fluid Therapy and Hemodynamic Monitoring
Be certain fingers or toes are visible whenever extremity is used for peripheral IV or arterial line.
Secure catheter or needle with transparent dressing and tape to promote easy visualization of site.
Assess site hourly for signs of ischemia, infiltration, and inadequate perfusion (check capillary refill, pulses, color).
Avoid use of restraints (e.g., arm boards); if used, check that they are secured safely and not restricting circulation or movement (check for pressure areas).
Use commercial IV protector (e.g., I.V. House) with minimal tape.

VLBW infants it may also occur in the creases of the neck, wrists, and ankles and around wounds. Zinc deficiency is most likely to appear in preterm infants with inadequate zinc intake, an ileostomy, short-bowel syndrome, or chronic diarrhea. Suspicious lesions are reported to the practitioner so that zinc supplements can be prescribed.

Skin injuries have been reported during the use of phototherapy blankets. Caution is warranted in using these products in ELBW infants or infants who are at risk for skin breakdown.

Administration of Medications

Administration of therapeutic agents such as drugs, ointments, IV infusions, and oxygen requires judicious handling and meticulous attention to detail. The computation, preparation, and administration of drugs in minute amounts often require collaboration between nurses, physicians, and pharmacists to reduce the chance for error. In addition, the immaturity of an infant's detoxification mechanisms and inability to demonstrate symptoms of toxicity (e.g., signs of auditory nerve involvement from ototoxic drugs such as gentamicin) complicate drug therapy and require that nurses be particularly alert for signs of adverse reaction (see Administration of Medication, Chapter 22).

Nurses should be aware of the hazards of administering bacteriostatic and hyperosmolar solutions to infants. Benzyl alcohol, a common preservative in bacteriostatic water and saline, has been shown to be toxic to newborns, and products containing this preservative should not be used to flush IV catheters, to dilute or reconstitute medications, or as an anesthetic to start IVs. It is recommended that medications with preservative such as benzyl alcohol be avoided whenever possible. *Nurses must read labels carefully to detect the presence of preservatives in any medication to be administered to an infant.*

Hyperosmolar solutions present a potential danger to preterm infants. Hyperosmolar solutions given orally to infants can produce clinical, physiologic, and morphologic alterations, the most serious of which is NEC. Oral and parenteral medications should be sufficiently diluted to prevent complications related to hyperosmolality.

There has been heightened awareness of the impact of medication errors and subsequent poor outcomes for high-risk neonates. Nurses, physicians, and pharmacists must work in cooperation to implement strategies in the NICU environment to eradicate medication errors. Technology alone has not proved to be the solution; therefore nurses must be extremely vigilant when administering medications to preterm and high-risk infants.

Developmental Outcome

Much attention has been focused on the effects of early developmental intervention on both normal and preterm infants. Infants respond to a great variety of stimuli, and the atmosphere and activities of the NICU are overstimulating. Consequently, infants in the NICU are subjected to *inappropriate* stimulation that can be harmful. For example, the noise level that results from monitoring equipment, alarms, and general unit activity has been correlated with the incidence of intracranial hemorrhage, especially in the ELBW or VLBW infant. Personnel should reduce noise-generating activities, such as closing doors (including incubator portholes), listening to loud radios, talking loudly, and handling equipment (e.g., trash containers). Byers, Waugh, and Lowman (2006) suggest monitoring sound levels in the nursery to address problem areas. Nursing care activities, such as taking vital signs, changing the infant's position, weighing, and changing diapers, are associated with frequent periods of hypoxia, oxygen desaturation, and elevated intracranial pressure. The more immature the infant, the less able he or she is to habituate to a single procedure, such as taking an oscillometric BP, without becoming overstimulated.

Twenty-four-hour surveillance of sick infants implies maximum visibility and often bright lights. Units should establish a night-day sleep pattern by either darkening the room, covering cribs with blankets, or placing eye patches over the infant's eyes at night. Infants need scheduled rest periods during which the lights are dimmed, the incubators are covered with blankets, and the infants are not disturbed for handling of any kind (Holditch-Davis, Blackburn, and VandenBerg, 2003). Sleep periods should be undisturbed for at least 50 minutes to allow complete sleep cycles.

Infants' eyes should be shielded from bright procedure lights to prevent potential harm. Many experts suggest that the human face, especially the parent's, is the best visual stimulus and that visual stimuli be kept to a minimum early in development. Developmental care, accentuating the infant's unique ability to achieve behavioral state organization, is tailored to the developmental level and tolerance of each infant based on a comprehensive behavioral assessment. During the early stages of development (especially before 33 weeks of gestation), external stimulation produces uncoordinated, random activity, such as jerky limb extension, hyperflexion, and irregular vital signs. At this stage infants need to have *minimum* environmental stimulation. Using the developmental model of supportive care, the nurse closely monitors physiologic and behavioral signs to promote organization and well-being of the high-risk infant during handling. Softly calling the infant by name and then gently placing a hand on the body signal care is beginning and alleviate the abrupt interruption that precedes caregiving. Infants are handled with slow, controlled movements (some infants are unstable if moved abruptly), and their random movements are controlled with limbs held flexed close to their bodies during turning or other position changes. This **containment** or **facilitated tucking** may also be used before invasive procedures such as heel stick to alleviate distress. **Blanket swaddling** and **nesting** or containment have been shown to decrease physiologic and behavioral stress during routine care procedures such as bathing, weighing, and heel stick. A nest constructed by placing blanket rolls underneath the bed sheet helps infants maintain an attitude of flexion when prone or side lying.

Although it must be individually adjusted, **skin-to-skin contact (kangaroo care)** and short periods of gentle massage can help reduce stress in preterm infants. Regular passive skin-to-skin contact between parents (mother or father) and LBW infants has been shown to alleviate stress. The parent wears a loose-fitting, open-front top that has a modified marsupial-like pocket carrier for the infant. The undressed (except for

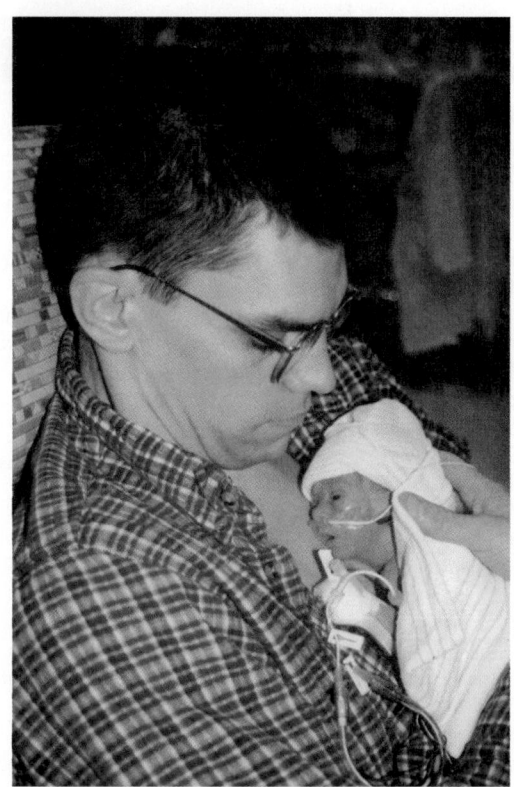

FIG. 9-10 ■ Father providing skin-to-skin (kangaroo) care. (Courtesy Judy Meyr, St Louis.)

diaper) infant is placed in a vertical position on the parent's bare chest, which permits direct eye contact, skin-to-skin sensations, and close proximity (Fig. 9-10). Skin-to-skin contact between parent and infant, in addition to being a safe and effective method for VLBW infant-parent acquaintance, can have a positive healing effect for the mother with a high-risk pregnancy. Mothers may experience psychologic healing related to preterm delivery and regain the mothering role through early skin-to-skin contact with their VLBW infants. Additional benefits of skin-to-skin care include earlier contact with mechanically ventilated infants, maintenance of neonatal thermal stability and oxygen saturation, increased feeding vigor, maintenance of organized state, and minimal untoward effects of being held (Conde-Agudelo, Diaz-Rossello, and Belizan, 2000; Anderson, 1999; Dodd, 2005). In full-term newborns, skin-to-skin contact has a strong analgesic effect during procedures such as heel lance (Ludington-Hoe, Hosseini, and Torowicz, 2005). LBW infants receiving skin-to-skin contact with breastfeeding mothers maintained higher oxygen saturation and were less likely to have desaturations below 90%, and their mothers were more likely to continue breastfeeding both in the hospital and for 1 month after discharge. Kangaroo care of preterm infants fosters appropriate neurobehavioral development by promoting stability of heart and respiratory function, minimizes purposeless movements, offers maternal proximity for attention, improves the infant's behavioral state, and permits self-regulating behaviors (McCain, Ludington-Hoe, Swinth, and others, 2005).

Cobedding of twins (or **multiples**) is another developmental intervention that has been implemented in neonatal intensive care and newborn nurseries to provide a better en-

TABLE 9-2

Signs of Stress or Fatigue in Neonates

SUBSYSTEM	SIGNS OF STRESS
Autonomic	Physiologic instability
Respiratory	Tachypnea, pauses, gasping, sighing
Color	Mottled, flushed, dusky, pale or gray
Visceral	Hiccups, gagging, choking, spitting up, grunting and straining as if having a bowel movement, coughing, sneezing, yawning
Autonomic	Tremors, startles, twitches
Motor	Fluctuating tone; lack of control over movement, activity, and posture
Flaccidity	Low tone in trunk; limp, floppy upper and lower extremities; limp, drooping jaw (gape face)
Hypertonicity	Arm or leg extensions, arm(s) outstretched with fingers splayed in salute gesture, fingers stiffly outstretched, trunk arching, neck hyperextended
Hyperflexion	Trunk, extremities, fisting
Activity	Squirming; frantic, diffuse activity or little or no activity or responsiveness
State	Disorganized quality to state behaviors, including available states, maintenance of state control, and transition from one state to another
Sleep	Whimpering sounds, facial twitching, irregular respirations, fussing, grimacing, restless appearance
Awake	Glazed, unfocused look, staring, worried or pained expression, hyperalert or panicked appearance, eye roving, crying, cry-face, actively averting gaze or closing eyes, irritability, prolonged awake periods, inconsolability, frenzy
	Abrupt or rapid state changes
Other state-related behaviors and attention-interaction	Efforts to attend to and interact with environmental stimulation eliciting signs of stress and disorganized subsystem functioning
Autonomic	Physiologic instability of varying degrees with autonomic, respiratory, color, and visceral responses
Motor	Fluctuating tone, increased motor activity, progressively frantic diffuse activity if stimulation continues
State	Roving eyes, gaze averting, glazed unfocused look, or worried, panicked expression, weak cry, cry-face, irritability
	Closed eyes and sleeplike withdrawal
	Abrupt state changes
	Signs of stress when presented with more than one type of stimulus at a time

Data from Als H: Toward a synactive theory of development: promise for the assessment and support of infant individuality, *Infant Mental Health J* 3(4):229-243, 1982; Als H: A synactive model of neonatal behavior organization: framework for the assessment of neurobehavioral development in the premature infant and for support of infants and parents in the neonatal intensive care environment, *Phys Occup Ther Pediatr* 6:3-55, 1986; Hunter JG: The neonatal intensive care unit. In Case-Smith J, Allen AS, Pratt PN, editors: *Occupational therapy for children*, ed 4, St Louis, 2001, Mosby.

vironment for neonatal growth and development (Altimier and Lutes, 2001; DellaPorta, Aforismo, and Butler-O'Hara, 1998). Cobedding involves placing twins or other multiples together in the same crib or incubator. Preliminary data from a multicenter study indicate that twins who are cobedding have improved thermoregulation, have significantly fewer apnea and bradycardia episodes, gain weight more quickly than their single counterparts, and have decreased length of stay. Parental satisfaction is also significantly greater with cobedded newborns. One major concern with cobedding is cross-transmission of infection between the neonates, but increased infection rates have not occurred with cobedding (LaMar and Dowling, 2006).

Additional research studies have confirmed the beneficial effects of developmental care with preterm infants. In addition to requiring fewer days of mechanical ventilation, preterm infants who received individualized developmental care had shorter hospital stays; a significant decrease in complications such as intraventricular hemorrhage and bronchopulmonary dysplasia; less need for sedation when critically ill; improved neurodevelopmental scores at 9, 18, and 36 months of life; and a decrease in feeding intolerance (Symington and Pinelli, 2003; Westrup, Sizun, and Lagercrantz, 2007).

The arena of developmental care for preterm infants has expanded to include a wide variety of interventions such as infant massage, soothing soft music, recordings of parents reading stories, positioning to enhance self-regulatory abili-

ties, enhancement of hand-to-mouth activities, uninterrupted sleep periods, decreased environmental light and noise, and even the use of stuffed animals to facilitate infant positioning. As a result of such interventions, parents may perceive the NICU environment as less threatening. Active participation in providing such an environment for their special infant also involves the parents in the provision of daily care when the newborn is critically ill and cannot be fed or held.*

When infants have reached sufficient developmental organization and stability, interventions are designed and implemented to support their growing abilities. Nurses and parents become adept at learning to read infants' behavioral cues and supplying appropriate interventions (Table 9-2). Clues include both approach and avoidance behaviors. **Approach behaviors** that are supported and enhanced include tongue extension, hand clasp, hand-to-mouth movements, sucking, looking, and cooing. Signs of stress or fatigue that signal the infant's need for "time-out" are described in Table 9-2.

When infants are recovering and are free of support systems, medically stable, and on room air or smaller amounts of oxygen, they are assessed to document behavioral state organization and ability to self-regulate. When the infant is stable and mature enough to begin developmental intervention, activities

---

*A resource for parents interested in developmental care products is Children's Medical Ventures, 275 Longwater Drive, Norwell, MA 02061; (888) 766-8443; http://www.childmed.com.

nursingcareguidelines

Developmental Interventions

GENERAL GUIDELINES
Individualize interventions for each infant.
Offer stimulus only during periods of alertness.
Begin one type of stimulus at a time.
Provide intervention for short periods.
Space periods according to infant's tolerance.
Continually assess infant's response to developmental interventions.
Titrate interventions according to infant's cues.
Terminate stimulation if infant displays evidence of overstimulation (see Table 9-2).
Provide 50-minute uninterrupted sleep periods.
Handle to promote or maintain behavioral organization, providing for flexion, containment, firm pressure, grasp, and nonnutritive sucking.

TACTILE
Stroke skin slowly and gently in head-to-toe direction (assess tolerance first).
Provide alternate textures (e.g., satin, velvet).
Provide firm boundaries: foot bracing, blankets, "nesting."
Encourage skin-to-skin (kangaroo) holding by parents and siblings as tolerated.
Containment holding in cupped palms of hand provides nesting and comfort.

AUDITORY
Reduce noise levels.
Mother's voice is the best.
Maintain 50 dB with maximum 55 dB for only 10 minutes per hour.
Play tape of parents' and siblings' voices.
Softly play simple, soothing music, recording of womb sounds, or music box for short periods only.*
Call infant by name at each interaction.

VESTIBULAR
Position with limbs and trunk in flexion, with hands to face at midline.
Slowly change position during handling; avoid quick position changes.
Side-to-side slow movement is preferred over rocking.
Place in sling (hammock) and rock.
Close infant's fist around cloth toy.
Lift head to upright position, tip to right and then to left, stopping at midline (only with stable, more mature infants).
Avoid rapid horizontal to vertical movements in ill infant to minimize intracranial pressure and autonomic consequences—desaturation, apnea, bradycardia.

OLFACTORY
Pass open container or a cotton gauze dipped in breast milk or formula under nose.
Place cloth doll that has been in close contact with mother' skin in the infant's bed—avoid perfumes, scented soaps, powders.
Use a pacifier dipped in mother's breast milk during gavage feeding for nonnutritive sucking.

GUSTATORY
Place infant's hand or a pacifier in mouth when sucking movements are observed or during gavage feeding.
Place one or two drops of milk in infant's mouth with each tube feeding.
Provide nonnutritive suckling at mother's breast.

VISUAL
Reduce light levels and protect eyes from direct lights such as examination or procedure lights.
Place photographs of parents and siblings in visual range (19 to 22 cm [7.5 to 8.5 inches]) in en face position (maintain for short periods when awake and alert; constant picture in close proximity may be too much stimulus).
Initiate eye contact; repeat as tolerated once the infant reaches equivalent of 30 weeks of gestation. Monitor carefully for stress responses.

*Suggested infant relaxation music: *Heartbeat Lullabies* by Terry Woodford. Available from Baby-Go-To-Sleep Center, Audio Therapy Innovations, Inc., PO Box 550, Colorado Springs, CO 80901; (800) 537-7748; http://www.babygotosleep.com.

are individualized according to each infant's cues, temperament, state, behavioral organization, and particular needs. Intervention periods are short (e.g., 2 to 3 minutes of voices, 5 minutes of quiet music). Hearing and vestibular interventions are initiated earlier than visual stimulation. One type of intervention at a time is applied to document the infant's tolerance and response (see Nursing Care Guidelines box). An intervention program for convalescing infants includes parents and siblings early in the infant's hospitalization; teaching parents to be responsive to the infant's individual cues is an important function of the NICU nurse. Parents, siblings, and health care providers are encouraged to adhere to the established developmental care plan to avoid disruption in sleep-wake cycles and minimize inappropriate stimuli.

Developmental care of the preterm neonate is an ongoing process in the NICU and is incorporated into the daily care given to each infant. The nurse is cognizant of the preterm infant's developmental needs, temperament, and newborn state, as well as environmental conditions that adversely affect the infant; nursing care is planned accordingly to enhance optimum physical, psychosocial, and neurologic development.

This task is often difficult to accomplish when invasive treatments or interventions are required to stabilize the critically ill neonate.

Family Support and Involvement

Professional health workers often are so absorbed in the lifesaving physical aspects of care that they ignore the emotional needs of infants and their families. The significance of early parent-child interaction and infant stimulation has been documented by reliable research. Nurses, aware of these infant and family needs, must incorporate activities that facilitate family interaction into the nursing care plan.

The birth of a preterm infant is an unexpected and stressful event for which families are emotionally unprepared. They find themselves simultaneously coping with their own needs, the needs of their infant, and the needs of their family (especially when there are other children). To compound the situation, their infant's precarious condition engenders an atmosphere of apprehension and uncertainty. They are faced with multiple crises and overwhelming feelings of responsibility, helplessness, and frustration.

All parents have some anxieties about the outcome of a pregnancy, but after a preterm birth the concern is heightened regarding both the viability and the normalcy of their infant. Mothers may see their infant only briefly before the newborn is removed to the intensive care unit or even to another hospital, leaving them with just the recollection of the infant's very small size and unusual appearance. They often feel alone or lost on the mother-baby unit, belonging neither with mothers who have lost their infants nor with those who have delivered healthy, full-term infants. The staff and physicians are often guarded in discussing the infant's condition; mothers are continually expecting to hear that their infant has died, and they are sensitive to the anxieties of other mothers and staff members. Going home without their infant only compounds their feelings of disappointment, failure, and deprivation.

When an infant is to be transported from the hospital, the parents need a description of the facility where the infant is going. They need to know the location, reputation, and nature of the facility and the care that the infant is expected to receive. The name of the infant's physician and the telephone number of the nursery should be given to them, and unfamiliar terms such as *neonatologist, ventilator, infusion,* and *incubator* should be explained. Explanations are kept simple, and parents are given the opportunity to ask questions. If booklets are available that describe the facility, they are given to the family.

Perhaps most important, the parents should have some contact with the infant before the transport. Being able to see, touch, and (if possible) hold their infant may help decrease the parents' anxiety. Often a photograph, or even a videotape, of their infant can serve as tangible evidence of the newborn's existence until the parents are able to travel to the regional facility. When possible, it is often advisable to transfer the mother to the same institution as her infant.

Parents need to be informed of their infant's progress and reassured that the infant is receiving proper care. They need to understand the smallest aspects of the infant's condition and treatment. Parents need a realistic, honest, and direct assessment of the situation. Using nonmedical terminology, moving at a pace that is comfortable for parents to assimilate the information, and avoiding lengthy technical explanations facilitate communication with family members. Psychologic tasks that must be accomplished by parents during their infant's care are presented in Box 9-2.

Facilitating Parent-Infant Relationships

Because of their physiologic instability, infants are separated from their mothers immediately and surrounded by a complex, impenetrable barrier of glass windows, mechanical equipment, and special caregivers. There is some evidence indicating that the emotional separation that accompanies the physical separation of mothers and infants may interfere with the normal maternal-infant attachment process discussed in Chapter 8. Maternal attachment is a cumulative process that begins before conception, strengthens by significant events during pregnancy, and matures through maternal-infant contact during the neonatal period and infancy.

When an infant is sick, the necessary physical separation appears to be accompanied by an emotional estrangement by the parents, which may seriously damage the capacity for parenting their infant. This detachment is further hampered by

---

BOX 9-2

Psychologic Tasks of Parents of a High-Risk Infant

- Work through the events surrounding labor and delivery.
- Acknowledge that the infant's life is endangered and begin the anticipatory grieving process.
- Confront and recognize feelings of inadequacy and guilt in not delivering a healthy child.
- Adapt to the neonatal intensive care environment.
- Resume parental relationships with the sick infant and initiate the caregiving role.
- Prepare to take the infant home.

Modified from Siegel R, Gardner SL, Merenstein GB: Families in crisis: theoretical and practical considerations. In Merenstein GB, Gardner SL, editors: *Handbook of neonatal intensive care,* ed 6, St Louis, 2006, Mosby.

---

the tenuous nature of the infant's condition. When survival is in doubt, parents may be reluctant to establish a relationship with their infant. They prepare themselves for the infant's death while continuing to hope for recovery. This **anticipatory grief** (see Chapter 18) and hesitancy to embark on a relationship are evidenced by behaviors such as delay in giving the infant a name, reluctance in visiting the nursery (or when they do visit, focusing on equipment and treatments rather than on their infant), and hesitancy to touch or handle the infant when given the opportunity.

Family-centered care of high-risk newborns includes encouraging and facilitating parental involvement rather than isolating parents from their infant and associated care. This is particularly important in relation to mothers; to reduce the effects of physical separation, mothers are united with their newborn at the earliest opportunity.

Preparing the parents to see their infant for the first time is a nursing responsibility. The nurse prepares parents for their infant's appearance, the equipment attached to the child, and the general atmosphere of the unit. The initial encounter with the intensive care unit is a stressful experience, and the frightening array of people, equipment, and activity is likely to be overwhelming. A book of photographs or pamphlets describing the NICU environment (infants in incubators or under radiant warmers, monitors, mechanical ventilators, and IV equipment) provides a useful and nonthreatening introduction to the NICU.

Parents are encouraged to visit their infant as soon as possible. Even if they saw the infant at the time of transport or shortly after birth, the infant may have changed considerably, especially if a number of medical and equipment requirements are associated with the infant's hospitalization. At the bedside the nurse should explain the function of each piece of equipment and the role it plays in facilitating recovery. Explanations may often need to be patiently repeated because parents' anxiety over the infant's condition and the surroundings may prevent them from really "hearing" what is being said. When possible, some items related to therapy can be removed; for example, phototherapy can be temporarily discontinued and eye patches removed to permit eye-to-eye contact.

Parents appreciate the support of a nurse during the initial visit with their infant, but they may also appreciate some time alone with the infant for a short while. It is important during the early visits to emphasize the positive aspects of their infant's behavior and development so that parents can focus on their infant as an individual rather than on the equipment that surrounds the child. For example, the nurse may describe the infant's spontaneous behaviors during care, such as the grasp reflex and spontaneous movement, or make comments about the infant's biologic functions. Most institutions have open visiting policies so that parents and siblings may visit their infant as often as they wish.

Parents vary greatly in the degree to which they are able to interact with their infant. Some may wish to touch or hold their infant during the first visit, whereas others may not feel comfortable enough to even enter the nursery. These reactions depend on a variety of prenatal and postnatal factors, such as the parity of the mother and her preparation before birth; the infant's size, condition, and physical appearance; and the type of treatment the infant is receiving. It is essential to recognize that the individualized pacing and quality of the interactions are more important than an early onset of these interactions. Parents may not be receptive to early and extended infant contact because they need time to adjust to the impact of an infant with birth problems and must be helped to grieve before they can accept their infant.

The parents' inability to focus on their infant is a clue for the nurse to assist the parents in expressing feelings of guilt, anxiety, helplessness, inadequacy, anger, and ambivalence. Nurses can help parents deal with these distressing feelings and recognize that they are normal responses shared by other parents. It is important to point out and reinforce the positive aspects of parents' behavior and interactions with their infant.

Most parents feel shaky and insecure about initiating interaction with their infant. Nurses can sense parents' level of readiness and offer encouragement in these initial efforts. Parents of preterm infants follow the same acquaintance process as do parents of term infants. They may quickly proceed through the process or may require several days, or even weeks, to complete the process. Parents begin by touching their infant's extremities with their fingertips and poking the infant tenderly, and then proceed to caresses and fondling (Figs. 9-11 and 9-12). Touching is the first act of communication between parents and child. Parents need to be prepared for their infant's exaggerated and generalized startle responses to touch so that they will not interpret these as negative reactions to their overtures. It may be necessary to limit tactile stimuli when the infant is critically ill and labile, but the nurse can offer other options such as speaking softly or sitting at the bedside.

Parents of acutely ill preterm infants may express feelings of helplessness and lack of control. Involving the parent in some type of caregiving activity, no matter how minor it may seem to the nurse, enables the parent to "take on" a more active role. Examples of such caregiving for the acutely ill infant who cannot be held and is seemingly not responding positively include moistening the infant's lips with a small amount of sterile water on a cotton-tipped swab or slipping the diaper from under the infant when it is wet or soiled.

Eventually, parents begin to endow their infant with an identity—as part of the family. When an infant no longer appears as a foreign object and begins to take on aspects of family members, such as the father's chin or the sister's nose, nurses can facilitate this incorporation. Parents are encouraged to bring in clothes, a toy, a stuffed animal, or a family snapshot for their infant, and the nurse can help parents set goals for themselves and for the infant. Parents may become

FIG. 9-11 ■ Father interacting with newborn receiving intensive care.

FIG. 9-12 ■ Mother and father interacting with their preterm infant. (Photo courtesy E. Jacobs, Texas Children's Hospital, Houston.)

involved by reading a children's storybook or nursery rhymes in a soft, soothing voice. Some families tape record the parents' voices telling or reading stories and play the tapes when the infant is able to cope with such stimuli. Feeding schedules are discussed, and parents are encouraged to visit at times when they can become involved in the care of their infant (Fig. 9-13).

Throughout the parent-infant acquaintance process, the nurse listens carefully to what the parents say to assess their concerns and their progress toward incorporating their infant into their lives. The manner in which parents refer to their infant and the questions they ask reveal their worries and feelings and can serve as valuable clues to future relationships with the infant. The alert nurse is attuned to these subtle indications of parents' needs, which provide guidelines for nursing intervention. Often all that the parents need is reassurance that they will have the support of the nurse during caregiving

FIG. 9-13 ■ Father feeding preterm infant. (Photo courtesy E. Jacobs, Texas Children's Hospital, Houston.)

FIG. 9-14 ■ Siblings visiting in the NICU. (Photo courtesy E. Jacobs, Texas Children's Hospital, Houston.)

activities and that the behaviors about which they are concerned are normal reactions and will disappear as the infant matures.

Parents need guidance in their relationships with their infant and assistance in their efforts to meet their infant's physical and developmental needs. The nursing staff must help parents understand that their preterm infant offers few behavioral rewards and show them how to accept small rewards from their infant. The infant's reactions and behaviors are explained to parents, who take their infant's jerky, rejective behavior personally. They need reassurance that these behaviors are not a reflection on their parenting skills. Parents are taught to recognize their infant's cues regarding stimulation, handling, and other interaction, especially aversive behaviors that indicate a need for rest. Nurses need to include parents in planning their infant's care and sensory stimulation materials, such as a music box or recording.

Above all, nurses must encourage and reinforce parents during their caregiving activities and interactions with their infant to promote healthy parent-child relationships. It is also helpful for the parents to have contact and communication with a consistent group of nurses. This decreases the different information given to parents and often instills confidence that, although the parents cannot be at their infant's bedside 24 hours a day, there are competent and caring nurses whom they may call to inquire about the infant's status. Periodic parent conferences involving the staff caring for the child serve to clarify misunderstandings or problems related to the infant's condition.

Siblings. In the past, concerns about sibling visitation in the NICU focused on fears of infection and disruption of nursing routines. These fears have not been substantiated, and sibling visits should be a part of the normal operation of NICUs (Fig. 9-14). Clearly defined policies and procedures should be developed to facilitate sibling visitation (American Academy of Pediatrics and American College of Obstetricians and Gynecologists, 2007; Moore, Coker, DuBuisson, and others, 2003).

The birth of a preterm infant is a difficult time for siblings, who rely on the support of understanding parents. When the happy anticipation is changed to sadness, worry, and altered routines, siblings are bewildered and deprived of their parents' attention. They know something is wrong, but they have only a dim understanding of what it is. Concern about the negative effects on visiting siblings of seeing the ill newborn has not been confirmed. Children have not hesitated to approach or touch the infant, and children younger than 5 years of age have been less reluctant than older children; in addition, there have been no measurable differences between previsit and postvisit behaviors.

The potential benefits of sibling visits must be weighed against exposure of the child to the environment of the NICU. Children must be prepared for the unfamiliar NICU atmosphere, but contact with the infant appears to have a positive effect on siblings by helping them deal with the reality rather than the bizarre fantasies that are characteristic of young children. Such visits also help to bond the family as a unit.

Support Groups. Parents need to feel that they are not alone. Parent support groups have been of immeasurable value to families of infants in the NICU. Some groups consist of parents who have infants in the hospital and share the same anxieties and concerns. Other groups include parents who have had infants in the NICU and who have dealt with the crisis effectively. The groups are usually under the leadership of a staff person and involve physicians, nurses, and social workers, but the parents can offer other parents something that no one else can provide.

An excellent resource for parents of preterm infants is the book by J. Zaichkin, *Newborn Intensive Care: What Every Parent Needs to Know* (2002). This resource has technical and anecdotal information regarding different problems facing preterm infants, common treatments and therapies, preparation for home discharge, and home care for the preterm infant. Another resource for parents wanting more information about kangaroo care is by S.M. Ludington-Hoe, *Kangaroo Care: The Best You Can Do to Help Your Preterm Infant* (1993).

Discharge Planning and Home Care

Parents become apprehensive and excited as the time for discharge approaches. They have many concerns and insecurities regarding the care of their infant. They fear that the child may still be in danger, that they will be unable to recognize signs of distress or illness in their infant, and that the infant may not yet be ready for discharge. Nurses need to begin early to assist parents in acquiring or increasing their skills in the care of their infant. Appropriate instruction must be provided and sufficient time allowed for the family to assimilate the information and learn the continuing special care requirements. Where rooming-in or other live-in arrangements are available, parents can stay for a few days and nights and assume the care of their infant under the supervision and support of the nursery staff.

There should be appropriate medical and nursing follow-up and referrals to services that can benefit the family, including developmental follow-up. Parents of preterm infants should also be given adequate information about immunizations with other discharge planning information. Most home health agencies provide nursing supervision, counseling, and referrals for nursing visits. With the trend toward early discharge, many hospital-based home health care agencies become involved in the follow-up and care of the NICU "graduate" in the home. For the parents of an infant being discharged with equipment such as an oxygen tank, apnea monitor, or even a ventilator, discharge planning requires multidisciplinary collaborative practice to ensure that the family has not only the appropriate resources, but also the available assistance for dealing with the infant's needs. Many communities have organized support groups, including those discussed previously, those designed for parents of infants who require special care because of specific defects or disabilities, and those for parents of multiple births.

Car seat safety is an essential aspect of discharge planning, and infants younger than 37 weeks of gestation should have a period of observation in an appropriate car seat to monitor for possible apnea, bradycardia, and decreased Sao_2 (American Academy of Pediatrics, 1999) (see Community Focus box). Several models can be adapted for small infants with the placement of blanket rolls on each side of the infant to support the head and trunk. For adequate support without slumping, the seat back–to-crotch strap distance must be 14 cm (5.5 inches) or less; a small rolled blanket may be placed between the crotch strap and the infant to reduce slouching. The distance from the lower harness strap to the seat bottom should be 25.5 cm (10 inches) or less to decrease the potential for the harness straps to cross the infant's ears (Howard-Salsman, 2006). The rear-facing position provides support for the head, neck, and back, thereby reducing the stress to the neck and spinal cord in a vehicle crash. An infant who cannot tolerate a semireclining position in a standard car seat may be placed in a car bed restraint. Car seat manufacturers must specify recommended minimum and maximum weights for the occupant; therefore it is important to check the manufacturer's recommendations before purchasing a car seat for a smaller infant. Additional guidelines are available from the American Academy of Pediatrics (2002), including a videotape for the safe transportation of preterm and LBW infants. (See Chapter 10 for a discussion of infant car restraints and the American Academy of Pedi-

COMMUNITY FOCUS

Preterm and Near-Term Infant Car Seat Evaluation

The American Academy of Pediatrics recommends that infants born before 37 weeks of gestation be evaluated for apnea, bradycardia, or oxygen desaturation episodes before hospital discharge. The Academy suggests that facilities develop policies for the implementation of a program of evaluation; however, there are few evidence-based practice recommendations published to date delineating specific requirements for such a program. Based on the available literature, suggestions for providing a car seat evaluation of infants born before 37 weeks of gestation include:

- Use the parents' car seat for the evaluation.
- Perform the evaluation 1 to 7 days before the infant's anticipated discharge.
- Secure infant in car seat per guidelines using blanket rolls on side.
- Set pulse oximeter low alarm at 88% (arbitrary).
- Set heart rate low alarm limit at 80 beats/min and apnea alarm at 20 seconds (cardiorespiratory monitor).
- Leave the infant undisturbed in car seat for 60 minutes *or* for the time period parents state it takes to arrive at their home.
- Document infant's tolerance to car seat evaluation.
- An episode of desaturation, bradycardia, or apnea (20 seconds or more) constitutes a failure, and evaluation by the practitioner must occur before discharge.
- Repeat the test after 24 hours once modifications are made to the car seat, car bed, or infant's position in either restraint system.
- It is recommended that a certified car seat technician place the infant in the car seat (or bed) if a failure occurs (see National Highway Traffic Safety Administration website* for car seat inspection station).
- The technician will demonstrate appropriate positioning of the infant in the restraint device to the parents and have the parents do a return demonstration.
- Document the interventions, the infant's tolerance, and the parents' return demonstration.

Modified from American Academy of Pediatrics: Safe transportation of premature and low birth weight infants, *Pediatrics* 97(5):758-760, 1996; American Academy of Pediatrics: Transporting children with special health care needs, *Pediatrics* 104(4):988-992, 1999.
*http://www.nhtsa.dot.gov.

atrics website* for a complete list of appropriate car seats for infants.)

An important part of discharge planning and care of the preterm infant is nutrition for continued growth; thus choice of feeding must be carefully addressed. Human milk should be fortified according to the infant's corrected age and physiologic needs. An enriched postdischarge formula (usually 22 kcal/oz) is required for preterm infants born at less than 36 weeks to meet appropriate growth standards (Lucas, Fewtrell, Morley, and others, 2001; Carver, Wu, Hall, and others, 2001). Full-term infant formulas are not considered adequate for proper growth in preterm infants.

Knowing that staff members are available for telephone or personal contact when the parents take the infant home provides a measure of security to anxious parents. Many NICU facilities maintain a policy of open communication between

___
*http://www.aap.org.

ETHICAL CASE STUDY	Preterm Infant

ETHICAL DECISION MAKING MODEL	Britt is a 6½-month-old infant in the neonatal intensive care unit (NICU). He was born at 28 weeks of gestation and as a result has numerous health problems, including postnecrotizing enterocolitis, short-bowel syndrome and subsequent ileostomy, chronic lung disease and ventilator dependency with a tracheostomy, grade III periventricular hemorrhage, partial blindness from retinopathy of prematurity, and bilateral hearing deficit that will eventually require hearing aids. Britt is dependent on intravenous total parenteral nutrition for nutrition and fluids. Britt's parents are Josh and Debi; they are 22 and 23 years old, respectively, and have another child, Darlene, who is 22 months old. Darlene was also a preemie and has various health care needs, including tube feedings through a skin-level feeding tube, atopy, and recurrent urinary tract infections due to reflux. The parents are only able to visit the NICU every other week because they live 120 miles from the hospital and cannot take off work because of financial problems. The extended family has no relationship with the parents because of a recent squabble over money loaned by the grandparents, which the parents have been unable to repay.
Evaluate the Issue	Britt has had 19 cardiac arrests, 3 of which occurred within the last 48 hours, and he has responded to drugs and higher ventilator and oxygen settings but shows signs of gradual decline in mental alertness and ability to maintain adequate cardiorespiratory and metabolic function. The nursing staff are concerned about Britt's quality of life and have suggested that the next time he "codes," the physician allow him to die a natural death. Britt's parents are unable to visit at this time but have requested by telephone conference that all available means be employed to keep Britt alive; they want to bring him home soon to be with the rest of the family. They further indicate that they have a lot of faith in a Higher Being and that Britt will soon be healed. Several nurses have refused to care for Britt because they "cannot stand to see him suffer."
Treat All Involved with Respect	The parents' concerns regarding Britt's condition and resuscitation efforts should be objectively addressed in person with a conference of nursing, medical, social worker, and perhaps clergy or spiritual advisors close to the family. Britt's mother has expressed strong guilt feelings regarding his illness and their inability to care for him as they care for Darlene. The extended family has instilled additional guilt over the financial situation and the parents' inability to visit Britt on a regular basis. The nurses must realize the parents' guilt over not being able to completely care for Britt as they have cared for Darlene.
Hear All Sides	The nurses must first consider the parents' views on Britt's health status. It is important to evaluate the parents' perception of Britt's health status and that of the daughter, Darlene. Are there parallels that may be drawn between the two children's course of illness? What considerations have the parents given to home care of Britt and Darlene? Does the family have religious beliefs that preclude allowing the child to die without further intervention? Do the parents fully understand the essence of Britt's health status?
Initiate Action	Which of the following actions is most appropriate for the nursing staff to take at this time? ■ Tell the parents that Britt is going to die regardless of resuscitation efforts and that his death is the best solution to prevent further suffering. ■ Persuade the primary care practitioner to request a Do Not Resuscitate order from the parents. ■ Enlist the assistance of the parents' pastor (or spiritual advisor) to help the family see the reality of Britt's suffering and eventual death. ■ Contact the local hospice facility for end-of-life care for Britt and the family.
Consider the Outcome	A number of ethical issues must be considered in this case. One dilemma the parents are facing is the deteriorating health and possible death of a child they have formed a bond with and have loved for 6½ months. The second ethical dilemma facing the parents is their religious belief about Britt's healing. The lack of support from extended family further complicates the situation. An ethical dilemma the nurses face is the issue of whether Britt has what would be considered a positive quality of life or experiences pain and suffering as a result of his deteriorating physical status.

staff and parents both during the infant's hospitalization and after discharge. It is the responsibility of the NICU staff to make certain that parents are prepared to care for their infant, both emotionally and physically. At the same time, it is important that parents establish a trusting relationship with the infant's primary care provider in the community before discharge from the acute care facility.

Neonatal Loss

The precarious nature of many high-risk infants makes death a real and ever-present possibility (see Ethical Case Study). Although infant mortality has been reduced sharply with improved technology, the mortality rate is still greatest during

the neonatal period. Nurses in the NICU are the persons who must prepare the parents for an inevitable death, provide end-of-life care for the infant and family, and facilitate a family's grieving process after an expected or unexpected death.

The loss of an infant has special meaning for the grieving parents. It represents a loss of a part of themselves (especially for mothers), a loss of the potential for immortality that offspring represent, and the loss of the dream child that has been fantasized throughout the pregnancy. There is often a sense of emptiness and failure. In addition, when an infant has lived for such a short time, there may be few, if any, pleasant memories to serve as a basis for the identification and idealization that are part of the resolution of a loss.

To help parents understand that the death is a reality, it is important that they be encouraged to hold their infant before death and, if possible, be present at the time of death so that their infant can die in their arms if they choose. Many who deny the need to hold the infant later regret the decision.

Parents are given the opportunity to actually "parent" the infant in any manner they wish or are able to do before and after the death. This may include seeing, touching, holding, caressing, and talking to their infant privately; the parents may also wish to bathe and dress the infant. If parents are hesitant about seeing their dead infant, it is advisable to keep the body in the unit for a few hours, since many parents change their minds after the initial shock of the death.

Parents may need to see and hold the infant more than once—the first time to say "hello" and the last time to say "good-bye." If parents wish to see the infant after the body has been taken to the morgue, the infant should be retrieved, wrapped in a blanket, rewarmed in a radiant warmer, and taken to the mother's room or other private place. The nurse should stay with the parents and provide them an opportunity for private time alone with their dead infant. Individual grief responses of the mother and father should be recognized and handled appropriately; gender differences and cultural and religious beliefs will affect the parents' grief responses.

Some neonatal units have a hospice approach for families with infants for whom the decision has been made to not prolong life and who are receiving only palliative care. A special "family" room is set aside and contains all supportive equipment needed for the care of the infant. It also provides a homelike atmosphere for the family. All hospice services are available to the family, and the infant remains under the care and supervision of a primary nurse on the NICU staff. (See Chapter 18 for further discussion of hospice care.)

A photograph of the infant taken before or after death is highly desirable. Parents may wish to have a special family portrait taken with the infant and other family members; this often helps personalize and make the experience more tangible. The parents may not wish to see the photograph at the time of death, but the chance to refer to it later will help make their infant seem more real, which is a part of the normal grief process. A photograph of their infant being held by the hand or touched by an adult offers a more positive image than a morgue type of photograph. A bereavement or memory packet can be given to the grieving parents and family; it may include the infant's handprints and footprints, a lock of hair, the bedside name card, name tags, armbands, and, as appropriate to the family's religious beliefs, a certificate of baptism.

Naming the deceased infant is an important step in the grieving process. Some parents may hesitate to give the newborn a name that had been chosen during the pregnancy for their special "baby." However, having a tangible person for whom to grieve is an important component of the grieving process.

A primary nurse who is familiar to the family should be present during the discussion about the dead or dying infant. The nurse should talk with parents openly and honestly about funeral arrangements, since few parents have had experience with this aspect of death. Many funeral homes now offer inexpensive arrangements for these special cases. Someone from the NICU should take the responsibility for acquiring this type of information. It is often helpful to parents for the NICU to have a list of local funeral homes, services offered, and prices. Families need to be informed of the options available, but a funeral is preferable because the ritual provides an opportunity for parents to feel the support of friends and relatives. A member of the clergy of the appropriate faith may be notified if the parents wish. Issues regarding an autopsy or organ donation (when appropriate) are approached in a multidisciplinary fashion (primary practitioner and primary nurse) with respect, sensitivity to cultural and religious beliefs, tact, and consideration of the family's wishes. (For additional suggestions for helping families who experience neonatal loss, see Grief and Perinatal Loss in Merenstein and Gardner, 2006, and Jansen, 2003.)

Before the parents leave the hospital, they are given the telephone number of the unit (if they do not have it) and invited to call any time they have any further questions. Many intensive care units make it a point to contact the parents several weeks after a neonatal death to assess the parents' coping mechanisms, evaluate the grieving process, and provide support as needed. Several organizations are available to offer support and understanding to families who have lost a newborn; these organization include the Compassionate Friends,* Aiding Mothers and Fathers Experiencing Neonatal Death (AMEND),† and Share Pregnancy and Infant Loss Support, Inc.‡ (See also Chapter 18 for further discussion of the family and the grief process.)

Nurses who care for critically ill infants also experience grief; NICU nurses may feel helpless and sorrowful. It is important that such grief be allowed and that nurses attend the funeral or memorial service as a part of working through the grief process. Nurses may fear that showing emotion is unprofessional and that the expression of grief indicates "loss of control." These fears are unfounded. Studies have demonstrated that to continue to be effective managers and providers of care, nurses must be allowed to grieve and support each other through the process (Gardner, Hauser, and Merenstein, 2006).

Baptism. Because many Christian parents wish to have their child baptized if death is anticipated or is a decided possibility, this becomes a nursing responsibility. Whenever possible, it is most desirable that a representative of the parents' faith (e.g., a Roman Catholic priest or a Protestant minister) perform such a ritual. When death is imminent, a nurse or a physician can perform the baptism by simply pouring water on the infant's forehead (a medicine dropper is a convenient means) while repeating the words, "I baptize you in the name of the Father and of the Son and of the Holy Spirit." This includes a birth of any gestational age, particularly when the parents are Roman Catholic.

When the parents' faith is uncertain, a conditional baptism can be carried out by saying, "If you are capable of receiving baptism, I baptize you in the name of the Father and of the Son and of the Holy Spirit." The baptism is recorded in the infant's chart, and a notice is placed on the crib or incubator. Parents are informed at the first opportunity.

---

*PO Box 3696, Oakbrook, IL 60522-3696; (630) 990-0010, (877) 969-0010; http://www.compassionatefriends.org.

†Contact Maureen Connelly, 4324 Berrywick Terrace, St. Louis, MO 63128; (314) 487-7582; e-mail: info@amendgroup.com[0]; http://www.amendgroup.com.

‡(800) 821-6819, (636) 947-6164; http://www.nationalshareoffice.com; offers a variety of services for grieving parents and family members.

BOX 9-3
Etiology of Preterm Birth

MATERNAL FACTORS
Socioeconomic:
- Malnutrition
- Age
- Race

Chronic medical conditions:
- Heart disease
- Renal disease
- Diabetes
- Hypertension

Behavioral:
- Substance abuse
- Smoking
- Poor or absent prenatal care

FACTORS RELATED TO PREGNANCY
Multiple pregnancy
Low body mass index (<19.8 kg/m²) (Ramsey and Goldenberg, 2006)
Abruptio placentae or placenta previa
Incompetent cervix
Premature rupture of membranes or chorioamnionitis
Polyhydramnios or oligohydramnios
Infection

FETAL FACTORS
Chromosomal abnormalities
Congenital anomalies

UNKNOWN FACTORS

HIGH RISK RELATED TO DYSMATURITY

PRETERM INFANTS

Prematurity accounts for the largest number of admissions to an NICU. Immaturity of most organ systems places infants at risk for a variety of neonatal complications (e.g., hyperbilirubinemia, respiratory distress syndrome). The actual cause of prematurity is not known in most instances (Box 9-3). The incidence of prematurity is lowest in the middle to high socioeconomic classes, in which pregnant women are generally in good health, are well nourished, and receive prompt and comprehensive prenatal care. The incidence is highest in the lower socioeconomic class, in which a combination of deleterious circumstances is present. Other factors, such as multiple pregnancies, pregnancy-induced hypertension, and placental problems that interrupt the normal course of gestation before completion of fetal development, are responsible for a large number of preterm births.

The outlook for preterm infants is largely, but not entirely, related to the state of physiologic and anatomic immaturity of the various organs and systems at the time of birth. Infants at term have advanced to a state of maturity sufficient to allow a successful transition to the extrauterine environment. Preterm infants must make the same adjustments but with functional immaturity proportional to the stage of development reached at the time of birth. The degree to which infants are prepared for extrauterine life can be predicted to some extent by birth weight and estimated gestational age (see Clinical Assessment of Gestational Age, Chapter 8).

Within the last decade infants previously designated as being preterm yet who were born between 34 and 36⁶⁄₇ weeks' gestation have been labeled as being near-term or late-preterm infants. Such infants have some of the same risk factors as those born before 34 weeks' gestation, but physical characteristics and adaptation to extrauterine life are variable. Late-preterm infants have metabolic and physical immaturity that places them at risk for greater mortality and morbidity than term infants (Engle, Tomashek, Wallman, and others, 2007). In the following sections the discussion of the preterm infant continues to apply to all infants who are born before a completed gestational age of 37 weeks. Because prematurity now encompasses a wider age, weight, and physiologic maturity range, physical characteristics described may also vary; such descriptions are generalized for description purposes.

Diagnostic Evaluation

Preterm infants have a number of distinct characteristics at various stages of development. Identification of these characteristics provides valuable clues to the gestational age and hence to the infant's physiologic capabilities. The general, outward physical appearance changes as the fetus progresses to maturity. Characteristics of skin, general attitude (or posture) when supine, appearance of hair, and amount of subcutaneous fat provide cues to a newborn's physical development. Observation of spontaneous, active movements and response to stimulation and passive movement contributes to the assessment of neurologic status. The appraisal is made as soon as possible after admission to the nursery, since much of the observation and management of infants depends on this information.

On inspection, preterm infants are very small and appear scrawny because they have only minimal subcutaneous fat deposits (or none in some cases) and have a proportionately large head in relation to the body, which reflects the cephalocaudal direction of growth. The skin is bright pink (often translucent, depending on the degree of immaturity), smooth, and shiny, with small blood vessels clearly visible underneath the thin epidermis. The fine lanugo hair is abundant over the body (depending on gestational age) but is sparse, fine, and fuzzy on the head. The ear cartilage is soft and pliable, and the soles and palms have minimal creases, resulting in a smooth appearance. The bones of the skull and the ribs feel soft, and the eyes may be closed. Male infants have few scrotal rugae, and the testes are undescended; in females the labia and clitoris are prominent. Fig. 9-15 compares the features of full-term and preterm infants.

In contrast to full-term infants' overall attitude of flexion and continuous activity, preterm infants may be inactive and listless. The extremities maintain an attitude of extension and remain in any position in which they are placed. Reflex activity is only partially developed—sucking is absent, weak, or ineffectual; swallow, gag, and cough reflexes are absent or weak; and other neurologic signs are absent or diminished. Physiologically immature, preterm infants are unable to maintain body temperature, have limited ability to excrete solutes in the urine, and have increased susceptibility to infection. A pliable thorax, immature lung tissue, and an immature regulatory center lead to periodic breathing, hypoventilation, and frequent periods of apnea. They are more susceptible to biochemical alterations such as hyperbilirubinemia and hypoglycemia, and they have a higher extracellular water content that

PRETERM   TERM

Posture—The preterm infant lies in a "relaxed attitude," limbs more extended; the body size is small, and the head may appear somewhat larger in proportion to the body size. The term infant has more subcutaneous fat tissue and rests in a more flexed attitude.

Ear—The preterm infant's ear cartilages are poorly developed, and the ear may fold easily; the hair is fine and feathery, and lanugo may cover the back and face. The mature infant's ear cartilages are well formed, and the hair is more likely to form firm, separate strands.

Sole—The sole of the foot of the preterm infant appears more turgid and may have only fine wrinkles. The mature infant's sole (foot) is well and deeply creased.

Female genitalia—The preterm female infant's clitoris is prominent, and labia majora are poorly developed and gaping. The mature female infant's labia majora are fully developed, and the clitoris is not as prominent.

Male genitalia—The preterm male infant's scrotum is undeveloped and not pendulous; minimal rugae are present, and the testes may be in the inguinal canals or in the abdominal cavity. The term male infant's scrotum is well developed, pendulous, and rugated, and the testes are well down in the scrotal sac.

Scarf sign—The preterm infant's elbow may be easily brought across the chest with little or no resistance. The mature infant's elbow may be brought to the midline of the chest, resisting attempts to bring the elbow past the midline.

FIG. 9-15 ■ Clinical and neurologic examinations comparing preterm and full-term infants. (Data from Pierog SH, Ferrara A: *Medical care of the sick newborn,* ed 2, St Louis, 1976, Mosby.)

NEUROLOGIC EVALUATION

PRETERM   TERM

Grasp reflex—The preterm infant's grasp is weak; the term infant's grasp is strong, allowing the infant to be lifted up from the mattress.

Heel-to-ear maneuver—The preterm infant's heel is easily brought to the ear, meeting with no resistance. This maneuver is not possible in the term infant, since there is considerable resistance at the knee.

FIG. 9-15, cont'd ▪ Clinical and neurologic examinations comparing preterm and full-term infants. (Data from Pierog SH, Ferrara A: *Medical care of the sick newborn,* ed 2, St Louis, 1976, Mosby.)

renders them more vulnerable to fluid and electrolyte derangements. Preterm infants exchange fully half of their extracellular fluid volume every 24 hours as compared with one seventh of the volume in adults.

The soft cranium is subject to characteristic unintentional deformation caused by positioning from one side to the other on a mattress. The head looks disproportionately longer from front to back, is flattened on both sides, and lacks the usual convexity seen at the temporal and parietal areas. This positional molding is often a concern to parents and may influence the parents' perception of the infant's attractiveness and their responsiveness to the infant. Positioning the infant on a waterbed or gel mattress can reduce or minimize cranial molding.

Neurologic impairment (such as intraventricular hemorrhage) and serious sequelae correlate with the size and gestational age of infants at birth and with the severity of neonatal complications. The greater the degree of immaturity, the greater the degree of potential disability. A greater incidence of cerebral palsy, attention deficit hyperactivity disorder (ADHD), visual-motor deficits, and altered intellectual functioning is observed in preterm than in full-term infants. However, behavioral development can be enhanced when families are provided with support and infants are referred to appropriate services for neurologic and developmental interventions. Parental interest and involvement are important variables in the developmental progress of infants.

Therapeutic Management

When delivery of a preterm infant is anticipated, the intensive care nursery is alerted and a team approach implemented. Ideally, a neonatologist, an advanced practice nurse, a staff nurse, and a respiratory therapist are present for the delivery.

Infants who do not require resuscitation are immediately transferred in a heated incubator to the NICU, where they are weighed and where IV lines, oxygen therapy, and other therapeutic interventions are initiated as needed. Resuscitation is conducted in the delivery area until infants can be safely transported to the NICU.

Subsequent care is determined by the infant's status. The general care of the preterm infant differs from that of the full-term infant primarily in the areas of respiratory support, temperature regulation, nutrition, susceptibility to infection, activity intolerance, and other consequences of physical immaturity.

Nursing Care Management

The nursing care, like the therapeutic management, is individualized for each infant. See appropriate discussions under Nursing Care of the High-Risk Newborn and Family for additional details of care.

POSTTERM INFANTS

Infants born of a gestation that extends beyond 42 weeks as calculated from the mother's last menstrual period (or by gestational age assessment) are considered to be postterm, or postmature, regardless of birth weight. This constitutes 3.5% to 15% of all pregnancies. The cause of delayed birth is unknown. Some infants are appropriate for gestational age but show the characteristics of progressive placental dysfunction. These infants display characteristics such as absence of lanugo, little if any vernix caseosa, abundant scalp hair, and long fingernails. The skin is often cracked, parchment-like, and desquamating. A common finding in postterm infants is a wasted physical appearance that reflects intrauterine deprivation. Depletion of subcutaneous fat gives them a thin, elongated appearance. The little vernix caseosa that remains in the skinfolds may be stained a deep yellow or green, which is usually an indication of meconium in the amniotic fluid.

There is a significant increase in fetal and neonatal mortality in postterm infants as compared with those born at term. They are especially prone to fetal distress associated with the decreasing efficiency of the placenta, macrosomia, and meconium aspiration syndrome. The greatest risk occurs during the stresses of labor and delivery, particularly in infants of **primigravidas,** or women delivering their first child. Close surveillance with fetal assessment and induction of labor is usually recommended when infants are significantly overdue.

HIGH RISK RELATED TO PHYSIOLOGIC FACTORS

HYPERBILIRUBINEMIA

The term **hyperbilirubinemia** refers to an excessive level of accumulated bilirubin in the blood and is characterized by **jaundice,** or **icterus,** a yellowish discoloration of the skin, sclerae, and nails. Hyperbilirubinemia is a common finding in the newborn and in most instances is relatively benign. However, in extreme cases, it can indicate a pathologic state.

Hyperbilirubinemia may result from increased unconjugated or conjugated bilirubin. The unconjugated form or indirect hyperbilirubinemia (Table 9-3) is the type most commonly seen in newborns. The following discussion of

TABLE 9-3

Comparison of Major Types of Unconjugated Hyperbilirubinemia*

PHYSIOLOGIC JAUNDICE	BREASTFEEDING-ASSOCIATED JAUNDICE (EARLY ONSET)	BREAST MILK JAUNDICE (LATE ONSET)	HEMOLYTIC DISEASE
CAUSE Immature hepatic function plus increased bilirubin load from red blood cell (RBC) hemolysis	Decreased milk intake related to fewer calories consumed by infant before mother's milk is well established; enterohepatic shunting	Possible factors in breast milk that prevent bilirubin conjugation; Less frequent stooling	Blood antigen incompatibility causing hemolysis of large numbers of RBCs; Liver unable to conjugate and excrete excess bilirubin from hemolysis
ONSET After 24 hours (preterm infants, prolonged)	Second to fourth day	Fifth to seventh day	During first 24 hours (levels increase >5 mg/dl/day)
PEAK 72-90 hours	Third to fifth day	Tenth to fifteenth day	Variable
DURATION Declines on fifth to seventh day	Variable	May remain jaundiced for 3-12 weeks or more	Depends on severity and treatment
THERAPY Increase frequency of feedings and avoid supplements. Evaluate stooling pattern. Monitor transcutaneous bilirubin (TcB) or total serum bilirubin (TSB) level. Perform risk assessment (see Fig. 9-16, A). Use phototherapy if bilirubin levels increase significantly or significant hemolysis is present (see Fig. 9-16, B).	Breastfeed frequently (10-12 times/day); avoid supplements such as water, dextrose water, or formula. Evaluate stooling pattern; stimulate as needed. Perform risk assessment (see Fig. 9-16, A). Use phototherapy if bilirubin levels increase significantly or significant hemolysis is present (see Fig. 9-16, B). If phototherapy is instituted, evaluate benefits and harm of temporarily discontinuing breastfeeding; additional assessments may be required. Assist mother with maintaining milk supply; feed expressed milk as appropriate. After discharge, follow up according to hour of discharge (see p. 277).	Increase frequency of breastfeeding; use no supplementation such as glucose water; cessation of breastfeeding is not recommended. Perform risk assessment (see Fig. 9-16, A). Consider performing additional evaluations: glucose 6-phosphate dehydrogenase, direct and indirect serum bilirubin, family history, and others as necessary. May include home phototherapy with a temporary (10-12 hour) discontinuation of breastfeeding; a subsequent TSB may be drawn to evaluate a drop in serum levels. Assist mother with maintenance of milk supply and reassurance regarding her milk supply and therapy. Use formula supplements only at practitioner's discretion.	Monitor TcB or TSB level. Perform risk assessment (see Fig. 9-16, A). Postnatal—Use phototherapy; administer intravenous immunoglobulin per protocol; if severe, perform exchange transfusion. Prenatal—Perform transfusion (fetus). Prevent sensitization (Rh incompatibility) of Rh-negative mother with Rh₀(D) immune globulin (RhIG). If mother is breastfeeding, assist with maintenance and storage of milk; may bottle feed expressed milk as appropriate to therapy. Minimize maternal-infant separation, and encourage contact as appropriate.

*Table depicts patterns of jaundice in term infants; patterns in preterm infants will vary according to factors such as gestational age, birth weight, and illness.

hyperbilirubinemia is limited to unconjugated hyperbilirubinemia.

Pathophysiology

Bilirubin is one of the breakdown products of the hemoglobin that results from red blood cell (RBC) destruction. When RBCs are destroyed, the breakdown products are released into the circulation, where the hemoglobin splits into two fractions: heme and globin. The globin (protein) portion is used by the body, and the heme portion is converted to **unconjugated bilirubin,** an insoluble substance bound to albumin.

In the liver the bilirubin is detached from the albumin molecule and, in the presence of the enzyme **glucuronyl transferase,** is conjugated with glucuronic acid to produce a highly soluble substance, **conjugated bilirubin,** which is then excreted into the bile. In the intestine, bacterial action reduces the conjugated bilirubin to urobilinogen, the pigment that gives stool its characteristic color. Most of the reduced bilirubin is excreted through the feces; a small amount is eliminated in the urine.

Normally the body is able to maintain a balance between the destruction of RBCs and the use or excretion of by-products. However, when developmental limitations or a pathologic process interferes with this balance, bilirubin accumulates in the tissues to produce jaundice. Possible causes of hyperbilirubinemia in the newborn are:

- Physiologic (developmental) factors (prematurity)
- An association with breastfeeding or breast milk
- Excess production of bilirubin (e.g., hemolytic disease, biochemical defects, bruises)
- Disturbed capacity of the liver to secrete conjugated bilirubin (e.g., enzyme deficiency, bile duct obstruction)
- Combined overproduction and undersecretion (e.g., sepsis)
- Some disease states (e.g., hypothyroidism, galactosemia, infant of a diabetic mother)
- Genetic predisposition to increased production (Native Americans, Asians)

The most common cause of hyperbilirubinemia is the relatively mild and self-limited **physiologic jaundice,** or **icterus neonatorum.** Unlike hemolytic disease of the newborn (HDN) (see p. 281), physiologic jaundice is not associated with any pathologic process. Although almost all newborns experience elevated bilirubin levels, only about half demonstrate observable signs of jaundice.

Two phases of physiologic jaundice have been identified in full-term infants. In the first phase, bilirubin levels of formula-fed Caucasian and African-American infants gradually increase to a peak by day of life 3 to 4, with a subsequent rapid decrease in serum levels for 2 to 3 days; in the second phase, serum bilirubin levels gradually decrease to less than 1 mg/dl over 1 to 2 weeks (Blackburn, 2007). This pattern varies according to racial group, method of feeding (breast vs bottle), and gestational age. In term breastfed infants, serum bilirubin levels peak later than those in formula-fed infants and at higher levels (7 to 14 mg/dl); in term breast-fed infants, the gradual decline in serum bilirubin levels may occur over 2 to 4 weeks, and in some cases may last as long as 6 weeks (Blackburn, 2007).

As noted above, infants of Asian descent (as well as Native Americans) have mean bilirubin levels almost twice those seen in Caucasians or African Americans. An increased incidence of hyperbilirubinemia is seen in newborns from certain geographic areas, particularly areas around Greece. These populations may have glucose-6-phosphate dehydrogenase (G6PD) deficiency, which can cause hemolytic anemia.

On average, newborns produce twice as much bilirubin as do adults because of higher concentrations of circulating erythrocytes and a shorter life span of RBCs (only 70 to 90 days, in contrast to 120 days in older children and adults). In addition, the liver's ability to conjugate bilirubin is reduced because of limited production of glucuronyl transferase. Newborns also have a lower plasma-binding capacity for bilirubin because of reduced albumin concentrations as compared with older children. Normal changes in hepatic circulation after birth may contribute to excess demands on liver function.

Normally, conjugated bilirubin is reduced to **urobilinogen** by the intestinal flora and excreted in feces. However, the sterile and less motile newborn bowel is initially less effective in excreting urobilinogen. In the newborn intestine the enzyme β-glucuronidase is able to convert conjugated bilirubin into the unconjugated form, which is subsequently reabsorbed by the intestinal mucosa and transported to the liver. This process, known as **enterohepatic circulation,** or **shunting,** is accentuated in the newborn and is thought to be a primary mechanism in physiologic jaundice (Blackburn, 2007). Feeding (1) stimulates peristalsis and produces more rapid passage of meconium, thus diminishing the amount of reabsorption of unconjugated bilirubin; and (2) introduces bacteria to aid in the reduction of bilirubin to urobilinogen. Colostrum, a natural cathartic, facilitates meconium evacuation.

Breastfeeding is associated with an increased incidence of jaundice as a result of two distinct processes. **Breastfeeding-associated jaundice (early-onset jaundice)** begins at 2 to 4 days of age and occurs in approximately 12% to 35% of breast-fed newborns (Blackburn, 2007). The jaundice is related to the process of breastfeeding and probably results from decreased caloric and fluid intake by breast-fed infants before the milk supply is well established, since fasting is associated with decreased hepatic clearance of bilirubin (Porter and Dennis, 2002). Reduced fluid intake results in dehydration, which also concentrates the bilirubin in the blood.

Breast milk jaundice (late-onset jaundice) begins at age 5 to 7 days and occurs in 2% to 4% of breast-fed infants (Blackburn, 2007). Rising levels of bilirubin peak during the second week and gradually diminish. Despite high levels of bilirubin that may persist for 3 to 12 weeks, these infants are well. The jaundice may be caused by factors in the breast milk (pregnanediol, fatty acids, and β-glucuronidase) that either inhibit the conjugation or decrease the excretion of bilirubin. Less frequent stooling by breast-fed infants may allow for extended time for reabsorption of bilirubin from stools.

Diagnostic Evaluation

The degree of jaundice is determined by serum bilirubin measurements. Normal values of unconjugated bilirubin are 0.2 to 1.4 mg/dl. In the newborn, levels must exceed 5 mg/dl before jaundice (icterus) is observable. It is important to note, however, that the evaluation of jaundice is not based solely on serum bilirubin levels, but also on the timing of the appearance of clinical jaundice; gestational age at birth; age in days since birth; family history, including maternal Rh factor; evidence of hemolysis; feeding method; infant's physiologic status; and the progression of serial serum bilirubin levels. The following criteria are indicators of pathologic jaundice that, when present,

FIG. 9-16 ■ A, Nomogram for designation of risk in 2840 well newborns at 36 or more weeks of gestational age with birth weight of 2000 g (4.4 pounds) or more, or 35 or more weeks of gestational age and birth weight of 2500 g (5.5 pounds) or more, based on the hour-specific serum bilirubin values. (This nomogram should not be used to represent the natural history of neonatal hyperbilirubinemia.) B, Guidelines for phototherapy in hospitalized infants of 35 or more weeks' gestation. (A, From Bhutani VK, Johnson L, Sivieri EM: Predictive ability of a predischarge hour-specific serum bilirubin for subsequent significant hyperbilirubinemia in healthy term and near-term newborns, *Pediatrics* 103(1):6-14, 1999. B, From American Academy of Pediatrics, Subcommittee on Hyperbilirubinemia: Management of hyperbilirubinemia in the newborn infant 35 or more weeks of gestation, *Pediatrics* 114(1):297-316, 2004.)

warrant further investigation as to the cause of the jaundice. It is not an all-inclusive list; other factors are also evaluated:

■ Appearance of jaundice within 24 hours of birth
■ Persistent jaundice over 2 weeks in a full-term formula-fed infant
■ Total serum bilirubin levels over 12.9 mg/dl (term infant) or over 15 mg/dl (preterm infant); upper limit for breast-fed infant: 15 mg/dl
■ Increase in serum bilirubin by 5 mg/dl/day

■ Direct bilirubin exceeding 1.5 to 2 mg/dl
■ Total serum bilirubin level over 95th percentile for age (in hours) on hour-specific nomogram (Fig. 9-16)

Noninvasive monitoring of bilirubin via cutaneous reflectance measurements (**transcutaneous bilirubinometry [TcB]**) allows for repetitive estimations of bilirubin and, when used correctly, may decrease the need for invasive monitoring (Thayyil and Marriott, 2005). The new TcB monitors provide accurate measurements within 2 to 3 mg/dl in most neonatal populations at serum levels below 15 mg/dl (American Academy of Pediatrics, 2004). TcB monitors must be used according to published guidelines as a screening tool, not as a predictor of need for therapy; multiple readings over time at a consistent site (e.g., sternum or forehead) are of more value than a single reading. After phototherapy has been initiated, TcB is no longer useful as a screening tool.

The use of hour-specific serum bilirubin levels to predict newborns at risk for rapidly rising levels has now become an official recommendation by the American Academy of Pediatrics (2004) for the monitoring of healthy neonates of 35 weeks of gestation or older before discharge from the hospital. The use of a nomogram with three levels (high, intermediate, or low risk) of rising total serum bilirubin values assists in the determination of which newborns might need further evaluation after discharge (Bhutani, Johnson, and Sivieri, 1999; Bhutani, Johnson, and Keren, 2004) (see Fig. 9-16, *A*). The hour-specific bilirubin risk nomogram is used to determine the infant's risk for developing hyperbilirubinemia requiring medical treatment or closer screening. Risk factors recognized to place infants in the high-risk category include gestational age of less than 38 weeks, breastfeeding, a sibling who had significant jaundice, and jaundice appearing before discharge (American Academy of Pediatrics, 2004).

It is also recommended that healthy near-term and term infants (older than 34⅞ weeks) receive follow-up care and assessment of bilirubin within 3 days of discharge if discharged at less than 24 hours and a risk assessment with TcB or the hour-specific nomogram. Newborns discharged at 24 to 47.9 hours should receive follow-up evaluation within 4 days (96 hours), and those discharged between 48 and 72 hours should receive follow-up within 5 days (American Academy of Pediatrics, 2004). The serum bilirubin may be obtained at the time of the metabolic screening, thus precluding the need for additional blood sampling. The newest guidelines for monitoring and treating neonatal hyperbilirubinemia are published extensively elsewhere, and the reader is referred to the American Academy of Pediatrics (2004) reference for an in-depth overview of management guidelines.

End-tidal carbon monoxide (ETCO) levels (measured in exhaled breath) may be of value in determining the presence of hemolysis and the rate of heme degradation and bilirubin production in some infants; these determinations may be useful in determining the need for surveillance during the first week of life (American Academy of Pediatrics, 2004). ETCO measurements are reported to have limited value in neonates whose mothers smoked during pregnancy and in neonates with G6PD deficiency (Steffensrud, 2004).

Complications. Unconjugated bilirubin is highly toxic to neurons; therefore an infant with severe jaundice is at risk of developing **bilirubin encephalopathy**, a syndrome of severe brain damage resulting from the deposition of unconjugated bilirubin in brain cells. **Kernicterus** describes the yellow staining of the brain cells that may result in bilirubin encephalopathy (Sgro, Shah, and Campbell, 2005). The damage occurs when the serum concentration reaches toxic levels, regardless of cause. There is evidence that a fraction of unconjugated bilirubin crosses the blood-brain barrier in neonates with physiologic hyperbilirubinemia. When certain pathologic conditions exist in addition to elevated bilirubin levels, there is an increase in the permeability of the blood-brain barrier to

unconjugated bilirubin and, thus, potential irreversible damage. The exact level of serum bilirubin required to cause damage is not yet known.

Multiple factors contribute to bilirubin neurotoxicity; therefore *serum bilirubin levels alone do not predict the risk of brain injury.* Factors that enhance the development of bilirubin encephalopathy include metabolic acidosis, lowered serum albumin levels, intracranial infections such as meningitis, and abrupt fluctuations in BP. In addition, any condition that increases the metabolic demands for oxygen or glucose (e.g., fetal distress, hypoxia, hypothermia, hypoglycemia) also increases the risk of brain damage at lower serum levels of bilirubin.

The signs of bilirubin encephalopathy are those of CNS depression or excitation. Prodromal symptoms consist of decreased activity, lethargy, irritability, hypotonia, and seizures. Later these subtle findings are followed by development of athetoid cerebral palsy, mental retardation, and deafness (Sgro, Shah, and Campbell, 2005). Those who survive may eventually show evidence of neurologic damage, such as mental retardation, ADHD, delayed or abnormal motor movement (especially ataxia or athetosis), behavior disorders, perceptual problems, or sensorineural hearing loss.

Therapeutic Management

The primary goals in the treatment of hyperbilirubinemia are to prevent bilirubin encephalopathy and, as in any blood group incompatibility, to reverse the hemolytic process (p. 281). The main form of treatment involves the use of phototherapy. Exchange transfusion is generally used for reducing dangerously high bilirubin levels that occur with hemolytic disease.

The pharmacologic management of hyperbilirubinemia with phenobarbital has centered primarily on the infant with hemolytic disease, and phenobarbital is most effective when given to the mother several days before delivery. Phenobarbital promotes (1) hepatic glucuronyl transferase synthesis, which increases bilirubin conjugation and hepatic clearance of the pigment in bile; and (2) protein synthesis, which may increase albumin for more bilirubin binding sites. However, the use of phenobarbital in either the antenatal or the postnatal period has not proved to be as effective as other treatments in reducing bilirubin. Bilirubin production in the newborn can be decreased by inhibiting heme oxygenase—an enzyme needed for heme breakdown (to biliverdin)—with **metalloporphyrins,** especially tin protoporphyrin and tin mesoporphyrin. The use of heme-oxygenase inhibitors provides a preventive approach to hyperbilirubinemia (Bhutani, Gourley, Adler, and others, 2000; Drummond and Kappas, 2004).

Healthy near-term and full-term infants with jaundice may also benefit from early initiation of feedings and frequent breastfeeding. These preventive measures are aimed at promoting increased intestinal motility, decreasing enterohepatic shunting, and establishing normal bacterial flora in the bowel to effectively enhance the excretion of unconjugated bilirubin.

Phototherapy consists of the application of fluorescent light to the infant's exposed skin (Fig. 9-17). Light promotes bilirubin excretion by **photoisomerization,** which alters the structure of bilirubin to a soluble form **(lumirubin)** for easier excretion.

Studies indicate that blue fluorescent light is more effective than white fluorescent in reducing bilirubin. However, be-

FIG. 9-17 ■ **A,** Infant receiving phototherapy; note nested boundaries for comfort and eye protection. **B,** Newborn laying on BiliBlanket, which may be used with overhead lights to provide intensive phototherapy. (Courtesy E. Jacobs, Texas Children's Hospital, Houston.)

cause blue light alters the infant's coloration, the normal light of fluorescent bulbs in the spectrum of 420 to 460 nm is often preferred so that the infant's skin can be better observed for color (jaundice, pallor, cyanosis) or other conditions. For phototherapy to be effective, the infant's skin must be fully exposed to an adequate amount of the light source. When serum bilirubin levels are rapidly increasing or approximating critical levels, double or intensive phototherapy is recommended. Intensive phototherapy with a higher irradiance is considered to be more effective than standard phototherapy for rapid reduction of serum bilirubin levels (Beachy, 2007). The color of the infant's skin does not influence the efficacy of phototherapy. Best results occur within the first 24 to 48 hours of treatment. Phototherapy alone is not effective in the management of hyperbilirubinemia when levels are at a critical level or are rising rapidly; it is designed primarily for the treatment of moderate hyperbilirubinemia.

An alternative to traditional phototherapy "bililights" is the **fiberoptic blanket** or **panel** (Wallaby, BiliBlanket), which consists of a light-generating illuminator; a bundle of plastic fibers affixed to a panel that distributes the energy; and a soft, disposable, light-permeable cover to protect the infant. The blanket delivers therapeutic light consistently and continuously to the infant and achieves the same photoisomerization as conventional phototherapy. The fiberoptic blanket is especially suited for home phototherapy. The portable blanket permits more infant-parent interaction and better temperature control because the infant can be covered. It also eliminates the need for using eye patches (*if eyes are not exposed to a direct light source*).

A Cochrane review of 24 studies indicated that conventional phototherapy was more effective at lowering serum bilirubin values than fiberoptic lights alone; when two fiberoptic devices were used simultaneously in preterm infants, the therapy was as effective as conventional therapy at reducing serum bilirubin. Combination phototherapy (fiberoptic and conventional) was found to be more effective than conventional therapy alone. The authors further concluded that fiberoptic phototherapy is a safe and effective alternative to conventional therapy in preterm infants. The authors also pointed out that no trials were available to show that fiberoptic therapy is more effective than conventional phototherapy (Mills and Tudehope, 2005).

The American Academy of Pediatrics (2004) practice parameter guidelines provide suggestions for initiating phototherapy (see Fig. 9-16, *B*) and for implementing exchange transfusion in healthy, term infants.

Some clinicians believe that preterm infants have a higher risk of developing pathologic jaundice at lower serum bilirubin levels than do healthy, term infants because of associated illness factors that may increase the entry of bilirubin into the brain; however, research has failed to confirm this belief (Cashore, 2000). Until further research is completed, the recommendations for starting phototherapy in infants of 36 weeks of gestation is at levels of 14.6 mg/dl; for those at 32 weeks, levels of 8.8 mg/dl; for those at 28 weeks, levels of 5.8 mg/dl; and for 24 week infants, 4.7 mg/dl (Maisels and Watchko, 2003). However, each infant should be carefully evaluated with other illness and risk factors in mind, rather than depending on absolute values for all infants in a specific group.

Phototherapy has not been found to cause long-term adverse effects. The effectiveness of treatment is determined by a decrease in total serum bilirubin levels. Concurrently, the infant's total physical status is assessed continually because the suppression of jaundice by phototherapy may mask signs of sepsis, hemolytic disease, or hepatitis.

Recommendations for prevention and management of early-onset jaundice in breast-fed infants include encouraging frequent breastfeeding, preferably every 2 hours; avoiding glucose water, formula, or water supplementation; and monitoring for early stooling. The infant's weight, voiding, and stooling should be evaluated along with the breastfeeding pattern (Lawrence and Lawrence, 2005). Parents are taught to evaluate the number of voids and evidence of adequate breastfeeding once the infant is home and are encouraged to bring the newborn to the hospital, clinic, or primary care practitioner if there are indications of hyperbilirubinemia (Wheeler, 2000).

Bilirubin levels are monitored in late-onset jaundice, and treatment options vary. If the serum bilirubin levels remain above 16 mg/dl for more than 24 hours, obtain a bilirubin reading 2 hours after breastfeeding, which may then be interrupted for 10 to 12 hours (provide fluid and calories during this time with supplementation) and repeat levels drawn; with a serum bilirubin level decrease of 2 mg/dl or more, the infant may resume breastfeeding if levels are below 15 mg/dl.

nursingprocess | The Newborn with Jaundice

ASSESSMENT

Assess for signs of clinical jaundice. See further assessments on p. 279.

DIAGNOSIS (PROBLEM IDENTIFICATION)

After the nursing assessment, a number of nursing diagnoses may be evident. Additional nursing diagnoses that may apply include:

- Risk for Impaired Parent-Infant Attachment
- Interrupted Breastfeeding
- Risk for Deficient Fluid Volume
- Risk for Impaired Skin Integrity
- Interrupted Family Processes

PLANNING

Expected outcomes include:

- Infant will receive appropriate therapy as needed to reduce serum bilirubin levels.
- Infant will experience no complications from therapy.
- Mother-infant dyad will achieve successful breastfeeding.
- Family will receive emotional support.
- Family will be prepared for home phototherapy (if prescribed).

IMPLEMENTATION

Numerous nursing interventions are discussed on pp. 279-281.

EVALUATION

The effectiveness of nursing interventions for the family and infant with jaundice is determined by continual reassessment and evaluation of care based on the following guidelines:

- Observe skin color; review bilirubinometric and/or laboratory findings.
- Evaluate feedings and elimination pattern.
- Check placement of eye shields; observe skin for signs of dehydration; monitor infant's temperature.
- Interview family members and observe parent-infant interactions.

In the event that levels do not drop significantly, further evaluation is necessary (Lawrence and Lawrence, 2005). Parents should be offered the option of continuing breastfeeding, since no harmful effects have been found in healthy, term infants with bilirubin levels less than 20 mg/dl who continue to consume human milk. Based on these findings, Maisels (2005) suggests that, when feasible, phototherapy be implemented without the interruption of breastfeeding. Home phototherapy and continued breastfeeding are another option. Phototherapy as a treatment for hyperbilirubinemia is further discussed on pp. 279-280.

Prognosis. Early recognition and treatment of hyperbilirubinemia prevent unnecessary medical therapies, parent-infant separation, breastfeeding disruption and possibly failure, and severe brain damage (bilirubin encephalopathy). The characteristic impaired neurologic functions associated with bilirubin encephalopathy include athetosis (involuntary writhing movements), sensorineural hearing loss, paralytic gaze palsy, and other gaze abnormalities. Motor skills are delayed, and dental enamel hypoplasia may also occur.

Nursing Care Management

The nursing care of the infant with jaundice is discussed in the Nursing Process box and in the following section.

Part of the routine physical assessment includes observing for evidence of jaundice at regular intervals. Jaundice is most reliably assessed by observing the infant's skin color from head to toe and the color of the sclerae and mucous membranes. Applying direct pressure to the skin, especially over bony prominences such as the tip of the nose or the sternum, causes blanching and allows the yellow stain to be more pronounced. For dark-skinned infants, the color of the sclerae, conjunctiva, and oral mucosa is the most reliable indicator. Also, bilirubin (especially at high levels) is not uniformly distributed in skin. The nurse observes the infant in natural daylight for a true assessment of color.

The TcB is a useful screening device and is used to detect neonatal jaundice in full-term infants. Because phototherapy reduces the accuracy of the instrument, its value is limited to assessments made before the initiation of phototherapy. Institutions in which the device is used set up their own criteria based on their experience with their particular instrument. Blood samples are also taken for the measurement of bilirubin in the laboratory.

With short hospital stays, jaundice may appear after discharge. A careful history from the parents may reveal significant familial patterns of hyperbilirubinemia (older siblings of the infant). Other considerations in assessment include the ethnic origin of the family (e.g., higher incidence in Asian infants); type of delivery (e.g., induction of labor); and infant characteristics such as weight loss after birth, gestational age, sex, and the presence of any bruising. The method and frequency of feeding are assessed.

NURSINGALERT

Evidence of jaundice that appears before the infant is 24 hours of age is an indication for assessing bilirubin levels.

NURSINGTIP

While blood is drawn, phototherapy lights are turned off. Blood is transported in a covered tube to avoid a false reading as a result of bilirubin destruction in the test tube.

Prevention of jaundice may be possible with early introduction of feedings and frequent nursing without supplementation. Every effort is made to provide an optimum thermal environment to reduce metabolic needs.

Phototherapy. The infant who receives phototherapy is placed nude under the light source and repositioned frequently to expose all body surface areas to the light. After phototherapy has been initiated, frequent serum bilirubin levels (every 6 to 12 hours) are necessary because visual assessment of jaundice is no longer considered valid.

Several precautions are instituted to protect the infant during phototherapy. The infant's eyes are shielded by an opaque mask to prevent exposure to the light (see Fig. 9-17). The eye shield should be properly sized and correctly positioned to cover the eyes completely but prevent any occlusion of the nares. The infant's eyelids are closed before the mask is applied, since the corneas may become excoriated if they come in contact with the dressing. On each nursing shift the eyes are checked for evidence of discharge, excessive pressure on the lids, or corneal irritation. Eye shields are removed during feedings, which provide the opportunity for visual and sensory stimulation.

Infants who are in an open crib must have a protective Plexiglas shield between them and the fluorescent lights to minimize the amount of undesirable ultraviolet light reaching their skin and to protect them from accidental bulb breakage. Their temperature is closely monitored to prevent hyperthermia or hypothermia. Maintaining the infant in a flexed position with rolled blankets along the sides of the body helps maintain heat and provides comfort.

Accurate charting is another important nursing responsibility and includes (1) times that phototherapy is started and stopped, (2) proper shielding of the eyes, (3) type of fluorescent lamp (by manufacturer), (4) number of lamps, (5) distance between surface of lamps and infant (should be no less than 18 inches), (6) use of phototherapy in combination with an incubator or open bassinet, (7) photometer measurement of light intensity according to hospital protocol, and (8) occurrence of side effects.

Minor side effects for which the nurse should be alert include loose, greenish stools; transient skin rashes; hyperthermia; increased metabolic rate; dehydration; electrolyte disturbances, such as hypocalcemia; and priapism. To prevent or minimize these effects, the temperature is monitored to detect early signs of hypothermia or hyperthermia, and the skin is observed for evidence of dehydration and drying, which can lead to excoriation and breakdown. Oily lubricants or lotions are not used on the skin in order to prevent increased tanning or a "frying" effect. Full-term infants receiving phototherapy may require additional fluid volume to compensate for insensible and intestinal fluid loss. Because phototherapy enhances the excretion of unconjugated bilirubin through the bowel, loose stools may indicate accelerated bilirubin removal. Frequent stooling can cause perianal irritation; therefore meticulous skin care, especially keeping the skin clean and dry, is essential.

After phototherapy is permanently discontinued, there is often a subsequent increase in the serum bilirubin level, often called the **rebound effect;** this is usually transient and resolves without resuming therapy; however, a follow-up serum bilirubin level should be checked.

Family Support. Parents need reassurance concerning their infant's progress. All the procedures are explained to familiarize them with the benefits and risks. Parents need to be reassured that the naked infant under the bilirubin light is warm and comfortable. Eye shields are removed when the parents are visiting to facilitate the attachment process. The parents can be reassured that the neonate is accustomed to darkness after months of intrauterine existence and benefits a great deal from auditory and tactile stimulation (see Family Focus box).

FAMILY FOCUS

Phototherapy and Parent-Infant Interaction

The traditional use of phototherapy has evoked concerns regarding a number of psychobehavioral issues, including parent-infant separation, potential social isolation, decreased sensorineural stimulation, altered biologic rhythms, altered feeding patterns, and activity changes. Parental anxiety is greatly increased, particularly at the sight of the newborn blindfolded and under special lights. The interruption of breastfeeding for phototherapy is a potential deterrent to successful maternal-infant attachment and interaction. Because research has demonstrated that bilirubin catabolism occurs primarily within the first few hours of the initiation of phototherapy, there is increased support for the periodic removal of the infant from treatment for feeding and holding. Intermittent phototherapy may be just as effective as continuous therapy when used correctly. The benefits of stopping phototherapy for parental feeding and holding outweigh concerns related to the clearance of bilirubin in the healthy full-term newborn with mild to moderate hyperbilirubinemia. Home phototherapy offers an additional opportunity to foster parent-infant attachment.

The initiation of any treatment requires **informed consent** by the parents for the therapy prescribed; however, in the case of phototherapy considerable anxiety may rightfully occur when words such as *kernicterus* and *brain damage* are used to describe possible effects of nontreatment. It is imperative that nurses remain sensitive to parents' feelings and information needs during this process; an important nursing intervention is assessment of the parents' understanding of the treatment involved and clarification of the nature of the therapy.

One of the most important nursing interventions is recognition of breastfeeding jaundice. Lack of familiarity among health professionals has caused many newborns prolonged hospitalization, termination of breastfeeding, and unnecessary phototherapy. Care of the new mother may include supporting successful and frequent breastfeeding. Parents also need reassurance of the benign nature of the jaundice and encouragement to resume breastfeeding if temporary cessation is prescribed. In some situations jaundice may increase the risk of parents discontinuing breastfeeding and developing the **vulnerable child syndrome**—a belief that their child has suffered a "close call" and is vulnerable to serious injury (see Critical Thinking Exercise).

Discharge Planning and Home Care. With short hospital stays, mothers and infants may be discharged before evidence of jaundice is present. It is important for the nurse to discuss signs of jaundice with the mother, since any clinical symptoms will probably appear at home. Home visits within 2 to 3 days after discharge to evaluate feeding and elimination patterns and jaundice are becoming routine for many health care organizations.

If home phototherapy is instituted, the hospital or home health care nurse or medical equipment company representative is usually responsible for teaching family members and assessing their abilities to implement the treatment safely. General guidelines for home care preparation and education are discussed in Chapter 20. Written instructions and supervision of care—especially the application of eye shields, if needed—are essential. The minor side effects of phototherapy

CRITICAL THINKING EXERCISE

Jaundice

A full-term, 5-day-old newborn is brought to the minor emergency department late in the evening for evaluation of newborn jaundice. A home health nurse visited earlier in the day and drew a serum bilirubin by heel stick; the results were total bilirubin 14.6 mg/dl, direct bilirubin 0.9 mg/dl. The father is concerned because a home health care worker mentioned that the newborn might develop brain damage if the bilirubin levels were to increase to high levels. The mother is breastfeeding every 2 to 3 hours, and the newborn has had four wet diapers and three semiliquid stools over the past 18 hours. The newborn's birth weight was 2834 g (6.2 pounds), and her current weight (nude) is 2722 g (6 pounds). On examination the infant is active and alert, with visibly jaundiced skin and sclerae, intact reflexes, and strong suck reflex. The history reveals no prenatal or delivery complications. Apgar scores at 1 and 5 minutes were 8 and 9, respectively, and the initial assessment did not reveal any problems. The mother's blood type is A positive, and the direct Coombs test is negative. The newborn was discharged from the birth hospital on the second day of life in apparent good health.

QUESTIONS

1. Evidence—Is there sufficient evidence to draw any conclusions about the newborn's condition at this time?
2. Assumptions—Describe some underlying assumptions about the following:
   a. Newborn jaundice in healthy full-term infant
   b. Serum bilirubin levels and the newborn's age in days; other pertinent laboratory values (may refer to Fig. 9-16)
   c. Nutritional and excretory function and relation to bilirubin metabolism
   d. The physical status of the infant per assessment data
3. What implications and priorities for nursing care can be drawn at this time?
4. Does the evidence objectively support your argument (conclusion)?
5. Are there alternative perspectives to your argument? What are they?

are reviewed, and parents may need instruction in taking axillary temperatures and recording times and amounts of feedings and the number of wet diapers and stools. Regardless of how benign the disorder or the therapy, these parents need support and understanding. Measures should be taken to assist the mother in achieving successful breastfeeding, including consultation with a lactation specialist on an outpatient basis. Siblings also benefit from an explanation of the therapy to allay fears or misconceptions.

In jaundice associated with breastfeeding, follow-up blood studies are usually required to assess the progress of the jaundice. If temporary cessation of breastfeeding is prescribed, mothers should be taught to pump the breasts every 3 to 4 hours to maintain lactation; the expressed milk is frozen for use after breastfeeding is resumed.

HEMOLYTIC DISEASE OF THE NEWBORN

Hyperbilirubinemia in the first 24 hours of life is most often the result of HDN (erythroblastosis fetalis), an abnormally rapid rate of RBC destruction. Anemia caused by this destruction stimulates the production of RBCs, which in turn provides increasing numbers of cells for hemolysis. Major causes of increased erythrocyte destruction are isoimmunization (primarily Rh) and ABO incompatibility.

Blood Incompatibility

The membranes of human blood cells contain a variety of **antigens,** also known as **agglutinogens,** substances capable of producing an immune response if recognized by the body as foreign. The reciprocal relationship between antigens on RBCs and antibodies in the plasma causes **agglutination** (clumping). In other words, antibodies in the plasma of one blood group (except the AB group, which contains no antibodies) produce agglutination when mixed with antigens of a different blood group. In the **ABO blood group system** the antibodies occur naturally. In the **Rh system** the person must be exposed to the Rh antigen before significant antibody formation takes place and causes a sensitivity response known as **isoimmunization.**

Rh Incompatibility (Isoimmunization). The Rh blood group consists of several antigens (with D being the most prevalent). For simplicity, only the terms **Rh positive** (presence of antigen) and **Rh negative** (absence of antigen) are used in this discussion. The presence or absence of the naturally occurring Rh factor determines the blood type.

Ordinarily, no problems are anticipated when the Rh blood types are the same in both mother and fetus or when the mother is Rh positive and the infant is Rh negative. Difficulty may arise when the mother is Rh negative and the infant is Rh positive. Although the maternal and fetal circulations are separate, fetal RBCs (with antigens foreign to the mother) sometimes gain access to the maternal circulation through minute breaks in the placental vessels. The mother's natural defense mechanism responds to these alien cells by producing anti-Rh antibodies.

Under normal circumstances, this process of isoimmunization has no effect during the first pregnancy with an Rh-positive fetus because the initial sensitization to Rh antigens rarely occurs before the onset of labor. However, with the increased risk of fetal blood being transferred to the maternal circulation during placental separation, maternal antibody production is stimulated. During a subsequent pregnancy with an Rh-positive fetus, these previously formed maternal antibodies to Rh-positive blood cells may enter the fetal circulation, where they attack and destroy fetal erythrocytes (Fig. 9-18). Multiple gestations, abruptio placentae, placenta previa, manual removal of the placenta, and cesarean delivery increase the incidence of transplacental hemorrhage and subsequent isoimmunization (Moise, 2002).

Because the condition begins in utero, the fetus attempts to compensate for the progressive hemolysis and anemia by accelerating the rate of erythropoiesis. As a result, immature RBCs (**erythroblasts**) appear in the fetal circulation; hence the term **erythroblastosis fetalis.**

There is wide variability in the development of maternal sensitization to Rh-positive antigens. Sensitization may occur during the first pregnancy if the woman had previously received an Rh-positive blood transfusion. No sensitization may occur in situations in which a strong placental barrier prevents transfer of fetal blood into the maternal circulation. In approximately 10% to 15% of sensitized mothers, there is no hemolytic reaction in the newborn. In addition, some Rh-negative women, even though exposed to Rh-positive fetal blood, are immunologically unable to produce antibodies to the foreign antigen (Neal, 2001).

FIRST PREGNANCY

Rh-negative mother | Antibodies

Normal Rh-positive infant | Sensitization

A

SECOND PREGNANCY

Sensitized mother | Erythroblastosis fetalis

B

FIG. 9-18 ■ Development of maternal sensitization to Rh antigens. **A,** Fetal Rh-positive erythrocytes enter maternal system. Maternal anti-Rh antibodies are formed. **B,** Anti-Rh antibodies cross placenta and attack fetal erythrocytes.

| TABLE 9-4 |
| Potential Maternal-Fetal ABO Incompatibilities |

MATERNAL BLOOD GROUP	INCOMPATIBLE FETAL BLOOD GROUP
O	A or B
B	A or AB
A	B or AB

In the most severe form of erythroblastosis fetalis, **hydrops fetalis,** the progressive hemolysis causes fetal hypoxia; cardiac failure; generalized edema (anasarca); and effusions into the pericardial, pleural, and peritoneal spaces. The fetus may be delivered stillborn or in severe respiratory distress. The administration of maternal Rh₀(D) immune globulin (RhIG), early intrauterine detection of isoimmunization by ultrasonography, and subsequent treatment by fetal blood transfusions have dramatically improved the outcome of affected fetuses (Moise, 2002).

ABO Incompatibility. Hemolytic disease can also occur when the major blood group antigens of the fetus are different from those of the mother. The major blood groups are A, B, AB, and O. In the North American Caucasian population, 46% have type O blood, 42% have type A blood, 9% have type B blood, and 3% have type AB blood.

The presence or absence of antibodies and antigens determines whether agglutination will occur. Antibodies in the plasma of one blood group (except the AB group, which contains no antibodies) will produce agglutination (clumping) when mixed with antigens of a different blood group. Naturally occurring antibodies in the recipient's blood cause agglutination of a donor's RBCs. The agglutinated donor cells become trapped in peripheral blood vessels, where they hemolyze, releasing large amounts of bilirubin into the circulation.

The most common blood group incompatibility in the neonate is between a mother with O blood group and an infant with A or B blood group (see Table 9-4 for possible ABO

incompatibilities). Naturally occurring anti-A or anti-B antibodies already present in the maternal circulation cross the placenta and attack the fetal RBCs, causing hemolysis. Usually the hemolytic reaction is less severe than in Rh incompatibility. Unlike the Rh reaction, ABO incompatibility may occur in the first pregnancy. The risk of significant hemolysis in subsequent pregnancies is higher when the first pregnancy is complicated by ABO incompatibility (Sarici, Yurdakok, Serdar, and others, 2002).

Clinical Manifestations

Jaundice may appear shortly after birth (during the first 24 hours) in the newborn affected by HDN, and serum levels of unconjugated bilirubin rise rapidly. Anemia results from the hemolysis of large numbers of erythrocytes, and hyperbilirubinemia and jaundice result from the liver's inability to conjugate and excrete the excess bilirubin. Most newborns with HDN are not jaundiced at birth. However, hepatosplenomegaly and varying degrees of hydrops may be evident. If the infant is severely affected, signs of anemia (notably, marked pallor) and hypovolemic shock are apparent. Hypoglycemia may occur as a result of pancreatic cell hyperplasia.

Diagnostic Evaluation

Early identification and diagnosis of Rh D sensitization are important in the management and prevention of fetal complications. A maternal antibody titer (**indirect Coombs test)** should be drawn at the first prenatal visit. Genetic testing allows early identification of paternal zygosity at the *RHD* gene locus, thus allowing earlier detection of the potential for isoimmunization and avoiding further maternal or fetal testing (Moise, 2002). Amniocentesis can be used to test the fetal blood type of a woman whose antibody screen is positive; the use of polymerase chain reaction may determine the fetal blood type and presence of maternal antibodies. The fetal hemoglobin and hematocrit can also be measured (Moise, 2002). Chorionic villus sampling has drawbacks that preclude its use, including possible spontaneous abortion of the fetus and fetomaternal hemorrhage, which would essentially make the situation worse. With either method, if the fetus is found to be Rh negative, no further treatment is required.

Ultrasonography is considered an important adjunct in the detection of isoimmunization; alterations in the placenta, umbilical cord, and amniotic fluid volume, as well as the presence of fetal hydrops, can be detected with high-resolution ultrasonography and allow early treatment before the development of erythroblastosis. Doppler ultrasonography of fetal middle cerebral artery peak velocity has been used to detect and measure fetal hemoglobin and, subsequently, fetal anemia (Moise, 2002). Erythroblastosis fetalis caused by Rh incompatibility can also be monitored by evaluating rising anti-Rh antibody titers in the maternal circulation or by testing the optical density of amniotic fluid (delta OD_{450} test), since bilirubin discolors the fluid (Mari, 2000).

The disease in the newborn is suspected on the basis of the timing and appearance of jaundice (see Table 9-3) and can be confirmed postnatally by detecting antibodies attached to the circulating erythrocytes of affected infants (**direct Coombs test or direct antiglobulin test**). The Coombs test may be performed on cord blood samples from infants born to Rh-negative mothers if there is a history of incompatibility or further investigation is warranted.

Therapeutic Management

The primary aim of therapeutic management of isoimmunization is prevention. Postnatal therapy is usually phototherapy for mild cases and exchange transfusion for more severe forms. Although phototherapy may control bilirubin levels in mild cases, the hemolytic process may continue, causing severe anemia between 7 and 21 days of life.

Prevention of Rh Isoimmunization. The administration of RhIG, a human gamma globulin concentrate of anti-D, to all unsensitized Rh-negative mothers after delivery or abortion of an Rh-positive infant or fetus prevents the development of maternal sensitization to the Rh factor. The injected anti-Rh antibodies are thought to destroy (by subsequent phagocytosis and agglutination) fetal RBCs passing into the maternal circulation before they can be recognized by the mother's immune system. Because the immune response is blocked, anti-D antibodies and memory cells (which produce the primary and secondary immune responses, respectively) are not formed (Blackburn, 2007; Shaw, 2003). The inhibition of memory cell formation is especially important because memory cells provide long-term immunity by initiating a rapid immune response after the antigen is reintroduced (McCance and Huether, 2002).

To be effective, RhIG (such as RhoGAM) must be administered to unsensitized mothers within 72 hours (but possibly as long as 3 to 4 weeks) after the first delivery or abortion and repeated after subsequent pregnancies or losses. The administration of RhIG at 26 to 28 weeks of gestation further reduces the risk of Rh isoimmunization. RhIG is not effective against existing Rh-positive antibodies in the maternal circulation.

Preliminary studies have demonstrated the effectiveness of IV immunoglobulin (IVIG) at decreasing the severity of RBC destruction (hemolysis) in HDN and subsequent development of jaundice; IVIG administered to the neonate is believed to attack the maternal cells that destroy neonatal RBCs, slowing the progression of bilirubin production (Mundy,

2005). This therapy, often used in conjunction with phototherapy, may decrease the necessity for exchange transfusion.

> **NURSINGALERT**
>
> RhIG is administered intramuscularly, not intravenously, and only to Rh-negative women with a negative Coombs test—never to the newborn or father.

Intrauterine Transfusion. Infants of mothers already sensitized may be treated by intrauterine transfusion, which consists of infusing blood into the umbilical vein of the fetus. The need for therapy is based on the antenatal diagnosis of isoimmunization by determining the optical density of amniotic fluid (by amniocentesis) as an index of fetal hemolysis or by serial ultrasonography, which may detect the presence of fetal hydrops as early as 16 weeks of gestation. With the advance of ultrasound technology, fetal transfusion may be accomplished directly via the umbilical vein, infusing type O Rh-negative packed RBCs to raise the fetal hematocrit to 40% to 50%; fetal movement and transfusion risks are minimized by administering vecuronium bromide for temporary fetal paralysis. The frequency of intrauterine transfusions may vary according to institution and fetal hydropic status yet may be as often as every 2 weeks until the fetus reaches pulmonary maturity at approximately 37 to 38 weeks of gestation (Moise, 2002). The use of intraperitoneal blood transfusions is employed less commonly for isoimmunization because of higher associated fetal risks; however, it may be used for cases in which intravascular access is impossible.

Exchange Transfusion. Exchange transfusion, in which the infant's blood is removed in small amounts (usually 5 to 10 ml at a time) and replaced with compatible blood (such as Rh-negative blood), is a standard mode of therapy for treatment of severe hyperbilirubinemia and is the treatment of choice for hyperbilirubinemia and hydrops caused by Rh incompatibility. Exchange transfusion removes the sensitized erythrocytes, lowers the serum bilirubin level to prevent bilirubin encephalopathy, corrects the anemia, and prevents cardiac failure. Indications for exchange transfusion in full-term infants may include a rapidly increasing serum bilirubin level and hemolysis despite intensive phototherapy. The criteria for exchange transfusions in preterm infants vary according to associated illness factors. The American Academy of Pediatrics (2004) practice parameter guidelines provide recommendations for initiating phototherapy and for exchange transfusion in infants at 35 weeks of gestation or more. An infant born with hydrops fetalis or signs of cardiac failure is a candidate for immediate exchange transfusion with fresh whole blood.

For exchange transfusion, fresh whole blood is typed and crossmatched to the mother's serum. The amount of donor blood used is usually double the blood volume of the infant, which is approximately 85 ml/kg body weight, but is limited to no more than 500 ml. The two-volume exchange transfusion replaces approximately 85% of the neonate's blood.

An exchange transfusion is a sterile surgical procedure. A catheter is inserted into the umbilical vein and threaded into the inferior vena cava. Depending on the infant's weight, 5 to 10 ml of blood is withdrawn within 15 to 20 seconds, and the same volume of donor blood is infused over 60 to 90 seconds. If the blood has been **citrated** (addition of citrate phosphate dextrose adenine to prevent coagulation), calcium gluconate may be given after the infusion of each 100 ml of donor's blood to prevent hypocalcemia.

Prognosis. The severe anemia of isoimmunization may result in stillbirth, shock, congestive heart failure, or pulmonary or cerebral complications such as cerebral palsy. As a result of early detection and intrauterine treatment, erythroblastotic newborns are seen less often and exchange transfusions for the condition are less common. Despite the availability of effective preventive measures, Rh HDN continues to cause significant fetal morbidity and mortality in the United States.

Nursing Care Management

The initial nursing responsibility is recognizing jaundice. The possibility of hemolytic disease can be anticipated from the prenatal and perinatal history. Prenatal evidence of incompatibility and a positive Coombs test result are cause for increased vigilance for early signs of jaundice in an infant.

If an exchange transfusion is required, the nurse prepares the infant and the family and assists the practitioner with the procedure. The infant receives nothing by mouth (is NPO) during the procedure; therefore a peripheral infusion of dextrose and electrolytes is established. The nurse documents the blood volume exchanged, including the amount of blood withdrawn and infused; the time of each procedure; and the cumulative record of the total volume exchanged. Vital signs, monitored electronically, are evaluated frequently and correlated with the removal and infusion of blood. If signs of cardiac or respiratory problems occur, the procedure is stopped temporarily and resumed after the infant's cardiorespiratory function stabilizes. The nurse also observes for signs of blood transfusion reaction and maintains the infant's blood glucose levels and fluid balance.

Throughout the procedure attention must be given to the infant's thermoregulation. Hypothermia increases oxygen and glucose consumption, causing metabolic acidosis. Not only do these consequences hinder the infant's overall physical ability to withstand the long procedure, but they also inhibit the binding capacity of albumin and bilirubin and the hepatic enzymatic reactions, thus increasing the risk of kernicterus. Conversely, hyperthermia damages the donor erythrocytes, elevating the free potassium content and predisposing the infant to cardiac arrest.

The exchange transfusion is performed with the infant in a radiant warmer. However, the infant is usually covered with sterile drapes that may prevent the radiant heat from sufficiently warming the skin. The blood may also be warmed (using specially designed devices, *never* a microwave oven) before infusion.

After the procedure is completed, the nurse inspects the umbilical site for evidence of bleeding. The catheter may remain in place in case repeated exchanges are required.

> **NURSINGALERT**
>
> Signs of blood exchange transfusion reaction include tachycardia or bradycardia, respiratory distress, dramatic change in BP, temperature instability, and generalized rash.

Family Support. Parents often feel guilty because they think they have caused the blood incompatibility. Parents should never be made to feel responsible or negligent. They are encouraged to verbalize their thoughts. Actions that were taken to prevent any problems, such as frequent antepartum examinations and blood tests, should be referred to and praised.

METABOLIC COMPLICATIONS

The high-risk infant is subject to a variety of complications related to physiologic function and the transition to extrauterine life. Prominent among these are fluid and electrolyte derangements, hypoglycemia, and hypocalcemia. These complications often occur concurrently with or as a secondary result of other neonatal disorders and may therefore be difficult to differentiate from other conditions. The major characteristics of hypoglycemia and hypocalcemia are outlined in Table 9-5.

RESPIRATORY DISTRESS SYNDROME

Respiratory distress is a name applied to respiratory dysfunction in neonates and is primarily a disease related to developmental delay in lung maturation. The terms **respiratory distress syndrome (RDS)** and **hyaline membrane disease** are most often applied to this severe lung disorder, which not only is responsible for more infant deaths than any other disease, but also carries the highest risk in terms of long-term respiratory and neurologic complications (see Chapter 23 for a discussion of acute RDS). It is seen almost exclusively in preterm infants. The disorder is rare in drug-exposed infants or infants who have been subjected to chronic intrauterine stress (e.g., maternal preeclampsia or hypertension). Respiratory distress of a nonpulmonary origin in neonates may also be caused by sepsis, cardiac defects (structural or functional), exposure to cold, airway obstruction (atresia), intraventricular hemorrhage, hypoglycemia, metabolic acidosis, acute blood loss, and drugs. Pneumonia in the neonatal period is respiratory distress caused by bacterial or viral agents and may occur alone or as a complication of RDS.

Pathophysiology

Preterm infants are born before the lungs are fully prepared to serve as efficient organs for gas exchange. This appears to be a critical factor in the development of RDS. The effects of lung immaturity are compounded by the presence of more cartilage in the chest wall, leading to increased compliance of the chest wall, which collapses inward in response to less compliant (stiffer) lung tissue.

There is evidence of fetal respiratory activity before birth. The lungs make feeble respiratory movements, and fluid is excreted through the alveoli. Because the final unfolding of the alveolar septa, which increases the surface area of the lungs, occurs during the last trimester of pregnancy, preterm infants are born with numerous underdeveloped and many uninflatable alveoli. Pulmonary blood flow is limited as a result of the collapsed state of the fetal lungs—poor vascular development in general and an immature capillary network in particular. Because of increased pulmonary vascular resistance, the major portion of fetal blood is shunted from the lungs by way of the ductus arteriosus and foramen ovale.

At birth, infants must initiate breathing and keep the previously fluid-filled lungs inflated with air. At the same time, the pulmonary capillary blood flow must be increased approximately tenfold to provide for adequate lung perfusion and to alter the intracardiac pressure that closes the fetal cardiac structures. Most full-term infants successfully accomplish these adjustments, but preterm infants with respiratory distress are unable to do so. Although numerous fac-

TABLE 9-5
Metabolic Complications

HYPOGLYCEMIA	HYPOCALCEMIA
DEFINITION Blood glucose concentration significantly lower than that in the majority of infants of the same age and weight (usually <45 mg/dl)	Abnormally low levels of calcium in circulating blood
TYPE **Increased or impaired glucose utilization**—Large or normal-size infants who appear to suffer from hyperinsulinism; infants born to women with diabetes; infants with increased metabolic demands such as those with cold stress, sepsis, or after resuscitation; infants with enzymatic or metabolic endocrine defects **Decreased glucose stores**—Small or growth-restricted infants, preterm infants	**Early onset**—Appears in first 48 hours; appears in preterm infants who experienced perinatal hypoxia or sometimes in infant of diabetic mother **Late onset**—Cow's milk–induced hypocalcemia (neonatal tetany); apparent after first 3-4 days (high phosphorus/calcium ratio of cow's milk depresses parathyroid activity, reducing serum calcium levels); infants with intestinal malabsorption, hypoparathyroidism, or hypomagnesemia
CLINICAL MANIFESTATIONS Vague, often indistinguishable from other newborn conditions **Cerebral signs**—Jitteriness, tremors, twitching, weak or high-pitched cry, lethargy, limpness, apathy, convulsions, and coma **Other**—Cyanosis, apnea, rapid irregular respirations, sweating, eye rolling, poor feeding Signs often transient but recurrent	**Early onset**—Jitteriness, apnea, cyanotic episodes, edema, high-pitched cry, abdominal distention **Late onset**—Twitching, tremors, seizures
SCREENING Bedside monitoring or serum blood glucose for all infants at risk	At-risk infants or those who are symptomatic
LABORATORY DIAGNOSIS Plasma glucose concentrations <47-50 mg/dl (2.6-2.8 mmol/L) in any newborn regardless of gestational age at birth	Serum calcium <7.8-8 mg/dl (1.95-2.0 mmol/L) in full-term infant or Ionized calcium <4.4 mg/dl (1.1 mmol/L)
TREATMENT Early feeding in normoglycemic infants (preventive); intravenous (IV) glucose administration if breastfeeding or formula feedings not tolerated or glucose level extremely low	**Early onset**—Increased formula feedings; administration of calcium supplements (sometimes) **Late onset**—Administration of calcium gluconate orally or intravenously (slowly); vitamin D Correct hypoparathyroidism
NURSING Identify infants at risk or with hypoglycemia. Reduce environmental factors that predispose to hypoglycemia (e.g., cold stress, respiratory distress). Administer IV glucose as prescribed. Initiate early breastfeeding or formula feedings in healthy infant. Ensure adequate intake of carbohydrate (breast milk or formula).	Identify infants at risk or with hypocalcemia. Administer calcium as prescribed.* Observe for signs of acute hypercalcemia (e.g., vomiting, bradycardia). Manipulate environment to reduce stimuli that might precipitate a seizure or tremors (e.g., picking up infant suddenly, sudden jarring of crib).

***Nursing Alert:** Calcium preparations should *never* be administered by bolus rapid infusion in infants.

tors are involved, immaturity of the surfactant system plays a central role.

Surfactant is a surface-active phospholipid secreted by the alveolar epithelium. Acting much like a detergent, this substance reduces the surface tension of fluids that line the alveoli and respiratory passages, resulting in uniform expansion and maintenance of lung expansion at low intraalveolar pressure. Immature development of these functions produces consequences that seriously compromise respiratory efficiency. Deficient surfactant production causes unequal inflation of alveoli on inspiration and the collapse of alveoli on end expiration. Without surfactant, infants are unable to keep their lungs inflated and therefore exert a great deal of effort to reexpand the alveoli with each breath. With increasing exhaustion, infants are able to open fewer and fewer alveoli. This inability to maintain lung expansion produces widespread atelectasis.

In the absence of alveolar stability (normal functional residual capacity) and with progressive atelectasis, pulmonary vascular resistance (PVR) increases, whereas with normal lung expansion it would decrease. Consequently, there is hypoperfusion to the lung tissue, with a decrease in effective pulmonary blood flow. The increase in PVR causes partial reversion to the fetal circulation, with a right-to-left shunting of blood through the persisting fetal communications—the ductus arteriosus and foramen ovale.

Inadequate pulmonary perfusion and ventilation produce hypoxemia and hypercapnia. Pulmonary arterioles, with their thick muscular layer, are markedly reactive to diminished oxygen concentration. Thus a decrease in oxygen tension causes vasoconstriction in the pulmonary arterioles that is further enhanced by a decrease in blood pH. This vasoconstriction contributes to a marked increase in PVR. In normal ventilation with increased oxygen concentration, the ductus arteriosus constricts and the pulmonary vessels dilate to decrease PVR.

Prolonged hypoxemia activates anaerobic glycolysis, which produces increased amounts of lactic acid. An increase in lactic acid causes metabolic acidosis; inability of the atelectatic lungs to blow off excess carbon dioxide produces respiratory acidosis. Acidosis causes further vasoconstriction. With deficient pulmonary circulation and alveolar perfusion, partial pressure of oxygen in arterial blood continues to fall, pH falls, and the materials needed for surfactant production are not circulated to the alveoli.

BOX 9-4

Clinical Manifestations of Respiratory Distress Syndrome

Tachypnea (up to 80 to 120 breaths/min) initially*
Dyspnea
Pronounced intercostal or substernal retractions (Fig. 9-19)
Fine inspiratory crackles
Audible expiratory grunt
Flaring of the external nares
Cyanosis or pallor

*Not all infants born with respiratory distress syndrome will manifest these characteristics; the very low–birth-weight and extremely low–birth-weight infant may have respiratory failure and shock at birth because of physiologic immaturity.

Diagnostic Evaluation

The diagnosis of RDS is made on the basis of clinical manifestations (Box 9-4) and radiographic studies. Radiographic findings characteristic of RDS include (1) a diffuse granular pattern over both lung fields that closely resembles ground glass and represents alveolar atelectasis and (2) dark streaks, or bronchograms, within the ground glass areas that represent dilated, air-filled bronchioles. It is important to distinguish between RDS and pneumonia in infants with respiratory distress. The extent of respiratory function and acid-base balance is determined by blood gas analysis. Criteria for visually evaluating the degree of respiratory distress are illustrated in Fig. 9-19. Pulse oximetry and carbon dioxide monitoring, as well as pulmonary function studies, assist in differentiating pulmonary and extrapulmonary illness and are used in the management of RDS.

Therapeutic Management

The treatment of RDS involves immediate establishment of adequate oxygenation and ventilation and supportive care and measures required for any preterm infant, as well as those instituted to prevent further complications associated with preterm birth. The supportive measures most crucial to a favorable outcome are to:

- Maintain adequate ventilation and oxygenation
- Maintain acid-base balance
- Maintain a neutral thermal environment
- Maintain adequate tissue perfusion and oxygenation
- Prevent hypotension
- Maintain adequate hydration and electrolyte status

Nipple and gavage feedings are contraindicated in any situation that creates a marked increase in respiratory rate be-

FIG. 9-19 ■ Criteria for evaluating respiratory distress. (Modified from Silvermann WA, Anderson DH: A controlled clinical trial of effects of water mist on obstructive respiratory signs, death rate, and necropsy findings among premature infants, *Pediatrics* 17:1, 1956.)

cause of the greater hazards of aspiration. Nutrition is provided by parenteral therapy during the acute stage of the disease, while minimal enteral feeding is provided to enhance maturation of the neonate's gastrointestinal system.

The administration of **exogenous surfactant** to preterm neonates with RDS has become an accepted and common therapy in most neonatal centers worldwide. Numerous clinical trials involving the administration of exogenous surfactant to infants with or at high risk for RDS demonstrate improvements in blood gas values and ventilator settings, decreased incidence of pulmonary air leaks, intraventricular hemorrhage, decreased deaths from RDS, and an overall decreased infant mortality rate (Merrill and Ballard, 2003; Stevens and Sinkin, 2007). The overall rates of some associated comorbidities (bronchopulmonary dysplasia, NEC, patent ductus arteriosus) have not decreased with surfactant replacement. Exogenous surfactant is derived from a natural source (e.g., porcine, bovine) or from the production of artificial surfactant.

Complications seen with surfactant administration include pulmonary hemorrhage and mucous plugging. Surfactant therapy is also being investigated for use in infants with meconium aspiration, infectious pneumonia, sepsis, persistent pulmonary hypertension, and lung hypoplasia concomitant with congenital diaphragmatic hernia (Finer, 2004; Stevens and Sinkin, 2007). Surfactant may be administered at birth as a preventive or prophylactic treatment of RDS or later on in the course of RDS as a rescue treatment. Surfactant is administered via an ET tube directly into the infant's trachea. Nursing responsibilities with surfactant administration include assistance in the delivery of the product, collection and monitoring of arterial blood gases, scrupulous monitoring of oxygenation with pulse oximetry, and assessment of the infant's tolerance of the procedure. After surfactant is absorbed, there is usually an increase in respiratory compliance that requires adjustment of ventilator settings to decrease mean airway pressure and prevent overinflation or hyperoxemia. Suctioning is usually delayed for an hour or so (depending on the type of surfactant and unit protocol) to allow maximum effects to occur. Research is in progress to investigate the possibility of delivering an aerosolized surfactant (Mazela, Merritt, and Finer, 2007). This method would decrease the problems associated with current delivery systems (contamination of the airway, interruption of mechanical ventilation, and loss of the drug in the ET tubing from reflux).

The goals of oxygen therapy are to provide adequate oxygen to the tissues, prevent lactic acid accumulation resulting from hypoxia, and at the same time avoid the potentially negative effects of oxygen and barotrauma. Numerous methods have been devised to improve oxygenation (Table 9-6). All require that the gas be warmed and humidified before entering the respiratory tract. If the infant does not require mechanical ventilation, oxygen can be supplied by nasal cannula or via nasal prongs in conjunction with continuous positive airway pressure (CPAP) (see Oxygen Therapy, Chapter 22). If oxygen saturation of the blood cannot be maintained at a satisfactory level and the carbon dioxide level ($Paco_2$) rises, infants will require ventilatory assistance.

TABLE 9-6
Common Methods for Assisted Ventilation in Neonatal Respiratory Distress

METHOD	DESCRIPTION	HOW PROVIDED
CONVENTIONAL METHODS		
Continuous positive airway pressure (CPAP)	Provides constant distending pressure to airway in spontaneously breathing infant	Nasal prongs Endotracheal tube Face mask Nasal cannula
Positive end-expiratory pressure (PEEP)*	Provides increased end-expiratory pressure during expiration and between mandatory breaths, which prevents alveolar collapse; maintains residual airway pressure	Endotracheal intubation and either volume-limited or pressure-limited ventilator
Intermittent mandatory ventilation (IMV)*	Allows infant to breathe spontaneously at own rate but provides mechanical cycled respirations and pressure at regular preset intervals	Endotracheal intubation and ventilator
Synchronized intermittent mandatory ventilation (SIMV)	Mechanically delivered breaths are synchronized to the onset of spontaneous patient breaths; assist/control mode facilitates full inspiratory synchrony; involves signal detection of onset of spontaneous respiration from abdominal movement, thoracic impedance, and airway pressure or flow changes	Patient-triggered infant ventilator with signal detector and assist/control mode; endotracheal tube
Volume guarantee ventilation	Delivers a predetermined volume of gas using an inspiratory pressure that varies according to the infant's lung compliance (often used in conjunction with SIMV)	Volume guarantee ventilator with flow sensor; endotracheal tube
ALTERNATIVE METHODS		
High-frequency oscillation (HFO)	Application of high-frequency, low-volume, sine-wave flow oscillations to airway at rates between 480 and 1200 breaths/min	Variable-speed piston pump (or loudspeaker, fluidic oscillator); endotracheal tube
High-frequency jet ventilation (HFJV)	Uses a separate, parallel, low-compliant circuit and injector port to deliver small pulses or jets of fresh gas deep into airway at rates between 250 and 900 breaths/min	May be used alone or with low-rate IMV; endotracheal tube

*Also referred to as conventional ventilation (vs high-frequency ventilation [HFV]).

Prevention. The most successful approach to prevention of RDS is prevention of preterm delivery, especially in elective early delivery and cesarean section. Improved methods for assessing the maturity of the fetal lung by amniocentesis, although not a routine procedure, allow a reasonable prediction of adequate surfactant formation. Because estimation of a delivery date can be miscalculated by as much as 1 month, such tests are particularly valuable when scheduling an elective cesarean section. The combination of maternal steroid administration before delivery and surfactant administration postnatally seems to have a synergistic effect on neonatal lungs, with the net result being a decrease in infant mortality, decreased incidence of intraventricular hemorrhage, fewer pulmonary air leaks, and fewer problems with pulmonary interstitial emphysema and RDS.

Prognosis. RDS is a self-limiting disease. Before the use of surfactant, infants typically experienced a period of deterioration (approximately 48 hours) and, in the absence of complications, improved by 72 hours. Often heralded by the onset of diuresis, this improvement was attributed primarily to increased production and greater availability of surfactant. With the administration of surfactant, lung compliance begins to improve almost immediately, resulting in lower oxygen requirements and a decreased need for ventilatory support (Stevens and Sinkin, 2007).

Infants with RDS who survive the first 96 hours have a reasonable chance of recovery. However, complications of RDS include associated respiratory conditions and problems associated with prematurity: patent ductus arteriosus and congestive heart failure, intraventricular hemorrhage, bronchopulmonary dysplasia, retinopathy of prematurity, pneumonia, air leak syndrome, sepsis, NEC, and neurologic sequelae.

Nursing Care Management

Care of infants with RDS involves all of the observations and interventions previously described for high-risk infants. In addition, the nurse is concerned with the complex problems related to respiratory therapy and the constant threat of hypoxemia and acidosis that complicates the care of patients in respiratory difficulty.

The respiratory therapist, an important member of the neonatal intensive care team, is often responsible for the maintenance of respiratory equipment. Although it may be the respiratory therapist's responsibility to regulate the apparatus, nurses should understand the equipment and be able to recognize when it is not functioning correctly. The most essential nursing function is to observe and assess the infant's response to therapy. Continuous monitoring and close observation are mandatory because an infant's status can change rapidly and because oxygen concentration and ventilation parameters are prescribed according to the infant's blood gas measurements and pulse oximetry readings.

Changes in oxygen concentration are based on these observations. The amount of oxygen administered, expressed as the fraction of inspired air (Fio_2), is determined on an individual basis according to pulse oximetry or direct or indirect measurement of arterial oxygen concentration. Capillary samples collected from the heel (see Chapter 22 for procedure) are useful for pH and $Paco_2$ determinations but *not* for oxygenation status. Continuous transcutaneous or pulse oximetry readings are recorded at least hourly. Blood sampling is per-

formed after ventilator changes for the acutely ill infant and thereafter when clinically indicated.

> **NURSINGALERT**
> Suctioning is not an innocuous procedure (it may cause bronchospasm, bradycardia resulting from vagal nerve stimulation, hypoxia, or increased intracranial pressure, predisposing the infant to intraventricular hemorrhage) and should never be carried out on a routine basis. Improper suctioning technique can also cause infection, airway damage, or even pneumothoraces.

Mucus may collect in the respiratory tract as a result of the infant's pulmonary condition. Secretions interfere with gas flow and predispose the infant to obstruction of the passages, including the ET tube. Suctioning should be performed only when necessary and should be based on individual infant assessment, which includes auscultation of the chest, evidence of decreased oxygenation, excess moisture in the ET tube, or increased infant irritability. During suctioning a variety of techniques can be used to minimize complications, including the use of a closed suctioning system (Cifuentes, Segars, and Carlo, 2003).

When nasopharyngeal passages, the trachea, or the ET tube is being suctioned, the catheter should be inserted gently but quickly; intermittent suction is applied as the catheter is withdrawn. It is imperative that the time the airway is obstructed by the catheter be limited to no more than 5 seconds, because continuous suction removes air from the lungs along with the mucus. It is recommended that the "two-person" suctioning procedure be used on infants who are acutely ill and who do not tolerate any procedure without profound decreases in oxygen saturation, BP, and heart rate. The object of suctioning an artificial airway is to maintain patency of that airway, not the bronchi. Suction applied beyond the ET tube can cause traumatic lesions of the trachea. The use of in-line suction catheters may decrease airway contamination and hypoxia.

The most advantageous positions for facilitating an infant's open airway are on the side with the head supported in alignment by a small folded blanket or, when on the back, positioned to keep the neck slightly extended. With the head in the "sniffing" position, the trachea is opened at its maximum; hyperextension reduces the tracheal diameter in neonates.

Inspection of the skin is part of routine infant assessment. Position changes and the use of water pillows are helpful in guarding against skin breakdown.

Mouth care is especially important when infants are receiving nothing by mouth, and the problem is often aggravated by the drying effect of oxygen therapy. Drying and cracking can be prevented by good oral hygiene using sterile water. Irritation to the nares or mouth that occurs from appliances used to administer oxygen (e.g., nasal CPAP) may be reduced by the use of a water-soluble ointment.

The nursing care of an infant with RDS is a demanding role; meticulous attention must be given to subtle changes in the infant's oxygenation status. The importance of attention to detail cannot be overemphasized, particularly in regard to medication administration. (See Nursing Care Plan.)

RESPIRATORY COMPLICATIONS

The newborn infant is vulnerable to a variety of pulmonary complications, some requiring oxygen therapy (Table 9-7). For example, the preterm infant is subject to periods of apnea, and in term, near-term, and postterm infants, intrauterine stress often causes the fetus to pass meconium, which may be aspirated before or during birth. Oxygen therapy, although lifesaving, is not without its hazards. Positive pressure introduced by mechanical apparatus has created an increase in the incidence of ruptured alveoli and subsequent **pneumothorax and bronchopulmonary dysplasia (chronic lung disease).** The use of nasal CPAP decreases the incidence of adverse effects associated with intubation and positive pressure ventilation in preterm infants with RDS (Davis and Henderson-Smart, 2003). **Retinopathy of prematurity** is observed almost exclusively in preterm infants and is related primarily to prematurity and oxygen therapy (Tables 9-8 and 9-9). There is some evidence to support the resuscitation of asphyxiated newborns with 21% oxygen rather than 100% oxygen; preliminary studies demonstrate no significant neurologic morbidities at 18 to 24 months in newborns resuscitated with 21% oxygen (Saugstad, Ramji, Irani, and others, 2003; Saugstad, 2007). Proponents for room air resuscitation suggest there are

fewer complications associated with oxidative stress and hyperoxemia when room air is administered (Vento and Saugstad, 2006). The 2005 American Heart Association Neonatal Resuscitation Guidelines recommend the initiation of neonatal resuscitation using either supplemental oxygen that is less than 100% oxygen or room air (no supplemental oxygen); if the neonate does not improve within 90 seconds, the use of supplemental oxygen is recommended. Pulse oximetry is recommended to monitor the infant's oxygenation status during resuscitation and to prevent excessive use of oxygen in preterm infants (American Heart Association, American Academy of Pediatrics, 2006). Large multicenter studies are still needed to determine the optimum concentration of oxygen for resuscitation of neonates.

Inhaled nitric oxide (INO) and **extracorporeal membrane oxygenation (ECMO)** are additional therapies used in the treatment of respiratory distress and respiratory failure in neonates. INO is used in term and near-term infants with conditions such as persistent pulmonary hypertension, meconium

Text continued on p. 294

nursingcareplan | The High-Risk Infant with Respiratory Distress Syndrome

Nursing Diagnosis	Patient Outcomes	Nursing Interventions	Rationale
Ineffective Breathing Pattern related to pulmonary, neurologic vascular, alveolar, and muscular immaturity	High-risk infant will maintain patent airway and ventilatory status adequate for oxygenation.	Position to facilitate airway expansion and prevent collection of secretions (prone position may be preferred in preterm infant to increase chest expansion and oxygenation).	To allow oxygen entry into bronchial tree and alveoli
CHILD'S/FAMILY'S DEFINING CHARACTERISTICS *(Subjective and Objective Data)*	**THE FOLLOWING NOC CONCEPTS APPLY TO THESE OUTCOMES**	Closely monitor for deviations from desired breathing pattern—pulse oximetry, arterial blood gases, clinical signs of poor oxygenation, grunting, nasal flaring, apnea, tachypnea, retractions, cyanosis.	To facilitate proper oxygenation by implementing appropriate therapy such as supplemental oxygen, mechanical ventilation, or change of position
Decreased inspiratory and expiratory pressure	Respiratory Status: Ventilation Respiratory Status: Gas Exchange Tissue Perfusion: Pulmonary	Monitor vital signs for change in condition or status such as decreased cardiac output (poor perfusion, mottling, deteriorating ventilation status).	To implement appropriate therapy such as suctioning, supplemental oxygen, or vasopressor drugs
Decreased minute ventilation Use of accessory muscles to breathe Nasal flaring Grunting Apnea Tachypnea Altered chest excursion Respiratory rate: <20 or >60 breaths/min		Assist with exogenous surfactant administration and monitor patient tolerance or change in status.	To increase alveolar expansion and enhance oxygen–carbon dioxide exchange
		Suction oropharynx, nasopharynx, trachea, or endotracheal tube only as necessary and based on respiratory assessment.	To remove secretions that may interfere with adequate ventilation and oxygenation
		Perform gentle chest percussion, vibration, and postural drainage based on assessed need and infant tolerance.	To facilitate drainage and removal of secretions

THE FOLLOWING NIC CONCEPTS APPLY TO THESE INTERVENTIONS

Vital Signs Monitoring
Newborn Monitoring
Acid-Base Management
Airway Management
Chest Physiotherapy
Oxygen Therapy
Airway Suctioning
Energy Management
Respiratory Monitoring

Continued

nursingcareplan | The High-Risk Infant with Respiratory Distress Syndrome—cont'd

Nursing Diagnosis	Patient Outcomes	Nursing Interventions	Rationale
Ineffective Thermoregulation related to immature neurologic and metabolic temperature control **CHILD'S/FAMILY'S DEFINING CHARACTERISTICS** *(Subjective and Objective Data)* Reduction in body temperature below normal range Slow capillary refill Cool skin Increased respiratory rate Tachycardia	Infant will maintain stable body temperature (specify range for age). **THE FOLLOWING NOC CONCEPT APPLIES TO THESE OUTCOMES** Thermoregulation: Newborn	Place newborn in a thermally controlled incubator or radiant warmer. Place knitted or cloth cap on head. Use environmental controls for decreasing body heat loss—plastic heat shield, increased ambient temperature, servo control on warmer or incubator. Monitor axillary temperature as often as necessary or per unit protocol. Check temperature of newborn in relation to environmental temperature and temperature of heating element. Monitor vital signs and skin color, perfusion, pulses, and respiratory status. Monitor for signs of hyperthermia (flushing, tachycardia, altered level of consciousness) and hypothermia (decreased activity; respiratory distress [deterioration]; cool, mottled extremities). Monitor serum glucose levels as necessary or per unit protocol. **THE FOLLOWING NIC CONCEPTS APPLY TO THESE INTERVENTIONS** Environmental Management Hypothermia Treatment	To control environmental temperature and keep infant's temperature stable To prevent heat loss from exposed scalp To regulate body temperature within acceptable range and minimize heat loss To detect necessity for environmental temperature regulation and to determine infant's response to environmental thermoregulation To detect change in thermoregulatory status, which may indicate a significant disease process such as sepsis To detect changes in status that require additional intervention for stabilization To prevent untoward effects of hyperthermia (fluctuating cerebral perfusion, apnea, increased metabolism with decreased available glucose for vital functions) or hypothermia (increased glucose utilization, lactic acidosis, respiratory compromise) To ensure euglycemia is maintained

Nursing Diagnosis	Patient Outcomes	Nursing Interventions	Rationale
Risk for Impaired Parent-Infant Attachment **CHILD'S/FAMILY'S DEFINING CHARACTERISTICS** *(Subjective and Objective Data)* **Risk Factors** Separation Preterm infant Physical barriers	Parent(s) will form emotional bond or attachment with newborn. **THE FOLLOWING NOC CONCEPT APPLIES TO THESE OUTCOMES** Parent-Infant Attachment	Encourage parent(s) to hold and make eye contact with newborn as physical status allows. Encourage parent-newborn skin-to-skin contact in delivery room as condition of newborn allows. Explain to parents the newborn's illness in simple terms and expectations for recovery. Encourage parents to name newborn. Encourage parent participation in newborn care activities such as touching infant, expressing and storing maternal breast milk, and talking to infant. **THE FOLLOWING NIC CONCEPTS APPLY TO THESE INTERVENTIONS** Infant Care Breastfeeding Assistance Anxiety Reduction Parent Education: Infant	To minimize effects of physical separation from newborn To facilitate parent-infant interaction that is meaningful and comforting To enhance parental knowledge and decrease potential fear of unknown regarding infant's survival and recovery To provide child individual identity To facilitate parental involvement in attaining the role of parents and decrease feelings of helplessness

TABLE 9-7

Respiratory Complications

DESCRIPTION	CLINICAL MANIFESTATIONS	THERAPEUTIC MANAGEMENT	NURSING CARE MANAGEMENT
MECONIUM ASPIRATION SYNDROME (MAS)			
Aspiration of amniotic fluid containing meconium into fetal or newborn trachea in utero or at first breath	Meconium stained at birth Tachypnea Hypoxia Acidemia Hyperventilation (early) Hypoventilation (later)	Suction hypopharynx at birth. Intubate and suction trachea (as needed). Monitor for respiratory distress; manage with supplemental oxygen. Prevent acidosis and hypoxemia. May use exogenous surfactant, inhaled nitric oxide, or extracorporeal membrane oxygenation (ECMO)	See Nursing Care Management, Respiratory Distress Syndrome (p. 288).
APNEA OF PREMATURITY			
Lapse of spontaneous breathing for 20 seconds or longer, which may or may not be followed by bradycardia, oxygen desaturation, and color change	Persistent apneic spells	Observe for apnea. Check for thermal stability. Administer caffeine (or, less commonly, theophylline). Administer nasal continuous positive airway pressure (CPAP).	Provide continuous electronic monitoring (respiratory and heart rates). Observe for presence of respirations. Observe color. Provide gentle tactile stimulation. Suction nose and oropharynx if still apneic. Apply artificial ventilation with bag-valve-mask and with sufficient pressure to lift rib cage. Assess for and manage any precipitating factors (e.g., temperature instability, abdominal distention, ambient oxygen). Observe for signs of caffeine toxicity: tachycardia (rate 180-190 beats/min) and (later) vomiting, restlessness, irritability. Assess skin (with use of nasal CPAP) for breakdown, irritation at nasal septum.
PNEUMOTHORAX			
Presence of extraneous air in pleural space as a result of alveolar rupture	Tachypnea or apnea Systemic hypotension Sudden or persistent oxygen desaturation Grunting, nasal flaring Retractions Absent or diminished breath sounds Shift in point of maximum impulse of heart sounds Bradycardia, cyanosis	Evacuate trapped air in pleural space through needle aspiration or insertion of chest tube.	Maintain close vigilance of infants with respiratory distress or those on assisted ventilation. Provide appropriate care of chest drainage apparatus. Ensure emergency needle aspiration setup is available.
BRONCHOPULMONARY DYSPLASIA (BPD)			
Pathologic process related to alveolar damage from lung disease, prolonged exposure to mechanical ventilation, high peak inspiratory pressures and oxygen, and immature alveoli and respiratory tract	Dyspnea Barrel chest Inability to wean from oxygen or mechanical ventilation after course of respiratory distress syndrome (surfactant deficiency) Wheezing	Prevention: Administer maternal steroids; administer exogenous surfactant postnatally. Provide early detection with pulmonary function tests. Use synchronized or volume guarantee ventilation, decreased inspiratory pressures, or nasal CPAP. Prevent air leaks. Use high-frequency ventilation. Prevent or control respiratory or systemic infections. Diagnosis established: Support respiratory efforts. Maintain adequate oxygenation and avoid hypoxemia. Administer diuretics, bronchodilators. Provide supplemental oxygen in hospital or home.	Provide individualized developmental care and enhancement. Provide opportunities for additional rest during feedings. Observe for signs of fluid overload or pulmonary edema. Assist with home oxygen therapy as needed. Assess susceptibility to upper respiratory tract infections and need for frequent hospitalization for respiratory dysfunction. Provide increased caloric density (feedings) with human milk fortifier, protein supplements, microlipids, and glucose polymers.

TABLE 9-8

Cardiovascular and Hematologic Complications

DESCRIPTION	CLINICAL MANIFESTATIONS	THERAPEUTIC MANAGEMENT	NURSING CARE MANAGEMENT
PATENT DUCTUS ARTERIOSUS (PDA)			
Failure of ductus arteriosus to close at birth, resulting in shunting of oxygenated blood from aorta through open ductus arteriosus into pulmonary artery, increasing workload on left side of heart and increasing pulmonary vascular congestion (see Chapter 25)	Decreased Po_2 Increased Pco_2 Recurrent apnea Bounding peripheral pulses Systolic or continuous murmur	Regulate parenteral fluids. Provide respiratory support. Administer indomethacin or ibuprofen or perform surgical ductal ligation.	See Nursing Care of the High-Risk Newborn and Family (p. 250).
PERSISTENT PULMONARY HYPERTENSION OF THE NEWBORN (PPHN)			
Severe pulmonary hypertension and large right-to-left shunt through foramen ovale and ductus arteriosus	Hypoxia Marked cyanosis Tachypnea with grunting and retractions Decreased peripheral pulses and prolonged capillary refill (poor perfusion) Shock	Regulate intravenous (IV) fluids. Provide supplemental oxygen and assisted ventilation. Administer vasodilators. Maintain acid-base balance. Prevent hypoxemia and hypercarbia. Administer inhaled nitric oxide or extracorporeal membrane oxygenation (ECMO).	See Nursing Care of the High-Risk Newborn and Family (p. 250) and Respiratory Distress Syndrome (p. 284). Provide nursing care to reduce stress to infant, especially noxious stimuli that cause increased oxygen demands. Decrease physical manipulation and disturbance.
ANEMIA			
Hemoglobin (<14 mg/dl) inadequate to carry oxygenated blood to tissues Anemia commonly occurs in ill preterm infants as a result of increased blood sampling and deficient erythropoiesis	Pallor Apnea Tachycardia Diminished activity Poor feeder Poor weight gain Respiratory distress—grunting, nasal flaring, intercostal retractions Respiratory difficulty	Administer volume expanders for hypovolemia at birth (e.g., normal saline). Transfuse with packed red blood cells (RBCs) or administer recombinant human erythropoietin.	Use microsamples for blood tests. Monitor amount of blood drawn for tests. Administer recombinant human erythropoietin as prescribed. Administer iron supplements as prescribed.
POLYCYTHEMIA OR HYPERVISCOSITY SYNDROME			

Venous hematocrit 65% results in venous stasis in vital organs and risk for microthrombus development	High incidence of:
	    Cardiovascular symptoms (PPHN, cyanosis, apnea)
	    Seizures
	    Hyperbilirubinemia
	    Gastrointestinal abnormalities
		Implement partial exchange transfusion with blood product or appropriate volume expander.
		Provide appropriate therapy for associated problems.
			See Nursing Care of the High-Risk Newborn and Family (p. 250) and Hyperbilirubinemia (p. 274).

VITAMIN K DEFICIENCY BLEEDING (FORMERLY HEMORRHAGIC DISEASE OF THE NEWBORN)			
Bleeding disorder resulting from transient deficiency of vitamin K–dependent blood factors; newborn's sterile gut does not produce adequate amounts of vitamin K	Oozing blood from umbilicus or circumcision Bloody or black stools Hematuria Ecchymoses	Administer prophylactic vitamin K.	Administer vitamin K via intramuscular route.

TABLE 9-9
Sensory and Neurologic Complications

DESCRIPTION	CLINICAL MANIFESTATIONS	THERAPEUTIC MANAGEMENT	NURSING CARE MANAGEMENT
RETINOPATHY OF PREMATURITY (ROP)			
Severe vascular constriction in the immature retinal vasculature, followed by hypoxemia in the retina, which in turn stimulates abnormal vascular proliferation of retinal capillaries into the hypoxic area; as retinal veins dilate and multiply in the direction of the lens, retinal detachment may occur if untreated Multifactorial etiology—preterm birth is major risk factor	Progressive vascular growth of retina Eventual blindness if not treated Diagnosed by ophthalmologic examination	Prevent preterm birth. Provide early screening and detection in infants born at <28 weeks of gestation and weight <1500 g (3.3 pounds). Decrease exposure to bright, direct lighting; although exposure to bright light has not been proven to contribute to ROP, such exposure is undesirable from a neurobehavioral developmental perspective. Use supplemental oxygen judiciously, and monitor oxygen blood levels carefully; prevent wide fluctuations in oxygen blood levels (hyperoxia and hypoxia). Arrest vascular proliferation process—cryotherapy or laser photocoagulation; surgical repair of detached retina.	See Nursing Care of the High-Risk Newborn and Family (p. 250). Provide preventive care by closely monitoring blood oxygen levels, responding promptly to saturation alarms, and preventing fluctuations in blood oxygen levels. Provide postoperative pain management when surgery is indicated. Provide parental education and support. Provide nursing care using principles of individualized developmental care.
HYPOXIC-ISCHEMIC BRAIN INJURY			
Nonprogressive neurologic (brain) impairment caused by intrauterine or postnatal asphyxia resulting in hypoxemia or cerebral ischemia Hypoxic-ischemic encephalopathy (HIE)—the resultant cellular damage causes the clinical manifestations	Appears within first 6-12 hours after hypoxic episode Seizures Abnormal muscle tone (usually hypotonia) Disturbance of sucking and swallowing Apneic episodes Stupor or coma Muscular weakness in hips and shoulders (full term), lower limb weakness (preterm)	Prevent hypoxia. Provide supportive care. Provide adequate ventilation. Maintain cerebral perfusion. Prevent cerebral edema. Treat underlying cause. Administer antiseizure drugs.	See Nursing Care of the High-Risk Newborn and Family (p. 250). Observe for signs that indicate cerebral hypoxia. Monitor ventilatory and intravenous therapy. Observe for and manage seizures. Support family. Provide guidelines for family management of mild to severe neurologic damage.
GERMINAL MATRIX/INTRAVENTRICULAR HEMORRHAGE (GM/IVH)			

Hemorrhage into and around ventricles caused by ruptured vessels as a result of an event that increases cerebral blood flow to area	Sudden deterioration in condition if bleed is large
	Most bleeds initially asymptomatic
	Tense, bulging anterior fontanel
	Neurologic signs:
	  Twitching
	  Stupor
	  Apnea
	  Seizures
	Evident on cranial ultrasonography or tomography
		Supportive care:
		  Provide ventilatory support.
		  Maintain oxygenation.
		  Regulate fluid and electrolytes, acid-base balance.
		  Suppress or prevent seizures.
		  Provide ventricular shunting or drainage.
			See Nursing Care of the High-Risk Newborn and Family (p. 250).
			Prevent increased cerebral blood pressure.
			Avoid events that may increase or decrease cerebral blood flow (e.g., pain, unnecessary stimulation, endotracheal suctioning, hypoxia, hyperosmolar drugs, rapid volume expansion).
			Elevate head of bed 20-30 degrees; keep head in midline.
			Support family.
			Monitor for posthemorrhagic hydrocephalus after diagnosis.
			Provide developmental care and enhancement.

INTRACRANIAL HEMORRHAGE Subdural Subarachnoid Intracerebellar	Sudden decrease in hematocrit Change in sensorium Poor feeding See Chapter 28	See Chapter 28	Same as for GM/IVH

aspiration syndrome (see Table 9-7), pneumonia, sepsis, and congenital diaphragmatic hernia to decrease or reverse pulmonary hypertension, pulmonary vasoconstriction, acidosis, and hypoxemia. Nitric oxide is a colorless, highly diffusible gas that can be administered through the ventilator circuit blended with oxygen. INO therapy may be used in conjunction with surfactant replacement therapy, high-frequency ventilation, or ECMO. INO has not proved to be significantly effective in decreasing rates of bronchopulmonary dysplasia or in improving survival rates in preterm infants (Barrington and Finer, 2007).

ECMO may be used in the management of term infants with acute severe respiratory failure for the same conditions as those mentioned for INO. This therapy involves a modified heart-lung machine, although in ECMO the heart is not stopped and blood does not entirely bypass the lungs. Blood is shunted from a catheter in the right atrium or right internal jugular vein by gravity to a servo-regulated roller pump, pumped through a membrane lung where it is oxygenated and through a small heat exchanger, then returned to the systemic circulation via a major artery such as the carotid artery to the aortic arch. ECMO provides oxygen to the circulation; allows the lungs to "rest"; and decreases pulmonary hypertension and hypoxemia in such conditions as persistent pulmonary hypertension of the newborn, congenital diaphragmatic hernia, sepsis, meconium aspiration, and severe pneumonia.

CARDIOVASCULAR COMPLICATIONS

The most serious cardiovascular disorders of the newborn are the congenital heart defects. Other conditions that occur in the newborn period are usually related to prematurity (e.g., anemia, patent ductus arteriosus) or other diseases (e.g., respiratory distress). Some of these disorders are outlined in Table 9-8.

CEREBRAL COMPLICATIONS

Cerebral injury in newborn infants is not uncommon. Newborn infants are particularly vulnerable to ischemic injury caused by variable (both increased and decreased) cerebral blood flow subsequent to asphyxia, and preterm infants, with a fragile cerebrovascular network, are highly prone to periventricular or intraventricular hemorrhage. Fragility and increased permeability of capillaries and prolonged prothrombin time predispose the preterm infant to trauma when delicate structures are subjected to the forces of labor. The more common cerebral complications are outlined in Table 9-9.

The highest incidence of abnormal neurologic findings occurs in infants with intracranial hemorrhage and VLBW. Major neurologic problems, such as cerebral palsy, seizures, and hydrocephalus, are usually diagnosed in the first 2 years of life. Less severe deficits, such as learning disorders, ADHD, and fine and gross motor incoordination, may not be diagnosed until preschool or even school age. Cerebral palsy is one of the most common neurologic deficits in survivors of prematurity (see Chapter 32).

NEONATAL SEIZURES

Seizures in the neonatal period are usually the clinical manifestation of a serious underlying disease. The most common cause of seizures for term and preterm neonates is hypoxic ischemic encephalopathy secondary to perinatal asphyxia (Volpe, 2001). Although not life threatening as an isolated

---

BOX 9-5
Causes of Neonatal Seizures

METABOLIC
Hypoglycemia, hyperglycemia
Hypocalcemia
Hypernatremia, hyponatremia
Hypomagnesemia
Pyridoxine deficiency
Aminoacidurias (e.g., phenylketonuria, maple syrup urine disease)
Hyperammonemia

TOXIC
Uremia
Bilirubin encephalopathy (kernicterus)

PRENATAL INFECTIONS
Toxoplasmosis
Syphilis
Cytomegalovirus
Herpes simplex
Hepatitis

POSTNATAL INFECTIONS
Bacterial meningitis
Viral meningoencephalitis
Sepsis
Brain abscess

TRAUMA AT BIRTH
Hypoxic brain injury
Intracranial hemorrhage
Subarachnoid, subdural hemorrhage
Intraventricular hemorrhage

MALFORMATIONS
Central nervous system agenesis
Hydroencephalopathy
Tuberous sclerosis

MISCELLANEOUS
Narcotic withdrawal
Degenerative disease
Benign familial neonatal seizures

---

entity, seizures constitute a medical emergency because they signal a disease process that may produce irreversible brain damage. Consequently, it is imperative to recognize a seizure and its significance so that the cause, as well as the seizure, can be treated (Box 9-5).

The features of neonatal seizures are different from those observed in the older infant or child. For example, the well-organized, generalized tonic-clonic seizures seen in older children are rare in infants, especially preterm infants. The newborn brain, with its immature anatomic and physiologic status and less cortical organization, is unable to allow ready development and maintenance of a generalized seizure. Instead, signs of seizures in newborns, especially preterm neonates, are subtle and include findings such as lip smacking, tongue thrusting, eye rolling, and arching (Volpe, 2001).

Jitteriness or tremulousness in the newborn is a repetitive shaking of an extremity or extremities that may be observed with crying, occur with changes in sleeping state, or are elicited with stimulation. Jitteriness is relatively common in newborns, and in a mild degree may be considered normal during the first 4 days of life. Jitteriness can be distinguished from seizures by several characteristics:

- Jitteriness is not accompanied by ocular movement as are seizures.
- The dominant movement in jitteriness is tremor, whereas seizure movement is clonic jerking that cannot be stopped by flexion of the affected limb.
- Jitteriness is highly sensitive to stimulation, whereas seizures are not.

Jitteriness may be a sign of hypoglycemia, and infants with jitteriness should have a blood glucose level evaluated.

A **tremor** is defined as repetitive movements of both hands (with or without movement of legs or jaws) at a frequency of 2 to 5 per second and lasting more than 10 minutes. It is common in newborn infants and has a variety of causes, including neurologic damage, hypoglycemia, and hypocalcemia. In most instances tremors are of no pathologic significance.

Neonatal seizures can be divided into four major types. These classifications are outlined in order of frequency in Table 9-10 and consist of clonic, tonic, subtle, and myoclonic seizures (Volpe, 2001). Clonic, multifocal clonic, and migratory clonic seizures are more common in term infants.

Diagnostic Evaluation

Early evaluation and diagnosis of seizures are urgent. In addition to a careful physical examination, the pregnancy and family histories are investigated for familial and prenatal causes. Blood is drawn for glucose and electrolyte examination, and cerebrospinal fluid may be obtained for testing of cell count and differential, protein, glucose, and culture. Electroencephalography may help identify subtle seizures but is less helpful in establishing a diagnosis. Other diagnostic procedures, such as computed tomography, magnetic resonance imaging, and cerebral ultrasound, may be indicated. A video electroencephalogram may be used to identify seizure activity in some newborns. More extensive metabolic testing may be needed when initial test results do not provide a diagnosis or the history is suggestive of an inherited metabolic disorder.

Therapeutic Management

Treatment is directed toward prevention of cerebral damage and involves correction of metabolic derangements, respiratory and cardiovascular support, and suppression of the seizure activity. The underlying cause is treated (e.g., glucose infusion for hypoglycemia, calcium for hypocalcemia, antibiotics for infection). If needed, respiratory support is provided for hypoxia, and anticonvulsants may be administered, especially when the other measures fail to control the seizures. Phenobarbital, given intravenously or orally, has been the drug of choice and is used if seizures are severe and persistent. Other drugs that may be used are phenytoin (Dilantin), lorazepam, and diazepam (Valium).

A newer drug, fosphenytoin sodium, is a water-soluble prodrug and has been designed to replace phenytoin. Fosphenytoin metabolizes to form phenytoin in the body yet can easily be diluted or mixed in dextrose and normal saline and may be given via IV or intramuscular routes. In addition, fosphenytoin does not cause pain during IV administration.

TABLE 9-10
Classifications of Neonatal Seizures

TYPE	CHARACTERISTICS
Clonic	Slow rhythmic jerking movements
	Approximately 1-3 per second
Focal	Involves face, upper or lower extremities on one side of body
	May involve neck or trunk
	Infant is conscious during event
Multifocal	May migrate randomly from one part of the body to another
	Movements may start at different times
Tonic	Extension, stiffening movements
Generalized	Extensions of all four limbs (similar to decerebrate rigidity)
	Upper limbs maintained in a stiffly flexed position (resembles decorticate rigidity)
Focal	Sustained posturing of a limb
	Asymmetric posturing of trunk or neck
Subtle	May develop in either full-term or preterm infants but is more common in preterm
	Often overlooked by inexperienced observers
	Signs:
	Horizontal eye deviation
	Repetitive blinking or fluttering of the eyelids, staring
	Sucking or other oral-buccal-lingual movements
	Arm movements that resemble rowing or swimming
	Leg movements described as pedaling or bicycling
	Apnea (common)
	Signs may appear alone or in combination
Myoclonic	Rapid jerks that involve flexor muscle groups
Focal	Involves upper extremity flexor muscle group
	No electroencephalogram (EEG) discharges observed
Multifocal	Asynchronous twitching of several parts of the body
	No associated EEG discharges observed
Generalized	Bilateral jerks of upper and lower limbs
	Associated with EEG discharges

Modified from Volpe J: Neonatal seizures. In Volpe J: *Neurology of the newborn*, ed 4, Philadelphia, 2001, Saunders.

Nursing Care Management

The major nursing responsibilities in the care of infants with seizures are to recognize when the infant is having a seizure so that therapy can be instituted, to carry out the therapeutic regimen, and to observe the response to the therapy and any further evidence of seizures or other symptomatology. Assessment and other aspects of care are the same as for all high-risk infants. Parents need to be informed of their infant's status, and the nurse should reinforce and clarify the practitioner's explanations. The infant's behaviors need to be interpreted for the parents, and the infant's responses to the treatment must be anticipated and their significance explained. Parents are encouraged to visit their infant and perform the parenting activities consistent with the care plan. Seizures are a frightening phenomenon and generate a great deal of anxiety and fear, which is easily compounded by the justifiable concern of the staff. Providing support and guidance is an important nursing function.

HIGH RISK RELATED TO INFECTIOUS PROCESSES

SEPSIS

Sepsis, or **septicemia,** refers to a generalized bacterial infection in the bloodstream. Neonates are highly susceptible to infection as a result of diminished nonspecific (inflammatory) and specific (humoral) immunity, such as impaired phagocytosis, delayed chemotactic response, minimal or absent immunoglobulin A and immunoglobulin M (IgA and IgM), and decreased complement levels. Because of the infant's poor response to pathogenic agents, there is usually no local inflammatory reaction at the portal of entry to signal an infection, and the resulting symptoms tend to be vague and nonspecific. Consequently, diagnosis and treatment may be delayed.

Breastfeeding has a protective benefit against infection and should be promoted for all newborns. It is of particular benefit to the high-risk neonate. Colostrum contains agglutinins that are effective against gram-negative bacteria.

Sepsis in the neonatal period can be acquired prenatally across the placenta from the maternal bloodstream or during labor from ingestion or aspiration of infected amniotic fluid. Prolonged rupture of the membranes always presents a risk for this type from maternal-fetal transfer of pathogenic organisms. In utero transplacental transfer can occur with organisms and viruses such as cytomegalovirus, toxoplasmosis, and *Treponema pallidum* (syphilis), which cross the placental barrier during the latter half of pregnancy. Intrapartum infection may occur via contact with an infected mother; examples of such infections include herpesvirus and HIV.

Early-onset sepsis (less than 3 days after birth) is acquired in the perinatal period; infection can occur from direct contact with organisms from the maternal gastrointestinal and genitourinary tracts. The most common infecting organism is *Escherichia coli*, whereas group B streptococci (GBS) rates remain low (Stoll, Hansen, Higgins, and others, 2005). *E. coli*, which may be present in the vagina, accounts for approximately half of all cases of sepsis caused by gram-negative organisms. GBS is an extremely virulent organism in neonates, with a high (50%) death rate in affected infants. Other bacteria noted to cause early-onset infection include *Haemophilus influenzae, Citrobacter* and *Enterobacter* organisms, coagulase-negative staphylococci, and *Streptococcus viridans* (Stoll, Hansen, Higgins, and others, 2005). Other pathogens that are harbored in the vagina and may infect the infant include gonococci, *C. albicans,* herpes simplex virus (type II), and chlamydia.

Late-onset sepsis (1 to 3 weeks after birth) is primarily nosocomial, and the offending organisms are usually staphylococci, *Klebsiella* organisms, enterococci, *E. coli,* and *Pseudomonas* or *Candida* species (Stoll, Hansen, Fanaroff, and others, 2002). Coagulase-negative staphylococci, considered to be primarily a contaminant in older children and adults, is commonly found to be the cause of septicemia in ELBW and VLBW infants. Bacterial invasion can occur through sites such as the umbilical stump; the skin; mucous membranes of the eye, nose, pharynx, and ear; and internal systems such as the respiratory, nervous, urinary, and gastrointestinal systems.

Postnatal infection is acquired by cross-contamination from other infants, personnel, or objects in the environment. Bacteria that are commonly called "water bugs" (because they are able to grow in water) are found in water supplies, humidifying apparatus, sink drains, suction machines, and most respiratory equipment. Organisms such as coagulase-negative staphylococci, which usually colonize the skin, may infect indwelling venous and arterial catheters used for infusions, blood sampling, and monitoring of vital signs. Neonatal sepsis is most common in the infant at risk, particularly the preterm infant or the infant born after a difficult or traumatic labor and delivery, who is least capable of resisting such bacterial invasion. These organisms are often transmitted by personnel from person to person or object to person by poor hand washing and inadequate housecleaning.

Diagnostic Evaluation

Diagnosis of sepsis is often based on suspicion of presenting clinical signs and symptoms. Because sepsis is so easily confused with other neonatal disorders, the definitive diagnosis is established by laboratory and radiographic examination. Isolation of the specific organism is always attempted through cultures of blood, urine, and cerebrospinal fluid. Blood studies may show signs of anemia, leukocytosis, or leukopenia. Leukopenia is usually an ominous sign because of its frequent association with high mortality. An elevated number of immature neutrophils, decreased or increased total neutrophils, and changes in neutrophil morphology also suggest an infectious process in the neonate. Other diagnostic data that are helpful in the determination of neonatal sepsis include C-reactive protein and interleukins, specifically interleukin-6 (Volante, Moretti, Pisani, and others, 2004; Laborada, Rego, Jain, and others, 2003).

Prevention

Several measures are important in the prevention of both early- and late-onset infection. Programs to screen pregnant women for GBS colonization (culture-based) and treatment of those women in labor have dramatically reduced the incidence of GBS infection in the neonate (Centers for Disease Control and Prevention, 2002b). Screening programs for other maternal infections, including hepatitis B and human immunodeficiency virus (HIV), have also been recommended. Breastfeeding by mothers infected with HIV is not recommended because the virus may be transmitted in breast milk.

Nursery procedures aimed at minimizing the risk of nosocomial infections include the practice of good hand-washing techniques, appropriate isolation precautions where indicated, and the adoption of recommended standards for spacing of infant beds.

Therapeutic Management

In addition to the institution of vigorous therapeutic measures, early recognition (Box 9-6) and diagnosis are essential to increase the infant's chance for survival and reduce the likelihood of permanent neurologic damage. Antibiotic therapy is initiated before laboratory results are available for confirmation and identification of the exact organism. Treatment consists of circulatory support, respiratory support, aggressive administration of antibiotics, and immunotherapy.

Supportive therapy usually involves administration of oxygen (if respiratory distress or hypoxia is evident), careful regulation of fluids, correction of electrolyte or acid-base imbalance, and temporary discontinuation of oral feedings. Blood transfusions may be needed to correct anemia and shock, and electronic monitoring of vital signs and regulation of the thermal environment are mandatory.

BOX 9-6
Manifestations of Neonatal Sepsis

GENERAL SIGNS
Infant generally "not doing well"
Poor temperature control—hypothermia, hyperthermia (rare)

CIRCULATORY SYSTEM
Pallor, cyanosis, or mottling
Cold, clammy skin
Hypotension
Edema
Irregular heartbeat—bradycardia, tachycardia

RESPIRATORY SYSTEM
Irregular respirations, apnea, or tachypnea
Cyanosis
Grunting
Dyspnea
Retractions

CENTRAL NERVOUS SYSTEM
Diminished activity—lethargy, hyporeflexia, coma
Increased activity—irritability, tremors, seizures
Full fontanel
Increased or decreased tone
Abnormal eye movements

GASTROINTESTINAL SYSTEM
Poor feeding
Vomiting
Diarrhea or decreased stooling
Abdominal distention
Hepatomegaly
Hemoccult-positive stools

HEMATOPOIETIC SYSTEM
Jaundice
Pallor
Petechiae, ecchymosis
Splenomegaly

Antibiotic therapy is continued for 7 to 10 days if cultures are positive, discontinued in 48 to 72 hours if cultures are negative and the infant is asymptomatic, and most often administered via IV infusion. Antifungal and antiviral therapies are implemented as appropriate, depending on causative agents.

Prognosis. The prognosis for neonatal sepsis is variable. Severe neurologic and respiratory sequelae may occur in ELBW and VLBW infants as a result of early-onset sepsis. Late-onset sepsis and meningitis may also result in poor outcomes for immunocompromised neonates. The trend in antenatal diagnosis of maternal GBS and subsequent maternal and neonatal treatment with antibiotic therapy has decreased the incidence of early-onset GBS disease by 70% (0.5 cases per 1000 live births in 1999), although rates of late-onset perinatal GBS disease remained constant (Centers for Disease Control and Prevention, 2002b). New rapid tests for identification of maternal GBS at delivery have been developed, but the sensitivity and specificity of these tests are still being evaluated

(Aziz, Baron, D'Souza, and others, 2005); a vaccine to prevent perinatal GBS is still some years from being available.

Nursing Care Management

Nursing care of the infant with sepsis involves observation and assessment as outlined for any high-risk infant. Recognition of the existing problem is of paramount importance; it is usually the nurse who observes and assesses infants and identifies that "something is wrong" with them. Awareness of the potential modes of infection transmission also helps the nurse identify those at risk for developing sepsis. Much of the care of infants with sepsis involves the medical treatment of the illness. Knowledge of the side effects of the specific antibiotic and proper regulation and administration of the drug are vital.

Prolonged antibiotic therapy poses additional hazards for affected infants. Antibiotics predispose the infant to growth of resistant organisms and superinfection from fungal or mycotic agents, such as *C. albicans*. Nurses must be alert for evidence of such complications. Nystatin oral suspension is swabbed on the buccal mucosa for prophylaxis against oral candidiasis.

A number of specimens may be needed to help identify the cause and source of the infection. It is recommended that the fully flexed position be avoided for obtaining spinal fluid and that the side-lying position (modified with neck extension) or sitting position be used instead. Continual cardiorespiratory and pulse oximetry monitoring provides an ongoing assessment of the infant's condition during the procedure.

Part of the total care of infants with sepsis is to decrease any additional physiologic or environmental stress. This includes providing an optimum thermoregulated environment and anticipating potential problems such as dehydration or hypoxia. Precautions are implemented to prevent the spread of infection to other newborns, but to be effective, activities must be carried out by all caregivers. Proper hand washing, the use of disposable equipment (e.g., linens, catheters, feeding supplies, IV equipment), disposal of excretions (e.g., vomitus, stool), and adequate housekeeping of the environment and equipment are essential. Because nurses are the most consistent caregivers involved with sick infants, it is usually their responsibility to see that standard precautions are maintained by everyone.

Another aspect of caring for infants with sepsis involves observation for signs of complications, including meningitis and septic shock, a severe complication caused by toxins in the bloodstream.

> **NURSINGALERT**
> Artificial and long natural fingernails worn by nurses have been associated with serious neonatal infection and morbidity from *Pseudomonas aeruginosa* (Moolenaar, Crutcher, San Joaquin, and others, 2000) and *Klebsiella* organisms in the NICU (Gupta, Della-Latta, Todd, and others, 2004).

NECROTIZING ENTEROCOLITIS

NEC is an acute inflammatory disease of the bowel with increased incidence in preterm infants. Three factors appear to play an important role in the development of NEC: intestinal ischemia, colonization by pathogenic bacteria, and substrate (formula feeding) in the intestinal lumen. The precise cause of NEC is still uncertain, but it appears to occur in infants whose gastrointestinal tract has suffered vascular compromise. Intestinal ischemia of unknown etiology, immature gastrointestinal host defenses, bacterial proliferation, and feeding substrate are now believed to have a multifactorial role in the etiology of NEC. Prematurity remains the most prominent risk factor in the development of NEC.

The damage to mucosal cells lining the bowel wall is great. Diminished blood supply to these cells causes their death in large numbers; they stop secreting protective, lubricating mucus; and the thin, unprotected bowel wall is attacked by proteolytic enzymes. Thus the bowel wall continues to swell and break down; it is unable to synthesize protective IgM, and the mucosa is permeable to macromolecules (e.g., exotoxins), which further hampers intestinal defenses. Gas-forming bacteria invade the damaged areas to produce **pneumatosis intestinalis,** the presence of gas in the submucosal or subserosal surfaces of the bowel.

A consistent relationship has been observed between the development of NEC and enteric feeding of hypertonic substances (e.g., formula, hyperosmolar medications). It is unclear whether this connection is a result of the formula imposing a stress on an ischemic bowel, serving as a substrate for bacterial growth, or both.

Diagnostic Evaluation

Radiographic studies show a sausage-shaped dilation of the intestine that progresses to marked distention and the characteristic pneumatosis intestinalis—"soapsuds," or the bubbly appearance of thickened bowel wall and ultralumina. There may be air in the portal circulation or free air observed in the abdomen, indicating perforation. Laboratory findings may include anemia, leukopenia, leukocytosis, metabolic acidosis, and electrolyte imbalance. In severe cases coagulopathy (disseminated intravascular coagulation) or thrombocytopenia may be evident. Organisms are often cultured from blood, although bacteremia or septicemia may not be prominent early in the course of the disease.

Therapeutic Management

Treatment of NEC begins with prevention. Oral feedings may be withheld for at least 24 to 48 hours from infants who are believed to have suffered birth asphyxia. Breast milk is the preferred enteral nutrient because it confers some passive immunity (IgA), macrophages, and lysozymes.

Minimal enteral feedings (trophic feeding, gastrointestinal priming) have gained acceptance with no evidence of increased incidence of NEC. However, a meta-analysis of feeding studies found that, although minimal enteral feedings resulted in a reduction in days to full enteral feeds, an increased risk for NEC could not be ruled out (Tyson and Kennedy, 2005).

The role of probiotics such as *Lactobacillus acidophilus* and *Bifidobacterium infantis* administered with enteral feedings for the prevention of NEC has yet to be fully explored to advocate widespread use in all VLBW infants. In some studies probiotics decreased the incidence of NEC (Bin-Nun, Bromiker, Wilschanski, and others, 2005; Hung-Chih, Bai-Horng, An-Chyi, and others, 2005).

Medical treatment of confirmed NEC consists of discontinuation of all oral feedings; institution of abdominal decompression via nasogastric suction; administration of IV antibiotics; and correction of extravascular volume depletion,

electrolyte abnormalities, acid-base imbalances, and hypoxia. Replacing oral feedings with parenteral fluids decreases the need for oxygen and circulation to the bowel. Serial abdominal radiographic films (every 6 to 8 hours in the acute phase) are taken to monitor for possible progression of the disease to intestinal perforation.

Prognosis. With early recognition and treatment, medical management is increasingly successful. If there is progressive deterioration under medical management or evidence of perforation, surgical resection and anastomosis are performed. Extensive involvement may necessitate surgical intervention and establishment of an ileostomy, jejunostomy, or colostomy. Sequelae in surviving infants include short-bowel syndrome (see Chapter 24), colonic stricture with obstruction, fat malabsorption, and failure to thrive secondary to intestinal dysfunction. A variety of surgical interventions for NEC are available and depend on the extent of bowel necrosis, associated illness factors, and infant stability. Intestinal transplantation has been successful in some former preterm infants with NEC-associated short-bowel syndrome who had already developed life-threatening total parenteral nutrition–related complications. Transplantation may be a lifesaving option for infants who previously faced high morbidity and mortality (Kato, Mittal, Nishida, and others, 2003).

Nursing Care Management

Nursing responsibilities begin with the prompt recognition of the early warning signs of NEC. Because the signs are similar to those observed in many other disorders of the newborn, nurses must constantly be aware of the possibility of this disease in infants who are at high risk for developing NEC (Box 9-7).

When the disease is suspected, the nurse assists with diagnostic procedures and implements the therapeutic regimen. Vital signs, including BP, are monitored for changes that might indicate bowel perforation, septicemia, or cardiovascular shock, and measures are instituted to prevent possible transmission to other infants. It is especially important to avoid rectal temperatures because of the increased danger of perforation. To avoid pressure on the distended abdomen and to facilitate continuous observation, infants are often left undiapered and positioned supine or on the side.

> **NURSINGTIP**
>
> Observe for indications of early development of NEC by checking the appearance of the abdomen for distention (measuring abdominal girth, measuring residual gastric contents before feedings, and listening for bowel sounds) and performing all routine assessments for high-risk neonates.

Conscientious attention to nutritional and hydration needs is essential, and antibiotics are administered as prescribed. The time at which oral feedings are reinstituted varies considerably but is usually at least 7 to 10 days after diagnosis and treatment. Feeding is usually re-established using human milk, if available.

Because NEC is an infectious disease, one of the most important nursing functions is control of infection. Strict hand washing is the primary barrier to spread, and confirmed multiple cases are isolated. Persons with symptoms of a gastrointestinal disorder should not care for these or any other infants.

BOX 9-7
Clinical Manifestations of Necrotizing Enterocolitis

NONSPECIFIC CLINICAL SIGNS	SPECIFIC SIGNS
Lethargy	Distended (often shiny) abdomen
Poor feeding	Blood in the stools or gastric contents
Hypotension	Gastric retention
Vomiting	Localized abdominal wall erythema or induration
Apnea	Bilious vomitus
Decreased urinary output	
Unstable temperature	
Jaundice	

BOX 9-8
Clinical Manifestations of Infants of Diabetic Mothers

- Large for gestational age
- Very plump and full faced
- Abundant vernix caseosa
- Plethora
- Listlessness and lethargy
- Large placenta and umbilical cord (Wharton jelly)
- Possibly meconium stained at birth

The infant who requires surgery requires the same careful attention and observation as any infant with abdominal surgery, including ostomy care (as applicable). This disorder is one of the most common reasons for performing ileostomies on newborns. Throughout the medical and surgical management of infants with NEC, the nurse is continually alert to signs of complications, such as septicemia, disseminated intravascular coagulation, hypoglycemia, and other metabolic derangements.

HIGH RISK RELATED TO MATERNAL CONDITIONS

The health of the fetus and newborn may be affected by a number of maternal conditions; essentially, any condition affecting the mother also has the potential for negatively affecting the health of the newborn. **Pregnancy-induced hypertension** or **HELLP (hemolysis, elevated liver enzymes, low platelets) syndrome** may cause preterm delivery, intrauterine growth restriction (IUGR), asphyxia, and death if it is not detected early and appropriate interventions implemented. It is not within the scope of this text to elaborate on the pathophysiology and treatment of these conditions; however, the reader is referred to any one of the excellent maternity texts available for a detailed discussion of these conditions.

INFANTS OF DIABETIC MOTHERS

Before insulin therapy, few women with diabetes were able to conceive; for those who did, the mortality rate for both mother and infant was high. The morbidity and mortality of infants of diabetic mothers (IDMs) have been significantly reduced as a result of effective control of maternal diabetes and an increased understanding of fetal disorders. Because infants born to women with gestational diabetes mellitus are at risk for the same complications as IDMs, the following discussion of IDMs includes infants born to women with gestational diabetes mellitus.

The severity of the maternal diabetes affects infant survival. Severity of maternal diabetes is determined by the duration of the disease before pregnancy; age of onset; extent of vascular complications; and abnormalities of the current pregnancy, such as pyelonephritis, diabetic ketoacidosis, pregnancy-induced hypertension, and noncompliance. *The single most important factor influencing fetal well-being is the euglycemic status of the mother.* It has been found that reasonable metabolic control that begins before conception and continues during the first weeks of pregnancy can prevent malformation in an IDM. Elevated levels of hemoglobin A1c during the first trimester appear to be associated with a higher incidence of congenital malformations.

Hypoglycemia may appear a short time after birth and in IDMs is associated with increased insulin activity in the blood (see also Table 9-5, p. 285). The serum glucose level that corresponds to clinical hypoglycemia have not been well defined. Because some infants experience metabolic complications at higher levels than previously thought, some researchers recommend that serum glucose levels be maintained above 45 mg/dl (2.5 mmol/L) in infants with abnormal clinical symptoms, and as high as 50 or 60 mg/dl in other infants (Deshpande and Ward, 2005; Cornblath, Hawdon, Williams, and others, 2000).

Hypoglycemia in the IDM is related to hypertrophy and hyperplasia of the pancreatic islet cells, and thus is a transient state of hyperinsulinism. High maternal blood glucose levels during fetal life provide a continual stimulus to the fetal islet cells for insulin production (glucose easily passes the placental barrier from maternal to fetal side; insulin, however, does not cross the placental barrier). This sustained state of hyperglycemia promotes fetal insulin secretion that ultimately leads to excessive growth and deposition of fat, which probably accounts for the infants who are large for gestational age, or macrosomic. When the neonate's glucose supply is removed abruptly at the time of birth, the continued production of insulin soon depletes the blood of circulating glucose, creating a state of hyperinsulinism and hypoglycemia within ½ to 4 hours, especially in infants of mothers with poorly controlled diabetes (formerly class C diabetes or beyond [class D through R]). Precipitous drops in blood glucose levels can cause serious neurologic damage or death.

IDMs have a characteristic appearance (Box 9-8). Infants of mothers with advanced diabetes may be small for gestational age, may have IUGR, or may be appropriate for gestational age because of the maternal vascular (placental) involvement. There is an increase in congenital anomalies in IDMs in addition to a high susceptibility to hypoglycemia, hypocalcemia, hypomagnesemia, polycythemia, hyperbilirubinemia, cardiomyopathy, hypomagnesemia, and RDS. Hyperinsulinemia and hyperglycemia in the diabetic mother may be factors in reducing fetal surfactant synthesis, thus contributing to the development of RDS. Although large, these infants may be delivered before term as a result of maternal complications or increased fetal size.

Therapeutic Management

The most effective management of IDMs is careful monitoring of serum glucose levels and observation for accompanying complications such as RDS. The infants are examined for the presence of any anomalies or birth injuries, and blood studies for determination of glucose, calcium, hematocrit, and bilirubin are obtained on a regular basis. Studies confirm the importance of maintaining serum glucose levels above 50 mg/dl (2.8 mmol/L) in hyperinsulinemic infants with hypoglycemia to prevent serious neurologic sequelae (Cowett and Loughead, 2002).

Because the hypertrophied pancreas is so sensitive to blood glucose concentrations, the administration of oral glucose may trigger a massive insulin release, resulting in rebound hypoglycemia. Therefore feedings of breast milk or formula begin within the first hour after birth, provided that the infant's cardiorespiratory condition is stable. Approximately half of these infants do well and adjust without complications. Infants born to mothers with uncontrolled diabetes may require IV dextrose infusions. Oral and IV intake may be titrated to maintain adequate blood glucose levels. Frequent blood glucose determinations are needed for the first 2 to 4 days of life to assess the degree of hypoglycemia present at any given time. Testing blood taken from the heel with calibrated portable reflectance meters (e.g., glucometers) is a simple and effective screening evaluation that can then be confirmed by laboratory examination.

Nursing Care Management

The nursing care of IDMs involves early examination for congenital anomalies, signs of possible respiratory or cardiac problems, maintenance of adequate thermoregulation, early introduction of carbohydrate feedings as appropriate, and monitoring of serum blood glucose levels (see Evidence-Based Practice box). The latter is of particular importance because many hypoglycemic infants may remain asymptomatic. IV glucose infusion requires careful monitoring of the site and the neonate's reaction to therapy; high glucose concentrations (>12.5%) should be infused via a central line instead of a peripheral site.

Because macrosomic infants are at risk for problems associated with a difficult delivery, they are monitored for birth injuries such as brachial plexus injury and palsy, fractured clavicle, and phrenic nerve palsy. Additional monitoring of the infant for problems associated with this condition (polycythemia, hypocalcemia, poor feeding, and hyperbilirubinemia) is also a vital nursing function.

There is some evidence that IDMs have an increased risk of acquiring type 2 diabetes and metabolic syndrome in childhood or early adulthood (Boney, Verma, Tucker, and others, 2005); therefore nursing care should also focus on healthy lifestyle and prevention later in life with IDMs.

DRUG-EXPOSED INFANTS*

Maternal habits hazardous to the fetus and neonate include drug addiction, smoking, and alcohol abuse. Occasional withdrawal reactions have been reported in neonates of mothers who use to excess such drugs as barbiturates, alcohol, amphetamines, or antidepressants. Serious reactions are seen in neonates whose mothers abuse psychoactive drugs or are treated with methadone.

---

*Note that the term *addiction* is often associated with behaviors whereby the person seeks the drug(s) to experience a high or euphoria, escape from reality, or satisfy a personal need. Newborns who have been exposed to drugs in utero are not addicted in a behavioral sense, yet they may experience mild to strong physiologic signs as a result of the exposure. Therefore, to say that an infant born to a mother who uses substances is addicted is incorrect; *drug-exposed newborn* is a better term, which implies intrauterine drug exposure.

Narcotics, which have a low molecular weight, readily cross the placental membrane and enter the fetal system. Illicit substances may also be transmitted to the newborn through breast milk. When the mother is a habitual user of opiates, especially heroin or methadone, the unborn child may also become chemically dependent or passively addicted to the drug, which places such infants at risk during the perinatal and early neonatal periods. **Neonatal abstinence syndrome (NAS)** is the term used to describe the set of behaviors exhibited by the infant exposed to chemical substances in utero.

Clinical Manifestations

Throughout this section, unless otherwise noted, the information presented refers to drug-exposed neonates in general, regardless of which drug they have been exposed to.

The adverse effects of exposure of the fetus to drugs are varied. They include transient behavioral changes such as alterations in fetal breathing movements or irreversible effects such as fetal death, IUGR, structural malformations, or mental retardation. Determining the specific effects of individual drugs on the fetus is made difficult by polydrug use, which is common; errors or omissions in reporting drug use; and variations in the strength, purity, and types of additives found in street drugs. Maternal conditions such as poverty, malnutrition, and comorbid conditions such as sexually transmitted infections further compound the difficulty in identifying the presence and consequences of intrauterine drug exposure. Most infants who are exposed to drugs in utero may demonstrate no immediate untoward effects and appear normal at birth. Infants exposed only to heroin may begin to exhibit signs of drug withdrawal within 12 to 24 hours. If mothers have been taking methadone, the signs appear somewhat later—anywhere from 1 or 2 days to 2 to 3 weeks or more after birth. The clinical manifestations may fall into any one or all of the following categories: CNS, gastrointestinal, respiratory, and autonomic nervous system signs (Greene and Goodman, 2003). The manifestations become most pronounced between 48 and 72 hours of age and may last from 6 days to 8 weeks, depending on the severity of the withdrawal (Box 9-9). Although these infants suck avidly on fists and display an exaggerated rooting reflex, they are poor feeders with uncoordinated and ineffectual sucking and swallowing reflexes.

Not all infants of narcotic-addicted mothers will show signs of withdrawal. Because of irregular and varying degrees of drug use, quality of drug, and mixed drug usage by the mother, some infants display mild or variable manifestations. Most manifestations are the vague, nonspecific signs characteristic of all infants in general; therefore it is important to differentiate between drug withdrawal and other disorders before specific therapy is instituted. Other conditions (e.g., hypocalcemia, hypoglycemia, sepsis) often coexist with the drug withdrawal. Additional signs seen in drug-exposed newborns include loose stools; tachycardia; fever; projectile vomiting; crying; nasal stuffiness; and generalized perspiration, which is unusual in newborns.

Diagnostic Evaluation

Newborn urine, hair, or meconium sampling may be required to identify drug exposure and implement appropriate early interventional therapies aimed at minimizing the consequences of intrauterine drug exposure. Meconium sampling for fetal drug exposure is reported to provide more screening

Glucose Water Feedings in the Newborn Period

ASK THE QUESTION   Is 5% dextrose in water (D_5W) feeding an appropriate substitute for breast milk or formula in the newborn?

SEARCH FOR EVIDENCE

Search Strategies   Articles since 1980; key terms: newborn hypoglycemia, dextrose water feedings, newborn serum glucose, newborn feeding, sterile water feeding of newborn

Databases Used   Medline, PubMed, Ovid CINAHL

CRITICALLY ANALYZE THE EVIDENCE

No systematic or randomized clinical trials evaluating the oral administration of D_5W vs infant formula, water, or breast milk were found in the literature surveyed. Seven key articles and two textbooks were selected for this review.

- Noerr (2001) indicates that formula and breast milk or colostrum are ideal for the newborn who is asymptomatic (for hypoglycemia) and able to tolerate oral feedings; the free fatty acids from the breakdown of fat in formula or breast milk decrease peripheral glucose use and decrease the effect of insulin to suppress hepatic glucose production.
- Hashim and Guillet (2002) suggest that infants be fed a carbohydrate source to maintain a steady state rise in glucose. They recommend that D_5W be avoided because it may lead to rapid increases and subsequent falls in serum glucose levels.
- Blackburn (2003) suggests that early feedings with a carbohydrate source initially increases blood glucose levels; this increase is accompanied by subsequent increase in plasma insulin levels and the development of cyclic changes in insulin and blood glucose levels in full-term infants; animal studies suggest that D_5W, if aspirated, is just as dangerous as formula.
- The American Academy of Pediatrics and American College of Obstetricians and Gynecologists (2007) do not recommend routine supplementation with D_5W for infants receiving phototherapy.
- Eidelman (2001) recommends the initiation of breastfeeding within the first 30 to 60 minutes of birth for the healthy term infant and suggests that feedings with water or dextrose water are unnecessary and counterproductive.
- Initial feedings of sterile water or glucose water in newborns were historically recommended by physicians in newborns on the premise that the infant's propensity to spit up and possibly aspirate the feeding source into the lungs was less likely to compromise the infant's respiratory status if the aspirate was water (or dextrose water) instead of formula, breast milk, or colostrum. Wakayama, Wilkins, and Kimura (1988) suggested that initial feedings of infant formula after surgical repair for inguinal hernia did not significantly increase the incidence of aspiration.
- Sperling and Menon (2004) indicate that the initiation of milk feedings in the full-term infant induces ketogenesis, thus sparing glucose for brain consumption and facilitating gluconeogenesis.

- Hoseth, Joergensen, Ebbesen, and others (2000) found that healthy, AGA, full-term, breast-fed infants (n = 223) were not at risk for developing hypoglycemia. Diwakar and Sasidhar (2002) had similar findings in 200 exclusively breast-fed healthy full-term, AGA infants. Blackburn (2003) suggests that healthy breast-fed infants have a higher number of ketone bodies than formula-fed infants; this alternate source of energy (ketone bodies) enables the healthy full-term infant to maintain a steady state serum glucose level while breastfeeding is being established.
- The physiologic effects of early milk intake (breast milk or formula) in the healthy newborn include the stimulation of gut maturation, promotion of intestinal mucosa integrity, and release of intestinal enzymes that enhance motility and perfusion (Blackburn, 2003). There is evidence that sterile water and dextrose water feedings do not promote intestinal maturation; these are primarily from studies in newborns who are jaundiced.

APPLY THE EVIDENCE: NURSING IMPLICATIONS

Currently no evidence exists to support the practice of oral dextrose water feedings in healthy AGA newborns as a substitute for breast milk or formula even to treat mild, asymptomatic, transient hypoglycemia. Likewise, only physiologic evidence supports the practice of early oral feedings of breast milk, formula, or colostrum in healthy newborns.

References

American Academy of Pediatrics and American College of Obstetricians and Gynecologists: *Guidelines for perinatal care*, ed 6, Elk Grove Village, Ill, 2007, The Academy.

Blackburn ST: Maternal, fetal, and neonatal physiology: a clinical perspective, ed 2, St Louis, 2003, Saunders.

Diwakar KK, Sasidhar MV: Plasma glucose levels in term infants who are appropriate size for gestation and exclusively breast fed, *Arch Dis Child Fetal Neonatal Educ* 87(1): F46-F48, 2002.

Eidelman AI: Hypoglycemia and the breastfed neonate, *Pediatr Clin North Am* 48(2):377-387, 2001.

Hashim MJ, Guillet R: Common issues in the care of sick neonates, *Am Fam Physician* 66(9):1685-1692, 2002.

Hoseth E, Joergensen A, Ebbesen F, and others: Blood glucose levels in a population of healthy, breast fed, term infants of appropriate size for gestational age, *Arch Dis Child Fetal Neonatal Educ* 83(2):F117-F119, 2000.

Noerr B: State of the science: neonatal hypoglycemia, *Adv Neonat Care* 1(1):4-21, 2001.

Sperling MA, Menon RK: Differential diagnosis and management of neonatal hypoglycemia, *Pediatr Clin North Am* 51(3):703-723, 2004.

Wakayama Y, Wilkins S, Kimura K: Is 5% dextrose in water a proper choice for initial postoperative feeding in infants? *J Pediatr Surg* 23(7):644-666, 1988.

---

accuracy than urine, since drug metabolites accumulate in meconium (Kandall, 1999). Urine toxicology screening has less accuracy, since it reflects only recent substance intake by the mother (Huestis and Choo, 2002). Meconium and hair testing for drug metabolites has the advantages of being noninvasive, more accurate, and easy to collect. One study examining urine, hair, and meconium samples for drug use found that, although all of these tests were reliable to a greater or lesser degree, the single most reliable method for determining prenatal drug use was a careful history collected by an experienced interviewer (Eyler, Behnke, Wobie, and others, 2005).

Therapeutic Management

The treatment of the drug-exposed infant initially consists of early identification through maternal history, presenting symptoms of NAS, or toxicology screening when substance abuse is strongly suspected. Early identification and intervention are essential to prevent further adverse effects; early dis-

BOX 9-9

Signs of Withdrawal in the Neonate

NEUROLOGIC
Irritability
Seizures
Hyperactivity
High-pitched cry
Tremors
Exaggerated Moro reflex
Hypertonicity of muscles

GASTROINTESTINAL
Poor feeding
Diarrhea
Dehydration
Vomiting
Frantic, uncoordinated sucking
Gastric residuals

AUTONOMIC
Diaphoresis
Fever
Mottled skin
Nasal stuffiness

MISCELLANEOUS
Disrupted sleep patterns
Diaphoresis
Tachypnea (>60 breaths/min)
Excoriations (knees, face)
Temperature instability

charge from the birth institution should be postponed until further assessment of the maternal situation and establishment of a treatment plan for the mother and infant. Drug therapies to decrease withdrawal effects include parenteral or oral administration of phenobarbital, chlorpromazine, clonidine, diazepam, methadone, and morphine. A combination of these drugs may be necessary to treat infants exposed to multiple drugs in utero, and careful attention should be given to possible adverse effects of the treatment drugs (Johnson, Gerada, and Greenough, 2003).

Prognosis. The prognosis for drug-exposed infants depends on the type and amount of drug(s) taken by the mother and the stage(s) of fetal development in which the drug was taken. The overall mortality of infants born to narcotic-addicted mothers is increased, but with early recognition, proper treatment, and long-term follow-up, the morbidity and mortality associated with drug exposure are decreased.

Often, drug-exposed infants will exhibit poor brain and body growth at birth; however, at times, infants will not exhibit any signs that indicate exposure to harmful agents and their condition may therefore be overlooked until symptoms appear later in life. Drug-exposed infants may have chronic feeding problems; irritability; abnormal neurologic responses; abnormal parent-infant interactions; developmental and cognitive delays; learning disabilities; and behavioral problems, including ADHD.

Nursing Care Management

One of the key factors in the treatment of drug-exposed neonates is early identification of substance abuse in the pregnant woman so treatment can be initiated and side effects minimized. This is especially problematic from a social and legal standpoint because the pregnant woman is often aware of the consequences of admitting to substance abuse and may therefore be less likely to readily admit to the problem for fear of social and legal repercussions. If the mother has had good prenatal care, the practitioner is aware of the problem and may have instituted therapy before delivery. However, a number of mothers deliver their infants without the benefit of

adequate care, and the condition is unknown to health care personnel at the time of delivery.

The degree of withdrawal is closely related to the amount of drug the mother has habitually taken, the length of time she has been taking the drug, and her drug level at the time of delivery. The most severe symptoms are observed in the infants of mothers who have taken large amounts of drugs over a long period. In addition, the nearer to the time of delivery that the mother takes the drug, the longer it takes the child to develop withdrawal, and the more severe the manifestations. The infant may not exhibit withdrawal symptoms until 7 to 10 days after delivery, by which time most newborns have been discharged from the birth center and caregivers are less likely to recognize signs of irritability and poor feeding as withdrawal, thus predisposing the newborn to abuse or neglect. The infant may be at further risk for subsequent abuse or neglect because of home conditions that preclude adequate newborn care and follow-up.

After the presence of NAS is identified in an infant, nursing care is directed toward treatment of the presenting signs, decreasing stimuli that may precipitate hyperactivity and irritability (e.g., dimming the lights, decreasing noise levels), providing adequate nutrition and hydration, and promoting maternal-infant relationships. Appropriate individualized developmental care is implemented to facilitate self-consoling and self-regulating behaviors. Irritable and hyperactive infants have been found to respond to physical comforting, movement, and close contact. Wrapping infants snugly and rocking and holding them tightly limits their ability to self-stimulate. Arranging nursing activities to reduce the amount of disturbance helps decrease exogenous stimulation.

Breastfeeding is encouraged in mothers who are not using illicit substances, are negative for HIV infection, and are compliant with a methadone program; breastfeeding promotes maternal-infant bonding, and small quantities of methadone passed through breast milk have not proved to be harmful.

The **Neonatal Abstinence Scoring System** has been developed to monitor infants in an objective manner and evaluate their response to clinical and pharmacologic interventions (Kandall, 1999; Finnegan, 1985). This system is also designed to assist nurses and other health care workers in evaluating the severity of the infant's withdrawal symptoms. Another tool that may be used to evaluate withdrawal behavior and treatment in newborns is the **Neonatal Withdrawal Inventory** developed by Zahorodny, Rom, Whitney, and others (1998); it is important to note that neither of these tools is specific to preterm infants and may not be representative of withdrawal behaviors in such infants (Marcellus, 2002).

The **Neonatal Intensive Care Unit Network Neurobehavioral Scale (NNNS)** is a comprehensive neurologic and behavioral assessment tool that may be used to identify newborns at risk as a result of intrauterine drug exposure. The tool measures stress or abstinence, state, neurologic status, and muscle tone in the context of the newborn's medical condition at the time of examination. The NNNS may be used for medically stable newborns who are at least 30 weeks of gestation and up to 48 weeks of corrected or conceptional age (Lester, Tronick, and Brazelton, 2004).

Loose stools, poor intake, and regurgitation after feeding predispose these infants to malnutrition, dehydration, and electrolyte imbalance. In addition, these infants burn up energy with continual activity and increased oxygen consumption at the cellular level. Frequent weighing, careful monitoring of intake and output and electrolytes, and additional caloric supplementation may be necessary. Hyperactive infants must be protected from skin abrasions on the knees, toes, and cheeks that are caused by rubbing on bed linens while in a prone position (awake). Monitoring and recording the activity level and its relationship to other activities, such as feeding and preventing complications, are important nursing functions.

A valuable aid to anticipating problems in the newborn is recognizing substance abuse in the mother. Unless the mother is enrolled in a methadone rehabilitation program, she seldom risks calling attention to her habit by seeking prenatal care. Consequently, infants and mothers are exposed to the additional hazards of obstetric and medical complications. Moreover, the nature of substance use and addiction makes the user susceptible to disorders such as infection (hepatitis B, HIV), foreign body reaction, and the hazards of inadequate nutrition and preterm birth. Methadone treatment does not prevent withdrawal reaction in neonates, but the clinical course may be modified. Also, the intensive psychologic support of mothers is a factor in the treatment and reduction of perinatal mortality. Experience has indicated that mothers are usually anxious and depressed, lack confidence, have a poor self-image, and have difficulty with interpersonal relationships. They may have a psychologic need for the pregnancy and an infant.

Initial symptoms or the recurrence of withdrawal symptoms may develop after discharge from the hospital; therefore it is important to establish rapport and maintain contact with the family so that they return for treatment if this occurs. The demands of the drug-exposed infant on the caregiver are enormous and unrewarding in terms of positive feedback. The infants are difficult to comfort, and they cry for long periods, which can be especially trying for the caregiver after the infant's discharge from the hospital. Long-term follow-up to evaluate the status of the infant and family is very important. Sudden infant death syndrome and HIV infection are observed more commonly in infants born to users of methadone and heroin.

Many problems arise in relation to the disposition of infants of drug-dependent mothers. Those who advocate separation of mothers and children argue that the mothers are not capable of assuming responsibility for their infant's care, that child care is frustrating to them, and that their existence is too disorganized and chaotic. Others encourage the maternal-infant bond and recommend a protected environment such as a therapeutic community, a halfway house, or continuous ongoing, supportive services in the home after discharge. Careful evaluation and the cooperative efforts of a variety of health professionals are required whether the choice is foster home placement or supportive follow-up care of mothers who keep their infants.

Alcohol Exposure

Alcohol ingestion during pregnancy is associated with both short- and long-term effects on the fetus and newborn. The quantity of alcohol required to produce fetal effects is unclear, but it is known that infants born to heavy drinkers have twice the risk of congenital abnormalities than those born to moderate drinkers (Stoll, 2007). Alcohol withdrawal can occur in neonates, particularly when maternal ingestion occurs near the time of delivery (Greene and Goodman, 2003). Signs and symptoms include jitteriness, increased tone and reflex responses, and irritability. Seizures are also common. The incidence of **fetal alcohol syndrome (FAS)** in the United States is about 2 per 1000 population (Stoll, 2007). FAS is based on minimal criteria of signs in each of three categories: prenatal and postnatal growth restriction; CNS malfunctions, including mental retardation; and craniofacial features such as microcephaly, small eyes or short palpebral fissures, thin upper lip, flat midface, and an indistinct philtrum. Neurologic problems in FAS children include some degree of IQ deficit, ADHD, diminished fine motor skills, and poor speech. These children have been shown to lack inhibition, have no stranger anxiety, and lack appropriate judgment skills

Infants who do not display the signs of FAS but are born to mothers who are also heavy alcohol drinkers have significantly more tremors, hypertonia, restlessness, excessive mouthing movements, crying, and inconsolability than infants of substance-abusive mothers who do not consume alcohol during pregnancy. An added concern regarding substance abuse is that many of the mothers often use several drugs, such as tranquilizers, sedatives, amphetamines, phencyclidine, marijuana, and other psychotropic agents.

Cocaine Exposure

Cocaine, a commonly used illicit drug used in the United States, has multiple modes of use. However, use of the relatively inexpensive and easily administered "crack" form is increasing, especially among women of childbearing age (Cambell, 2003). Because crack vaporizes at relatively low temperatures, it is smoked and absorbed in large quantities through pulmonary vasculature. The drug readily crosses the placenta, placing the fetus at risk (Malanga and Kosofsy, 1999).

Cocaine is a CNS stimulant and peripheral sympathomimetic. Legally it is classified as a narcotic, but it is not an opioid. The effects on the fetus are secondary to maternal effects—increased BP, decreased uterine blood flow, and increased vascular resistance. Consequently, the fetus suffers decreased blood flow and oxygenation because of placental and fetal vasoconstriction. Researchers have concluded that variables such as the mother's lack of prenatal care; poor nutrition; and use of tobacco, alcohol, and other drugs during pregnancy compound the effects of cocaine exposure in the infant (Askin and Diehl-Jones, 2001; Tronick and Beeghly, 1999).

Infants may appear normal, or they may show neurologic problems at birth that may continue during the neonatal period. In much of the research literature, these findings were transient, and there has been variable evidence demonstrating permanent sequelae. Either of two types of behavior may emerge as a result of cocaine effects on fetal development: neurobehavioral depression or excitability. The behaviors of the depressed infant include lethargy, poor suck, hypotonia, weak cry, and difficulty in arousing. The behaviors of the excitable neonate may include a high-pitched cry, hypertonicity, rigidity, irritability, inability to be consoled, and intolerance to a change in routine (Chiriboga, Brust, Bateman, and others, 1999; Chiriboga, Kuhn, and Wasserman, 2007). Other behaviors may include frequent startling, poorly defined awake state, sleeping difficulties, and persistent primitive reflexes. Some infants develop late onset of symptoms (2 to 8 weeks). They may become irritable and hypertonic, experience sleep-wake disruptions, and demonstrate an inability to tolerate change; they may also be slightly febrile. However, many of the findings cited above have been refuted in other studies (Eyler and Behnke, 1999; Tronick and Beeghly, 1999).

The adverse effects on the cocaine-exposed neonate are related to dose-response. The higher the dose, the more effects are noted, such as IUGR, hypertonia, and decreased fetal head growth (Chiriboga, Brust, Bateman, and others, 1999).

Sequelae of prenatal cocaine exposure include a smaller head circumference, decreased birth length, and decreased weight. Head growth may be one of the best predictors of long-term development (Bateman and Chiriboga, 2000). Other neonatal effects of cocaine exposure include increased incidence of gastroschisis, genitourinary anomalies, and periventricular and intraventricular hemorrhage. Some studies found that long-term sequelae for newborns exposed to cocaine include lower language, motor, and cognitive scores and an increased risk for learning disabilities (Singer, Arendt, Minnes, and others, 2002; Koren, Nulman, Rovet, and others, 1998; Morrow, Culbertson, Accornero, and others, 2006); however, one study revealed no significant differences in the total or verbal IQ scores but did note an increased risk of specific cognitive impairments (Singer, Minnes, Short, and others, 2004). Arendt, Angelopoulos, Salvator, and others (1999) noted that the fine and gross motor development indexes in 2-year-old children who were exposed to cocaine prenatally were lower than in the control group. Some researchers noted that the exposed children may be affected emotionally rather than intellectually. In a study of first-grade students, Delaney-Black, Cobington, Templin, and others (1998) concluded that the children who were exposed to cocaine prenatally were rated by their teachers as having more behavior problems than the control group.

One study using the Brazelton Neonatal Assessment Scale showed that cocaine-exposed infants scored low in response to arousal, auditory, and visual stimuli (Eyler, Behnke, and Conlon, 1998). However, other studies have not found significant differences between affected infants and others (Frank, Jacobs, Beeghly, and others, 2002; Richardson, Hamel, and Goldschmidt, 1996; Messinger, Bauer, Das, and others, 2004).

Therapeutic Management. Treatment of these infants is similar to that for other drug-exposed infants: reduction of external stimuli, supportive treatment aimed at alleviating symptoms, and, at times, mild sedation.

Nursing Care Management. Nursing care of cocaine-exposed infants is the same as that for other drug-exposed infants. Because they have increased flexor tone, these infants respond to swaddling in a semiflexed position (Askin and Diehl-Jones, 2001). Positioning, infant massage, and limited tactile stimulation have been shown to be effective interventions. Effects of the drug from breast milk have been reported (Kandall, 1999); therefore mothers should be cautioned regarding this hazard to their infants.

Referral to early intervention programs, including child health care, parental drug treatment, individualized developmental care, and parenting education, is essential in promoting the optimum outcome for these children. Because these children often live in an impoverished environment, they are at high risk for cognitive delays, lack of child health care, and inadequate nutrition and would benefit from an early intervention program.

Methamphetamine Exposure

The fetal and neonatal effects of maternal use of methamphetamines in pregnancy are not well known but appear to be dose related (Smith, Yonekura, Wallace, and others, 2003). LBW, preterm birth, and perinatal mortality may be consequences of higher doses used throughout pregnancy. In addition, a higher incidence of cleft lip and palate and cardiac defects has been reported in infants exposed to methamphetamines in utero (Plessinger, 1998).

Methamphetamine use has increased significantly in the past 10 years in certain regions of the United States. In Smith, Yonekura, Wallace, and others' (2003) study, 63% of pregnant women using methamphetamines reported using the drug throughout the pregnancy. A higher incidence of preterm delivery and placental abruption was associated with methamphetamine use. In addition, fetal growth restriction (small for gestational age) was slightly higher in methamphetamine-exposed offspring; however, 80% of these neonates' mothers also had significant alcohol and tobacco use.

Study reports vary in the time of clinical manifestations of withdrawal from this drug; one study did not identify any signs of withdrawal in the first 3 days after birth, but long-term data were not collected (Smith, Yonekura, Wallace, and others, 2003). A study of infants exposed to methamphetamine in utero showed that such infants had significantly smaller head circumferences and birth weights than those not exposed; in addition, the exposed infants exhibited withdrawal signs of agitation, vomiting, and tachypnea, which were not observed in the unexposed infants (Chomchai, Na Manorom, Watanarungasan, and others, 2004). After birth, infants may experience bradycardia or tachycardia that resolves as the drug is cleared from the system. Lethargy may continue for several months, along with frequent infections and poor weight gain. Emotional disturbances and delays in gross and fine motor coordination may be seen during early childhood.

The long-term effects of methamphetamine exposure on children living in households where the product is manufactured are not known, but there are early reports of burns in exposed children and concerns regarding the effects of the toxic by-products of methamphetamine production on small children. Skin rashes and respiratory illnesses are common problems seen in methamphetamine-exposed children, but physical neglect and speech and language developmental delays are of significant concern as well (Crocker, 2005).

Marijuana Exposure

Marijuana has replaced cocaine as the most common illicit drug used by women ages 18 to 44 years (nonpregnant and pregnant) in the United States (Ebrahim and Gfoerer, 2004). Marijuana crosses the placenta. Its use during pregnancy may result in a shortened gestation and a higher incidence of IUGR (Wagner, Katikaneni, Cox, and others, 1998). A strong association has been reported between the use of marijuana and a decrease in fetal growth and infant birth weight and length (Hurd, Wang, Anderson, and others, 2005). Other investigators have found a higher incidence of meconium staining (Bandstra and Accornero, 2006). Compounding the issue of the effects of marijuana, especially among women ages 18 to 30 years (Ebrahim and Gfoerer, 2004), is multidrug use, which combines the harmful effects of marijuana, tobacco, alcohol, opiates, and cocaine. Long-term follow-up studies on exposed infants are needed.

MATERNAL INFECTIONS

The range of pathologic conditions produced by infectious agents is large, and the difference between the maternal and fetal effects caused by any one agent is also great. Some maternal infections, especially during early gestation, can result in fetal loss or malformations because the fetus's ability to handle infectious organisms is limited and the fetal immunologic system is unable to prevent the dissemination of infectious organisms to the various tissues.

Not all prenatal infections produce teratogenic effects. Furthermore, the clinical picture of disorders caused by transplacental transfer of infectious agents is not always well defined. Some microbial agents can cause remarkably similar manifestations, and it is not uncommon to test for all when a prenatal infection is suspected. This is the so-called **TORCH complex,** an acronym for:

T—*Toxoplasmosis*
O—*Other* (e.g., hepatitis B)
R—*Rubella*
C—*Cytomegalovirus* infection
H—*Herpes* simplex

To determine the causative agent in a symptomatic infant, tests are performed to rule out each of these infections. The *O* category may involve testing for several viral infections (e.g., hepatitis B, varicella zoster, measles, mumps, HIV, syphilis, and human parvovirus). Bacterial infections are not included in the TORCH workup because they are usually identified by clinical manifestations and readily available laboratory tests. Gonococcal conjunctivitis (ophthalmia neonatorum) and chlamydial conjunctivitis have been significantly reduced by prophylactic measures at birth (see Chapter 8). The major maternal infections, their possible effects, and specific nursing considerations are outlined in Table 9-11.

TABLE 9-11

Infections Acquired from Mother Before, During, or After Birth*

FETAL OR NEWBORN EFFECT	COMMENTS AND NURSING CARE MANAGEMENT†
HUMAN IMMUNODEFICIENCY VIRUS (HIV)	
No apparent significant clinical manifestations are apparent at birth General pediatric manifestations include lymphadenopathy; failure to thrive; splenomegaly; diarrhea; parotitis; CNS disease, including microcephaly; oral candidiasis; cardiomyopathy; and recurrent opportunistic infections Early diagnosis and aggressive treatment greatly diminish the manifestations cited above	**Transmitted**—Transplacentally; during vaginal delivery; potentially in breast milk **Prevention**—Interventions to decrease incidence of maternal-child transmission: 1. Cesarean section before onset of labor and rupture of membranes 2. Antiretroviral treatment of oral zidovudine (and other antivirals in HAART regimen) to mother during pregnancy, IV administration of zidovudine during labor, and oral administration to newborn and for the first 6 weeks of life 3. Complete avoidance of breastfeeding (American Academy of Pediatrics, 2006a) **Recommended treatment**—See the U.S. Department of Health and Human Service's AIDS Info website‡ for specific treatment recommendations other than those listed above
CHICKENPOX (VARICELLA-ZOSTER VIRUS [VZV])	
Intrauterine exposure (during first or early second trimester)—congenital varicella syndrome: limb dysplasia, microcephaly, cortical atrophy, chorioretinitis, cataracts, cutaneous scars, other anomalies, auditory nerve palsy, mental retardation Potentially severe symptoms (rash, fever) and higher mortality in infant whose mother develops varicella 5 days before to 2 days after delivery, depending on transplacental transfer of IgG antibodies specific to varicella zoster	**Transmitted**—First trimester (congenital varicella syndrome); perinatal period (infection) **Treatment**—Exposed infants: varicella zoster immune globulin (VariZIG) or IVIG to infants born to mothers with onset of disease 5 days before delivery or within 48 hours after delivery; consider acyclovir in hospitalized preterm infants (see American Academy of Pediatrics, 2006a, for recommendations) Institute isolation precautions in newborn born to mother with varicella up to 21-28 days (latter time if newborn received VariZIG) after birth (if hospitalized) **Prevention**—Universal immunization of all children with varicella (Var) vaccine

CNS, Central nervous system; *IgG,* immunoglobulin G; *IV,* intravenous; *IVIG,* intravenous immunoglobulin; *HAART,* highly active antiretroviral therapy; *HBsAg,* hepatitis B surface antigen.
*This table is not an exhaustive representation of all perinatally transmitted infections. For further information regarding specific diseases or treatment not listed here, refer to American Academy of Pediatrics, Committee on Infectious Diseases, Pickering L, editor: *Red book: 2006 report of the Committee on Infectious Diseases,* ed 27, Elk Grove Village, Ill, 2006, The Academy.
†Isolation precautions depend on institutional policy (see Infection Control, Chapter 22).
‡http://www.aidsinfo.nih.gov.

Continued

TABLE 9-11

Infections Acquired from Mother Before, During, or After Birth—cont'd

FETAL OR NEWBORN EFFECT	COMMENTS AND NURSING CARE MANAGEMENT†
CHLAMYDIA INFECTION (CHLAMYDIA TRACHOMATIS) Conjunctivitis, trachoma, pneumonia	**Transmitted**—Last trimester or perinatal period **Prevention**—Standard ophthalmic prophylaxis for gonococcal ophthalmia neonatorum (topical antibiotics, silver nitrate, or povidone-iodine) is not effective in treatment or prevention of chlamydia conjunctivitis **Treatment**—Oral erythromycin 14 days for conjunctivitis; pneumonia: treat with oral azithromycin, erythromycin, or oral sulfonamide; trachoma: topical erythromycin, tetracycline or sulfacetamide ointment
ENTEROVIRUS (NONPOLIO)—GROUP A AND B COXSACKIEVIRUS, ECHOVIRUS, ENTEROVIRUS Nonspecific; many signs may mimic bacterial sepsis Additional manifestations may include poor feeding, common cold, stomatitis, herpangina, pneumonia, rash, encephalitis, vomiting, diarrhea, fever, arrhythmias, congestive heart failure, lethargy, seizures, conjunctivitis, hemorrhagic conjunctivitis, meningeal involvement	**Transmitted**—Peripartum **Treatment**—Supportive; IVIG in life-threatening neonatal infections
CYTOMEGALOVIRUS (CMV) Variable manifestation from asymptomatic to severe Microcephaly, intrauterine growth restriction, cerebral calcifications, chorioretinitis Jaundice, hepatosplenomegaly Petechial or purpuric rash Neurologic sequelae—seizure disorders, sensorimotor deafness, mental retardation	Infection acquired at birth, shortly thereafter, or via human milk is not associated with clinical illness in healthy term infants **Transmitted**—Transplacentally; at birth through infected birth canal; postnatal consumption of CMV-positive breast milk Preterm infants at greater risk for illness when infected via breast milk Virus detected in urine or tissue by electron microscopy Pregnant women advised to take appropriate prevention precautions; since virus is spread primarily via urine and saliva, avoid contact with secretions; standard precautions are sufficient for health care workers **Treatment**—IV antivirals such as ganciclovir given to newborn
ERYTHEMA INFECTIOSUM (PARVOVIRUS B19) Fetal hydrops and death from anemia and heart failure; early exposure (first trimester exposure) Anemia from later exposure No teratogenic effects established Ordinarily, low risk of ill effect to fetus	**Transmitted**—Transplacentally First trimester infection most serious effects **Treatment**—Supportive care Fetal hydrops may be treated with intrauterine blood transfusions Pregnant health care workers should not care for patients who might be highly contagious (e.g., child with parvovirus-associated aplastic crisis) Routine exclusion of pregnant women from workplace where disease is occurring is not recommended
GONOCOCCAL DISEASE (NEISSERIA GONORRHOEAE) Ophthalmitis, scalp abscesses, vaginitis Disseminated—neonatal gonococcal arthritis, septicemia, meningitis	**Transmitted**—Last trimester or perinatal period **Prevention**—Apply prophylactic medication to eyes at time of birth Obtain smears for culture Consider testing for *C. trachomatis*, congenital syphilis, and HIV in neonate with positive gonococcal disease **Treatment**—Ceftriaxone, not penicillin, due to increase in penicillin-resistant *N. gonorrhoeae*
HEPATITIS B VIRUS May be asymptomatic at birth Acute hepatitis, changes in liver function	**Transmitted**—Transplacentally (rare, <2% of perinatal infections); contaminated maternal fluids or secretions during delivery **Treatment**—Hepatitis B immune globulin (HBIG) to all infants (regardless of birth weight) of HBsAg-positive mothers within 12 hours of birth; in addition, administer hepatitis B vaccine (monovalent) at separate site See American Academy of Pediatrics (2006a) for additional preterm infant considerations **Prevention**—Universal immunization of all infants with hepatitis B vaccine (see Immunizations, Chapter 10)

CNS, Central nervous system; *IgG*, immunoglobulin G; *IV*, intravenous; *IVIG*, intravenous immunoglobulin; *HAART*, highly active antiretroviral therapy; *HBsAg*, hepatitis B surface antigen.
*This table is not an exhaustive representation of all perinatally transmitted infections. For further information regarding specific diseases or treatment not listed here, refer to American Academy of Pediatrics, Committee on Infectious Diseases, Pickering L, editor: *Red book: 2006 report of the Committee on Infectious Diseases*, ed 27, Elk Grove Village, Ill, 2006, The Academy.
†Isolation precautions depend on institutional policy (see Infection Control, Chapter 22).

TABLE 9-11

Infections Acquired from Mother Before, During, or After Birth—cont'd

FETAL OR NEWBORN EFFECT	COMMENTS AND NURSING CARE MANAGEMENT†
LISTERIOSIS (LISTERIA MONOCYTOGENES) Maternal infection associated with abortion, preterm delivery, and fetal death; amnionitis during labor and brown-stained amniotic fluid may occur. Preterm birth, sepsis, and pneumonia seen in early-onset disease; late-onset disease usually manifested as meningitis Late-onset infection occurs after first week of life usually as meningitis	**Transmitted**—Transplacentally, by ascending infection or exposure at delivery **Treatment**—Treat infected newborn with antibiotics (ampicillin and gentamicin)
RUBELLA, CONGENITAL (RUBELLA VIRUS) Congenital rubella syndrome Eye defects—cataracts (unilateral or bilateral), microphthalmia, retinitis, glaucoma CNS signs—microcephaly, seizures, severe mental retardation Congenital heart defects—patent ductus arteriosus Auditory—high incidence of delayed hearing loss Intrauterine growth restriction Hyperbilirubinemia, meningitis, thrombocytopenia, hepatomegaly, and dermal erythropoiesis (blueberry muffin lesions) Interstitial pneumonitis Milder forms of disease may have few visible manifestations or may be asymptomatic	**Transmitted**—First trimester; early second trimester **Prevention**—Pregnant women should avoid contact with all affected persons, including infants with rubella syndrome Emphasize vaccination of all unimmunized prepubertal children, susceptible adolescents, and women of childbearing age (nonpregnant) Caution women against pregnancy for at least 3 months after vaccination
SYPHILIS, CONGENITAL (TREPONEMA PALLIDUM) Stillbirth, prematurity, hydrops fetalis May be asymptomatic at birth and in first few weeks of life, or may have multisystem manifestations: hepatosplenomegaly, lymphadenopathy, hemolytic anemia, and thrombocytopenia Copper-colored maculopapular cutaneous lesions (usually after first few weeks of life), mucous membrane patches, hair loss, nail exfoliation, snuffles (syphilitic rhinitis), profound anemia, poor feeding, pseudoparalysis of one or more limbs, dysmorphic teeth (older child)	**Transmitted**—Transplacentally; can be anytime during pregnancy or at birth Most severe form of syphilis **Treatment**—IV penicillin§ Diagnostic evaluation dependent on maternal serology testing and infant symptoms (see American Academy of Pediatrics, 2006a) Treated infants should be evaluated at 1, 2, 4, 6, and 12 months of age
TOXOPLASMOSIS (TOXOPLASMA GONDII) May be asymptomatic at birth (70%-90% of cases) or have maculopapular rash, lymphadenopathy, hepatosplenomegaly, jaundice, thrombocytopenia Hydrocephaly, cerebral calcifications, chorioretinitis (classic triad) Microcephaly, seizures, mental retardation, deafness Encephalitis, myocarditis, hepatosplenomegaly, anemia, jaundice, diarrhea, vomiting, purpura	**Transmitted**—Throughout pregnancy Newborn of mother with positive HIV status and previous toxoplasmosis infection should be evaluated for congenital toxoplasmosis Predominant host for organism is cats May be transmitted through cat feces, poorly cooked or raw infected meats **Prevention**—Caution pregnant women to avoid contact with cat feces (e.g., emptying cat litter boxes) Maternal treatment to decrease fetal infection: spiramycin (in the United States, available only from the USDA) **Treatment**—If not fetal infection or immunocompromised: sulfonamides (Septra, Bactrim), pyrimethamine (Daraprim), folinic acid (leucovorin) If infant immunocompromised, see American Academy of Pediatrics (2006a)

†Isolation precautions depend on institutional policy (see Infection Control, Chapter 22).
§See also Centers for Disease Control and Prevention: Sexually transmitted diseases treatment guidelines, 2006, *MMWR Recomm Rep* 55(RR-11):1-94, 2006.

Nursing Care Management

One of the major goals in care of infants suspected of having an infectious disease is identification of the causative organism. Until the diagnosis is established, standard precautions are implemented according to institutional policy. In suspected cytomegalovirus and rubella infections, pregnant personnel are cautioned to avoid contact with the infant. Herpes simplex is easily transmitted from one infant to another; therefore risk of cross-contamination is reduced or eliminated by wearing gloves for patient contact. The American Academy of Pediatrics' *Red Book: 2006 Report of the Committee on Infectious Diseases* (2006a) provides guidelines for the type and duration of precautions for most bacterial and viral exposures. Careful hand washing is the most important nursing intervention in reducing the spread of any infection.

Specimens need to be obtained for laboratory examinations, and the infant and parents need to be prepared for diagnostic procedures. When possible, long-term disabilities are prevented by early evaluation and implementation of therapy. The family is taught any special handling techniques needed for the care of their infant and signs of complications or possible sequelae. If sequelae are inevitable, the family will need assistance in determining how they can best cope with the problems, such as assistance with home care, referral to appropriate agencies, or placement in an institution for care. The major goal of nursing care is prevention of these disorders with provision of adequate prenatal care for the expectant mother and precautions regarding exposure to teratogenic infections.

CONGENITAL ANOMALIES*

An appreciation of the basic mechanisms involved in morphogenesis is essential to the understanding of congenital anomalies. **Morphogenesis** (the study of cell differentiation and development) is a genetically controlled set of events that occurs in precisely timed sequence during embryonic and fetal life. Some of the determinants of normal morphogenesis include the proper migration of cells, a well-timed mitotic rate, and controlled cell death by apoptosis. Disturbances in any of these factors may result in abnormal morphogenesis that can be expressed as various patterns of structural defects (Jones, 2006):

Malformation—Results from deficient formation of tissues. *Example:* Ventricular septal defects

Deformation—Results from the action of mechanical forces on a normal tissue. These forces may be extrinsic to the developing embryo, such as uterine constraints (especially common during the second trimester of development), or intrinsic, resulting from consequences of a primary malformation. *Example:* Arthrogryposes, or contraction of the lower limbs

Disruption—Results from the breakdown of previously normal tissue. *Example:* Amnion disruption sequence (amniotic band sequence)

Dysplasia—Results from abnormal organization of cells within a tissue. *Example:* Hamartomas

Malformations can be classified according to the defect in morphogenesis, including incomplete morphogenesis, development of accessory tissue, or functional defects. Incomplete morphogenesis may result from lack of development (e.g., vas deferens agenesis, or the absence of vas deferens), hypoplasia (e.g., micrognathia, or poorly developed chin), incomplete separation (e.g., syndactyly, or fused digits), incomplete closure (e.g., cleft palate), or persistence of earlier location (e.g., cryptorchidism, or undescended testes). Development of accessory tissue may result in abnormalities such as polydactyly (supernumerary digits), and functional defects may be the cause of contractures, such as clubfoot.

Congenital anomalies, or **birth defects,** can be identified prenatally, at birth, or at any point after birth. About 2% to 3% of all births are associated with a major congenital anomaly. Accurate identification of such defects may provide a valuable clue for the presence of or potential for a genetic disorder (Box 9-10).

Overall, genetic disorders can be classified as **chromosomal abnormalities** (numeric and structural changes in the normal chromosome pattern), **gene substitutions** or **alterations** (single-gene and polygenic disorders), and **complex** (or **multifactorial**) **disorders** (those that result from interactions between the individual's genetic predisposition and environmental factors). Chromosomal abnormalities account for approximately 25% of all major birth defects, and single-gene disorders account for approximately 20%. In addition, expo-

*Miguel F. da Cunha, PhD, revised this section.

> **BOX 9-10**
>
> ## Assessment Clues to Genetic Disorders*
>
> **Major or minor birth defects (anomalies) and dysmorphic features**—Cardiac defect, ear or eye abnormalities, micrognathia, forehead prominence, low-set hairline on forehead or nape of neck, wide-set eyes, epicanthal folds, low-set ears
>
> **Growth abnormalities**—Short stature, overgrowth, asymmetric growth, intrauterine growth restriction, postnatal growth delay
>
> **Skeletal abnormalities**—Limb abnormalities, asymmetry, scoliosis, pectus excavatum, hyperextensible joints, hypotonic or hypertonic muscle tone, pectus excavatum, finger or joint abnormalities
>
> **Vision or hearing problems**—Coloboma of the iris, cat's eye, hearing loss, vision loss
>
> **Metabolic disorders**—Unusual odor of breath, urine, or stool; coarse facial features
>
> **Sexual development abnormalities**—Ambiguous genitalia, small penis, delayed onset of puberty, primary amenorrhea, precocious sexual development, large testicles
>
> **Skin disorders**—Unusual pigmentation, café-au-lait spots, dry and scaly skin, skin tumors, sparse hair, absent or unusual teeth
>
> **Recurrent infection or immunodeficiency**—Ear infections, pneumonia
>
> Developmental and speech delays or loss of milestones:
>
> - **Cognitive delays**—Learning disabilities, mild to severe mental retardation
> - **Behavioral disorders**—Hyperactivity, attention deficit disorder, autistic-like behavior, aggressive behavior
>
> *Suggests genetic etiology if two or more findings are present.

sure to known **teratogens** (agents that cause congenital anomalies) accounts for about 5% of major birth defects. The etiology of the remaining 50% is currently unknown. However, many of these idiopathic birth defects occur in families in patterns similar to complex diseases such as diabetes mellitus and mental illnesses, indicating a possible multifactorial or even polygenic etiology (Nussbaum, McInnes, and Willard, 2004).

The types of malformations that can result from genetic or prenatal environmental causes can be **major structural abnormalities** with serious medical, surgical, or quality-of-life consequences, or they can be **minor anomalies** or **normal variants** with no serious consequences, such as a sacral dimple, an extra nipple, or a single simian crease of the hand. Malformations can occur in isolation, such as congenital heart defect, or multiple anomalies may be present. A recognized pattern of malformations resulting from a single specific cause is called a **syndrome** (e.g., Turner syndrome and FAS).

The identification of a genetic etiology for a birth defect has important implications for knowing:

Diagnosis—What is the disorder?
Etiology—What caused it?
Prognosis—What are possible consequences?
Therapy—What can be done?
Recurrence risk—Will it happen again?
Prenatal diagnosis—Is testing available for future pregnancies?

Establishing a diagnosis helps the family and health care team to develop an awareness of the findings that may be seen with the disorder and to initiate early intervention strategies, including genetic counseling for the parents and extended family. For example, children with DiGeorge, or 22q11 deletion, syndrome may be diagnosed through the identification of the combination of velopharyngeal incompetence and cardiac defects. After the diagnosis of a chromosome microdeletion disorder is made, evaluation for immune function and renal abnormalities can be initiated. Cognitive, speech, and language delays are commonly seen in children with this disorder, and enrollment in early childhood intervention programs should be arranged as soon after diagnosis as possible.

GENETIC ETIOLOGY OF CONGENITAL ANOMALIES
Chromosomal Abnormalities

Chromosomal abnormalities are deviations in either number or structure of chromosomes, and the consequences in either situation can usually be observed in the affected individual. **Numeric chromosomal abnormalities** can result from the addition of one chromosome to each of the existing pair. Human somatic cells are diploid, with a chromosome complement of 2n = 46. Gametes, both ova and spermatozoa, are haploid cells, with 23 chromosomes each (n = 23). The addition of one haploid complement (23 chromosomes) to a diploid cell will mean that all pairs will now have acquired one chromosome each and are no longer pairs, but "trios." The cell is now a triploid cell (3n = 69). This type of configuration, in which one chromosome was equally added to each pair, is termed **euploidy,** and is designated by the suffix *-ploidy.* Such an enormous increase in chromosome number (46 to 69) represents a large gene imbalance and will likely not be compatible with life. Deviations in chromosome number that are compatible with life, in spite of resulting in physical or developmental abnormalities, usually involve the gain of one (or few) chromosomes, which are added to an existing pair (only that particular pair becomes a trio). In this case, the chromosome number will increase from the typical 46 to 47 (or 48) through an *unequal* addition of one (or few) chromosomes to only that specific pair. This unequal addition of one (or few) chromosomes is termed **aneuploidy** and is designated by the suffix *-somy.*

The most common type of aneuploidy, from a clinical perspective, is the **trisomies.** A type of aneuploidy that results from the loss of one member of a chromosome pair is termed a **monosomy.** The only monosomy that is compatible with life is Turner syndrome, which results from the loss of one of the X chromosomes in women.

Most chromosomal abnormalities in number and structure result from abnormal cell division during germ cell formation or early cell division in the zygote. **Structural abnormalities** usually involve some degree of chromosome breakage. Fragments broken off a chromosome can be lost (**deletion**), may rearrange in abnormal configurations, or may attach to another chromosome (**translocation**). If the rearrangement of fragments between two chromosomes is reciprocal, that is, without loss of genetic material, the resulting configuration is termed a **balanced translocation.** An individual with a balanced translocation is usually normal in appearance and function but may potentially transmit to the developing offspring the translocation in an unbalanced form, resulting in spontaneous abortion or a child with **congenital abnormalities.** Therefore referral for genetic counseling is recommended for individuals found to have a translocation.

Both numeric and structural abnormalities of autosomes and sex chromosomes account for a variety of disorders of infancy and childhood. A few are associated with a group of characteristics that clearly indicate the precise chromosomal anomaly (Table 9-12). The most common is Down syndrome, which is caused by a trisomy of chromosome 21 (see Chapter 19 for a further discussion of Down syndrome). Other known viable autosomal trisomies involve chromosomes 18 (Edwards syndrome) and 13 (Patau syndrome). Although the prognosis for survival after birth is poor, some children have lived for several years. Abnormalities of sex chromosomes are discussed in Chapter 17.

Single-Gene Defects

Single-gene disorders are caused by a mutation or change in a single gene. A single allele of that gene on a chromosome or two alleles of the same (**homologous**) gene pair on both chromosomes may undergo mutations. For example, one of many genetic variants of cystic fibrosis is caused when two matched pairs of genes on chromosomes 7 carry the cystic fibrosis gene mutation. However, Marfan syndrome occurs when a mutation in the fibrillin gene occurs on one chromosome 15. Single-gene disorders are individually rare, but collectively play a significant role in human disease. It is estimated that 6% to 8% of hospitalized children have a single-gene disorder.

Multifactorial Inheritance

Some congenital anomalies are caused by multifactorial inheritance. The concept of multifactorial inheritance has acquired new and expanded importance with the identification of **complex disorders.** These are disease processes for which the individual has a certain genetic predisposition, but the expression of the gene (disease) depends on its interaction with environmental stimuli. Cleft lip and palate, neural tube defects, and congenital heart defects are some examples of conditions caused by multifactorial inheritance.

DEFECTS CAUSED BY CHEMICAL AGENTS

Prenatal environmental influences from chemicals such as alcohol, medications, or drugs; infectious disease; or radiation or other environmental influences may be regarded as nongenetic causes of congenital anomalies because these effects can produce congenital structural, functional, or growth defects. An agent that produces congenital malformations or increases their incidence is called a **teratogen.**

The relationship of the fetal and maternal circulations allows for the interchange of chemical substances across the placental membrane. Many drugs have been suspected of producing congenital malformations, and some have been definitely implicated. Some of the most recognized teratogenic drugs include alcohol, tobacco, antiepileptic medications, isotretinoin (Accutane), lithium, cocaine, and diethylstilbestrol (Table 9-13).

The extent to which chemical agents affect the unborn child depends on the interplay of several factors: the nature of the agent and its accessibility to the fetus, the gestational age at which exposure occurred, the level and duration of the dosage, and the genetic makeup of the fetus. For example, fetal exposure to valproic acid in the first 3 months of pregnancy may result in congenital anomalies such as neural tube defects, congenital heart defects, and distinctive facial features. The limited metabolic capabilities of the fetal liver and its immature enzyme and transport systems render the unborn child ill equipped for maintaining homeostasis when chemical disturbances are imposed by the mother or the environment. This includes both substances produced by the mother in re-

TABLE 9-12
Common Chromosomal Abnormalities

ABNORMALITY, CHROMOSOME NOTATION, AND APPROXIMATE INCIDENCE	MAJOR CLINICAL MANIFESTATIONS
TRISOMY 21 (DOWN SYNDROME) 47,XY or XX, 21$^+$ (free trisomy) 46,XY or XX, t(14;21)$^+$ (translocation) 46,XY or XX/47,XY or XX, 21$^+$ (mosaic) **Incidence**—1:800 live births*†	Brachycephaly with flat occiput; epicanthal folds; small ears, nose, and mouth with protruding tongue; muscular hypotonia; broad, short hands with stubby fingers and transverse palmar crease; broad, stubby feet with wide space between big and second toes; cardiac defects; mental retardation; variable life expectancy
TRISOMY 18 (EDWARDS SYNDROME) 47,XY or XX, 18$^+$ **Incidence**—1:7500 live births*	Deformed and low-set ears; micrognathia; rocker-bottom feet; overlapping (index over third) fingers; prominent occiput; hypertelorism; failure to thrive and early death; mental retardation
TRISOMY 13 (PATAU SYNDROME) 47,XY or XX, 13$^+$ **Incidence**—1:22,700 live births*	Multiple anomalies, including cleft lip and palate (frequently bilateral); ear malformations; microphthalmia; polydactyly; eye defects; mental retardation; early death
KLINEFELTER SYNDROME 47,XXY (or multiple X, Y) **Incidence**—1:1000 live male births*	Male phenotype, small testes with decreased androgen production, infertility, well-developed genitalia, sparse facial hair, female pubic hair pattern; slightly taller than normal males (longer legs); gynecomastia frequent; voice may not change at puberty **Infrequent abnormalities**—Scoliosis, pectus excavatum, fifth finger clinodactyly, dental anomalies, cardiac anomalies, pulmonary diseases, varicose veins **Intellectual development**—Normal to borderline (IQ 85), language delay
TURNER SYNDROME 45,X0 **Incidence**—1:4000 live female births*	Female phenotype, ovarian dysgenesis (streak gonads), short stature, decreased estrogens, infertility, delayed sexual development, webbing of the neck, low posterior neckline, neonatal lymphedema, cubitus valgus, short fourth metacarpals, "shield" chest, divergent nipples, sex chromatin negative, coarctation of the aorta, urinary tract abnormalities, fetal cystic hygroma or hydrops, normal intellectual development

*Data from Nussbaum RL, McInnes RR, Willard HF: *Thompson and Thompson genetics in medicine*, ed 6 (Rev Print), Philadelphia, 2004, Saunders.
†Risk related to maternal age: age 30 years = 1:900; age 35 years = 1:385; age 40 years = 1:100; age 45 years and over = 1:25. From Nussbaum, McInnes, and Willard (2004).

sponse to a disease state (such as diabetes) and exogenous substances ingested or inhaled by the mother.

The teratogenic effect of drugs is not believed to have an effect on developing tissue until day 15 of gestation, when tissue differentiation begins to take place. Before that time, drugs usually have little effect because they are believed to have an insignificant affinity for undifferentiated tissue. Also, until implantation takes place, at approximately 7 days after conception, the embryo is not exposed to maternal blood that contains the drug. However, some drugs may affect the uterine lining, making it unsuitable for implantation. Drugs administered between days 15 and 90 may produce an effect if the tissue for which the drug has an affinity is in the process of differentiation at that time. After 90 days, when differentiation is complete, most fetal tissues are believed to be relatively resistant to teratogenic effects of drugs. However, the impact on ongoing neurologic development is not known.

Nursing Care Management

Expectant mothers are cautioned against ingesting any medication without first consulting a practitioner. To help ensure that fewer women will inadvertently take some chemical that might be harmful to the fetus, labels on medications are now required to include information regarding the possible teratogenic effects of the drug. All women of childbearing age should be educated regarding the effects of chemicals, especially alco-

hol, on the unborn fetus. FAS is an irreversible condition but is completely preventable. The March of Dimes* and Centers for Disease Control and Prevention† have information about prevention tips, and the Genetic Alliance‡ has information about support groups for families of children with FAS. Genetic counseling is recommended for women who have a concern about a possible teratogen during pregnancy.

FYI

One drug recognized for its carcinogenic effect is diethylstilbestrol. Large doses of this hormone, given to pregnant women in the United States between 1938 and 1971 to prevent abortion, cause adenocarcinoma of the vagina in a significant proportion of the female offspring when they reach adolescence and early adulthood.

INBORN ERRORS OF METABOLISM

Inborn errors of metabolism (IEMs) constitute a large number of inherited diseases caused by the absence or deficiency of a substance essential to cellular metabolism, usually an enzyme.

---

*1275 Mamaroneck Ave., White Plains, NY 10605; (914) 997-4488; http://www.marchofdimes.com.
†http://www.cdc.gov.
‡4301 Connecticut Ave. NW, Suite 404, Washington, DC 20008; http://www.geneticalliance.org.

TABLE 9-13	
Congenital Effects of Maternal Alcohol Ingestion and Tobacco Smoking	
FETAL OR NEWBORN EFFECTS	**COMMENTS AND NURSING CARE MANAGEMENT**
ALCOHOL (FETAL ALCOHOL SYNDROME [FAS] OR ALCOHOL-RELATED BIRTH DEFECTS [ARBD])	

Features vary—infant may not display physical features; involves three main categories:
  Growth failure in utero, including microcephaly
  Midfacial dysmorphic features
  Central nervous system (CNS) involvement, including cognitive impairment, irritability, hyperactivity, hypertonia, and behavioral problems
Facial features include hypoplastic maxilla, micrognathia, short palpebral fissures, thinned upper lip, hypoplastic philtrum, short, upturned nose. One or a combination of these features present in infancy or later.
Children or adults who demonstrate cognitive, behavioral, and psychosocial problems without physical features and growth delay are referred to as having FAE (fetal alcohol effects) or alcohol-related neurodevelopmental disorder (ARND).
Affected infants may display nonspecific signs such as irritability, lethargy, difficulty establishing respirations, seizures, tremors, poor suck reflex, abdominal distention. Birth defects may occur but are less common.
Diagnosis is made more difficult by lack of a single biologic marker and may be made based on maternal history of alcohol ingestion.
	Quantity of alcohol consumed is not the determinant; rather, it is the amount consumed in excess of the liver's ability to detoxify alcohol. Free alcohol has an affinity for brain tissue; hence the CNS symptoms. Ethanol by-products also contribute to toxicity, as do other substances consumed in addition to alcohol and poor maternal self-care.
	Effects of alcohol on CNS are not reversible.
	FAS (ARBD) is the leading cause of preventable mental retardation in the United States.
	Early intervention with mother is aimed at minimizing fetal effects, education, and involvement in prevention and treatment counseling.
	Early intervention with newborn focuses on reducing the effects of alcohol exposure on growing child, especially in relation to cognitive deficits and learning disabilities.
	Treatment in neonatal period is similar to that of drug-exposed infants and should involve extensive assessment and individualized developmental care.
	Provide resources to help decrease or eliminate alcohol intake. *During Your Pregnancy: Tips for Giving Up Alcohol* is available from the March of Dimes.*
	Further information is available at National Organization on Fetal Alcohol Syndrome† and Centers for Disease Control and Prevention.‡

MATERNAL TOBACCO SMOKING	
Smoking is associated with significant birth weight deficits; positive dose-response relationship is related to size of fetus. Two active substances—nicotine and cotinine—are higher in newborns of mothers who smoke than in mothers who do not. Postnatal growth deficits occur, as do deficits in emotional and behavioral development in the growing child. Maternal smoking is associated with an increased risk of sudden infant death syndrome, respiratory tract illnesses in childhood, and childhood learning deficits.	Counseling regarding fetal and postnatal effects should be made available to all pregnant women, and they are encouraged to stop smoking. Smoking cessation during pregnancy decreases chance of fetal complications. Encourage pregnant woman to enroll in a smoking cessation program. Evaluate polydrug use in conjunction with smoking. Increased incidence of perinatal complications leading to preterm birth includes abruptio placentae, placenta previa, and premature rupture of membranes. Provide resources to help eliminate smoking. *During Your Pregnancy: Tips to Quit* is available from the March of Dimes*

*http://www.marchofdimes.com.
†900 17th St. NW, Suite 910, Washington, DC 20006; (202) 785-4585; http://www.nofas.org.
‡Fetal Alcohol Syndrome Branch, Division of Birth Defects, Child Development and Disability and Health, Centers for Disease Control and Prevention, Atlanta, http://www.cdc.gov/ncbddd/fas.

When the normal metabolic process is interrupted as a result of a missing enzyme, an accumulation of substances precedes the interruption, the end product of the process is absent, or the process takes an alternate metabolic pathway. The consequence is manifested as an illness. Most IEMs are characterized by abnormal protein, carbohydrate, or fat metabolism.

Newborn screening for IEMs varies from state to state, but all states test for phenylketonuria (PKU) and congenital hypothyroidism and the majority test for galactosemia.* The purpose of screening is to identify children who may have a condition that benefits from early identification and treatment to prevent mental retardation. The screening test is most reliable if the blood sample is taken after the infant has ingested a source of protein for 24 hours. Because of early discharge of newborns, recommendations for screening include (1) collecting the initial specimen as close as possible to discharge or no later than 7 days, (2) obtaining a subsequent sample by 2 weeks of age if the initial specimen is collected before the newborn is 24 hours old, and (3) designating a primary care provider to all newborns before discharge for adequate newborn screening follow-up (Kaye, Committee on Genetics, Accurso, and others, 2006). A new screening test, tandem mass spectrometry, has the potential for identifying more than 20 IEMs in addition to the standard IEMs. With tandem mass spectrometry, earlier identification of IEMs may prevent further developmental delays and morbidities in affected children (Schultze, Lindner, Kohlmüller, and others, 2003).

A major concern is that a significantly large number of infants are *not* rescreened for PKU after early discharge and are at risk for a missed or delayed diagnosis of PKU. Special consideration must be given to screening infants born at home who have no hospital contact. It is always necessary to confirm the screening results with diagnostic testing.

CONGENITAL HYPOTHYROIDISM

Congenital hypothyroidism (CH) may have a number of causes and can be either permanent or transient. Transient CH is frequently associated with maternal Graves disease that

*Because newborn screening varies by state and policies change frequently, a good resource is the National Newborn Screening and Genetics Resource Center, http://genes-r-us.uthscsa.edu.

BOX 9-11
Clinical Manifestations of Congenital Hypothyroidism

BIRTH*
Poor feeding
Lethargy
Prolonged jaundice (>2 weeks)
Respiratory difficulties
Cyanosis
Constipation
Bradycardia
Hoarse cry
Large anterior and posterior
  fontanels
Postterm
Birth weight over 4000 g
  (8.8 pounds)

AGES 6 TO 9 WEEKS†
Depressed nasal bridge
Short forehead
Puffy eyelids

Large tongue
Thick, dry, mottled skin
Coarse, dry, lusterless hair
Abdominal distention
Umbilical hernia
Hyporeflexia
Bradycardia
Hypothermia
Hypotension
Anemia
Widely patent cranial sutures

OLDER CHILD
Short stature
Obesity
Varying degrees of intellectual
  deficits
Abnormal tendon reflexes
Slow, awkward movements

*Clinical manifestations may not be obvious at birth, possibly because of maternal transfer of thyroid hormone to fetus. Manifestations may be delayed in infants with certain types of familial hypothyroidism and in breast-fed infants (may show once weaned).
†If untreated, classical features.

was treated with antithyroid drugs. The majority of cases are sporadic (nonhereditary), but approximately 15% of all cases are transmitted as an autosomal dominant trait. The most common pathogenesis is thyroid dysgenesis, mostly with unknown causes. Worldwide, the most common cause of CH resulting in endemic cretinism is iodine deficiency. However, no matter what the cause, the manifestations (Box 9-11) and management are similar. In some conditions the thyroid deficiency is severe and manifestations develop early; in others, the symptoms may be delayed for months or years. Early detection and prompt initiation of treatment are essential, since their delay will result in various degrees of mental retardation, in which the IQ loss has a direct relationship to the time treatment is initiated. If treatment is implemented from 0 to 3 months of age, the mean IQ attained is 89 (range: 64 to 107); if treatment begins at 3 to 6 months, mean IQ will reach 71 (range: 36 to 96); treatment initiated after 6 months of age will result in a mean IQ of 54 (range: 25 to 80).

Results of screening tests in the United States indicate that CH occurs in approximately 1 in 4000 to 1 in 3000 newborns (Kaye, Committee on Genetics, Accurso, and others, 2006). It affects all races and ethnicities, but it is more prevalent among Hispanic and American Indian or Alaskan Native people (1 in 2000 to 1 in 700 newborns) and less prevalent among African Americans (1 in 3200 to 1 in 17,000 newborns). Infants with Down syndrome have a much higher rate of either permanent or transient forms of the disorder (approximately 1 in 140 newborns) (Kaye, Committee on Genetics, Accurso, and others, 2006). Also, a higher incidence of other congenital abnormalities has been observed in infants with CH. In addition, many preterm infants have transient hypothyroidism (hypothyroxinemia) at birth as a result of hypothalamic and pituitary immaturity. Some screening programs target both primary (thyroid-based) and secondary (pituitary-based) hypothyroidism.

Diagnostic Evaluation

Because CH is one of the most common preventable causes of mental retardation, early diagnosis and treatment of this disease are essential interventions. Neonatal screening consists of an initial filter paper blood spot thyroxine (T_4) measurement followed by measurement of thyroid-stimulating hormone (TSH) in specimens with low T_4 values.

Tests are mandatory in all U.S. states and U.S. territories. Although a blood sample obtained by heel stick for the spot test is best obtained between 2 and 6 days of age, specimens are usually taken within the first 24 to 48 hours or before discharge as part of a concurrent screen for other metabolic defects. Early screening can result in overdiagnosis (false positives) but is preferable to missing the diagnosis.

Screening results that show a low level of T_4 (<6 mcg/dl) and a high level of TSH (>60 μU/ml) indicate CH and the need for further tests to determine the cause of the disease (see Appendix C for values). Additional tests include serum measurement of T_4, triiodothyronine (T_3), resin uptake, free T_4, and thyroid-bound globulin. Tests of thyroid gland function (thyroid scan and uptake) usually involve oral administration of a radioactive isotope of iodine (^{131}I) and measurement of iodine uptake by the thyroid, usually within 24 hours. In CH, protein-bound iodine, T_4, T_3, and free T_4 levels are low and thyroid uptake of ^{131}I is decreased. Skeletal radiography is used to assess age.

In the newborn, thyroid function studies are elevated in comparison with values in older children; therefore it is important to document the timing of the tests. In preterm and sick full-term infants, thyroid function tests are usually lower than in the healthy full-term infant; a repeat T_4 and TSH may be evaluated after 30 weeks (corrected age) in newborns born before that time and after resolution of the acute illness in the sick full-term infant.

Therapeutic Management

Treatment involves lifelong thyroid hormone replacement therapy as soon as possible after diagnosis to abolish all signs of hypothyroidism and reestablish normal physical and mental development. The drug of choice is synthetic levothyroxine sodium (Synthroid, Levothroid). Regular measurement of thyroxine levels is important in ensuring optimum treatment. Bone-age surveys are also performed to ensure optimum growth.

Prognosis. If treatment is started shortly after birth, normal physical growth and intelligence are possible. The most significant factor adversely affecting eventual intellectual development appears to be inadequate treatment, which may be related to noncompliance. On the other hand, prolonged overtreatment can result in future temperament disorders, and close monitoring of adequate hormone replacement is essential, especially in the first 2 to 3 years of life (Selva, Harper, Downs, and others, 2005).

Nursing Care Management

The most important nursing objective is early identification of the disorder. Nurses caring for neonates must be certain that screening is performed, especially in infants who are preterm, discharged early, or born at home. Approximately 10% of cases are detected only by a second screening at 2 to 6 weeks of age. Nurses in community health need to be aware of the

FIG. 9-20 ■ Metabolic error and consequences in phenylketonuria.

earliest signs of the disorder. Parental remarks about an unusually "quiet and good" baby and demonstrated symptoms such as prolonged jaundice, constipation, and umbilical hernia should lead to a suspicion of hypothyroidism, which requires a referral for specific tests.

After the diagnosis is confirmed, parents need an explanation of the disorder and the necessity of lifelong treatment. The child should be referred to a pediatric endocrinologist for care. The importance of compliance with the drug regimen for the child to achieve normal growth and development must be stressed (American Academy of Pediatrics, 2006b). Because the drug is tasteless, it can be crushed and added to formula, water, or food. If a dose is missed, twice the dose should be given the next day. Unless there are maternal contraindicative factors, breastfeeding is acceptable in infants with hypothyroidism. Parents also need to be aware of signs indicating overdose, such as a rapid pulse, dyspnea, irritability, insomnia, fever, sweating, and weight loss. Ideally, they should know how to count the pulse and be instructed to withhold a dose and consult their practitioner if the pulse rate is above a certain value. Signs of inadequate treatment are fatigue, sleepiness, decreased appetite, and constipation.

If the diagnosis was delayed past early infancy, the chance of permanent mental retardation is great. Parents need the same guidance in caring for their child as do others who have an offspring with cognitive impairment (see Chapter 19). They need an opportunity to discuss their feelings regarding late recognition of the disorder. Although treatment will not reverse the intellectual deficit, it may prevent further damage.

Genetic counseling is important for the rare families where the etiology of CH is thyroid dyshormonogenesis, which is inherited in an autosomal recessive manner (see Genetic Evaluation and Counseling, p. 316).

PHENYLKETONURIA

PKU, an inborn error of metabolism inherited as an autosomal recessive trait (the *PAH* gene is located on chromosome 12q24), is caused by a deficiency or absence of the enzyme needed to metabolize the essential amino acid **phenylalanine.** Classic PKU is at one end of a spectrum of conditions known as **hyperphenylalaninemia.** Because rarer forms are a result of a deficiency in other enzymes and are diagnosed and treated differently, the following discussion of PKU is limited to the severe, classic form.

In PKU the hepatic enzyme **phenylalanine hydroxylase,** which normally controls the conversion of phenylalanine to tyrosine, is deficient. This results in the accumulation of phenylalanine in the bloodstream and urinary excretion of abnormal amounts of its metabolites, the phenyl acids (Fig. 9-20). One of these **phenylketones, phenylacetic acid,** gives urine the characteristic musty odor associated with the disease. Another is **phenylpyruvic acid,** which is responsible for the term **phenylketonuria.**

Tyrosine, the amino acid produced by the metabolism of phenylalanine, is absent in PKU. Tyrosine is needed to form the pigment melanin and the hormones epinephrine and thyroxine. Decreased melanin production results in similar phenotypes of most individuals with PKU: blond hair, blue eyes, and fair skin that is particularly susceptible to eczema and other dermatologic problems. Children with a genetically darker skin color may be red haired or brunette.

The prevalence of PKU varies widely in the United States due to the fact that different states have different definition criteria for what constitutes hyperphenylalaninemia and PKU. The reported figures for PKU range from 1 per 19,000 to 1 per 13,500 live births. The disease has a wide variation of incidence by ethnic groups. The disease is most prevalent among individuals of Northern European ancestry, as well as American Indians and Alaskan Natives, whereas African-American, Hispanic, Jewish, and Asian individuals account for the lowest frequencies (Hellekson, 2001). Among African Americans, for instance, the incidence of PKU is 1 per 50,000 live births (McPhee and Ganong, 2006).

Clinical manifestations in untreated PKU include failure to thrive (growth failure); frequent vomiting; irritability; hyperactivity; and unpredictable, erratic behavior. Mental retardation is thought to be caused by the accumulation of phenylalanine and presumably by decreased levels of the neurotransmitters dopamine and tryptophan, which affect the normal development of the brain and CNS, resulting in defective myelinization, cystic degeneration of the gray and white matter, and disturbances in cortical lamination. Older children commonly display bizarre or schizoid behavior patterns such as fright reactions, screaming episodes, head banging, arm biting, disorientation, failure to respond to strong stimuli, and catatonia-like positions.

Diagnostic Evaluation*

The objective in diagnosing and treating the disorder is to prevent mental retardation. Every newborn in the United States should be screened for PKU. The most commonly used test for screening newborns is the **Guthrie blood test,** a bacterial inhibition assay for phenylalanine in the blood. *Bacillus subtilis,* present in the culture medium, grows if the blood contains an excessive amount of phenylalanine. If performed properly, this test detects serum phenylalanine levels greater than 4 mg/dl (normal value is 1.6 mg/dl), but it will not quantify the results. Other methods for testing include quantitative fluorometric assay and tandem mass spectrometry, which will give an absolute value. Only fresh heel blood, not cord blood, can be used for the test.

NURSINGALERT

Avoid "layering" the blood specimen on the special Guthrie paper. Layering is placing one drop of blood on top of the other or overlapping the specimen. This practice results in a falsely high reading, or false positive, which will lead the newborn screening department to call the family and physician to arrange for a diagnostic blood phenylalanine test to determine whether the newborn truly has PKU. Best results are obtained by collecting the specimen with a pipette from the heel stick and spreading the blood uniformly over the blot paper.

Because of the possibility of variant forms of hyperphenylalaninemia, PKU cofactor variant screen should be performed in all children diagnosed with PKU.

---

*Always refer patient to a genetic metabolic specialist. For a reference list, visit the American Society of Human Genetics website, http://www.ashg.org.

Therapeutic Management*

Treatment of PKU involves restricting phenylalanine in the diet. Because the genetic enzyme is intracellular, systemic administration of phenylalanine hydroxylase is of no value. Phenylalanine cannot be eliminated, since it is an essential amino acid in tissue growth. Therefore dietary management must meet two criteria: (1) meet the child's nutritional need for optimum growth and (2) maintain phenylalanine levels within a safe range (2 to 6 mg/dl in neonates and children up to 12 years, 2 to 10 mg/dl through adolescence, and 2 to 15 mg/dl in adults) (Kaye, Committee on Genetics, Accurso, and others, 2006).

Professionals agree that infants with PKU who have blood phenylalanine levels higher than 10 mg/dl should be started on treatment to establish metabolic control as soon as possible, ideally by 7 to 10 days of age (Kaye, Committee on Genetics, Accurso, and others, 2006). The daily amounts of phenylalanine are individualized for each child and require frequent changes on the basis of appetite, growth and development, and blood phenylalanine and tyrosine levels.

Because all natural food proteins contain phenylalanine and will be limited, the diet must be supplemented with a specially prepared phenylalanine-free formula (e.g., Phenex-1 for infants or Phenex-2 for children and adults).† The phenylalanine-free formula is an amino acid–modified formula essential in the low phenylalanine diet to provide the appropriate protein, vitamins, minerals, and calories for optimal growth and development. Because tyrosine becomes an essential amino acid, the phenylalanine-free formula supplies an adequate amount, but in some cases additional supplementation may be needed. The phenylalanine-free amino acid–modified formula for infants has all the nutrients necessary for adequate infant growth. Because of the low phenylalanine content of breast milk, total or partial breastfeeding may be possible with close monitoring of phenylalanine levels (Lawrence and Lawrence, 2005).

It is interesting to recall that when treatment for PKU was first instituted, it was believed that phenylalanine withdrawal during only the first 3 years of age would suffice to avoid mental retardation and other deleterious manifestations of PKU. However, most clinicians now agree that to achieve optimal metabolic control and outcome, a restricted phenylalanine diet, including medical foods and low-protein products, most likely will be medically required for virtually all individuals with classic PKU for their entire life (Kaye, Committee on Genetics, Accurso, and others, 2006). Such life-time reduction of phenylalanine intake is necessary to prevent neuropsychologic and cognitive deficits, since even a mild hyperphenylalaninemia (20 mg/dl) would produce such effects. To evaluate the effectiveness of dietary treatment, frequent monitoring of blood phenylalanine and tyrosine levels is necessary.

Phenylalanine levels greater than 6 mg/dl in mothers with PKU affect the normal embryologic development of the fetus, including mental retardation, cardiac defects, and LBW. It is

---

*For more information, contact American Society of Human Genetics, 9650 Rockville Pike, Bethesda, MD 20814; (301) 634-7300, (866) HUM-GENE; http://www.ashg.org.
†A resource for dietary management is Acosta PB, Yannicelli S: *The Ross metabolic formula system nutrition support protocols,* ed 4, Columbus, Ohio, 2001, Abbott Nutrition; (800) 227-5767; http://abbottnutrition.com.

recommended that phenylalanine levels below 6 mg/dl be achieved at least 3 months before conception in women with PKU (Kaye, Committee on Genetics, Accurso, and others, 2006).

Prognosis. Although many individuals with treated PKU manifest no cognitive and behavioral deficits, many comparisons of individuals with PKU to controls show lower performance on IQ tests, with larger differences in other cognitive domains; however, their performance is still in the average range. Evidence for differences in behavioral adjustment is inconsistent despite anecdotal reports suggesting greater risk for internalizing psychopathology and attention disorders. In addition, there are insufficient data on the effects of phenylalanine restriction over many decades of life (Kaye, Committee on Genetics, Accurso, and others, 2006). Recent data suggest that treatment with tetrahydrobiopterin in addition to the phenylalanine-restricted diet may be beneficial to PKU patients (Matalon, Michaels-Matalon, Koch, and others, 2005). Total bone mineral density is considerably lower in children who are on a low-phenylalanine diet, even though calcium, phosphorus, and magnesium intakes are higher than normal.

Nursing Care Management

The principal nursing considerations involve teaching the family regarding the dietary restrictions. Although the treatment may sound simple, the task of maintaining such a strict dietary regimen is demanding, especially for older children and adolescents. In addition, mothers of children with PKU may have to spend many hours preparing special foods such as low-phenylalanine snacks. However, in one study mothers of children with PKU reported experiencing considerably less stress than those with mitochondrial disease (Read, 2003). Foods with low phenylalanine levels (e.g., vegetables; fruits; juices; some cereals, breads, and starches) must be measured to provide the prescribed amount of phenylalanine. High-protein foods, such as meat and dairy products, are eliminated from the diet. The sweetener aspartame (NutraSweet) should be avoided because it is composed of two amino acids, aspartic acid and phenylalanine, and if used will decrease the amount of natural phenylalanine that is prescribed for the day. However, medications that use aspartame as the sweetener may be used if no other nonaspartame medications are available, since the content of the artificial sweetener is minimal or can be counted in the total daily phenylalanine allowance.

Maintaining the diet during infancy presents few problems. Solid foods such as cereal, fruits, and vegetables are introduced as usual to the infant. Difficulties arise as the child gets older. Studies show a gradual decline in diet compliance with consequent increases in blood phenylalanine levels during early adolescence and young adulthood (Walter and White, 2004).

A decreased appetite and refusal to eat may reduce intake of the calculated phenylalanine requirement. The child's increasing independence may inhibit absolute control of what he or she eats. Either factor can result in decreased or increased phenylalanine levels. During the school years, peer pressure becomes a major force in deterring the child from eating the prescribed foods or abstaining from high-protein foods such as milkshakes or ice cream. Limitations of this diet are best illustrated by an example: a quarter-pound ham-

burger may provide a 2-day phenylalanine allowance for a school-age child.

The assistance of a registered dietitian is essential. Parents need a basic understanding of the disorder and practical suggestions regarding food selection and preparation.* Meal planning is based on weighing the food on a gram scale; a less accurate method is the exchange list. As soon as children are old enough, usually by early preschool, they should be involved in the daily calculation, menu planning, and formula preparation. Using a computer, voice-activated calculator, cards, or colored beads can help children keep track of the daily allowance of phenylalanine foods. A system of goal setting, self-monitoring, contracts, and rewards can promote compliance in adolescents.

Preparation of the phenylalanine-free formula can present some challenges. The formula tends to be lumpy; mixing the powder with a small amount of water to make a paste, then adding the rest of the required liquid, helps alleviate this problem. A blender or mixer dissolves the powder more easily; a rechargeable hand mixer can be used when traveling. Although the taste is virtually impossible to camouflage, many new products are on the market today. Some of the complete formulas are chocolate, vanilla, strawberry, and orange flavored. Incomplete formulas are also available that do not contain the vitamins and minerals and are plain tasting; these can be added to cold foods instead of mixing as a formula. Formula bars are convenient for the active adolescent. Formula capsules are also available, but the patient would need to take 20 or more capsules per day.

Family Support.† In addition to the problem related to a child with a chronic disorder (see Chapter 18), the parents have the burden of knowing that they are carriers of the defect. Genetic counseling is especially important to inform the parents that prenatal testing is now available to detect the presence of the defective gene in heterozygotes. Counseling is also important for adults with PKU to inform them that all their offspring will be carriers for PKU (see Genetic Evaluation and Counseling, p. 316, and Family Focus box).

GALACTOSEMIA

Galactosemia is a rare autosomal recessive disorder that results from various gene mutations leading to three distinct enzymatic deficiencies. The most common type of galactosemia (**classic galactosemia**) results from a deficiency of a hepatic enzyme, **galactose 1-phosphate uridyltransferase (GALT)**, and affects approximately 1 of 50,000 births. The other two varieties of galactosemia involve deficiencies in the enzymes galactokinase (GALK) and galactose 4′-epimerase (GALE); these are extremely rare disorders. All three enzymes (GALT, GALK, and GALE) are involved in the conversion of galactose into glucose.

As galactose accumulates in the blood, several organs are affected. Hepatic dysfunction leads to cirrhosis, resulting in

---

*A helpful resource is Schuett V, editor: *Low protein cookery for phenylketonuria,* ed 3, Madison, Wis, 1997, University of Wisconsin Press; Madison, WI 53715.
†National support groups include the National Coalition for PKU and Allied Disorders, http://www.pku-allieddisorders.org; and the Children's PKU Network, which offers a variety of support services; contact at 3790 Via de la Valle, Suite 120, Del Mar, CA 92014; (800) 377-6677; e-mail: PKUnetwork@aol.com; http://www.pkunetwork.org.

FAMILY FOCUS

Supporting Families

I am a registered nurse and the mother of a child diagnosed with PKU; I also have three siblings with PKU. As a parent, I was devastated when I received a phone call informing me that my son's blood level of phenylalanine was high and that he has PKU. The nurse attempted to comfort me by saying that she understood how I felt and what I was going through. I wanted to scream, "No, you don't know how I feel and what I am going through!" but didn't because I realized she thought she was helping me. It is so important for nurses to be aware of what they say when parent(s) face a crisis such as the diagnosis of chronic disease in their child. It is often best to say nothing at all. A sincere "I'm sorry" can also mean a lot.

—*L.E., RN*

jaundice in the infant by the second week of life. The spleen subsequently becomes enlarged as a result of portal hypertension. Cataracts are usually recognizable by 1 or 2 months of age; cerebral damage, manifested by the symptoms of lethargy and hypotonia, is evident soon afterward. Infants with galactosemia appear normal at birth, but within a few days of ingesting milk (which has a high lactose content), they begin to experience vomiting and diarrhea, leading to weight loss. *E. coli* sepsis is also a common presenting clinical sign. Death during the first month of life is not infrequent in untreated infants. Occasionally classic galactosemia is seen with milder, chronic manifestations, such as failure to thrive, feeding difficulty, and developmental delay. This presentation is more frequent among African-American children with galactosemia (Kaye, Committee on Genetics, Accurso, and others, 2006).

Diagnostic Evaluation

Diagnosis is made on the basis of the infant's history, physical examination, galactosuria, increased levels of galactose in the blood, and decreased levels of GALT activity in erythrocytes. The infant may display characteristics of malnutrition; signs of dehydration, decreased muscle mass, and decreased body fat may be evident (Askin and Diehl-Jones, 2003). Newborn screening for this disease is required in most states. Heterozygotes can also be identified, since heterozygotic individuals have significantly lower levels of the essential enzyme.

Therapeutic Management

During infancy, treatment consists of eliminating all milk and lactose-containing formula, including breast milk. Traditionally, lactose-free formulas are used, with soy-protein formula being the feeding of choice; however, recent research suggests that elemental formula (galactose-free) may be more beneficial than soy formulas (Zlatunich and Packman, 2005). As the infant progresses to solids, only foods low in galactose should be consumed. Certain fruits are high in galactose, and some dietitians recommend that they be avoided. Food lists should be given to the family to ensure appropriate foods are chosen.

If galactosemia is suspected, supportive treatment and care are implemented, including monitoring for hypoglycemia, liver failure, bleeding disorders, and *E. coli* sepsis.

Prognosis. Follow-up studies of children treated from birth or within the first 2 months of life after symptoms appear have found long-term complications, such as ovarian dysfunction, cataracts, abnormal speech, cognitive impairment, growth retardation, and motor delay (Lashley, 2002). These findings have revealed that eliminating sources of galactose does not significantly improve the outcome. New therapeutic strategies, such as enhancing residual transferase activity, replacing depleted metabolites, or using gene replacement therapy, are needed to improve the prognosis for these children.

Nursing Care Management*

Nursing interventions are similar to those for PKU, except that dietary restrictions are easier to maintain because many more foods are allowed. However, reading food labels carefully for the presence of any form of lactose, especially dairy products, is mandatory.

GENETIC EVALUATION AND COUNSELING

Genetic counseling is a communication process concerned with the human problems associated with the occurrence, or risk of occurrence, of a genetic disorder in a family. It involves relaying information about the diagnosis, treatment options, recurrence risk, and availability of prenatal diagnosis. With the completion of the Human Genome Project, the international project to determine the total genetic information in humans, a new era of human genetics is unfolding (International Human Genome Sequencing Consortium, 2004), and it will lead to a better understanding of specifically how genetic variation contributes to health and disease. It is essential that nurses master the basic principles of heredity, understand how heredity contributes to disorders, and be aware of the types of genetic testing available (Table 9-14).

Nurses frequently encounter children with genetic diseases and families in which there is a risk that a disorder may be transmitted to or occur in an offspring. It is a responsibility of nurses to be alert to situations in which persons could benefit from a genetic evaluation and counseling (see Nursing Care Guidelines box), to be aware of the local genetic resources, to aid the family in finding services, and to offer support and care for children and families affected by genetic conditions. Local genetic clinics can be located through several sites; for example, GeneTests,† a publicly funded medical genetics information resource developed for physicians and other health care providers, is available at no cost to all interested persons. Another resource is the National Society of Genetic Counselors,‡ which lists genetic counselors by states in the United States.

Maintaining contact with the family or referring the family to an agency that can provide a sustained relationship, usually the public health agency in their locality, is one of the most important aspects in the care of the patient and family. In a disorder that requires conscientious diet management, such as PKU or galactosemia, it is important to make certain that the family understands and follows the advice. A vital role for

---

*Information and support for parents can be found at the American Liver Foundation, http://www.liverfoundation.org; and at Parents of Galactosemic Children, Inc., PO Box 2401, Mandeville, LA 74070-2401; (866) 900-PGC1; http://www.galactosemia.org.
†http://www.genetests.org.
‡http://www.nsgc.org.

TABLE 9-14

Types of Genetic Testing

TEST AND METHOD	SPECIMEN	INDICATION	COMMENTS
Chromosome analysis (karyotyping)	Blood, skin, amniocytes, bone marrow	Detection of chromosomal abnormality, sex determination, cancer classification	Almost 100% accuracy for whole or partial chromosomal abnormality; will not detect microdeletions or duplication (submicroscopic chromosome segments), single-gene defects, or multifactorial disorders
Fluorescence in situ hybridization (FISH)	Blood, skin, amniocytes, bone marrow	Detection of microdeletion or duplications of chromosome segments (not visible by chromosome analysis)	A technique that is a cross between chromosome analysis and single-gene DNA tests
Direct DNA mutation detection (polymerase chain reaction, Southern blot, gene sequencing)	Blood, skin, amniocytes	Detection of gene mutation(s) in affected individual for diagnosis, in unaffected carrier, or for presymptomatic diagnosis	Gene location must be mapped, and disease-producing mutations must be characterized; can test single individual
Indirect DNA linkage studies (restriction length fragment polymorphisms, microsatellites, genetic markers)	Blood	Prediction of carrier, or presymptomatic status based on inheritance of same chromosome segment as in known affected individual	Must test several family members, including 1-2 confirmed affected individuals, for testing to be valid
Biochemical	Blood, skin, amniotic fluid, muscle biopsy, urine, stool, cerebrospinal fluid	Detection of metabolic pathway errors, enzyme defects, prenatal neural tube or ventral wall defect	Results may be difficult to interpret if partial pathway error or modified substrate is present Maternal serum α-fetoprotein levels screen for neural tube or ventral wall defects

DNA, Deoxyribonucleic acid.

nursingcareguidelines

Common Indications for Referral

- Previous child with multiple congenital anomalies; mental retardation; or an isolated birth defect, such as neural tube defect, cleft lip, or cleft palate
- Family history of a hereditary condition, such as cystic fibrosis, fragile X syndrome, or diabetes
- Prenatal diagnosis for advanced maternal age or other indication
- Consanguinity
- Teratogen exposure, such as to occupational chemicals, medications, alcohol
- Repeated pregnancy loss or infertility
- Newly diagnosed abnormality or genetic condition
- Before undertaking genetic testing and after receiving results, particularly when testing for susceptibility to late-onset disorders, such as cancer or neurologic disease
- As follow-up for a positive newborn test, as with phenylketonuria, or a heterozygote screening test, such as Tay-Sachs disease

From Nussbaum R, McInnes R, Willard H: *Thompson and Thompson genetics in medicine,* ed 6, Philadelphia, 2004, Saunders.

nurses is to advocate for the child and family as they make their way through the various specialty clinics. This is especially important for families who are more vulnerable because of cognitive, hearing, language, or financial issues and those who otherwise may have difficulty accessing health services. Nurses can reinforce the genetic information or arrange for additional genetic counseling if a family has additional questions or misunderstandings.

One of the current ethical concerns is the testing of healthy children for carrier status of a genetic condition that either will not have adverse consequences until adulthood or only has reproductive implications. The American Academy of Pediatrics' (2001) policy statement does not support the broad use of carrier testing or screening in children or adolescents. When there is no clear medical benefit to testing in childhood, the child should be permitted to wait until adulthood to choose whether or not to be tested. Genetic counseling is recommended to help the family weigh all of the issues.

PSYCHOLOGIC ASPECTS OF GENETIC DISEASE

The diagnosis of a genetic disorder in a child can be a life-altering experience for families. They may have to reassess their perception of "self" and the loss of the dream of the perfect baby. Parents may change educational, employment, and reproductive plans after the diagnosis of a genetic disorder in their child.

Families may need to have the genetic information repeated several times. Families may also encounter ethical or moral dilemmas regarding genetic evaluation and testing options, as well as potential involvement of other family members. Nurses are pivotal caregivers in assessing the family's understanding of the genetic disorder, psychologic responses, and coping mechanisms. Nurses may help families by providing support and attempting to alleviate possible feelings of guilt, and by helping the family make the best possible adjustment to the disorder.

It is important to stress that there is nothing shameful about an inherited or congenital defect and to emphasize any appropriate remedy. The thought of a hereditary disorder often creates intrafamily strife, hostility, and marital disharmony, sometimes to the point of family disintegration. Relatives may change reproductive plans after the diagnosis of a genetic disorder in a member, or the decision to reproduce may be postponed indefinitely on the basis of a disorder in a relative, even a remote one. Although people may understand the information on an intellectual level, they may still harbor fears on an emotional level. Nurses can help the family identify their personal strengths and offer them information about local and national support groups. (The Genetic Alliance* is a nonprofit organization that has a database of support groups for genetic conditions.) Finally, it is important to keep in mind that the infant or child has the same basic needs after the diagnosis of a genetic disorder as he or she had before the diagnosis.

_____
*http://www.geneticalliance.org.

KEY POINTS

■ Birth injuries are usually transient and may involve soft tissue, bone, or nervous tissue.

■ High-risk neonates are those newborn infants, regardless of gestational age or birth weight, who have a greater than average chance of morbidity or mortality because of conditions or circumstances associated with birth and adjustment to extrauterine life.

■ Appropriate developmental care for preterm infants focuses on individualized neurobehavioral assessment, planning, diagnosis, intervention, and reevaluation to foster appropriate growth and maturation in a potentially harmful environment.

■ Parents are encouraged to interact with their high-risk infant and gradually assume care of the infant as allowed by the infant's condition.

■ Because of their immature physical status, preterm infants need special attention to promote respiratory efforts, maintain body temperature, maintain fluid and electrolyte balance, prevent infection, and provide adequate nutrition for growth.

■ Jaundice is a common transient problem in the newborn that results from RBC breakdown that exceeds the ability of the immature liver to metabolize and excrete.

■ Preterm infants are subject to a number of complications, including apnea, sepsis, RDS, NEC, and intraventricular hemorrhage.

■ Sepsis is a serious condition with generalized nonspecific manifestations that requires immediate intervention involving systemic antibiotics and observation for associated complications.

■ Maternal conditions that may pose health risks in the neonatal period include maternal diabetes, perinatal infections, and substance abuse.

■ Chromosomal disorders are caused by abnormalities in either chromosomal structure or number.

■ Some of the most significant IEMs in the neonatal period include CH, PKU, and galactosemia. Specific population-based newborn screening for IEMs should take place in situations where the incidence of other IEMs is prevalent. Severe cognitive delays can result if these conditions are undiagnosed and untreated.

■ Genetic counseling is directed toward providing individuals and families with information needed to make decisions about a course of action appropriate to them.

■ Although no cure for genetic disease is presently available, various therapeutic measures are used to modify the basic defect.

??? answers to CRITICAL THINKING EXERCISE

JAUNDICE

1. Yes, there are sufficient data to arrive at some possible conclusions.
2. a. See text, pp. 274-281.
   b. Levels are within acceptable limits based on available data; based on available data, ABO incompatibility–related hemolysis is not evident but may warrant further investigation.
   c. Oral intake is adequate; urine and stool output is appropriate.
   d. The assessment of behavior and reflexes indicates no particular concerns; the newborn seems to be healthy.
3. No immediate intervention to reduce bilirubin is warranted at this time, although the treatment is a medical decision. Nursing care should focus on alleviating parents' concerns regarding condition of infant, who appears to be healthy, and address their concerns about the misinformation on the potential for brain damage (which is a nonexistent problem at this point). Encourage the mother to continue breastfeeding on demand and observe the infant's activity levels, intake, and urinary and stool output. Emphasize that jaundice and hyperbilirubinemia are transient conditions of the newborn. At this point a follow-up appointment should be scheduled with the primary practitioner in 24 hours to monitor the bilirubin level, address the parents' concerns, and monitor the infant's weight.
4. Yes—the infant's laboratory data and physical assessment data support these conclusions. Additionally, knowledge about physiologic hyperbilirubinemia of the newborn supports these conclusions. Phototherapy does not seem warranted at this time based on the available data.
5. One might question the need to interrupt breastfeeding; however, this does not seem necessary at this point. The available data do not point to a pathologic process; however, some may elect to obtain further laboratory data (complete blood count, reticulocyte count).

REFERENCES

Alster TS, Railan D: Laser treatment of vascular birthmarks, *J Craniofac Surg* 17(4):720-723, 2006.

Altimier L, Lutes L: Cobedding multiples, *Newborn Infant Nurs Rev* 1(4):205-206, 2001.

American Academy of Pediatrics, Committee on Infectious Diseases, Pickering L, editor: *Red book: 2006 report of the Committee on Infectious Diseases,* ed 27, Elk Grove, Ill, 2006a, The Academy.

American Academy of Pediatrics: Update on newborn screening and treatment for congenital hypothyroidism, *Pediatrics* 117(6):2290-2303, 2006b.

American Academy of Pediatrics: Breastfeeding and the use of human milk, *Pediatrics* 115(2):496-506, 2005a.

American Academy of Pediatrics, Task Force on Sudden Infant Death Syndrome: The changing concept of sudden infant death syndrome: diagnostic coding shifts, controversies regarding the sleeping environment, and new variables to consider in reducing risk, *Pediatrics* 116(5):1245-1255, 2005b.

American Academy of Pediatrics, Subcommittee on Hyperbilirubinemia: Management of hyperbilirubinemia in the newborn infant 35 or more weeks of gestation (clinical practice guideline), *Pediatrics* 114(1):297-316, 2004.

American Academy of Pediatrics, Committee on Injury and Poison Prevention: Selecting and using the most appropriate car safety seats for growing children: guidelines for counseling parents, *Pediatrics* 109(3):550-553, 2002.

American Academy of Pediatrics, Committee on Bioethics: Ethical issues with genetic testing in pediatrics, *Pediatrics* 107(6):1451-1455, 2001.

American Academy of Pediatrics: Safe transportation of newborns at hospital discharge, *Pediatrics* 104(4):986-987, 1999.

American Academy of Pediatrics and American College of Obstetricians and Gynecologists: *Guidelines for perinatal care,* ed 6, Elk Grove Village, Ill, 2007, The Academy.

American Heart Association: Guidelines for cardiopulmonary and emergency cardiovascular care, part 13, Neonatal resuscitation guidelines, *Circulation* 112(24 Suppl):IV118-IV195, 2005.

American Heart Association, American Academy of Pediatrics: 2005 American Heart Association guidelines for cardiopulmonary resuscitation and emergency cardiovascular care of pediatric and neonatal patients: neonatal resuscitation guidelines, *Pediatrics* 117(5):e1029-e1038, 2006.

Anderson GC: Kangaroo care of the premature infant. In Goldson E, editor: *Nurturing the premature infant: developmental interventions in the neonatal intensive care nursery,* New York, 1999, Oxford University Press.

Arendt R, Angelopoulos J, Salvator A, and others: Motor development of cocaine-exposed children at age two years, *Pediatrics* 103(1):86-92, 1999.

Askin DF, Diehl-Jones B: Liver, part III, Pathophysiology of liver dysfunction, *Neonatal Netw* 22(3):5-15, 2003.

Askin DF, Diehl-Jones B: Cocaine: effects of in utero exposure on the fetus and newborn, *J Perinat Neonatal Nurs* 14(4):83-102, 2001.

Aziz N, Baron EJ, D'Souza H, and others: Comparison of rapid intrapartum screening methods for group B streptococcal vaginal colonization, *J Matern Fetal Neonatal Med* 18(4):225-229, 2005.

Bandstra ES, Accornero VH: Infants of substance abusing mothers. In Martin RJ, Fanaroff AA, Walsh MC, editors: *Fanaroff and Martin's neonatal-perinatal medicine: diseases of the fetus and infant,* ed 8, St Louis, 2006, Mosby.

Barrington KJ, Finer NN: Inhaled nitric oxide for preterm infants: a systematic review, *Pediatrics* 120(5):1088-1099, 2007.

Bateman DA, Chiriboga CA: Dose-response effect of cocaine on newborn head circumference, *Pediatrics* 106(3):e33, 2000.

Beachy JM: Investigating jaundice in the newborn, *Neonatal Netw* 26(5):327-333, 2007.

Beauman SS, Swanson A: Neonatal infusion therapy: preventing complications and improving outcomes, *Newborn Infant Nurs Rev* 16(4):193-201, 2006.

Bhutani VK, Gourley GR, Adler S, and others: Noninvasive measurement of total serum bilirubin in a multiracial predischarge newborn population to assess the risk of severe hyperbilirubinemia, *Pediatrics* 106(2):e17, 2000.

Bhutani VK, Johnson LH, Keren R: Diagnosis and management of hyperbilirubinemia in the term neonate: for a safer first week, *Pediatr Clin North Am* 51(4):843-861, 2004.

Bhutani VK, Johnson L, Sivieri EM: Predictive ability of a predischarge hour-specific serum bilirubin for subsequent significant hyperbilirubinemia in healthy term and near-term newborns, *Pediatrics* 103(1):6-14, 1999.

Bin-Nun A, Bromiker R, Wilschanski M, and others: Oral probiotics prevent necrotizing enterocolitis in very low birth weight neonates, *J Pediatr* 147(2):143-146, 2005.

Blackburn ST: *Maternal, fetal, and neonatal physiology: a clinical perspective,* ed 3, Philadelphia, 2007, Saunders.

Blake WW, Murray JA: Heat balance. In Merenstein GB, Gardner SL, editors: *Handbook of neonatal intensive care,* ed 6, St Louis, 2006, Mosby.

Boney CM, Verma A, Tucker R, and others: Metabolic syndrome in childhood: association with birth weight, maternal obesity, and gestational diabetes mellitus, *Pediatrics* 115(3):e290-e296, 2005.

Boo NY, Foong KW, Mahdy ZA, and others: Risk factors associated with subaponeurotic haemorrhage in full-term infants exposed to vacuum extraction, *Br J Obstet Gynaecol* 112:1516-1521, 2005.

Brown ZA, Wald A, Morrow RA, and others: Effect of serologic status and cesarean delivery on transmission rates of herpes simplex virus from mother to infant, *JAMA* 289:203-209, 2003.

Byers JF, Waugh WR, Lowman LB: Sound level exposure of high-risk infants in different environmental conditions, *Neonatal Netw* 25(1):25-32, 2006.

Cambell S: Prenatal cocaine exposure and neonatal/infant outcomes, *Neonatal Netw* 22(1):19-21, 2003.

Carver JD, Wu PY, Hall RT, and others: Growth of preterm infants fed nutrient-enriched or term formula after hospital discharge, *Pediatrics* 107(4):683-689, 2001.

Cashore WJ: Bilirubin and jaundice in the micropremie, *Clin Perinatol* 27(1):171-179, 2000.

Centers for Disease Control and Prevention: *Enterobacter sakazakii* infections associated with the use of powdered infant formula—Tennessee, 2001, *MMWR* 51(14):98-300, 2002a.

Centers for Disease Control and Prevention: Prevention of perinatal group B streptococcal disease: revised guidelines, *MMWR* 51(RR11):1-22, 2002b.

Chiriboga CA, Brust JC, Bateman D, and others: Drug-response effect on fetal cocaine exposure on newborn neurologic function, *Pediatrics* 103(1):79-85, 1999.

Chiriboga CA, Kuhn L, Wasserman GA.: Prenatal cocaine exposures and dose-related cocaine effects on infant tone and behavior, *Neurotoxicol Teratol* 29(3):323-330, 2007.

Chomchai C, Na Manorom N, Watanarungasan P, and others: Methamphetamine abuse during pregnancy and its impact on neonates born at Siriraj Hospital, Bangkok, Thailand, *Southeast Asian J Trop Med Public Health* 35(1):228-231, 2004.

Cifuentes J, Segars AH, Carlo W: Respiratory system management and complications. In Kenner C, Lott J, editors: *Comprehensive neonatal nursing: a physiologic perspective,* ed 3, Philadelphia, 2003, Saunders.

Conde-Agudelo A, Diaz-Rossello JL, Belizan JM: Kangaroo mother care to reduce morbidity and mortality in low birthweight infants, *Cochrane Neonatal Review,* 2000, retrieved June 20, 2007, from http://www. nichd.nih.gov/cochraneneonatal/Vickers/Vickers.htm.

Conlon JD, Drolet BA: Skin lesions in the neonate, *Pediatr Clin North Am* 51(4):863-888, vii-viii, 2004.

Cornblath M, Hawdon JM, Williams A, and others: Controversies regarding definition of neonatal hypoglycemia: suggested operational thresholds, *Pediatrics* 105(5):1141, 2000.

Cowett RM, Loughead JL: Neonatal glucose metabolism: differential diagnoses, evaluation, and treatment of hypoglycemia, *Neonatal Netw* 21(4):9-19, 2002.

Crocker E: Meth's burning issues, *Nurse Week, Heartland Ed* 6(8):22-23, 2005.

Davis PG, Henderson-Smart DJ: Nasal continuous positive airways pressure immediately after extubation for preventing morbidity in preterm infants, *Cochrane Database Syst Rev* (2):CD000143, 2003.

Delaney-Black V, Cobington C, Templin T, and others: Prenatal cocaine exposure and child behavior, *Pediatrics* 102(4):945-950, 1998.

DellaPorta K, Aforismo D, Butler-O'Hara M: Cobedding of twins in the neonatal intensive care, *Pediatr Nurs* 24(6):529-531, 1998.

Deshpande S, Ward Platt M: The investigation and management of neonatal hypoglycaemia, *Semin Fetal Neonatal Med* 10(4):351-361, 2005.

Dodd VL: Implications of kangaroo care for growth and development in preterm infants, *J Obstet Gynecol Neonatal Nurs* 34(2):218-232, 2005.

Dohil MA, Baugh WP, Eichenfield LF: Vascular and pigmented birthmarks, *Pediatr Clin North Am* 47(4):783-812, 2000.

Doumouchtsis SK, Arulkumaran S: Head injuries after instrumental vaginal deliveries, *Curr Opin Obstet Gynecol* 18(2):129-134, 2006.

Drummond GS, Kappas A: Chemoprevention of severe neonatal hyperbilirubinemia, *Semin Perinatol* 28(5):365-368, 2004.

Ebrahim SH, Gfoerer J: Pregnancy-related substance use in the United States during 1996-1998, *Obstet Gynecol* 101(2):374-379, 2003.

Edwards WH, Conner JM, Soll RF, and others: The effect of prophylactic ointment therapy on nosocomial sepsis rates and skin integrity in infants with birth weights of 501 to 1000 g, *Pediatrics* 113(5):1195-1203, 2004.

Engle WA: A recommendation for the definition of "late preterm" (near-term) and the birth weight–gestational age classification system, *Semin Perinatol* 30(1):2-7, 2006.

Engle WA, Tomashek KM, Wallman C, and others: Late-preterm infants: a population at risk, *Pediatrics* 120(6):1390-1401, 2007.

Eyler FD, Behnke M: Early development of infants exposed to drugs prenatally, *Clin Perinatol* 26(1):107-150, 1999.

Eyler FD, Behnke M, Conlon M: Birth outcome from a prospective, matched study of prenatal crack/cocaine use, part II, Interactive and dose effects on neurobehavioral assessment, *Pediatrics* 101(2):237-241, 1998.

Eyler FD, Behnke M, Wobie K, and others: Relative ability of biologic specimens and interviews to detect prenatal cocaine use, *Neurotoxicol Teratol* 27(4):677-687, 2005.

Finer NN: Surfactant use for neonatal lung injury: beyond respiratory distress syndrome, *Paediatr Respir Rev* 5(Suppl A):S289-S297, 2004.

Finnegan LP: Neonatal abstinence. In Nelson N, editor: *Current therapy in neonatal perinatal medicine 1985-1986,* Toronto, 1985, Decker.

Forsythe SJ: *Enterobacter sakazakii* and other bacteria in powdered infant milk formula, *Maternal Child Nutrition* 1(1):44-50, 2005.

Frank DA, Jacobs RR, Beeghly M, and others: Level of prenatal cocaine exposure and scores on the Bayley Scales of Infant Development: modifying effects of caregiver, early intervention, and birth weight, *Pediatrics* 110(6):1143-1152, 2002.

Gardner SL, Hauser P, Merenstein GB: Grief and perinatal loss. In Merenstein GB, Gardner SL, editors: *Handbook of neonatal intensive care,* ed 6, St Louis, 2006, Mosby.

Gardner SL, Snell BJ, Lawrence RA: Breastfeeding the neonate with special needs. In Merenstein GB, Gardner SL, editors: *Handbook of neonatal intensive care,* ed 6, St Louis, 2006, Mosby.

Gray L, Watt L, Blass EM: Skin-to-skin contact is analgesic in healthy newborns, *Pediatrics* 105(1):110-111, 2000; retrieved July 1, 2007, from http://www.pediatrics.org/cgi/content/full/105/1/e14.

Greene CM, Goodman MH: Neonatal abstinence syndrome: strategies for care of the drug-exposed infant, *Neonatal Netw* 22(4):15-25, 2003.

Gupta A, Della-Latta P, Todd B, and others: Outbreak of extended-spectrum beta-lactamase-producing *Klebsiella pneumoniae* in a neonatal intensive care unit linked to artificial nails, *Infect Control Hosp Epidemiol* 25(3):210-215, 2004.

Hellekson KL: Practice guidelines: NIH consensus statement on phenylketonuria, *Am Fam Physician* 63(7):1430-1432, 2001.

Holditch-Davis D, Blackburn ST, VandenBerg K: Newborn and infant neurobehavioral development. In Kenner C, Lott J, editors: *Comprehensive neonatal nursing: a physiologic perspective,* Philadelphia, 2003, Saunders.

Howard-Salsman KD: Car seat safety for high-risk infants, *Neonatal Netw* 25(2):117-129, 2006.

Hudic I, Fatusic Z, Sinanovic O, and others: Etiological risk factors for brachial plexus palsy, *J Matern Fetal Neonatal Med* 19(10):655-661, 2006.

Huestis MA, Choo RE: Drug abuse's smallest victims: in utero drug exposure, *Forensic Sci Int* 128(1-2):20-30, 2002.

Hung-Chih L, Bai-Horng S, An-Chyi C, and others: Oral probiotics reduce the incidence and severity of necrotizing enterocolitis in very low birth weight infants, *Pediatrics* 115(1):1-4, 2005.

Hurd YL, Wang X, Anderson V, and others: Marijuana impairs growth in mid-gestation fetuses, *Neurotoxicol Teratol* 27(2):221-229, 2005.

International Human Genome Sequencing Consortium: Finishing the euchromatic sequence of the human genome, *Nature* 431:931-945, 2004.

Jansen JL: A bereavement model for the intensive care nursery, *Neonatal Netw* 22(3):17-23, 2003.

Johnson CB: Head, eyes, ears, nose, mouth and neck assessment. In Tappero EP, Honeyfield ME, editors: *Physical assessment of the newborn: a comprehensive approach to the art of physical assessment,* ed 3, Santa Rosa, Calif, 2003, NICU Ink.

Johnson K, Gerada C, Greenough A: Treatment of neonatal abstinence syndrome, *Arch Dis Child Fetal Neonatal Educ* 88(1):F2-F5, 2003.

Jones KL: Smith's recognizable patterns of human malformation, ed 4, Philadelphia, 2006, Saunders.

Joyner B, Soto MA, Adam HM: Brachial plexus injury, *Pediatr Rev* 27(6):238-239, 2006.

Kandall SR: Treatment strategies for drug-exposed neonates, *Clin Perinatol* 26(1):231-243, 1999.

Kato T, Mittal N, Nishida S, and others: The role of intestinal transplantation in the management of babies with extensive gut resections, *J Pediatr Surg* 38(2):145-149, 2003.

Kaye CI, Committee on Genetics, Accurso F, and others: Newborn screening fact sheets, *Pediatrics* 118(3):e934-e963, 2006.

Kenner C: Resuscitation and stabilization of the newborn. In Kenner C, Lott JW, editors: *Comprehensive neonatal nursing,* ed 3, Philadelphia, 2003, Saunders.

Kimberlin DW: Herpes simplex virus infections of the newborn, *Semin Perinatol* 31(1):19-25, 2007.

Kimberlin DW: Herpes simplex virus infections in neonates and early childhood, *Semin Pediatr Infect Dis* 16:271-281, 2005.

Kirkpatrick JM, Alexander J, Cain RM: Recovering urine from diapers: are test results accurate? *MCN* 22(2):96-102, 1997.

Kliegman RM: The relationship of neonatal feeding practices and the pathogenesis and prevention of necrotizing enterocolitis, *Pediatrics* 111(3):671-672, 2003.

Koren G, Nulman I, Rovet J, and others: Long-term neurodevelopmental risks in children exposed in utero to cocaine: the Toronto adoption study, *Ann NY Acad Sci* 846:306-312, 1998.

Laborada G, Rego M, Jain A, and others: Diagnostic value of cytokines and C-reactive protein in the first 24 hours of neonatal sepsis, *Am J Perinatol* 20(8):491-501, 2003.

LaMar K, Dowling DA: Incidence of infection for preterm twins cared for in cobedding in the neonatal intensive-care unit, *J Obstet Gynecol Neonatal Nurs* 35(2):193-198, 2006.

Lashley FR: Newborn screening: new opportunities and new challenges, *Newborn Infant Nurs Rev* 2(4):228-242, 2002.

Lawrence RA, Lawrence RM: *Breastfeeding: a guide for the medical profession,* ed 6, St Louis, 2005, Mosby.

Lester BM, Tronick EZ, Brazelton TB: The Neonatal Intensive Care Unit Network Neurobehavioral Scale procedures, *Pediatrics* 113(3 Suppl):641-667, 2004.

L'Herault J, Petroff L, Jeffrey J: The effectiveness of a thermal mattress in stabilizing and maintaining body temperature during the transport of very low–birth weight newborns, *Appl Nurs Res* 14(4):210-219, 2001.

Lucas A, Fewtrell MS, Morley R, and others: Randomized trial of nutrient-enriched formula versus standard formula for postdischarge preterm infants, *Pediatrics* 108(3):703-711, 2001.

Ludington-Hoe SM, Hosseini R, Torowicz DL: Skin-to-skin contact (kangaroo care) analgesia for preterm infant heel stick, *AACN Clin Issues* 16(3):373-387, 2005.

Lund CH, Kuller JM: Assessment and management of the integumentary system. In Kenner C, Lott JW, editors: *Comprehensive neonatal nursing,* ed 3, Philadelphia, 2003, Saunders.

Maisels MJ: Jaundice. In MacDonald MG, Seshia MMK, Mullett MD, editors: *Avery's neonatology,* Philadelphia, 2005, Lippincott.

Maisels MJ, Watchko JF: Treatment of jaundice in low birthweight infants, *Arch Dis Child Fetal Neonatal Educ* 88(6):F459-F463, 2003.

Malanga CJ, Kosofsy BE: Mechanism of action of drugs of abuse on the developing fetal brain, *Clin Perinatol* 26(1):17-37, 1999.

Mangurten HH: Birth injuries. In Martin RJ, Fanaroff AA, Walsh MC, editors: *Fanaroff and Martin's neonatal-perinatal medicine: diseases of the fetus and infant,* ed 8, St Louis, 2006, Mosby.

Marcellus L: Care of substance-exposed infants: the current state of practice in Canadian hospitals, *J Perinat Neonatal Nurs* 16(3):51-68, 2002.

Mari G: Noninvasive diagnosis by Doppler ultrasonography of fetal anemia due to maternal red-cell isoimmunization, *N Engl J Med* 342(1):9-14, 2000.

Matalon R, Michaels-Matalon K, Koch R, and others: Response of patients with phenylketonuria in the US to tetrahydrobiopterin, *Mol Genet Metab* 86(Suppl 1):S17-S21, 2005.

Mazela J, Merritt TA, Finer NN: Aerosolized surfactants, *Curr Opin Pediatr* 19(2):155-162, 2007.

McCain GC: An evidence-based guideline for introducing oral feeding to healthy preterm infants, *Neonatal Netw* 22(5):45-50, 2003.

McCain GC, Ludington-Hoe SM, Swinth JY, and others: Heart rate variability responses of a preterm infant to kangaroo care, *J Obstet Gynecol Neonatal Nurs* 34(6):689-694, 2005.

McCall EM, Alderdice FA, Halliday HL, and others: Interventions to prevent hypothermia at birth in preterm and/or low birthweight babies, *Cochrane Database Syst Rev* (1):CD004210, 2005.

McCance K, Huether S: *Pathophysiology: the biological basis for disease in infants and children,* ed 5, St Louis, 2006, Mosby.

McPhee SJ, Ganong, WF: *Pathophysiology of disease: an introduction to clinical medicine,* ed 5, New York, 2006, Lang Medical Books.

Merenstein GB, Gardner SL: *Handbook of neonatal intensive care,* ed 6, St Louis, 2006, Mosby.

Merrill J, Ballard R: Pulmonary surfactant for neonatal respiratory disorders, *Curr Opin Pediatr* 15(2):149-154, 2003.

Messinger DS, Bauer CR, Das A, and others: The maternal lifestyle study: cognitive, motor, and behavioral outcomes of cocaine-exposed and opiate-exposed infants through three years of age, *Pediatrics* 113(6):1677-1685, 2004.

Mills JF, Tudehope D: Fibreoptic phototherapy for neonatal jaundice, *Cochrane Database Syst Rev* (1):CD002060, 2005.

Moise KJ: Management of rhesus alloimmunization in pregnancy, *Obstet Gynecol* 100(3):600-611, 2002.

Moolenaar RL, Crutcher JM, San Joaquin VH, and others: A prolonged outbreak of *Pseudomonas aeruginosa* in a neonatal intensive care unit: did staff fingernails play a role in disease transmission? *Infect Control Hosp Epidemiol* 21(2):80-85, 2000.

Moore KA, Coker K, DuBuisson AB, and others: Implementing potentially better practices for improving family-centered care in neonatal intensive care units: successes and challenges, *Pediatrics* 111(4):e450-e460, 2003.

Morrow CE, Culbertson JL, Accornero VH, and others: Learning disabilities and intellectual functioning in school-aged children with prenatal cocaine exposure, *Dev Neuropsychol* 30(3):905-931, 2006.

Mundy CA: Intravenous immunoglobulin in the management of hemolytic disease of the newborn, *Neonatal Netw* 24(6):17-24, 2005.

Neal JL: RhD isoimmunization and current management modalities, *J Obstet Gynecol Neonatal Nurs* 30(6):589-607, 2001.

Nussbaum RL, McInnes RR, Willard HF: *Thompson and Thompson genetics in medicine*, ed 6 (rev reprint), Philadelphia, 2004, Saunders.

Paige PL, Moe PC: Neurologic disorders. In Merenstein GB, Gardner SL, editors: *Handbook of neonatal intensive care*, ed 6, St Louis, 2006, Mosby.

Parker LA, Montrowl SJ: Neonatal herpes infection: a review, *Newborn Infant Nurs Rev* 4(1):62-69, 2004.

Pinelli J, Symington A: Non-nutritive sucking for promoting physiologic stability and nutrition in preterm infants, *Cochrane Database Syst Rev* (4): CD001071, 2005.

Plessinger M: Prenatal exposure to amphetamines, *Obstet Gynecol Clin North Am* 25(1):119-138, 1998.

Polak JD, Ringler N, Daugherty B: Unit based procedures: impact on the incidence of nosocomial infections in the newborn intensive care unit, *Newborn Infant Nurs Reviews* 4(1):38-45, 2004.

Porter ML, Dennis BL: Hyperbilirubinemia in the term newborn, *Am Fam Physician* 65(4):599-606, 613-614, 2002.

Premji SS, Paes B, Jacobson K, and others: Evidence-based feeding guideline for very low birth-weight infants, *Adv Neonatal Care* 2(1):5-18, 2002.

Price AE, Ditaranto P, Yaylali I, and others: Botulinum toxin type A as an adjunct to the surgical treatment of the medial rotation deformity of the shoulder in birth injuries of the brachial plexus, *J Bone Joint Surg Br* 89(3):327-329, 2007.

Putta LV, Spencer JP: Assisted vaginal delivery using the vacuum extractor, *Am Fam Physician* 62(6):1316-1320, 2000.

Ramsey PS, Goldenberg PL: Obstetric management of prematurity. In Martin RJ, Fanaroff AA, Walsh MC, editors: *Fanaroff and Martin's neonatal-perinatal medicine: diseases of the fetus and infant*, ed 8, St Louis, 2006, Mosby.

Read CY: The demands of biochemical genetic disorders: a survey of mothers of children with mitochondrial disease or phenylketonuria, *J Pediatr Nurs* 18(3):181-186, 2003.

Reynolds RM, Thureen PJ: Special circumstances: trophic feeds, necrotizing enterocolitis and bronchopulmonary dysplasia, *Semin Fetal Neonatal Med* 12(1):64-70, 2007.

Richardson GA, Hamel SC, Goldschmidt L, and others: The effects of prenatal cocaine use on neonatal neurobehavioral status, *Neurotoxicol Teratol* 18(5):519-528, 1996.

Sarici SU, Yurdakok M, Serdar MA, and others: An early (sixth-hour) serum bilirubin measurement is useful in predicting the development of significant hyperbilirubinemia and severe ABO hemolytic disease in a selective high-risk population of newborns with ABO incompatibility, *Pediatrics* 109(4):e53, 2002.

Saugstad OD: Optimal oxygenation at birth and in the neonatal period, *Neonatology* 91(4):319-322, 2007.

Saugstad OD, Ramji S, Irani SF, and others: Resuscitation of newborn infants with 21% or 100% oxygen: follow-up at 18 and 24 months, *Pediatrics* 112(2):296-300, 2003.

Schanler RJ, Shulman RJ, Lau C, and others: Feeding strategies for premature infants: randomized trial of gastrointestinal priming and tube-feeding method, *Pediatrics* 103(2):434-439, 1999.

Schultze A, Lindner M, Kohlmüller D, and others: Expanded newborn screening for inborn errors of metabolism by electrospray ionization–tandem mass spectrometer: results, outcomes, and implications, *Pediatrics* 111(6):1399-1406, 2003.

Selva KA, Harper A, Downs A, and others: Neurodevelopmental outcomes in congenital hypothyroidism: comparison of dose and time to reach target T4 and TSH, *J Pediatr* 147:775-780, 2005.

Sgro M, Shah V, Campbell D: *Canadian Paediatric Surveillance Program: Challenge of early discharge: newborn assessment for jaundice*, 2005, retrieved June 28, 2007, from http://www.cps.ca/English/Surveillance/CPSP/Resources/NHS.htm.

Shaw N: Assessment and management of the hematologic system. In Kenner C, Lott J, editors: *Comprehensive neonatal nursing: a physiologic perspective*, ed 3, Philadelphia, 2003, Saunders.

Singer LT, Arendt R, Minnes S, and others: Cognitive and motor outcomes of cocaine-exposed infants, *JAMA* 287(15):1952-1960, 2002.

Singer LT, Minnes S, Short E, and others: Cognitive outcomes of preschool children with prenatal cocaine exposure, *JAMA* 291(20):2448-2456, 2004.

Smith L, Yonekura ML, Wallace T, and others: Effects of prenatal methamphetamine exposure on fetal growth and drug withdrawal symptoms in infants born at term, *J Devel Behav Pediatr* 24(1):17-23, 2003.

Steffensrud S: Hyperbilirubinemia in term and near-term infants: kernicterus on the rise? *Newborn Infant Nurs Rev* 4(4):191-202, 2004.

Stevens TP, Sinkin RA: Surfactant replacement therapy, *Chest* 131(5):1577-1582, 2007.

Stoll BJ, Hansen N, Fanaroff AA, and others: Late-onset sepsis in very low birth weight neonates: the experience of the NICHD Neonatal Research Network, *Pediatrics* 110(2 Pt 1):285-291, 2002.

Stoll BJ, Hansen NI, Higgins RD, and others: Very low birth weight preterm infants with early onset neonatal sepsis: the predominance of gram-negative infections continues in the National Institute of Child Health and Human Development Neonatal Research Network, 2002-2003, *Pediatr Infect Dis J* 24(7):635-639, 2005.

Stoll BJ: Metabolic disturbances. In Behrman R: *Nelson textbook of pediatrics*, ed 18, Philadelphia, 2007, Saunders.

Symington A, Pinelli J: Developmental care for promoting development and preventing morbidity in preterm infants (Cochrane Review). In *The Cochrane Library*, Issue 1, 2003, Oxford, Update Software.

Tappero E: Musculoskeletal system assessment. In Tappero E, Honeyfield MA: *Physical assessment of the newborn*, ed 3, Santa Rosa, Calif, 2003, NICU Ink.

Thayyil S, Marriott L: Can transcutaneous bilirubinometry reduce the need for serum bilirubin estimations in term and near term infants? *Arch Dis Child* 90(12):1311-1312, 2005.

Tronick EZ, Beeghly M: Prenatal cocaine exposure, child development, and the compromising effects of cumulative risk, *Clin Perinatol* 26(1):151-171, 1999.

Tyson JE, Kennedy KA: Trophic feedings for parenterally fed infants, *Cochrane Database Syst Rev* (3):CD000504, 2005.

Uchil D, Arulkumaran S: Neonatal subgaleal hemorrhage and its relationship to delivery by vacuum extraction, *Obstet Gynecol Surv* 58:687-693, 2003.

Uhing MR: Management of birth injuries, *Pediatr Clin North Am* 51(4):1169-1186, 2004.

Vento M, Saugstad O: Oxygen therapy. In Martin RJ, Fanaroff AA, Walsh MC, editors: *Fanaroff and Martin's neonatal-perinatal medicine: diseases of the fetus and infant*, ed 8, St Louis, 2006, Mosby.

Volante E, Moretti S, Pisani F, and others: Early diagnosis of bacterial infection in the neonate, *J Matern Fetal Med* 16(Suppl 2):13-16, 2004.

Volpe JJ: *Neurology of the newborn*, ed 4, Philadelphia, 2001, Saunders.

Wagner C, Katikaneni LD, Cox TH, and others: The impact of prenatal drug exposure on the neonate, *Obstet Gynecol Clin North Am* 25(1):169-194, 1998.

Walter JH, White FJ: Blood phenylalanine control in adolescents with phenylketonuria, *Int J Adolesc Med Health* 16(1):41-45, 2004.

Westrup B, Sizun J, Lagercrantz H: Family-centered developmental supportive care: a holistic and humane approach to reduce stress and pain in neonates, *J Perinatol* 27(Suppl 1):S12-S18, 2007.

Wheeler BJ: Kernicterus: ancient history or ongoing threat? *Mother Baby J* 5(2):21-30, 2000.

Witt C: Skin assessment. In Tappero EP, Honeyfield ME, editors: *Physical assessment of the newborn*, ed 3, Petaluma, Calif, 2003, NICU Ink.

Zahorodny W, Rom C, Whitney W, and others: The neonatal withdrawal inventory: a simplified score of newborn withdrawal, *Devel Behav Pediatr* 19(2):89-93, 1998.

Zlatunich CO, Packman S: Galactosaemia: early treatment with an elemental formula, *J Inherit Metab Dis* 28:163-168, 2005.

Health Promotion of the Infant and Family

DAVID WILSON

CHAPTER OUTLINE

PROMOTING OPTIMAL GROWTH AND DEVELOPMENT, 323
Biologic Development, 323
Proportional Changes, 323
Maturation of Systems, 323
Fine Motor Development, 325
Gross Motor Development, 325
Psychosocial Development: Developing a Sense of Trust (Erikson), 327
Cognitive Development: Sensorimotor Phase (Piaget), 327
Development of Body Image, 330
Social Development, 331
Attachment, 331
Language Development, 332
Play, 333
Temperament, 334
Childrearing Practices Related to Temperament, 335

Coping with Concerns Related to Normal Growth and Development, 335
Separation and Stranger Fear, 335
Alternate Child Care Arrangements, 335
Limit Setting and Discipline, 341
Thumb Sucking and Use of a Pacifier, 342
Teething, 342
Infant Shoes, 343
PROMOTING OPTIMAL HEALTH DURING INFANCY, 343
Nutrition, 343
The First 6 Months, 344
The Second 6 Months, 345
Selection and Preparation of Solid Foods, 345
Introduction of Solid Foods, 346
Weaning, 347
Sleep and Activity, 347
Sleep Problems, 347
Dental Health, 349

Immunizations, 350
Schedule for Immunizations, 350
Recommendations for Routine Immunizations, 351
Recommendations for Selected Immunizations, 359
Reactions, 359
Contraindications and Precautions, 359
Administration, 359
Injury Prevention, 365
Aspiration of Foreign Objects, 365
Suffocation, 368
Motor Vehicle Injuries, 369
Falls, 370
Poisoning, 370
Burns, 371
Drowning, 372
Bodily Damage, 372
Nurse's Role in Injury Prevention, 372
Anticipatory Guidance—Care of Families, 374

LEARNING OBJECTIVES

On completion of this chapter the reader will be able to:

- Identify the major biologic, psychosocial, cognitive, and social developments during the first year.
- Relate parent-child attachment, separation anxiety, and stranger fear to developmental achievements during infancy.

- Provide anticipatory guidance to parents regarding common parental concerns during infancy.
- Provide parents with feeding recommendations for infants.
- Outline immunization requirements during infancy.

- List general contraindications, precautions, and administration routes for childhood immunizations.
- Provide anticipatory guidance to parents regarding injury prevention based on the infant's developmental achievements.

PROMOTING OPTIMAL GROWTH AND DEVELOPMENT

BIOLOGIC DEVELOPMENT

At no other time in life are physical changes and developmental achievements as dramatic as during infancy. All major body systems undergo progressive maturation, and there is concurrent development of skills that increasingly allow infants to respond to and cope with the environment. Acquisition of these fine and gross motor skills occurs in an orderly head-to-toe and center-to-periphery (cephalocaudal-proximodistal) sequence.

Proportional Changes

During the first year, especially the initial 6 months, **growth** is very rapid. Infants gain 150 to 210 g (about 5 to 7 ounces) weekly until approximately age 5 to 6 months, when the birth weight has at least doubled. An average weight for a 6-month-old child is 7.3 kg (16 pounds). Weight gain slows during the second 6 months. By 1 year of age the infant's birth weight has tripled, for an average weight of 9.75 kg (21.5 pounds). Infants who are breast-fed beyond 4 to 6 months of age typically gain less weight than those who are bottle-fed, yet head circumference is more than adequate. Dewey (2001) attributes the decreased weight gain seen in breast-fed infants to self-regulation of energy intake. This self-regulation of intake with breastfeeding (vs formula feeding) is believed to have further significance in the development of childhood obesity and subsequent cardiovascular disease (Grummer-Strawn, Mei, and Centers for Disease Control and Prevention, 2004; Schack-Nielsen and Michaelsen, 2006).

Height increases by 2.5 cm (1 inch) a month during the first 6 months and also slows during the second 6 months. Increases in length occur in sudden spurts, rather than in a slow, gradual pattern. Average height is 65 cm (25.5 inches) at 6 months and 74 cm (29 inches) at 12 months. By 1 year the birth length has increased by almost 50%. This increase occurs mainly in the trunk, rather than in the legs and contributes to the characteristic physique of the infant.

Head growth is also rapid. During the first 6 months head circumference increases approximately 1.5 cm (0.6 inch) per month, but the rate of growth declines to only 0.5 cm (0.2 inch) monthly during the second 6 months. The average size is 43 cm (17 inches) at 6 months and 46 cm (18 inches) at 12 months. By 1 year, head size has increased by almost 33%. Closure of the cranial sutures occurs, with the posterior fontanel fusing by 6 to 8 weeks of age and the anterior fontanel closing by 12 to 18 months of age (average 14 months).

Expanding head size reflects the growth and differentiation of the **nervous system.** By the end of the first year the brain has increased in weight about two and one half times. Maturation of the brain is exhibited in the dramatic developmental achievements of infancy (see Table 10-2). Primitive reflexes are replaced by voluntary, purposeful movement, and new reflexes that influence motor development appear.

The **chest** assumes a more adult contour, with the lateral diameter becoming larger than the anteroposterior diameter. The chest circumference approximately equals the head circumference by the end of the first year. The **heart** grows less rapidly than does the rest of the body. Its weight is usually doubled by 1 year of age in comparison with body weight, which triples during the same period. The size of the heart is still large in relation to the chest cavity; its width is approximately 55% of the chest width.

Maturation of Systems

Other organ systems also change and grow during infancy. The **respiratory rate** slows somewhat (see inside back cover) and is relatively stable. Respiratory movements continue to be abdominal. Several factors predispose the infant to more severe and acute respiratory problems than older children. The close proximity of the trachea to the bronchi and its branching structures rapidly transmits an infectious agent from one anatomic location to another. The short, straight eustachian tube closely communicates with the ear, allowing infection to ascend from the pharynx to the middle ear. In addition, the inability of the immune system to produce **immunoglobulin**

A (**IgA**) in the mucosal lining provides less protection against infection in infancy than during later childhood.

The **heart rate** slows (see inside back cover), and the rhythm is often **sinus arrhythmia** (rate increases with inspiration and decreases with expiration). Blood pressure also changes during infancy (see inside back cover). Systolic pressure rises during the first 2 months as a result of the increasing ability of the left ventricle to pump blood into the systemic circulation. Diastolic pressure decreases during the first 3 months, then gradually rises to values close to those at birth. Fluctuations in blood pressure occur during varying states of activity and emotion.

Significant **hematopoietic changes** occur during the first year (see Appendix C). Fetal hemoglobin (HgbF) is present for the first 5 months, with adult hemoglobin steadily increasing through the first half of infancy. Fetal hemoglobin results in a shortened survival of red blood cells and thus a decreased number of red blood cells. A common result at 2 to 3 months of age is **physiologic anemia.** High levels of fetal hemoglobin are thought to depress the production of erythropoietin, a hormone released by the kidney that stimulates red blood cell production.

Maternally derived iron stores are present for the first 5 to 6 months and gradually diminish, which also accounts for lowered hemoglobin levels toward the end of the first 6 months. The occurrence of physiologic anemia is not affected by an adequate supply of iron. However, when erythropoiesis is stimulated, iron supplies are necessary for the formation of hemoglobin.

The **digestive processes** are relatively immature at birth. Although term newborn infants have some limitations in digestive function, studies indicate that human milk has properties that partially compensate for decreased digestive enzymatic activity, thus enabling the breast-fed infant to receive optimal nutrition during the first several months of life. Saliva is secreted in small amounts, but the majority of the digestive processes do not begin functioning until age 3 months, when drooling is common because of the poorly coordinated swallowing reflex. The enzyme **amylase** (also called **ptyalin**) is present in small amounts but usually has little effect on the foodstuffs because of the small amount of time the food stays in the mouth. Gastric digestion in the stomach consists primarily of the action of hydrochloric acid and rennin, an enzyme that acts specifically on the casein in milk to cause the formation of **curds**—coagulated semisolid particles of milk. The curds cause the milk to be retained in the stomach long enough for digestion to occur.

Digestion also takes place in the duodenum, where pancreatic enzymes and bile begin to break down protein and fat. Secretion of the pancreatic enzyme **amylase,** which is needed for digestion of complex carbohydrates, is deficient until about the fourth to sixth month of life. **Lipase** is also limited, and infants do not achieve adult levels of fat absorption until 4 to 5 months of age. **Trypsin** is secreted in sufficient quantities to catabolize protein into polypeptides and some amino acids.

The immaturity of the digestive processes is evident in the appearance of stools. During infancy, solid foods (e.g., peas, carrots, corn, raisins) are passed incompletely broken down in the feces. An excess quantity of fiber easily disposes the child to loose, bulky stools.

During infancy the stomach enlarges to accommodate a greater volume of food. By the end of the first year the infant is able to tolerate three meals a day and an evening bottle and may have one or two bowel movements daily. However, with any type of gastric irritation the infant is vulnerable to diarrhea, vomiting, and dehydration (see Chapter 24).

The **liver** is the most immature of all the gastrointestinal organs throughout infancy. The ability to conjugate bilirubin and secrete bile is achieved after the first couple of weeks of life. However, the capacities for gluconeogenesis, formation of plasma protein and ketones, storage of vitamins, and deamination of amino acids remain relatively immature for the first year of life.

Maturation of the suckling, sucking, and swallowing reflexes and the eruption of **teeth** (see Teething, p. 342) parallel the changes in the gastrointestinal tract and prepare the infant for the introduction of solid foods.

The **immunologic system** undergoes numerous changes during the first year. The full-term newborn receives significant amounts of maternal immunoglobulin G (IgG), which, for approximately 3 months, confers immunity against antigens to which the mother was exposed. During this time the infant begins to synthesize IgG; approximately 40% of adult levels are reached by 1 year of age. Significant amounts of immunoglobulin M (IgM) are produced at birth, and adult levels are reached by 9 months of age. Secretory IgA is not present at birth but is found in saliva and tears by 2 to 5 weeks. IgA is present in large amounts in colostrum; IgA confers protection to the mucous membranes of the gastrointestinal tract (Lawrence and Lawrence, 2005) against many bacteria, such as *Escherichia coli,* and viruses such as rubella, poliovirus, and the enteroviruses. The development of the mucosa-associated lymphoid tissue (MALT) occurs during infancy; in part this system is believed to prevent colonization and passage of bacteria across the infant's mucosal barrier (Lawrence and Lawrence, 2005). The function and quantity of T lymphocytes, lymphokines, interferon-γ, interleukins, tumor necrosis factor-α, and complement are reduced in early infancy, thus preventing optimal response to certain bacteria and viruses. The production of IgA and immunoglobulins D and E (IgD and IgE) is much more gradual, and maximum levels are not attained until early childhood.

There is evidence that **vernix caseosa,** a white oily substance that coats the term infant's body and is often found in abundance in creases of the axilla and groin, has innate immunologic properties that serve to protect the newborn from infection (Narendran and Hoath, 2006). The epidermis of the full-term infant undergoes maturation during the first month of life; the newborn's skin acts as a barrier to infection, assists in thermal regulation, and prevents transepidermal water loss in term infants.

During infancy, **thermoregulation** becomes more efficient; the ability of the skin to contract and of muscles to shiver in response to cold increases. The peripheral capillaries respond to changes in ambient temperature to regulate heat loss. The capillaries constrict in response to cold, conserving core body temperature and decreasing potential evaporative heat loss from the skin surface. The capillaries dilate in response to heat, decreasing internal body temperature through evaporation, conduction, and convection. Shivering (**thermogenesis**) causes the muscles and muscle fibers to contract, generating metabolic heat, which is distributed throughout the body. Increased adipose tissue during the first 6 months insulates the body against heat loss.

A shift in the **total body fluid** occurs; at birth 75% of the term infant's body weight is water, and there is an excess of extracellular fluid. As the percentage of body water decreases, so does the amount of extracellular fluid—from 40% at term to 20% in adulthood. The high proportion of extracellular fluid, which is composed of blood plasma, interstitial fluid, and lymph, predisposes the infant to a more rapid loss of total body fluid and, consequently, dehydration.

The immaturity of the **renal structures** also predisposes the infant to dehydration and electrolyte imbalance. Complete maturity of the kidney occurs during the latter half of the second year, when the cuboidal epithelium of the glomeruli becomes flattened. Before this time the filtration capacity of the glomeruli is reduced. Urine is voided frequently and has a low specific gravity (1.000 to 1.010).

Auditory acuity is at adult levels during infancy. Visual acuity begins to improve, and binocular fixation is established. **Binocularity,** or the fixation of two ocular images into one cerebral picture (**fusion),** begins to develop by 6 weeks of age and should be well established by age 4 months. **Depth perception (stereopsis)** begins to develop by age 7 to 9 months but may not be fully mature until 2 or 3 years of age, thus increasing the infant's and younger toddler's risk of falling.

Fine Motor Development

Fine motor behavior includes the use of the hands and fingers in the **prehension** (grasp) of an object. Grasping occurs during the first 2 to 3 months as a reflex and gradually becomes voluntary. At 1 month of age the hands are predominantly closed, and by 3 months they are mostly open. By this time infants demonstrate a desire to grasp an object, but they "grasp" it more with the eyes than with the hands. If a rattle is placed in the hand, the infant will actively hold onto it. By 4 months of age the infant regards both a small pellet and the hands and then looks from the object to the hands and back again. By 5 months the infant is able to voluntarily grasp an object.

By 6 months of age infants have increased manipulative skill. They hold their bottle, grasp their feet and pull them to their mouth, and feed themselves a cracker. By 7 months they transfer objects from one hand to the other, use one hand for grasping, and hold a cube in each hand simultaneously. They enjoy banging objects and will explore the movable parts of a toy.

Gradually the **palmar grasp** (using the whole hand) is replaced by a **pincer grasp** (using the thumb and index finger). By 8 to 10 months of age the infant uses a crude pincer grasp and by 11 months has progressed to a neat pincer grasp (Fig. 10-1). By 10 months of age the pincer grasp is sufficiently established to enable infants to pick up a raisin and other finger foods. They can deliberately let go of an object and will offer it to someone. By 11 months they put objects into a container and like to remove them. By age 1 year, infants try to build a tower of two blocks but fail.

Gross Motor Development

Head Control. The full-term newborn can momentarily hold the head in midline and parallel when the body is suspended ventrally and can lift and turn the head from side to

FIG. 10-1 ■ Crude pincer grasp at 8 to 10 months. (Photo by Paul Vincent Kuntz, Texas Children's Hospital, Houston.)

side when prone (see Fig. 8-7). This is not the case when the infant is lying prone on a pillow or soft surface; infants do not have the head control to lift their head out of the depression of the object and therefore risk suffocation in the prone position early in infancy (see Sudden Infant Death Syndrome, Chapter 11). Marked head lag is evident when the infant is pulled from a lying to a sitting position. By 3 months of age infants can hold their head well beyond the plane of the body. By 4 months of age infants can lift the head and front portion of the chest approximately 90 degrees above the table, bearing their weight on the forearms. Only slight head lag is evident when the infant is pulled from a lying to a sitting position, and by 4 to 6 months head control is well established (Figs. 10-2 and 10-3).

> **NURSINGALERT**
>
> Any child who displays head lag at 6 months of age should have a developmental and neurologic evaluation.

Rolling Over. Newborns may roll over accidentally because of their rounded back. The ability to willfully turn from the abdomen to the back occurs around 5 months, and the ability to turn from the back to the abdomen occurs at approximately 6 months. Infants put to sleep on their side may easily roll over to a prone (face-down) position, thus placing them at higher risk for sudden infant death syndrome (SIDS). It is therefore important to place infants in a supine position for sleep. While the infant is awake, a prone position is acceptable to enhance achievement of milestones such as head control, crawling, creeping, and turning over. It is noteworthy that the parachute reflex (Fig. 10-4), a protective response to falling, appears at approximately 7 months.

> **NURSINGALERT**
>
> In the first several months, before the infant can roll over, the head should be positioned on alternating sides to prevent positional plagiocephaly (when asleep or awake in the supine position) (see Chapter 11).

Sitting. The ability to sit follows progressive head control and straightening of the back (Fig. 10-5). For the first 2

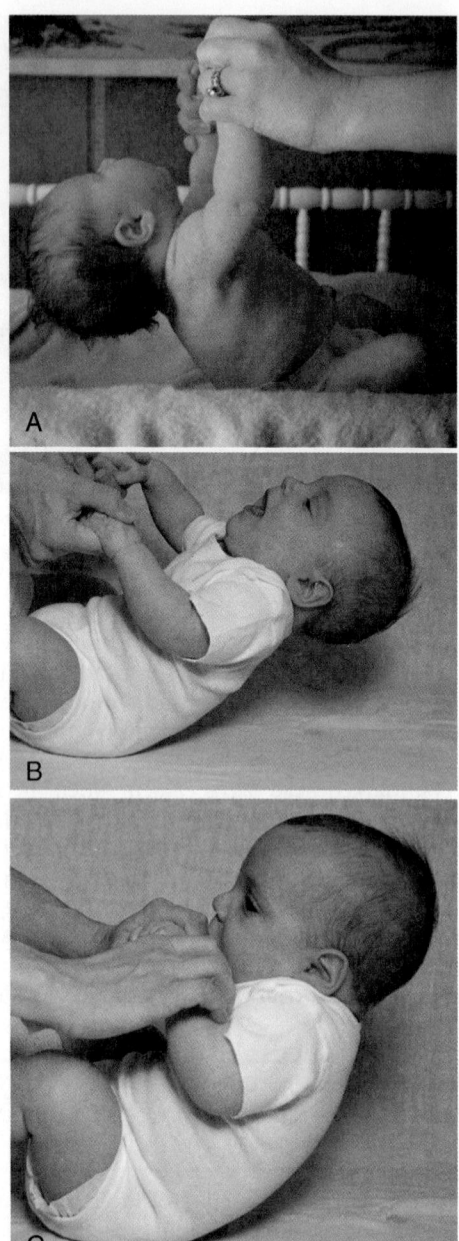

FIG. 10-2 ■ Head control while pulled to sitting position. A, Complete head lag at 1 month. B, Partial head lag at 2 months. C, Almost no head lag at 4 months.

FIG. 10-3 ■ Head control while prone. A, Infant momentarily lifts head at 1 month. B, Infant lifts head and chest 90 degrees and bears weight on forearms at 4 months. C, Infant lifts head, chest, and upper abdomen and can bear weight on hands at 6 months. Note how this position facilitates turning from abdomen to back.

to 3 months the back is uniformly rounded. The convex cervical curve forms at approximately 3 to 4 months of age, when head control is established. The convex lumbar curve appears when the child begins to sit, at about age 4 months. As the spinal column straightens, the infant can be propped in a sitting position. By age 7 months infants can sit alone, leaning forward on their hands for support. By age 8 months they can sit well while unsupported and begin to explore their surroundings in this position rather than in a lying position. By 10 months they can maneuver from a prone to a sitting position.

Locomotion. Locomotion involves acquiring the ability to bear weight, propel forward on all four extremities, stand upright with support, cruise by holding onto furniture, and finally, walk alone (Fig. 10-6). Following a cephalocaudal pattern, infants 4 to 6 months old have increasing coordination in their arms. Initial locomotion results in infants propelling themselves backward by pushing with the arms. By 6 to 7 months of age they are able to bear all their weight on their legs with assistance. **Crawling** (propelling forward with belly on floor) progresses to **creeping** on hands and knees (with belly off floor) by 9 months. At this time they stand while holding onto furniture and can pull themselves to the standing position, but they are unable to maneuver back down except by falling. By 11 months they walk while holding onto furniture or with both hands held, and by age 1 year they may

FIG. 10-4 ■ Parachute reflex. (Photo by Paul Vincent Kuntz, Texas Children's Hospital, Houston.)

be able to walk with one hand held. A number of infants attempt their first independent steps by their first birthday.

PSYCHOSOCIAL DEVELOPMENT: DEVELOPING A SENSE OF TRUST (ERIKSON)

Erikson's phase I (birth to 1 year) is concerned with **acquiring a sense of trust** while **overcoming a sense of mistrust.** The trust that develops is a trust of self, of others, and of the world. Infants "trust" that their feeding, comfort, stimulation, and caring needs will be met. The crucial element for the achievement of this task is the quality of both the parent (caregiver)–child relationship and the care the infant receives. The provision of food, warmth, and shelter by itself is inadequate for the development of a strong sense of self. The infant and parent must jointly learn to satisfactorily meet their needs for mutual regulation of frustration to occur. When this synchrony fails to develop, mistrust is the eventual outcome.

Failure to learn **delayed gratification** leads to mistrust. Mistrust can result from either too much or too little frustration. If parents always meet their children's needs before the children signal their readiness, infants will never learn to test their ability to control the environment. If the delay is prolonged, infants will experience constant frustration and eventually mistrust others in their efforts to satisfy them. Therefore consistency of care is essential.

The trust acquired in infancy provides the foundation for all succeeding phases. Trust allows infants a feeling of physical comfort and security, which assists them in experiencing unfamiliar, unknown situations with a minimum of fear. Erikson has divided the first year of life into two oral-social stages. During the first 3 to 4 months, food intake is the most important social activity in which the infant engages. The newborn can tolerate little frustration or delay of gratification. Primary **narcissism** (total concern for oneself) is at its height.

However, as bodily processes such as vision, motor movements, and vocalization become better controlled, infants use more advanced behaviors to interact with others. For example, rather than cry, infants may put their arms up to signify a desire to be held. The next social modality involves a mode of reaching out to others through **grasping.** Grasping is initially reflexive, but even as a reflex it has a powerful social meaning for the parents. The reciprocal response to the infant's grasping is the parents' holding on and touching. There is pleasurable tactile stimulation for both the child and the parents.

Tactile stimulation is extremely important in the total process of acquiring trust. The degree of mothering skill, the quantity of food, or the length of sucking does not determine the quality of the experience. Rather, it is the total nature of the quality of the interpersonal relationship that influences the infant's formulation of trust.

During the second stage the more active and aggressive modality of **biting** occurs. Infants learn that they can hold onto what is their own and can more fully control their environment. During this stage infants may be confronted with one of their first conflicts. If they are breastfeeding, they quickly learn that biting causes the mother to become upset and withdraw the breast. Yet biting also brings internal relief from teething discomfort and a sense of power or control.

This conflict may be solved in a variety of ways. The mother may wean the infant from the breast and begin bottle feeding, or the infant may learn to bite substitute nipples, such as a pacifier, and retain pleasurable breastfeeding. The successful resolution of this conflict strengthens the mother-child relationship because it occurs at a time when infants are recognizing the mother as the most significant person in their life.

COGNITIVE DEVELOPMENT: SENSORIMOTOR PHASE (PIAGET)

The theory most commonly used to explain **cognition,** or the ability to know, is that of Piaget. The period from birth to 24 months is termed the **sensorimotor phase** and is composed of six stages; however, because this discussion is concerned with ages birth to 12 months, only the first four stages are discussed. The last two stages occur during the toddler period of 12 to 24 months and are discussed in Chapter 12.

During the sensorimotor phase, infants progress from reflexive behaviors to simple repetitive acts to imitative activity. Three crucial events take place during this phase. The first event involves **separation,** in which infants learn to separate themselves from other objects in the environment. They realize that others besides themselves control the environment and that certain readjustments must take place for mutual satisfaction to occur. This coincides with Erikson's concept of the formation of trust.

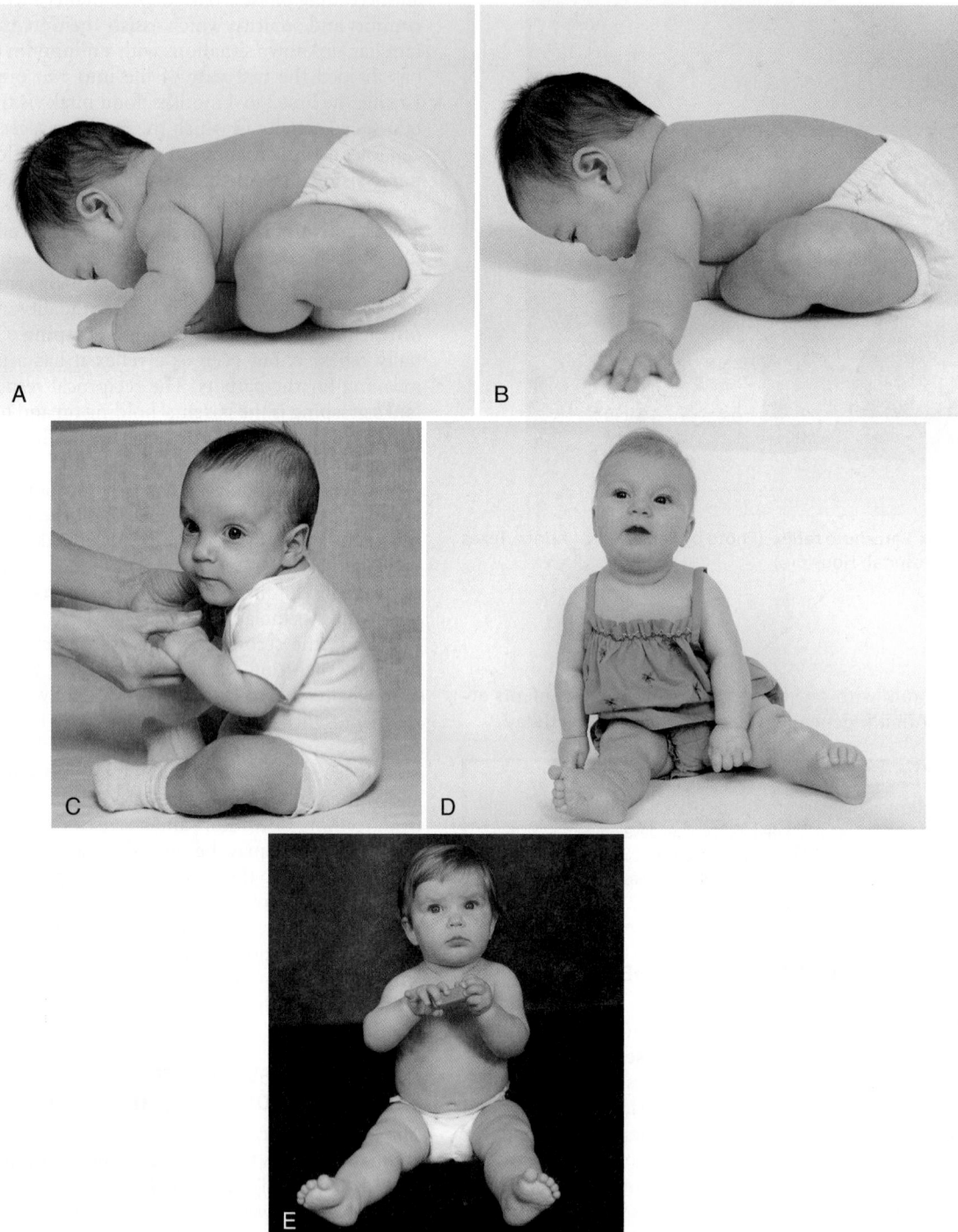

FIG. 10-5 ■ Development of sitting. **A,** Back is completely rounded, and infant has no ability to sit upright at 1 month. **B,** At 2 months, infant exhibits more control; back is still rounded, but infant can try to pull up with some head control. **C,** Back is rounded only in lumbar area, and infant is able to sit erect with good head control at 4 months. **D,** Infant can sit alone, leaning on hands for support, at 7 months. **E,** Infant sits without support at 8 months. Note the transferring of objects that occurs at 7 months. (**B, D,** and **E** photos by Paul Vincent Kuntz, Texas Children's Hospital, Houston.)

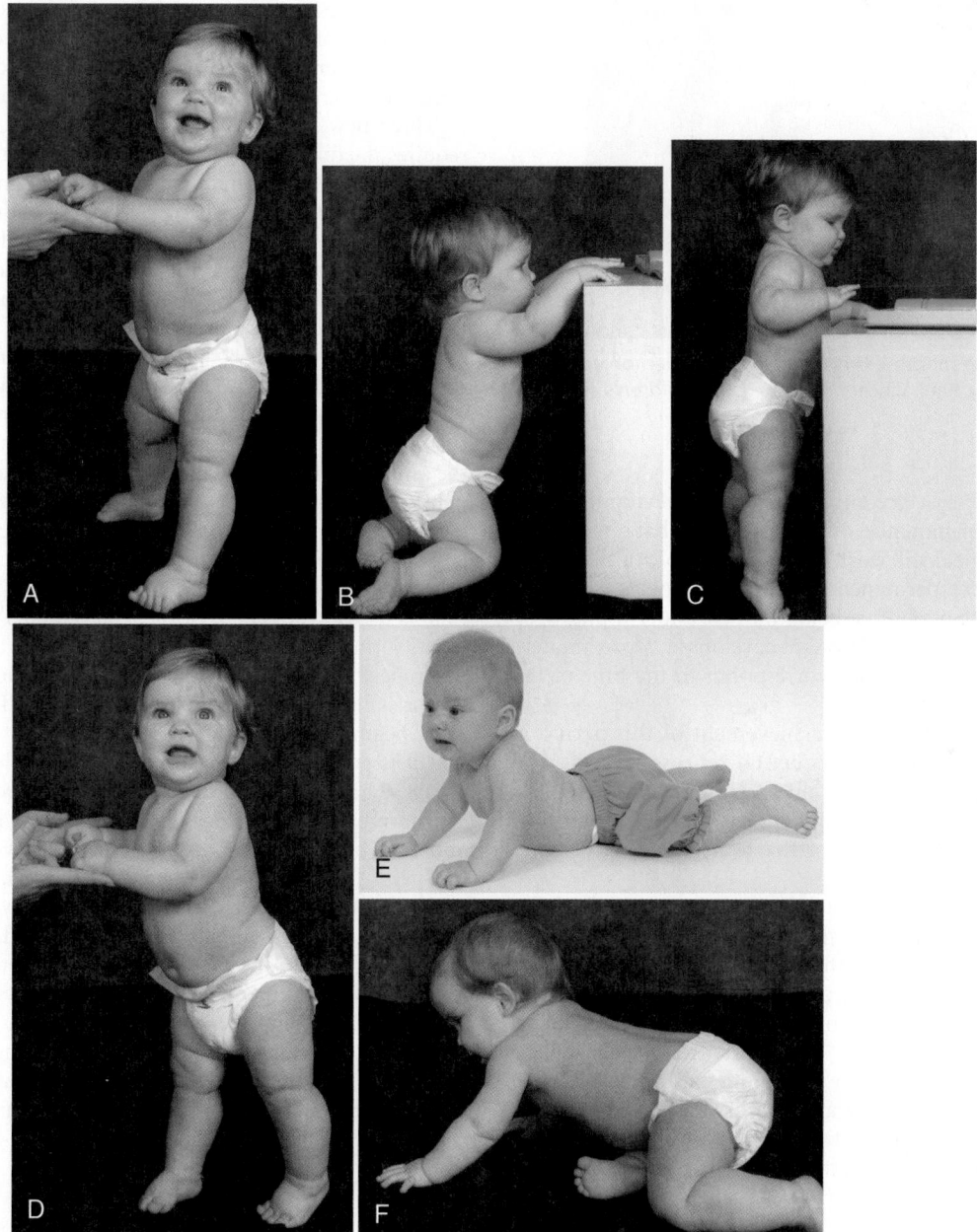

FIG. 10-6 ■ Development of locomotion. **A,** Infant bears full weight on feet by 7 months. **B,** Infant can maneuver from sitting to kneeling position. **C,** Infant can stand holding onto furniture at 9 months. **D,** While standing, infant takes deliberate step at 10 months. **E,** Infant crawls with abdomen on floor and pulls self forward at about 7 months, and then, **F,** creeps on hands and knees at 9 months. (Photos by Paul Vincent Kuntz, Texas Children's Hospital, Houston.)

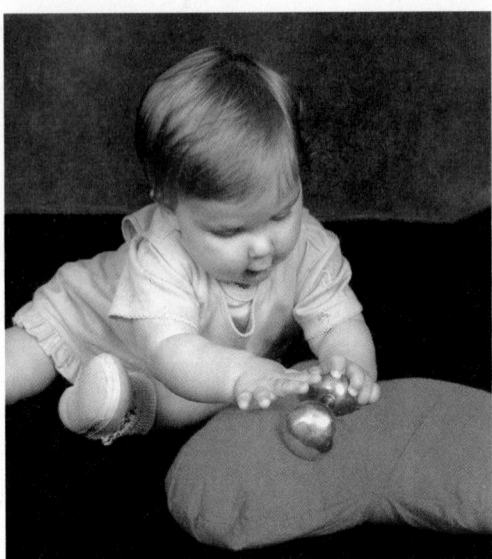

FIG. 10-7 ■ Nine-month-old is able to find hidden object under pillow. (Photo by Paul Vincent Kuntz, Texas Children's Hospital, Houston.)

The second major accomplishment is achieving the concept of **object permanence,** or the realization that objects that leave the visual field still exist. A typical example of the development of object permanence is when infants are able to pursue objects they observe being hidden under a pillow or behind a chair (Fig. 10-7). This skill develops at approximately 9 to 10 months of age, which corresponds to the time of increased locomotion skills.

The last major intellectual achievement of this period is the ability to use **symbols,** or **mental representation.** The use of symbols allows the infant to think of an object or situation without actually experiencing it. The recognition of symbols is the beginning of the understanding of time and space.

The first stage, from birth to 1 month, is identified by the infant's **use of reflexes.** At birth the infant's individuality and temperament are expressed through the physiologic reflexes of sucking, rooting, grasping, and crying. The repetitious nature of the reflexes is the beginning of associations between an act and a sequential response. When infants cry because they are hungry, a nipple is put in the mouth, and they suck, feel satisfaction, and sleep. They are assimilating this experience while perceiving auditory, tactile, and visual cues. This experience of perceiving certain patterns, or "ordering," provides a foundation for the subsequent stages.

The second stage, **primary circular reactions,** marks the beginning of the replacement of reflexive behavior with voluntary acts. During the period from 1 to 4 months, activities such as sucking or grasping become deliberate acts that elicit certain responses. The beginning of accommodation is evident. Infants incorporate and adapt their reactions to the environment and recognize the stimulus that produced a response. Previously they would cry until the nipple was brought to the mouth. Now they associate the nipple with the sound of the parent's voice. They accommodate this new piece of information and adapt by ceasing to cry when they hear the voice—before receiving the nipple. What is taking place is realization of causality and recognition of an orderly sequence of events. The environment is taken in with all of the senses and with whatever motor ability is present.

The **secondary circular reactions** stage is a continuation of primary circular reactions and lasts until 8 months of age. In this stage the primary circular reactions are repeated and prolonged for the response that results. Grasping and holding now become shaking, banging, and pulling. Shaking is performed to hear a noise, not solely for the pleasure of shaking. The quality and quantity of an act become evident. "More" or "less" shaking produces different responses. Causality, time, deliberate intention, and separateness from the environment begin to develop.

Three new processes of human behavior occur. **Imitation** requires the differentiation of selected acts from several events. By the second half of the first year, infants can imitate sounds and simple gestures. **Play** becomes evident as they take pleasure in performing an act after they have mastered it. Much of infants' waking hours are absorbed in sensorimotor play. **Affect** (outward manifestation of emotion and feeling) is seen as infants begin to develop a sense of permanence. During the first 6 months infants believe that an object exists only for as long as they can visually perceive it. In other words: out of sight, out of mind. Affect to external objects is evident when the object continues to be present or remembered even though it is beyond the range of perception. Object permanence is a critical component of parent-child attachment and is seen in the development of stranger anxiety at 6 to 8 months of age (see p. 332).

During the fourth sensorimotor stage, **coordination of secondary schemas and their application to new situations,** infants use previous behavioral achievements primarily as the foundation for adding new intellectual skills to their expanding repertoire. This stage is largely transitional. Increasing motor skills allow for greater exploration of the environment. They begin to discover that hiding an object does not mean that it is gone, but that removing an obstacle will reveal the object. This marks the beginning of intellectual reasoning. Furthermore, they can experience an event by observing it, and they begin to associate symbols with events (e.g., "bye-bye" with "Mommy or Daddy goes to work"), but the classification is purely their own. In this stage they learn from the object itself; this is in contrast to the second stage, in which infants learn from the type of interaction between objects or individuals. Intentionality is further developed in that infants now actively attempt to remove a barrier to the desired (or undesired) action (see Fig. 10-7). If something is in their way, they attempt to climb over it or push it away. Previously an obstacle would cause them to give up any further attempt to achieve the desired goal.

DEVELOPMENT OF BODY IMAGE

The development of body image parallels sensorimotor development. Infants' kinesthetic and tactile experiences are the first perceptions of their body, and the mouth is the principal area of pleasurable sensations. Other parts of the body are primarily objects of pleasure—the hands and fingers to suck and the feet to play with. As physical needs are met, they feel comfort and satisfaction with their body. Messages conveyed by the caregivers reinforce these feelings. For example, when infants smile, they receive emotional satisfaction from others who smile back.

Achieving the concept of object permanence is basic to the development of self-image. By the end of the first year infants recognize that they are distinct from their parents. At the same

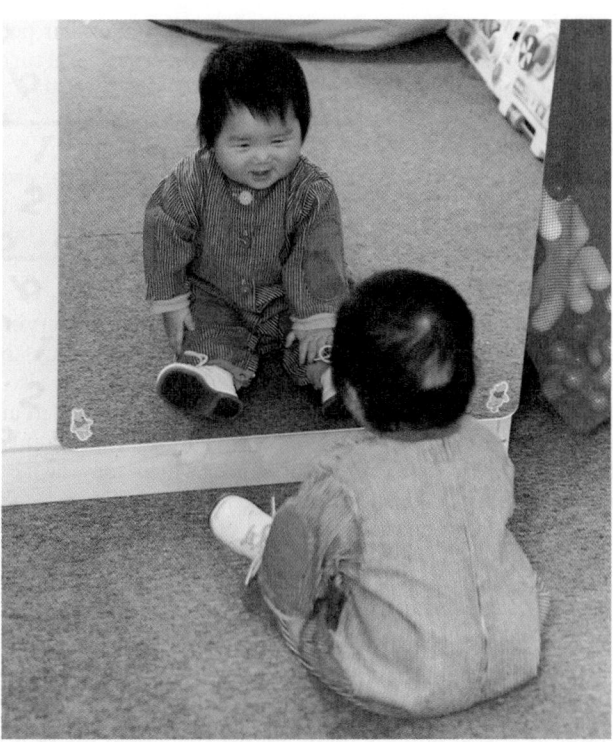

FIG. 10-8 ■ Nine-month-old infant enjoying own image in mirror.

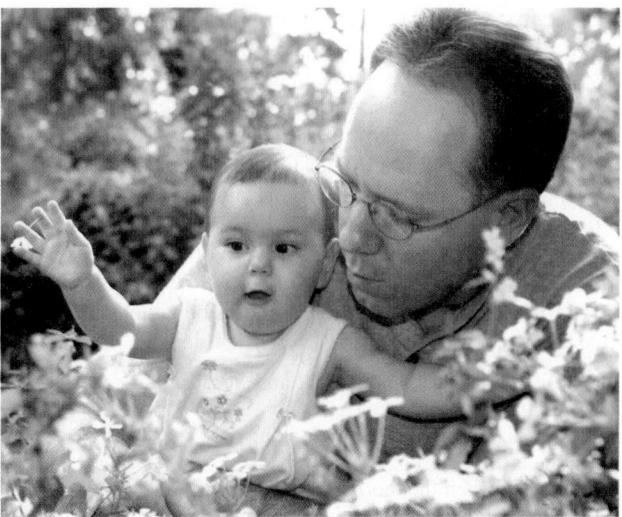

FIG. 10-9 ■ Infancy is an important time for attachment to significant others. (Photo by Paul Vincent Kuntz, Texas Children's Hospital, Houston.)

time, they have increasing interest in their image, especially in the mirror (Fig. 10-8). As motor skills develop, they learn that parts of the body are useful; for example, the hands bring objects to the mouth, and the legs help them move to different locations. All these achievements transmit messages to them about themselves. Therefore it is important to transmit positive messages to infants about their bodies.

SOCIAL DEVELOPMENT

Infants' social development is initially influenced by their reflexive behavior, such as the grasp, and eventually depends primarily on the interaction between them and the principal caregivers. **Attachment** to the parent is increasingly evident during the second half of the first year. In addition, tremendous strides are made in communication and personal-social behavior. Whereas crying and reflexive behavior are methods to meet one's needs in the neonatal period, the social smile is an early step in social communication. This has a profound effect on family members and is a tremendous stimulus for evoking continued responses from others. By 4 months infants laugh aloud.

Play is a major socializing agent and provides stimulation needed to learn from and interact with the environment. By age 6 months infants are very personable. They play games such as peek-a-boo when their head is hidden in a towel, they signal their desire to be picked up by extending their arms, and they show displeasure when a toy is removed or their face is washed.

Attachment

The importance of human physical contact to infants cannot be overemphasized. Parenting is not an instinctual ability but a learned, acquired process. The attachment of parent and child, which often begins before birth and assumes even more importance at birth (see Chapter 8), continues during the first year (Fig. 10-9). In the following discussion of attachment, the term *mother* is used in the broad context of the consistent caregiver with whom the child relates more than anyone else. However, with society's changing social climate and sex-role stereotypes, this person may well be the father or a grandparent. Studies on paternal-infant attachment demonstrate that stages similar to maternal attachment occur and that fathers are more involved in child care when mothers are employed (although mothers continue to do the majority of infant care). Additional research has shown that inexperienced, first-time fathers are as capable as experienced fathers of developing a close attachment with their infants. Studies of fathers of high-risk infants demonstrate that fathers experience feelings of love and affection toward their offspring during the newborn period; fathers in one study verbalized more positive feelings of love and affection toward the newborn when they were able to have close physical contact such as holding the child (Sullivan, 1999). Children who had insecure attachment to their teenage mothers were found to have a strong attachment to the grandmother who was also a primary caretaker (Patterson, 1997). With many single-parent families in existence, a grandmother (or other significant caretaker) may become the primary caretaker. It is important for nurses to recognize that infant-parent attachments may be present or absent in situations wherein caretaker roles are less well defined by those involved.

Attachment progresses during infancy, with the child assuming an increasingly significant role. Two components of cognitive development are required for attachment: (1) the ability to discriminate the mother from other individuals, and (2) the achievement of object permanence. Both these processes prepare the infant for an equally important aspect of attachment: separation from the parent. **Separation-individuation** should occur as a harmonious, parallel process with emotional attachment.

During the formation of attachment to the parent, the infant progresses through four distinct but overlapping stages.

For the first few weeks infants respond indiscriminately to anyone. Beginning at approximately 8 to 12 weeks of age, they cry, smile, and vocalize more to the mother than to anyone else but continue to respond to others, whether familiar or not. At approximately 6 months of age, infants show a distinct preference for the mother. They follow her more, cry when she leaves, enjoy playing with her more, and feel most secure in her arms. About 1 month after showing attachment to the mother, many infants begin attaching to other members of the family, most often the father.

Infants acquire other developmental behaviors that influence the attachment process. These include:

■ Differential crying, smiling, and vocalization (more to the mother than to anyone else)
■ Visual-motor orientation (looking more at the mother, even if she is not close)
■ Crying when the mother leaves the room
■ Approaching through locomotion (crawling, creeping, or walking)
■ Clinging (especially in the presence of a stranger)
■ Exploring away from the mother while using her as a secure base

Reactive attachment disorder (RAD) is a psychologic and developmental problem that stems from maladaptive or absent attachment between the infant and parent and may persist into childhood and even adulthood (Wilson, 2001; Zeanah and Fox, 2004). Two different patterns of RAD have emerged: the emotionally withdrawn–inhibited pattern and an indiscriminate-disinhibited pattern (Zeanah and Fox, 2004). Signs of RAD are usually seen before the age of 5 years in infants who had insecure attachments to the mother or other primary caretaker (American Psychiatric Association, 2002). The child may manifest behaviors such as not being cuddly with parents, failing to make eye contact with significant others, having poor impulse control, and being destructive to self and others. Maltreated and orphaned children often are diagnosed with this complex disorder. Without early intervention, some of these children fail to develop a conscience and suffer from an antisocial personality disorder that may lead to criminal acts.

Separation Anxiety. Between ages 4 and 8 months the infant progresses through the first stage of separation-individuation and begins to have some awareness of self and mother as separate beings. At the same time, object permanence is developing, and the infant is aware that the parent can be absent. Therefore separation anxiety develops and is manifested through a predictable sequence of behaviors.

During the early second half of the first year, infants protest when placed in their crib, and a short time later they object when the mother leaves the room. Infants may not notice the mother's absence if they are absorbed in an activity. However, when they realize her absence, they protest. From this point on, they become alert to her activities and whereabouts. By 11 to 12 months they are able to anticipate her imminent departure by watching her behaviors, and they begin to protest *before* she leaves. At this point many parents learn to postpone alerting the child to their departure until just before leaving.

Stranger Fear. As infants demonstrate attachment to one person, they correspondingly exhibit less friendliness to others. Between ages 6 and 8 months, fear of strangers and stranger anxiety become prominent and are related to infants' ability to discriminate between familiar and unfamiliar people. Behaviors such as clinging to the parent, crying, and turning away from the stranger are common.

> **NURSING ALERT**
>
> Be alert to parents' reports about maternal postpartum depression and infant crying, since these concerns may indicate a stressed mother-infant relationship.

Language Development

The infant's first means of verbal communication is crying. Crying as a biologic sign conveys a message of urgency and signals displeasure, such as hunger. However, crying is also a social event that affects the development of the parent-infant relationship—either by its absence, which usually has a positive effect on parents, or its presence, which may evoke a negative response or persuade parents to minister to the child's physical or emotional needs.

In the first few weeks of life, crying has a reflexive quality and is mostly related to physiologic needs. Infants cry for 1 to 1½ hours a day up to 3 weeks of age and then build up to 2, and even 4, hours by 6 weeks. Crying tends to decrease by 12 weeks. It is thought that the increase in crying for no apparent reason during the first few months may be related to the discharge of energy and the maturational changes in the central nervous system. At the end of the first year, infants cry for attention, from fear (especially stranger fear), and from frustration, usually in response to their developing but inadequate motor skills.

Vocalizations heard during crying eventually become syllables and words (e.g., the "mama" heard during vigorous crying). Infants vocalize as early as 5 to 6 weeks of age by making small throaty sounds. By 2 months they make single vowel sounds such as *ah, eh,* and *uh.* By 3 to 4 months the consonants *n, k, g, p,* and *b* are added, and the infants coo, gurgle, and laugh aloud. By 8 months they imitate sounds, add the consonants *t, d,* and *w,* and combine syllables (e.g., "dada"), but they do not ascribe meaning to the word until 10 to 11 months of age (see Family Focus box). By 9 to 10 months they comprehend the meaning of the word "no" and obey simple commands. By age 1 year they can say three to five words with meaning. Because language development is based on expressive skills (ability to make thoughts, ideas, and desires known to others) and receptive skills (ability to understand the words being spoken), it is important that infants are exposed to expressive speech and that infants with delays in achieving milestones are carefully evaluated for potential hearing loss. (See Universal Newborn Hearing Screening, Chapter 8.)

> **FAMILY FOCUS**
>
> ### Child's Developing Language Skills
>
> During the acquisition of new language skills the child temporarily may stop using other recently learned sounds or words. This is often distressing for parents, who have waited in anticipation for the words "dada" or "mama," because these sounds are commonly replaced by other vocalizations and may not be repeated for several weeks. Nurses can reassure parents that the child will again say these special words, and with increased meaning.

Play

Play during infancy represents the various social modalities observed during cognitive development. The activity of infants is primarily narcissistic and revolves around their own body. As discussed under Development of Body Image (p. 330), body parts are primarily objects of play and pleasure.

During the first year, play becomes more sophisticated and interdependent. From birth to 3 months, infants' responses to the environment are global and largely undifferentiated. Play is dependent; pleasure is demonstrated by a quieting attitude (1 month), a smile (2 months), or a squeal (3 months). From 3 to 6 months, infants show more discriminate interest in stimuli and begin to play alone with a rattle or a soft stuffed toy or with someone else. There is much more interaction during play. By 4 months of age they laugh aloud, show preference for certain toys, and become excited when food or a favorite object is brought to them. They recognize an image in a mirror, smile at it, and vocalize to it.

By 6 months to 1 year, play involves sensorimotor skills. Actual games such as peek-a-boo and pat-a-cake are played. Verbal repetition and imitation of simple gestures occur in response to demonstration. Play is much more selective, not only in terms of specific toys, but also in terms of "playmates." Although play is solitary or one sided, infants choose with whom they will interact. At 6 to 8 months they usually refuse to play with strangers. Parents are definite favorites, and infants know how to attract their attention. At 6 months they extend the arms to be picked up, at 7 months cough to make their presence known, at 10 months pull the parent's clothing, and at 12 months call them by name. This represents a tremendous advance from the newborn who signaled biologic needs by crying to express displeasure.

Stimulation is as important for psychosocial growth as food is for physical growth. Knowledge of developmental milestones allows nurses to guide parents regarding proper play for infants. It is not sufficient to place a mobile over a crib and toys in a playpen for a child's optimum social, emotional, and intellectual development. Play must provide interpersonal contact and recreational and educational stimulation. Infants need to be *played with,* not merely *allowed to play.* Although the type of play infants engage in is called **solitary,** this is a figurative, not literal, term to denote one-sided play. The type of toys given to the child is much less important than the quality of personal interaction that occurs.

Table 10-1 lists play activities appropriate for the developmental level of the infant in view of motor, language, and personal-social achievements. Although the activities are grouped according to the major mode of stimulation provided, there is overlap in many instances. In addition, play activities suggested for one age-group may be appropriate for older infants but inappropriate for younger infants.

TABLE 10-1			
Play During Infancy			
VISUAL STIMULATION	**AUDITORY STIMULATION**	**TACTILE STIMULATION**	**KINETIC STIMULATION**
SUGGESTED ACTIVITIES **Birth–1 Month** Look at infant at close range. Hang bright, shiny object within 20-25 cm (8-10 inches) of infant's face and in midline. Hang mobiles with black-and-white designs.	Talk to infant; sing in soft voice. Play music box, tape, or compact disc. Have ticking clock or metronome nearby.	Hold, caress, cuddle. Keep infant warm. May like to be swaddled.	Rock infant; place in cradle.
Age 2-3 Months Provide bright objects. Make room bright with pictures or mirrors. Take infant to various rooms while doing chores. Place infant in infant seat for vertical view of environment (use a safe surface).	Talk to infant. Include in family gatherings. Expose to various environmental noises other than those of home. Use rattles, wind chimes.	Caress infant while bathing, at diaper change. Comb hair with a soft brush. Give massage.	Use stroller for walks. Use infant swing. Take in car for rides. Exercise body by moving extremities in swimming motion. Use cradle gym.
Age 4-6 Months Place infant in front of unbreakable mirror. Give brightly colored toys to hold (small enough to grasp).	Talk to infant; repeat sounds infant makes. Laugh when infant laughs. Call infant by name. Place rattle or bell in hand.	Give infant soft squeeze toys of various textures. Allow to splash in bath. Place nude on soft, furry rug and move extremities.	Use swing or stroller. Bounce infant in lap while holding in standing position. Support infant in sitting position; let infant lean forward to balance self. Place infant on floor to crawl, roll over, sit.

Continued

TABLE 10-1
Play During Infancy—cont'd

VISUAL STIMULATION	AUDITORY STIMULATION	TACTILE STIMULATION	KINETIC STIMULATION
SUGGESTED ACTIVITIES—cont'd **Age 6-9 Months**			
Give infant large toys with bright colors, movable parts, and noisemakers. Play peek-a-boo, especially hiding face in a towel. Make funny faces to encourage imitation. Give ball of yarn or string to pull apart.	Call infant by name. Repeat simple words such as "dada," "mama," "bye-bye." Speak clearly. Name parts of body, people, and foods. Tell infant what you are doing. Use "no" only when necessary. Give simple commands. Show how to clap hands, bang a drum.	Let infant play with fabrics of various textures. Have bowl with foods of different sizes and textures to feel. Let infant "catch" running water. Encourage "swimming" in large bathtub or shallow pool. Give wad of sticky tape to manipulate.	Hold upright to bear weight and bounce. Pick up, say "up." Put down, say "down." Place toys out of reach; encourage infant to get them. Play pat-a-cake.
Age 9-12 Months			
Show infant large pictures in books. Take infant to places where there are animals, many people, different objects (e.g., shopping center). Play ball by rolling it to child, demonstrate "throwing" it back. Demonstrate building a two-block tower.	Read infant simple nursery rhymes. Point to body parts and name each one. Imitate sounds of animals.	Give infant finger foods of different textures. Let infant mess and squash food. Let infant feel cold (ice cube) or warm objects; say what temperature each is. Let infant feel a breeze (fan blowing).	Give large push-pull toys. Place furniture in a circle to encourage cruising.
SUGGESTED TOYS **Birth–6 Months**			
Nursery mobiles Unbreakable mirrors See-through crib bumpers Contrasting colored sheets	Music boxes Musical mobiles Crib dangle bells Small-handled clear rattle	Stuffed animals Soft clothes Soft or furry quilt Soft mobiles	Rocking crib or cradle Infant swing
Age 6-12 Months			
Various colored blocks Nested boxes or cups Books with rhymes and bright pictures Strings of big beads Simple take-apart toys Large ball Cup and spoon Large puzzles Jack-in-the-box	Rattles of different sizes, shapes, tones, and bright colors Squeaky animals and dolls Records with light, rhythmic music	Soft, different-texture animals and dolls Sponge toys, floating toys Squeeze toys Teething toys Books with textures or objects, such as fur and zipper	Activity box for crib Push-pull toys Wind-up swing

TEMPERAMENT

The infant's temperament or behavioral style influences the type of interaction that occurs between the child and parents, especially the mother, and other family members (see Temperament, Chapter 5). In assessing a child's temperament, it is the parents' perception of the child and the degree of fit between their expectations and the child's actual temperament that are important. The more dissonance, or lack of harmony, between the child's temperament and the parent's ability to accept and deal with the behavior, the more risk for subsequent parent-child conflicts.

Although most behavioral researchers agree there is a strong biologic component to temperament, researchers also suggest that temperament may be modified by the environment, particularly the family (Wilson, White, Cobb, and others, 2000). Family interaction with the infant is perceived as a circular process wherein each family member affects the others and the family as a unit. With these concepts in mind, the nurse has an important role in helping the family understand the infant's temperament as it relates to family dynamics and the eventual well-being of the child and family unit (Wilson, White, Cobb, and others, 2000).

The **Revised Infant Temperament Questionnaire (RITQ)** can be used as a screening tool with parents (Carey and McDevitt, 1978). The questionnaire focuses on nine temperament variables, but the 95 questions relate specifically to activities such as sleep, feeding, play, diapering, and dressing. The scores from the RITQ help identify the child's temperamental style. Use of the RITQ is well accepted by parents and should be accompanied by an adequate explanation of the results. In discussing the results, it is best to avoid descriptors such as "difficult"; instead, infants can be described in terms of characteristics such as "intense" or "less predictable." The Early Infancy Temperament Questionnaire is a 76-item parent questionnaire that was adapted from the RITQ to specifically evaluate temperament characteristics of infants 1 to 4 months old, whereas the RITQ is best suited for infants 4 months old and older (Medoff-Cooper, Carey, and McDevitt, 1993).

With knowledge of the infant's temperament, nurses are better able to (1) provide parents with background information that will help them see their child in a better perspective, (2) offer a more organized picture of their child's behavior and possibly reveal distortions in their perceptions of the behavior, and (3) guide parents regarding appropriate childrearing techniques.

Childrearing Practices Related to Temperament

Most parents realize that their infant is born with unique characteristics, and few parents of difficult infants need to be told of the challenge of caring for them. However, few parents are aware of the significance of the temperamental characteristics and of constructive approaches to dealing with them. The following are examples of interventions that promote more positive parenting of infants with different temperament styles.*

"Difficult" children may respond better to scheduled feedings and structured caregiving routines than to demand feedings and frequent changes in daily routines. These children sleep less and may need more structured approaches to bedtime to prevent bedtime problems. "Highly distractible" children may require additional soothing measures such as swinging, rocking, or being carried in a pack that the parent wears across the chest or back. Children with "high activity" levels require vigilant watching, and parents need to take extra precautions in safeguarding the home. These children benefit from increased opportunities for gross motor activity to constructively channel their energy.

The child who is "slow to warm up" may demonstrate more stranger fear than other children and may require gradual and frequent preparation for new situations, such as substitute child care. Even the "easy child" can present problems in that the parents may need reminders to feed the child who sleeps for prolonged intervals and rarely cries. They may need to "retrain" the child because of the ease of developing habits such as keeping the child up late or sleeping with the youngster, which may later become troublesome.

Appropriate counseling based on awareness of the child's temperament can greatly enhance the quality of interaction between parents and infant. Even just letting parents know that "difficult" traits are innate can relieve feelings of guilt and incompetence.

Because of the complexity of the developmental process during the first 12 months, Table 10-2 is presented to help

organize and clarify the data already discussed. Although all milestones are important, some represent essential integrative aspects of development that lay the foundation for achievement of more advanced skills. These essential milestones are designated by a square (■) in the table. The table represents the average monthly age at which various skills are attained. It must be remembered that, although the sequence is the same, the rate will vary among children.

COPING WITH CONCERNS RELATED TO NORMAL GROWTH AND DEVELOPMENT
Separation and Stranger Fear

A number of fears can appear during infancy. However, the fear that causes parents the most concern is fear related to strangers and separation. Although erroneously interpreted by some as a sign of undesirable, antisocial behavior, stranger fear and separation anxiety are important components of a strong, healthy parent-child attachment. Nevertheless, this period can present difficulties for the parent and child. Parents may be more confined to the home because the infant violently protests having baby-sitters. To accustom the infant to new people, parents are encouraged to have close friends or relatives visit often. This provides other persons with whom the child is comfortable and can give parents time for themselves.

Infants also need opportunities to safely experience strangers. Usually toward the end of the first year, infants begin to venture away from the parent and demonstrate curiosity about strangers. If allowed to explore at their own rate, many infants eventually "warm up." If parents hold the child away from their face, the infant can observe while maintaining close physical contact.

The best approach for the stranger (including nurses) is to talk softly; meet the child at eye level (to appear smaller); maintain a safe distance from the infant; and avoid sudden, intrusive gestures, such as holding the arms out and smiling broadly.

Parents also may wonder whether they should encourage the child's clinging, dependent behavior, especially if there is pressure from others who view this as "spoiling" (see following discussion). Parents need to be reassured that such behavior is healthy, desirable, and necessary for the child's optimal emotional development. If parents can reassure the infant of their presence, the infant will learn to realize that they are still there even if not physically present. Talking to infants when leaving the room, allowing them to hear one's voice on the telephone, and using transitional objects (e.g., a favorite blanket or toy) reassures them of the parent's continued presence.

Alternate Child Care Arrangements

For many parents, especially working mothers, locating safe and competent child care facilities for the infant is an increasingly difficult problem—one that is compounded by the number of mothers working outside the home. Over the past 40 years there have been variable shifts in child care arrangements; whereas the majority of children are cared for in group centers or other settings, there are increasingly more children being cared for in home settings.

The basic types of care are in-home care, either in the parents' or caregivers' home (family daycare), and center-based care, usually in a daycare center. **In-home care** may consist of a full-time baby-sitter who lives in the home, a full-time baby-sitter who comes to the home, cooperative arrangements such

---

*Recommended resources for parents are Turecki SK, Tonner L: *The difficult child,* New York, 2000, Bantam Books; and Chess S, Thomas A: *Know your child: an authoritative guide for today's parents,* Lanham, MD, 1996, Jason Aronson.

Text continued on p. 340

TABLE 10-2
Growth and Development During Infancy

PHYSICAL	GROSS MOTOR	FINE MOTOR
AGE 1 MONTH Weight gain of 150-210 g (5-7 ounces) weekly for first 6 months Height gain of 2.5 cm (1 inch) monthly for first 6 months Head circumference increases by 1.5 cm (0.5 inch) monthly for first 6 months Primitive reflexes present and strong Doll's eye reflex and dance reflex fading Obligatory nose breathing (most infants)	■ Assumes flexed position with pelvis high but knees not under abdomen when prone (at birth, knees flexed under abdomen) ■ Can turn head from side to side when prone; lifts head momentarily from bed (see Fig. 10-3, A) Has marked head lag, especially when pulled from lying to sitting position (see Fig. 10-2, A) Holds head momentarily parallel and in midline when suspended in prone position Assumes asymmetric tonic neck flex position when supine When held in standing position, body is limp at knees and hips In sitting position, back is uniformly rounded, with absence of head control	Hands predominantly closed Grasp reflex strong Hand clenches on contact with rattle
AGE 2 MONTHS Posterior fontanel closed Crawling reflex disappears	■ Assumes less flexed position when prone—hips flat, legs extended, arms flexed, head to side Less head lag when pulled to sitting position (see Fig. 10-2, B) Can maintain head in same plane as rest of body when held in ventral suspension When prone, can lift head almost 45 degrees off table When moved to sitting position, head is held up but bends forward (see Fig. 10-5, B) Assumes symmetric tonic neck position intermittently	Hands often open Grasp reflex fading
AGE 3 MONTHS Primitive reflexes fading	Able to hold head more erect when sitting, but still bobs forward Has only slight head lag when pulled to sitting position Assumes symmetric body positioning Able to raise head and shoulders from prone position to a 45- to 90-degree angle from table; bears weight on forearms When held in standing position, able to bear slight fraction of weight on legs Regards own hand	■ Actively holds rattle but will not reach for it Grasp reflex absent Hands kept loosely open Clutches own hand; pulls at blankets and clothes
AGE 4 MONTHS Drooling begins Moro, tonic neck, and rooting reflexes have disappeared	■ Has almost no head lag when pulled to sitting position (see Fig. 10-2, C) ■ Balances head well in sitting position (see Fig. 10-5, C) Back less rounded, curved only in lumbar area Able to sit erect if propped up Able to raise head and chest off surface to angle of 90 degrees (see Fig. 10-3, B) Assumes predominant symmetric position ■ Rolls from back to side	■ Inspects and plays with hands; pulls clothing or blanket over face in play Tries to reach objects with hand but overshoots Grasps object with both hands Plays with rattle placed in hand, shakes it, but cannot pick it up if dropped Can carry objects to mouth
AGE 5 MONTHS Beginning signs of tooth eruption Birth weight doubles	No head lag when pulled to sitting position When sitting, able to hold head erect and steady Able to sit for longer periods when back is well supported Back straight When prone, assumes symmetric positioning with arms extended ■ Can turn over from abdomen to back When supine, puts feet to mouth	■ Able to grasp objects voluntarily Uses palmar grasp, bidextrous approach Plays with toes Takes objects directly to mouth Holds one cube while regarding a second one

■ Milestones that represent essential integrative aspects of development that lay the foundation for the achievement of more advanced skills.
*Degree of visual acuity varies according to vision measurement procedure used.

SENSORY	VOCALIZATION	SOCIALIZATION AND COGNITION
■ Able to fixate on moving object in range of 45 degrees when held at a distance of 20-25 cm (8-10 inches) Visual acuity approaches 20/100* Follows light to midline Quiets when hears a voice	Cries to express displeasure Makes small, throaty sounds Makes comfort sounds during feeding	Is in sensorimotor phase—stage I, use of reflexes (birth–1 month), and stage II, primary circular reactions (1-4 months) Watches parent's face intently as she or he talks to infant
Binocular fixation and convergence to near objects beginning When supine, follows dangling toy from side to point beyond midline Visually searches to locate sounds Turns head to side when sound is made at level of ear	■ Vocalizes, distinct from crying Crying becomes differentiated Coos Vocalizes to familiar voice	■ Demonstrates social smile in response to various stimuli
■ Follows objects to periphery (180 degrees) ■ Locates sound by turning head to side and looking in same direction Begins to have ability to coordinate stimuli from various sense organs	■ Squeals aloud to show pleasure Coos, babbles, chuckles Vocalizes when smiling "Talks" a great deal when spoken to Less crying during periods of wakefulness	Displays considerable interest in surroundings Ceases crying when parent enters room Can recognize familiar faces and objects, such as feeding bottle Shows awareness of strange situations
Able to accommodate to near objects Binocular vision fairly well established Can focus on a 1.25 cm (0.5 inch) block Beginning eye-hand coordination	Makes consonant sounds *n, k, g, p, b* ■ Laughs aloud Vocalization changes according to mood	Is in stage III, secondary circular reactions Demands attention by fussing; becomes bored if left alone Enjoys social interaction with people Anticipates feeding when sees bottle or mother if breastfeeding Shows excitement with whole body, squeals, breathes heavily Shows interest in strange stimuli Begins to show memory
Visually pursues a dropped object Is able to sustain visual inspection of an object Can localize sounds made below ear	Squeals Makes cooing vowel sounds interspersed with consonant sounds (e.g., *ah-goo*)	Smiles at mirror image Pats bottle or breast with both hands More enthusiastically playful, but may have rapid mood swings Is able to discriminate strangers from family Vocalizes displeasure when object is taken away Discovers parts of body

Continued

TABLE 10-2

Growth and Development During Infancy—cont'd

PHYSICAL	GROSS MOTOR	FINE MOTOR
AGE 6 MONTHS Growth rate may begin to decline Weight gain of 90-150 g (3-5 ounces) weekly for next 6 months Height gain of 1.25 cm (0.5 inch) monthly for next 6 months ■ Teething may begin with eruption of two lower central incisors ■ Chewing and biting occur	When prone, can lift chest and upper abdomen off surface, bearing weight on hands (see Fig. 10-3, C) When about to be pulled to a sitting position, lifts head Sits in high chair with back straight Rolls from back to abdomen When held in standing position, bears almost all of weight Hand regard absent	Resecures a dropped object Drops one cube when another is given Grasps and manipulates small objects Holds bottle Grasps feet and pulls to mouth
AGE 7 MONTHS Eruption of upper central incisors	When supine, spontaneously lifts head off surface ■ Sits, leaning forward on both hands (see Fig. 10-5, D) When prone, bears weight on one hand Sits erect momentarily Bears full weight on feet (see Fig. 10-6, A) When held in standing position, bounces actively	■ Transfers objects from one hand to the other (see Fig. 10-5, E) Has unidextrous approach and grasp Holds two cubes more than momentarily Bangs cubes on table Rakes at a small object
AGE 8 MONTHS Begins to show regular patterns in bladder and bowel elimination Parachute reflex appears (see Fig. 10-4)	■ Sits steadily unsupported (see Fig. 10-5, E) Readily bears weight on legs when supported; may stand holding onto furniture Adjusts posture to reach an object	Has beginning pincer grasp using index, fourth, and fifth fingers against lower part of thumb Releases objects at will Rings bell purposely Retains two cubes while regarding third cube Secures an object by pulling on a string Reaches persistently for toys out of reach
AGE 9 MONTHS Eruption of upper lateral incisor may begin	Creeps on hands and knees Sits steadily on floor for prolonged time (10 minutes) Recovers balance when leaning forward but cannot do so when leaning sideways ■ Pulls self to standing position and stands holding onto furniture (see Fig. 10-6, B and C)	■ Uses thumb and index finger in crude pincer grasp (see Fig. 10-1) Preference for use of dominant hand now evident Grasps third cube Compares two cubes by bringing them together
AGE 10 MONTHS Labyrinth-righting reflex is strongest when infant is in prone or supine position; is able to raise head	Can change from prone to sitting position Stands while holding onto furniture; sits by falling down Recovers balance easily while sitting While standing, lifts one foot to take a step (see Fig. 10-6, D)	Crude release of an object beginning Grasps bell by handle

■ Milestones that represent essential integrative aspects of development that lay the foundation for the achievement of more advanced skills.

SENSORY	VOCALIZATION	SOCIALIZATION AND COGNITION
Adjusts posture to see an object Prefers more complex visual stimuli Can localize sounds made above ear Will turn head to the side, then look up or down	▪ Begins to imitate sounds ▪ Babbling resembles one-syllable utterances—*ma, mu, da, di, hi* Vocalizes to toys, mirror image Takes pleasure in hearing own sounds (self-reinforcement)	Recognizes parents; begins to fear strangers Holds arms out to be picked up Has definite likes and dislikes Begins to imitate (cough, protrusion of tongue) Excites on hearing footsteps ▪ Briefly searches for a dropped object (object permanence beginning) Frequent mood swings, from crying to laughing, with little or no provocation
▪ Can fixate on very small objects Responds to own name Localizes sound by turning head in a curving arch Beginning awareness of depth and space Has taste preferences	▪ Produces vowel sounds and chained syllables—*baba, dada, kaka* Vocalizes four distinct vowel sounds "Talks" when others are talking	▪ Increasing fear of strangers; shows signs of fretfulness when parent disappears Imitates simple acts and noises Tries to attract attention by coughing or snorting Plays peek-a-boo Demonstrates dislike of food by keeping lips closed Exhibits oral aggressiveness in biting and mouthing Demonstrates expectation in response to repetition of stimuli
	Makes consonant sounds *t, d, w* Listens selectively to familiar words Utterances signal emphasis and emotion Combines syllables, such as *dada*, but does not ascribe meaning to them	Increasing anxiety over loss of parent, particularly mother, and fear of strangers Responds to word "no" Dislikes dressing, diaper change
Localizes sounds by turning head diagonally and directly toward sound Depth perception increasing	Responds to simple verbal commands Comprehends "no-no"	Parent (mother) is increasingly important for own sake Shows increasing interest in pleasing parent Begins to show fears of going to bed and being left alone Puts arms in front of face to avoid having it washed
	▪ Says "dada," "mama" with meaning Comprehends "bye-bye" May say one word (e.g., "hi," "bye," "no")	Inhibits behavior to verbal command of "no-no" or own name Imitates facial expressions; waves bye-bye Extends toy to another person but will not release it ▪ Develops object permanence Repeats actions that attract attention and cause laughter Pulls clothes of another to attract attention Plays interactive games such as pat-a-cake Reacts to adult anger; cries when scolded Demonstrates independence in dressing, feeding, locomotive skills, and testing of parents Looks at and follows picture in a book

Continued

TABLE 10-2

Growth and Development During Infancy—cont'd

PHYSICAL	GROSS MOTOR	FINE MOTOR
AGE 11 MONTHS Eruption of lower lateral incisor may begin	When sitting, pivots to reach toward back to pick up an object ■ Cruises or walks holding onto furniture or with both hands held	Explores objects more thoroughly (e.g., clapper inside bell) Has neat pincer grasp Drops object deliberately for it to be picked up Puts one object after another into a container (sequential play) Able to manipulate an object to remove it from tight-fitting enclosure
AGE 12 MONTHS ■ Birth weight tripled ■ Birth length increased by 50% Head and chest circumference equal (head circumference 46 cm [18 inches]) Has 6-8 deciduous teeth Anterior fontanel almost closed Landau reflex fading Babinski reflex disappears Lumbar curve develops; lordosis evident during walking	■ Walks with one hand held Cruises well ■ May attempt to stand alone momentarily; may attempt first step alone Can sit down from standing position without help	Releases cube in cup Attempts to build two-block tower but fails Tries to insert a pellet into a narrow-necked bottle but fails Can turn pages in a book, many at a time

■ Milestones that represent essential integrative aspects of development that lay the foundation for the achievement of more advanced skills.

---

as exchange baby-sitting, or family daycare. A licensed **small family childcare home** typically provides care and protection for up to six children for part of a 24-hour day and does not include informal arrangements such as exchange baby-sitting or caregivers in the child's own home. The six children may include the family daycare provider's own children younger than 5 years of age living in the home. **Large family childcare homes** may provide care for eight to twelve children. Unfortunately, many family daycare homes operate without a license and may care for large numbers of infants without adequate staff and facilities.

Child center-based care usually refers to a licensed daycare facility that provides care for six or more children, for 6 or more hours in a 24-hour day. **Work-based group care** is another option that is becoming increasingly popular as employers recognize the benefit of providing high-quality and convenient child care to their employees. **Sick-child care** may also be available for times when the youngster is ill. Such programs are often located in community hospitals or in work settings.

A major nursing responsibility is guiding parents in locating suitable facilities that have a well-qualified staff. State licensing agencies can help parents identify daycare centers that accept children of specific age-groups and are convenient to home and work. Their records are available to the public and provide reports from the health, safety, and fire departments; periodic evaluations from the licensing agency; complaints filed against the center; and qualification of the center's employees. State-licensed programs are supposed to abide by established standards, which represent the minimum require-

ments and safeguards. However, enforcement of the standards is sometimes inadequate.

Early childhood programs may also belong to a voluntary accreditation system sponsored by National Association for the Education of Young Children, which serves as a model for optimum care.* References from other parents are also helpful, provided that they have investigated the center carefully and have remained involved with the agency's activities.

Guidelines for selecting child care facilities are discussed under Preschool and Kindergarten Experience, Chapter 13. The same conscientious attention should be applied to locating competent baby-sitters. References from other employers are essential, and there is no substitute for observing the interaction between the individual and the child. Although very young infants need little if any preparation for the introduction of a new caregiver, older infants may benefit from a

---

*Information about accreditation criteria and procedures of the NAEYC Academy for Early Childhood Program Accreditation is available from the National Association for the Education of Young Children, 1313 L St. NW, Suite 500, Washington, DC 20005; (800) 424-2460 or (202) 232-8777; http://www.naeyc.org. These criteria are excellent guidelines for evaluating child care facilities. Other resources are (1) *Child Care: What's Best for Your Family* and a number of other child care articles and pamphlets from American Academy of Pediatrics, 141 Northwest Point Blvd., Elk Grove Village, IL 60007; (847) 434-4000; http://aap.org; to access online, enter the Medem Network, http://www.medem.com, then enter "Medical Library" for pamphlet titles; (2) *Parent's Guide to Day Care*, available from National Association of Pediatric Nurse Practitioners, 20 Brace Road, Suite 200, Cherry Hill, NJ 08034-2634; (856) 857-9700; fax: (856) 857-1600[0]; http://www.napnap.org; and (3) Child Care Aware, (800) 424-2246; http://www.childcareaware.org.

SENSORY	VOCALIZATION	SOCIALIZATION AND COGNITION
	Imitates definite speech sounds	Experiences joy and satisfaction when a task is mastered
		Reacts to restrictions with frustration
		Rolls ball to another on request
		Anticipates body gestures when a familiar nursery rhyme or story is being told (e.g., holds toes and feet in response to "This little piggy went to market")
		Plays games up-down, "so big," or peek-a-boo
		Shakes head for "no"
Discriminates simple geometric forms (e.g., circle)	■ Says three to five words besides "dada," "mama"	Shows emotions such as jealousy, affection (may hug or kiss on request), anger, fear
Amblyopia may develop with lack of binocularity	Comprehends meaning of several words (comprehension always precedes verbalization)	Enjoys familiar surroundings and explores away from parent
Can follow rapidly moving object	Recognizes objects by name	Is fearful in strange situation; clings to parent
Controls and adjusts response to sound; listens for sound to recur	Imitates animal sounds	May develop habit of "security blanket" or favorite toy
	Understands simple verbal commands (e.g., "Give it to me," "Show me your eyes")	Has increasing determination to practice locomotor skills
		■ Searches for an object even if it has not been hidden, but searches only where object was last seen

gradual placement to reduce stranger anxiety. At all times the parent should have the right to visit the child, and regular conferences should be established to review the child's progress.

One of the areas that is increasingly important in selecting child care is the center's health practices; however, parents often do not check the center for health and safety features. Evidence shows that children, especially those under age 3 years in daycare centers, have more illnesses—especially diarrhea, otitis media, respiratory tract infections (especially if the caregiver smokes), hepatitis A, meningitis, and cytomegalovirus—than children cared for in their home. The strongest predictor of risk of illness is the number of unrelated children in the room. Proactive infection control measures and education of staff have been effective in reducing the incidence of upper respiratory tract infections, diarrhea, and rotavirus. It has been reported that families who have children in out-of-home child care lose an estimated 13 days of work per year as a result of infections (Brady, 2005). Parents should inquire about the center's policy regarding the attendance and care of sick children.

Limit Setting and Discipline

As infants' motor skills advance and mobility increases, parents are faced with the need to set safe limits to protect the child and establish a positive and supportive parent-child relationship (see Nurse's Role in Injury Prevention, p. 372). Although there are numerous disciplinary techniques, some are more appropriate for this age than others. An effective approach used in disciplining a child is the use of time-out. The

basic principles are the same as those discussed in Chapter 3, except that the place for time-out needs to be commensurate with the child's abilities. For example, the playpen is better for most infants than a chair. Although parents may be concerned about instituting discipline during infancy, it is important to stress that the earlier effective disciplinary methods are employed, the easier it is to continue these approaches.

Parents must recognize the infant's cognitive and behavioral limitations; adequate protection from hazards must be implemented because infants and toddlers do not understand a cause-and-effect relationship between dangerous objects and physical harm. Additionally, parents may need reassurance that their infant's behavior is exploratory in nature, not oppositional (at this age) and primarily centered on the infant's basic needs of warmth, love, food, security, and comfort. Parents may verbalize that comforting the infant too much or meeting its needs will result in a spoiled child; there is no substantial evidence that meeting the infant's basic needs will result in such behaviors later in life. Children will innately test limits and explore during the exploratory phase of growth; instead of discouraging exploration, parents should provide safe alternatives, put dangerous household items away, and give children consistent discipline and nurturing.

Effective teaching for injury prevention optimally begins in infancy by helping parents understand the nature of their child's normal development. It must be reiterated continually that infants cry because a need is not being met, not to intentionally irritate an adult. The fussy or irritable infant is a potential victim of shaken baby syndrome (or other bodily harm), since adults and caretakers may not understand the nature of the infant's crying.

Thumb Sucking and Use of a Pacifier

Sucking is the infant's chief pleasure and may not be entirely satisfied by breastfeeding or bottle feeding. It is such a strong need that infants who are deprived of sucking, such as those with a cleft lip repair, will suck on their tongue. Some newborns are born with sucking blisters on their hands from in utero sucking activity. The benefits of nonnutritive sucking in *preterm* infants include increased weight gain, decreased length of stay, and improved pain management (Pinelli and Symington, 2000; Pinelli, Symington, and Ciliska, 2002). There is currently no evidence that pacifier use and nonnutritive sucking in *preterm* infants has any effect on the initiation and length of breastfeeding. Nonnutritive sucking should not be withheld from *preterm* infants, especially when performed in conjunction with the use of concentrated sucrose for pain management.

Pacifier use, particularly in the early days after birth and in the birth hospital, has gained considerable attention in the scientific literature. Some experts now state that "nontherapeutic" pacifier use should be discouraged, since there are no known benefits to its use other than for nonnutritive sucking and for managing pain.

Biancuzzo (2003) suggests that it cannot be stated with absolute certainty that pacifier use is bad in every situation but warns there is potential harm in the use of pacifiers based on available evidence. Furthermore, she admonishes health care workers to be informed regarding potential harm in pacifier use and to inform parents of the potential. Lawrence and Lawrence (2005), as well as other experts in breastfeeding, recommend that health care workers not introduce pacifiers to breast-fed infants unless at the request of the parent. Pacifier use is not recommended as part of the Baby-Friendly Hospital Initiative. (See Box 8-5, p. 230.)

A review of studies by the Joanna Briggs Institute (2005) found an association between pacifier use in infancy and a reduction in breastfeeding and exclusive breastfeeding. However, the authors concluded that pacifier use did not cause a reduction in breastfeeding; rather it was a "marker for socioeconomic, demographic, psychosocial and cultural factors that determine pacifier use and breastfeeding." In addition, the researchers examined studies related to pacifier use and prevention of SIDS; infants put to sleep with a pacifier had a *reduced* risk of SIDS. Because of the limited number of studies correlating pacifier use and increased risk of infections or dental malocclusion, the authors were unable to make any recommendations for or against pacifier use in relation to these practices (Joanna Briggs Institute, 2005).

The American Academy of Pediatrics (2005) recommends limited pacifier use in infants, citing the strong evidence for pacifier use and its protective effect in SIDS reduction; the exact mechanism involved in the protection for SIDS is not known. Still, pacifier use should not replace actual feeding or suckling; prohibiting pacifier use will not absolutely ensure an increase in the length of breastfeeding; and there should be an emphasis on allowing the infant to control the pace, frequency, and termination of feeding rather than allowing the pacifier (or anything else) to become the focus of the interaction.

To decrease dependence on nonnutritive sucking in young infants, sucking pleasure can be increased by prolonging feeding time. Also, the parent's excessive use of the pacifier to calm the child should be explored. It is not unusual for parents to place a pacifier in the infant's mouth as soon as crying begins, thus reinforcing a pattern of distress-relief.

The effect of continual pacifier use on early speech and language development is unknown, but the pacifier may decrease the child's desire to imitate sounds and affect intelligibility. Parents need to be alerted that continual dependence on a pacifier may influence social and speech development.

If the child uses a pacifier, safety considerations in purchasing one must be stressed. Parents should be cautioned against altering a pacifier, thus making it more dangerous (see Aspiration of Foreign Objects, p. 365).

During infancy and early childhood there is no need to restrain nonnutritive sucking of the fingers. Malocclusion may occur if thumb sucking persists past 4 to 6 years of age, or when the permanent teeth erupt. Pacifiers may be perceived by some parents as less damaging because they are discarded by 2 to 3 years of age, whereas thumb sucking may persist well into school-age years. Both pacifier use and thumb sucking may also have significant cultural variations.

Thumb sucking reaches its peak at age 18 to 20 months and is most prevalent when the child is hungry, tired, or feeling insecure. Persistent thumb sucking in a listless, apathetic child always warrants investigation. It may be a sign of an emotional problem between parent and child or of boredom, isolation, and lack of stimulation.

Teething

One of the more difficult periods in the infant's (and parents') life is the eruption of the deciduous (primary) teeth, often referred to as *teething*. The age of tooth eruption shows considerable variation among children, but the order of their appearance is fairly regular and predictable (Fig. 10-10). The first primary teeth to erupt are the lower central incisors, which appear at approximately 6 to 10 months of age (average 8 months). These are followed closely by the upper central incisors.

> **NURSING TIP**
>
> A quick guide to assessment of deciduous teeth during the first 2 years is: Age of the child in months − 6 = Number of teeth. For example: 8 months of age − 6 = 2 teeth at this time.

Teething is a physiologic process; some discomfort is common as the crown of the tooth breaks through the periodontal membrane. Some children show minimum evidence of teething, such as drooling, swollen gums, increased finger sucking, or biting on hard objects. Others are very irritable, have difficulty sleeping, and refuse to eat. Generally, signs of illness such as fever, vomiting, or diarrhea are not symptoms of teething but of illness and may warrant further investigation (Macknin, Piedmonte, Jacobs, and others, 2000). Anderson (2004) suggests that frequent waking periods are related to environmental, behavioral, or developmental changes rather than teething. The author also cautions parents (and health care workers) to not overdiagnose teething; the ill-appearing child or child with a temperature over 38° C (100.4° F) should be evaluated by the practitioner.

Because teething pain is a result of inflammation, cold is soothing. Giving the child a frozen teething ring or an ice cube wrapped in a washcloth helps relieve the inflammation. Sev-

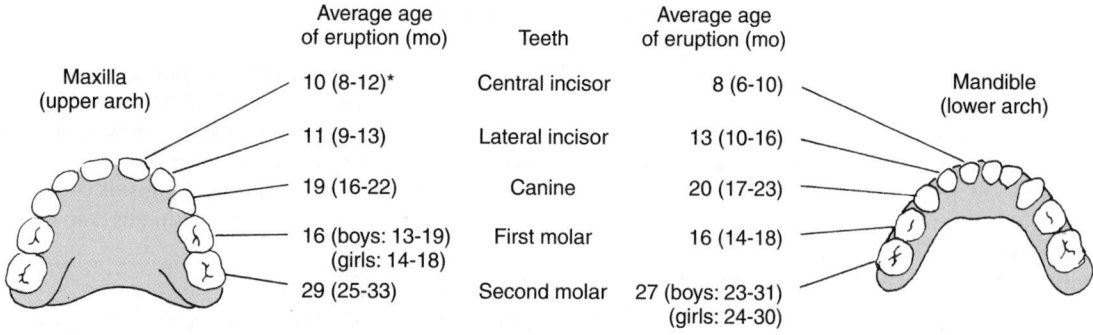

Maxilla (upper arch)	Average age of eruption (mo)	Teeth	Average age of eruption (mo)	Mandible (lower arch)
	10 (8-12)*	Central incisor	8 (6-10)	
	11 (9-13)	Lateral incisor	13 (10-16)	
	19 (16-22)	Canine	20 (17-23)	
	16 (boys: 13-19) (girls: 14-18)	First molar	16 (14-18)	
	29 (25-33)	Second molar	27 (boys: 23-31) (girls: 24-30)	

FIG. 10-10 ■ Sequence of eruption of primary teeth. *Range represents ±1 standard deviation, or 67% of subjects studied. (Data from McDonald RE, Avery DR: *Dentistry for the child and adolescent,* ed 6, St Louis, 1994, Mosby.)

eral nonprescription topical anesthetic ointments are available, such as Baby Ora-Jel, although parents and health care workers should be aware of the risks of using topical anesthetic products (absorption rates vary in infants) (Anderson, 2004). The active ingredient in most of them is benzocaine. If such products are used, parents are advised to apply them correctly. In the event of persistent irritability that affects sleeping and feeding, systemic analgesics such as acetaminophen or ibuprofen can be given (if age appropriate) for no more than 3 days (Anderson, 2004); however, parents should know that this is a temporary measure and should contact the practitioner if symptoms persist or if the child's condition changes.

> **NURSINGALERT**
>
> The use of teething powders or procedures such as cutting or rubbing the gums with aspirin are discouraged, since ingestion of the powder, infection or irritation of the tissue, and ingestion or aspiration of the aspirin can occur. Hard candy may cause accidental choking or aspiration and should be avoided at this age.

Infant Shoes

Many parents are unaware of the types of shoes that are appropriate for the older infant and buy expensive infant shoes because of misleading advertising claims. Inflexible shoes that have hard soles can be detrimental by delaying walking, aggravating intoeing or outtoeing, and impeding the development of supportive foot muscles. Therefore counseling parents regarding footwear should begin when infants are 6 months old—well before they are walking.

It is helpful to begin by explaining to parents that changes in the feet occur during infancy and early childhood as locomotion and weight bearing progress. At birth the feet are flat because the arches are protected by fat pads on the soles. As the bones in the arches develop, the pads disappear and the feet begin to assume a mature shape. A normal arch is determined by proper alignment of all the bones and development of the surrounding musculature, not by the height of the arch.

When children begin walking, the main reason for shoes is protection. To provide protection, the shoe should retain its fit; be made of durable material with a smooth interior and few construction seams to irritate the skin; and be soft and flexible, especially in the toe area. A high-top shoe is not necessary for support but may be helpful in keeping the foot in the shoe. A good infant-toddler shoe is one that can easily be

bent in half by squeezing the heel and toe with the thumb and index finger (Wall, 2000).

A good shoe conforms to the anatomic shape of the foot, with a rounded toe and sufficient toe room. During weight bearing there should be the space of at least half the width of the thumbnail, or 1.25 cm (0.5 inch), between the end of the longest toe and the shoe. Roomy and square-toed socks allow for proper growth and alignment. Inexpensive but well-constructed athletic shoes or soft-leather moccasin-type shoes are suggested as adequate footgear for walking infants.

Even if the shoes are fitted properly, frequent changes are needed to accommodate the infant's rapidly growing feet. Shoe size changes at approximately 3-month intervals between 12 and 36 months; during this time the child's foot should be measured every 3 months. Curled toes when shoes are removed and redness and irritation of the skin on the bottom of the toes indicate the need for a larger size.

PROMOTING OPTIMAL HEALTH DURING INFANCY

NUTRITION

Ideally, discussion of optimal nutrition should begin prenatally with a discussion regarding maternal intake of adequate nutrition in the form of a balanced diet and adequate amounts of protein, vitamins, and minerals, all of which have an impact on the growing fetus. Nurses should encourage and provide information for parents to discuss the options of breastfeeding or bottle feeding the infant well in advance of the delivery date. The choice for either is highly individual and is discussed in Chapter 8. This section is primarily concerned with infant nutrition during the months when growth needs and developmental milestones ready the child for the introduction of solid foods.

Despite adequate availability of optimal nutrient sources, concern remains that infants are not being fed appropriately. These practices may have far-reaching, long-term health consequences, affecting infants and, as they grow, children and adults. Certain chronic health conditions have been linked to feeding practices in infancy. Nurses must continue to be proactive in teaching parents about what constitutes appropriate infant nutrition and nutritional habits, which provide the opportunity to grow and develop into a healthy child and adult.

Health care professionals have recently become more aware of the use of complementary and alternative medical therapies in children that may not be as beneficial as touted in various media sources. One concern is children's intake of megavitamins and herbs; parents may assume that the word *natural* in reference to ingredients means the product is safe, when this may not be the case. One report recently cited the home administration of star anise tea to treat colic as the cause of adverse neurologic reactions in seven infants (Ize-Ludlow, Ragone, Bruck, and others, 2004). It is important for nurses to be aware of the effects, availability, and practice of complementary therapies and to be able to cogently discuss their use with parents (Loman, 2003; Niggemann and Grüber, 2003).

The First 6 Months

Human milk is the most desirable complete diet for the infant during the first 6 months. The normal infant receiving breast milk from a well-nourished mother usually requires no specific vitamin or mineral supplements, with a few exceptions. The American Academy of Pediatrics (2003) recommends that all infants (including those exclusively breast-fed) receive a daily supplement of 200 IU of vitamin D beginning in the first 2 months of life to prevent rickets and vitamin D deficiency. If the infant is being exclusively breast-fed after 4 to 6 months (when fetal iron stores are depleted), iron supplementation, which may be accomplished with iron-fortified cereal, is recommended to offset the decrease in iron available in human milk at this time and to enhance erythropoiesis. Infants who are breast-fed or bottle-fed do not require additional fluids, especially water or juice, during the first 4 months of life. Excessive intake of water in infants may result in water intoxication, failure to thrive, and hyponatremia.

Employed mothers can continue breastfeeding with guidance and encouragement. Mothers are encouraged to set realistic goals for employment and breastfeeding, with accurate information regarding the costs, risks, and benefits of available feeding options. Barriers encountered by working breastfeeding mothers include lack of employer or co-worker support, unavailable or inadequate facilities for pumping and storing milk, and insufficient time allowed to pump during work (Rojjanasrirat, 2004). Important themes that emerged in the study by Rojjanasrirat (2004) of working breastfeeding mothers included support (emotional, informational, and instrumental), attitude, and psychologic distress.

Many mothers may find that a program of breast pumping when away from home and bottle feeding the infant the expressed milk with or without formula supplementation is successful. Expressed breast milk may be stored in the refrigerator (4° C [39° F]) without danger of bacterial contamination for up to 5 days (Lawrence and Lawrence, 2005). Although feeding the infant at home may occur on a demand basis, pumping milk away from home may be needed every 3 to 4 hours to maintain adequate supply. Breast milk may be expressed by hand or pump (manual or electric) and stored in an appropriate air-tight glass or plastic container. Expressed breast milk may be frozen (−18° C [0° F] or lower) for up to 12 months (depending on the type of freezer used), but care should be taken to prevent freezer burn (see Appendix P, protocol no. 8, in Lawrence and Lawrence, 2005, for further guidelines on storing and freezing human milk). Health care workers and new mothers may find the booklet "Working and Breastfeeding—Can You Do It? Yes, You Can!"

(available in English and Spanish) by Johnson & Johnson helpful.*

In addition to efficient breast pumping, mothers also need child care by a trusted individual or agency and support and assistance from significant others. As with all breastfeeding mothers, these women must have proper nutrition and rest for adequate lactation. Maternal fatigue is considered the biggest threat to successful breastfeeding in employed mothers.

> **NURSINGALERT**
>
> Warming expressed milk in a microwave decreases the availability of antiinfective properties and vitamin C and causes a separation of milk layers, which affects fat content (Lawrence and Lawrence, 2005). To prevent oral burns from uneven warming of the milk, breast milk should never be thawed or rewarmed in a microwave oven. To thaw the frozen milk, either place container under a lukewarm water bath (<40.5° C [105° F]) or place in refrigerator overnight.

An acceptable alternative to breastfeeding is commercial iron-fortified formula. Like human milk, it supplies all nutrients needed by the infant for the first 6 months. Unmodified whole cow's milk, low-fat cow's milk, skim milk, other animal milks, and imitation milks are not acceptable as a major source of nutrition for infants because of their limited digestibility, increased risk of contamination, and lack of components needed for appropriate growth. Whole milk can cause iron deficiency anemia in infants, possibly as a result of occult gastrointestinal blood loss. Pasteurized whole cow's milk is deficient in iron, zinc, and vitamin C and has a high renal solute load, which makes it undesirable for infants less than 12 months of age (American Academy of Pediatrics, 2004).

> **NURSINGALERT**
>
> Whole cow's milk should not be introduced to infants until after 1 year of age (American Academy of Pediatrics, 2004).

> **NURSINGALERT**
>
> Dietary fat in infants under 6 months should not be restricted unless on specific medical advice. Substituting skim or low-fat milk is unacceptable, since the essential fatty acids are inadequate and the solute concentration of protein and electrolytes, such as sodium, is too high.

> **NURSINGALERT**
>
> Microwaving of bottles and baby food is not recommended because of uneven heating, which may cause burns to the mouth and tongue.

The amount of formula per feeding and the number of feedings per day vary among infants. Infants being fed on demand usually determine their own feeding schedule, but some infants may need a more planned schedule based on average feeding patterns to ensure sufficient nutrients. In general, the number of feedings decreases from six at 1 month of age to four or five at 6 months. Regardless of the number of feedings, the total amount of formula ingested will usually

---

*Developed by National Healthy Mothers, Healthy Babies Coalition, 2000 N. Beauregard St., 6th floor, Alexandria, VA 22311; (703) 837-4792; http://www.hmhb.org.

level off at about 32 ounces (946 ml) per day. Water supplementation is not recommended for healthy infants because it may lead to water intoxication (American Academy of Pediatrics, 2004).

> **NURSINGALERT**
>
> Bottled water for mixing powdered or concentrated formula is a relatively safe alternative to tap water, but parents should carefully read the label on the water for ingredients and not assume that it is sterile (Morin, 2007).

The addition of solid foods before 4 to 6 months of age is not recommended. During the early months solid foods are not compatible with the ability of the gastrointestinal tract and infant's nutritional needs. Feeding solids to young infants exposes them to food antigens that may produce food protein allergy. There is now ample evidence that early introduction of foods other than maternal milk in the first 6 months of life predisposes children to an increased risk for food allergy development; foods known to be allergenic (e.g., peanuts, eggs, fish, seafood) should be introduced later than 12 months according to the child's risk for atopy (Fiocchi, Assa'ad, Bahna, and others, 2006).

Developmentally, infants are not ready for solid food. The extrusion (protrusion) reflex is strong and often causes them to push food out of the mouth. Infants instinctively suck when given food. Because of their limited motor abilities, infants are unable to deliberately push food away or avoid feeding. Therefore early introduction of solids is a type of forced feeding that may lead to excessive weight gain and increased predisposition to allergies and iron deficiency anemia. Parents should be cautioned concerning the excessive use of juices and nonnutritive drinks such as fruit-flavored drinks or carbonated beverages (soda or pop) during this period. Many juices and nonnutritive drinks, although readily available to consumers, do not provide sufficient and appropriate caloric intake for infants less than 12 months of age; such drinks may replace the nutrients in breast milk or formula and lead to growth or health problems. Fruit juices are not required in the first 6 months; there are no studies demonstrating benefits of giving fruit juice to infants.

The Second 6 Months

During the second half of the first year, human milk or formula should optimally continue to be the primary source of nutrition. Fluoride supplementation should begin, depending on the infant's intake of fluoride (in formula mixed with tap water or bottled water [containing fluoride] as appropriate) (see Dental Health, p. 349). If breastfeeding is discontinued, a commercial iron-fortified formula should be substituted. Follow-up or transition formulas marketed for older infants offer no special advantages over other infant formulas and provide excessive protein (American Academy of Pediatrics, 2004).

The major change in feeding habits is the addition of solid foods to the infant's diet. Physiologically and developmentally, the infant 4 to 6 months of age is in a transition period. By this time the gastrointestinal tract has matured sufficiently to handle more complex nutrients and is less sensitive to potentially allergenic foods. Tooth eruption is beginning and facilitates biting and chewing. The extrusion reflex has disappeared, and swallowing is more coordinated to allow the infant to accept solids easily. Head control is well developed, which permits infants to sit with support and purposely turn the head away to communicate lack of interest in food. Voluntary grasping and improved eye-hand coordination gradually allow infants to pick up finger foods and feed themselves. Their increasing sense of independence is evident in their desire to hold the bottle and try to "help" during feeding.

Selection and Preparation of Solid Foods

The choice of solid foods to introduce first is variable but should meet the reasons for feeding solids, such as supplying nutrients not found in formula or breast milk. Iron-fortified infant cereal is generally introduced first because of its high iron content (7 mg/3 Tbsp of prepared dry cereal). Commercially prepared ready-to-serve dry cereals for infants include rice, barley, oatmeal, and high-protein cereals; rice is usually suggested as an initial food because of its easy digestibility and low allergenic potential. Cereals such as cream of farina are not used, since infant commercial cereals are a better source of iron. Some of the commercial baby cereals are combined with fruit. There is little nutritional benefit from these preparations, and they are more expensive. New foods should be added one at a time; therefore parents should avoid cereal combinations when beginning a new grain.

Infant cereal (iron fortified) may be mixed with expressed breast milk or water until whole milk is given. After 6 months of age, small amounts of fruit juices can be mixed with the dry cereal; the vitamin C content of the juice enhances the absorption of iron in the cereal. Because of their benefit as a source of iron, infant cereals should be continued until the child is 18 months of age.

Fruit juice can be offered from a cup for its rich source of vitamin C and as a substitute for milk for one feeding a day. Large quantities of certain juices (e.g., apple, pear, prune, sweet cherry, peach, grape) are avoided because they may cause abdominal pain, diarrhea, or bloating in some children. Avoid fruit-flavored drinks, which may be marketed as juices but contain high concentrations of complex sugars. White grape juice (no more than 5 oz/day) is reported to be better absorbed and safe for infants this age without causing gastrointestinal distress (Calamaro, 2000). Some researchers have found fruit juice, particularly apple juice, to exacerbate colic and diarrhea, possibly because of carbohydrate malabsorption (Duro, Rising, Cedillo, and others, 2002; Moukarzel, Lesicka, and Ament, 2002). The American Academy of Pediatrics (2001b, 2006a) recommends that fruit juice intake not exceed 4 to 6 ounces per day and that juices not be given to infants less than 4 to 6 months old. Because vitamin C is naturally destroyed by heat, juice is not warmed. Juice containers are always kept covered and refrigerated to prevent further vitamin loss.

The addition of other foods is arbitrary. A common sequence is to introduce strained fruits followed by vegetables and, finally, meats; however, some clinicians prefer to add vegetables before fruit. If foods are introduced early, citrus fruits, meats, and eggs are delayed until after 6 months of age because of their potential to result in allergy. At 6 months, foods such as a cracker or zwieback can be offered as finger and teething foods. By 8 to 9 months, junior foods and nutritious finger foods such as firmly cooked vegetable, raw pieces of fruit, or cheese can be given. By 1 year, well-cooked table foods are served.

The introduction of solid foods into the infant's diet at this age is primarily for taste and chewing experience. The majority of the infant's caloric needs are derived from the primary milk source (human or formula); therefore solids should not be perceived as a substitute for milk until the child is older than 12 months. Portion sizes may vary according to the infant's taste. In general, 1 tablespoon per year of age (i.e., ½ to ¾ tablespoon for most infants under 12 months) is adequate for most infants. In most cases 2 tablespoons may be served, but because of the infant's focus on the texture and feel of the food, smaller amounts will be consumed. Another reason for smaller portions is the concern over feeding habits in early childhood and obesity; early feeding of smaller portions may help prevent the "clean your plate" or "eat all your food or you can't get down from the table" concepts, which are known to contribute to overeating in later life. The addition of solid foods to the exclusively breast-fed infant's diet does not significantly increase overall caloric intake or weight gain (Dewey, 2001).

Commercially prepared baby foods are the most common type of food served to infants in the United States. They are convenient but sometimes contain added salt or sugar and can be relatively expensive. An alternative is to prepare baby foods at home, which is a simple and inexpensive process. Fruits and vegetables can be steamed in a small amount of water and pureed in a blender or food processor. Many of them, such as ripe banana, can be mashed fine with a fork. Fruits such as apples or pears require little or no water in the cooking process. Vegetables such as carrots, potatoes, or string beans require additional water in the cooking and blending process.

Parents are cautioned to avoid reliance on foods and supplements marketed as iron- or vitamin-fortified as primary sources of minerals. Instead encourage parents to offer the child a variety of fruits, vegetables, and whole grains, including those known to naturally be rich in iron (Fox, Reidy, Novak, and others, 2006).

Introduction of Solid Foods

When the spoon is first introduced, infants often push it away and appear dissatisfied. Some patience and skill are required to overcome this initial response. Food that is placed on the

FAMILY-CENTERED CARE

Feeding During the First Year

BIRTH TO 6 MONTHS (BREASTFEEDING OR BOTTLE FEEDING)
Breastfeeding
Most desirable complete diet for first half of year.*
Requires supplements of vitamin D (200 IU/day).

Formula
Iron-fortified commercial formula is a complete food for the first half of the year.*
Requires fluoride supplements (0.25 mg) when the concentration of fluoride in the drinking water is below 0.3 ppm after 6 months of age.
Evaporated milk formula requires supplements of vitamin C, iron, and fluoride (in accordance with the fluoride content of the local water supply after 6 months of age).

AGE 6 TO 12 MONTHS (SOLID FOODS)
May begin to add solids by 5 to 6 months of age.
First foods are strained, pureed, or finely mashed.
Finger foods such as teething crackers, raw fruit, or vegetables can be introduced by 6 to 7 months.
Chopped table food or commercially prepared junior foods can be started by 9 to 12 months.
With the exception of cereal, the order of introducing foods is variable; a recommended sequence is fruit, then vegetables, and then meat.
Introduce one food at a time, usually at intervals of 4 to 7 days, to identify food allergies.
Introduce solids when infant is hungry.
Begin spoon feeding by pushing food to back of tongue because of infant's natural tendency to thrust tongue forward.
Use small spoon with straight handle; begin with 1 or 2 teaspoons of food; gradually increase to 2 to 3 tablespoons per feeding.
As the quantity of solids increases, decrease the quantity of milk to prevent overfeeding. Limit formula or milk to approximately 960 ml (32 ounces) daily, and fruit juice to less than 180 ml (6 ounces) daily.
Never introduce foods by mixing them with the formula in the bottle.

Cereal—Start at 4 to 6 Months of Age
Introduce commercially prepared iron-fortified infant cereals and administer daily until 18 months.
Rice cereal is usually introduced first because of its low allergenic potential.
Parents can discontinue supplemental iron once cereal is given.

Fruits and Vegetables—Start at 6 to 8 Months of Age
Applesauce, bananas, and pears are usually well tolerated.
Avoid fruits and vegetables marketed in cans that are not specifically designed for infants because of variable and sometimes high lead content and addition of salt, sugar, or preservatives.
Offer fruit juice only from a cup, not a bottle, to reduce the development of nursing caries.

Meat, Fish, and Poultry—Start at 8 to 10 Months of Age
Avoid fatty meats.
Prepare by baking, broiling, steaming, or poaching.
Include organ meats such as liver, which has a high iron, vitamin A, and vitamin B complex content.
If soup is given, be certain all ingredients are familiar to child's diet.
Avoid commercial meat-vegetable combinations because protein is low.

Eggs and Cheese—Start at 12 Months of Age
Serve egg yolk hard boiled and mashed, soft cooked, or poached.
Introduce egg white in small quantities (1 teaspoon) toward end of first year to detect an allergy.
Use cheese as a substitute for meat and as finger food.

*Breastfeeding or commercial formula feeding for up to 12 months of age is recommended. After 1 year, whole cow's milk can be given.

front of the tongue and pushed out is simply scooped up and refed. As infants become accustomed to the spoon, they will more eagerly accept the food and eventually open the mouth in anticipation (or keep it closed in dislike). Because the first introduction of food is a new experience, spoon feeding should be attempted after ingestion of some breast milk or formula to associate this activity with a pleasurable and satisfying experience. Trying to introduce a food after the entire milk feeding is generally useless because the infant is satiated and has no inclination to try something new.

After several spoon feedings, food can be introduced at the beginning of a meal. It is best to introduce many foods during the first year, when the infant is more likely to eat them because of a hearty appetite resulting from a rapid growth rate. During the toddler years eating becomes less of an adventure, and strong food preferences emerge.

One food item is introduced at intervals of 4 to 7 days to allow for identification of food allergies. New foods are fed in small amounts, from 1 teaspoon to a few tablespoons. As the amount of solid food increases, the quantity of milk is decreased to less than 1 L/day to prevent overfeeding.

Because feeding is a learning process, as well as a means of nutrition, new foods are given alone to allow the child to learn new tastes and textures. Food should not be mixed in the bottle and fed through a nipple with a large hole. This deprives the child of the pleasure of learning new tastes and developing a discriminating palate. It can also cause problems with poor chewing of food later in life because of lack of experience. Guidelines for the introduction of new foods are given in the Family-Centered Care box.

Introducing solid foods can be an exciting time for parent and child. Most infants are good eaters and enjoy eating from a spoon and later feeding themselves. However, the transition from "parent doing it" to "baby doing it" can be a trying experience, particularly for those who value a clean house or who view cleaning up the mess as a waste of time. Finger foods such as soft fruits or vegetables are just as good as playthings as food; they can be squeezed, smeared, squashed, and thoroughly painted on oneself, others, and the environment. However, all of this is part of learning, and mastery follows many accidents.

Weaning

Defined as the process of giving up one method of feeding for another, **weaning** usually refers to relinquishing the breast or bottle for a cup. In Western societies this is generally regarded as a major task for infants and is often seen as a potentially traumatic experience. It is psychologically significant because the infant is required to give up a major source of oral pleasure and gratification.

There is no one time for weaning that is best for every child, but generally most infants show signs of readiness during the second half of the first year. They have learned that good things come from a spoon. It is recommended that weaning be accomplished with the infant's needs as a guide (Lawrence and Lawrence, 2005). Their increasing desire for freedom of movement may lessen their desire to be held close for feedings. They are acquiring more control over their actions and can easily manipulate a cup to their lips (even if it is held upside down!). Imitation becomes a powerful motivator by age 8 or 9 months, and they enjoy using a cup or glass like others do.

Weaning should be gradual by replacing one bottle or breastfeeding session at a time. The nighttime feeding is usually the last feeding to be discontinued. It is advisable to never allow a child to take a bottle of milk to bed—this is a major cause of nursing caries in deciduous teeth. If breastfeeding is terminated before 5 or 6 months of age, weaning should be to a bottle to provide for the infant's continued sucking needs. If discontinued later, weaning can be directly to a cup, especially by age 12 to 14 months. Any sweet liquid, such as fruit juice, should be given in a cup, and not at bedtime.

SLEEP AND ACTIVITY

Sleep patterns vary among infants, with active infants typically sleeping less than placid children. Generally, by 3 to 4 months of age most infants have developed a nocturnal pattern of sleep that lasts 9 to 11 hours. The total daily sleep is approximately 15 hours. The number of naps per day varies, but infants may take one or two naps by the end of the first year. Breast-fed infants usually sleep for shorter periods, with more frequent waking, especially during the night, compared with bottle-fed infants (Quillin and Glenn, 2004); average total sleep for 4-week-old infants in this study was 14 hours. Because of the trend toward breastfeeding, sleep norms such as those previously described, which were based primarily on bottle-fed infants, may not be relevant.

Most infants are naturally active and need no encouragement to be mobile. Problems can arise when devices such as playpens, strollers, commercial swings, and mobile walkers are used excessively. These items restrict movement and prevent infants from exploring and developing gross motor skills. Contrary to popular belief, mobile walkers do not enhance coordination and are dangerous if tipped over or placed near stairs. The American Academy of Pediatrics (2001a) recommended a ban on the sale of infant walkers because of the large number of injuries. Newer models of infant walkers have been designed to decrease infant injuries (see Falls, p. 370).

Sleep Problems

A number of sleep problems are identified in small children. The two major categories are the **dyssomnias:** the child has trouble either falling or staying asleep at night, or has difficulty staying awake during the day. The second category, **parasomnias,** are characterized as confusional arousals, sleepwalking, sleep terrors, nightmares, and rhythmic movement disorders; these typically occur in children 3 to 8 years old (Dahl, 1998) and decline in incidence as the child matures (Davis, Parker, and Montgomery, 2004). This discussion focuses on minor sleep issues in infants such as refusal to go to sleep or frequent waking during the night (Table 10-3). Other sleep disturbances such as obstructive sleep apnea and sleep terrors are discussed elsewhere in this text.

Concerns regarding sleep are common during infancy (see Cultural Awareness box). Sometimes these concerns are as basic as parents' questioning whether the infant needs additional sleep. In this case it is best to investigate the reason for their concern, stressing the individual needs of each child. Infants who are active during wakeful periods and growing normally are sleeping a sufficient amount of time.

Sleep problems in early infancy have also been positively correlated with higher maternal depression scores (Hiscock and Wake, 2001; Hawkins-Walsh, 2003) and poorer general and mental health in both mother and father (Martin, Hiscock,

TABLE 10-3

Selected Sleep Disturbances During Infancy and Early Childhood

DISORDER AND DESCRIPTION	MANAGEMENT
NIGHTTIME FEEDING Child has a prolonged need for middle-of-night bottle or breastfeeding. Child goes to sleep at breast or with a bottle. Awakenings are frequent (may be hourly). Child returns to sleep after feeding; other comfort measures (e.g., rocking or holding) are usually ineffective.	Increase daytime feeding intervals to 4 hours or more (may need to be done gradually). Offer last feeding as late as possible at night; may need to gradually reduce amount of formula or length of breastfeeding. Offer no bottles in bed. Put to bed awake. When child is crying, check at progressively longer intervals each night; reassure child but do not hold, rock, take to parent's bed, or give bottle or pacifier.
DEVELOPMENTAL NIGHT CRYING Child age 6 to 12 months with undisturbed nighttime sleep now awakes abruptly; may be accompanied by nightmares.	Reassure parents that this phase is temporary. Enter room immediately to check on child but keep reassurances brief. Avoid feeding, rocking, taking to parent's bed, or any other routine that may initiate trained night crying.
REFUSAL TO GO TO SLEEP Child resists bedtime and comes out of room repeatedly. Nighttime sleep may be continuous, but frequent awakenings and refusal to return to sleep may occur and become a problem if parent allows child to deviate from usual sleep pattern.	Evaluate if hour of sleep is too early (child may resist sleep if not tired). Assist parents in establishing consistent before-bedtime routine and enforcing consistent limits regarding child's bedtime behavior. If child persists in leaving bedroom, close door for progressively longer periods. Use reward system with child to provide motivation.
TRAINED NIGHT CRYING (INAPPROPRIATE SLEEP ASSOCIATIONS) Child typically falls asleep in place other than own bed (e.g., rocking chair or parent's bed) and is brought to own bed while asleep; on awakening, cries until usual routine is instituted (e.g., rocking).	Put child in own bed when awake. If possible, arrange sleeping area separate from other family members. When child is crying, check at progressively longer intervals each night; reassure child but do not resume usual routine.
NIGHTTIME FEARS Child resists going to bed or wakes during the night because of fears. Child seeks parent's physical presence and falls asleep easily with parent nearby, unless fear is overwhelming.	Evaluate if hour of sleep is too early (child may fantasize when nothing to do but think in dark room). Calmly reassure the frightened child; keeping a night-light on may be helpful. Use reward system with child to provide motivation to deal with fears. Avoid patterns that can lead to additional problems (e.g., sleeping with child or taking child to parent's room). If child's fear is overwhelming, consider desensitization (e.g., progressively spending longer periods of time alone; consult professional help for protracted fears). Distinguish between nightmares and sleep terrors (confused partial arousals).

Modified from Ferber R: Behavioral "insomnia" in the child, *Psychiatr Clin North Am* 10(4):641-653, 1987.

Hardy, and others, 2007); therefore nurses must discuss infant sleep problems with the mother (and family) in addition to other developmental aspects of newborn care.

When a sleeping problem is presented, a careful assessment is essential. Charting sleep habits both before and after interventions is also an important strategy. Questions regarding the frequency and duration of waking, the usual bedtime routine, the number of nighttime feedings, the perceived problem (e.g., how much disruption the behavior generates), and the attempted interventions are important in planning effective approaches designed for the specific sleep problem. A common suggestion given for any type of sleep problem, "Let the child cry until he or she falls asleep," is very difficult to implement and is inappropriate for certain conditions. After the parents relent and console the child, they have only reinforced the crying.

Another approach to night crying is known as **graduated extinction.** This involves letting the child cry for progressively longer times between brief parental interventions that consist only of reassurance—not rocking, holding, or using a bottle or pacifier. For example, the parents may check on the child every 5 minutes (of crying) during the first night and progressively extend this interval by 5 minutes on successive nights (Ferber and Kryger, 1995).

Families who cannot tolerate unexpected crying spells while everyone else is asleep can try the two-step approach. Graduated extinction is used during naps and at bedtime until the parents retire. If the child cries during the night, the parents use comforting measures. However, after the child is partially trained, step 2 is initiated—the use of graduated extinction at all times.

Children who learn to fall asleep on their own at bedtime have longer sustained sleep periods than those who fall asleep with a parent present (Davis, Parker, and Montgomery, 2004). In addition, comforting children outside their own bed at night once they awaken was associated with poor sleep con-

CULTURAL AWARENESS

The Family Bed

Cosleeping, or sharing the "family bed," in which parents allow the children to sleep with them, is a relatively common and accepted practice, especially among African-American, Hispanic, and Asian families such as the Japanese (Schachter, Fuchs, Bijer, and others, 1989). One survey indicates the practice is growing in some parts of the United States, especially among young (<18 years of age) African-American and Asian women in the Southern states; infants in the survey who coslept with an adult were less than 8 weeks old (Willinger, Ko, Hoffman, and others, 2003). Other groups that practice cosleeping include (1) single parents, whose need for company may encourage this practice; (2) working parents, who desire the closeness at night that was lost during the day; and (3) parents who have had an issue about sleep or separation in their own past (Brazelton, 1990).

Ball (2003) reported a positive relationship between parent-infant bed sharing and increased frequency of breastfeeding in the United Kingdom. The Academy of Breastfeeding Medicine (2003) suggests there is insufficient data to prevent parents from cosleeping and emphasizes that parents be informed of the risks and benefits of cosleeping. Despite initial popular belief that cosleeping would prevent sudden infant death syndrome (SIDS), no scientific evidence supports this theory (American Academy of Pediatrics, 2000); however, there is evidence that the infant sleeping in the same room as the mother reduces the risk for SIDS (American Academy of Pediatrics, 2005). There is evidence of an increase in the number of infant deaths by suffocation associated with bed sharing and the use of adult beds, particularly in infants less than 3 months old (Drago and Dannenberg, 1999). A study from Scotland indicates that the risk for SIDS when bed sharing is significantly increased for infants less than 11 weeks of age (Tappin, Ecob, and Brooke, 2005). Other studies have correlated higher incidences of SIDS and infant cosleeping with maternal smoking, cosleeping with multiple family members, maternal overweight, soft bedding, and unintentional asphyxiation resulting from adult intoxication (overlaying)

(American Academy of Pediatrics, 2000, 2005; Hauck, Herman, Donovan, and others, 2003; Carroll-Pankhurst and Mortimer, 2001; Person, Lavezzi, and Wolf, 2002; McGarvey, McDonnell, Chong, and others, 2003).

One of the difficulties in interpreting the available data on the studies of infant-parent cosleeping to date is the terminology used (Mesich, 2005). At times parents may place the infant to sleep in the adult bed, then carry the child to her or his own bed after a time (although some experts advise this does not help the child sleep through the night). In some cases a breastfeeding mother may wish to have the infant with her in an adult bed for feeding and comfort, and then place the child in a crib or bassinette. Whether these incidents constitute cosleeping in the larger studies that identified cosleeping as a risk factor for SIDS is not clear. Further studies must clearly define the terminology of cosleeping. As Willinger, Ko, Hoffman, and others (2003) point out, further studies on infant cosleeping are needed to clarify the issues because the practice is not only growing but also has cultural meaning in some populations. In a recent article, Mesich (2005) encouraged nurses to become familiar with the various studies and terminology regarding parent cosleeping to counsel parents effectively.

The latest recommendation for cosleeping from the American Academy of Pediatrics is that the infant's crib or bassinette be placed in close proximity to the mother's bed and that the infant be placed in the adult bed only for breastfeeding purposes, then placed to sleep in his or her own crib (American Academy of Pediatrics, 2005). Other recommendations included avoidance of soft bedding, overheating the infant, prone or side position to sleep, maternal smoking in pregnancy and second-hand smoke exposure for the infant, and placing the infant to sleep on a couch or armchair (American Academy of Pediatrics, 2005).

Population-based studies of infant cosleeping and SIDS are currently in progress; until evidence-based data are available to support or condemn the practice, parents should carefully evaluate the options available for sharing the family bed with infants, particularly under conditions known to place the infant at high risk for asphyxiation.

---

solidation. Feeding the 5-month-old after awakening at night has been associated with fewer consecutive sleep hours (Touchette, Petit, Paquet, and others, 2005). The authors of this study recommend parental presence at bedtime until the child is drowsy, then placing the child in his or her own bed for a night's sleep.

The best way to prevent sleep problems is to encourage parents to establish bedtime rituals that do not foster problematic patterns. One of the most constructive is placing infants awake in their own crib. When infants are accustomed to falling asleep somewhere else, such as in their parent's arms, and then being transferred to their crib, they awaken in unfamiliar surroundings and are unable to fall asleep until the routine is repeated. Also, the bed should be used for sleeping only—not as a playpen. It is advisable not to hang playthings over or on the bed; in this way the child associates the bed with sleep, not with activity. Although the interventions described previously and in Table 10-3 are usually successful, it is much easier to prevent the problem with appropriate counseling during the early months of the infant's life.

DENTAL HEALTH

Good infant dental hygiene begins with appropriate maternal dental health prior to and during the pregnancy and counseling during early infancy regarding dietary intake for the promotion

of optimum oral hygiene (Douglass, Douglass, and Silk, 2004). Parents are counseled early regarding the risk of feeding practices that increase the risk of poor dental health. Some of these, as previously mentioned, include avoiding propping the milk bottle, giving the milk bottle in the bed, or giving fruit juices in a bottle, especially before 6 months of age.

Once the primary teeth erupt, cleaning should begin. The teeth and gums are initially cleaned by wiping with a damp cloth; toothbrushing is too harsh for the tender gingiva. The caregiver can stabilize the infant by cradling the child with one arm and using the free hand to cleanse the teeth. Oral hygiene can be made pleasant by singing or talking to the infant. It is recommended that the infant have an oral health examination by 6 months of age from a qualified pediatric health practitioner. Infants at high risk for dental caries should be seen by a dentist between 6 months and 1 year of age (American Academy of Pediatric Dentistry, 2006). It is generally recommended that a small, soft-bristled toothbrush be used as more teeth erupt and the infant adjusts to the routine of cleaning. Water is preferred to toothpaste, which the infant will swallow (and if the toothpaste is fluoridated, the infant will ingest excessive amounts of fluoride).

Fluoride, an essential mineral for building caries-resistant teeth, is needed beginning at 6 months of age if the infant does not receive water with adequate fluoride content. The Ameri-

Case Study—Immunizations

Keeping Current on Vaccine Recommendations

It is much easier to keep current if you know where to look for the official recommendations of the American Academy of Pediatrics and the Centers for Disease Control and Prevention's (CDC's) Advisory Committee on Immunization Practices (ACIP). The primary sources are publications and the Internet. You can also contact each organization to request information:

American Academy of Pediatrics
141 Northwest Point Blvd.
Elk Grove Village, IL 60007
(847) 434-4000
Fax: (847) 434-8000
http://www.aap.org

Centers for Disease Control and Prevention
1600 Clifton Road NE
Atlanta, GA 30333
(404) 639-3311
http://www.cdc.gov
Information Hotline: (800) 232-4636 (English and Spanish)
International Travel Hotline: (877) 394-8747
Vaccines and immunizations: http://www.cdc.gov/vaccines

The CDC now offers a valuable resource tool for parents and clinicians online. The tool will print out an individualized vaccination schedule with dates associated with each vaccination based on the child's date of birth. Clinicians can use this tool for children under 5 years of age to serve as a reminder for parents. Nurses should note that the personalized tool is based on the current immunization schedule and may need to be adjusted with the yearly updates from the American Academy of Pediatrics and ACIP. The tool is available at http://www2a.cdc.gov/nip/kidstuff/newscheduler_le.

The American Academy of Pediatrics' **Report of the Committee on Infectious Diseases,** known as the **Red Book,** is an authoritative source of information on vaccines and other important pediatric infectious diseases (American Academy of Pediatrics, 2006b). However, it lacks an in-depth review and reference list of controversial issues. The recommendations in the *Red Book* first appear in the journal *Pediatrics* or the *AAP News.* Typically, the most recent immunization schedule appears in the January issue of the journal.

A publication of the CDC, *Morbidity and Mortality Weekly Report* (MMWR), contains comprehensive reviews of the literature and important background data regarding vaccine efficacy and side effects. To receive an electronic copy, send an e-mail message to listserv@listserv.cdc.gov. The body content should read: *SUBscribe mmwr-toc.* Electronic copy also is available from the CDC's website at http://www.cdc.gov or from the CDC's file transfer protocol server at ftp://ftp.cdc.gov.

Immunofacts—Immunization Gateway: Your Vaccine Fact-Finder at http://www.immunofacts.com provides direct links to all of the best vaccine resources on the Internet.

Vaccine information statements (VISs) are available by calling your state or local health department. They can also be downloaded from the **Immunization Action Coalition's** website at http://www.immunize.org/vis or the CDC's website at http://www.cdc.gov/vaccines/pubs/vis/default.htm. Several language translations are available. The Immunization Action Coalition has various publications for parents and older children (adolescents) on different immunizations and in several languages.

can Academy of Pediatric Dentistry recommends fluoride supplementation begin at 6 months. The fluoride dosage has been decreased from earlier recommendations because of an increased occurrence of dental fluorosis from excessive fluoride ingestion. The latest recommendation is to give children 6 months to 3 years of age 0.25 mg of fluoride daily if water fluoride content is less than 0.3 ppm (parts per million) (American Academy of Pediatric Dentistry, 2006). If bottled water is used to reconstitute powdered or concentrated formula, it should either be fluoride free or contain low levels of fluoride (American Dental Association, 2007).

Dietary considerations are also important because habits begun during infancy tend to continue into later years. Foods with concentrated sugar are used sparingly (if at all) in the infant's diet. The practice of coating pacifiers with honey or using commercially available hard-candy pacifiers is discouraged. Besides being cariogenic, honey also may cause infant botulism, and parts of the candy pacifier can be aspirated (see Aspiration of Foreign Objects, p. 365). Parents need to be counseled regarding the detrimental effects of frequent and prolonged bottle feeding or breastfeeding during sleep, when the sweet milk or other fluid, such as juice, bathes the teeth, producing nursing caries. In addition, carbonated beverages should be avoided in infancy. (See also Chapter 12 for a more extensive discussion of dental care, including nursing caries.)

IMMUNIZATIONS

One of the most dramatic advances in pediatrics has been the decline of infectious diseases during the twentieth century because of the widespread use of immunization for preventable diseases. Although many of the immunizations can be given to individuals of any age, the recommended primary schedule begins during infancy and, with the exception of boosters, is completed during early childhood. Therefore health promotion during infancy includes a discussion of childhood immunizations for diphtheria, tetanus, and pertussis (DTaP, using acellular pertussis); poliovirus; measles, mumps, and rubella (MMR); *Haemophilus influenzae* type b (Hib); hepatitis B virus (HepB); hepatitis A virus (HepA); meningococcal; pneumococcal conjugate vaccine (PCV); influenza; rotavirus vaccine; and chickenpox (varicella). Selected vaccines generally reserved for children considered at high risk for the disease are discussed here and as appropriate throughout the text. (See also Communicable Diseases, Chapter 14, for a discussion of several of the diseases for which vaccines are available.)

Schedule for Immunizations

In the United States two organizations—the Advisory Committee on Immunization Practices of the Centers for Disease Control and Prevention, and the Committee on Infectious Diseases of the American Academy of Pediatrics—govern the recommendations for immunization policies and procedures. In Canada, recommendations are from the National Advisory Committee on Immunization under the authority of the minister of health and Public Health Agency of Canada. The policies of each committee are *recommendations,* not rules, and they change as a result of advances in the field of immunology. Nurses need to keep informed of the latest advances and changes in policy (see Community Focus box).

In the United States the recommended age for beginning primary immunizations of infants is within 2 weeks of birth or, in special circumstances, at birth (Fig. 10-11, *A*). Infants born preterm should receive the full dose of each vaccine at the appropriate chronologic age. Recommended schedules for children not immunized during infancy are included in Fig. 10-12. Table 10-4 describes Canadian immunization schedules for children.

Children who began primary immunizations at the recommended age but fail to receive all of the doses do not need to begin the series again but instead receive only the missed doses. For situations in which there is doubt that the child will return for immunizations according to the optimum schedule, any of the recommended vaccines can be administered simultaneously. Parenteral vaccines are given in separate syringes in different injection sites (American Academy of Pediatrics, 2006b). The product brand names, routes of administration, and manufacturers for the principal childhood vaccinations are listed in Table 10-7.

Recommendations for Routine Immunizations

Hepatitis A Virus (HAV). HAV has been recognized as a significant child health problem, particularly in communities where widespread childhood hepatitis A immunization is not recommended. HAV is spread by the fecal-oral route and from person-to-person contact, by ingestion of contaminated food or water, and rarely by blood transfusion. The illness has an abrupt onset, with fever, malaise, anorexia, nausea, abdominal discomfort, dark urine, and jaundice being the most common clinical signs of infection. In children under 6 years of age the disease may be asymptomatic, and jaundice is rarely evident.

HAV vaccine is now recommended for all children beginning at age 1 year (i.e., 12 months to 23 months); the second dose in the two-dose series may be administered no sooner than 6 months after the first dose. Since the implementation of widespread childhood HepA vaccination, infection rates among children ages 5 to 14 years have declined significantly (Centers for Disease Control and Prevention, 2006a). For further information see footnote 9 in Fig. 10-11, *A*.

Hepatitis B Virus (HBV). HBV is an important pediatric disease because HBV infections that occur during childhood and adolescence can lead to fatal consequences from cirrhosis or liver cancer during adulthood. Up to 90% of infants infected perinatally and 25% to 50% of children infected before age 5 years become HBV carriers. In addition, the incidence of HBV infection increases rapidly during adolescence (American Academy of Pediatrics, 2006b). Past immunization strategies targeted several high-risk groups, including health care workers and others in contact with blood and body fluids, recipients of certain blood products (such as those with hemophilia), heterosexuals with multiple partners, sexually active homosexual and bisexual men, intravenous drug abusers, immigrants from countries in which HBV is widespread, and children born to mothers who are hepatitis B surface antigen (HBsAg)–positive.

To improve immunization rates, current recommendations include vaccinations for all newborns. Both full-term and preterm infants born to mothers whose HBsAg status is positive should receive HepB, 0.5 ml, within 12 hours of birth. If the mother's HBsAg status is unknown, her blood should be drawn for HBsAg status determination; if she is positive, the infant should receive hepatitis B immune globulin (HBIG), 0.5 ml, as soon as possible but no later than age 1 week. Because the immune response to HepB is not optimum in newborns weighing less than 2000 g (4.4 pounds), the first HepB dose should be given to such infants at 1 month, as long as the mother's HBsAg status is negative (American Academy of Pediatrics, 2006b). Only the single-antigen (monovalent) HepB should be given as the first dose (see also Fig. 10-11, *A*, footnote 1).

In the late 1990s HepB contained small amounts of mercury (thimerosal) as a preservative, which generated concern regarding possible mercury poisoning in infants and led to a subsequent decrease in hepatitis B immunization rates in newborns. However, a preservative-free HepB (Recombivax HB, pediatric-adolescent formulation) is available, and the Centers for Disease Control and Prevention (2005a) strongly recommends that HepB immunization occur in newborns before discharge from the birth hospital. To date, studies have not found any association between thimerosal in vaccines and neurologic developmental disorders such as autism spectrum disorder (Parker, Schwartz, Todd, and others, 2004; Heron, Golding, and ALSPAC Study Team, 2004). The American Academy of Pediatrics (2006b) also encourages immunization of all children by age 11 years.

The vaccine is given intramuscularly in the vastus lateralis muscle in newborns or in the deltoid muscle for toddlers and children. Regardless of age, the dorsogluteal site is avoided because it has been associated with low antibody seroconversion rates, indicating a reduced immune response (Zuckerman, Cockcroft, and Zuckerman, 1992). No data exist regarding the seroconversion when the ventrogluteal site is used. The vaccine can be safely administered simultaneously at a separate site with DTaP, MMR, and Hib vaccines.

Diphtheria. Although cases of diphtheria are rarely seen in the United States, the disease can result in significant morbidity. Respiratory manifestations include respiratory nasopharyngitis or obstructive laryngotracheitis with upper airway obstruction. The cutaneous manifestations of the disease include vaginal, otic, conjunctival, or cutaneous lesions, which are primarily seen in the tropics (American Academy of Pediatrics, 2006b). Diphtheria vaccine is commonly administered (1) in combination with tetanus and pertussis vaccines (DTaP) or DTaP and Hib vaccines for children younger than 7 years of age, (2) in combination with a conjugate Hib vaccine (see Fig. 10-11, *A*, footnote 4), (3) in a combined vaccine with tetanus (DT) for children younger than 7 years of age who have some contraindication to receiving pertussis vaccine, or (4) as a single antigen when combined antigen preparations are not indicated.

Although the diphtheria vaccine does not produce absolute immunity, protective antitoxin persists for 10 years or more when given according to the recommended schedule, and boosters are given every 10 years for life (see discussion below for adolescent diphtheria and acellular pertussis and tetanus toxoid recommendation). Several vaccines contain diphtheria toxoid (Hib, meningococcal, pneumococcal), but this does not confer immunity to the disease.

Tetanus. Tetanus vaccine comes in three forms: tetanus toxoid, tetanus immunoglobulin (TIG) (human), and tetanus antitoxin (equine antitoxin). However, tetanus antitoxin is no longer available in the United States. Tetanus toxoid is used for

Text continued on p. 356

For those who fall behind or start late, see the catch-up schedule

Vaccine ▼ Age ►	Birth	1 month	2 months	4 months	6 months	12 months	15 months	18 months	19–23 months	2–3 years	4–6 years
Hepatitis B[1]	HepB	HepB		see footnote 1		HepB					
Rotavirus[2]			Rota	Rota	Rota						
Diphtheria, Tetanus, Pertussis[3]			DTaP	DTaP	DTaP	see footnote 3	DTaP				DTaP
Haemophilus influenzae type b[4]			Hib	Hib	Hib[4]	Hib					
Pneumococcal[5]			PCV	PCV	PCV	PCV				PPV	
Inactivated Poliovirus			IPV	IPV		IPV					IPV
Influenza[6]						Influenza (Yearly)					
Measles, Mumps, Rubella[7]						MMR					MMR
Varicella[8]						Varicella					Varicella
Hepatitis A[9]						HepA (2 doses)				HepA Series	
Meningococcal[10]										MCV4	

Range of recommended ages

Certain high-risk groups

This schedule indicates the recommended ages for routine administration of currently licensed childhood vaccines, as of December 1, 2007, for children aged 0 through 6 years. Additional information is available at www.cdc.gov/vaccines/recs/schedules. Any dose not administered at the recommended age should be administered at any subsequent visit, when indicated and feasible. Additional vaccines may be licensed and recommended during the year. Licensed combination vaccines may be used whenever any components of the combination are indicated and other components of the vaccine are not contraindicated and if approved by the Food and Drug Administration for that dose of the series. **Providers should consult the respective Advisory Committee on Immunization Practices statement for detailed recommendations, including for high risk conditions:** http://www.cdc.gov/vaccines/pubs/ACIP-list.htm. Clinically significant adverse events that follow immunization should be reported to the Vaccine Adverse Event Reporting System (VAERS). Guidance about how to obtain and complete VAERS form is available at www.vaers.hhs.gov or by telephone, 800-822-7967.

1. Hepatitis B vaccine (HepB). *(Minimum age: birth)*
At birth:
- Administer monovalent HepB to all newborns prior to hospital discharge.
- If mother is hepatitis B surface antigen (HBsAg)-positive, administer HepB and 0.5 mL of hepatitis B immune globulin (HBIG) within 12 hours of birth.
- If mother's HBsAg status is unknown, administer HepB within 12 hours of birth. Determine the HBsAg status as soon as possible and if HBsAg-positive, administer HBIG (no later than age 1 week).
- If mother is HBsAg-negative, the birth dose can be delayed, **in rare cases,** with a provider's order and a **copy of the mother's** negative HBsAg laboratory report in the infant's medical record.

After the birth dose:
- The HepB series should be completed with either monovalent HepB or a combination vaccine containing HepB. The second dose should be administered at age 1–2 months. The final dose should be administered no earlier than age 24 weeks. Infants born to HBsAg-positive mothers should be tested for HBsAg and antibody to HBsAg after completion of at least 3 doses of a licensed HepB series, at age 9–18 months (generally at the next well-child visit).

4-month dose:
- It is permissible to administer 4 doses of HepB when combination vaccines are administered after the birth dose. If monovalent HepB is used for doses after the birth dose, a dose at age 4 months is not needed.

2. Rotavirus vaccine (Rota). *(Minimum age: 6 weeks)*
- Administer the first dose at age 6–12 weeks.
- Do not start the series later than age 12 weeks.
- Administer the final dose in the series by age 32 weeks. Do not administer any dose later than age 32 weeks.
- Data on safety and efficacy outside of these age ranges are insufficient.

3. Diphtheria and tetanus toxoids and acellular pertussis vaccine (DTaP). *(Minimum age: 6 weeks)*
- The fourth dose of DTaP may be administered as early as age 12 months, provided 6 months have elapsed since the third dose.
- Administer the final dose in the series at age 4–6 years.

4. Haemophilus influenzae type b conjugate vaccine (Hib). *(Minimum age: 6 weeks)*
- If PRP-OMP (PedvaxHIB® or ComVax® [Merck]) is administered at ages 2 and 4 months, a dose at age 6 months is not required.
- TriHIBit® (DTaP/Hib) combination products should not be used for primary immunization but can be used as boosters following any Hib vaccine in children age 12 months or older.

5. Pneumococcal vaccine. *(Minimum age: 6 weeks for pneumococcal conjugate vaccine [PCV]; 2 years for pneumococcal polysaccharide vaccine [PPV])*
- Administer one dose of PCV to all healthy children aged 24–59 months having any incomplete schedule.
- Administer PPV to children aged 2 years and older with underlying medical conditions.

6. Influenza vaccine. *(Minimum age: 6 months for trivalent inactivated influenza vaccine [TIV]; 2 years for live, attenuated influenza vaccine [LAIV])*
- Administer annually to children aged 6–59 months and to all close contacts of children aged 0–59 months.
- Administer annually to children 5 years of age and older with certain risk factors, to other persons (including household members) in close contact with persons in groups at higher risk, and to any child whose parents request vaccination.
- For healthy nonpregnant persons (those who do not have underlying medical conditions that predispose them to influenza complications) ages 2–49 years, either LAIV or TIV may be used.
- Children receiving TIV should receive 0.25 mL if age 6-35 mos or 0.5 mL if age 3 years or older.
- Administer 2 doses (separated by 4 weeks or longer) to children younger than 9 years who are receiving influenza vaccine for the first time or who were vaccinated for the first time last season, but only received one dose.

7. Measles, mumps, and rubella vaccine (MMR). *(Minimum age: 12 months)*
- Administer the second dose of MMR at age 4–6 years. MMR may be administered before age 4–6 years, provided 4 weeks or more have elapsed since the first dose.

8. Varicella vaccine. *(Minimum age: 12 months)*
- Administer second dose at age 4–6 years; may be administered 3 months or more after first dose.
- Don't repeat second dose if administered 28 days or more after first dose.

9. Hepatitis A vaccine (HepA). *(Minimum age: 12 months)*
- HepA is recommended for all children aged 1 yr (i.e., aged 12–23 months). The 2 doses in the series should be administered at least 6 months apart.
- Children not fully vaccinated by age 2 years can be vaccinated at subsequent visits.
- HepA is recommended for certain other groups of children, including in areas where vaccination programs target older children.

10. Meningococcal vaccine. *(Minimum age: 2 years for meningococcal conjugate vaccine (MCV4) and for meningococcal polysaccharide vaccine (MPSV4))*
- MCV4 is recommended for children aged 2–10 years with terminal complement deficiencies or anatomic or functional asplenia and certain other high-risk groups. Use of MPSV4 is also acceptable.
- Persons who received MPSV4 3 or more years prior and remain at increased risk for meningococcal disease should be vaccinated with MCV4.

The Recommended Immunization Schedules for Persons Aged 0–18 Years are approved by the Advisory Committee on Immunization Practices (www.cdc.gov/vaccines/recs/acip), the American Academy of Pediatrics (http://www.aap.org), and the American Academy of Family Physicians (http://www.aafp.org).

DEPARTMENT OF HEALTH AND HUMAN SERVICES • CENTERS FOR DISEASE CONTROL AND PREVENTION • SAFER • HEATHIER • PEOPLE™

A

FIG. 10-11 ■ Recommended immunization schedules for persons aged 0 to 6 years **(A)** and 7 to 18 years **(B)**—United States, 2008. (From Centers for Disease Control and Prevention: Recommended immunization schedules for persons aged 0-18 years—United States, 2008. *MMWR* 56[51 and 52]:Q1-Q4, 2007.)

For those who fall behind or start late, see the green bars and the catch-up schedule

Vaccine ▼ Age ►	7-10 years	11-12 years	13-18 years
Diphtheria, Tetanus, Pertussis[1]	*see footnote 1*	**Tdap**	**Tdap**
Human Papillomavirus[2]	*see footnote 2*	**HPV (3 doses)**	**HPV Series**
Meningococcal[3]	**MCV4**	**MCV4**	**MCV4**
Pneumococcal[4]	**PPV**		
Influenza[5]	**Influenza (Yearly)**		
Hepatitis A[6]	**HepA Series**		
Hepatitis B[7]	**HepB Series**		
Inactivated Poliovirus[8]	**IPV Series**		
Measles, Mumps, Rubella[9]	**MMR Series**		
Varicella[10]	**Varicella Series**		

Legend:
- Range of recommended ages
- Catch-up immunization
- Certain high-risk groups

This schedule indicates the recommended ages for routine administration of currently licensed childhood vaccines, as of December 1, 2007, for children aged 7–18 years. Additional information is available at www.cdc.gov/vaccines/recs/schedules. Any dose not administered at the recommended age should be administered at any subsequent visit, when indicated and feasible. Additional vaccines may be licensed and recommended during the year. Licensed combination vaccines may be used whenever any components of the combination are indicated and other components of the vaccine are not contraindicated and if approved by the Food and Drug Administration for that dose of the series. **Providers should consult the respective Advisory Committee on Immunization Practices statement for detailed recommendations, including for high risk conditions:** http://www.cdc.gov/vaccines/pubs/ACIP-list.htm. Clinically significant adverse events that follow immunization should be reported to the Vaccine Adverse Event Reporting System (VAERS). Guidance about how to obtain and complete VAERS form is available at www.vaers.hhs.gov or by telephone, 800-822-7967.

1. Tetanus and diphtheria toxoids and acellular pertussis vaccine (Tdap). *(Minimum age: 10 years for BOOSTRIX® and 11 years for ADACEL™)*
- Administer at age 11–12 years for those who have completed the recommended childhood DTP/DTaP vaccination series and have not received a tetanus and diphtheria toxoids (Td) booster dose.
- 13–18 year olds who missed the 11–12 year Tdap or received Td only, are encouraged to receive one dose of Tdap 5 years after the last Td/DTaP dose.

2. Human papillomavirus vaccine (HPV). *(Minimum age: 9 years)*
- Administer the first dose of the HPV vaccine series to females at age 11–12 years.
- Administer the second dose 2 months after the first dose and the third dose 6 months after the first dose.
- Administer the HPV vaccine series to females at age 13–18 years if not previously vaccinated.

3. Meningococcal vaccine.
- Administer MCV4 at age 11–12 years and at age 13–18 years if not previously vaccinated. MPSV4 is an acceptable alternative.
- Administer MCV4 to previously unvaccinated college freshmen living in dormitories.
- MCV4 is recommended for children aged 2-10 years with terminal complement deficiencies or anatomic or functional asplenia and certain other high-risk groups.
- Persons who received MPSV4 3 or more years prior and remain at increased risk for meningococcal disease should be vaccinated with MCV4.

4. Pneumococcal polysaccharide vaccine (PPV).
- Administer PPV to certain high-risk groups.

5. Influenza vaccine.
- Administer annually to all close contacts of children aged 0–59 months.
- Administer annually to persons with certain risk factors, health-care workers, and other persons (including household members) in close contact with persons in groups at higher risk.

- Administer 2 doses (separated by 4 weeks or longer) to children younger than 9 years who are receiving influenza vaccine for the first time or who were vaccinated for the first time last season, but only received one dose.
- For healthy nonpregnant persons (those who do not have underlying medical conditions that predispose them to influenza complications) ages 2–49 years, either LAIV or TIV may be used.

6. Hepatitis A vaccine (HepA).
- The 2 doses in the series should be administered at least 6 months apart.
- HepA is recommended for certain other groups of children, including in areas where vaccination programs target older children.

7. Hepatitis B vaccine (HepB).
- Administer the 3-dose series to those who were not previously vaccinated.
- A 2-dose series of Recombivax HB® is licensed for children aged 11–15 years.

8. Inactivated poliovirus vaccine (IPV).
- For children who received an all-IPV or all-oral poliovirus (OPV) series, a fourth dose is not necessary if the third dose was administered at age 4 years or older.
- If both OPV and IPV were administered as part of a series, a total of 4 doses should be administered, regardless of the child's current age.

9. Measles, mumps, and rubella vaccine (MMR).
- If not previously vaccinated, administer 2 doses of MMR during any visit, with 4 or more weeks between the doses.

10. Varicella vaccine.
- Administer 2 doses of varicella vaccine to persons younger than 13 years of age at least 3 months apart. Do not repeat the second dose, if administered 28 or more days following the first dose.
- Administer 2 doses of varicella vaccine to persons aged 13 years or older at least 4 weeks apart.

The Recommended Immunization Schedules for Persons Aged 0–18 Years are approved by the Advisory Committee on Immunization Practices (www.cdc.gov/vaccines/recs/acip), the American Academy of Pediatrics (http://www.aap.org), and the American Academy of Family Physicians (http://www.aafp.org).

DEPARTMENT OF HEALTH AND HUMAN SERVICES • CENTERS FOR DISEASE CONTROL AND PREVENTION
SAFER • HEALTHIER • PEOPLE™

B

FIG. 10-11, cont'd ■ Recommended immunization schedules for persons aged 0 to 6 years **(A)** and 7 to 18 years **(B)**—United States, 2008. (From Centers for Disease Control and Prevention: Recommended immunization schedules for persons aged 0-18 years—United States, 2008. *MMWR* 56[51 and 52]:Q1-Q4, 2007.)

The table below provides catch-up schedules and minimum intervals between doses for children whose vaccinations have been delayed. A vaccine series does not need to be restarted, regardless of the time that has elapsed between doses. Use the section appropriate for the child's age.

CATCH-UP SCHEDULE FOR PERSONS AGED 4 MONTHS–6 YEARS

Vaccine	Minimum Age for Dose 1	Minimum Interval Between Doses			
		Dose 1 to Dose 2	Dose 2 to Dose 3	Dose 3 to Dose 4	Dose 4 to Dose 5
Hepatitis B[1]	Birth	4 weeks	8 weeks (and 16 weeks after first dose)		
Rotavirus[2]	6 wks	4 weeks	4 weeks		
Diphtheria, Tetanus, Pertussis[3]	6 wks	4 weeks	4 weeks	6 months	6 months[3]
Haemophilus influenzae type b[4]	6 wks	4 weeks if first dose administered at younger than 12 months of age / 8 weeks (as final dose) if first dose administered at age 12-14 months / No further doses needed if first dose administered at 15 months of age or older	4 weeks[4] if current age is younger than 12 months / 8 weeks (as final dose)[4] if current age is 12 months or older and second dose administered at younger than 15 months of age / No further doses needed if previous dose administered at age 15 months or older	8 weeks (as final dose) This dose only necessary for children aged 12 months–5 years who received 3 doses before age 12 months	
Pneumococcal[5]	6 wks	4 weeks if first dose administered at younger than 12 months of age / 8 weeks (as final dose) if first dose administered at age 12 months or older or current age 24–59 months / No further doses needed for healthy children if first dose administered at age 24 months or older	4 weeks if current age is younger than 12 months / 8 weeks (as final dose) if current age is 12 months or older / No further doses needed for healthy children if previous dose administered at age 24 months or older	8 weeks (as final dose) This dose only necessary for children aged 12 months–5 years who received 3 doses before age 12 months	
Inactivated Poliovirus[6]	6 wks	4 weeks	4 weeks	4 weeks[6]	
Measles, Mumps, Rubella[7]	12 mos	4 weeks			
Varicella[8]	12 mos	3 months			
Hepatitis A[9]	12 mos	6 months			

CATCH-UP SCHEDULE FOR PERSONS AGED 7–18 YEARS

Vaccine	Minimum Age for Dose 1	Dose 1 to Dose 2	Dose 2 to Dose 3	Dose 3 to Dose 4	
Tetanus, Diphtheria/ Tetanus, Diphtheria, Pertussis[10]	7 yrs[10]	4 weeks	4 weeks if first dose administered at younger than 12 months of age / 6 months if first dose administered at age 12 months or older	6 months if first dose administered at younger than 12 months of age	
Human Papillomavirus[11]	9 yrs	4 weeks	12 weeks		
Hepatitis A[9]	12 mos	6 months			
Hepatitis B[1]	Birth	4 weeks	8 weeks (and 16 weeks after first dose)		
Inactivated Poliovirus[6]	6 wks	4 weeks	4 weeks	4 weeks[6]	
Measles, Mumps, Rubella[7]	12 mos	4 weeks			
Varicella[8]	12 mos	4 weeks if first dose administered at age 13 years or older / 3 months if first dose administered at younger than 13 years of age			

1. Hepatitis B vaccine (HepB).
- Administer the 3-dose series to those who were not previously vaccinated.
- A 2-dose series of Recombivax HB® is licensed for children aged 11–15 years.

2. Rotavirus vaccine (Rota).
- Do not start the series later than age 12 weeks.
- Administer the final dose in the series by age 32 weeks.
- Do not administer a dose later than age 32 weeks.
- Data on safety and efficacy outside of these age ranges are insufficient.

3. Diphtheria and tetanus toxoids and acellular pertussis vaccine (DTaP).
- The fifth dose is not necessary if the fourth dose was administered at age 4 years or older.
- DTaP is not indicated for persons aged 7 years or older.

4. Haemophilus influenzae type b conjugate vaccine (Hib).
- Vaccine is not generally recommended for children aged 5 years or older.
- If current age is younger than 12 months and the first 2 doses were PRP-OMP (PedvaxHIB® or ComVax® [Merck]), the third (and final) dose should be administered at age 12–15 months and at least 8 weeks after the second dose.
- If first dose was administered at age 7–11 months, administer 2 doses separated by 4 weeks plus a booster at age 12–15 months.

5. Pneumococcal conjugate vaccine (PCV).
- Administer one dose of PCV to all healthy children aged 24–59 months having any incomplete schedule.
- For children with underlying medical conditions administer 2 doses of PCV at least 8 weeks apart if previously received less than 3 doses or 1 dose of PCV if previously received 3 doses.

6. Inactivated poliovirus vaccine (IPV).
- For children who received an all-IPV or all-oral poliovirus (OPV) series, a fourth dose is not necessary if third dose was administered at age 4 years or older.

- If both OPV and IPV were administered as part of a series, a total of 4 doses should be administered, regardless of the child's current age.
- IPV is not routinely recommended for persons aged 18 years and older.

7. Measles, mumps, and rubella vaccine (MMR).
- The second dose of MMR is recommended routinely at age 4–6 years but may be administered earlier if desired.
- If not previously vaccinated, administer 2 doses of MMR during any visit with 4 or more weeks between the doses.

8. Varicella vaccine.
- The second dose of varicella vaccine is recommended routinely at age 4–6 years but may be administered earlier if desired.
- Do not repeat the second dose in persons younger than 13 years of age if administered 28 or more days after the first dose.

9. Hepatitis A vaccine (HepA).
- HepA is recommended for certain groups of children, including in areas where vaccination programs target older children. See MMWR 2006;55(No. RR-7):1–23.

10. Tetanus and diphtheria toxoids vaccine (Td) and tetanus and diphtheria toxoids and acellular pertussis vaccine (Tdap).
- Tdap should be substituted for a single dose of Td in the primary catch-up series or as a booster if age appropriate; use Td for other doses.
- A 5-year interval from the last Td dose is encouraged when Tdap is used as a booster dose. A booster (fourth) dose is needed if any of the previous doses were administered at younger than 12 months of age. Refer to ACIP recommendations for further information. See MMWR 2006;55(No. RR-3).

11. Human papillomavirus vaccine (HPV).
- Administer the HPV vaccine series to females at age 13–18 years if not previously vaccinated.

Information about reporting reactions after immunization is available online at http://www.vaers.hhs.gov or by telephone via the 24-hour national toll-free information line 800-822-7967. Suspected cases of vaccine-preventable diseases should be reported to the state or local health department. Additional information, including precautions and contraindications for immunization, is available from the National Center for Immunization and Respiratory Diseases at http://www.cdc.gov/vaccines or telephone, 800-CDC-INFO (800-232-4636).

DEPARTMENT OF HEALTH AND HUMAN SERVICES ● CENTERS FOR DISEASE CONTROL AND PREVENTION ● SAFER • HEALTHIER • PEOPLE

FIG. 10-12 ■ Catch-up immunization schedule for persons aged 4 months to 18 years who start late or who are more than 1 month behind. (From Centers for Disease Control and Prevention: Recommended immunization schedules for persons aged 0-18 years—United States, 2008. MMWR 56[51 and 52]:Q1-Q4, 2007.)

TABLE 10-4

Recommended Immunization Schedules: Canada, 2006

A. INFANTS AND CHILDREN

AGE AT VACCINATION	DTaP-IPV[a]	Hib[b]	MMR[c]	Var[d]	HB[e]	Pneu–C-7[f]	Men-C[g]	Tdap[h]	Inf[i]
Birth					X				
2 months	X	X				X	X		
4 months	X	X				X	(X)		
6 months	X	X			Infancy	X	X		X
12 months			X	X	3 doses	X 12-15 months	X if not yet given		6-23 months
18 months	X	X	X or		or				1-2 doses
4-6 years	X		X						
14-16 years					X Preteen/teen 2-3 doses		X if not yet given	X	X

B. CHILDREN <7 YEARS OF AGE NOT IMMUNIZED IN EARLY INFANCY

TIMING	DTaP-IPV	Hib	MMR	VaR	HB	Pneu–C-7	Men-C	Tdap
First visit	X	X	X	X	X	X	X	
2 months later	X	(X)	X		X	(X)	(X)	
2 months later	X					(X)		
6-12 months later	X	(X)			X			
4-6 years of age	(X)							
14-16 years of age								X

C. CHILDREN 7 YEARS OF AGE UP TO 17 YEARS OF AGE NOT IMMUNIZED IN EARLY INFANCY

TIMING	Tdap	IPV[j]	MMR	Var	HB	Men-C
First visit	X	X	X	X	X	X
2 months later	X	X	X	(X)	(X)	
6-12 months later	X	X			X	
10 years later	X					

Modified from Public Health Agency of Canada: *Canadian immunization guide,* ed 7, Ottawa, Ontario, Canada, 2006, The Agency.

Parentheses imply that these doses may not be required, depending on the age of the child or adult.

[a]**Diphtheria, tetanus, acellular pertussis, and inactivated polio virus vaccine (DTaP-IPV):** DTaP-IPV (±Hib) vaccine is the preferred vaccine for all doses in the vaccination series, including completion of the series in children who have received ≥1 dose of DPT (whole cell) vaccine (e.g., recent immigrants). In schedules A and B, the 4- to 6-year dose can be omitted if the fourth dose was given after the fourth birthday.

[b]*Haemophilus influenzae* **type b conjugate vaccine (Hib):** The Hib schedule shown is for the *Haemophilus* b capsular polysaccharide–polyribosylribitol phosphate (PRP) conjugated to tetanus toxoid (PRP-T). For catch up, the number of doses depends on the age at which the schedule is begun. Not usually required past age 5 years.

[c]**Measles, mumps, and rubella vaccine (MMR):** A second dose of MMR is recommended for children at least 1 month after the first dose for the purpose of better measles protection. For convenience, options include giving it with the next scheduled vaccination at 18 months of age or at school entry (4-6 years) (depending on the provincial/territorial policy) or at any intervening age that is practical. In the catch-up schedule (B), the first dose should not be given until the child is ≥12 months old. MMR should be given to all susceptible adolescents and adults.

[d]**Varicella vaccine (Var):** Children aged 12 months to 12 years should receive 1 dose of varicella vaccine. Susceptible individuals ≥13 years of age should receive 2 doses at least 28 days apart.

[e]**Hepatitis B vaccine (HB):** Hepatitis B vaccine can be routinely given to infants or preadolescents, depending on the provincial/territorial policy. For infants born to chronic carrier mothers, the first dose should be given at birth (with hepatitis B immunoglobulin); otherwise, the first dose can be given at 2 months of age to fit more conveniently with other routine infant immunization visits. The second dose should be administered at least 1 month after the first dose, and the third at least 2 months after the second dose, but these may fit more conveniently into the 4- and 6-month immunization visits. A 2-dose schedule for adolescents is an option.

[f]**Pneumococcal conjugate vaccine–7-valent (Pneu–C-7):** Recommended for all children <2 years of age. The recommended schedule depends on the age of the child when vaccination is begun.

[g]**Meningococcal C conjugate vaccine (Men-C):** Recommended for children <5 years of age, adolescents, and young adults. The recommended schedule depends on the age of the individual, and the conjugate vaccine used. At least 1 dose in the primary infant series should be given after 5 months of age. If the provincial/territorial policy is to give Men-C to persons ≥12 months of age, 1 dose is sufficient.

[h]**Diphtheria, tetanus, acellular pertussis vaccine—adult/adolescent formulation (Tdap):** A combined adsorbed "adult type" preparation for use in people ≥7 years of age; contains less diphtheria toxoid and pertussis antigens than preparations given to younger children and is less likely to cause reactions in older people.

[i]**Influenza vaccine (Inf):** Recommended for all children 6-23 months of age and all persons ≥65 years of age. Previously unvaccinated children <9 years of age require 2 doses of the current season's vaccine with an interval of ≥4 weeks. The second dose within the same season is not required if the child received ≥1 doses of influenza vaccine during the previous influenza season.

[j]**Inactivated polio virus (IPV)**

routine primary immunization, usually in one of the combinations listed for diphtheria, and provides protective antitoxin levels for approximately 10 years.

Tetanus and diphtheria toxoids along with acellular pertussis vaccine (Tdap–adolescent formulation) is now recommended for children 11 to 12 years who have completed the recommended DTaP/DTP vaccine series yet have not received the tetanus (Td) booster dose. Adolescents who are 13 to 18 years of age and have not received the Td/Tdap booster should receive a single Tdap booster provided the routine DTaP/DTP childhood immunization series has been previously received. It is recommended that subsequent Td boosters be administered every 10 years (American Academy of Pediatrics, 2006b) (see Fig. 10-11, *B,* footnote 1). Boostrix (Tdap) is currently licensed for children 10 to 18 years of age, whereas Adacel (Tdap) is licensed for individuals 11 to 64 years of age.

For wound management, passive immunity is available with TIG. In persons with a history of two previous doses of tetanus toxoid, a booster dose of the toxoid can be given. Separate syringes and different sites are used when tetanus toxoid and TIG are given concurrently. Table 10-5 summarizes the recommended procedure for tetanus prophylaxis in wound management.

For children over 7 years who require wound prophylaxis, tetanus immunization may be accomplished by administering Td (adult-type diphtheria and tetanus toxoids). In the event that TIG is not available, the equine antitoxin (not available in the United States) may be administered after appropriate testing for sensitivity; the antitoxin is administered in a separate syringe and at a separate intramuscular site if given concurrently with tetanus toxoid.

Pertussis. Pertussis vaccine is recommended for all children 6 weeks through 6 years of age (up to the seventh birthday) who have no neurologic contraindications to its use. Concerns over outbreaks of the disease in the past decade have prompted discussion about vaccinating infants and adults; many cases of pertussis have been seen in children less than 6 months or persons over 7 years, both categories for which pertussis vaccination was not previously recommended (Centers for Disease Control and Prevention, 2005c). The tetanus and diphtheria toxoids and acellular pertussis vaccine (Tdap) is now recommended at age 11 to 12 years for children who have completed the DTaP/DTP childhood series; the Tdap is also recommended for adolescents 13 to 18 years who have not received a tetanus booster (Td) or Tdap dose and have completed the childhood DTaP/DTP series (American Academy of Pediatrics, 2006b).

Currently, two forms of pertussis vaccine are available in the United States. The **whole-cell pertussis vaccine** is prepared from inactivated cells of *Bordetella pertussis* and contains multiple antigens. In contrast, the **acellular pertussis** vaccine contains one or more immunogens derived from *B. pertussis.* The highly purified acellular vaccine is associated with fewer local and systemic reactions than those occurring with the whole-cell vaccine in children of similar age. The acellular pertussis vaccine is recommended by the American Academy of Pediatrics (2006b) for the first three immunizations and is usually given at 2, 4, and 6 months of age with diphtheria and tetanus (DTaP). Four forms of acellular pertussis vaccine are currently licensed for use in infants: Tripedia, Daptacel, Pediarix, and Infanrix (diphtheria, tetanus toxoid, and acellular pertussis conjugate). TriHIBit may be used for the fourth dose after three doses of DTaP and after a primary series of any Hib vaccine. Either the acellular or whole-cell vaccine may be given for the fourth and fifth doses, but the acellular is preferred. It is also recommended that the first three DTaP vaccinations be from the same manufacturer; the fourth dose may be from a different manufacturer. The child who has received one or more whole-cell vaccines may complete the series of five with the acellular vaccine.

Health care workers under age 65 who have potential exposure to children or adults with pertussis should be given the Tdap booster Adacel every 10 years; in addition, health care workers should take the necessary protective precautions against droplet contamination (wear procedural or surgical masks and practice hand washing). The diagnosis of pertussis may be missed or delayed in unvaccinated infants, who often are seen with respiratory distress and apnea without the typical cough (Centers for Disease Control and Prevention, 2005c). Additional guidelines for prevention and treatment of pertussis among health care workers and close contacts are found in the Centers for Disease Control and Prevention report (2006b).

Polio. An all-IPV (inactivated poliovirus vaccine) schedule for routine childhood polio vaccination is now recommended for children in the United States. All children should receive four doses of IPV at 2 months, 4 months, 6 to 18

TABLE 10-5

Guide to Tetanus Prophylaxis in Routine Wound Management

HISTORY OF ADSORBED TETANUS TOXOID (DOSES)	CLEAN, MINOR WOUNDS		ALL OTHER WOUNDS*	
	Td OR Tdap†	TIG	Td OR Tdap†	TIG‡
Unknown or <3	Yes	No	Yes	Yes
3§	No‖	No	No¶	No

Data from American Academy of Pediatrics, Committee on Infectious Diseases, Pickering L, editor: *Red book: 2006 report of the Committee on Infectious Diseases,* ed 27, Elk Grove Village, Ill, 2006, The Academy.
Td, Tetanus, diphtheria; *Tdap,* booster tetanus toxoid, reduced diphtheria toxoid, and acellular pertussis; *TIG,* tetanus immune globulin.
*Such as, but not limited to, wounds contaminated with dirt, feces, soil, and saliva; puncture wounds; avulsions; and wounds resulting from missiles, crushing, burns, and frostbite.
†Tdap is preferred to Td for adolescents who never have received Tdap. Td is preferred to tetanus toxoid (TT) for adolescents who received Tdap previously or when Tdap is not available.
‡Intravenous immune globulin should be used when TIG is not available.
§If only three doses of fluid toxoid have been received, then a fourth dose of toxoid, preferably an adsorbed toxoid, should be given.
‖Yes, if 10 years since last dose.
¶Yes, if 5 years since last dose. (More frequent boosters are not needed and can accentuate side effects.)

months, and 4 to 6 years of age (American Academy of Pediatrics, 2006b).

The change from the exclusive use of oral polio vaccine (OPV) to the exclusive use of IPV is related to the rare risk of vaccine-associated polio paralysis (VAPP) from OPV. The exclusive use of IPV eliminates the risk of VAPP but is associated with an increased number of injections and increased cost. Since IPV usage was instituted in the United States in 2000, no new cases of VAPP have occurred. Pediarix is a combination vaccine containing DTaP, hepatitis B, and IPV; this may be used as the primary immunization beginning at 2 months of age (American Academy of Pediatrics, 2006b).

Measles. The measles (rubeola) vaccine is given at 12 to 15 months of age. During the course of measles outbreaks, the vaccine can be given any time after 6 months of age, followed by a second inoculation after age 12 months. The second measles immunization is recommended at 4 to 6 years of age (at school entry) but may be given earlier provided that 4 weeks have lapsed since the administration of the previous dose. Revaccination should occur by 11 to 12 years of age if the measles vaccine was not administered at school entry (4 to 6 years). Any child who is vaccinated before 12 months of age should receive two additional doses beginning at 12 to 15 months and separated by at least 4 weeks (American Academy of Pediatrics, 2006b). Revaccination should include all individuals born after 1956 who have not received two doses of measles vaccine after 12 months of age. Individuals born before this date are thought to be immune from exposure to natural measles virus. Because of the continuing occurrence of measles in older children and young adults, potentially susceptible adolescents and young adults should be identified and immunized if two doses of measles vaccine have not been administered previously or the person had a confirmed case of the illness.

Mumps. Mumps virus vaccine is recommended for children at 12 to 15 months of age and is typically given in combination with measles and rubella. It should not be administered to infants younger than 12 months because persisting maternal antibodies can interfere with the immune response. Because of continued occurrence of the disease, especially in children 10 to 19 years of age, mumps immunization is recommended for all individuals born after 1957 who may be susceptible to mumps (i.e., those who have no history of having had the disease or vaccine and who have no laboratory evidence of immunity).

Rubella. Rubella is a relatively mild infection in children, but in a pregnant woman the actual infection presents serious risks to the developing fetus. Therefore the aim of rubella immunization is actually protection of the unborn child rather than the recipient of the immunization.

Rubella immunization is recommended for all children at 12 to 15 months of age and is administered in a combined form with measles and mumps vaccine. Increased emphasis should also be placed on vaccinating all unimmunized prepubertal children and susceptible adolescents and adult women in the childbearing age-group. Because the live attenuated virus may cross the placenta and theoretically present a risk to the developing fetus, rubella vaccine is currently not given to any pregnant woman.

Haemophilus influenzae Type b. Hib conjugate vaccines protect against a number of serious infections caused by Hib, especially bacterial meningitis, epiglottitis, bacterial pneumonia, septic arthritis, and sepsis (Hib is not associated with the viruses that cause influenza, or "flu"). Hib vaccines that are currently available include PedvaxHIB and Comvax, which are combination vaccines; and HibTITER and ActHIB (see Table 10-7). These conjugate vaccines connect Hib to a nontoxic form of another organism, such as meningococcal protein or diphtheria protein. There is no antibody response to these nontoxic proteins, but they significantly improve the antibody response to Hib, especially in infants. The use of combination vaccines provides equivalent immunogenicity and decreases the number of injections an infant receives; however, it is important that they be given to the appropriate-age child.

When possible, the Hib conjugate vaccine used at the first vaccination should be used for all subsequent vaccinations in the primary series. The DTaP/Hib combination vaccine (TriHIBit) should not be used for the first three doses at 2, 4, or 6 months but may be used as a booster after any Hib vaccine. All Hib vaccines are administered by intramuscular injection using a separate syringe and at a site separate from any concurrent vaccinations.

> **NURSING ALERT**
>
> The use of meningococcal and diphtheria proteins in combination vaccines does not mean the child has received adequate immunization for meningococcal or diphtheria illnesses; the child must be given the appropriate vaccine for that specific disease.

Varicella. Administration of the cell-free live-attenuated varicella vaccine (Varivax) is recommended for any susceptible child (who lacks proof of varicella vaccination or a reliable history of varicella infection). The first dose of varicella vaccine is recommended for children ages 12 to 15 months; to ensure adequate protection, a second varicella vaccine is recommended for children at 4 to 6 years of age (American Academy of Pediatrics, 2007).

A single dose of 0.5 ml should be given by subcutaneous injection. Children 13 years of age or older who are susceptible should receive two doses administered at least 4 weeks apart (American Academy of Pediatrics, 2006b). The vaccine should be kept frozen in the lyophilic form (stable particles that readily go into solution) and used within 30 minutes of being reconstituted to ensure viral potency. Varicella vaccine may be administered simultaneously with MMR. However, separate syringes and injection sites should be used. If they are not administered simultaneously, the interval between administration of varicella vaccine and MMR should be at least 1 month. Varicella vaccine may also be given simultaneously with DTaP, IPV, HepB, or Hib (American Academy of Pediatrics, 2006b).

The varicella vaccine is reported to be effective in preventing varicella for at least 11 years (American Academy of Pediatrics, 2006b).

Pneumococcal. A seven-valent *Streptococcus pneumoniae* conjugate vaccine (PCV7, or Prevnar) has been used for children under 2 years of age since 2000. Streptococcal pneumococci are responsible for a number of bacterial infections in children under 2 years, which may cause serious morbidity and mortality. Among these are generalized infections such as septicemia and meningitis or localized infections such as otitis media, sinusitis, and pneumonia. These illnesses are particularly problematic in children who attend daycare facilities (the incidence in daycare children is two or three times higher than in children not attending out-of-home daycare) and in those who are immunocompromised.

The vaccine is administered at 2, 4, and 6 months, with a fourth dose at 12 to 15 months of age; children 7 to 11 months old may receive three doses as long as they are 6 to 8 weeks apart and a fourth dose at 12 to 15 months; children 12 to 23 months who have not been immunized with the pneumococcal vaccine may be given two doses, 6 to 8 weeks apart. PCV7 is also recommended for all children under 24 months and in older children (24 to 59 months) with sickle cell disease; functional or anatomic asplenia; nephrotic syndrome or chronic renal failure; conditions associated with immunosuppression, such as solid organ transplantation, drug therapy, or cytoreduction therapy (including long-term systemic corticosteroid therapy); diabetes mellitus; cochlear implants; congenital immunodeficiency; human immunodeficiency virus (HIV) infection; cerebrospinal fluid leaks; chronic cardiovascular disease (e.g., congestive heart failure or cardiomyopathy); chronic pulmonary disease (e.g., emphysema or cystic fibrosis, but not asthma); chronic liver disease (e.g., cirrhosis); or exposure to living environments or social settings in which the risk of invasive pneumococcal disease or its complications is very high (e.g., Alaskan Native, African-American, and certain Native American populations) (American Academy of Pediatrics, 2006b). Low-birth-weight infants (≤1500 g [3.3 pounds]) should receive the vaccine when they reach a chronologic age of 6 to 8 weeks regardless of calculated gestational age. The PCV7 vaccine may be administered in conjunction with all other immunizations in a separate syringe and at a separate intramuscular site.

The PPV (pneumococcal polysaccharide [23-valent] vaccine) is not recommended for children younger than 24 months who do not have one of the high-risk conditions described previously. One dose of PPV is recommended in children older than 23 months who have one of the high-risk conditions after primary immunization with PCV7. (See American Academy of Pediatrics, 2006b, Tables 3-48 and 3-49 for PCV7 and PPV schedule.)

Influenza. The influenza vaccine is now recommended annually for children 6 months and older. The vaccine should be administered annually to children 5 years of age and older with risk factors (including asthma, cardiac disease, HIV, diabetes, and sickle cell disease), health care workers, and other persons in close contact (including household members) with persons in groups at high risk. It is also recommended that close contacts in households with children ages 0 to 5 months receive the trivalent inactivated influenza vaccine because of the high rate of influenza-related hospitalization. Influenza vaccine (trivalent inactivated influenza vaccine) may be given to any healthy children 6 to 59 months old, since this age-group is at particular risk for influenza-related hospitalizations. Children who have a reported anaphylactic hypersensitivity to eggs should not receive the vaccine.

The vaccine is administered in early fall before the flu season begins and is repeated yearly for ongoing protection. The intramuscular vaccine is administered as two separate doses 2 weeks apart in first-time recipients under the age of 8 years. The dose is 0.25 ml for children ages 3 months to 35 months and 0.5 ml for children 3 years and above. The vaccine may be given simultaneously with other vaccines but at a separate site (American Academy of Pediatrics, 2006b). The vaccine is administered yearly because different strains of influenza are used each year in the manufacture of the vaccine.

FluMist, a live attenuated influenza vaccine, is an acceptable alternative to the intramuscular trivalent vaccine in specific age-groups. The vaccine is given nasally as two doses 4 weeks apart in healthy persons ages 2 to 49 years.

Meningococcal. Invasive meningococcal disease continues to be the cause of high morbidity in children in the United States. Infants younger than 1 year of age are particularly susceptible, yet the highest fatalities occur in adolescents (approximately 20%). There is also evidence that the risk of meningococcal infections is high in college freshmen living in dormitories. Meningococcal infections are also responsible for significant morbidities, including limb or digit amputation, skin scarring, hearing loss, and neurologic disabilities (American Academy of Pediatrics, 2006b).

Neisseria meningitidis is the leading cause of bacterial meningitis in the United States. It is now recommended that children receive the quadrivalent conjugate vaccine MCV4 (Menactra) at the 11- to 12-year visit. Menactra was recently approved for use in children 2 to 10 years of age.

The vaccine protects against meningococcal disease caused by serogroups A, C, Y, and W-135 and should also be administered to adolescents at high school entry or 15 years of age (whichever comes first) who have not been previously immunized for meningococcal disease, college freshmen living in dormitories, and pediatric patients 11 years and older who are at increased risk of meningococcal disease (adolescents with asplenia or complement deficiencies and HIV). The MCV4 vaccine is also recommended for adolescents ages 11 to 18 years traveling to countries where meningococcal infections are prevalent. MCV4 is administered as an intramuscular injection (0.5 ml) and may be administered in conjunction with other vaccines in a separate syringe and at a separate site.

There have been recent concerns regarding reports of an association between Menactra and cases of Guillain-Barré syndrome in vaccinated persons ages 11 to 19 years of age; onset of symptoms occurred within 2 to 23 days of vaccination. A preliminary survey by the Centers for Disease Control and Prevention (2006c) indicates there are insufficient data to change the 2005 recommendation for adolescents, college freshmen residing in dormitories, and other high-risk populations.

The meningococcal vaccine Menomune (A, C, Y, W-135; MPSV4), which has been available since the early 1980s, may be used for children 2 to 10 years of age and MCV4 for children over 10 years. The MCV4 is recommended over the MPSV4 for children aged 2 to 10 years who are at increased risk for meningitis (American Academy of Pediatrics, 2008). MPSV4 may be administered subcutaneously conjointly with other vaccines in a separate syringe at a separate site. It is unknown whether future recommendations for booster immunization with MCV4 will be necessary (American Academy of Pediatrics, 2006b).

Immunization with MCV4 is contraindicated in persons with hypersensitivity to any components of the vaccine, including diphtheria toxoid, and to rubber latex (part of vial stopper).

Recommendations for Selected Immunizations

Two additional vaccines are recommended for children and adolescents at high risk for particular diseases. In February 2006 a new rotavirus vaccine, RotaTeq, received a license from the U.S. Food and Drug Administration (FDA) for distribution in the United States. A second rotavirus vaccine, Rotarix, is licensed for use in Europe, and application to the FDA for use in the United States was made in late 2007. Rotavirus is one of the leading causes of severe diarrhea in infants and young children. A previous rotavirus vaccine was removed from the market in the late 1990s because of its association with intussusception. The new oral rotavirus vaccine is licensed for administration to infants at 6 to 12 weeks of age, with two additional doses administered at 4- to 10-week intervals but not after 32 weeks of age; the dose is 2 ml, and the product must be protected from light until administration (US Food and Drug Administration, 2006) (see Fig. 10-11, *A*).

A quadrivalent human papillomavirus (HPV) vaccine, Gardasil, has been approved and is recommended for female children and adolescents to prevent HPV-related cervical cancer. The vaccine is administered intramuscularly in three separate doses; the first dose in the series may be given at 11 to 12 years of age (minimum age 9 years), while the second dose is administered 2 months after the first, with the third dose being given 6 months after the first dose (Centers for Disease Control and Prevention, 2007b) (see Fig. 10-11, *B*).

Immunizations that may be used in older children and adolescents in the future and that are being evaluated include vaccines for preventing diseases such as herpes simplex virus, human cytomegalovirus, and Epstein-Barr virus. A vaccine for respiratory syncytial virus is currently being tested in animal models with apparent success. Others, such as the rabies vaccine, are discussed elsewhere in this text.

Reactions

Vaccines for routine immunizations are among the safest and most reliable drugs available. However, minor side effects do occur after many of the immunizations, and, rarely, a serious reaction may result from the vaccine.

With inactivated antigens, such as DTaP, side effects are most likely to occur within a few hours or days of administration and are usually limited to local tenderness, erythema, and swelling at the injection site; low-grade fever; and behavioral changes (drowsiness, fretfulness, eating less, prolonged or unusual cry). Rarely, more severe reactions may occur, especially with pertussis (see Table 10-6). Reactions to DTaP tend to be more severe if they occurred with a previous immunization.

Hib vaccine is one of the safest vaccines available but may be associated with low-grade fever and mild local reactions at the site of injection, which resolve rapidly. Fever (temperature >38.5° C [101.3° F]) may rarely occur.

A number of inactive components are incorporated in vaccines to enhance their effectiveness and safety. Some of these components include preservatives, stabilizers, adjuvants, antibiotics, and purified culture medium proteins to enhance effectiveness. A child may react to the preservative in the vaccine rather than the vaccine component; an example of this is the HepB vaccine, which is prepared from yeast cultures. Yeast hypersensitivity would preclude one from receiving that particular vaccine (Schuval, 2003). Trace amounts of neomycin are used to decrease bacterial growth within certain vaccine preparations, and persons with documented anaphylactic reactions to neomycin should avoid those vaccines. Most vaccine preparations now contain vial stoppers with a synthetic rubber to prevent latex allergy reactions. In the event that an individual has a severe reaction to a vaccine and subsequent immunizations are required, an allergist may be consulted to determine the best course of action (Schuval, 2003).

A commonly observed reaction includes localized erythema and induration, which may occur when the vaccine is not administered deeply enough into the muscle. This reaction can be prevented by ensuring that needle length is appropriate for the child's muscle size. Although many vaccine preparations are commercially available in prepackaged form, the enclosed needle may not be of adequate length to penetrate the muscle in certain children (see Atraumatic Care box, p. 360, and Administration, below).

Unlike the inactivated antigens, live attenuated virus vaccines such as MMR multiply for days or weeks, and unfavorable reactions and vaccine-associated disorders can occur for 30 to 60 days. These reactions are usually mild, although reactions to rubella tend to be more troublesome in older children and adults.

Contraindications and Precautions

Nurses need to be aware of the reasons for withholding immunizations—both for the child's safety in terms of avoiding reactions and for the child's maximum benefit from receiving the vaccine. Unfounded fears and lack of knowledge regarding contraindications can needlessly prevent a child from having protection from life-threatening diseases. Issues that have surfaced regarding vaccines include the misconception that administering combination vaccines may overload the child's immune system; the combined vaccines have undergone rigorous study in relation to side effects and immunogenicity rates following administration.

Parents must be given appropriate information regarding vaccine safety, benefits, and risks so they can make informed decisions regarding vaccinations for their children (Koslap-Petraco and Parsons, 2003; Fredrickson, Davis, Arnold, and others, 2004). The advantage of widespread media coverage on television and the Internet is that information is readily available at any given moment; the disadvantage may rest in the fact that information—rather, misinformation—from questionable sources is also readily available and may influence parents to make decisions that may have deleterious consequences for their children's health. In one survey, parents' fear of side effects was the most commonly expressed (52%) reason for vaccination refusal; other common reasons included the belief that the disease was not harmful (26%), religious beliefs (28%), and philosophical reasons (26%) (Fredrickson, Davis, Arnold, and others, 2004). The contraindications to the usual childhood vaccines are presented in Table 10-6. See also Family-Centered Care box.

Administration

The principal precautions in administering immunizations include proper storage of the vaccine to protect its potency and institution of recommended procedures for injection. The nurse must be familiar with the manufacturer's directions

Text continued on p. 363

ATRAUMATIC CARE

Immunizations

Needle length is an important factor and must be considered for each individual child; fewer reactions to immunizations are observed when the vaccine is given deep into the muscle rather than into subcutaneous tissue. Contrary to previous belief, deep intramuscular tissue has a better blood supply and fewer pain receptors than adipose tissue, thus providing an optimum site for immunizations with fewer side effects (Zuckerman, 2000). To minimize local reactions from vaccines:

- Recommended needle length for newborn to 2 months is ⅝ inch.
- Select a needle of adequate length (2.5 cm [1 inch] in infants) to deposit the antigen deep in the muscle mass.
- Toddlers and older children require a needle length of ⅝ to 1 inch for deltoid, or 1 to 1¼ inches for vastus lateralis (Schechter, Zempsky, Cohen, and others, 2007).
- Adolescents require a needle length of 1 to 2 inches in deltoid or vastus lateralis (Schechter, Zempsky, Cohen, and others, 2007).
- Inject into the vastus lateralis or ventrogluteal muscle; the deltoid may be used in children 18 months of age or older.
- Use an air bubble to clear the needle after injecting the vaccine (theoretically beneficial but unproved).

To minimize pain:

- Apply the topical anesthetic EMLA (lidocaine-prilocaine) to the injection site and cover with an occlusive dressing for at least 1 hour.*
- Apply the topical anesthetic LMX4 (4% lidocaine) to the injection site 30 minutes before the injection; there is no evidence that an occlusive dressing is required except to prevent ingestion or accidental application to the eyes in infants (Wong, 2003). To date, the studies for LMX4 have only discussed pain from procedures such as venipuncture, not injections.

- Apply a vapocoolant spray (e.g., ethyl chloride or FluoriMethane) directly to the skin or to a cotton ball, which is placed on the skin for 15 seconds immediately before the injection (Reis and Holubkov, 1997).
- There is evidence that a concentrated oral sucrose solution (24%) and nonnutritive sucking (pacifier) decrease the pain related to minor invasive procedures in neonates (Stevens, Johnston, Franck, and others, 1999; Stevens, Yamada, and Ohlsson, 2001). Most studies have focused on heel lance, venipuncture, and circumcision (neonatal period), but one institution has incorporated a neonatal oral sucrose pain protocol for painful procedures, including injections (Thompson, 2005). Therefore it is recommended that a concentrated oral sucrose solution (1 to 2 ml) be administered orally 2 minutes before the injection, during the injection, and up to 3 minutes after the procedure to decrease neonatal pain with immunizations.
- In preschool children, use distraction, such as telling the child to "take a deep breath and blow and blow and blow until I tell you to stop."
- Two studies in adult patients receiving intramuscular injections documented a decrease in pain sensation at the time of the injection when manual pressure was applied to the site before the injection; pressure was applied for 10 seconds in both studies (Barnhill, Holbert, Jackson, and others, 1996; Chung, Ng, and Wong, 2002). To date, there are no published studies involving the use of this technique in children.

NOTE: Changing the needle on the syringe after drawing up the vaccine and before injecting it has not been shown to decrease local reactions. In children 4 to 6 years of age, the administration of sequential injections or simultaneous injections of vaccines did not alter their perceptions of distress, but parents preferred the simultaneous method (Horn and McCarthy, 1999).
*The use of the EMLA patch before administration of diphtheria-tetanus–acellular pertussis–inactivated poliovirus–*Haemophilus influenzae* type b (DTaP-IPV-Hib) and hepatitis B vaccines did not decrease antibody titers in immunized infants and was effective in reducing pain in 6-month-old children (Halperin, Halperin, McGrath, and others, 2002). The EMLA patch is no longer commercially available in the United States.

FAMILY-CENTERED CARE

Communicating with Parents About Immunizations

- Provide accurate and user-friendly information on vaccines (the necessity for each one, the disease each prevents, potential adverse effects).
- Realize that the parent is expressing concern for the child's health.
- Acknowledge the parent's concerns in a genuine, empathetic manner.
- Tailor the discussion to the needs of the parent.
- Avoid judgmental or threatening language.
- Be knowledgeable about the benefits of individual vaccines, the common adverse effects, and how to minimize those effects.
- Give the parent the vaccine information statement (VIS) beforehand and be prepared to answer any questions that may arise.
- Help the parent make an informed decision regarding the administration of each vaccine.

- Be flexible and provide parents options regarding the administration of multiple vaccines, especially in infants, who must receive multiple injections at 2, 4, and 6 months (i.e., allow parents to space the vaccinations at different visits to decrease the total number of injections at each visit; make provisions for office visits for immunization purposes only [does not incur a practitioner fee except for administration of vaccine], provided the child is healthy).
- Involve the parent in minimizing the potential adverse effects of the vaccine (e.g., administering an appropriate dose of acetaminophen 45 minutes before administering the vaccine [as warranted]; applying EMLA [lidocaine-prilocaine] or LMX4 [4% lidocaine] to the injection sites before administration; following up to check on the child if untoward reactions have occurred in the past or parent is especially anxious about the child's well-being).
- Respect the parent's ultimate wishes.

Data from Coyer SM: Understanding parental concerns about immunizations, *J Pediatr Health Care* 16(4):193-196, 2002; Fredrickson DD, Davis TC, Bocchini JA: Explaining the risks and benefits of vaccines to parents, *Pediatr Ann* 30(7):400-406, 2001; and Rosenthal P: Overcoming skepticism toward vaccines: a look at the real benefits and risks, *Consult Pediatr* 4(Suppl):S3-S7, 2004.

TABLE 10-6

Contraindications and Precautions to Vaccinations[a]

TRUE CONTRAINDICATIONS	PRECAUTIONS[b]	NOT CONTRAINDICATIONS (VACCINES MAY BE ADMINISTERED)
GENERAL FOR ALL VACCINES (DTaP, IPV, MMR, Hib, HepB, VARICELLA, PCV, HepA, INFLUENZA, MENINGOCOCCAL)		
Anaphylactic reaction to vaccine contraindication to further doses of that vaccine Anaphylactic reaction to vaccine contraindication to use of vaccines containing that substance Moderate or severe illnesses with or without fever		Mild to moderate local reaction (soreness, redness, swelling) after a dose of injectable antigen Mild acute illness with or without low-grade fever Current antimicrobial therapy Convalescent phase of illnesses Prematurity (same dosage and indications as for normal, full-term infants) Recent exposure to infectious disease History of penicillin or other nonspecific allergies or family history of such allergies
DIPHTHERIA, TETANUS, AND PERTUSSIS OR ACELLULAR PERTUSSIS VACCINE (DTP OR DTaP)		
Encephalopathy within 7 days of administration of previous dose of DTaP	Fever of 40.5° C (105° F) within 48 hours after vaccination with prior dose of DTaP Collapse or shocklike state (hypotonic-hyporesponsive episode) within 48 hours of receiving prior dose of DTaP Seizures within 3 days of receiving prior dose of DTaP[c] Persistent, inconsolable crying lasting 3 hours within 48 hours of receiving prior dose of DTaP	Temperature of <40.5° C (105° F) after previous dose of DTaP Family history of seizures[c] Family history of sudden infant death syndrome Family history of adverse event after DTaP administration
DIPHTHERIA, TETANUS (DT, Td)		
Severe allergic reaction after a previous dose or to a vaccine component	GBS 6 weeks after previous dose of tetanus toxoid–containing vaccine Moderate or severe acute illness with or without fever	Same as DTaP or DTP
INACTIVATED POLIOVIRUS VACCINE (IPV)		
Anaphylactic reaction to neomycin or streptomycin	Pregnancy	Breastfeeding Diarrhea
MEASLES, MUMPS, RUBELLA VACCINE (MMR)		
Pregnancy Known altered immunodeficiency (hematologic and solid tumors, congenital immunodeficiency, and long-term immunosuppressive therapy)	Recent immunoglobulin administration Immunoglobulin products and MMR should not be given simultaneously; if unavoidable, give at different sites and revaccinate or test for seroconversion in 3 months; if immunoglobulin is given first, MMR should not be given for at least 3-6 months, depending on dose; if MMR is given first, immunoglobulin should not be given for 2 weeks Thrombocytopenia or thrombocytopenic purpura	Simultaneous tuberculosis skin testing[d] Breastfeeding Pregnancy of mother of recipient Immunodeficient family member or household contact Infection with HIV Nonanaphylactic reactions to eggs or neomycin Consider MMR for mildly symptomatic HIV-infected children (see American Academy of Pediatrics, 2006b)
HAEMOPHILUS INFLUENZAE TYPE B VACCINE (Hib)		
None identified		History of Hib disease

Modified from American Academy of Pediatrics, Committee on Infectious Diseases, Pickering L, editor: *Red book: 2006 report of the Committee on Infectious Diseases*, ed 27, Elk Grove Village, Ill, 2006, The Academy.

HIV, Human immunodeficiency virus; *GBS*, Guillain-Barré syndrome; *PPD*, purified protein derivative; *LAIV*, live-attenuated influenza vaccine.

[a]This information is based on the recommendations of Advisory Committee on Immunization Practices (ACIP) and those of Committee on Infectious Diseases (Red Book committee) of American Academy of Pediatrics. Sometimes these recommendations vary from those contained in manufacturer's package inserts. For more detailed information, consult published recommendations of ACIP and American Academy of Pediatrics and manufacturer's package inserts.

[b]Events or conditions listed as precautions, although not contraindications, should be carefully reviewed. Benefits and risks of administering a specific vaccine to an individual under the circumstances should be considered. If risks are believed to outweigh benefits, vaccination should be withheld; if benefits are believed to outweigh risks (e.g., during an outbreak or foreign travel), vaccination should be administered. Whether and when to administer DTaP to children with proven or suspected underlying neurologic disorders should be decided on individual basis. It is prudent on theoretic grounds to avoid vaccinating pregnant women.

[c]Acetaminophen given before administering DTaP and thereafter every 4 hours for 24 hours should be considered for children with personal history or family history of convulsions in siblings or parents.

[d]Measles vaccination may temporarily suppress tuberculin reactivity. If testing cannot be done the day of MMR vaccination, the test should be postponed for 4 to 6 weeks.

Continued

TABLE 10-6

Contraindications and Precautions to Vaccinations—cont'd

TRUE CONTRAINDICATIONS	PRECAUTIONS[b]	NOT CONTRAINDICATIONS (VACCINES MAY BE ADMINISTERED)
HEPATITIS B VIRUS VACCINE (HepB)		
Anaphylactic reaction to common baker's yeast	Preterm birth[e]	Pregnancy
VARICELLA VACCINE		
Severe allergic reaction after a previous dose or to a vaccine component (e.g., neomycin or gelatin) Infection with HIV Known altered immunodeficiency (hematologic and solid tumors, congenital immunodeficiency, and long-term immunosuppressive therapy) Pregnancy Children receiving corticosteroids	Recent immune globulin administration (see *Measles* in American Academy of Pediatrics, 2006b) Family history of immunodeficiency	Breastfeeding
PNEUMOCOCCAL VACCINE (PCV)		
Severe allergic reaction after a previous dose or to a vaccine component	Moderate or severe acute illness with or without fever A child who has received pneumococcal polysaccharide vaccine (PPV) previously should wait at least 2 months before receiving PCV	Minor illnesses with or without fever Mild upper respiratory tract infection Allergic rhinitis
ROTAVIRUS VACCINE		
Severe allergic reaction after a previous dose or to a vaccine component Infants born to HIV-positive mother Known or suspected weakened immune system caused by radiation; drugs; or conditions such as leukemia, blood disorders, cancer	Altered immunocompetence Moderate to severe acute gastroenteritis Moderate to severe febrile illness Chronic gastrointestinal diseases Intussusception	Pregnancy Previous history of rotavirus infection; history of intussusception; temperature 38° C (100.5° F); close contact with immunocompromised person(s); blood transfusion or immunoglobulins within previous 42 days
INFLUENZA VACCINE (INACTIVATED/LIVE-ATTENUATED)[f]		
Severe allergic reaction after a previous dose or to a vaccine component, including eggs Egg hypersensitivity LAIV should not be administered to persons taking salicylates, with known or suspected immunodeficiency, with a history of GBS, or with a reactive airway disease or other chronic disorder considered high risk for severe influenza	GBS within 6 weeks after previous influenza immunization	Pregnancy
MENINGOCOCCAL VACCINE		
MCV4—Allergy to vaccine components, including diphtheria toxoid, and possible reaction to latex stopper; history of GBS		Pregnancy
MPSV4—Allergy to vaccine components		Pregnancy

HIV, Human immunodeficiency virus; *GBS,* Guillain-Barré syndrome; *PPD,* purified protein derivative; *LAIV,* live-attenuated influenza vaccine.
[b]Events or conditions listed as precautions, although not contraindications, should be carefully reviewed. Benefits and risks of administering a specific vaccine to an individual under the circumstances should be considered. If risks are believed to outweigh benefits, vaccination should be withheld; if benefits are believed to outweigh risks (e.g., during an outbreak or foreign travel), vaccination should be administered. Whether and when to administer DTaP to children with proven or suspected underlying neurologic disorders should be decided on individual basis. It is prudent on theoretic grounds to avoid vaccinating pregnant women.
[e]Birth weight <2000 g (4.4 pounds) and unknown or hepatitis B surface antigen (HBsAg)–positive mother is not a contraindication for vaccination.
[f]See James JM, Zeiger RS, Lester MR, and others: Safe administration of influenza vaccine to patients with egg allergies, *J Pediatr* 133(5):624-628, 1998.

TABLE 10-6

Contraindications and Precautions to Vaccinations—cont'd

TRUE CONTRAINDICATIONS	PRECAUTIONS[b]	NOT CONTRAINDICATIONS (VACCINES MAY BE ADMINISTERED)
TETANUS (BOOSTER TOXOID), REDUCED DIPHTHERIA TOXOID, ACELLULAR PERTUSSIS ADSORBED (TDaP)		
Serious reaction to any vaccine component History of encephalopathy (e.g., coma, prolonged seizures) within 7 days of administration of a pertussis vaccine that is not attributable to another identifiable cause	GBS 6 weeks after previous dose of a tetanus toxoid vaccine Progressive neurologic disorder, uncontrolled epilepsy, or progressive encephalopathy until the condition has stabilized	Temperature 40.5° C (105° F) within 48 hours after DTP/DTaP immunization not attributable to another cause Collapse or shocklike state within 48 hours after DTP/DTaP immunization Persistent crying lasting 3 hours or longer, occurring within 48 hours after DTP/DTaP immunization Convulsions with or without fever, occurring within 3 days after DTaP/DTP immunization History of entire limb swelling reaction after pediatric DTaP/DTP or Td immunization that was not an Arthus hypersensitivity reaction Stable neurologic disorder, including well-controlled seizures, history of seizure disorder, and cerebral palsy Brachial neuritis Latex allergy other than anaphylactic allergies (e.g., history of contact to latex gloves) Immunosuppression, including persons with HIV Antibiotic use Intercurrent minor illness
HUMAN PAPILLOMAVIRUS VACCINE		
Pregnancy Hypersensitivity to yeast or any vaccine component		Immunosuppressed female Minor acute illness Lactation

[b]Events or conditions listed as precautions, although not contraindications, should be carefully reviewed. Benefits and risks of administering a specific vaccine to an individual under the circumstances should be considered. If risks are believed to outweigh benefits, vaccination should be withheld; if benefits are believed to outweigh risks (e.g., during an outbreak or foreign travel), vaccination should be administered. Whether and when to administer DTaP to children with proven or suspected underlying neurologic disorders should be decided on individual basis. It is prudent on theoretic grounds to avoid vaccinating pregnant women.

for storage and reconstitution of the vaccine. For example, if the vaccine is to be refrigerated, it should be stored on a center shelf, not in the door, where frequent temperature increases from opening the refrigerator can alter the vaccine's potency. For protection against light, the vial can be wrapped in aluminum foil. Periodic checks are established to ensure that no vaccine is used after its expiration date.

The DTaP vaccines contain the adjuvant alum to retain the antigen at the injection site and prolong the stimulatory effect. Because subcutaneous or intracutaneous injection of the adjuvant can cause local irritation, inflammation, or abscess formation, attention to excellent intramuscular injection technique must be used (see Atraumatic Care box, p. 360, and Table 10-7).

One of the most important features of injecting vaccines is adequate penetration of the muscle for deposition of the drug intramuscularly and not subcutaneously. The use of appropriate needle length is an essential component of administering vaccines. In two studies, the use of longer needles significantly decreased the incidence of localized edema and tenderness when vaccines were administered to a group of infants (Diggle and Deeks, 2000; Diggle, Deeks, and Pollard, 2006) (see Intramuscular Administration, Chapter 22).

The total series requires several injections, and every attempt is made to rotate the sites and administer the injections as painlessly as possible (see Intramuscular Administration, Chapter 22). When two or more injections are given at separate sites, the order of injections is arbitrary. Because allergic reactions can occur after injection of vaccines, appropriate precautions are taken (see Anaphylaxis, Chapter 25).

Nurses often administer vaccines and thus have the responsibility for adequately informing parents of the nature, prevalence, and risks of the disease; the type of immunization product to be used; the expected benefits and the risk of side effects of the vaccine; and the need for accurate immunization records. Referring to immunizations as "baby shots" and limiting the discussion to vague statements about the vaccines are unacceptable practices.

Another important nursing responsibility is accurate documentation. Each child should have an immunization record for parents to keep, especially for families who move frequently. Although immunization rates have increased significantly, health professionals should use every opportunity to encourage complete immunization of all children (see Community Focus box). Blank immunization records may be downloaded from a number of websites, including the Im-

TABLE 10-7

Product Brand Names for Principal Childhood Vaccine Types

PRODUCT	BRAND NAME (MANUFACTURER, DISTRIBUTOR)	ROUTE
DTaP—Diphtheria and tetanus toxoids and acellular pertussis vaccine	Infanrix (GKS) Tripedia (SP) Daptacel (SP)	Intramuscular
Tdap—Tetanus (booster toxoid), reduced diphtheria toxoid, acellular pertussis adsorbed	Boostrix (booster for ages 10-18 years) (GKS) Adacel (booster for ages 11 to 64) (SP)	Intramuscular
DTaP-Hib—Diphtheria and tetanus toxoids and acellular pertussis and *Haemophilus influenzae* type b vaccine	TriHIBit* (ActHIB Hib reconstituted with Tripedia DTaP) (SP) Pediarix (DTaP, HepB, IPV) (GKS)	Intramuscular
DTwP—Diphtheria and tetanus toxoids and whole-cell pertussis vaccine	No trade name (SP)	Intramuscular
HepA—Hepatitis A vaccine	Havrix (GKS) Vaqta (MRK) Twinrix (HepA and HepB—ages 18 and above) (GKS)	Intramuscular
HepB—Hepatitis B vaccine	Engerix-B (GKS) Recombivax HB (MRK)	Intramuscular
Hib—*H. influenzae* type b conjugate vaccine		
HbOC—Oligosaccharides conjugated to diphtheria CRM_{197} toxin protein	HibTITER (Wyeth)	Intramuscular
PRP-OMP—Polyribosylribitol phosphate polysaccharide conjugated to a meningococcal outer membrane protein	PedvaxHIB (MRK)	Intramuscular
PRP-T—Polyribosylribitol phosphate polysaccharide conjugated to tetanus toxoid	ActHIB (SP)	Intramuscular
Hib-HepB—*H. influenzae* type b and hepatitis B vaccine	Comvax (Hib component = PRP-OMP) (MRK)	Intramuscular
Hib/DTaP/IPV	Pentacel (SP)—pending FDA licensure	
IPV—Trivalent inactivated polio vaccine (killed Salk type)	IPOL (SP)	Intramuscular or subcutaneous
MMR—Measles, mumps, rubella vaccine	M-M-R$_{II}$ (MRK)	Subcutaneous
MMRV—Measles, mumps, rubella, and varicella virus vaccine live	ProQuad (MRK)	Subcutaneous
PCV—Pneumococcal conjugate vaccine	Prevnar (Wyeth)	Intramuscular
PPV—Pneumococcal polysaccharide vaccine	Pneumovax 23 (MRK)	Intramuscular
TIV (influenza)—Trivalent inactivated influenza vaccine	Fluvirin (Novartis) Fluzone (SP) Fluarix (GKS)	Intramuscular
MCV4 (meningococcal conjugate)—Quadrivalent, groups A, C, Y, and W-135	Menactra (SP)	Intramuscular
MPSV4 (meningococcal polysaccharide)—Groups A, C, Y, and W-135	Menomune (SP)	Subcutaneous
Influenza—live attenuated (LAIV)	FluMist (MedImmune)	Intranasal
Varicella live vaccine	Varivax (MRK)	Subcutaneous
Rotavirus	RotaTeq (MRK) Rotarix (GKS)—pending FDA licensure	Oral
Human papillomavirus vaccine (quadrivalent)	Gardasil (MRK)	Intramuscular

Modified from American Academy of Pediatrics: Combination vaccines for childhood immunization: recommendations of the Advisory Committee on Immunization Practices (ACIP), the American Academy of Pediatrics (AAP), and the American Academy of Family Physicians (AAFP), *Pediatrics* 103(5):1072, 1999; American Academy of Pediatrics, Committee on Infectious Diseases, Pickering L, editor: *Red book: 2006 report of the Committee on Infectious Diseases*, ed 27, Elk Grove Village, Ill, 2006, The Academy; Centers for Disease Control and Prevention: Quadrivalent human papillomavirus vaccine, *MMWR* 56(RR-2):1-24, 2007; and US Food and Drug Administration: Biological license application supplement: noteworthy approvals. In *FDA News*, Rockville, Md, Feb 3, 2006, The Administration, retrieved Jan 2, 2008 from http://www.fda.gov/cber/appr2007/2007Lsup.htm.

GKS, GlaxoKlineSmith; *MRK*, Merck & Co.; *SP*, Sanofi Pasteur.

*TriHIBit is licensed only for the fourth dose in the vaccination series, recommended at ages 15-18 months.

munization Action Coalition,* which has vaccine information and records in a number of languages.

The following information is documented on the medical record: day, month, and year of administration; manufacturer and lot number of vaccine; and the name, address, and title of the person administering the vaccine. Additional data to record are the site and route of administration and evidence

that the parent or legal guardian gave informed consent before the immunization was administered. Any adverse reactions after the administration of any vaccine are reported to the **Vaccine Adverse Event Reporting System.***

An additional source of vaccine information that must be given to parents (by law; National Childhood Vaccine Injury

---

*http://www.immunize.org.

---

*For information call (800) 822-7967 or visit http://www.fda.gov/cber/vaers/vaers.htm.

COMMUNITY FOCUS

Improving Immunization Rates Among Children and Adolescents

Strategies that may increase compliance include giving parents vaccine information at the time of the newborn's discharge, mailing reminder cards, making immunization services readily available, removing barriers to vaccination (such as long waiting times and appointment-only systems), and taking every opportunity to immunize children when they enter a health care facility (such as emergency departments, clinics, private offices, and hospitals).

Despite improvements in vaccination rates among infants and young children, adolescents are often incompletely immunized. An immunization update is an important part of adolescent preventive care, especially at 11 to 12 years of age. With the exception of pregnant teenagers, all adolescents should receive a second dose of the measles, mumps, and rubella (MMR) vaccine unless they have documentation of two MMR vaccinations after the first 12 months of life. Two doses of varicella vaccine are recommended for persons 13 years of age or older; these should be administered at least 4 weeks apart. All adolescents who have not previously completed the three-dose series of the hepatitis B vaccine should initiate or complete the series at age 11 to 12 years.

Adolescents ages 11 to 12 years and no later than 16 years should receive a dose of the tetanus and diphtheria toxoids and acellular pertussis (TdaP) vaccine if they have received the primary series of vaccinations and if no dose was received during the previous 5 years.

Hepatitis A vaccine should be given to all adolescents who have not yet been vaccinated for hepatitis A and to those who are traveling or living in countries where the hepatitis A virus is endemic or in communities with high rates of hepatitis A, chronic liver disease, intravenous drug users, or men who have sex with other men. Adolescents who have chronic disorders or underlying medical conditions that place them at high risk for complications associated with the disease, such as influenza, should receive the appropriate vaccines (see p. 359). The meningococcal vaccine (MCV4) is now recommended for all older children (ages 11 and older) and adolescents who have not previously received the polysaccharide meningococcal vaccine (MPSV4); they should be vaccinated before or when entering college, especially if planning to live in a college dormitory.

Finally, the human papillomavirus (HPV) vaccine may be offered to girls 11 to 12 years of age to prevent cervical cancer. The vaccine is given in a series of three intramuscular injections, with the second dose 2 months after the first, and the third and final dose 6 months after the first. Adolescents 13 to 18 years of age may also complete the three-dose series if not previously immunized for HPV.

Act, 1986) before the administration of given vaccines is the **vaccine information statement (VIS)** for the particular vaccine being administered. Practitioners are required to fully inform families of the risks and benefits of the vaccines. VISs are designed to provide updated information to the adult vaccinee or parents or legal guardians of children being vaccinated regarding the risks and benefits of each vaccine. Questions regarding the information in the VISs should be answered by the practitioner. VISs are available for the following vaccines: anthrax, tetanus, diphtheria, pertussis, MMR, IPV, varicella, Hib, influenza, meningococcal, pneumococcal, rabies, smallpox, yellow fever, Japanese encephalitis, rotavirus, human papillomavirus, typhoid, HPV, HepA, and HepB. An updated VIS should be provided, and docu-

mentation in the patient's chart should state that the VIS was given and include the publication date of the VIS. VISs are available from state or local health departments or from the Immunization Action Coalition* and Centers for Disease Control and Prevention.†

In response to the concerns of manufacturers, practitioners, and parents of children with serious vaccine-associated injuries, the **National Childhood Vaccine Injury Act** of 1986 and the **Vaccine Compensation Amendments** of 1987 were passed. Basically, these laws are designed to provide fair compensation for children who are inadvertently injured and provide greater protection from liability for vaccine manufacturers and providers.

One survey found that a large percentage (65%) of children under the age of 2 years were not fully immunized in a large health maintenance organization population, perhaps because of the lack of coordinated immunization information. In addition, the study found that more than 51% had at least one immunization error and more than 20% had an unnecessary or incorrect immunization based on current recommendations (Mell, Ogren, Davis, and others, 2005). Therefore recommendations are in place to improve the overall effectiveness of the national vaccination program. It has been suggested that local or national computerized registries and improved record tracking systems be established to improve communication; additional recommendations include improving provider knowledge of immunization status and contraindications for administering vaccines and simplifying the immunization guidelines (Lee and Bernstein, 2005).

INJURY PREVENTION

Injuries are a major cause of death during infancy, especially for children 6 to 12 months old. According to a Canadian survey (Pickett, Streight, Simpson, and others, 2003), the top leading causes of injury to infants were falls, ingestion injuries, and burns. The three leading cause of accidental death injury in infants were suffocation, motor vehicle–related injuries, and drowning (Centers for Disease Control and Prevention, 2007a). Constant vigilance, awareness, and supervision are essential as the child gains increased locomotor and manipulative skills that are coupled with an insatiable curiosity about the environment. Box 10-1 lists the major developmental achievements of each period during infancy and the appropriate injury prevention plan.

Aspiration of Foreign Objects

Asphyxiation by foreign material in the respiratory tract, combined with mechanical suffocation, is one of the leading causes of fatal injury in children younger than 1 year. Both food and nonfood items are among the most common foreign bodies ingested and found in the gastrointestinal tract (Agran, Anderson, Winn, and others, 2003). The size, shape, and consistency of foods or objects are important determinants of fatal obstruction. For example, small spheric or cylindric and pliable objects (less than 3.2 cm [1.25 inches]) are more likely to completely obstruct the airway. Unfortunately, common household items can be deadly to infants.

As soon as infants have the ability to find their mouth, they are vulnerable to aspiration of small objects, such as those left

---

*http://www.immunize.org/vis.
†http://www.cdc.gov/vaccines/pubs/vis/default.htm.

BOX 10-1

Injury Prevention During Infancy

BIRTH TO 4 MONTHS

Major Developmental Accomplishments

Exhibits involuntary reflexes (e.g., crawling reflex may propel infant forward or backward; startle reflex may cause the body to jerk)

May roll over

Has increasing eye-hand coordination and voluntary grasp reflex

Injury Prevention

Aspiration

Aspiration is not as great a danger to this age-group, but parents should begin practicing safeguarding early (see under Age 4 to 7 Months).

Never shake baby powder directly on infant; place powder in hand and then on infant's skin; store container closed and out of infant's reach.

Hold infant for feeding; do not prop bottle.

Know emergency procedures for choking.

Use pacifier with one-piece construction and loop handle.

Burns

Install smoke detectors in home.

Use caution when warming formula in microwave oven; always check temperature of liquid before feeding.

Check bathwater.

Do not pour hot liquids when infant is close by, such as sitting on lap.

Beware of cigarette ashes that may fall on infant.

Do not leave infant in sun for more than a few minutes; keep skin covered.

Wash flame-retardant clothes according to label directions.

Use cool-mist vaporizers.

Do not leave child in parked car.

Check surface heat of car restraint before placing child in seat.

Suffocation and Drowning

Keep all plastic bags stored out of infant's reach; discard large plastic garment bags after tying in a knot.

Do not cover mattress with plastic.

Use firm mattress and loose blankets, with no pillows.

Make certain crib design follows federal regulations and mattress fits snugly—crib slats 2.375 inches (6 cm) apart.*

Position crib away from other furniture and away from radiators.

Do not tie pacifier on a string around infant's neck.

Remove bibs at bedtime.

Never leave infant alone in bath.

Do not leave infant under 12 months alone on adult or youth mattress or "beanbag" type seats.

Motor Vehicles

Transport infant in federally approved, rear-facing car seat, preferably in back seat.†

Do not place infant on seat (of car) or in lap.

Do not place child in a carriage or stroller behind a parked car.

Do not place infant or child in front passenger seat with an air bag.

Do not leave infant unattended in car, especially in environmental temperatures above 70° F.

Falls

Always raise crib rails.

Never leave infant alone on a raised, unguarded surface.

When in doubt as to where to place child, use floor.

Restrain child in infant seat, and never leave child unattended while the seat is resting on a raised surface.

Avoid using a high chair until child can sit well with support.

Poisoning

Poisoning is not as great a danger to this age-group, but parents should begin practicing safeguards early (see under Age 4 to 7 Months).

Bodily Damage

Keep sharp or jagged objects such as knives and broken glass out of child's reach.

Keep diaper pins closed and away from infant.

AGE 4 TO 7 MONTHS

Major Developmental Accomplishments

Rolls over

Sits momentarily

Grasps and manipulates small objects

Resecures a dropped object

Has well-developed eye-hand coordination

Can focus on and locate very small objects

Has prominent mouthing (oral fixation)

Can push up on hands and knees

Crawls backward

Injury Prevention

Aspiration

Keep buttons, beads, syringe caps, and other small objects out of infant's reach.

Keep floor free of any small objects.

Do not feed infant hard candy, nuts, food with pits or seeds, or whole or circular pieces of hot dog.

Exercise caution when giving teething biscuits, since large chunks may be broken off and aspirated.

Do not feed infant while he or she is lying down.

Inspect toys for removable parts.

Keep baby powder, if used, out of reach.

Avoid storing large quantities of cleaning fluid, paints, pesticides, and other toxic substances.

Discard used containers of poisonous substances.

Do not store toxic substances in food or drink containers.

Discard used button-size batteries; store new batteries in safe area.

Know telephone number of local poison control center ([800] 222-1222) (usually listed in front of telephone directory).

Suffocation

Keep all latex balloons out of reach.

Remove all crib toys that are strung across crib or playpen when child begins to push up on hands or knees or is 5 months old.

Burns

Keep water faucets out of reach.

Place hot objects (cigarettes, candles, incense) on high surface out of child's reach.

Limit exposure to sun; apply sunscreen.

Falls

Restrain in a high chair.

Keep crib rails raised to full height.

Motor Vehicles

See under Birth to 4 Months.

*Information on many items such as cribs or walkers is available from U.S. Consumer Product Safety Commission, (800) 638-2722; http://www.cpsc.gov.
†See footnote on p. 370.

BOX 10-1
Injury Prevention During Infancy—cont'd

AGE 4 TO 7 MONTHS—cont'd
Injury Prevention—cont'd
Poisoning
Make certain that paint for furniture or toys does not contain lead.
Place toxic substances on a high shelf or in locked cabinet.
Hang plants or place on high surface rather than on floor.
Know telephone number of local poison control center ([800] 222-1222) (usually listed in front of telephone directory).

Bodily Damage
Give toys that are smooth and rounded, preferably made of wood or plastic.
Avoid long, pointed objects as toys.
Avoid toys that are excessively loud.
Keep sharp objects out of infant's reach.

AGE 8 TO 12 MONTHS
Major Developmental Accomplishments
Crawls or creeps
Stands, holding onto furniture
Stands alone
Cruises around furniture
Walks
Climbs
Pulls on objects
Throws objects
Is able to pick up small objects; has pincer grasp
Explores by putting objects in mouth
Dislikes being restrained
Explores away from parent
Increasingly understands simple commands and phrases

Injury Prevention
Aspiration
Keep small objects off floor, off furniture, and out of reach of children.
Take care in feeding solid table food to give very small pieces.
Do not use beanbag toys or allow child to play with dried beans.
See also under Age 4 to 7 Months.

Bodily Damage
See under Age 4 to 7 Months.
Avoid placing televisions or other large objects on top of furniture, which may be overturned when infant pulls self to standing position.

Falls
Avoid walkers, especially near stairs.*
Ensure that furniture is sturdy enough for child to pull self to standing position and cruise.
Fence stairways at top and bottom if child has access to either end.*
Dress infant in safe shoes and clothing (soles that do not "catch" on floor, tied shoelaces, pant legs that do not touch floor).

Suffocation and Drowning
Keep doors of ovens, dishwashers, refrigerators, coolers, and front-loading clothes washers and dryers closed at all times.
If storing an unused large appliance, such as a refrigerator, remove the door.
Supervise contact with inflated balloons; immediately discard popped balloons, and keep uninflated balloons out of reach.
Fence swimming pools and other bodies of standing water such as decorative fountains; lock gate to swimming pools so only adult can access.
Always supervise when near any source of water, such as cleaning buckets, drainage areas, toilets.
Keep bathroom doors closed.
Eliminate unnecessary pools of water.
Keep one hand on child at all times when in tub.

Poisoning
Administer medications as a drug, not as a candy.
Do not administer medications unless prescribed by a practitioner.
Return medications and poisons to safe storage area immediately after use; replace caps properly if a child-protector cap is used.
Have poison control center number ([800] 222-1222) on telephone and refrigerator.

Burns
Place guards in front of or around any heating appliance, fireplace, or furnace.
Keep electrical wires hidden or out of reach.
Place plastic guards over electrical outlets; place furniture in front of outlets.
Keep hanging tablecloths out of reach (child may pull down hot liquids or heavy or sharp objects).

*Information on many items such as cribs or walkers is available from U.S. Consumer Product Safety Commission, (800) 638-2722; http://www.cpsc.gov.

within reach or removable parts of objects that may on initial inspection appear safe. **Toys** are one of the leading sources for asphyxiation; therefore all toys must be carefully inspected for potential danger. Rattles, for example, have small beads in them to produce noise. A broken or cracked rattle can be dangerous because the beads can easily be aspirated while the infant has the toy in the mouth. Stuffed animals are another potentially dangerous toy if any of the parts, such as the eyes or nose, are removable buttons or plastic pieces. An active infant can grab a low-hanging mobile and quickly chew off a small piece. As soon as the infant crawls or plays on the floor, the floor must be kept free of any small articles that can be picked up and swallowed, such as coins.

When infant **clothes** are purchased, the type of closure is important. A front button can easily be pulled off and swal-

lowed. Safety pins for diapers are kept closed and away from the dressing table. Even though a young infant may not search for them, practicing this good habit from the beginning prevents future injuries.

Food items are also a very common cause of aspiration in children, and the most common offenders are hot dogs, candy, nuts, and grapes. When new foods are given to the child, nuts, hard candies, marshmallows, large amounts of peanut butter, or fruits with pits or seeds are avoided. When traveling (especially in airplanes) or entertaining, parents must keep snack foods such as peanuts and popcorn away from young children. If given to young children, hot dogs must be cut into small, irregular pieces rather than served whole or sliced into sections, since their size (diameter), round shape, and consistency allow for complete occlusion of the airway. Perhaps the most dangerous foods are dried beans, which, if aspirated, enlarge when they come in contact with the wet mucosa and block the airway.

Pacifiers can also be dangerous because the entire object may be aspirated if it is small, or the nipple and shield may become detached from the handle and become lodged in the pharynx. Improvised pacifiers, such as those made in hospitals from a padded nipple, also present dangers. The nipple may separate from the plastic collar and be aspirated. In addition, parents may continue to offer this pacifier to the infant at home. To prevent the hazards of improvised pacifiers, hospitals should use only safe commercial types. Pacifiers should not be altered from their original shape to encourage or discourage usage. Candy pacifiers pose dangers because the candy portion can dislodge from the circular base and be aspirated. To be safe, pacifiers should have:

- Sturdy, one-piece construction with material that is nontoxic, flexible, and firm but not brittle
- An easily grasped handle
- A mouthguard that cannot be separated from the nipple, has two ventilating holes, and is too large to be aspirated
- No detachable ribbon or string
- A label warning against tying the pacifier around the infant's neck

Using a syringe to accurately measure and dispense oral liquid medications to young children has become common practice. However, the **syringe cap** is a potential aspiration hazard. As a precaution, keep parts of medication devices out of the reach of children and use a syringe designed for childhood medication administration.

Even safety devices can be dangerous. To prevent tampering, items (such as baby food jars) may be covered with a plastic oversleeve. The **tear-down strip** can be aspirated and is very difficult to locate because it is clear.

Another hazardous substance if aspirated is **baby powder,** which is usually a mixture of talc (hydrous magnesium silicate) and other silicates. Although the use of talc has been discouraged, it is a common baby care product that can cause severe and often fatal aspiration pneumonia. One of the factors involved in talc aspiration is the similar appearance of baby powder containers and nursing bottles. Talc containers often become favorite playthings and are placed in the mouth. Improperly using powder by sprinkling it directly on the skin creates a cloud of talc dust that is easily inhaled. Parents are advised of the danger of baby powder and are discouraged from using it. If they prefer to use a powder, a cornstarch preparation can be substituted (see Diaper Dermatitis, Chapter 30). Whenever a powder is used, it is placed in the hand and then applied to the skin, never shaken directly from the container to the skin. The container is kept closed and immediately stored in a safe place, especially away from curious toddlers, who often imitate caregiving activities and may shake it on the infant.

Suffocation

Schnitzer (2006) indicates that almost 67% of injury deaths in infants are due to suffocation. Mechanical suffocation includes suffocation by covering of the airway (i.e., mouth and nose); by pressure on the throat and chest; and by exclusion of air, such as by refrigerator entrapment. Nonfood items cause the majority of deaths in young children. **Latex balloons,** whether partially inflated, uninflated, or popped, are the lead-

ing cause of pediatric choking deaths from children's products. They should be kept away from infants and young children. Even the practice of inflating latex gloves to amuse children in health care settings may pose a danger, especially if the child is latex sensitive. Future deaths may be avoided by changing balloon design and materials and substituting Mylar or paper balloons. In addition, the accessibility of the plastic linings of diapers used on the infant or on dolls is especially dangerous to young children.

The type of **bed** or **crib** poses a number of hazards. An infant who is placed in a bed under tucked-in blankets and sheets can be caught under them and unable to wriggle free. Baby pillows filled with plastic foam beads that make them resemble small beanbags are dangerous; very young infants are suffocated when the pillow contours to the face and blocks the airway. There are potential dangers in adults sleeping with an infant because of the possibility of their rolling over and smothering the child (overlaying), especially when alcohol, tobacco, or recreational drugs are involved. Studies of sudden and unexpected infant deaths have shown that such infants were found in unsafe sleeping positions (prone or on soft bedding surface) or were placed to sleep in a bed, sofa, or chair not intended for infant sleeping. Another common cause of infant suffocation was wedging between a bed or mattress and a wall and oronasal obstruction by a plastic bag.

> **NURSINGALERT**
> Encourage adults to:
> - Blow up balloons for children
> - Closely supervise children's balloon play
> - Pick up and dispose of broken balloon pieces
> - Warn older children of dangers of chewing or sucking on balloons
> - Substitute Mylar or paper balloons for latex balloons

Infant strangulation may occur if the infant's head becomes caught between the crib slats and mattress or objects close to the crib. Suffocation deaths are not confined to cribs; ill-fitting mattresses in adult or youth beds, bunk beds, and waterbeds have also been reported. According to U.S. federal regulation, the distance between crib slats should not be more than 2.375 inches (6 cm), roughly the width of three adult fingers. Mattresses and bumper pads should fit snugly against the slats. A general rule is that the mattress is too small if two adult fingers can be placed between the mattress and crib or bed side. A temporary solution is to place large, rolled towels in the space to create a snug fit.

Corner post extensions on cribs are another source of strangulation. Children have died when their clothing caught on raised corner posts as they climbed out of the crib. Voluntary manufacturing standards state that corner post extensions not exceed 0.0625 inch (0.16 cm). However, the safety of any extension is questionable. Decorative extensions need to be removed from cribs. Ideally, information regarding correct crib design should be given prenatally, before parents have purchased or borrowed a crib.*

Mesh-sided playpens and cribs can result in death if the sides are left in the lowered position. Infants have suffocated when they fell off the edge of the mattress and the head or

---

*A number of parent education pamphlets—such as *Crib Safety Tips* and *Is Your Used Crib Safe?*—are available in English and Spanish from the U.S. Consumer Product Safety Commission, 4330 East West Highway, Bethesda, MD 20814; (800) 638-2772; http://www.cpsc.gov.

chest was compressed between the floorboard and mesh side. Parents should be advised of this danger and encouraged to always keep the sides locked securely in the up position whenever the child is in the playpen or crib.

The crib should be positioned away from large furniture, since children who crawl out of the crib may become caught between the two objects. Cribs should also be located away from windows, where any type of drape or blind cords (split or single) can become wrapped around the infant's neck.

Another cause of suffocation is **plastic bags.** Large plastic bags used over garments are lightweight and can easily and quickly be wrapped around the head of an active infant or pressed against the face. For this reason, pillows and mattresses should not be covered with plastic. Older infants may play with a plastic bag and accidentally pull it over their heads. Because plastic is nonporous, suffocation occurs in a matter of minutes.

Bibs are removed at bedtime, and objects such as pacifiers are never hung on a string around the infant's neck. This is a common practice in some cultures that can be remedied by tying a *short* string to a pacifier and pinning the string to the child's shirt. Toys that have strings attached, such as a telephone, or toys that are tied to cribs or playpens can be hazards because the string can become wrapped around the child's neck or the child can become entrapped in the toy. As a precaution, all cords should be less than 30 cm (12 inches) long. Crib toys should be hung high enough that the infant cannot become entangled in them and should no longer be used after the child is able to reach them.

If applied too loosely or left unfastened, restraining straps can be a hazard. For example, a child may slide off a high chair beneath the tray and become strangled on the loose strap. All straps should be fastened securely.

Motor Vehicle Injuries

Automobile injuries are the leading cause of accidental death in children between the ages of 1 and 9 years (Centers for Disease Control and Prevention, 2007a). A significant number of nonfatal vehicle-related injuries in children between 1 and 4 years of age occur as a result of back-over injuries while playing in a driveway (Centers for Disease Control and Prevention, 2005b). However, many infants are injured or die from improper restraint within the vehicle, most often while riding on the lap of another occupant. Reports indicate that child restraint use decreases with increasing age of children and increasing number of occupants. Lack of proper child restraint continues to be a major factor in fatal accidents involving children. All infants must be secured in a federally approved restraint rather than held or placed on the seat of the car. There is no safe alternative.

Infant restraints are designed either as an infant-only model or as a convertible infant-toddler model (Fig. 10-13). Either restraint is a semireclined seat when facing the *rear* of the car. A rear-facing car seat provides the best protection for the disproportionately heavy head and weak neck of a young child. This position minimizes the stress on the neck by spreading the forces of a frontal crash over the entire back, neck, and head; the spine is supported by the back of the car seat. If the seat were faced forward, the head would whip forward because of the force of the crash, creating enormous stress on the neck. One recent study has shown that children from birth to 23 months experienced fewer injuries when rid-

FIG. 10-13 ■ Convertible seat in forward-facing position for older infants and toddlers.

ing in rear-facing car restraints (Henary, Sherwood, Crandall, and others, 2007). The findings suggest that guidelines may soon be revised to recommend a rear-facing car restraint position in children over 1 year of age.

The restraint is anchored to the vehicle with the vehicle's seat belt or LATCH (lower anchors and tethers for children) system, and the restraint has a harness system for securing the infant (see Fig. 12-11). The five-point harness system provides the most effective support for infant restraint; the three-point harness system secures only the upper body. Many infant seats have a plastic base that can be left in the car; the seat latches or clicks into the base so that the base does not have to be installed each time the car seat is removed. The LATCH system provides car seat anchors between the front cushion and backrest so the seat belt does not have to be used. Some automobiles have tether anchors for rear-facing infant-only seats as well. Although many infant restraints can be recliners, they are used in the car only in the position specified by the manufacturer.

> **NURSINGALERT**
>
> Infants should face the rear from birth to 9070 g (20 pounds) and as close to 1 year of age as possible. If the child weighs 20 pounds but is not 1 year old, the rear-facing position is still recommended.

Severe injuries and deaths in children have occurred from air bags deploying on impact in the front passenger seat. The back seat is the safest area of the car for children. For restraints to be effective, they must be used properly. Dressing the infant in an outfit with sleeves and legs allows the harness to hold the child securely in the seat. A small blanket or towel rolled tightly can be placed on either side of the head to minimize movement and keep the infant's hips against the back of the seat. Padding between the infant's legs and crotch is added to prevent slouching. Thick, soft padding is not placed under the infant or behind the back because during the impact the padding will compress, leaving the harness straps loose. Preterm infants being discharged home from the hospital should be placed in an appropriate car seat restraint as it would be placed in the car and the infant's heart rate and oxygen saturation monitored for a minimum of 1 hour and maximum of 3 hours (depending on the length of the trip to the home) to detect any potential problems with airway occlusion. (See Community Focus, p. 268, for preterm infant restraint; for further discussion of car seat restraints, see Chapter 12.)

Falls

Residential injuries, especially falls, accounted for the highest incidence of unintentional injuries to children seen in emergency departments in the United States (Phelan, Khoury, Kalkwarf, and others, 2005). Falls are most common after 4 months of age when the infant has learned to roll over, but they can occur at any age. The best advice is never to place a child of any age unattended on a raised surface.

When in doubt, the safest place is the floor. Even though young infants cannot climb over a partially raised crib rail, it is best to form a habit of raising the rail all the way, since someday that infant will be able to climb out. Crib sides should have a latching device that cannot be easily released.

Another danger area for falling is the **changing table,** which is usually high and narrow. Although these tables have a restraining belt, children are never left unattended, even when restrained. The best way to avoid the need to leave the child unattended is to arrange the area with all necessary articles within easy reach so the child's safety can be ensured. During the latter half of the first year, infants usually resist dressing and diapering and may be difficult to manage; therefore changing clothes may need to take place on a larger safe surface such as a clean floor.

Infant seats, high chairs, mobile walkers, and swings present additional opportunities for falls. If the **infant seat** is placed on a table, the child should never be left unrestrained or unattended. The same rule is essential for other baby equipment, particularly when the child has learned to crawl and to stand up. Small infants can slip through a high chair if a protective harness is not used. The danger of falls from being unrestrained also applies to shopping carts. **High chairs** are designed for older infants who can sit well and who are tall enough to have the tray at the level of their chest or abdomen.

Infant walkers (mobile) are responsible for a number of different types of injuries that occur because the walker tipped over or fell down stairs. Parents need to be warned of these dangers and encouraged to keep a constant vigil on their child's activities. The American Academy of Pediatrics (2001a) does not recommend the use of mobile infant walkers. The use of older-model mobile walkers in particular should be discouraged. In response to the large number of accidents and deaths associated with infant walkers, several manufacturers modified these products to prevent falls down stairs. The new

models should have a label or sign indicating "meets new safety standard," must be wider than 36 inches, or must have a braking mechanism to stop the walker. Infant walkers may still pose a risk for climbing up to reach dangerous objects and should be carefully supervised. One alternative is to use a stationary play station with a seat similar to a walker. There is no evidence that infant walkers help infants walk sooner.

After infants are mobile, they should not be allowed to crawl unsupervised on any raised surface, near stairs, or near any water reservoir. Gates should be used at the *bottom* and *top of stairs,* since both present dangers to the crawling and climbing infant. However, certain types of gates can present hazards. Freestanding enclosures constructed of crisscrossed wood slats that expand and contract can trap the head or neck when children attempt to climb over them. If these types of gates are used, they must be securely fastened to prevent mobility of the slats.

Even when the environment is made safe, infants may sometimes literally trip over their own feet from **clothing.** Slippery socks; hard, slick soles on shoes or rubber soles that can catch, especially on a carpet; and long pants or pajama bottoms can easily upset a child's balance. Such dangers need to be pointed out to parents, especially when infants are taking their first steps.

An alarming number of small children fall out of windows and are hurt; this is especially common with windows such as bay windows that have wide ledges for children to sit on. Window screens should not be perceived as fall-prevention devices; rather, window guards should be installed to prevent falls from any window, regardless of the height. Furniture should be kept away from windows so children cannot climb onto the furniture and access the window.

Poisoning

Poisoning is one of the major causes of death in children younger than 5 years of age. The highest incidence occurs in the 2-year-old group, with the second highest incidence occurring in 1-year-old children. Infants who do not crawl are relatively free from danger of poisonous agents by virtue of immobility. However, after locomotion begins, danger from poisoning is present almost everywhere. There are more than 500 toxic substances in the average home, with approximately one third of all poisonings occurring in the kitchen.

The major reason for ingestion of poisons is **improper storage.** To protect the infant, toxic agents should not be placed on a low shelf, table, or floor. Drugs that are kept in a purse pose additional dangers; if the handbag is given to infants to play with, they may open it and ingest the drug. Another unrecognized hazard occurs during diaper changes, when infants are near many toxic substances such as ointments, creams, oils, and talc. Common household over-the-counter medications such as acetaminophen and cold and cough preparations, cosmetics and personal care products, and cleaning products are also sources of childhood poisoning (Wilkerson, Northington, and Fisher, 2005).

Plants are another source of poisoning for infants. Plants are commonly placed on the floor, and the leaves or flowers are attractive and easy to pull off. More than 700 species of plants are known to have caused illness or death.

Another danger is ingestion of the **button-sized batteries** used in devices such as hearing aids, calculators, watches, and

*An air bag safety fact sheet is available from the American Academy of Pediatrics, 141 Northwest Point Blvd., Elk Grove Village, IL 60007; (847) 434-4000; fax: (847) 434-8000; http://www.aap.org; for car seats, http://www.aap.org/family/carseatguide.htm. Information is also available from the Insurance Institute for Highway Safety, 1005 N. Glebe Road, Suite 800, Arlington, VA 22201; (703) 247-1500; fax: (703) 247-1588; http://www.highwaysafety.org. The National Highway Traffic Safety Administration, http://www.nhtsa.dot.gov, also provides child passenger safety and air bag safety information for parents.

cameras. Because they are bright and shiny, they are attractive to children. However, they can cause severe morbidity, even death, if lodged in the esophagus. The strong alkali in a battery can leak and cause a severe caustic burn. As a precaution, small batteries must be safely stored and discarded where young children cannot easily retrieve them.

Not all poisonings result from ingestion. **Inhalation** is another possible route, such as inhaling chlorine vapors from household cleaning or pool supplies. The production of methamphetamines, a common central nervous system stimulant also known as ice, speed, or crystal, involves a number of chemicals that may be toxic alone (by contact or ingestion) or during the production (cooking) of the drug itself. Methamphetamine laboratories are commonly located in household areas where children may be exposed to harmful inhalants; children are also at risk for burns from being in an area where methamphetamine is being cooked, since explosions are not uncommon. Children should be protected from environments in which inhaled toxins exist (for a discussion of passive or second-hand tobacco smoke, see Chapter 23).

The only sure way to prevent poisoning is to remove toxic agents, which means placing containers out of the infant's reach or contact. Because crawling infants soon become climbing toddlers, it is best to keep all toxic agents, especially drugs, in a locked cabinet. Special plastic hooks can be attached to the inside of cabinet doors to keep them securely closed. Firm thumb pressure is required to unlatch the hook, and small children are usually unable to manipulate them. Locks are best, but for frequently used cleaning agents, such as those often kept under a kitchen sink, hooks are a practical alternative.

With several hundred toxic substances in each house, locking up all potentially toxic substances can present a problem; however, careful planning can help. A large surplus of cleaning agents, furniture polishes, laundry additives, paints, insecticides, and solvents should be avoided. Used poison containers should be promptly discarded and not used to store another poison without adequately marking the package. Potentially hazardous substances should not be stored in any type of food container. A popular container used to store toxic liquids is a soda, or pop, bottle. A child who is unaware of the dangerous contents is vulnerable to poisoning. Parents should know the location of local poison control centers and call them in the event of a suspected poisoning. Emergency measures for poisoning are discussed in Chapter 14.

Burns

Scalding from water that is too hot; excessive sunburn; and burns from house fires, electrical wires, sockets, and heating elements such as radiators, registers, and floor furnaces cause a significant number of deaths and many more injuries in infants. The infant's skin is particularly sensitive to irritation, and the mechanisms for temperature perception are not completely developed. As a general precaution, all homes should have smoke alarms installed near the bedroom areas and on each level of the building.

Scald burns from **hot tap water** can be prevented by lowering the water heater to a safe temperature of 49° C (120° F). In addition, the bathwater should be checked before the infant is immersed. Scalds can also occur from bathing infants in the kitchen sink when the garbage disposal, occluded with debris,

causes the draining dishwasher effluent to back up into the sink. The temperature of the effluent from a dishwasher is typically that of the maximum water temperature of the household water heater, but many dishwashers are equipped with heating elements that heat water to a temperature that is even higher. As a precaution, instruct caregivers to avoid bathing small children in the kitchen sink while the dishwasher is running.

If baby food is warmed in a **microwave oven,** it must be checked before feeding because the container may remain cool while the contents are hot. The handles of cooking pots should be turned toward the back of the stove. When the infant is underfoot, pouring hot liquids and cooking with hot oil are avoided. Hanging tablecloths are also placed out of the infant's reach to prevent pulling hot items off the table.

Sunburn can be a source of a first- or second-degree burn. Exposure to direct sunlight should be avoided for the first 6 months. When infants are in the sun, the body, especially the face and head, should be covered. Sunscreen can be used on older infants but should be used on small areas of the body and sparingly in infants younger than 6 months (see Sunburn, Chapter 30). Although dark-skinned infants burn less readily, their thin skin also can become sunburned and needs protection.

Electrical outlets should be covered with protective plastic caps that prevent the child from sucking on the outlet or putting objects such as hairpins into it. Live wires are placed out of reach so that curious infants cannot chew on them and break the rubber coating. Infants should not be allowed to play near television sets, stereo units, or other appliances, whether these units are turned on or off, because infants cannot determine when the appliance is safe.

Any **heat-producing element** should have a guard placed in front of it. Fireplaces should be well screened because they are appealing and within easy access. Small, portable heaters should be placed on a high surface. Floor furnaces should have barrier gates to prevent children from crawling or walking over them. Burning cigarettes, candles, and incense should be kept out of reach, and infants should not be held by a smoking adult because falling ashes are a hazard, especially to the eyes. Heated-mist vaporizers are a source of burns and should not be used. If humidity is needed, only cool-mist vaporizers are safe.

By law, all infant sleepwear must be flame retardant. Unfortunately, this does not apply to all **infant clothing.** Flame-retardant fabric must never be viewed as the ultimate protection against burns. Repeated washing reduces the flame-retardant properties, and the use of soap or bleach destroys the protection. If sleepwear is home sewn, parents are advised to look for specially treated, flame-retardant fabric.

Another type of thermal injury occurs when children are exposed to excessive heat during confinement in poorly ventilated **vehicles.** The practice of leaving the windows open a couple of inches is not protective. Parents are cautioned to never leave children in parked cars if the outside ambient temperature is above 27° C (80° F). A significant number of childhood deaths occur annually when a child is left unattended in a vehicle.

Children can also be burned by overheated metal hardware and vinyl seats in cars parked in the sun. As a precaution, the surface heat of car restraints should be determined before placing children in them. Covering the restraints and hardware (such as metal latches on seat belts) may be necessary to prevent skin burns. An additional safeguard is buying a light-colored restraint, which absorbs less heat.

Drowning

Drowning in this age-group can occur in just an inch or two of water. Consequently, infants should *always* be supervised in a bathtub or near a source of water such as a swimming pool, lake, toilet, or bucket. In a survey of drownings most infants younger than age 1 year drowned in a toilet, bathtub, or bucket (Lassman, 2002); 5-gallon buckets are particularly dangerous because the child may inadvertently fall in head first and, because of the weight of the upper body at this age, be unable to withdraw from the bucket. Organized swimming instruction is not recommended for children younger than 4 years of age because it may lead to a false sense of security. No infant can be expected to learn the elements of water safety or to react appropriately in an emergency. Therefore all young children need to be considered at risk when near water. Infants and toddlers are also at increased risk of infection and seizures from swallowing large amounts of water.

Bodily Damage

Injuries can occur in numerous ways. Sharp, jagged-edged objects can cause wounds in the skin. Long-pointed articles, such as the common toothpick or fork, can be poked into the eye or ear, causing serious damage. Such articles should be safely stored away from the infant's reach; forks are best avoided for self-feeding until the child has mastered the spoon, usually by age 18 months.

In addition to hazards such as aspiration, small articles can be placed in the ear or nose, and excessive noise from toys can result in sensorineural hearing loss. Although toys with the highest noise levels are model airplanes, air guns, and toy cap guns, even common squeaking toys used by young children may be harmful if placed close to the ear.

As children begin to pull themselves to a standing position, **heavy objects,** such as unsturdy furniture or any freestanding item (e.g., wrought iron fish tank stands, stereo equipment, or television), can be extremely dangerous if pulled down on top of the child. To prevent injury from furniture tipping over, televisions should be placed on lower furniture and as far back as possible. Angle braces or anchors can secure furniture to walls.

Even clothes and hair can present dangers to infants who cannot call attention to the problem. For example, constriction injuries can occur from excessively tight bands on socks or strands of hair or thread wrapped tightly around appendages, usually toes or fingers.

An alarming trend is the increasing number of infant deaths attributed to homicide. In one study 6.4% of 10,370 infant injury deaths occurred as a result of homicide (Brenner, Overpeck, Trumble, and others, 1999). Infant deaths that were previously attributed to SIDS now may be found to occur as a result of intentional harm. Specific interventions must be in place to protect infants from harm, especially in preventable situations.

Another commonly unrecognized danger to infants is animal attacks. As newcomers to the home, infants can provoke jealousy in animals such as dogs or cats or play with pets, unaware of the danger. Parents must be vigilant to protect the child from household pets and farm animals (see Animal Bites, Chapter 30).

Nurse's Role in Injury Prevention

The task of injury prevention begins to be appreciated only when the potential environmental dangers to which infants are vulnerable are considered. Injury prevention and parent education should be handled on a growth and developmental basis. It is simply impossible to completely protect infants and small children from all potential dangers without placing them in a sterile, impractical environment. However, a large percentage of childhood deaths continue to occur as a result of preventable injuries (Martin, Kochanek, Strobino, and others, 2005; Schnitzer, 2006). Nurses must be aware of the possible causes of injury in each age-group to provide anticipatory, preventive teaching. For example, the nurse should discuss guidelines for injury prevention during infancy (see Box 10-1) before the child reaches the susceptible age-group. Preventive teaching ideally begins during pregnancy.

Two thirds of all injuries to children occur in the home, and therefore the importance of safety cannot be overemphasized. The Family-Centered Care box summarizes a home safety checklist that can be presented to parents to increase their awareness of danger areas in the home and assist them in implementing safety devices and practices *before* their absence can inflict injury on infants. Hands-on displays such as cabinet latches or toilet seat locks can familiarize parents with inexpensive, commercial devices that can be used in the home to prevent injuries.

Injury prevention requires protection of the child and education of the caregiver. Nurses in ambulatory care settings, health maintenance centers, or visiting nurse agencies are in a most favorable position for injury education. This does not exclude nurses in inpatient facilities, who could use visiting times as an excellent opportunity for discussing this topic. Although early postpartum discharge may be restrictive for parent teaching, this is an excellent opportunity to introduce the family to infant safety and safety for other children as well. Parents should be encouraged to take an infant cardiopulmonary resuscitation (CPR) class to deal effectively with potential problems. This tool further empowers the parents to raise their new infant in the best environment possible.

One approach to teaching injury prevention is to relate why children in various age-groups are prone to specific types of injuries. Stressing prevention is just as important as emphasizing the *why* of the injury. However, injury prevention must also be practical. Asking parents for their ideas leads to realistic suggestions that can be followed. For instance, bathroom cleaning agents, cosmetics, and personal care items can be placed on a top shelf in the linen closet, and towels or sheets can be stored on the lower shelves and floor.

If an injury has occurred, the nurse should not be too quick to admonish the parent. Injuries do not always indicate neglect. It is a difficult task to watch children carefully without overprotecting or unnecessarily confining them. Small falls help children learn the dangers of heights. Touching a hot object once can emphasize to the child the pain of a burn. Allowing children to explore while maintaining consistent, age-appropriate limits is sound advice.

Parents need to remember that infants and young children cannot anticipate danger or understand when it is or is not present. Additionally, infants have no cognitive concept of

FAMILY-CENTERED CARE

Child Safety Home Checklist

SAFETY: FIRE, ELECTRICAL, BURNS

- ❏ Guards in front of or around any heating appliance, fireplace, or furnace (including floor furnace)*
- ❏ Electrical wires hidden or out of reach*
- ❏ No frayed or broken wires; no overloaded sockets
- ❏ Plastic guards or caps over electrical outlets; furniture in front of outlets*
- ❏ Hanging tablecloths out of reach, away from open fires*
- ❏ Smoke detectors tested and operating properly
- ❏ Kitchen matches stored out of child's reach*
- ❏ Large, deep ashtrays throughout house (if used)
- ❏ Small stoves, heaters, and other hot objects (cigarettes, candles, coffee pots, slow cookers) placed where they cannot be tipped over or reached by children
- ❏ Hot water heater set at 49° C (120° F) or lower
- ❏ Pot handles turned toward back of stove, center of table
- ❏ No loose clothing worn near stove
- ❏ No cooking or eating hot foods or liquids with child standing nearby or sitting in lap
- ❏ All small appliances, such as iron, turned off, disconnected, and placed out of reach when not in use
- ❏ Cool, not hot, mist vaporizer used
- ❏ Fire extinguisher available on each floor and checked periodically
- ❏ Electrical fuse box and gas shutoff accessible
- ❏ Family escape plan in case of a fire practiced periodically; fire escape ladder available on upper-level floors
- ❏ Telephone number of fire or rescue squad and address of home with nearest cross street posted near phone

SAFETY: SUFFOCATION AND ASPIRATION

- ❏ Small objects stored out of reach*
- ❏ Toys inspected for small removable parts or long strings*
- ❏ Hanging crib toys and mobiles placed out of reach
- ❏ Plastic bags stored away from young child's reach; large plastic garment bags discarded after tying in knots*
- ❏ Mattress or pillow not covered with plastic or in manner accessible to child*
- ❏ Crib design according to federal regulations (crib slats less than 2.375 inches [6 cm] apart) with snug-fitting mattress*†
- ❏ Crib positioned away from other furniture or windows*
- ❏ Portable playpen gates up at all times while in use*
- ❏ Accordion-style gates not used*
- ❏ Bathroom doors kept closed and toilet seats down*
- ❏ Faucets turned off firmly*
- ❏ Pool fenced with locked gate
- ❏ Proper safety equipment at poolside
- ❏ Electronic garage door openers stored safely and garage door adjusted to rise when door strikes object
- ❏ Doors of ovens, trunks, dishwashers, refrigerators, and front-loading clothes washers and dryers kept closed*
- ❏ Unused appliance, such as a refrigerator, securely closed with lock or doors removed*

- ❏ Food served in small, noncylindric pieces*
- ❏ Toy chests without lids or with lids that securely lock in open position*
- ❏ Buckets and wading pools kept empty when not in use*
- ❏ Clothesline above head level
- ❏ At least one member of household trained in basic life support (cardiopulmonary resuscitation), including first aid for choking

SAFETY: POISONING

- ❏ Toxic substances, including batteries, placed on a high shelf, preferably in locked cabinet
- ❏ Toxic plants hung or placed out of reach*
- ❏ Excess quantities of cleaning fluid, paints, pesticides, drugs, and other toxic substances not stored in home
- ❏ Used containers of poisonous substances discarded where child cannot obtain access
- ❏ Telephone number of local poison control center ([800] 222-1222) and home address with nearest cross street posted near phone
- ❏ Medicines clearly labeled in childproof containers and stored out of reach
- ❏ Household cleaners, disinfectants, and insecticides kept in their original containers, separate from food and out of reach
- ❏ Smoking in areas away from children

SAFETY: FALLS

- ❏ Nonskid mats, strips, or surfaces in tubs and showers
- ❏ Exits, halls, and passageways in rooms kept clear of toys, furniture, boxes, or other items that could be obstructive
- ❏ Stairs and halls well lighted, with switches at both top and bottom
- ❏ Sturdy handrails for all steps and stairways
- ❏ Nothing stored on stairways
- ❏ Treads, risers, and carpeting in good repair
- ❏ Glass doors and walls marked with decals
- ❏ Safety glass used in doors, windows, and walls
- ❏ Gates on top and bottom of staircases and elevated areas, such as porch, fire escape*
- ❏ Guardrails on upstairs windows with locks that limit height of window opening and access to areas such as fire escape*
- ❏ Crib side rails raised to full height; mattress lowered as child grows*
- ❏ Restraints used in high chairs, walkers, or other baby furniture; preferably walkers not used*
- ❏ Scatter rugs secured in place or used with nonskid backing
- ❏ Walks, patios, and driveways in good repair

SAFETY: BODILY INJURY

- ❏ Knives, power tools, and unloaded firearms stored safely or placed in locked cabinet
- ❏ Garden tools returned to storage racks after use
- ❏ Pets properly restrained and immunized for rabies
- ❏ Swings, slides, and other outdoor play equipment kept in safe condition
- ❏ Yard free of broken glass, nail-studded boards, other litter
- ❏ Cement birdbaths placed where young child cannot tip them over*
- ❏ Furniture anchored so child cannot pull down on top of self when climbing or pulling to stand.

*Safety measures are specific for homes with young children. All safety measures should be implemented in homes where children reside and visit frequently, such as those of grandparents or baby-sitters.
†Federal regulations are available from U.S. Consumer Product Safety Commission, (800) 638-2772; http://www.cpsc.gov.

cause and effect and therefore cannot relate meaning to experiences or potential dangers. A dead electrical wire may present no actual harm, but if the child is allowed to play with it, a poor behavior is enforced and will be practiced when the child encounters a live wire. Although it is always wise to explain why something is dangerous, it must be remembered that small children need to be physically removed from the situation.

It is not easy to teach safety, supervise closely, and refrain from saying "no" a hundred times a day. Parents become acutely aware of this dilemma as soon as the infant learns to crawl. Preventing injuries to children is usually the first reason for limit setting and discipline, but limits are also set to prevent damage to valuable household objects. When small children are in the home, dangerous objects must be removed or guarded and valuable articles placed out of reach.

When children are taught the meaning of "no," they should also be taught what "yes" means. Children should be praised for playing with suitable toys, their efforts at behaving or listening should be reinforced, and innovative and creative recreational toys should be provided for them. Infants love to tear paper and avidly pursue books, magazines, or newspapers left on the floor. Instead of always scolding them for destroying a valued book, parents should provide child-safe books (such as those constructed of fabric) for them to play with. If they enjoy pots and pans, a cabinet can be arranged with safe utensils for them to explore.

One additional factor must be stressed concerning injury prevention and education. Children are imitators; they copy what they see and hear. *Practicing safety teaches safety,* which applies to parents and their children and to nurses and their clients. Saying one thing but doing another confuses children and can lead to difficulties as the child grows older.

ANTICIPATORY GUIDANCE—CARE OF FAMILIES

Childrearing is no easy task; it presents challenges to both new parents and "seasoned" parents. With society's changing roles and mores, combined with a highly mobile population, there is little stability for traditional role models and time-honored methods of raising children. As a result, parents look to professionals for guidance. Nurses are in an advantageous position to render assistance and suggestions. Every phase of a child's life has its particular traumas—toilet training for toddlers, unexplained fears for preschoolers, and identity crises for adolescents. For parents of an infant, some challenges center around dependency, discipline, increased mobility, and safety. Major areas for parental guidance during the first year are listed in the Family-Centered Care box.

FAMILY-CENTERED CARE

Guidance During Infant's First Year

FIRST 6 MONTHS
Teach car safety with use of federally approved restraint, facing rearward, in the middle of the back seat—not in a seat with an air bag.
Understand each parent's adjustment to newborn, especially mother's postpartum emotional needs.
Teach care of infant and help parents understand his or her individual needs and temperament and that the infant expresses wants through crying.
Reassure parents that infant cannot be spoiled by too much attention during the first 4 to 6 months.
Encourage parents to establish a schedule that meets needs of child and themselves.
Help parents understand infant's need for stimulation in environment.
Support parents' pleasure in seeing child's growing friendliness and social response, especially smiling.
Plan anticipatory guidance for safety.
Stress need for immunization.
Prepare for introduction of solid foods.

SECOND 6 MONTHS
Prepare parents for child's "stranger anxiety."
Encourage parents to allow child to cling to them and avoid long separation from either.
Guide parents concerning discipline because of infant's increasing mobility.
Encourage use of negative voice and eye contact rather than physical punishment as a means of discipline.
Encourage showing most attention when infant is behaving well, rather than when infant is crying.
Teach injury prevention because of child's advancing motor skills and curiosity.
Encourage parents to leave child with suitable caregiver to allow some free time.
Discuss readiness for weaning.
Explore parents' feelings regarding infant's sleep patterns.

KEY POINTS

- Biologic development of the child encompasses proportional changes; sensory changes, including binocularity and depth perception; maturation of biologic systems; fine motor development; and gross motor development.
- In Erikson's theory of psychosocial development, the period from birth to 1 year is concerned with acquiring a sense of trust while overcoming a sense of mistrust.
- Piaget's theory of cognitive development, as it applies to the infant, focuses on the sensorimotor phase, which includes the use of reflexes, primary circular reactions, secondary circular reactions, and coordination of secondary schemas and their application to new situations.
- Development of body image begins in infancy; by 1 year of age infants recognize that they are distinct from their parents.
- Social development of the infant is guided by attachment, language development, personal-social behavior, and participation in play.
- Temperament influences the type of interaction that occurs between the child and parents and siblings.
- Parents are faced with many concerns, including infant fears, daycare, limit setting and discipline, thumb sucking and pacifier use, teething, and choice of infant shoes.
- Breast milk is the most desirable food for the infant during the first 6 months; formula is an acceptable alternative, followed by gradual introduction of solid food during the second 6 months. Whole milk is not recommended until after 12 months.
- Solids may be introduced between 4 and 6 months, beginning with iron-fortified rice cereal.
- Common sleep problems that develop during infancy—and that are easily prevented—are associated with night crying and feeding. Nurses should instruct the parents, after careful assessment, in strategies to deal with the specific problem.

- Cleaning the teeth regularly and appropriate dietary intake promote good dental health.
- Recommended routine immunizations include those for HAV and HBV, diphtheria, tetanus, pertussis, polio, measles, mumps, rubella, varicella (chickenpox), pneumococcal, meningococcal, influenza, and *H. influenzae* type b.

- Recommended immunizations for selected groups of children include rotavirus and the HPV vaccine.
- Because injuries are a major cause of death during infancy, parents should be alerted to the risks related to aspiration of foreign objects, suffocation, falls, poisoning, burns, motor vehicle injuries, and bodily damage, as well as preventive actions needed to make the environment safe for infants.

REFERENCES

Academy of Breastfeeding Medicine: *Clinical protocol: guideline on co-sleeping and breastfeeding,* 2003, The Academy, retrieved Jan 1, 2007 from http://www.bfmed/org/ace-files/protocol/cosleeping.pdf.

Agran PF, Anderson C, Winn D, and others: Rates of pediatric injuries by 3-month intervals for children 0 to 3 years of age, *Pediatrics* 111(6): e683-e692, 2003.

American Academy of Pediatric Dentistry: Guideline on infant oral health care. In *AAPD Reference Manual 2005-2006,* retrieved Jan 1, 2008, from http://www.aapd.org/media/Policies_Guidelines/G_InfantOralHealthCare.pdf.

American Academy of Pediatrics, Committee on Infectious Diseases: Recommended immunization schedule for children and adolescents—United States, 2007, *Pediatrics* 119(1):207-208, 2007.

American Academy of Pediatrics: Dietary recommendations for children and adolescents: a guide for practitioners, *Pediatrics* 117(2):544-559, 2006a.

American Academy of Pediatrics, Committee on Infectious Diseases, Pickering L, editor: *Red book: 2006 report of the Committee on Infectious Diseases,* ed 27, Elk Grove Village, Ill, 2006b, The Academy.

American Academy of Pediatrics, Committee on Infectious Diseases: Recommended immunization schedules for children and adolescents—United States, 2008, *Pediatrics* 121(1):219-220, 2008.

American Academy of Pediatrics, Task Force on Sudden Infant Death Syndrome: The changing concept of sudden infant death syndrome: diagnostic coding shifts, controversies regarding the sleeping environment, and new variables to consider in reducing risk, *Pediatrics* 116(5):1245-1255, 2005.

American Academy of Pediatrics, Committee on Nutrition: *Pediatric nutrition handbook,* ed 5, Elk Grove Village, Ill, 2004, The Academy.

American Academy of Pediatrics: Prevention of rickets and vitamin D deficiency: new guidelines for vitamin D intake, *Pediatrics* 111(4):908-910, 2003.

American Academy of Pediatrics, Committee on Injury and Poison Prevention: Injuries associated with infant walkers, *Pediatrics* 108(3):790-792, 2001a.

American Academy of Pediatrics, Committee on Nutrition: The use and misuse of fruit juice in pediatrics, *Pediatrics* 107(5):1210-1213, 2001b.

American Academy of Pediatrics, Task Force on Infant Sleep Position and Sudden Infant Death Syndrome: Changing concepts of sudden infant death syndrome: implications for infant sleeping environment and sleep position, *Pediatrics* 105(3):650-656, 2000.

American Dental Association: For the dental patient . . . infants, formula and fluoride, *J Am Dent Assoc* 138(1):132, 2007.

American Psychiatric Association: *Reactive attachment disorder (position statement),* Washington, DC, 2002, The Association; retrieved June 2007 from http://www.psych.org/edu/other_res/lib_archives/archives/200205.pdf.

Anderson JE: "Nothing but the tooth": dispelling myths about teething, *Contemp Pediatr* 21(7):75-83, 2004.

Ball HL: Breastfeeding, bed sharing, and infant sleep, *Birth* 30(3):181-188, 2003.

Barnhill BJ, Holbert MD, Jackson NM, and others: Using pressure to decrease the pain of intramuscular injections, *J Pain Symptom Manage* 12(1):52-58, 1996.

Biancuzzo M: Breastfeeding the newborn: clinical strategies for nurses, ed 2, St Louis, 2003, Mosby.

Brady MT: Infectious disease in pediatric out-of-home child care, *Am J Infect Control* 33(5):276-285, 2005.

Brazelton T: Parent-infant cosleeping revisited, *Brazelton Center Newslett* vol 2, 1990.

Brenner RA, Overpeck MD, Trumble AC, and others: Deaths attributable to injuries in infants, United States, 1983-1991, *Pediatrics* 103(5):968-974, 1999.

Calamaro CJ: Infant nutrition in the first year of life: tradition or science? *Pediatr Nurs* 26(2):211-215, 2000.

Carroll-Pankhurst C, Mortimer EA: Sudden infant death syndrome, bedsharing, parental weight, and age at death, *Pediatrics* 107(3):530-536, 2001.

Carey WB, McDevitt SC: Revision of the infant temperament questionnaire, *Pediatrics* 61(5):735-739, 1978.

Centers for Disease Control and Prevention: Fatal injuries among children by race and ethnicity—United States, 1999-2002, *MMWR* 56(SS-5):1-16, 2007a.

Centers for Disease Control and Prevention: Quadrivalent human papillomavirus vaccine, *MMWR* 56(RR-2):1-24, 2007b.

Centers for Disease Control and Prevention: Prevention of hepatitis A through active or passive immunization, *MMWR* 55(RR-7):1-23, 2006a.

Centers for Disease Control and Prevention: Preventing tetanus, diphtheria, and pertussis among adults: use of tetanus toxoid, reduced diphtheria toxoid, and acellular pertussis vaccine, *MMWR* 55(RR-17):1-33, 2006b.

Centers for Disease Control and Prevention: Update: Guillain-Barré syndrome among recipients of Menactra meningococcal conjugate vaccine—United States, June 2005–September 2006, *MMWR* 55(41):1120-1124, 2006c.

Centers for Disease Control and Prevention: A comprehensive immunization strategy to eliminate transmission of hepatitis B virus infection in the United States, *MMWR* 54(RR-16):1-23, 2005a.

Centers for Disease Control and Prevention: Nonfatal motor-vehicle-related backover injuries among children—United States, 2001-2003, *MMWR* 54(06):144-146, 2005b.

Centers for Disease Control and Prevention: Outbreaks of pertussis associated with hospitals—Kentucky, Pennsylvania, and Oregon, 2003, *MMWR* 54(03):67-71, 2005c.

Chung JWY, Ng WMY, Wong TKS: An experimental study on the use of manual pressure to reduce pain in intramuscular injections, *J Clin Nurs* 11:457-461, 2002.

Dahl RE: The development and disorders of sleep, *Adv Pediatr* 45:73-90, 1998.

Davis KF, Parker K, Montgomery GL: Sleep in infants and young children, part 2, Common sleep problems, *J Pediatr Health Care* 18(3):130-137, 2004.

Dewey KG: Nutrition, growth, and complementary feeding of the breastfed infant, *Pediatr Clin North Am* 48(1):87-104, 2001.

Diggle L, Deeks J: Effect of needle length on incidence of local reactions to routine immunizations in infants aged 4 months: randomized controlled trial, *BMJ* 321(7266):931-993, 2000.

Diggle L, Deeks JJ, Pollard AJ: Effect of needle size and immunogenicity and reactogenicity of vaccines in infants: a randomized controlled trial, *BMJ* 333(7568):571, 2006.

Douglass JM, Douglass AB, Silk HJ: A practical guide to infant oral health, *Am Fam Physician* 70(11):2113-2120, 2004.

Drago DA, Dannenberg AL: Infant mechanical suffocating deaths in the United States, 1980-1997, *Pediatrics* 103(5):e59, 1999.

Duro D, Rising R, Cedillo M, and others: Association between infantile colic and carbohydrate malabsorption from fruit juices in infancy, *Pediatrics* 109(5):797-805, 2002.

Ferber R, Kryger M: *Principles and practice of sleep medicine in the child,* Philadelphia, 1995, Saunders.

Fiocchi A, Assa'ad A, Bahna S, and others: Food allergy and the introduction of solid foods to infants: a consensus document, *Ann Allergy Asthma Immunol* 97(1):10-20, 2006.

Fox MK, Reidy K, Novak T, and others: Sources of energy and nutrients in the diets of infants and toddlers, *J Am Diet Assoc* 106(1 Suppl 1):S28-S42, 2006.

Fredrickson DD, Davis TC, Arnold CL, and others: Childhood immunization refusal: provider and parent perceptions, *Fam Med* 36(6):431-438, 2004.

Grummer-Strawn LM, Mei Z, Centers for Disease Control and Prevention Pediatric Nutrition Surveillance System: Does breastfeeding protect against pediatric overweight? Analysis of longitudinal data from the Centers for Disease Control and Prevention Pediatric Nutrition Surveillance System, *Pediatrics* 113(2):e81-e86, 2004.

Halperin BA, Halperin SA, McGrath P, and others: Use of lidocaine-prilocaine patch to decrease intramuscular injection pain does not adversely affect the antibody response to diphtheria–tetanus–acellular pertussis–inactivated poliovirus–*Haemophilus influenzae* type b conjugate and hepatitis B vaccines in infants from birth to 6 months of age, *Pediatr Infect Dis* 21(5):399-405, 2002.

Hauck FR, Herman SM, Donovan M, and others: Sleep environment and the risk of sudden infant death syndrome in an urban population: the Chicago Infant Mortality Study, *Pediatrics* 111(5 part 2):1207-1214, 2003.

Hawkins-Walsh E: A behavioural infant sleep intervention resolved sleep problems, *Evidence-Based Nurs* 6(1):10-12, 2003.

Henary B, Sherwood CP, Crandall JR, and others: Car safety for children: rear facing for best protection, *Inj Prev* 13(6):398-402, 2007.

Heron J, Golding J, ALSPAC Study Team: Thimerosal exposure in infants and developmental disorders: a prospective cohort study in the United Kingdom does not support a causal association, *Pediatrics* 114(3):577-583, 2004.

Hiscock H, Wake M: Infant sleep problems and postnatal depression: a community-based study, *Pediatrics* 107(6):1317-1322, 2001.

Horn MI, McCarthy AM: Children's responses to sequential versus simultaneous immunization injections, *J Pediatr Health Care* 13(1):18-23, 1999.

Ize-Ludlow D, Ragone S, Bruck IS, and others: Neurotoxicities in infants seen with the consumption of star anise tea, *Pediatrics* 114(5):e653, 2004.

Joanna Briggs Institute: Evidence based practice information sheet for health professionals: early childhood pacifier use in relation to breastfeeding, SIDS, infection, and malocclusion, *Best Practice* 9(3):1-6, 2005.

Koslap-Petraco MB, Parsons T: Communicating the benefits of combination vaccines to parents and health care providers, *J Pediatr Health Care* 17(2):53-57, 2003.

Lassman J: Water safety, *J Emerg Nurs* 28(3):241-243, 2002.

Lawrence RA, Lawrence RM: *Breastfeeding: a guide for the medical profession,* ed 6, St Louis, 2005, Mosby.

Lee MS, Bernstein HH: Immunizations, neonatal jaundice and animal-induced injuries, *Curr Opin Pediatr* 17(3):418-429, 2005.

Loman DG: The use of complementary and alternative health care practices among children, *J Pediatr Health Care* 17(2):58-63, 2003.

Macknin ML, Piedmonte M, Jacobs J, and others: Symptoms associated with infant teething: a prospective study, *Pediatrics* 105(4):747-752, 2000.

Martin J, Hiscock H, Hardy P, and others: Adverse associations of infant and child sleep problems and parent health: an Australian population study, *Pediatrics* 119(5):947-955, 2007.

Martin JA, Kochanek KD, Strobino DM, and others: Annual summary of vital statistics—2003, *Pediatrics* 115(3):619-634, 2005.

McGarvey C, McDonnell M, Chong A, and others: Factors relating to the infant's last sleep environment in sudden infant death syndrome in the Republic of Ireland, *Arch Dis Child* 88(12):1058-1064, 2003.

Medoff-Cooper B, Carey WB, McDevitt SC: The early infancy temperament questionnaire, *J Dev Behav Pediatr* 14(4):230-235, 1993.

Mell LK, Ogren DS, Davis RL, and others: Compliance with national immunization guidelines for children younger than 2 years, 1996-1999, *Pediatrics* 115(2):461-468, 2005.

Mesich HM: Mother-infant co-sleeping: understanding the debate and maximizing infant safety, *MCN* 30(1):30-37, 2005.

Morin K: Infant nutrition: what about water softeners and bottled water for babies? *MCN* 32(1):57, 2007.

Moukarzel AA, Lesicka H, Ament ME: Irritable bowel syndrome and nonspecific diarrhea in infancy and childhood—relationship with juice carbohydrate malabsorption, *Clin Pediatr* 41(3):145-150, 2002.

Narendran V, Hoath SB: The skin. In Martin RJ, Fanaroff AA, Walsh MC, editors: *Fanaroff and Martin's neonatal-perinatal medicine,* ed 8, St Louis, 2006, Mosby.

Niggemann B, Grüber C: Side-effects of complementary and alternative medicine, *Allergy* 58(8):707-716, 2003.

Parker SK, Schwartz B, Todd J, and others: Thimerosol-containing vaccines and autistic spectrum disorder: a critical review of published original data, *Pediatrics* 114(3):793-804, 2004.

Patterson DL: Adolescent-mothering: child-grandmother attachment, *J Pediatr Nurs* 12(4):228-237, 1997.

Person TL, Lavezzi WA, Wolf BC: Cosleeping and sudden unexpected death in infancy, *Arch Pathol Lab Med* 126(3):343-345, 2002.

Phelan KJ, Khoury J, Kalkwarf H, and others: Residential injuries in U.S. children and adolescents, *Pub Health Rep* 120(1):63-70, 2005.

Pickett W, Streight S, Simpson K, and others: Injuries experienced by infant children: a population-based epidemiological analysis, *Pediatrics* 111(4 pt 1):e365-e370, 2003.

Pinelli J, Symington A: Non-nutritive sucking for promoting physiologic stability and nutrition in preterm infants, *Cochrane Database Syst Rev* (2):CD001071, 2000.

Pinelli J, Symington A, Ciliska D: Nonnutritive sucking in high-risk infants: benign intervention or legitimate therapy? *J Obstet Gynecol Neonatal Nurs* 31(5):582-591, 2002.

Quillin SI, Glenn LL: Interaction between feeding method and co-sleeping on maternal-newborn sleep, *J Obstet Gynecol Neonatal Nurs* 33(5):580-588, 2004.

Reis EC, Holubkov R: Vapocoolant spray is equally effective as EMLA cream in reducing immunization pain in school-aged children, *Pediatrics* 100(6):1025, 1997.

Rojjanasrirat W: Working women's breastfeeding experiences, *MCN* 29(4):222-227, 2004.

Schachter F, Fuchs ML, Bijer PE, and others: Cosleeping and sleep problems in Hispanic-American urban young children, *Pediatrics* 84(3):522-530, 1989.

Schack-Nielsen L, Michaelsen KF: Breast feeding and future health, *Curr Opin Nutr Metab Care* 9(3):289-296, 2006.

Schechter NL, Zempsky WT, Cohen LL, and others: Pain reduction during pediatric immunizations: evidence-based review and recommendations, *Pediatrics* 119(5):e1184-e1198, 2007.

Schnitzer PG: Prevention of unintentional childhood injuries, *Am Fam Physician* 74(11):1864-1869, 2006.

Schuval S: Avoiding allergic reactions to childhood vaccines (and what to do when they occur), *Contemp Pediatr* 22(4):29-49, 53, 2003.

Stevens B, Johnston C, Franck L, and others: The efficacy of developmentally sensitive interventions and sucrose for relieving procedural pain in very low birth weight neonates, *Nurs Res* 48(1):35-43, 1999.

Stevens B, Yamada J, Ohlsson A: Sucrose for analgesia in newborn infants undergoing painful procedures. In *Cochrane Database Syst Rev* (4):CD001069, 2001.

Sullivan JR: Development of father-infant attachment in fathers of preterm infants, *Neonatal Netw* 18(7):33-39, 1999.

Tappin D, Ecob R, Brooke H: Bedsharing, room-sharing, and sudden infant death syndrome in Scotland: a case-controlled study, *J Pediatr* 147(1):32-37, 2005.

Thompson DG: Utilizing an oral sucrose solution to minimize neonatal pain, *J Spec Pediatr Nurs* 10(1):3-10, 2005.

Touchette E, Petit D, Paquet J, and others: Factors associated with fragmented sleep at night across early childhood, *Arch Pediatr Adolesc Med* 159(3):242-249, 2005.

US Food and Drug Administration: FDA approves new vaccine to prevent rotavirus gastroenteritis in infants. In *FDA News,* Rockville, Md, Feb 3, 2006, The Administration, retrieved Jan 1, 2008, from http://www.fda.gov/bbs/topics/news/2006/NEW01307.html

Wall EJ: Practical primary pediatric orthopedics, *Nurs Clin North Am* 35(1):95-113, 2000.

Wilkerson R, Northington LD, Fisher W: Ingestion of toxic substances by infants and children: what we don't know can hurt, *Crit Care Nurs* 25(4):35-44, 2005.

Willinger M, Ko CW, Hoffman HJ, and others: Trends in infant bed sharing in the United States, 1993-2000: the National Infant Sleep Position study, *Arch Pediatr Adolesc Med* 157(1):33-39, 2003.

Wilson ME, White MA, Cobb B, and others: Family dynamics, parental-fetal attachment and infant temperament, *J Adv Nurs* 31(1):204-210, 2000.

Wilson S: Attachment disorders: review and current status, *J Psychol* 135(1):37-51, 2001.

Wong DL: Topical local anesthetics: two products for pain relief during minor procedures, *Am J Nurs* 103(6):42-45, 2003.

Zeanah CH, Fox NA: Temperament and attachment disorders, *J Clin Child Adolesc Psychol* 33(1):82-87, 2004.

Zuckerman JN, Cockcroft A, Zuckerman AJ: Site of injection for vaccination, *BMJ* 305(6862):1158, 1992.

Zuckerman J: The importance of injecting vaccines into muscle, *BMJ* 321(7271):1237-1238, 2000.

11

Health Problems of Infants

DAVID WILSON

CHAPTER OUTLINE

NUTRITIONAL DISORDERS, 378
Vitamin Imbalances, 378
Complementary and Alternative
  Medicine, 379
Mineral Imbalances, 379
Vegetarian Diets, 379
Nursing Care Management, 380
Protein-Energy Malnutrition, 381
  Kwashiorkor, 383
  Marasmus, 383

Food Sensitivity, 384
  Cow's Milk Allergy, 386
  Lactose Intolerance, 387
FEEDING DIFFICULTIES, 395
Regurgitation and "Spitting Up," 395
Paroxysmal Abdominal Pain (Colic), 395
Growth Failure (Failure to Thrive), 396

POSITIONAL PLAGIOCEPHALY, 400
**DISORDERS OF UNKNOWN
ETIOLOGY, 401**
Sudden Infant Death Syndrome, 401
Apnea and Apparent Life-Threatening
  Event, 404

LEARNING OBJECTIVES

On completion of this chapter the reader will be able to:

- Identify children at increased risk of developing nutritional disorders.
- Outline a nutritional counseling plan for vitamin or mineral deficiency or excess.
- Outline a dietary plan for parents when the infant is sensitive to cow's milk.

- List measures that can be used to alleviate colic.
- Plan nursing care that meets the physical and emotional needs of the child and family with growth failure.

- Provide nursing care that meets the immediate and long-term needs of the family that has lost a child from sudden infant death syndrome.
- Identify the stresses and needs of the family whose child is being home monitored for apnea.

RELATED TOPICS and ADDITIONAL RESOURCES

 IN TEXT

Anaphylaxis, Ch. 25
Asthma, Ch. 23
Cardiopulmonary Resuscitation, Ch. 23
Chronic Illness, Disability, or End-of-Life
  Care for Child and Family, Ch. 18
Gastroesophageal Reflux, Ch. 24
Iron Deficiency Anemia, Ch. 26
Neonatal Loss, Ch. 9
Nutritional Assessment, Ch. 6
Obesity, Ch. 17
Provide Optimum Nutrition (Newborn),
  Ch. 8

 COMPANION CD

Case Study—Health Problems of Infants
NCLEX Review Questions

evolve

evolve.elsevier.com/Wong/essentials/

NCLEX Review Questions
Nursing Care Plan—The Child with
  Growth Failure
WebLinks

 **WONG'S CLINICAL MANUAL
OF PEDIATRIC NURSING, 7th Ed**

Patient and Family Education—Home Apnea
  Monitoring, p. 574; Infant
  Cardiopulmonary Resuscitation for the
  Layperson, p. 576

NUTRITIONAL DISORDERS

An American Academy of Pediatrics (2006a) report endorses the Dietary Guidelines for Americans introduced in 2005, yet part of the report highlights the dietary changes that have occurred in households across the United States. These changes include increased dependence on meals not cooked in the home; increased consumption of snack foods; decreased daily activity among children; and poor nutritional intake of a well-balanced source of foods such as fruits, vegetables, and fiber, which could lead to increases in cardiovascular disease. Micronutrient intakes in adolescents are also reported to be substantially below recommended dietary reference intake (DRI) values. Others reported an increased dependence on fortified foods and supplements in toddlers to meet nutritional requirements, rather than meeting such needs with a wide variety of fruits, vegetables, and whole grains (Fox, Reidy, Novak, and others, 2006).

The findings of these studies and other similar reports are important for nurses who work with infants and children. Nurses must endeavor to promote healthy nutrition habits early in the child's life through proper education of families and children about healthy lifestyle habits, including diet and exercise for health promotion and prevention of morbidities associated with poor micronutrient intake and sedentary lifestyle.

VITAMIN IMBALANCES

Although true vitamin deficiencies are rare in the United States, subclinical deficiencies are commonly seen in population subgroups in which either maternal or child dietary intake of foods containing adequate amounts of vitamins is imbalanced. **Vitamin D–deficiency rickets,** once rarely seen because of the widespread commercial availability of vitamin D–fortified milk, increased before the turn of the century. Populations at risk include:

- Children exclusively breast-fed by mothers with an inadequate intake of vitamin D or who are breast-fed longer than 6 months without adequate maternal vitamin D intake or supplementation
- Children with dark skin pigmentation who are exposed to minimal sunlight because of socioeconomic, religious, or cultural beliefs or housing in urban areas with high levels of pollution
- Children with diets that are low in sources of vitamin D and calcium
- Individuals who use milk products not supplemented with vitamin D (e.g., yogurt, raw cow's milk) as the primary source of milk

The American Academy of Pediatrics (2003c) now recommends that infants who are exclusively breast-fed begin to receive 200 IU of vitamin D by age 2 months. Furthermore, children who have minimal sun exposure, do not consume at least 500 ml of vitamin D–fortified milk, or are not taking a vitamin supplement with vitamin D should take vitamin D supplements daily to prevent rickets and vitamin D deficiency. The 200 IU of vitamin D may be obtained by taking a multivitamin supplement containing 400 IU vitamin D per ml or per tablet (American Academy of Pediatrics, 2003c). Inadequate maternal ingestion of cobalamin (vitamin B_{12}) may contribute to infant neurologic impairment when exclusive breastfeeding (past 6 months) is the only source of the infant's nutrition (Centers for Disease Control and Prevention, 2003).

Children may also be at risk secondary to disorders or their treatment. For example, vitamin deficiencies of the fat-soluble vitamins A and D may occur in malabsorptive disorders. Preterm infants may develop rickets in the second month of life as a result of inadequate intake of vitamin D, calcium, and phosphorus. Children receiving high doses of salicylates may have impaired vitamin C storage. Environmental tobacco smoke exposure has been implicated in decreased concentrations of ascorbate in children; therefore increased intake of sources of vitamin C should be encouraged even in children minimally exposed to environmental tobacco smoke (Preston, Rodriguez, and Rivera, 2006; Preston, Rodriguez, Rivera, and others, 2003). Children with chronic illnesses resulting in anorexia, decreased food intake, or possible nutrient malabsorption as a result of multiple medications should be carefully evaluated for adequate vitamin and mineral intake in some form (parenteral or enteral).

Children with sickle cell disease are reported to have suboptimal intakes (according to DRI recommendations) of vitamins E and D, folate, calcium, and fiber, which decrease significantly with increasing age. Poor dietary intake was a significant factor in the study's findings (Kawchak, Schall, Zemel, and others, 2007).

Vitamin A deficiency has been reported with increased morbidity and mortality in children with measles. However, a Cochrane review of studies wherein a single dose of vitamin A was administered to children with measles found no decrease in mortality. Children with measles under the age of 2 years who received two doses of vitamin A (200,000 IU) on consecutive days did have decreased mortality rates and a reduced rate of pneumonia-specific mortality (Huiming, Chaomin, and Meng, 2005). Complications from diarrhea and infections are often increased in infants and children with vitamin A deficiency. The American Academy of Pediatrics (2006b) recommends that vitamin A supplementation be considered in children hospitalized with measles and associated complications (diarrhea, croup, pneumonia), especially children between the ages of 6 months and 2 years. Although scurvy (caused by a deficiency of vitamin C) is rare in developed countries, cases have been reported in children who were fed an organic diet deficient in vegetables and fruits (Burk and Molodow, 2007).

An excessive dose of a vitamin is generally defined as 10 or more times the recommended dietary allowance (RDA), although the fat-soluble vitamins, especially A and D, tend to cause toxic reactions at lower doses. With the addition of vitamins to commercially prepared foods, the potential for hypervitaminosis has increased, especially when combined with the excessive use of vitamin supplements. Hypervitaminosis of A and D presents the greatest problems, since these fat-soluble vitamins are stored in the body. High intakes of vitamin A have been linked to physeal growth arrest, which can lead to osteoporosis, fracture, and metaphyseal irregularity (Saltzman and King, 2007). Vitamin D is the most likely of all vitamins to cause toxic reactions in relatively small overdoses. The water-soluble vitamins, primarily niacin, B_6, and C, can also cause toxicity. Poor outcomes in infants, namely a fatal hypermagnesemia, have been associated with megavitamin therapy with high doses of magnesium oxide (McGuire, Kulkarni, and Baden, 2000), and severe anemia and thrombocytopenia have resulted from megadoses of vitamin A (Perrotta, Nobili, Rossi, and others, 2002).

One vitamin supplement that is recommended for all women of childbearing age is a daily dose of 0.4 mg of folic acid, the usual RDA. Folic acid taken before conception and during early pregnancy can reduce the risk of neural tube defects such as spina bifida by as much as 70%. Drugs such as oral contraceptives and antidepressants may decrease folic acid absorption; thus adolescent females taking such medications should consider supplementation.

Deficiencies and excesses of vitamins A, B complex, C, D, E, and K are summarized in Table 11-1, and the RDAs and DRIs are listed in Appendix G. General nursing care management is discussed below, and specific interventions are presented in Table 11-1.

COMPLEMENTARY AND ALTERNATIVE MEDICINE

The misuse or overuse of vitamins as a part of **complementary and alternative medicine (CAM)** places some children at risk for health problems. One survey found that a relatively small group of parents routinely gave their children megavitamin therapy; however, the researcher recommends further research to ascertain a more realistic number of children using multivitamin preparations (Loman, 2003). Sawni, Ragothaman, Thomas, and others (2007) noted that of persons reportedly using CAM, the most common CAM remedies used in children seen in the emergency department were home or folk remedies (59%), herbs (41%), prayer for healing (14%), and massage therapy (10%). A survey in a WIC (Women, Infants, and Children) clinic found that child herbal use was common, especially among Hispanic children attending the clinic. Some of the herbs used by the children in the survey (St. John's wort, dong quai, and kava) have questionable safety (Lohse, Stotts, and Priebe, 2006).

There is concern among health care workers that terms often used to market supplements such as megavitamins may mislead parents regarding the actual benefits (or harm) of such therapies. The intention herein is not to discredit the use of CAM such as vitamin supplements; rather, it is to ensure safety and efficacy in children who may experience inadvertent harm. The use of various herbal therapies, or intake of herbs, is also becoming more popular; many of these have been a part of medicine since early days and are beneficial in some cases.

There are reports of an increase in the use of herbs by lactating mothers to increase breast milk supply. The **galactogogues** fenugreek, blessed thistle, fennel, and chaste tree have been purported to increase maternal milk supply, yet few studies support the efficacy or the safety of these herbs in breastfeeding infants; fenugreek has been the most widely studied, yet it may have adverse effects such as colic and diarrhea in breastfeeding infants (Conover and Buehler, 2004; Lawrence and Lawrence, 2005). For a discussion of galactogogues, including those mentioned above, see Appendix P in Lawrence and Lawrence (2005).

Herbs known to have adverse effects in children include ephedra, comfrey, and pennyroyal; some herbs may not be harmful taken alone but may counteract or potentiate prescription medications when taken together (Loman, 2003). Parents should be fully informed of the use of herbs to ensure that there is more benefit than potential harm in the ingredient being used. Health care workers also need to be knowledgeable of the benefits or potential harm in herbs to appropriately counsel parents and address their concerns. Little

research has been performed in children on many over-the-counter herbal medicines, yet some herbs are known to cause harm in children (Kemper and Gardiner, 2004; Lanski, Greenwald, Perkins, and others, 2003; Loman, 2003). Parents should be cautioned not to exceed the upper limits of vitamin intake according to the new DRI (see p. 380 and Appendix G).*

MINERAL IMBALANCES

A number of minerals are essential nutrients. The **macrominerals** refer to those with daily requirements greater than 100 mg and include calcium, phosphorus, magnesium, sodium, potassium, chloride, and sulfur. **Microminerals,** or **trace elements,** have daily requirements of less than 100 mg and include several essential minerals and those whose exact role in nutrition is still unclear. The greatest concern with minerals is deficiency, especially of iron, calcium, phosphorus, magnesium, and zinc. Low levels of zinc can cause nutritional failure to thrive.

The regulation of mineral balance in the body is a complex process. Dietary extremes of mineral intake can cause a number of mineral-mineral interactions that could result in unexpected deficiencies or excesses. For example, excessive amounts of one mineral, such as zinc, can result in a deficiency of another mineral, such as copper, even if sufficient amounts of copper are ingested. Thus megadose intake of one mineral may cause an inadvertent deficiency of another essential mineral by blocking its absorption in the blood or intestinal wall, or by competing with binding sites on protein carriers needed for metabolism.

Deficiencies can also occur when various substances in the diet interact with minerals. For example, iron, zinc, and calcium can form insoluble complexes with **phytates** or **oxalates** (substances found in plant proteins), which impair the bioavailability of the mineral. This type of interaction is important in vegetarian diets because plant foods such as soy are high in phytates. Contrary to popular opinion, spinach is not an ideal source of iron or calcium because of its high oxalate content.

Children with certain illnesses are at greater risk for growth failure, especially in relation to bone mineral deficiency as a result of the treatment of the disease, decreased nutrient intake, or decreased absorption of necessary minerals. Those at risk for such deficiencies include children who are receiving or have received radiation and chemotherapy for cancer; children with human immunodeficiency virus (HIV), sickle cell disease, cystic fibrosis, gastrointestinal malabsorption, or nephrosis; and very low–birth-weight preterm infants.

Deficiencies and excesses of the essential macrominerals and microminerals are summarized in Table 11-2. General nursing care management is discussed on p. 380, and specific interventions are discussed in the table.

VEGETARIAN DIETS

Vegetarian diets have become increasingly popular in the United States because people are concerned about hypertension; cholesterol; obesity; cardiovascular disease; cancer of the stomach, intestine, and colon; and the influence of the animal

*Helpful websites for health care and consumer information concerning herbs are National Center for Complementary and Alternative Medicine, http://www.nccam.nih.gov; American Botanical Council, http://www.herbalgram.org; and Herb Research Foundation, http://www.herbs.org.

rights movement. In one survey, adolescent vegetarians were more likely than nonvegetarians to meet the *Healthy People 2010* objectives for overall nutrient consumption (Perry, McGuire, Neumark-Sztainer and others, 2002). The American Dietetic Association and Dietitians of Canada (2003) issued a statement endorsing vegetarian diets for adults and children; the statement further notes that well-planned vegetarian diets are adequate for all stages of the life cycle and promote normal growth. Children and adolescents on vegetarian diets have the potential for lifelong healthy diets and have been shown to have lower intakes of cholesterol, saturated fat, and total fat and higher intakes of fruits, fiber, and vegetables than nonvegetarians (American Dietetic Association and Dietitians of Canada, 2003).

The major types of vegetarianism are:

Lacto-ovo vegetarians, who exclude meat from their diet but consume dairy products and rarely fish.
Lactovegetarians, who exclude meat and eggs but drink milk.
Pure vegetarians (vegans), who eliminate any food of animal origin, including milk and eggs.
Macrobiotics, who are even more restrictive than pure vegetarians, allowing only a few types of fruits, vegetables, and legumes.
Semi-vegetarians, who consume a lacto-ovo vegetarian diet with some fish and poultry. This is an increasingly popular form of vegetarianism and poses little or no nutritional risk to infants unless dietary fat and cholesterol intake is severely restricted.

Many individuals who are concerned about healthy diets subscribe to vegetarian diets that may not be typified by the above categories. Therefore during nutritional assessment it is necessary to clearly list exactly what the diet includes and excludes.*

The major deficiencies that may occur in the stricter vegan diets are inadequate protein for growth; inadequate calories for energy and growth; poor digestibility of many of the bulky natural, unprocessed foods, especially for infants; and deficiencies of vitamin B_6, niacin, riboflavin, vitamin D, iron, calcium, and zinc. Strict vegan diets also require supplements of vitamin B_{12} and vitamin D. Vitamin D is essential if exposure to sunlight is inadequate (<5 to 15 min/day on the hands, arms, and face of light-skinned persons; slightly more in darker pigmented individuals) or in persons who are dark-skinned or who live in northern latitudes or cloudy or smoky areas. Many of these deficiencies can be avoided in children who are not consuming 100% of the RDA of vitamins and minerals with a multivitamin-mineral supplement (Dunham and Kollar, 2006).

Evaluate for iron deficiency anemia and rickets in children on strict vegetarian and macrobiotic diets; this may occur as a result of consuming plant foods such as unrefined cereals, which impair the absorption of iron, calcium, and zinc. Other factors that affect iron absorption are listed in Box 11-1.

NURSING CARE MANAGEMENT

Identification of adequacy of nutrient intake is the initial nursing goal and requires assessment based on a dietary history and physical examination for signs of deficiency or excess

---

> ### BOX 11-1
> ### Factors That Affect Iron Absorption
>
> **INCREASE**
> Acidity (low pH)—Administer iron between meals (gastric hydrochloric acid)
> Ascorbic acid (vitamin C)—Administer iron with juice, fruit, or multivitamin preparation
> Vitamin A
> Calcium
> Tissue (cellular) need
> Meat, fish, poultry
> Cooking in cast iron pots
>
> **DECREASE**
> Alkalinity (high pH)—Avoid any antacid preparation
> Phosphates—Milk is unfavorable vehicle for iron administration
> Phytates—Found in cereals
> Oxalates—Found in many fruits and vegetables (plums, currants, green beans, spinach, sweet potatoes, tomatoes)
> Tannins—Found in tea, coffee
> Tissue (cellular) saturation
> Malabsorptive disorders
> Disturbances that cause diarrhea or steatorrhea
> Infection

(see Nutritional Assessment, Chapter 6). After assessment data are collected, this information is evaluated against standard intakes to identify areas of concern. The Institute of Medicine (IOM) (2000) has developed guidelines for nutritional intake that encompass the **RDAs** yet extend their scope to include additional parameters related to nutritional intake. The **DRIs*** are composed of four categories. These include estimated average requirements (EARs) for age and gender categories, tolerable upper-limit (UL) nutrient intakes that are associated with a low risk of adverse effects, adequate intakes (AIs) of nutrients, and new standard RDAs. The new guidelines present information about lifestyle factors that may affect nutrient function, such as caffeine intake and exercise, and about how the nutrient may be related to chronic disease. An important factor in the development of the DRIs that affects children, particularly infants 0 to 6 months, is that the AIs are based on the nutrient intake of full-term, healthy, breast-fed infants (by well-nourished mothers), which now represents the gold standard for infant nutrition in this age-group.

The American Heart Association (AHA) (2005) (see also Gidding, Dennison, Birch, and others, 2005) Dietary Guidelines, patterned after the 2005 Dietary Guidelines for Americans, may also be used to encourage healthy dietary intakes designed to decrease obesity and cardiovascular risk factors and subsequent cardiovascular disease, which is now known to occur in young children as well as adults. The AHA Guidelines have been endorsed by the American Academy of Pediatrics (2006a), yet it is important to note that these guidelines are for children ages 2 years and older. The guidelines encourage a variety of fruits, vegetables, whole grains, and low-fat

---

*Further information regarding vegetarian diets may be found at the Vegetarian Resource Group, PO Box 1463, Baltimore, MD 21203; (410) 366-8343; http://www.vrg.org.

*For information on the DRIs go to IOM website, http://www.iom.edu, and click on the link for Food and Nutrition; or call (202) 334-2352.

MyPyramid: Sample Serving Sizes

Grain group—1 slice of bread; 1 ounce of ready-to-eat cereal; ½ cup of cooked cereal, rice, or pasta

Vegetable group—1 cup of raw leafy vegetable; ½ cup of other vegetable, cooked or chopped raw; ¾ cup of vegetable juice

Fruit group—1 medium apple, banana, or orange; ½ cup of chopped, cooked, or canned fruit; ¾ cup of fruit juice

Milk group—2 cups of milk or yogurt, ½ ounces of natural cheese, 1 ounce of processed cheese

Meat group—2 to 3 ounces of cooked lean meat, poultry, or fish; ½ cup of cooked dry beans, 1 egg, or 2 tablespoons of peanut butter count as 1 ounce of lean meat

dairy and nonfat dairy products, in addition to fish, beans, and lean meat.

MyPyramid, developed by the U.S. Department of Agriculture, replaces the Food Guide Pyramid as a guide for adult and childhood nutrition. This interactive dietary guide aims to simplify food choices designed to decrease fat and empty calorie intake and increase consumption of grains and vegetables. The MyPyramid for Kids (Fig. 11-1) incorporates examples of exercise for children as well as suggested serving sizes. The Internet version of MyPyramid for Kids* offers an interactive game for children (Blast Off). Suggested serving sizes for the five food groups are listed in Box 11-2.

A vegetarian food guide pyramid (rainbow for Canadian vegetarians) developed by the American Dietetic Association and Dietitians of Canada includes guidelines for meeting the minimum recommendations for nutrients, including protein, iron, zinc, calcium, vitamin D, riboflavin, and iodine. The new food guide can be adapted to different types of vegetarian diets according to specific needs (American Dietetic Association and Dietitians of Canada, 2003; Messina, Melina, and Mangels, 2003).

Achieving a nutritionally adequate vegetarian diet is not difficult (except with the strictest diets), but it requires careful planning and knowledge of nutrient sources. For children the lacto-ovo vegetarian diet is nutritionally adequate; however, the vegan diet requires supplementation with vitamins D and B_{12} for children ages 2 to 12 years. Infants should be breast-fed for the first 6 months and preferably for 1 year, be introduced to some solid foods after about 4 to 6 months, and receive iron-fortified cereal for at least 18 months. Vitamin B_{12} supplementation is recommended if the breastfeeding mother's intake of the vitamin is inadequate or if she is not on vitamin supplements (Dunham and Kollar, 2006). The introduction of solids for vegetarian infants may occur using the same guidelines as for other children (see p. 346). The American Dietetic Association and Dietitians of Canada (2003) recommend iron supplementation in infants exclusively breast-fed after 4 to 6 months by vegetarian mothers and no dietary fat restrictions in vegetarian children younger than 2 years. The use of vitamin C juices (in moderate amounts, not as a milk substitute) with foods high in iron will further improve iron absorption. Breast milk from vegetarian mothers can be deficient in vita-

min B_{12}; supplementation of both mother and child is advisable. If cow's or human milk or commercial infant formula is not given, fortified soy formula is recommended. A variety of foods should be introduced during the early years to ensure a well-balanced intake.

To ensure sufficient protein in the diet, foods with incomplete proteins (those that do not have all the essential amino acids) must be eaten at the same meal with other foods that supply the missing amino acids. The three basic combinations of foods consumed by vegetarians that generally provide the appropriate amounts of essential amino acids are:

1. Grains (cereal, rice, pasta) and legumes (beans, peas, lentils, peanuts)
2. Grains and milk products (milk, cheese, yogurt)
3. Seeds (sesame, sunflower) and legumes

Additional dietary considerations for young children are found in Chapters 12 and 14.

PROTEIN-ENERGY MALNUTRITION

Malnutrition continues to be a major health problem in the world today, particularly in children under 5 years of age. Lack of food, however, is not always the primary cause for malnutrition. In many developing and underdeveloped nations, diarrhea (gastroenteritis) is a major factor in malnutrition. Additional factors are bottle-feeding (in poor sanitary conditions), inadequate knowledge of proper child care practices, parental illiteracy, economic and political factors, climate conditions, cultural and religious food preferences, and simply the lack of adequate food. Müller and Krawinkel (2005) point out that poverty is the underlying cause of malnutrition. The most extreme forms of malnutrition, or **protein-energy malnutrition (PEM),** are kwashiorkor and marasmus.

In the United States milder forms of PEM are seen as a result of primary malnutrition, although the classic cases of marasmus and kwashiorkor may also occur. Unlike developing countries, where the main reason for PEM is inadequate food, in the United States PEM occurs despite ample dietary supplies (see Growth Failure [Failure to Thrive], p. 396). PEM may also be seen in persons with chronic health problems such as cystic fibrosis, renal dialysis, and gastrointestinal malabsorption; in the elderly who have chronic malnutrition; or in persons with acute illnesses such as prolonged, untreated anorexia nervosa. Kwashiorkor has been reported in the United States in children fed only a rice beverage diet (Rice Dream) and few solid foods (Katz, Mahlberg, Honig, and others, 2005). The rice drink contains 0.13 g of protein per ounce (compared with the 0.5 g found in human milk and infant formulas) and is an inadequate source of nutrition for children. Other reported cases of kwashiorkor in developed countries involved infants who were fed nonstandard infant diets such as flour water, corn porridge, molasses, and nondairy creamer (Katz, Mahlberg, Honig, and others, 2005). Kwashiorkor has also been reported in the United States when infants have been fed inappropriate food as a result of parental (caretaker) nutritional ignorance, a perceived cow milk–based formula intolerance, family social chaos, or cow's milk intolerance (Liu, Howard, Mancini, and others, 2001). It is therefore important that health care workers not assume that PEM cannot occur in developed countries; a comprehensive dietary history should be obtained in any child with clinical features resembling PEM.

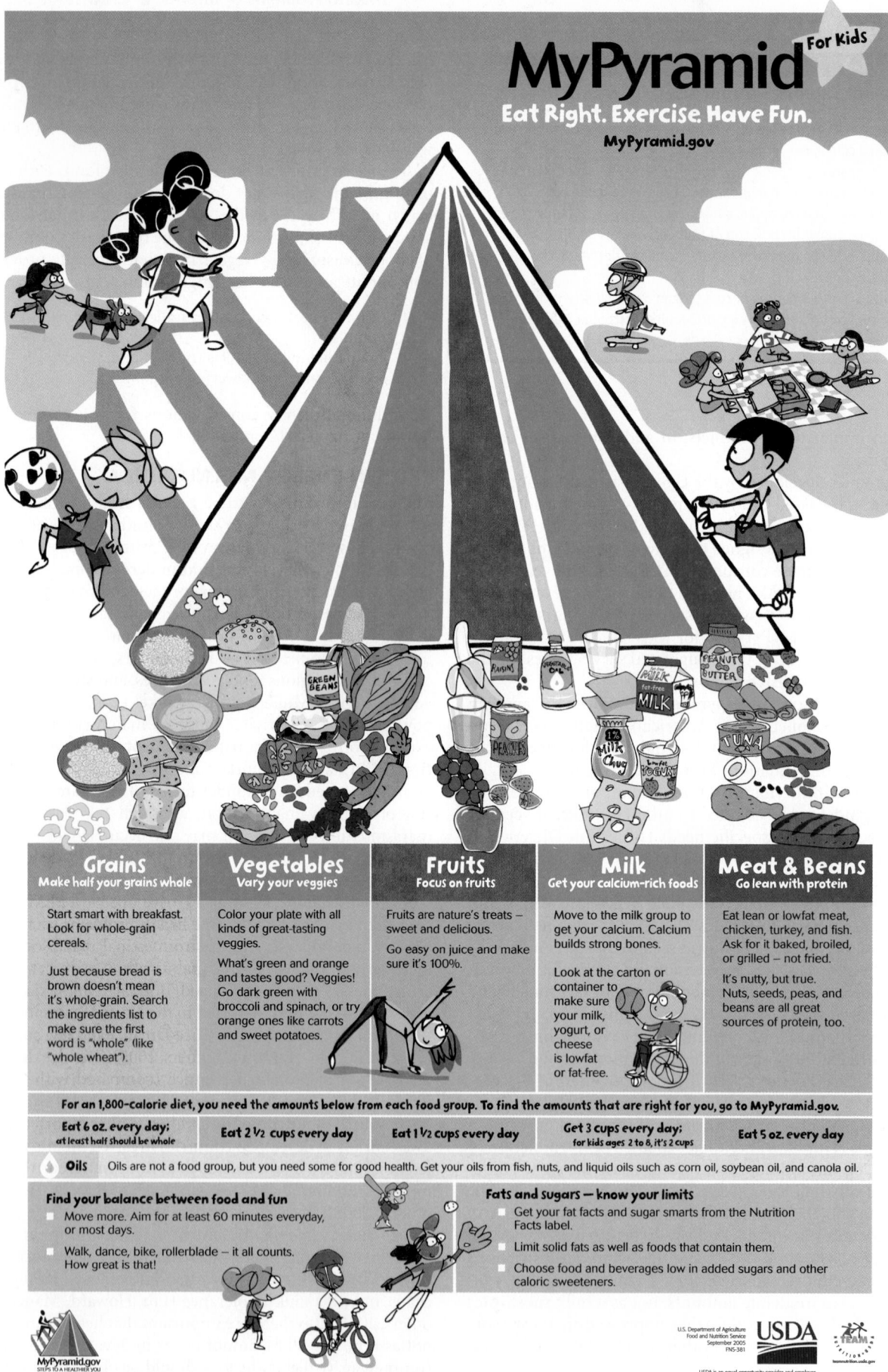

FIG. 11-1 ■ MyPyramid for Kids. (From Food and Nutrition Service, US Department of Agriculture: *MyPyramid for kids* [FNS-381], Washington, DC, April 19, 2005, The Service, available online at http://www.mypyramid.gov.)

Kwashiorkor

Kwashiorkor has been defined in the past as primarily a deficiency of protein with an adequate supply of calories. A diet consisting mainly of starch grains or tubers provides adequate calories in the form of carbohydrates but an inadequate amount of high-quality proteins. Some evidence, however, supports a multifactorial etiology, including cultural, psychologic, and infective factors that may interact to place the child at risk for kwashiorkor. Penny (2003) suggests that kwashiorkor may result from the interplay of nutrient deprivation and infectious or environmental stresses, which produce an imbalanced response to such insults. Kwashiorkor often occurs subsequent to an infectious outbreak of measles and dysentery. There is further evidence that oxidative stress occurs in children with kwashiorkor, resulting in free radical damage, which may precipitate cellular changes resulting in edema and muscle wasting (Penny, 2003). The role of the essential fatty acid arachidonic acid in lipid metabolism, altered leukotriene production, and oxidative stress in kwashiorkor has yet to be fully understood, yet arachidonic acid seems to have an interactive role in its development (Penny, 2003).

Taken from the Ga language (Ghana), the word *kwashiorkor* means "the sickness the older child gets when the next baby is born" and aptly describes the syndrome that develops in the first child, usually between 1 and 4 years of age, when weaned from the breast after the second child is born.

The child with kwashiorkor has thin, wasted extremities and a prominent abdomen from edema (ascites). The edema often masks the severe muscular atrophy, making the child appear less debilitated than he or she actually is. The skin is scaly and dry and has areas of depigmentation. Several dermatoses may be evident, partly resulting from the vitamin deficiencies. Permanent blindness often results from the severe lack of vitamin A. Mineral deficiencies are common, especially iron, calcium, and zinc. Acute zinc deficiency is a common complication of severe PEM and results in skin rashes, loss of hair, impaired immune response and susceptibility to infections, digestive problems, night blindness, changes in affective behavior, defective wound healing, and impaired growth. Its depressant effect on appetite further limits food intake. The hair is thin, dry, coarse, and dull. Depigmentation is common, and patchy alopecia may occur.

Diarrhea (persistent diarrhea malnutrition syndrome) commonly occurs from a lowered resistance to infection and further complicates the electrolyte imbalance. Low levels of cytokines (protein cells involved in the primary response to infection) have been reported in children with kwashiorkor, suggesting that such children have a blunted immune response to infection. A large number of fatalities in children with kwashiorkor occur in those who develop HIV infection. Gastrointestinal disturbances occur, such as fatty infiltration of the liver and atrophy of the acini cells of the pancreas. Anemia is also a common finding in malnourished children. Protein deficiency increases the child's susceptibility to infection, which eventually results in death. Fatal deterioration may be caused by diarrhea and infection or by circulatory failure.

Marasmus

Marasmus results from general malnutrition of both calories and protein. It is a common occurrence in underdeveloped countries during times of drought, especially in cultures where adults eat first; the remaining food is often insufficient in quality and quantity for the children.

Marasmus is usually a syndrome of physical and emotional deprivation and is not confined to geographic areas where food supplies are inadequate. It may be seen in children with failure to thrive in whom the cause is not solely nutritional but primarily emotional. Marasmus may be seen in infants as young as 3 months of age if breastfeeding is not successful and there are no suitable alternatives. **Marasmic kwashiorkor** is a form of PEM in which clinical findings of both kwashiorkor and marasmus are evident; the child has edema, severe wasting, and stunted growth. In marasmic kwashiorkor the child suffers from inadequate nutrient intake and superimposed infection. Fluid and electrolyte disturbances, hypothermia, and hypoglycemia are associated with a poor prognosis.

Marasmus is characterized by gradual wasting and atrophy of body tissues, especially of subcutaneous fat. The child appears to be very old, with loose and wrinkled skin, unlike the child with kwashiorkor, who appears more rounded from the edema. Fat metabolism is less impaired than in kwashiorkor, so that deficiency of fat-soluble vitamins is usually minimal or absent. In general, the clinical manifestations of marasmus are similar to those seen in kwashiorkor with the following exceptions: with marasmus there is no edema from hypoalbuminemia or sodium retention, which contributes to a severely emaciated appearance; no dermatoses caused by vitamin deficiencies; little or no depigmentation of hair or skin; moderately normal fat metabolism and lipid absorption; and smaller head size and slower recovery after treatment.

The child is fretful, apathetic, withdrawn, and so lethargic that prostration frequently occurs. Intercurrent infection with debilitating diseases such as tuberculosis, parasitosis, HIV, and dysentery is common.

Therapeutic Management

The treatment of PEM includes providing a diet with high-quality proteins, carbohydrates, vitamins, and minerals. When PEM occurs as a result of persistent diarrhea (see also Diarrhea, Chapter 24), three management goals are identified:

1. Rehydration with an oral rehydration solution that also replaces electrolytes
2. Administration of medications such as antibiotics and antidiarrheals
3. Provision of adequate nutrition by either breastfeeding or a proper weaning diet

Local protocols are employed in developing countries to deal with PEM. Penny (2003) proposes a three-phase treatment protocol: (1) acute or initial phase in the first 2 to 10 days, involving initiation of treatment for oral rehydration, diarrhea, intestinal parasites, prevention of hypoglycemia and hypothermia, and subsequent dietary management; (2) recovery or rehabilitation (2 to 6 weeks), focusing on increasing dietary intake and weight gain; and (3) follow-up phase, focusing on care after discharge in an outpatient setting to prevent relapse and promote weight gain, provide developmental stimulation, and evaluate cognitive and motor deficits. In the acute phase care is taken to prevent fluid overload; the child is observed closely for signs of food or fluid intolerance. The refeeding syndrome may occur if intake progresses too rapidly; cardiac failure may cause sudden death in the child who has been malnourished and refed too rapidly.

Vitamin and mineral supplementation are required in most cases of PEM; vitamin A, zinc, and copper are recommended; iron supplementation is not recommended until the child is able to tolerate a steady food source. In addition, the child is observed for signs of skin breakdown, which should be treated to prevent infection. Breastfeeding is encouraged if the mother and child are able to do so effectively; in some cases partial supplementation with a modified cow's milk–based formula may be necessary (Penny, 2003). In severely malnourished children a modest energy food source is given initially followed by a high protein and energy food source; severely malnourished children will not tolerate a high energy and protein source initially. A number of food sources may be provided to treat PEM and include oral rehydration solutions (ReSoMal), amino acid–based elemental food, and ready-to-feed foods that do not require the addition of water (to minimize contaminated water consumption); parenteral and oral antibiotics are often part of the standard treatment for PEM (Ciliberto, Sandige, Ndekha, and others, 2005; Amadi, Mwiya, Chomba, and others, 2005).

Nursing Care Management

Because PEM appears early in childhood, primarily in children 6 months to 2 years of age, and is associated with early weaning, low protein diet, delayed introduction of complementary foods, and frequent infections (Müller and Krawinkel, 2005), it is essential that nursing care focus on prevention of PEM through parent education about feeding practices during this crucial period. Breastfeeding (provided the mother is HIV-free) is the optimal method of feeding for the first 6 months. The immune properties naturally found in breast milk not only nourish the infant but aid in the prevention of opportunistic infections, which may contribute to PEM. Provision of essential physiologic needs, such as appropriate nutrient intake, protection from infection, adequate hydration, skin care, and restoration of physiologic integrity, is paramount. Additional nursing care focuses on education about and administration of childhood vaccinations to prevent illness, promotion of maternal nutrition and well-being for the lactating mother, encouragement and participation in well-child visits for infants and toddlers, and education regarding sanitation practices to prevent childhood gastrointestinal diseases.

Poor skin integrity further increases the chance of infections, hypothermia, water loss, and skin breakdown. Tube feedings may be required in infants too weak to breastfeed or bottle feed. Oral rehydration with an approved oral rehydration solution is commonly used in cases of PEM where diarrhea and infection are not immediately life threatening.

It is imperative that nurses be at the forefront in educating and reinforcing healthy nutrition habits in parents of small children to prevent malnutrition. Because children with marasmus may suffer from emotional starvation as well, care should be consistent with care of the child with failure to thrive (pp. 396-400).

FOOD SENSITIVITY

Food sensitivity is a general term that includes any type of adverse reaction to food or food additives. Food sensitivities can be divided into two broad categories:

1. **Food allergy or hypersensitivity,** which refers to reactions involving immunologic mechanisms, usually immunoglobulin E (IgE); the reactions may be immediate or delayed and mild or severe, such as an anaphylactic reaction.
2. **Food intolerance,** which refers to reactions involving known or unknown nonimmunologic mechanisms; lactose intolerance is an example of a reaction that looks like allergy but is caused by deficiency of the enzyme lactase.

This classification is not universally accepted, however; therefore the terms *food sensitivity, hypersensitivity, allergy,* and *intolerance* are often used interchangeably. The American Academy of Allergy, Asthma, and Immunology further suggests defining food-induced reactions according to the following: adverse food reactions, food hypersensitivity (allergy), food anaphylaxis, food intolerance, food idiosyncrasy, food toxicity or poisoning, anaphylactoid reaction to food, pharmacologic food reaction, and metabolic food reaction (American Academy of Pediatrics, 2004).

The clinical manifestations of food hypersensitivity may be divided as follows (American Academy of Pediatrics, 2004):

Systemic—Anaphylactic, failure to thrive
Gastrointestinal—Abdominal pain, vomiting, cramping, diarrhea
Respiratory—Cough, wheezing, rhinitis, infiltrates
Cutaneous—Urticaria, rash, atopic dermatitis

Food hypersensitivities usually occur either as an immunoglobulin E (IgE)–mediated or non-IgE-mediated immune response; some toxic reactions may occur as a result of a toxin found within the food (Sampson, 2004). Food allergy is caused by exposure to **allergens,** usually proteins (but not the smaller amino acids) that are capable of inducing IgE antibody formation (sensitization) when ingested. **Sensitization** refers to the initial exposure of an individual to an allergen, resulting in an immune response; subsequent exposure induces a much stronger response that is clinically apparent. Consequently, food hypersensitivity typically occurs after the food has been ingested one or more times. The most common food allergens are listed in Box 11-3.

Allergies in general demonstrate a genetic component: children who have one parent with allergy have a 50% or greater risk of developing allergy; children who have both parents with allergy have up to a 100% risk of developing allergy. Allergy with a hereditary tendency is referred to as **atopy.** Some infants with atopy can be identified at birth from elevated levels of IgE in cord blood.

Deaths have been reported in children who suffered an anaphylactic reaction to food. Onset of the reactions occurred shortly after ingestion (5 to 30 minutes). In most of the children the reactions did not begin with skin signs, such as hives, red rash, and flushing, but rather mimicked an acute asthma attack (wheezing, decreased air movement in airways, dyspnea). Children with food anaphylaxis should be watched closely because a biphasic response has been recorded in a number of cases in which there is an immediate response, apparent recovery, then acute recurrence of symptoms (Sampson, 2003). Parents, teachers, and child daycare workers should be educated regarding signs and symptoms of food hypersensitivity reactions. People with food sensitivity should avoid unfamiliar foods and restaurants that do not disclose food ingredients. New labeling guidelines require that food additives such as spices and flavoring be clearly labeled on commercially sold, store-bought foods. Hidden ingredients in

BOX 11-3

Hyperallergenic Foods and Sources

Nuts*—Some chocolates, candy, baked goods, cherry soda (may be flavored with a nut extract), walnut oil

Eggs*—Mayonnaise, creamy salad dressing, baked goods, egg noodles, some cake icing, meringue, custard, pancakes, French toast, root beer

Wheat*—Almost all baked goods, wieners, bologna, pressed or chopped cold cuts, gravy, pasta, some canned soups

Legumes—Peanuts,* peanut butter or oil, beans, peas, lentils

Fish or shellfish*—Cod liver oil, pizza with anchovies, Caesar salad dressing, any food fried in same oil as fish

Soy*—Soy sauce, teriyaki or Worcestershire sauce, tofu, baked goods using soy flour or oil, soy nuts, soy infant formulas or milk, soybean paste, tuna packed in vegetable oil, many margarines

Chocolate—Cola beverages, cocoa, chocolate-flavored drinks

Milk—Ice cream, butter, margarine (if it contains dairy products), yogurt, cheese, pudding, baked goods, wieners, bologna, canned creamed soups, instant breakfast drinks, powdered milk drinks, milk chocolate

Buckwheat—Some cereals, pancakes

Pork, chicken—Bacon, wieners, sausage, pork fat, chicken broth

Strawberries, melon, pineapple—Gelatin, syrups

Corn—Popcorn, cereal, muffins, cornstarch, corn meal, corn bread, corn tortilla

Citrus fruits—Orange, lemon, lime, grapefruit; any of these in drinks, gelatin, juice, or medicines

Tomatoes—Juice, some vegetable soups, spaghetti, pizza sauce, catsup

Spices—Chili, pepper, vinegar, cinnamon

*Most common allergens.

---

nursingcareguidelines

Preventing Atopy in Children

IDENTIFY CHILDREN AT RISK
Family history of allergy
Increased immunoglobulin E in cord blood and postnatal serum
Dry, flaky skin

PRENATAL PRECAUTIONS (LAST TRIMESTER)
Avoid any known food allergens
Avoid milk and other dairy products, peanuts, and eggs
Minimize ingestion of other hyperallergenic foods (see Box 11-3)

POSTNATAL PRECAUTIONS
Breast milk (preferred), extensively hydrolyzed formula (Nutramigen, Pregestimil, or Alimentum), or amino acid formula (Neocate or EleCare) exclusively for at least 6 months
No solid food for first 6 months
No whole cow's milk, substitution milks, or soy formula for 12 months
Avoid hen's eggs until 24 months; peanut, tree nuts, fish, and seafood for 36 months; and chocolate for first 12 to 18 months
One new food added at 5-day intervals to identify possible reaction
Read commercial food product label carefully for ingredients, preservatives

ENVIRONMENTAL CONTROL
Limited exposure to dust mites, molds, furry animals, latex products, and second-hand cigarette smoke

Data from Johnstone D: Strategy for intervention of food allergy in infants, *Int Pediatr* 4(4):319-325, 1989; Zeiger RS, Heller S, Mellon M, and others: Effectiveness of dietary manipulation in the prevention of food allergy in infants, *J Allergy Clin Immunol* 78(1 pt 2):224-238, 1986; Wood RA: Prospects for the prevention of allergy in children, *Curr Opin Pediatr* 8(6):601-605, 1995; Fiocchi A, Assa'ad A, Bahna S, and others: Food allergy and the introduction of solid foods to infants: a consensus document, *Ann Allergy Asthma Immunol* 97(1):10-20, 2006.

---

prepared foods have been implicated as a potential source of food hypersensitivity.

Other symptoms of anaphylaxis to food allergens include wheezing, cough, dyspnea, urticaria, abdominal cramps, vomiting, diarrhea, a drop in systemic blood pressure or shock, and, in small preverbal children, restlessness, urticaria, irritability, listlessness, and unresponsiveness. **Oral allergy syndrome** occurs when a food allergen is ingested (commonly fruits and vegetables) and there is subsequent edema and pruritus involving the lips, tongue, palate, and throat; recovery from symptoms is usually rapid. **Immediate gastrointestinal hypersensitivity** is an IgE-mediated reaction to a food allergen, and reactions include nausea, abdominal pain, cramping, diarrhea, vomiting, anaphylaxis, or all of these. Additional food hypersensitivities seen in young children include allergic eosinophilic gastritis, allergic eosinophilic gastroenterocolitis, dietary protein enterocolitis (or milk protein intolerance), and dietary protein proctitis.

Although the reason is unknown, many children "outgrow" their food allergies; children may outgrow milk and egg allergies, but peanut allergies may persist. Children who are allergic to more than one food may develop tolerance to each food at different times. Because of the tendency to lose the hypersensitivity, allergic foods should be reintroduced into the diet after a period of abstinence (usually a year or more) to evaluate whether the food can be safely added to the diet. However, foods that are associated with severe anaphylactic reactions will continue to present a lifelong risk and must be avoided. Because children with food allergies (usually two or more) are at risk for inadequate nutrient intake and growth failure, it is recommended that they have an annual nutritional assess-

ment to prevent such problems (Christie, Hine, Parker, and others, 2002).

Breastfeeding is now considered to be a primary strategy for avoiding atopy in families with known food sensitivities; however, there is some evidence that cow's milk protein is transferred via breast milk. The breastfeeding mother is encouraged to avoid foods such as peanuts, tree nuts, fish, and shellfish during the first 6 months of breastfeeding. In addition, supplementation, if required, is best with hydrolysated or amino acid formulas, *not soy* formulas. Additional recommendations to decrease the incidence of food allergies in children at higher risk for allergies is to avoid introduction of selected complementary and solid foods: dairy products should not be introduced until 12 months of age; hen's eggs at 24 months; and peanut, tree nuts, fish, and seafood at 36 months (Fiocchi, Assa'ad, Bahna and others, 2006). The strategies listed in the Nursing Care Guidelines box are those recommended by most authorities for infants with a family history of atopy.*

---

*Further information for parents of infants with food allergies is available from the American Academy of Allergy, Asthma, and Immunology, 555 E. Wells St., Suite 1100, Milwaukee, WI 53202; (414) 272-6071; http://www.aaaai.org. Additional helpful websites for information on food allergy include MedlinePlus (sponsored by U.S. National Library of Medicine and National Institutes of Health), http://medlineplus.gov; Food Allergy and Anaphylaxis Network, (800) 929-4040, http://www.foodallergy.org; National Institute of Allergy and Infectious Diseases, http://www3.niaid.nih.gov; and http://www.allergicchild.com.

NURSINGALERT

Sampson (2003) suggests that indications for the administration of intramuscular epinephrine in a child with a life-threatening anaphylactic reaction, or one who is experiencing severe symptoms, include any one of the following: itching sensation or tightness in throat; hoarseness; "barky" cough; difficulty swallowing; dyspnea; wheezing; cyanosis; respiratory arrest; mild dysrhythmia or mild hypotension; severe bradycardia, hypotension, or cardiac arrest; or loss of consciousness.

Children with extremely sensitive food allergies should wear medical identification such as a bracelet and have an injectable epinephrine cartridge (EpiPen) readily available and know how to use it. It is also helpful for the child to have a copy of the individualized written treatment plan on hand for prompt diagnosis and treatment (such plans can be downloaded from http://www.foodallergy.org and completed by the practitioner).

Cow's Milk Allergy

Cow's milk allergy (CMA) (also referred to as cow's milk protein allergy [CMPA] or cow milk protein intolerance [CMPI]) is a multifaceted disorder representing adverse systemic and local gastrointestinal reactions to cow's milk protein. (This discussion is centered on cow's milk protein found in commercial infant formulas; whole milk is not recommended for infants younger than the age of 12 months.) The hypersensitivity may be manifested within the first 4 months of life through a variety of signs and symptoms that may appear within 45 minutes of milk ingestion or after a period of several days (Box 11-4). In infants who are highly sensitive to the protein, even a small amount of cow's milk protein may induce anaphylactic reaction. Cases of contamination of non-cow milk–based infant formula during the manufacturing process resulting in severe reactions have been documented (Levin, Motala, and Lopata, 2005). The diagnosis may initially be made from the history, although the history alone is not diagnostic; the timing and diversity of clinical manifestations vary greatly. For example, CMA may be manifested as colic (see p. 395), diarrhea, vomiting, gastrointestinal bleeding, gastroesophageal reflux, chronic constipation, or sleeplessness in an otherwise healthy infant.

The incidence of CMA is reported to range from 2% to 7.5% in developed countries, although the percentage may appear to be higher because of parental report of symptoms rather than actual confirmation of CMA (Host, 2002; Salvatore and Vandenplas, 2002).

Diagnostic Evaluation. A number of diagnostic tests may be performed, including stool analysis for blood (both frank and occult bleeding can occur from the colitis), serum IgE levels, skin-prick or scratch testing, and radioallergosorbent test (measures IgE antibodies to specific allergens in serum by radioimmunoassay). Both skin and radioallergosorbent testing help identify the offending food, but the results are not always conclusive.

The most definitive diagnostic strategy is elimination of milk in the diet, followed by challenge testing after improvement of symptoms. A clinical diagnosis is made when symptoms improve after removal of milk from the diet and two or more challenge tests produce symptoms (Ewing and Allen, 2005). Challenge testing involves reintroducing small quantities of milk in the diet to detect resurgence of symptoms; at times challenge testing involves the use of a placebo so that the

---

BOX 11-4

Common Clinical Manifestations of Cow's Milk Sensitivity

GASTROINTESTINAL	OTHER SIGNS AND SYMPTOMS
Diarrhea	Eczema
Vomiting	Excessive crying
Colic	Pallor (from anemia secondary to chronic blood loss in gastrointestinal tract)
Abdominal pain	
RESPIRATORY	
Rhinitis	
Bronchitis	
Asthma	
Wheezing	
Sneezing	
Coughing	
Chronic nasal discharge	

---

parent is unaware of (or "blind" to) the timing of allergen ingestion. A double-blind placebo-controlled food challenge is the gold standard for diagnosing food allergies such as CMA, yet it may not be used very often for diagnosing CMA because of the expense, time involved, and risk for further exposure and anaphylactic reaction (Ewing and Allen, 2005).

Therapeutic Management. Treatment of CMA is elimination of cow's milk–based formula and all other dairy products. For infants fed cow's milk formula, this primarily involves changing the formula to a casein hydrolysate milk formula, or extensively hydrolyzed formula (Pregestimil, Nutramigen, or Alimentum), in which the protein has been broken down into its amino acids through enzymatic hydrolysis. Although the American Academy of Pediatrics (2004) recommends the use of hydrolyzed formulas for CMA, many practitioners may start a soy formula instead. Approximately 10% of infants who are sensitive to cow's milk protein will also demonstrate sensitivity to soy (Assa'ad, 2006), yet soy is less expensive than protein hydrolysate formula. An intolerance to soy is reported to be higher in infants under age 6 months, with a family history of atopy, and with severe gastrointestinal symptoms (Ewing and Allen, 2005). Other choices for children who are intolerant to cow's milk–based formula are the amino acid–based formulas Neocate or EleCare, yet their cost is a major consideration. Goat's milk is not an acceptable substitute because it cross-reacts with cow's milk protein, is deficient in folic acid, and is unsuitable as the only source of calories. Anaphylactic reaction to goat's milk has been noted in an infant who was also allergic to cow's milk (Pessler and Nejat, 2004). Infants who are breast-fed but have symptoms of cow's milk hypersensitivity are treated by eliminating all peanuts and tree nuts from the lactating mother's diet, and possibly eggs and milk (American Academy of Pediatrics, 2004). If maternal dairy intake is restricted, vitamin D and calcium supplementation should be considered to prevent deficiency. Infants are maintained on the milk-free diet for 1 or 2 years, after which time small quantities of milk are reintroduced; eggs and fish may be introduced at 3 years of age.

Nursing Care Management. The principal nursing objectives are to prevent and reduce exposure of infants to cow's milk protein by encouraging exclusive breastfeeding in the first 6 months of life, or even up to 12 months if there is a high risk for atopy. In addition, nurses have an important role in the identification of potential CMA, appropriate counseling of parents regarding signs and symptoms of CMA, and the use of substitute formulas that are appropriate for infants with diagnosed CMA. Parents need much reassurance regarding the needs of nonverbal infants with such an array of symptoms. Endless nights of lost sleep and a crying infant may promote feelings of parenting inadequacy and role conflict, thus aggravating the situation. Nurses can reassure parents that many of these symptoms are common and the reasons are often never found, yet the child does achieve appropriate growth and development; acute symptoms are reported to the practitioner for further evaluation. The protein hydrolysate (partially hydrolyzed and extensively hydrolyzed) formulas tend to be less palatable and more expensive than milk-based formulas. Consequently, the child's reluctance to accept the new formula may be a problem. This can be overcome by adding nonnutritive, hypoallergenic flavor packets or by introducing the formula gradually over a few days using 1 ounce of new formula to 7 ounces of old formula, then 2 to 6 ounces, 3 to 5 ounces, and as needed. Parents also need to be reassured that the infant will receive complete nutrition from the new formula and will suffer no ill effects from the absence of cow's milk.

Once solid foods are started, parents need guidance in avoiding milk products (see Box 11-3), although many children reportedly outgrow cow's milk protein sensitivity by 3 to 4 years of age (Fiocchi and Martelli, 2006).

Lactose Intolerance

Lactose intolerance refers to at least four different entities that involve a deficiency of the enzyme **lactase,** which is needed for the hydrolysis or digestion of lactose in the small intestine; lactose is hydrolyzed into glucose and galactose. **Congenital lactase deficiency** occurs soon after birth after the newborn has consumed lactose-containing milk (human milk or commercial formula). This inborn error of metabolism involves the complete absence or severely reduced presence of lactase, is rare, and requires lifelong lactose-free or extremely reduced lactose diet.

Primary lactase deficiency, sometimes referred to as **late-onset lactase deficiency,** is the most common type of lactose intolerance and is manifested usually after 4 or 5 years of age, although the time of onset is variable. Ethnic groups with a high incidence of lactase deficiency include Asians, southern Europeans, Arabs, Israelis, and African Americans, whereas Scandinavians tend to have the lowest. Lactose malabsorption manifests as lactose intolerance and is characterized by an imbalance between the ability for lactase to hydrolyze the ingested lactose and the amount of lactose ingested (Heyman and American Academy of Pediatrics Committee on Nutrition, 2006).

Secondary lactase deficiency may occur secondary to damage of the intestinal lumen, which decreases or destroys the enzyme lactase. Cystic fibrosis; sprue; celiac disease; kwashiorkor; or infections such as giardiasis, HIV, or rotavirus may cause a temporary or permanent lactose intolerance.

Developmental lactase deficiency refers to the relative lactase deficiency observed in preterm infants of less than 34 weeks gestation (Heyman and American Academy of Pediatrics Committee on Nutrition, 2006).

The primary symptoms of lactose intolerance include abdominal pain, bloating, flatulence, and diarrhea after the ingestion of lactose. The onset of symptoms occurs within 30 minutes to several hours of lactose consumption. Lactose intolerance is often perceived as an allergy, and in several studies with reports of acute gastrointestinal symptoms ascribed to lactose intolerance, measurement of lactase activity is normal (Goldberg, Folta, and Must, 2002).

Lactose intolerance may be diagnosed on the basis of the history and improvement with a lactose-reduced diet. The breath hydrogen test is used to positively diagnose the condition. Breath samples in lactose-deficient individuals will yield a higher percentage of hydrogen (20 ppm [parts per million] or more above baseline). In infants lactose malabsorption may be diagnosed by evaluating fecal pH and reducing substances; fecal pH in infants is usually lower than in older children, but an acidic pH may indicate malabsorption (Heyman and American Academy of Pediatrics Committee on Pediatrics, 2006).

Treatment of lactose intolerance is elimination of offending dairy products; however, some advocate decreasing amounts of dairy products rather than total elimination, especially in small children (Heyman and American Academy of Pediatrics Committee on Nutrition, 2006; Goldberg, Folta, and Must, 2002). In infants, lactose-free or low-lactose formula offers no special advantages over lactose-containing formula except in the severely malnourished (Heyman and American Academy of Pediatrics Committee on Pediatrics, 2006)

One concern is that dairy avoidance in children and adolescents with lactose intolerance will contribute to reduced bone mineral density and osteoporosis (Sibley, 2004). There is evidence that dietary lactose enhances calcium absorption and that lactose-free diets may negatively affect bone mineralization (Heyman and American Academy of Pediatrics Committee on Nutrition, 2006). It has been suggested that individuals with lactose maldigestion who do not experience lactose intolerance symptoms continue to consume small amounts of dairy products with meals to prevent reduced bone mass density and subsequent osteoporosis (Sibley, 2004). There is evidence that **probiotics** (food preparations containing microorganisms such as *Lactobacillus,* which alter the gastrointestinal microflora and thus are beneficial to the host) improve lactose intolerance when live cultures are fermented in dairy products (Zeisel and Erickson, 2003). The positive attributes of probiotics for those with lactose maldigestion include delayed gastrointestinal transit (slower than milk), positive effects on intestinal and colonic microflora, and a reduction of maldigestion symptoms (de Vrese, Stegelmann, Richter, and others, 2001).

Most people are able to tolerate small amounts of lactose even in the presence of deficient lactase activity (Heyman and American Academy of Pediatrics Committee on Nutrition, 2006; Goldberg, Folta, and Must, 2002) and should be encouraged to continue their intake of dairy products in small amounts to obtain much-needed nutrients. Milk taken at meals may be better tolerated than when taken alone (see Family-Centered Care box). Pretreated milk (with microbial-derived lactase) is reported to be effective in improving lactose absorption. Because dairy products are a major source of calcium and vitamin D, supplementation of these nutrients is needed to prevent deficiency. Yogurt contains inactive lactase

FAMILY-CENTERED CARE

Controlling Symptoms of Lactose Intolerance

- In infants substitute lactose-free or soy-based formula for cow's milk–based formula or human milk.
- Limit milk consumption to one to two glasses per day.
- Drink milk with other foods rather than alone.
- Eat hard cheese, cottage cheese, or yogurt instead of drinking milk.
- Use enzyme tablets (Lactaid, Lactrase, Dairy Ease) to metabolize the lactose in milk or supplement the body's own lactase (add tablets to milk or sprinkle on dairy products such as ice cream).
- Eat small amounts of dairy foods daily to help colonic bacteria adapt to ingested lactose.
- Include a probiotic (yogurt or cultured [fermented] milk) in meal or as a snack that has *Lactobacillus* or *Bifidobacterium* organisms.
- Take a calcium supplement if unable to consume any dairy products such as cheese.

enzyme, which is activated by the temperature and pH of the duodenum; this lactase activity substitutes for the lack of endogenous lactase. Fresh, plain yogurt may be tolerated better than frozen or flavored yogurt; hard cheeses, lactase-treated dairy products, and lactase tablets taken with dairy products are also viable options. An important distinction between lactose intolerance and food hypersensitivity is that lactose intolerance will not manifest as an anaphylactic-type reaction.

Nursing Care Management. Nursing care is similar to the interventions discussed for CMA: explaining the dietary restrictions to the family; identifying alternate sources of calcium such as yogurt and calcium supplementation; explaining the importance of supplementation; and discussing sources of lactose, especially hidden sources such as its use as a bulk agent in certain medications, and ways of controlling the symptoms (see Family-Centered Care box). Parents are advised to check with the pharmacist regarding this possibility when obtaining medication.

Text continued on p. 395

TABLE 11-1

Vitamins and Their Nutritional Significance*

PHYSIOLOGIC FUNCTIONS AND SOURCES	RESULTS OF DEFICIENCY OR EXCESS	NURSING CARE MANAGEMENT
VITAMIN A (RETINOL)† **Functions** Necessary component in formation of pigment rhodopsin (visual purple) Formation and maintenance of epithelial tissue Normal bone growth and tooth development Needed for growth and spermatogenesis Involved in thyroxine formation Antioxidant **Sources** **Natural form**—Liver, kidney, fish oils, milk and nonskim milk products, egg yolk **Provitamin A (carotene)**—Carrots, sweet potatoes, squash, apricots, spinach, collards, broccoli, cabbage, artichokes	**Deficiency** Night blindness Keratinization (hardening and scaling) of epithelium Xerophthalmia (hardening and scaling of cornea and conjunctiva) Phrynoderma (toad skin) Drying of respiratory, gastrointestinal, and genitourinary tracts Defective tooth enamel Delayed growth Impaired bone formation Decreased thyroxine formation Decreased resistance to infections **Excess** **Early signs**—Irritability, anorexia, pruritus, fissures at corners of nose and lips, dry skin **Later signs**—Hepatomegaly, jaundice, retarded growth, poor weight gain, thickening of the cortex of long bones with pain and fragility, hard tender lumps in extremities and occiput of the skull Can cause birth defects if excessive maternal intake NOTE: Overdose results from ingestion of large quantities of the vitamin only, not the provitamin; large amounts of carotene (carotenemia) cause yellow or orange discoloration of the skin (not the sclera, urine, or feces as in jaundice) but none of the above symptoms.	**Deficiency** Encourage foods rich in vitamin A, such as whole cow's milk (after 12 months). As milk consumption decreases, encourage foods rich in vitamin A. Ensure adequate intake in preterm infants. Advise parents of safe use of supplements in child with measles. It may play a role in prevention of severity of bronchopulmonary dysplasia in preterm infants (affects growth of respiratory tract epithelial cells). **Excess** Emphasize correct use of vitamin supplements and potential hazards of excess. Evaluate child's dietary habits to calculate approximate intake; if excessive, remove supplemental source (e.g., daily feeding of liver). Advise parents of the benign nature of carotenemia; treatment is avoidance of excess pigmented fruits or vegetables, especially carrots; skin color returns to normal in 2 to 6 weeks.

RDA, Recommended dietary allowance; *PUD,* peptic ulcer disease.
*This listing is not intended to be all inclusive.
†Fat soluble.

Vitamins and Their Nutritional Significance—cont'd

PHYSIOLOGIC FUNCTIONS AND SOURCES	RESULTS OF DEFICIENCY OR EXCESS	NURSING CARE MANAGEMENT
VITAMIN B₁ (THIAMINE)‡ **Functions** Coenzyme (with phosphorus) in carbohydrate metabolism Needed for healthy nervous system Digestion and normal appetite **Sources** Pork, beef, liver, legumes, nuts, whole or enriched grains and cereals, green vegetables, fruits, milk, brown rice	**Deficiency** **Gastrointestinal**—Anorexia, constipation, indigestion **Neurologic**—Apathy, fatigue, emotional instability, polyneuritis, tenderness of calf muscles, partial anesthesia, muscle weakness, paresthesia, hyperesthesia, decreased or absent tendon reflexes, convulsions, coma (in infants) **Cardiovascular**—Palpitations, cardiac failure, peripheral vasodilation, edema **Excess** Headache Irritability Insomnia Weakness	**Deficiency: Vitamin B Complex** Encourage foods rich in B vitamins. Stress proper cooking and storage techniques to preserve potency, such as minimum cooking of vegetables in small amount of liquid, storage of milk in opaque container. Encourage fortified breakfast cereals and soy milk (which contain vitamin B₁₂) for persons on strict vegetarian diets. Dairy products and eggs contain vitamin B₁₂, if these are allowed. Otherwise, supplementation may be required. Evaluate need for vitamin supplements when dieting, when using unfortified goat's milk exclusively for infant feeding (deficient in folic acid), or when the breastfeeding mother is a strict vegetarian (vitamin B₁₂). **Excess** Emphasize correct use of vitamin supplements and potential hazards of excess. Individuals with malabsorption syndrome or being treated with hemodialysis or peritoneal dialysis may have increased need for thiamine.
VITAMIN B₂ (RIBOFLAVIN)‡ **Functions** Coenzyme (with phosphorus) in carbohydrate, protein, and fat metabolism Maintains healthy skin, especially around mouth, nose, and eyes **Sources** Milk and its products, eggs, organs (liver, kidney, heart), enriched cereals, some green leafy vegetables,§ legumes	**Deficiency** Ariboflavinosis **Lips**—Cheilosis (fissures at corners of lips), perlèche (inflammation at corners of lips) **Tongue**—Glossitis **Nose**—Irritation and cracks at nasal angle **Eyes**—Burning, itching, tearing, photophobia, blurred vision, corneal vascularization, cataracts **Skin**—Seborrheic dermatitis, delayed wound healing and tissue repair **Excess** Paresthesia, pruritus	Same as vitamin B complex
NIACIN (NICOTINIC ACID, NICOTINAMIDE)‡ **Functions** Coenzyme (with riboflavin) in protein and fat metabolism Needed for healthy nervous system and skin and for normal digestion May lower cholesterol **Sources** Meat, poultry, fish, peanuts, beans, peas, whole or enriched grains (except corn and rice) Milk and its products are sources of tryptophan (60 mg tryptophan = 1 mg niacin).	**Deficiency** Pellagra (rash, diarrhea, mental status changes, stomatitis) **Oral**—Stomatitis, glossitis **Cutaneous**—Scaly dermatitis on exposed areas **Gastrointestinal**—Anorexia, weight loss, diarrhea, fatigue **Neurologic**—Apathy, anxiety, confusion, depression, dementia **Excess** Release of histamine, a vasodilator (flushing, decreased blood pressure, increased cerebral blood flow; aggravates asthma) Dermatologic problems (pruritus, rash, hyperkeratosis, acanthosis nigricans) Increased gastric acidity (aggravates PUD) Hepatotoxicity Increased serum uric acid levels Elevated plasma glucose levels Certain cardiac arrhythmias	Same as vitamin B complex **Excess** If used as hypolipidemic agent, stress safe storage to prevent child's accidental ingestion.

‡Water soluble.
§Green leafy vegetables include spinach, broccoli, kale, turnip greens, mustard greens, collards, dandelion greens, and beet greens.

Continued

| TABLE 11-1

Vitamins and Their Nutritional Significance—cont'd

PHYSIOLOGIC FUNCTIONS AND SOURCES	RESULTS OF DEFICIENCY OR EXCESS	NURSING CARE MANAGEMENT
VITAMIN B$_6$ (PYRIDOXINE)‡ **Functions** Coenzyme in protein and fat metabolism Needed for formation of antibodies and hemo-globin Needed for utilization of copper and iron Aids in conversion of tryptophan to niacin **Sources** Meats, especially liver and kidney, cereal grains (wheat, corn), yeast, soybeans, peanuts, tuna, chicken, salmon	**Deficiency** Scaly dermatitis Weight loss Anemia Retarded growth Irritability Seizures Peripheral neuritis **Excess** Peripheral nervous system toxicity (unsteady gait, numb feet and hands, clumsiness of hands, sometimes perioral numbness) May cause PUD or seizures	Same as vitamin B complex **Deficiency** Stress proper cooking and storing techniques to preserve potency. Cook food covered in small amount of water. Do not soak food in water. Store in light-resistant container.
FOLIC ACID (FOLACIN; REDUCED FORM CALLED FOLINIC ACID OR CITROVORUM FACTOR)‡ **Functions** Coenzyme for single-carbon transfer (purines, thymine, hemoglobin) Necessary for formation of red blood cells May prevent neural tube defects (i.e., myelomeningocele) and facial clefts (cleft lip and palate) **Sources** Green leafy vegetables, beets, cabbage, asparagus, liver, kidneys, nuts, eggs, whole grain cereals, legumes, bananas	**Deficiency** Macrocytic anemia Bone marrow depression Glossitis Intestinal malabsorption Growth failure **Excess** Rare because megadoses not available over the counter May cause insomnia and irritability	Same as vitamin B complex **Deficiency** Stress proper cooking and storing techniques to preserve potency: Cook food covered in small amount of water. Do not soak food in water. Store in light-resistant container. Women of childbearing age should supplement to prevent neural tube defects and orofacial clefts.
VITAMIN B$_{12}$ (COBALAMIN)‡ **Functions** Coenzyme in protein synthesis; indirect effect on formation of red blood cells (particularly on formation of nucleic acids and folic acid metabolism) Needed for normal functioning of nervous tissue **Sources** Meat, liver, kidney, fish, shellfish, poultry, milk, eggs, cheese, nutritional yeast, sea vegetables	**Deficiency** Pernicious anemia (one form of deficiency from absence of intrinsic factor in gastric secretions) General signs of severe anemia Lemon-yellow tinge to skin Spinal cord degeneration Delayed brain growth **Excess** Rare	Same as vitamin B complex **Deficiency** Consider fortified foods or supplements in persons over 50 years of age to meet RDA because malabsorption of food-bound vitamin B$_{12}$ is common.
VITAMIN C (ASCORBIC ACID)‡ **Functions** Essential for collagen formation Increases absorption of iron for hemoglobin formation Enhances conversion of folic acid to folinic acid Affects cholesterol synthesis and conversion of proline to hydroxyproline Probably a coenzyme in metabolism of tyrosine and phenylalanine May play role in hydroxylation of adrenal steroids May have stimulating effect on phagocytic activity of leukocytes and formation of antibodies Antioxidant agent (spares other vitamins from oxidation)	**Deficiency** Scurvy **Skin**—Dry, rough, petechiae, perifollicular hyperkeratotic papules (raised areas around hair follicles) **Musculoskeletal**—Bleeding muscles and joints, pseudoparalysis from pain, swelling of joints, costochondral beading (scorbutic rosary) **Gums**—Spongy, friable, swollen, bleed easily, bluish red or black, teeth loosen and fall out **General disposition**—Irritable, anorexic, apprehensive, in pain, refuses to move, assumes semi-froglike position when supine (scorbutic pose) Signs of anemia Decreased wound healing Increased susceptibility to infection	**Deficiency** Encourage foods rich in vitamin C. Evaluate child's diet for sources of vitamin, especially when cow's milk is principal source of nutrition. Tobacco smokers require an additional 35 mg/day; nonsmokers exposed to second-hand smoke should make sure they meet RDA. Stress proper cooking and storage techniques to preserve potency: Wash vegetables quickly; do not soak in water. Cook vegetables in covered pot with minimum water and for short time; avoid copper or cast iron cookware. Do not add baking soda to cooking water. Use fresh fruits and vegetables as soon as possible; store in refrigerator. Store juice in airtight, opaque container. Wrap cut fruit or eat soon after exposing to air.

RDA, Recommended dietary allowance; *PUD*, peptic ulcer disease.
‡Water soluble.

TABLE 11-1

Vitamins and Their Nutritional Significance—cont'd

PHYSIOLOGIC FUNCTIONS AND SOURCES	RESULTS OF DEFICIENCY OR EXCESS	NURSING CARE MANAGEMENT
Sources Citrus fruits, strawberries, tomatoes, potatoes, cabbage, broccoli, cauliflower, spinach, papaya, mango, cantaloupe, watermelon, enriched fruit juice	**Excess** Diarrhea Increased excretion of uric acid and acidification of urine (may cause urate precipitation and formation of oxalate stones) Hemolysis Impaired leukocytosis activity Damage to beta cells of pancreas and decreased insulin production Reproductive failure "Rebound scurvy" from withdrawal of large amounts	**Excess** Emphasize correct use of vitamin supplement and potential hazards of excess. Identify groups at risk for excessive vitamin C supplements (e.g., those with thalassemia or those receiving anticoagulant or aminoglycoside antibiotic therapy)
VITAMIN D₂ (ERGOCALCIFEROL) AND VITAMIN D₃ (CHOLECALCIFEROL)† **Functions** Absorption of calcium and phosphorus and decreased renal excretion of phosphorus **Sources** Direct sunlight Cod liver oil, herring, mackerel, salmon, tuna, sardines Enriched food sources—Milk, milk products, enriched cereals, margarine, breads, many breakfast drinks	**Deficiency** Rickets **Head**—Craniotabes (softening of cranial bones, prominence of frontal bones), deformed shape (skull flat and depressed toward middle), delayed closure of fontanels **Chest**—Rachitic rosary (enlargement of costochondral junction of ribs), Harrison groove (horizontal depression in lower portion of rib cage), pigeon chest (sharp protrusion of sternum) **Spine**—Kyphosis, scoliosis, lordosis **Abdomen**—Pot belly, constipation **Extremities**—Bowing of arms and legs, knock knee, saber shins, instability of hip joints, pelvic deformity, enlargement of epiphyses at ends of long bones **Teeth**—Delayed calcification, especially of permanent teeth **Rachitic tetany**—Seizures **Excess** **Acute**—Vomiting, dehydration, fever, abdominal cramps, bone pain, seizures, coma **Chronic**—Lassitude, mental slowness, anorexia, failure to thrive, thirst, urinary urgency, polyuria, vomiting, diarrhea, abdominal cramps, bone pain, pathologic fractures **Calcification of soft tissue**—Kidneys, lungs, adrenal glands, vessels (hypertension), heart, gastric lining, tympanic membrane (deafness) Osteoporosis of long bones Elevated serum levels of calcium and phosphorus	**Deficiency** Encourage foods rich in vitamin D, especially fortified whole cow's milk (>12 months of age). Encourage use of vitamin D supplement by age 2 months in all infants (see text). Observe for possibility of overdose from supplements. If prescribed, supervise proper use of orthoses (splints and braces). Same as vitamin A; may include low-calcium diet during initial therapy **Excess** Same as vitamin A; may include low-calcium diet during initial therapy
VITAMIN E (TOCOPHEROL)† **Functions** Production of red blood cells and protection from hemolysis Muscle and liver integrity Coenzyme factor in tissue respiration Minimizes oxidation of polyunsaturated fatty acids and vitamins A and C in intestinal tract and tissues **Sources** Vegetable oils, wheat germ oil, milk, egg yolk, fish, whole grains, nuts, legumes, spinach, broccoli	**Deficiency** Hemolytic anemia from hemolysis caused by shortened life of red blood cells, especially in preterm infants; focal necrosis of tissues **Excess** Little is known; less toxic than other fat-soluble vitamins	**Deficiency** Initiate early feeding in preterm infants; may need supplementation. Potential role as antioxidant in immune function, prevention of or limiting the severity of retinopathy and prevention of hemolytic anemia, bronchopulmonary dysplasia, and intracranial hemorrhage.

†Fat soluble.

Continued

TABLE 11-1

Vitamins and Their Nutritional Significance—cont'd

PHYSIOLOGIC FUNCTIONS AND SOURCES	RESULTS OF DEFICIENCY OR EXCESS	NURSING CARE MANAGEMENT
VITAMIN K† **Functions** Catalyst for production of prothrombin and blood-clotting factors II, VII, IX, and X by the liver **Sources** Pork, liver, green leafy vegetables, cabbage, tomatoes, egg yolk, cheese	**Deficiency** Hemorrhage **Excess** Hemolytic anemia in individuals who are deficient in glucose 6-phosphate dehydrogenase	**Deficiency** Administer prophylactically to all newborns. Other indications include intestinal disease, lack of bile, prolonged antibiotic therapy; may be used in management of blood-clotting time when anticoagulants such as warfarin (Coumadin) and dicumarol (bishydroxycoumarin), which are vitamin K antagonists, are used.

RDA, Recommended dietary allowance; *PUD*, peptic ulcer disease.
†Fat soluble.

TABLE 11-2

Minerals and Their Nutritional Significance*

PHYSIOLOGIC FUNCTIONS AND SOURCES	RESULTS OF DEFICIENCY OR EXCESS	NURSING CARE MANAGEMENT
CALCIUM† **Functions** Bone and tooth development and maintenance (in combination with phosphorus) Muscle contractions, especially the heart Blood clotting Absorption of vitamin B_{12} Enzyme activation Nerve conduction Integrity of intracellular cement substances and various membranes **Sources** Dairy products, egg yolk, sardines, canned salmon with bones, green leafy vegetables‡ (except spinach), soybeans, dried beans, peas	**Deficiency** Rickets Tetany Impaired growth, especially of bones and teeth Osteoporosis **Excess** Drowsiness, extreme lethargy Impaired absorption of other minerals (iron, zinc, manganese) Calcium deposits in tissues (renal failure)	**Deficiency** Encourage foods rich in calcium, especially dairy products. Give vitamin D supplements in infants beginning by age 2 months (see text). Caution that oxalates in leafy vegetables (spinach), oxalates in chocolates, and a high phosphorus intake (especially from carbonated beverages) can decrease calcium absorption. Discourage use of whole cow's milk in newborns and infants under 12 months because the phosphorus/calcium ratio favors excretion of calcium. Advise against diets that restrict dairy products unless adequate supplementation is followed. **Excess** Emphasize correct use of calcium supplements, especially the possible interaction between megadoses of calcium and resulting deficiency states of other minerals.
CHLORIDE† **Functions** Acid-base and fluid balance Enzyme activation in saliva Component of hydrochloric acid in stomach **Sources** Salt, meat, eggs, dairy products, many prepared and preserved foods	**Deficiency** Acid-base disturbances (hypochloremic alkalosis, dehydration); occurs mostly in combination with sodium loss **Excess** Acid-base disturbance	Deficiency and excess are unusual; most diets supply adequate chloride (usually in combination with sodium). Disease states such as excessive vomiting may require chloride replacement.

*This listing is not intended to be all inclusive.
†Macrominerals—required intake >100 mg/day.
‡Green leafy vegetables include spinach, broccoli, kale, turnip greens, mustard greens, collards, dandelion greens, and beet greens.

TABLE 11-2		

Minerals and Their Nutritional Significance—cont'd

PHYSIOLOGIC FUNCTIONS AND SOURCES	RESULTS OF DEFICIENCY OR EXCESS	NURSING CARE MANAGEMENT
COPPER§ **Functions** Production of hemoglobin Essential component of several enzyme systems **Sources** Organ meats, oysters, nuts, seeds, legumes, corn oil margarine	**Deficiency** Anemia, leukopenia, neutropenia **Excess** Severe vomiting and diarrhea Hemolytic anemia	**Deficiency** Emphasize the correct use of any vitamin supplement with mineral because deficiency from inadequate food sources is less likely than from excess intake of other minerals, especially zinc and possibly iron. **Excess** Cooking acid foods in unlined copper pots can lead to chronic and toxic accumulation of copper.
FLUORIDE§ **Functions** Formation of caries-resistant teeth Strong bone development **Sources** Fluoridated water and foods or beverages prepared with fluoridated water, fish, tea	**Deficiency** Increased susceptibility to tooth decay **Excess** Fluorosis (mottling or pitting of enamel) Severe bone deformities	Fluoride has the narrowest range of safe and adequate intake; therefore stress the importance of storing supplements in a safe area. **Deficiency** In areas with optimally fluoridated water, encourage sufficient intake to supply recommended amount of fluoride. In areas of unfluoridated water or when ready-to-use formula, powder formula, bottled water, or breast milk is used, stress the importance of fluoride supplements (age appropriate). **Excess** In areas with excess fluoride in the water, consider the use of bottled water (without fluoride) in drinking and cooking to reduce the fluoride intake to safe levels.
IODINE§ **Functions** Production of thyroid hormone Normal reproduction **Sources** Seafood, kelp, iodized salt, sea salt, enriched bread, milk (from dairy processing); medications including amiodarone, povidone-iodine, and prenatal vitamins	**Deficiency** Goiter (enlarged thyroid from decreased thyroxine formation) **Excess** Thyrotoxicosis, goiter, hypothyroidism	**Deficiency** Encourage use of iodized salt for individuals living far from the sea. **Excess** If iodine preparations are in the home, stress the importance of safe storage.
IRON **Functions** Formation of hemoglobin and myoglobin Essential part of several enzymes and proteins **Sources** Liver, especially pork, followed by calf, beef, and chicken; kidney, red meat, poultry, shellfish, whole grains, iron-enriched infant formula and cereal, enriched cereals and bread, legumes, nuts, seeds, green leafy vegetables (except spinach), dried fruits, potatoes, molasses, tofu, prune juice	**Deficiency** Anemia (See Chapter 26.) **Excess** Hemosiderosis (excess iron storage in various tissues of the body, especially the spleen, liver, lymph glands, heart, and pancreas) Hemochromatosis (excess iron storage with cellular damage)	**Deficiency** Discourage excessive milk consumption, especially more than 1 L/day (milk is a poor source of iron). If iron supplements are prescribed, teach parents factors that affect absorption. **Excess** Stress the importance of storing iron supplements in a safe area.

§Microminerals or trace elements—required intake <100 mg/day.

Continued

TABLE 11-2		

Minerals and Their Nutritional Significance—cont'd

PHYSIOLOGIC FUNCTIONS AND SOURCES	RESULTS OF DEFICIENCY OR EXCESS	NURSING CARE MANAGEMENT
MAGNESIUM† **Functions** Bone and tooth formation Production of proteins Nerve conduction to muscles Activation of enzymes needed for carbohydrate and protein metabolism **Sources** Whole grains, nuts, soybeans, meat, green leafy vegetables (uncooked), tea, cocoa, raisins	**Deficiency** Tremors, spasm Irregular heartbeat Muscular weakness Lower extremity cramps Convulsions, delirium **Excess** Nervous system disturbances caused by imbalance in calcium/magnesium ratio	Deficiency and excess are unusual, except in disease states such as prolonged vomiting or diarrhea or kidney dysfunction, where replacement may be needed.
PHOSPHORUS† **Functions** Bone and tooth development (in combination with calcium) Involved in numerous chemical reactions, including protein, carbohydrate, and fat metabolism Acid-base balance **Sources** Dairy products, eggs, meat, poultry, legumes, carbonated beverages	**Deficiency** Weakness, anorexia, malaise, bone pain **Excess** Produces secondary calcium deficiency from disturbed calcium/phosphorus ratio	**Deficiency** Dietary deficiency is uncommon, although prolonged use of antacids can produce deficiency, in which case supplementation is recommended. To preserve calcium/phosphorus ratio in newborns, discourage use of whole cow's milk.
POTASSIUM† **Functions** Acid-base and fluid balance (major intracellular fluid cation) Nerve conduction Muscular contraction, especially the heart Release of energy **Sources** Bananas, citrus fruit, dried fruits, meat, fish, bran, legumes, peanut butter, potatoes, coffee, tea, cocoa	**Deficiency** Cardiac arrhythmias Muscular weakness Lethargy Kidney and respiratory failure Heart failure **Excess** Cardiac arrhythmias Respiratory failure Mental confusion Numbness of extremities	Dietary deficiency and excess are unlikely, although disease states such as prolonged nausea and vomiting or the use of diuretics can result in hypokalemia; in such instances, encourage replacement with supplements of rich food sources, such as bananas.
SELENIUM§ **Functions** Antioxidant, especially protective of vitamin E Protects against toxicity of heavy metals Associated with fat metabolism **Sources** Seafood, organs, egg yolk, whole grains, chicken, meat, tomatoes, cabbage, garlic, mushrooms, milk	**Deficiency** Keshan disease (cardiomyopathy in children; found in China) **Excess** Eye, nose, and throat irritation Increased dental caries Liver and kidney degeneration	Deficiency and excess are uncommon in North America, although selenium deficiency can occur in patients receiving prolonged total parenteral alimentation; in these instances, supplementation is required.

†Macrominerals—required intake >100 mg/day.
§Microminerals or trace elements—required intake <100 mg/day.

TABLE 11-2
Minerals and Their Nutritional Significance—cont'd

PHYSIOLOGIC FUNCTIONS AND SOURCES	RESULTS OF DEFICIENCY OR EXCESS	NURSING CARE MANAGEMENT
SODIUM† **Functions** Acid-base and fluid balance (major extracellular fluid cation) Cell permeability; absorption of glucose Muscle contraction **Sources** Table salt, seafood, meat, poultry, numerous prepared foods	**Deficiency** Dehydration Hypotension Convulsions Muscle cramps **Excess** Edema Hypertension Intracranial hemorrhage	**Deficiency** Deficient intake is rare, although losses secondary to nausea, vomiting, excessive sweating, and use of diuretics can occur and require replacement. **Excess** Encourage parents to limit excessive use of salt in preparing foods and to limit commercial foods with high sodium content, such as smoked meats.
ZINC§ **Functions** Component of about 100 enzymes Synthesis of nucleic acids and protein in immune system and coagulation Release of vitamin A from liver Improved wound healing with vitamin C Normal taste sensitivity **Sources** Seafood (especially oysters), meat, poultry, eggs, wheat, legumes	**Deficiency** Loss of appetite Diminished taste sensation Delayed healing **Skin lesions**—Erythematous, crusted lesions around body orifices Alopecia Diarrhea Growth failure Delayed sexual maturity **Excess** Vomiting and diarrhea Malaise, dizziness Anemia, gastric bleeding Impaired absorption of calcium and copper	Emphasize correct use of zinc supplements and the possible interaction with other minerals. **Deficiency** Encourage food sources rich in zinc, especially protein. Caution that fiber, phytates, oxalates, tannins (in tea or coffee), iron, and calcium adversely affect zinc absorption. Recognize groups at risk for zinc deficiency, such as vegetarians and Hispanics, whose diets may have restricted or low meat content and high fiber and phytate content; and patients with malabsorption syndromes.

†Macrominerals—required intake >100 mg/day.
§Microminerals or trace elements—required intake <100 mg/day.

FEEDING DIFFICULTIES
REGURGITATION AND "SPITTING UP"

The return of small amounts of food after a feeding is a common occurrence during infancy. It should not be confused with vomiting, which can be associated with a number of disturbances that may be insignificant or serious. Regurgitation is usually benign, although persistent regurgitation necessitates medical evaluation to rule out gastroesophageal reflux (see Chapter 24). For clarification the terms are defined as:

Regurgitation—Return of undigested food from the stomach, usually accompanied by burping
Spitting up—Dribbling of unswallowed formula from the infant's mouth immediately after a feeding

The normal occurrence of regurgitation or spitting up should be explained to parents, especially to those who are unduly concerned about it. Regurgitation can be reduced by some simple measures, such as frequent burping during and after feeding, minimum handling during and after feeding, and positioning the child on the right side with the head slightly elevated after feeding. The inconvenience of spitting up can be managed with the use of absorbent bibs on the infant and protective cloths on the parent.

Sometimes frequent dribbling of formula causes excoriation of the corners of the mouth, chin, and neck. Keeping the area dry promotes healing but can be difficult to maintain. Helpful suggestions include applying a thin film of petrolatum or A&D ointment to the affected areas after cleansing and using absorbent nonplastic-lined terry-cloth bibs, which are changed frequently.

PAROXYSMAL ABDOMINAL PAIN (COLIC)

Colic is reported to occur in 5% to 30% of all infants (Neu and Robinson, 2003), yet has no particular affinity in regard to the gender, race, or socioeconomic status of the infant and family (Ellett, 2003). The condition is generally described as paroxysmal abdominal pain or cramping that is manifested by loud crying and drawing the legs up to the abdomen. Other definitions include variables such as duration of cry greater than 3 hours a day, occurring more than 3 days per week, and parental dissatisfaction with the child's behavior. Some studies report an increase in symptoms (fussiness and crying) in the late afternoon or evening; however, in some infants the onset of symptoms occurs at another time. Colic is more common in young infants under the age of 3 months than in older infants, and infants with "difficult" temperaments are more likely to be colicky. Despite the obvious behavioral indications of pain, the child tolerates breast milk or some type of infant formula well, gains weight, and usually thrives. There is no evidence of a residual effect of colic on older children, except perhaps a strained parent-child relationship in some cases; in other words, infants who are colicky grow up to be normal children and adults.

Among the theories that have been investigated as potential causes are too rapid feeding, overeating, swallowing excessive air, improper feeding technique (especially in positioning and burping), and emotional stress or tension between parent and child. Although all of these may occur, there is no evidence that one factor is consistently present. In some infants colic may be a sign of CMA or cow's milk intolerance, and eliminating cow's milk products from the infant's diet and the diet of lactating mothers can reduce the symptoms; in some infants soy milk may cause the same discomfort as cow's milk. Parental smoking, strained parent-infant interaction, lactase deficiency, difficult infant temperament, difficulty regulating emotions, central nervous system immaturity, and neurochemical dysregulation in the brain have also been proposed as potential causes of colic (Ellett, 2003; Neu and Robinson, 2003). A positive association between consumption of fruit juices (carbohydrate malabsorption) and colic has been demonstrated in some cases (Duro, Rising, Cedillo, and others, 2002). The final consensus of most experts who study colic is that it is multifactorial in nature and that no single treatment for every colicky infant will be effective in alleviating the symptoms.

Therapeutic Management

Management of colic should begin with an investigation of possible organic causes, such as CMA, intussusception, or other gastrointestinal problem. If a sensitivity to cow's milk is strongly suspected, a trial substitution of another formula such as an extensively hydrolyzed (Nutramigen, Alimentum, Pregestimil), whey hydrolysate, or amino acid (Neocate, EleCare) formula is warranted. Soy formulas are usually avoided because of the possibility of sensitivity to soy protein as well.

The use of drugs, including sedatives, antispasmodics, antihistamines, and antiflatulents, is sometimes recommended. The most commonly used sedatives are phenobarbital, hydroxyzine hydrochloride (Atarax), and chloral hydrate. Simethicone (Mylicon) may also help allay the symptoms of colic. However, in most controlled studies none of these drugs completely reduced the symptoms of colic. Herbal (chamomile) tea offered at the onset of crying and up to three times daily has proved effective in relieving the symptoms of colic in some infants (Weizman, Alkrinawi, Goldfarb, and others, 1993); however, parents are to be cautioned regarding the unknown safety of this treatment (Crotteau, Wright, and Eglash, 2006). Behavioral interventions have not proved effective at reducing symptoms of colic but have helped parents deal with the crying infant in a more positive manner. The addition of lactase to infant formula has produced mixed results as far as abatement of overall symptoms.

An extensive review of a wide variety of interventions for colic indicates there are no specific safe remedies to alleviate symptoms of colic in every infant; dietary changes such as eliminating cow's milk protein from the lactating mother's diet and behavioral interventions were shown to be effective in helping parents reduce stimulation and respond to the infant's crying, yet these interventions are perceived only as moderately effective (Joanna Briggs Institute, 2004).

Nursing Care Management

The initial step in managing colic is to take a thorough, detailed history of the usual daily events. Areas that should be stressed include (1) the infant's diet; (2) the diet of the breast-feeding mother; (3) the time of day when crying occurs; (4) the relationship of the crying to feeding time; (5) the presence of specific family members during the crying and habits of family members, such as smoking; (6) activity of the mother or usual caregiver before, during, and after the crying; (7) characteristics of the cry (duration, intensity); (8) measures used to relieve the crying and their effectiveness; and (9) the infant's stooling, voiding, and sleeping patterns. Of special emphasis is a careful assessment of the feeding process via demonstration by the parent.

If cow's milk sensitivity is suspected, breastfeeding mothers should follow a milk-free diet for a minimum of 3 to 5 days in an attempt to reduce symptoms in the infant. Mothers need to be cautioned that some nondairy creamers may contain calcium caseinate, a cow's milk protein. If a milk-free diet is helpful, lactating mothers may need calcium supplements to meet the body's requirement. Bottle-fed infants may improve with the same dietary modifications as for the child with CMA (see p. 386).

Perhaps the most important nursing intervention (once the diagnosis of colic is established) is reassurance of both parents that they are not doing anything wrong and that the infant is not experiencing any physical or emotional harm. Parents, especially mothers, become easily frustrated with the infant's crying and perceive this as a sign that there is something horribly wrong. An empathetic, gentle, and reassuring attitude, in addition to suggestions about remedies for treatment, will help allay parents' anxieties, which are usually exacerbated by loss of sleep and preoccupation over the infant's welfare. Other support persons and extended family members may be enlisted to help support the parents during this time of difficulty.

When no cause can be identified, helping parents understand the infant's crying behavior and modifying parent interventions to promptly attend to the infant's needs can decrease the length of fussiness and crying. Other approaches for managing colic are listed in the Family-Centered Care box. Parents are encouraged to try as many of these approaches as possible, because not all are effective for every infant. One author suggests that a problem-solving discussion with the parents, in addition to acknowledgment that the infant has colic, is an optimal strategy for helping parents manage the infant with colic until a cure is found (Ellett, 2003).

GROWTH FAILURE (FAILURE TO THRIVE)

Growth failure, or failure to thrive (FTT), is a sign of inadequate growth resulting from inability to obtain or use calories required for growth. FTT has no universal definition, although one of the more common parameters is a weight (and sometimes height) that falls below the 5th percentile for the child's age. Another definition of FTT includes a weight for age (height) z value of less than -2.0 (a z value is a standard deviation value that represents anthropometric data normal-

FAMILY-CENTERED CARE

Managing the Colicky Infant

- Place infant prone over a covered hot-water bottle, heated towel, or covered heating pad.
- Massage infant's abdomen.
- Respond immediately to the crying.
- Change infant's position frequently; walk with child's face down and with body across parent's arm, with parent's hand under infant's abdomen, applying gentle pressure (Fig. 11-2).
- Use a front carrier for transporting infant.
- Swaddle infant tightly with a soft, stretchy blanket.
- Place infant in an electric (or wind-up) infant swing.
- Take infant for car rides or outside for a change in environment.
- Use bottles that minimize air swallowing (curved bottle or inner collapsible bag).
- Use a commercial device* in the crib that stimulates the vibration and sound of a car ride or plays soothing "noise," in utero sounds, or music.†
- Provide smaller, frequent feedings; burp infant during and after feedings using the shoulder position or sitting upright, and place infant in an upright seat after feedings.
- Introduce a pacifier for added sucking.
- In breast-fed infants, mother should avoid all milk products for a trial period.
- If household members smoke, avoid smoking near infant; preferably confine smoking activity to outside of home.
- Give appropriate dose of acetaminophen elixir or suppository if suggested by health professional; not recommended for daily use.
- If nothing reduces the crying, place infant in crib and allow to cry; periodically hold and comfort child and put down again.
- Maintain a brief diary of the time of day the crying starts; events going on in household; time, amount and type of last feeding; length of crying; and characteristics of cry. Although this will not stop the crying, it may help the practitioner identify a possible cause.

*Sweet Dreems, Inc., Sleep Tight Order Department, (800) NO COLIC, (800) 662-6542; http://www.colic.com.
†Suggested infant relaxation music: *Heartbeat Lullabies* by Terry Woodford. Available from Baby-Go-To-Sleep Center, Audio Therapy Innovations, Inc., PO Box 550, Colorado Springs, CO 80901; (800) 537-7448; website: http://www.babygotosleep.com.

FIG. 11-2 ■ The "colic carry" may be comforting to an infant with colic. (Photo by Paul Vincent Kuntz, Texas Children's Hospital, Houston.)

2. **Nonorganic failure to thrive (NFTT)**—A definable cause that is unrelated to disease. NFTT is most often the result of psychosocial factors, such as inadequate nutritional information by the parent; deficiency in maternal care or a disturbance in maternal-child attachment; or a disturbance in the child's ability to separate from the parent, leading to food refusal to maintain attention.
3. **Idiopathic failure to thrive**—Unexplained by the usual organic and environmental etiologies but may also be classified as NFTT. Both categories of NFTT account for the majority of cases of FTT.

izing for sex and age with greater precision than growth percentile curves [Markowitz and Duggan, 2003]). A third way to define FTT is a weight curve that crosses more than 2 percentile lines on the National Center for Health Statistics growth charts after previous achievement of a stable growth pattern. Growth measurements alone are not used to diagnose children with FTT. Rather, the finding of a pattern of persistent deviation from established growth parameters is cause for concern. In addition to lack of consensus on the precise definition of FTT, there are those who advocate for a change in terminology; thus, terms such as *growth failure* and *pediatric undernutrition* are used in the literature for failure to thrive (Locklin, 2005).

Traditionally the three general categories of failure to thrive have been as follows:

1. **Organic failure to thrive**—Result of a physical cause, such as congenital heart defects, neurologic lesions, microcephaly, chronic renal failure, gastroesophageal reflux, malabsorption syndrome, endocrine dysfunction, cystic fibrosis, or acquired immunodeficiency syndrome (AIDS).

Some experts, however, suggest that the above classifications are too simplistic because most cases of growth failure have mixed causes; they suggest that FTT be classified according to pathophysiology for the following categories: (1) inadequate caloric intake—incorrect formula preparation, neglect, food fads, excessive juice consumption, poverty, behavioral problems affecting eating, or central nervous system problems affecting intake; (2) inadequate absorption—cystic fibrosis, celiac disease, vitamin or mineral deficiencies, biliary atresia, or hepatic disease; (3) increased metabolism—hyperthyroidism, congenital heart defects, or chronic immunodeficiency; and (4) defective utilization—genetic anomaly such as trisomy 21 or 18, congenital infection, or metabolic storage diseases (Krugman and Dubowitz, 2003). The etiology of growth failure is often multifactorial and involves a combination of infant organic disease, dysfunctional parenting behaviors, subtle neurologic or behavioral problems, and disturbed parent-child interactions (Block, Krebs, and American Academy of Pediatrics Committee on Child Abuse and Neglect and Committee on Nutrition, 2005).

Other factors that can lead to inadequate infant caloric intake include:

Poverty—Lack of funds to buy sufficient food; diluting formula to extend available supply

Health or childrearing beliefs—Fad diets; excessive concern with preventing conditions such as obesity, hypercholesterolemia, or nursing caries; strict use of scheduled feedings

Inadequate nutritional knowledge—Cultural confusion of newly arrived immigrants who are unaware of appropriate food selections in American markets; parents with cognitive impairment

Family stress—Overwhelming involvement with another chronically ill child; any number of other stresses (financial, marital, excessive parenting and employment responsibilities, depression, chemical abuse, acute grief)

Feeding resistance—Result of nonoral nutritional therapy early in life

Insufficient breast milk—Result of a number of different causes (fatigue, illness, poor release of milk, insufficient glandular tissue, lack of maternal confidence)

In the following discussion, *FTT* is used to describe any child with growth failure, whether it be organic, nonorganic, a combination of both, or of unknown etiology.

Diagnostic Evaluation

Diagnosis is initially made from evidence of growth failure. If FTT is recent, the weight, but not the height, is below accepted standards (usually the 5th percentile); if FTT is longstanding, both weight and height are low, indicating chronic malnutrition. Perhaps as important as anthropometric measurements are a complete health and dietary history (including perinatal history), physical examination for evidence of organic causes, developmental assessment, and family assessment. A dietary intake history, either a 24-hour food intake or a history of food consumed over a 3- to 5-day period, is also essential. In addition, the child's activity level, parental height, perceived food allergies, and dietary restrictions should be explored. An assessment of household organization and mealtime behaviors and rituals is important in the collection of pertinent data. Other tests (lead toxicity, anemia, stool-reducing substances, occult blood, ova and parasites, alkaline phosphatase, and zinc levels) are selected only as indicated to rule out organic problems. In most cases laboratory studies are of little diagnostic value, and hospitalization is avoided except in extreme FTT (American Academy of Pediatrics, 2004). To prevent the overuse of diagnostic procedures, FTT should be considered early in the differential diagnosis. To avoid the social stigma of FTT during the early investigative phase, many health care workers use the term *growth delay* (or *failure*) until the actual cause is established.

Therapeutic Management

The primary management of FTT is aimed at reversing the cause of the growth failure. If malnutrition is severe, the initial treatment is directed at reversing the malnutrition. The goal is to provide sufficient calories to support "catch-up" growth—a rate of growth greater than the expected rate for age. Any co-existing medical problems are treated.

In most cases of FTT a multidisciplinary team of physician, nurse, dietitian, child life specialist, occupational therapist, pediatric feeding specialist, and social worker or mental health professional is needed to deal with the multiple problems. Ef-

forts are made to relieve any additional stresses on the family by offering referrals to welfare agencies or supplemental food programs. In some cases family therapy may be required; temporary placement in a foster home may relieve the family's stress, protect the child, and allow the child some stability if insurmountable obstacles are preventing appropriate family function. Behavior modification aimed at mealtime rituals (or lack thereof) and family social time may be required. Hospitalization admission is indicated for (1) evidence (anthropometric) of severe acute malnutrition, (2) child abuse or neglect, (3) significant dehydration, (4) caretaker substance abuse or psychosis, and (5) outpatient management that does not result in weight gain (American Academy of Pediatrics, 2004; Block, Krebs, and American Academy of Pediatrics Committee on Child Abuse and Neglect and Committee on Nutrition, 2005).

Prognosis

The prognosis for FTT is related to the cause. There are few long-term studies that provide sufficient data for children with FTT; however, some studies indicate that children who had FTT as infants had shorter heights, lower weights, and lower scores on measures of psychomotor development than peers (Rudolf and Logan, 2005). The authors of the analysis caution widespread generalization of these findings. Factors related to poor prognosis are severe feeding resistance, lack of awareness in and cooperation from the parent(s), low family income, low maternal educational level, adolescent mother, and early age of onset of FTT. Because later cognitive and motor function is affected by malnourishment in infancy, many of these children may be below normal in intellectual development, have poorer language development and less well-developed reading skills, attain lower social maturity, and have a higher incidence of behavioral disturbances. Such findings indicate that a long-term plan and follow-up care are needed for the optimum development of these children.

Nursing Care Management

Caring for the child with FTT presents many nursing challenges, whether treatment takes place in the hospital, clinic, or home. Providing a positive feeding environment, teaching the parents successful feeding strategies, and supporting the child and family are essential components of care.

Nurses play a critical role in the diagnosis of FTT through their assessment of the child, parents, and family interactions. Knowledge of the characteristics of children with FTT and their families is essential in helping identify these children and hastening the confirmation of a correct diagnosis (Box 11-5). Accurate assessment of initial weight and height and daily weight, as well as recording of all food intake, is mandatory. The nurse documents the child's feeding behavior and the parent-child interaction during feeding, other caregiving activities, and play. An excellent feeding observation instrument is the Nursing Child Assessment Satellite Training (NCAST) Feeding Scale, which is designed to assess the feeding interaction of infants up to 12 months of age (Barnard, Hammond, Booth, and others, 1993).* (See Nutritional Assessment, Chapter 6.)

---

*Training is required to use the feeding scale. For information, contact Jean F. Kelly, PhD, Executive Director, NCAST-AVENUW, University of Washington, PO Box 357920, Seattle, WA 98195; (206) 543-8528; e-mail: ncast@u.washington.edu; http://www.ncast.org.

Clinical Manifestations of Failure to Thrive

- Growth failure (see p. 397 for definitions)
- Developmental delays—social, motor, adaptive, language
- Undernutrition
- Apathy
- Withdrawn behavior
- Feeding or eating disorders, such as vomiting, feeding resistance, anorexia, pica, rumination
- No fear of strangers (at age when stranger anxiety is normal)
- Avoidance of eye contact
- Wide-eyed gaze and continual scan of the environment ("radar gaze")
- Stiff and unyielding, or flaccid and unresponsive
- Minimal smiling

A feature of many children with FTT is their irregularity (low rhythmicity) in activities of daily living. Some children with FTT may typify the "difficult" temperament pattern. However, another type is the passive, sleepy, lethargic infant who does not wake up for feedings. Parents who have been advised to adhere to "demand feeding schedules" may be unsure of whether to wake the child or let the child sleep. Because of their inexperience and lack of guidance, parents may develop a pattern of infrequent feeding that is inadequate to meet the infant's nutritional needs. Such a pattern is particularly detrimental with the breastfeeding infant, for whom frequent nursing is essential to an adequate milk supply.

Some parents are at increased risk for attachment problems because of (1) isolation and social crisis; (2) inadequate support systems, such as teenage and single mothers; and (3) poor parenting role models as a child. Other factors that should be considered are lack of education; physical and mental health problems such as physical and sexual abuse, depression, or drug dependence; immaturity, especially in adolescent parents; and lack of commitment to parenting, such as giving priority to entertainment or employment. Often these parents and their families are under stress and in multiple chronic emotional, social, and financial crises.

Because part of the difficulty between parent and child is dissatisfaction and frustration, the child should have a primary core of nurses (Fig. 11-3). The nurses caring for the child can learn to perceive the child's cues and reverse the cycle of dissatisfaction, especially in the area of feeding. Depending on the cause of FTT, children may be treated on an outpatient basis.

Because many of these children are responding to stimuli that have led to the negative feeding patterns, the first goal is to structure the feeding environment to encourage eating. Initially staff members and a feeding specialist may need to feed these children to assess thoroughly the difficulties encountered during the feeding process and to devise strategies that eliminate or minimize such problems. General guidelines for the feeding process are outlined in the Nursing Care Guidelines box.

Four primary goals in the nutritional management of FTT are to (1) correct nutritional deficiencies and achieve ideal weight for height, (2) allow for catch-up growth, (3) restore optimum body composition, and (4) educate the parents or

FIG. 11-3 ■ A consistent nurse is important in developing trust in infants with failure to thrive.

nursingcareguidelines

Feeding Children with Failure to Thrive

Provide a primary core of staff to feed the child. The same nurses are able to learn the child's cues and respond consistently.

Provide a quiet, unstimulating atmosphere. A number of these children are very distractible, and their attention is diverted with minimal stimuli. Older children do well at a feeding table; younger children should always be held.

Maintain a calm, even temperament throughout the meal. Negative outbursts may be commonplace in this child's habit formation. Limits on eating behavior definitely need to be provided, but they should be stated in a firm, calm tone. If the nurse is hurried or anxious, the feeding process will not be optimized.

Talk to the child by giving directions about eating. "Take a bite, Lisa" is appropriate and directive. The more distractible the child, the more directive the nurse should be to refocus attention on feeding. Positive comments about feeding are actively given.

Be persistent. This is perhaps one of the most important guidelines. Parents often give up when the child begins negative feeding behavior. Calm perseverance through 10 to 15 minutes of food refusal will eventually diminish negative behavior. Although forced feeding is avoided, "strictly encouraged" feeding is essential.

Maintain a face-to-face posture with the child when possible. Encourage eye contact and remain with the child throughout the meal.

Introduce new foods slowly. Often these children have been exclusively bottle-fed. If acceptance of solids is a problem, begin with pureed food and, once accepted, advance to junior and regular solid foods.

Follow the child's rhythm of feeding. The child will set a rhythm when the previous conditions are met.

Develop a structured routine. Disruption in their other activities of daily living has great impact on feeding responses, so bathing, sleeping, dressing, playing, and feeding are structured. The nurse should feed the child in the same way and place as often as possible. The length of the feeding should also be established (usually 30 minutes).

primary caregivers regarding the child's nutritional requirements and appropriate feeding methods (Corrales and Utter, 2005; Maggioni and Lifshitz, 1995). To increase caloric intake in formula-fed infants, supplements such as Polycose or medium-chain triglycerides may be added slowly. Other carbohydrate additives include fortified rice cereal and vegetable oil. Because vitamin and mineral deficiencies may occur, multivitamin supplementation, including zinc and iron, is recommended. The consumption of fruit juices should be minimized in infants under 6 months. Usually only in extreme cases of malnourishment are tube feedings or intravenous therapy required.

Besides attending to the physical needs of the child, the interdisciplinary team must plan care for appropriate developmental stimulation. After an approximate developmental age is established, a planned program of play is begun. Ideally a child life specialist is involved to implement and supervise the stimulation program. Every effort is made to teach the parent how to play and interact with the child.

Nursing care of these children involves a family systems approach. In other words, for the entire family to become healthy, each member must be helped to change. Care of the parents is aimed at helping them increase their feelings of self-esteem through positive, successful parenting skills. Initially this necessitates providing an environment in which they feel welcomed and accepted. Because these parents are often distrustful of authority figures, it may take some time before they develop any trust toward the nurse. One approach is to empathize with the parent about the difficulties of childrearing. For example, the nurse may state that many parents find adjusting to parenthood a trying time or that the demands of caring for an infant can become overwhelming.

The nurse teaches infant care techniques to the parents through example and demonstration rather than by lecturing. As the nurse perceives the infant's cues, he or she emphasizes these to the parents. For example, during a feeding the nurse might comment that the infant is still hungry because the child sucks vigorously and looks at the nurse. When the infant is satisfied, the nurse points out that the infant is signaling this by releasing the strong suck, closing the eyes, and breathing deeply and more slowly.

Plans are made to implement these interventions at home. A home health referral is made, and if a foster grandparent was included, this person should also visit the family. Social agencies that can provide financial or housing assistance to lessen the stress of everyday life are also contacted.

POSITIONAL PLAGIOCEPHALY

Since the Back to Sleep campaign began in 1992 advocating nonprone sleeping for infants to prevent sudden infant death syndrome (SIDS), an increase in the incidence of positional plagiocephaly has been observed (American Academy of Pediatrics, 2005; Littlefield, Saba, and Kelly, 2004). The term *plagiocephaly* connotes an oblique or asymmetric head; *positional plagiocephaly, deformational plagiocephaly*, or *nonsynostotic plagiocephaly* implies an acquired condition that occurs as a result of cranial molding during infancy (American Academy of Pediatrics, 2003b; Hummel and Fortado, 2005). Because the infant's sutures are not closed, the skull is pliable and, when the infant is placed on the back to sleep, the posterior occiput flattens over time (Fig. 11-4, *A*); a typical bald spot will develop, which is usually transient. As a result of prolonged pressure on one side of the skull, that side becomes misshapen; mild facial asymmetry may develop. The sternocleidomastoid muscle may tighten on the preferential side, and torticollis may also develop. Congenital or acquired torticollis may cause plagiocephaly; this discussion centers only on plagiocephaly caused by supine sleeping position.

Diagnostic Evaluation

The diagnosis of positional plagiocephaly may be made on physical examination of the infant's head; the infant's head is viewed frontally and from above. The typical infant's head shape will resemble a parallelogram, with unilateral flattening of the occiput, frontal and parietal bossing, a prominent cheekbone, and an anterior ear displacement (American Academy of Pediatrics, 2003b). An evaluation of neck movement and range of motion is also made to determine the presence of torticollis. In most cases skull films and further radiologic studies (computed tomographic scan) are used only to rule out craniosynostosis or other cranial deformity that may affect brain growth.

Therapeutic Management

Treatment of torticollis and plagiocephaly initially involved exercises to loosen the tight muscle and switching head position sides during feeding, carrying, and sleep. If the plagiocephaly is not resolved within 4 to 8 weeks of physical therapy, a customized helmet may be worn to decrease the pressure on the affected side of the skull (Biggs, 2003). If no improvement occurs with physical therapy or a molded helmet over a given period, the infant may be referred to a pediatric neurosurgeon or craniofacial surgeon (American Academy of Pediatrics, 2003b). In one study repositioning was not found to be as helpful in reducing plagiocephaly as was the use of an orthotic helmet (see Fig. 11-4, *B*); those treated with a helmet were older and had a longer treatment period, leading the authors to conclude that early detection and orthotic intervention were likely to be more successful (Graham, Gomez, Halberg, and others, 2005).

Nursing Care Management

Minor skull flattening is not considered significant, but parents should be taught to prevent plagiocephaly by altering the infant's head position during sleep. Infants should be placed prone on a firm surface during awake time (tummy time), which prevents plagiocephaly and facilitates development of upper shoulder girdle strength; the latter helps in the progressive development of movements such as rolling over and starting to rise up on all fours, which are precursors to crawling and eventually walking. Despite the perceived increase in the incidence of positional plagiocephaly, the supine sleeping position is still recommended because it has led to a significant decrease in loss of infant lives from SIDS (American Academy of Pediatrics, 2005). Additional measures to prevent plagiocephaly include avoiding excessive time spent in car restraint seats or infant seats and bouncers. Alternating the infant's head position for sleep times can also prevent unilateral molding. When a nurse or parent notices plagiocephaly, a consultation with the primary practitioner is recommended to evaluate the head shape and ascertain the need for early intervention.

Nurses are in a unique position in well-child care settings to encourage parents to follow guidelines for preventing pla-

FIG. 11-4 ■ **A,** Plagiocephaly. **B,** Helmet used to correct plagiocephaly. (Courtesy Dr. Gerardo Cabrera-Meza, Department of Neonatology, Baylor College of Medicine, Houston.)

giocephaly, to demonstrate alternating head placement for sleeping, to demonstrate sternocleidomastoid muscle exercises (as appropriate to the condition), and to encourage tummy time for infants during awake periods. Most important, nurses should continue to encourage parents to place the infant in a supine sleep position despite the development of plagiocephaly. Parents should not become so alarmed by plagiocephaly that they abandon supine sleeping position for the infant but should consult with the practitioner for further advice.

DISORDERS OF UNKNOWN ETIOLOGY
SUDDEN INFANT DEATH SYNDROME

Sudden infant death syndrome (SIDS) is defined as the sudden death of an infant younger than 1 year of age that remains unexplained after a complete postmortem examination, including an investigation of the death scene and a review of the case history. Since 1992, the incidence of SIDS in the United States has decreased by 53% to an all-time low of 0.57 per 1000 live births in 2002 (American Academy of Pediatrics, 2005). The dramatic decrease is attributed to the Back to Sleep campaign.* SIDS is the third leading cause of infant deaths (birth to 12 months) and the first leading cause of postneonatal (between 1 month and 12 months) deaths. SIDS claimed

---

*Back to Sleep materials may be ordered by contacting National Institute of Child Health and Human Development, Back to Sleep, 31 Center Dr., Building 31, Room 2A32, Bethesda, MD 20892; (800) 505-CRIB; fax: (301) 984-1473; http://www.nichd.nih.gov/sids.

the lives of 2162 infants in 2003 (Heron and Smith, 2007). Table 11-3 summarizes the major epidemiologic characteristics of SIDS.

Etiology

Numerous theories have been proposed regarding the etiology of SIDS; however, the cause remains unknown. One compelling hypothesis is that SIDS is related to a brainstem abnormality in the neurologic regulation of cardiorespiratory control. Abnormalities include prolonged sleep apnea, increased frequency of brief inspiratory pauses, excessive periodic breathing, and impaired arousal responsiveness to increased carbon dioxide or decreased oxygen. However, sleep apnea is not the cause of SIDS. The vast majority of infants with apnea do not die, and only a minority of SIDS victims have documented **apparent life-threatening events (ALTEs)** (see Apnea and Apparent Life-Threatening Event, p. 404). Numerous studies indicate that there is no association between SIDS and any childhood vaccine.

A genetic predisposition to SIDS has been postulated as a cause. In one study a genetic mutation on chromosome 6q 22.1-22.31 was positively linked to a syndrome of SIDS and dysgenesis of the testis (Puffenberger, Hu-Lince, Parod, and others, 2004).

Maternal smoking during pregnancy has emerged in numerous epidemiologic studies as a major factor in SIDS, and tobacco smoke in the infant's environment after birth has also been shown to have a possible relationship with the incidence of SIDS (American Academy of Pediatrics, 2005). Recent data

TABLE 11-3	
Epidemiology of Sudden Infant Death Syndrome (SIDS)	
FACTORS	**OCCURRENCE**
Incidence	0.57:1000 live births (2002)
Peak age	2 to 3 months; 95% occur by 6 months; infants born preterm died from SIDS at mean age of 6 weeks later than mean age of death from SIDS for term infants
Sex	Higher percentage of males affected
Time of death	During sleep
Time of year	Increased incidence in winter
Racial	Greater incidence in African Americans, Native Americans, and Hispanics. In 2001 SIDS in African Americans was 2.5 times higher than in Caucasians; prone positioning rates were also higher in African Americans in 2001 (21% in African Americans vs 11% in Caucasians)
Socioeconomic	Increased occurrence in lower socioeconomic class
Birth	Higher incidence in:
	Preterm infants, especially infants of extremely and very low birth weight
	Multiple births*
	Neonates with low Apgar scores
	Infants with central nervous system disturbances and respiratory disorders such as bronchopulmonary dysplasia
	Increasing birth order (subsequent siblings as opposed to firstborn child)
	Infants with a recent history of illness
Sleep habits	Highest risk associated with prone position; use of soft bedding; overheating (thermal stress); cosleeping with adult, especially on sofa, or noninfant bed
	Infants cosleeping with adult at higher risk if <11 weeks old
Feeding habits	Lower incidence in breast-fed infants
Pacifier	Lower incidence in infants put to sleep with pacifier
Siblings	May be greater incidence of SIDS in siblings
Maternal	Young age; cigarette smoking, especially during pregnancy; poor prenatal care; substance abuse (heroin, methadone, cocaine); a few studies have shown an increased risk in infants exposed to second-hand environmental tobacco smoke

Data from American Academy of Pediatrics, Task Force on Sudden Infant Death Syndrome: The changing concept of sudden infant death syndrome: diagnostic coding shifts, controversies regarding the sleeping environment, and new variables to consider in reducing risk, *Pediatrics* 116(5):1245-1255, 2005; American Academy of Pediatrics, Task Force on Infant Sleep Position and Sudden Infant Death Syndrome: Changing concepts of sudden infant death syndrome: implications for infant sleeping environment and sleep position, *Pediatrics* 105(3):650-656, 2000.
*Although a rare event, simultaneous death of twins from SIDS can occur.

show that exposure to tobacco smoke increased an infant's risk for SIDS 1.9 times over infants not exposed; 59% of SIDS deaths in smoke-exposed infants were attributed to maternal smoking (Anderson, Johnson, and Batal, 2005). It has been postulated that 12% of all SIDS deaths could be prevented with prenatal maternal smoking cessation (Pollack, 2001). One mechanism that has been proposed as a link between maternal smoking and SIDS is a decrease in the infant's ability to arouse to auditory stimuli in mothers who smoked prenatally (Franco, Groswasser, Hassid, and others, 1999). Increased nicotine concentrations in lung tissue were found in children who died from SIDS compared with a group of control children (McMartin, Platt, Hackman, and others, 2002).

Cosleeping, or an infant sharing a bed with an adult or older child on a noninfant bed, has been reported to have a positive association with SIDS. One survey found a high association between infant deaths, nonstandard beds (sofa, day bed), and bed sharing; a large percentage of infants were found dead on their backs when bed sharing, suggesting suffocation (Unger, Kemp, Wilkins, and others, 2003). A study from Scotland indicates that the risk for SIDS when bed sharing is significantly increased for infants less than 11 weeks of age (Tappin, Ecob, and Brooke, 2005). Other studies have correlated higher incidences of SIDS and infant cosleeping with maternal smoking, cosleeping with multiple family members, maternal overweight, soft bedding, and unintentional asphyxiation resulting from adult intoxication (overlaying) (American

Academy of Pediatrics, 2000, 2005; Hauck, Herman, Donovan, and others, 2003; Carroll-Pankhurst and Mortimer, 2001; Person, Lavezzi, and Wolf, 2002; McGarvey, McDonnell, Chong, and others, 2003).

A study by Hauck, Herman, Donovan, and others (2003) found that bed sharing and SIDS correlated positively only in cases where the infant was sleeping with someone other than the parent; a high number of SIDS cases involved sleeping on a sofa.

Cosleeping with infants in the age range when most SIDS deaths occur has not been shown to be preventive. The latest recommendation for cosleeping from the American Academy of Pediatrics is that the infant's crib or bassinette be placed in close proximity to the mother's bed and that the infant be placed in the adult bed only for breastfeeding, then placed to sleep in his or her own crib once the feeding session is completed (American Academy of Pediatrics, 2005).

Mesich (2005) notes that the current scientific literature fails to provide definitive guidance regarding mother-infant sleeping together in relation to safety or nonsafety; certain sleep environments (prone sleeping, tobacco smoke exposure, soft bedding, noninfant bed surface, use of certain drugs by cosleeper, and thermal stress), however, are known to increase the risk for SIDS. (See also Cultural Awareness box, p. 349.)

Studies from countries other than the United States link sleep habits with an increased risk of SIDS. Prone sleeping may cause oropharyngeal obstruction or affect thermal balance or arousal state. One study found that healthy full-term infants had significantly impaired arousal from active and quiet sleep states when sleeping prone (Horne, Ferens, Watts, and others, 2001). Rebreathing of carbon dioxide by infants in the prone position is also a possible cause for SIDS. Infants sleeping prone and on soft bedding may not be able to move their heads to the side, thus increasing the risk of suffocation and lethal rebreathing. Evidence from other countries and the United States shows an increased incidence of SIDS in infants placed in a side-lying position; thus the side-lying position is no longer recommended for infants sleeping at home, daycare, or hospitals (unless medically indicated).

Soft bedding such as waterbeds, sheepskins, beanbags, pillows, or quilts should be avoided for infant sleeping surfaces. Bedding items such as stuffed animals or toys should be removed from the crib while the infant is asleep. Most preterm infants being discharged from the hospital should be placed in a supine sleeping position unless special factors predispose them to airway obstruction. One postulated cause of SIDS has been suggested to be a prolonged Q-T interval; however, at the time of this writing no strong evidence supports universal testing of newborns for prolonged Q-T interval or to support this as a cause of SIDS (American Academy of Pediatrics, 2005).

One study indicated that breastfeeding during the first 16 weeks of life decreased the likelihood of SIDS (Alm, Wennergren, Norvenius, and others, 2002). Some studies have found pacifier use in infants to be a protective factor against the occurrence of SIDS; the data for pacifier use in this population of infants (first year of life) is said to be more compelling than data linking pacifier use to the development of dental complications and the inhibition of breastfeeding (American Academy of Pediatrics, 2005). Therefore recent American Academy of Pediatrics (2005) recommendations are to use a pacifier at naptime and bedtime, use pacifier only if infant is breastfeeding successfully, use no sweetened coating on the pacifier, and avoid forcing the infant to use the pacifier.

The American Academy of Pediatrics (2005) recommends that healthy infants be placed to sleep in the supine (on the back) position. There is an increased risk of SIDS in infants placed in the side-lying position, primarily because of their ability to turn to a prone position; therefore, the side-lying sleep position is no longer recommended.

Although the etiology is unknown, autopsies reveal consistent pathologic findings such as pulmonary edema and intrathoracic hemorrhages that confirm the diagnosis of SIDS. Consequently, autopsies should be performed on all infants suspected of dying of SIDS, and the findings should be shared with the parents as soon as possible after the death.

Whether subsequent siblings of one SIDS infant are at increased risk for SIDS is unclear. Even if the increased risk is correct, families have a 99% chance that their subsequent child will *not* die of SIDS. A review of recurrent sibling deaths attributed to SIDS in England failed to ascertain a precise risk of recurrence; previous studies suggested a recurrence risk range of 1.7 to 10.1, yet the researchers concluded the studies had too many methodologic flaws to draw any firm conclusions (Bacon, Hall, Stephenson, and others, 2007). Others report recurrence risks for a SIDS death in a family with a previous infant SIDS death range from 2% to 6% (American Academy of Pediatrics, 2005). Home monitoring is not recommended for this group of children, but it is often used by practitioners and may even be requested by parents. Monitoring is best initiated on an individual basis.

Nursing Care Management

Nurses have a vital role in preventing SIDS by educating families about the risk of prone sleeping position in infants from birth to 6 months of age, the use of appropriate bedding surfaces, maternal smoking, and the dangers of cosleeping on noninfant surfaces with adults or other children. Additionally nurses have an important role in modeling behaviors for parents to foster the implementation of practices that decrease the risk of SIDS: placing infants in a supine sleeping position in the hospital and limiting pacifier use to naps and bedtime only; data indicate that a small percentage of nurses still place healthy infants in a side-lying position in the hospital (Bullock, Mickey, Green, and others, 2004; Thompson, 2005). Statistics for infants being placed in a prone sleeping position in the United States decreased from 70% in 1992 to 13% in 2004 (American Academy of Pediatrics, 2005). Nurses must be proactive in further decreasing the incidence of SIDS; postpartum discharge planning, newborn discharges, follow-up home visits, well-baby clinic visits, and immunization visits provide an excellent opportunity to educate parents in these matters.

A concern of many health care workers is that infants placed on the back to sleep will aspirate emesis or mucus; yet studies fail to show an increase in infant deaths, spitting up during sleep, aspiration, asphyxia, or respiratory failure as a result of supine sleep positioning (Malloy, 2002; Tablizo, Jacinto, Parsley, and others, 2007).

Loss of a child from SIDS presents several crises with which the parents must cope. In addition to grief and mourning the death of their child, the parents must face a tragedy that was sudden, unexpected, and unexplained. The psychologic intervention for the family must deal with these additional variables. This discussion focuses primarily on the objectives of care for families experiencing SIDS, rather than on the process of grief and mourning, which is explored in Chapter 18.

> **NURSINGALERT**
>
> Research findings have important implications for practices that may reduce the risk of SIDS, such as avoiding smoking during pregnancy and near the infant; encouraging the supine sleeping position; avoiding soft, moldable mattresses, blankets, and pillows; discouraging bed sharing; encouraging breastfeeding; and avoiding overheating during sleep. The infant's head position should be varied to prevent flattening of the skull (positional plagiocephaly).

Finding the Infant. Usually it is the mother who finds the child dead in the crib. Typically the child is in a disheveled bed, with blankets over the head, and huddled in a corner. Frothy, blood-tinged fluid fills the mouth and nostrils, and the infant may be lying face down in the secretions, suggesting that he or she bled to death. The diaper is wet and full of stool, which is consistent with a cataclysmic type of death. The hands may be clutching the sheets, as if the child were in distress before death. The initial appearance of the child combined with the shock of such an unexpected event adds to the horror that the parents must face.

The parent who finds the infant initially must deal with her or his initial shock, panic, grief, questions of the other siblings, and the decision of where to find help. The first persons to arrive may be the police and ambulance attendants. Ideally, they will handle the situation by asking few questions; giving no indication of wrongdoing, abuse, or neglect; making sensitive judgments concerning any resuscitation efforts for the child; and comforting the members of the family as much as possible. These individuals should be properly informed about SIDS to recognize its characteristic signs and tell parents that their child probably died of a condition called sudden infant death syndrome, which cannot be predicted or prevented. A compassionate, sensitive approach to the family during the first few minutes can help spare them some of the overwhelming guilt and anguish that commonly follow this type of death.

Arriving at the Emergency Department. The first contact that nurses typically have with these families is in the emergency department, when the infant is seen by a physician to be pronounced dead. Usually there is no attempt at resuscitation. During the time in the emergency department several aspects warrant special consideration. Parents are asked only factual questions, such as when they found the infant, how he or she looked, and whom they called for help. Any remarks that may suggest responsibility, such as why they did not check on the child earlier, why they did not hear the infant cry out, whether the head was buried in a blanket, or whether other siblings were jealous of this child, are avoided.

A review of 60 studies shows that parents experiencing perinatal death perceive health care workers' responses as having a significant impact on the parents' grieving process; many health care workers' behaviors were perceived as thoughtless or insensitive. The findings suggest that nurses and physicians would benefit from more bereavement training (Gold, 2007).

The discussion of an autopsy should be presented at this time, emphasizing that a diagnosis cannot be confirmed until the postmortem examination is completed. If the mother was breastfeeding, she needs information about abrupt discontinuation of lactation.

Another important aspect of compassionate care for these parents is allowing them to say good-bye to their child. A debriefing session may help health care workers who dealt with the family and deceased infant to cope with feelings that are often engendered when a SIDS victim is brought into the acute care facility. Comprehensive guidelines have been published for health professionals involved in SIDS investigations to assist the family and at the same time to determine that the infant's death was not the result of other factors such as child maltreatment (American Academy of Pediatrics, 2001).

Returning Home. When the parents return home, they should be visited by a competent, qualified professional as soon after the death as possible. Printed material that contains excellent information about SIDS (available from several qualified organizations*) should be provided.

Ideally, the number of visits and plans for subsequent intervention need to be flexible. For example, the siblings may

initially appear accepting of the explanation and well adjusted but may later refuse to go to sleep or ask questions about graves or funerals, indicating their need for further help in dealing with the death. Parents facing the question of a subsequent child will need support. Both the birth of a subsequent child and the survival of that child, especially past the age of death of the previous child, are important transitional stages for parents.

Because the mourning process continues for at least a year or more, referrals to other parents who have lost a child to SIDS should be considered. The practitioner should be available to answer parents' questions regarding the infant's death, which may persist for months to years later until there is some resolution of the loss of the child.

APNEA AND APPARENT LIFE-THREATENING EVENT

Apnea is defined as a cessation of breathing for 20 seconds. **Apnea of infancy** is defined as an unexplained respiratory pause of 20 seconds or more, or pauses of less than 20 seconds that are accompanied by pallor, cyanosis, bradycardia, or hypotension in the term infant. The latter is a distinct entity from apnea of prematurity (see Chapter 9). An **apparent life-threatening event (ALTE),** formerly referred to as aborted SIDS death or near-miss SIDS, generally refers to an event that is sudden and frightening to the observer, in which the infant exhibits a combination of apnea, change in color (pallor, cyanosis, redness), change in muscle tone (usually hypotonia), choking, gagging, or coughing, and which usually involves a significant intervention and even cardiopulmonary resuscitation (CPR) by the caregiver who witnesses the event (National Institutes of Health Consensus Development Conference, 1987). The definition of ALTE may include apnea, but ALTE may occur without apnea (Silvestri and Weese-Mayer, 2003).

Apnea during infancy can be a symptom of any one of many disorders, including sepsis, seizures or other neurologic disorder, upper or lower airway infection or abnormality, gastroesophageal reflux, hypoglycemia or other metabolic problems, impaired regulation of breathing during sleep or feeding, or a result of intentional harm by an adult caregiver. Delayed ventilatory responses to hypercapnia and hypoxia were observed in one study of 69 infants with apnea of infancy (Katz-Salamon, 2004). Abusive head injury has been reported in a small percentage (2.5%) of children with ALTE (Altman, Brand, Forman, and others, 2003). Intentional suffocation and Munchausen syndrome by proxy cases have also been reported with ALTE (Hall and Zalman, 2005). However, in about half the cases no cause is identified.

Infants with a history of ALTEs may be at increased risk for SIDS, but these children constitute only approximately 7% to 12% of all SIDS victims. Most infants with ALTE are less than 6 months of age, and although there has been a significant decrease in SIDS since 1992, the incidence of ALTE has not changed (Hall and Zalman, 2005). A diagnosis of apnea of infancy or idiopathic ALTE is often made when no cause is found.

Results from the Collaborative Home Infant Monitoring Evaluation study found that apnea and bradycardia occurred at conventional and extreme alarm thresholds in all groups of infants studied: siblings of SIDS infants, infants with ALTEs, symptomatic (of apnea and bradycardia) and asymptomatic

---

*American SIDS Institute, 509 Augusta Dr., Marietta, GA 30067; (800) 232-SIDS, (770) 426-8746; http://www.sids.org; First Candle, 1314 Bedford Ave., Suite 210, Baltimore, MD 21208; (800) 221-7437; http://www.sidsalliance.org; National Sudden Infant Death Resource Center, Georgetown University, Box 571272, Washington, DC 20057-1272; (866) 866-7437, (202) 687-7466; http://www.sidscenter.org.

preterm infants weighing less than 1750 g (3.8 pounds) at birth, and healthy term infants. The researchers concluded that many infants experience apnea and bradycardia in each of these groups yet do not die (Jobe, 2001; Ramanathan, Corwin, Hunt, and others, 2001). Furthermore, it was reported that apnea does not appear to be an immediate precursor to SIDS and that cardiorespiratory monitoring is not an effective tool for identifying infants at greater risk for SIDS (American Academy of Pediatrics, 2003a).

Diagnostic Evaluation

An essential component of the diagnostic process includes a detailed description of the event—who witnessed the event, where the infant was during the event, and what, if any, activities were involved (such as during or after a feeding, riding in a car seat restraint, presence of siblings or any minor children, what clothing the infant was wearing). In addition, a prenatal and postnatal history must be obtained. A short period of observation in the emergency department may be appropriate to observe the infant's respiratory pattern and response to feeding. A careful evaluation of the preterm infant in a car restraint is essential; upper airway occlusion and subsequent apnea and cyanosis may occur if the infant is not positioned properly. Reported diagnoses in infants with ALTE include a neurologic event such as a seizure (30% of cases seen); gastrointestinal problem, including gastroesophageal reflux (50%); respiratory conditions (20%); and metabolic, cardiac, or child abuse (each <5%). In some cases, multiple diagnoses may be made (Hall and Zalman, 2005).

In the event that an underlying diagnosis such as those mentioned previously is not established, home monitoring may be recommended. The most commonly used monitoring is continuous recording of cardiorespiratory patterns (cardiopneumogram, or pneumocardiogram). Four-channel pneumocardiograms (or multichannel pneumogram) monitor heart rate, respirations (chest impedance), nasal airflow, and oxygen saturation. A more sophisticated test, polysomnography (sleep study), also records brain waves, eye and body movements, esophageal manometry, and end-tidal carbon dioxide measurements. However, none of these tests can predict risk. Some children with normal results may still have subsequent apneic episodes.

Therapeutic Management

The treatment of the infant with an ALTE depends on the underlying condition (see above). Treatment of recurrent apnea (without an underlying organic problem) usually involves continuous home monitoring of cardiorespiratory rhythms and in some cases the use of methylxanthines (respiratory stimulant drugs, such as theophylline or caffeine). The decision to discontinue the monitoring is based on the infant's clinical condition. A general guideline for discontinuation is when infants with ALTEs have gone 2 or 3 months without significant numbers of episodes requiring intervention.

Newer home apnea monitors allow download of information that assists the practitioner in the decision about when home monitoring may be discontinued. It is imperative to remember, however, that the home apnea monitor will not predict or prevent SIDS deaths. Furthermore, impedance-based monitors detect chest wall movement and will not detect obstructive apnea unless the episode involves significant bradycardia (see Family-Centered Care box).

FAMILY-CENTERED CARE

Using Apnea Monitors

Use the monitor as instructed by the practitioner or home monitor equipment company.

Do not adjust the monitor to eliminate false alarms. Adjustments could compromise the monitor's effectiveness.

Place the monitor on a firm surface away from the crib and drapes; plug power cord directly into a wall socket with a three-pronged outlet.

Do not sleep in the same bed as the monitored infant.

Keep pets and children away from the monitor and infant.

Keep the monitor away from possible electrical interferences such as appliances (e.g., electric blankets, televisions, air conditioners, remote telephones).

Be aware that strong signals from nearby radio and television stations, airports, ham radios, cellular phones, or police stations could interfere with the monitor. Check for interference if the monitor is to be operated in these areas.

Check the monitor several times a day to be sure the alarm is working and that it can be heard from room to room. Be certain the caregiver can reach the monitor quickly (in less than 30 seconds).

Periodically check the monitor's breath detection indicator and battery or charger connections.

Read the monitor's user manual carefully; report problems promptly.

Inform community utility and rescue squads of home monitoring as appropriate.

Keep emergency numbers near phones in the home.

Practice safety precautions:
- Remove leads when infant is not attached to the monitor.
- Unplug the power cord from the electrical outlet when the cord is not plugged into the monitor.
- Use safety covers on electrical outlets to prevent children from inserting objects into a socket.

Data primarily from US Food and Drug Administration: *Safety alert: important tips for apnea monitor users*, Rockville, Md, 1990, US Department of Health and Human Services.

Nursing Care Management

The diagnosis of an ALTE engenders great anxiety and concern in parents, and the institution of home monitoring presents additional physical and emotional burdens. Parents of infants on home apnea monitors report experiencing emotional distress, especially depression and hostility, during the first few weeks after hospital discharge (Abendroth, Moser, Dracup, and others, 1999). For parents of a SIDS victim who have a new infant on home apnea monitoring, the anxiety is compounded by the uncertainty of the future of the living child and grief for the lost child. Home apnea monitoring may offer some predictability and control over the current child's survival through the period of uncertainty. If monitoring is required, the nurse can be a major source of support to the family in terms of education about the equipment, observation of the infant's status, and immediate intervention during apneic episodes, including CPR. Several reports indicate that the first week to month after discharge is the most stressful for parents, particularly when the rate of false alarms is high (Bennett, 2002). To help the family cope with the numerous procedures they must learn, adequate preparation before discharge and written instructions are essential. In the first few weeks after discharge, parents may benefit by having a practi-

FIG. 11-5 ■ Placement of electrodes or belt for apnea monitoring. In small infants, one fingerbreadth may be used.

tioner readily available to answer questions regarding false alarms and for other technical assistance (Abendroth, Moser, Dracup, and others, 1999).

Several types of home monitors are available and are set up by either a home monitor equipment company or home health staff. Nurses, especially those involved in the care at home, must become familiar with the equipment, including its advantages and disadvantages. Safety is a major concern because monitors can cause electrical burns and electrocution. The following precautions are recommended:

■ Remove leads from infant when not attached to monitor.
■ Unplug power cord from electrical outlet when cord is not plugged into monitor.
■ Use safety covers on electrical outlets to discourage children from inserting objects into a socket.

Siblings should also be supervised when near the infant and taught that the monitor is not a toy. Other safety practices include informing local utility and rescue squads of the home monitoring in case of an emergency. Telephone numbers for these services should be posted near all telephones in the home.

NURSING ALERT

If the infant is apneic, gently stimulate the trunk by patting or rubbing it. If the infant is prone, turn to the back and flick the feet. If there is still no response, begin CPR and activate the emergency medical service—"Call 911!" Never vigorously shake the child. No more than 10 to 15 seconds are spent on stimulation before implementing CPR.

Caregivers need detailed information regarding proper attachment of the electrodes to the infant's chest with impedance monitors that detect chest movement. The electrodes are placed in the midaxillary line, at a space one or two fingerbreadths below the nipple. For home use, electrodes attached to a belt that is placed around the child's trunk are preferred (Fig. 11-5). The belt is positioned so that the electrodes contact the skin in the same area. Monitors may have memory chips that allow for event recording, which can be an effective

tool in evaluating the use of the monitor, events immediately before and after the event, and reported frequency of alarms.

Monitors are effective only if they are used. They do not prevent death but alert the caregiver to the ALTE in time to intervene. The need to use the monitor and to respond appropriately to alarms must be stressed. Noncompliance can result in the infant's death.

Family Support. Many of the stresses observed during the monitoring period are characteristic of those of families with chronically ill children. The child with an apnea or cardiorespiratory monitor may have additional health care needs such as a gastrostomy, tracheostomy, ostomy, and myriad medications or treatments that exacerbate the parents' stress. Parents report increased stress, including concern for the child's survival, fear of incompetence in assuming home responsibility, inadequate respite care, lack of time for other children and spouse, social isolation from friends and extended family, constant work, and fatigue. The monitored child is at risk for vulnerable child syndrome, which may lead to lack of parental separation and preferential treatment, causing further family disruption (Bennett, 2002). To deal with these potential effects, nurses need to employ the same interventions as those discussed for children with chronic illness (see Chapter 18) and be aware of the need for referral when difficulties are suspected.

To lessen the continuous responsibility of monitoring, other family members, such as grandparents, should be taught how to manipulate the equipment, read and interpret the signals, and administer CPR. They are encouraged to stay with the infant for regular periods to allow parents respite. Support groups of other families who have successfully completed monitoring can also be of benefit. Because baby-sitters are difficult to locate, support group members or nursing students may be potential sources of qualified caregivers.

KEY POINTS

■ Common nutritional disorders of infancy and early childhood may result from vitamin and mineral deficiency or excess, some types of vegetarian diets, protein-energy malnutrition, and food intolerance.

■ Food consumption varies among vegetarians; therefore, a detailed dietary intake is essential for planning adequate intakes, particularly in children and pregnant and lactating women.

■ Protein-energy malnutrition may occur as a complication of underlying disease, lack of parental education about infant nutrition, inappropriate management of food allergy, or incorrect preparation of formula.

■ Food intolerance encompasses food allergies and food sensitivities, which can have a number of systemic and local clinical manifestations. CMA and lactose intolerance may occur in some children.

■ Treatment of colic may involve a change in infant feeding practices, correction of a stressful environment, behavior modification, and support of the parent.

■ Growth failure or FTT may occur in children who have a chronic illness, or it may occur in a family environment wherein healthy infant feeding practices are poorly managed or understood; FTT is not always associated with a pattern of disturbed maternal-infant relationship.

- Positional plagiocephaly can be easily prevented by allowing the awake infant to have periods of tummy time and by alternating the infant's head position during sleep.
- SIDS is the third leading cause of infant death in the United States.
- Factors that place the infant at high risk for SIDS include prone sleeping position, soft bedding, sleeping in a noninfant bed with an adult or older child, and maternal prenatal smoking.

- The primary nursing responsibility in care associated with sudden infant death is educating the family of newborns about the risks for SIDS, modeling appropriate behaviors in the hospital such as placing the infant in a supine sleep position, and providing emotional support of the family who has experienced a SIDS loss.
- Infants with ALTEs are carefully evaluated for clues to the underlying cause.
- Home apnea or cardiorespiratory monitors do not prevent SIDS.

REFERENCES

Abendroth D, Moser DK, Dracup K, and others: Do apnea monitors decrease emotional distress in parents of infants at high risk for cardiopulmonary arrest? *J Pediatr Health Care* 13(2):50-57, 1999.

Alm B, Wennergren G, Norvenius SG, and others: Breast-feeding and the sudden infant death syndrome in Scandinavia, 1992-1995, *Arch Dis Child* 86(6):400-402, 2002.

Altman RL, Brand DA, Forman S, and others: Abusive head injury as a cause of apparent life-threatening events in infancy, *Arch Pediatr Adolesc Med* 157(10):1011-1015, 2003.

Amadi B, Mwiya M, Chomba E, and others: Improved nutritional recovery on an elemental diet in Zambian children with persistent diarrhoea and malnutrition, *J Trop Pediatr* 51(1):5-10, 2005.

American Academy of Pediatrics: Dietary recommendations for children and adolescents: a guide for practitioners, *Pediatrics* 117(2):544-559, 2006a.

American Academy of Pediatrics, Committee on Infectious Diseases, Pickering L, editor: *Red book: 2006 report of the Committee on Infectious Diseases,* ed 27, Elk Grove Village, Ill, 2006b, The Academy.

American Academy of Pediatrics, Task Force on Sudden Infant Death Syndrome: The changing concept of sudden infant death syndrome: diagnostic coding shifts, controversies regarding the sleeping environment, and new variables to consider in reducing risk, *Pediatrics* 116(5):1245-1255, 2005.

American Academy of Pediatrics, Committee on Nutrition: *Pediatric nutrition handbook,* ed 5, Elk Grove Village, Ill, 2004, The Academy.

American Academy of Pediatrics, Committee on Fetus and Newborn: Apnea, sudden infant death syndrome, and home monitoring, *Pediatrics* 111(4):914-917, 2003a.

American Academy of Pediatrics: Prevention and management of positional skull deformities in infants (clinical report), *Pediatrics* 112(1):199-202, 2003b.

American Academy of Pediatrics: Prevention of rickets and vitamin D deficiency: new guidelines for vitamin D intake, *Pediatrics* 111(4):908-910, 2003c.

American Academy of Pediatrics, Committee on Child Abuse and Neglect: Distinguishing sudden infant death syndrome from child abuse fatalities, *Pediatrics* 107(2):437-441, 2001.

American Academy of Pediatrics, Task Force on Infant Sleep Position and Sudden Infant Death Syndrome: Changing concepts of sudden infant death syndrome: implications for infant sleeping environment and sleep position, *Pediatrics* 105(3):650-656, 2000.

American Dietetic Association and Dietitians of Canada: Position of the American Dietetic Association and Dietitians of Canada: vegetarian diets, *J Am Diet Assoc* 103(6):748-765, 2003.

American Heart Association: *Dietary recommendations for children,* 2005, retrieved Jan 3, 2008, from http://www.americanheart.org/presenter.jhtml?identifier=3033999.

Anderson ME, Johnson DC, Batal HA: Sudden infant death syndrome and prenatal maternal smoking: rising attributed risk in the Back to Sleep era, *BMC Med* 3(1):4, 2005.

Assa'ad AH: Gastrointestinal food allergy and intolerance, *Pediatr Ann* 35(10):718-726, 2006.

Bacon CJ, Hall DBM, Stephenson TJ, and others: How common is repeat sudden infant death syndrome? *Arch Dis Child* June 12, 2007, doi 10.1136/adc.2006.113969.

Barnard K, Hammond MA, Booth CL, and others: Measurement and meaning of parent-child interaction. In Morrison F, Lord C, Keating D, editors: *Applied developmental psychology,* vol 3, New York, 1993, Academic Press.

Bennett AD: Home apnea monitoring for infants: a discussion of primary care issues, *Adv Nurs Pract* 10(3):48-53, 2002.

Biggs WS: Diagnosis and management of positional head deformity, *Am Fam Physician* 67(9):1953-1956, 2003.

Block RW, Krebs NF, American Academy of Pediatrics Committee on Child Abuse and Neglect and Committee on Nutrition: Failure to thrive as a manifestation of child neglect, *Pediatrics* 116(5):1234-1237, 2005.

Bullock LFC, Mickey K, Green J, and others: Are nurses acting as role models for the prevention of SIDS? *MCN* 29(3):172-177, 2004.

Burk CJ, Molodow R: Infantile scurvy: an old diagnosis revisited with a modern dietary twist, *Am J Clin Dermatol* 8(2):103-106, 2007.

Carroll-Pankhurst C, Mortimer EA: Sudden infant death syndrome, bedsharing, parental weight, and age of death, *Pediatrics* 107(3):530-536, 2001.

Centers for Disease Control and Prevention: Neurologic impairment in children associated with maternal dietary deficiency of cobalamin—Georgia, 2001, *MMWR* 52(4):61-64, 2003.

Christie L, Hine RJ, Parker JG, and others: Food allergies in children affect nutrient intake and growth, *J Am Diet Assoc* 102(11):1648-1651, 2002.

Ciliberto MA, Sandige H, Ndekha MJ, and others: Comparison of a home-based therapy with ready-to-use therapeutic food with standard therapy in the treatment of malnourished Malawin children: a controlled, clinical effectiveness trial, *Am J Clin Nutr* 81(4):864-870, 2005.

Conover E, Buehler BA: Use of herbal agents by breastfeeding women may affect infants, *Pediatr Ann* 33(4):235-240, 2004.

Corrales KM, Utter SL: Growth failure. In Samour PQ, King K, editors: *Handbook of pediatric nutrition,* ed 3, Sudbury, Mass, 2005, Jones & Bartlett.

Crotteau CA, Wright ST, Eglash A: What is the best treatment for infants with colic? *J Fam Pract* 55(7):634-636, 2006.

De Vrese M, Stegelmann A, Richter B, and others: Probiotics: compensation for lactase insufficiency, *Am J Clin Nutr* 73(2 Suppl):421S-429S, 2001.

Dunham L, Kollar L: Vegetarian eating for children and adolescents, *J Pediatr Health Care* 20(1):27-34, 2006.

Duro D, Rising R, Cedillo M, and others: Association between infantile colic and carbohydrate malabsorption from fruit juices in infancy, *Pediatrics* 109(5):797-805, 2002.

Ellett MLC: What is known about colic? *Gastroenterol Nurs* 26(2):60-65, 2003.

Ewing WM, Allen PJ: The diagnosis and management of cow milk protein intolerance in the primary care setting, *Pediatr Nurs* 31(6):486-492, 2005.

Fiocchi A, Assa'ad A, Bahna S, and others: Food allergy and the introduction of solid foods to infants: a consensus document, *Ann Allergy Asthma Immunol* 97(1):10-20, 2006.

Fiocchi A, Martelli A: Dietary management of food allergy, *Pediatr Ann* 35(10):755-763, 2006.

Fox M, Reidy K, Novak T, and others: Sources of energy and nutrients in the diets of infants and toddlers, *J Am Diet Assoc* 106(1 Suppl 1):S28-S42, 2006.

Franco P, Groswasser J, Hassid S, and others: Prenatal exposure to cigarette smoking is associated with a decrease in arousal in infants, *J Pediatr* 135(1):34-38, 1999.

Gidding SS, Dennison BA, Birch LL, and others: Dietary recommendations for children and adolescents: a guide for practitioners: consensus statement from the American Heart Association, *Circulation* 112(13):2061-2075, 2005.

Gold KJ: Navigating care after a baby dies: a systematic review of parent experiences with health providers, *J Perinatol* 27(4):230-237, 2007.

Goldberg JP, Folta SC, Must A: Milk: can a "good" food be so bad? *Pediatrics* 110(4):826-831, 2002.

Graham JM, Gomez M, Halberg A, and others: Management of deformational plagiocephaly: repositioning versus orthotic therapy, *J Pediatr* 146(2):258-262, 2005.

Hall KL, Zalman B: Evaluation and management of apparent life threatening events in children, *Am Fam Physician* 71(12):2301-2308, 2005.

Hauck FR, Herman SM, Donovan M, and others: Sleep environment and the risk of sudden infant death syndrome in an urban population: the Chicago Infant Mortality Study, *Pediatrics* 111(5):1207-1214, 2003.

Heron MP, Smith BL: Deaths: leading causes for 2003, *Natl Vital Stat Rep* 55(10):1-92, 2007.

Heyman MB, American Academy of Pediatrics Committee on Nutrition: Lactose intolerance in infants, children, and adolescents, *Pediatrics* 118(3):1279-1286, 2006.

Horne RS, Ferens D, Watts AM, and others: The prone sleeping position impairs arousability in term infants, *J Pediatr* 138(6):793-795, 2001.

Host A: Frequency of cow's milk allergy in childhood, *Ann Allergy Asthma Immunol* 89(6 Suppl 1):33-37, 2002.

Huiming Y, Chaomin W, Meng M: Vitamin A for treating measles in children, *Cochrane Database Syst Rev* (4):CD001479, 2005.

Hummel P, Fortado D: Impacting infant head shapes, *Adv Neon Care* 5(6):329-342, 2005.

Institute of Medicine, Food and Nutrition Board: *Dietary reference intakes: applications in dietary assessment,* Washington, DC, 2000, National Academy Press.

Joanna Briggs Institute: Best practice information sheet: the effectiveness of interventions for infant colic, *Best Practice* 8(2):1-6, 2004.

Jobe AH: What do home monitors contribute to the SIDS problem? (editorial), *JAMA* 285(17): 2244-2245, 2001.

Katz KA, Mahlberg MA, Honig PJ, and others: Rice nightmare: kwashiorkor in two Philadelphia-area infants fed Rice Dream beverage, *J Am Acad Dermatol* 52(5 Suppl 1):S69-S72, 2005.

Katz-Salamon M: Delayed chemoreceptor responses in infants with apnoea, *Arch Dis Child* 89(3):261-266, 2004.

Kawchak DA, Schall JI, Zemel BS, and others: Adequacy of dietary intake declines with age in children with sickle cell disease, *J Am Diet Assoc* 107(5):843-848, 2007.

Kemper KJ, Gardiner P: Herbal medicines. In Behrman RE, Kliegman RM, Jenson HB, editors: *Nelson textbook of pediatrics,* ed 17, Philadelphia, 2004, Saunders.

Krugman SD, Dubowitz H: Failure to thrive, *Am Fam Physician* 68(5):879-886, 2003.

Lanski SL, Greenwald M, Perkins A, and others: Herbal therapy in a pediatric emergency department population: expect the unexpected, *Pediatrics* 111(5 pt 1):981-985, 2003.

Lawrence RA, Lawrence RM: *Breastfeeding: a guide for the medical profession,* ed 6, St Louis, 2005, Mosby.

Levin ME, Motala C, Lopata AL: Anaphylaxis in a milk-allergic child after ingestion of soy formula cross-contaminated with cow's milk protein, *Pediatrics* 116(5):1223-1225, 2005.

Littlefield TR, Saba NM, Kelly KM: On the current incidence of deformational plagiocephaly: an estimation based on prospective registration at a single center, *Semin Pediatr Neurol* 11(4):301-304, 2004.

Liu T, Howard RM, Mancini AJ, and others: Kwashiorkor in the United States: fad diets, perceived and true milk allergy, and nutritional ignorance, *Arch Dermatol* 137(5):630-636, 2001.

Locklin M: The redefinition of failure to thrive from a case study perspective, *Pediatr Nurs* 31(6):474-479, 495, 2005.

Lohse B, Stotts JL, Priebe JR: Survey of herbal use by Kansas and Wisconsin WIC participants reveals moderate, appropriate use and identifies herbal education needs, *J Am Diet Assoc* 106(2):227-237, 2006.

Loman DG: The use of complementary and alternative health care practices among children, *J Pediatr Health Care* 17(2):58-63, 2003.

Maggioni A, Lifshitz F: Nutritional management of failure to thrive, *Pediatr Clin North Am* 42(4):791-809, 1995.

Malloy MH: Trends in postneonatal aspiration deaths and reclassification of sudden infant death syndrome: impact of the "Back to Sleep" program, *Pediatrics* 109(4):661-665, 2002.

Markowitz R, Duggan C: Failure to thrive: malnutrition in the pediatric setting. In Walker WA, Watkins JB, Duggan C, editors: *Nutrition in pediatrics,* ed 3, Hamilton, Ontario, 2003, Decker.

McGarvey C, McDonnell M, Chong A, and others: Factors relating to the infant's last sleep environment in sudden infant death syndrome in the Republic of Ireland, *Arch Dis Child* 88(12):1058-1064, 2003.

McGuire JK, Kulkarni MS, Baden HP: Fatal hypermagnesemia in a child treated with megavitamin/megamineral therapy, *Pediatrics* 105(2):414, 2000.

McMartin KI, Platt MS, Hackman R, and others: Lung tissue concentrations of nicotine in sudden infant death syndrome, *J Pediatr* 140(2):205-209, 2002.

Mesich HM: Mother-infant co-sleeping: understanding the debate and maximizing infant safety, *MCN* 30(1):30-37, 2005.

Messina V, Melina V, Mangels AR: A new food guide for North American vegetarians, *J Am Diet Assoc* 103(6):771-775, 2003.

Müller O, Krawinkel M: Malnutrition and health in developing countries, *CMAJ* 173(3):279-286, 2005.

National Institutes of Health Consensus Development Conference on Infantile Apnea and Home Monitoring, Sept 29 to Oct 1, 1986, *Pediatrics* 79(2):292-299, 1987.

Neu M, Robinson JA: Infants with colic: their childhood characteristics, *J Pediatr Nurs* 18(1):12-20, 2003.

Penny ME: Protein-energy malnutrition: pathophysiology, clinical consequences, and treatment. In Walker WA, Watkins JB, Duggan C, editors: *Nutrition in pediatrics,* ed 3, Hamilton, Ontario, 2003, Decker.

Perrotta S, Nobili B, Rossi F, and others: Infant hypervitaminosis A causes severe anemia and thrombocytopenia: evidence of a retinol-dependent bone marrow cell growth inhibition, *Blood* 99(6):2017-2022, 2002.

Perry CL, McGuire MT, Neumark-Sztainer D, and others: Adolescent vegetarians: how well do their dietary patterns meet the *Healthy People 2010* objectives? *Arch Pediatr Adolesc Med* 156(5):426-427, 2002.

Person TLA, Lavezzi WA, Wolf BC: Cosleeping and sudden unexpected death in infancy, *Arch Pathol Lab Med* 126(3):343-345, 2002.

Pessler F, Nejat M: Anaphylactic reaction to goat's milk in a cow's milk-allergic infant, *Pediatr Allergy Immunol* 15(2):183-185, 2004.

Pollack HA: Sudden infant death syndrome, maternal smoking during pregnancy and effectiveness of smoking cessation intervention, *Am J Public Health* 91(3):432-436, 2001.

Preston AM, Rodriguez C, Rivera CE: Plasma ascorbate in a population of children: influence of age, gender, vitamin C intake, and smoke exposure, *PR Health Sci J* 25(2):137-142, 2006.

Preston AM, Rodriguez C, Rivera C, and others: Influence of environmental tobacco smoke on vitamin C status in children, *Am J Clin Nutr* 77(1):167-172, 2003.

Puffenberger EG, Hu-Lince D, Parod JM, and others: Mapping of sudden infant death with dysgenesis of the testis syndrome (SIDDT) by a SNP genome scan and identification of TSPYL loss of function, *Proc Natl Acad Sci USA* 101(32):11689-11694, 2004.

Ramanathan R, Corwin MJ, Hunt DE, and others: Cardiorespiratory events recorded on home monitors: comparison of healthy infants with those at increased risk for SIDS, *JAMA* 285(17):2199-2243, 2001.

Rudolf MCJ, Logan S: What is the long term outcome for children who fail to thrive? A systematic review, *Arch Dis Child* 90(9):925-931, 2005.

Saltzman MD, King EC: Central physeal arrests as a manifestation of hypervitaminosis A, *J Pediatr Orthop* 27(3):351-353, 2007.

Salvatore S, Vandenplas Y: Gastroesophageal reflux and cow milk allergy: is there a link? *Pediatrics* 110(5):972-984, 2002.

Sampson HA: Update on food allergy, *J Allergy Clin Immunol* 113(5):805-819, 2004.

Sampson HA: Anaphylaxis and emergency treatment, *Pediatrics* 111(6 Pt 3):1601-1608, 2003.

Sawni A, Ragothaman R, Thomas RL, and others: The use of complementary/alternative therapies among children attending an urban pediatric emergency department, *Clin Pediatr* 46(1):36-41, 2007.

Sibley E: Carbohydrate intolerance, *Curr Opin Gastroenterol* 20(2):162-167, 2004.

Silvestri JM, Weese-Mayer D: Disorders of respiratory control: apnea and SIDS. In Rudolph CD, Rudolph AM, Hostetter MK, editors: *Rudolph's pediatrics,* ed 21, New York, 2003, McGraw-Hill.

Tablizo MA, Jacinto P, Parsley D, and others: Supine sleeping position does not cause clinical aspiration in neonates in hospital newborn nurseries, *Arch Pediatr Adolesc Med* 161(5):507-510, 2007.

Tappin D, Ecob R, Brooke H: Bedsharing, roomsharing, and sudden infant death syndrome in Scotland: a case-control study, *J Pediatr* 147(1):32-37, 2005.

Thompson DG: Safe sleep practices for hospitalized infants, *Pediatr Nurs* 31(5):400-403, 409, 2005.

Unger B, Kemp JS, Wilkins D, and others: Racial disparity and modifiable risk factors among infants dying suddenly and unexpectedly, *Pediatrics* 111(2):e127-e131, 2003.

Weizman Z, Alkrinawi S, Goldfarb D, and others: Efficacy of herbal tea preparation in infantile colic, *J Pediatr* 122(4):650-652, 1993.

Zeisel SH, Erickson KE: Dietary supplements (nutraceuticals). In Walker WA, Watkins JB, Duggan C, editors: *Nutrition in pediatrics,* ed 3, Hamilton, Ontario, 2003, Decker.

Health Promotion of the Toddler and Family

DAVID WILSON

CHAPTER OUTLINE

PROMOTING OPTIMAL GROWTH
AND DEVELOPMENT, 410
Biologic Development, 410
  Proportional Changes, 410
  Sensory Changes, 410
  Maturation of Systems, 410
  Gross and Fine Motor Development, 411
Psychosocial Development, 411
  Developing a Sense of Autonomy
    (Erikson), 411
Cognitive Development: Sensorimotor
  and Preoperational Phase (Piaget), 412
Spiritual Development, 413
Development of Body Image, 414
Development of Gender Identity, 415

Social Development, 415
  Language, 415
  Personal-Social Behavior, 416
  Play, 416
Coping with Concerns Related to Normal
  Growth and Development, 417
  Toilet Training, 417
  Sibling Rivalry, 420
  Temper Tantrums, 421
  Negativism, 421
  Regression, 422
PROMOTING OPTIMAL HEALTH DURING
TODDLERHOOD, 422
Nutrition, 422
  Nutritional Counseling, 422
  Dietary Guidelines, 423

Sleep and Activity, 424
Dental Health, 424
  Regular Dental Examinations, 424
  Removal of Plaque, 424
  Fluoride, 425
  Low-Cariogenic Diet, 426
Injury Prevention, 426
  Motor Vehicle Injuries, 428
  Drowning, 431
  Burns, 431
  Poisoning, 432
  Falls, 433
  Aspiration and Suffocation, 433
  Bodily Damage, 433
  Terrorism and Violence, 434
Anticipatory Guidance—Care of
  Families, 434

LEARNING OBJECTIVES

On completion of this chapter the
reader will be able to:

- Identify the major biologic, psychosocial,
  cognitive, and social developments during
  the toddler years.
- Relate separation anxiety and negativism
  to developmental tasks.

- Recognize readiness for toilet training
  and offer parents guidelines.
- Provide parents with information to
  prepare toddlers for the birth of a sibling.
- Provide parents with guidelines for
  handling temper tantrums.

- Provide parents with feeding
  recommendations.
- Outline a preventive dental hygiene plan
  for toddlers.
- Provide anticipatory guidance to parents
  regarding injury prevention based on the
  toddler's developmental achievements.

RELATED TOPICS and ADDITIONAL RESOURCES

 IN TEXT

Animal Bites, *Ch. 30*
Childhood Mortality, *Ch. 1*
Dental Problems, *Ch. 15*
Enuresis, *Ch. 17*
Family Influences on Child Health
    Promotion, *Ch. 3*
Fears, *Ch. 13*
Growth and Development, *Ch. 5*
Ingestion of Injurious Agents, *Ch. 14*
Injury Prevention, *Ch. 10* (Infant); *Ch. 13*
    (Preschooler)
Limit Setting and Discipline, *Ch. 10*
Moral Development, *Ch. 13*

Promote Parent-Infant Bonding
    (Attachment), *Ch. 8*
Sleep Problems, *Ch. 10* (Infant); *Ch. 13*
    (Preschooler)
Social, Cultural, and Religious Influences on
    Child Health Promotion, *Ch. 4*
Spiritual Development, *Ch. 13*
Stress in Childhood, *Ch. 5*

 COMPANION CD

Case Study—Toilet Training/Toddler
    Development
NCLEX Review Questions
Pediatric Assessment Video Clips

 evolve
evolve.elsevier.com/Wong/essentials/

NCLEX Review Questions
Pediatric Assessment Video Clips
Skills—Car Seat Safety; Instructing Families
    in Child Safety
WebLinks

**WONG'S CLINICAL MANUAL
OF PEDIATRIC NURSING, 7th Ed**

Guidelines for Automobile Safety Seats,
    p. 237
Patient and Family Education—Caring for
    the Choking Child, *p. 582;* Caring for
    Your Child's Teeth, *p. 507*

PROMOTING OPTIMAL GROWTH AND DEVELOPMENT

At times the term *terrible twos* is used to describe the toddler years, the period from 12 to 36 months of age. It is a time of intense exploration of the environment as children attempt to find out how things work and how to control others through temper tantrums, negativism, and obstinacy. Although this can be a challenging time for parents and child as each learns to know the other better, it is an extremely important period for developmental achievement and intellectual growth.

BIOLOGIC DEVELOPMENT
Proportional Changes

Physical growth slows considerably during toddlerhood. The average **weight** gain is 1.8 to 2.7 kg (4 to 6 pounds) per year. The average weight at 2 years is 12 kg (26.5 pounds). The birth weight is quadrupled by 2½ years of age. The rate of increase in **height** also slows. The usual increment is an addition of 7.5 cm (3 inches) per year and occurs mainly in elongation of the legs rather than the trunk. The average height of a 2-year-old is 86.6 cm (34 inches). In general, adult height is about twice the 2-year-old child's height. Accurate measurement of height and weight during the toddler years should reveal a steady growth curve that is *steplike* in nature rather than linear (straight), which is characteristic of the growth spurts during the early childhood years.

The rate of increase in **head circumference** slows somewhat by the end of infancy, and head circumference is usually equal to chest circumference by 1 to 2 years of age. The usual total increase in head circumference during the second year is 2.5 cm (1 inch). Then the rate of increase slows until at age 5 years the increase is less than 1.25 cm (0.5 inch) per year. The anterior fontanel closes between 1 and 1½ years of age.

Chest circumference continues to increase in size and exceeds head circumference during the toddler years. The chest's shape also changes as the transverse, or lateral, diameter exceeds the anteroposterior diameter. After the second year the chest circumference exceeds the abdominal measurement, which, in addition to the growth of the lower extremities, makes the child appear taller and leaner. However, the toddler retains a squat, "pot-bellied" appearance because of the less developed abdominal musculature and short legs. The legs retain a slightly bowed or curved appearance during the second year from the weight of the relatively large trunk.

Sensory Changes

Visual acuity of 20/40 is considered acceptable during the toddler years. Full binocular vision is well developed, and any evidence of persistent strabismus requires professional attention as early as possible to prevent amblyopia. Depth perception continues to develop, but because of the child's lack of motor coordination, falls from heights continue to be a persistent danger.

The senses of **hearing, smell, taste,** and **touch** become increasingly well developed, coordinated with each other, and associated with other experiences. All of the senses are used to explore the environment. Toddlers will visually inspect an object by turning it over; they may taste it, smell it, and touch it several times before they are satisfied with their investigation. They will shake it to see if it makes noise and vigorously test its durability.

Another example of the integrated function of the senses is the toddler's development of specific **taste preferences.** The child is much less likely than infants to try a new food because of its appearance, texture, or smell, not just its taste.

Maturation of Systems

Most of the physiologic systems are relatively mature by the end of toddlerhood. Volume of the **respiratory tract** and growth of associated structures continue to increase during early childhood, lessening some of the factors that predisposed the child to frequent and serious infections during infancy. The internal structures of the ear and throat continue to be short and straight, and the lymphoid tissue of the tonsils and adenoids continues to be large. As a result, otitis media, tonsillitis, and upper respiratory tract infections are common. The respiratory and heart rates slow, and the blood pressure increases (see inside back cover). Respirations continue to be abdominal.

Under conditions of moderate variation in temperature, the toddler rarely has the difficulties of the young infant in maintaining **body temperature.** The mature functioning of the renal system serves to conserve fluid under times of stress, decreasing the risk of dehydration.

The **digestive processes** are fairly complete by the beginning of toddlerhood. The acidity of the gastric contents continues to increase and has a protective function, since it is capable of destroying many types of bacteria. Stomach capacity increases to allow for the usual schedule of three meals a day.

One of the more prominent changes of the gastrointestinal system is the voluntary control of elimination. With complete myelination of the spinal cord, control of the anal and urethral sphincters is gradually achieved. The physiologic ability to control the sphincters probably occurs somewhere between ages 18 and 24 months. Bladder capacity also increases considerably. By 14 to 18 months of age the child is able to retain urine for up to 2 hours or longer.

The **defense mechanisms** of the skin and blood, particularly phagocytosis, are much more efficient in toddlers than in infants. The production of antibodies is well established. However, many young children demonstrate a sudden increase in colds and minor infections when they enter preschool or other group situations, such as daycare, because of their exposure to pathogens.

Rapid growth in **neurobehavioral organization** contributes to greater regularity of sleep-wake cycles, the diminishing of crying and unexplained fussiness, and the enhanced predictability in mood. Valuable stimulants of early brain development include the various interactions (talking, singing, and playing) between the toddler and caregivers. Adequate nutrition; protection from environmental toxins such as lead, various drugs, and stress; and promotion of good health care all contribute to healthy brain growth.

Gross and Fine Motor Development

The major **gross motor skill** during the toddler years is the development of locomotion. By 12 to 13 months of age toddlers walk alone using a wide stance for extra balance, and by 18 months they try to run but fall easily. Between 2 and 3 years of age, refinement of the upright, biped position is evident in improved coordination and equilibrium. At age 2 years, toddlers can walk up and down stairs, and by age 2½ years they can jump using both feet, stand on one foot for a second or two, and manage a few steps on tiptoe. By the end of the second year they can stand on one foot, walk on tiptoe, and climb stairs with alternate footing.

Fine motor development is demonstrated in increasingly skillful manual dexterity. For example, by age 12 months toddlers are able to grasp a very small object but are unable to release it at will. At 15 months they can drop a raisin into a narrow-necked bottle. Casting or throwing objects and retrieving them become almost obsessive activities at about 15 months. By 18 months of age toddlers can throw a ball overhand without losing their balance. By 2 years of age toddlers use their hands to build towers, and by 3 years of age they draw circles on paper.

Mastery of gross and fine motor skills is evident in all phases of the child's activity, such as play, dressing, language comprehension, response to discipline, social interaction, and propensity for injuries. Activities occur less in isolation and more in conjunction with other physical and mental abilities to produce a purposeful result. For example, the toddler walks to reach a new location, releases a toy to pick it up or to choose a new one, and scribbles to look at the image produced. The possibilities of the exploration, investigation, and manipulation of the environment—and its hazards—are endless.

PSYCHOSOCIAL DEVELOPMENT

Toddlers are faced with the mastery of several important tasks. If the need for basic trust has been satisfied, they are ready to give up dependence for control, independence, and autonomy. Some of the specific tasks to be dealt with include:

- Differentiation of self from others, particularly the mother
- Toleration of separation from parent
- Ability to withstand delayed gratification
- Control over bodily functions
- Acquisition of socially acceptable behavior
- Verbal means of communication
- Ability to interact with others in a less egocentric manner

Mastery of these goals is only begun during late infancy and the toddler years; tasks such as developing interpersonal relationships with others may not be completed until adolescence. However, crucial foundations for successful completion of such developmental tasks are laid during these early formative years.

Developing a Sense of Autonomy (Erikson)

According to Erikson, the developmental task of toddlerhood is acquiring a sense of **autonomy** while overcoming a sense of **doubt** and **shame.** As infants gain trust in the predictability and reliability of their parents, environment, and interaction with others, they begin to discover that their behavior is their own and that it has a predictable, reliable effect on others. Although they realize their will and control over others, they are confronted with the conflict of exerting autonomy and relinquishing the much-enjoyed dependence on others. Exerting their will has definite negative consequences, whereas retaining dependent, submissive behavior is generally rewarded with affection and approval. However, continued dependence creates a sense of doubt regarding their potential capacity to control their actions. This doubt is compounded by a sense of shame for feeling this urge to revolt against others' will and a fear that they will exceed their own capacity for manipulating the environment. Skillful monitoring and balance of controls by parents allows a growing rate of realistic successes and the emergence of autonomy.

Just as the infant has the social modalities of grasping and biting, the toddler has the newly gained modality of holding on and letting go. To hold on and let go is evident with the use of the hands, mouth, eyes, and, eventually, the sphincters, when toilet training is begun. These social modalities are expressed constantly in the child's play activities, such as throwing objects; taking objects out of boxes, drawers, or cabinets; holding on tighter when someone says, "No, don't touch"; and refusing or spitting out food as taste preferences become very strong.

Several characteristics, especially negativism and ritualism, are typical of toddlers in their quest for autonomy. As toddlers attempt to express their will, they often act with **negativism,** the persistent negative response to requests. The words "no" or "me do" can be the sole vocabulary. Emotions become strongly expressed, usually in rapid mood swings. One minute, toddlers can be engrossed in an activity, and the next minute they might be angry because they are unable to manipulate a toy or open a door. If scolded for doing something wrong, they can have a temper tantrum and almost instantaneously pull at the parent's legs to be picked up and comforted. Understanding and coping with these swift changes is often difficult for parents. Many parents find the negativism exasperating and, instead of dealing constructively with it, give in to it, which further threatens children in their search for learning acceptable methods of interacting with others (see Temper Tantrums and Negativism, p. 421).

In contrast to negativism, which frequently disrupts the environment, **ritualism,** the need to maintain sameness and reliability, provides a sense of comfort. Toddlers can venture out with security when they know that familiar people, places, and routines still exist. One can easily understand why any change in the daily routine represents such a threat to these children. Without comfortable rituals, they have little opportunity to exert autonomy. Consequently, dependency and regression occur (see Regression, p. 422).

Erikson focuses on the development of the **ego,** which may be thought of as reason or common sense, during this phase of psychosocial development. The child struggles to deal with the impulses of the **id** and attempts to tolerate frustration and learn socially acceptable ways of interacting with the environment. The ego is evident as the child is able to tolerate delayed gratification. Toddlers also have a rudimentary beginning of the **superego,** or conscience, which is the incorporation of the morals of society and the process of acculturation.

With the development of the ego, children further differentiate themselves from others and expand their sense of trust within themselves. But as they begin to develop awareness of their own will and capacity to achieve, they also become aware of their ability to fail. This ever-present awareness of potential failure creates doubt and shame. Successful mastery of the task of autonomy necessitates opportunities for self-mastery while withstanding the frustration of necessary limit setting and delayed gratification. Opportunities for self-mastery are present in appropriate play activities, toilet training, the crisis of sibling rivalry, and successful interactions with significant others (Fig. 12-1).

COGNITIVE DEVELOPMENT: SENSORIMOTOR AND PREOPERATIONAL PHASE (PIAGET)

The period from 12 to 24 months of age is a continuation of the final two stages of the sensorimotor phase. During this time the cognitive processes develop rapidly and at times seem similar to those of mature thinking. However, reasoning skills are still primitive and need to be understood to effectively deal with the typical behaviors of a child of this age.

Tertiary Circular Reactions. In the fifth stage of the sensorimotor phase (13 to 18 months of age), the child uses active experimentation to achieve previously unattainable goals. Newly acquired physical skills are increasingly important for the function they serve rather than for the acts themselves. The child incorporates the old learning of secondary

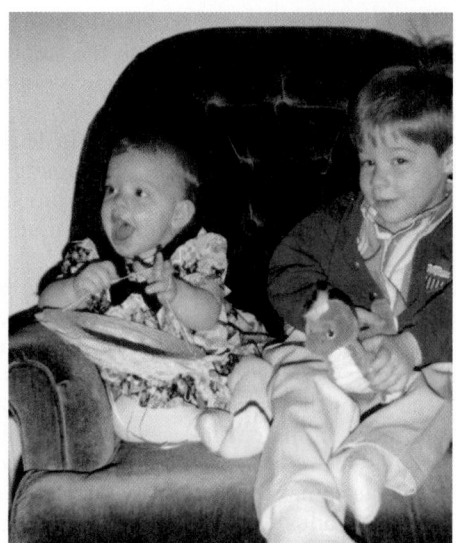

FIG. 12-1 ■ Toddlers begin socializing with significant others such as siblings as a part of development.

circular reactions with new skills and applies the combined knowledge to new situations, with emphasis on the results of the experimentation. In this way there is the beginning of rational judgment and intellectual reasoning. During this stage there is further differentiation of oneself from objects. This is evident in the child's increasing ability to venture away from the parent and to tolerate longer periods of separation.

Awareness of a **causal relationship** between two events is apparent. After flipping a light switch, toddlers are aware that a reciprocal response occurs. However, they are not able to transfer that knowledge to new situations. Therefore every time they see what appears to be a light switch, they must reinvestigate its function. Such behavior demonstrates the beginning of categorizing data into distinct classes and subclasses. There are innumerable examples of this type of behavior as toddlers continuously explore the same object each time it appears in a new place.

Because classification of objects is still rudimentary, the appearance of an object denotes its function. For example, if the child's toys are stored in a paper bag or large container, that toy receptacle is no different from the garbage pail or laundry basket. If allowed to turn over the toy receptacle, the child will just as quickly do the same to other similar containers because, in the child's mind, there is no difference. Expecting the child to judge which receptacles are permissible to explore and which are not is inappropriate for this age-group. Instead, the forbidden object, such as the garbage pail, should be placed out of reach.

The discovery of objects as objects leads to the awareness of their spatial relationships. Children are able to recognize different shapes and their relationship to each other. For example, they can fit slightly smaller boxes into each other (nesting) and can place a round object into a hole, even if the board is turned around, upside down, or reversed. Children are also aware of space and the relationship of their body to dimensions such as height. They will stretch, stand on a low stair or stool, and pull a string to reach an object.

Object permanence has also advanced. Although they still cannot find an object that has been invisibly displaced or

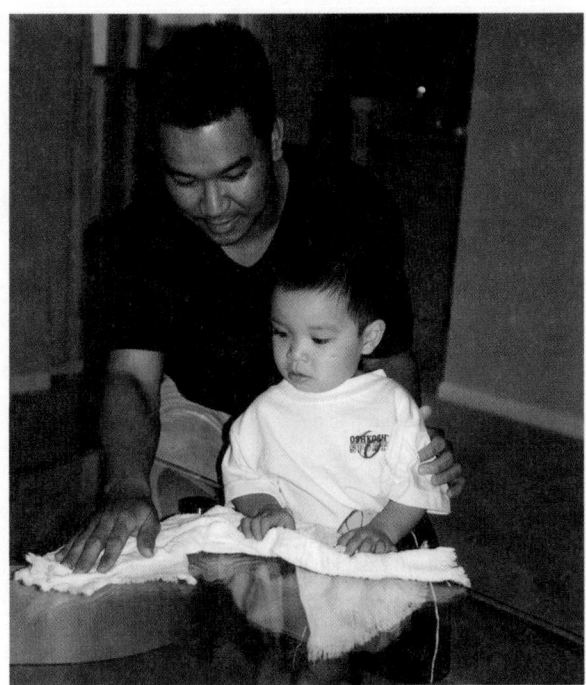

FIG. 12-2 ■ Domestic mimicry is common during toddlerhood.

moved from under one pillow to another without their seeing the change, toddlers are increasingly aware of the existence of objects behind closed doors, in drawers, and under tables. Parents are usually acutely aware of this developmental achievement and find high places and locked cabinets the only places inaccessible to toddlers.

Invention of New Means Through Mental Combinations. From ages 19 to 24 months the child is in the final sensorimotor stage. During this stage the child completes the more primitive, autistic-like thought processes of infancy and is prepared for the more complex mental operations that occur during the phase of preoperational thought. One of the most dramatic achievements of this stage is in the area of object permanence. Children will now actively search for an object in several potential hiding places. In addition, they can infer a cause when only experiencing the effect. They can infer that an object was hidden in any number of places even if they only saw the original hiding place.

Imitation displays deeper meaning and understanding. There is greater symbolization to imitation. The child is acutely aware of others' actions and attempts to copy them in gestures and in words. **Domestic mimicry** (imitating household activities) and sex-role behavior become increasingly common during this period and during the second year. Identification with the parent of the same gender becomes apparent by the second year and represents the child's intellectual ability to differentiate different models of behavior and to imitate them appropriately (Fig. 12-2).

The conception of time is still embryonic, but children have some sense of timing in terms of anticipation, memory, and the limited ability to wait. They may listen to the command, "Just a minute," and behave appropriately. However, their sense of timing is exaggerated—1 minute can seem like an hour. Toddlers' limited attention spans also indicate their sense of immediacy and concern for the present.

Preoperational Phase. At approximately 2 years of age the child enters the preconceptual phase of cognitive development, which lasts until about age 4 years. The preconceptual phase is a subdivision of the preoperational phase, which spans ages 2 to 7 years. The preconceptual phase is primarily one of transition that bridges the purely self-satisfying behavior of infancy and the rudimentary socialized behavior of latency. **Preoperational thought** implies that children cannot think in terms of **operations**—the ability to manipulate objects in relation to each other in a logical fashion. Rather, toddlers think primarily on the basis of their perception of an event. Problem solving is based on what they see or hear directly rather than on what they recall about objects and events. Several characteristics are unique to preoperational thought (Box 12-1).

Within the second year the child increasingly uses language symbolically and is concerned with the "why" and "how" of things. For example, a pencil is "something to write with," and food is "something to eat." However, such mental symbolization is closely associated with prelogical reasoning. For instance, a needle is "something that hurts." Such painful experiences take on new significance because memory is associated with the specific event, and fears are likely to develop, such as resistance to people who wear colored uniforms or rooms that look like the practitioner's office. Because of the vulnerability of these early years, it is essential to prepare children for any new experience, whether it is a new baby-sitter or a visit to the dentist.

SPIRITUAL DEVELOPMENT

Spiritual development in children is often discussed in terms of the child's developmental level because the evolution of spirituality often parallels cognitive development (Elkins and Cavendish, 2004). The child's family and environment strongly influence the child's perception of the world around him or her, and this often includes spirituality. Furthermore, family values, beliefs, customs, and expressions of these will influence the child's perception of his or her spiritual self (Elkins and Cavendish, 2004). The relationship between spirituality, illness in childhood, and nursing has been studied in the context of suffering, terminal illness such as cancer, and end-of-life care. In the past two decades there has been an increased interest in and focus on spiritual care in adults and children as further understanding of the influence of one's spirituality on health, illness, and well-being has progressed.

Toddlers learn about God through the words and the actions of those closest to them. They have only a vague idea of God and religious teachings because of their immature cognitive processes; however, if God is spoken about with reverence, young children associate God with something special. During this period the assignment of powerful religious symbols and images is strongly influenced by the manner in which it is presented; therein lies the potential for the development of guilt and fear or, conversely, love and companionship with religious symbols (Roehlkepartain, King, Wagener, and others, 2006).

Toddlers begin to assimilate behaviors associated with the divine (folding hands in prayer). Routines such as saying prayers before meals or at bedtime can be important and comforting. Because toddlers tend to find solace in ritualistic behavior and routines, they incorporate routines associated with religious practices into their behavioral patterns, without

BOX 12-1

Characteristics of Preoperational Thought

Egocentrism—Inability to envision situations from perspectives other than one's own
  Example—If a person is positioned between the toddler and another child, the toddler, who is facing the person, will explain that both children can see the middle person's face. The young child is unable to realize that the other person views the middle person from a different perspective, the back.
  Implication—Avoid moralizing about "why" something is wrong if it requires an understanding of someone else's feelings or opinion. Telling a child to stop hitting because hitting hurts the other person is often ineffective because, to the aggressor, it feels good to hit someone else. Instead, emphasize that hitting is not allowed.

Transductive reasoning—Reasoning from the particular to the particular
  Example—Child refuses to eat a food because something previously eaten did not taste good.
  Implication—Accept child's reasoning; offer refused food at different time.

Global organization—Reasoning that changing any one part of the whole changes the entire whole
  Example—Child refuses to sleep in room because location of bed is changed.
  Implication—Accept child's reasoning; use same bed position or introduce change slowly.

Centration—Focusing on one aspect rather than considering all possible alternatives
  Example—Child refuses to eat a food because of its color, even though its taste and smell are acceptable.
  Implication—Accept child's reasoning.

Animism—Attributing lifelike qualities to inanimate objects
  Example—Child scolds stairs for making child fall down.
  Implication—Join child in the "scolding." Keep frightening objects out of view.

Irreversibility—Inability to undo or reverse the actions initiated physically
  Example—When told to stop doing something, such as talking, child is unable to think of positive activity.
  Implication—State requests or instructions positively (e.g., "Be quiet.").

Magical thinking—Believing that thoughts are all-powerful and can cause events
  Examples—Child wishes someone died; then if the person dies, child feels at fault because of the "bad" thought that made the death happen.
    ■ Calling children "bad" because they did something wrong makes children feel as if they are bad.
  Implication—Clarify that thoughts do not make things happen and that child is not responsible.
    ■ Use "I" messages rather than "you" messages to communicate thoughts, feelings, expectations, or beliefs without imposing blame or criticism. Emphasize that the act is bad, not the child.

Inability to conserve—Inability to understand the idea that a mass can be changed in size, shape, volume, or length without losing or adding to the original mass (instead, children judge what they see by the immediate perceptual clues given to them)
  Example—If two lines of equal length are presented in such a way that one appears longer than the other, child will state that one line is longer even if child measures both lines with a ruler or yardstick and finds that each has the same length.
  Implication—Change the most obvious perceptual clue to reorient child's view of what is seen.
    ■ Give medicine in a small medicine cup, rather than a large cup, because the child will imagine that the large vessel contains more liquid. If child refuses the medicine in the small cup, pour it into a large cup, since the liquid will appear to be less in a tall, wide container.
    ■ Give a large, flat cookie rather than a thick, small one, or do the reverse with meat or cheese; child will usually eat larger size of favorite food and smaller size of less favorite food.

understanding all the implications of the rituals until later. Near the end of toddlerhood, when children use preoperational thought, there is some advancement of their understanding of God. Religious teachings, such as reward or fear of punishment (heaven or hell) and moral development (see Chapter 5), may influence their behavior (Fosarelli, 2003).

DEVELOPMENT OF BODY IMAGE

As in infancy, the development of body image closely parallels cognitive development. Developing psychologic understanding provides greater self-awareness, and young children learn to answer the question "Who am I?" During the second year, children recognize themselves in a mirror and make verbal references to themselves ("Me big"). With increasing motor ability, toddlers recognize the usefulness of body parts and gradually learn their names. They also learn that certain parts of the body have various meanings; for example, during toilet training the genitalia become significant and cleanliness is emphasized. By 2 years of age they recognize gender differences and refer to themselves by name and then by pronoun. Gender identity is developed by age 3 years. Also by this time the child begins to remember events with reference to their personal significance, forming an autobiographic memory

that helps to establish a continuous identity throughout life's events (Thompson, 2001).

After they begin preoperational thought, toddlers can use symbols to represent objects, but their thinking may lead to inaccuracies. For example, if someone who is pregnant is called "fat," they will describe all "fat" women as having babies. They begin to recognize words used to describe physical appearance, such as *pretty, handsome,* or *big boy.* Such expressions eventually influence how children view their own bodies.

Although little research has been done on body-image development in young children, it is evident that body integrity is poorly understood and that intrusive experiences are threatening (Dahlquist, Busby, Slifer, and others, 2002). For example, toddlers forcefully resist procedures such as examining the ear or mouth or taking a rectal temperature. Toddlers also have unclear body boundaries and may associate nonviable parts, such as feces, with essential body parts. This can be seen in a toddler who is upset by flushing the toilet and watching the stool disappear.

Nurses can assist parents in fostering a positive body image in their child by encouraging them to avoid negative labels, such as "skinny arms" or "chubby legs"—self-perceptions that can last a lifetime. Body parts, especially those related to elimination and reproduction, should be called by their correct names. Respect for the body should be practiced.

DEVELOPMENT OF GENDER IDENTITY

Just as toddlers explore their environment, they also explore their bodies and find that touching certain body parts is pleasurable. Masturbation can occur and involves manual stimulation of genitals and posturing movements against objects. Other demonstrations of sensual activities include rocking, sucking on fingers and toes, swinging, and hugging people and toys. During the activity the child may perspire, and the activity may be difficult to interrupt. If performed in public, the behavior should be ignored. The child should be taught that it is more acceptable to perform the behavior in private (Meyer, 2002).

Children in this age-group are learning vocabulary associated with anatomy, elimination, and reproduction. Certain associations between words and functions become significant and can influence future sexual attitudes. For example, if parents refer to the genitalia as dirty, especially in the context of elimination, this association between "genitalia" and "dirty" may be transferred to sexual functions.

Sex-role differences become obvious to children and are evident in much of their imitative play. A sense of maleness or femaleness, **gender identity,** is formed by age 3 years. Early attitudes are formed about affectionate behaviors between adults from observing parental and other adult sexual or sensual activities. (See also Sex Education, Chapter 13.) The quality of relationships with parents is important to the child's capacity for sexual and emotional relationships later in life (DeLamater and Friedrich, 2002).

SOCIAL DEVELOPMENT

A major task of the toddler period is differentiation of self from significant others, usually the mother. The differentiation process consists of two phases: **separation,** the children's emergence from a symbiotic fusion with the mother; and **individuation,** those achievements that mark children's expression of their individual characteristics in the environment. Although the process begins during the latter half of infancy, the major achievements occur during the toddler years.

Toddlers have an increased understanding and awareness of object permanence and some ability to withstand delayed gratification and tolerate moderate frustration. As a result, toddlers react differently to strangers than do infants. The appearance of unfamiliar persons does not represent such a significant threat to their attachment to mother. They have learned from experience that parents exist when physically absent. Repetition of events such as going to bed without the parents but waking to find them there again reinforces the reliability of such brief separations. Consequently, toddlers are able to venture away from their parents for brief periods because of the security of knowing that the parents will be there when they return. Verbal and visual reassurance from the parent gradually replaces some of the previous need to be physically close for comfort.

According to Harpaz-Rotem and Bergman (2006), the separation-individuation phase encompasses the phenomenon of **rapprochement;** as the toddler separates from the mother and begins to make sense of experiences in the environment, he or she is drawn back to the mother for assistance

FIG. 12-3 ■ Transitional objects, such as a warm and fuzzy stuffed animal, are sources of security to a toddler.

in verbally articulating the meaning of the experiences. Developmentally the term *rapprochement* means the child moves away and returns for reassurance. If the mother's response to the toddler is inappropriate, the toddler may experience insecurity and confusion.

Transitional objects, such as a favorite blanket or toy, provide security for children, especially when they are separated from parents, dealing with a new stress, or just fatigued (Fig. 12-3). Security objects often become so important to toddlers that they refuse to let them be taken away. Such behavior is normal; there is no need to discourage this tendency. During separations, such as daycare, hospitalization, or even staying overnight with a relative, transitional objects should be provided to minimize any fear or loneliness.

Learning to tolerate and master brief periods of separation is an important developmental task for children in this age-group. In addition, it is a necessary component of parenting, since brief periods of separation allow parents to restore their energy and patience and to minimize directing their irritations and frustrations at the children.

Language

The most striking characteristic of language development during early childhood is the increasing level of comprehension. Although the number of words acquired—from about four at 1 year of age to approximately 300 at age 2 years—is notable, *the ability to comprehend and understand speech is much greater than the number of words the child can say.* Bilingual children can also achieve their early linguistic milestones in each of the languages at the same time and produce a substantial number of semantically corresponding words in each of their two languages from the very first words or signs (Petitto, Katerlos, Levy, and others, 2001).

At age 1 year the child uses one-word sentences or holophrases. The word "up" can mean "pick me up" or "look up there." For the child the one word conveys the meaning of a sentence, but to others it may mean many things or nothing. At this age about 25% of the vocalizations are intelligible. By the age of 2 years the child uses multiword sentences by stringing together two or three words, such as the phrases "mama go bye-bye" or "all gone," and approximately 65% of the speech is understandable. By 3 years the child puts words together into simple sentences, begins to master grammatical rules (syntax development), and acquires five or six new words daily.

Gestures precede or accompany each of the language milestones up to 30 months of age (putting phone to ear, pointing). After sufficient language development, gestures phase out and the pace of word learning increases (Bates and Dick, 2002).

Personal-Social Behavior

One of the most dramatic aspects of development in the toddler is personal-social interaction. Personal-social behaviors are evident in such areas as dressing, feeding, playing, and establishing self-control. Parents frequently wonder why their manageable, docile, lovable infant has turned into a determined, strong-willed, volatile little tyrant. In addition, the tyrant of the terrible twos can swiftly and unpredictably revert back to the adorable infant. All of this is part of growing up, as toddlers acquire a more sophisticated awareness that others' feelings and desires can be different from their own. Through interactions with caregivers, the child is able to explore these differences and their consequences.

Toddlers are developing skills of independence, which are evident in all areas of behavior. By 15 months children feed themselves, drink well from a covered cup, and manage a spoon with considerable spilling. By 2 years they use a spoon well, and by 3 years they may be using a fork. Between ages 2 and 3 years they eat with the family and like to help with chores such as setting the table or removing dishes from the dishwasher, but they lack table manners and may find it difficult to sit through the family's entire meal.

In dressing, toddlers also demonstrate strides in independence. The 15-month-old child helps by putting the arm or foot out for dressing and pulls shoes and socks off. The 18-month-old child removes gloves, helps with pullover shirts, and may be able to unzip. By age 2 years the toddler removes most articles of clothing and puts on socks, shoes, and pants without regard for right or left and back or front. Help is still needed to fasten clothes.

Toddlers also begin to develop concern for the feelings of others and develop an understanding of how adult expectations for behavior apply to specific situations (e.g., causing a sibling to cry while playing rough) (Thompson, 2001). As their understanding is fostered, they are able to develop control. Age-appropriate discipline contributes to healthy social and emotional development. Positive reinforcement, redirection, and time-out are appropriate for most toddlers. Social and emotional problems can develop in the youngest children. Early screening and intervention promote more positive outcomes as the young child grows and develops.

Play

Play magnifies the toddler's physical and psychosocial development. Interaction with people becomes increasingly important. The solitary play of infancy progresses to **parallel play**—the toddler plays alongside, not with, other children. Although sensorimotor play is still prominent, there is much less emphasis on the exclusive use of one sensory modality. The toddler inspects the toy, talks to the toy, tests its strength and durability, and invents several uses for it. **Imitation** is one of the most

FIG. 12-4 ■ Young children enjoy dressing up.

distinguishing characteristics of play and enriches children's opportunity to engage in fantasy. With less emphasis on gender-stereotyped toys, play objects such as dolls, carriages, dollhouses, balls, dishes, cooking utensils, child-size furniture, trucks, and dress-up clothes are suitable for both genders (Fig. 12-4); however, boys may be more interested than girls in activities related to trucks, trailers, men, and building blocks, whereas girls may prefer doll-related activities.

Increased locomotive skills make push-pull toys, straddle trucks or cycles, a small gym and slide, balls of various sizes, and riding toys appropriate for the energetic toddler. Finger paints, thick crayons, chalk, blackboard, paper, and puzzles with large, simple pieces use the child's developing fine motor skills. Interlocking blocks in various sizes and shapes provide hours of fun and, during later years, are useful objects for creative and imaginative play. The most educational toy is the one that fosters the interaction of an adult with a child in supportive, unconditional play. Toys are never substitutes for the attention of devoted caregivers, but toys can enhance these interactions (Glassy, Romano, and Committee on Early Childhood, 2003).

Certain aspects of play are related to emerging linguistic abilities. Talking is a form of play for toddlers, who enjoy musical toys such as age-appropriate cassette tape players, "talking" dolls and animals, and toy telephones. Appropriate children's television programs are excellent for children in this age-group, who learn to associate words with visual images. However, total media time should be limited to 1 to 2 hours of quality programming per day (American Academy of Pediatrics, 2001). Toddlers also enjoy "reading" stories from a picture book and imitating the sounds of animals.

Tactile play is also important for the exploring toddler. Water toys, a sandbox with pail and shovel, finger paints, soap bubbles, and clay provide excellent opportunities for creative and manipulative recreation. Adults sometimes forget the fascination of feeling textures such as slippery cream, mud, or pudding; catching air bubbles; squeezing and reshaping clay; or smearing paints. These types of unstructured activities are as important as educational play to allow children freedom of expression.

Selection of appropriate toys must involve safety factors, especially in relation to size and sturdiness. The oral activity of toddlers puts them at risk for aspirating small objects or ingesting toxic substances. Parents need to be especially vigilant of toys played with in other children's homes or those of older siblings. Toys are a potential source of serious bodily damage to toddlers, who may have the physical strength to manipulate them but not the knowledge to appreciate their danger (Stephenson, 2005) (see Family-Centered Care box: Toy Safety, Chapter 5). Government agencies do not inspect and police all toys on the market. Therefore adults who purchase play equipment, supervise purchases, or allow children to use play equipment need to evaluate its safety, including toys that are gifts or those that are purchased by the children themselves. Adults should also be alert to notices of toys determined to be defective and recalled by the manufacturers. Parents and health care workers can obtain information on a variety of recalled products and can report potentially dangerous toys and child products to the U.S. Consumer Product Safety Commission* or, in Canada, the Canadian Toy Testing Council.† Printable tips on toy safety are also available from Safe Kids Worldwide.‡

NURSINGALERT

Remind parents to request toddler toys when purchasing children's meals at fast-food restaurants.

Table 12-1 summarizes the major features of growth and development for the age-groups of 15, 18, 24, and 30 months.

COPING WITH CONCERNS RELATED TO NORMAL GROWTH AND DEVELOPMENT
Toilet Training

One of the major tasks of toddlerhood is toilet training. Anticipatory guidance and clinical intervention for families surrounding toilet training should begin during routine well-child visits before the child's developmental readiness to toilet train. Preparation and education reveal and allay misconceptions; lead to the development of appropriate expectations; and provide information, guidance, and support to parents for managing this potentially frustrating process.

Voluntary control of the anal and urethral sphincters is achieved sometime after the child is walking, probably between ages 18 and 24 months. However, complex psychophysiologic factors are required for readiness. The child must be able to recognize the urge to let go and hold on and be able to communicate this sensation to the parent. In addition, some motivation is probably involved in the desire to please the parent by holding on, rather than pleasing oneself by letting go.

Schmitt (2004) notes that comparative studies over the past five decades indicate that children in the 1990s in the United States were toilet trained at a later age (18 months in the 1960s vs 36 months in the 1990s); one possible contributing factor is the availability and convenience of disposable diapers.

Five markers signal a child's readiness to toilet train: bladder readiness, bowel readiness, cognitive readiness, motor readiness, and psychologic readiness (Schmitt, 2004). Accord-

nursingcareguidelines

Assessing Toilet Training Readiness
PHYSICAL READINESS
Voluntary control of anal and urethral sphincters, usually by 18 to 24 months of age
Ability to stay dry for 2 hours; decreased number of wet diapers; waking dry from nap
Regular bowel movements
Gross motor skills of sitting, walking, and squatting
Fine motor skills to remove clothing

MENTAL READINESS
Recognizes urge to defecate or urinate
Verbal or nonverbal communicative skills to indicate when wet or has urge to defecate or urinate
Cognitive skills to imitate appropriate behavior and follow directions

PSYCHOLOGIC READINESS
Expresses willingness to please parent
Able to sit on toilet for 5 to 10 minutes without fussing or getting off
Curiosity about adults' or older sibling's toilet habits
Impatience with soiled or wet diapers; desire to be changed immediately

PARENTAL READINESS
Recognizes child's level of readiness
Willing to invest the time required for toilet training
Absence of family stress or change, such as a divorce, moving, new sibling, or imminent vacation

ing to some experts, physiologic and psychologic readiness is not complete until ages 22 to 30 months (Schum, Kolb, McAuliffe, and others, 2002); however, Schmitt (2004) emphasizes that parents should begin preparing the child for toilet training earlier than 30 months. By this time the child has mastered the majority of essential gross motor skills, can communicate intelligibly, is in less conflict with parents in terms of self-assertion and negativism, and is aware of the ability to control the body and please the parent. There is no universal right age to begin toilet training or an absolute deadline to complete training. One of the nurse's most important responsibilities is to help parents identify the readiness signs in their child (see Nursing Care Guidelines box).* On average, girls are developmentally ready to begin toilet training 2 to 2½ months before boys (Schum, Kolb, McAuliffe, and others, 2002).

Nighttime bladder control normally takes several months to years after daytime training begins. This is because the sleep cycle needs to mature so the child can awake in time to urinate. Few children will have night wetting episodes after daytime dryness is totally achieved; however, those children who do not have nighttime dryness by the age of 6 years are likely to require intervention (Mercer, 2003).

Case Study—Toilet Training/Toddler Development

TABLE 12-1

Growth and Development During the Toddler Years

PHYSICAL	GROSS MOTOR	FINE MOTOR
AGE 15 MONTHS Steady growth in height and weight Head circumference 48 cm (19 inches) Weight 11 kg (24 pounds) Height 78.7 cm (31 inches)	Walks without help (usually since age 13 months) Creeps up stairs Kneels without support Cannot walk around corners or stop suddenly without losing balance without support Cannot throw ball without falling Runs clumsily; falls often	Constantly casting objects to floor Builds tower of two cubes Holds two cubes in one hand Releases a pellet into a narrow-necked bottle Scribbles spontaneously Uses cup well but often rotates spoon before it reaches mouth
AGE 18 MONTHS Picky eater as a result of decreased growth needs and need to assert independence Anterior fontanel closed Physiologically able to control sphincters	Assumes standing position Walks up stairs with one hand held Pulls and pushes toys Jumps in place with both feet Seats self on chair Throws ball overhand without falling	Builds tower of three or four cubes Release, prehension, and reach well developed Turns pages in a book two or three at a time In a drawing, makes stroke imitatively Manages spoon without rotation
AGE 24 MONTHS Head circumference 49-50 cm (19.5-20 inches) Chest circumference exceeds head circumference Lateral diameter of chest exceeds anteroposterior diameter Usual weight gain of 1.8-2.7 kg (4-6 pounds) per year Usual gain in height of 10-12.5 cm (4-5 inches) per year Adult height approximately double height at 2 years of age Primary dentition of 16 teeth May demonstrate readiness for beginning daytime control of bowel and bladder	Goes up and down stairs alone with two feet on each step Runs fairly well, with wide stance Picks up object without falling Kicks ball forward without overbalancing	Builds tower of six or seven cubes Aligns two or more cubes like a train Turns pages of book one at a time In drawing, imitates vertical and circular strokes Turns doorknob, unscrews lid
AGE 30 MONTHS Birth weight quadrupled Primary dentition (20 teeth) completed May have daytime bowel and bladder control	Jumps with both feet Jumps from chair or step Stands on one foot momentarily Takes a few steps on tiptoe	Builds tower of eight cubes Adds chimney blocks to train of block Good hand-finger coordination; holds crayon with fingers rather than fist In drawing, imitates vertical and horizontal strokes; makes two or more strokes for cross; draws circles

Bowel training is usually accomplished before bladder training because of its greater regularity and predictability. There is a stronger sensation for defecation than for urination, and the sensation of defecation can be brought to the child's attention. A well-balanced diet that includes dietary fiber helps keep stool soft and supports the development and maintenance of regular bowel movements.

A number of techniques can be helpful when initiating training, and cultural differences should be considered. Parents should begin the readiness phase of toilet training by teaching the child about how the body functions in relation to voiding and having a stool. Schmitt (2004) suggests that parents talk about how adults and animals perform such functions on a routine basis. Another suggestion is to make toilet training as easy and simple as possible. The selection of the child's clothing is an important consideration, as is the potty chair or use of the toilet. A freestanding potty chair

allows children a feeling of security. Planting the feet firmly on the floor also facilitates defecation. Another option is a portable seat attached to the regular toilet, which may ease the transition from potty chair to regular toilet (Fig. 12-5). Placing a small bench under the feet helps stabilize the child's position. It is probably best to keep the potty in the bathroom and to let the child observe the excreta being flushed down the toilet to associate these activities with usual practices. If a potty chair is not available, having the child sit facing the toilet tank provides added support. Practice sessions should be limited to 5 to 8 minutes, and a parent should stay with the child, practicing sanitary habits after every session. Children should be praised for cooperative behavior and successful evacuation. Dressing children in easily removed clothing; using training pants, "pull-on" diapers, or underwear; and encouraging imitation by watching others are other helpful suggestions.

SENSORY	LANGUAGE	SOCIALIZATION
Able to identify geometric forms; places round object into appropriate hole Binocular vision well developed Displays an intense and prolonged interest in pictures	Uses expressive jargon Says four to six words, including names "Asks" for objects by pointing Understands simple commands May use head-shaking gesture to denote "no" Uses "no" even while agreeing to the request Uses common gestures such as putting cup to mouth when empty	Tolerates some separation from parent Less likely to fear strangers Beginning to imitate parents, such as cleaning house (sweeping, dusting), folding clothes May discard bottle Kisses and hugs parents; may kiss pictures in a book
	Says 10 or more words Points to a common object, such as a shoe or ball, and to two or three body parts Forms word combinations Forms gesture-word combinations (points while naming) Forms gesture-gesture combinations	Expresses emotions; has temper tantrums Great imitator (domestic mimicry) Takes off gloves, socks, and shoes, and unzips zippers Temper tantrums may be more evident Beginning awareness of ownership ("my toy") May develop dependence on transitional objects, such as security blanket
Accommodation well developed in geometric discrimination; able to insert square block into oblong space	Has a vocabulary of approximately 300 words Uses two- or three-word phrases Uses pronouns "I," "me," "you" Understands directional commands Gives first name; refers to self by name Verbalizes need for toileting, food, or drink Talks incessantly Able to remember and imitate arbitrary sequences of manual actions and gestures	Stage of parallel play Has sustained attention span Temper tantrums decreasing Pulls people to show them something Increased independence from parent Dresses self in simple clothing Develops visual recognition and verbal self-reference ("Me big") Develops awareness that feelings and desires of others may be different and begins to explore implications and consequences
	Gives first and last name Refers to self by appropriate pronoun Uses plurals Names one color	Separates more easily from parent In play, helps put things away; can carry breakable objects; pushes with good steering Begins to notice sex differences; knows own sex May attend to toilet needs without help except for wiping Emotions expand to include pride, shame, guilt, embarrassment

When the child begins to experience regular daytime dryness, parents may experiment with underwear during the day. Daytime accidents are common, particularly during periods of intense activity. Young children become so engrossed in play activity that, if they are not reminded, they will wait until it is too late to reach the bathroom. Therefore frequent reminders and trips to the toilet are necessary. Parents often forget to plan ahead when the toddler is being toilet trained; before trips outside the house it is important to remind the child to at least try to urinate to decrease the chance of needing to use the toilet while the car is stuck in traffic.

As the child masters each step of toileting (discussion, undressing, going, wiping, dressing, flushing, and hand washing), he or she gains a sense of accomplishment that parents should reinforce. If the parent-child relationship becomes strained, both may need a break to focus on enjoyable activities together. Regression may coincide with a stressful family situation or the child being pushed too hard and too fast. Regression is a normal part of toilet training and does not mean failure but should be viewed as a temporary setback to a more comfortable place for the child.

NURSING ALERT

Once the child has been successfully toilet trained for bladder control, sudden wetting accidents and frequent urinating urges may require further investigation for a possible urinary tract infection (UTI), especially in girls. Younger children often have a UTI without accompanying fever or painful urination.

Daycare providers also play a role in the support and education of parents regarding toilet training practices. It is important for parents to inform all caregivers of their individual family values and the child's specific needs when planning for training away from home. Ensuring consistency in care of the

FIG. 12-5 ■ A, Sitting in reverse fashion on a regular toilet provides additional security to a young child. **B,** Children may begin toilet training sitting on a small potty chair.

toddler, as well as ensuring healthy practices in a sanitary environment, allows for safe and effective toilet practices in all settings.

Sibling Rivalry

Children have a natural jealousy and resentment toward a new child in the family or toward other children in the family when a parent turns his or her attention from them and interacts with their brother or sister; this is referred to as **sibling rivalry.**

The arrival of a new infant represents a crisis for even the best-prepared toddlers. They do not hate or resent the infant, but the changes that this additional sibling produces, especially the separation from mother during the birth. The parents now share their love and attention with someone else, the usual routine is disrupted, and toddlers may lose their crib or room—all at a time when they thought they were in control of their world. Sibling rivalry tends to be most pronounced in the firstborn, who experiences **dethronement** (loss of sole parental attention). It also seems to be most difficult for young children, particularly in terms of mother-child interaction.

Preparation of children for the birth of a sibling is individual, but dictated to some extent by age. Time for toddlers is a vague concept. Tomorrow could be yesterday or next week, and a month from now could be never. Preparing children too soon for the birth may lessen their interest by the time the event occurs. A good time to start talking about the baby is when toddlers become aware of the pregnancy and the changes taking place in the home in anticipation of the new member.

Toddlers need to have a realistic idea of what the newborn will be like. Telling them that a new playmate will come home soon sets up unrealistic expectations. Rather, parents should stress the activities that will take place when the baby arrives

home, such as diapering, bottle feeding or breastfeeding, bathing, and dressing. At the same time, parents should emphasize which routines will stay the same, such as reading stories or going to the park. If toddlers have had no contact with an infant, it is a good idea to introduce them to one, if feasible. Providing a doll with which toddlers can imitate parental behaviors is another excellent strategy. They can tend to the doll's needs (diapering, feeding) at the same time the parent is performing similar activities for the infant.

A new sibling in the home is stressful, so any additional stresses for the toddler should be avoided or minimized. For example, moving the toddler to a regular bed or to a different room should be done well in advance of the infant's arrival.

Pregnancy is an abstraction for toddlers. They need concrete illustrations of how the baby is growing inside the mother. It is an excellent opportunity for introducing aspects of reproduction in simple terms that the child can comprehend. Seeing simple pictures of the uterus and fetus and feeling the fetus move help the child feel involved in the experience. Children also benefit from classes for siblings that may be part of prenatal sessions.

When the new baby arrives, toddlers keenly feel the changed focus of attention. Visitors may initiate problems when they inadvertently shower the infant with attention and presents while neglecting the older child. Parents can minimize this by alerting visitors to the toddler's needs, having small presents on hand for the toddler, and including the child in the visit as much as possible. The toddler can also help with the care of the newborn by getting diapers and doing other small tasks (Fig. 12-6).

How children exhibit jealousy is complex. Some will hit the infant, push the child off the mother's lap, or pull the bottle or breast from the infant's mouth. For this reason, infants must

FIG. 12-6 ■ To minimize sibling rivalry, parents should include the toddler during caregiving activities.

be protected by parental supervision of the interaction between the siblings. More often, however, the expressions of hostility and resentment are more subtle and covert. Toddlers may verbally express a wish that the infant "go back inside mommy," or they will revert to more infantile forms of behavior, such as demanding a bottle, soiling their underpants, clinging for attention, using baby talk, or aggressively acting out toward others. The latter is particularly common in preschoolers, who may seem accepting of the new sibling at home but behave poorly in daycare or preschool. This is a form of displacement that says, "I can't let my parents know how I feel, so I will tell you."

Temper Tantrums

Temper tantrums are nearly universal during toddlerhood as independence is established and more complex tasks are attempted that may overwhelm the child emotionally. Toddlers may assert their independence by violently objecting to discipline. They may lie down on the floor, kick their feet, and scream at the top of their lungs. Some have learned the effectiveness of holding their breath until the parent relents. Although holding one's breath may cause fainting from the lack of oxygen, the accumulation of carbon dioxide will stimulate the respiratory control center, resulting in no physical harm. Rarely, breath-holding spells can involve symmetric tonic-clonic movements, which can be frightening to parents; the child recovers quickly once the spell is over, and there is no residual damage (Stein, 2003). Tantrums are an indication of the child's inability to control emotions; toddlers are particularly prone to tantrums because their strong drive for mastery and autonomy is frustrated by adult figures or lack of motor and cognitive skills (Needlman, Howard, and Zuckerman, 1995).

The best approach toward tapering temper tantrums requires consistency and developmentally appropriate expectations and rewards. Ensuring consistency among all caregivers in expectations, prioritizing what rules are important, and developing consequences that are reasonable for the child's level of development help manage the behavior. For example, a popular time for a tantrum is before bed. Active toddlers often have trouble slowing down and, when placed in bed, resist staying there. Parents can reinforce consistency and expectations by stating, "After this story it is bedtime." Starting at 18 months, time-outs work well for managing temper tantrums.

During tantrums, parents should ignore the behavior, provided the behavior is not injurious to the child, such as violently banging the head on the floor. They should continue to be present to provide a feeling of control and security to the child once the tantrum has subsided. At this time a toy or a favorite activity can be substituted for the request (see also Limit Setting and Discipline, Chapter 3). During periods of no tantrums, parents can practice developmentally appropriate positive reinforcement.

Other suggestions for handling tantrums include (Needlman, Howard, and Zuckerman, 1995):

- Offering the child options instead of an "all or none" position
- Picking one's battles carefully and ignoring small skirmishes over unimportant issues
- Giving comfort once the child is able to control emotions but not giving in to the original request
- Praising the child for positive behavior when he or she is not having a tantrum

Temper tantrums are common during the toddler years and essentially represent normal developmental behaviors. However, temper tantrums can be signs of serious problems. Nurses should be alert to situations that require further evaluation.

Negativism

One of the more difficult aspects of rearing children in this age-group is their persistent "no" response to every request. The negativism is not an expression of being stubborn or insolent, but a necessary assertion of self-control. Children test limits to gain understanding of the world and to learn to modify their behavior to fit the expectations of society. Negativism begins to subside as most children prepare to enter kindergarten.

One method of dealing with the negativism is to reduce the opportunities for a "no" answer. Asking the child, "Do you want to go to sleep now?" is an example of a question that will almost certainly be answered with an emphatic "no." Instead, tell the child that it is time to go to sleep and proceed accordingly. In their attempt to exert control, children like to make choices. When confronted with appropriate choices, such as "You may have a peanut butter and jelly sandwich or chicken noodle soup for lunch," they are more likely to choose one rather than automatically say no. However, if their response is negative, parents should make the choice for the child.

Nurses working with children and parents can assist parents in understanding this concept by role modeling. For example, when the nurse approaches the toddler for taking vital signs, instead of asking "Can I listen to your heart?" the nurse can say, "I am going to listen to your heart." Because of normal developmental behavior, the toddler is first going to resist attempts at taking vital signs because it is an intrusion on her body. Second, the toddler is most likely going to answer "no," not because he or she necessarily fears the procedure itself, but because of the tendency to answer all questions with a negative response. If the nurse asks the question and the toddler says "no" but the nurse proceeds anyway, the toddler starts to mistrust the nurse's actions, since they contradict his or her words.

Regression

The retreat from one's present pattern of functioning to past levels of behavior is referred to as **regression.** It usually occurs in instances of discomfort or stress when one attempts to conserve psychic energy by reverting to patterns of behavior that were successful in earlier stages of development. Regression is common in toddlers, since almost any additional stress hinders their ability to master present developmental tasks. Any threat to their autonomy, such as illness, hospitalization, separation from a parent, disruption of established routines, or adjustment to a new sibling, represents a need to revert to earlier forms of behavior, such as increased dependency; refusal to use the potty chair; temper tantrums; demand for the bottle or pacifier; and loss of newly learned motor, language, social, and cognitive skills.

At first, such regression appears acceptable and comfortable for children, but the loss of newly acquired achievements is frightening and threatening, since children are aware of their helplessness. Parents become concerned about regressive behavior and frequently, in their efforts to deal with it, force the child to cope with an additional source of stress: the pressure to live up to expected standards. Brazelton (1999) suggests that these predictable times of regression, or **touchpoints,** are an opportunity to prepare parents for the next step in their child's development.

When regression does occur, the best approach is to ignore it while praising existing patterns of appropriate behavior. Regression is a child's way of saying, "I can't cope with this present stress and perfect this skill as well, but I will if given patience and understanding." For this reason, it is advisable not to attempt new areas of learning when an additional crisis is present or expected, such as beginning toilet training shortly before a sibling is born or during a brief period of hospitalization.

PROMOTING OPTIMAL HEALTH DURING TODDLERHOOD

NUTRITION

From 12 to 18 months of age, the growth rate slows, decreasing the child's need for calories, protein, and fluid. However, the requirements for protein (1.2 g/kg) and calories (102 kcal/kg) are still relatively high to meet the demands for muscle tissue growth and high activity level. The requirements for most vitamins and minerals increase slightly during toddlerhood. The need for minerals such as iron, calcium, and phosphorus may be difficult to meet, considering the characteristic food habits of children in this age-group.

At approximately 18 months of age, most toddlers manifest this decreased nutritional need with a decreased appetite, a phenomenon known as **physiologic anorexia.** They become picky, fussy eaters with strong taste preferences. They may eat large amounts one day and almost nothing the next. Toddlers are increasingly aware of the nonnutritive function of food: the pleasure of eating, the social aspect of mealtime, and the control of refusing food. They are influenced by factors other than taste when choosing food. If a family member refuses to eat something, toddlers are likely to imitate that response. If the plate is overfilled, they are likely to push it away, overwhelmed by its size. If food does not appear or smell appetizing, they will probably not agree to try it. In essence, mealtime is more closely associated with psychologic components than with nutritional ones.

The ritualism of this age also dictates certain principles in feeding practices. Toddlers like to have the same dish, cup, or spoon every time they eat. They may reject a favorite food simply because it is served in a different dish. If one food touches another, they often refuse to eat it. Mixed foods, such as stews or casseroles, are rarely favorites. Because toddlers have unpredictable table manners, it is best to use plastic dishes and cups, for both economic and safety reasons. For some children a regular mealtime schedule also contributes to their desire and need for predictability and ritualism.

Developmentally, by 12 months of age most children are eating many of the same foods prepared for the rest of the family. Some may have mastered using a cup with occasional spilling, although most cannot adeptly use a spoon until 18 months of age or later and generally prefer using their fingers.

Nutritional Counseling

The emphasis on preventing childhood obesity and subsequent cardiovascular disease in the United States has prompted a number of changes in dietary recommendations for children and adults alike. It is now recognized that lifetime eating habits may be established in early childhood, and health care workers are increasingly emphasizing the role of food selection choices, exercise, stress reduction, and other lifestyle choices (tobacco and alcohol use) on the quality of adult life and survival. Conditions such as obesity and cardiovascular disease can be prevented by encouraging healthy eating habits in toddlers and their families.

If food is used as a reward or sign of approval, a child may overeat for nonnutritive reasons. If food is forced and mealtime is consistently unpleasant, the usual pleasure associated with eating may not develop. Mealtimes should be enjoyable rather than times for discipline or family arguments. The social aspect of mealtime may be distracting for young children; therefore an earlier feeding hour may be appropriate. Young children are unable to sit through a long meal and become restless and disruptive. This is particularly common when children are brought to the table just after active play. Calling them in from play 15 minutes before mealtime allows them ample opportunity to get ready for eating while settling down their active minds and bodies.

The method of serving food also takes on more importance during this period. Toddlers need to have a sense of control and achievement in their abilities. Giving them large, adult-size portions can overwhelm them. In general, what is eaten is much more significant than how much is consumed. Small amounts of meat and vegetables supply greater food value than a large consumption of bread or potato. Serving sizes need to be appropriate for age (Box 12-2). Young children tend to like less spicy, bland food, although this is a cul-

BOX 12-2

Sample Menu for Toddlers Based on MyPyramid for Kids*

BREAKFAST
½ cup dry, unsweetened cereal
½ cup orange juice
2 ounces low-fat milk†

SNACK
½-1 whole banana

LUNCH
1 slice cheese
2 teaspoons all-fruit preserves
1 slice whole-wheat bread
2 tablespoons peas
2 ounces low-fat milk†

SNACK
2 graham crackers
2 ounces low-fat milk†

DINNER
1 chicken leg, roasted without skin
¼-½ cup macaroni and cheese
2 tablespoons green beans, cooked
2 tablespoons carrots, cooked
2-3 ounces low-fat milk†

SNACK
½ cup frozen yogurt

TOTAL (PER DAY)
Bread, cereal, rice, pasta: 6 ounces
Vegetable: 2½ cups
Fruit (vitamin A and C sources): 1½ cups
Milk, yogurt, cheese, pudding: 2 cups
Meat, poultry, fish, dried beans, eggs, nuts: 5 ounces

*Use fats, oils, and sweets sparingly; obtain oils from fish or liquid oils such as corn oil, soybean oil, and canola oil. Increase fluids with servings of water. Serving sizes are minimums for nutritional adequacy. Many children eat more. Menu is based on an 1800-calorie diet.
†Substitute whole milk if child is younger than 24 months.

turally determined preference. Substitutions can be provided for foods that they do not enjoy, although parents need not cater to all of their desires. Frequent nutritious snacks can replace a meal. **Grazing**—nibbling and snacking—is a good way to ensure proper nutrition, provided that appropriate foods are offered.

NURSING TIP

A general guide to serving sizes for toddlers is 1 tablespoon of solid food per year of age, or one fourth to one third of the adult portion size.
- Use the tablespoon guide for easily measured foods such as vegetables or rice.
- Use the fraction guide for bread or milk.

Mastication skills continue to mature, putting children at risk for choking; therefore large round foods (hot dogs, grapes, peas, carrots, popcorn, fruit gel snacks) should be avoided until the child is able to chew them effectively. Active play while eating should be discouraged to prevent choking. Appetite and food preferences are sporadic. Often the interest in food parallels a growth spurt, so that periods of good eating are interspersed with phases of poor eating. If exposed to the same food every day, a young toddler does not learn how to manage the complex sensory information needed to eat new, more difficult foods (vegetables with a different texture vs pureed, slippery fruits). To help prevent "food jags," it is recommended that parents present food in various physical forms. The child may need to progress to eating new foods in a stepwise fashion: visually tolerating the food, interacting with the food, smelling the food, touching the food, tasting, and then eating the food.

Many authorities consider this period of picky eating to be a developmental phase and stress that most toddlers will consume the necessary amount of food required for growth (Cathey and Gaylord, 2004). It has also been suggested that parents plan a nutritionally balanced week instead of day because of the way toddlers will restrict food intake in their effort to exert control over their environment (Morin, 2007).

Dietary Guidelines

Dietary guidelines are necessary to promote adequate energy and nutrient intake to support physical, emotional, psychologic, and cognitive development. A number of new dietary guidelines have been developed to address the issue of childhood obesity, sedentary lifestyles, and increase in cardiovascular disease mortality in the United States. Guidelines such as the 2005 American Heart Association Dietary Guidelines* provide suggestions for children ages 2 years and up and are discussed in Chapter 11. In addition, Chapter 11 discusses the Dietary Reference Intakes developed by the Institute of Medicine and the food guide pyramids MyPyramid and MyPyramid for Kids (see Fig. 11-1), developed by the U.S. Department of Agriculture (2005), which provide dietary guidelines for proper food selection and serving sizes tailored to the child's level of activity and lifestyle.

Nutrition during toddlerhood involves a transition as a young toddler is weaned off milk- or formula-based diets. Milk intake, the chief source of calcium and phosphorus, should average two or three servings (24 to 30 ounces) a day. More than a quart of milk consumption daily considerably limits the intake of solid foods, resulting in a deficiency of dietary iron and other nutrients. After 2 years of age children can be given no-fat or low-fat milk to reduce daily total fat to less than 30% of calories, saturated fatty acids to less than 10% of calories, and cholesterol to less than 300 mg. Other measures to reduce dietary fat include using lean meats, fat-modified products (such as low-fat cheese), and low-fat cooking. Because less fat in children's diet can also mean fewer calories and nutrients, caregivers must know what kinds of food to choose. *Trans* fatty acids and saturated fats, however, should be avoided (Allen and Myers, 2006).

Iron-fortified cereals and iron-rich foods are recommended for all children beyond 6 months of age. Parents should be encouraged to provide an iron-rich diet that includes heme and nonheme iron sources (red meats, poultry, fish, green leafy vegetables, dried fruit, beans) and limit

*http://www.americanheart.org/presenter.jhtml?identifier=3033999.

whole-milk consumption. Iron supplementation may be necessary in some cases.

Calcium and vitamin D are essential for healthy bone development. Adequate intake of calcium for the child 1 to 3 years of age is 500 mg. Whole milk, cheese, yogurt, legumes (beans), and vegetables (broccoli, collard greens, kale) are good sources for calcium. Popular calcium-fortified foods include waffles, cereals and cereal bars, orange juice, and some white breads. Adequate vitamin D intake is essential to prevent rickets; it is now recommended that children and adolescents have an intake of at least 200 IU of vitamin D daily. Multivitamin preparations containing 400 IU of vitamin D (by tablet or liquid) are adequate if food intake is poor or exposure to sunlight is minimal; commercially available vitamin D vitamin tablets contain too much vitamin D for children at this time (American Academy of Pediatrics, 2003). Sources of vitamin D include fish, fish oils, and egg yolks. Fortified cereals, dairy products, and meat are also good sources of zinc and vitamin E.

It is recommended by the American Heart Association (2005) that toddlers have 1 cup of fruit each day. Vitamin C enhances iron absorption. Toddlers should consume approximately 4 to 6 ounces of juice per day. It tastes good to toddlers and is readily available. A 6-ounce glass of fruit juice equals one fruit serving; however, juices lack the fiber of whole fruit and should not be a substitution for whole fruit. High intake of juice can contribute to diarrhea, overnutrition or undernutrition, and the development of caries; thus only 4 to 6 ounces of 100% fruit juice per day are recommended (American Academy of Pediatrics, 2004a). Fruit-flavored drinks advertised as juices may not actually contain 100% juice and should be avoided.

Fat restriction, other than *trans* fatty acids and saturated fats, is not appropriate for toddlers. Thirty percent of calories should come from fat. Whole milk is recommended as a source of fat until 2 years of age.

SLEEP AND ACTIVITY

Total sleep decreases only slightly during the second year and averages about 12 hours a day. Most children take one nap a day but may relinquish this habit by the end of the second or third year. Children reach an adult pattern of sleep by 3 years of age (Howard and Wong, 2001).

Sleep problems are common, especially going to bed and falling asleep, and are a response to fears and awareness of separation. Fears can be provoked by a child's daily stressors such as pressure to toilet train, moves, sibling birth, experiences of loss, or separation from parents. Establishing a regular bedtime and routine is helpful, and providing transitional objects, such as a favorite stuffed animal or blanket, can ease the child's insecurity at bedtime (see Fig. 12-3). Toddlers no longer sleeping in a crib may come out of their rooms after being put to bed. Limit prolonged bedtime rituals by defining a length of time and set of activities (one more story, one more drink). Toddlers who are too immature to respond to the measures identified may need their doorway gated.

A toddler's activity level is high, and there is rarely a problem with too little physical exercise, provided inappropriate restrictions are not instituted. With increasing numbers of young children being cared for outside the home, attention to

the kinds of activity provided is important. For example, children with high activity levels may benefit from an environment in which outdoor play is encouraged. Neurodevelopment is necessary for the developing child to participate in activities.

DENTAL HEALTH
Regular Dental Examinations

The American Academy of Pediatric Dentistry (2006) now recommends that every child have an oral health examination by a practitioner by 6 months of age; if the child is in a high-risk category for caries, it is recommended that an initial visit to a dentist or pedodontist (pediatric dentist) occur by age 6 months or within 6 months of the eruption of the first tooth. Every child should have an established dental home by the age of 12 months (American Academy of Pediatric Dentistry, 2006). Initial visits to the dentist should be nontraumatizing. Because toddlers react negatively to new and potentially frightening experiences, the initial visit can center around meeting the dentist, seeing the equipment, and sitting in the chair. If the child is cooperative, the dentist may just look at the teeth but reserve a more thorough examination for another visit. Modeling, in which the child observes procedures performed on the parent or a cooperative sibling, can also be effective.

Removal of Plaque

Oral hygiene measures should be implemented according to the suggested schedule noted above to remove **plaque,** soft bacterial deposits that adhere to the teeth and cause **dental caries** (decay or cavities) and **periodontal** (gum) **disease.** Poor oral hygiene and poor dietary habits are associated with the development of caries in children.

The most effective methods for plaque removal are brushing and flossing. Several brushing techniques exist, although there is no universal agreement regarding the best method. One that is suitable for cleaning the primary teeth is the scrub method. The tips of the bristles are placed firmly at a 45-degree angle against the teeth and gums and moved back and forth in a vibratory motion. The ends of the bristles should be wiggling but not moving forcefully back and forth, which can damage the gums and enamel. All the surfaces of the teeth are cleaned in this manner except the lingual (inner) surfaces of the anterior teeth. To clean these surfaces, the toothbrush is placed vertical to the teeth and moved up and down. Only a few teeth are brushed at one time, using six to eight strokes for each section. A systematic approach is used so that all surfaces are thoroughly cleaned (Fig. 12-7).

For young children the most effective cleaning is done by parents (Fig. 12-8). Several positions can be used that facilitate access to the mouth and help stabilize the head for comfort:

- Stand with child's back toward adult. (When done in front of a bathroom mirror, both child and adult can see what is being done in the mirror.)
- Sit on a couch or bed with child's head resting in adult's lap.
- Sit on the floor or a stool with child's head resting between adult's thighs.

With all positions, use one hand to cup the chin and one to brush the teeth. For easier access to back teeth, hold the mouth partially open.

FIG. 12-7 ■ Young children can participate in toothbrushing, but parents need to brush all of the child's teeth thoroughly.

FIG. 12-8 ■ The most effective cleaning of teeth is done by parents.

NURSINGTIP

- To encourage children to open their mouth, ask them to "tweet like a bird" to brush the front teeth and to "roar like a lion" to brush the back teeth.
- Sing, tell stories, or talk to children during teeth cleaning to prevent boredom.

For effective cleaning, a small toothbrush with soft, rounded, multitufted nylon bristles that are short and uniform in length is recommended. Nylon bristles dry more rapidly after use and retain their shape better than natural bristles. Toothbrushes are replaced as soon as the bristles are frayed or bent. With young children, brushing may be more easily accomplished using only water, since many children dislike the foam from toothpaste and the foam interferes with visibility. There is also the danger of swallowing fluoridated toothpaste (see following discussion under Fluoride). Introduce toothpaste around 2 years of age and allow children to select the flavor they like to encourage the brushing habit. Use a pea-sized amount of toothpaste (apply across the narrow width of the toothbrush, rather than along its length, to decrease the chance of applying an excessive amount).

After the teeth have been cleaned, the teeth are flossed to remove plaque and debris from between the teeth and below the gum margin, where brushing is ineffective. Because young children do not have the dexterity to manipulate the dental floss, parents must perform the procedure.

A disclosing agent is helpful in identifying those areas of the teeth where plaque accumulates. It also helps motivate children to clean their teeth because plaque is difficult to see. After cleaning, the mouth is inspected to ensure that all traces of plaque have been removed. Where plaque remains, the teeth are rebrushed.

Ideally, the teeth should be cleaned after each meal and especially before bedtime, and the child should be given nothing to eat or drink after the night brushing except water. At those times when brushing is impractical, the "swish-and-swallow" method of cleaning the mouth is taught: with a mouthful of water the child rinses the mouth and swallows, repeating the procedure three or four times.*

Fluoride

Fluoride supplementation should be considered for any child over the age of 6 months whose drinking water is deficient in fluoride. Supplementation based on fluoride concentration of water supply less than 0.3 ppm (parts per million) is 0.25 mg for a child 6 months to 3 years of age and 0.5 mg for a child 3 to 6 years of age (American Academy of Pediatric Dentistry, 2006).

Fluoride, a mineral, is found in water, foods, or drinks in which fluoridated water was used as part of the processing system. Because the water fluoridation process and manufacturing of fluoride toothpaste are almost impossible to standardize in the United States, the dosage of fluoride supplements has been lowered to reduce the incidence of fluorosis (Table 12-2). Increased fluoride ingestion leads to enamel protein retention, hypomineralization of the enamel and dentin, and disturbance of crystal formation. The effects caused by this change range from barely discernible white fiberlike lines or spots to gray-brown stains or pitted areas. Parents should be cautioned against regular use of fluoridated water or beverages such as bottled water containing fluoride if the community water supply already has an adequate amount of fluoride.

*More detailed information can be obtained from the American Academy of Pediatric Dentistry, http://www.aapd.org.

TABLE 12-2

Fluoride Supplementation*

	WATER FLUORIDE CONTENT (ppm)	
AGE	0.3	0.3-0.6
Birth–6 months	0	0
6 months–3 years	0.25	0
3-6 years	0.50	0.25
6-16 years	1.00	0.50

From American Academy of Pediatric Dentistry: Guideline on fluoride therapy. In *AAPD reference manual 2005-2006,* 2006.
ppm, Parts per million.
*Fluoride daily doses are given in milligrams.

FIG. 12-9 ■ Nursing caries. (Courtesy Bruce Carter, DDS, Texas Children's Hospital, Houston.)

Low-Cariogenic Diet

Diet is critical to developing good teeth because the carious process depends primarily on fermentable sugars, especially sucrose. Refined table sugar, honey, molasses, corn syrup, and dried fruits such as raisins are highly cariogenic. Complex carbohydrates, such as breads, potatoes, and pasta, also contribute to caries because they lower the plaque pH.

Ideally, highly cariogenic foods, especially those containing complex sugars, should be eliminated. However, because this is impractical, some suggestions can be helpful. First, *the frequency with which sugar is consumed is more important than the total amount eaten.* Therefore, when sweets are eaten, they are less damaging if consumed immediately after a meal rather than as a snack between meals. When sweets are served as the dessert, the teeth can be cleaned afterward, decreasing the amount of time the sugar is in the mouth.

Second, the form of sugar (sucrose) is important. The more cariogenic foods are those that are sticky or hard, since they remain in the mouth longer. Consequently, sucking on lollipops is more cariogenic than eating a chocolate bar. Sometimes the source of the sugar is "hidden," as in numerous prescription and nonprescription drugs and in many popular cereals, including the "all-natural" variety. Reading food labels is essential in eliminating sources of sucrose.

Some snacks do not contribute to tooth decay. Aged cheeses, such as cheddar, may alter the pH and retard bacterial growth. Sugarless gum chewed after eating may actually protect against cavities by stimulating saliva that neutralizes acid. The artificial sweeteners saccharin, aspartame, and Splenda are noncariogenic; sorbitol has low cariogenic potential.

A special form of tooth decay in infants and young toddlers is **nursing caries** (also called **nursing bottle caries** or **bottle-mouth caries**), which occurs when the child is routinely given a bottle of milk or juice at nap or bedtime or uses the bottle as a pacifier while awake (Fig. 12-9). The practice of coating pacifiers in honey can also contribute to caries, and honey may be a potential source of botulism in infants (see Chapter 32). As the sweet liquid pools in the mouth, the teeth are bathed for several hours in this cariogenic environment. The maxillary (upper) incisors and molars are affected most, since the mandibular (lower) incisors are protected by the lower lip, tongue, and saliva. Severely decayed teeth may require the application of stainless steel bands to preserve the spacing until the permanent teeth erupt.

Prevention involves eliminating the bedtime bottle completely, feeding the last bottle before bedtime, substituting a bottle of water for milk or juice, not using the bottle as a pacifier, and never coating pacifiers in sweet substances. Juice in bottles, especially commercially available ready-to-use bottles, is discouraged; these beverages are especially damaging because the sugar is more readily converted to acid. Juice should always be offered in a cup to avoid prolonging the bottle-feeding habit. Toddlers should be encouraged to drink from a cup at the first birthday and weaned from a bottle by 14 months of age. Nurses are in an excellent position to counsel parents regarding the dangers of this habit and other aspects of dental care.*

INJURY PREVENTION

Injuries cause more deaths in children between the ages of 1 and 4 years than in any other childhood age-group except adolescence. Agran, Anderson, Winn, and others (2003) found that the highest rate of childhood injury was in children ages 15 to 17 months; the next highest rates were in children 15 years and older. The injury death rate has remained relatively unchanged during the past decade; however, the corresponding rates from all other causes of death combined have declined significantly. Traumatic injury is the leading cause of childhood hospitalization, and infants and younger children are at higher risk because of small size and inability to protect themselves (Dowd, Keenan, and Bratton 2002). Child protection (adapting environment, society regulations and laws) and parent and child education are key determinants in injury prevention.

A major factor in the critical increase of injuries during early childhood is the unrestricted freedom achieved through locomotion combined with an unawareness of danger within the environment. Specific categories of injuries and appropriate prevention are best understood by associating them with the major developmental achievements of young children (Table 12-3). The discussions of injuries in Chapters 1 and 10 are also relevant to safety concerns at this age.

*Sources of information about nursing caries and other aspects of child dental health include the National Institute of Dental and Craniofacial Research, National Institutes of Health, Bethesda, MD 20892-2190; (301) 402-7364; http://www.nidcr.nih.gov; American Academy of Pediatric Dentistry, 211 E. Chicago Ave., Suite 1700, Chicago, IL 60611; (312) 337-2169; http://www.aapd.org; American Dental Association, 211 E. Chicago Ave., Chicago, IL 60611; (312) 440-2500; http://www.ada.org; and Canadian Dental Association, 1815 Alta Vista Drive, Ottawa, Ontario K1G 3Y6; (613) 523-1770; http://www.cda-adc.ca.

TABLE 12-3

Injury Prevention During Early Childhood

DEVELOPMENTAL ABILITIES RELATED TO RISK OF INJURY	INJURY PREVENTION

MOTOR VEHICLES
Walks, runs, and climbs
Able to open doors and gates
Can ride tricycle
Can throw ball and other objects
	Use federally approved car restraint per manufacturer's recommendations for weight and height.
	Supervise child while playing outside.
	Do not allow child to play on curb or behind a parked car.
	Do not permit child to play in pile of leaves, snow, or large cardboard container in trafficked area.
	Supervise tricycle riding; have child wear helmet.
	Limit playing in driveways with parked cars or provide physical barriers limiting access.
	Lock fences and doors if not directly supervising children.
	Teach child to obey pedestrian safety rules:
	    Obey traffic regulations; cross only at crosswalks and only when traffic signal indicates it is safe.
	    Stand back a step from the curb until it is time to cross.
	    Look left, right, and left again and check for turning cars before crossing street.
	    Use sidewalks; when there is no sidewalk, walk on the left, facing traffic.
	    Wear light colors at night and attach fluorescent material to clothing.

DROWNING Able to explore if left unsupervised Has great curiosity Helpless in water; unaware of its danger; depth of water has no significance	Supervise closely when near any source of water, including buckets. Never, under any circumstance, leave unsupervised in bathtub. Keep bathroom doors closed and lid down on toilet. Have fence around swimming pool and lock gate.*
BURNS Able to reach heights by climbing, stretching, and standing on toes Pulls objects Explores any holes or opening Can open drawers and closets Unaware of potential sources of heat or fire Plays with mechanical objects	Turn pot handles toward back of stove. Place electric appliances, such as coffee maker and popcorn machine, toward back of counter. Place guardrails in front of radiators, fireplaces, or other heating elements. Store matches and cigarette lighters in locked or inaccessible area; discard carefully. Place burning candles, incense, hot foods, and cigarettes out of reach. Do not let tablecloth hang within child's reach. Do not let electric cord from iron or other appliance hang within child's reach. Cover electrical outlets with protective plastic caps. Keep electrical wires hidden or out of reach. Do not allow child to play with electrical appliance, wires, or lighters. Stress danger of open flames; teach what "hot" means. Always check bathwater temperature; adjust water heater temperature to 49° C (120° F) or lower; do not allow children to play with faucets. Apply a sunscreen when child is exposed to sunlight (all year round).
POISONING Explores by putting objects in mouth Can open drawers, closets, and most containers Climbs Cannot read labels Does not know safe dose or amount	Place all potentially toxic agents out of reach or in a locked cabinet, including cosmetics, personal care items, cleaning products, pesticides, medications. Caution against eating nonedible items, such as plants. Replace medications or poisons immediately in locked cabinet; replace child-guard caps promptly. Administer medications as a drug, not as a candy. Do not store large surplus of toxic agents. Promptly discard empty poison containers; never reuse to store a food item or other poison. Teach child not to play in trash containers. Never remove labels from containers of toxic substances. Know number of nearest poison control center: **(800) 222-1222.**

*Detailed guidelines for safety barriers for pools may be found at http://www.cpsc.gov/CPSCPUB/PUBS/Pool.pdf.

Continued

TABLE 12-3

Injury Prevention During Early Childhood—cont'd

DEVELOPMENTAL ABILITIES RELATED TO RISK OF INJURY	INJURY PREVENTION
FALLS Able to open doors and some windows Goes up and down stairs Depth perception unrefined	Use window guards—do not rely on screens to stop falls. Place gates at top and bottom of stairs. Keep doors locked or use child-proof doorknob covers at entry to stairs, high porch, or other elevated area, including laundry chute. Ensure safe and effective barriers on porches, balconies, decks. Remove unsecured or scatter rugs. Apply nonskid decals in bathtub or shower. Keep crib rails fully raised and mattress at lowest level. Place carpeting under crib and in bathroom. Keep large toys and bumper pads out of crib or playpen (child can use these as "stairs" to climb out), then move to youth bed when child is able to climb out of crib. Avoid using mobile walker, especially near stairs. Dress in safe clothing (soles that do not "catch" on floor, tied shoelaces, pant legs that do not touch floor). Keep child restrained in vehicle; never leave unattended in vehicle or shopping cart. Never leave child unattended in high chair. Supervise at playgrounds; select play areas with soft ground cover and safe equipment.
CHOKING AND SUFFOCATION Puts things in mouth May swallow hard or inedible pieces of food	Avoid large, round chunks of meat, such as whole hot dogs (slice lengthwise into short pieces). Avoid fruit with pits, fish with bones, hard candy, chewing gum, nuts, popcorn, grapes, marshmallows. Choose large, sturdy toys without sharp edges or small removable parts. Discard old refrigerators, ovens, and so on, and remove the door. Install smoke and carbon monoxide alarms; change batteries every 6 months. Develop a fire escape plan for the entire family and have drills. Keep automatic garage door transmitter in an inaccessible place. Select safe toy boxes or chests without heavy, hinged lids. Keep venetian blind cords out of child's reach. Remove drawstrings from clothing; shorten essential drawstrings to 15.15 cm (6 inches) or less. Avoid contact with round, hollow, semirigid plastic items such as half a plastic ball.

BODILY DAMAGE
Still clumsy in many skills
Easily distracted from tasks
Unaware of potential danger from strangers or other people
	Avoid giving sharp or pointed objects—such as knives, scissors, or toothpicks—especially when walking or running.
	Do not allow lollipops or similar objects in mouth when walking or running.
	Teach safety precautions (e.g., to carry knife or scissors with pointed end away from face).
	Store all dangerous tools, garden equipment, and firearms in locked cabinet.
	Be alert to danger of unsupervised animals and household pets.
	Use safety glass on large glassed areas, such as sliding glass doors.
	Teach child name, address, and phone number and to ask for help from appropriate people (cashier, security guard, policeman) if lost; have identification on child (sewn in clothes, inside shoe).
	Teach stranger safety:
	    Avoid personalized clothing in public places.
	    Never go with a stranger.
	    Tell parents if anyone makes child feel uncomfortable in any way.
	    Always listen to child's concerns regarding others' behavior.
	    Teach child to say "no" when confronted with uncomfortable situations.

Motor Vehicle Injuries

Motor vehicle injuries cause more accidental deaths in all pediatric age-groups after age 1 year than any other type of injury or disease and are responsible for almost half of all accidental deaths among children ages 1 to 4 years. Many of the deaths are caused by injuries within the car when restraints have not been used or have been used improperly. Unrestrained children riding in the vehicle's front seat are at highest risk for injury (Durbin, Chen, Smith, and others, 2005). Approved restraints properly installed and applied can prevent many fatalities and injuries (Schnitzer, 2006; American Academy of Pediatrics, 2007). Motor vehicle back-over injuries and deaths, along with deaths or serious injury resulting from heat stroke when left in a car, account for a large number

FIG. 12-10 ■ A, Automobile booster seat. Note placement of shoulder strap (away from neck and face). B, Locking clip used with free-sliding lap/shoulder belt to keep the belt in a tight-holding position.

of motor vehicle–related injuries in children (Centers for Disease Control and Prevention, 2005; McLaren, Null, and Quinn, 2005).

Car Restraints. Five types of restraints are available: (1) infant-only devices, (2) convertible models for both infants and toddlers, (3) boosters, (4) shoulder-lap safety belts, and (5) devices for children with special needs (see Chapter 18). Some vehicles have manufacturer-installed seats that convert to child car restraints.

The infant-type restraints are discussed in Chapter 10; the convertible restraints and boosters are included here. The **convertible restraint** is suitable for infants in the rearward-facing position and for toddlers in the forward-facing position (Fig. 12-10, *A*). The transition point for switching to the forward-facing position is defined by the manufacturer but is generally at a body weight of at least 9 kg (20 pounds) and 1 year of age. Infants who weigh 20 pounds before 1 year of age should continue to ride rear-facing (American Academy of Pediatrics, 2007). One recent study has shown that children from birth to 23 months experienced fewer injuries when riding in rear-facing car restraints (Henary, Sherwood, Crandall, and others, 2007). The findings suggest that guidelines may be revised in the future to recommend a rear-facing car restraint position in children over 1 year of age.

Convertible safety seats should be used until the child weighs at least 13.6 kg (30 pounds) or more regardless of age and as long as the child fits properly into the seat (American Academy of Pediatrics, 2007). The restraint consists of a molded hard plastic or metal frame with energy-absorbing padding and a special harness system designed to hold the child firmly in the seat and distribute the forces to body areas that can withstand the impact.

Convertible restraints use different types of harness systems: a **five-point harness** that consists of a strap over each shoulder, one on each side of the pelvis, and one between the legs (all five come together at a common buckle), as well as a **padded overhead shield** that uses shoulder straps attached to a shield that is held in place by a crotch strap. In some seats a **T-shield,** a padded triangular shield, attaches to shoulder straps to keep the child safely restrained. With both the infant and toddler restraints, it is important not to add extra blankets, head cushions, or padding between the child and the restraint straps that did not come as original equipment because

these "add-ons" create spaces of air between the child and the restraint and decrease support for the back, head, and neck. Cars with free-sliding latch plates on the lap or shoulder belt require the use of a metal locking clip to keep the belt in a tight-holding position. The locking clip is threaded onto the belt above the latch plate (Fig. 12-10, *B*). If parents have newer cars with automatic lap and shoulder belts, they need to have additional lap belts installed to properly secure the restraint.

Booster seats are not restraint systems like the convertible devices because they depend on the vehicle belts to hold the child and booster seat in place. Three booster models have been approved by the National Highway Traffic Safety Administration: the high-back belt-positioning seat, which provides head and neck support for the child riding in a vehicle seat without a head rest; the no-back belt-positioning seat, which should be used only if the vehicle seat has a head rest; and a combination seat, which converts from a forward-facing toddler seat to a booster seat. This last model is equipped with a harness for use by toddlers; the harness may be removed and a shoulder-lap belt used when the child outgrows the harness. Booster seats are used for children who are less than 145 cm (4 feet, 9 inches) tall and who weigh more than 18 kg (40 pounds), typically those between 4 and 8 years of age. A booster seat should be used until the child is able to sit against the back of the seat with feet hanging down and legs bent at the knees. The belt-positioning booster model raises a child higher in the seat, moving the shoulder part of the belt off the neck and the lap portion of the belt off the abdomen onto the pelvis. Children who outgrow the convertible restraint may still be able to ride safely in a booster seat until the midpoint of the head is higher than the vehicle seat back.

Children should use specially designed car restraints until they are 145 cm (4 feet, 9 inches) in height or are 8 to 12 years old (American Academy of Pediatrics, 2007). **Shoulder-lap safety belts** should be worn low on the hips, snug, and not on the abdominal area. Children should be taught to sit up straight to allow for proper fit. The shoulder belt is used only if it does not cross the child's neck or face.

Shoulder-only automatic belts are designed to protect adults. Children should use the manual shoulder belts in the rear seat. Air bags do not take the place of child safety seats or seat belts and can be lethal to young children. The safest area of the car for children is the back seat. Children who must ride

FAMILY-CENTERED CARE

Using Car Safety Restraints

- Read manufacturer's directions and follow them exactly.
- Start using car seat when child is infant so he or she will be accustomed to riding restrained.
- Provide favorite toy, stuffed animal, or snack for child while in car seat.
- Anchor car safety seat securely to car's anchoring system and apply harness snugly to child.*
- Do not start the car until everyone is properly restrained.
- Always use the restraint, even for short trips.
- If car seat is vinyl and used in hot car, cover with cloth to prevent skin burns.
- If child begins to climb out or undo the harness, firmly say, "No." It may be necessary to stop the car to reinforce the expected behavior. Use rewards, such as stars or stickers, to encourage cooperation.
- Encourage child to help attach buckles, straps, and shields, but always double-check fastenings.
- Decrease boredom on long trips. Keep soft toys in the car for quiet play; talk to child; point out objects and teach child about them. Stop periodically. If child wishes to sleep, make certain child stays in the restraint.
- Insist that others who transport children also follow these safety rules.

*A free car seat restraint inspection may be obtained from a SafeKids inspector. Check for local inspection SafeKids clinics or access website for information: http://www.safekids.org.

FIG. 12-11 ■ LATCH (Lower Anchors and Tethers for Children) universal child safety seat system. **A,** Flexible two-point attachment with top tether. **B,** Rigid two-point attachment with top tether. **C,** Top tether. (Courtesy US Department of Transportation, National Highway Traffic Safety Administration.)

in the passenger side of the front seat with an air bag should be positioned as far back as possible.

Built-in seats are available in some cars and vans. They may be used for children who are at least 1 year of age and weigh at least 9 kg (20 pounds). Built-in seats eliminate installation problems. However, weight and height limits vary. Reinforce that owners must verify with vehicle manufacturers details about built-in seats.

For any restraint to be effective, it must be used consistently and properly. Examples of misuse include misrouting the vehicle seat belt through the restraint; failing to use the vehicle seat belt to secure the restraint; failing to use a tether strap; failing to use the restraint's harness system; and incorrectly positioning the child, especially by facing infants forward instead of rearward. To address these issues, nurses must stress correct use of car restraints and rules that ensure compliance (see Family-Centered Care box). Children riding in car safety seats are generally much better behaved than children left unrestrained, which can be a major benefit to parents and should be emphasized as an additional advantage of restraints. Additional information about child safety restraints is available from various sources.*

The LATCH (Lower Anchors and Tethers for Children) universal child safety seat system was implemented as a requirement starting in 2002 for all new automobiles and child safety seats. This system provides uniform anchorage consist-

ing of two lower anchorages and one upper anchorage in the rear seat of the vehicle (Fig. 12-11). When used appropriately, the top anchor (tether) strap prevents the child from pitching forward in a crash. If the tether strap is not used, up to 90% of the restraint's protection is lost. Instructions for proper installation of the tether strap and permanent bracket are included with the car restraint. New child safety seats will have a hook, buckle, strap, or other connector that attaches to the anchorage. Seat belts will no longer be used to anchor child safety seats to newer vehicles. The first phase requires all new cars to have an upper anchorage. After fall 2002, all new cars were required to have the entire LATCH system.

Children with special needs may require a restraint system that secures them appropriately in the event of a crash. Ex-

*American Academy of Pediatrics, 141 Northwest Point Blvd., Elk Grove Village, IL 60007; (847) 434-4000; http://www.aap.org; and local division of traffic safety or National Highway Traffic Safety Administration, 1200 New Jersey Ave. SE, West Building, Washington, DC 20590; (888) 327-4236; http://www.nhtsa.dot.gov.

amples of such devices include car bed restraints for infants who cannot tolerate a semireclining position and specially adapted molded-plastic chairs for children who have spica casts.* The E-Z-On vest is a special safety harness for larger children with poor trunk control. Additional safety restraints and a listing of distributors are available at the SafetyBeltSafe U.S.A. website.† See also Chapter 9 for discussion of preterm infants being discharged home and car seat evaluation.

Other Car-Related Injuries. Injuries may also occur during sudden stops when objects are left unrestrained. On sudden impact, a loose ball becomes a projectile missile. Therefore all items should be secured or stored in the trunk or behind a barrier such as netting in vans and wagons.

Children older than 3 years of age are often involved in pedestrian traffic injuries. Because of their gross motor skills of walking, running, and climbing and their fine motor skills of opening doors and fence gates, they are likely to be in hazardous areas when unsupervised. Unaware of danger and unable to approximate the speed of a car, they are hit by moving vehicles. Running after a ball, riding a tricycle, and playing behind a parked car are common activities that may result in a vehicular tragedy.

Toddlers playing in driveways or farmyards are at risk of back-over injury from vehicles in reverse gear. From 2001 to 2003, 7475 children 1 to 14 years of age were involved in motor vehicle back-over (nonfatal) injuries; the highest incidence of injuries occurred in driveways or parking lots, and most children injured were pedestrians (as opposed to riding a bicycle or tricycle) (Centers for Disease Control and Prevention, 2005). A precaution when children are playing in driveways is attaching to the tricycle a pole with a bright flag that is high enough to be visible through an automobile's back window. Another safeguard is the use of a device that beeps when the vehicle is driven in reverse to alert children to the oncoming car, van, tractor, or truck. Some models now come equipped with rearview motion cameras so the driver can see the driveway clearly while backing out.

Preventing vehicular injuries involves protecting and educating children and adults about the danger of moved or parked vehicles. Children should never ride in the open back of a truck; the danger of falls can be compounded by another vehicle striking the child or by the truck rolling over. In addition, leaving children unsupervised in a parked vehicle, especially in a private driveway, provides an opportunity for the child to release the brake or put the car in gear. Children in bicycle-towed trailers or bicycle-mounted child seats can also be injured by collisions or falls.

One type of injury that has become more commonplace occurs when children crawl into an open trunk and pull it closed. Asphyxia may occur in such cases; therefore car trunks should not be left open when children are not being supervised. Some cars are equipped with a safety switch that can be activated from inside the trunk to open a closed trunk door.

Another automobile-related hazard for toddlers is overheating (hyperthermia) and subsequent death when left in a vehicle in hot weather (>27° C [80° F]). Small children dissipate heat poorly, and an increase in body temperature can cause death in a few hours. In 2003 a total of 42 children died as a result of overheating when left alone in a parked car; in 2004 the total number of child deaths was 35 (McLaren, Null, and Quinn, 2005). It is estimated that with the ambient temperature at 22° to 35.5° C (72° to 96° F), the vehicle interior temperature rises by 10.5° to 11° C (19° to 20° F) for each 10 minutes, even with a window cracked (Null, 2007). In a recent study of 171 child fatalities from overheating in a car, 50% of adults who left a child in a car either forgot or were unaware that the child was still in the car. A significant number of those children (32) were left by family members who intended to take the child to daycare but forgot the child in the car at the workplace; 22 children were left in the car by a daycare worker or driver (Guard and Gallagher, 2005). Parents are cautioned against leaving infants in a vehicle alone for *any reason*.

Preventing vehicular injuries involves protecting and educating children about the danger of moving or parked vehicles. Although preschool children are too young to be trusted to always obey, the parent should emphasize looking for moving vehicles before crossing the street, recognizing the stop and go colors of traffic lights, and following traffic officers' signals. Physical barriers limiting children from playing near vehicles help prevent these injuries. Most important, what is preached must be practiced. Children learn through imitation, and consistency reinforces learning.

Drowning

Drowning, not including drowning from water transportation, ranks second among boys and third among girls ages 1 to 4 years as a cause of accidental death. With well-developed skills of locomotion, toddlers are able to reach potentially dangerous areas, such as bathtubs, toilets, buckets, swimming pools, hot tubs, and ponds or lakes. The toddler's intense drive for exploration and investigation, combined with an unawareness of the danger of water and her or his helplessness in water, makes drowning always a viable threat. It is also one category of injury that results in death within minutes, diminishing the chance for rescue and survival. Close adult supervision of children when near any source of water is essential; many drownings in this age-group occur when a supervising adult becomes distracted. Teaching swimming and water safety can be helpful but cannot be regarded as sufficient protection. Pool fencing, although critical, does not always deter the fast-moving child (see Table 12-3).

Burns

Burns rank second among girls and third among boys in this age-group as a cause of accidental death. Toddlers' ability to climb, stretch, and reach objects above their head makes any hot surface a potential source of danger. Scalds from children pulling pots on top of themselves are a major source of burns. As a precaution, pot handles should be turned toward the back of the stove.

Other sources of heat, such as radiators, fireplaces, accessible furnaces, kerosene heaters, or wood-burning stoves, should have guards placed in front of them. Portable electric heaters must be placed in a high area, well out of reach of climbing young children. Hair curling irons may also be easily reached and can burn hands of curious toddlers.

Hot objects such as candles, incense, cigarettes, pots of tea or coffee, or irons must be placed away from children. The flame of a candle and the smoke of a cigarette invite investigation. Flame burns represent one of the most fatal types of burns and commonly occur when children play with matches

*Britax Hippo by Snug Seat.
†http://www.carseat.org.

FIG. 12-12 ■ Special plastic caps in electrical sockets prevent young fingers from exploring dangerous areas.

FIG. 12-13 ■ Children are most likely to ingest substances that are on their level, such as cleaning agents stored under sinks, rat poison, plants, or diaper pail deodorants.

and accidentally set themselves (and the home) on fire. To prevent flame burns, matches and lighters must be stored safely away from children, and parents need to teach children the dangers of playing with such objects. In addition, all homes, apartments, or any type of dwelling where people sleep should have smoke detectors installed to alert the occupants of a fire. A safety plan for immediate escape is also essential.

Electrical burns represent an immediate danger to children. Young toddlers may explore outlets with conductive articles and wires by mouthing them. Since water is an excellent conductor, the chance for a severe circumoral electrical burn is great. Electrical outlets should have protective guards plugged into them when not in use (Fig. 12-12) or be made inaccessible by having furniture placed in front of them when feasible.

Scald burns are the most common type of thermal injury in children. A scalding burn is often caused by high-temperature tap water, which children come in contact with as a result of turning on the hot-water faucet, falling into a bathtub of hot water, pulling hot pots onto themselves, or suffering deliberate abuse. Limiting household water temperatures to less than 49° C (120° F) is highly recommended. At this temperature it takes 10 minutes of exposure to the water to cause a full-thickness burn. Conversely, water temperatures of 54° C (130° F), the usual setting of most water heaters, expose household members to the risk of full-thickness burns within 30 seconds. Nurses can help prevent such burns by advising parents of this common household danger and recommending that they readjust the water heater to a safe temperature.

Sunburns are a year-round concern. Children spend a large amount of time outdoors. Their increased mobility makes it difficult to prevent sun exposure. Sunburn can be prevented by applying a sunscreen with a sun protection factor (SPF) of 15 or greater, dressing in protective clothing (wide-brimmed hat, protective cotton clothing with a tight weave), and avoiding sun exposure between 10 AM and 2 PM.

Poisoning

Toddlers are at the highest risk for poisoning. Mouthing activity continues to be prevalent after 1 year of age, and exploring objects by tasting them is part of children's curious investigation. The toddlers' curiosity and inability to understand logical consequences further place them at risk for ingesting harmful substances. Many household products, medications, and plants can be poisonous if swallowed, if in contact with the skin or eyes, or if inhaled (Shannon, 2000). Although in many instances poisoning does not result in death, it may cause significant morbidity, such as esophageal stricture from lye ingestion. Toddlers are able to climb most heights, open most drawers or closets, and unscrew most lids. By trial and error, younger children also manage to undo tops of bottles, plastic containers, aerosol cans, and jars, including those with child-resistant lids. Newer forms of drugs, such as transdermal patches and cough-suppressant lozenges, have created additional dangers, since they are not packaged with safety caps and the lozenges look like candy.

The major reason for poisoning is improper storage (Fig. 12-13). The guidelines suggested in Chapter 10 apply to children in this age-group as well. However, unlike the infant, who is confined to certain heights and unable to unlatch inventive locks, young children manage to find access to many high-level, tight-security places. For this age-group only a locked cabinet is safe.

Emergency and preventive measures for accidental poisoning are discussed in Chapter 14. Parents should have ready access to the telephone number for the poison control center and be prepared to act on the advice of the center.*

Falls

Falls are still a hazard to children in this age-group, although by the later part of early childhood, gross and fine motor skills are well developed, decreasing the incidence of falls down stairs or from chairs. However, playground injuries are common. Children need to be taught safety at play areas, such as no horseplay on high slides or jungle gyms, *sitting* on swings, and staying away from moving swings (Purvis and Hirsch, 2003). Passive prevention includes placement of grass, sand, or wood chips under play equipment. Swing seats should be made of plastic, canvas, or rubber and have smooth or rounded edges. Slides should have inclines of no more than 30 degrees, have evenly spaced rungs for climbing, and have protective "tunnels."

The climbing and running of the typical toddler are complicated by the child's total disregard and lack of appreciation for danger. Gates must be placed at both ends of stairs. Accessible windows must have window guards, not screens, to prevent falls to the ground below. Falling from open windows is a major cause of accidental death in urban, lower socioeconomic groups. Doors leading to stairwells or porches must be locked, since preschoolers can easily open them. A convenient type of lock is a sliding bar or hook that can be attached to the door and frame at a level higher than the child can reach; such locks also have safety clasps or devices that prevent children from being able to open them. Falls from balconies, porches, decks, and bleachers are all possible for the active toddler. Rails need to be sized appropriately, since most children younger than 6 years can slip through a 6-inch opening and none older than 1 year can usually pass through a 4-inch opening.

Cribs and vehicles are other sources of falls. To avoid injury, crib rails should be fully raised, the mattress should be kept at the lowest position, and toys or bumper pads that may be used as steps to climb out should be removed. Ideally, the floor under the crib should be carpeted. Once children reach a height of 89 cm (35 inches), they should sleep in a bed rather than a crib. If a bunk bed is selected, parents should be aware of possible dangers: falls from the top bed and from the ladder, and head entrapment between the mattress and guardrail or between the supporting mattress slats.

Children can fall from high chairs, shopping carts, carriages, car seats, and strollers if not properly restrained or because of a change in balance created by weighting the object down with heavy objects (Powell, Jovtis, and Tanz, 2002). Therefore proper restraint and adequate supervision are essential. Children, especially older infants who are mobile, should not be placed in an infant seat on top of a shopping cart, since the infant seat may fall off the cart; the safest place for an infant seat is inside the cart's bed.

---

*The national toll-free telephone number for poison control centers is (800) 222-1222. This number provides everyone in the United States with free access—24 hours a day, 7 days a week—to their regional poison center. For some tips on preventing poisoning in your home, see the TIPP slip, "Protect your Child . . . Prevent Poisoning," available at http://www.aap.org/family/poistipp.htm.

Aspiration and Suffocation

Foreign body aspiration is most common during the second year of life. Usually by 1 year of age children chew well, but they may have difficulty with large pieces of food, such as meat and whole hot dogs, and with hard foods, such as nuts. Young children cannot discard pits from fruit or bones from fish. It takes practice to learn how to chew gum without swallowing it. Gel snacks that are sealed in plastic wrappers can also be difficult to manage, and the plastic wrapper can be aspirated. Therefore parents must implement the same precautions as discussed for infants regarding food selection (see Chapter 10).

Play objects for toddlers must still be chosen with an awareness of danger from small parts. Large, sturdy toys without sharp edges or removable parts are safest. Small plastic toys such as Legos can cause choking or can be aspirated; such plastic items often do not appear on radiographic films. Balloons, coins, paper clips, pins, bells, button batteries, pull-tabs on cans, thumbtacks, nails, screws, jewelry (especially pierced earrings), and all types of pins are common household objects that can cause significant harm if swallowed or aspirated. Because of the danger of aspiration, parents should be taught emergency procedures for choking (see Airway Obstruction, Chapter 23).

Suffocation from causes seen during infancy is less frequent, but old refrigerators, ovens, and other large appliances are an ever-present threat. Toddlers can climb inside these appliances and, if they close the door behind them, can be trapped inside. Removing all doors before discarding or storing old appliances prevents such tragic deaths. Toddlers may also suffocate when unsafe toy box lids accidentally close on their head or neck

Hollow, semirigid, hemispherical or ellipsoidal objects can form suction and cupping around a small child's face, causing complete airway obstruction. Several different types of objects have been involved with such incidents, including toys, components of toys, and containers (Nakamura, Pollack-Nelson, and Chidekel, 2003).

Because some of the older heating systems and hot water heaters may emit carbon monoxide, which is undetectable by human smell, houses should have a carbon monoxide detector in addition to a smoke detector.

Bodily Damage

Toddlers are still clumsy in many of their skills and can seriously harm themselves when walking while holding a sharp or pointed object or having food or objects such as spoons in their mouths. Preventing such occurrences is the best approach with toddlers. With preschoolers, teaching safety is most important. The child should be taught that, when walking with a pointed object such as a knife or scissors, the pointed end is held away from the face. Dangerous garden or workshop equipment and all firearms should be stored in a locked cabinet (Crawley-Coha, 2002). Power lawn mowers and weed eaters are especially dangerous because they can throw rocks and other solid items (projectiles), and young children should not be allowed in an area where such tools are in use; nor should they be taken for a ride on a mower or allowed to operate the device (Robertson, 2003).

Safety education should include respect for firearms and their appropriate use including nonpowder guns, such as air guns, rifles (BB and pellet), and paintball guns, which can cause serious penetrating injuries (Darras, 2002; Laraque and Committee on Injury, Violence, and Poison Prevention, 2004). Firearm safety devices such as a trigger locks and personalized locks should be used to prevent unintentional firing of guns and subsequent injuries or fatalities (Meadows-Oliver, 2003). In addition, the child should be warned of and protected against potential danger from animals. (See Bodily Damage, Chapter 10; Animal Bites, Chapter 30.)

Household safety should be practiced and includes the usual precautions recommended for any age-group (see Family-Centered Care box: Child Safety Home Checklist, Chapter 10). An additional safeguard for young children is the use of safety glass in doors, windows, and tabletops and the application of decals on glassed doors or windows to reduce the likelihood of running through glass. Also, children should not be allowed to run, jump, wrestle, or play ball near glass structures.

Another cause of death by traumatic injury is electrically operated garage doors. Young children playing in the garage may become trapped under the door. Although the automatic doors (only available in models built since 1993) should reverse when striking an object, they may not do so when hitting a flexible object or one that is very close to the ground. Precautions include placing controls where they are inaccessible to children, such as high on a wall and in a locked car, and instructing children not to run under a closing garage door. Periodically the door should be checked to determine whether it returns after striking an object and whether the limit settings meet manufacturer recommendations. Additional safety precautions include having an automatic eye near ground level of the door frame, which prevents the door from closing when an object is detected at the door opening.

A discussion of bodily damage must also include alerting the parent to threats to the child's well-being from adults or other children who might take advantage of the toddler who cannot protect himself or herself. Because toddlers are often not able to verbalize emotions and feelings or may not understand inappropriate touching behavior by a family member or friend, it is important for parents to protect children by not leaving them in situations where there is a potential for bodily harm. The "stranger danger" concept is still important to teach, yet statistics show that personal harm more often comes from a relative or family friend who is not considered a stranger. Therefore it is important to discuss appropriate and inappropriate touching (what feels comfortable and what does not) in a manner that will not frighten or overwhelm the child. Child abductions can be prevented with close adult supervision; additional safeguards include screening for risk factors for missing children such as divorce, family discord, and substance abuse (American Academy of Pediatrics, 2004b). Encourage parents to have a current, high-quality picture of the child. The goal is not to induce fear about such events but to make nurses and parents aware so they can take steps to keep each child safe from bodily harm.

Terrorism and Violence

During a time of national conflict and struggle, terrorism, violence, and fear afflict young developing minds. Emergency preparedness and anticipatory guidance are the responsibility of all health care professionals. The immature emotional and physical developmental stage of toddlers makes them unable to distinguish reality from fantasy. Fears and anxiety can be exhibited in separation anxiety and sleep problems. Children who recently mastered toileting may develop secondary enuresis. Providing easy, clear answers to questions at an age-appropriate level and allaying children's fears foster security and comfort. Supporting a sense of control and developmentally appropriate activities, limiting television viewing, and ensuring a feeling of safety in home and community can assist children in coping with such crises. The websites for the American Academy of Pediatrics,* the U.S. Department for Homeland Security,† and the American Red Cross‡ offer a wealth of information for clinicians, families, and children.

ANTICIPATORY GUIDANCE—CARE OF FAMILIES

Understanding toddlers is fundamental to successful childrearing. Nurses, particularly those in ambulatory or child health centers, are in a favorable position to assist parents in facilitating the tasks and meeting the needs of children in this age-group. Prevention yields better results than treatment. Anticipatory guidance is paramount if one wishes to prevent future problems (see Family-Centered Care box).

Advice is sometimes not the sole answer. Actual assistance, such as being available for home visiting or telephone consulting, should be part of the nurse's flexible repertoire of interventions. Whether parents are experiencing the dilemmas of rearing a first or a subsequent child, they benefit from sharing their feelings, frustrations, and satisfactions. They need adult companionship, freedom from childrearing responsibilities, and periodic separations from their children. Part of a nurse's responsibility is to provide opportunities for parents to express their feelings and to meet their physical, mental, and spiritual needs.

*http://www.aap.org.
†http://www.dhs.gov/index.shtm.
‡http://www.redcross.org.

KEY POINTS

- The toddler stage, extending from 12 to 36 months, is a period of intense exploration of the environment.
- Biologic development during the toddler years is characterized by the acquisition of fine and gross motor skills that allow children to master a wide variety of activities.
- Although most of the physiologic systems are mature by the end of toddlerhood, development of certain areas of the brain is still occurring, allowing for greater intellectual capacity.
- Locomotion is the major gross motor skill acquired during toddlerhood, followed by increased eye-hand coordination.
- Specific tasks in the psychosocial development of a toddler include differentiating self from others, tolerating separation from parent, coping with delayed gratification, controlling bodily functions, acquiring socially acceptable behavior, communicating verbally, and interacting with others in a less egocentric manner.
- According to Erikson, the major developmental task of toddlerhood is acquiring a sense of autonomy while overcoming a sense of doubt and shame.

FAMILY-CENTERED CARE

Guidance During Toddler Years

AGES 12 TO 18 MONTHS

Prepare parents for expected behavioral changes of toddler, especially negativism and ritualism.

Assess present feeding habits and encourage gradual weaning from bottle and increased intake of solid foods.

Stress expected feeding changes of physiologic anorexia, food fads and strong taste preferences, need for scheduled routine at mealtimes, inability to sit through an entire meal, and lack of table manners.

Assess sleep patterns at night, particularly habit of a bedtime bottle, which is a major cause of dental caries, and procrastination behaviors that delay hour of sleep.

Prepare parents for potential dangers of the home, particularly motor vehicle injuries, poisoning, and falling injuries; give appropriate suggestions for safeproofing the home.

Discuss need for firm but gentle discipline and ways to deal with negativism and temper tantrums; stress positive benefits of appropriate discipline.

Emphasize importance for both child and parents of brief, periodic separations.

Discuss new toys that use developing gross and fine motor, language, cognitive, and social skills.

Emphasize need for dental supervision, types of basic dental hygiene at home, and food habits that predispose to caries; stress importance of supplemental fluoride.

AGES 18 TO 24 MONTHS

Stress importance of peer companionship in play.

Explore need for preparation for additional sibling; stress importance of preparing child for new experiences.

Discuss present discipline methods, their effectiveness, and parents' feelings about child's negativism; stress that negativism is important aspect of developing self-assertion and independence and is not a sign of spoiling.

Discuss signs of readiness for toilet training; emphasize importance of waiting for physical and psychologic readiness.

Discuss development of fears, such as darkness or loud noises, and of habits, such as security blanket or thumb sucking; stress normalcy of these transient behaviors.

Prepare parents for signs of regression in time of stress.

Assess child's ability to separate easily from parents for brief periods under familiar circumstances.

Allow parents to express their feelings of weariness, frustration, and exasperation; be aware that it is often difficult to love toddlers at times when they are not asleep!

Point out some of the expected changes of the next year, such as longer attention span, somewhat less negativism, and increased concern for pleasing others.

AGES 24 TO 36 MONTHS

Discuss importance of imitation and domestic mimicry and need to include child in activities.

Discuss approaches toward toilet training, particularly realistic expectations and attitude toward accidents.

Stress uniqueness of toddlers' thought processes, especially through their use of language, poor understanding of time, causal relationships in terms of proximity of events, and inability to see events from another's perspective.

Stress that discipline still must be structured and concrete and that relying solely on verbal reasoning and explanation leads to injuries, confusion, and misunderstanding.

Discuss investigation of preschool or daycare center toward completion of second year.

■ In Piaget's sensorimotor and preoperational phases of development, the toddler experiments by incorporating the old learning of secondary circular reactions with new skills and applies this knowledge to new situations. There is the beginning of rational judgment, an understanding of causal relationships, and discovery of objects as objects. Preoperational thought is characterized by egocentricism, centration, global organization of thought processes, animism, and irreversibility.

■ Language is the major cognitive achievement in toddlerhood.

■ The most striking characteristic of language development during early childhood is the increasing level of comprehension.

■ Development of body image occurs with increasing motor ability, at which point toddlers recognize the importance and capacity of body parts.

■ The two phases of differentiation of self from significant others are separation and individuation.

■ Parental concerns during the toddler years include toilet training, coping with sibling rivalry, limit setting and discipline, dealing with temper tantrums, negativism, and regression.

■ Effective discipline techniques for toddlers include reward, ignoring or extinction, and time-out.

■ Nutrition is important at this stage because eating habits established in toddlerhood tend to have long-term effects.

■ Regular dental examinations, fluoride supplementation, removal of plaque, and provision of a low-cariogenic diet promote optimum dental health.

■ Because of increased locomotion, toddlers are at high risk for sustaining injuries. Fatal injuries are primarily a result of motor vehicle accidents, drownings, and burns.

REFERENCES

Agran PF, Anderson C, Winn D, and others: Rates of pediatric injuries by 3-month intervals for children 0 to 3 years of age, *Pediatrics* 111(6 Pt 1): e683-e692, 2003.

Allen RE, Myers AL: Nutrition in toddlers, *Am Fam Physician* 74(9):1527-1532, 1533-1534, 2006.

American Academy of Pediatric Dentistry: Guideline on infant oral health care. In *AAPD reference manual 2005-2006,* 2006, retrieved Jan 11, 2008, from http://www.aapd.org/media/Policies_Guidelines/G_InfantOralHealthCare.pdf.

American Academy of Pediatrics: *Car safety seats: a guide for families 2007,* 2007, retrieved Aug 1, 2007, from http://www.aap.org/family/carseatguide.htm.

American Academy of Pediatrics, Committee on Nutrition: *Pediatric nutrition handbook,* ed 5, Elk Grove Village, Ill, 2004a, The Academy.

American Academy of Pediatrics: The pediatrician's role in the prevention of missing children, *Pediatrics* 114(4):1100-1105, 2004b.

American Academy of Pediatrics: Prevention of rickets and vitamin D deficiency: new guidelines for vitamin D intake, *Pediatrics* 111(4):908-910, 2003.

American Academy of Pediatrics, Committee on Public Health: Children, adolescents, and television, *Pediatrics* 107(2):423-426, 2001.

American Heart Association: *Dietary recommendations for children,* 2005, retrieved Jan 3, 2008, from http://www.americanheart.org/presenter.jhtml?identifier=3033999.

Bates E, Dick F: Language, gesture, and the developing brain, *Dev Psychobiol* 40:293-310, 2002.

Brazelton TB: How to help parents of young children: the touchpoints model, *J Perinatol* 19(6 pt 2):S6-S7, 1999.

Cathey M, Gaylord N: Picky eating: a toddler's continuing approach to mealtime, *Pediatr Nurs* 30(2):101-107, 2004.

Centers for Disease Control and Prevention: Nonfatal motor-vehicle-related backover injuries among children—United States, 2001-2003, *MMWR* 54(06):144-146, 2005.

Crawley-Coha T: Childhood injury: a status report, part 2, *J Pediatr Nurs* 17(2):133-138, 2002.

Dahlquist LM, Busby SM, Slifer KJ, and others: Distraction for children of different ages who undergo repeated needle sticks, *J Pediatr Oncol Nurs* 19(1):22-34, 2002.

Darras KM: Firearm safety: an essential primary care issue, *Adv Nurs Pract* 10(2):51-54, 2002.

DeLamater J, Friedrich WN: Human sexual development, *J Sex Res* 39(1):10-14, 2002.

Dowd DM, Keenan HT, Bratton SL: Epidemiology and prevention of childhood injuries, *Crit Care Med* 30(11):S385-S392, 2002.

Durbin DR, Chen I, Smith R, and others: Effects of seating position and appropriate restraint use on the risk of injury to children in motor vehicle crashes, *Pediatrics* 115(3):e305-e309, 2005.

Elkins M, Cavendish R: Developing a plan for pediatric spiritual care, *Holistic Nurs Pract* 18(4):179-184, 2004.

Fosarelli P: Children and the development of faith: implications for pediatric practice, *Contemp Pediatr* 20(1):85-98, 2003.

Glassy D, Romano J, and Committee on Early Childhood, Adoption, and Dependent Care: Selecting appropriate toys for young children: the pediatrician's role, *Pediatrics* 111(4):911-913, 2003.

Guard A, Gallagher SS: Heat related deaths in young children in parked cars: an analysis of 171 fatalities in the United States, 1995-2002, *Inj Prev* 11(1):33-37, 2005.

Harpaz-Rotem I, Bergman A: On an evolving theory of attachment: rapprochement-theory of a developing mind, *Psychoanal Study Child* 61:170-189, 2006.

Henary B, Sherwood CP, Crandall JR, and others: Car safety for children: rear facing for best protection, *Inj Prev* 13(6):398-402, 2007.

Howard BJ, Wong J: Sleep disorders, *Pediatr Rev* 22(10):327-342, 2001.

Laraque D, Committee on Injury, Violence, and Poison Prevention: Injury risk of nonpowder guns, *Pediatrics* 114(5):1357-1361, 2004.

McLaren C, Null J, Quinn J: Heat stress from enclosed vehicles: moderate ambient temperatures cause significant temperature rise in enclosed vehicles, *Pediatrics* 116(1):e109-e112, 2005.

Meadows-Oliver M: Firearm safety devices, *J Pediatr Health Care* 17(3):157-158, 2003.

Mercer R: Treating nocturnal enuresis, *Adv Nurs Pract* 11(2):26-31, 2003.

Meyer TL: Unveiling the secrecy behind masturbation, *Pediatr Rev* 23(4):148-149, 2002.

Morin K: Infant nutrition: toddlers: start off on the right foot, *MCN* 32(2):122, 2007.

Nakamura SW, Pollack-Nelson C, Chidekel AS: Suction-type suffocation incidents in infants and toddlers, *Pediatrics* 111(1):e12-e16, 2003.

Needlman R, Howard B, Zuckerman B: Helping parents get beyond the terrible 2's, *Patient Care* 29(1):52-61, 1995.

Null J: *Hyperthermia deaths of children in vehicles,* 2007, San Francisco State University, retrieved July 2007 from http://www.ggweather.com/heat.

Petitto LA, Katerlos M, Levy BG, and others: Bilingual signed and spoken language acquisition from birth: implications for the mechanisms underlying early bilingual language acquisition, *J Child Lang* 28(2):453-496, 2001.

Powell EC, Jovtis E, Tanz RR: Incidence and description of stroller related injuries to children, *Pediatrics* 110(5):e62, 2002.

Purvis JM, Hirsch SA: Playground injury prevention, *Clin Orthop* 409:11-19, 2003.

Robertson WW: Power lawnmower injuries, *Clin Orthop* 409:37-42, 2003.

Roehlkepartain EC, King PE, Wagener LM, and others, editors: *The handbook of spiritual development in childhood and adolescence,* Thousand Oaks, Calif, 2006, Sage.

Schmitt BD: Toilet training: getting it right the first time, *Contemp Pediatr* 21(3):105-108, 111-112, 115-116, 2004.

Schnitzer PG: Prevention of unintentional childhood injuries, *Am Fam Physician* 74(11):1864-1869, 2006.

Schum TR, Kolb TM, McAuliffe TL, and others: Sequential acquisition of toilet-training skills: a descriptive study of gender and age differences in normal children, *Pediatrics* 109(3):e48, 2002.

Shannon M: Ingestion of toxic substances by children, *N Engl J Med* 342(3):186-191, 2000.

Stein MT: Difficult behavior: temper tantrums to conduct disorders. In Rudolph CD, Rudolph AM, Hostetter MK, editors: *Rudolph's pediatrics,* ed 21, New York, 2003, McGraw-Hill.

Stephenson M: Danger in the toy box, *J Pediatr Health Care* 19(3):187-189, 2005.

Thompson RA: Caring for infants and toddlers, *Future Child* 11(1):21-33, 2001.

US Department of Agriculture: *Steps to a healthier you: MyPyramid,* retrieved June 2007 from http://www.mypyramid.gov/index.html.

13

Health Promotion of the Preschooler and Family

REBECCA A. MONROE

CHAPTER OUTLINE

PROMOTING OPTIMAL GROWTH AND DEVELOPMENT, 438
Biologic Development, 438
  Gross and Fine Motor Skills, 438
Psychosocial Development, 438
  Developing a Sense of Initiative (Erikson), 438
Cognitive Development, 439
  Preoperational Phase (Piaget), 439
Moral Development, 439
  Preconventional or Premoral Level (Kohlberg), 439

Spiritual Development, 439
Development of Body Image, 440
Development of Sexuality, 440
Social Development, 440
  Language, 440
  Personal-Social Behavior, 440
  Play, 441
Coping with Concerns Related to Normal Growth and Development, 442
  Preschool and Kindergarten Experience, 442
  Sex Education, 443

Fears, 446
Stress, 446
Aggression, 447
Speech Problems, 447
PROMOTING OPTIMAL HEALTH DURING THE PRESCHOOL YEARS, 447
Nutrition, 447
Sleep and Activity, 448
  Sleep Problems, 449
Dental Health, 450
Injury Prevention, 450
Anticipatory Guidance—Care of Families, 450

LEARNING OBJECTIVES

On completion of this chapter the reader will be able to:
- Identify the major biologic, psychosocial, cognitive, moral, spiritual, and social developments that occur during the preschool years.
- List the benefits of imaginary playmates.
- Prepare preschoolers for preschool or daycare experience.

- Provide parents with guidelines for sex education.
- Provide parents with guidelines for dealing with a child's fears, stresses, aggression, and sleep problems.
- Recognize the causes of stuttering during the preschool years.

- Offer parents suggestions for preventing speech problems.
- Recognize feeding patterns of preschoolers.
- Provide anticipatory guidance to parents regarding injury prevention based on the preschooler's developmental achievements.

RELATED TOPICS and ADDITIONAL RESOURCES

 IN TEXT

Cognitive Development (Piaget), *Ch. 5*
Injury Prevention, *Ch. 10*
Limit Setting and Discipline, *Ch. 3*
School Phobia, *Ch. 17*
Sibling Rivalry, *Ch. 12*
Television, *Ch. 5*
Working Mothers, *Ch. 3*

 Companion CD

Case Study—Sleep Problems
Critical Thinking Exercise—Imitative Play
NCLEX Review Questions
Pediatric Assessment Video Clips

evolve

evolve.elsevier.com/Wong/essentials/

NCLEX Review Questions
Pediatric Assessment Video Clips
WebLinks

 WONG'S CLINICAL MANUAL OF PEDIATRIC NURSING, 7th Ed

Sleep Assessment, *p. 139*

PROMOTING OPTIMAL GROWTH AND DEVELOPMENT

The combined biologic, psychosocial, cognitive, spiritual, and social achievements during the **preschool period** (3 to 5 years of age) prepare preschoolers for their most significant change in lifestyle: entrance into school. Their control of bodily functions, experience of brief and prolonged periods of separation, ability to interact cooperatively with other children and adults, use of language for mental symbolization, and increased attention span and memory prepare them for the next major period: the school years. Successful achievement of previous levels of growth and development is essential for preschoolers to refine many of the tasks that were mastered during the toddler years.

BIOLOGIC DEVELOPMENT

The rate of physical growth slows and stabilizes during the preschool years. The average **weight** is 14.5 kg (32 pounds) at 3 years, 16.7 kg (36.8 pounds) at 4 years, and 18.7 kg (41.5 pounds) at 5 years. The average weight gain per year remains approximately 2 to 3 kg (4.5 to 6.5 pounds).

Growth in **height** also remains steady, with a yearly increase of 6.5 to 9 cm (2.5 to 3.5 inches), and generally occurs by elongation of the legs rather than of the trunk. The average height is 95 cm (37.5 inches) at 3 years, 103 cm (40.5 inches) at 4 years, and 110 cm (43.5 inches) at 5 years.

Physical proportions no longer resemble those of the squat, pot-bellied toddler. The preschooler is slender but sturdy, graceful, agile, and posturally erect. There is little difference in physical characteristics according to gender, except as dictated by such factors as dress and hairstyle.

Most organ systems can adjust to moderate stress and change. During this period, most children are toilet trained. For the most part, motor development consists of increases in strength and refinement of previously learned skills, such as walking, running, and jumping. However, muscle development and bone growth are still far from mature. Excessive activity and overexertion can injure delicate tissues. Good posture, appropriate exercise, and adequate nutrition and rest are essential for optimal development of the musculoskeletal system.

Gross and Fine Motor Skills

Walking, running, climbing, and jumping are well established by age 36 months. Refinement in eye-hand and muscle coordination is evident in several areas. At age 3, the preschooler rides a tricycle, walks on tiptoe, balances on one foot for a few seconds, and broad jumps. By age 4, the child skips and hops proficiently on one foot (Fig. 13-1) and catches a ball reliably. By age 5, the child skips on alternate feet, jumps rope, and begins to skate and swim.

Fine motor development is evident in the child's increasingly skillful manipulation, such as in drawing and dressing. These skills provide readiness for learning and independence for entry into school.

PSYCHOSOCIAL DEVELOPMENT
Developing a Sense of Initiative (Erikson)

After preschoolers have mastered the tasks of the toddler period, they are ready to face the developmental endeavors of the preschool period. Erikson maintained that the chief psychosocial task of this period is acquiring a sense of **initiative**.

FIG. 13-1 ▪ A 4-year-old child has sufficient balance to stand or hop on one foot.

🌐 CULTURAL AWARENESS

Learning Sociocultural Mores

Developing a conscience implies learning the sociocultural mores of the family's heritage. Depending on the type of attitudes conveyed, children will learn not only appropriate behaviors, but also tolerant, biased, or prejudicial values concerning their ethnic, religious, and social background and those of other groups. Much of this influence may remain dormant until they associate with children or adults of a different heritage. Then, depending on the particular group, they may be accepted or ostracized for their attitudes.

Children are in a stage of energetic learning. They play, work, and live to the fullest and feel a real sense of accomplishment and satisfaction in their activities. Conflict arises when children overstep the limits of their ability and inquiry and experience a sense of **guilt** for not having behaved appropriately. Feelings of guilt, anxiety, and fear may also result from thoughts that differ from expected behavior.

A particularly stressful thought is wishing one's parent dead. As a sense of rivalry or competition develops between the child and same-sex parent, the child may think of ways to get rid of the interfering parent. In most situations, this rivalry is resolved when the child strongly identifies with the same-sex parent and peers during the school years. However, if that parent dies before the identification process is completed, the preschooler may be overwhelmed with feelings of guilt for having wished and therefore "caused" the death. Clarifying for children that wishes cannot and do not make events occur is essential in helping them overcome their guilt and anxiety.

Development of the **superego,** or **conscience,** begins toward the end of the toddler years and is a major task for preschoolers (see Cultural Awareness box). Learning right from wrong and good from bad is the beginning of morality (see Moral Development).

COGNITIVE DEVELOPMENT

One of the tasks related to the preschool period is readiness for school and scholastic learning. Many of the thought processes of this period are crucial for achieving such readiness, and it is intentional that the child begins school between ages 5 and 6 rather than at an earlier age.

Preoperational Phase (Piaget)

Piaget's cognitive theory does not include a period specifically for children who are 3 to 5 years old. The **preoperational phase** covers the age span from 2 to 7 years and is divided into two stages: the **preconceptual phase,** ages 2 to 4, and the phase of **intuitive thought,** ages 4 to 7. One of the main transitions during these two phases is the shift from totally egocentric thought to social awareness and the ability to consider other viewpoints. However, egocentricity is still evident. (For a review of the characteristics of preoperational thought, see Chapter 12.)

Language continues to develop during the preschool period. Speech remains primarily a vehicle of egocentric communication. Preschoolers assume that everyone thinks as they do and that a brief explanation of their thinking makes the entire thought understood by others. Because of this self-referenced, egocentric verbal communication, it is often necessary to explore and understand the young child's thinking through other, nonverbal approaches. For children in this age-group, the most enlightening and effective method is **play,** which becomes the child's way of understanding, adjusting to, and working out life's experiences.

Preschoolers increasingly use language without comprehending the meaning of words, particularly concepts of right and left, causality, and time. Children may use the concepts correctly but only in the circumstances in which they have learned them. For example, they may know how to put on shoes by remembering that the buckle is always on the outside of the foot. However, if different shoes have no buckles, they cannot reason which shoe fits which foot. In other words, they do not understand the concept of *right and left.*

Superficially, **causality** resembles logical thought. Preschoolers explain a concept as they heard it described by others, but their understanding is limited. An example is the concept of time. Because **time** is still incompletely understood, the child interprets it according to his or her own frame of reference, such as "A long time means until Christmas." Consequently, time is best explained in relationship to an event, such as "Your mother will visit you after you finish your lunch." Avoiding words such as *yesterday, tomorrow, next week,* or *Tuesday* to express when an event is expected to occur and instead associating time with expected daily events help children learn about temporal relationships while increasing their trust in others' predictions.

Preschoolers' thinking is often described as **magical thinking.** Because of their egocentrism and transductive reasoning, they believe that thoughts are all-powerful. Such thinking places them in the vulnerable position of feeling guilty and responsible for bad thoughts, which may coincide with the

occurrence of a wished event. Their inability to logically reason the cause and effect of illness or an injury makes it especially difficult for them to understand such events.

> **NURSING ALERT**
>
> Counseling children whose parents are going through a divorce or separation should involve a discussion with the child about her or his role. Because of magical thinking, the child may believe he or she wished the other parent away. The child should be reassured that this is not the case.

Preschoolers believe in the power of words and accept their meaning literally. An example of this type of thinking is calling children "bad" because they did something wrong. In the preschooler's mind, calling them bad means they are a bad person; thus it is better to say that their actions were bad by saying, for example, "That was a bad thing to do."

MORAL DEVELOPMENT
Preconventional or Premoral Level (Kohlberg)

Young children's development of moral judgment is at the most basic level. They have little, if any, concern about why something is wrong. They behave because of the freedom or restriction that is placed on actions. In the **punishment and obedience orientation,** children (ages about 2 to 4 years) judge whether an action is good or bad depending on whether it results in reward or punishment. If children are punished for it, the action is bad. If they are not punished, the action is good, regardless of the meaning of the act. For example, if parents allow hitting, the child will perceive that hitting is good because it is not associated with punishment.

From approximately 4 to 7 years of age, children are in the stage of **naive instrumental orientation,** in which actions are directed toward satisfying their needs and, less frequently, the needs of others. They have a concrete sense of justice and fairness during this period of development.

SPIRITUAL DEVELOPMENT

Children's knowledge of faith and religion is learned from significant others in their environment, usually from parents and their religious beliefs and practices (Fosarelli, 2003). However, young children's understanding of spirituality is influenced by their cognitive level. Preschoolers have a concrete concept of a God with physical characteristics, often like an imaginary friend. They understand simple Bible stories and memorize short prayers, but their understanding of the meaning of these rituals is limited. Preschoolers benefit from concrete representations of religious practices, such as picture Bible books and small statues, such as those of the Nativity scene. They will imitate the religious practices of their parents without fully understanding the significance of these acts.

Development of the conscience is strongly linked to spiritual development. At this age, children are learning right from wrong and behaving correctly to avoid punishment. Wrongdoing provokes feelings of guilt, and preschoolers often misinterpret illness as a punishment for real or imagined transgressions. It is important that children view God as one who bestows unconditional love, rather than as a judge of good or bad behavior. Observing religious traditions and participating in a religious community can help children cope during stressful periods, such as illness, hospitalization, and other traumatic events (Barnes, Plotnikoff, Fox, and others, 2000).

In many religious faiths, cultural practices and religion are closely intertwined (McEvoy, 2003) and are an important part of the child's and family's life (see Box 4-2).

DEVELOPMENT OF BODY IMAGE

The preschool years play a significant role in the development of body image. With increasing comprehension of language, preschoolers recognize that individuals have undesirable and desirable appearances. They recognize differences in skin color and racial identity and are vulnerable to learning prejudices and biases. They are aware of the meaning of words such as *pretty* or *ugly,* and they reflect the opinions of others regarding their own appearance. By 5 years of age, children compare their size with that of their peers and can become conscious of being large or short, especially if others refer to them as "so big" or "so little" for their age. In one study, negative associations between weight status and self-concept were identified in girls as young as 5 years of age (Davison and Birch, 2001).

Despite the advances in body image development, preschoolers have poorly defined body boundaries and little knowledge of their internal anatomy. Intrusive experiences are frightening, especially those that disrupt the integrity of the skin, such as injections and surgery. They fear that if their skin is "broken," all of their blood and "insides" can leak out. Therefore bandages are critical to "keep everything from coming out."

DEVELOPMENT OF SEXUALITY

Sexual development during these years is an important phase in a person's overall sexual identity and beliefs. Preschoolers are forming strong attachments to the opposite-sex parent while identifying with the same-sex parent. **Sex-typing,** or the process by which an individual develops the behavior, personality, attitudes, and beliefs appropriate for his or her culture and sex, occurs through several mechanisms during this period. Probably the most powerful mechanisms are childrearing practices and imitations. Gender identification is a result of complex prenatal and postnatal psychologic factors, as well as biologic or genetic factors, and that most children are aware of their gender and the expected sets of related behaviors by 1½ to 2½ years of age.

As sexual identity develops beyond gender recognition, modesty may become a concern. Sex-role imitation and "dressing up" like Mommy or Daddy are important activities. Attitudes and responses of others to role-playing can condition the child to views of self or others. For example, comments such as "Boys shouldn't play with dolls" can influence a boy's self-concept of masculinity.

Sexual exploration may be more pronounced now than ever before, particularly in terms of exploring and manipulating the genitalia. Questions about sexual reproduction may come to the forefront in the preschooler's search for understanding (see Sex Education, p. 443, and in Chapter 15).

SOCIAL DEVELOPMENT

During the preschool period, the **separation-individuation process** is completed. Preschoolers have overcome much of the anxiety associated with strangers and the fear of separation of earlier years. They relate to unfamiliar people easily and tolerate brief separations from parents with little or no protest. However, they still need parental security, reassurance, guidance, and approval, especially when entering preschool or elementary school. Prolonged separation, such as that imposed by illness and hospitalization, is difficult, but preschoolers respond to anticipatory preparation and concrete explanation. They can cope with changes in daily routine much better than toddlers, although they may develop more imaginary fears. Preschoolers gain security and comfort from familiar objects, such as toys, dolls, or photographs of family members. They are able to work through many of their unresolved fears, fantasies, and anxieties through play, especially if guided with appropriate play objects (e.g., dolls, puppets) that represent family members, health care professionals, and other children.

Language

During the preschool years, language becomes more sophisticated and complex. Both cognitive ability and environment—particularly, consistent role models—influence vocabulary, speech, and comprehension. Language becomes a major mode of communication and social interaction, and its development during the preschool period sets the stage for later success in school (Needlman, 2004) (Fig. 13-2). Vocabulary increases dramatically, from 300 words at age 2 to more than 2100 words at the end of 5 years. Sentence structure, grammatical usage, and intelligibility also advance to a more adult level. Through language, preschool children learn to express feelings of frustration or anger without acting them out.

Children between the ages of 3 and 4 years form sentences of about three or four words and include only the most essential words to convey a meaning. Such speech is often termed **telegraphic** for its brevity. Three-year-old children ask many questions and use plurals, correct pronouns, and the past tense of verbs. They name familiar objects, such as animals, parts of the body, relatives, and friends. They can give and follow simple commands. They talk incessantly, regardless of whether anyone is listening or answering them. They enjoy musical or talking toys or dolls and imitate new words proficiently.

From ages 4 to 5 years, preschoolers use longer sentences of four or five words and use more words to convey a message, such as prepositions, adjectives, and a variety of verbs. They follow simple directional commands, such as "Put the ball on the chair," but can carry out only one request at a time. They answer questions such as "What do you do when you are hungry?" by describing the appropriate action. The pattern of asking questions is at its peak, and children will usually repeat a question until they receive an answer.

By age 6, children can use all parts of speech correctly, except for deviations from the rule. They can define simple things by describing their use, shape, or general category of classification, rather than simply describing their outward appearance. For example, they define a ball as "round," "something you bounce," or "a toy," rather than only describing its color. They can give some opposites, such as "If Mommy is a woman, Daddy is a man." They can also describe an object according to its composition, such as "A spoon is made of metal."

Personal-Social Behavior

The pervasive ritualism and negativism of toddlerhood gradually diminish during the preschool years. Although self-assertion is still a major theme, preschoolers demonstrate

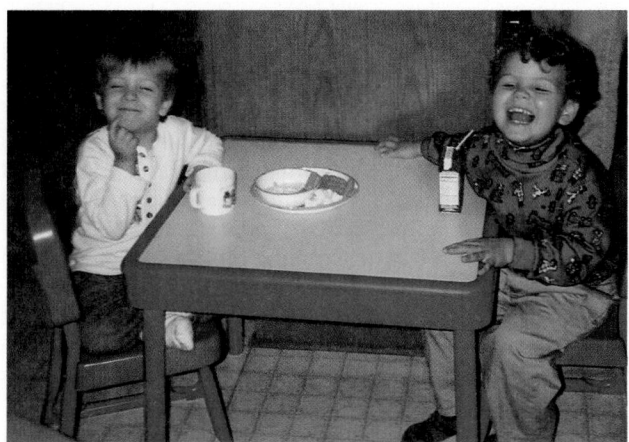

FIG. 13-2 ■ Preschool children enjoy friends and often use nonverbal messages to communicate.

FIG. 13-3 ■ Most preschoolers are able to dress themselves but need help with more difficult items of clothing.

their sense of autonomy differently. They are able to verbalize their request for independence and perform independently because of their much-refined physical and cognitive development. By 4 or 5 years of age, they need little if any assistance with dressing, eating, or toileting (Fig. 13-3). They can also be trusted to obey warnings of danger, although 3- or 4-year-old children may exceed their boundaries at times.

They are also much more sociable and willing to please. They have internalized many of the standards and values of the family and culture. However, by the end of early childhood they begin to question parental values and compare them with those of their peer group and other authority figures. As a result, they may be less willing to abide by the family's code of conduct. Preschoolers become increasingly aware of their position and role within the family. Although this is a more secure age for experiencing the addition of another sibling, relinquishing the position of only or youngest is still difficult and requires special parental attention to prevent feelings of desertion and resentment (Brazelton and Sparrow, 2001) (see Sibling Rivalry, Chapter 12).

Play

Various types of play are typical of this period, but preschoolers especially enjoy **associative play**—group play in similar or identical activities but without rigid organization or rules. Play should provide for physical, social, and mental development.

Play activities for physical growth and refinement of motor skills include jumping, running, and climbing. Tricycles, wagons, gym and sports equipment, sandboxes, wading pools, and activities at water parks can help develop muscles and coordination (Fig. 13-4). Activities such as swimming and skating teach safety as well as muscle development and coordination. Children involved in the work of play do not require expensive toys and gadgets to keep them entertained but often enjoy playing with common household items such as a broom handle or even items adults consider junk (boxes, sticks, rocks, and dirt). The imaginative mind of the preschooler enjoys playing for play's sake.

Manipulative, constructive, creative, and educational toys provide for quiet activities, fine motor development, and self-expression. Easy construction sets, large blocks of various sizes and shapes, a counting frame, alphabet or number flash

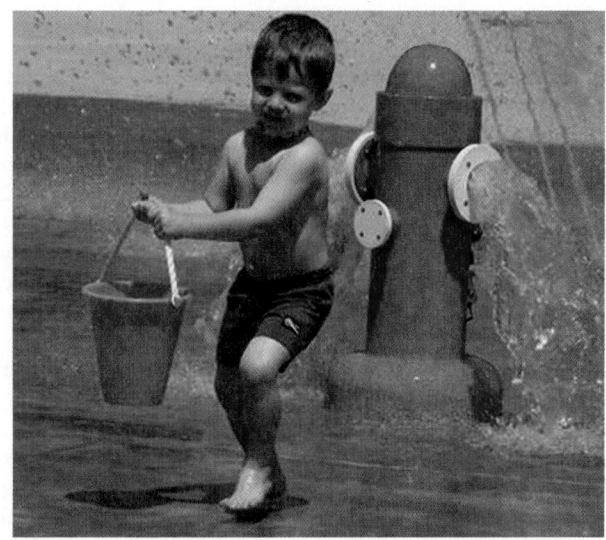

FIG. 13-4 ■ Preschoolers enjoy play activities that promote motor skills such as jumping and running. Water play is an exciting activity for preschoolers.

cards, paints, crayons, simple carpentry tools, musical toys, illustrated books, simple sewing or handicraft sets, large puzzles, and clay are suitable toys. Electronic games and computer programs are especially valuable in helping children learn basic skills, such as letters and simple words.

Probably the most characteristic and pervasive preschool activity is **imitative, imaginative,** and **dramatic play.** Dress-up clothes, dolls, housekeeping toys, dollhouses, play store toys, telephones, farm animals and equipment, village sets, trains, trucks, cars, planes, hand puppets, and medical kits

FIG. 13-5 ■ Imaginative and imitative play is typical of preschoolers.

provide hours of self-expression (Fig. 13-5). Probably at no other time is the reproduction of adult behavior so faithful and absorbing as in 4- and 5-year-old children. Toward the end of the preschool period, children are less satisfied with make-believe or pretend objects and enjoy doing the actual activity, such as cooking and carpentry.

Television and videos also have their place in children's play, although each should be only one part of children's total repertoire of social and recreational activities. Parents and other caregivers should supervise the selection of programs, watch and discuss programs with their children, schedule limited time for television viewing, and set a good example of television viewing (Yalçin, Türul, Naçar, and others, 2002; American Academy of Pediatrics, 2001a). Children also enjoy and learn from educational programs; however, television viewing may limit time spent in other meaningful activities such as reading, physical activity, and socialization (American Academy of Pediatrics, 2001a).

Television can become an interactive activity when adults view programs with children and discuss program content. In one study, viewing educational programs as preschoolers was associated with higher grades, more book reading, greater emphasis on achievement, increased creativity, and less aggression in adolescent years (Anderson, Huston, Schmitt, and others, 2001). The researchers emphasize that the content of television viewing appeared more important than the amount viewed.

Play is so much a part of the young child's life that reality and fantasy become blurred. Make-believe is reality during play and only becomes fantasy when the toys are put away or the dress-up clothes are removed. It is no wonder that **imaginary playmates** are so much a part of this age period. The appearance of imaginary companions usually occurs between ages 2½ and 3 years, and for the most part, such playmates are relinquished when the child enters school. The birth order and number of siblings may influence the creation of imaginary companions, with firstborn and only children being more likely to create imaginary playmates (Gleason, Sebanc, and Hartup, 2000).

Imaginary companions serve many purposes: they become friends in times of loneliness, they accomplish what the child is still attempting, and they experience what the child wants to forget or remember. It is not unusual for the "friend" to have myriad vices and to be blamed for wrongdoing. Sometimes the child hopes to escape punishment by saying, "My friend George broke the glass." At other times, the child may fantasize that the companion misbehaved and play the role of the parent. This becomes a way of assuming control and authority in a safe situation.

Parents often worry about the imaginary playmates, not realizing how normal and useful they are. Parents need to be reassured that the child's fantasy is a sign of health that helps differentiate make-believe and reality. Parents can acknowledge the presence of the imaginary companion by calling him or her by name and even agreeing to simple requests such as setting an extra place at the table, but they should not allow the child to use the playmate to avoid punishment or responsibility. For example, if the child blames the companion for messing up a room, parents need to state clearly that the child is the only one they see; therefore the child is responsible for cleaning up.

Children also benefit from play that occurs between them and a parent. **Mutual play** fosters development from birth through the school years and provides enriched opportunities for learning. Through mutual play, parents can provide tactile and kinesthetic experiences, can maximize verbal and language abilities, and can offer praise and encouragement for exploration of the world. In addition, mutual play encourages positive interactions between the parent and child, strengthening their relationship.*

Table 13-1 summarizes the major developmental achievements for children 3, 4, and 5 years of age.

COPING WITH CONCERNS RELATED TO NORMAL GROWTH AND DEVELOPMENT
Preschool and Kindergarten Experience

Some children are home schooled, but many children attend some type of early childhood program, usually preschool or a daycare center. Group care has become commonplace with the large number of parents currently employed outside the home (see Alternate Child Care Arrangements, Chapter 10). The effects of early education and stimulation on children have increasingly gained recognition. (For a discussion of the effects of daycare on young children, see Working Mothers, Chapter 3.) Because social development widens to include age-mates and other significant adults, preschool provides an excellent vehicle for expanding children's experiences with others. It is also excellent preparation for entrance into elementary school.

In preschool or daycare centers, children are exposed to opportunities for learning group cooperation; adjusting to sociocultural differences; and coping with frustration, dissatisfaction, and anger. If activities are tailored to provide mastery and achievement, children increasingly have feelings of success, self-confidence, and personal competence. Whether structured learning is imposed is less important than the social climate, type of guidance, and attitude toward the chil-

---

*Recommended books for suggestions on mutual play include *Quick and Fun Learning Activities* books, by Teacher Created Resources, 6421 Industry Way, Westminster, CA 92683; (800) 662-4321; http://www.teachercreated.com.

dren that is fostered by the teacher or leader. With a teacher who is aware of preschoolers' developmental abilities and needs, children will learn from the activity that is provided. Most programs incorporate a daily schedule of quiet play, active outdoor activity, group activities such as games and projects, creative or free play, and snack and rest periods. Preschool is particularly beneficial for children who lack a peer-group experience, such as an only child, and for children from impoverished homes.

One of the issues that parents face is the child's readiness for preschool or kindergarten. There are no absolute indicators for school readiness, but the child's social maturity, especially attention span, is as important as his or her academic readiness. Using a developmental screening tool that addresses cognitive (especially language), social, and physical milestones can identify children who may benefit from diagnostic testing and early intervention programs before starting school. Parents play an integral role in their children's school readiness. They should promote a positive attitude toward learning, read to their children, encourage their children to participate in a variety of activities to explore their talents, and choose appropriate child care or preschool programs (Jellinek, Patel, and Froehle, 2002).

Nurses and other health care workers can guide parents in selecting enriched social and educational early intervention programs, schools, and child care centers. Careful selection of early childhood education is intrinsic to future learning and development. Licensed and regulated programs are mandated to abide by established standards, which represent minimum requirements and safeguards. Regulation is important to protect children from harm and to promote the conditions essential for a child's healthy development and learning. The National Association for the Education of Young Children serves as the model for optimal care of small children.*

Areas for parents to evaluate include the facility's daily program, teacher qualifications, staff-to-student ratio, discipline policy, environmental safety precautions, provision of meals, sanitary conditions, adequate indoor and outdoor space per child, and fee schedule. References from other parents help in evaluating a facility, but personal observation of the facility is recommended. Encourage parents to meet the director and some of the employees at a few facilities to make an informed choice.

Evaluation of the facility's health practices is extremely important. Children in daycare centers have more illnesses than children not in daycare centers, especially gastrointestinal tract infections; respiratory tract infections; and hepatitis A, varicella-zoster virus, and cytomegalovirus infections (Rafanello, 2001). Nurses play an important role in infection control. Not only can they advise parents regarding the evaluation of a facility's sanitary practices, but they can also take an active part in educating staff in measures to minimize transmission of infection (Fig. 13-6).

Children need preparation for the preschool or kindergarten experience. For young children it represents a change from

---

*Information about accreditation criteria and procedures of the NAEYC Academy for Early Childhood Program Accreditation is available from the National Association for the Education of Young Children, 1313 L St. NW, Suite 500, Washington, DC 20005; (800) 424-2460 or (202) 232-8777; http://www.naeyc.org. These criteria are excellent guidelines for evaluating preschools or daycare centers.

FIG. 13-6 ■ Thorough hand washing is the single most effective method of preventing infection.

their usual home environment and prolonged separation from parents. Before children begin school, parents should present the idea as exciting and pleasurable. Talking to children about activities such as painting, building with blocks, or enjoying swings and other outdoor equipment allows children to fantasize about the forthcoming event in a positive manner. When the first day of school arrives, parents should behave confidently. Such behavior requires parents to have resolved their own feelings regarding the experience.

Parents should introduce their child to the teacher and the facility. In some instances, it is helpful for parents to remain with the child for at least part of the first day until the child is comfortable and at ease. Other specific actions that can help reduce separation anxiety include providing the school with detailed information about the child's home environment, such as familiar routines, favorite activities, food preferences, names of siblings or pets, and personal habits. Such information helps the child feel familiar in the strange surroundings. When schools automatically request this information, the parent has a valuable clue to evaluating the quality of the program because the request represents the staff's awareness of each child's needs. Transitional objects, such as a favorite toy, may also help the child bridge the gap from home to school.

Sex Education

Preschoolers have assimilated a tremendous amount of information during their short lifetimes. Although their thinking may not be mature, they search constantly for explanations and reasons that are logical and reasonable to them. The word "why" seems to supplant the word "no," which was common in toddlerhood. It is only natural that as they learn about "me," they will also want to know "why me" and "how me." Questions such as "Where do babies come from?" are as casual as "What makes it rain?" or "Who is that?" It is the *way* in

TABLE 13-1
Growth and Development During Preschool Years

PHYSICAL	GROSS MOTOR	FINE MOTOR	LANGUAGE
AGE 3 YEARS			
Usual weight gain of 1.8-2.7 kg (4-6 pounds) Average weight of 14.5 kg (32 pounds) Usual gain in height of 7.5 cm (3 inches) per year Average height of 95 cm (37.5 inches) May have achieved nighttime control of bowel and bladder	Rides tricycle Jumps off bottom step Stands on one foot for a few seconds Goes up stairs using alternate feet; may still come down using both feet on step Broad jumps May try to dance, but balance may not be adequate	Builds tower of 9-10 cubes Builds bridge with three cubes Adeptly places small pellets in narrow-necked bottle In drawing, copies a circle, imitates a cross, names what has been drawn; cannot draw stick figure but may make circle with facial features	Has vocabulary of about 900 words Uses primarily telegraphic speech Uses complete sentences of three or four words Talks incessantly regardless of whether anyone is paying attention Repeats sentence of six syllables Asks many questions Can prepare simple meals, such as cold cereal and milk
AGE 4 YEARS			
Pulse and respiration rates decrease slightly Growth rate is similar to that of previous year Average weight of 16.7 kg (36.8 pounds) Average height of 103 cm (40.5 inches) Length at birth is doubled Maximum potential for development of amblyopia	Skips and hops on one foot Catches ball reliably Throws ball overhead Walks down stairs using alternate footing	Uses scissors successfully to cut out picture following outline Can lace shoes but may not be able to tie bow In drawing, copies a square, traces a cross and diamond, adds three parts to stick figure	Has vocabulary of 1500 words or more Uses sentences of four or five words Questioning is at peak Tells exaggerated stories Knows simple songs May be mildly profane if associates with older children Obeys four prepositional phrases, such as *under, on top of, beside, in back of,* or *in front of* Names one or more colors Comprehends analogies, such as, "If ice is cold, fire is _____."
AGE 5 YEARS			
Pulse and respiration rates decrease slightly Average weight of 18.7 kg (41.5 pounds) Average height of 110 cm (43.5 inches) Eruption of permanent dentition may begin Handedness is established (about 90% are right-handed)	Skips and hops on alternate feet Throws and catches ball well Jumps rope Skates with good balance Walks backward with heel to toe Jumps from height of 12 inches and lands on toes Balances on alternate feet with eyes closed	Ties shoelaces Uses scissors, simple tools, or pencil very well In drawing, copies a diamond and triangle; adds seven to nine parts to stick figure; prints a few letters, numbers, or words, such as first name	Has vocabulary of about 2100 words Uses sentences of six to eight words, with all parts of speech Names coins (e.g., nickel, dime) Names four or more colors Describes drawing or pictures with much comment and enumeration Knows names of days of week, months, and other time-associated words Knows composition of articles, such as "A shoe is made of _____." Can follow three commands in succession

which questions about procreation are answered that conditions children, even the youngest, to separate these questions from others about their world.

Two rules govern answering sensitive questions about topics such as sex. The first is to *find out what children know and think.* By investigating the theories children have produced as a reasonable explanation, parents can not only give correct information, but also help children understand why their explanation is inaccurate. Another reason for ascertaining what the child thinks before offering any information is that the "unasked for" answer may be given. For example, 4-year-old Sally asked her father, "Where did I come from?" Both parents quickly took this inquiry as a clue for offering sex education. After the explanation, Sally exclaimed, "I don't know about all

SOCIALIZATION	COGNITION	FAMILY RELATIONSHIPS
Dresses self almost completely if helped with back buttons and told which shoe is right or left Pulls on shoes Has increased attention span Feeds self completely Can help to set table; can dry dishes without breaking any May have fears, especially of dark and going to bed Knows own gender and gender of others Play is parallel and associative; begins to learn simple games, but often follows own rules; begins to share	Is in preconceptual phase Is egocentric in thought and behavior Has beginning understanding of time; uses many time-oriented expressions, talks about past and future as much as about present, pretends to tell time Has improved concept of space, as demonstrated by understanding of prepositions and ability to follow directional command Has beginning ability to view concepts from another perspective	Attempts to please parents and conform to their expectations Is less jealous of younger sibling; may be opportune time for birth of additional sibling Is aware of family relationships and sex-role functions Boys tend to identify more with father or other male figure Has increased ability to separate easily and comfortably from parents for short periods
Very independent Tends to be selfish and impatient Aggressive physically as well as verbally Takes pride in accomplishments Has mood swings Shows off dramatically, enjoys entertaining others Tells family tales to others with no restraint Still has many fears Play is associative Imaginary playmates are common Uses dramatic, imaginative, and imitative devices Sexual exploration and curiosity demonstrated through play, such as being "doctor" or "nurse"	Is in phase of intuitive thought Causality is still related to proximity of events Understands time better, especially in terms of sequence of daily events Unable to conserve matter Judges everything according to one dimension, such as height, width, or order Immediate perceptual clues dominate judgment Is beginning to develop less egocentrism and more social awareness May count correctly but has poor mathematic concept of numbers Obeys because parents have set limits, not because of understanding of right or wrong	Rebels if parents expect too much, such as impeccable table manners Takes aggression and frustration out on parents or siblings Do's and don'ts become important May have rivalry with older or younger siblings; may resent older sibling's privileges and younger sibling's invasion of privacy and possessions May "run away" from home Identifies strongly with parent of opposite sex Is able to run simple errands outside the home
Less rebellious and quarrelsome than at age 4 years More settled and eager to get down to business Not as open and accessible in thoughts and behavior as in earlier years Independent but trustworthy, not foolhardy; more responsible Has fewer fears; relies on outer authority to control world Eager to do things right and to please; tries to "live by the rules" Has better manners Cares for self totally, occasionally needing supervision in dress or hygiene Not ready for concentrated close work or small print because of slight farsightedness and still unrefined eye-hand coordination Play is associative; tries to follow rules but may cheat to avoid losing	Begins to question what parents think by comparing them with age-mates and other adults May notice prejudice and bias in outside world Is more able to view other's perspective, but tolerates differences rather than understanding them May begin to show understanding of conservation of numbers through counting objects regardless of arrangement Uses time-oriented words with increased understanding Very cautious about factual information regarding world	Gets along well with parents May seek out parent more often than at age 4 years for reassurance and security, especially when entering school Begins to question parents' thinking and principles Strongly identifies with parent of same sex, especially boys with their fathers Enjoys activities such as sports, cooking, and shopping with parent of same sex

that! All I know is Mary came from New York, and I want to know where I was born."

The second rule for giving information is to *be honest*. It is true that much of the correct information will be forgotten or misunderstood by the preschooler, but the correct information can be restated until the child absorbs and comprehends the facts. Even though the correct anatomic words may be hard to

pronounce or even more difficult to remember, they become foundational content for explaining other concepts later on.

Honesty does not imply imparting to children every fact of life or allowing excessive permissiveness in sexual curiosity. When children ask one question, they are looking for one answer. When they are ready, they will ask about the other "unfinished" parts of the story. Sooner or later they will wonder how the "sperm meets the egg" and "how the baby gets out," but during this period, it is best to wait until they ask.

Regardless of whether children are given sex education, they will engage in games of sexual curiosity and exploration. At about 3 years of age, children are aware of the anatomic differences between the sexes and are concerned with how the other "works." This is not really "sexual" curiosity because many children are still unaware of the reproductive function of the genitalia. Their curiosity is for the eliminative function of the anatomy. Little boys wonder how girls can urinate without a penis, so they watch girls go to the bathroom. Because they cannot see anything but the stream of urine coming out, they want to observe further. "Doctor play" is often a game invented for just such investigation. Little girls are no less curious about boys' anatomy. It is intriguing to closely inspect this "thing" that girls do not have.

One question that parents often have is how to handle such sexual curiosity. A positive approach is to neither condone nor condemn the sexual curiosity but to express that if children have questions, they should ask the parents; the parents should then encourage them to engage in some other activity. In this way, children can be helped to understand that there are ways that their sexual curiosity can be satisfied other than through playing investigative games. This in no way condemns the act but stresses alternate methods to seek solutions and answers. Allowing children unrestricted permissiveness only intensifies their anxiety and concern, since exploring and searching usually yield little evidence to satisfy their curiosity.

Many excellent books on sex education are available for preschool children at public libraries. The Sexuality Information and Education Council of the United States,* local chapters of the Planned Parenthood Federation of America,† and the American Academy of Pediatrics‡ have bibliographies of suggested reading material. Parents should read the book themselves *before* giving or reading it to a child.

Another concern for some parents is **masturbation,** or self-stimulation of the genitalia. This occurs at any age for a variety of reasons and, if not excessive, is normal and healthy. It is most common at 4 years of age and during adolescence. For preschoolers, it is a part of sexual curiosity and exploration. If parents are concerned about their children masturbating, it is essential for nurses to investigate the circumstances associated with the activity because it may be an expression of anxiety, boredom, or unresolved conflicts. Children who openly and publicly masturbate are inviting a reaction, such as discipline, punishment, or criticism. They may be overwhelmed by their sexual feelings and are asking others to help them channel them into more constructive outlets. Masturbation, like other forms of sex play, is a private act, and parents should emphasize this to children when teaching them socially acceptable behavior.

Fears

A great number and variety of real and imagined fears are present during the preschool years, including fear of the dark, being left alone (especially at bedtime), animals (particularly large dogs), ghosts, sexual matters (castration), and objects or persons associated with pain. The exact cause of children's fears is unknown. Parents often become perplexed about handling the fears because no amount of logical persuasion, coercion, or ridicule will send away the ghosts, boogeymen, monsters, and devils. Inappropriate television viewing by preschoolers may increase fears and anxieties because of the inability to separate reality-based experiences from fantasy portrayed on television.

The concept of **animism,** ascribing lifelike qualities to inanimate objects, helps explain why children fear objects. For example, a child may refuse to use the toilet after watching a television commercial in which the toilet bowel is portrayed as turning into a monster and swallowing a child.

Preschoolers also experience fear of annihilation. Because of poorly defined body boundaries and improved cognitive abilities, young children develop concerns related to loss of body parts. They fear losing body parts with certain medical procedures such as an intravenous insertion or cast application on a limb and may see these procedures as real threats to their existence.

The best way to help children overcome their fears is by actively involving them in finding practical methods to deal with the frightening experience. This may be as simple as keeping a night-light on in the child's bedroom for assurance that no monsters lurk in the dark. Exposing children to the feared object in a safe situation also provides a type of conditioning, or **desensitization.** For instance, children who are afraid of dogs should never be forced to approach or touch one, but they may be gradually introduced to the experience by watching other children play with the animal. This type of modeling, with others demonstrating fearlessness, can be effective if the child is allowed to progress at his or her own rate.

Usually by 5 or 6 years of age, children relinquish many of their fears. Explaining the developmental sequence of fears and their gradual disappearance may help parents feel more secure in handling preschoolers' fears. Sometimes fears do not subside with simple measures or developmental maturation. When children experience severe fears that disrupt family life, professional help is required.

Stress

Although for parents the preschool years generally are less troublesome than toddlerhood, this period of life presents children with many unique stresses. Some, such as fears, are innate and stem from preschoolers' unique understanding of the world. Others are imposed, such as beginning school. Although minimal amounts of stress are beneficial during the early years to help children develop effective coping skills, excessive stress is harmful. Young children are especially vulnerable because of their limited capacity to cope. Expression of frustration, fear, or anxiety is hampered by inadequate expressive language.

To help parents deal with stress in their child's life, they must be aware of signs of stress (see Stress in Childhood, Chapter 5) and be helped to identify the source. Any number of stressors may be present, such as the birth of a sibling, marital discord, divorce and separation, relocation, or illness.

The best approach to dealing with stress is prevention—monitoring the amount of stress in children's lives so that levels do not exceed their coping ability. In many instances, struc-

*130 W. 42nd St., Suite 350, New York, NY 10036; (212) 819-9770; fax: (212) 819-9776; http://www.siecus.org.
†434 W. 33rd St., New York, NY 10001; (212) 541-7800 or (800) 230-7526; fax: (212) 245-1845; http://www.plannedparenthood.org.
‡American Academy of Pediatrics, 141 Northwest Point Blvd., Elk Grove Village, IL 60007; (888) 227-1770; fax: (847) 228-1281; http://www.aap.org.

turing children's schedules to allow rest and preparing them for change, such as entering school, are sufficient measures.

Aggression

The term **aggression** refers to behavior that attempts to hurt a person or destroy property. Aggression differs from anger, which is a temporary emotional state, but anger may be expressed through aggression. Hyperaggressive behavior in preschoolers is characterized by unprovoked physical attacks on other children and adults, destruction of others' property, frequent intense temper tantrums, extreme impulsivity, disrespect, and noncompliance. Aggression is influenced by a complex set of biologic, sociocultural, and familial variables. Factors that tend to increase aggressive behavior are gender, frustration, modeling, and reinforcement.

Evidence indicates that gender differences exist and that boys are more aggressive than girls (Bendersky, Bennett, and Lewis, 2006). **Frustration,** or the continual thwarting of self-satisfaction by disapproval, humiliation, punishment, or insults, can lead children to act out against others as a means of release. Especially if they fear their parents, these children will displace their anger on others, particularly peers and other authority figures. This type of aggression often applies to the child who is well behaved at home but a discipline problem at school or a bully among playmates.

Modeling, or imitating the behavior of significant others, is a powerful influencing force in preschoolers. Children who see their parents as physically abusive are observing behavior that they come to know as acceptable and therefore may exhibit this behavior with others (Gershoff, 2002). Another aspect of modeling is the "double standard" for acceptable conduct. For example, in some families, aggression is synonymous with masculinity, and boys are encouraged to defend themselves. Television is also a significant source for modeling at this age. Numerous studies have found a positive correlation between viewing violent programs and developing aggression; therefore parents need encouragement to supervise programs viewed by their preschool children, especially those with aggressive tendencies (Brown and Hamilton-Giachritsis, 2005). The American Academy of Pediatrics (2001a) offers a list of recommendations for healthy television viewing.

Reinforcement can also shape aggressive behavior. Sometimes the reward for aggression is negative (e.g., punishment), yet reinforcing because it brings attention. For example, children who are ignored by a parent until they hit a sibling or the parent learn that this act garners attention.

When children exhibit extreme behaviors, such as aggression, parents may be concerned about the need for professional help. Generally, the difference between "normal" and "problematic" behavior is not the behavior itself but its **quantity** (number of occurrences), **severity** (interference with social or cognitive functioning), **distribution** (different manifestations), **onset** (when behavior started), and **duration** (at least 4 weeks).*

Speech Problems

The most critical period for speech development occurs between 2 and 4 years of age. During this period, children are using their rapidly growing vocabulary faster than they can produce the words. Failure to master sensorimotor integrations results in **stuttering** or **stammering** as children try to say the word they are already thinking about. This dysfluency in speech pattern is a *normal* characteristic of language development in children ages 2 to 5 years, affects boys more frequently, and usually resolves during childhood (National Institute on Deafness and Other Communication Disorders, 2002). When parents or other significant persons place undue emphasis on a child's dysfluency, an abnormal speech pattern may develop. The National Institute on Deafness and Other Communication Disorders (2002) encourages parents and caregivers of children who stutter to speak slowly and clearly, refrain from correcting or criticizing the child's speech, resist completing the child's sentences, and take time to listen attentively.

The best therapy for speech problems is prevention and early detection. Common causes of speech problems are hearing loss, developmental delay, autism, and lack of verbal or psychosocial stimulation (Feldman, 2005). Referral for further evaluation and treatment may be necessary to prevent a problem from interfering with learning. Anticipatory preparation of parents for expected developmental norms may allay caregiver concerns.

Children pressured into producing sounds ahead of their developmental level may develop **dyslalia** (articulation problems) or revert to using infantile speech. Prevention involves educating parents regarding the usual achievement of speech production during childhood. The **Denver Articulation Screening Exam** is an excellent tool for assessing articulation skills in the child and for explaining to parents the expected progression of sounds (see Appendix A).

PROMOTING OPTIMAL HEALTH DURING THE PRESCHOOL YEARS*

NUTRITION

Nutritional requirements for preschoolers are fairly similar to those for toddlers (Story, Holt, and Sofka, 2002). The requirement for calories per unit of body weight continues to decrease slightly to 90 kcal/kg, for an average daily intake of 1800 calories. Fluid requirements may also decrease slightly to approximately 100 ml/kg/day but depend on the activity level, climatic conditions, and state of health. Protein requirements increase with age, and the recommended intake for preschoolers is 13 to 19 g/day (0.45 to 0.67 oz/day) (Food and Nutrition Board, 2003).

The American Academy of Pediatrics recommends the following fat intake levels for children over the age of 2 years: saturated fatty acid consumption should be less than 10% of total caloric intake, and total fat over several days should be no more than 30% and no less than 20% of total caloric intake (Kleinman, 2004). Evidence is increasing that the incidence of coronary heart disease, obesity, and chronic health problems such as diabetes mellitus can be influenced by early eating patterns (Barlow and Expert Committee, 2007). Research supports the efficacy of limiting fat intake, and negative health effects have not been reported (Johnson, 2000). Preschoolers may have a decreased fat intake with substitutes such as soy-enriched foods without affecting overall food taste, energy, and nutrient value (Endres, Barter, Theodora, and others,

---

*Information on child development and behavior can be obtained through Developmental Behavioral Pediatrics Online, http://www.dbpeds.org.

*For a more comprehensive understanding, the reader is urged to review Promoting Optimal Health During Toddlerhood, Chapter 12.

2003). Parents and others who provide soy substitutes should ensure that the products are vitamin enriched and low in fat content (Endres, Barter, Theodora, and others, 2003).

It is important that all diets contain adequate nutrients such as calcium. The recommendation for daily calcium intake for children 1 to 3 years of age is 500 mg, and the recommendation for children 4 to 8 years of age is 800 mg (Food and Nutrition Board, 2003). Milk and dairy products are excellent sources of calcium and vitamin D (fortified). Low-fat milk may be substituted so the quantity of milk may remain the same while limiting fat intake overall.

Excessive consumption of fruit juices has been associated with adverse health effects such as dental caries and gastrointestinal symptoms; therefore the American Academy of Pediatrics (2001c) recommends limiting the intake of fruit juice to 4 to 6 oz/day for children ages 1 to 6 years. Parents should be educated regarding nonnutritious fruit drinks, which usually contain less than 10% fruit juice, yet are often advertised as healthy and nutritious; sugar content is dramatically increased and often precludes an adequate intake of milk by the child. While counseling parents regarding moderation in fruit juice consumption, providers should offer suggestions for more appropriate sources of nutrients such as ascorbic acid, folate, and potassium. In young children, intake of carbonated beverages that are acidic or that contain high amounts of sugar is also known to contribute to dental caries; large amounts of nonnutritive calories in such beverages may also displace or preclude intake of nutrients necessary for growth.

MyPyramid for Kids is appropriate for preschoolers (see Chapter 6 and Fig. 11-1). This new system is comprehensive and applicable to children as young as 2 years of age. The foods depicted are those commonly eaten by children in this age-group, and the illustrations emphasize the importance of physical activity. Parents and caregivers can provide opportunities for children to learn to like a variety of nutritious foods by exposing them to these foods. The importance of role-modeling by parents cannot be overemphasized in regard to food intake and dietary habits; if the parent will not eat a particular food or if their dietary habits are poor, children are likely to develop the same habits.

> **NURSING ALERT**
> Obesity has increased over the past several decades in young children. Efforts to provide a healthy diet and to encourage physical activity should begin early to help children achieve optimal health (Spear, Barlow, Ervin, and others, 2007; Johnson, 2000).

Some preschoolers still have food habits that are typical of toddlers, such as food fads and strong taste preferences. When children reach 4 years of age, they seem to enter another period of finicky eating, which is generally characteristic of the more rebellious behavior of children in this age-group. As with the toddler, small portions should be offered of each item being served. The practice of having the child remain at the table until the "plate is clean" should be avoided because this may contribute to overeating and the development of poor eating habits that contribute to poor health later in life. By age 5 years, children are more agreeable to trying new foods, especially if they are encouraged by an adult who allows them to help with food preparation or experiment with a new taste or different dish (Fig. 13-7). Mealtimes can become battle-

FIG. 13-7 ■ Preschool-age children enjoy helping adults and are more likely to try new foods if they can assist in the preparation.

grounds if parents expect perfect table manners.* Usually the 5-year-old child is ready for the "social" side of eating, but the 3- or 4-year-old child still has difficulty sitting quietly through a long family meal.

The amount and variety of foods consumed by young children vary greatly from day to day. Consequently, parents sometimes worry about the quantity and quality of food preschoolers consume. In general, the quality is much more important than the quantity, a fact that should be stressed during nutritional counseling.

One way to lessen parental concern is advising parents to keep a weekly record of everything the child eats. In particular, the parents can measure the amount of food, such as setting aside a half cup of vegetables and serving the child from this premeasured amount, to provide a more accurate estimate of food intake at each meal. When parents look at the food chart at the end of the week, they are usually amazed by how much the child has consumed. In general, preschoolers consume only slightly more than toddlers, or about half an adult's portion.

SLEEP AND ACTIVITY

Sleep patterns vary widely, but the average preschooler sleeps about 12 hours a night and infrequently takes daytime naps. Waking during the night is common throughout early childhood and may be related to social rather than developmental factors (Thiedke, 2001). Motor activity levels continue to be high and allow preschoolers to explore their environment, begin learning physical games and sports, and interact with others. Sedentary activities, such as television and video or computer games, are increasingly appealing and can become an unhealthy substitute for active play.

Preschoolers' increased gross motor abilities and coordination allow them to engage in many physical activities, if only at a novice level. Whether young children should begin formalized training in an activity at this early age is controversial. Training programs must consider the child's physical and psychologic immaturity, and readiness to participate in organized

---
*An excellent resource for parents related to mealtimes with toddlers and preschoolers is Satter E: *How to get your kid to eat . . . but not too much,* Palo Alto, Calif, 1987, Bull Publishing.

TABLE 13-2

Comparison of Nightmares to Sleep Terrors

NIGHTMARES	SLEEP TERRORS
DESCRIPTION	
A scary dream; takes place during rapid eye movement (REM) sleep and is followed by full waking	A partial arousal from very deep (state IV, non-REM) sleep
TIME OF DISTRESS	
After the dream is over, child wakes and cries or calls, not during the nightmare itself	During the terror itself, child screams and thrashes; afterward is calm
TIME OF OCCURRENCE	
In the second half of the night, when dreams are most intense	Usually 1-4 hours after falling asleep, when non-REM sleep is deepest
CHILD'S BEHAVIOR	
Crying in younger children, fright in all; these behaviors persist even though the child is awake	Initially child may sit up, thrash, or run in a bizarre manner, with eyes bulging, heart racing, and profuse perspiring; may cry, scream, talk, or moan; there is apparent fright, anger, or obvious confusion, which disappears when child is fully awake
RESPONSIVENESS TO OTHERS	
Is aware of and reassured by another's presence	Is not very aware of another's presence, is not comforted, and may push person away and scream and thrash more if held or restrained
RETURN TO SLEEP	
May be considerably delayed because of persistent fear	Usually rapid; often difficult to keep child awake
DESCRIPTION OF DREAM	
Yes (if old enough)	No memory of a dream or of yelling or thrashing
INTERVENTIONS	
Accept dream as real fear. Sit with child; offer comfort, assurance, and sense of protection. Avoid taking child to own bed. Consider professional counseling for recurrent nightmares unresponsive to above approaches.	Observe child for a few minutes, *without interfering,* until child becomes calm or wakes fully. Intervene only if necessary to protect child from injury. Guide child back to bed if needed. Stress to parents that sleep terrors are a normal, common phenomenon in preschoolers that require relatively little intervention.

Modified from Ferber R: *Solve your child's sleep problems,* New York, 1985, Simon & Schuster.

sports should be determined individually. The decision to participate should be based on the child's, not the parent's, motivation and enjoyment. The American Academy of Pediatrics (2001b) encourages free play and a variety of physical activities; however, the academy also supports organized play when it is developmentally appropriate and occurs in a nonthreatening, fun, and safe environment.

Sleep Problems

The preschool years are a prime time for sleep disturbances. As toddlers and preschoolers cope with autonomy, separation, and object permanence, they begin to have more sleep problems (Thiedke, 2001). Some have trouble going to sleep, especially after so much activity and stimulation during the day. Others may develop bedtime fears, wake during the night, or have nightmares or sleep terrors. Still others may prolong the inevitable through elaborate rituals.

Recommendations for handling a sleep disturbance are offered only *after* a thorough assessment of the problem. Cultural traditions may dictate sleep practices that are contrary to certain well-accepted professional recommendations; therefore parents may not perceive a particular sleep practice as a problem (see Cultural Awareness box in Chapter 10, p. 349).

Interventions differ greatly; for example, **nightmares** (frightening dreams that are followed by full arousal) and **sleep terrors** (partial arousal from deep, nondreaming sleep) require different approaches (Table 13-2).

For children who delay going to bed, a recommended approach involves counseling parents about the importance of a consistent bedtime ritual and emphasizing the normalcy of this type of behavior in young children. Parents should ignore attention-seeking behavior and not take the child into the parents' bed or allow the child to stay up past a reasonable hour. Other measures that may be helpful include keeping a light on in the room, providing transitional objects such as a favorite toy, or leaving a drink of water by the bed.

Helping children slow down *before* bedtime also reduces the resistance to going to bed. One strategy is to establish limited rituals that signal readiness for bed, such as a bath or story. Parents can reinforce the pattern by stating, "After this story, it is bedtime," and consistently carrying out the routine. If anticipated extra stimulation, such as having visitors arrive at bedtime, disrupts this routine, it is advisable to settle children in bed beforehand. Television viewing before bedtime may cause bedtime resistance and delay sleep.

DENTAL HEALTH

By the beginning of the preschool period, the eruption of the deciduous (primary) teeth is complete. Dental care is essential to preserve these temporary teeth and to teach good dental habits (see Chapter 12). Although preschoolers' fine motor control is improved, they still require assistance and supervision with brushing, and flossing should be performed by parents. Professional care and prophylaxis, especially fluoride supplements (if needed), should be continued. Routine dental care should be well established during preschool years and is recommended at 6- to 12-month intervals depending on the family history, the child's dental development, and the presence or absence of dental caries (Martof, 2001). For children cared for away from home, parents should be encouraged to monitor the dental care provided by others, including minimizing cariogenic foods in the diet. Trauma to teeth during this period is not uncommon, and prompt evaluation by a dentist is warranted if oral trauma occurs. Preservation of the space previously occupied by an avulsed tooth is necessary for proper eruption of the secondary tooth.

INJURY PREVENTION

Because of improved gross and fine motor skills, coordination, and balance, preschoolers are less prone to falls than are toddlers. They tend to be less reckless; listen more to parental rules; and are aware of potential dangers, such as hot objects, sharp instruments, and dangerous heights. Putting objects in the mouth as part of exploration has all but ceased, although accidental poisoning is still a danger. Pedestrian motor vehicle injuries increase because of activities such as playing in the parking lot, driveway, or street; riding tricycles, bicycles, and other play vehicles; running after balls; or forgetting safety regulations when crossing streets.

In general, the guidelines suggested for injury prevention in Table 12-3 apply to children in this age-group as well. However, emphasis is now on **education** concerning safety and potential hazards, in addition to appropriate protection. This period is an excellent time to start enforcing the use of safety items such as bicycle helmets to prevent head trauma; children are less likely to warm to the idea later in life because of peer pressure. Because preschoolers are great imitators, it is essential that parents set a good example by "practicing what they preach." Children quickly observe discrepancies in what they are told to do and what they see others do. Establishing habits at this time, such as wearing protective equipment, can create long-term safety behaviors.

ANTICIPATORY GUIDANCE—CARE OF FAMILIES

The preschool years present fewer childrearing difficulties than do earlier years, and this stage of development is facilitated by appropriate anticipatory guidance in the areas already discussed (see Family-Centered Care box). There is a shift in childrearing practices from protection to education. Whereas injury prevention previously focused on safeguarding the immediate environment, with less emphasis on reasoning, now the protective guardrails or electrical outlet caps

---

FAMILY-CENTERED CARE

Guidance During Preschool Years

AGE 3 YEARS

Prepare parents for child's increasing interest in widening relationships.

Encourage enrollment in preschool.

Emphasize importance of setting limits.

Prepare parents to expect exaggerated tension-reduction behaviors, such as need for a "security blanket."

Encourage parents to offer child choices.

Prepare parents to expect marked changes at 3½ years, when child becomes insecure, and exhibits emotional extremes.

Prepare parents for normal dysfluency in speech and advise them to avoid focusing on the pattern.

Prepare parents to expect extra demands on their attention as a reflection of child's emotional insecurity and fear of loss of love.

Warn parents that the equilibrium of a 3-year-old will change to the aggressive, out-of-bounds behavior of a 4-year-old.

Inform parents to anticipate a more stable appetite with more food selections.

Stress need for protection and education of child to prevent injury (see Injury Prevention, Chapter 12).

AGE 4 YEARS

Prepare parents for more aggressive behavior, including motor activity and offensive language.

Prepare parents to expect resistance to parental authority.

Explore parental feelings regarding child's behavior.

Suggest some type of respite for primary caregivers, such as placing child in preschool for part of the day.

Prepare parents for child's increasing sexual curiosity.

Emphasize the importance of realistic limit setting on behavior and appropriate disciplinary techniques.

Prepare parents for the highly imaginative 4-year-old who indulges in "tall tales" (to be differentiated from lies) and develops imaginary playmates.

Prepare parents to expect nightmares or an increase in them.

Provide reassurance that a period of calmness begins at 5 years of age.

AGE 5 YEARS

Inform parents to expect a tranquil period at 5 years of age.

Help parents prepare children for entrance into school environment.

Make certain that immunizations are up to date before child enters school.

Suggest that unemployed parental caregivers consider own activities when children begin school.

Suggest swimming lessons for the child.

---

may replaced by verbal explanations of why danger exists and how to avoid it.

During this period, an emotional transition between parent and child occurs. Although children are still attached to their parents and accept all their values and beliefs, they are nearing the period of life when they will question previous teachings and prefer the companionship of peers. Entry into school marks a separation from home for parents, as well as for children. Parents may need help in adjusting to this change, particularly if one parent has focused his or her daily activities primarily on home responsibilities. All family members must adjust to changes, which is part of the process of growth and development.

KEY POINTS

- The preschool years consist of the period from 3 to 5 years of age, a time that is considered critical for emotional and psychologic development.
- Biologic development in the preschool period is characterized by mature body systems and refinement in gross and fine motor behavior, as evidenced by participation in activities such as running, riding a tricycle, and drawing.
- According to Erikson, acquiring a sense of initiative is the chief psychosocial task of the preschooler. Development of the superego occurs during this period, and conscience begins to emerge.
- According to Piaget, the preschool age is characterized by intuitive or prelogical thinking and a move toward logical thought processes through advanced, complex learning, language, and understanding of causality.
- The seeds of moral development are planted during the preschool period. According to Kohlberg, these children are in the stage of naive instrumental orientation, in which they are concerned with satisfying their own needs and, less frequently, the needs of others.
- Social development includes further separation-individuation; more sophisticated language; greater independence; and more complex, imaginative forms of play.
- Areas of special concern to parents during the preschool period are the preschool and kindergarten experience, sex education, fears, stress, and speech problems.
- In selecting an early learning program, parents should inquire about daily activities, teacher qualifications, accreditation, student-staff ratio, safety, meals, fees, and health practices.
- Two rules that govern how parents answer questions about sex and other sensitive issues are to find out what the child knows and to be honest.
- Fears constitute a great part of the preschool period; fear of objects or potential annihilation and parent-induced fears are common.
- Preschool aggression may result from frustration, modeling behavior, and reinforcement.
- Hesitancy or dysfluency in speech patterns is a normal characteristic of language development. Speech problems can occur when parents express excessive concern over this pattern.
- Health promotion continues to be directed toward proper nutrition, adequate sleep, proper dental care, and injury prevention.

REFERENCES

American Academy of Pediatrics, Committee on Public Education: Children, adolescents, and television, *Pediatrics* 107(2):423-426, 2001a.

American Academy of Pediatrics, Committee on Sports Medicine and Fitness and Committee on School Health: Organized sports for children and preadolescents, *Pediatrics* 107(6):1459-1462, 2001b.

American Academy of Pediatrics, Committee on Nutrition: The use and misuse of fruit juices in pediatrics, *Pediatrics* 107(5):1210-1213, 2001c.

Anderson DR, Huston AC, Schmitt KL, and others: Early childhood television viewing and adolescent behavior: the recontact study, *Monogr Soc Res Child Dev* 66(1):I-VIII, 1-147, 2001.

Barlow SE, Expert Committee: Expert committee recommendations regarding the prevention, assessment, and treatment of child and adolescent overweight and obesity: summary report, *Pediatrics* 120(Suppl 4):S164-S192, 2007.

Barnes LL, Plotnikoff GA, Fox K, and others: Spirituality, religion, and pediatrics: intersecting worlds of healing, *Pediatrics* 104(6):899-908, 2000.

Bendersky M, Bennett D, Lewis M: Aggression at age 5 as a function of prenatal exposure to cocaine, gender, and environmental risk, *J Pediatr Psychol Adv Access* 31(1):71-84, 2006.

Brazelton TB, Sparrow JD: *Touchpoints 3 to 6: your child's emotional and behavioral development,* Cambridge, Mass, 2001, Da Capo Press.

Brown KD, Hamilton-Giachritsis C: The influence of violent media on children and adolescents: a public-health approach, *Lancet* 365(9460):702-710, 2005.

Davison KK, Birch LL: Weight status and self-concept in young girls, *Pediatrics* 107(1):46-53, 2001.

Endres J, Barter S, Theodora P, and others: Soy-enhanced lunch acceptance by preschoolers, *J Am Diet Assoc* 103(3):346-351, 2003.

Feldman HM: Evaluation and management of language and speech disorders in preschool children, *Pediatr Rev* 26(4):131-142, 2005.

Food and Nutrition Board: *Dietary reference intakes: guiding principles for nutrition labeling and fortification,* Washington, DC, 2003, National Academies Press.

Fosarelli P: Children and the development of faith: implications for pediatric practice, *Contemp Pediatr* 20(1):85-98, 2003.

Gershoff ET: Corporal punishment by parents and associated child behaviors and experiences: a meta-analytic and theoretical review, *Psychol Bull* 128(4):539-579, 2002.

Gleason TR, Sebanc AM, Hartup WW: Imaginary companions of preschool children, *Dev Psychol* 36(4):419-428, 2000.

Jellinek M, Patel BP, Froehle MC, editors: *Bright futures in practice: mental health,* vol 1, Arlington, Va, 2002, National Center for Education in Maternal and Child Health.

Johnson RK: Changing eating and physical activity patterns of U.S. children, *Proc Nutr Soc* 59(2):295-301, 2000.

Kleinman RE, editor: *Pediatric nutrition handbook,* ed 5, Elk Grove Village, Ill, 2004, American Academy of Pediatrics.

Martof A: Consultation with the specialist: dental care, *Pediatr Rev* 22(1):13-15, 2001.

McEvoy M: Culture and spirituality as an integrated concept in pediatric care, *MCN* 28(1):39-43, 2003.

McEvoy M: An added dimension to the pediatric health maintenance visit: the spiritual history, *J Pediatr Health Care* 14(5):216-220, 2000.

National Institute on Deafness and Other Communication Disorders: *Stuttering,* 2002, National Institutes of Health, retrieved March 2007 from http://www.nidcd.nih.gov/health/voice/stutter.

Needlman R: Growth and development: preschool years. In Behrman RE, Kliegman RM, Jenson HB, editors: *Nelson textbook of pediatrics,* ed 17, Philadelphia, 2004, Saunders.

Rafanello D: Controlling the spread of infectious disease in child care programs, *Healthy Child Care Am,* Winter, pp. 1-11, 2001.

Spear BA, Barlow SE, Ervin C, and others: Recommendations for treatment of child and adolescent overweight and obesity, *Pediatrics* 120(Suppl 4):S254-S288, 2007.

Story M, Holt K, Sofka D, editors: *Bright futures in practice: nutrition,* ed 2, Arlington, Va, 2002, National Center for Education in Maternal and Child Health.

Thiedke CC: Sleep disorders and sleep problems in childhood, *Am Fam Physician* 63(2):277-284, 2001.

Yalçin SS, Türul B, Naçar N, and others: Factors that affect television viewing time in preschool and primary schoolchildren, *Pediatr Int* 44(6):622-627, 2002.

14

Health Problems of Toddlers and Preschoolers

DAVID WILSON, LISA CREAMER, AND FAYE BLAIR

CHAPTER OUTLINE

INFECTIOUS DISORDERS, 453
Communicable Diseases, 453
Conjunctivitis, 464
Stomatitis, 465
INTESTINAL PARASITIC DISEASES, 466
General Nursing Care Management, 466
Giardiasis, 466
Enterobiasis (Pinworms), 468
INGESTION OF INJURIOUS AGENTS, 469
Principles of Emergency Treatment, 470
  Assessment, 473
  Gastric Decontamination, 473
  Prevention of Recurrence, 474

Heavy Metal Poisoning, 475
Lead Poisoning, 475
  Causes of Lead Poisoning, 476
  Screening for Lead Poisoning, 478
CHILD MALTREATMENT, 480
Child Neglect, 480
  Types of Neglect, 480
Emotional Abuse, 480
Physical Abuse, 480
  Shaken Baby Syndrome, 481
  Munchausen Syndrome by Proxy, 481
  Factors Predisposing to Physical Abuse, 481

Sexual Abuse, 482
  Characteristics of Abusers and Victims, 482
  Initiation and Perpetuation of Sexual Abuse, 482
Nursing Care of the Maltreated Child, 483
  Caregiver-Child Interaction, 485
  History and Interview, 485
  Physical Assessment, 486
Nursing Care Plan: The Child Who Is Maltreated, 489

LEARNING OBJECTIVES

On completion of this chapter the reader will be able to:

- Describe the major characteristics of communicable diseases of childhood.
- List three principles of nursing care of children with communicable disease.
- Describe the nursing care of the child with conjunctivitis.
- Distinguish between aphthous stomatitis and herpetic gingivostomatitis.

- Outline a teaching plan designed to prevent transmission of intestinal parasites.
- Identify the principles in the emergency treatment of poisoning.
- Name four sources of lead in the environment.

- Describe the nursing care of the child with lead poisoning.
- State three factors thought to be associated with child abuse.
- State four areas of the history that should arouse suspicion of abuse.
- Describe the nursing care of the abused child.

RELATED TOPICS and ADDITIONAL RESOURCES

 IN TEXT

Collection of Specimens, *Ch. 22*
Compliance, *Ch. 22*
Controlling Elevated Temperatures, *Ch. 22*
Growth Failure (Failure to Thrive), *Ch. 11*
Health Practices, *Ch. 4*
Immunizations, *Ch. 10*
Infection Control, *Ch. 22*
Pain Assessment; Pain Management, *Ch. 7*
Pertussis (Whooping Cough), *Ch. 23*
Poisoning, *Ch. 12*
Posttraumatic Stress Disorder, *Ch. 17*
Seizure Disorders, *Ch. 28*
Sexual Assault (Rape), *Ch. 17*

Skin Lesions, *Ch. 30*
Stool Specimens, *Ch. 22*

 COMPANION CD

Case Studies—Chickenpox; Child Abuse;
 Salicylate Ingestion; Behaviors Indicative
 of Future Child Abuse; Varicella in Spite
 of Vaccine; Bacterial Conjunctivitis;
 Ingestion of an Injurious Agent; Heavy
 Metal Poisoning
Critical Thinking Exercises—Poisoning;
 Conjunctivitis
NCLEX Review Questions

 evolve
evolve.elsevier.com/Wong/essentials/

NCLEX Review Questions
Nursing Care Plan—The Child Who Is
 Maltreated

**WONG'S CLINICAL MANUAL
OF PEDIATRIC NURSING, 7th Ed**

Nursing Care Plan—The Child with Toxic
 Ingestion or Inhalation, *p. 498*

INFECTIOUS DISORDERS
COMMUNICABLE DISEASES

The incidence of childhood communicable diseases has declined significantly since the advent of immunizations. Serious complications resulting from such infections have been further reduced with the use of antibiotics and antitoxins. However, infectious diseases do occur, and nurses must be familiar with the infectious agent to recognize the disease and to institute appropriate preventive and supportive interventions (Table 14-1). (See also Chapter 30 for a discussion of nursing care for dermatologic conditions.)

Nursing Care Management

The more common communicable diseases of childhood, their therapeutic management, and specific nursing care are described in Table 14-1. The following is a general discussion of nursing care management for communicable diseases. The nursing process for care of the child with a communicable disease is outlined in the Nursing Process box.

Identification of the infectious agent is of primary importance to prevent exposure to susceptible individuals. Nurses in ambulatory care settings, child care centers, and schools are often the first persons to see signs of a communicable disease, such as a rash or sore throat. The nurse must operate under a high index of suspicion for common childhood diseases to identify potentially infectious cases and to recognize diseases that require medical intervention. An example is the common complaint of sore throat. Although most often a symptom of a minor viral infection, it can signal diphtheria or a streptococcal infection, such as scarlet fever. Each of these bacterial conditions requires appropriate medical treatment to prevent serious sequelae.

Text continued on p. 462

nursingprocess | The Child with Communicable Disease

ASSESSMENT
Assess for signs and symptoms of a communicable disease and its consequences. (See Table 14-1 for discussion of specific communicable diseases.)

DIAGNOSIS (PROBLEM IDENTIFICATION)
After a thorough assessment, several nursing diagnoses are evident:
- Risk for Infection related to susceptible host and infectious agents
- Pain related to skin lesions, malaise
- Impaired Social Interaction related to isolation from peers
- Risk for Impaired Skin Integrity related to scratching from pruritus
- Interrupted Family Processes related to child with an acute illness

PLANNING
Expected patient outcomes include:
- Child will not spread the infection to others.
- Child will not experience complications.
- Child will have minimum discomfort.
- Child and family will receive adequate emotional support.

IMPLEMENTATION
Numerous intervention strategies are discussed on pp. 453-464.

EVALUATION
The effectiveness of nursing interventions for the child with a communicable disease is determined by continual assessment and evaluation of care based on the following guidelines:
- Observe or inquire about family members' use of control measures; observe for signs of disease in household contacts.
- Monitor vital signs, especially temperature; inquire about the identification of high-risk contacts and appropriate isolation of the contacts; observe or inquire about compliance with antibiotic or antiviral therapy.
- Inquire about effectiveness of comfort measures.
- Interview family and child regarding their feelings and concerns, especially when child returns to school.

Case Study—Varicella in Spite of Vaccine

TABLE 14-1

Communicable Diseases of Childhood

DISEASE

CHICKENPOX (VARICELLA) (FIG. 14-1)

Agents—Varicella-zoster virus (VZV)

Source—Primary secretions of respiratory tract of infected persons; to a lesser degree, skin lesions (scabs not infectious)

Transmissions—Direct contact, droplet (airborne) spread, and contaminated objects

Incubation period—2-3 weeks, usually 14-16 days

Period of communicability—Probably 1 day before eruption of lesions (prodromal period) to 6 days after first crop of vesicles when crusts have formed

FIG. 14-1 ■ Chickenpox (varicella). **A,** Progression of disease. **B,** Simultaneous stages of lesions in chickenpox. **C,** Clinical view. (**C,** From Habif TP: *Clinical dermatology: a color guide to diagnosis and therapy,* ed 4, St Louis, 2004, Mosby.)

DIPHTHERIA

Agent—*Corynebacterium diphtheriae*

Source—Discharges from mucous membranes of nose and nasopharynx, skin, and other lesions of infected person

Transmission—Direct contact with infected person, a carrier, or contaminated articles

Incubation period—Usually 2-5 days, possibly longer

Period of communicability—Variable; until virulent bacilli are no longer present (identified by three negative cultures); usually 2 weeks but as long as 4 weeks

ADLs, Activities of daily living; *IVIG,* intravenous immune globulin.

CLINICAL MANIFESTATIONS	THERAPEUTIC MANAGEMENT AND COMPLICATIONS	NURSING CARE MANAGEMENT
Prodromal stage—Slight fever, malaise, and anorexia for first 24 hours; rash highly pruritic; begins as macule, rapidly progresses to papule and then vesicle (surrounded by erythematous base; becomes umbilicated and cloudy; breaks easily and forms crusts); all three stages (papule, vesicle, crust) present in varying degrees at one time **Distribution**—Centripetal, spreading to face and proximal extremities but sparse on distal limbs and less on areas not exposed to heat (i.e., from clothing or sun) **Constitutional signs and symptoms**—Elevated temperature from lymphadenopathy, irritability from pruritus	**Specific**—Antiviral agent acyclovir (Zovirax); varicella-zoster immune globulin (VariZIG) or IVIG after exposure in high-risk children **Supportive**—Diphenhydramine hydrochloride or antihistamines to relieve itching; skin care to prevent secondary bacterial infection **Complications**—Secondary bacterial infections (abscesses, cellulitis, necrotizing fasciitis, pneumonia, sepsis) Encephalitis Varicella pneumonia (rare in normal children) Hemorrhagic varicella (tiny hemorrhages in vesicles and numerous petechiae in skin) Chronic or transient thrombocytopenia **Preventive**—Childhood immunization. Disease does not confer immunity.	Maintain standard, airborne, and contact precautions if hospitalized until all lesions are crusted; for immunized child with mild breakthrough varicella, isolate until no new lesions are seen. Keep child in home away from susceptible individuals until vesicles have dried (usually 1 week after onset of disease), and isolate high-risk children from infected children. Administer skin care: give bath and change clothes and linens daily; administer topical calamine lotion; keep child's fingernails short and clean; apply mittens if child scratches. Keep child cool (may decrease number of lesions). Lessen pruritus; keep child occupied. Remove loose crusts that rub and irritate skin. Teach child to apply pressure to pruritic area rather than scratching it. Avoid use of aspirin (possible association with Reye syndrome).
Vary according to anatomic location of pseudomembrane **Nasal**—Resembles common cold, serosanguineous mucopurulent nasal discharge without constitutional symptoms; may have frank epistaxis **Tonsillar-pharyngeal**—Malaise; anorexia; sore throat; low-grade fever; pulse increased above expected for temperature within 24 hours; smooth, adherent, white or gray membrane; lymphadenitis possibly pronounced ("bull's neck"); in severe cases, toxemia, septic shock, and death within 6-10 days **Laryngeal**—Fever, hoarseness, cough, with or without previous signs listed; potential airway obstruction; apprehensive; dyspneic retractions; cyanosis	Equine antitoxin (usually intravenously); preceded by skin or conjunctival test to rule out sensitivity to horse serum Antibiotics (penicillin G procaine or erythromycin) in addition to equine antitoxin Complete bed rest (prevention of myocarditis) Tracheostomy for airway obstruction Treatment of infected contacts and carriers **Complications**—Toxic cardiomyopathy (second to third week) Toxic neuropathy **Preventive**—Childhood immunization Disease does not confer immunity.	Follow standard and droplet precautions until two cultures are negative for *C. diphtheriae*; use contact precautions with cutaneous manifestations. Administer antibiotics in timely manner. Participate in sensitivity testing; have epinephrine available. Administer complete care to maintain bed rest. Use suctioning as needed. Observe respiration for signs of obstruction. Administer humidified oxygen as prescribed.

Continued

TABLE 14-1

Communicable Diseases of Childhood—cont'd

DISEASE

FIG. 14-2 ■ Erythema infectiosum. (From Habif TP: *Clinical dermatology: a color guide to diagnosis and therapy,* ed 4, St Louis, 2004, Mosby.)

ERYTHEMA INFECTIOSUM (FIFTH DISEASE) (FIG. 14-2)
Agent—Human parvovirus (HPV) B19
Source—Infected persons, mainly school-age children
Transmission—Respiratory secretions and blood, blood products
Incubation period—4-14 days; may be as long as 21 days
Period of communicability—Uncertain but before onset of symptoms in children with aplastic crisis

EXANTHEM SUBITUM (ROSEOLA INFANTUM) (FIG. 14-3)
Agent—Human herpesvirus type 6 (HHV-6; rarely HHV-7)
Source—Possibly acquired from saliva of healthy adult person; entry via nasal, buccal, or conjunctival mucosa
Transmission—Year round; no reported contact with infected individual in most cases (virtually limited to children under 3 years but peak age is 6-15 months)
Incubation period—Usually 5-15 days
Period of communicability—Unknown

FIG. 14-3 ■ Roseola infantum. (From Habif TP: *Clinical dermatology: a color guide to diagnosis and therapy,* ed 4, St Louis, 2004, Mosby.)

ADLs, Activities of daily living; *IVIG,* intravenous immune globulin.

CLINICAL MANIFESTATIONS	THERAPEUTIC MANAGEMENT AND COMPLICATIONS	NURSING CARE MANAGEMENT
Rash appears in three stages: I—Erythema on face, chiefly on cheeks ("slapped face" appearance); disappears by 1-4 days II—About 1 day after rash appears on face, maculopapular red spots appear, symmetrically distributed on upper and lower extremities; rash progresses from proximal to distal surfaces and may last a week or more III—Rash subsides but reappears if skin is irritated or traumatized (sun, heat, cold, friction) In children with aplastic crisis, rash usually absent and prodromal illness includes fever, myalgia, lethargy, nausea, vomiting, and abdominal pain Child with sickle cell disease may have concurrent vaso-occlusive crisis	**Symptomatic and supportive**—Antipyretics, analgesics, antiinflammatory drugs Possible blood transfusion for transient aplastic anemia **Complications**—Self-limited arthritis and arthralgia (arthritis may become chronic); more common in adult women May result in serious complications (anemia, hydrops) or fetal death if mother infected during pregnancy (primarily second trimester) Aplastic crisis in children with hemolytic disease or immunodeficiency Myocarditis (rare)	Isolation of child is not necessary, except hospitalized child (immunosuppressed or with aplastic crises) suspected of HPV infection is placed on respiratory isolation and standard precautions. Pregnant women need not be excluded from workplace where HPV infection is present; they should not care for patients with aplastic crises. Explain low risk of fetal death to those in contact with affected children; assist with routine fetal ultrasound for detection of fetal hydrops.
Persistent high fever for 3-4 days in child who appears well Precipitous drop in fever to normal with appearance of rash **Rash**—Discrete rose-pink macules or maculopapules appearing first on trunk, then spreading to neck, face, and extremities; nonpruritic; fades on pressure; lasts 1-2 days **Associated signs and symptoms**—Cervical and postauricular lymphadenopathy, inflamed pharynx, cough, coryza	Nonspecific Antipyretics to control fever **Complications**—Recurrent febrile seizures (possibly from latent infection of central nervous system that is reactivated by fever) Encephalitis (rare)	Teach parents measures for lowering temperature (antipyretic drugs); ensure adequate parental understanding of specific antipyretic dosage to prevent accidental overdose. If child is prone to seizures, discuss appropriate precautions and possibility of recurrent febrile seizures.

Continued

| **TABLE 14-1**
Communicable Diseases of Childhood—cont'd

DISEASE

FIG. 14-4 ■ Measles (rubeola). **A,** Progression of disease. **B,** Exanthem first appears at the hairline and spreads from head to toe over 3 days. **C,** Measles ultimately involves the palms and soles. (B and C, From Zitelli BJ, Davis HW: *Atlas of pediatric physical diagnosis,* ed 5, St Louis, 2007, Mosby; courtesy Michael Sherlock, MD, Lutherville, Md.)

MEASLES (RUBEOLA) (FIG. 14-4)
Agent—Virus
Source—Respiratory tract secretions, blood, and urine of infected person
Transmission—Usually by direct contact with droplets of infected person; primarily in the winter
Incubation period—10-20 days
Period of communicability—From 4 days before to 5 days after rash appears, but mainly during prodromal (catarrhal) stage

MUMPS
Agent—Paramyxovirus
Source—Saliva of infected persons
Transmission—Direct contact with or droplet spread from an infected person
Incubation period—14-21 days
Period of communicability—Most communicable immediately before and after swelling begins

PERTUSSIS (WHOOPING COUGH)
Agent—*Bordetella pertussis*
Source—Discharge from respiratory tract of infected persons

ADLs, Activities of daily living; *IVIG,* intravenous immune globulin.

CLINICAL MANIFESTATIONS	THERAPEUTIC MANAGEMENT AND COMPLICATIONS	NURSING CARE MANAGEMENT
Prodromal (catarrhal) stage—Fever and malaise, followed in 24 hours by coryza, cough, conjunctivitis, Koplik spots (small, irregular red spots with a minute, bluish white center first seen on buccal mucosa opposite molars 2 days before rash); symptoms gradually increasing in severity until second day after rash appears, when they begin to subside **Rash**—Appears 3-4 days after onset of prodromal stage; begins as erythematous maculopapular eruption on face and gradually spreads downward; more severe in earlier sites (appears confluent) and less intense in later sites (appears discrete); after 3-4 days assumes brownish appearance, and fine desquamation occurs over area of extensive involvement **Constitutional signs and symptoms**—Anorexia, abdominal pain, malaise, generalized lymphadenopathy	**Preventive**—Childhood immunization Vitamin A supplementation (see p. 464) **Supportive**—Bed rest during febrile period; antipyretics Antibiotics to prevent secondary bacterial infection in high-risk children **Complications**—Otitis media Pneumonia (bacterial) Obstructive laryngitis and laryngotracheitis Encephalitis (rare but has high mortality)	Maintain isolation until fifth day of rash; if child is hospitalized, institute droplet precautions. Encourage rest during prodromal stage; provide quiet activity. **Fever**—Instruct parents to administer antipyretics; avoid chilling; if child is prone to seizures, institute appropriate precautions. **Eye care**—Dim lights if photophobia present; clean eyelids with warm saline solution to remove secretions or crusts; keep child from rubbing eyes. **Coryza, cough**—Use cool-mist vaporizer; protect skin around nares with layer of petrolatum; encourage fluids and soft, bland foods. **Skin care**—Keep skin clean; use tepid baths as necessary.
Prodromal stage—Fever, headache, malaise, and anorexia for 24 hours, followed by "earache" that is aggravated by chewing **Parotitis**—By third day, parotid gland(s) (either unilateral or bilateral) enlarges and reaches maximum size in 1-3 days; accompanied by pain and tenderness; other exocrine glands (submandibular) may also be swollen	**Preventive**—Childhood immunization **Symptomatic and supportive**—Analgesics for pain and antipyretics for fever Intravenous fluid if needed for child who refuses to drink or vomits because of meningoencephalitis **Complications**—Sensorineural deafness Postinfectious encephalitis Myocarditis Arthritis Hepatitis Epididymoorchitis Oopharitis Pancreatitis Sterility (extremely rare in adult males) Meningitis	Maintain isolation during period of communicability; institute droplet and contact precautions during hospitalization. Encourage rest and decreased activity during prodromal phase until swelling subsides. Give analgesics for pain; if child is unwilling to swallow pills or tablets medication, use elixir form. Encourage fluids and soft, bland foods; avoid foods requiring chewing. Apply hot or cold compresses to neck, whichever is more comforting. To relieve orchitis, provide warmth and local support with tight-fitting underpants.
Catarrhal stage—Begins with symptoms of upper respiratory tract infection, such as coryza, sneezing, lacrimation, cough, and low-grade fever; symptoms continue for 1-2 weeks, when dry, hacking cough becomes more severe	**Preventive**—Immunization; current belief is that childhood immunizations for pertussis do not confer lifelong immunity to adolescents and adults; therefore a pertussis booster is recommended for adolescents (see Fig. 10-11)	Maintain isolation during catarrhal stage; if child is hospitalized, institute droplet precautions.

Continued

TABLE 14-1

Communicable Diseases of Childhood—cont'd

DISEASE

PERTUSSIS (WHOOPING COUGH)—cont'd

Transmission—Direct contact or droplet spread from infected person; indirect contact with freshly contaminated articles

Incubation period—6-20 days; usually 7-10 days

Period of communicability—Greatest during catarrhal stage before onset of paroxysms

FIG. 14-5 ■ Rubella (German measles). **A,** Progression of rash. **B,** Clinical view. (**B,** From Zitelli BJ, Davis HW: *Atlas of pediatric physical diagnosis,* ed 5, St Louis, 2007, Mosby; courtesy Michael Sherlock, MD, Lutherville, Md.)

POLIOMYELITIS

Agent—Enteroviruses, three types: type 1, most frequent cause of paralysis, both epidemic and endemic; type 2, least frequently associated with paralysis; type 3, second most frequently associated with paralysis

Source—Feces and oropharyngeal secretions of infected persons, especially young children

Transmission—Direct contact with persons with apparent or inapparent active infection; spread via fecal-oral and pharyngeal-oropharyngeal routes

Vaccine-acquired paralytic polio may occur as a result of the live oral polio vaccination (no longer available in the United States)

Incubation period—Usually 7-14 days, with range of 5-35 days

Period of communicability—Not exactly known; virus present in throat and feces shortly after infection and persists for about 1 week in throat and 4-6 weeks in feces

RUBELLA (GERMAN MEASLES) (FIG. 14-5)

Agent—Rubella virus

Source—Primarily nasopharyngeal secretions of person with apparent or inapparent infection; virus also present in blood, stool, and urine

Incubation period—14-21 days

Period of communicability—7 days before to about 5 days after appearance of rash

Constitutional signs and symptoms—Occasionally low-grade fever, headache, malaise, and lymphadenopathy

CLINICAL MANIFESTATIONS	THERAPEUTIC MANAGEMENT AND COMPLICATIONS	NURSING CARE MANAGEMENT
Paroxysmal stage—Cough most common at night, consists of short, rapid coughs followed by sudden inspiration associated with a high-pitched crowing sound or "whoop"; during paroxysms, cheeks become flushed or cyanotic, eyes bulge, and tongue protrudes; paroxysm may continue until thick mucous plug is dislodged; vomiting frequently follows attack; stage generally lasts 4-6 weeks, followed by convalescent stage Infants under 6 months may not have characteristic whoop cough, but have difficulty maintaining adequate oxygenation with amount of secretions, frequent vomiting of mucus and formula or breast milk Pertussis may occur in adolescents and adults with varying manifestations; cough and whoop may be absent; however, as many as 50% of adolescents may have a cough for up to 10 weeks (American Academy of Pediatrics, 2006); additional symptoms in adolescents include difficulty breathing and posttussive vomiting (See also Chapter 10, Immunizations, for discussion of pertussis immunization schedule)	Antimicrobial therapy (e.g., erythromycin, clarithromycin, azithromycin) **Supportive**—Hospitalization sometimes required for infants, children who are dehydrated, or those who have complications Increased oxygen intake and humidity Adequate fluids Intensive care and mechanical ventilation if needed for infants <6 months **Complications**—Pneumonia (usual cause of death in younger children) Atelectasis Otitis media Seizures Hemorrhage (scleral, conjunctival, epistaxis; pulmonary hemorrhage in neonate) Weight loss and dehydration Hernias (umbilical and inguinal) Prolapsed rectum Complications reported among adolescents include syncope, sleep disturbance, rib fractures, incontinence, and pneumonia (American Academy of Pediatrics, 2006)	Obtain nasopharyngeal culture for diagnosis. Encourage oral fluids; offer small amount of fluids frequently. Ensure adequate oxygenation during paroxysms; position infant on side to decrease chance of aspiration with vomiting. Provide humidified oxygen; suction as needed to prevent choking on secretions. Observe for signs of airway obstruction (increased restlessness, apprehension, retractions, cyanosis). Encourage compliance with antibiotic therapy for household contacts. Encourage adolescents to obtain pertussis booster (Tdap) (see also Immunizations, Chapter 10). Use standard precautions and mask in health care workers exposed to children with persistent cough and high suspicion of pertussis.
May be manifested in three different forms: **Abortive or inapparent**—Fever, uneasiness, sore throat, headache, anorexia, vomiting, abdominal pain; lasts a few hours to a few days **Nonparalytic**—Same manifestations as abortive but more severe, with pain and stiffness in neck, back, and legs **Paralytic**—Initial course similar to nonparalytic type, followed by recovery and then signs of central nervous system paralysis	**Preventive**—Childhood immunization **Supportive**—Complete bed rest during acute phase Mechanical or assisted ventilation in case of respiratory paralysis Physical therapy for muscles after acute stage **Complications**—Permanent paralysis Respiratory arrest Hypertension Kidney stones from demineralization of bone during prolonged immobility	Administer mild sedatives as necessary to relieve anxiety and promote rest. Participate in physiotherapy procedures (use of moist hot packs and range-of-motion exercises). Position child to maintain body alignment and prevent contractures or skin breakdown; use footboard or appropriate orthoses to prevent footdrop; use pressure mattress for prolonged immobility. Encourage child to perform ADLs to capability; promote early ambulation with assistive devices; administer analgesics for maximum comfort during physical activity; give high-protein diet and bowel management for prolonged immobility. Observe for respiratory paralysis (difficulty in talking, ineffective cough, inability to hold breath, shallow and rapid respirations); report such signs and symptoms to practitioner.
Prodromal stage—Absent in children, present in adults and adolescents; consists of low-grade fever, headache, malaise, anorexia, mild conjunctivitis, coryza, sore throat, cough, and lymphadenopathy; lasts 1-5 days, subsides 1 day after appearance of rash **Rash**—First appears on face and rapidly spreads downward to neck, arms, trunk, and legs; by end of first day, body is covered with discrete, pinkish red maculopapular exanthema; disappears in same order as it began and is usually gone by third day	**Preventive**—Childhood immunization No treatment necessary other than antipyretics for low-grade fever and analgesics for discomfort **Complications**—Rare (arthritis, encephalitis, or purpura); most benign of all childhood communicable diseases; greatest danger is teratogenic effect on fetus	Reassure parents of benign nature of illness in affected child. Use comfort measures as necessary. Avoid contact with pregnant woman. Monitor rubella titer in pregnant adolescent.

Continued

TABLE 14-1

Communicable Diseases of Childhood—cont'd

	DISEASE
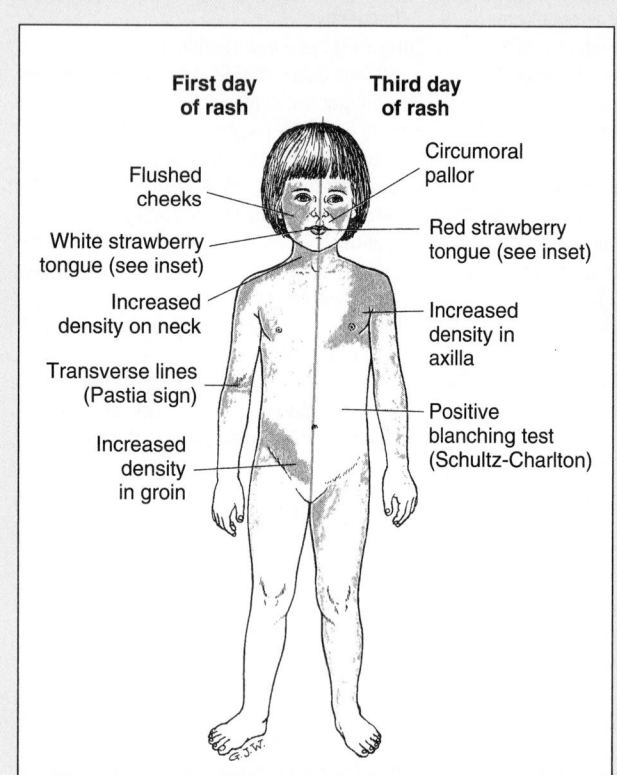

FIG. 14-6 ■ Scarlet fever. | **SCARLET FEVER (FIG. 14-6)**
Agent—Group A β-hemolytic streptococci
Source—Usually from nasopharyngeal secretions of infected persons and carriers
Transmission—Direct contact with infected person or droplet spread; indirectly by contact with contaminated articles or ingestion of contaminated milk or other food
Incubation period—2-5 days, with range of 1-7 days
Period of communicability—During incubation period and clinical illness, approximately 10 days; during first 2 weeks of carrier phase, although may persist for months

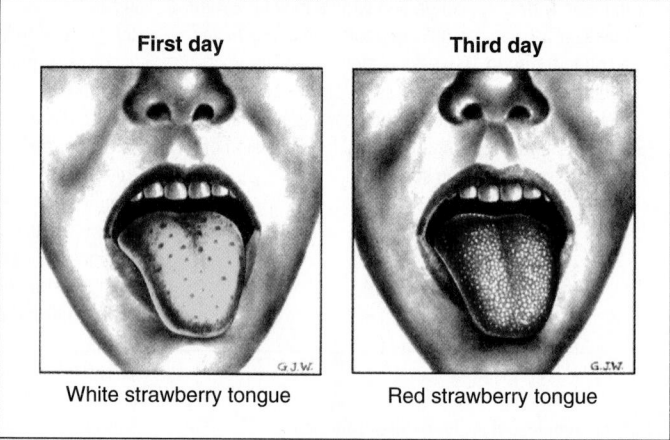 |

ADLs, Activities of daily living; *IVIG,* intravenous immune globulin.

When a communicable disease is suspected, it is important to assess:

- Recent exposure to a known case
- **Prodromal symptoms** (symptoms that occur between early manifestations of the disease and its overt clinical syndrome) or evidence of constitutional symptoms, such as a fever or rash (see Table 14-1)
- Immunization history
- History of having the disease

Immunizations are available for many diseases, and infection usually confers lifelong immunity; therefore the possibility of many infectious agents can be eliminated based on these two criteria.

Prevent Spread. Prevention consists of two components: prevention of the disease and control of its spread to others. **Primary prevention** rests almost exclusively on immunization. (The nurse's role in immunization of children is discussed in Chapter 10.)

Control measures to prevent spread of disease should include techniques to reduce risk of cross-transmission of infectious organisms between patients and to protect health care workers from organisms harbored by patients. If the child is hospitalized, the facility's policies for infection control are followed (see Chapter 22). The most important procedure is

hand washing. Persons directly caring for the child or handling contaminated articles must wash their hands and practice effective standard precautions in care of their patients.

The child is instructed to practice good hand-washing technique after toileting and before eating. For those diseases spread by droplets, the nurse instructs parents in measures to reduce airborne transmission. The child who is old enough should use a tissue to cover the face during coughing or sneezing; otherwise, the parent should cover the child's mouth with a tissue and then discard it. The usual hygiene measures of not sharing eating and drinking utensils are stressed to the family.

> **NURSINGALERT**
>
> If a child is admitted to the hospital with an undiagnosed exanthema, strict transmission-based precautions (contact, airborne, and droplet) and standard precautions are instituted until a diagnosis is confirmed. Childhood communicable diseases requiring these precautions include diphtheria, chickenpox, measles, tuberculosis, adenovirus, *Haemophilus influenzae* type b, influenza, mumps, *Mycoplasma pneumoniae* infection, pertussis, plague, streptococcal pharyngitis, pneumonia, or scarlet fever (American Academy of Pediatrics, 2006).

Prevent Complications. Although most children recover without difficulty, certain groups are at risk for serious, even fatal, complications from communicable diseases,

CLINICAL MANIFESTATIONS	THERAPEUTIC MANAGEMENT AND COMPLICATIONS	NURSING CARE MANAGEMENT
Prodromal stage—Abrupt high fever, pulse increased out of proportion to fever, vomiting, headache, chills, malaise, abdominal pain, halitosis **Enanthema**—Tonsils enlarged, edematous, reddened, and covered with patches of exudates; in severe cases appearance resembles membrane seen in diphtheria; pharynx is edematous and beefy red; during first 1-2 days tongue is coated and papillae become red and swollen (white strawberry tongue); by fourth or fifth day white coat sloughs off, leaving prominent papillae (red strawberry tongue); palate is covered with erythematous punctate lesions **Exanthema**—Rash appears within 12 hours after prodromal signs; red pinhead-sized punctate lesions rapidly become generalized but are absent on face, which becomes flushed with striking circumoral pallor; rash more intense in folds of joints; by end of first week desquamation begins (fine, sandpaper-like on torso; sheetlike sloughing on palms and soles), which may be complete by 3 weeks or longer	Full course of penicillin (or erythromycin in penicillin-sensitive children) or oral cephalosporin Antibiotic therapy for newly diagnosed carriers (nose or throat cultures positive for streptococci) **Supportive**—Rest during febrile phase, analgesics for sore throat; antipruritics for rash if bothersome **Complications**—Peritonsillar and retropharyngeal abscess Sinusitis Otitis media Acute glomerulonephritis Acute rheumatic fever Polyarthritis (uncommon)	Institute standard and droplet precautions until 24 hours after initiation of treatment. Ensure compliance with oral antibiotic therapy; intramuscular benzathine penicillin G [Bicillin] may be given. Encourage rest during febrile phase; provide quiet activity during convalescent period. Relieve discomfort of sore throat with analgesics, gargles, lozenges, antiseptic throat sprays, and inhalation of cool mist. Encourage fluids during febrile phase; avoid irritating liquids (certain citrus juices) or rough foods (chips); when child is able to eat, begin with soft diet. Advise parents to consult practitioner if fever persists after beginning therapy. Discuss procedures for preventing spread of infection—discard toothbrush; avoid sharing drinking and eating utensils.

especially the viral diseases chickenpox and erythema infectiosum (EI) (fifth disease) caused by **human parvovirus (HPV) B19.** Most healthy children are less likely to become infected from either of these viruses compared with children with **immunodeficiency**—those receiving steroid or other immunosuppressive therapy, those with a generalized malignancy such as leukemia or lymphoma, or those with an immunologic disorder—who are at risk for viremia from replication of the **varicella-zoster virus (VZV)*** in the blood. VZV is so named because it causes two distinct diseases: **varicella (chickenpox)** and **zoster (herpes zoster** or **shingles).** Varicella occurs primarily in children younger than 15 years of age. However, it leaves the threat of herpes zoster, an intensely painful varicella that is localized to a single **dermatome** (body area innervated by a particular segment of the spinal cord). In children the dermatomes most likely affected by herpes zoster are the cervical and sacral dermatomes (Leung, Robson, and Leong, 2006). Immunocompromised patients and healthy infants younger than 1 year of age (who also have reduced immunity) are at a higher risk for reactivation of VZV causing

herpes zoster, probably as a result of a deficiency in cellular immunity (Chen, George, Woodruff, and others, 2002). Complications of herpes zoster virus in children include secondary bacterial infection, depigmentation, and scarring; postherpetic neuralgia in children is uncommon (Leung, Robson, and Leong, 2006).

Children with hemolytic disease, such as sickle cell disease, are at risk for aplastic anemia from EI. HPV B19 infects and lyses red blood cell precursors, thus interrupting the production of red blood cells. Therefore the virus may precipitate a severe aplastic crisis in patients who need increased red blood cell production to maintain normal red blood cell volumes; thrombocytopenia and neutropenia may also occur as a result of HPV B19 infection. The fetus has a relatively high rate of red blood cell production and an immature immune system; it may develop severe anemia and hydrops as a result of maternal HPV infection. Fetal death rates as a result of HPV B19 have been estimated to be between 2% and 6% (American Academy of Pediatrics, 2006).

> **NURSINGALERT**
>
> Children at risk for contracting these communicable diseases are referred to the practitioner immediately in case of known exposure or outbreaks.

---

*Educational materials may be obtained from the VZV Research Foundation, 1201 Lexington Ave., Suite 204, New York, NY 10028; (212) 222-3390; http://www.vzvfoundation.org; or GlaxoSmithKline, 3030 Cornwallis Road, Research Triangle Park, NC 27709; (800) 825-5249; http://us.gsk.com.

In the past decade there has been an increase in the cases of pertussis, particularly in infants less than 6 months old and in children 10 to 14 years of age. Early clinical manifestations of pertussis in infants may include gagging, coughing, emesis, and apnea; the typical "whoop" associated with the disease is absent (American Academy of Pediatrics, 2006). In older children the disease may manifest as a common cold (see Table 14-1). There is now a recommendation that children ages 11 to 18 receive a booster pertussis vaccine (Tdap) to prevent the disease (see Immunizations, Chapter 10). Because pertussis is contagious, especially among close household members, pertussis should be identified early and treatment initiated for the child and those who have been exposed. Azithromycin (for infants under 1 month) and erythromycin are administered to infants and children with pertussis (American Academy of Pediatrics, 2006).

Prevention of complications from diseases such as diphtheria, pertussis, and scarlet fever requires compliance with antibiotic therapy. With oral preparations the need to complete the entire course of therapy is stressed (see Compliance, Chapter 22). The use of varicella-zoster immune globulin (VariZIG) or immune globulin intravenous (IGIV) is recommended for children who are immunocompromised, who have no previous history of varicella, and who are likely to contract the disease and have complications as a result (American Academy of Pediatrics, 2006). The antiviral agent acyclovir (Zovirax) may be used to treat varicella infections in susceptible immunocompromised persons; it is effective in decreasing the number of lesions; shortening the duration of fever; and decreasing itching, lethargy, and anorexia. Oral acyclovir should be considered for susceptible pregnant women, immunocompromised children without a history of varicella disease, newborns whose mother had varicella within 5 days before delivery or within 48 hours after delivery, and hospitalized preterm infants with significant varicella exposure (American Academy of Pediatrics, 2006).

Evidence suggests that vitamin A supplementation reduces both morbidity and mortality in measles and that all children with severe measles should be given vitamin A supplements. A single oral dose of 200,000 IU for children at least 1 year old (use half that dose for children 6 to 12 months of age) is recommended. The higher dose may be associated with vomiting and headache for a few hours. The dose should be repeated the next day and at 4 weeks for children with ophthalmologic evidence of vitamin A deficiency (American Academy of Pediatrics, 2006).

> **NURSINGALERT**
>
> Although the risk of vitamin A toxicity from these doses (they are 100 to 200 times the recommended dietary allowance) is relatively low, nurses should instruct parents on safe storage of the drug. Ideally, vitamin A should be dispensed in the age-appropriate unit dose to prevent excessive administration and possible toxicity.

Provide Comfort. Many communicable diseases cause skin manifestations that are bothersome to the child. The chief discomfort from most rashes is itching, and measures such as cool baths (usually without soap) and lotions (e.g., calamine) are helpful.

> **NURSINGALERT**
>
> When lotions with active ingredients such as diphenhydramine in Caladryl are used, they are applied sparingly, especially over open lesions, where excessive absorption can lead to drug toxicity. These lotions should be used with caution in children who are simultaneously receiving an oral antihistamine. Cooling the lotion in the refrigerator beforehand often makes it more soothing on the skin than at room temperature.

To avoid overheating, which increases itching, children should wear lightweight, loose, nonirritating clothing and keep out of the sun. If the child persists in scratching, the nails are kept short and smooth; mittens and clothes with long sleeves or legs may be needed. For severe itching, antipruritic medication, such as diphenhydramine (Benadryl) or hydroxyzine (Atarax), may be required, especially when the child has trouble sleeping because of itching. Loratadine, cetirizine, and fexofenadine do not cause drowsiness and may be preferred for urticaria during the day.

An elevated temperature is common, and both antipyretic medicine (acetaminophen or ibuprofen) and environmental manipulation are implemented (see Controlling Elevated Temperature, Chapter 22). The acetaminophen is effective in lowering the fever but does not significantly reduce the symptoms of itching, anorexia, abdominal pain, fussiness, or vomiting.

A sore throat, another frequent symptom, is managed with lozenges, saline rinses (if the child is old enough to cooperate), and analgesics. Because most children are anorectic during an illness, bland foods and increased liquids are usually preferred. During the early stages of the disease, children voluntarily curtail their activity, and although bed rest is beneficial, it should not be imposed unless specifically indicated. During periods of irritability, quiet activity (e.g., reading, music, television, video games, puzzles, coloring) helps distract children from the discomfort.

Support Child and Family. Most communicable diseases are benign, but may produce considerable concern and anxiety for parents. Often the occurrence of a disease such as chickenpox is the first time the child is acutely uncomfortable. Parents need assistance to cope with manifestations of the illness, such as intense itching. The family and child need reassurance that recovery is generally rapid. However, visible signs of the dermatosis may be present for some time after the child is well enough to resume usual activities.

> **NURSINGALERT**
>
> The occurrence of a communicable disease provides the opportunity to ask parents about the child's immunization status and reinforce the benefits of vaccines for children.

CONJUNCTIVITIS

Acute conjunctivitis (inflammation of the conjunctiva) occurs from a variety of causes that are typically age related. In newborns conjunctivitis can occur from infection during birth, most often from *Chlamydia trachomatis* (inclusion conjunctivitis) or *Neisseria gonorrhoeae*. These organisms, as well as herpes simplex virus (HSV), cause serious ocular damage. In infants recurrent conjunctivitis may be a sign of nasolacrimal (tear) duct obstruction. A chemical conjunctivitis may occur within 24 hours of instillation of neonatal ophthalmic prophylaxis; the clinical features include mild lid edema and a sterile, nonpurulent eye discharge (Fuloria and Kreiter, 2002).

BOX 14-1

Clinical Manifestations of Conjunctivitis

BACTERIAL CONJUNCTIVITIS ("PINK EYE")
Purulent drainage
Crusting of eyelids, especially on awakening
Inflamed conjunctiva
Swollen lids

VIRAL CONJUNCTIVITIS
Usually occurs with upper respiratory tract infection
Serous (watery) drainage
Inflamed conjunctiva
Swollen lids

ALLERGIC CONJUNCTIVITIS
Itching
Watery to thick, stringy discharge
Inflamed conjunctiva
Swollen lids

CONJUNCTIVITIS CAUSED BY FOREIGN BODY
Tearing
Pain
Inflamed conjunctiva
Usually only one eye affected

In children the usual causes of conjunctivitis are viral, bacterial, allergic, or related to a foreign body. Bacterial infection accounts for most instances of acute conjunctivitis in children. Diagnosis is made primarily from the clinical manifestations (Box 14-1), although cultures of purulent drainage may be needed to identify the specific cause.

Therapeutic Management

Treatment of conjunctivitis depends on the cause. Viral conjunctivitis is self-limiting, and treatment is limited to removal of the accumulated secretions. Bacterial conjunctivitis has traditionally been treated with topical antibacterial agents such as polymyxin and bacitracin (Polysporin), sodium sulfacetamide (Sulamyd), or trimethoprim and polymyxin (Polytrim). However, in one study of children with acute infective conjunctivitis treated by placebo vs topical chloramphenicol, there was little difference in cure rates; the authors concluded that most children will get better without antibiotic treatment (Rose, Harnden, Brueggemann, and others, 2005). Fluoroquinolones, approved for children ages 1 year and older, are viewed by ophthalmologists as the best ophthalmic antimicrobial agents available (Lichtenstein, Rinehart, and Levofloxacin Bacterial Conjunctivitis Study Group, 2003). Drops may be used during the day and an ointment at bedtime because the ointment preparation remains in the eye longer. Ointments are usually not used in the daytime because they blur vision. Corticosteroids are avoided because they reduce ocular resistance to bacteria.

Nursing Care Management

Nursing care includes keeping the eye clean and properly administering ophthalmic medication. Accumulated secretions are always removed by wiping from the inner canthus downward and outward, away from the opposite eye. Warm, moist compresses, such as a clean washcloth wrung out with hot tap water, are helpful in removing the crusts. Compresses are *not* kept on the eye because an occlusive covering promotes bacterial growth. Medication is instilled immediately after the eyes have been cleaned and according to correct procedure (see Chapter 22).

Prevention of infection in other family members is an important consideration with bacterial conjunctivitis. The child's washcloth and towel are kept separate from those used by others. Tissues used to clean the eye are discarded. The child should refrain from rubbing the eye and is instructed in good hand-washing technique.

NURSING ALERT

Signs of serious conjunctivitis include reduction or loss of vision, ocular pain, photophobia, exophthalmos (bulging eyeball), decreased ocular mobility, corneal ulceration, and unusual patterns of inflammation (e.g., the perilimbal flush associated with iritis or localized inflammation associated with scleritis). If a patient has any of these signs, refer him or her immediately to an ophthalmologist (Lederman and Lederman, 2003).

STOMATITIS

Stomatitis is inflammation of the oral mucosa, which may include the buccal (cheek) and labial (lip) mucosa, tongue, gingiva, palate, and floor of the mouth. It may be infectious or noninfectious and may be caused by local or systemic factors. In children aphthous stomatitis and herpetic stomatitis are typically seen. Children with immunosuppression and those receiving chemotherapy or head and neck radiotherapy are at high risk for developing mucosal ulceration and herpetic stomatitis.

Aphthous stomatitis (aphthous ulcer, canker sore) is a benign but painful condition whose cause is unknown. Its onset is usually associated with mild traumatic injury (biting the cheek, hitting the mucosa with a toothbrush, or a mouth appliance rubbing on the mucosa), allergy, or emotional stress. The lesions are painful, small, whitish ulcerations surrounded by a red border. They are distinguished from other types of stomatitis by healthy adjacent tissues, absence of vesicles, and no systemic illness. The ulcers persist for 4 to 12 days and heal uneventfully.

Herpetic gingivostomatitis (HGS) is caused by HSV, most often type 1, and may occur as a primary infection or recur in a less severe form known as **recurrent herpes labialis** (commonly called *cold sores* or *fever blisters*). The primary infection usually begins with a fever; the pharynx becomes edematous and erythematous; and vesicles erupt on the mucosa, causing severe pain (Fig. 14-7). Cervical lymphadenitis often occurs, and the breath has a distinctly foul odor. In the recurrent form the vesicles appear on the lips, usually singly or in groups. The precipitating factors for the cold sores include emotional stress, trauma (often related to dental procedures), immunosuppression, or exposure to excessive sunlight. The disease can last 5 to 14 days, with varying degrees of severity.

Stomatitis may occur as a manifestation of hand-foot-and-mouth disease and herpangina; both manifest with scattered vesicles on the buccal mucosa and are commonly caused by the nonpolio enteroviruses (primarily coxsackieviruses). Children with either hand-foot-and-mouth or herpangina often have poor intake as a result of the mouth sores.

FIG. 14-7 ■ Primary gingivostomatitis. (Reproduced with permission of the Wellcome Foundation, Ltd.)

Therapeutic Management

Treatment for all types of stomatitis is aimed at relief of symptoms, primarily pain. Acetaminophen and ibuprofen are usually sufficient for mild cases, but with more severe HGS, stronger analgesics such as codeine may be needed. Topical anesthetics are helpful and include over-the-counter preparations such as Orabase, Anbesol, and Kank-A. Lidocaine (Xylocaine Viscous) can be prescribed for the child who can keep 1 teaspoon of the solution in the mouth for 2 to 3 minutes and then expectorate the drug. A mixture of equal parts of diphenhydramine elixir and Maalox (aluminum and magnesium hydroxide) provides mild analgesia, antiinflammatory properties, and a protective coating for the lesions. Sucralfate can also be used as a coating agent for oral mucous membranes. Specific treatment for children with severe cases of HGS is the use of antiviral agents such as acyclovir (Faden, 2006).

Nursing Care Management

The chief nursing goals for children with stomatitis are relief of pain and prevention of spread of the herpes virus. Analgesics and topical anesthetics are used as needed to provide relief, especially before meals to encourage food and fluid intake. For younger infants and toddlers who cannot swish and swallow, the diphenhydramine and Maalox solution may be applied with a cotton-tipped applicator before feedings to minimize pain. Educating parents regarding the use of these medications is important to maintain adequate hydration in the child whose mouth is too sore to take liquids. Drinking bland fluids through a straw is helpful in avoiding the painful lesions. Mouth care is encouraged; the use of a very soft bristle toothbrush or disposable foam-tipped toothbrush provides gentle cleaning near ulcerated areas.

Careful hand washing is essential when caring for children with HGS. Because the infection is autoinoculable, children should keep their fingers out of the mouth; contaminated hands can infect other body parts. Very young children may require elbow restraints to ensure compliance. Articles placed in the mouth are cleaned thoroughly. Newborns and individuals with immunosuppression should not be exposed to infected children.

> **NURSING ALERT**
>
> When examining herpetic lesions, wear gloves. The virus easily enters breaks in the skin and can cause herpetic whitlow of the fingers.

Because herpes infection is often associated with sexual transmission, the nurse should explain to parents and older children that HGS is usually caused by type 1 HSV, the type not associated with sexual activity.

INTESTINAL PARASITIC DISEASES

Intestinal parasitic diseases, including helminths (worms) and protozoa, constitute the most frequent infections in the world. In the United States the incidence of intestinal parasitic disease, especially giardiasis, has increased among young children who attend daycare centers. Young children are especially at risk because of typical hand-mouth activity and uncontrolled fecal activity.

Intestinal parasitic diseases in humans are caused by various infecting organisms. This discussion is limited to the two most common parasitic infections among children in the United States: giardiasis and pinworms. Table 14-2 describes the outstanding features of selected helminths that belong to the family of nematodes.

GENERAL NURSING CARE MANAGEMENT

Nursing responsibilities related to intestinal parasitic infections involve assistance with identification of the parasite, treatment of the infection, and prevention of initial infection or reinfection. Identification of the organism is accomplished by laboratory examination of substances containing the worm, its larvae, or ova. Most are identified by examining fecal smears from the stools of persons suspected of harboring the parasite. Fresh specimens are best for revealing parasites or larvae; therefore collected specimens should be taken directly to the laboratory for examination. If this is not feasible, the specimen is placed in a container with a preservative. Parents need clear instructions on obtaining an adequate sample and the number of samples required (see Stool Specimens, Chapter 22). In most parasitic infections, examination of other family members, especially children, may be carried out to identify those who are similarly affected.

After the diagnosis is confirmed and appropriate treatment is planned, parents need further explanation and reinforcement. Compliance in terms of drug therapy and other measures, such as thorough hand washing, is essential for eradication of the parasite. The family needs to understand the nature of transmission and that in some cases the medication must be repeated in 2 weeks to 1 month to kill organisms hatched since initial treatment.

The nurse's most important function is preventive education of children and families regarding hygiene and health habits. Thorough hand washing before eating or handling food and after using the toilet is the most important precautionary method. Other preventive practices are listed in the Community Focus box.

GIARDIASIS

Giardiasis is caused by the protozoan *Giardia lamblia* (also called *Giardia intestinalis, Giardia duodenalis,* and *Lamblia intestinalis*). It is the most common intestinal parasitic pathogen in the United States. Child care centers and institutions providing care for persons with developmental disabilities are common sites for urban giardiasis, and the children may pass cysts for months. Giardiasis should also be considered in those with a history of recent travel to an endemic area (Pickering, 2004).

The potential for transmission is great, because the **cysts**—the nonmotile stage of the protozoa—can survive in the environment for months. Chief modes of transmission are person to person; contaminated water, especially in mountain lakes and streams and swimming or wading pools frequented by diapered infants; food; and animals, especially puppies. In

TABLE 14-2
Selected Intestinal Parasites

CLINICAL MANIFESTATIONS	COMMENTS
ASCARIASIS—*ASCARIS LUMBRICOIDES* (COMMON ROUNDWORM)	
Light infections—Asymptomatic	Transferred to mouth by way of contaminated food, fingers, or toys
Heavy infections—Anorexia, irritability, nervousness, enlarged abdomen, weight loss, fever, intestinal colic	Largest of the intestinal helminths
Severe infections—Intestinal obstruction, appendicitis, perforation of intestine with peritonitis, obstructive jaundice, lung involvement (pneumonitis)	Affects principally young children 1-4 years of age Prevalent in warm climates
HOOKWORM DISEASE—*NECATOR AMERICANUS*	
Light infections in well-nourished individuals—No problems	Transmitted by discharging eggs on the soil, which are picked up, causing infection from direct skin contact with contaminated soil
Heavier infections—Mild to severe anemia, malnutrition	Recommend wearing shoes, although children playing in contaminated soil expose many skin surfaces
May be itching and burning followed by erythema and a papular eruption in areas to which the organism migrates	
STRONGYLOIDIASIS—*STRONGYLOIDES STERCORALIS* (THREADWORM)	
Light infection—Asymptomatic	Transmission is same as for hookworm except autoinfection common
Heavy infection—Respiratory signs and symptoms; abdominal pain, distention; nausea and vomiting; diarrhea (large, pale stools, often with mucus)	Older children and adults affected more often than young children Severe infections may lead to severe nutritional deficiency
Threat to life in children with weakened immunologic defenses	
VISCERAL LARVA MIGRANS—*TOXOCARA CANIS* (DOGS) **INTESTINAL TOXOCARIASIS—*TOXOCARA CATI* (CATS)**	
Depends on reactivity of infected individual	Transmitted by direct contamination of hands from contact with dog, cat, or objects or by ingestion of soil
May be asymptomatic except for eosinophilia	Keep dogs and cats away from areas where children play; sandboxes especially important transmission areas
Specific diagnosis difficult	Periodic deworming of diagnosed dogs and cats Control of dog and cat population
TRICHURIASIS—*TRICHURIS TRICHIURA* (WHIPWORM)	
Light infections—Asymptomatic	Transmitted from contaminated soil, vegetables, toys, and other objects
Heavy infections—Abdominal pain and distention, diarrhea	Most frequent in warm, moist climates Occurs most often in undernourished children living in unsanitary conditions

COMMUNITY FOCUS

Preventing Intestinal Parasitic Disease

- Always wash hands and fingernails with soap and water before eating and handling food and after toileting.
- Avoid placing fingers in mouth and biting nails.
- Discourage children from scratching bare anal area.
- Use superabsorbent disposable diapers to prevent leakage.
- Change diapers as soon as soiled and dispose of diapers in closed receptacle out of children's reach.
- Do not rinse cloth or disposable diapers in toilet.
- Disinfect toilet seats and diaper-changing areas; use dilute household bleach (10% solution) or ammonia (Lysol) and wipe clean with paper towels.

- Drink only treated water or bottled water, especially if camping.
- Wash all raw fruits and vegetables and food that has fallen on the floor.
- Avoid growing foods in soil fertilized with human or untreated animal excreta.
- Teach children to defecate only in a toilet, not on the ground.
- Keep dogs and cats away from playgrounds or sandboxes.
- Avoid swimming in pools frequented by diapered children.
- Wear shoes outside.

children, person-to-person transmission is the most likely cause. Although individuals infected with giardiasis may be asymptomatic, common symptoms include abdominal cramps and diarrhea (Box 14-2).

Diagnosis of giardiasis may be made by microscopic examination of stool specimens or duodenal fluid, or by identi-fication of *G. lamblia* antigens in these specimens by techniques such as enzyme immunoassay (EIA). Because the *Giardia* organisms live in the upper intestine and are excreted in a highly variable pattern, repeated microscopic examination of stool specimens may be required to identify **trophozoites** (active parasites) or cysts. Duodenal specimens are ob-

BOX 14-2
Clinical Manifestations of Giardiasis

Infants and young children:
- Diarrhea
- Vomiting
- Anorexia
- Growth failure (failure to thrive), if chronic exposure

Children older than 5 years of age:
- Abdominal cramps
- Intermittent loose stools
- Constipation

Stools that are malodorous, watery, pale, and greasy

Spontaneous resolution of most infections in 4 to 6 weeks

Rare, chronic form:
- Intermittent loose, foul-smelling stools
- Possibility of abdominal bloating, flatulence, sulfur-tasting belches, epigastric pain, vomiting, headache, and weight loss

FIG. 14-8 ▪ Prevention of giardiasis, especially in daycare centers, requires sanitary practices during diaper changes, such as discarding paper diapers in a covered receptacle, changing paper covers on the diaper-changing surface, and having facilities for hand washing nearby. NOTE: Soiled cloth diapers and clothing should be stored in a plastic bag for transport home.

tained by direct aspiration, biopsy, or the **string** test. In the string test, the child swallows a gelatin capsule with a nylon string attached. Several hours later, the string is withdrawn and the contents are sent for laboratory analysis. With the availability of EIA techniques to identify *Giardia* antigens in stool specimens, other tests are being used less often.

Therapeutic Management

The drugs of choice for treatment of giardiasis are metronidazole (Flagyl), tinidazole (Tindamax), and nitazoxanide (Alinia). Tinidazole is said to have an 80% to 100% cure rate after a single dose (American Academy of Pediatrics, 2006). Metronidazole and tinidazole have a metallic taste as well as gastrointestinal side effects, including nausea and vomiting. Nitazoxanide has no bitter taste and should be taken with food to avoid gastrointestinal symptoms. Albendazole is also used to treat the disease and reportedly has fewer side effects than metronidazole (American Academy of Pediatrics, 2006).

Nursing Care Management

The most important nursing consideration is prevention of giardiasis and education of parents, child care center staff, and those who are entrusted with the daily care of small children. Attention to meticulous sanitary practices, especially during diaper changes, is essential (see Community Focus box and Fig. 14-8). Nurses can play an important role in educating parents of small children and daycare staff regarding appropriate sanitation practices (see Preschool and Kindergarten Experience, Chapter 13). In addition young children who are infected or who have diarrhea should be discouraged from swimming in community or private pools until they are infection-free. Lakes and streams may contain high numbers of *Giardia* spore cysts, which can be swallowed in the water. Children are discouraged from swimming in stagnant bodies of water, and in water where there are known infected children swimming when there is a high chance of swallowing water. *Giardia* organisms are said to be resistant to chlorine (Hlavsa, Watson, and Beach, 2005). Parents are encouraged to take small children to the restroom frequently when swimming, to avoid letting children in diapers in swimming areas, and to change diapers away from the water source (see also

Centers for Disease Control information on recreational water illnesses*). After children are infected, family education regarding drug administration is essential.

ENTEROBIASIS (PINWORMS)

Enterobiasis, or pinworms, caused by the nematode *Enterobius vermicularis,* is the most common helminthic infection in the United States. It is universally present in temperate climatic zones and may infect more than 30% of all children at any one time. Crowded conditions, such as in classrooms and daycare centers, favor transmission.

Infection begins when the eggs are ingested or inhaled (the eggs float in the air). The eggs hatch in the upper intestine, then mature and migrate through the intestine. After mating, adult females migrate out the anus and lay eggs (American Academy of Pediatrics, 2006). The movement of the worms on skin and mucous membrane surfaces causes intense itching. As the child scratches, eggs are deposited on the hands and underneath the fingernails. The typical hand-to-mouth activity of young children makes them especially prone to reinfection. Pinworm eggs persist in the indoor environment for 2 to 3 weeks, contaminating anything they contact, such as toilet seats, doorknobs, bed linen, underwear, and food. Except for the intense rectal itching associated with pinworms, the clinical manifestations are nonspecific (Box 14-3).

Diagnostic Evaluation

Diagnosis is most commonly made from the tape test (see Nursing Care Management). Repeated tests to collect eggs may be necessary, and if there is a possibility that other fam-

---

*http://www.cdc.gov/healthyswimming.

BOX 14-3
Clinical Manifestations of Pinworms

Intense perianal itching (principal symptom); evidence of itching in young children includes:
- General irritability
- Restlessness
- Poor sleep
- Bed-wetting
- Distractibility
- Short attention span

Perianal dermatitis and excoriation secondary to itching

If worms migrate, possible vaginal (vulvovaginitis) and urethral infection

the chance of ova collecting under the nails, dressing children in one-piece sleeping outfits, and daily showering rather than tub bathing. Families should be informed that recurrence is common. Repeated infections should be treated in the same manner as the first one.

INGESTION OF INJURIOUS AGENTS

Since the passage of the Poison Prevention Packaging Act of 1970, which requires that certain potentially hazardous drugs and household products be sold in child-resistant containers, the incidence of poisonings in children has decreased dramatically. However, despite these advances, poisoning remains a significant health concern, with most cases (51% in 2004) occurring in children younger than 6 years of age. Although pharmaceuticals such as analgesics, cough and cold preparations, topical preparations, antibiotics, vitamins, gastrointestinal preparations, hormones, and antihistamines are frequently the agents of poisonings, children may be poisoned by a variety of substances. The most frequently ingested poisons include (Watson, Litovitz, Rodgers, and others, 2005; Litovitz, Klein-Schwartz, White, and others, 2000; Powers, 2000):

- Cosmetics and personal care products (perfume, cologne, aftershave)*
- Cleaning products (hypochlorite ["household"] bleach, pine oil disinfectants)
- Plants (nontoxic gastrointestinal irritants, oxalates) (Box 14-4)
- Foreign bodies, toys, and miscellaneous substances (desiccants, thermometers, bubble-blowing solutions)

Many poisonings reflect the ready accessibility of the product in the home, where more than 90% of poisonings occur, although a significant number take place elsewhere, such as in a grandparent's or friend's home, in a school, or in a health care facility.

ily members may be infected, a tape test should be performed on them.

Therapeutic Management

The drugs available for treatment of pinworms include mebendazole (Vermox), pyrantel pamoate (Pin-Rid, Antiminth), and albendazole. The drug of choice is mebendazole, which is safe, effective, and convenient, with few side effects. However, it is not recommended for children younger than 2 years of age. If pyrvinium pamoate is prescribed, parents are advised that the drug stains stool and vomitus bright red, as well as clothing or skin that comes in contact with the drug; it is available without prescription and should not be used in children under 2 years without consulting the primary practitioner. Because pinworms are easily transmitted, all household members are treated. The dose of antiparasitic medication should be repeated in 2 weeks to completely eradicate the parasite and prevent reinfection.

Nursing Care Management

Nursing care is directed at identifying the parasite, eradicating the organism, and preventing reinfection. Parents need clear, detailed instructions for the **tape test.** A loop of transparent (not "frosted" or "magic") tape, sticky side out, is placed around the end of a tongue depressor, which is then firmly pressed against the child's perianal area. A convenient, commercially prepared tape is also available for this purpose. Pinworm specimens are collected in the morning as soon as the child awakens and *before* the child has a bowel movement or bathes. The procedure may need to be performed on 3 or more consecutive days before eggs are collected. Parents are instructed to place the tongue blade in a glass jar or loosely in a plastic bag so that it can be brought in for microscopic examination. For specimens collected in the hospital, practitioner's office, or clinic, the tape is placed smoothly on a glass slide, sticky side down, for examination.

Adherence to the drug regimen is usually excellent because the duration of treatment is typically only one dose. However, the family is reminded of the need to take a second dose in 2 weeks to ensure eradication of the eggs.

To prevent reinfection, washing all clothes and bed linens in hot water and vacuuming the house may be recommended. However, there is little documentation on the effectiveness of these measures, since pinworms survive on many surfaces. Helpful suggestions include hand washing after toileting and before eating, keeping the child's fingernails short to minimize

NURSING ALERT

The following five commonly used and easily available drugs (first four are over-the-counter products) can cause serious or fatal consequences if as little as ¼ teaspoon or ½ tablet is ingested: methyl salicylate, camphor, topical imidazolines (sympathomimetics such as those contained in Visine, Afrin, and Clear Eyes), benzocaine, and diphenoxylate-atropine (Lomotil and others). Stress to parents the importance of keeping such drugs away from children. If these agents are ingested, advise parents to seek medical treatment immediately. Emesis should not be induced at home.

The developmental characteristics of young children predispose them to poisoning by ingestion. Infants and toddlers explore their environment through oral experimentation. Because the sense of taste is not discriminating at this age, many unpalatable substances are ingested. In addition, toddlers and preschoolers are developing autonomy and initiative, which increase their curiosity and noncompliant behavior. Imitation is also a powerful motivator, especially when combined with lack of awareness of danger.

This section is primarily concerned with the immediate emergency treatment of ingestion of injurious agents. Specific management of corrosive, hydrocarbon, acetaminophen, salicylate, iron, and plant poisoning is summarized in Box 14-5.

*The most common substances in each category are in parentheses. Substances ingested are not necessarily most toxic but often readily available.

BOX 14-4
Poisonous and Nonpoisonous Plants

**POISONOUS PLANTS
(TOXIC PARTS)**
Apple (leaves, seeds)
Apricot (leaves, stem, seed pits)
Azalea (all parts)
Buttercup (all parts)
Castor (bean or seeds—extremely toxic)
Cherry (wild or cultivated) (twigs, seeds, foliage)
Daffodil (bulbs)
Dumbcane (dieffenbachia) (all parts)
Elephant ear (all parts)
English ivy (all parts)
Foxglove (leaves, seeds, flowers)
Holly (berries and leaves)
Hyacinth (bulbs)
Ivy (leaves)
Mistletoe* (berries, leaves)
Oak tree (acorn, foliage)
Philodendron (all parts)
Plum (pit)
Poinsettia† (leaves)
Poison ivy, poison oak (leaves, stems, sap, fruit, smoke from burning plants)
Pokeweed, pokeberry (roots, berries, leaves [when eaten raw])

Pothos (all parts)
Rhubarb (leaves)
Tulip (bulbs)
Water hemlock (all parts)
Wisteria (seeds, pods)
Yew (all parts)

NONPOISONOUS PLANTS
African violet
Aluminum plant
Asparagus fern
Begonia
Boston fern
Christmas cactus
Coleus
Gardenia
Grape ivy
Jade plant
Piggyback begonia
Piggyback plant
Prayer plant
Rubber tree
Snake plant
Spider plant
Swedish ivy
Wax plant
Weeping fig
Zebra plant

*Eating one or two berries or leaves is probably nontoxic.
†Mildly toxic if ingested in massive quantities.

Because of the importance of lead poisoning among young children, ingestion of lead is discussed separately. Appropriate suggestions for poison prevention are discussed on p. 474 and in Chapter 12.

PRINCIPLES OF EMERGENCY TREATMENT

A poisoning may or may not require emergency intervention, but in every instance medical evaluation is necessary to initiate appropriate action. Parents are advised to call the **poison control center (PCC)** *before* initiating any intervention. The local PCC telephone number (usually listed in the front of the telephone directory) should be posted near each phone in the house* (see Critical Thinking Exercise and Emergency Treatment box).

Based on the initial telephone assessment, the PCC counsels the parents to begin treatment at home or to take the child to an emergency facility. When a call is taken, the name and telephone number of the caller is recorded to reestablish contact if the connection is interrupted. Because most poisonings are managed in the home, expert advice is essential in minimizing adverse effects. When the exact quantity or type of ingested toxin is not known, admission to a health care facility

*Also available by calling (800) 222-1222 or online at American Association of Poison Control Centers, http://www.aapcc.org.

??? CRITICAL THINKING EXERCISE

Poisoning
Mrs. Berry, a neighbor, calls you. She is upset because her 2-year-old son has eaten several chewable multivitamins with iron. She asks you if she should give her son ipecac. What should you advise her to do?

QUESTIONS
1. Evidence—Is there sufficient evidence to formulate an answer for Mrs. Berry?
2. Assumptions—Describe some underlying assumptions about the following:
   a. What is the best initial response when a child ingests a potentially poisonous substance?
   b. What is ipecac?
   c. What are the dangers involved in the use of ipecac?
3. What is the priority for nursing care at this time?
4. Does the evidence support your conclusion?
5. What alternative perspectives might you have?

emergencytreatment

Poisoning
1. **Assess the victim:**
   - Initiate cardiorespiratory support if needed (Airway, Breathing, Circulation).
   - Take vital signs; reevaluate routinely.
   - Treat associated complications.
2. **Terminate exposure:**
   - Empty mouth of pills, plant parts, or other material.
   - Flush eyes continuously with normal saline (or room-temperature tap water at home) for 15 to 20 minutes.
   - Flush skin and wash with soap and a soft cloth; remove contaminated clothes, especially if a pesticide, acid, alkali, or hydrocarbon is involved.
   - Bring victim of an inhalation poisoning into fresh air.
3. **Identify the poison:**
   - Question the victim and witnesses.
   - Look for environmental clues (empty container, nearby spill, odor on breath) and save all evidence of poison (container, vomitus, urine).
   - Be alert to signs and symptoms of potential poisoning in absence of other evidence, including symptoms of ocular or dermal exposure.
   - Call poison control center or other competent emergency facility for immediate advice regarding treatment.
4. **Prevent poison absorption:**
   - Place child in side-lying, sitting, or kneeling position with head below chest to prevent aspiration.
   - Administer activated charcoal if ordered (unless used repeatedly, usual dose is 1 g/kg unless amount of toxin is known), administer drug antidote, or perform gastric lavage.

BOX 14-5

Selected Poisonings in Children

CORROSIVES (STRONG ACIDS OR ALKALIS)

Drain, toilet, or oven cleaners
Electric dishwasher detergent (liquid, because of higher pH, is more hazardous than granular)
Mildew remover
Batteries
Clinitest tablets
Denture cleaners
Bleach

Clinical Manifestations

Severe burning pain in mouth, throat, and stomach
White, swollen mucous membranes; edema of lips, tongue, and pharynx (respiratory obstruction)
Violent vomiting (hemoptysis)
Drooling and inability to clear secretions
Signs of shock
Anxiety and agitation

Comments

Household bleach is a frequently ingested corrosive but rarely causes serious damage.
Liquid corrosives cause more damage than granular preparations.

Treatment

Inducing emesis is contraindicated (vomiting redamages the mucosa).
Contact poison control center (PCC) immediately. If PCC or medical advice and treatment not immediately available, it may be appropriate to dilute corrosive with water or milk (usually no more than 120 ml [4 ounces]).
Do not neutralize. Neutralization can cause an exothermic reaction (which produces heat and causes increased symptoms or produces a thermal burn in addition to a chemical burn).
Maintain patent airway as needed.
Administer analgesics.
Do not allow oral intake.
Esophageal stricture may require repeated dilations or surgery.

HYDROCARBONS

Gasoline
Kerosene
Lamp oil
Mineral seal oil (found in furniture polish)
Lighter fluid
Turpentine
Paint thinner and remover (some types)

Clinical Manifestations

Gagging, choking, and coughing
Nausea
Vomiting
Alterations in sensorium, such as lethargy
Weakness
Respiratory symptoms of pulmonary involvement
- Tachypnea
- Cyanosis
- Retractions
- Grunting

Comments

Immediate danger is aspiration (even small amounts can cause bronchitis and chemical pneumonia).
Gasoline, kerosene, lighter fluid, mineral seal oil, and turpentine cause severe pneumonia.

Treatment

Inducing emesis is generally contraindicated
Gastric decontamination and emptying are questionable, even when the hydrocarbon contains a heavy metal or pesticide; if gastric lavage must be performed, a cuffed endotracheal tube should be in place before lavage because of a high risk of aspiration.
Symptomatic treatment of chemical pneumonia includes high humidity, oxygen, hydration, and antibiotics for secondary infection.

ACETAMINOPHEN

Clinical Manifestations

Occurs in four stages:
1. Initial period (2 to 4 hours after ingestion)
   - Nausea
   - Vomiting
   - Sweating
   - Pallor
2. Latent period (24 to 36 hours)
   - Patient improves
3. Hepatic involvement (may last up to 7 days and be permanent)
   - Pain in right upper quadrant
   - Jaundice
   - Confusion
   - Stupor
   - Coagulation abnormalities
4. Patients who do not die in hepatic stage gradually recover.

Comments

Most common accidental drug poisoning in children.
Occurs from acute ingestion.
Toxic dose is 150 mg/kg or greater in children.
Because of multiple formulations and concentrations, chronic acetaminophen toxicity is a significant problem.
Parents should be counseled to read product packaging carefully and to consult a health care professional to avoid inappropriate dosing (Abruzzi and Stork, 2002).

Treatment

Antidote *N*-acetylcysteine (Mucomyst) can usually be given orally but is first diluted in fruit juice or soda because of the antidote's offensive odor.
Given as 1 loading dose and usually 17 maintenance doses in different dosages.
May be given intravenously, but use is investigational.

Continued

BOX 14-5

Selected Poisonings in Children—cont'd

ASPIRIN (ACETYLSALICYLIC ACID [ASA])
Clinical Manifestations
Acute poisoning
- Nausea
- Disorientation
- Vomiting
- Dehydration
- Diaphoresis
- Hyperpnea
- Hyperpyrexia
- Oliguria
- Tinnitus
- Coma
- Convulsions

Chronic poisoning
- Same as above but subtle onset (often mistaken for viral illness)
- Dehydration, coma, and seizures may be more severe
- Bleeding tendencies

Comments
May be caused by acute ingestion (severe toxicity occurs with 300 to 500 mg/kg).
May be caused by chronic ingestion (i.e., 100 mg/kg/day for 2 or more days); can be more serious than acute ingestion.
Time to peak serum salicylate level can vary with enteric aspirin or the presence of concretions (bezoars).

Treatment
Hospitalization for severe toxicity
Emesis, lavage, activated charcoal, or cathartic
Lavage will not remove concretions of ASA
Activated charcoal important early in ASA toxicity
Sodium bicarbonate transfusions are used to correct metabolic acidosis, and urinary alkalinization may be effective in enhancing elimination; urinary alkalinization is difficult to achieve
Be aware of the risk for fluid overload and pulmonary edema
External cooling for hyperpyrexia
Anticonvulsants
Oxygen and ventilation for respiratory depression
Vitamin K for bleeding
In severe cases, hemodialysis (not peritoneal dialysis)

IRON
Mineral supplement or vitamin containing iron

Clinical Manifestations
Occurs in five stages:
1. Initial period (½ to 6 hours after ingestion; if child does not develop gastrointestinal symptoms in 6 hours, toxicity is unlikely)
   - Vomiting
   - Hematemesis
   - Diarrhea
   - Hematochezia (bloody stools)
   - Gastric pain

2. Latency (2 to 12 hours): patient improves
3. Systemic toxicity (4 to 24 hours)
   - Metabolic acidosis
   - Fever
   - Hyperglycemia
   - Bleeding
   - Shock
   - Death (may occur)
4. Hepatic injury (48 to 96 hours)
   - Seizures
   - Coma
5. Rarely, pyloric stenosis develops at 2 to 5 weeks

Comments
Factors related to frequency of iron poisoning include:
- Widespread availability
- Packaging of large quantities in individual containers
- Lack of parental awareness of iron toxicity
- Resemblance of iron tablets to candy (e.g., M&Ms)

Toxic dose is based on the amount of elemental iron in various salts (sulfate, gluconate, fumarate), which ranges from 20% to 33%; ingestions of 60 mg/kg are considered dangerous.

Treatment
Emesis or lavage
For toxic doses lavage may be necessary for all chewable tablets or liquids if spontaneous vomiting has not occurred
Chelation therapy with deferoxamine in severe intoxication (may turn urine a red to orange color)
If intravenous deferoxamine is given too rapidly, hypotension, facial flushing, rash, urticaria, tachycardia, and shock may occur; stop the infusion, maintain the intravenous line with normal saline, and notify the practitioner immediately

PLANTS
Plants listed in Box 14-4

Clinical Manifestations
Depends on type of plant ingested
May cause local irritation of oropharynx and entire gastrointestinal tract
May cause respiratory, renal, and central nervous system symptoms
Topical contact with plants can cause dermatitis

Comments
Some of most frequently ingested substances
Rarely cause serious problems, although some plant ingestions can be fatal
Can also cause choking and allergic reactions

Treatment
Induce emesis
Wash from skin or eyes
Supportive care as needed

with pediatric emergency treatment services for laboratory evaluation and surveillance is critical during the time after ingestion.

Assessment

The first and most important principle in dealing with a poisoning is to treat the child first, not the poison. This requires an immediate concern for life support. Vital signs are taken, and respiratory or circulatory support is instituted as needed. The child's condition is routinely reevaluated. Because shock is a complication of several types of household poisons, particularly corrosives, measures to reduce the effects of shock, beginning with the ABCs (airway, breathing, circulation) of resuscitation, are important. Establishing and maintaining vascular access for rapid intravascular volume expansion is vital in the treatment of pediatric shock.

The emergency department nurse's responsibility is to be prepared for immediate intervention with all of the necessary equipment. Because time and speed are critical factors in recovery from serious poisonings, anticipation of potential problems and complications may mean the difference between life and death.

Gastric Decontamination

In general, the immediate treatment is to remove the ingested poison by adsorbing the toxin with activated charcoal, performing gastric lavage, or increasing bowel motility (catharsis). Because of continuing controversy regarding the use of these methods, each toxic ingestion should be treated individually (Abruzzi and Stork, 2002). Specific antidotes may be administered for certain poisonings. **Syrup of ipecac,** an emetic that exerts its action through irritation of the gastric mucosa and by stimulation of the vomiting center, is no longer recommended for immediate treatment of poison ingestion (American Academy of Clinical Toxicology and European Association of Poisons Centres and Clinical Toxicologists, 2004b; American Academy of Pediatrics, 2003). The American Academy of Pediatrics (2003) recommends that existing ipecac in the home be disposed of safely and that the first action for a caregiver of a child who may have ingested a toxic substance is to consult the local PCC. If the PCC cannot be reached, the child should be taken to the nearest emergency department.

NURSING ALERT

Syrup of ipecac is not recommended for poison treatment intervention in the home (American Academy of Pediatrics, 2003).

Ipecac is contraindicated because it may cause prolonged vomiting (up to 12 hours), which makes it relatively contraindicated in ingestions that may cause sedation, coma, or seizures (Powers, 2000). Medications such as calcium channel blockers and benzodiazepines either produce a rapid onset of adverse symptoms (e.g., sedation, seizures, coma) or exaggerate the vagal response induced by gagging, which can lead to significant bradycardia. Under either circumstance, uncontrolled vomiting becomes an undesirable and unsafe event.

No emetic or other substance should be given at home without consultation with a PCC or physician.

If the child is admitted to an emergency facility, **gastric lavage** may be performed to empty the stomach of the toxic agent; however, this procedure is associated with serious complications (gastrointestinal perforation, hypoxia, aspiration) and it is no longer recommended in all cases of ingestion. There is no conclusive evidence that gastric lavage decreases morbidity (Criddle, 2007; Heard, 2005). In addition, gastric lavage may be of little use if used beyond 1 hour of ingestion (Heard, 2005). Conditions that may be appropriate for the use of gastric lavage include presentation within 1 hour of ingestion of a toxin, ingestion in patient who has decreased gastrointestinal motility, the ingestion of a toxic amount of sustained-release medication, and a massive or life-threatening amount of poison (Criddle, 2007). When gastric lavage is used, the patient requires a protected airway, possible sedation, and the largest-diameter tube that can be inserted to facilitate passage of gastric contents.

A more commonly used method of gastrointestinal decontamination is the use of **activated charcoal,** an odorless, tasteless, fine black powder that adsorbs many compounds, creating a stable complex. Activated charcoal may replace ipecac as the home remedy of choice (Bond, 2002), but the American Academy of Pediatrics (2003) suggests it is premature to recommend the administration of activated charcoal in the home. Activated charcoal is mixed with water or a saline cathartic to form a slurry. Slurries are neither gritty nor distasteful but resemble black mud. To increase the child's acceptance of activated charcoal, the nurse should mix it with diet soda and serve it through a straw in an opaque container with a cover (such as a disposable coffee cup and lid) or an ordinary cup covered with aluminum foil or placed inside a small paper bag. In one small study, healthy adolescents preferred the taste of activated charcoal mixed with Coca-Cola or chocolate milk mixture instead of water (Cheng and Ratnapalan, 2007). For small children a nasogastric tube may be required to administer activated charcoal.

Potential complications from the use of activated charcoal include aspiration (usually in patients with impaired gag reflexes), constipation, and intestinal obstruction (in multiple doses). Superactivated charcoal products for gastric decontamination are reported to be more palatable and just as effective (Criddle, 2007; Heard, 2005). Cathartics, such as sorbitol, sodium, or magnesium, may be administered to stimulate evacuation of the bowel, thus decreasing systemic absorption of the poison and aiding in the removal of the charcoal. Many commercial preparations of activated charcoal contain cathartics. However, the use of cathartics is controversial, and the American Academy of Clinical Toxicology and European Association of Poisons Centres and Clinical Toxicologists (2004a) do not recommend their use in children. The Evidence-Based Practice box reviews recent literature on the use of gastric lavage in comparison to activated charcoal when a child has ingested poison.

In a minority of poisonings, specific **antidotes** are available to counteract the poison. They are highly effective and should be available in all emergency facilities. The supply of antidotes should be checked routinely and replaced as used or according to expiration dates. Antidotes available to treat toxin ingestion include N-acetylcysteine for acetaminophen poisoning, oxygen for carbon monoxide inhalation, naloxone for opioid overdose, flumazenil (Romazicon) for benzodiazepines (diazepam [Valium], midazolam [Versed]) overdose, digoxin immune Fab (Digibind) for digoxin toxicity, amyl nitrate for cyanide, and antivenin for certain poisonous bites.

Gastric Lavage in Children
Curt Roberts and Danna Salinas

ASK THE QUESTION What is the effect of gastric lavage in reducing systemic absorption of toxic substances compared with the administration of activated charcoal or forced emesis?

SEARCH FOR EVIDENCE

Search Strategies Keywords included gastric lavage, gastric decontamination, activated charcoal, and toxic ingestion. Searches were limited to English articles with human subjects.

Databases Used PubMed, STAT!Ref, UpToDateOnline, CINAHL, EMBASE, D.A.R.E, Cochrane Library, National Guideline Clearinghouse (AHRQ)

CRITICALLY ANALYZE THE EVIDENCE

Eddleston, Juszczak, and Buckley (2003) recently completed a review of the literature to determine whether gastric lavage pushes poisons beyond the pylorus to assist with faster elimination of toxins from the body. The review examined two studies designed to measure movement of substances through the stomach and into the small intestine after gastric lavage. One study randomized 40 patients to gastric emptying by forced emesis or gastric lavage and maintained a control group of 20 patients in whom gastric emptying was not necessary. Either radiopaque pellets or radiolabeled water was used as a marker. There were no significant differences in the number of pellets in the small bowel between the emesis group and the control group or between the gastric lavage group and the control group. The second study consisted of five volunteers who were subjected to gastric lavage on three occasions. Less poison was found in the small bowel after gastric lavage than after no intervention. The researchers concluded there was no evidence that gastric lavage drives toxins into the small intestine.

Other studies have demonstrated that gastric lavage is equivalent to forced emesis as a method of gastric emptying (American Academy of Clinical Toxicology and European Association of Poisons Centres and Clinical Toxicologists, 1999, 2005; Smilkstein, 2002). A randomized crossover study with 12 volunteers who ingested paracetamol 50 mg/kg 1 hour after a standard meal demonstrated that activated charcoal administered within 1 hour of ingestion was more effective than gastric lavage followed by charcoal because there was a delay in administration of the activated charcoal (Christophersen, Levin, Hoegberg, and others, 2002). Forced emesis was superior to gastric lavage when the goal was to remove large particles and fragments. However, the literature supports that gastric emptying has limited benefit in gastrointestinal decontamination because administration of activated charcoal appears to be more effective (American Academy of Clinical Toxicology and European Association of Poisons Centres and Clinical Toxicologists, 1999, 2005; Smilkstein, 2002).

Numerous complications are reported with both gastrointestinal lavage and activated charcoal. Complications of orogastric or nasogastric intubation include esophageal tears or perforation, nasal injury, oropharyngeal injury, gastric perforation, and inadvertent tracheal intubation (American Academy of Clinical Toxicology and European Association of Poisons Centres and Clinical Toxicologists, 1999, 2005; Smilkstein, 2002; Caravati, Knight, Linscott, and others, 2001). Neither the American Academy of Clinical Toxicology nor the European Association of Poisons Centres and Clinical Toxicologists (2005) has recommended the routine use of gastric lavage in the management of toxic ingestions since 1997. Contraindications to the administration of charcoal also exist, including in patients who have ingested corrosive materials and in those at risk for hemorrhage or perforation due to structural abnormalities or recent surgery.

APPLY THE EVIDENCE: NURSING IMPLICATIONS

Gastric lavage has little or no effect in reducing absorption, especially when used as an intervention more than 1 hour after ingestion. Single-dose or multidose activated charcoal is most effective when administered within 1 hour of ingestion but may have an effect up to 4 hours after ingestion, depending on the substance. Administration of activated charcoal should not be delayed by the use of forced emesis or gastric lavage.

References

American Academy of Clinical Toxicology, European Association of Poisons Centres and Clinical Toxicologists: Position paper: single-dose activated charcoal, *J Toxicol Clin Toxicol* 43:61-87, 2005.

American Academy of Clinical Toxicology, European Association of Poisons Centres and Clinical Toxicologists: Position statement and practice guidelines on the use of multi-dose activated charcoal in the treatment of acute poisoning, *J Toxicol Clin Toxicol* 37(6):731-751, 1999.

Caravati EM, Knight HH, Linscott MS, and others: Esophageal laceration and charcoal mediastinum complicating gastric lavage, *J Emerg Med* 20(3):273-276, 2001.

Christophersen AB, Levin D, Hoegberg LCG, and others: Activated charcoal alone or after gastric lavage: a simulated large paracetamol intoxication, *Br J Clin Pharmacol* 53(3):312-317, 2002.

Eddleston M, Juszczak E, Buckley N: Does gastric lavage really push poisons beyond the pylorus? A systematic review of the evidence, *Ann Emerg Med* 42(3):359-364, 2003.

Smilkstein MJ: Techniques used to prevent gastrointestinal absorption of toxic compounds. In Goldfrank LR, Flomenbaum NE, Lewin NA, and others, editors: *Goldfrank's toxicologic emergencies*, ed 7, New York, 2002, McGraw-Hill.

Prevention of Recurrence

The ultimate objective is to prevent poisonings from occurring or recurring. One effective counseling method is first to discuss the difficulties of constantly watching and safeguarding young children (see Family Focus box). In this way the challenging task of raising children can lead to a discussion of injury prevention as part of the parental role. This approach also incorporates contributory causes for the incident, such as inadequate support systems; marital discord; discipline techniques (especially use of physical punishment); parental dis-

tress; or any disruption in the family or family activities, such as vacations, moves, visitors, illnesses, or births. A visit to the home, especially after repeat poisonings, is recommended as part of the follow-up care to assess hazards, including family factors, and to evaluate appropriate injury-proofing measures. One method of identifying risk areas is to ask specific questions or to have the parent complete a questionnaire designed to isolate factors that predispose children to poisoning. Another approach is to encourage parents to bend down to the child's eye level and survey the home environment for poten-

FAMILY FOCUS

Poisoning

A poisoning is more than a physical emergency for the child—it usually represents an emotional crisis for the parents, particularly in terms of guilt, self-reproach, and insecurity in the parenting role. The emergency department is no place to admonish the family for negligence, lack of appropriate supervision, or failure to injury-proof the home. Rather, it is a time to calm and support the child and parents, while unaccusingly exploring the circumstances of the injury. If the nurse prematurely attempts to discuss ways of preventing such an incident from recurring, the parents' anxiety will block out any suggestions or offered guidance. Therefore it is preferable for the nurse to delay the discussion until the child's condition is stabilized or, if the child is discharged immediately after emergency treatment, to make a public health referral or send a packet of information.

COMMUNITY FOCUS

Poison Prevention

- Assess possible contributing factors in occurrence of injury, such as discipline, parent-child relationship, developmental ability, environmental factors, and behavior problems.
- Institute anticipatory guidance for possible future injuries based on child's age and developmental level.
- Initiate referral to appropriate agency to evaluate home environment and need for injury-proofing measures.
- Provide assistance with environmental manipulation, such as lead removal, when necessary.
- Educate parents regarding safe storage of toxic substances.
- Advise parents to take drugs out of sight of children.
- Teach children the hazards of ingesting nonfood items.
- Advise parents against using plants for teas or medicine.
- Discuss problems of discipline and children's noncompliance and offer strategies for effective discipline.
- Instruct parents regarding correct administration of drugs for therapeutic purposes and to discontinue drug if there is evidence of mild toxicity.
- Advise parents to contact the poison control center ([800] 222-1222) or practitioner immediately when a poisoning occurs.
- Tell them to post number of regional poison control center with emergency phone list by telephone.
- They should include by the telephone the home address with nearest cross street in case an ambulance is needed. (In an emergency, family members may not remember the house address, and baby-sitters may not be aware of the information.)

tial hazards. Have the parents try to open cabinets and reach shelves to access poisons.

Passive measures (those that do not require active participation) have been the most successful in preventing poisoning and include using child-resistant closures and limiting the number of tablets in one container. However, these measures alone are not sufficient to prevent poisoning, since most toxic agents in the home do not have safety closures. Therefore, **active measures** (those that require participation) are essential. Guidelines for preventing the occurrence or recurrence of a poisoning are listed in the Community Focus box.

HEAVY METAL POISONING

Heavy metal poisoning can occur from the ingestion of a variety of substances, the most common being lead. Other sources that are important in terms of children are iron and mercury. **Mercury toxicity,** a rare form of heavy metal poisoning, has occurred in children from a variety of sources, such as broken thermometers or thermostats, broken fluorescent light bulbs, disk batteries, topical medications, gas regulators, cathartics, and interior latex house paint (Clifton, 2007; Etzel, 2001). Elemental mercury (also called metallic mercury or quicksilver) is nontoxic if ingested and if the gastrointestinal tract is healthy (e.g., has no fistulas). However, mercury is volatile at room temperature and enters the bloodstream after it is inhaled, causing toxicity (tremors, memory loss, insomnia, gingivitis, diarrhea, anorexia, weight loss). The classic form of mercury poisoning is called **acrodynia** (or "painful extremities").

NURSING ALERT

Mercury thermometers are no longer recommended because, if they are broken, the inhaled vapors can cause toxicity. To prevent inhalation, spilled mercury must be cleaned up quickly, using disposable towels and rubber gloves and washing the hands well after removing the spill.

Heavy metals have an affinity for certain essential tissue chemicals, which must remain free for adequate cell functioning. When metals are bound to these substances, cellular enzyme systems are inactivated. Treatment involves **chelation,** use of a chemical compound that combines with the metal for rapid and safe excretion.

LEAD POISONING ✗   *[handwritten: Normal lead in Blood should be 0-10.]*

Poisoning from lead has been a problem throughout history and throughout the world. In the United States the problem began in the early 1900s, when white lead was added to paints and when tetraethyl lead was added to gasoline as an antiknock compound. Lead content in paint was decreased in 1950, and in 1978 the use of lead in household paint was banned. The use of lead in paint and leaded gasoline has been banned in the United States. After this change in policy, the average blood lead level (BLL) in the United States for people ages 1 to 74 years dropped from 12.8 mcg/dl in 1980 to 1.9 mcg/dl in 1999 (American Academy of Pediatrics, 2005). Yet because lead does not decompose or break down into smaller particles, lead deposited in the past is still present in soil near heavily trafficked areas. Coupled with deteriorating lead-based paint falling from the exterior of nearby houses, soil becomes a significant pathway by which lead poisoning can occur. Bare soil used as a play area contributes to the lead exposure of young children, since lead-contaminated dust is tracked into the home.   *[handwritten: Chicago]*

A child does not need to eat loose paint chips to be exposed to the toxin; normal hand-to-mouth behavior, coupled with the presence of lead dust in the environment, is the usual method of poisoning (American Academy of Pediatrics, 2005; Erickson and Thompson, 2005). Cultural practices may also lead to pediatric ingestion of substances containing lead, especially when these are brought in from other countries. Children of Hispanic origin are believed to be at higher risk for lead poisoning as a result of exposure to culturally related items   *[handwritten: Lake Forest-a lot of older homes.]*

[handwritten: Affects nervous system, iron, lead in mouth, in bones (xray-black lines)]

[sidebar: Case Study—Heavy Metal Poisoning]

BOX 14-6
Sources of Lead*

Lead-based paint in deteriorating condition
Lead solder
Lead crystal
Battery casings
Lead fishing sinkers
Lead curtain weights
Lead bullets
Some of these may contain lead:
- Ceramic ware
- Water
- Pottery
- Pewter
- Dyes
- Industrial factories
- Vinyl mini-blinds
- Playground equipment
- Collectible toys
- Some imported toys or children's metal jewelry
- Artists' paints
- Pool cue chalk

Occupations and hobbies involving lead:
- Battery and aircraft manufacturing
- Lead smelting
- Brass foundry work
- Radiator repair
- Construction work
- Bridge repair work
- Painting contracting
- Mining
- Ceramics work
- Stained-glass making
- Jewelry making

*The U.S. Consumer Product Safety Commission issues alerts and recalls for products that contain lead and may unexpectedly pose a hazard to young children. Additional information may be obtained from Alliance for Healthy Homes, http://www.afhh.org.

CULTURAL AWARENESS

Sources of Lead

In some cultures the use of traditional ethnic remedies that contain lead may increase children's risk of lead poisoning. These remedies include:

Azarcon (Mexico)—For digestive problems; a bright orange powder; usual dose is 0.25 to 1 teaspoon, often mixed with oil, milk, or sugar or sometimes given as a tea; sometimes a pinch is added to a baby bottle or tortilla dough for preventive purposes

Greta (Mexico)—A yellow-orange powder, used in the same way as azarcon

Paylooah (Southeast Asia)—Used for rash or fever; an orange-red powder given as 0.5 teaspoon straight or in a tea

Surma (India)—Black powder applied to the inner lower eyelid that is used as a cosmetic to improve eyesight

Unknown ayurvedic (Tibet)—Small, gray-brown balls used to improve slow development; two balls given orally three times a day

Tamarindo jellied, fruit candy (Mexico)—Fruit candy packaged in paper wrappers that contain high lead levels

Lozeena (Iraq)—A bright orange powder used to color meat and rice

Modified from Centers for Disease Control and Prevention: Lead poisoning associated with use of traditional ethnic remedies—California, 1991-1992, *MMWR* 42(27):521-524, 1993; Centers for Disease Control and Prevention: Lead poisoning associated with imported candy and powdered food coloring—California and Michigan, *MMWR* 47(48):1041-1043, 1998; Centers for Disease Control and Prevention: Childhood lead poisoning associated with tamarind candy and folk remedies—California, 1992-2000, *MMWR* 51(31):684-686, 2002.

---

that contain lead (Erickson and Thompson, 2005). Other risk factors for having an elevated BLL include poverty, age less than 6 years, dwelling in urban areas, and living in older rental homes where lead decontamination may not be a priority. Children of immigrants and internationally adopted children may have been exposed to sources of lead before arrival in the United States and should also be carefully evaluated for lead exposure (Woolf, Goldman, and Bellinger, 2007). Any child, however, is at risk for becoming lead poisoned if hazardous conditions for lead are present in their environment.

Causes of Lead Poisoning

Although there are numerous sources of lead (Box 14-6), in most instances of acute childhood lead poisoning, the source is nonintact lead-based paint in an older home or lead-contaminated bare soil in the yard. Microparticles of lead gain entrance into a child's body through ingestion or inhalation and, in the case of an exposed pregnant woman, by placental transfer. When measured, a mother's lead level is nearly the same as that of her unborn child. A level of lead not harmful to an adult woman can be harmful to the fetus.

Inhalation exposure usually occurs during renovation and remodeling activities in the home, whereas ingestion happens

during normal day-to-day play and mouthing activities. Sometimes a child will actually swallow loose chips of lead-based paint because it has a sweet taste. Water and food may also be contaminated with lead.

Because of family, cultural, or ethnic traditions, a source of lead may be a routine part of life for a child. Nurses must educate themselves about the practices of their patients and identify when such products may be a source of lead. The use of pottery or dishes containing lead may be an issue, as may the use of folk remedies for stomachaches or the use of some cosmetics (see Cultural Awareness box). Some hobbies and occupations of adult family members may contribute to lead hazards carried into the household on clothes, shoes, or skin (American Academy of Pediatrics, 2005). Nurses are often in a position to observe or elicit information about these practices and educate families about their potential harm.

Pathophysiology and Clinical Manifestations

Lead can affect any part of the body, including the renal, hematologic, and neurologic systems (Fig. 14-9). Of most concern for young children is the developing brain and nervous system, which are more vulnerable than those of an older child or adult. Lead in the body moves via an equilibration process between the blood, the soft tissues and organs, and the bones and teeth. Lead ultimately settles in the bones and teeth, where it remains inert and in storage. This makes up the largest portion of the body burden, approximately 75% to 90%. At the cellular level it competes with molecules of calcium, interfering with the regulating action of calcium.

The neurologic system is of most concern when young children are exposed to lead. The developing brain is especially vulnerable. Lead disrupts the biochemical processes and may have a direct effect on the release of neurotransmitters,

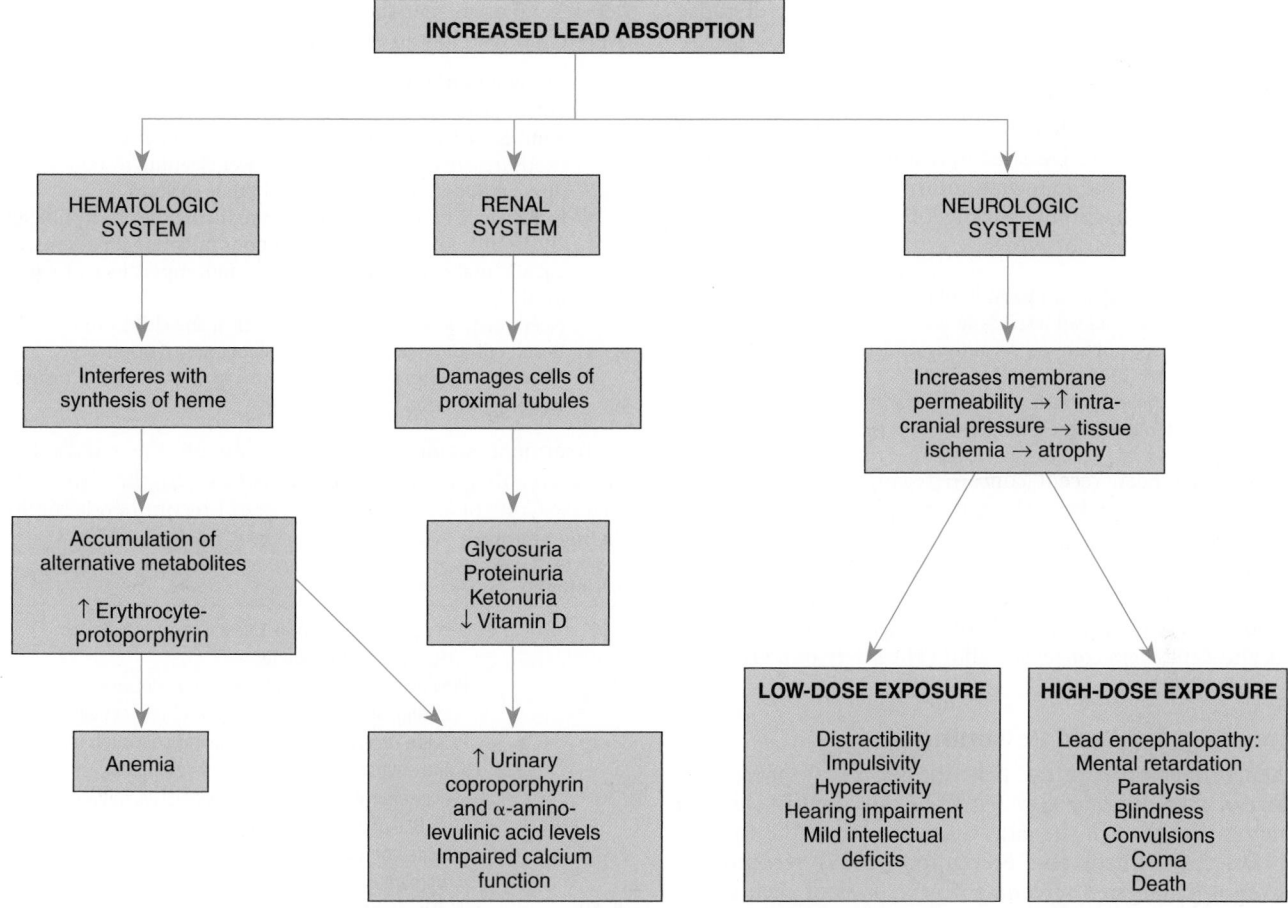

FIG. 14-9 ■ Main effects of lead on body systems.

may cause alterations in the blood-brain barrier, and may interfere with the regulation of synaptic activity (Lidsky and Schneider, 2006).

There is a relationship between anemia and lead poisoning. Children who are iron deficient absorb lead more readily than those with sufficient iron stores. Lead can interfere with the binding of iron onto the heme molecule. This sometimes creates a picture of anemia, even though the child is not iron deficient. Lead toxicity to the erythrocytes leads to the release of the enzyme erythrocyte protoporphyrin (EP). Because EP is not sensitive to BLLs of less than about 16 to 25 mcg/dl, it is no longer used as a screening test. Therefore the BLL test is currently used for screening and diagnosis. However, elevation of the EP level (above 35 mcg/dl of whole blood) is a good indicator of toxicity from lead and reflects the length of exposure and body burden of lead in the individual child.

Although adults have been shown to suffer adverse renal effects from occupational lead exposure, few studies document renal effects in children at other than extremely high lead levels. One can hypothesize that lead can affect the renal integrity of children as well as adults. Therefore the renal system of a child is still considered a potential target for the harmful effects of lead.

The lead levels identified in children have declined since the initiation of screening for children at risk for lead poisoning. With earlier intervention, the most prevalent effects have changed. Since the late 1960s, children have rarely died

of lead poisoning, and seizures or mental retardation have become less likely. However, even mild and moderate lead poisoning can cause a number of cognitive and behavioral problems in young children, including aggression, hyperactivity, impulsivity, delinquency, disinterest, and withdrawal. Long-term neurocognitive signs of lead poisoning include developmental delays, lowered intelligence quotient (IQ), reading skill deficits, visual-spatial problems, visual-motor problems, learning disabilities, and lower academic success. Physical growth and reproductive efficiency may also be adversely affected by chronic lead toxicity (Woolf, Goldman, and Bellinger, 2007).

NURSING ALERT

Acute signs of lead poisoning include nausea, vomiting, constipation, anorexia, and abdominal pain. Additional clinical manifestations are hypophosphatemia, glycosuria, and aminoaciduria (Erickson and Thompson, 2005).

Diagnostic Evaluation

Children with lead poisoning rarely have symptoms, even at levels requiring chelation therapy. A diagnosis of lead poisoning is based only on the lead testing of a venous blood specimen from a venipuncture. The collection process is important. Blood must be collected carefully to avoid contamination by lead on the skin. The level of concern for an elevated BLL has dropped from 80 mcg/dl in 1950 to 10 mcg/dl today (American Academy of Pediatrics, 2005).

Anticipatory Guidance

Anticipatory guidance lends support to primary prevention efforts. The Centers for Disease Control and Prevention (2005) recommends that the following information be made available to families beginning during prenatal care, at 3 to 6 months, and at 1 year of age:

- Hazards of lead-based paint in older housing
- Ways to control lead hazards safely
- Hazards accompanying repainting and renovation of homes built before 1978
- Other exposure sources, such as traditional remedies, that might be relevant for a family

There has been recent concern regarding imported toys and other items children play with that have been found to contain lead. Parents should carefully evaluate the source (manufacturer) of every toy or item and not assume it is safe just because it is sold on the U.S. market. The U.S. Consumer Product Safety Commission* is an excellent resource for parents and caretakers concerned about the safety of a given toy or product.

Screening for Lead Poisoning

When primary prevention fails, the secondary prevention effort of screening for elevated BLLs can identify children much earlier than in the past. Guidelines from the Centers for Disease Control and Prevention (2005) recommend universal or targeted screening on the basis of each state's determination of need. This need is established using blood lead surveillance and other risk factor data collected over time to establish the status and risk of children throughout the state. In areas without available data, universal screening is recommended.

Universal screening should be done at ages 1 and 2 years. Any child between the ages of 3 and 6 years who has not been previously screened should also be tested. Any child with risk factors should be screened more often.

Targeted screening is acceptable when an area has been determined by existing data to have less risk. Children should be screened when they live in a high-risk geographic area or are members of a group determined to be at risk (e.g., Medicaid recipients), or if their family cannot answer "no" to the following personal risk questions:

- Does your child live in or regularly visit a house that was built before 1950?
- Does your child live in or regularly visit a house built before 1978 with recent or ongoing renovations or remodeling within the past 6 months?
- Does your child have a sibling or playmate who has or did have lead poisoning?

Therapeutic Management

The degree of concern, urgency, and need for medical intervention changes as the lead level increases. Education is one of the most important elements of the treatment process. The Centers for Disease Control and Prevention (2005) has identi-

*http://www.cpsc.gov.

fied several areas that should be discussed with the family of every child who has an elevated BLL (10 mcg/dl):

- The child's BLL and what it means
- Potential adverse health effects of an elevated BLL
- Sources of lead exposure and suggestions on how to reduce exposure, such as importance of wet cleaning to remove lead dust on floors, window sills, and other surfaces
- Importance of good nutrition in reducing the absorption and effects of lead; for persons with poor nutritional patterns, adequate intake of calcium and iron and importance of regular meals
- Need for follow-up testing to monitor the child's BLL
- Results of an environmental investigation if applicable
- Hazards of improper removal of lead paint (dry sanding, scraping, or open-flame burning)

Treatment actions vary depending on the child's BLL. Based on a diagnosis from a venous BLL test, the Centers for Disease Control and Prevention (2002) recommends the following actions:

BLL (mcg/dl)	Action
<10	Reassess or rescreen in 1 year. If exposure status changes, do this sooner.
10-14	Provide family with lead poisoning education, follow-up testing, and social service referral if necessary.
15-19	Provide family with lead poisoning education (dietary and environmental), follow-up testing, and social service referral as needed; if BLL persists, initiate actions for BLL of 20 to 44 mcg/dl.
20-44	Provide coordination of care, clinical management, environmental investigation, and lead hazard control.
45-69	Within 48 hours, provide coordination of care and clinical management, including treatment, environmental investigation, and lead hazard control. The child must not remain in a lead-hazardous environment if resolution is to occur.
≥70	*Immediately* provide medical treatment and begin coordination of care, clinical management, environmental investigation, and lead hazard control.

Chelation Therapy. Chelation is the term used for removing lead from circulating blood and, theoretically, some lead from organs and tissues. It is unclear whether chelation affects lead stores in bones. Although not an antidote in the truest sense, it does serve a similar purpose in that the toxic substance or poison is removed from the body. However, chelation does not counteract any effects of the lead. Because lead in circulating blood (the compartment most readily accessed by the chelator) is such a small part of the total body burden, the equilibration process will cause blood lead to rise again after treatment.

Historically two chelating agents have been used consistently: calcium disodium edetate ($CaNa_2EDTA$ or calcium EDTA) and succimer (Chemet, *meso*-2,3 dimercaptosuccinic acid [DMSA]). British antilewisite (BAL, dimercaprol, dimercaptopropanol) is used in conjunction with EDTA. All the agents have potential toxic side effects and contraindications. Renal, hepatic, and hematologic parameters must be monitored.

Because of the equilibration process between blood, soft tissues, and other sites in the body, there is often a rebound of the BLL after chelation. After the body burden of lead is re-

COMMUNITY FOCUS

Reducing Blood Lead Levels

- Make certain child does not have access to peeling paint or chewable surfaces painted with lead-based paint, especially window sills and wells.
- If a house was built before 1960 (possibly before 1980) and has hard-surface floors, wet mop them at least once per week. Wipe other hard surfaces (e.g., window sills, baseboards). If there are loose paint chips in an area, such as a window well, use a wet disposable cloth to pick up and discard them. Do not vacuum hard-surfaced floors or window sills or wells, since this spreads dust. Use vacuum cleaners with agitators to remove dust from rugs rather than vacuum cleaners with suction only. If a rug is known to contain lead dust and cannot be washed, it should be discarded.
- Wash and dry child's hands and face frequently, especially before eating.
- Wash toys and pacifiers frequently.
- If soil around home is or is likely to be contaminated with lead (e.g., if home was built before 1960 or is near a major highway), plant grass or other ground cover; plant bushes around outside of house so that child cannot play there.
- During remodeling of older homes, follow correct procedures. Be certain children and pregnant women are not in the home, day or night, until process is completed. After deleading, thoroughly clean house, using cleaning solution to damp mop and dust before inhabitants return.

- In areas where lead content of water exceeds the drinking water standard and a particular faucet has not been used for 6 hours or more, "flush" the cold-water pipes by running the water until it becomes as cold as it will get (30 seconds to more than 2 minutes). The more time water has been sitting in pipes, the more lead it may contain.
- *Use only cold water* for consumption (drinking, cooking, and especially for reconstituting powder infant formula). Hot water dissolves lead more quickly than cold water and thus contains higher levels of lead. It is all right to use first-flush water for nonconsumption uses.
- Have water tested by a competent laboratory. This action is especially important for apartment dwellers; flushing may not be effective in high-rise buildings or in other buildings with lead-soldered central piping.*
- Do not store food in open cans, particularly if cans are imported.
- Do not use pottery or ceramic ware that was inadequately fired or is meant for decorative use for food storage or service. Do not store drinks or food in lead crystal.
- Avoid folk remedies or cosmetics that contain lead.
- Make certain that home exposure is not occurring from parental occupations or hobbies. Household members employed in occupations such as lead smelting should shower and change into clean clothing before leaving work. Construction and lead abatement workers may also bring home lead contaminants.
- Ensure child eats regular meals, since more lead is absorbed on an empty stomach.
- Ensure child's diet contains sufficient iron and calcium and not excessive fat.

Modified from Centers for Disease Control and Prevention: *Preventing lead poisoning in young children,* Atlanta, 1991, The Centers.
*For more information, contact the county or state department of health or environment for information on local water quality. For general information on lead, call the EPA Safe Drinking Water Hotline, (800) 426-4791, http://www.epa.gov; National Lead Information Center, 422 S. Clinton Ave., Rochester, NY 14620; (800) 424-LEAD (5323); http://www.epa.gov/lead/pubs/nlic.htm; Water Quality Association, (630) 505-0160; http://www.wqa.org; or NSF International, (877) 867-3435; http://www.nsf.org.

duced enough to stabilize the BLL, rebound will cease. Multiple chelation treatments may be necessary. Adequate hydration is essential during therapy because the chelates are excreted via the kidneys.

BAL must not be used in the presence of a glucose 6-phosphate dehydrogenase (G6PD) deficiency or peanut allergy, nor should it be given in conjunction with iron. It is never used as a single-agent therapy, only in conjunction with EDTA. It must be given only at a deep intramuscular site. EDTA should be given intravenously over several hours or, when necessary to restrict fluids, may be given intramuscularly.

Succimer is given orally over a 19-day course of treatment. The capsule is opened and sprinkled on a small amount of food or may be swallowed whole. Adverse effects include nausea, vomiting, diarrhea, loss of appetite, rash, elevated liver function tests, and neutropenia. Because the chelates are excreted via the kidneys, adequate hydration is essential.

An oral chelating agent, D-penicillamine, is sometimes used to treat lead poisoning, but low doses should be used in children and monitoring of renal function and blood counts during administration is essential (Woolf, Goldman, and Bellinger, 2007).

Prognosis. Although most of the pathophysiologic effects of lead are reversible, the most serious consequences of both high and low lead exposure are the effects on the central nervous system. In children with lead encephalopathy, perma-

nent brain damage can result in mental retardation, behavior changes, possible paralysis, and seizures. However, moderate-to low-dose exposure may also cause permanent neurologic deficits. Increased distractibility, short attention span, impulsivity, reading disabilities, and school failure have been associated with lead exposure (Markowitz, 2000). There is some evidence that treatment of moderate levels of lead poisoning can result in cognitive improvement (American Academy of Pediatrics, 2005).

Nursing Care Management

The primary nursing goal in lead poisoning is to prevent the child's initial or further exposure to lead. For children with low-level exposure, this requires identifying the sources of lead in the environment. Careful history taking is the most useful and most valuable tool and should concentrate on the personal risk questions (see p. 478). Suggestions for reducing lead in the child's environment are listed in the Community Focus box.

Children who must undergo chelation therapy are prepared for the injections, and all efforts are made to reduce injection pain. Chelating agents are administered deeply into a large muscle mass (see Atraumatic Care box). To lessen the pain from EDTA, the local anesthetic procaine is injected with the drug. Rotation of sites is essential to prevent the formation of painful areas of fibrotic tissue. Because EDTA

ATRAUMATIC CARE

Lead Chelation Therapy

To lessen the pain from intramuscular injection of calcium disodium edetate (CaNa₂EDTA or calcium EDTA), the local anesthetic procaine is injected with the drug. Apply topical anesthetic cream such as eutectic mixture of local anesthetic (e.g., lidocaine-prilocaine [EMLA]) or LMX4 (4% lidocaine) over the puncture site before the injection of EDTA and British antilewisite (BAL) (time per manufacturer's guidelines). Administer intravenous EDTA whenever possible.

and lead are toxic to the kidneys, records are kept of intake and output, and the results of urinalysis are assessed to monitor renal functioning.

> **NURSING ALERT**
>
> Use extreme caution with chelating agents. Incidences of child death from hypocalcemia have been recorded when Na₂EDTA was substituted for CaNa₂EDTA and used as a chelating agent (Centers for Diseases Control and Prevention, 2006).

> **NURSING ALERT**
>
> Calcium EDTA is always administered when there is adequate urinary output. Children receiving the drug intramuscularly must be able to maintain adequate oral intake of fluids.

Discharge planning for children with lead poisoning must include thorough education of families regarding safety from lead hazards, clear instructions regarding medication administration and follow-up, and confirmation that the child will be discharged to a home without lead hazards. Although caution must be used to avoid alarming parents unnecessarily, it is important that they know the risk implications for their child's behavior and cognitive functions. Nurses should observe the development and behavior of children who are hospitalized. Any concerns that are identified should be thoroughly evaluated. Referral to a child development or speech and language specialist may be indicated.

As in any situational crisis, parents need support and understanding if their child is treated for lead poisoning. Many families at the highest risk for lead poisoning have the fewest resources to comply with measures such as relocation or removing lead from the environment where the child experiences exposure.

CHILD MALTREATMENT

The broad term **child maltreatment** includes intentional physical abuse or neglect, emotional abuse or neglect, and sexual abuse of children, usually by adults. It is one of the most significant social problems affecting children. In 2005, Child Protective Services (CPS) agencies in the United States confirmed that an estimated 900,000 children were victims of child maltreatment. Of the confirmed cases, 17% suffered physical abuse, 9% sexual abuse, 63% neglect, and 7% emotional abuse. In 2005, estimates indicated that 1460 children died as a result of child abuse and neglect (US Department of Health and Human Services, 2007). Reported statistics only partially represent the actual incidence of child maltreatment, since many cases are believed to go unreported.*

CHILD NEGLECT

Child neglect is the most common form of maltreatment. More than half of all reported cases are associated with deprivation of necessities, and 40% of deaths from maltreatment are in this group (US Department of Health and Human Services, 2007). **Neglect** is generally defined as the failure of a parent or other person legally responsible for the child's welfare to provide for the child's basic needs and an adequate level of care.

Important contributing factors for child neglect are lack of knowledge of child's needs, lack of resources, and caretaker substance abuse. For example, neglectful parents often demonstrate poor parenting skills. They may be unaware that an infant needs to be fed every 3 to 4 hours, may not know what to feed the child, and may have insufficient funds to buy food. An equally serious lack of knowledge is failure to recognize emotional nurturing as an essential need of children. (See also Growth Failure [Failure to Thrive], Chapter 11.)

Types of Neglect

Neglect takes many forms and can be classified broadly as physical or emotional maltreatment. **Physical neglect** involves the deprivation of necessities, such as food, clothing, shelter, supervision, medical care, and education. **Emotional neglect** generally refers to failure to meet the child's needs for affection, attention, and emotional nurturance. Neglect may also include lack of intervention for or fostering of maladaptive behavior, such as delinquency or substance abuse.

EMOTIONAL ABUSE

Emotional abuse, an even more difficult aspect of maltreatment to define, refers to the deliberate attempt to destroy or significantly impair a child's self-esteem or competence. Emotional abuse may take the following forms: rejecting, isolating, terrorizing, ignoring, corrupting, verbally assaulting, or overpressuring the child (Nelms, 2001).

PHYSICAL ABUSE *Scalding & Accidental Scalding*

The deliberate infliction of physical injury on a child, usually by the child's caregiver, is termed **physical abuse.** Legal definitions of physical abuse are defined in state and federal statutes. The federal definition of abuse is "any recent act or failure to act that results in imminent risk of serious harm, death, serious physical or emotional harm of a child (less than 18 years of age) by a parent or caretaker who is responsible for the child's welfare" (Child Abuse Prevention and Treatment Act, 1996, Public Law 104-235). Minor physical injury is responsible for more reported cases of maltreatment than major physical injury, but major physical abuse causes more deaths. Despite the importance of the problem, a universally accepted definition of what constitutes minor and major physical abuse does not exist. Rather, each state in the United States defines abuse according to its individual reporting laws.

Bites

---

*Additional information is available from the Child Welfare Information Gateway, Children's Bureau/ACYF, 1250 Maryland Ave. SW, Eighth Floor, Washington, DC 20024; (703) 835-7565 or (800) 394-3366; http://www.childwelfare.gov.

Case Study—Child Abuse

Shaken Baby Syndrome

retinal hemorrhage

Shaken baby syndrome (SBS) is a serious form of child abuse caused by violent shaking of infants and young children. This violent shaking would be easily recognized by others as dangerous (American Academy of Pediatrics, 2001) and is most often a result of the caregiver's frustration with crying (Castiglia, 2001). Every year in America an estimated 1200 to 1400 children are shaken; of these victims, 25% to 30% die as a result of their injuries and the rest have life-long complications (National Center on Shaken Baby Syndrome, 2007).

It is important to understand what happens in SBS. Infants have a large head-to-body ratio, weak neck muscles, and a large amount of water in the brain. Violent shaking causes the brain to rotate within the skull, resulting in shearing forces tearing blood vessels and neurons. The characteristic injuries that occur are intracranial bleeding (subdural and subarachnoid hematomas) and retinal hemorrhages, but they may also include fractures of the ribs and long bones. Most often there are no signs of external injury. SBS is often not an isolated event. In one study 45% of the children with inflicted traumatic brain injury caused by shaking showed some evidence of prior injury (Ewing-Cobb, Kramar, Prasad, and others, 1998).

Victims of SBS can be seen with a variety of symptoms, from generalized flulike symptoms to unresponsiveness with impending death (Miehl, 2005). Many of the presenting symptoms, such as vomiting, irritability, poor feeding, and listlessness, are often mistaken for common infant and childhood ailments. In more severe forms, presenting symptoms may include seizures, posturing, alterations in level of consciousness, apnea, bradycardia, or death. The long-term outcomes of SBS include seizure disorder; visual impairments, including blindness; developmental delays; hearing loss; cerebral palsy; and mild to profound mental, cognitive, and motor impairments (Walls, 2006). Nurses can take an active role in prevention of SBS by teaching all caregivers about crying and techniques to cope with inconsolable crying (Carbaugh, 2004).

> **NURSINGALERT**
>
> Nurses should stress to parents the danger of shaking infants (shaking can cause SBS). Education must include coping mechanisms for caring for children with inconsolable crying.

Munchausen Syndrome by Proxy

Munchausen syndrome by proxy (MSBP), also known as factitious disorder by proxy or medical child abuse, is a rare but serious form of child abuse in which caretakers deliberately exaggerate or fabricate histories and symptoms or induce symptoms. This form of child maltreatment may include physical, emotional, and psychologic abuse for the gratification of the caretaker. In most cases the perpetrator is the biologic mother, with some degree of health care knowledge and training. Health care providers can become easily misled and unknowingly enable the perpetrator (Leider, Irving, Mauricio, and others, 2005). As a result of the history of symptoms provided by the caretaker, the child endures painful and unnecessary medical testing and procedures. Common symptoms reported by the caretaker include seizures, nausea and vomiting, diarrhea, and altered mental status; they are usually witnessed only by the perpetrator.

Considerations when determining whether a child is a victim of MSBP include:

- Is the child's condition consistent with the reported history?
- Does diagnostic evidence support reported history?
- Has anyone other than the caretaker witnessed the symptoms?
- Is treatment being provided primarily because of the caretaker's demands?

The resolution of symptoms after separation from the perpetrator confirms the diagnosis.

Factors Predisposing to Physical Abuse

The causes of child abuse are multifaceted. Child maltreatment occurs across all socioeconomic, religious, cultural, racial, and ethnic groups (Goldman, Salus, Wolcott, and others, 2003). Three risk factors are commonly identified in child abuse: parental characteristics, characteristics of the child, and environmental characteristics. However, no single factor or group of factors is predictive of abuse. Rather, the interaction of these factors is thought to increase the risk of abuse occurring in a particular family.

Parental Characteristics. Certain identified characteristics occur more frequently in parents who abuse their children and are therefore considered risk factors. Younger parents more often are abusers of their children. One-parent families are at higher risk for abuse, and in single-parent families that include an unrelated partner, the partner is frequently the abuser.

Abusive families are often more socially isolated and have fewer supportive relationships. These parents are often from low-income circumstances, with concurrent undereducation and substance abuse problems. With little or no available support system and concurrent stressors imposed by the child or environment, these parents are vulnerable to additional crises of any nature and may strike out at the child to release their increasing frustration and anxiety.

Other factors identified in abusive parents include low self-esteem and little knowledge of appropriate parenting skills. Parenting skills are learned behaviors, and parents who grew up with poor parental role models may have difficulty parenting their own children. Approximately, one third of parents who were maltreated as children will subject their children to similar maltreatment (Gara, Allen, Herzog, and others, 2000).

Characteristics of the Child. The onus for child abuse is always on the abuser; however, some characteristics are common in children who are abused. Children from birth to 3 years of age are at highest risk for being abused (US Department of Health and Human Services, 2007). Infants and small children require constant attention and must have all their needs met by others. This can result in parental or caretaker fatigue with resultant striking out at the child with physical force, shaking the child, or ignoring the child's needs.

The physical and emotional demands placed on the parents or caretaker of an unwanted, brain-damaged, hyperactive, or physically disabled child may overwhelm them, resulting in abuse. Disabled children may not understand that abusive behaviors are not appropriate, so do not tell others or defend themselves. Preterm infants may be at risk for maltreatment because of failure of parent-child bonding during early infancy, increased physical needs, or irritability. One child in the family may be singled out in an abusive family. Removing that child from the home often places the other siblings at risk for abuse. Therefore no child is safe if left in the abusive environment unless the parents can be helped to learn new parenting skills and to meet their needs and release their frustration through alternatives other than attacking their children.

Environmental Characteristics. The environment is a significant part of the potential abusive situation. A typical environment is one of chronic stress, including problems of divorce, poverty, unemployment, poor housing, frequent relocation, alcoholism, and drug addiction. Increased exposure between children and parents, such as that which occurs in crowded living conditions, also increases the likelihood of abuse.

Although most reporting of abuse has been from lower socioeconomic populations, as stated before, child abuse is not a problem of any one societal group. Stresses imposed by poverty predispose lower socioeconomic families to abusive situations, and abuse in these groups is more apt to be reported. However, concealed crises may also be present in upper-class families. Families who have substitute caregivers such as day-care providers and baby-sitters may also be at risk for child abuse, especially if the family has not fully evaluated the caregiver. Nurses need to be aware of all these factors to identify the less obvious examples of child abuse and neglect.

SEXUAL ABUSE

Sexual abuse is one of the most devastating types of child maltreatment, and estimates indicate that it has increased significantly during the past decade (US Department of Health and Human Services, 2007). Child sexual abuse constitutes approximately 10% of officially substantiated child maltreatment cases. Some of the apparent increase can be attributed to increased awareness (Putnam, 2003).

As with all forms of child maltreatment, no universal definition for sexual abuse exists. Definitions of sexual abuse cover a range of acts, including involvement of children in sexual acts they do not understand, that they cannot give consent to, or that violate social taboos (Finkel and DeJong, 2001). The Child Abuse and Prevention Act (Public Law 93-247) defines **sexual abuse** as "the use, persuasion, or coercion of any child to engage in sexually explicit conduct (or any simulation of such conduct) or producing any visual depiction of such conduct, or rape, molestation, prostitution, or incest with children."

Sexual abuse includes the following types of sexual maltreatment (see also Sexual Assault [Rape], Chapter 17):

Incest—Any physical sexual activity between family members; blood relationship is not required (abusers can include stepparents, unrelated siblings, grandparents, uncles, and aunts); does not include sexual relations between legally sanctioned partners, such as spouses

Molestation—A vague term that includes "indecent liberties," such as touching, fondling, kissing, single or mutual masturbation, or oral-genital contact

Exhibitionism—Indecent exposure; usually exposure of the genitalia by an adult male to children or women

Child pornography—Arranging and photographing, in any media, sexual acts involving children, alone or with adults or animals, regardless of consent by the child's legal guardian; also may denote distribution of such material in any form, with or without profit

Child prostitution—Involving children in sex acts for profit and usually with changing partners

Pedophilia—Literally means "love of child" and does not denote a type of sexual activity but the preference of an adult for prepubertal children as the means of achieving sexual excitement

Characteristics of Abusers and Victims

Anyone, including siblings and mothers, can be sexual abusers, but a typical abuser is a man whom the victim knows. Offenders come from all levels of society. Adults comprise 80% of offenders of sexual abuse, with the remaining 20% being adolescents and preadolescents (Johnson, 2003). Most sexual abuse is committed by men and by persons known to the child, with family members constituting up to two thirds of the perpetrators (Christian, Lavell, and DeJong, 2000). Many offenders hold full-time jobs, are active in community affairs, and do not have prior criminal records (Finkel and DeJong, 2001). Offenders often are employed in or volunteer for positions that will bring them into contact with young girls and boys such as teaching or coaching. Child sexual abuse may be generational unless discovered and stopped (Johnson, 2003). Offenders may commit many assaults before being caught.

Incestuous relationships between father or stepfather and daughter are generally prolonged, and the victims are usually reluctant to report the situation because of fear of retaliation and fear that they will not be believed. Typically, incestuous relationships begin later than other forms of child abuse. The eldest daughter is usually abused, but in her absence another sister may be substituted. Sibling incest may also occur. Sexual abuse by relatives with a strong emotional bond with the victim is the most devastating to the child.

Boys are also victims of both intrafamilial and extrafamilial abuse. Male victims are much less likely to report abuse, and they may suffer much greater emotional harm from incestuous relationships, especially between mother and son, than female victims. Boys are likely to be subjected to anal penetration and oral-genital contact; to have subtle physical findings; and to be abused by a father, stepfather, or mother's boyfriend.

Considerable evidence exists to show that at least 20% of American women and 5% to 10% of American men experienced some form of sexual abuse as children. Race and socioeconomic status do not seem to be major risk factors. Significant risk factors for child sexual abuse include parental unavailability, lack of emotional closeness and flexibility, social isolation, emotional deprivation, and communication difficulties. Approximately 20% to 25% of child sexual abuse cases involve penetration or oral-genital contact. The mean age of vulnerability is 9 years, with a range from infancy to 17 years of age (Berlinger and Elliott, 2002).

Initiation and Perpetuation of Sexual Abuse

The cycle of sexual abuse often starts insidiously, unless it involves an isolated attack, such as rape. Often offenders spend time with the victims to gain their trust before initiating any sexual contact. Most victims are then pressured into being an accessory to the sexual activity through various means (Box 14-7) and may be unaware that sexual activity is part of the offer. Children may not reveal the truth for fear that their parents would not believe them, especially if the offender is a trusted member of the family. Some fear they will be blamed for the situation, and many young children with limited vocabulary have difficulty describing the activity when they do have the courage or opportunity to reveal the abuse.

Methods Used to Pressure Children into Sexual Activity

- The child is offered gifts or privileges.
- The adult misrepresents moral standards by telling the child that it is "okay to do."
- Isolated and emotionally and socially impoverished children are enticed by adults who meet their needs for warmth and human contact.
- The successful sex offender pressures the victim into secrecy regarding the activity by describing it as a "secret between us" that other people may take away if they find out.
- The offender plays on the child's fears, including fear of punishment by the offender, fear of repercussions if the child tells, and fear of abandonment or rejection by the family.

nursingcareguidelines

Talking with Children Who Reveal Abuse
- Provide a private time and place to talk.
- Do not promise not to tell; tell them that you are required by law to report the abuse.
- Do not express shock or criticize their family.
- Use their vocabulary to discuss body parts.
- Avoid using any leading statements that can distort their report.
- Reassure them that they have done the right thing by telling.
- Tell them that the abuse is not their fault, that they are not bad or to blame.
- Determine their immediate need for safety.
- Let the child know what will happen when you report.

Incest most frequently occurs between fathers and daughters, but may be between grandfather and granddaughter or brother and sister. Brother-sister incest has been found to be just as damaging as father-daughter abuse (Cyr, Wright, McDuff, and others, 2002). Victims may take years to disclose this abuse. However, not all incestuous relationships follow this pattern of silence. Reports of father-daughter incest during child custody conflicts have become more common and have raised serious concerns regarding the possibility of false accusation. Rather than tolerating or denying the child's sexual abuse, the other parent (usually the mother) is typically the chief accuser.

NURSING CARE OF THE MALTREATED CHILD

A critical responsibility of health professionals is identifying abusive situations as early as possible. The characteristics that may predispose members of some families to commit abuse can serve as a framework for assessing vulnerability but are never predictive of actual abuse. A careful, detailed history and interview combined with a thorough physical examination are the diagnostic tools needed to identify abuse. Nurses have a special role because they may be the first person to see the child and parent and are the consistent caregivers if the child is hospitalized (see Nursing Care Guidelines box).

During the interview with the child and family, the nurse must be careful to avoid biasing the child's retelling of the events. Some experts suggest that health professionals limit the interview to the child's physical and mental health concerns and leave topics of the family's social, legal, or other problems to the police or CPS (McClain, Giardet, Lahoti, and others, 2000). If this is not possible, an effort should be made to coordinate the interview process so that all pertinent health care professionals can be present.

NURSINGALERT
Nurses must be aware of their biases regarding child abuse. Nurses are often less likely to report abuse when the child is female and from a middle-income, as opposed to lower-income, family; are significantly less comfortable dealing with sexual abuse, abuse of infants, and fathers as the abusers; and experience greater discomfort when dealing with abusers of children with disabilities than with abusers of children without disabilities.

Warning Signs of Abuse

- Physical evidence of abuse or neglect, including previous injuries
- Conflicting stories about the "accident" or injury from the parents or others
- Cause of injury blamed on sibling or other party
- An injury inconsistent with the history, such as a concussion and broken arm from falling off a bed
- History inconsistent with child's developmental level, such as a 6-month-old turning on the hot water
- A complaint other than the one associated with signs of abuse (e.g., a chief complaint of a cold when there is evidence of first- and second-degree burns)
- Inappropriate response of caregiver, such as an exaggerated or absent emotional response, refusal to sign for additional tests or agree to necessary treatment, excessive delay in seeking treatment, or absence of the parents for questioning
- Inappropriate response of child, such as little or no response to pain, fear of being touched, excessive or lack of separation anxiety, or indiscriminate friendliness to strangers
- Child's report of physical or sexual abuse
- Previous reports of abuse in the family
- Repeated visits to emergency facilities with injuries

Recognition of abuse or neglect necessitates a familiarity with both physical and behavioral signs that suggest maltreatment (Boxes 14-8 and 14-9). No one indicator can be used to diagnose maltreatment. It is a pattern or combination of indicators that should arouse suspicion and further investigation. It is important to note that some situations may be misinterpreted as abuse; for example, bleeding disorders, osteogenesis imperfecta, sudden infant death syndrome (SIDS), and cultural practices such as cupping or coin rubbing (see Health Practices, Chapter 4) may mimic physical abuse. Unintentional injuries, such as burns from metal buckles on car seats, bruising from seat belts, or spiral fractures from a twist and fall injury, may also be wrongly diagnosed as abuse. Normal variants, such as Mongolian spots and congenital anomalies of genitalia, can be mistaken for abuse.

BOX 14-9

Clinical Manifestations of Potential Child Maltreatment

PHYSICAL NEGLECT
Suggestive Physical Findings
Growth failure

Signs of malnutrition, such as thin extremities, abdominal distention, lack of subcutaneous fat

Poor personal hygiene

Unclean or inappropriate dress

Evidence of poor health care, such as delayed immunization, untreated infections, frequent colds

Frequent injuries from lack of supervision

Suggestive Behaviors
Dull and inactive affect; excessively passive or sleepy

Self-stimulatory behaviors, such as finger sucking or rocking

Begging or stealing food

Absenteeism from school

Substance abuse

Vandalism or shoplifting

EMOTIONAL ABUSE AND NEGLECT
Suggestive Physical Findings
Growth failure

Eating or feeding disorder

Enuresis

Sleep disorder

Suggestive Behaviors
Self-stimulatory behaviors, such as biting, rocking, sucking

During infancy, lack of social smile and stranger anxiety

Withdrawal from environment and people

Unusual fearfulness

Antisocial behavior, such as destructiveness, stealing, cruelty to animals or people

Extremes of behavior, such as overcompliant and passive, or aggressive and demanding

Lags in emotional and intellectual development, especially language

Suicide attempts

PHYSICAL ABUSE
Suggestive Physical Findings
Bruises and welts (may be in various stages of healing)
- On face, lips, mouth, back, buttocks, thighs, or areas of torso
- Regular patterns descriptive of object used, such as belt buckle, hand, wire hanger, chain, wooden spoon, squeeze or pinch marks
- May be present in various stages of healing

Burns
- On soles, palms, back, or buttocks
- Patterns descriptive of object used, such as round cigar or cigarette burns; sharply demarcated areas from immersion in scalding water; rope burns on wrists or ankles from being bound; burns in the shape of an iron, radiator, or electric stove burner
- Absence of "splash" marks and presence of symmetric burns
- Stun gun injury: lesions circular, fairly uniform (up to 0.5 cm), and paired about 5 cm apart

Fractures and dislocations
- Skull, nose, or facial structures
- Injury denoting type of abuse, such as spiral fracture or dislocation from twisting of an extremity or whiplash from shaking the child
- Multiple new or old fractures in various stages of healing

Lacerations and abrasions
- On backs of arms, legs, torso, face, or external genitalia
- Unusual symptoms, such as abdominal swelling, pain, and vomiting from punching
- Descriptive marks such as from human bites or pulling out of hair

Chemical
- Unexplained repeated poisoning, especially drug overdose
- Unexplained sudden illness, such as hypoglycemia from insulin administration

Suggestive Behaviors
Wary of physical contact with adults

Apparent fear of parents or going home

Lying very still while surveying environment

Inappropriate reaction to injury, such as failure to cry from pain

Lack of reaction to frightening events

Apprehensive when hearing other children cry

Indiscriminate friendliness and displays of affection

Superficial relationships

Acting-out behavior, such as aggression, to seek attention

Withdrawal behavior

SEXUAL ABUSE
Suggestive Physical Findings
Bruises, bleeding, lacerations, or irritation of external genitalia, anus, mouth, or throat

Torn, stained, or bloody underclothing

Pain on urination or pain, swelling, and itching of genital area

Penile discharge

Sexually transmitted disease, nonspecific vaginitis

Difficulty in walking or sitting

Unusual odor in the genital area

Recurrent urinary tract infections

Presence of sperm

Pregnancy in young adolescent

Suggestive Behaviors
Sudden emergence of sexually related problems, including excessive or public masturbation, age-inappropriate sexual play, promiscuity, or overtly seductive behavior

Withdrawn behavior, excessive daydreaming

Preoccupation with fantasies, especially in play

Poor relationships with peers

Sudden changes, such as anxiety, loss or gain of weight, clinging behavior

In incestuous relationships, excessive anger at mother for not protecting daughter

Regressive behavior, such as bed-wetting or thumb sucking

Sudden onset of phobias or fears, particularly fears of the dark, men, strangers, or particular settings or situations (e.g., undue fear of leaving the house or staying at the daycare center or the baby-sitter's house)

Running away from home

Substance abuse, particularly of alcohol or mood-elevating drugs

Profound and rapid personality changes, especially extreme depression, hostility, and aggression (often accompanied by social withdrawal)

Rapidly declining school performance

Suicidal attempts or ideation

Caregiver-Child Interaction

The nurse can use the initial contact with the family to assess the interaction between the caregiver and the child. Caregivers who seem indifferent to or unsupportive of the child should cause concern. Observations of the caregivers should include emotional support for the child, attentiveness to the child's needs, and concern for the child's injury. Although caregivers and children may vary in responses to a stressful event, an unusual caregiver-child relationship should be noted and factored into the overall evaluation of the child. Certain behavioral responses of the parents to their child and to the interviewer should alert the nurse to the possibility of maltreatment. Abusive parents may have difficulty showing concern toward their child. They may be unable or unwilling to comfort the child. Abusers may blame the child for the injuries or belittle him or her for being clumsy or stupid. When interacting with the health care workers, the parents may become hostile or uncooperative. During the child's hospitalization they may not participate in the child's care and may show little concern for his or her progress, eventual discharge, or need for follow-up care.

Abused children's responses to their parents or the injury may also support the suspicion of abuse. Although no one pattern is typical, extremes of behavior may be observed. Children may be unresponsive to the parent or excessively clinging and intolerant of separation. They may be overly attached to the abusive parent, possibly in the hope of preventing any upset that may precipitate anger and another attack. During care of the injury, children may be passive and accepting of the discomfort or uncooperative and fearful of any physical contact. They may avoid eye contact. Some children maintain a wary watchfulness of all strangers; some shy away from strangers as if frightened; others are unusually affectionate and outgoing.

History and Interview

Child Physical Abuse. It is often difficult to differentiate child maltreatment from accidental injuries. Caregivers whose history of events may be deceptive or incomplete or children who are nonverbal may make the assessment more complex. A purposeful, skilled history and appropriate interview questions will help the nurse to ensure the right course of action. Knowledge of mechanism of injury and child development is essential. Cases of abuse are often detected because the child or caregiver history of events is inconsistent with physical findings. Children who are verbal can often give a history of the injury. Separating the child from the caregiver may provide a more reliable history. It is important to ask nonleading, open-ended questions. The history should include a narrative of the injury from both caregiver and child (if verbal). Date, time, and location where injury took place along with who was present at time of the injury are essential questions. Family history for bleeding or bone disorders is important. Areas of history that are concerning for abuse are outlined in Box 14-8.

Neglect and Emotional Abuse. Each child may manifest different responses to neglect depending on the situation and developmental age. The goal of the interview is to determine if the child is in a safe environment and if the caregiver has the skills and resources to care for the child. It is often difficult to determine whether the circumstances constitute poor parenting skills or true neglect. Behaviors suggestive of abuse or neglect are found in Box 14-9.

Sexual Abuse. An essential component to identifying sexual abuse is the interview. Several dynamics may impede the child's revelation of sexual abuse. Child sexual abuse is often perpetrated by someone known to the children, including family members. In some cases the children may have been sworn to secrecy. They may have been told that no one will believe them or their family would be harmed if they tell someone about the abuse. Small children may imitate behaviors they have had perpetrated on themselves or have seen others do. The nurse must be able to recognize normal, age-related sexual curiosity and self-stimulating behaviors. Typically, children do not act out specific details of the sexual act or perform intrusive acts on others unless they have sexual knowledge beyond their normal age-related development (Johnson, 2003).

Children's reports of sexual abuse may vary from contradictory stories to unwavering versions of the experience. Stories that sound contradictory may reflect the child's experiences in several instances of abuse. Also, children who repeatedly tell identical facts may have been prompted to do so. Increasing evidence suggests that the types of interrogation children are exposed to after reports of sexual abuse shape their thinking. To avoid biasing the interaction, nurses must be skillful interviewers when questioning children who may be victims of abuse. Medical records should include verbatim statements made by the child and interviewer that reflect appropriate nonleading questions and statements (Hornor, 2001; McClain, Giradet, Lahoti, and others, 2000). The child may not be emotionally ready to discuss the abuse. Establishing rapport with the child is essential to gaining his or her trust. Interviews should not be rushed. Engaging the child in play activities while encouraging conversation may help the child discuss the abuse. It may take several interviews or psychologic counseling for the child to be forthcoming about the abuse. Information regarding the last sexual contact is important because it determines the need for a forensic evaluation. Forensic testing should be considered for children who have been sexually abused within the past 72 to 96 hours.

Unfortunately, there is no typical profile of the victim, and there must be a high index of suspicion to identify these children. Physical signs vary and may include any of those listed for sexual abuse. The victim may exhibit various behavioral manifestations, but none of these behaviors is diagnostic. When abused children exhibit these behaviors, the signs may be incorrectly attributed to the normal stresses of childhood, especially in older school-age children or adolescents. Even signs considered most predictive of sexual abuse, such as certain genital findings, sexually inappropriate behavior for age, enactment of adult sexual activity, and intense focus on sexual activity (e.g., masturbation), do not always indicate that sexual abuse has occurred. Conversely, abused children may not demonstrate more knowledge of sexual activity than nonabused children. However, one difference in the abused children's explanation of sexual activity may be unusual affective responses. For example, abused children may have an increased incidence of sleep disorders, temper tantrums, and depression (Calam, Horne, Glasgow, and others, 1998).

NURSING ALERT

When children report potentially sexually abusive experiences, their reports need to be taken seriously, but also cautiously, to avoid alarming the child or falsely accusing someone.

Physical Assessment

Child Physical Abuse. The goal of the physical assessment for child physical abuse is identification of all injuries. A systems approach ensures the whole body is evaluated. In instances of severe abuse and injuries, the assessment should begin with a rapid assessment of airway, breathing, circulation, and neurologic systems. A systematic head-to-toe examination follows. Attention to areas often overlooked, such as the scalp, behind the ears, and the lingual frenulum, is essential. An exterior examination of the genitalia and the child's posterior surface should be completed.

Record the location and a detailed description of all injuries. Note color, size, and location of all bruising. Burn documentation should include location, pattern, demarcation lines, and presence of eschar or blisters. Diagrams of the injuries using a body diagram form are helpful. If available, photographs of the injuries using a measurement tool should be obtained.

Not all forms of physical abuse have obvious signs. Intraabdominal organ injury from blunt trauma to the abdomen can occur without signs of external abdominal bruising. Nurses should consider intraabdominal injury in infants and children who have any other signs of abuse.

> **NURSINGALERT**
> Incompatibility between the history and the injury is probably the most important criterion on which to base the decision to report suspected abuse.

All evidence collected must adhere to strict guidelines for legal purposes; chain of custody must be appropriately maintained with local law enforcement personnel. Documentation on the chain of custody form should include names of persons collecting or receiving evidence (such as photographs and DNA samples), type of evidence collected or received, and date of receipt (Kaczor, Pierce, Makoroff, and others, 2006).

Neglect and Emotional Abuse. Neglect from deprivation of necessities is easier to identify than emotional neglect or abuse because physical signs are usually evident. Assessment of the child's height, weight, nutritional status, hygiene, and age-appropriate interactions is important for the overall picture of potential neglect. Emotional maltreatment may be readily suspected, but it is difficult to substantiate. Physical signs are often nonspecific, and nurses must rely on behavioral indicators, which range from depression to acting-out behavior, to help identify a possibly abusive situation. Any persistent and unexplained change in the child's behavior is an important clue to possible emotional abuse.

Sexual Abuse. Identifying instances of sexual abuse is particularly difficult because, often, few if any obvious physical indications of the activity exist. Physical signs vary and may include any of those listed in Box 14-9 for sexual abuse. The goal of the physical examination is to document genital findings. In most cases, the genital examination is normal, which does not mean that sexual abuse did not occur. Fondling or genital-to-genital contact without penetration may leave no physical findings. Forensic evidence collection should be considered for any child with known or suspected sexual contact within 72 hours. Forensic evidence obtained directly from a prepubertal victim's body diminishes greatly after 24 hours, with the best chance for evidence collection coming from bed linens or the child's underwear (Christian, Lavelle,

DeJong, and others, 2000). The female genital examination should include a description of the vulva, hymen, and surrounding tissue. Abnormal findings of concern are injuries to the posterior vulva or the lower half of the hymeneal ring, or abrasions, bruising, or bleeding of the genital or anal tissue. It is often helpful to use a magnifying instrument (colposcope) to detect subtle injuries. There are many variants of normal findings for female genital anatomy, so it is recommended that the examination be done by a practitioner experienced with these types of cases. Contrary to popular myth, the size of the hymenal opening is not predictive of the likelihood of sexual abuse (Christian and Rubin, 2002). For male victims, presence of swelling, abrasions, or bruising of the genital tissue is of concern for abuse. The anal area should be examined for symmetry, tone, fissures, or scars. Genital tissue heals quickly and most often without scars. Therefore, unless seen within a few days of injury, the genital tissue may appear normal. In addition, the vaginal and anal mucosa is elastic; therefore penetration without disruption of tissue is possible. This defies another myth that there is always evidence of female virginity. Consideration should be given to the collection of specimens for determining the presence of sexually transmitted diseases, which may have been contracted during the sexual contact.

A number of nursing diagnoses are prominent in the nursing care of the maltreated child and family, and others specific to individual cases become evident. The most common nursing diagnoses are outlined in the Nursing Process box. The expected outcomes are described in the Nursing Care Plan on p. 489.

Nursing Care Management

Protect Child from Further Abuse. Initially, identification of instances of suspected abuse or neglect is essential. The nurse may come in contact with abused children in an emergency department, practitioner's office, home, daycare center, or school.

> **NURSINGALERT**
> The priority is to remove the child from the abusive situation to prevent further injury.

All states and provinces in North America have laws for mandatory reporting of child maltreatment. Suspected child abuse is reported to the local authorities.* Referrals usually come to the state child welfare department and are assigned to a caseworker in an agency such as CPS. After a referral has been made, a caseworker is assigned to investigate the report. Based on the findings, the child is left in the home or temporarily removed.

A court proceeding may be necessary before the child can be placed outside the home or when parental rights are to be terminated. When the courts are involved, they usually require firsthand testimony by the referring parties. Nurses may be subpoenaed to appear in court, or their notes may be introduced as evidence in court hearings. Accurate and factual documentation is essential. Behaviors are described, not interpreted, and are recorded daily to establish a progress record (see Nursing Care Guidelines box). Conversations among the

---

*Telephone numbers are usually listed under Child Abuse in the business white pages of the local directory, or call the emergency child abuse hotline: (800) 422-4453 ([800] 4-A-CHILD).

nursingprocess | The Child Who Is Maltreated

ASSESSMENT
Assess for signs and symptoms of child maltreatment, including negligence or suspected maltreatment. (See Box 14-9 and the defining characteristics in the Nursing Care Plan, p. 489.)

DIAGNOSIS (PROBLEM IDENTIFICATION)
Following a thorough assessment, several nursing diagnoses are evident (see Nursing Care Plan, p. 489). Other possible nursing diagnoses include:
- Altered Parenting related to child, caregiver, or situational characteristics that precipitate abusive behavior
- Altered Family Processes
- Powerlessness
- Altered Protection
- Rape-Trauma Syndrome

PLANNING
Expected patient outcomes include:
- The child will be in a safe environment.
- The child and family will receive adequate support and referrals.
- The child will express feelings about returning home or going to foster care.
- The child will engage in positive relationships with caregivers.
- Parents will be knowledgeable of the child's physical and developmental needs.
- Caregivers are familiar with and access community agencies for support and education.

IMPLEMENTATION
Numerous intervention strategies are discussed on pp. 483-488.

EVALUATION
The effectiveness of nursing interventions for the family and the maltreated child are determined by continual assessment and evaluation of care based on the following guidelines:
- Observe child for physical and behavioral evidence of abuse; observe child's reactions to health professionals; if child is hospitalized, check staffing patterns for schedule of consistent group of nurses caring for child.
- Interview parents regarding their knowledge of child's physical and developmental needs.
- Interview child regarding feelings about returning home or placement outside the home.
- Investigate community programs aimed at preventing child maltreatment.

---

nurse, child, and parent are recorded verbatim as much as possible.

Support Child. Children suspected of being abused are often hospitalized for medical management of their injuries and to allow further assessment of their safety needs. The needs of these children are the same as those of any hospitalized child. The child should be treated as a child with the usual physical needs, developmental tasks, and play interests—not as a victim of abuse. The goal of the nurse-child relationship is to provide a role model for the parents in helping them to relate positively and constructively to their child and to foster a therapeutic environment for the child in his or her reprieve from the abusing situation.

Support Family. The nurse also encourages the child's relationship with nonoffending parents. The nurse does not become a substitute parent, but rather acts as a role model for parents in helping them to relate positively and constructively to their child. When parental ignorance of childrearing practices has played a part in the abuse, the nurse can educate the parent regarding children's physical and emotional needs. Because of the parents' own childrearing, they may not be aware of nonviolent methods of discipline, such as time-out. They may also need help in dealing with their frustration so that they do not vent anger on the child. Because these parents may be sensitive to criticism, teaching is implemented through demonstration and example rather than through lecturing. Any competent parenting abilities they demonstrate are praised to promote their sense of parental adequacy.

Family members are advised to encourage the child to resume normal activities and observe the child for signs of distress (see Posttraumatic Stress Disorder, Chapter 17). Children

nursingcareguidelines

Recording Assessment Data in Suspected Abuse

HISTORY OF INJURY
Date, time, and place of occurrence
Sequence of events with recorded times
Presence of witnesses, especially person caring for child at time of incident
Time lapse between occurrence of injury and initiation of treatment
Interview with child when appropriate, including verbal quotations and information from drawing or other play activities
Interview with parent, witnesses, or other significant persons, including verbal quotations
Description of parent-child interactions (verbal interactions, eye contact, touching, parental concern)
Name, age, and condition of other children in home (if possible)

PHYSICAL EXAMINATION
Location, size, shape, and color of bruises; approximate location, size, and shape on drawing of body outline
Distinguishing characteristics, such as a bruise in the shape of a hand or a round burn (possibly caused by cigarette)
Symmetry or asymmetry of injury; presence of other injuries
Degree of pain; any bone tenderness
Evidence of past injuries; general state of health and hygiene
Developmental level of child; screening test (see Developmental Assessment, Chapter 5)

express their feelings primarily through behavior. Parents should be alert for changes in behavior that indicate distress resulting from the incident, such as remaining in the house, refusing to go to school, changing sleeping patterns, and increasing frequency of nightmares. Children are encouraged to talk about these feelings and nightmares because the more they talk about the experience, the more they are able to gain control over it.

Referral to appropriate social service agencies is also essential. Many abusive parents live in poverty, and the daily stresses imposed by their circumstances are overwhelming. Resources for financial aid, improved housing, and child care should be sought. Self-help groups also provide important services. Groups such as **Parents Anonymous*** (a group for parents who have abused or fear that they may abuse their child, but only in terms of physical abuse, not sexual abuse) and **Parents United International, Inc.**† (a group devoted to helping sexually abused families), are accepting and nonjudgmental.

Plan for Discharge. Discharge planning should begin as soon as possible after the legal disposition for placement, which may be temporary foster home placement, return to the parents, or permanent termination of parental rights. The latter is the most drastic solution, but it is necessary in situations of life-threatening abuse. Whenever children are sent to a foster home or juvenile institution, they must be allowed an opportunity to express their feelings. No matter how severe the abuse, they usually mourn the loss of their parents. They need help to understand why they must not return home and that this new home is in no way a punishment. Whenever possible, foster parents are encouraged to visit in the hospital, and the nurse should take an active role in helping these new parents understand the child. It is unfortunate that some abused children live in torment as they are sent from one foster home to another, sometimes enduring worse circumstances than those that existed in their original home. Only through constant evaluation of the placement residence and the child's adjustment to a new environment can the vicious circle of abuse, abandonment, and neglect be stopped.

Prevent Abuse. Prevention of child maltreatment has been an extremely difficult goal. Programs aimed at identifying potential abusers and instituting supportive intervention before the occurrence of an abusive act have met with variable success. However, nurses have played an important role in such programs. For example, home visiting by nurses to primiparas who were either teenagers, unmarried, or of low socioeconomic status was noted to be an effective preventive measure (Eckenrode, Ganzel, Henderson, and others, 2000; McMillian, 2000). The nurses provided information on normal child growth and development and routine health care needs, served as informal support persons, and referred families to appropriate services when a need for assistance was identified.

Such programs provide models for reducing factors that increase the risk of abuse. Nurses in a variety of settings can implement similar activities. For example, nurses in prenatal

clinics can prepare expectant families for parenthood. Nursery and postpartum nurses can foster the attachment process by encouraging parents to hold and look at their infant, as well as teaching coping mechanisms for prolonged crying. Nurses in neonatal intensive care units can minimize the effects of separation by encouraging parents to visit and can help parents become comfortable caring for their child. Nurses in ambulatory settings can teach parents appropriate methods of bathing, feeding, toileting, disciplining, and preventing injuries, while stressing the normal needs and developmental characteristics of children. Nurses must be sensitive to parental needs for attention, reassurance, and reinforcement, and refer parents to community services and self-help groups.

Unlike preventive efforts for neglect and physical abuse, which have been aimed at the potential offender, **prevention of child sexual abuse** has centered on education of children to protect themselves. Materials are available for parents that describe sexual abuse and its prevention.* Supporting parental qualities of respect, affection, empathy, and ability to set boundaries and providing high-quality child care and education comprise the true preventive approach to sexual abuse. Helpful games such as "What if the baby-sitter wants to wrestle and hug but tells you to keep it a secret?" can be used to explore dangerous situations in advance and help children learn the importance of saying "no." They need reassurance that no matter what the other person says or does, the parents want to know about it and will not punish them. Even if children participate in the activity before telling the parents, they must be reassured that it was not their fault.

It is equally important to teach children safety in terms of potential risk situations. Several suggestions for parents regarding protecting and educating children against possible molestation are presented in the Family-Centered Care box. The nurse is frequently in a position to discuss the topic of abuse with parents and to provide guidance. In addition, parents need to be made aware that "nice" people, including friends and relatives, can be offenders; parents should carefully observe how others act toward the child. A sudden change in the child's behavior and a response such as "I don't like Uncle anymore" are clues to investigate the relationship. In the event of any doubt, further solitary encounters with this person and the child should be prevented. It is sometimes to the child's great misfortune that parents do not take certain comments seriously, such as "He hugs me too tight" or "I don't want to go with him." Casual parental statements such as "He just loves you" or "You do whatever adults tell you to do" can place children in jeopardy. Health professionals must alert parents to such dangers and guide them toward an appreciation of the problem, providing concrete guidelines toward child education and protection (see Nursing Care Plan).

*675 West Foothill Blvd., Suite 220, Claremont, CA 91711; (909) 621-6184; http://www.parentsanonymous.org.
†615 15th Street, Modesto, CA, 95354; (209) 572-3446; http://www.parentsunited.info.

*Sources of information are Prevent Child Abuse America, 500 N. Michigan Ave., Suite 200, Chicago, IL 60611; (312) 663-3520 or (800) Children; http://www.preventchildabuse.org; Kempe Children's Center, 1825 Marion St., Denver, CO 80218; (303) 864-5300, http://www.kempecenter.org; American Humane, 63 Inverness Drive East, Englewood, CO 80112; (303) 792-9900; http://www.americanhumane.org; and Child Welfare Information Gateway, Children's Bureau/ACYF, 1250 Maryland Ave. SW, Eighth Floor, Washington, DC 20024; (703) 835-7565 or (800) 394-3366; http://www.childwelfare.gov.

nursingcareplan | The Child Who Is Maltreated

Nursing Diagnosis	Expected Patient Outcomes	Nursing Interventions	Rationale
Risk for Trauma related to child, caregiver(s), environment	Child will not experience any maltreatment.	Observe child for physical and behavioral evidence of abuse.	To detect abuse and protect the child
CHILD'S/FAMILY'S DEFINING CHARACTERISTICS *(Subjective and Objective Data)*	Child and family will receive adequate support. Child will be protected from further abuse.	Report suspicions to appropriate authorities.	To comply with laws requiring health care providers to report suspicions of maltreatment to child protective services
Physical Neglect Growth failure (failure to thrive) Malnutrition Poor hygiene Poor health care Frequent injuries	Child will be able to express feelings about returning to home or foster home. Child and family, including foster parents if appropriate, will be prepared for discharge.	Assist in removing child from unsafe environment. Refer family to social agencies.	To prevent further injury or neglect To provide assistance for physical needs to help prevent physical neglect To provide counseling and education so that parents learn appropriate parenting skills
Emotional Neglect Growth failure (failure to thrive) Enuresis Sleep disorders	**THE FOLLOWING NOC CONCEPTS APPLY TO THESE OUTCOMES** Abuse Support	Collaborate with multidisciplinary team.	To involve several disciplines providing expertise in prevention of future neglect or abuse
Physical Abuse Bruises Burns Fractures or dislocation Lacerations Intracranial hemorrhage	Abuse Recovery: Physical Abuse Recovery: Sexual Anxiety Self-Control Fear Self-Control Coping	Keep factual, objective records of child and parental behaviors. Be aware of signs for continued abuse or neglect.	To provide essential documentation that clearly specifies the physical findings of the examination To prevent further injury or neglect
Sexual Abuse Torn or bloody underclothing Bruises, bleeding, lacerations of external genitalia, anus, mouth, or throat Genital discharge or odor Recurrent urinary tract infection	Personal Safety Behavior Safe Home Environment	Help parents identify circumstances that precipitate an abused act. Assist families with realizing abuse or neglect has occurred.	To promote more effective parenting skills To help parents recognize abuse as a family problem and seek assistance
		THE FOLLOWING NIC CONCEPTS APPLY TO THESE INTERVENTIONS Abuse Protection Support: Child Coping Enhancement Environment Management: Violence Prevention	

Nursing Diagnosis	Expected Patient Outcomes	Nursing Interventions	Rationale
Fear/Anxiety related to negative interpersonal interaction, repeated maltreatment, powerlessness, potential loss of parents	Child will exhibit minimum fear and anxiety.	Provide consistent caregiver during hospitalization.	To promote trust
CHILD'S/FAMILY'S DEFINING CHARACTERISTICS *(Subjective and Objective Data)*	Child will engage in positive relationships with caregivers. Child will grieve loss of parent.	Demonstrate acceptance of child.	To minimize feelings of shame and guilt
Withdrawn and depressed Change in behavior Inappropriate responses Fear of strangers Lack of engagement with others May not cry or ask for food when hungry No response to painful interventions	**THE FOLLOWING NOC CONCEPTS APPLY TO THESE OUTCOMES** Anxiety Self-Control Fear Self-Control Coping	Praise child's abilities. Treat child as one with a specific physical problem, not as "abused" victim. Avoid asking too many questions. Use play to communicate. Encourage child to talk about feelings. Provide private time and place to talk. Help child grieve for loss of parents if parental rights are terminated. Encourage introduction of foster parents before placement if possible.	To promote self-esteem To promote self-esteem and minimize feelings of guilt To avoid upsetting child or interfering with interrogation To allow child to communicate thoughts and feelings To facilitate coping To foster trust To help child express feelings because child may be attached to parents despite the abuse To give child time to adjust
		THE FOLLOWING NIC CONCEPTS APPLY TO THESE INTERVENTIONS Active Listening Calming Technique Counseling Presence Therapeutic Play Distraction	

FAMILY-CENTERED CARE

Preventing or Dealing with Sexual Abuse of Children

Sexual assault of children is much more common than most people realize. It may be preventable if children have good preparation. *To provide protection and preparation:*

- Pay careful attention to who is around children. (Unwanted touch may come from someone liked and trusted.)
- Back up a child's right to say no.
- Encourage communication by taking seriously what children say.
- Take a second look at signals of potential danger.
- Refuse to leave children in the company of those not trusted.
- Include information about sexual assault when teaching about safety.
- Provide specific definitions and examples of sexual assault.
- Remind children that even "nice" people sometimes do mean things.
- Urge children to tell about *anybody* who causes them to be uncomfortable.
- Prepare children to deal with bribes, threats, and possible physical force.
- Virtually eliminate secrets between children and parents.
- Teach children how to say no, ask for help, and control who touches them and how.
- Model self-protective and limit-setting behavior for children.

Should it ever become necessary to help a child recover from a sexual assault:

- Listen carefully to understand the child.
- Support the child for telling through praise, belief, sympathy, and lack of blame.
- Know local resources and choose help carefully.
- Provide opportunities to talk about the assault.
- Provide opportunities for the entire family to go through a recovery process.

Sexual assault affects everyone. To help deal with this social problem:

- Provide care and support to those who have been victimized.
- Recognize that offenders may not change behavior even with intervention.
- Organize neighborhood programs to support each other's efforts to protect children.
- Encourage schools to provide information about sexual assault as a problem of health and safety.
- Organize community groups to support educational treatment and law enforcement programs.

Modified from Adams C, Fay J: *No more secrets: protecting your child from sexual assault,* San Luis Obispo, Calif, 1981, Impact.

KEY POINTS

- Common infectious disorders during early childhood include communicable diseases, intestinal parasitic infections, conjunctivitis, and stomatitis.
- Nursing goals in the treatment of a communicable disease are identification, prevention of transmission, provision of comfort, and prevention of complications.
- Intestinal parasitic diseases constitute the most common infections in the world; giardiasis and enterobiasis are the most widespread parasitic infections among children in the United States.
- Although the incidence of poisoning has decreased in the past 30 years as a result of more stringent packaging regulations, childhood poisoning remains a serious health concern.

- The major principles of treatment for poisoning include assessment and the ABCs of resuscitation (airway, breathing, and cardiovascular supportive measures), minimization of poison absorption, prevention of complications, family support, and prevention of recurrence.
- Communication with the area poison control center is essential in the treatment of any poisoning.
- Acetaminophen poisoning is the most common accidental drug poisoning among children and occurs primarily from acute overdose.
- The most important factor contributing to lead poisoning is its availability in the child's environment. Lead-based paint is the most toxic source of lead.
- Because of increasing awareness of the detrimental effects of low levels of lead on the developing nervous system, acceptable BLLs have been decreasing and now are at less than 10 mcg/dl.
- Child maltreatment may take the form of physical abuse or neglect, emotional abuse or neglect, or sexual abuse.
- Parental, child, and environmental characteristics are criteria that may predispose children to maltreatment.
- Identification of abuse entails securing evidence of maltreatment, taking a history pertaining to the incident, and assessing parental and child behaviors.
- The reported incidence of sexual abuse has increased in the past decade; common forms are incest, molestation, rape, exhibitionism, child pornography, child prostitution, and pedophilia.

answers to CRITICAL THINKING EXERCISE

POISONING

1. Yes, there is sufficient evidence to formulate an answer for Mrs. Berry.
2. a. When a child ingests a poisonous substance, the initial goal is to limit the absorption of the poison in the gastrointestinal system and enhance elimination. Specific actions that are taken to limit absorption and enhance elimination of poisons are to administer an agent that neutralizes the poison such as activated charcoal. Multiple administrations of activated charcoal may also enhance excretion of the poison through the gastrointestinal tract, thus limiting absorption.
   b. Ipecac is an emetic that induces vomiting by producing an irritant effect on the gastric mucosa. In the past, ipecac was recommended for home treatment of some cases of ingestion. However, ipecac is no longer recommended for routine home treatment of poisoning.
   c. Ipecac induces emesis, which may predispose the child to aspiration if level of consciousness is affected. In addition, emesis may be prolonged beyond the desired time when oral hydration is desirable. In the event that hydrocarbons or corrosive substances are ingested, inducing vomiting with ipecac may cause esophageal damage and aspiration into the lungs.
3. The first priority for nursing care is to advise Mrs. Berry to call the poison control center immediately to obtain guidance. Each ingestion is treated individually, and information from the poison control center is essential to determine the most appropriate action. The most toxic ingredient in a chewable multivitamin is iron, which produces symptoms after several hours. Therefore treatment, if needed, should begin long before symptoms appear.
4. Yes, there is sufficient information to formulate an answer for Mrs. Berry.
5. This situation is straightforward, and the response is easily derived from the information. No alternative perspectives are apparent at this time.

REFERENCES

Abruzzi G, Stork CM: Pediatric toxicological concerns, *Emerg Med Clin North Am* 20(1):223-247, 2002.

American Academy of Clinical Toxicology, European Association of Poisons Centres and Clinical Toxicologists: Position paper: cathartics, *J Toxicol* 42(3):243-253, 2004a.

American Academy of Clinical Toxicology, European Association of Poisons Centres and Clinical Toxicologists: Position paper: ipecac syrup, *J Toxicol* 42(2):133-143, 2004b.

American Academy of Pediatrics, Committee on Infectious Diseases, Pickering L, editor: *Red book: 2006 report of the Committee on Infectious Diseases,* ed 27, Elk Grove Village, Ill, 2006, The Academy.

American Academy of Pediatrics, Committee on Environmental Health: Lead exposure in children: prevention, detection, and management, *Pediatrics* 116(4):1036-1046, 2005.

American Academy of Pediatrics, Committee on Injury, Violence, and Poison Prevention: Poison treatment in the home, *Pediatrics* 112(5):1182-1185, 2003.

American Academy of Pediatrics, Committee on Child Abuse and Neglect: Shaken baby syndrome: rotational cranial injuries (technical report), *Pediatrics* 108(1):206-210, 2001.

Berlinger L, Elliott D: Sexual abuse of children. In Myers J, Berliner L, Briere J, and others, editors: *APSAC handbook on child maltreatment,* ed 2, Thousand Oaks, Calif, 2002, Sage Publications.

Bond GR: Activated charcoal in the home: helpful and important or simply a distraction? *Pediatrics* 109(1):145-146, 2002.

Calam R, Horne L, Glasgow D, and others: Psychological disturbances and child sexual abuse: a follow-up study, *Child Abuse Negl* 22(9):901-913, 1998.

Carbaugh SF: The long road home: understanding shaken baby syndrome, *Adv Neonatal Care* 4:105-117, 2004.

Castiglia R: Shaken baby syndrome, *J Pediatr Health Care* 15(2):78-80, 2001.

Centers for Disease Control and Prevention: Deaths associated with hypocalcemia from chelation therapy—Texas, Pennsylvania, and Oregon, 2003-2005, *MMWR* 55(08):204-207, 2006.

Centers for Disease Control and Prevention: *Statewide plan for childhood blood lead screening,* Atlanta, 2005, The Centers.

Centers for Disease Control and Prevention: *Managing elevated blood lead levels among young children: recommendations from the Advisory Committee on Childhood Lead Poisoning Prevention,* Atlanta, 2002, The Centers.

Chen TM, George S, Woodruff CA, and others: Clinical manifestations of varicella-zoster virus infection, *Dermatol Clin* 20(2):267-282, 2002.

Cheng A, Ratnapalan S: Improving the palatability of activated charcoal in pediatric patients, *Pediatr Emerg Care* 23(6):384-386, 2007.

Christian C, Lavelle J, DeJong A, and others: Forensic evidence findings in prepubertal victims of sexual assault, *Pediatrics* 106:100-104, 2000.

Christian CW, Rubin DM: Sexual abuse. In Giardino AP, Giardino ER, editors: *Recognition of child abuse for the mandated reporter,* St Louis, 2002, G.W. Medical Publishing.

Clifton JC: Mercury exposure and public health, *Pediatr Clin North Am* 54(2):237-269, 2007.

Criddle LM: An overview of pediatric poisonings, *AACN Adv Crit Care* 18(2):109-118, 2007.

Cyr M, Wright J, McDuff P, and others: Intrafamilial sexual abuse: brother-sister incest does not differ from father-daughter incest and stepfather-stepdaughter incest, *Child Abuse Neglect* 26(9):957-973, 2002.

Eckenrode J, Ganzel B, Henderson C, and others: Preventing child abuse and neglect with a program of nurse home visitation: the limiting effects of domestic violence, *JAMA* 284(11):1385-1391, 2000.

Erickson L, Thompson T: A review of a preventable poison: pediatric lead poisoning, *J Soc Pediatr Nurs* 10(4):171-182, 2005.

Etzel RA: Indoor air pollutants in homes and schools, *Pediatr Clin North Am* 48(5):1153-1165, 2001.

Ewing-Cobb L, Kramer L, Prasad M, and others: Neuroimaging, physical, and developmental findings after inflicted and noninflicted traumatic brain injury in young children, *Pediatrics* 102:300-307, 1998.

Faden H: Management of primary herpetic gingivostomatitis in young children, *Pediatr Emerg Care* 22(4):268-269, 2006.

Finkel MA, DeJong AR: Medical findings in child sexual abuse. In Reece RM, Ludwig S, editors: *Child abuse medical diagnosis and management,* Philadelphia, 2001, Lippincott Williams & Wilkins.

Fuloria M, Kreiter S: The newborn examination, part I, Emergencies and common abnormalities involving the skin, head, neck, chest, and respiratory and cardiovascular systems, *Am Fam Physician* 65(1):61-68, 2002.

Gara MA, Allen LA, Herzog EP, and others: The abused child as parent: the structure and content of physically abused mothers' perceptions of their babies, *Child Abuse Negl* 24(5):627-639, 2000.

Goldman J, Salus MK, Wolcott D, and others: What factors contribute to child abuse and neglect? In *A coordinated response to child abuse and neglect: the foundation for practice,* 2003, Child Welfare Information Gateway, retrieved June 4, 2007, from http://www.childwelfare.gov/pubs/usermanuals/foundation/foundatione.cfm.

Heard K: Gastrointestinal decontamination, *Med Clin North Am* 89(6):1067-1078, 2005.

Hlavsa MC, Watson JC, Beach MJ: Giardiasis surveillance—United States, 1998-2002, *MMWR* 54(SS1):9-16, 2005.

Hornor G: Repeated sexual abuse allegations: a problem for primary care providers, *J Pediatr Health Care* 15(2):71-76, 2001.

Johnson M: Child sexual abuse. In Thomas DO, Bernardo LM, Herman B, editors: *Core curriculum for pediatric emergency nursing,* Sudbury, Mass, 2003, Jones & Bartlett.

Kaczor K, Pierce MC, Makoroff K, and others: Bruising and physical child abuse, *Clin Pediatr Emerg Med* 7(3):153-160, 2006.

Lederman C, Lederman M: Ophthalmologic emergencies. In Crain EF, Gershel JC, editors: *Clinical manual of emergency pediatrics,* ed 4, New York, 2003, McGraw-Hill.

Leider HS, Irving SY, Mauricio R, and others: Munchausen syndrome by proxy: a case report, *AACN Clin Issues* 16(2):178-184, 2005.

Leung AK, Robson WL, Leong AG: Herpes zoster in childhood, *J Pediatr Health Care* 20(5):1783-1785, 2006.

Lichtenstein SJ, Rinehart M, Levofloxacin Bacterial Conjunctivitis Study Group: Efficacy and safety of 0.5% levofloxacin ophthalmic solution for the treatment of bacterial conjunctivitis in pediatric patients, *J AAPOS* 7(5):317-324, 2003.

Lidsky TI, Schneider JS: Adverse effects of childhood lead poisoning: the clinical neuropsychological perspective, *Environ Res* 100(1):284-293, 2006.

Litovitz T, Klein-Schwartz W, White S, and others: 1999 Annual report of the American Association of Poison Control Centers toxic exposure surveillance system, *Am J Emerg Med* 18(5):517-574, 2000.

Markowitz M: Lead poisoning, *Pediatr Rev* 21(10):327-335, 2000.

McClain N, Giardet R, Lahoti S, and others: Evaluation of sexual abuse in the pediatric patient, *J Pediatr Health Care* 14(3):93-102, 2000.

McMillian H: Child maltreatment: what we know in the year 2000, *Can J Psychiatry* 45(8):702-709, 2000.

Miehl NJ: Shaken baby syndrome, *J Forensic Nurs* 1(3):111-117, 2005.

National Center on Shaken Baby Syndrome: *Shaken baby syndrome: medical facts,* 2007, retrieved July 12, 2007, from http://www.dontshake.com/Audience.aspx?categoryID=8&PageName=MedicalFactsAnswers.htm.

Nelms BC: Emotional abuse: helping prevent the problem, *J Pediatr Health Care* 15(3):103-104, 2001.

Pickering LK: Giardiasis and balantidiasis. In Behrman RE, Kliegman R, Jenson HB, editors: *Nelson textbook of pediatrics,* ed 17, Philadelphia, 2004, Saunders.

Powers K: Diagnosis and management of common toxic ingestions and inhalations, *Pediatr Ann* 29(6):330-342, 2000.

Putnam FW: Ten year update review: child sexual abuse, *J Am Acad Child Adolesc Psychiatry* 42(3):269-278, 2003.

Rose PW, Harnden A, Brueggemann AB, and others: Chloramphenicol treatment for acute infective conjunctivitis in children in primary care: a randomized double-blind placebo-controlled trial, *Lancet* 366(9479):37-43, 2005.

US Department of Health and Human Services, Administration on Children, Youth and Families: *Child maltreatment 2005,* Washington, DC, 2007, US Government Printing Office, retrieved June 4, 2007, from http://www.acf.hhs.gov/programs/cb/pubs/cm05/index.htm.

Walls C: Shaken baby syndrome education: a role for nurse practitioners working with families of small children, *J Pediatr Health Care* 20(5):304-310, 2006.

Watson WA, Litovitz TL, Rodgers GC, and others: 2004 Annual report of the American Association of Poison Control Centers Toxic Exposure Surveillance System, *Am J Emerg Med* 23(5):589-666, 2005.

Woolf AD, Goldman R, Bellinger DC: Update on clinical management of childhood lead poisoning, *Pediatr Clin North Am* 54(2):271-294, 2007.

http://evolve.elsevier.com/Wong/essentials/

15

Health Promotion of the School-Age Child and Family

CHERYL C. RODGERS

CHAPTER OUTLINE

PROMOTING OPTIMAL GROWTH
AND DEVELOPMENT, 493
Biologic Development, 493
    Proportional Changes, 493
    Maturation of Systems, 493
    Prepubescence, 494
Psychosocial Development: Developing a
    Sense of Industry (Erikson), 494
Cognitive Development (Piaget), 495
Moral Development (Kohlberg), 495
Spiritual Development, 496
Social Development, 497
    Social Relationships and Cooperation, 497
    Relationships with Families, 498
    Play, 498

Developing a Self-Concept, 499
    Developing a Body Image, 500
Coping with Concerns Related to Normal
    Growth and Development, 500
    School Experience, 500
    Latchkey Children, 500
    Limit Setting and Discipline, 501
    Dishonest Behavior, 501
    Stress and Fear, 504
PROMOTING OPTIMAL HEALTH DURING
THE SCHOOL YEARS, 504
Nutrition, 504
Sleep and Rest, 505

Exercise and Activity, 505
    Sports, 505
    Acquisition of Skills, 506
Dental Health, 506
    Dental Problems, 506
Sex Education, 507
    Nurse's Role in Sex Education, 507
School Health, 508
Injury Prevention, 508
Anticipatory Guidance—Care of
    Families, 509

LEARNING OBJECTIVES

On completion of this chapter the reader will be able to:
- Describe the physical, cognitive, and moral changes that take place during the middle childhood years.
- Describe ways to help a child develop a sense of accomplishment.

- Demonstrate an understanding of the changing interpersonal relationships of school-age children.
- Discuss the role of the peer group in the socialization of the school-age child.
- Discuss the role of schools in the development and socialization of the school-age child.

- Outline an appropriate health teaching plan for the school-age child.
- Plan a sex education session for a group of school-age children.
- Identify the causes and discuss the preventive aspects of injury in middle childhood.

RELATED TOPICS and ADDITIONAL RESOURCES

 IN TEXT

Childhood Mortality, *Ch. 1*
Dental Health, *Ch. 12*
Eating Disorders, *Ch. 17*
Growth and Development, *Ch. 5*
Health Problems of School-Age Children
  and Adolescents, *Ch. 17*
Immunizations, *Ch. 10*
Physical and Developmental Assessment
  of the Child, *Ch. 5 and Ch. 6*

Psychosocial History, *Ch. 6*
Limit Setting and Discipline, *Ch. 3*
Traumatic Injury, *Ch. 31*

 Companion CD

Case Study—Injury Prevention
Critical Thinking Exercise—Injury Prevention
NCLEX Review Questions
Pediatric Assessment Video Clips

evolve.elsevier.com/Wong/essentials/

NCLEX Review Questions
Pediatric Assessment Video Clips
WebLinks

**WONG'S CLINICAL MANUAL
OF PEDIATRIC NURSING, 7th Ed**

Guidelines for Automobile Safety Seats,
  p. 237

PROMOTING OPTIMAL GROWTH AND DEVELOPMENT

The segment of the life span that extends from age 6 to approximately age 12 has a variety of labels, each of which describes an important characteristic of the period. These middle years are most often referred to as **school-age** or the **school years.** This period begins with entrance into the school environment, which has a significant impact on development and relationships.

Physiologically the middle years begin with the shedding of the first deciduous tooth and end at puberty with the acquisition of the final permanent teeth (with the exception of the wisdom teeth). Before 5 or 6 years of age, children have progressed from helpless infants to sturdy, complicated individuals with an ability to communicate, conceptualize in a limited way, and become involved in complex social and motor behaviors. Physical growth is also rapid during the preschool-age years. In contrast, the period of middle childhood, between the rapid growth of early childhood and the prepubescent growth spurt, is a time of gradual growth and development with more even progress in both physical and emotional aspects.

BIOLOGIC DEVELOPMENT

During middle childhood, growth in height and weight assumes a slower but steady pace as compared with the earlier years. Between ages 6 and 12, children will grow an average of 5 cm (2 inches) per year to gain 30 to 60 cm (1 to 2 feet) in height and will almost double their weight, increasing 2 to 3 kg (4.5 to 6.5 pounds) per year. The average 6-year-old child is about 116 cm (45.7 inches) tall and weighs about 21 kg (46 pounds); the average 12-year-old child is about 150 cm (59 inches) tall and weighs approximately 40 kg (88 pounds). During this period, girls and boys differ little in size, although boys tend to be slightly taller and somewhat heavier than girls. Toward the end of the school-age years, both boys and girls begin to increase in size, although most girls begin to surpass boys in both height and weight, to the acute discomfort of both girls and boys.

Proportional Changes

School-age children are more graceful than they were as preschoolers, and they are steadier on their feet. Their body proportions take on a slimmer look, with longer legs, varying body proportion, and a lower center of gravity. Posture improves over that of the preschool period to facilitate locomotion and efficiency in using the arms and trunk. These proportions make climbing, bicycle riding, and other activities easier. Fat gradually diminishes, and its distribution patterns change, contributing to the thinner appearance of the child during the middle years.

Accompanying the skeletal lengthening and fat diminution is an increase in the percentage of body weight represented by muscle tissue. By the end of this age period, both boys and girls double their strength and physical capabilities, and their steady and relatively consistent development of coordination increases their poise and skill. However, this increased strength can be misleading. Although strength increases, muscles are still functionally immature when compared with those of the adolescent, and they are more readily damaged by muscular injury caused by overuse.

The most pronounced changes that indicate increasing maturity in children are a decrease in head circumference in relation to standing height, a decrease in waist circumference in relation to height, and an increase in leg length in relation to height. These observations often provide a clue to a child's degree of physical maturity and have proved useful in predicting readiness for meeting the demands of school. There appears to be a correlation between physical indications of maturity and success in school.

Specific physiologic and anatomic characteristics are typical of children in middle childhood. Facial proportions change as the face grows faster in relation to the remainder of the cranium. The skull and brain grow very slowly during this period and increase little in size. Because all of the primary (deciduous) teeth are lost during this age span, middle childhood is sometimes known as the **age of the loose tooth** (Fig. 15-1). The early years of middle childhood, when the new secondary (permanent) teeth appear too large for the face, are known as the **ugly duckling stage.**

Maturation of Systems

Maturity of the gastrointestinal system is reflected in fewer stomach upsets, better maintenance of blood glucose levels, and an increased stomach capacity, which permits retention of food for longer periods. The school-age child does not need to be fed as carefully, as promptly, or as frequently as the pre-

FIG. 15-1 ■ Middle childhood is the stage of development when deciduous teeth are shed.

school-age child. Caloric needs are less than they were in the preschool years.

Physical maturation is evident in other body tissues and organs. **Bladder capacity,** although differing widely among individual children, is generally greater in girls than in boys. The **heart** grows more slowly during the middle years and is smaller in relation to the rest of the body than at any other period of life. Heart and respiratory rates steadily decrease and blood pressure increases from ages 6 to 12 (see inside back cover).

The **immune system** becomes more competent in its ability to localize infections and to produce an antibody-antigen response. However, children have several infections in the first 1 to 2 years of school because of increased exposure to other children.

Bones continue to ossify throughout childhood but yield to pressure and muscle pulls more readily than with mature bones. Children need ample opportunity to move around, but they should observe caution in carrying heavy loads. For example, they should shift books or tote bags from one arm to the other. Backpacks distribute weight more evenly than tote bags.

Wider differences between children are observed at the end of middle childhood than at the beginning. These differences become increasingly apparent and, if they are extreme or unique, may create emotional problems. The associated characteristics of height and weight relationships, rapid or slow growth, and other important features of development should be explained to children and their families. Physical maturity is not necessarily correlated with emotional and social maturity. Seven-year-old children who look like 10-year-old children will, in fact, think and act like 7-year-old children. To expect behaviors appropriate for the older age is unrealistic and can be detrimental to their development of competence and self-esteem. Conversely, to treat 10-year-old children who look young physically as though they were younger is an equal disservice to them.

Prepubescence

Preadolescence is the period of approximately 2 years that begins at the end of middle childhood and ends with the thirteenth birthday. Because puberty signals the beginning of the development of secondary sex characteristics, **prepubescence** typically occurs during preadolescence.

Toward the end of middle childhood the discrepancies in growth and maturation between boys and girls become apparent. On the average, there is a difference of approximately 2 years between girls and boys in the age of onset of pubescence. This is a period of rapid growth in height and weight, especially for girls.

There is no universal age at which children assume the characteristics of prepubescence. The first physiologic signs appear at about 9 years of age (particularly in girls) and are usually clearly evident in 11- to 12-year-old children. Although preadolescent children do not want to be different, variability in physical growth and physiologic changes between children of the same sex and between the two sexes is often striking at this time. This variability, especially in relation to the onset of secondary sexual characteristics, is of great concern to the preadolescent. Either early or late appearance of these characteristics is a source of embarrassment and uneasiness to both sexes.

Preadolescence is a period of considerable overlapping of developmental characteristics of both middle childhood and early adolescence. However, several unique characteristics set this period apart from others. Generally, puberty begins at 10 years in girls and 12 years in boys, but can be normal for either sex after the age of 8 years. Boys experience little visible sexual maturation during preadolescence.

PSYCHOSOCIAL DEVELOPMENT: DEVELOPING A SENSE OF INDUSTRY (ERIKSON)

Freud described middle childhood as the **latency period,** a time of tranquility between the Oedipal phase of early childhood and the eroticism of adolescence. During this time children experience relationships with same-sex peers following the indifference of earlier years and preceding the heterosexual fascination that occurs for most boys and girls in puberty.

Successful mastery of Erikson's first three stages of psychosocial development is important in terms of development of a healthy personality. Successful completion of these stages requires a loving environment within a stable family unit. These experiences prepare the child to engage in experiences and relationships beyond the intimate family group.

A **sense of industry,** or a **stage of accomplishment,** is achieved somewhere between age 6 and adolescence. School-age children are eager to develop skills and participate in meaningful and socially useful work. They acquire a sense of personal and interpersonal competence; receive the systematic instruction prescribed by their individual cultures; and develop the skills needed to become useful, contributing members of their social communities.

Interests expand in the middle years, and with a growing sense of independence, children want to engage in tasks that can be carried through to completion (Fig. 15-2). They gain satisfaction from independent behavior in exploring and manipulating their environment and from interaction with peers. Often the acquisition of skills provides a way to achieve success in social activities. Reinforcement in the form of grades, material rewards, additional privileges, and recognition provides encouragement and stimulation.

A sense of accomplishment also involves the ability to cooperate, to compete with others, and to cope effectively with people. Middle childhood is the time when children learn the

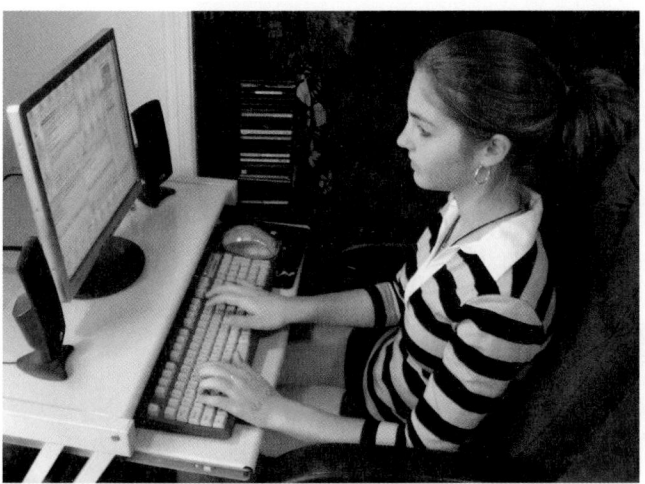

FIG. 15-2 ■ School-age children are motivated to complete tasks working alone.

value of doing things with others and the benefits derived from division of labor in the accomplishment of goals. Peer approval is a strong motivating power.

The danger inherent in this period of development is the occurrence of situations that might result in a sense of **inferiority.** Children with physical and mental limitations may be at a disadvantage in the acquisition of certain skills. When the reward structure is based on evidence of mastery, children who are incapable of developing these skills risk feeling inadequate and inferior. Even children without chronic disabilities may experience feelings of inadequacy in some areas. No child is able to do everything well, and children must learn that they will not be able to master every skill they attempt. All children, even children who usually have positive attitudes toward work and their own abilities, will feel some degree of inferiority when they encounter specific skills that they cannot master.

Children need and want real achievement. Children achieve a sense of industry when they have access to tasks that need to be done and they are able to complete the tasks well despite individual differences in their innate capacities and emotional development.

COGNITIVE DEVELOPMENT (PIAGET)

When children enter the school years, they begin to acquire the ability to relate a series of events to mental representations that can be expressed both verbally and symbolically. This is the stage Piaget describes as **concrete operations,** when children are able to use thought processes to experience events and actions. The rigid, egocentric view of the preschool years is replaced by mental processes that allow children to see things from another's point of view.

During this stage, children develop an understanding of relationships between things and ideas. They progress from making judgments based on what they see (**perceptual thinking**) to making judgments based on what they reason (**conceptual thinking**). They are able to master symbols and to use their memories of past experiences to evaluate and interpret the present.

One cognitive task of school-age children is mastering the concept of **conservation** (Fig. 15-3). At an early age (about 5 to 7 years), children grasp the concept of reversibility of numbers as a basis for simple mathematics problems (e.g.,

$2 + 4 = 6$ and $6 - 4 = 2$). They learn that simply altering their arrangement in space does not change certain properties of the environment, and they are able to resist perceptual cues that suggest alterations in the physical state of an object. For example, they recognize that changing the shape of a substance such as a lump of clay does not alter its total mass. They no longer perceive a tall, thin glass of water as containing a greater volume than a short, wide glass; they can distinguish between the weight of items regardless of their size. They recognize that size is not necessarily related to weight or volume. There is a developmental sequence in children's capacity to conserve matter. Conservation of mass usually is accomplished first, weight some time later, and volume last.

School-age children also develop **classification** skills. They can group and sort objects according to the attributes they share, place things in a sensible and logical order, and hold a concept in mind while making decisions based on that concept. Another characteristic of middle childhood is that children derive enjoyment from classifying and ordering their environment. They become occupied with collections of objects, such as stickers, shells, dolls, cars, cards, and stuffed animals. They may even begin to order friends and relationships (e.g., best friend, second best friend).

They develop the ability to understand relational terms and concepts, such as bigger and smaller; darker and paler; heavier and lighter; to the right of and to the left of; first, last, and intermediate relationships; and more than and less than. They view family relationships in terms of reciprocal roles (e.g., to be a brother, one must have a sibling).

School-age children learn the alphabet and the world of symbols called *words,* which can be arranged in terms of structure and their relationship to the alphabet. They learn to tell time, to see the relationship of events in time (history) and places in space (geography), and to combine time and space relationships (geology and astronomy).

The **ability to read** is acquired during the school years and becomes the most significant and valuable tool for independent inquiry. Children's capacity to explore, imagine, and expand their knowledge is enhanced by reading.

MORAL DEVELOPMENT (KOHLBERG)

As children move from egocentrism to more logical patterns of thought, they also move through stages in the development of conscience and moral standards. Young children do not believe that standards of behavior come from within themselves but that rules are established and set down by others. During the preschool years children adopt and internalize the moral values of their parents. They learn standards for acceptable behavior, act according to these standards, and feel guilty when they violate them. Although children 6 or 7 years of age know the rules and behaviors expected of them, they do not understand the reasons behind them. Rewards and punishments guide their judgment; a "bad act" is one that breaks a rule or causes harm. Young children believe that what other people tell them to do is right and that what they themselves think is wrong. Consequently, children 6 or 7 years old may interpret accidents or misfortunes as punishment for "bad" acts.

Older school-age children are able to judge an act by the intentions that prompted it rather than just its consequences. Rules and judgments become less absolute and authoritarian, and begin to be founded on the needs and desires of others. For older children, a rule violation is likely to be viewed in

Liquids:
Conserving child recognizes that each glass contains the same amount of liquid. Usually attained at age 5 to 7 years.

Mass (continuous substance): Conserving child recognizes that each object contains the same amount of dough. Usually attained at age 5 to 7 years.
Weight:
Conserving child recognizes that each object weighs the same. Usually attained at age 9 to 10 years.

Number:
Conserving child recognizes that each row contains the same number of marbles. Usually attained at age 5 to 7 years.

Length:
Conserving child recognizes that the two pencils are still of equal length. Usually attained at age 6 to 7 years.

Area:
Conserving child recognizes that the amount of uncovered area remains the same on each sheet. Usually attained at age 9 to 10 years.

Volume (water displacement): Conserving child recognizes that water levels are the same, since only the shape of the clay has changed. Pieces of clay displace the same volume of liquid. Usually attained at age 9 to 12 years.

Two identical glasses filled to the same level have equal amounts of liquid.

Contents of one glass poured into different-shaped glass—liquid of unequal height.

Two identical balls of play dough have equal mass and weight.

One ball is rolled into a flattened "pancake" shape.

Two rows of marbles have equal number and equal length.

Two rows of marbles have equal number, but one is increased in length.

Two pencils of equal length are aligned so that they are of equal length.

One pencil is moved to a different position and is no longer aligned with the other.

Two identical sheets of paper are covered by the same number of stamps, leaving the same amount of uncovered space.

The stamps are rearranged on one sheet.

Identical balls of clay are placed in identical glasses, displacing the same amount of liquid.

One ball of clay is removed and altered in shape, but will displace an equal amount when replaced in the liquid.

FIG. 15-3 ■ Common examples that demonstrate the child's ability to conserve (ages are only approximate).

relation to the total context in which it appears. The situation, as well as the morality of the rule itself, influences reactions. Although younger children judge an act only according to whether it is right or wrong, older children take into account a different point of view. They are able to understand and accept the concept of treating others as they would like to be treated.

SPIRITUAL DEVELOPMENT

Children at this age think in concrete terms, but are avid learners and have a great desire to learn about their God. They picture God as human and use adjectives such as "loving" and "helping" to describe their deity. They are fascinated by the concepts of hell and heaven, with a developing conscience and concern about rules. They may fear going to hell for misbe-

FIG. 15-4 ■ School-age children enjoy engaging in activities with a "best friend."

havior. School-age children want and expect to be punished for misbehavior and, when given the option, tend to choose a punishment that "fits the crime." However, they may view illness or injury as a punishment for a real or imagined misdeed. The beliefs and ideals of family and religious persons are more influential than those of their peers in matters of faith.

School-age children begin to learn the difference between the natural and the supernatural but have difficulty understanding symbols. Consequently, religious concepts must be presented to them in concrete terms. Prayer or other religious rituals comfort them, and if these activities are a part of their daily lives, they can help them cope with threatening situations. Their petitions to their God in prayers tend to be for tangible rewards. Although younger children expect their prayers to be answered, as they get older, they begin to recognize that this does not always occur and become less concerned when prayers are not answered. They are able to discuss their feelings about their faith and how it relates to their lives (see Cultural Awareness box).

SOCIAL DEVELOPMENT

One of the most important socializing agents in the school-age years is the peer group. In addition to parents and the schools, the peer group conveys a substantial amount of information to its members. Peer groups have a culture of their own, with secrets, traditions, and codes of ethics that promote feelings of solidarity and detachment from adults. Through peer relationships, children learn how to deal with dominance and hostility, how to relate to persons in positions of leadership and authority, and how to explore ideas and the physical environment.

Peer group identification is an important factor in gaining independence from parents. The aid and support of the group provide the child with enough security to risk the moderate parental rejection brought about by small victories in the development of independence.

A child's concept of the appropriate sex role is also influenced by relationships with peers. During the early school years few gender differences exist in the play experiences of children. Both girls and boys share games and other activities. However, in the later school years the differences in the play of boys and girls becomes more marked.

Social Relationships and Cooperation

Daily relationships with peers provide important social interactions for school-age children. For the first time, children join group activities with unrestrained enthusiasm and steady participation. Previous interactions were limited to short periods under considerable adult supervision. With increased skills and wider opportunities, children become involved with one or more peer groups in which they can gain status as respected members.

Valuable lessons are learned from daily interaction with age-mates. First, children learn to appreciate the numerous and varied points of view that are represented in the peer group. As children interact with peers who see the world in ways that are somewhat different from their own, they become aware of the limits of their own point of view. Because age-mates are peers and are not forced to accept each other's ideas as they are expected to accept those of adults, other children have a significant influence on decreasing the egocentric outlook of the child. Consequently, children learn to argue, persuade, bargain, cooperate, and compromise to maintain friendships.

Second, children become increasingly sensitive to the social norms and pressures of the peer group. The peer group establishes standards for acceptance and rejection, and children are often willing to modify their behavior to be accepted by the group. The need for peer approval becomes a powerful influence toward conformity. Children learn to dress, talk, and behave in a manner acceptable to the group. A variety of roles, such as class joker or class hero, may be assumed by individual children to gain approval from the group.

Third, the interaction among peers leads to the formation of intimate friendships between same-sex peers. The school-age period is the time when children have "best friends" with whom they share secrets, private jokes, and adventures; they come to one another's aid in times of trouble. In the course of these friendships children also fight, threaten each other, break up, and reunite. These relationships, in which the child experiences love and closeness for a peer, may be important as a foundation for relationships in adulthood (Fig. 15-4).

Clubs and Peer Groups. One of the outstanding characteristics of middle childhood is the formation of formalized groups, or clubs. A prominent feature of these groups is the rigid rules imposed on the members. There is exclusiveness in the selection of persons who have the privilege of joining. Acceptance in the group is often determined on a pass-fail basis according to social or behavioral criteria. Conformity is the core of the group structure. There are often secret codes, shared interests, and special modes of dress, and each child must abide by a standard of behavior established by the members. Conforming to the rules provides children with feelings of security and relieves them of the responsibility of making decisions. By merging their identities with those of their peers, children are able to move from the family group to an outside group as a step toward seeking further independence. Peer groups and clubs allow children to substitute conformity to a peer group for conformity to a family at a time when children are still too insecure to function independently.

During the early school years, groups are usually small and loosely organized, with changing membership and no formal structure. The clubs and groups usually do not display elements of cooperation and order that are seen in groups of older children. In general, girls' groups are less formalized than boys' are, and although there may be a mixture of both sexes in the early school years, the groups of later school years are composed predominantly of children of the same sex. Common interests are the basis around which the group is structured.

Peer-group identification and association are essential to a child's socialization. Poor relationships with peers and a lack of group identification can contribute to bullying. **Bullying** is any recurring activity that is intended to harm or bother someone where there is a perceived imbalance of power between the aggressor(s) and the victim (Glew, Fan, Katon, and others, 2005). Bullying occurs most frequently at school during unstructured times, with recess being the most common opportunity for bullying, followed by gym classes, lunchrooms, hallways, and buses (Glew, Fan, Katon, and others, 2005). Bullies may be from any ethnic, racial, or socioeconomic group. They are generally defiant toward adults, antisocial, and likely to break school rules. They have little anxiety, strong self-esteem, and dominant personalities; may come from homes where parental involvement and nurturing are lacking; and may experience or witness violence or abuse at home (Lyznicki, McCaffree, and Robinowitz, 2004). Boys who bully tend to use physical force, whereas girls who bully employ psychologic methods such as ostracism or rumors. Bullying by boys is more common than by girls. Children who are targeted for bullying often have characteristics different from the group norm (i.e., children who are short or obese; have facial deformities; or have attention deficit hyperactivity disorder, mental retardation, or other developmental disabilities) (Vessey, Carlson, and David, 2003).

The long-term consequences of bullying are significant. Chronic bullies seem to continue their behaviors into adulthood, negatively influencing their ability to develop and maintain relationships. Victims of bullying often feel socially rejected and can fear school, which can develop into school phobia or long-term problems of depression and low self-esteem (Vreeman and Carroll, 2007). School personnel play an important role in implementing antibullying interventions in the elementary schools before bullying becomes a part of the school culture (Glew, Fan, Katon, and others, 2005).

There are also dangers in peer-group attachments that are too strong. Peer pressures force some children to take risks or engage in behaviors that are against their better judgment. A child's membership in a gang is associated with marked increases in serious delinquent behavior (Dishion, Nelson, and Yasui, 2005). Peer-group activities that result in unlawful or criminal **gang violence** are increasing in the United States. An integration of family-centered and school-based programs is needed to reduce the influences for children to become affiliated with gangs (Dishion, Nelson, and Yasui, 2005).

Relationships with Families

Although the peer group is influential and necessary to normal child development, parents are the primary influence in shaping the child's personality, setting standards for behavior, and establishing value systems. Family values usually take precedence over peer value systems. Although children may appear to reject parental values while testing the new values of the peer group, ultimately they retain and incorporate into their own value systems the parental values they have found to be of worth.

In the middle school years, children want to spend more time in the company of peers and they often prefer peer-group activities to family activities. This can be disturbing to parents. Children become intolerant and critical of their parents, especially when their parents' ways deviate from those of the group. They discover that parents can be wrong, and they begin to question the knowledge and authority of their parents who were previously considered to be all-knowing and all-powerful.

Although increased independence is the goal of middle childhood, children are not prepared to abandon all parental control. They need and want restrictions placed on their behavior, and they are not prepared to cope with all the problems of their expanding environment. They feel more secure knowing there is an authority figure to implement controls and restrictions. Children may complain loudly about restrictions and try to break down parental barriers, but they are uneasy if they succeed in doing so. They respect adults who prevent them from acting on every urge. Children view this behavior as an expression of love and concern for their welfare.

Children also need their parents as adults, not as friends. Sometimes parents, hurt by their children's rejection, attempt to maintain their love and gratitude by assuming the role of "pals." Children need the stable, secure strength provided by mature adults to whom they can turn during troubled relationships with peers or stressful changes in their world. With a secure base in a loving family, children are able to develop the self-confidence and maturity needed to break loose from the group and stand independently.

Play

Play takes on new dimensions that reflect a new stage of development in the school years. Play involves increased physical skill, intellectual ability, and fantasy. In addition, children develop a sense of belonging to a team or club by forming groups and cliques.

Rules and Rituals. The need for conformity in middle childhood is strongly manifested in the activities and games of school-age children. In the preschool years, children's games were either invented for them or played in the company of a friend or an adult. Now children begin to see the need for rules, and their games have fixed and unvarying rules that may be bizarre and extraordinarily rigid. Part of the enjoyment of the game is knowing the rules because knowing means belonging. Conformity and ritual permeate their play and are also evident in their behavior and language. Childhood is full of chants and taunts, such as "Eeeny, meeny, miney, mo," "Last one is a rotten egg," and "Step on a crack, break your mother's back." Children derive a sense of pleasure and power from such sayings, which have been handed down with few changes through generations.

Team Play. A more complex form of play that evolves from the need for peer interaction is team games and sports. A referee, umpire, or person of authority may be required so that the rules can be followed more accurately. Team play teaches children to modify or exchange personal goals for goals of the group; it also teaches them that division of labor is an effective strategy for attaining a goal. Children learn about competition and the importance of winning—an attribute highly valued in the United States.

Team play can also contribute to children's social, intellectual, and skill growth. Children work hard to develop the skills needed to become team members, to improve their contribution to the group, and to anticipate the consequences of their behavior for the group. Team play helps stimulate cognitive growth because children are called on to learn many complex rules, make judgments about those rules, plan strategies, and assess the strengths and weaknesses of members of their own team and members of the opposing team.

Quiet Games and Activities. Although play at this age is highly active, school-age children also enjoy quiet and solitary activities. The middle years are the time for collections, which constitute another ritual. Young school-age children's collections are an odd assortment of unrelated objects in messy, disorganized piles. Collections of later school years are more orderly; selective; and organized in scrapbooks, on shelves, or in boxes.

School-age children become fascinated with complex board, card, or computer games that they can play alone, with a best friend, or with a group. As in all games, adherence to the rules is fanatic. Disagreements over rules can cause much discussion and argument, but are easily resolved by reading the rules of the game.

The newly acquired skill of reading becomes increasingly satisfying as school-age children expand their knowledge of the world through books (Fig. 15-5). School-age children never tire of stories and, as with preschool children, love to have stories read aloud. Sewing, cooking, carpentry, gardening, and creative activities such as painting are other activities enjoyed. Many creative skills such as music and art, as well as athletic skills such as swimming, karate, dancing, and skating, are learned during these years and continue to be enjoyed into adolescence and adulthood (Fig. 15-6).

Ego Mastery. Play affords children the means to acquire mastery over themselves, their environment, and others. Through play, children can feel as big, as powerful, and as skillful as their imaginations will allow. They can also feel in control and attain vicarious mastery and power over whomever and whatever they choose. School-age children still need the opportunity to use large muscles in exuberant outdoor play and the freedom to exert their newfound autonomy and initiative. They need space in which to exercise large muscles and to deal with tensions, frustrations, and hostility. Physical skills practiced and mastered in play help them develop a feeling of personal competence, which contributes to a sense of accomplishment and provides status in their peer group.

DEVELOPING A SELF-CONCEPT

The term **self-concept** refers to a conscious awareness of self-perceptions, such as one's physical characteristics, abilities, values, self-ideals and expectancy, and idea of self in relation to others. It also includes one's body image, sexuality, and self-esteem. Although primary caregivers continue to exert influ-

FIG. 15-5 ■ Selecting a book with the assistance of an adult.

FIG. 15-6 ■ School-age children take pride in learning new skills.

ence on children's self-evaluation, the opinions of peers and teachers provide valuable input during middle childhood. With the emphasis on skill building and broadened social relationships, children are continually engaged in the process of self-evaluation.

Significant adults can often manage to unobtrusively manipulate the environment so that children experience success. Each small success increases a child's self-image. The more positive children feel about themselves, the more confident they will be in trying for success in the future. All children profit from feeling that they are in some way special to a significant adult. A positive self-concept makes children feel likeable, worthwhile, and capable of significant contributions. These feelings lead to self-respect, self-confidence, and happiness. Negative feelings lead to self-doubt.

Developing a Body Image

School-age children have a relatively accurate and positive perception of their physical selves, but in general they like their physical selves less as they grow older. The head appears to be the most important part of the school-age child's perceived image of self, with hair and eye color the characteristics used most frequently to describe the physical self.

Body image is influenced, but not solely determined, by significant others. The number of significant others influencing one's perception of the physical self increases with age. Children are acutely aware of their own body, the bodies of their peers, and those of adults. They are also aware of deviations from the norm. It is important that children learn about bodily functions and that adults provide correct information.

Physical impairments, such as hearing or visual defects, ears that "stick out," or birthmarks, assume great importance. Increasing awareness of these differences, especially when accompanied by unkind comments and taunts from others, may cause a child to feel inferior and less desirable. This is especially true if the defect interferes with the child's ability to participate in games and activities.

Table 15-1 summarizes the major developmental achievements of the school-age years.

COPING WITH CONCERNS RELATED TO NORMAL GROWTH AND DEVELOPMENT
School Experience

School serves as the agent for transmitting the values of society to each succeeding generation of children. School is also the setting for relationships with peers. After the family, schools are the second most important socializing agent in the lives of children.

Entrance into school causes a sharp break in the structure of the child's world. For many children it is their first experience in conforming to a group pattern imposed by an adult who is not a parent and who has responsibility for too many children to be constantly aware of each child as an individual. Children want to go to school and usually adapt to the new conditions with little difficulty. Successful adjustment is related to the child's physical and emotional maturity and the parent's readiness to accept the separation associated with school entrance. Unfortunately, some parents express their unconscious attempts to delay the child's maturity by clinging behavior, particularly with their youngest child.

By the time they enter school, most children have a fairly realistic concept of what school involves. They receive information regarding the role of a student from parents, siblings, playmates, and the media. In addition, most children have had some experience with daycare, preschool, or kindergarten. Middle-class children have fewer adjustments to make and less to learn about expected behavior, since schools tend to reflect dominant middle-class customs and values. If the child has attended a preschool program, the focus of the preschool program also affects the child's adjustment. Some preschool programs provide custodial care only, whereas others emphasize emotional, social, and intellectual development.

Classmates have a significant impact on the socialization of children. School is the first time that most children become members of a large group of individuals their own age. Peer relationships become increasingly important and influential as children proceed through school. The specific influence exerted by the peer group depends on the background, interests, and abilities of the individual child.

Teachers. Children respond best to teachers who possess the characteristics of a warm, loving parent. Teachers in the early grades perform many of the activities formerly assumed by the parent, such as recognizing the child's personal needs (e.g., the need to go to the bathroom, need for help with clothing) and helping to develop their social behavior (e.g., manners).

Teachers, like parents, are concerned about the child's psychologic and emotional welfare. Although the functions of teachers and parents differ, both place constraints on behavior and both are in a position to enforce standards of conduct. However, the teacher's primary responsibility involves stimulating and guiding children's intellectual development, as opposed to providing for their physical welfare beyond the school setting.

Teachers serve as models that children try to emulate. Children seek their teachers' approval and avoid their disapproval. The teacher is a significant person in the life of the early schoolchild, and hero worship of a teacher may extend into late childhood and preadolescence. Teachers who make supportive statements that reassure or commend children, use accepting and clarifying statements that help children refine ideas and feelings, and provide assistance that aids children with their own problem solving contribute to the development of a positive self-concept in the school-age child.

Parents. Parents share responsibility for helping children achieve their maximum potential. Parents can supplement the school program in numerous ways (see Family-Centered Care box). Cultivating responsibility is the goal of parental assistance. Being responsible for schoolwork helps children learn to keep promises, meet deadlines, and succeed at their jobs as adults. Responsible children may occasionally ask for help (e.g., with a spelling list), but usually they prefer to think through their work by themselves. Excessive pressure or lack of encouragement from parents may inhibit the development of these desirable traits.

Latchkey Children

The term **latchkey children** is used to describe children in elementary school who are left to care for themselves before or after school without the supervision of an adult. The increasing numbers of single-parent families and working mothers, together with the lack of available child care, have created a stress-provoking situation for many school-age children. Some of these children may have a chronic illness as well.

FAMILY-CENTERED CARE

Helping Children in School
GENERAL GUIDELINES
Be supportive—provide companionship; share ideas and thoughts.

Be positive—every child should experience some success each day.

Share an interest in reading—use the library; discuss books they are reading.

Support and encourage activity rather than passivity.

Encourage originality—help children make their own projects from discarded articles or other available materials.

Foster the development of hobbies and collections.

Encourage children to wonder and reflect during free time.

Encourage family experiences and trips to places of interest.

Encourage questions—help children discover sources for information or places to explore and investigate.

Stimulate creative thinking and problem solving—help children try out new solutions to problems without fear of making mistakes.

Use rewards rather than punishment.

SPECIFIC GUIDELINES
Meet the teacher at the beginning of school and plan to visit the school to see what is taught and expected.

Send the child to school every day. Teachers are concerned when parents make other plans for their children; it conveys the impression that school is unimportant.

Demonstrate an interest in what the child is learning.

Demonstrate an interest in content and growth more than in grades.

Make it clear to the child that schoolwork is between the child and the teacher; teacher and child should set goals for better school performance to allow the child to feel responsible for school successes and failures.

Take advantage of situations that support and reinforce school learning.

Share information with teachers that will help them understand the child better.

Communicate with the teacher if there appears to be a problem; avoid waiting for a scheduled conference.

Provide a quiet, well-lit area for study that is safe from interruption; do not allow television or radio.

Avoid dictating a study time, but do enforce rules, such as no television until homework is done; accept the child's word that work is complete.

Help with homework should focus on explaining the question, not giving the answer.

Teach the child to break large tasks (e.g., a report) into smaller, manageable tasks spread over the allotted time rather than attempt the entire project the night before it is to be completed.

Limit home tutoring to special circumstances, such as when the teacher requests parental assistance after a child's prolonged absence.

Request special help for children with learning problems.

Support the school staff by showing respect for both the school system and the teacher, at least in the child's presence.

Inadequate adult supervision after school leaves children at greater risk for injury and delinquent behavior. In some instances outside activities are curtailed and relationships with peers may be significantly diminished. Latchkey children may feel more lonely, isolated, and fearful than children who have someone to care for them. To cope with their fears and anxieties while alone, these children may devise strategies such as hiding, playing the television at loud volume, or using pets for comfort.

Many communities and persons concerned about the welfare of latchkey children are trying to help these children and their parents deal with this potentially serious problem. Some communities and employers have implemented after-school programs or telephone "hotlines" that provide check-in and reassurance for children. Nurses should be aware of these community services and encourage parents to teach self-help skills to these children.

Limit Setting and Discipline
Many factors influence the amount and manner of discipline and limit setting imposed on school-age children. Some of these factors are the parents' psychosocial maturity, the parents' childhood and childrearing experiences, the children's temperament, the context of the children's misconduct, and the children's response to rewards and punishments. When children develop an ability to see a situation from another's point of view, they are also able to understand the effects of their reactions on others and themselves.

Discipline should take place in a positive, supportive environment with the use of strategies to instruct and guide desired behaviors and eliminate undesired behaviors (Ateah, 2003). Reasoning is an effective technique for middle school–age children. With advancing cognitive skills, they are able to benefit from more complex disciplinary strategies. For example, withholding privileges, requiring compensation, imposing penalties, and contracting can be used with great success. Problem solving is the best approach to limit setting, and children themselves can be included in the process of determining appropriate disciplinary measures.

Dishonest Behavior
During middle childhood, children may engage in what is considered to be antisocial behavior. Previously well-behaved children may engage in lying, stealing, and cheating. Such behaviors are disturbing and challenging to parents.

Lying can occur for a number of reasons. By the time children enter school, they still "tell stories," often exaggerating a story or situation as a means of impressing their family or friends. However, during middle childhood, children become able to distinguish between fact and fantasy. If children do not develop this characteristic, parents need to teach them what is real and what is make-believe.

Young children may lie to escape punishment or to get out of some difficulty even when their misbehavior is evident. Older children may lie to meet expectations set by others to which they have been unable to measure up. However, most children know that lying and cheating are wrong, and they are concerned when it is observed in their friends. They are quick to tell on others when they detect cheating.

Parents need to be reassured that all children lie occasionally and that sometimes children may have difficulty separating fantasy from reality. Parents should be helped to understand the importance of being truthful in their relationships with children.

Cheating is most common in young children 5 to 6 years of age. They find it difficult to lose at a game or contest, so they may cheat to win. They have not yet realized that this behavior is wrong, and they do it almost automatically. This behavior usually disappears as they mature. However, because children model observed behaviors, parents need to be aware of their own behavior. When parents set examples

TABLE 15-1	
Growth and Development During School-Age Years	
PHYSICAL AND MOTOR	**MENTAL**
AGE 6 YEARS	
Height and weight gain continues slowly	Develops concept of numbers
Weight 16-26.3 kg (35.5-58 pounds)	Can count 13 pennies
Height 106.7-122 cm (42-48 inches)	Knows whether it is morning or afternoon
Central mandibular incisors erupt	Defines common objects such as fork and chair in terms of their use
Loses first tooth	Obeys three commands in succession
Gradual increase in dexterity	Knows right and left hands
Active age; constant activity	Says which is pretty and which is ugly of a series of drawings of faces
Often returns to finger feeding	Describes the objects in a picture rather than simply enumerating them
More aware of hand as a tool	Attends first grade
Likes to draw, print, color	
Vision reaches maturity	
AGE 7 YEARS	
Begins to grow at least 5 cm (2 inches) in height per year	Notices that certain items are missing from pictures
Weight 17.7-30 kg (39-66.5 pounds)	Can copy a diamond
Height 112-130 cm (44-51 inches)	Repeats three numbers backward
Maxillary central incisors and lateral mandibular incisors erupt	Develops concept of time; reads ordinary clock or watch correctly to nearest quarter hour; uses clock for practical purposes
More cautious in approaches to new performances	Attends second grade
Repeats performances to master them	More mechanical in reading; often does not stop at the end of a sentence; skips words such as "it," "the," and "he"
Jaw begins to expand to accommodate permanent teeth	
AGES 8 TO 9 YEARS	
Continues to gain 5 cm (2 inches) in height per year	Gives similarities and differences between two things from memory
Weight 19.5-39.5 kg (43-87 pounds)	Counts backward from 20 to 1; understands concept of reversibility
Height 117-142 cm (46-56 inches)	Repeats days of the week and months in order; knows the date
Lateral incisors (maxillary) and mandibular cuspids erupt	Describes common objects in detail, not merely their use
Movement fluid; often graceful and poised	Makes change out of a quarter
Always on the go; jumps, chases, skips	Attends third and fourth grades
Increased smoothness and speed in fine motor control; uses cursive writing	Reads more; may plan to wake up early just to read
Dresses self completely	Reads classic books, but also enjoys comics
Likely to overdo; hard to quiet down after recess	More aware of time; can be relied on to get to school on time
More limber; bones grow faster than ligaments	Can grasp concepts of parts and whole (fractions)
	Understands concepts of space, cause and effect, nesting (puzzles), conservation (permanence of mass and volume)
	Classifies objects by more than one quality; has collections
	Produces simple paintings or drawings
AGES 10 TO 12 YEARS	
Weight 24.5-58 kg (54-128 pounds)	Writes brief stories
Height 127-162.5 cm (50-64 inches)	Attends fifth to seventh grades
Posture is more similar to an adult's; will overcome lordosis	Writes occasional short letters to friends or relatives on own initiative
Remainder of teeth will erupt and tend toward full development (except wisdom teeth)	Uses telephone for practical purposes
	Responds to magazine, radio, or other advertising
Girls—Pubescent changes may begin to appear; body lines soften and round out	Reads for practical information or own enjoyment—stories or library books of adventure or romance, animal stories
Boys—Slow growth in height and rapid weight gain; may become obese in this period	

of honesty, children are more likely to conform to these standards.

As with other ethically related behavior, **stealing** is not unexpected in the younger child. Between 5 and 8 years of age, children's sense of property rights is limited, and they tend to take something simply because they are attracted to it or to take money for what it will buy. They are equally likely to give away something valuable that belongs to them. When young children are caught and punished, they are penitent—they "didn't mean to" and "promise to never do it again"—but they are likely to repeat the performance the following day. Often they not only steal but also lie about their behavior or attempt

ADAPTIVE	PERSONAL-SOCIAL
At table, uses knife to spread butter or jam on bread	Can share and cooperate better
At play, cuts, folds, pastes paper; sews crudely if needle is threaded	Has great need for children of own age
Takes bath without supervision; performs bedtime activities alone	Will cheat to win
Reads from memory; enjoys oral spelling game	Often engages in rough play
Likes table games, checkers, simple card games	Often jealous of younger brother or sister
Giggles a lot	Does what adults are seen doing
Sometimes steals money or attractive items	May have occasional temper tantrums
Has difficulty owning up to misdeeds	Is a boaster
Tries out own abilities	Is more independent, probably influence of school
	Has own way of doing things
	Increases socialization
Uses table knife for cutting meat; may need help with tough or difficult pieces	Is becoming a real member of the family group
Brushes and combs hair acceptably without help	Takes part in group play
Likes to help and have a choice	Boys prefer playing with boys; girls prefer playing with girls
Is less resistant and stubborn	Spends a lot of time alone; does not require a lot of companionship
Makes use of common tools such as hammer, saw, screwdriver	Is easy to get along with at home
Uses household and sewing utensils	Likes the reward system
Helps with routine household tasks such as dusting, sweeping	Dramatizes
Assumes responsibility for share of household chores	Is more sociable
Looks after all of own needs at table	Is better behaved
Buys useful articles; exercises some choice in making purchases	Is interested in boy-girl relationships but will not admit it
Runs useful errands	Goes about home and community freely, alone or with friends
Likes pictorial magazines	Likes to compete and play games
Likes school; wants to answer all the questions	Shows preference in friends and groups
Is afraid of failing a grade; is ashamed of bad grades	Plays mostly with groups of own sex but is beginning to mix
Is more critical of self	Develops modesty
Takes music and sport lessons	Compares self with others
	Enjoys organizations, clubs, and group sports
Makes useful tools or does easy repair work	Loves friends; talks about them constantly
Cooks or sews in small way	Chooses friends more selectively; may have a "best friend"
Raises pets	Enjoys conversation
Washes and dries own hair; is responsible for a thorough job of cleaning hair, but may need reminding to do so	Develops beginning interest in opposite sex
Is sometimes left alone at home for an hour or so	Is more diplomatic
Is successful in looking after own needs or those of other children left in his or her care	Likes family; family really has meaning
	Likes mother and wants to please her in many ways
	Demonstrates affection
	Likes father, who is admired and may be idolized
	Respects parents

to justify it with excuses. It is seldom helpful to trap children into admission by asking directly if they committed the offense. Children do not take responsibility for these behaviors until the end of middle childhood.

Children steal for several reasons. Young children may lack a sense of property rights, attempt to acquire a specific object to bribe favors from other children, have a strong desire to own a coveted item, or have a desire for revenge to "get back at someone" (usually a parent for unfair treatment). Older children may steal to supplement an inadequate allowance. Stealing can be an indication that something is seriously wrong or lacking in the child's life. For example, children may steal to make up for love or another satisfaction that they feel is lacking. In most situations it is wise not to attempt to attach a hidden or deep meaning to the stealing. An admonition, together with an appropriate and reasonable punishment, such as having the older child pay back the money or return the stolen items, takes care of most cases. Most children can be taught to respect the property rights of others with little difficulty despite numerous temptations and opportunities. If children's personal rights are respected, they are likely to respect the rights of others. Some children simply need more time to learn the rules regarding private property.

Stress and Fear

Children today experience significant amounts of stress, which can cause long-term adjustment and health problems. Stress in childhood comes from a variety of sources such as conflict within the family, interpersonal relationships, poverty, and chronic illness. The school environment and participation in multiple organized activities can be additional sources of stress. The demands from coaches and parents, in addition to school requirements and pressure from teachers to do well on proficiency testing, can cause unrealistic expectations on the school-age child (Ryan-Wenger, Sharrer, and Campbell, 2005). In addition, with the increased exposure to sexuality and provocative clothing and behaviors, children of this age-group may feel pressured to have a girlfriend or boyfriend, which their maturity level cannot handle and which causes additional stress (Ryan-Wenger, Sharrer, and Campbell, 2005).

The increasing violence in society has also spilled over into the school setting. In the present information age, in which tragedy is broadcast daily in the media, children come to school knowing more about the latest world events than any previous generation of children. In addition, today's children are often personally aware of violence in their families or communities. Many children know other children who have been killed or children who have brought weapons to school. School-age children can be victims of teasing, bullying, and physical abuse in the school environment (Nansel, Overpeck, Haynie, and others, 2003).

To help children cope with stress, parents, teachers, and health care providers need to frequently reassure children that they are safe, have honest and open communication, encourage children to express their feelings, and promote a daily routine (Nansel, Overpeck, Haynie, and others, 2003). Adults must recognize signs that indicate a child is undergoing stress, identify the source of the stress promptly, and refer those children who need specialized treatment.

> **NURSINGALERT**
>
> The nurse who observes the following signs of stress in a child should explore the situation further:
> - Stomach pains or headache
> - Changes in sleep patterns or nightmares
> - Bed-wetting
> - Changes in eating habits
> - Aggressive or stubborn behavior
> - Withdrawal or reluctance to participate
> - Regression to earlier behaviors (e.g., thumb sucking)
> - Trouble concentrating or changes in academic performance

Children 7 to 12 years of age are capable of identifying their own physiologic responses to stress with terms that have meaning to them. Some words or phrases used by children to describe their body's reaction to stress include *tight muscles, hot* or *red in the face, tingling, chills or goose bumps, shakiness, heart beating fast, headache,* and *stomachache* (Sharrer and Ryan-Wenger, 2002). Children should be taught to recognize these signs as indicators of stress and to use techniques to manage their stress. Children can learn relaxation techniques such as deep-breathing exercises, progressive relaxation of muscle groups, and positive imagery to immediately reduce stress (Mortweet and Christophersen, 2004). Encouraging them to "blow off steam" through physical activity reduces tension and anxiety. Children can be encouraged to observe effective coping strategies in others and adopt them for their own use (Mortweet and Christophersen, 2004). When an effective strategy has been developed for one situation, parents can show the child how to transfer the coping strategy or technique to other situations.

In addition to stress, school-age children experience a wide variety of fears, including fear of the dark, excessive worry about past behavior, self-consciousness, social withdrawal, and an excessive need for reassurance. These fears are considered normal for children this age. During the middle-school years, children become less fearful of body safety than they were as preschoolers, but they still fear being hurt, being kidnapped, or having to undergo surgery. They also fear death and are fascinated by all the aspects of death and dying. The fears of noises, darkness, storms, and dogs lessen, but new fears related predominantly to school and family bother children during this time.

PROMOTING OPTIMAL HEALTH DURING THE SCHOOL YEARS

NUTRITION

Although caloric needs are diminished in relation to body size during middle childhood, resources are being laid down at this time for the increased growth needs of adolescence. Parents and children need to be aware of the value of a balanced diet to promote growth because children usually eat what their family members eat. The quality of the child's diet depends on the family's pattern of eating.

Likes and dislikes established at an early age continue in middle childhood, although preferences for single foods subside, and children develop a taste for a variety of foods. However, the easy availability of fast-food restaurants, the influence of the mass media, and the temptation of "junk food" make it easy for children to fill up on empty calories. Foods that do not promote growth, such as sugars, starches, and excess fats, are common in the school-age child's diet. The easy availability of high-calorie foods, combined with the tendency toward more sedentary activities, has also contributed to an epidemic of childhood obesity. This problem is discussed further in Chapter 17.

Parents are unable to monitor what their children eat when they are away from home. A parent may pack a lunch for school but be unaware of how much is eaten, traded, sold, or thrown away. Nutrition education can and should be integrated in the curriculum throughout the school years. Important aspects of nutrition education include the U.S. Food and Drug Administration's MyPyramid; elements of a wholesome diet; and how food products are grown, processed, and prepared. However, the school cafeteria may not always provide healthy, nutritious meals. The school nurse can take an active role in nutrition education by working with teachers to plan and implement units on nutrition instruction and by working with parents and children to give nutritional guidance.

SLEEP AND REST

The amount of sleep and rest required during middle childhood is highly individualized. The amount of sleep depends on the child's age, activity level, and state of health. The growth rate slows in the school-age years, and less energy is expended in growth than during preceding years.

School-age children usually do not require a nap, and they sleep approximately 11 hours at age 5 years and 9.25 hours at age 12 years during the night (Carno, Hoffman, Carcillo, and others, 2003). Although fewer bedtime problems occur during these years, occasional difficulties are still associated with the bedtime ritual. Usually children 6 or 7 years old exhibit few bedtime problems, and encouraging quiet activity before bedtime, such as coloring or reading, facilitates the task of going to bed. However, most children in middle childhood must be reminded frequently to go to bed; 8- to 9-year-old children and 11-year-old children are particularly resistant. Often these children are unaware that they are tired; if they are allowed to remain up later than usual, they are fatigued the following day. Sometimes, bedtime resistance can be resolved by allowing a later bedtime as the child gets older. Twelve-year-old children usually offer no resistance at bedtime; some even retire early to read a book or listen to music.

EXERCISE AND ACTIVITY

The improved capabilities and adaptability of the school-age child permit greater speed and effort in motor activities. Larger, stronger muscles permit longer and increasingly strenuous play without exhaustion. School-age children acquire the coordination, timing, and concentration that are required to participate in adult-type activities, but they may lack the strength, stamina, and control of the adolescent and adult. They can engage in a greater amount of physical activity during the school years. However, parents, teachers, and coaches must remember that, although children this age are large and appear strong, they may not be ready for strenuous competitive athletics.

All growing children need regular exercise and opportunities for satisfying experiences consistent with individual likes and dislikes. Appropriate activities during the school-age years include running, jumping rope, swimming, roller skating, ice skating, dancing, and bicycle riding. Positive reinforcement achieved by experiencing increasingly smooth, rhythmic, and efficient use of the body conditions the child toward regular physical activity. Exercise is essential for muscle development and tone, refinement of balance and coordination, increased strength and endurance, and stimulation of body functions and metabolic processes. Children need ample space to run, jump, skip, and climb, in addition to safe indoor and outdoor facilities and equipment. Most children have abundant energy and need little encouragement to engage in physical activity. Children with disabling conditions or those who hesitate to become involved in active play (such as obese children) require special assessment and help so that activities appeal to them and are compatible with their limitations while also meeting their developmental needs.

FIG. 15-7 ■ The activities engaged in by school-age children vary according to interest and opportunity. **A,** Little League competitors. **B,** Playing tug-of-war.

Sports

Considerable controversy surrounds the trend toward early participation in competitive athletics and the amount and type of competitive sports that are appropriate for children in the elementary grades. The current view is that virtually every child is suited for some sport, and authorities do not discourage participation if children are matched to the type of sport appropriate to their abilities and to their physical and emotional constitution. School-age children enjoy competition (Fig. 15-7). However, teachers and coaches must understand the physical limitations of children this age and teach them the proper techniques and safety measures needed to avoid injuries. A safe and appropriate sport can be identified for even the most unskilled and uncompetitive child, including children with chronic illnesses and mental retardation. Common activities for school-age children include baseball, soccer, gymnastics, and swimming. Equipment must be maintained in safe condition, and protective apparatus should be worn to prevent serious injury (see Traumatic Injury, Chapter 31).

During the school-age years girls have the same basic body structure as boys and have a similar response to systematic exercise training. However, at puberty, boys become larger and have more muscle mass, and at this stage, it is usually recommended that girls compete only against other girls. Before puberty there is no essential difference in strength and size between girls and boys, making these precautions unnecessary.

Preadolescence is a time to teach fundamental motor skills; develop fitness in a practical, safe, and gradual manner; and promote healthy attitudes and values. Activities should include both practice sessions and unstructured play; the actual game or event should be managed in a manner that stresses mastery of the sport and enhancement of self-image rather than winning or pleasing others. All children should have an opportunity to participate, and special ceremonies should recognize all participants, not just individuals who excel in sports or athletics.

Acquisition of Skills

School-age children demonstrate increasing fine motor abilities and complex artistic skills. Handedness is well established by the beginning of the school years, and children make great strides in writing and drawing during this period. It is a time of energetic and vibrant creative productivity. With the tools of language and reading, children create poems, stories, and plays. With more advanced fine motor skills, they are able to master an unlimited variety of handicrafts, such as ceramics, needlework, wood carving, and beadwork. They avidly pursue these skills in solitude; with a friend; or through organized groups such as boys' or girls' clubs or special interest groups that use crafts or other activities as a means to occupy, entertain, and educate children.

School-age children are capable of assuming responsibility for their own needs, although their distaste for soap and water and "dress" clothes is legendary. School-age children can and want to assume their share of household tasks, which usually are related to the male and female roles that have been defined by their culture. Many children also assume responsibility for tasks outside the home, such as baby-sitting, mowing lawns, or paper routes.

DENTAL HEALTH

The first permanent (secondary) teeth erupt at about 6 years of age, beginning with the 6-year molar, which erupts posterior to the deciduous molars. Other permanent teeth appear in approximately the same order as eruption of the primary teeth (see Teething, Chapter 10) and follow shedding of the deciduous teeth (Fig. 15-8). With the appearance of the second permanent (12-year) molar, most permanent teeth are present. Permanent dentition is more advanced in girls than in boys.

Because the permanent teeth erupt during the school-age years, dental hygiene and regular attention to dental caries are important parts of health supervision during this period (see Dental Health, Chapter 12). Correct brushing techniques should be taught or reinforced, and the role that fermentable carbohydrates play in production of dental caries should be emphasized. It is important to be alert to possible malocclusion problems that may result from irregular eruption of permanent teeth and that may impair function. Regular dental supervision and continued fluoride supplementation are integral parts of the health maintenance program.

The most effective means of preventing dental caries is proper oral hygiene. Children should be taught to perform their own dental care with the supervision and guidance of the parents. Parents should learn the correct brushing technique with their children, and they should monitor their child's efforts until the child can assume full responsibility.

Teeth should be brushed after meals, after snacks, and at bedtime. Children who brush their teeth frequently and become accustomed to the feel of a clean mouth at an early age

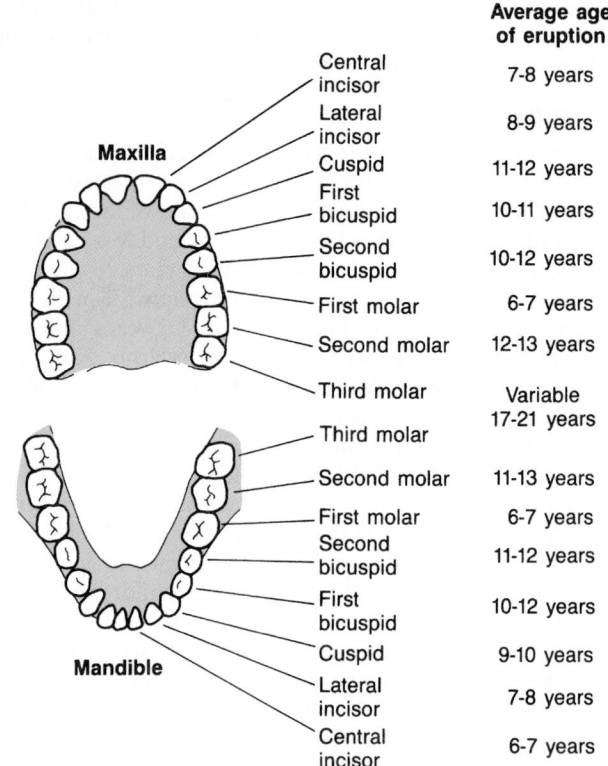

	Average age of eruption
Maxilla Central incisor	7-8 years
Lateral incisor	8-9 years
Cuspid	11-12 years
First bicuspid	10-11 years
Second bicuspid	10-12 years
First molar	6-7 years
Second molar	12-13 years
Third molar	Variable 17-21 years
Third molar	
Second molar	11-13 years
First molar	6-7 years
Second bicuspid	11-12 years
First bicuspid	10-12 years
Cuspid	9-10 years
Mandible Lateral incisor	7-8 years
Central incisor	6-7 years

FIG. 15-8 ■ Sequence of eruption of secondary teeth. (Data from McDonald RE, Avery DR: *Dentistry for the child and adolescent,* ed 6, St Louis, 1994, Mosby.)

usually maintain the habit throughout life. For the school-age child with mixed and permanent dentition, the best toothbrush is one with soft nylon bristles and an overall length of about 21 cm (6 inches). Several methods of brushing have been described and recommended for children, but there is no conclusive evidence that one method is superior to another. Thorough cleaning is more important than the specific technique used. The dentist should assess factors such as the manipulative skills and special needs of the child, and suggest the most appropriate brushing technique and regimen. Flossing follows brushing. Parents should perform the flossing until children acquire the manual dexterity required (usually at about 8 or 9 years of age).

Dental Problems

Limited or inadequate dental care results in the most common dental problems: dental caries, malocclusion, and periodontal disease. Trauma, especially tooth avulsion, is another important dental problem. All of these conditions benefit from early intervention to prevent tooth loss.

Dental caries (cavities) is the principal oral problem in children and adolescents. Reducing the incidence and consequences of dental caries is extremely important in childhood. If untreated, dental caries can result in total destruction of the involved teeth. The prevalence rate of caries increases steadily across the life span; 18% of children ages 2 to 4 years have caries, whereas 52% of children ages 6 to 8 years have caries (American Academy of Pediatrics, 2000).

Dental caries is a multifactorial disease involving susceptible teeth, cariogenic microflora, and an appropriate oral environment. The incidence of lesions and the likelihood of progressive invasion vary considerably and depend on a number of factors being present in the right combination. Because many children are exposed to health care but not dental care, oral inspection is an integral part of the physical assessment of every child. If there is any evidence of dental caries or other unhealthy dental state, the child should be referred for dental services. An alarming number of children do not receive regular dental supervision, and a significant number reach adulthood without dental examinations or treatment by a dentist.

Periodontal disease, an inflammatory and degenerative condition involving the gums and tissues supporting the teeth, often begins in childhood and accounts for a significant amount of tooth loss in adulthood. The more common periodontal problems are **gingivitis** (simple inflammation of the gums) and **periodontitis** (inflammation of the gums and loss of connective tissue and bone in the supporting structures of the teeth).

Gingivitis, the most prevalent periodontal disease, is a reversible inflammatory disease that can begin in early childhood and is most often associated with the buildup of plaque on the teeth. Changes take place in the plaque bacteria, in both the type and number of organisms, causing them to release destructive exotoxins, enzymes, and other noxious agents. These substances produce an inflammatory reaction in the gingival tissues, causing the gums to become red, edematous, tender, and subject to bleeding at the slightest irritation. Management is directed toward prevention by conscientious brushing and flossing, including the use of fluoride. The child should see the dentist at any signs of inflammation or irritation.

Malocclusion occurs when teeth of the upper and lower dental arches do not approximate in the proper relationships. As a result, the physiologic function of chewing is less effective and the cosmetic effect is displeasing. Teeth that are uneven, crowded, or overlapping are unable to meet their counterparts in the opposite jaw in the appropriate relationships and may be predisposed to disease in later years.

Orthodontic treatment is most successful when it is started in the late school-age or early teenage years, after the last primary teeth have been shed and before growth ceases. However, referral should be made as soon as malocclusion is evident, since some deformities can be corrected at an earlier age.

Dental injury may occur in childhood and includes fractures of varying degrees of severity, chipping, dislocation, or avulsion. All tooth injuries require prompt treatment by a competent dentist to prevent permanent displacement or loss. Delayed examination and diagnosis of tooth damage can result in infection or pulp involvement. Because it can affect the remaining teeth, replacement of the lost tooth is needed to maintain normal alignment and position of the other teeth.

A tooth that is **avulsed** (exarticulated, or "knocked out") should be replanted by the child, parent, or nurse and stabilized as soon as possible so that the blood supply to the tooth can be reestablished and the tooth kept alive (see Emergency Treatment box). A tooth that is replanted within 15 minutes has a 98% survival rate (Krause-Parello, 2005). Avulsed primary teeth are usually not reimplanted.

As with all injuries to the mouth, an avulsed tooth causes a large amount of bleeding, which is frightening to children and their families; therefore the nurse or anyone faced with dental trauma should be prepared to provide support and reassurance during the dental trauma.

---

emergencytreatment

Avulsed Permanent Tooth

Recover tooth.
Hold tooth by crown; avoid touching root area.
If tooth is dirty, rinse it gently under running water or saline; be certain to insert stopper in sink or basin (to avoid tooth loss).

TO REIMPLANT TOOTH

Insert tooth into socket; be certain that the lip-side (or convex surface) is facing front.
Have child maintain tooth in place by slowly biting down on a piece of gauze.
Transport child to dentist immediately.
Avoid sudden stops or sharp turns to prevent dislodging tooth.

IF RELUCTANT TO REIMPLANT TOOTH

Place avulsed tooth in suitable medium for transport:
- Cold milk
- Saliva—under child's or parent's tongue

If child is holding tooth in the mouth, avoid sudden stops to prevent swallowing tooth.
DON'T FORGET TO TAKE THE TOOTH.

SEX EDUCATION

Many children experience some form of sex play during or before preadolescence as a response to normal curiosity, not as a result of love or sexual urges. Children are experimentalists by nature, and sex play is incidental and transitory. Any adverse emotional consequences or guilt feelings depend on how the behavior is managed by the parents, if it is discovered, or whether children view their actions as wrong in the eyes of significant persons, particularly the parents.

The child's attitude toward sex is acquired indirectly at an early age. Initial curiosity about differences in body structure between boys and girls and between children and adults arises in the preschool years. Middle childhood is an ideal time for formal sex education, and many authorities believe that the topic is best presented from a life span approach. Information about sexual maturation and the process of reproduction minimizes the child's uncertainty, embarrassment, and feelings of isolation that often accompany puberty.

An important component of ongoing sex education is effective communication with parents. If parents either repress the child's sexual curiosity or avoid dealing with it, the sexual information that the child receives may be acquired almost entirely from peers. When peers are the primary source of sexual information, it is transmitted and exchanged in secret conversation and contains a large amount of misinformation.

Nurse's Role in Sex Education

No matter where nurses practice, they can provide information on human sexuality to both parents and children. To discuss the topic adequately, nurses must have an understanding of the physiologic aspects of sexuality; knowledge of the cultural and societal values; and an awareness of their own attitudes, feelings, and biases about sexuality.

When presenting sexual information to school-age children, nurses should treat sex as a normal part of growth and development. Questions should be answered honestly, matter-of-factly, and to the same extent as questions about other topics. Answers should be at the child's level of understanding. There may be times when boys and girls should be taught content separately.

Children need help to differentiate sex and sexuality. Exercises on clarifying values, identifying role models, engaging in problem-solving skills, and practicing responsibility are important to prepare children for early adolescence and puberty. In addition, children need explanations of sexual information that is provided via the media or jokes. Information concerning pregnancy; contraceptives; and sexually transmitted diseases, including human immunodeficiency virus and human papillomavirus, should be presented in simple, accurate terms.

Preadolescents need precise and concrete information that will allow them to answer questions such as "What if I start my period in the middle of class?" or "How can I keep people from telling I have an erection?" It is important to tell children what they want to know and what they can expect to happen as they become mature sexually.

During encounters with parents, nurses can be open and available for questions and discussion. They can set an example by the language they use in discussing body parts and their function and by the way in which they deal with problems that have emotional overtones, such as exploratory sex play and masturbation. Parents need help to understand normal behaviors and to view sexual curiosity in their children as a part of the developmental process. Assessing the parents' level of knowledge and understanding of sexuality provides cues to their need for supplemental information that will prepare them for the increasingly complex explanations they will need to provide as their children grow older.

SCHOOL HEALTH

Child health maintenance is ultimately the responsibility of the parents; however, the public schools and health departments in the United States have contributed to the improvement of child health by providing a healthful school environment, health services, and health education that emphasize sound health practices. Most of these functions constitute major components of community health services and involve large amounts of public funds and large numbers of health professionals, including nurses.

A school health program is involved in ongoing health maintenance through assessment, screening, and referral activities. Routine health services provided by most schools include health appraisal, emergency care, safety education, communicable disease control, counseling, and follow-up care. Health education of school-age children is directed toward providing knowledge of health and influencing habits, attitudes, and conduct in relation to health and injury prevention.

Traditionally, school nurses were viewed as the individuals who detected diseases in the school, applied bandages, and cared for students who were ill or injured. Although these functions remain important parts of the school nurse's job, the role has expanded considerably in recent years. Today, school nurses manage and coordinate all the care required by regular students and students with special health care needs. In many settings, school health services have enlarged into family health centers that meet the needs of not only school-

age children, but also their families and the community. In these settings, school nurse practitioners provide health care that includes assessment of physical, psychomedical, psychoeducational, behavioral, and learning problems, as well as comprehensive well-child care (Hackbarth and Gall, 2005).

The passage of the Education for All Handicapped Children Act and its amendments (Public Laws 94-142 and 99-457) mandated the integration of children with chronic illness or disability into the least restrictive environments, including regular classrooms whenever possible. School nurses are responsible for the medical and nursing needs of these children while they are in the school setting. School nurses develop, implement, and evaluate individualized health care plans for these children. Unfortunately, not all schools have a school nurse, and the use of unlicensed assistive personnel (UAP) is increasing. In many schools, nurses are faced with the task of delegating to and supervising UAP (Potter and Grant, 2004). Delegation and supervision of UAP requires skillful nursing assessment, effective communication, and professional judgment.

INJURY PREVENTION

Because school-age children have developed more refined muscular coordination and control and can apply their cognitive capacities to their behavior, the number of injuries in middle childhood is diminished compared with the number in early childhood. The most common cause of severe injury and death in school-age children is motor vehicle accidents—

FIG. 15-9 ■ The right size bike is important; the child should be able to sit on the bike and place the balls of both feet on the ground. The foot should comfortably reach and manipulate the pedal in the down position. Wearing a protective helmet is mandatory. The helmet should be positioned so it sits low on the forehead and parallel to the ground when the head is held upright. It should not rock back and forth or shift from side to side. The strap should fasten securely under the chin.

Critical Thinking Exercise—Injury Prevention

either as a pedestrian or passenger (Schnitzer, 2006). It is important that nurses continue to emphasize three automobile safety measures that have been found to reduce the severity of injuries: effective car restraint systems, door-lock mechanisms, and appropriate passenger-seating locations in the motor vehicle. The American Academy of Pediatrics advises health professionals and parents that the rear vehicle seat is the safest place for children under the age of 13 years (Durbin, Chen, Smith, and others, 2005).

The school-age child's desire for riding bicycles increases the risk of injury on streets. Other serious injuries include accidents on skateboards, roller skates, in-line skates, scooters, and other sports equipment. All-terrain vehicles (ATVs), popular with children younger than 16 years of age, are unstable, difficult to handle, and responsible for an increasing number of childhood injuries. The Consumer Product Safety Commission has outlined ATV recommendations that include free driver training, no passengers, use of helmets, no roadway traveling, and adult supervision for children under the age of 16 years (Humphries, Stone, Stapczynski, and others, 2006).

Most injuries occur in or near the home or school. The most effective means of prevention is education of the child and family regarding the hazards of risk taking and the improper use of equipment. Safety helmets, protective eye and mouth shields, and protective padding are strongly recommended for children engaging in active sports, even though they may not be required equipment. Falls from bicycles, ATVs, and skating devices are the cause of a significant number of head injuries in school-age children. Because head injury is the major cause of bicycle-related fatalities, the most important aspect of bicycle safety is to encourage the rider to wear a protective helmet (Fig. 15-9) (Khambalia, MacArthur, and Parkin, 2005).

Physically active school-age children are also highly susceptible to cuts and abrasions, and the incidence of childhood fractures, strains, and sprains is high. Trampoline injuries are highest in children 5 through 14 years and account for numerous fractures, sprains, and head injuries. Trampolines in the home environment, routine physical education classes, or outdoor playgrounds are not recommended for children of any age (Nysted and Drogset, 2006). Serious injuries are discussed elsewhere in the book: burns (Chapter 30), eye trauma (Chapter 19), near-drowning (Chapter 28), and head injuries (Chapter 28). The prevalence of injuries depends on the dangers present in the environment, the protection offered by adults, and the behavior patterns of the children. Table 15-2 lists characteristics of the school-age child that make them prone to injury and suggestions for injury prevention. Family-Centered Care boxes provide guidelines for bicycle, skateboard, and in-line skate safety and guidance during the school years.

ANTICIPATORY GUIDANCE—CARE OF FAMILIES

Parents of the school-age child must share their child's time with the increasingly important peer group. Experiences with the peer group prepare school-age children for the broader world of relationships and increased independence from their parents. Parents must learn to provide support as unobtrusively as possible without feeling rejected, hurt, or angry. The nurse can help parents of the school-age child by providing anticipatory guidance and reassurance throughout this period (see Family-Centered Care box).

FAMILY-CENTERED CARE

Bicycle Safety

- Always wear a properly fitted bicycle helmet that is approved by the U.S. Consumer Product Safety Commission (CPSC); encourage parents to look for the CPSC approval sticker on the inside liner of the helmet.
- Replace a helmet every 5 years or sooner if manufacturer recommends it. **Never use a damaged or outgrown helmet.**
- Ride bicycles with traffic and away from parked cars.
- Ride single file.
- Walk bicycles through busy intersections only at crosswalks.
- Give hand signals well in advance of turning or stopping.
- Keep as close to the curb as practical.
- Watch for drain grates, potholes, soft shoulders, loose dirt, or gravel.
- Keep both hands on handlebars, except with signaling.
- Never ride double on a bicycle.
- Do not carry packages that interfere with vision or control; do not drag objects behind bike.
- Watch for and yield to pedestrians.
- Watch for cars backing up or pulling out of driveways; be especially careful at intersections.
- Look left, right, then left before turning into traffic or roadway.
- Never hitch a ride on a truck or other vehicle.
- Learn rules of the road and respect for traffic officers.
- Obey all local ordinances.
- Wear shoes that fit securely while riding.
- Wear light colors at night and attach fluorescent material to clothing and bicycle.
- Equip bicycle with proper lights and reflectors.
- Be certain the bicycle is the correct size for rider (see Fig. 15-9).
- Have bicycle inspected to ensure good mechanical condition.
- Children riding as passengers must wear appropriate-size helmets and sit in specially designed protective seats.

Modified from American Academy of Pediatrics, Committee on Injury and Poison Prevention: Bicycle helmets, *Pediatrics* 108(4):1030-1032, 2001.

FAMILY-CENTERED CARE

Skateboard and In-Line Skate Safety

- Children younger than 5 years of age should not use skateboards or in-line skates because they are not developmentally prepared to protect themselves from injury. Children ages 6 to 10 years should use these only with close adult supervision.
- Children who ride skateboards or in-line skates should wear helmets and other protective equipment, especially on knees, wrists, and elbows, to prevent injury.
- Skateboards and in-line skates should never be used near traffic. Their use should be prohibited on streets and highways. Activities that bring skateboards together (e.g., "catching a ride") are especially dangerous.
- Some types of use, such as riding homemade ramps on hard surfaces, may be particularly hazardous.

Data from American Academy of Pediatrics, Committee on Injury and Poison Prevention: Skateboard injuries, *Pediatrics* 109(3):542-543, 2002; and American Academy of Pediatrics, Committee on Injury and Poison Prevention: In-line skating injuries in children and adolescents, *Pediatrics* 117(5):1846-1847, 2006.

TABLE 15-2

Injury Prevention During School-Age Years

DEVELOPMENTAL ABILITIES RELATED TO RISK OF INJURY	INJURY PREVENTION
MOTOR VEHICLE ACCIDENTS Is increasingly involved in activities away from home Is excited by speed and motion Is easily distracted by environment Can be reasoned with	Educate child regarding proper use of seat belts while a passenger in a vehicle. Maintain discipline while a passenger in a vehicle (e.g., keep arms inside, do not lean against doors, do not interfere with driver). Remind parents and children that no one should ride in the bed of a pickup truck. Emphasize safe pedestrian behavior. Insist on child wearing safety apparel (e.g., helmet) when applicable, such as riding bicycle, motorcycle, moped, or all-terrain vehicle (see Family-Centered Care box, p. 509).
DROWNING Is apt to overdo May work hard to perfect a skill Has cautious, but not fearful, gross motor actions Likes swimming	Teach child to swim. Teach basic rules of water safety. Select safe and supervised places to swim. Check sufficient water depth for diving. Swim with a companion. Use an approved flotation device. Advocate for legislation requiring fencing around pools. Learn cardiopulmonary resuscitation.
BURNS Has increasing independence Is adventurous Enjoys trying new things	Make certain home has smoke detectors. Set water heaters to 48.9° C (120° F) to avoid scald burns. Instruct child in behavior in areas involving contact with potential burn hazards (e.g., gasoline, matches, bonfires or barbecues, lighter fluid, firecrackers, cigarette lighters, cooking utensils, chemistry sets). Instruct child to avoid climbing or flying kite around high-tension wires. Instruct child in proper behavior in the event of fire (e.g., fire drills at home and school). Teach child safe cooking (use low heat; avoid any frying; be careful of steam burns, scalds, or exploding foods, especially from microwaving).
POISONING Adheres to group rules May be easily influenced by peers Has strong allegiance to friends	Educate child regarding hazards of taking nonprescription drugs and chemicals, including aspirin and alcohol. Teach child to say "no" if offered illegal or dangerous drugs or alcohol. Keep potentially dangerous products in properly labeled receptacles, preferably out of reach.

BODILY DAMAGE
Has increased physical skills
Needs strenuous physical activity
Is interested in acquiring new skills and perfecting attained skills
Is daring and adventurous, especially with peers
Frequently plays in hazardous places
Confidence often exceeds physical capacity
Desires group loyalty and has strong need for friends' approval
Delights in physical activity
Takes risks
Is likely to overdo
Growth in height exceeds muscular growth and coordination
	Help provide facilities for supervised activities.
	Encourage playing in safe places.
	Keep firearms safely locked up except under adult supervision.
	Teach proper care of, use of, and respect for devices with potential danger (e.g., power tools, firecrackers).
	Teach children not to tease or surprise dogs, invade their territory, take dogs' toys, or interfere with dogs' feeding.
	Stress eye, ear, or mouth protection when using potentially hazardous objects or devices or when engaging in potentially hazardous sports.
	Do not permit use of trampolines except as part of supervised training.
	Teach safety regarding use of corrective devices (glasses); if child wears contact lenses, monitor duration of wear to prevent corneal damage.
	Stress careful selection, use, and maintenance of sports and recreation equipment, such as skateboards and in-line skates (see Family-Centered Care box, p. 509).
	Emphasize proper conditioning, safe practices, and use of safety equipment for sports or recreational activities.
	Caution against engaging in hazardous sports, such as those involving trampolines.
	Use safety glass and decals on large glassed areas, such as sliding glass doors.
	Use window guards to prevent falls.
	Teach name, address, and phone number and emphasize that child should ask for help from appropriate people (e.g., cashier, security guard, police) if lost; have identification on child (e.g., sewn in clothes, inside shoe).
	Teach stranger safety:
	    Avoid personalized clothing in public places.
	    Caution child to never go with a stranger.
	Have child tell parents if anyone makes child feel uncomfortable in any way.
	Always listen to child's concerns regarding others' behavior.
	Teach child to say "no" when confronted by uncomfortable situations.

FAMILY-CENTERED CARE

Guidance During School Years

AGE 6 YEARS
Prepare parents to expect strong food preferences and frequent refusal of specific food items.

Prepare parents to expect increasingly ravenous appetite.

Prepare parents for emotionality as child experiences erratic mood changes.

Help parents anticipate continued susceptibility to illness.

Teach injury prevention and safety, especially bicycle safety.

Encourage parents to respect child's need for privacy and to provide a separate bedroom for child, if possible.

Prepare parents for child's increasing interests outside the home.

Help parents understand the need to encourage child's interactions with peers.

AGES 7 TO 10 YEARS
Prepare parents to expect improvement in health with fewer illnesses, but warn them that allergies may increase or become apparent.

Prepare parents to expect an increase in minor injuries.

Emphasize caution in selecting and maintaining sports equipment and reemphasize safety.

Prepare parents to expect increased involvement with peers and interest in activities outside the home.

Emphasize the need to encourage independence while maintaining limit setting and discipline.

Prepare mothers to expect more demands at 8 years.

Prepare fathers to expect increasing admiration at 10 years; encourage father-child activities.

Prepare parents for prepubescent changes in girls.

AGES 11 TO 12 YEARS
Help parents prepare child for body changes of pubescence.

Prepare parents to expect a growth spurt in girls.

Make certain child's sex education is adequate with accurate information.

Prepare parents to expect energetic but stormy behavior at 11 years, becoming more even-tempered at 12 years.

Encourage parents to support child's desire to "grow up" but to allow regressive behavior when needed.

Prepare parents to expect an increase in child's masturbation.

Instruct parents that the amount of rest the child needs may increase.

Help parents educate child regarding experimentation with potentially harmful activities.

HEALTH GUIDANCE
Help parents understand the importance of regular health and dental care for the child.

Encourage parents to teach and model sound health practices, including diet, rest, activity, and exercise.

Stress the need to encourage children to engage in appropriate physical activities.

Emphasize providing a safe physical and emotional environment.

Encourage parents to teach and model safety practices.

KEY POINTS

- Middle childhood, also known as the school years, is the period of life that extends from 6 to 12 years of age.

- Although growth is slower than in previous years, there is a steady gain in height and weight, with maturation of body systems; primary teeth are lost and replaced by permanent teeth.

- A major task during the middle school years is developing a sense of industry or accomplishment (Erikson).

- Piaget's period of concrete operations refers to the school-age period, when children are able to use their thought processes to experience events and actions and make judgments based on reasoning.

- The child develops a conscience and is able to understand and adhere to rules and standards set by others.

- Entertaining different points of view, becoming sensitive to social norms, and forming peer friendships are important features of social development during the school years.

- Cooperative play, team activities, and the acquisition of skills are prime elements of play during the school years; rules and rituals assume greater importance.

- Parental concerns during middle childhood include lying, cheating, stealing, and school achievement.

- The availability of junk foods, irregular family meals, and schedules of working parents often interfere with optimal nutrition.

- Dental care is important during this time; potential dental problems include caries, periodontal disease, malocclusion, and dental injury.

- Increased socialization and media exposure make the school years an ideal time for sex education.

- School health programs ideally include health appraisal, emergency care, safety education, communicable disease control, counseling, guidance, and health education with adjustment to individual student needs.

- Injury prevention is directed toward safety education, provision of safe play areas and equipment, and well-supervised sports activities.

REFERENCES

American Academy of Pediatrics, Pediatrics Collaborative Care Program: *Oral health risk assessment training for pediatricians and other child health professionals*, Rockville, Md, 2000, National Institutes of Health.

Ateah CA: Disciplinary practices with children: parental sources of information, attitudes, and educational needs, *Issues Compr Pediatr Nurs* 26:89-101, 2003.

Carno MA, Hoffman LA, Carcillo JA, and others: Developmental stages of sleep from birth to adolescence, common childhood sleep disorders: overview and nursing implications, *J Pediatr Nurs* 18(4):274-283, 2003.

Dishion TJ, Nelson SE, Yasui M: Predicting early adolescent gang involvement from middle school adaptation, *J Clin Child Adolesc Psychol* 34(1):62-73, 2005.

Durbin DR, Chen I, Smith R, and others: Effects of seating position and appropriate restraint use on the risk of injury to children in motor vehicle crashes, *Pediatrics* 115(3):305-309, 2005.

Glew GM, Fan MY, Katon W, and others: Bullying, psychosocial adjustment, and academic performance in elementary school, *Arch Pediatr Adolesc Med* 159:1026-1031, 2005.

Hackbarth D, Gall GB: Evaluation of school-based health center programs and services: the whys and hows of demonstrating program effectiveness, *Nurs Clin North Am* 40(4):711-724, 2005.

Humphries RL, Stone CK, Stapczynski JS, and others: An assessment of pediatric all-terrain vehicle injuries, *Pediatr Emerg Care* 22(7):491-494, 2006.

Khambalia A, MacArthur C, Parkin PC: Peer and adult companion helmet use is associated with bicycle helmet use by children, *Pediatrics* 116(4):939-942, 2005.

Krause-Parello CA: Tooth avulsion in the school setting, *J School Nurs* 21(5):279-282, 2005.

Lyznicki JM, McCaffree MA, Robinowitz CB: Childhood bullying: implications for physicians, *Am Fam Physician* 70(9):1723-1728, 2004.

Mortweet SL, Christophersen E: Coping skills for the angry/impatient/clamorous child: a home/office practicum, *Contemp Pediatr* 21(6):43-45, 2004.

Nansel TR, Overpeck, MD, Haynie DL, and others: Relationships between bullying and violence among US youth, *Arch Pediatr Adolesc Med* 157(4):348-353, 2003.

Nysted M, Drogset JO: Trampoline injuries, *Br J Sports Med* 40:984-987, 2006.

Potter P, Grant E: Understanding RN and unlicensed assistive personnel working relationships in designing care delivery strategies, *J Nurs Admin* 34(1):19-24, 2004.

Ryan-Wenger NA, Sharrer VW, Campbell KK: Changes in children's stressors over the past 30 years, *Pediatr Nurs* 31(4):282-288, 2005.

Schnitzer PG: Prevention of unintentional childhood injuries, *Am Fam Physician* 74(11):1864-1869, 2006.

Sharrer VW, Ryan-Wenger NA: School-age children's self-reported stress symptoms, *Pediatr Nurs* 28(1):21-27, 2002.

Vessey JA, Carlson K, David J: Helping children who are being teased and bullied, *Nurs Spectrum* 13:16-18, 2003.

Vreeman RC, Carroll AE: A systematic review of school-based interventions to prevent bullying, *Arch Pediatr Adolesc Med* 161(1):78-88, 2007.

Health Promotion of the Adolescent and Family

LINDA M. KOLLAR

CHAPTER OUTLINE

PROMOTING OPTIMAL GROWTH AND DEVELOPMENT, 514
Biologic Development, 514
  Hormonal Changes of Puberty, 514
  Sexual Maturation, 515
  Physical Growth, 515
  Physiologic Changes, 518
Psychosocial Development: Developing a Sense of Identity (Erikson), 518
Cognitive Development (Piaget), 519
Moral Development (Kohlberg), 519
Spiritual Development, 520
Social Development, 520
  Relationships with Parents, 520
  Relationships with Peers, 520
  Interests and Activities, 521

Adolescent Sexuality, 522
Development of Self-Concept and Body Image, 523
  Responses to Puberty, 524
PROMOTING OPTIMAL HEALTH DURING ADOLESCENCE, 524
Immunizations, 526
Nutrition, 526
  Eating Habits and Behavior, 527
Sleep and Rest, 528
Exercise and Activity, 528
Dental Health, 528
Personal Care, 528
  Vision, 528
  Hearing, 529
  Posture, 529

Body Art, 529
Tanning, 529
Stress Reduction, 529
Sexuality Education and Guidance, 530
Injury Prevention, 531
  Motor Vehicle–Related Injuries, 532
  Firearms, 532
  Sports Injuries, 532
Anticipatory Guidance—Care of Families, 532

LEARNING OBJECTIVES

On completion of this chapter the reader will be able to:

- Describe the physical changes that occur at puberty.
- Discuss the reactions of the adolescent to physical changes that take place at puberty.

- Demonstrate an understanding of the processes by which the adolescent develops a sense of identity.
- Discuss the significance of the changing interpersonal relationships and the role of the peer group during adolescence.
- Outline a health teaching plan for adolescents.

- Plan a sexuality education session for a group of adolescents.
- Identify the causes and discuss the preventive aspects of injuries during adolescence.

PROMOTING OPTIMAL GROWTH AND DEVELOPMENT

Adolescence is a period of transition between childhood and adulthood—a time of rapid physical, cognitive, social, and emotional maturation as the boy prepares for manhood and the girl prepares for womanhood (see Cultural Awareness box). The precise boundaries of adolescence are difficult to define, but this period is customarily viewed as beginning with the gradual appearance of secondary sex characteristics at about 11 or 12 years of age and ending with cessation of body growth at 18 to 20 years.

Several terms are used to refer to this stage of growth and development. **Puberty** refers to the maturational, hormonal, and growth process that occurs when the reproductive organs begin to function and the secondary sex characteristics develop. This process is sometimes divided into three stages: **prepubescence,** the period of about 2 years immediately before puberty when the child is developing preliminary physical changes that herald sexual maturity; **puberty,** the point at which sexual maturity is achieved, marked by the first menstrual flow in girls but by less obvious indications in boys; and **postpubescence,** a 1- to 2-year period following puberty during which skeletal growth is completed and reproductive functions become fairly well established. **Adolescence,** which literally means, "to grow into maturity," is generally regarded as the psychologic, social, and maturational process initiated by the pubertal changes. It involves three distinct subphases: **early adolescence** (ages 11 to 14), **middle adolescence** (ages 15 to 17), and **late adolescence** (ages 18 to 20). The term **teenage years** is used synonymously with *adolescence* to describe ages 13 through 19.

BIOLOGIC DEVELOPMENT

The physical changes of puberty are primarily the result of hormonal activity under the influence of the central nervous system, although all aspects of physiologic functioning are mutually interacting. The obvious physical changes are noted in increased physical growth and in the appearance and development of secondary sex characteristics; less obvious are physiologic alterations and neurogonadal maturity, accompanied by the ability to procreate. Physical distinction between the sexes is made on the basis of distinguishing characteristics. **Primary sex characteristics** are the external and internal organs that carry out the reproductive functions (e.g., ovaries,

uterus, breasts, penis). **Secondary sex characteristics** are the changes that occur throughout the body as a result of hormonal changes (e.g., voice alterations, development of facial and pubertal hair, fat deposits), but that play no direct part in reproduction.

Hormonal Changes of Puberty

The events of puberty are caused by hormonal influences and controlled by the anterior pituitary (adenohypophysis) in response to a stimulus from the hypothalamus. Stimulation of the gonads has a dual function:

1. Production and release of gametes—production of sperm in the male and maturation and release of ova in the female
2. Secretion of sex-appropriate hormones—estrogen and progesterone from the ovaries (female) and testosterone from the testes (male)

The ovaries, testes, and adrenals secrete sex hormones. These hormones are produced in varying amounts by both sexes throughout the life span. The adrenal cortex is responsible for the small amounts secreted before the pubescent years, but the sex hormone production that accompanies maturation of the gonads is responsible for the biologic changes observed during puberty.

Estrogen, the feminizing hormone, is found in low quantities during childhood. This hormone is secreted in slowly increasing amounts until about age 11 years. In males this gradual increase continues through maturation. In females the onset of estrogen production in the ovary causes a pronounced increase that continues until about 3 years after the onset of menstruation, at which time it reaches a maximum level that continues throughout the reproductive life of the female.

Androgens, the masculinizing hormones, are also secreted in small and gradually increasing amounts up to about 7 or 9 years of age, at which time there is a more rapid increase in both sexes, especially boys, until about age 15 years. These hormones appear to be responsible for most of the rapid growth changes of early adolescence. With the onset of testicular function, the level of androgens (principally **testosterone**) in males increases over that in females and continues to increase until a maximum is attained at maturity.

Sexual Maturation

The visible evidence of sexual maturation is achieved in an orderly sequence, and the state of maturity can be estimated on the basis of the appearance of these external manifestations. The age at which these changes are observed and the time required to progress from one stage to another may vary among children. The time from the appearance of breast buds to full maturity may be 1½ to 6 years for adolescent girls. It may take 2 to 5 years for male genitalia to reach adult size. The stages of development of secondary sex characteristics and genital development have been defined as a guide for estimating sexual maturity and are referred to as the **Tanner stages.** The usual sequence of appearance of maturational changes is presented in Box 16-1.

Sexual Maturation in Girls. In most girls the initial indication of puberty is the appearance of breast buds, an event known as **thelarche,** which occurs between 9 and 13½ years of age (Fig. 16-1). This is followed in approximately 2 to 6 months by growth of pubic hair on the mons pubis, known as **adrenarche** (Fig. 16-2). In a minority of normally developing girls, however, pubic hair may precede breast development.

The initial appearance of menstruation, or **menarche,** occurs about 2 years after the appearance of the first pubescent changes, approximately 9 months after attainment of peak height velocity, and 3 months after attainment of peak weight velocity. Menarche has been related to a critical gain in body fat content (more fat content, earlier menarche), although this is controversial. The normal age range of menarche is usually 10½ to 15 years, with the average age being 12 years, 9½ months for North American girls. Ovulation and regular menstrual periods usually occur 6 to 14 months after menarche. Girls may be considered to have **pubertal delay** if breast development has not occurred by age 13 or if menarche has not occurred within 4 years of the onset of breast development.

Sexual Maturation in Boys. The first pubescent changes in boys are testicular enlargement accompanied by thinning, reddening, and increased looseness of the scrotum (Fig. 16-3). These events usually occur between 9½ and 14 years of age. Early puberty is also characterized by the initial appearance of pubic hair. Penile enlargement begins, and testicular enlargement and pubic hair growth continue throughout midpuberty. During this period there is also increasing muscularity, early voice changes, and development of early facial hair. Temporary breast enlargement and tenderness, **gynecomastia,** are common during midpuberty, occurring in up to one third of boys.

BOX 16-1
Usual Sequence of Maturational Changes

GIRLS
Breast changes
Rapid increase in height and weight
Growth of pubic hair
Appearance of axillary hair
Menstruation (usually begins 2 years after first signs)
Abrupt deceleration of linear growth

BOYS
Enlargement of testicles
Growth of pubic hair, axillary hair, hair on upper lip, hair on face and elsewhere on body (facial hair usually appears about 2 years after appearance of pubic hair)
Rapid increase in height
Changes in the larynx and consequently the voice (usually take place along with growth of penis)
Nocturnal emissions
Abrupt deceleration of linear growth

The spurts in height and weight occur concurrently toward the end of midpuberty. For most boys, breast enlargement disappears within 2 years. By late puberty there is a definite increase in the length and width of the penis, testicular enlargement continues, and first ejaculation occurs. Axillary hair develops, and facial hair extends to cover the anterior neck. Final voice changes occur secondary to the growth of the larynx. Concerns about **pubertal delay** should be considered for boys who exhibit no enlargement of the testes or scrotal changes by 13½ to 14 years of age, or if genital growth is not complete 4 years after the testicles begin to enlarge.

Physical Growth

A constant phenomenon associated with sexual maturation is a dramatic increase in growth. The final 20% to 25% of height is achieved during puberty, and most of this growth occurs during a 24- to 36-month period—the adolescent **growth spurt.** This accelerated growth occurs in all children but, as in other areas of development, is highly variable in age of onset, duration, and extent. The growth spurt begins earlier in girls, usually between ages 9½ and 14½ years; on average it begins between ages 10½ and 16 years in boys. During this period, the average boy gains 10 to 30 cm (4 to 12 inches) in height and 7 to 30 kg (15.5 to 66 pounds) in weight. The average girl, in whom the growth spurt is slower and less extensive, gains 5 to 20 cm (2 to 8 inches) in height and 7 to 25 kg (15.5 to 55 pounds) in weight. Growth in height typically ceases 2 to 2½ years after menarche in girls and at age 18 to 20 years in boys.

This increase in size is acquired in a characteristic sequence. Growth in length of the extremities and neck precedes growth in other areas, and because these parts are the first to reach adult length, the hands and feet appear larger than normal during adolescence. Increases in hip and chest breadth take place in a few months, followed several months later by an increase in shoulder width. These changes are followed by increases in length of the trunk and depth of the chest. This sequence of changes is responsible for the characteristic long-legged, gawky appearance of the early adolescent child.

Stage 2
(pubertal)

Stage 3

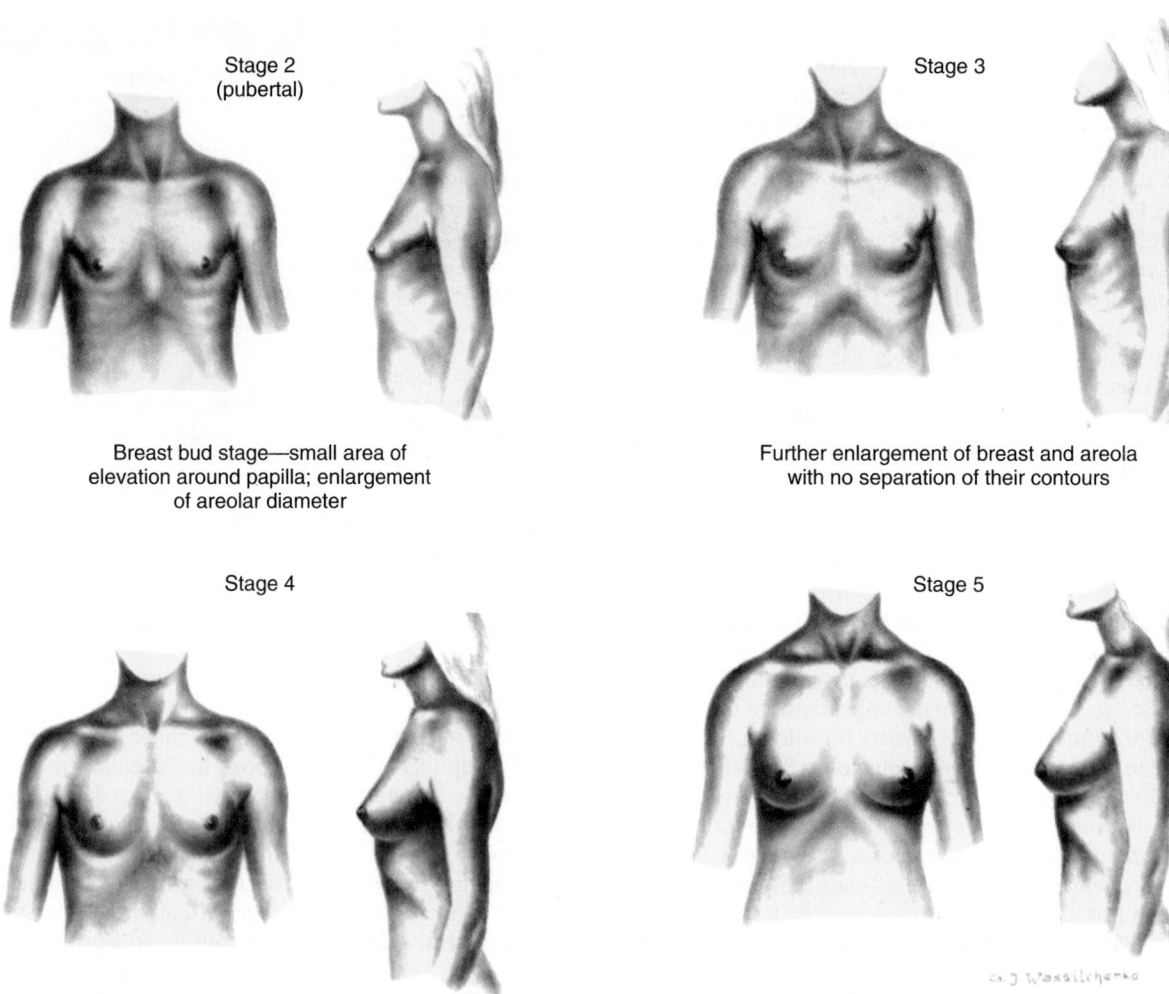

Breast bud stage—small area of
elevation around papilla; enlargement
of areolar diameter

Further enlargement of breast and areola
with no separation of their contours

Stage 4

Stage 5

Projection of areola and papilla
to form a secondary mound (may
not occur in all girls)

Mature configuration; projection of papilla
only caused by recession of areola
into general contour

FIG. 16-1 ■ Development of breasts in girls—average age span, 9 to 13½ years. Stage 1 (prepubertal—elevation of papilla only) is not shown. (Modified from Marshall WA, Tanner JM: Variations in pattern of pubertal changes in girls, *Arch Dis Child* 44(235):291-303, 1969; and Daniel WA, Paulshock BZ: A physician's guide to sexual maturity, *Patient Care* 13:122-124, 1979.)

Sex Differences in General Growth Patterns. Sex differences in general growth and distribution patterns are apparent in skeletal growth, muscle mass, adipose tissue, and skin. **Skeletal growth** differences between boys and girls are apparently a function of hormonal effects at puberty and are evident primarily in limb length. The earlier cessation of growth in girls is caused by epiphyseal unity under the potent effect of estrogen secretion, and the hormonal effect on female bone growth is much stronger than the similar effect of testosterone in boys. In boys the prolonged growth period before puberty and the less rapid epiphyseal closure are reflected in their greater overall height and longer arms and legs. Other skeletal differences are increased shoulder width in boys and broader hip development in girls.

Hypertrophy of the laryngeal mucosa and enlargement of the larynx and vocal cords occur in both boys and girls to produce **voice changes.** Girls' voices become slightly deeper and considerably fuller, but the effect in boys is striking. The change in the voice of adolescent boys occurs between Tanner

stages 3 and 4, with the voice often shifting uncontrollably from deep to high tones in the middle of a sentence. The average lengthening of the vocal cords is 10.9 mm (0.4 inch) for boys and 4.2 mm (0.17 inch) for girls.

Growth of **lean body mass,** principally muscle, which tends to occur after the bone growth spurt, takes place steadily during adolescence. Lean body mass is both quantitatively and qualitatively greater in boys than in girls at comparable stages of pubertal development. Muscle development, under the influence of androgenic hormones, increases steadily. Muscles become remarkably well developed in boys, whereas in girls, muscle mass increase is proportionate to general tissue growth.

Nonlean body mass, primarily fat, is also increased but follows a less orderly pattern. There may be a transient increase in subcutaneous fat just before the skeletal growth spurt, especially in boys. This is followed 1 to 2 years later by a modest to marked decrease, which is again more marked in boys. Later, variable amounts of fat are deposited to fill out and contour the mature physique in patterns characteristic of

Stage 1
(prepubertal)

No pubic hair; essentially the same as
during childhood; no distinction between
hair on pubis and over the abdomen

Stage 2

Sparse growth of long, straight, downy, and
slightly pigmented hair extending along labia;
between stages 2 and 3 begins to appear on pubis

Stage 3

Hair darker, coarser, and curly and
spread sparsely over entire pubis in
the typical female triangle

Stage 4

Pubic hair denser, curled, and adult in distribution
but less abundant and restricted to the pubic area

Stage 5

Hair adult in quantity, type, and pattern
with spread to inner aspect of thighs

FIG. 16-2 ■ Growth in pubic hair in girls—average age span for stages 2 through 5: 9 to 13½ years. (Modified from Marshall WA, Tanner JM: Variations in pattern of pubertal changes in girls, *Arch Dis Child* 44(235):291-303, 1969; and Daniel WA, Paulshock BZ: A physician's guide to sexual maturity, *Patient Care* 13:122-124, 1979.)

Stage 1
(prepubertal)

No pubic hair; essentially the same as
during childhood; no distinction between
hair on pubis and over the abdomen

Stage 2 (pubertal)

Initial enlargement of scrotum and testes;
reddening and textural changes of scrotal skin;
sparse growth of long, straight, downy, and
slightly pigmented hair at base of penis

Stage 3

Initial enlargement of penis, mainly in
length; testes and scrotum further enlarged;
hair darker, coarser, and curly and spread
sparsely over entire pubis

Stage 4

Increased size of penis with growth in diameter and
development of glans; glans larger and broader; scrotum
darker; pubic hair more abundant with curling but
restricted to pubic area

Stage 5

Testes, scrotum, and penis adult in size and shape;
hair adult in quantity and type with spread to inner
surface of thighs

FIG. 16-3 ■ Developmental stages of secondary sex characteristics and genital development in boys—average age span, 9½ to 14 years. (Modified from Marshall WA, Tanner JM: Variations in pattern of pubertal changes in girls, *Arch Dis Child* 44(235):291-303, 1969; and Daniel WA, Paulshock BZ: A physician's guide to sexual maturity, *Patient Care* 13:122-124, 1979.)

the adolescent's sex, particularly in the regions over the thighs, hips, and buttocks and around the breast tissue. It should be noted, however, that pediatric obesity is steadily on the increase in the United States, and obesity can change the timing and sequence of puberty. Girls with thelarche as the first sign of puberty have earlier menarche and greater body fat and body mass index (BMI) at menarche than girls with adrenarche as the first pubertal sign. This may have long-term effects for increased risk of adult adiposity and obesity (Biro, Lucky, Simbarti, and others, 2003).

Hormonal influences during puberty cause acceleration in growth and maturation of the skin and its structural appendages. Sebaceous glands become extremely active at this time, especially those on the genitalia and in the "flush areas" of the body (i.e., face, neck, shoulders, upper back, and chest). This increased activity and the structural nature of the glands are extremely important in the pathogenesis of a common problem of puberty: acne (see Chapter 30). The eccrine sweat glands, present almost everywhere on the human skin, become fully functional and respond to emotional as well as thermal stimulation. Heavy sweating appears to be more pronounced in boys than in girls. The apocrine sweat glands, nonfunctional in childhood, reach secretory capacity during puberty. Unlike the eccrine sweat glands, the apocrine glands are limited in distribution and grow in conjunction with hair follicles in the axillae, around the areola of the breast, around the umbilicus, on the external auditory canal, and in the genital and anal regions. Apocrine glands secrete a thick substance as a result of emotional stimulation that, when acted on by surface bacteria, becomes highly odoriferous.

Body hair assumes characteristic distribution patterns and changes texture during puberty. Under the influence of gonadal and adrenal androgens, hair coarsens, darkens, and lengthens at sites related to secondary sex characteristics. Pubic and axillary hair appears in both sexes, although pubic hair is more extensive in males than in females. Beard, mustache, and body hair on the chest, upward along the linea alba, and sometimes on other areas (e.g., back and shoulders) appears in males and is androgen dependent. Extremity hair appears in varying amounts in both males and females but is also more prolific in the male.

Physiologic Changes

A number of physiologic functions are altered in response to some of the pubertal changes. The size and strength of the heart, blood volume, and systolic blood pressure increase, whereas the pulse rate and basal heat production decrease (see inside back cover). Blood volume, which has increased steadily during childhood, reaches a higher value in boys than in girls, a fact that may be related to the increased muscle mass in pubertal boys. Adult values are reached for all formed elements of the blood. Respiratory rate and basal metabolic rate, decreasing steadily throughout childhood, reach the adult rate in adolescence. Respiratory volume and vital capacity are increased, and to a far greater extent in males than in females. During this period, physiologic responses to exercise change drastically: performance improves, especially in boys, and the body is able to make the physiologic adjustments needed for normal functioning after exercise is completed. These capabilities are a result of the increased size and strength of muscles and the increased level of cardiac, respiratory, and metabolic functioning.

PSYCHOSOCIAL DEVELOPMENT: DEVELOPING A SENSE OF IDENTITY (ERIKSON)

Traditional psychosocial theory holds that the developmental crisis of adolescence leads to the formation of a **sense of identity**. Throughout childhood, individuals have been going through the process of identification as they concentrate on various parts of the body at specific times. During infancy children identify themselves as being separate from the mother, during early childhood they establish gender-role identification with the appropriate-sex parent, and in later childhood they establish who they are in relation to others. In adolescence they come to see themselves as distinct individuals, somehow unique and separate from every other individual.

Adolescence begins with the onset of puberty and extends to relative physical and emotional stability at or near graduation from high school. During this time the adolescent is faced with the crisis of **group identity vs alienation.** In the period that follows, the individual strives to attain autonomy from the family and develop a sense of **personal identity** as opposed to **role diffusion.** A sense of group identity appears to be essential to the development of a personal identity. Young adolescents must resolve questions concerning relationships with a peer group before they are able to resolve questions about who they are in relation to family and society.

Group Identity. During the early stage of adolescence, pressure to belong to a group is intensified. Teenagers find it essential to belong to a group from which they can derive status. Belonging to a crowd helps adolescents establish the differences between themselves and their parents. They dress as the group dresses and wear makeup and hairstyles according to group criteria, all of which are different from those of the parental generation. Language, music, and dancing reflect a culture that is exclusive to the adolescent. When adults begin to emulate these fashions and interests, the style changes immediately. The evidence of adolescent conformity to the peer group and nonconformity to the adult group provides teenagers with a frame of reference for self-assertion and rejection of the identity of their parents' generation. To be different is to be unaccepted and alienated from the group.

Individual Identity. The quest for personal identity is part of the ongoing identification process. As adolescents establish identity within a group, they also attempt to incorporate multiple body changes into a concept of the self. Body awareness is part of self-awareness. In their search for identity, adolescents consider the relationships that have developed between themselves and others in the past, as well as the directions they hope to take in the future.

Significant others hold expectations for the behavior of the adolescent. Often these expectations or demands are persistent enough that individuals make certain decisions that they would not make if they were solely responsible for identity formation. Adolescents may find it too easy to slip into the roles expected by others without incorporating personal goals or questioning decisions. Thus individuals may become what parents or others wish them to be based on these premature decisions. Young persons might form a negative identity when society or their culture provides them with a self-image that is contrary to the values of the community. Labels such as "juvenile delinquent," "hoodlum," or "failure" are applied to certain adolescents, who then accept and live up to these labels with behaviors that validate and strengthen them.

??? CRITICAL THINKING EXERCISE

Discussing the Future

Jeremy, age 17, will be graduating from high school in the spring. His mother, a single parent, tells you that she is concerned because graduation is quickly approaching and Jeremy has made no plans for what he will do with his life after graduation. Whenever Jeremy mentions the topic, his mother tells him, "This is what you must do," and begins to outline the steps he must take. Jeremy just walks away. She asks, "What should I do?" What advice should you give Jeremy's mother?

QUESTIONS
1. Evidence—Is there sufficient evidence to draw any conclusions about what advice to give Jeremy's mother?
2. Assumptions—Describe an underlying assumption about each of the following issues:
   a. Adolescents and the search for personal identity
   b. The influence of others on the adolescent's search for personal identity
   c. Ways to communicate with adolescents
3. What implications and priorities for nursing care can be drawn at this time?
4. Does the evidence objectively support your argument (conclusion)?
5. Are there alternative perspectives to your arguments? What are they?

The process of evolving a personal identity is time-consuming and fraught with periods of confusion, depression, and discouragement. Determining an identity and a place in the world is a critical and perilous feature of adolescence (see Critical Thinking Exercise). However, as the pieces gradually shift and settle into place, a positive identity emerges. Role diffusion results when the individual is unable to formulate a satisfactory identity from the multiplicity of aspirations, roles, and identifications.

Sex-Role Identity. Adolescence is the time for consolidation of a sex-role identity. During early adolescence the peer group begins to communicate expectations regarding heterosexual relationships, and as development progresses, adolescents encounter expectations for mature sex-role behavior from both peers and adults. Expectations vary from culture to culture, among geographic areas, and among socioeconomic groups.

Emotionality. Adolescents vacillate in their emotional states between considerable maturity and childlike behavior. One minute they are exuberant and enthusiastic; the next minute they are depressed and withdrawn. Unpredictable but essentially normal, mood swings are common during this time. As the tension is relieved, emotion is brought under control and individuals retreat to review what has happened, to attempt to master their anger, and to grow in their ability to control their emotions and gain from the new experience. Because of these mood swings, adolescents are frequently labeled as unstable, inconsistent, and unpredictable. Little things can cause an emotional upheaval and, depending on the teenager's interpretation, can mean a great deal.

Teenagers are better able to control their emotions in later adolescence. They can approach problems more calmly and rationally, and although they are still subject to periods of sadness, their feelings are less vulnerable and they begin to demonstrate the more mature emotions of later adolescence. Whereas early adolescents react immediately and emotionally, older adolescents can control their emotions until socially acceptable times and places for expression present themselves. They are still subject to heightened emotion, and when it is expressed, their behavior reflects feelings of insecurity, tension, and indecision.

COGNITIVE DEVELOPMENT (PIAGET)

Cognitive thinking culminates with the capacity for **abstract thinking.** This stage, the period of **formal operations,** is Piaget's fourth and last stage. Adolescents are no longer restricted to the real and actual, which was typical of the period of concrete thought; now they are also concerned with the possible. They think beyond the present. Without having to center attention on the immediate situation, they can imagine a sequence of events that might occur, such as college and occupational possibilities; how things might change in the future, such as relationships with parents; and the consequences of their actions, such as dropping out of school. At this time their thoughts can be influenced by logical principles rather than just their own perceptions and experiences. They become increasingly capable of scientific reasoning and formal logic.

Adolescents are capable of mentally manipulating more than two categories of variables at the same time. For example, they can consider the relationship between speed, distance, and time in planning a trip. They can detect logical consistency or inconsistency in a set of statements and evaluate a system or set of values in a more analytic manner. For instance, they question the parent who insists on honesty in the youngster but at the same time cheats on an income tax report or expense account.

In adolescence, young people begin to consider both their own thinking and the thinking of others. They wonder what opinion others have of them, and they are able to imagine the thoughts of others. With this capacity comes the ability to differentiate between others' thoughts and their own and to interpret the thoughts of others more accurately. They are able to understand that few concepts are absolute or independent of other influencing factors. As they become aware that other cultures and communities have different norms and standards from their own, it becomes easier for them to accept members of these other cultures, and the decision to behave in their own culture in an accepted manner becomes a more conscious commitment.

MORAL DEVELOPMENT (KOHLBERG)

Although younger children merely accept the decisions or point of view of adults, adolescents, to gain autonomy from adults, must substitute their own set of morals and values. When old principles are challenged but new independent values have not yet emerged to take their place, young people search for a moral code that preserves their personal integrity and guides their behavior, especially in the face of strong pressure to violate the old beliefs. Their decisions involving moral dilemmas must be based on an **internalized set of moral principles** that provides them with the resources to evaluate the demands of the situation and to plan actions that are consistent with their ideals.

Late adolescence is characterized by serious questioning of existing moral values and their relevance to society and the individual. Adolescents can easily take the role of another. They understand duty and obligation based on reciprocal rights of others and the concept of justice that is founded on making amends for misdeeds and repairing or replacing what has been spoiled by wrongdoing. However, they seriously question established moral codes, often as a result of observing that adults verbally ascribe to a code but do not adhere to it.

SPIRITUAL DEVELOPMENT

As adolescents move toward independence from parents and other authorities, some begin to question the values and ideals of their families. Others cling to these values as a stable element in their lives as they struggle with the conflicts of this turbulent period. Adolescents need to work out these conflicts for themselves, but they also need support from authority figures or peers for their resolution.

Adolescents are capable of understanding abstract concepts and of interpreting analogies and symbols. They are able to empathize, philosophize, and think logically. Most teens search for ideals and speculate about illogical statements and conflicting ideologies. Their tendency toward introspection and emotional intensity often makes it difficult for others to know what they are thinking. They tend to keep their thoughts private, fearing that no one will understand these feelings that they perceive to be unique and special. However, they may reveal deep spiritual concerns. They need support and encouragement in their struggle for understanding and the freedom to question without censure.

Greater levels of religiosity and spirituality are associated with fewer high-risk behaviors and more health-promoting behaviors (Brown, 2001). Nurses play an important role for teens by providing an opportunity to discuss issues regarding spirituality.

SOCIAL DEVELOPMENT

To achieve full maturity, adolescents must free themselves from family domination and define an identity independent of parental authority. However, this process is fraught with ambivalence on the part of both teenagers and their parents. Adolescents want to grow up and to be free of parental restraints, but they are fearful as they try to comprehend the responsibilities that are linked with independence. Feelings of immortality and exemption from the consequences of risk-taking behavior, although viewed as negative, can serve an important developmental function at this time. These feelings give adolescents the courage to separate from their parents and become independent. Part of this emancipation involves developing social relationships outside the family that help teenagers identify their role in society. Adolescence is a time of intense sociability and often a time of equally intense loneliness. Acceptance by peers, a few close friends, and the secure love of a supportive family are requisites for interpersonal maturation.

Relationships with Parents

During adolescence the parent-child relationship changes from one of protection-dependency to one of **mutual affection and equality.** The process of achieving independence often involves turmoil and ambiguity as both parent and adolescent learn to play new roles and work toward this end while, at the same time, resolving the often painful series of rifts essential to establishing the ultimate relationship.

Most behavior observed in the adolescent is related to the struggle for independence and the external restrictions and checks that are placed on this spontaneous maturation process. On the one hand, adolescents are accepted as maturing preadults. They are allowed privileges heretofore denied, and they are provided with increasing responsibilities. On the other hand, because of their unpredictability and insecurity in evaluating situations and making sound judgments, they must conform to regulations and restrictions set by adults. This state of affairs is particularly exemplified by the struggle between parents and adolescents concerning the nightly curfew.

As teenagers assert their rights for grown-up privileges, they frequently create tensions within the home. They resist parental control, and conflicts can arise from almost any situation or any subject. Favorite topics of dispute include use of the home telephone, Internet use, the need for a personal cellular telephone, manners, dress, chores and duties, homework, disrespectful behavior, friendships, dating and relationships, money, automobiles, alcohol and other substance abuse, and time schedules. Present in these areas of conflict are the overriding arguments that "Everyone else has one" or is allowed the desired item or privilege and the ever-present assertions that "You don't understand me or trust me" and "You always treat me like a baby." Spoken or unspoken, parents' reactions consist of "Is this all the thanks I get for what I have done for you?"

Teenagers' earliest attempts to achieve emancipation from parental controls are manifested in a period of rejection of the parents. They absent themselves from home and family activities and spend an increasing amount of time with the peer group. They confide less in their parents, but parents continue to play an important role in the personal and health-related decision making of adolescents.

With advancing adolescence, teenagers become more competent, and with this competence comes a need for more autonomy. Although they may be psychologically prepared for independence, they are often thwarted in their efforts by lack of money or other parental barriers. Conflict arises in relation to the teenager's outside activities and the elements of privacy and trust. Parental monitoring remains important throughout adolescence and may have a direct influence on adolescent sexual and substance use behavior. Parents should be guided toward an authoritative style of parenting in which authority is used to guide the adolescent while allowing developmentally appropriate levels of freedom and providing clear, consistent messages regarding expectations. Authoritative style of parenting has been shown to have both immediate and long-term protective effects toward adolescent risk reduction (DeVore and Ginsburg, 2005). However, to gain the trust of adolescents, parents must respect their adolescent's privacy and show an honest and sincere interest in what the adolescent believes and feels (see Family Focus box).

Relationships with Peers

Although parents remain the primary influence in their lives, for the majority of teenagers, peers assume a more significant role in adolescence than they did during childhood. The peer group serves as a strong support to teenagers, individually and collectively, providing them with a sense of belonging and a feeling of strength and power. The peer group forms the transitional world between dependence and autonomy.

Communication with Adolescents: The Art of Listening

Conflicts between parents and their adolescents are often a result of a natural characteristic of parenthood: the desire to protect one's offspring—from harm or from simply doing something "stupid" or embarrassing or something they may later regret. Teenagers sometimes "bounce" their thoughts and ideas off adults. At times they really want some feedback; at other times they simply want to elicit a reaction.

I found it easy to listen openly, thoughtfully, and without interrupting when my teenagers' friends discussed troublesome topics. However, one day, when one of my own teenagers had a similar conversation with me, the parent part kicked in. I felt responsible and spoke my piece on the spot.

This brought communication to a halt and resulted in defensiveness. It was a long time before my child tried to talk to me about anything controversial again.

The next time one of my teenagers started a similar conversation, I decided to try to trick myself. Throughout the entire conversation, I told myself over and over again to act as if this were not my teenager, but rather someone else's child. I found this actually worked quite well, and I was able to listen without interrupting. I continue to use the system, sometimes with more success than at other times.

—Mother of four

Peer Group. Adolescents are usually social, gregarious, and group minded. Thus the peer group has an intense influence on adolescents' self-evaluation and behavior. To gain acceptance by a group, younger teenagers tend to conform completely in such things as mode of dress, hairstyle, taste in music, and vocabulary. Teenagers use the peer group as a yardstick of what is normal.

The school is psychologically important to adolescents as a focus of social life. Teenagers usually distribute themselves into a relatively predictable social hierarchy. They know to which groups they and others belong. A sense of school connectedness and optimal social connectedness is associated with positive outcomes for school completion, positive mood, and decreased high-risk behavior in adolescents (Bond, Butler, Thomas, and others, 2007). School connectedness is correlated with caring teachers and the absence of prejudice or discrimination from peers. A sense of school connectedness is less dependent on class size, attendance, academic preparation, and parental involvement (Maes and Lievens, 2003).

Within the larger groups are smaller, distinct, and exclusive crowds or cliques of selected close friends who are emotionally attached to one another. The selection is based on common tastes, interests, and background. Although cliques may become formalized, most remain informal and small. However, each has an identifying feature that proclaims its difference from others and its solidarity within itself, in much the same manner as the adolescent generation as a whole sets itself apart from the adult generation. Cliques are usually made up of one sex, and girls tend to be more cliquish than boys and to have a greater need for close friendships (Fig. 16-4). Within the intimacy of the group, adolescents

FIG. 16-4 ■ Teenagers like to gather in small groups.

gain support in learning about themselves, consideration for the feelings of others, and increased ego development and self-reliance.

To belong is of utmost importance; thus adolescents behave in a way that will ensure their establishment in a group. Adolescents are highly susceptible to social approval, acceptance, and demands. To be ignored or criticized by peers creates feelings of inferiority, inadequacy, and incompetence.

Best Friends. Personal friendships of the one-on-one variety usually develop between same-sex adolescents. This relationship is closer and more stable than it is in middle childhood, and it is important in the quest for identity. A best friend is the best audience on whom to try out possible roles and identities that an adolescent wants to test. Best friends may try a role together, each providing support for the other. Each cares about what the other thinks and feels. Because a sense of intimacy grows within a permanent relationship, the stability of this same-sex friendship is an important link in the progress toward an intimate relationship in young adulthood.

Interests and Activities

Adolescents spend a large amount of time engaging in leisure-time activities. As teenagers progress through the developmental stages of adolescence, these leisure-time activities move from being family centered to being peer centered. In addition to providing teenagers with fun and enjoyment, leisure-time activities assist in the development of social, physical, and cognitive skills. Leisure-time activities also allow teenagers the opportunity to learn to set priorities and structure their time (Fig. 16-5).

Today, many adolescents must learn to juggle their time between school, activities, and the responsibilities of a job. Adolescent work experiences provide many benefits, including time management, teamwork skills, and increased income. However, many jobs available to teenagers do not provide opportunities to apply the skills they learn in school, and jobs often have high demands for quick work with low rewards. Few apprentice opportunities are available for teenagers. It is generally recommended that adolescents limit their work to no more than 20 hours per week during the school year.

FIG. 16-5 ■ The cell phone allows adolescents to talk for hours with peers.

FIG. 16-6 ■ Heterosexual relationships are important for most adolescents.

ADOLESCENT SEXUALITY

Sexual activity rates have been decreasing for teens since the 1990s, including a decline in the rate among early adolescents (Santelli, Lindberg, Finer, and others, 2007). Among teenagers who have initiated sexual intercourse at an age younger than 14 years, the incidence of sexual abuse is high. In 2002 about half of all teenagers had had sexual intercourse at least once (Abma, Martinez, Mosher, and others, 2004). Teens engage in a wide range of sexual activity, including kissing and petting (fondling), oral sex, and vaginal and rectal sex. Data indicate that adolescents are engaging in sexual activity such as oral sex and delaying vaginal intercourse (Mosher, Chandra, and Jones, 2005); whether this is intended to preserve female virginity or to presumably avoid sexually transmitted disease or pregnancy is not known.

Adolescence represents a critical time in the development of sexuality. Hormonal, physical, cognitive, and social changes that occur during adolescence all have an impact on sexual development. Of all the developmental changes that affect adolescent sexuality, none is more obvious than the impact of puberty. Adolescents must come to terms with hormonal influences, physiologic manifestations such as menstruation and ejaculation, and physical changes such as breast and genital development. All these changes have a profound impact on the way teenagers perceive their bodies (i.e., body image). In addition to transitions in body image, increasing levels of pubertal hormones contribute to increased levels of sexual motivation among both boys and girls.

Changes in sexual motivations and feelings, happening at the same time as shifts in cognitive skills, contribute to painful conjectures ("Is what I'm feeling normal?"), self-conscious concern ("Am I good-looking enough?"), and hypothetical thinking ("What if she wants to have sex?"). The emergence of formal operational thinking also increases adolescents' decision-making capabilities concerning sexual issues. As they mature, teenagers become better able to think through potential risks and benefits of sexual behaviors before they engage in any behavior. Older adolescents may also be able to conceptualize more long-term consequences of present behaviors. One of the important tasks of adolescence is to incorporate sexuality successfully into close, intimate relationships. This task is made possible by the advanced cognitive abilities that emerge over the course of adolescence.

Part of adolescent identity formation involves the development of sexual identity. As they begin to integrate changes involved with puberty, young adolescents also develop emotional and social identities separate from their family's. For young adolescents, the process of sexual identity development usually involves forming close friendships with same-sex peers, with whom they may experiment sexually, often to satisfy curiosity. Sexual activity among young teenagers varies by gender. Masturbation provides an opportunity for sexual self-exploration; participation in this behavior is influenced by learned cultural attitudes and sex-role expectations.

Many teenagers begin to make a shift from relationships with same-sex peers to intimate relationships with members of the opposite sex during middle adolescence (Fig. 16-6). Opposite-sex relationships typically begin with peer activities involving both boys and girls. Pairing off as couples becomes more common as middle adolescence progresses. The type and degree of seriousness of partner relationships vary. Initial relationships are usually noncommittal, extremely mobile, and seldom characterized by any deep romantic attachments.

Sexual activity becomes more common during middle adolescence. The relationship between love and sexual expression is brought into focus during middle adolescence. Most young people oppose exploitation, pressure, or force in sex as well as sex solely for the sake of physical enjoyment without a personal relationship. Adolescents find it hard to believe that sex can exist without love; therefore they view each relationship as real love.

An integrated sexual identity often emerges during late adolescence as individuals incorporate sexual experiences, feelings, and knowledge. For most, this identity is consistent with their own physical and mental capacities and with societal limits and expectations. Most older adolescents identify themselves as being predominantly heterosexual or bisexual, with a smaller number self-identifying as homosexual and an even smaller group still unsure of their sexual orientation, although this varies somewhat by ethnicity (Saewyc, Bearinger, Heinz, and others, 1998; Russell, Seif, and Truong, 2001). Whatever their sexual orientation, most older teenagers possess the capacity to have intimate relationships that satisfy the emotional and sexual needs of both partners.

Sexual orientation is an important aspect of sexual identity. Sexual orientation is defined as a pattern of sexual arousal or romantic attraction toward persons of the opposite gender (heterosexual), of the same gender (homosexual, often called gay or lesbian), or of both genders (bisexual). Sexual orientation encompasses several dimensions, including attraction, fantasy, actual sexual behavior, and self-labeling or group affiliation. In individuals the direction and intensity of each dimension are not necessarily consistent with any of the others. For example, individuals may be attracted most strongly to their same gender, fantasize about both genders, have sexual activity only with the opposite gender, and identify as gay or lesbian. Other individuals may engage in same-gender sexual behavior, fantasize about both genders, but identify as heterosexual. As with all aspects of sexual identity, the dimensions of sexual orientation are influenced by cultural meaning and expectation, by gender, by peer groups, and by other environmental contexts.

Adolescence is the period during which individuals commonly begin to identify their sexual orientation as part of their developing sexual identity. However, this identification process can be profoundly influenced by cultural beliefs and values, by societal and family pressures, or by a lack of similar peers. The majority of adolescents eventually report an orientation toward exclusively heterosexual relationships. For adolescents whose orientation encompasses any same-gender dimensions, the identity process during adolescence can be complicated, especially when community norms disapprove of orientations other than heterosexual. Adolescents who have witnessed harassment or violence directed at gay, lesbian, and bisexual people, for example, may be reluctant to self-identify, even when their attractions and behaviors are exclusively same-gender or bisexual.

The development of sexual orientation as part of sexual identity includes several developmental milestones during late childhood and throughout adolescence. These milestones do not necessarily occur in the same order for everyone, nor are they completed in the same amount of time. They include (1) the realization of romantic or erotic attraction to people of one (or both) genders; (2) erotic daydreaming about one or both genders; (3) romantic partners or dates without sexual activity; (4) sexual activity with people of the preferred gender or gen-

CRITICAL THINKING EXERCISE

Discussing Sexual Orientation with Adolescents

John, a 17-year-old adolescent, comes into the school-based clinic and tells the nurse practitioner that he thinks he is homosexual. What is the most appropriate response for the nurse practitioner?

QUESTIONS
1. Evidence—Is there sufficient evidence to draw any conclusions about John's sexual orientation at this time?
2. Assumptions—Describe an underlying assumption about each of the following issues:
   a. Sexual orientation in adolescents
   b. Society's reaction to homosexuality
   c. Health care professionals and sexuality
3. What implications and priorities for nursing care can be drawn at this time?
4. Does the evidence support your argument (conclusion)?
5. Are there alternative perspectives to your arguments? What are they?

ders (also, for some teens, sexual activity with a nonpreferred gender, out of curiosity or through social pressure); (5) self-identification of the orientation that best fits one's current circumstances and understanding; (6) publicly self-identifying that orientation, usually to intimate friends and family first, then the wider social group; and (7) an intimate, committed sexual relationship with a person of the gender appropriate to one's orientation.

There is no evidence that gay, lesbian, or bisexual adults are more or less likely to create long-term, stable relationships than are heterosexual couples. It should be noted that bisexual adolescents and adults do not generally engage in sexual relationships with both genders concurrently; self-identification as bisexual usually refers to the ability to be attracted to either gender but does not imply that such a person requires partners of both genders, or that one must be equally attracted to and have sexual experience with both genders in order to be bisexual.

Although the order of these milestones varies greatly among adolescents, adolescents who identify as gay, lesbian, or bisexual tend to publicly self-identify later than heterosexual peers. Without positive gay, lesbian, or bisexual role models or a supportive peer group, sexual-minority teens can feel isolated, and they may not share their orientation with anyone for fear of rejection or violence. (See Critical Thinking Exercise.) When adolescents who would otherwise identify as bisexual can only find a peer group of gay and lesbian teens, they may focus on their same-gender dimensions of orientation and adopt the label of lesbian or gay; later, they may self-label as bisexual. Likewise, some gay and lesbian adolescents may first identify as heterosexual, then bisexual, before identifying as gay or lesbian.

DEVELOPMENT OF SELF-CONCEPT AND BODY IMAGE

The sudden growth that takes place in early adolescence creates feelings of confusion for adolescents. They have lost the security of a familiar body and feel uncomfortable with their altered body. Consequently, they may try to either hide their body or advertise it, or they may alternate between the two extremes. Teenagers are acutely aware of their appearance as they begin to acquire images of themselves as adults, but they see discrepancies between their ideal and actual skills and abilities.

Adolescents are continually comparing themselves with their peers and making judgments about their own normality based on these observations. Pubertal children feel most comfortable when they are just like their friends and age-mates. Perceived defects or deviations from the group average are threatening to their idealized image. Any blemish is likely to be magnified out of proportion, and any delay of the visible evidence of maturity is cause for worry. Unfortunately, this is also the time when the hormonal effect of the sebaceous glands produces acne, which creates problems for many adolescents. To the adolescent, even the most insignificant pimple may be viewed as a gross disfigurement. The advent of chronic disease or a permanent physical disability has special significance during adolescence and creates additional stresses for both adolescents with the condition and health care providers.

Experts have determined that the body image established during adolescence is the one that individuals retain throughout life. Much of adolescents' search for identity takes place before a mirror as they try to read from the reflected features just who they are and what they look like to other people. Adolescents practice facial expressions and postures, try out hair arrangements, worry about a pimple, and in other ways attempt to assess the best means to achieve a maximum effect—to reveal the "true self."

The self-concept becomes more differentiated as adolescents acquire a more complex picture of themselves, one that takes situational factors into account. The self-concept gradually becomes more individualized and more distinct from the concepts of others. Although younger teenagers describe themselves in terms of similarities with peers, as adolescence advances, young people describe themselves in terms of their special characteristics.

Responses to Puberty

The response to the physical changes of pubertal growth and development differs depending on the stage of development. Young adolescents become preoccupied with the rapid changes in their body and are interested in the anatomy, physiology, and function of their sexual organs. Boys must also confront the sexual feelings and tensions that accompany puberty, and the appearance of nocturnal emissions may be puzzling, troublesome, or embarrassing events. Unless the boy has been prepared in advance, he may find it difficult to discuss his feelings with his parents and may turn to his friends for information and guidance. Many girls also are concerned over the rapid changes in their body. Some girls perceive the increase in weight and associated fat deposition as evidence of obesity and may indulge in fad diets. Although many girls look forward to menstruation and take this event in stride, others may find the first menstrual period a distressing and frightening event. All teenagers, regardless of gender, are concerned with the question, "Am I normal?" To answer this question, they compare their body with the bodies of their peers and with images in the media. This leads to a great deal of uncertainty about their appearance and attractiveness.

If an adolescent does not enter puberty at the same time as his or her peers, considerable inner conflict may occur. Early-maturing girls and boys have higher rates of sexual risk-taking behaviors, delinquency, and substance abuse than their on-time peers (Costello, Sung, Worthman, and others, 2007; Lynne, Graber, Nichols, and others, 2007). Nurses who work with adolescents must provide teaching and health care interventions that are appropriate for the chronologic and cognitive development of the adolescent rather than the stage of physical maturation.

As growth and development proceed through middle adolescence, the rapid body changes diminish, and the adolescent has time to try to make the body more attractive. Adolescents strive to achieve the perfect body within their own cultural norms. The "right" clothes and hairstyle become very important. By late adolescence the heightened concern with body image has ended and is replaced with a general comfort with the body.

The changes that occur during the early, middle, and late phases of adolescence are summarized in Table 16-1.

PROMOTING OPTIMAL HEALTH DURING ADOLESCENCE

The major causes of morbidity and mortality in adolescence are not diseases, but health-damaging behaviors. New sources of morbidity in adolescence include injury, depression, violence, sexually transmitted diseases, and pregnancy; obesity may begin in childhood or adolescence, but the health consequences are more evident in early and middle adulthood. Health promotion for this age-group consists mainly of teaching and guidance to avoid risk-taking activities and health-damaging behaviors. Adolescence provides an opportunity for teenagers to incorporate healthy lifestyle behaviors that will benefit them not only during the teenage years, but also throughout the life span.

Effective health education for adolescents should incorporate a developmentally appropriate, multifaceted approach. Motivational interviewing has been shown to improve adherence to health care advice by using a collaborative approach (Gance-Cleveland, 2007). Education alone is not enough to change behavior. Effective programs must include opportunities to improve communication skills and enhance their social network to make more positive connections (Tuttle, Campbell-Heider, and David, 2006).

As adolescents develop, they are able to assume additional responsibility for their own health, including maintaining health practices, taking prescribed medications, keeping appointments, and performing procedures when necessary. Health professionals who work with adolescents should consider their increasing independence and responsibility while maintaining privacy and ensuring confidentiality (see Nursing Care Guidelines box and Critical Thinking Exercise). Parents should also respect their teenager's independence and move toward the role of consultant about health issues while maintaining some level of involvement throughout adolescence.

In response to changes in adolescent morbidity and mortality, the American Medical Association (1997) developed the **Guidelines for Adolescent Preventive Services (GAPS),** which provide a framework for health care providers to use in their clinical practice. The following discussion provides in-

TABLE 16-1

Growth and Development During Adolescence

EARLY ADOLESCENCE (11-14 YEARS)	MIDDLE ADOLESCENCE (15-17 YEARS)	LATE ADOLESCENCE (18-20 YEARS)
GROWTH		
Rapidly accelerating growth	Growth decelerating in girls	Physically mature
Reaches peak velocity	Stature reaches 95% of adult height	Structure and reproductive growth almost complete
Secondary sex characteristics appear	Secondary sex characteristics well advanced	
COGNITION		
Explores newfound ability for limited abstract thought	Developing capacity for abstract thinking	Established abstract thought
Clumsy groping for new values and energies	Enjoys intellectual powers, often in idealistic terms	Can perceive and act on long-range options
Comparison of "normality" with peers of same sex	Concern with philosophic, political, and social problems	Able to view problems comprehensively
		Intellectual and functional identity established
IDENTITY		
Preoccupied with rapid body changes	Modifies body image	Body image and gender-role definition nearly secured
Trying out various roles	Very self-centered; increased narcissism	Mature sexual identity
Measurement of attractiveness by acceptance or rejection of peers	Tendency toward inner experience and self-discovery	Phase of consolidation of identity
Conformity to group norms	Has a rich fantasy life	Stability of self-esteem
	Idealistic	Comfortable with physical growth
	Able to perceive future implications of current behavior and decisions; variable application	Social roles defined and articulated
RELATIONSHIPS WITH PARENTS		
Defining independence-dependence boundaries	Major conflicts over independence and control	Emotional and physical separation from parents completed
Strong desire to remain dependent on parents while trying to detach	Low point in parent-child relationship	Independence from family with less conflict
No major conflicts over parental control	Greatest push for emancipation; disengagement	Emancipation nearly secured
	Final and irreversible emotional detachment from parents; mourning	
RELATIONSHIPS WITH PEERS		
Seeks peer affiliations to counter instability generated by rapid change	Strong need for identity to affirm self-image	Peer group recedes in importance in favor of individual friendship
Upsurge of close, idealized friendships with members of the same sex	Behavioral standards set by peer group	Testing of romantic relationships against possibility of permanent alliance
Struggle for mastery takes place within peer group	Acceptance by peers extremely important—fear of rejection	Relationships characterized by giving and sharing
	Exploration of ability to attract opposite sex	
SEXUALITY		
Self-exploration and evaluation	Multiple plural relationships	Forms stable relationships and attachment to another
Limited dating, usually group	Internal identification of heterosexual, homosexual, or bisexual attractions	Growing capacity for mutuality and reciprocity
Limited intimacy	Exploration of "self appeal"	Dating as a romantic pair
	Feeling of "being in love"	May publicly identify as gay, lesbian, or bisexual
	Tentative establishment of relationships	Intimacy involves commitment rather than exploration and romanticism
PSYCHOLOGIC HEALTH		
Wide mood swings	Tendency toward inner experiences; more introspective	More constancy of emotion
Intense daydreaming	Tendency to withdraw when upset or feelings are hurt	Anger more likely to be concealed
Anger outwardly expressed with moodiness, temper outbursts, and verbal insults and name-calling	Vacillation of emotions in time and range	
	Feelings of inadequacy common; difficulty in asking for help	

nursingcareguidelines

Interviewing Adolescents

- Ensure confidentiality and privacy; interview adolescent without parents.
- Show concern for adolescent's perspective: "First, I'd like to talk about your main concerns" and "I'd like to know what you think is happening."
- Offer a nonthreatening explanation for the questions you ask: "I'm going to ask a number of questions to help me better understand your health."
- Maintain objectivity; avoid assumptions, judgments, and lectures.
- Ask open-ended questions when possible; move to more directive questions if necessary.
- Begin with less sensitive issues and proceed to more sensitive ones.
- Use language that both the adolescent and you understand. Clarify terms, such as "having sex."
- Restate: reflect back to adolescents what they have said, along with feelings that may be associated with their descriptions.

???? CRITICAL THINKING EXERCISE

Respecting Privacy

Jamie, a 17-year-old girl, arrives at the adolescent clinic with her mother, Mrs. S., for a routine history and physical examination with the nurse practitioner. As the nurse practitioner walks with Jamie to an examination room, Mrs. S. whispers to the nurse practitioner, "I need to speak with you in private." How should the nurse practitioner respond to Mrs. S.'s request?

QUESTIONS

1. Evidence—Is there sufficient evidence to formulate a response to Jamie's mother?
2. Assumptions—Describe an underlying assumption about each of the following topics:
   a. The role of the adolescent in health care
   b. The role of the parents in the health of their adolescent
   c. Adolescents and confidentiality
3. What priorities or implications for nursing care should be established at this time?
4. Does the evidence support your conclusion?
5. Are there alternative perspectives that you should consider? What are they?

formation on specific GAPS topics and recommendations related to screening, guidance, and immunizations.

IMMUNIZATIONS

An immunization update is an important part of adolescent preventive care. Obtaining a record of the teenager's prior immunizations is important. Adolescents 11 to 18 years of age should receive a single tetanus-diphtheria–acellular pertussis (Tdap) vaccine if they have received the recommended childhood series of DTaP immunizations. This vaccine is now recommended because of the increased incidence of pertussis seen in adolescents and adults who were immunized with the

DTaP series as young children. The adolescent who has received Td but not Tdap vaccine should also receive a single dose of the Tdap vaccine provided 5 years have elapsed between the Td and Tdap vaccination (American Academy of Pediatrics, 2006). Meningococcal vaccine (MCV4) should be given to adolescents 11 to 12 years of age or at 15 years of age if previous immunization with MPSV4 occurred in childhood and at least 3 to 5 years have passed since primary immunization. The MCV4 vaccine is now preferred over the MPSV4 vaccine (American Academy of Pediatrics, 2008).

The human papillomavirus (HPV) vaccine series is recommended only for girls based on research results at this time. Additional recommendations may be made for boys if it is determined to be safe and effective. The series may be started as early as 9 years of age, with the second and third doses at 2 months and 6 months, respectively.

With the exception of pregnant teenagers, all adolescents should receive a second measles-mumps-rubella (MMR) vaccine unless they have documentation of two MMR vaccinations during childhood.

All adolescents who have not previously received three doses of hepatitis B vaccine should be vaccinated against hepatitis B virus. The hepatitis A vaccine should be given to all adolescents as part of the routine immunization schedule; the two-dose series may be completed in childhood, and a catch-up schedule for those who have not been previously immunized is recommended. Annual influenza vaccination with either the live attenuated influenza vaccine or trivalent influenza vaccine is now encouraged for all children and adolescents. All adolescents should also be assessed for previous history of varicella infection or vaccination. Vaccination with the varicella vaccine is recommended for those with no previous history; for those with no previous infection or history, the varicella vaccine may be given in two doses 4 or more weeks apart to adolescents 13 years or older (American Academy of Pediatrics, 2008). (See also Immunizations, Chapter 10.)

NUTRITION

The rapid and extensive increase in height, weight, muscle mass, and sexual maturity of adolescence is accompanied by increased nutritional requirements. Because nutritional needs are closely related to the increase in body mass, the peak requirements occur in the years of maximum growth, during which the body mass almost doubles. The caloric and protein requirements during this time are higher than at almost any other time of life. As a result of this increased anabolic need, the adolescent is highly sensitive to caloric restrictions.

Current guidelines for caloric intake are provided by a number of sources. The Dietary Reference Intakes (DRIs) provide age-specific guidelines for nutrients (see Chapter 6). Another guideline, which was recently developed by the American Heart Association (2005), aims at promoting balanced nutrient intake in children and adolescents with an overall decrease in fat intake and discretionary calories or snacks that increase the propensity for obesity and cardiovascular disease. Caloric intake can be tailored to meet the adolescent's increased growth needs as well as activity level such as involvement in sports. The guidelines also encourage limiting sweetened beverage consumption and moderating caloric intake to activity levels.

Adolescents usually have sufficient intake of protein to meet their needs, except for those who limit their food intake because of economic problems or in an attempt to lose weight. There is a substantial increase in the need for the minerals calcium, iron, and zinc during periods of rapid growth: calcium for skeletal growth, iron for expansion of muscle mass and blood volume, and zinc for the generation of both skeletal and bone tissue. Girls with heavy or frequent menses may be especially susceptible to iron deficiency resulting from blood loss. Calcium intake from food sources is essential during adolescence to assist in the prevention of osteoporosis. Eventual bone mass is a balance between the amount of bone laid down during adolescence and the amount later lost with aging. Overall, osteoporosis is a result of polygenic and multiple environmental factors such as nutrition, economics, and exercise (Ongphiphadhanakul, 2007). Dietary intervention should promote the regular consumption of breakfast and a balanced intake of a variety of foods.

Eating Habits and Behavior

Eating and attitudes toward food are primarily family centered during early and middle childhood, and food habits are largely related to cultural and individual family preferences and patterns. With adolescence and the move toward independence, family influences on the child diminish. Children's interests, attitudes, and routines are altered as an increasing number of meals are eaten away from home. These changes are largely a result of the high value that teenagers place on peer acceptability and sociability. Their peers easily influence their eating habits.

Pressure for time and commitments to activities adversely affect the teenager's eating habits. Omitting breakfast or eating a breakfast that is nutritionally poor in quality is frequently a problem. Snacks, usually selected on the basis of accessibility rather than nutritional merit, become more and more a part of the habitual eating pattern during adolescence (Fig. 16-7). Excess intake of calories, sugar, fat, cholesterol, and sodium is common among adolescents and is found in all income and racial or ethnic groups and both genders. Inadequate intake of certain vitamins (folic acid, vitamin B_6, vitamin A) and minerals (iron, calcium, zinc) is also evident, particularly among girls and teenagers of low socioeconomic status. In combination with other factors, these dietary patterns could result in increased risk for obesity and chronic diseases such as heart disease, osteoporosis, and some types of cancer later in life. Girls, in particular, may be susceptible to iron deficiency at menarche. Maximum bone mass is also acquired during adolescence; therefore the calcium deposited during these years determines the risk of osteoporosis. Milk is usually passed over in favor of soft drinks.

Overeating or undereating during adolescence presents special problems. When they experience the normal increase in weight and fat deposition of the growth spurt, teenage girls often resort to dieting. The desire for a slim figure and a fear of becoming "fat" prompt teenage girls to embark on nutritionally inadequate reducing regimens that drain their energy and deprive their growing bodies of essential nutrients. They resort to diets on their own or with peers in an effort to conform. Many adopt current fad diets and are victims of food misinformation. Boys are less inclined to undereat. They are more concerned about gaining size and strength. However, they tend to eat foods high in calories but low in other essential nutrients.

Obesity is increasing among both children and adolescents in the United States. The obesity currently seen is not a result

FIG. 16-7 ■ Snacking on empty calories is common among adolescents, especially during inactivity.

of metabolic disturbances, but of poor dietary habits and increasingly sedentary lifestyles. Childhood obesity often results in obesity in adulthood. Adolescent obesity poses both immediate and long-term problems for adolescents. Obesity is directly linked to the development of cardiovascular disease and other chronic illnesses such as diabetes. Anorexia nervosa and bulimia nervosa also commonly occur during the adolescent and young adult years. If left untreated, these disorders, like obesity, can lead to considerable morbidity and mortality. The past two decades have revealed an increase in the overall portion size of foods. The largest portions for most foods are found at fast-food restaurants. However, portion sizes for desserts and hamburgers are the largest at home (Nielsen and Popkin, 2003). Lifestyle changes necessary for adolescents to lose weight require the involvement of family members who provide support and encourage active participation.

Nursing Care Management

Adolescents should receive at a minimum an annual assessment of weight, height, and BMI for age, plotted on a standard growth chart. Healthy dietary habits should be discussed with all adolescents. The frequency of eating at fast-food and other restaurants, consumption of sweetened beverages, and consumption of excessive portion sizes should be identified. In addition to food intake, the nurse should assess the level of physical activity and sedentary behaviors. Readiness to change; environmental supports and barriers; and family history of diabetes, heart disease, and early stroke must be considered when planning nutritional education and guidance. Nurses in the school setting can assist in advocating for comprehensive nutritional services for preschool through grade 12 students. Comprehensive nutrition education with access to nutritious meals and snacks and physical activity at school will begin to reverse the trend of childhood obesity (Briggs, Safaii, and Beall, 2003).

To help teenagers select a nutritious diet, it is best to begin with their present diet and actively involve them in the process. Adolescents do not respond well to judgmental attitudes and dislike lectures, but they do respond when their independence is respected and they are given the opportunity to make their own decisions regarding food choices.

In general, adolescents are body conscious and concerned about their appearance. Concrete messages about the relationship between an attractive appearance and the benefits of a healthy lifestyle are most effective. However, helping young persons arrive at a decision for change is more difficult than providing information. They respond best when the counselor provides straightforward information, uses instructional methods that actively involve them, talks *with* them and not *at* them, and listens to what they have to say.

SLEEP AND REST

Teenagers vary in their need for sleep and rest. Rapid physical growth, the tendency toward overexertion, and the overall increased activity of this age contribute to fatigue in adolescents. During growth spurts the need for sleep is increased. Their propensity for staying up late makes it difficult to arise in the morning, and they may sleep late at every opportunity. Adequate sleep and rest at this time are important to a total health regimen.

EXERCISE AND ACTIVITY

Although today's youth are less fit than children 20 years ago, adolescents probably spend more time and energy practicing and participating in sports activities than members of any other age-group. Many adolescents participate in sports within school settings (Fig. 16-8). School-based, health-oriented physical education may provide both immediate effects of the activity and sustained effects through encouragement of lifelong activity patterns. High schools continue to cut physical education classes, with only half of high school students attending physical education classes in 2005. Less than half of students attended these classes daily, and the majority of classes included only 20 minutes of exercise (Centers for Disease Control and Prevention, 2006a). To improve health outcomes, school-age children and adolescents should engage in 60 minutes or more of moderate to vigorous physical activity daily (Strong, Malina, Blimkie, and others, 2005).

FIG. 16-8 ■ Adolescents should be encouraged to participate in activities that contribute to lifelong physical fitness.

The practice of sports, games, and even dancing contributes significantly to growth and development, the education process, and better health. These activities provide exercise for growing muscles, interactions with peers, and a socially acceptable means of enjoying stimulation and conflict. In addition, competitive activities help the teenager in the process of self-appraisal and the development of self-respect and concern for others. Because physical fitness appears to be a major influence on one's lifelong health status, children should be encouraged to participate in activities that contribute to lifelong physical fitness. Nurses can encourage participation as a way to promote health and build self-esteem. However, adolescents should not be encouraged to engage in physical activities that are beyond their physical or emotional capacity (see Health Problems Related to Sports Participation, Chapter 17).

DENTAL HEALTH

Dental health should not be neglected during adolescence, although the rate of caries formation is not as great as in childhood. Dental care is an aspect of preventive care that is not received by substantial proportions of children in the United States. Pit and fissure sealants are a safe and effective technique for dental caries prevention. Early adolescence is usually when corrective orthodontic appliances are worn, and these are frequently a source of embarrassment and concern to the youngster. Reassurance regarding the temporary nature of the annoyance and anticipation of an improved appearance help adolescents tolerate the inconvenience. It is also important to reinforce the orthodontist's directions regarding use and care of the appliances and to emphasize careful attention to toothbrushing during this time (see also Chapters 12 and 15).

PERSONAL CARE

The body-conscious teenager is highly amenable to discussion and counseling about personal care and hygiene. Body changes associated with puberty bring special needs for cleanliness. The hyperactive sebaceous glands and newly functioning apocrine glands make frequent bathing or showering a necessity, and underarm deodorants assume an important place in personal care. The adolescent discovers that hair requires more frequent shampooing, and girls often have questions about hair removal, use of cosmetics, and menstrual hygiene. Peer group discussions center on the advantages of particular products or methods. Adolescents are continually bombarded with messages from the media regarding the best way to enhance their popularity and attractiveness. Nurses are in a position to help them evaluate the relative merits of commercial products.

Vision

Regular vision testing is an important part of health care and supervision during adolescence. During adolescence, visual refractive difficulties reach a peak that is not exceeded until the fifth decade of life. The increased demands of schoolwork make adequate vision essential for academic success. Consequently, teenagers are more likely to be referred for visual evaluation. The need for corrective lenses can create psychologic problems for teenagers if they believe that glasses spoil their appearance or do not fit their body image. Contact lenses may be a preferred solution; a variety of lenses are now available at fairly reasonable prices. For some, the impact of a visual defect, no matter how slight, may be stressful.

Hearing

Considerable concern has focused on current teenage practices that cause hearing damage. Cochlear damage from relatively continuous exposure to the loud sound levels of rock music has been documented. The popularity of personal music players with lightweight earphones that are inserted into the ear canal is of particular concern to health care professionals. When these units are used for extended periods, permanent hearing loss can occur. Although appeals for more judicious use are not always successful, teenagers should be informed of the risk. Efforts directed toward legislating legal limits to the noise exposure that can be achieved through the sets may be another possible solution. (See Chapter 19 for a discussion of noise-related hearing loss.)

Posture

Many adolescents demonstrate altered posture. Rapid skeletal growth is often associated with slower muscular growth, and as a result, some teenagers may appear awkward or slump and fail to stand or sit upright. However, some postural defects of adolescence require early medical intervention. Scoliosis is a defect of the spine that occurs frequently in adolescence and is more common in girls than in boys (see Idiopathic Scoliosis, Chapter 31). The majority of the cases are idiopathic, and the defect manifests as a painless curvature of the spine. Fortunately, most of these spinal curvatures will not require treatment. However, because there is no way to predict which curvatures will progress, all curvatures of the spine should be referred for further evaluation.

Body Art

Body art (piercing and tattooing) is an aspect of adolescent identity formation. The skin has become the latest source of parent-adolescent conflict. The adolescent often seeks body art as an expression of his or her personal identity and style. Tattoos may mark significant life events such as new relationships, births, and deaths. Piercing the ear, nose, nipple, eyebrow, navel, penis, or tongue may sometimes create a health problem. It is a nursing responsibility to caution girls and boys against having piercing performed by friends, parents, or themselves. Although in most cases piercings have few if any serious side effects, there is always a danger of complications such as infection, cyst or keloid formation, bleeding, dermatitis, or metal allergy. Using the same unsterilized needle to pierce body parts of multiple teenagers presents the same risk of human immunodeficiency virus (HIV), hepatitis C, and hepatitis B virus transmission as occurs with other needle-sharing activities.

A qualified operator using proper sterile technique should perform the procedure. This is especially important if a youngster has a history of diabetes, allergies, or skin disorders. Adolescents should be informed about the approximate time for healing after body piercing and the care of the pierced area during and after healing. Some body sites need extra precautions. For example, cartilage (ear, nose) has a poor blood supply and heals slowly and scars easily; nipple piercing puts the adolescent at risk for breast abscess. Finally, migration of the piercing is common with naval and other flat skin surface piercing. Piercing guns should not be used for piercing anything other than the earlobe because guns place the piercing too deeply.

It is estimated that 3% to 5% of people in Western society have a tattoo and that 13% of the population in the United States has at least one tattoo. Studies of distinct populations of young adults and adolescents report body art rates as high as 23% (Braverman, 2006). Professionals as well as amateur artists administer tattoos. The risk to the adolescent receiving a tattoo is low. The greatest risk is for the tattoo artist who comes in contact with the client's blood. Adolescents who are amateur tattoo artists benefit from discussions about standard precautions and the hepatitis B vaccination. Many states either have no regulations or do not enforce existing regulations of piercing and tattooing facilities. The local health department is a source of information about local regulatory requirements. The Centers for Disease Control and Prevention has an excellent website that outlines safety concerns for persons performing and receiving body art.*

Tanning

The quest for an attractive appearance leads many teenagers to excessive sunbathing and artificial means for tanning. However, this practice has serious long-term risks, and the adolescent should be educated regarding the detrimental effects of sunlight on the skin (see Sunburn, Chapter 30). Long-term effects include premature aging of the skin, increased risk of skin cancer, and, in susceptible individuals, phototoxic reactions.

The increasing popularity of artificial tanning has prompted concern from health professionals regarding the use of sunlamps and tanning machines. The long-term effects of tanning machines are similar to those of the sun; dermatologists do not recommend suntanning by this means. Those who insist on using tanning equipment should be warned that goggles must be worn in tanning booths to prevent serious corneal burning. Education on the use of sunscreens, including hypoallergenic products, with a sun protective factor (SPF) of at least 15 and a nonalcohol base without lanolin, parabens, or fragrance, is important. Broad-spectrum sunscreens that protect against both ultraviolet A and B (UV-A and UV-B) are the most effective. Self-tanning creams safely stimulate the appearance of a tan; however, teens using these products should be cautioned that sun protection is still required. Targeting health education messages to adolescents and incorporating educational components relating to sun protection behaviors in school health curricula and in health care visits will increase adolescent knowledge and awareness.

STRESS REDUCTION

The multiple changes occurring in adolescence can result in great stress (Fig. 16-9 and Box 16-2). Adolescents are faced with pressures from peers that often involve taking serious health risks, including pressures for sexual experimentation; use of drugs, alcohol, and cigarettes; and potentially dangerous physical activities.

Early-maturing girls and late-maturing children are especially sensitive to the stresses of being different from their peers. Many feel intense anxiety over their identity. Both early- and late-maturing children feel out of place among their classmates, but slow-maturing children appear to suffer the most pronounced inner turmoil and may be hesitant to voice their concerns. Slow-maturing adolescents need support and reassurance that they are not abnormal and need only be patient until the time comes when they, too, will mature physically.

---

*http://www.cdc.gov/Features/BodyArt.

FIG. 16-9 ■ Adolescents use being alone as a method of coping with stress. Health care professionals need to assess whether this indicates clinical depression.

BOX 16-2

Areas of Stress in Adolescence

- Body image
- Sexuality conflicts
- Scholastic pressures
- Competitive pressures
- Relationships with parents
- Relationships with siblings
- Relationships with peers
- Finances
- Decisions about present and future roles
- Career planning
- Ideologic conflicts

SEXUALITY EDUCATION AND GUIDANCE

Contemporary adolescents are constantly exposed to sexual symbolism and erotic stimulation from the mass media. At the same time, the development of primary and secondary sex characteristics and the increased sensitivity of the genitalia produce thoughts and fantasies about sexual relationships. Sexual aspects of interpersonal relationships become particularly important. Societal expectations push adolescents toward dating, and their own inner sex drive urges them toward exploration.

Our society continues to do a poor job of educating adolescents about pubertal growth and development. Omar, McElderry, and Zakharia (2003) found that 36% of boys and 2% of girls had never been spoken to about pubertal development or sexuality issues. Girls received education at a mean age of 13 years and boys at an average age of 15 years. A large portion of their knowledge relating to sex is acquired from peers, television, movies, and magazines. In addition, some information obtained from their parents may be inaccurate. As a result, the information they accumulate may be incomplete, inaccurate, riddled with cultural and moral judgments, and not very helpful.

The responsibility for providing sexuality education has been assumed by parents, schools, churches, community agencies such as Planned Parenthood Federation of America, Inc.,* and health professionals, especially nurses. Many adolescents perceive nurses, especially school nurses, as individuals who possess important information and who are willing to discuss sex with them. To be able to discuss the topic adequately, nurses must have not only an understanding of the physiologic aspects of sexuality and a knowledge of cultural and societal values, but also an awareness of their own attitudes, feelings, and biases about sexuality.

Comprehensive information about sexuality education is offered by the Sexuality Information and Education Council of the United States (SIECUS)† and the Sex Information and Education Council of Canada.‡ SIECUS maintains that every sexuality education program should present the topic from six aspects: biologic, social, health, personal adjustments and attitudes, interpersonal associations, and the establishment of values.

Whether nurses counsel young people on an individual basis, in mixed groups, or in groups segregated by gender makes little difference. Ideally, boys and girls should be able to discuss sexuality objectively with one another and in groups, but this is not always possible. The differences in the rate of maturation between boys and girls and between different members of the same sex often make it desirable to discuss certain aspects of sexuality in segregated groups. As a rule, the need for separate discussion groups diminishes as young people mature.

Sexuality education should consist of instruction concerning normal body functions and should be presented in a straightforward manner using correct terminology. When discussing sex and sexual activities, nurses should use simple but correct language, not street language, highly scientific terminology, or evasive jargon. Once they understand the meaning of biologic terms such as *uterus, testicles,* and *vagina,* most teenagers prefer to use them in their discussions.

Many girls arrive at menarche with ambivalent attitudes, myths, and illogical beliefs. Even girls adequately prepared for menstruation do not always understand its relationship to the total process of reproduction. Many are under the incorrect impression that the "safe" time for sexual intercourse is midway between menstrual periods.

Teenagers' curiosity and desire for information extend beyond the need for anatomic and physiologic knowledge. They need to know more than the mechanics of conception, pregnancy, and birth. Adolescents, girls in particular, want answers to questions such as "What is it like?" "Does it hurt?" "What happens when . . . ?" and "Is it all right if you . . . ?" Boys are often concerned about the fallacy that a relationship exists between penis size and sexual function. They need reassurance that masturbation is a normal and common practice, that some degree of homosexuality in early adolescence is not unusual, and that oral-genital relations can be normal substitutes for intercourse.

Teenagers need to discuss intercourse, alternative methods of sexual satisfaction, and how to resist peer pressure. With the

---

*434 West 33rd St., New York, NY 10001; (212) 541-7800; http://www.plannedparenthood.org.

†130 West 42nd St., Suite 350, New York, NY 10036; (212) 819-9770; http://www.siecus.org.

‡850 Coxwell Ave., Toronto, Ontario M4C 5R1; (416) 466-5304; http://www.sieccan.org.

BOX 16-3

Injury Prevention During Adolescence

DEVELOPMENTAL ABILITIES RELATED TO RISK OF INJURY

Need for independence and freedom

Testing independence

Age permitted to drive a motor vehicle (varies from state to state)

Inclination for risk taking

Feeling of indestructibility

Need for discharging energy, often at expense of logical thinking and other control mechanisms

Strong need for peer approval

Attempting hazardous feats

Peak incidence for practice and participation in sports

Access to more complex tools, objects, and locations

Can assume responsibility for own actions

INJURY PREVENTION

Motor or Nonmotor Vehicles

Pedestrian—Emphasize and encourage safe pedestrian behavior.
- At night, walk with a friend.
- If someone is following you, go to nearest place with people.
- Do not walk in secluded areas; take well-traveled walkways.

Passenger—Promote appropriate behavior while riding in a motor vehicle. Refuse to ride with an impaired person or one who is driving recklessly.

Driver—Provide competent driver education; encourage judicious use of vehicle; discourage drag racing or "playing chicken"; maintain vehicle in proper condition (brakes, tires, etc.).

Teach and promote safety and maintenance of two- and three-wheeled vehicles.

Promote and encourage wearing of safety apparel such as helmet, long trousers.

Reinforce the dangers of drugs, including alcohol, when operating a motor vehicle.

Drowning

Teach nonswimmer to swim.

Teach basic rules of water safety.
- Judicious selection of place to swim
- Sufficient water depth for diving
- Swimming with companion

Burns

Reinforce proper behavior in areas with burn hazards (gasoline, electric wires, fires).

Advise regarding excessive exposure to natural or artificial sunlight (ultraviolet burn).

Discourage smoking.

Encourage use of sunscreen.

Poisoning

Educate in hazards of drug use, including alcohol.

Falls

Teach and encourage general safety measures in all activities.

Bodily Damage

Promote acquisition of proper instruction in sports and use of sports equipment.

Instruct in safe use of and respect for firearms and other devices with potential danger (e.g., power tools, firecrackers).

Provide and encourage use of protective equipment when using potentially hazardous devices.

Promote access to or provision of safe sports and recreational facilities.

Be alert for signs of depression (potential suicide).

Discourage use of hazardous sports equipment (e.g., trampoline, surfboards).

Instruct regarding proper use of corrective devices (e.g., glasses, contact lenses, hearing aids).

Encourage and foster judicious application of safety principles and prevention.

---

increased incidence of sexually transmitted diseases, especially HIV infection, the topic of "safe sex," especially abstinence or the use of condoms, is essential. Role-playing can help teenagers learn effective approaches to dealing with difficult situations. Sex and sexuality cannot be taught without discussions of mature decision making, sexual responsibility, and values clarification. Adolescents may receive inaccurate and ambiguous messages regarding sexual behavior; for example, an adolescent may be told that abstinence from vaginal intercourse will prevent transmission of a sexually transmitted disease. Accurate and unbiased information regarding sexual practices should be provided in a setting wherein the adolescent feels comfortable asking questions without being degraded or made to feel uncomfortable for seeking information.

Adolescents need role models and life experiences with delayed gratification. Most important, they need problem-solving experience and decision-making skills so that they can anticipate the positive and negative outcomes of a decision. With this type of assistance, teenagers can become sexually responsible young adults.

INJURY PREVENTION

Physical injuries are the greatest single cause of death in the adolescent age-group and claim more lives than all other causes combined. The most vulnerable ages are the years 15 to 24, when accidental injuries account for about 60% of deaths in boys and 40% of deaths in girls. These figures remain fairly constant from year to year and are significant because almost all fatal injuries are preventable.

During adolescence, peak physical, sensory, and psychomotor function gives teenagers a feeling of strength and confidence that they have never experienced before, and the physiologic changes of puberty give impetus to many basic instinctual forces. One manifestation of this is an increase in energy that simply must be discharged through action, often at the expense of logical thinking and other control mechanisms. Their propensity for risk-taking behavior plus feelings of indestructibility makes adolescents especially prone to injuries. Some of the developmental characteristics of teenagers and injury prevention suggestions are outlined in Box 16-3.

Motor Vehicle–Related Injuries

The adolescent's newly acquired ability to drive and the normal developmental need for independence and freedom make the automobile an attractive part of an adolescent's life. Thirty-six percent of all teen deaths in the United States are the result of motor vehicle crashes (Centers for Disease Control and Prevention, 2006b). Many factors contribute to the higher rate of crashes among teen drivers, including lacking driving experience and maturity, following too closely, driving too fast, having other teen passengers in the car, and using alcohol (Williams and Ferguson, 2002). Because of the significant increase in the number of accidents when adolescents drive at night, many states have effectively enacted driving curfews, decreasing fatal crashes by 38% and crashes involving injury by 40% for adolescents (Baker, Chen, and Li, 2007).

Nurses should educate teenagers and their parents about the risk of driving while drinking alcohol or of riding in an automobile with a drunk driver. Many families arrange a no-questions-asked ride home to prevent an adolescent from riding with a drunk driver. Families should also require adolescents to log several hours of supervised practice driving before taking the car out alone. The major risk for death in a motor vehicle accident is failure to use a safety restraint. Teenage seatbelt use, especially among boys, is lower than adult seat belt use. Belt use as a passenger is low for adolescents even when the driver is an adult. Continued efforts to ensure teenage seat belt use should be focused at the individual educational level and through tough enforcement laws (Williams, McCartt, and Geary, 2003).

Other Vehicle Injuries. The increasing use of motorcycles, all-terrain vehicles (ATVs), jet skis, and snowmobiles has caused an increase in injuries among young people who are below the legal age for driving automobiles. Many adolescents ride bicycles without helmets and without lights at night, and the overwhelming majority of deaths from bicycle injuries (primarily head injuries) involve teenagers.

Firearms

Firearms are the major cause of intentional fatal injuries in the United States. Adolescence is the peak age for being either a victim or an offender in an injury involving a firearm. Gun carrying among adolescents is on the rise and is not limited to the stereotypic inner-city youth. Family members and acquaintances are a common source of guns for young people. Gun availability in the home is strongly linked to unintentional death and injury to children (Glatt, 2005). In addition, the presence of a gun in the home increases the risk of adolescent suicide and homicide. All families should be assessed for the presence of a gun in the home and informed of this risk. They must take preventive action to ensure that the guns are never loaded, that they are locked up in a safe place, and that ammunition is stored and locked up separately in a location accessible only to appropriate adults.

Nonpowder Firearms. Guns that do not use powder (e.g., air rifles, BB guns), although viewed as toys by many, account for almost as many injuries as powder guns. The regulations regarding nonpowder guns are relaxed; they can be purchased legally by adolescents and are labeled as suitable for children as young as 8 years of age. Few states regulate their use. Nurses should act as child advocates and urge passage of laws to regulate the sale of these potentially dangerous "toys."

Sports Injuries

Because the degree of physical maturation, size, coordination, and endurance varies greatly among adolescents of the same age, sports competition between young people who differ greatly in strength and agility is unfair and hazardous. Matching candidates for sports should be done relative to physical maturity, height, weight, and physical fitness and skills, particularly in a sport involving rigorous body contact. Age is a less important consideration.

Every sport has some potential for injury, whether one participates in serious competition or engages in the activity for pure enjoyment. Overuse injuries are common in adolescents and result in more time missed from the activity than fractures. A large number of severe or fatal injuries occur to youths who are not physically prepared for the activity. The increase in strength and vigor in adolescence may tempt adolescents to overextend themselves, especially boys who are urged on by teammates or are stimulated by the admiration of female observers. Injuries sustained in sports or recreational activities can involve any part of the body and range from relatively minor cuts, bruises, and abrasions to totally incapacitating central nervous system injuries or death. The leading cause of serious sports injuries among boys is participation in football, whereas most girls are injured while participating in gymnastics.

Nursing Care Management

Injury prevention is an ongoing part of nursing responsibility throughout the childhood years. Anticipatory guidance to parents and children regarding the expected problems and hazards related to growth and development does not end as children approach maturity. They need education in basic safety precautions, instruction in skills required in the performance of activities such as sports, instruction in handling motor vehicles, and information about using proper protective equipment and properly maintaining equipment. During adolescence, however, health and safety education and guidance are more effective when the young people are involved directly. Parents and health professionals can emphasize the importance of safety during performance of activities and the proper conditioning and preparation for sports.

Prevention can occur on a variety of levels. Safety advocacy, public policy changes, and legislation can curtail injuries. Examples of such approaches are laws that mandate wearing seat belts, using helmets while driving moving vehicles other than automobiles, keeping the legal drinking age at 21 years, and instituting curfews for teen drivers. In addition to improvements in the environment, health education for teenagers and significant adults is essential. Helping adolescents understand their need for engaging in risky behavior, exploring possible negative outcomes, and weighing possible alternatives are critical components of injury prevention.

ANTICIPATORY GUIDANCE—CARE OF FAMILIES

Both adolescents and their parents are often confused and perplexed about the changes and behavior of this stage of development. Parents need support and guidance to help them through this trying time. They need to understand the changes taking place and to accept the expected behaviors that accompany the process of detachment. Parents may need help to "let go" and to promote the changed relationship from one of dependence to one of mutuality (see Family-Centered Care and Family Focus boxes).

FAMILY-CENTERED CARE

Guidance During Adolescence

ENCOURAGE PARENTS TO:

Accept adolescent as a unique individual.

Respect adolescent's ideas, likes and dislikes, and wishes.

Be involved with school functions and attend adolescent's performances, whether it be a sporting event or a school play.

Listen and try to be open to teenager's views, even when they disagree with parental views.

Avoid criticism about no-win topics.

Provide opportunity for choosing options and accept natural consequences of these choices.

Allow young persons to learn by doing, even when choices and methods differ from those of adults.

Provide adolescent with clear, reasonable limits.

Clarify house rules and consequences for breaking them. Adhere to the rules (even though it hurts!!).

Let society's rules and consequences teach responsibility outside the home.

Allow increasing independence within limitations of safety and well-being.

Be available but avoid pressing teenager too far.

Respect adolescent's privacy.

Try to share adolescent's feelings of joy or sorrow.

Respond to feelings, as well as words.

Be available to answer questions, give information, and provide companionship.

Try to make communication clear.

Avoid comparisons with siblings.

Assist adolescent in selecting appropriate career goals and preparing for adult role.

Welcome adolescent's friends into the home and treat them with respect.

Provide unconditional love and acceptance.

Be willing to apologize when mistaken.

BE AWARE THAT ADOLESCENTS:

Are subject to turbulent, unpredictable behavior.

Are struggling for independence.

Are extremely sensitive to feelings and behavior that affect them.

May receive a different message from what was sent.

Consider friends extremely important.

Have a strong need "to belong."

FAMILY FOCUS

Family Rules for Adolescents

U.S. society does little to help adolescents mature and separate. Americans have remarkably few rites of passage that mark the stages of life. Few ceremonies and tests are practiced to determine eligibility for specific adult privileges. Obtaining a driver's license, graduating from high school, and reaching legal age for drinking are among the few milestones that exist. U.S. society also does not have many generally agreed-on social dictums. When is the right age to begin dating? What is a reasonable curfew? Should an 18-year-old be allowed to stay out all night? There are few areas of general agreement. Every family makes up its own rules, influenced, but uninstructed, by the society at large. Many families have great difficulty with this process.

Modified from Prothrow-Stith D: *Deadly consequences: how violence is destroying our teenage population and a plan to begin solving the problem*, New York, 1993, HarperCollins.

KEY POINTS

- Adolescence is considered as beginning with the gradual appearance of secondary sex characteristics at about 11 or 12 years of age and ending with cessation of body growth at 18 to 20 years.

- Biologic development during puberty is characterized by increased activity of the pituitary gland, which results in sexual maturity and the appearance of secondary sex characteristics.

- According to Erikson, the major developmental crisis of adolescence is establishing a sense of identity.

- Cognitive development in adolescence includes abstract thought, thinking beyond the present, logical reasoning, and a sense of idealism.

- Development of body image is closely tied to body changes and social interactions.

- According to Kohlberg's theory of moral development, adolescents begin to question existing moral values and learn to make choices.

- Spiritual development is characterized by the questioning of family values and ideals, a move to more philosophic thinking, and emphasis on personal religion.

- Adolescent relationships with parents may be strained, whereas the influence of the peer group increases and intimate relationships assume importance.

- Teenagers demonstrate a wide variety of interests, and their increased physical and cognitive skills allow them to engage in increasingly difficult and complex activities.

- Adolescents' emotions fluctuate.

- Nutritional needs, especially for calcium, zinc, and iron, may not be met by teenagers' eating habits, such as snacking and irregular mealtimes.

- Motor vehicle injuries are the primary cause of death from injury in the adolescent years.

answers to
CRITICAL THINKING EXERCISES

DISCUSSING THE FUTURE

1. Yes, there is sufficient information to arrive at a conclusion about what advice to give Jeremy's mother.

2. a. During adolescence, teens consider all their past relationships as they attempt to form their own personal identity. They attempt to formulate a satisfactory identity from a multiplicity of roles, aspirations, and identifications. The process of developing this identity is time-consuming and can be associated with confusion and discouragement.

   b. If significant others are too persistent and demand that adolescents make specific decisions or behave in definite ways, adolescents often make premature decisions and accept roles that do not incorporate their own personal goals or aspirations.

   c. Parents who communicate well with their teens have an open, nonjudgmental, nondictatorial manner. They demonstrate that they are available and willing to listen to their teenagers. However, they also wait until the teenager opens the discussion, and then they listen attentively and allow the teen to explore issues.

3. The nursing priority in this situation is to have the mother become more aware that Jeremy is not likely to discuss his concerns on a timetable, and that it is important for her to respect his point of view. Although Jeremy wants his mother's guidance and support, he does not want to be told what to do, and he needs an opportunity to express his own feelings and views. An example of appropriate advice to give Jeremy's mother might be: "Be open and available to Jeremy. Tell him what you think, but *not what to do.*"

4. Yes, the information about how teens formulate a personal identity and the principles of effective parent communication allow the nurse to formulate this response.

5. If Jeremy's mother changes her behavior and Jeremy still does not want to communicate and continues to withdraw from conversation, after a significant time the nurse might explore the possibility of counseling for Jeremy and his mother. Jeremy could be suffering from depression or some other condition that causes him to withdraw from conversation and interaction with his mother.

DISCUSSING SEXUAL ORIENTATION WITH ADOLESCENTS

1. No, there are insufficient data to arrive at a conclusion about John's sexual orientation. Further discussion with him is necessary before making any assumptions.

2. a. Studies of gay men and lesbians indicate that adolescence is the time when individuals become aware of same-sex attraction. Homosexual and bisexual youths are at risk for health-damaging behaviors such as early initiation of sexual behavior, substance abuse, suicide, and running away from home.

   b. Homosexual and bisexual youths are often confronted with the antihomosexual attitudes and values of society. It is this reaction of society that makes it difficult for homosexual and bisexual youths to grow up and become healthy physically and mentally.

   c. Health professionals who work with adolescents should consider the adolescent's increasing independence and responsibility while ensuring confidentiality.

3. The nurse's first priority in this situation is to give John permission to discuss his feelings about this topic. He has come to the nurse practitioner to discuss this matter, and he probably feels comfortable sharing this information with her. The nurse practitioner needs to be open and nonjudgmental in her interactions with John. He needs to know that the nurse practitioner will maintain confidentiality, ap-

preciate his feelings, and remain sensitive to his need to talk about this topic. An example of an appropriate response for the nurse practitioner might be: "John, tell me more about how you came to this conclusion."

4. Yes, the information about sexual orientation in adolescence and the role of the health care professional support this conclusion.

5. It might be appropriate for the nurse to gather information about John's support system and to determine the attitudes and values of John's family and peer group toward homosexuality. In addition to establishing a trusting relationship and effective communications with John, the nurse practitioner should make certain that John has a safe environment.

RESPECTING PRIVACY

1. Yes, there is sufficient evidence for the nurse to formulate a response to Jamie's mother.

2. a. As teenagers progress through adolescence, they are able to assume more responsibility for their own health. They can take prescribed medications, keep health care appointments, and discuss their care with health care professionals.

   b. Parents of adolescents should respect their teenager's independence while maintaining some level of involvement with their child. However, in matters of health care, they should gradually assume the role of a consultant and allow their child to take an increasingly active role in relating to health professionals.

   c. Health professionals who work with adolescents must consider the adolescent's increasing independence and responsibility while also maintaining privacy and ensuring confidentiality. In most adolescent clinics, health care professionals meet with the adolescent and the parent together, followed by individual time with both the adolescent and the parent.

3. The first priority for nursing care at this point is to reassure both Jamie and her mother that they will each have an opportunity to express their concerns to the nurse practitioner. Because Jamie is the nurse practitioner's patient and the setting is an adolescent clinic, the nurse practitioner should speak with Jamie first, after he or she has met briefly with Jamie and her mother together. An appropriate response by the nurse practitioner might be: "I would like to begin by speaking with both of you together, then spend some time with just you, Jamie, then with just you, Mrs. S." Knowing that her mother will also have an opportunity to express concerns, Jamie will likely be more open and may even say, "I know what my mother will tell you," and address the issue herself. This response will also demonstrate to Jamie that the nurse practitioner respects her privacy and will maintain confidentiality. If the nurse speaks with Jamie first, Jamie might think that her privacy is being violated and become distrustful of both the nurse practitioner and her mother. In addition, if the nurse practitioner speaks with Mrs. S. first, Jamie is likely to become defensive and spend her time trying to draw from the nurse practitioner what her mother said.

4. Yes, the information about adolescent growth and development and the roles of adolescents, their parents, and the health care professional support this conclusion.

5. The nurse practitioner should remember the circumstances under which she or he would not be able to maintain confidentiality. For example, if either Jamie or her mother share information indicating that Jamie is at risk for either self-destructive behavior (e.g., a suicide attempt) or maltreatment by others (child abuse), the nurse practitioner would not be able to maintain confidentiality. However, this does not seem to be the case based on the evidence presented at this point.

REFERENCES

Abma JC, Martinez GM, Mosher WE, and others: Teenagers in the United States: sexual activity, contraceptive use, and childbearing, 2002, *Vital Health Stats* 23(24):1-48, 2004.

American Academy of Pediatrics, Committee on Infectious Diseases: Recommended immunization schedules for children and adolescents—United States, 2008, *Pediatrics* 121(1):219-220, 2008.

American Academy of Pediatrics, Committee on Infectious Diseases, Pickering L, editor: *Red book: 2006 report of the Committee on Infectious Diseases,* ed 27, Elk Grove Village, Ill, 2006, The Academy.

American Heart Association: *Dietary recommendations for children and adolescents,* 2005, retrieved Jan 24, 2008, from http://www.americanheart.org/presenter.jhtml?identifier=3033999.

American Medical Association: *Guidelines for Adolescent Preventive Services (GAPS),* Chicago, 1997, The Association.

Baker SP, Chen L, Li G: *Nationwide review of graduated driver licensing,* Washington, DC, 2007, AAA Foundation for Traffic Safety.

Biro FM, Lucky AW, Simbarti LA, and others: Pubertal maturation in girls and the relationship to anthropometric changes: pathways through puberty, *J Pediatr* 142(6):643-646, 2003.

Bond L, Butler H, Thomas L, and others: Social and school connectedness in early secondary school as predictors of late teenage substance use, mental health, and academic outcomes, *J Adolesc Health* 40(4):357.e9-357.e18, 2007.

Braverman PK: Body art: piercing, tattooing, and scarification, *Adolesc Med* 17:505-519, 2006.

Briggs M, Safaii S, Beall DL: Nutrition services: an essential component of comprehensive school health programs, *J Am Diet Assoc* 103(4):505-514, 2003.

Brown J: Body and spirit: religion, spirituality and health among adolescents, *Adolesc Med* 12(3):509-523, 2001.

Centers for Disease Control and Prevention: *Welcome to WISQARS,* 2006b, retrieved Jan 24, 2008, from http://www.cdc.gov/ncipc/wisqars.

Centers for Disease Control and Prevention: Youth risk behavior surveillance—United States, 2005, *MMWR* 55(SS-5):1-108, 2006a.

Costello EJ, Sung, M, Worthman C, and others: Pubertal maturation and the development of alcohol use and abuse, *Drug Alcohol Depend* 88(4 Suppl 1):S50-S59, 2007.

DeVore ER, Ginsburg KR: The protective effects of good parenting on adolescents, *Curr Opin Pediatr* 17(4):460-465, 2005.

Gance-Cleveland B: Motivational interviewing: improving patient education, *J Pediatr Health* 21(2):81-88, 2007.

Glatt K: Child-to-child unintentional injury and death from firearms in the United States: what can be done? *J Pediatr Nurs* 10(6):448-452, 2005.

Lynne SD, Graber JA, Nichols TR, and others: Links between pubertal timing, peer influences and externalizing behaviors among urban students followed through middle school, *J Adolesc Health* 40(2):181.e7-13, 2007.

Maes L, Lievens J: Can the school make a difference? A multilevel analysis of adolescent risk and health behaviour, *Soc Sci Med* 56(3):517-529, 2003.

Mosher WD, Chandra A, Jones J: Sexual behavior and selected health measures: men and women 15-44 years of age, United States, 2002, *Adv Data,* Sep 15(362):1-55, 2005.

Nielsen SJ, Popkin BM: Patterns and trends in food portion sizes, 1977-1998, *JAMA* 289(4):450-453, 2003.

Omar H, McElderry D, Zakharia R: Educating adolescents about puberty: what are we missing? *Int J Adolesc Med Health* 15(1):79-83, 2003.

Ongphiphadhanakul B: Osteoporosis: the role of genetics and the environment, *Forum Nutr* 60:158-167, 2007.

Saewyc EM, Bearinger LH, Heinz PA, and others: Gender differences in health and risk behaviors among bisexual and homosexual adolescents, *J Adolesc Health* 23(3):181-188, 1998.

Santelli JS, Lindberg LD, Finer LB, and others: Explaining recent declines in adolescent pregnancy in the United States: the contribution of abstinence and improved contraceptive use, *Am J Pub Health* 97(1):150-156, 2007.

Strong WB, Malina RM, Blimkie CJ, and others: Evidence based physical activity for school-aged youth, *J Pediatr* 146:732-737, 2005.

Tuttle J, Campbell-Heider N, David TM: Positive adolescent life skills training for high-risk teens: results of a group intervention study, *J Pediatr Health* 20(3):184-191, 2006.

Williams AF, Ferguson SA: Rationale for graduated licensing and the risks it should address, *Inj Prevent* 6:9-16, 2002

Williams AF, McCartt AF, Geary L: Seatbelt use by high school students, *Inj Prevent* 9:25-28, 2003.

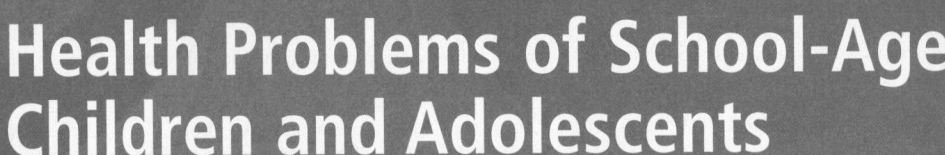

Health Problems of School-Age Children and Adolescents

LINDA M. KOLLAR AND DAVID WILSON

CHAPTER OUTLINE

PROBLEMS RELATED TO ELIMINATION, 537
Enuresis, 537
Encopresis, 538
HEALTH PROBLEMS RELATED TO SPORTS PARTICIPATION, 538
Overuse Syndromes, 538
  Stress Fractures, 539
Nurse's Role in Sports for Children and Adolescents, 539
ALTERED GROWTH AND MATURATION, 540
Sex Chromosome Disorders, 540
  Turner Syndrome, 540
  Klinefelter Syndrome, 540
DISORDERS RELATED TO THE REPRODUCTIVE SYSTEM, 541
Amenorrhea, 541
Dysmenorrhea, 541

Vaginitis, 542
Disorders of the Male Reproductive System, 542
Gynecomastia, 543
HEALTH PROBLEMS RELATED TO SEXUALITY, 543
Adolescent Pregnancy, 543
Contraception, 544
Sexually Transmitted Diseases, 547
Pelvic Inflammatory Disease, 547
Sexual Assault (Rape), 549
  Rape Trauma Syndrome, 550
EATING DISORDERS, 551
Obesity, 551
Anorexia Nervosa and Bulimia Nervosa, 556
DISORDERS WITH BEHAVIORAL COMPONENTS, 559
Attention Deficit Hyperactivity Disorder and Learning Disability, 559

Posttraumatic Stress Disorder, 562
School Phobia, 562
Recurrent Abdominal Pain, 562
Conversion Reaction, 563
Childhood Depression, 563
Childhood Schizophrenia, 564
SERIOUS HEALTH PROBLEMS OF LATER CHILDHOOD AND ADOLESCENCE, 564
Substance Abuse, 564
  Motivation, 564
  Types of Drugs Abused, 565
Suicide, 568
  Methods, 569
  Motivation, 570

LEARNING OBJECTIVES

On completion of this chapter the reader will be able to:
- Outline a care plan for the child or adolescent with a health problem.
- Demonstrate an understanding of the types, causes, and prevention of sports injuries in middle childhood and adolescence.

- Describe the most common causes of physical growth or maturation failure in later childhood.
- Demonstrate an understanding of common disorders of the male and female reproductive systems.
- Demonstrate an understanding of health problems related to adolescent sexuality.

- Outline a plan for discussing sexuality issues with adolescents.
- Outline a care plan for the child or adolescent with an eating disorder.
- Discuss the manifestations and nursing management of selected emotional or behavioral problems.

RELATED TOPICS and ADDITIONAL RESOURCES

 IN TEXT

Acne, *Ch. 30*
Congenital Anomalies, *Ch. 9*
Drug-Exposed Infants, *Ch. 9*
Growth Failure (Failure to Thrive), *Ch. 11*
Health Promotion of the Adolescent and
  Family, *Ch. 16*
Health Promotion of the School-Age Child
  and Family, *Ch. 15*
Human Immunodeficiency Virus and
  Acquired Immunodeficiency Syndrome,
  Ch. 26
Hypopituitarism, *Ch. 29*
Infection Control, *Ch. 22*

Obstructive Sleep-Disordered Breathing,
  Ch. 23
Physical Examination, *Ch. 6*
Precocious Puberty, *Ch. 29*
Sexual Abuse, *Ch. 14*
Traumatic Injury, *Ch. 31*

 COMPANION CD

Case Studies—Attention Deficit
  Hyperactivity Disorder; Teen Smoking
Critical Thinking Exercises—Obesity;
  Depression; Turner Syndrome
NCLEX Review Questions

 evolve

evolve.elsevier.com/Wong/essentials/

Critical Thinking Case Study—Obesity
NCLEX Review Questions
Nursing Care Plan—The Adolescent with an
  Eating Disorder
WebLinks

**WONG'S CLINICAL MANUAL
OF PEDIATRIC NURSING, 7th Ed**

Nursing Care Plan—The Adolescent with an
  Eating Disorder, *p. 395*

PROBLEMS RELATED TO ELIMINATION

ENURESIS

Enuresis (bed-wetting), or nocturnal enuresis, is a common and troublesome disorder that is defined as intentional or involuntary passage of urine into bed (usually at night) in children who are beyond the age when voluntary bladder control should normally have been acquired. The inappropriate voiding of urine must occur at least twice a week for at least 3 months, and the chronologic or developmental age of the child must be at least 5 years. The predominant symptom is urgency that is immediate and accompanied by acute discomfort, restlessness, and urinary frequency. Enuresis is more common in boys; nocturnal bed-wetting usually ceases between 6 and 8 years of age. Enuresis can also be defined as primary (bed-wetting in children who have never been dry for extended periods) or secondary (the onset of wetting after a period of established urinary continence). The passage of urine may occur only during nighttime sleep with the child remaining dry during the day (monosymptomatic); or it may be polysymptomatic, wherein the child has daytime urinary urgency, an occasional daytime accident, in conjunction with other conditions such as sleep apnea, urinary tract infection, neurologic impairment, constipation, or emotional stressors (Berry, 2006). The nocturnal, monosymptomatic type is most common. The condition may be particularly distressing to adolescents, who may refuse therapy. Although enuresis may occur during the daytime, the following discussion primarily focuses on nocturnal enuresis.

Before psychogenic factors are considered, organic causes that may be related to enuresis should be ruled out. These include structural disorders of the urinary tract; urinary tract infection; neurologic deficits; disorders that increase the normal output of urine, such as diabetes; and disorders that impair the concentrating ability of the kidneys, such as chronic renal failure or sickle cell disease. A bladder volume of 300 to 350 ml (10 to 12 ounces) is sufficient to hold a night's urine. Normal bladder capacity (in ounces) is the child's age plus 2. In other cases the enuresis is influenced by emotional factors, although it is doubtful that they are causative factors. Parents

report that these children sleep more soundly than other children; however, the depth of sleep has not been identified as the cause of nocturnal enuresis (Berry, 2006). Nocturnal enuresis has a strong familial tendency.

Therapeutic techniques used to manage nocturnal enuresis include medications, bladder training, restriction or elimination of fluids after the evening meal, interruption of sleep to void, and various devices designed to establish a conditioned reflex response to waken the child at the initiation of voiding (alarms).

Three types of drugs are used to treat enuresis: tricyclic antidepressants, antidiuretics, and anticholinergics. A drug used frequently to inhibit urination is the tricyclic antidepressant imipramine. Another anticholinergic drug, oxybutynin, reduces uninhibited bladder contractions and may be helpful for children with daytime urinary frequency. Desmopressin (DDAVP) nasal spray, an analog of vasopressin, reduces nighttime urinary output to a volume less than functional bladder capacity. Drugs are usually considered second-line management, and parents should be cautioned not to think that these agents will cure the condition; parents are also advised of the drug's side effects (Sethi, Bhargava, and Shipra, 2005).

Nursing Care Management

Regardless of the techniques used, the nurse can help both children and parents understand the problem of enuresis, the treatment plan, and the difficulties they may encounter in the process. The nurse can also provide consistent support and encouragement to help sustain both the child and the parents through the inconsistent and unpredictable treatment process. Parents need to understand that punishment is contraindicated because of its negative emotional impact and limited success in reducing the behavior. Positive reinforcement of the desired behavior may be beneficial (Sethi, Bhargava, and Shipra, 2005). Children need to believe that they are helping themselves, and they need to sustain feelings of confidence and hope.

Parents should also be taught to observe for side effects of any medications used. All children with primary enuresis should be encouraged to void before bedtime. Diapering should be avoided. Positive reinforcement in the form of keeping diaries to record dry nights has been effective in motivating children.

ENCOPRESIS

Encopresis is the repeated voluntary or involuntary passage of feces of normal or near-normal consistency in places not appropriate for that purpose according to the individual's own sociocultural setting. The event must occur at least once per month for at least 3 months, and the chronologic or developmental age of the child must be at least 4 years. The fecal incontinence must not be caused by any physiologic effect, such as a laxative, or a general medical condition.

Primary encopresis is identified by age 4 when the child has not achieved fecal continence. **Secondary encopresis** is fecal incontinence occurring in a child older than 4 years of age after a period of established fecal continence. The disorder is more common in boys than in girls.

One of the most common causes of encopresis is constipation, which may be precipitated by environmental change. Chronic, severe constipation has a tendency to impair the usual movement and contractions of the colon, which can lead to fecal obstruction. Abnormalities in the digestive tract (e.g., Hirschsprung disease, anorectal lesions, malformations, and rectal prolapse) and medical conditions such as hypothyroidism, hypokalemia, hypercalcemia, lead intoxication, myelomeningocele, cerebral palsy, muscular dystrophy, and irritable bowel syndrome are also associated with constipation, which can lead to encopresis (Coughlin, 2003). Children with encopresis often feel ashamed and may wish to avoid situations that might lead to embarrassment. School performance and attendance are affected as the child's offensive odor becomes a target for scorn and ridicule from classmates.

Therapeutic management consists of determining the cause of the soiling and using appropriate interventions to correct the problem. Diet, lubricants, and a toilet ritual that encourages the child to establish normal defecation are used. Fecal impaction is relieved by lubricants such as mineral oil; osmotic laxatives such as lactulose, sorbitol, or polyethylene glycol (PEG or MiraLAX); and magnesium hydroxide. Customary dosages are usually insufficient. Mineral oil should be avoided in children who have dysphagia or vomiting to prevent risk of aspiration. Dietary changes may be helpful, including elimination of milk and dairy products; consumption of increased amounts of high-fiber foods, such as fruits, vegetables, and cereals; and increased fluids. Behavioral therapy may be indicated to eliminate any fear that has developed as a result of painful defecation. Frequently, psychotherapeutic intervention with the child and the family becomes necessary.

Nursing Care Management

The nursing care of the child with encopresis involves education and support of the family and treatment of existing constipation. Education regarding the physiology of normal defecation, toilet training as a developmental process, and the treatment outlined for the particular family is essential to a successful outcome. Family counseling is directed toward reassurance that most problems resolve successfully, although relapses during periods of stress are possible (see Family Focus box).

FAMILY FOCUS

Helping Families Understand Encopresis
The prevailing attitude of nurses toward the family of a child with encopresis should be one of no-fault, thus relieving the guilt of both parents and child. Because parents and children are often reluctant to volunteer information, direct questioning about the soiling is more successful. Parents are usually relieved to know that other parents share this problem and are surprised to know that functional changes that take place as the condition develops make control of seepage impossible. Many parents complain that their children soil because they do not take time from play for a bowel movement. Actually, the children may be unaware of a prior sensation and unable to control the urge once it begins. They may be so accustomed to bowel accidents that they are unable to smell or feel it and even deny soiling when it occurs.

HEALTH PROBLEMS RELATED TO SPORTS PARTICIPATION

Every sport has the potential for injury to the participant—whether the adolescent engages in serious competition or participates for enjoyment. Serious injury occurs most often during rough contact sports or to persons who are not physically prepared for the activity. Injuries also occur when the children's or adolescents' bodies are not suited to the sport, when their muscles and body systems (respiratory and cardiovascular) are not conditioned to endure physical stress, or when they lack the insight and judgment to recognize that an activity exceeds their physical abilities. Rapidly growing bones, muscles, joints, and tendons are especially vulnerable to unusual strain. More injuries occur during recreational sports participation than during organized athletic competition.

The environment and the sports or recreational equipment can also present risks (Fig. 17-1). Children who participate in physical activity or sports do so in many different environments: indoors and outdoors, on floors, on the ground and snow, on or beneath water surfaces, and sometimes in free air space. Most of these activities also involve equipment, which children and adolescents may not be physically mature enough to manage safely. A common example of this would include skateboarding when the child or adolescent does not take safety precautions and perceives increased risk-taking as a part of the sport.

Acute overload injuries are those that occur suddenly during an activity and produce immediate symptoms. A blow or overstretching, twisting, or sudden stress to tissues can cause these injuries. For descriptions and management of traumatic injuries see Chapter 31.

OVERUSE SYNDROMES

To excel in sports, the young athlete is forced to train longer, harder, and earlier in life than previously. The rewards are an increased level of fitness, better performance, faster times, and the satisfaction of attaining a personal goal. With the increase in the number of children participating in sports year-round, more overuse injuries are being seen in the pediatric age-group (Lord and Winell, 2004).

The risk of overuse injury is always present and can be related to several factors: training errors, muscle-tendon imbal-

FIG. 17-1 ■ Football is an example of a strenuous collision sport.

ance, anatomic malalignment (e.g., femoral anteversion, excessive lumbar lordosis, tibial torsion), incorrect footwear or playing surface, an associated disease state, and growth (growth cartilage is less resistant to microtrauma). Athletes who run extensively frequently experience shin splints. The ligaments tear away from the tibial shaft, and this creates the pain. Ice, rest, and nonsteroidal antiinflammatory drugs (NSAIDs), such as ibuprofen or naproxen, are the usual treatment. Shin splints are rarely serious.

Chronic pain in athletes is often associated with overuse injury, which can occur at any level of athletic participation. The common feature in overuse injuries is the **repetitive microtrauma** that occurs to a particular anatomic structure (Lord and Winell, 2004). Performing the same movements time and time again can cause several types of injury:

- Frictional, or rubbing of one structure against another
- Tractional, or repeated pull on a ligament or tendon
- Cyclic, or repetitive loading of impact forces (stress fractures)

The end result is inflammation of the involved structure with complaints of pain, tenderness, swelling, and disability.

Bursae, tendons, muscles, ligaments, joints, and bones are all subject to overuse. Plantar fasciitis is common in athletes, and Osgood-Schlatter disease is seen in children who do a lot of jumping. The occurrence of overuse-type injuries, such as sore shoulders and strained elbows, may indicate that too much is being requested of the child in too short a period.

Stress Fractures

Given the intensity and duration of sports training, many young athletes suffer stress fractures, especially after a recent increase in training regimens. These fractures occur as a result of repeated muscle contraction and are seen most often in sports involving repetitive weight bearing such as running, gymnastics, and basketball. They occur less often in swimming (in the upper extremities). Tibial fractures are most common.

The most common symptom of stress fracture is a sharp, persistent, progressive pain or a deep, persistent dull ache located over the bone. Sometimes there is pain on impact (heel strike), but the most important clinical sign is pain over the

involved bony surface. Diagnosis is based on clinical observation. Plain radiographs are rarely diagnostic of stress fractures during the initial few weeks, since callus formation is not yet evident. Occasionally a bone scan may be needed and will indicate a "hot spot."

Therapeutic Management

Development of inflammation is common to all overuse syndromes; therefore management involves rest or alteration of activities, physical therapy, and medication. Rest is the primary therapy, usually interpreted as reduced activity and the use of alternative exercise—not bed rest or immobilization with casting. The main purpose is to alleviate the repetitive stress that initiated the symptoms. It is important to keep the child or adolescent mobile, and training can be continued. Alternative exercise is selected that maintains conditioning without aggravating the injury. For example, pool running (treading water in the deep end of a pool) can use the same movements as running but without the weight bearing; bicycling, swimming, and rowing are viable alternatives.

Other modalities include cryotherapy and cold whirlpool baths. Sometimes taping, bracing, splinting, and other orthoses are employed, depending on the injury. NSAIDs are often prescribed to reduce inflammation and pain. Topical medications are of questionable value.

NURSE'S ROLE IN SPORTS FOR CHILDREN AND ADOLESCENTS

Nurses are often involved in sports activities in the areas of preparation and evaluation for activities, prevention of injury, treatment of injuries, and rehabilitation after injury. Selecting an appropriate sport for both recreation and competition is a joint effort of the adolescent, parents, and health professionals. The best approach to counseling children, adolescents, and parents regarding sports participation is to encourage activities that are most likely to provide pleasure and physical benefits throughout childhood and into adulthood. Exposure to a variety of activities is better for young children than limiting them to one sport. Parents should be cautioned against overcommitting children to sports activities so they have time for other activities.

When children sustain athletic injuries, nurses are often responsible for instructions regarding care. Instructions (e.g., schedule for appointments, application of ice, any restrictions in activity) should be clear and accompanied by written directions. The importance of taking medications as prescribed is emphasized, especially if medications are needed for an extended period and if adherence is an issue. Medications given an hour before practice or competition may help children continue their activities.

Prevention of sports injuries is the most important aspect of athletic programs. Children should be suited to the activity; the environment and the equipment must be safe. Children should be prepared for the sport, especially if it requires strenuous or continuous physical exertion. Nurses, coaches, and athletic trainers must collaborate to ensure that safety measures are implemented. Stretching exercises, warm-up and cool-down activities, and appropriate training are requirements for safe participation. Protective measures such as pads, taping, and wrapping are also important to prevent injury. Finally, nurses must be aware of environmental safety risks.

ALTERED GROWTH AND MATURATION

The absence of physical or sexual maturation at a time when other children are experiencing positive evidence of sexual development and its associated spurt in growth and physical strength is an important concern to both the parents and their affected child. In most instances the delay in development is a simple physiologic or **constitutional delay** that represents one end of the normal genetically influenced variation of pubertal growth. These adolescents will go through a delayed but normal puberty and finally catch up, in their late teens, with their more rapidly developing age-mates. Growth delay may be proportionate or disproportionate; either require careful evaluation by a multidisciplinary team. Less benign causes of delayed development may be endocrine disorders such as growth hormone deficiency, a disease process such as human immunodeficiency virus (HIV) or chronic malabsorption, or a chromosomal abnormality such as Turner syndrome. Additional causes of delayed development include asthma, cystic fibrosis, malabsorption syndromes, cardiac anomalies, and chronic renal conditions. Skeletal disorders that affect growth in stature are those described as dwarfism. Most disorders are caused by congenital defects, such as achondroplasia, and by inborn errors of metabolism such as Hurler syndrome or Hunter syndrome.

The rate of maturation is important during the school years, but at puberty it assumes significant proportions to both teens and their parents. Girls or boys who lag behind their peers in physical maturation are painfully aware of their difference in growth. Adolescent girls with delayed maturation may feel out of place among companions whose hips and breasts are developing, feel cheated if they have not yet menstruated, and feel left out when their friends giggle and talk about boys. Adolescent boys with delayed maturation may feel inferior and small compared with their more muscular companions with whom they can no longer compete physically. Serial measurements of height and weight, as well as other anthropometric data, are obtained and plotted on standard growth charts to determine the pattern of growth and to compare the individual child with the norms for his or her age-group (Appendix B). When children are in the extremes of height ranges, it is important to compare their height with that of their parents and siblings.

Psychosocial, or *deprivation, dwarfism* is a stress-induced growth failure. It is defined as growth restriction in children older than 2 years of age that is caused by environmental (emotional) stress and is associated with a marked delay in physical growth, delayed developmental skills, and immature behavior. When these children are removed from the deprived environment, their growth proceeds at a normal or increased rate.

Management of growth delay in childhood and adolescence includes continued medical observation, attention to general health and nutrition, and psychologic support. Growth hormone is often recommended to treat growth hormone deficiency (see Hypopituitarism, Chapter 29).

Nursing Care Management

Deviation from the normal course of puberty is a significant concern for affected adolescents. For some adolescents, this concern assumes monumental proportions. Many cases of delayed development are caused by simple constitutional delay of puberty, and the child can be assured that normal development will eventually take place.

One difficulty related to a size that is incongruent with chronologic and mental age is the manner in which others relate to the child. People often respond to children with short stature as though they were younger than their age. Consequently, these children may react with babyish or juvenile behavior, thus establishing a circular pattern of behavior and response. Conversely, children who are tall or physically advanced for their age are frequently treated as though they were more advanced than their years. They are often considered clumsy, cognitively delayed, or immature when they perform according to the normal behavioral expectations for their age.

Listening to distressed adolescents and conveying interest and concern are important interventions. Slowly maturing adolescents need support and reassurance that they are unique individuals who have an important contribution to society that is equally as important as that of their peers. Counseling and therapy are individualized for each youth. Encouraging these children to focus on the positive aspects of their bodies and personalities and to adopt sound health practices and practice good grooming fosters a more positive self-image.

SEX CHROMOSOME DISORDERS

Most sex chromosome abnormalities are caused by an alteration in sex chromosome number (Table 17-1). The majority of these conditions are due to nondisjunction. An alteration in the number of sex chromosomes usually does not produce the profound defects that are associated with the autosomal disorders (trisomies). Intelligence may be normal or low normal, or the child may have some learning disabilities. Moderate or severe mental retardation is less common.

Turner Syndrome

Turner syndrome is caused by absence of one of the X chromosomes. Most girls who have this disorder have one X chromosome missing from all cells (45,XO). This disorder is often recognized at birth if the newborn has a webbed neck, low posterior hairline, widely spaced nipples, and edema of the hands and feet. This condition is often diagnosed in the preschool child because growth is restricted or delayed around 3 to 4 years of age. In some cases it may be diagnosed at puberty because of three features: short stature, delayed sexual development, and amenorrhea; individuals with Turner syndrome are generally infertile. They may also have difficulty with peer relationships and understanding social cues. They frequently exhibit behavioral problems, especially immature, socially isolated behavior. Diagnosis is confirmed on the basis of a negative sex chromatin test.

Therapy is individualized for these girls and consists primarily of female hormone treatment and psychologic counseling for both the child and parents. Linear growth can be increased by the administration of growth hormone if therapy is begun early. Estrogen therapy is initiated during the usual time for puberty to promote the development of secondary sex characteristics. Responses to estrogen therapy vary from girl to girl, but gradual feminization is accomplished to some degree in most individuals.

Klinefelter Syndrome

Klinefelter syndrome, the most common of all sex chromosome disorders, is caused by the presence of one or more additional X chromosomes and only one Y chromosome. Most males with this syndrome have a chromosome complement of 47,XXY. The

Common Sex Chromosome Disorders

SYNDROME	CHROMOSOMAL NOTATION	PHENOTYPE	FREQUENCY (LIVE BIRTHS)	CLINICAL MANIFESTATIONS
Turner	45,X or 45,XO	Female	1:10,000 female births	Short stature; webbed neck; low posterior hairline; shield-shaped chest with widely spaced nipples; sterile; no development of secondary sex characteristics; urinary tract abnormalities; normal intellectual development
Triple X, or superfemale	47,XXX (can also be 48,XXXX or 49,XXXXX)	Female	1:1000 female births	Normal female characteristics; usually tall; variable mental capacity and behavior; at risk for impaired language, learning difficulties; fertile
Jacob, XYY male	47,XYY (can also be 48,XYYY or mosaic)	Male	1:1000 male births	Usually normal sexual development; tendency to be tall with long head; poor coordination; offspring chromosomally normal; previously thought to have aggressive tendencies but well-controlled studies refuted this hypothesis
Klinefelter	47,XXY (or 48,XXYY, 48,XXXY, 49,XXXXY, and so on, mosaics)	Male	1:1000 male births	Tall with long legs; hypogenitalism; sterile; male secondary sex characteristics may be deficient; may demonstrate aberrant behavior; learning disabled; 80% have gynecomastia

disorder is infrequently diagnosed before puberty, at which time varying degrees of failure of adolescent virilization occur. Some males are not diagnosed until they appear for evaluation for infertility. All have absence of sperm in the semen (azoospermia), small testes, and defective development of secondary sex characteristics (gynecomastia, hypogonadism). In 80% of these boys there is a chromatin-positive buccal smear, and the extra chromosome is apparent on chromosome analysis.

Cognitive impairment is a frequent clinical finding and appears to be related to the number of X chromosomes. Boys may also have gross motor skill difficulties, a developmental language delay, poor verbal skills, reduced auditory memory, shyness, passivity, behavioral problems, and school difficulties. Therapy is directed toward enhancing the masculine characteristics through administration of testosterone.

Nursing Care Management

The nursing care of children with Turner or Klinefelter syndrome is primarily supportive. Nurses assist in the diagnosis, explain tests and therapies, and provide support and encouragement to the child and family. Because both disorders render the individual unable to reproduce, psychologic counseling is an important aspect of care. In young adults marriage and sexual relationships are possible, but alternative reproductive options, such as artificial insemination and adoption, should be discussed.

DISORDERS RELATED TO THE REPRODUCTIVE SYSTEM

AMENORRHEA

Menarche, or the first menstrual period, occurs relatively late in female pubertal development. Although girls vary in the onset and rate of progression of pubertal development, the sequence and tempo should be the same. When an adolescent is seen with a complaint of absence of menses, a careful history of the timing of her pubertal development will help to determine if there is a need for further evaluation or if reassurance is all that is necessary.

Primary amenorrhea is an absence of secondary sex characteristics and no uterine bleeding by 14 to 15 years of age, or absence of uterine bleeding with secondary sex characteristics by 16 years of age (Master-Hunter and Heiman, 2006). No uterine bleeding after attaining a sexual maturity rating of 5 on the Tanner scale (see Figures 16-1 and 16-2) for 1 year, or after breast development for 4 years, is also considered primary amenorrhea (American Academy of Pediatrics and American College of Obstetricians and Gynecologists, 2006). The cause of primary amenorrhea may be anatomic, hormonal, genetic, or idiopathic. A thorough patient and family history and physical examination will provide clues to the etiology.

Secondary amenorrhea is defined as the absence of menses for 6 months or at least three cycles after menstruation was previously established. Irregular menstrual cycles are common within the first year or two after menarche. These early cycles may be anovulatory, resulting in regular, irregular, or absent bleeding; however, cycle lengths outside the range of 21 to 45 days should be investigated (American Academy of Pediatrics and American College of Obstetricians and Gynecologists, 2006). Girls with a later onset of menarche will take longer to establish regular ovulatory cycles.

Pregnancy is the most common cause of secondary amenorrhea and should be ruled out in both types of amenorrhea, even if the adolescent denies sexual activity. Other factors that disturb the hypothalamic-pituitary-gonadal axis and cause secondary amenorrhea include physical or emotional stress; sudden environmental change; hyperthyroidism or hypothyroidism; polycystic ovary disease; chronic illness; extreme weight loss or gain; intensive exercise; anorexia nervosa or bulimia; ovarian disturbance; and extrinsic pharmacologic agents, especially phenothiazines, contraceptive steroids, and heroin.

DYSMENORRHEA

A certain amount of discomfort during the first day or two of the menstrual flow is extremely common. Most girls experience cramping, abdominal pain, backache, and leg ache, but in a few cases the pain is intolerable and incapacitating. **Pri-**

mary dysmenorrhea is painful menses not related to any pelvic disease. **Secondary dysmenorrhea** is defined as painful menses with a pathologic condition such as endometriosis, salpingitis, or congenital anomalies of the müllerian system.

Primary dysmenorrhea usually begins at the time of menarche or within 6 to 12 months. The pain begins with menstrual flow or hours before the onset of bleeding each month, usually continuing for 48 to 72 hours. The exact etiology is unknown, but the pain is clearly related to ovulatory cycles. The overproduction of uterine prostaglandins has been implicated; women with dysmenorrhea have higher levels of prostaglandins. Overproduction of vasopressin (a hormone that stimulates the contraction of muscular tissue) may also contribute to dysmenorrhea.

A careful history should include the onset of symptoms; the duration, type of pain, and relationship to menstrual flow; age at menarche; family history of dysmenorrhea; and sexual history. The nurse should also ask about previous treatments, including dosages of medications. Associated symptoms such as nausea, vomiting, diarrhea, and leg and back pain are helpful for diagnosis and treatment. Depending on the results of the history, the physical examination may include a gynecologic examination.

Therapeutic Management

First-line treatment for adolescents with dysmenorrhea is the administration of NSAIDs, which block the formation of prostaglandins for 2 to 3 days of the menstrual cycle. The girl should be instructed to begin the medication at the first sign of cramping or bleeding. Girls with regular menstrual cycles benefit from beginning the medication 1 or 2 days before the onset of their menses. The medications should be taken with food.

Cyclic estrogen therapy and oral contraceptives are also effective. Simple exercises such as pelvic rocking, assuming the knee-chest position, and breathing exercises may be beneficial. Adequate personal hygiene, participation in regular activities, and methods to decrease stress should be discussed with the adolescent. Dietary changes, supplements, and herbal medications are often used to treat dysmenorrhea. Randomized controlled clinical trials have demonstrated that vitamins B_1 and E are effective in the treatment of dysmenorrhea (Dennehy, 2006).

Nursing Care Management

All adolescent girls need reassurance that menstruation is a normal function. When nurses are asked for advice regarding menstrual problems, they have a valuable opportunity to engage in health teaching concerning menstrual physiology; hygiene; and the importance of a well-balanced diet, exercise, and general health maintenance. Health teaching can dispel myths about menstruation and femininity. When assessment indicates a potential problem and the need for evaluation, referral to an appropriate practitioner, health service, or clinic may be necessary.

One of the most difficult experiences facing the adolescent girl is the gynecologic examination. Whether it is her first experience or not, she is often filled with apprehension. Almost all adolescents are extremely self-conscious about their bodies and the changes taking place. They need continuing support in the form of anticipatory guidance regarding what to expect and suggestions of what to do to relax during the procedure. Most girls favor a semisitting position, which has the additional advantage of allowing eye contact during the procedure. Sometimes a pillow helps the patient feel more comfortable and less vulnerable. The provision of a mirror for the girl to see what is taking place if she so desires helps the examiner explain various aspects of anatomy. When possible, it is important to respect the adolescent's request for a female provider.

VAGINITIS

Vaginitis can be caused by physical, chemical, or infectious agents. Physical causes may include a forgotten tampon; chemical irritants include bubble bath, douching, deodorant pads, and tampons. Removing the offending material or discontinuing use of the irritating substance is usually all that is necessary to treat physical or chemical vaginitis. Infectious vaginitis can be caused by *Candida* fungi (yeast), *Trichomonas* protozoa parasites, or bacteria. Diagnosis is confirmed with microscopic evaluation of vaginal secretions or vaginal culture. Treatment varies depending on the infectious agent.

Health teaching is important in the prevention and management of vaginitis. Adolescent girls need reassurance that increased vaginal mucus can occur at the time of ovulation, before menstruation, or with sexual excitement. Many teenage girls mistake these variations as signs of infection. Girls should be taught to wipe from front to back after toileting and to realize that vaginitis can result from irritation, foreign objects, and sexual activity. Nurses should stress the importance of an evaluation to determine the exact cause.

DISORDERS OF THE MALE REPRODUCTIVE SYSTEM

Most obvious anomalies, such as hypospadias, hydrocele, phimosis, and cryptorchidism, are identified with corrective measures instituted during early childhood. The most frequent problems related to the reproductive organs in later childhood are:

- Infections, such as urethritis (see Urinary Tract Infection, Chapter 27)
- Hematuria
- Penile problems, such as nonretractable foreskin in uncircumcised males, carcinoma, and trauma
- Scrotal conditions, such as varicocele (elongation, dilation, and tortuosity of the veins superior to the testicle)
- Testicular torsion (a condition in which the testicle hangs free from its vascular structures, which can result in partial or complete venous occlusion with rotation)

Tumors of the testes are not common, but when manifested in adolescence, they are generally malignant and demand immediate evaluation. Testicular cancer is the most common solid tumor in males 15 to 34 years of age. The usual presenting symptom for testicular cancer is a heavy, hard, painless mass (either smooth or nodular) that is palpated on the testis. Treatment involves surgical removal of the affected testicle (orchiectomy) and possibly chemotherapy and radiation if metastasis has occurred.

Nursing Care Management

The adolescent boy is also self-conscious about his changing body and needs preparation for a genital examination. The most successful approach is to assume a matter-of-fact attitude

CRITICAL THINKING EXERCISE

Testicular Self-Examination

At a recent faculty meeting, Paul, the pediatric nurse practitioner who runs the school-based health clinic, presented his plan for a class on testicular self-examination (TSE) to be delivered to the sophomore boys. Several teachers questioned the value of providing such a class when there is limited time to deliver content relating to "routine academic subjects." What important issues regarding testicular cancer and TSE should Paul use to justify providing this class to the sophomore boys?

QUESTIONS
1. Evidence—Is there sufficient evidence to justify teaching sophomore boys about TSE?
2. Assumptions—Describe the underlying assumption about each of the following:
   a. Detection of testicular cancers in adolescence
   b. Usual presenting symptom of testicular cancer
   c. Knowledge of genital anatomy among adolescent boys
   d. Ways to teach adolescent boys about their anatomy
3. What priorities and implications for nursing care can be drawn at this time?
4. Does the evidence support your nursing intervention?
5. What alternative perspectives might you have?

toward the examination, explain precisely what will take place, and maintain a continuous commentary about what is being done and the findings at each phase of the examination.

The routine health assessment of every adolescent boy should include teaching about testicular cancer and how to perform a testicular self-examination (TSE) every month. This rare malignancy is curable if detected early. Nurses are in an ideal position to teach TSE in a manner that is respectful of the adolescent boy's anxieties and that promotes early treatment (see Critical Thinking Exercise).

The normal testicle is a firm organ with a smooth, egg-shaped contour; the epididymis is palpated as a raised swelling on the superior aspect of the testicle and should not be taken for an abnormality.

GYNECOMASTIA

The male breast, although not strictly part of the male reproductive system, responds to hormonal changes. Some degree of bilateral or unilateral breast enlargement occurs frequently in boys during puberty. It is estimated that approximately half of adolescent boys have transient gynecomastia, usually lasting less than 1 year, which subsides spontaneously with achievement of male development. A careful assessment of the pubertal stage at the onset of gynecomastia; medication history, including anabolic steroids; and the exclusion of renal, liver, thyroid, and endocrine disorders or dysfunction allow the examiner to reassure the adolescent that the changes are pubertal gynecomastia and that no further assessment is indicated.

If the condition persists or is extensive enough to cause embarrassment or to produce doubts about gender identity in the young boy, plastic surgery may be indicated for cosmetic and psychologic considerations. Administration of testosterone has no effect on breast development or regression and may aggravate the condition.

Nursing Care Management

Treatment usually consists of assurance to the adolescent and his parents that this is a benign and temporary situation. A physical examination with palpation is necessary to differentiate gynecomastia from increased adiposity caused by being overweight. Adolescents who are distressed about physical integrity and masculinity may benefit from the knowledge that this condition occurs in more than 50% of all adolescent boys.

HEALTH PROBLEMS RELATED TO SEXUALITY

It is estimated that by the time adolescents finish high school, more than half of them will have had at least one sexual experience with a member of the same or opposite gender (Mosher, Chandra, and Jones, 2005). Many serious health consequences are associated with adolescent sexual activity, including unplanned pregnancy and sexually transmitted diseases (STDs); additional health problems may arise from an increased number of sexual partners over time and incomplete education regarding sexual practices in adolescents. Health professionals must understand the issues related to adolescent sexual activity and the psychosocial dynamics that influence them.

ADOLESCENT PREGNANCY

In recent years the teenage pregnancy rate has shown a continual downward trend. Between 1990 and 2003, birth rates for teenagers 15 to 17 and 18 to 19 years of age declined nationally for all races. In 2005 the teenage birth rate decreased 2% (from 2004) to 40.4 births per 1000 women ages 15 to 19 (Hamilton, Martin, and Ventura, 2006). The decline over the past decade has been attributed to a drop in the number of repeat pregnancies and an increase in the use of condoms and long-term hormonal contraceptive methods among adolescents. However, adolescent birth rates still remain high in the United States compared with those in other developed countries (American Academy of Pediatrics, 2005a). The number of teens initiating sexual intercourse before the age of 15 has significantly decreased in the past 10 years (Anderson, Santelli, and Morrow, 2006). Teens who postpone the initiation of sexual intercourse decrease their risk for STDs, including HIV.

The reduction in teen pregnancy is an important national goal because of the risk for negative outcomes for both mother and child. A wide range of factors put an adolescent at risk for pregnancy, including having sex with an older partner, the type of contraception used; living in poverty; having a mother who was a teen parent; school failure; lack of access to confidential health care; and living in a poor community where access to education, health care, and work may not be optimal.

With better facilities available for care, the mortality associated with teenage pregnancies is decreasing, but morbidity remains high. Teenage girls and their unborn infants are at greater risk for complications of both pregnancy and delivery. The most frequent complications are premature labor and low-birth-weight infants, high neonatal mortality, iron deficiency anemia, fetopelvic disproportion, and prolonged labor. The pregnancies of adolescents less than 15 years old are more frequently complicated by obstetric problems and neonatal morbidity and mortality than those of adolescents ages 15 to 19. The increased risk has traditionally been thought to be related to incomplete growth and physiologic immaturity. However, pregnancy can take place only after the girl has achieved an advanced state of growth and sexual maturity. Therefore concerns are dietary habits, substance use (especially cigarettes), STDs, the effects of poverty, and a late onset of prenatal care.

Nursing Care Management

A pregnant teenager needs careful assessment by the nurse to determine the level of social support available to her and her partner. The adolescent needs to make many important decisions and may not have the life experience to know how to cope with this stress. Whenever possible, guidance from the adults in her life will be invaluable. Information about options to continue the pregnancy and parent the child, continue the pregnancy with adoption, or terminate the pregnancy with abortion should be given in a nonjudgmental manner. If the adolescent chooses to continue the pregnancy, prenatal care should be initiated as soon as possible. No matter what the teenager decides, nutrition information will be necessary.

CONTRACEPTION

Family planning services have developed and expanded during recent years, but the need for contraceptive services as part of the health care of adolescents remains great. The birth control pill and condom remain the most popular methods for adolescents; 3-month injectable contraception is more popular among lower-income adolescents. Adolescents commonly delay seeking contraceptive information. The typical interval from onset of sexual intercourse until the first visit for contraception is 1 year. A pregnancy scare is usually the precipitating event for the contraception appointment. Counseling about contraceptive options should be conducted in a manner that is consistent with the cognitive level of the adolescent. The adolescent should be given accurate information about the risks and benefits of each method before making a choice.

Many teenagers feel ambivalent regarding their sexual activity and avoid many contraceptives because their use seems too premeditated and implies that sex is planned rather than a spontaneous activity. Most of these girls believe that sex is all right if it is not planned. This may often play a role in adolescents delaying contraception, waiting for a relationship that is "close enough." A close relationship would allow the adolescents to accept and acknowledge their sexual activity.

The choice of a safe and effective contraceptive method must be suited to the individual (Table 17-2). The choice is based on preference after the adolescent is informed of the benefits and disadvantages. Motivation is necessary for most methods. For example, the pill is effective if used correctly, but the adolescent must remember to take the pill at approximately the same time every day. For many young women, a medroxyprogesterone injection (Depo-Provera) is an ideal choice because it is extremely effective and is administered every 12 weeks, but side effects such as weight gain and decreased bone mineralization may make it undesirable. Sexually active adolescents need to know that contraceptive devices other than condoms do not prevent STDs. Condom use is still important and must be discussed with all sexually and non–sexually active adolescents.

Confidentiality is a critical issue when discussing contraception with adolescents. Privacy is important to adolescents as they struggle to forge a personal identity and establish social relationships. Adolescents are particularly concerned about the judgments of others. The predominant belief among many health professionals is that parental notification is important but that the "parents' rights" view is not necessarily sensitive to the health needs and basic rights of youth. No evidence substantiates the belief that providing contraceptive guidance contributes to sexual irresponsibility and promiscuity.

TABLE 17-2

Advantages and Disadvantages of Contraceptive Methods in Adolescents

METHOD	ADVANTAGES	DISADVANTAGES
BEHAVIORAL METHODS		
Abstinence	100% effective in preventing sexually transmitted diseases (STDs) and pregnancy	Peer pressure to conform Relatively high failure rate from noncompliance
Withdrawal (coitus interruptus) Withdrawal of penis before ejaculation	No medical visit necessary	High failure rate Some seminal fluid often released before ejaculation Ejaculate at vaginal orifice may enter vagina No STD protection
Calendar method Refrain from intercourse during fertile period (time of ovulation)	Teaches adolescent girls about their menstrual cycle Encourages couple participation	High failure rate Requires a regular, predictable menstrual cycle (irregular menses are common for first 2 years after menarche) No STD protection
BARRIER METHODS		
Condom	Minimal side effects Easy to use Available without prescription Portable Provides protection against STDs	Requires consistent use Requires premeditated intent for sexual union May decrease sensation Misuse results in failure Decreased spontaneity

HIV, Human immunodeficiency virus.

TABLE 17-2

Advantages and Disadvantages of Contraceptive Methods in Adolescents—cont'd

METHOD	ADVANTAGES	DISADVANTAGES
BARRIER METHODS—cont'd *Male*—Penile covering to trap sperm	Spermicidal condoms increase effectiveness for pregnancy and STD prevention Inexpensive in comparison to female condom	Latex sensitivity or allergies in small percentage of people Improper use may lead to pregnancy or development of STD
Female—Inserted into vagina with base covering part of perineum; may be inserted 8 hours before intercourse	Female participation Made of polyurethane; no latex sensitivities and can be used with oil-based lubricants Provides protection from STDs	May be difficult to insert Coital dependent Noisy
Diaphragm Cervical covering to prevent sperm from reaching egg Must be used in conjunction with spermicidal jelly May be inserted 4-6 hours before intercourse If inserted early, should be checked for placement before coitus	Can be fitted in virgins Low failure rate when used correctly Few contraindications May be reused	High failure rate in adolescents because of inconvenience of use Requires consistent use Requires fitting and instruction by medical personnel Requires premeditated intent for sexual union Requires body awareness and comfort with touching oneself for insertion Little STD protection May increase incidence of urinary tract infection
Lea's shield Reusable vaginal contraceptive made of silicone; elliptical bowl placed in vagina up to 48 hours before sexual intercourse; removed 8 hours after intercourse	No latex allergies Reusable Very effective in nulliparous women Simple fitting	Less effective in women who have delivered a baby Requires prescription No STD protection More effective if spermicidal cream is used May increase incidence of urinary tract infection
Cervical cap Soft rubber dome with a firm but pliable rim; fits over base of the cervix close to the junction of the cervix and vaginal fornices	May be inserted hours before intercourse Insertion and removal similar to diaphragm	Available in only four sizes Must remain in place at least 6 hours after intercourse, but no more than 48 hours Not recommended for women with abnormal Papanicolaou test, history of toxic shock syndrome, or difficulty with proper fitting No STD protection
CHEMICALS **Spermicidal foam, jelly, cream, and suppositories** Substance inserted into vagina to kill sperm	Available without prescription Inexpensive Easy to use No major health concerns	High failure rate unless combined with condom Possible for sperm to be ejaculated directly into uterine os, bypassing spermicide in vagina Must be used shortly before coitus; therefore requires interruption of sexual experience Repeated sexual union requires repeated application Requires premeditated intent for sexual union Messy Nonoxynol-9 associated with increased transmission of HIV to females; should not be used with anal sex in male partner sex for same reason No STD protection.
HORMONAL METHODS **Oral contraceptives** Estrogen and progesterone-like compounds Inhibit ovulation by blocking release of gonadotropins from anterior pituitary gland	99% effective if used correctly Safe for adolescents Method of choice for most adolescents Administered by mouth Becomes a ritual not associated with sexual activity Regulates menses, decreases dysmenorrhea and acne, decreases menstrual flow Prevents ovarian and endometrial cancers Prevents functional ovarian cysts	Higher failure rate in adolescents than in older women Need to follow precise instructions; requires continued motivation, consistent use Requires prescription Price substantial for teenager No STD protection Possible side effects include headaches, missed or scanty periods, breakthrough bleeding, blood clot Increased rates of chlamydia

Continued

TABLE 17-2

Advantages and Disadvantages of Contraceptive Methods in Adolescents—cont'd

METHOD	ADVANTAGES	DISADVANTAGES
HORMONAL METHODS—cont'd		
Medroxyprogesterone acetate (Depo-Provera) Progestin that suppresses hormonal cycle and prevents ovulation Injection given every 3 months	No interruption of sex Invisible method	No STD protection Possible side effects include significant weight gain, decreased bone density, decreased high-density lipoproteins (HDLs), irregular menses or amenorrhea, decreased libido, depression Fertility perhaps delayed after discontinuation Must return to care provider every 3 months for injection Food and Drug Administration recommends discontinuation after 2 years because of decreased bone density
Ortho Evra transdermal system 4.5-cm square patch with norelgestromin and ethinyl estradiol Hormonal patch applied to skin weekly for 3 weeks per month Suppresses ovulation, thickens cervical mucus, and thins endometrium	88.2% effective in perfect users Simple to use Regular menstrual cycles Not associated with sexual activity Avoids first-pass metabolism, resulting in more constant levels	Not recommended for women >90 kg (198 pounds) Possible side effects include skin reaction at site, nausea, headache, dysmenorrhea, and breast tenderness Slight increase risk of blood clot formation over combination oral contraceptive pill Patch may be visible No STD protection
NuvaRing Etonogestrel plus ethinyl estradiol Soft flexible transparent ring placed in vagina for 3 weeks Suppresses ovulation	99.3% effective Immediate return to ovulation at discontinuation May leave in place during sexual intercourse Avoids first-pass metabolism, resulting in more constant levels No spermicide needed No vaginal erosion No weight gain	Device may be felt by female or partner during sexual intercourse Device may fall out Possible side effects include headache, vaginitis, leukorrhea, nausea, and breakthrough bleeding May have late withdrawal bleeding requiring placement of ring during menses No STD protection
Levonorgestrel intrauterine system (Mirena) T-shape intrauterine device that releases 20 mcg/d of levonorgestrel Inserted within 7 days of menses and remains in place for 5 years Thickens cervical mucus, inhibits sperm mobility and function	>99% effective Effectively prevents fertilization, resulting in low rates of ectopic pregnancy Reduced length and quantity of menstrual bleeding Reduced dysmenorrhea No weight gain	Risk of perforation at time of insertion 2%-12% expulsion rate Not recommended in nulliparous women or women not in monogamous relationships Possible side effects include abdominal pain, headache, vaginal discharge, and breast pain No STD protection
Letonogestrel implant (Implanon) 40 × 2 mm implanted rod Progestin-only method Suppresses ovulation	>99% effective Efficacy not user dependent Provides 3 years of protection Single rod insertion and removal Palpable but not visible after insertion	Irregular menstrual bleeding Other less common side effects include headache, vaginitis, weight gain (1.7 kg [3.7 pounds] at 2 years) No STD protection
EMERGENCY OR POSTCOITAL CONTRACEPTION		
Emergency contraception works in one of three ways: by suppressing or delaying ovulation, by preventing the meeting of sperm and egg, or by preventing implantation **Progestin-only pill given within 72 hours of intercourse** *or* **Insertion of a copper-releasing intrauterine device** up to 7 days after unprotected intercourse	Useful in unplanned sexual intercourse or contraceptive failure May be given in advance for emergency use Available without prescription for adults	No STD protection May cause nausea if combination method used May change timing of next menstrual cycle

HIV, Human immunodeficiency virus.

Nursing Care Management

Nurses are often involved in providing education about contraception. Such education is ideally combined with ongoing sex education. Although sexual abstinence is a highly desirable form of contraception for teenagers, nurses working with adolescents must recognize that teens feel multiple pressures to engage in sexual intercourse. Postponing sexual involvement requires effective communication and decision-making skills. Adolescents benefit from role-playing refusal skills and opportunities to practice making decisions in a safe environment. Information about safe sex must be provided, and role-playing how to discuss condom use with a partner is helpful to teenagers.

Education concerning contraception should be provided in both oral and written form. All available methods, including their benefits, disadvantages, and side effects, should be discussed. Concrete, concise language must be used, demonstrations of how to use the contraceptive should be provided, and adolescents should repeat all instructions in their own words. If teenagers are using oral contraceptive pills, they should be encouraged to use a daily activity as a reminder or cue to take the pill. A knowledgeable phone triage person should be available for questions and concerns. Parents or other important adults may be included in all discussions, with the adolescent's permission.

SEXUALLY TRANSMITTED DISEASES

Sexually active adolescents are at increased risk (compared with adults) for the acquisition of STDs. Physiologically, the adolescent girl's cervix has a large ectropion, which is composed of columnar epithelial cells that are much more susceptible to STDs, especially human papillomavirus (HPV) and *Chlamydia* infection. The adolescent's immune system also contributes to the increased risk because the adolescent has not had an opportunity to develop resistance to these organisms (Shrier, 2004). Behavioral factors contributing to increased risk include initiating sexual intercourse at an early age, high disease prevalence among sexual partners, and inconsistent use of barrier or other types of contraceptives. In addition, adolescents may participate in unprotected oral or anal sex in the belief that STDs cannot be transmitted through those activities (Shrier, 2004). A listing of common STDs is included in Table 17-3.

The rates of chlamydia and gonorrhea are reported to be highest among adolescent girls ages 15 to 19 years, and high rates of HPV exist in the adolescent population (Centers for Disease Control and Prevention, 2006a). Whereas much emphasis has been placed on prevention of HIV in the past decade, other STDs have received little attention in regards to prevention. Lack of awareness regarding one's susceptibility to STDs when engaged in unprotected sexual activity, be it oral, anal, or vaginal intercourse, is perhaps one of the greatest dangers adolescents face.

Therapeutic Management

Effective treatment of both males and females with an STD involves administration of the appropriate therapeutic agent. Treatment of sexual partners is also an essential part of therapy. Adolescents need help to develop strategies to inform their partner and to abstain from sex until both have completed treatment.

A totally effective prophylaxis against infection is not yet available; therefore preventive efforts must be directed toward finding and treating affected persons, locating and examining contacts of affected persons, educating young people regarding the facts of the disease and its spread, and encouraging the use of condoms in sexually active young people.

Nursing Care Management

Nursing responsibilities encompass all aspects of STD education, confidentiality, prevention, and treatment. Part of the sex education of young people should include providing information about these diseases, including their symptoms and treatment, and dispelling the myths associated with their mode of transmission. Many vulnerable adolescents are uninformed or misinformed about STDs.

Primary prevention efforts for STDs include encouraging abstinence and postponing sexual involvement; encouraging condom use; and ensuring vaccination for hepatitis A and B and HPV. Nurses play a role in secondary prevention by helping to identify early cases and referring adolescents for treatment. Nurses can also be involved in tertiary prevention by decreasing the medical and psychologic effects of STDs; conducting support groups for adolescents with HIV, herpes simplex virus, and HPV infections; and assisting pregnant adolescents in obtaining adequate prenatal screening and treatment of STDs.

PELVIC INFLAMMATORY DISEASE

Pelvic inflammatory disease (PID) is an infection of the upper genital tract (endometrium, fallopian tubes, and ovaries), most commonly caused by sexually transmitted bacteria, such as *Neisseria gonorrhoeae*, Chlamydia trachomatis, and a variety of other anaerobic bacteria.

The long-term effects of PID include infertility because of tubal scarring, ectopic pregnancy, and chronic abdominal pain. It is estimated that each year 1 million females of reproductive age experience an episode of PID, with approximately 20% of cases occurring in teenagers. Women under the age of 25 years have a one in eight chance of experiencing PID compared with those over age 25 years, whose risk is one in 80.

Presenting symptoms in the adolescent may be generalized, including fever; abdominal pain; urinary tract symptoms; and vague influenza-like manifestations, such as malaise, nausea, diarrhea, or constipation. A pelvic examination is indicated for every sexually active female who complains of lower abdominal pain to evaluate for the possibility of PID.

PID is of major concern to nurses because of its devastating effects on the reproductive tract. Approximately 25% of females experiencing PID may have short-term complications, such as acute abscess formation in the fallopian tubes (tubo-ovarian abscess), or long-term complications, such as chronic pelvic pain, dyspareunia (painful coitus), or adhesion formation. Most significant, however, is the increased risk for ectopic pregnancy or infertility, which results from tubal scarring.

Prevention is the primary concern of health care professionals. Barrier contraceptive methods, such as condoms, seem to offer the best protection for preventing STDs and PID. Sexually active female teenagers should be screened every 6 months to detect asymptomatic STDs, and treatment should be initiated to prevent PID and all associated complications.

TABLE 17-3
Selected Sexually Transmitted Diseases*

MANIFESTATIONS	THERAPY	NURSING CARE MANAGEMENT
GONORRHEA *(NEISSERIA GONORRHOEAE)*		
Male—Urethritis (dysuria with profuse yellow discharge, frequency, urgency, nocturia) or pharyngitis **Female**—Cervicitis (postpubertal); may be associated with discharge, dysuria, dyspareunia, vulvovaginitis (prepubertal), or pharyngitis	For uncomplicated urogenital and anorectal gonorrhea: 　Single intramuscular dose of ceftriaxone† *or* 　Single oral dose of cefixime	Instruct patient to abstain from sexual intercourse for 7 days after single-dose treatment, or until completion of a 7-day regimen. Find and treat sexual contacts. Educate young people regarding facts of the disease and its spread. Encourage use of condoms in sexually active young people.
CHLAMYDIA *(CHLAMYDIA TRACHOMATIS)*		
Male—Meatal erythema, tenderness, itching, dysuria, urethral discharge; or no symptoms **Female**—Mucopurulent cervical exudate with erythema, edema, congestion; or no symptoms	Azithromycin or doxycycline If pregnant—azithromycin	Same as above Rescreen women 3-4 months after treatment; repeat infection elevates risk for pelvic inflammatory disease (PID). Consider concomitant treatment of gonorrhea.
SYPHILIS *(TREPONEMA PALLIDUM)*		
Primary stage—Chancre, a hard, painless, red, sharply defined lesion with indurated base, raised border, eroded surface, and scanty yellow discharge; usually located on penis, vulva, or cervix **Secondary stage**—Systemic influenza-like symptoms and lymphadenopathy, rash; usually appears 1-3 weeks after healing of chancre	Penicillin G (parenteral—benzathine, aqueous procaine, or aqueous crystalline)	Instruct patients to use condoms to avoid spread or infection with other organisms. Identify sexual contacts of infected person(s). Test women in pregnancy and prior to delivery (VDRL and RPR). Evaluate newborn for presence of disease if mother is untreated.
HERPES PROGENITALIS (GENITAL HERPES SIMPLEX VIRUS [HSV])		
Small (usually painful) vesicles on genital area, buttocks, and thighs; itching usually initial symptom; when vesicles break, shallow, circular, extremely painful lesions remain	No known cure Acyclovir, famciclovir, or valacyclovir May need suppressive therapy for recurrences	Instruct patients to use condoms to avoid spread or infection with other organisms. Infection can be transmitted to infant during birth. Evaluate maternal history and observe infant for signs or symptoms. Cultures may be obtained in newborn.
TRICHOMONIASIS *(TRICHOMONAS VAGINALIS)*		
Pruritus and edema of external genitalia; foul-smelling, greenish vaginal discharge; sometimes postcoital bleeding May be asymptomatic, especially in males	Oral metronidazole or oral tinidazole Metronidazole may be given in single oral dose or 7-day regimen	Patient should not consume alcohol while taking medication and for at least 48 hours following last dose. Sexual partners should be treated.
HUMAN PAPILLOMAVIRUS (HPV)		
Warts found on any part of male or female genitalia	**Patient applied:** 　Podofilox solution (0.5%) or gel, or imiquimod (5%) cream **Provider applied:** 　Podophyllin resin 10%-25% in compound tincture of benzoin 　Freezing with liquid nitrogen or cryoprobe (cryotherapy) 　Trichloroacetic acid or bichloroacetic acid 80%-90% 　Laser therapy or intralesional interferon or surgical removal	An acceptable alternative is to forgo treatment and await spontaneous resolution. Treatments are usually painful; analgesics may be needed, and steroid cream may provide relief. Male partners should inform female partner of need for Papanicolaou testing. Vaccine available to females aged 9-18 years (see Chapter 10) for prevention of HPV.
ACQUIRED IMMUNODEFICIENCY SYNDROME (HUMAN IMMUNODEFICIENCY VIRUS)		
See Chapter 26.	Numerous antiviral medications to delay viral replication and progression of disease	See Chapter 26.

*Updated information on specific treatment of STDs may be accessed at http://www.cdc.gov/std/treatment.
†Centers for Disease Control and Prevention: Update to CDC's *Sexually transmitted disease treatment guidelines, 2006*: fluoroquinolones no longer recommended for treatment of gonococcal infections, *MMWR* 56(14):332-336, 2007.

Reinfection with *Chlamydia* organisms is associated with a higher incidence of PID. Females who have had a *Chlamydia* infection should be rescreened for *Chlamydia* 3 months after treatment.

SEXUAL ASSAULT (RAPE)

The adolescent girl is particularly vulnerable to sexual assault, and 75% of adolescents who are raped know their assailant (Clements, Speck, Crane, and others, 2004). Females are more likely to report these experiences than males (Neinstein, 2002). In each instance the victim is potentially subjected to serious physical or emotional harm. There is no typical victim. Sexual assault victims are of all ages, ethnic groups, and economic groups and are of either gender, although adolescents and children with a physical or developmental disability are more vulnerable to sexual abuse than their peers. Acquaintance rape is far more common than stranger rape; however, stranger rape is reported more often.

An understanding of the legal definitions of sexual assault, rape, acquaintance rape, and statutory rape is essential for the nurse to identify, treat, and manage adolescent victims (Box 17-1).

Statutory rape laws have been revised in many states across the country. The motivation for tougher laws and greater enforcement is to decrease teen pregnancy, increase male responsibility, and decrease welfare dependency. Traditionally, statutory rape laws have been concerned with the protection of girls. In the past 20 years, many laws have been rewritten to be gender neutral. Statutory rape laws require reporting to child protective services or local law enforcement. One risk of strict statutory rape enforcement is that girls may not seek health care for reproductive care, prenatal care, or domestic violence. Young people may fear not only for themselves, but also for their partner. However, sexual coercion of teens by adults remains a problem and results in STDs and adolescent pregnancy.

In the United States, it is illegal for anyone to have sexual intercourse with a child under the age of 12 years. These laws protect the health and safety of children incapable of protecting themselves. When consensuality is considered in statutory rape laws and cases, it implies that adolescents are morally and socially responsible for sexual contact that occurs with adults.

This does not afford adolescents the same protections provided to children under the age of 12 (Kandakai and Smith, 2007).

Nurses can obtain information about their state statutory rape reporting responsibilities from state or local child protective services agencies, legal counsel, rape crisis organizations, state or local law enforcement agencies, or the state nurses' association. The limits of confidentiality should be clearly reviewed with each adolescent patient before beginning the interview about sexual activity.

There has been a reported increase in the use of drug-facilitated sexual assaults. Older adolescents and young adults at parties, bars, and raves are at risk for having a drug slipped into their beverage when they are not looking. Substances most often referred to as "date rape" drugs are flunitrazepam (Rohypnol), a sedative-hypnotic benzodiazepine; γ-hydroxybutyric acid (GHB), a sleep aid; and ketamine, an anesthetic agent (Schwartz, Milteer, and LeBeau, 2000). However, alcohol is the most widely used drug in such assaults. These fast-acting drugs cause disinhibition, passivity, relaxation of muscles, and lasting amnesia. The victim wakes up in strange surroundings and realizes she has been sexually assaulted. She may not report the crime for days or weeks or may never report it. Acquaintance rape is frequently underreported because the victim may believe she contributed to the act in some way. The victim may not identify the experience as rape because it does not fit the standard concept.

Diagnostic Evaluation

The rape victim may exhibit a variety of reactions (Box 17-2), and the circumstances of the initial medical evaluation may be frightening and stressful. The initial contact with the rape

---

BOX 17-1
Definitions of Sexual Assaults

Sexual assault—Comprehensive term that includes various types of forced or inappropriate sexual activity. Sexual assault includes both physical and psychologic coercion as well as touch, penetration, and other sexual contact.

Rape—Forced sexual intercourse that occurs by physical force or psychologic coercion. Rape includes vaginal, anal, or oral penetration by body parts or inanimate objects.

Acquaintance rape (date rape)—Applied to situations in which the assailant and victim know each other.

Statutory rape—Consensual sexual contact by a person 18 years of age or older with a person under the age of consent or unable to consent because of developmental disability. Age of consent varies by state.

BOX 17-2
Clinical Manifestations of Rape Victims

MAY DISPLAY A VARIETY OF EMOTIONS AND BEHAVIORS:
Hysterical crying
Giggling
Agitation
Feelings of degradation
Anger and rage
Helplessness
Nervousness
Rapid mood swings
Appearing calm and controlled (masking inner turmoil)
Confused
Self-blame
Fear—of the rape and of injury

EVIDENCE OF PHYSICAL FORCE FROM:
Roughness
Nonbrutal beating (slapping)
Brutal beating (slugging, kicking, beating repeatedly with fists)
Choking or gagging

MEDICAL EXAMINATION PROVIDES EVIDENCE OF:
Penetration
Ejaculation
Use of force

victim must be supportive because the interrogation and associated activities have the potential to add to the trauma of the sexual assault. First of all, the victim needs to know that she (or he) is (1) all right and (2) not being blamed for the situation.

It is important to obtain a clear account of the circumstances of an alleged rape without forcing the victim to relive a painful experience. Information includes date, time, location, and an accurate description of any type of sexual contact. The physical examination is carried out as soon as possible, since physical evidence deteriorates rapidly. The victim should not bathe or shower before the examination.

NURSINGALERT

It is not uncommon for rape victims to delay seeking help, especially in cases of acquaintance or date rape. Nurses can be most supportive by acknowledging the painful and sometimes confusing feelings that surround such experiences and by focusing on the fact that the victim is seeking assistance now.

The young person is always told in advance in understandable terms exactly what to expect in the way of tests and procedures, and the explanation is accompanied by strong emotional support. The victim is examined thoroughly, including nongenital areas, for evidence of injury that might substantiate the use of force.

The forensic examination of a sexual assault victim must follow strict legal requirements. The medical record may provide key evidence for the legal case. Practitioners specially trained for rape examination should be used when possible. Nurses are often members of this group and are known as sexual assault nurse examiners (SANEs). Evaluation for STDs is an important part of the evaluation. All potential infection sites are tested to detect gonorrhea, chlamydia, and trichomoniasis. Blood samples for syphilis, hepatitis B virus, and HIV are obtained as a baseline (American Academy of Pediatrics, 2001a). The adolescent is reexamined at appropriate intervals (4 to 6 weeks for syphilis; 2 to 3 days for gonorrhea) to determine if a disease was acquired from the assailant.

Prophylactic treatment for chlamydia and gonorrhea is recommended. Female victims should be provided with emergency contraception. The recommendation for HIV prophylaxis varies depending on the geographic area, the circumstances of the assault, and the known HIV status of the perpetrator. The Centers for Disease Control and Prevention (2006a) maintains updates and recommendations for treatment of STDs incurred as a result of sexual assault.*

Therapeutic Management

Adolescents who have been raped arrive at the emergency department or practitioner's office under a variety of circumstances. They are usually brought by parents, friends, or police officers, but some may seek medical help on their own. It is advisable to obtain parental consent for examination, but the examination may be performed without parental consent if the adolescent is mature and the parents are unavailable. A female observer should be present during the history and examination of female victims who are examined by a male

FAMILY FOCUS

Supporting the Rape Victim's Parents
In addition to the needs of the adolescent rape victim, the nurse is also sensitive to the needs and reactions of the adolescent's parents. Some will be angry and blame the adolescent; others will feel guilty and embarrassed. Many reactions can be expected at the time of the incident, ranging from despair to extreme agitation. Frequently the parents require as much support and reassurance as the victim. Agitated, angry, or incapacitated parents are unable to provide support for their adolescent. Meeting their needs can foster their ability to support the teenager during the crisis.

practitioner. Whether a parent should be present during the examination is determined on an individual basis. The parent's presence is usually encouraged if the parent is supportive and the young person agrees.

Rape Trauma Syndrome

The term **rape trauma syndrome** refers to the victim's reaction to a sexual assault. The syndrome involves two phases: (1) the acute phase of disorganization of lifestyle and (2) a long-term process of reorganization. These phases encompass behavioral, somatic, and psychologic reactions to the stressful event. Counseling should begin immediately upon the adolescent's entrance into the emergency department with follow-up within the first 24 hours. Early intervention has been shown to be effective in decreasing the extent of rape trauma syndrome (Patel and Minshall, 2001).

Nursing Care Management

Many of the approaches that have been described for the sexually abused child (see Chapter 14) apply to the adolescent. Sexual assault is a devastating experience with long-lasting effects. The primary goal of nursing care is to avoid inflicting further stress on the adolescent, who is often angry, confused, frightened, embarrassed, and filled with self-blame. The nurse must do everything possible to reduce the stress of the interrogation and examination. Although most health professionals and law enforcement officers are sensitive to the needs of the adolescent and attempt to make the process as nonstressful as possible, the nurse should be alert to cues that indicate the victim is being overstressed.

Follow-up care of the rape victim is essential and extends over a long period. Aside from the universal need for emotional support, the needs of rape victims vary widely and depend on the nature of the incident, the victim's age when the rape occurred, the physical and emotional injuries sustained by the victim, the legal actions being considered as a result, the resources available for informal support, and the anticipated reactions of persons in the informal support network (see Family Focus box).*

EATING DISORDERS

OBESITY

Few problems in childhood and adolescence are so obvious to others, are so difficult to treat, and have such long-term effects on health as obesity. Several different definitions have been proposed for obesity and overweight. **Obesity** has been defined as an increase in body weight resulting from an excessive accumulation of body fat relative to lean body mass. **Overweight** refers to the state of weighing more than average for height and body build. Currently, the **body mass index (BMI)** measurement is recommended as the most accurate method for screening children and adolescents for obesity. The BMI measurement is strongly associated with subcutaneous and total body fat and also with skinfold thickness measurements. It is also highly specific for children with the greatest amount of body fat. Pediatric growth charts that include BMI for age and gender are available from Centers for Disease Control and Prevention.* Children with a BMI between the 85th and 95th percentiles are considered overweight, and obesity is defined by a BMI greater than the 95th percentile (Moran, 2003).

Regardless of the definition used, the number of overweight children in the United States is increasing and may be approaching epidemic status (Shulman, 2004). In children ages 6 to 11 years, the prevalence of childhood overweight remained fairly constant in the years 1963 and 1974 at approximately 4% and 5.5%, respectively. However, in the National Health and Nutrition Examination Survey, those numbers have steadily climbed to reach 16% in both 6- to 11-year-olds and 12- to 19-year-olds in 2001 to 2002; almost 32% of children ages 6 to 19 were at risk for overweight (Hedley, Ogden, Johnson, and others, 2004). African-American and Hispanic children and youth are disproportionately represented by a higher prevalence of overweight (21.5% and 21.8%, respectively) when compared with non-Hispanic Caucasian children (12.3%) (National Institute for Health Care Management Foundation, 2003). These numbers double if they include children defined as being at risk for overweight (>85th percentile on growth chart). A study of 9464 American Indian schoolchildren ages 5 to 18 years found that 39% were overweight, and a further review of tribes across the United States found that 30% to 46% of American Indians were at risk for overweight (>85th percentile) (Hardy, Harrell, and Bell, 2004).

Because adult obesity is associated with increased mortality and morbidity from a variety of complications, both physical and psychologic, adolescent obesity is a serious condition. Research indicates that overweight children and adolescents are at risk of continuing to be obese as adults, thereby experiencing the health and social consequences of obesity much earlier than children and adolescents of normal weight. Parental obesity increases the risk of overweight by twofold to threefold (Baker, Barlow, Cochran, and others, 2005). The probability that overweight school-age children will become obese adults is estimated at 50%, whereas the likelihood that overweight adolescents will become obese adults is estimated at 70% to 80% (National Institute for Health Care Management Foundation, 2003).

Obesity in childhood and adolescence has been related to elevated blood cholesterol, high blood pressure, respiratory disorders, orthopedic conditions (Taylor, Theim, Mirch, and

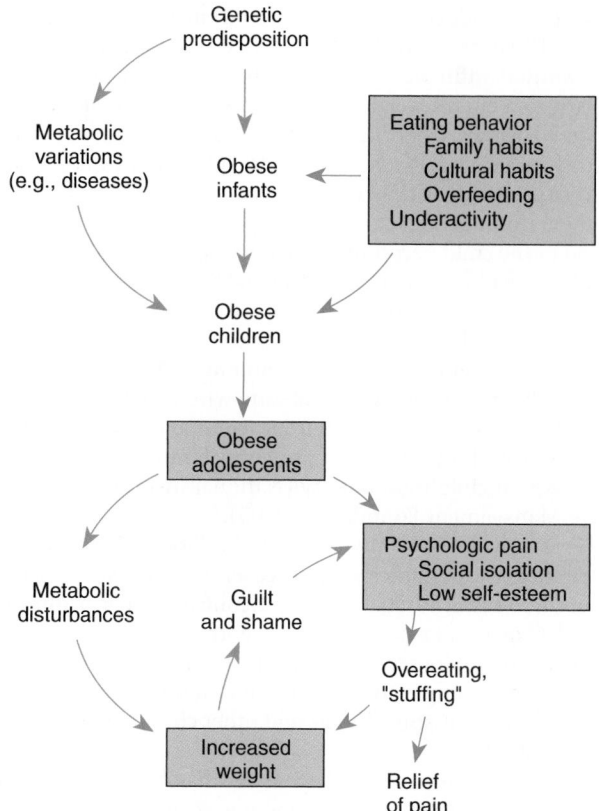

FIG. 17-2 ■ Complex relationships in obesity.

others, 2006), cholelithiasis, some types of adult-onset cancer (MacKenzie, 2000), nonalcoholic fatty liver disease (NAFLD) (Baker, Barlow, Cochran, and others, 2005; Angulo, 2002), and type 2 diabetes mellitus (Ehtisham, Barrett, and Shaw, 2000). The incidence of metabolic syndrome was 50% in a study group of overweight and obese adolescents (Weiss, Dziura, Burgert, and others, 2004). Common emotional consequences of obesity include poor body image, low self-esteem, social isolation, and feelings of depression and rejection (Sjöberg, Nilsson, and Leppert, 2005).

Etiology and Pathophysiology

Obesity results from a caloric intake that consistently exceeds caloric requirements and expenditure and may involve a variety of interrelated influences, including metabolic, hypothalamic, hereditary, social, cultural, and psychologic factors (Fig. 17-2). Because the etiology of obesity is multifactorial, the treatment requires multilevel interventions.

Birth weight is not a contributing factor in detection and prediction of childhood obesity; obese children do not have higher birth weights than nonobese children. There is, however, a high correlation between childhood adiposity and parental adiposity.

A balance between **energy intake** and **energy expenditure** is a critical factor in regulating body weight. Factors that raise energy intake or decrease energy expenditure by even small amounts can have a long-term impact on the development of overweight and obesity. For example, a positive balance of one serving of a sweetened juice or soft drink (about 120 kcal) per day would produce a 50 kg (110 pound) increase in body mass over a 10-year period (Hill, Wyatt, Reed, and others, 2003).

Familial influence is an epidemiologic consideration in regard to a child's weight. Twin studies suggest that approximately 50% to 70% of the tendency toward obesity is inherited (Kiess, Galler, Reich, and others, 2001). Twin studies have also suggested that this tendency is a combination of genetic and environmental factors. If both parents are lean, the likelihood of the child becoming overweight is just 9%. When both parents are obese, there is a 60% to 80% increase in the likelihood of the child becoming obese (Koeppen-Schomerus, Wardle, and Plomin, 2001). The specific influences of genes and environment within the developing child is not well defined. The increasing rates of obesity within genetically stable populations suggest that environmental and some perinatal factors (e.g., bottle feeding) are contributors to the current increases in childhood obesity (National Institute for Health Care Management Foundation, 2003).

Fewer than 5% of the cases of childhood obesity can be attributed to an underlying **disease.** Such diseases include hypothyroidism; adrenal hypercorticoidism; hyperinsulinism; and dysfunction or damage to the central nervous system as a result of tumor, injury, infection, or vascular accident. Obesity is a frequent complication of muscular dystrophy, paraplegia, Down syndrome, spina bifida, and other chronic illnesses that limit mobility.

A major focus of obesity research has been on **appetite regulation.** The expression of appetite is chemically coded in the hypothalamus by distinctive circuitry. Orexigenic substances produce signals that promote eating behaviors, and anorexigenic substances promote the cessation of eating behaviors. Feedback loops between signals have been identified where one signal peptide is able to alter the secretion of another signal peptide. No one signal has been identified as the gatekeeper of appetite. It is apparent that an entire network of signals, including their frequency and amplitude, is responsible for triggering eating behaviors.

There is little evidence to support a relationship between obesity and "**low metabolism.**" Small differences may exist in regulation of dietary intake or metabolic rate between obese and nonobese children that could lead to an energy imbalance and inappropriate weight gain, but these small differences are difficult to accurately quantify. No differences in basal metabolic rate, sleeping metabolic rate, respiratory quotient, heart rate, or total energy expenditure have been found in normal weight children with or without a familial predisposition to overweight (Baker, Barlow, Cochran, and others, 2005). In childhood, overeating is the dominant feature in obesity, whereas in adult life, reduced physical activity with normal intake is more likely.

The tendency toward obesity is manifested whenever **environmental conditions** are favorable to excessive caloric intake, such as an abundance of food, limited access to low-fat foods, reduced or minimum physical activity, and snacking combined with excessive television viewing. Family and cultural eating patterns, as well as psychologic factors, play an important role; many families and cultures consider fat to be an indication of good health. It is not uncommon for obese children to have families that emphasize large meals or admonish children for leaving food on their plates. Parents may have an exaggerated concept of the amount of food children require and expect them to eat more than they need. The

prevalence of obesity shows a marked difference between upper- and lower-class children, with differences often becoming apparent before 6 years of age. Lower socioeconomic groups have a greater prevalence of obesity, especially in girls. Physical activity may also be influenced by sociocultural factors.

Some **community factors** that influence activity patterns include unsafe neighborhoods that keep children from playing outside. Many communities lack affordable and accessible areas for low-income youth to be active, thus limiting opportunities for young people to participate in physical activities. Social policies also contribute to obesity. The increased availability of high-fat foods, pricing strategies that promote unhealthy food choices, and overzealous food advertising that targets children and adolescents with high-fat and high-sugar foods are some examples.

Institutional factors also influence patterns of obesity and decreased physical activity. Many school policies allow students to leave school for lunch. Vending machines in school often are filled with high-fat and high-calorie foods and soft drinks. Although well-balanced, nutritious school lunches may be available to students, they will often opt for less nutritious choices such as high-fat snacks.

Physical inactivity has also been identified as an important contributing factor in the development and maintenance of childhood overweight. There is little doubt that physical activity has decreased in elementary and secondary schools in the United States. Consequently, most of a child's physical activity must occur within the family or outside of school. Decreased physical activity within the family is a powerful influence on children, since children imitate their parents and other adults. Parental obesity and low levels of physical activity are correlated with decreased physical activity in children.

The growing attraction and availability of many sedentary activities, including television, video games, computers, and the Internet, have greatly influenced the amount of time that children spend participating in sedentary behaviors. A study conducted by the Kaiser Family Foundation demonstrated that children watch an average of 2½ hours of television per day, and that one in five kids watches TV for 5 hours or more every day (Rideout, Foehr, Roberts, and others, 1999). When combining television viewing with video games, it is estimated that children may spend as much as 6½ hours per day on various media, which takes time away from meaningful activities such as exercise and reading (American Academy of Pediatrics, 2001b).

Psychologic factors also affect eating patterns. In infancy, children experience relief from discomfort through feeding and learn to associate eating with a sense of well-being, security, and the comforting presence of a nurturing person. Eating is soon associated with the feeling of being loved. In addition, the pleasurable oral sensation of sucking provides a connection between emotions and early eating behavior. Many parents use food as a positive reinforcer for desired behaviors. This practice may become a habit, and the child may continue to use food as a reward, a comfort, and a means of dealing with depression or hostility. Many individuals eat when they are not hungry or in response to boredom, loneliness, sadness, depression, or tiredness. Difficulty in determining feelings of satiety can lead to weight problems and may compound the factor of eating in response to emotional rather than physical hunger cues.

Eating behaviors are closely related to memory. Memory and appetite are chemically encoded, with each individual having his or her own circuitry relating to eating behaviors. Like memory, the circuitry can be modified over time (Feldman, Friedman, and Sleisenger, 2002).

Diagnostic Evaluation

A careful history is obtained regarding the development of obesity, and a physical examination is performed to differentiate simple obesity from increased fat that results from organic causes. A family history of obesity, diabetes, coronary heart disease, and dyslipidemia should be obtained for all children who are overweight or at risk for overweight. Specific information from the patient and family about the effects of obesity on daily functioning—for example, problems with nighttime breathing and sleep, daytime sleepiness, pain in the joints, ability to keep up with family activities and peers at school—will be helpful. The physical examination should focus on identifying comorbid conditions and identifiable causes of obesity. For some, psychologic assessment, by interviews and standardized personality tests, may provide insight into the personality and emotional problems that contribute to obesity and that might interfere with therapy.

It is useful to estimate the degree of obesity to determine the component of body weight that can be modified. All the following methods have been used to assess obesity: BMI, body weight, weight-height ratios, weight-age ratios, hydrostatic (underwater) weight, skinfold measurements, bioelectrical analysis, computed tomography (CT), magnetic resonance imaging (MRI), and neutron activation. Each of these methods has advantages and disadvantages. Hydrostatic, or underwater, weighing provides the most accurate measurement of lean body weight.

BMI is currently considered the best method to assess weight in children and adolescents. The calculation is based on the individual's height and weight. In adults, BMI definitions are fixed measures without regard for sex and age. The BMI in children and adolescents varies to accommodate age- and gender-specific changes in growth. The formula for BMI calculation is:

$$\frac{\text{Weight in pounds} \div \text{Height in inches} \times 703}{\text{Height in inches}}$$

or

$$\frac{\text{Weight in kilograms}}{[\text{Height in meters}]^2}$$

BMI measures in children and adolescents are plotted on growth charts that enable heath care professionals to determine BMI-for-age for the patient (see Appendix B).

The initial assessment of obese children and adolescents should include screening to evaluate for comorbidities. The history is an important guide to determine the workup. A complete physical examination is important. Some areas to focus on include (1) skin for stretch markings and discolorations (e.g., acanthosis nigricans), (2) joints for swelling and evidence of pain, and (3) airway for evidence of obstruction and enlarged tonsils. Basic laboratory studies include a fasting lipid panel; fasting insulin level; fasting glucose hepatic enzymes, including γ-glutamyltransferase (GGT); and, in some institutions, hemoglobin A_{1c}. Other studies, such as a sleep study, metabolic studies, and radiographic evaluations, may be added based on the history and physical examination. These assess-

ments may determine whether the patient needs a referral to specialty services for more focused evaluation and treatment, such as endocrinology (insulin resistance, diabetes), hepatology (elevated liver enzymes, NAFLD), orthopedics (Blount disease), or pulmonary medicine (sleep-disordered breathing, continuous positive airway pressure).

Therapeutic Management

The best approach to the management of obesity is a preventive one. Early recognition and control measures are essential before the child or adolescent reaches an obese state. Health care providers must educate families about the medical complications of obesity, and families are encouraged to be involved in the treatment plan.

The treatment of obesity is difficult. Many approaches do not achieve long-term success. The average individual only loses about 5% to 10% of his or her weight with available therapies. Losing weight can have a significant positive effect on many comorbidities, but unfortunately the lost weight is frequently regained in a year or two (Yanovski and Yanovski, 2002).

Diet modification is an essential part of weight-reduction programs. Dietary counseling is directed toward improving the nutritional quality of the diet rather than on dietary restriction. Children should avoid fad diets. Most dietitians and nutrition experts recommend a diet with low-saturated fat, moderate total fat (≤30%), and five servings of fruits and vegetables, consistent with the MyPyramid* food guide for children. Also, promoting high-fiber foods and avoiding highly refined starches and sugars will decrease caloric intake. The Dietary Guidelines for Americans† may be used as a guide for caloric intake for adolescents concerned about weight control; these guidelines also emphasize daily exercise in weight management for children and adolescents. Many programs recommend using a food diary as a helpful tool to increase awareness of food choices and eating behaviors. The goal is to encourage the individual to make healthier choices in food selection and discourage eating food by habit or to appease boredom.

In patients with severe obesity, strict diets have been used, such as the protein-sparing modified fast, a hypocaloric, ketogenic diet that is designed to provide enough protein to minimize loss of lean body mass during weight loss. Such diets need to be closely monitored and should be used only with multidisciplinary teams that include a physician, nutritionist, and behavioral therapist. Generally, the diet consists of 1.5 to 2.5 g of protein per kilogram. The intake of carbohydrates is low enough to induce ketosis. The benefits of the diet are relatively rapid weight loss and anorexia induced by ketosis. Potential complications include protein losses, hypokalemia, hypoglycemia, inadequate calcium intake, and orthostatic hypotension. Potassium and calcium supplements and adequate calorie-free beverages can minimize these complications (Baker, Barlow, Cochran, and others, 2005). It is difficult to sustain such diets over the long term, and the long-term outcomes of using these diets have not been established.

Some drugs have been used to promote weight loss in children with certain conditions such as metformin in obese adolescents with insulin resistance and hyperinsulinism, octreo-

---

*http://www.mypyramid.gov/kids/index.html.
†http://www.health.gov/dietaryguidelines/dga2005/document/default.htm.

tide for hypothalamic obesity caused by intracranial tumors, growth hormone in children with Prader-Willi syndrome, and leptin for congenital leptin deficiency. The drug sibutramine, in addition to behavioral therapy, significantly reduced BMI and body weight more than placebo; however, the drug was associated with side effects (tachycardia and hypertension) (Berkowitz, Fujioka, Daniels, and others, 2006).

Bariatric surgery may be the only practical alternative for increasing numbers of severely overweight adolescents who have failed organized attempts to lose or maintain weight loss through conventional nonoperative approaches and who have serious life-threatening conditions. Some preliminary studies suggest that adolescents with severe obesity have successful weight loss up to 14 years after bariatric surgery; most adolescents were reported to have a significant change in lifestyle as a result of the weight loss after surgery (Sugerman, Sugerman, DeMaria, and others, 2003). Others suggest that bariatric surgery in adolescents is safe and they have fewer postoperative complications than adults, but the procedure is relatively uncommon in comparison to the number of adults having surgery for obesity (Tsai, Inge, and Burd, 2007). In general, bariatric surgery should be reserved for severely obese adolescents with comorbidities after careful consideration. Candidates for surgery should be referred to centers that offer a multidisciplinary team experienced in the management of childhood and adolescent obesity, and the surgery should be performed by surgeons who have participated in subspecialty training in bariatric medical and surgical care as detailed by the American College of Surgeons and the American Society for Metabolic and Bariatric Surgery.

Nursing Care Management

Nurses play a key role in the adherence and maintenance phases of many weight-reduction programs. Nurses assess, manage, and evaluate the progress of many overweight adolescents. They also play an important role in recognizing potential weight problems and assisting parents and adolescents in preventing obesity. The nursing process in the care of the adolescent with obesity or overweight is outlined in the Nursing Process box.

The presence of obesity may not be obvious from appearance alone. Regular assessment of height and weight and computation of the BMI facilitate early recognition. Children with a BMI greater than or equal to the 95th percentile for age and sex should receive in-depth medical assessment. Children with a BMI in the 85th to 95th percentile range should be evaluated for secondary complications, such as hypertension and hyperlipidemia, and family history (Greaser and Whyte, 2004). Evaluation includes a height and weight history of the adolescent and family members, eating habits, appetite and hunger patterns, and physical activities. A psychosocial history is also helpful in understanding the impact of obesity on the child's life.

Before initiating a treatment plan, it is important to be certain that the family is ready for change. Lack of readiness may result in failure, frustration, and reluctance to address the problem in the future. The nurse should explore with adolescents the reasons behind the desire to lose weight, since motivation to lose weight is the key to success. Adolescents need to take a personal responsibility for dietary habits and physical activity. Teens who are forced by their parents to seek help are

---

nursingprocess | **The Child or Adolescent Who Is Overweight or Obese**

ASSESSMENT
The nurse assists in determining the child or adolescent's body mass index, gathers appropriate anthropometric data, uses standardized growth charts to plot growth, and obtains a comprehensive health history. Further information that is appropriate to obtain in the assessment includes a 24-hour food intake history, family health history, and lifestyle practices that affect the child or adolescent's well-being. The health interview and nutritional assessment often provide clues and guidelines for further investigation.

DIAGNOSIS (PROBLEM IDENTIFICATION)
Several nursing diagnoses are identified after a thorough assessment:
- Situational Low Self-Esteem
- Imbalanced Nutrition: More Than Body Requirements
- Risk for Injury
- Risk-Prone Health Behavior
- Disturbed Personal Identity

PLANNING
Expected patient outcomes for the adolescent with an eating disorder include:
- Child or adolescent will develop a positive self-image.
- Adolescent will willingly engage in behaviors to reverse effects of cardiovascular disease.

- Healthy personal identity will be achieved.
- Healthy eating patterns will be adopted.
- Adolescent will assume control for changes in lifestyle designed to lose weight.
- Child or adolescent will remain injury free.

IMPLEMENTATION
Numerous intervention strategies are discussed on pp. 554-556.

EVALUATION
The effectiveness of nursing interventions is determined by continual reassessment and evaluation of nursing care based on the following observational guidelines:
- Perform nutritional assessment; measure weight; review diet and nutritional intake (e.g., log); interview adolescent regarding food and eating behaviors; observe eating behaviors.
- Interview adolescent regarding self-perceptions; observe behavior; confer with psychologist and other members of the interdisciplinary team regarding evidence of progress.
- Observe adolescent's behavior, and interview him or her regarding attitudes, concerns, and behaviors.

seldom motivated, become rebellious, and are unwilling to control their dietary intake.

Nutritional Counseling. Preventing an increase in body fat during growth is a realistic approach. This is often accomplished by adjusting three aspects of eating:

1. Reducing the quantity eaten by purchasing, preparing, and serving smaller portions
2. Altering the quality consumed by substituting low-calorie, low-fat foods for high-calorie foods (especially for snacks)
3. Altering situations by severing associations between eating and other stimuli, such as eating while watching television

The most successful diets are those that use ordinary foods in controlled portions rather than diets that require the avoidance of specific foods. Recently, low-carbohydrate diets such as the Atkins diet have been promoted for weight loss in adults and adolescents (Sondike, Copperman, and Jacobson, 2003). However, low-carbohydrate diets can result in ketosis, insulin resistance, and glucose intolerance. More research is needed to evaluate the long-term safety and efficacy of these diets for children and adolescents.

The nurse teaches adolescents and parents how to incorporate favorite foods into their diet and to select satisfying substitutes. The dieting teen should eat what the rest of the family eats, but less of it. When parents buy and prepare smaller amounts, they eliminate tempting second helpings and leftovers. To maintain a healthy diet, it is necessary to encourage the consumption of high-nutrient foods such as fruits, vegetables, whole grains, and low-fat dairy protein products. Calories and fat should be kept to a healthy level without being significantly restricted. To be successful, a dietary program should be nutritionally sound with sufficient satiety value, produce the desired weight loss, and be accompanied by nutrition education and continued support. Children and adolescents should not initiate a reduction diet without health assessment and counseling (Schwimmer, 2004).

Behavioral Therapy. Altering eating behavior and eliminating inappropriate eating habits are essential to weight reduction, especially in maintaining long-term weight control. Most behavioral modification programs include the following concepts:

- A description of the behavior to be controlled, such as eating habits
- Attempts to modify and control the stimuli that govern eating
- Development of eating techniques designed to control speed of eating
- Positive reinforcement for these modifications through a suitable reward system

Specific strategies to modify eating habits are included in Box 17-3.

Group Involvement. Commercial groups (e.g., Weight Watchers) or diet workshops composed primarily of adults may be helpful to some teenagers; however, a group of other adolescents is often more effective. Teenage groups include summer camps designed for obese young people and conducted by health professionals, school groups organized and led by a school nurse, and groups associated with special clinics.

These groups are concerned not only with weight loss but also with the development of a positive self-image and the encouragement of physical activity. Nutrition education, diet planning, and the improvement of social skills are essential components of these groups. Improvement is determined by positive changes in all aspects of behavior.

Family Involvement. There is a definite connection between family environment, interaction, and obesity. The nurse needs to educate parents in the purposes of the therapeutic measures and their role in management. The family needs nutrition education and counseling regarding the reinforcement plan, alterations in the food environment, and ways to maintain proper attitudes. They can support their child in efforts to change eating behaviors, food intake, and physical activity.

Physical Activity. Regular physical activity is incorporated into all weight-reduction programs. Any form of increased physical activity is beneficial, provided that the activities are age appropriate and enjoyable. Recommendations for physical activity need to consider the current health status and developmental level of the child or adolescent. The best choice for exercise is any form that is enjoyable and likely to be sustainable. Aerobic and endurance exercises help oxidize body fats. Light exercises like walking may provide an opportunity for the family to increase time together and increase caloric expenditure. Walking for 30 minutes each day and decreasing caloric intake by 500 calories per day may significantly reduce the risk of chronic disease. Weight training can increase basal metabolic rate and replace fat mass with muscle mass. However, weight training is not generally recommended for prepubertal children until they have reached physical and skeletal

---

BOX 17-3

Helpful Suggestions to Promote Healthy Eating Habits

1. Identify current eating patterns and behaviors by keeping a food diary to look for areas to change. Record everything eaten, including where, when, and associated activities.
2. Change eating patterns.
   - Choose sugar-free beverages or low-fat milk only.
   - Limit fast-food consumption to no more than once a week.
   - Do not skip meals.
   - Eat three meals and one or two snacks per day.
   - Try the plate method: one half plate of vegetables, one fourth plate of lean meat, and one fourth plate of starch or starchy vegetables (potatoes, peas).
   - Take second helpings of fruits and vegetables (not potatoes) only.
   - Avoid low-fat food (these are usually high in sugars).
   - Use whole grain breads, cereals, and pastas.
   - Pack your lunch for school.
   - Buy healthy foods for snacking.
3. Change the act of eating.
   - Eat meals at the family dinner table.
   - Avoid distractions (e.g., television).
   - Slow down; meals may last at least 20 to 30 minutes.
4. Substitute other activities for managing stress, such as hobbies, walking, listening to music, talking to friends on the phone, reading, playing a game.
5. Provide alternative rewards for reinforcement or accomplishments (e.g., CDs, movie, concert, new clothes, new games).
6. Think positively.
7. Enlist family involvement and support.

maturity. In prepubertal children increasing outdoor playtime is likely to be beneficial. Many children find exercise videos and treadmills boring and may not continue these activities. There are a great variety of physical activities to choose from that are likely to appeal to different people. Team sports and individual sports such as dance, bike riding, swimming, and karate are some. Limiting sedentary activities such as television viewing (while eating snacks!) is the most effective way to encourage physical activity (Robinson, 2001).

Prevention. Weight loss programs do not enjoy the success of therapeutic interventions for other disorders. Gradual accumulation of adipose tissue during childhood establishes a pattern of eating that is difficult to reverse in adolescence. Prevention of obesity should begin in early childhood with the development of healthy eating habits, regular exercise patterns, and a positive relationship between parents and children. Prevention of adolescent obesity is best accomplished by early identification of obesity in the preschool, school-age, and preadolescent periods. Health care professionals should encourage frequent health care visits for children who are overweight or obese and incorporate a dietary history and counseling into each well-infant, well-child, and well-adolescent visit.

ANOREXIA NERVOSA AND BULIMIA NERVOSA

Anorexia nervosa (AN) is an eating disorder characterized by a refusal to maintain a minimally normal body weight and by severe weight loss in the absence of obvious physical causes. Approximately 5% of adolescent females in the United States have AN, and 5% to 10% of all cases occur in males (American Academy of Pediatrics, 2003). The average age of onset is 13 years, but the disorder can occur as early as 10 years of age and as late as 25 years of age. Individuals with AN are described as perfectionists, academically high achievers, conforming, and conscientious. Typically, they have high energy levels, even with marked emaciation. Patients with AN may eventually develop bulimia (Mehler, 2001).

Bulimia (from the Greek meaning "ox hunger") refers to an eating disorder similar to AN. Bulimia nervosa (BN) is observed more commonly in older adolescent girls and young women; males with bulimia are less common. BN patients may be of average or slightly above average weight. BN is characterized by repeated episodes of binge eating followed by inappropriate compensatory behaviors, such as self-induced vomiting; misuse of laxatives, diuretics, or other medications; fasting; or excessive exercise (American Psychiatric Association, 2000). The binge behavior consists of secretive, frenzied consumption of large amounts of high-calorie (or "forbidden") foods during a brief time (usually less than 2 hours). The binge is counteracted by a variety of weight control methods **(purging)**. These binge-purge cycles are followed by self-deprecating thoughts, a depressed mood, and an awareness that the eating pattern is abnormal.

Although persons with BN have many issues in common with those who have other eating disorders, impulse control and satiety regulation are important problems in BN. Many individuals with BN begin with only occasional binges and purges "just for fun," enjoying the control over their weight while eating amounts of food that would normally produce obesity. As the condition progresses, the frequency of binges increases, the amount of food consumed increases, and they

gradually lose control over the binge-purge cycle. The frequency of binging can be anywhere from once per week to seven or eight times per day. Because persons with BN usually binge on high-calorie foods, especially sweets, ice cream, and pastries, insulin production is stimulated to cope with the added carbohydrates. When the food is vomited, the unused insulin stimulates hunger and the desire to eat.

A third eating disorder, identified as **EDNOS (eating disorder not otherwise specified)**, has components of both AN and BN with varying degrees of symptomatology that are not always characteristic of the established diagnostic criteria for AN and BN (American Dietetic Association, 2006). **Binge eating disorder (BED)** is a type of EDNOS. Persons with BED may diet in an attempt to control their weight but without the extreme weight-control compensatory practices of vomiting, laxative use, diuretics, and excessive exercise (American Dietetic Association, 2006; Forman, 2007).

Etiology and Pathophysiology

The etiology of these disorders remains unclear. There is a distinct psychologic component, and the diagnosis is based primarily on psychologic and behavioral criteria. Dieting appears to be common to the initiation of both AN and BN. The disorders appear to be caused by a combination of genetic, neurochemical, psychodevelopmental, and sociocultural factors. The dominant aspects of AN are a relentless pursuit of thinness and a fear of fatness, usually preceded by a period of mood disturbances and behavior changes.

Weight loss may be triggered by a typical adolescent crisis such as the onset of menstruation or a traumatic interpersonal incident that precipitates serious, out-of-control dieting. Situations of severe family stress (such as parental separation or divorce) or circumstances in which the adolescent perceives a lack of personal control (such as teasing at school, changing schools, or going to college) may precipitate a desire for control and the decision not to eat. Frequently, there is an exaggerated misinterpretation of the normal fat deposition characteristic of early adolescence or anxiety because of comments that the adolescent is putting on weight.

Many experts have associated the development of an eating disorder with family characteristics such as an adolescent perception of high parental expectations for achievement and appearance, difficulty managing conflict and poor communication styles, enmeshment and occasionally estrangement between family members, devaluation of the mother or the maternal role, and marital tension. Families struggling with an eating disorder have been characterized as often having difficulties responding positively to the changing physical and emotional needs of the adolescent. Family stress of any kind may become a significant factor in the development of an eating disorder (Forman, 2007).

Society's emphasis and the media's focus on tall, thin individuals may also play a role. Studies evaluating the possible association of eating disorders and sexual abuse have been conflicting. Childhood sexual abuse may be a factor in some cases of AN.

Patients with eating disorders commonly have psychiatric problems, including affective disorder, anxiety disorder, obsessive-compulsive disorder, and personality disorder. Adult women with eating disorders were found to have higher rates of obsessive-compulsive behavior traits in their child-

BOX 17-4

Clinical Manifestations of Anorexia Nervosa

- Severe and profound weight loss
- Secondary amenorrhea (if menarche attained)
- Primary amenorrhea (if menarche not attained)
- Sinus bradycardia
- Lowered body temperature
- Hypotension
- Intolerance to cold
- Dry skin and brittle nails
- Appearance of lanugo hair
- Thinning hair
- Abdominal pain
- Bloating
- Constipation
- Fatigue
- Lightheadedness
- Evidence of muscle wasting (cachectic appearance)
- Bone pain with exercise

BOX 17-5

Diagnostic Criteria for Anorexia Nervosa

1. Refusal to maintain body weight over a minimal normal weight for age and height (e.g., weight loss leading to maintenance of body weight less than 85% of that expected; or failure to make expected weight gain during period of growth, leading to body weight less than 85% of that expected)
2. Intense fear of gaining weight or becoming fat, even though underweight
3. Disturbance of body image, undue influence of shape or weight on evaluation, or denial of the seriousness of the current low body weight
4. In postmenarchal females, amenorrhea (i.e., the absence of at least three consecutive menstrual cycles); a woman is considered to have amenorrhea if her periods occur only after hormone (e.g., estrogen) administration

Specify type:

Restricting type—no regular bingeing or purging behavior (i.e., self-induced vomiting or the misuse of laxatives, diuretics, or enemas).

Binge eating/purging type—during the current episode of anorexia nervosa, the person has regularly engaged in binge eating or purging behavior (i.e., self-induced vomiting or the misuse of laxatives, diuretics, or enemas).

American Psychiatric Association: *Diagnostic and statistical manual of mental disorders*, ed 4 (text rev) (DSM-IV TR), Washington, DC, 2000, The Association.

hood. Patients with eating disorders have also been found to have higher reported rates of substance abuse, with alcohol problems being more common in those with BN than AN (Forman, 2007). It is important to note that many of the clinical findings are directly related to the state of starvation and improve with weight gain.

Many sports and artistic endeavors that emphasize leanness (e.g., ballet and running) and sports in which the scoring is partly subjective (e.g., skating and gymnastics) have been associated with a higher incidence of eating disorders such as AN. The term **female athlete triad,** characterized by disordered eating behavior, amenorrhea, and osteoporosis, has been applied to young women with restrictive eating disorders and amenorrhea (Rome, Ammerman, Rosen, and others, 2003).

A genetic role has been postulated for eating disorders; a significant number of young females with a first-degree relative having an eating disorder were at a significantly higher rate of having an eating disorder (Forman, 2007).

Diagnostic Evaluation

Diagnosis of AN is made on the basis of clinical manifestations (Box 17-4) and conformity to the criteria established by the American Psychiatric Association (2000) (Box 17-5). Diagnosis of BN is confirmed, according to the American Psychiatric Association's *Diagnostic and Statistical Manual of Mental Disorders* (2000) (Box 17-6), by at least two binge-eating episodes per week for the preceding 3 months.

A complete history and physical examination are important to rule out other causes for weight loss. The medical assessment of an eating disorder focuses on the complications of altered nutritional status and purging. A careful history assesses weight changes, dietary patterns, and the frequency and severity of purging and excessive exercise. The patient's weight and height should be measured and evaluated for appropriateness according to standard weight for height, age, and sex determined according to the percentile of his or her expected body weight or BMI.

Additional diagnostic measures may include a complete blood count to evaluate for anemia and other hematologic abnormalities; erythrocyte sedimentation rate or C-reactive protein to detect evidence of inflammation; electrolytes as well as calcium, magnesium, phosphorus, blood urea nitrogen, and

BOX 17-6

Diagnostic Criteria for Bulimia

1. Recurrent episodes of binge eating. An episode of binge eating is characterized by both of the following:
   - Eating, in a discrete period (e.g., within any 2-hour period), an amount of food that is definitely larger than most people would eat during a similar period and under similar circumstances
   - A sense of lack of control over eating during the episode (e.g., a feeling that one cannot stop eating or control what or how much one is eating)
2. Recurrent inappropriate compensatory behavior to prevent weight gain, such as self-induced vomiting; misuse of laxatives, diuretics, enemas, or other medications; fasting; or excessive exercise.
3. The binge eating and inappropriate compensatory behaviors both occur, on average, at least twice a week for 3 months.
4. Self-evaluation is unduly influenced by body shape and weight.
5. The disturbance does not occur exclusively during episodes of anorexia nervosa.

Specify type:

Purging type—During the current episode of bulimia nervosa, the person has regularly engaged in self-induced vomiting or the misuse of laxatives, diuretics, or enemas.

Nonpurging type—During the current episode of bulimia nervosa, the person has used other inappropriate compensatory behaviors, such as fasting or excessive exercise, but has not regularly engaged in self-induced vomiting or the misuse of laxatives, diuretics, or enemas.

American Psychiatric Association: *Diagnostic and statistical manual of mental disorders*, ed 4 (text rev) (DSM-IV TR), Washington, DC, 2000, The Association.

creatinine; urinalysis, including specific gravity; and bone density studies for osteopenia, which is commonly observed in patients with AN. In patients with prolonged amenorrhea, human chorionic gonadotropin (hCG) is assessed to determine the presence of pregnancy. Other tests for patients with amenorrhea include thyroid function tests and measurement of serum prolactin and follicle-stimulating hormone to help rule out prolactinoma (hormone-secreting pituitary tumor), hyperthyroidism, hypothyroidism, or ovarian failure. In addition, a comprehensive cardiac evaluation is often recommended in those with AN. Further diagnostic tests may be required based on the history and findings from above diagnostic tests.

Therapeutic Management

The treatment of AN involves four major goals:

1. Restoration of a healthy weight
2. Establishment of healthy eating patterns
3. Resolution of disturbed patterns of family interaction
4. Individual psychotherapy to correct deficits and distortions in psychologic functioning

Most adolescents are treated on an outpatient basis, but those with problems requiring immediate medical attention, such as severe malnutrition or electrolyte or psychiatric disturbances (severe depression or suicidal ideation), require hospitalization. A multidisciplinary team of dietitians, physicians, nurses, and counselors provide the interventions.

Persons with BN may benefit from cognitive behavioral therapy, other psychotherapy, antidepressant medications, or a combination of antidepressant medication and psychotherapy (Forman, 2007).

Nutrition Therapy. The most important goal is to treat any life-threatening malnutrition and to restore dietary stability and weight gain. This may require the administration of tube feedings or intravenous fluids if the malnutrition is severe. In most cases, it is best to reintroduce food and snacks slowly in a stepwise manner. A reasonable goal is to reach an eventual intake of 2000 to 3000 kcal per day and a weight gain of 0.22 to 0.45 kg (0.5 to 1 pound) per week (American Dietetic Association, 2006). When restoring nutrition, health professionals must avoid the **refeeding syndrome,** which consists of cardiovascular, neurologic, and hematologic complications that occur when nutritional replacement is given too rapidly. This syndrome can be avoided with slow refeeding and the addition of phosphorus when total body phosphorus is depleted. Treatment goal weights are individualized and based on age, height, stage of puberty, premorbid weight, and previous growth charts. In girls who have reached menarche, resumption of menses is an objective measure of return to biologic health.

Dietary interventions are combined with psychotherapy to improve the underlying psychologic misconceptions about weight loss. Another aspect of treatment is to relieve the anxiety related to eating and the depression that accompanies the disorder. The administration of antianxiety or antidepressant medications is beneficial. However, when these drugs are used, patients should be carefully monitored for cardiovascular side effects.

Psychotherapy. Behavioral interventions are often necessary to encourage patients to accomplish the desired caloric intake and weight gain. Weight restoration as an outpatient is accomplished with behavioral contracts negotiated between the therapists and patient. The goal is to increase the patient's feelings of control and responsibility toward achieving recovery. The contract can stipulate at what weight tube feedings will be implemented. Individual psychotherapy is aimed at helping the young person resolve the adolescent identity crisis, particularly as it relates to a distorted body image. If the disorder is related to a dysfunctional family situation, therapy is most successful when it is started soon after the onset of illness and directed toward disengagement and redirection of malfunctioning processes in the family.

Pharmacologic Therapy. Pharmacotherapy in the treatment of AN has been disappointing so far. The few studies that have been done have primarily evaluated medications' efficacy in the treatment of comorbid disorders such as obsessive-compulsive disorders and depression. Anxiolytic medications may be helpful before meals to relieve some patients' anxiety.

Tricyclic antidepressants and fluoxetine belong to a group of medications known as selective serotonin reuptake inhibitors (SSRIs), which have been more successful when used with BN. There is also some evidence that tricyclic antidepressants such as desipramine, imipramine, and amitriptyline; monoamine oxidase inhibitors; and buspirone are more effective compared with a placebo in decreasing binging and vomiting in patients with BN. Topiramate, an antiepileptic agent, and the selective serotonin antagonist ondansetron may have some benefit in treating BN.

Nursing Care Management

Nurses need to adopt and maintain a kind and supportive yet firm manner in managing the care of the adolescent with eating disorders without creating a passive-dependent attitude. The individual requires sustained support and reassurance to cope with ambivalent feelings related to body concept and the desire to be seen as cooperative, reliable, and worthy of receiving kindness. Encouraging the adolescent with education and activities that strengthen self-esteem facilitates the resocialization process and promotes social acceptance among peers.

It is important for nurses to be aware of the physical side effects of AN. Patients frequently limit their fluid intake. Urinary tract problems are common, and ketones and protein may be detected in the urine as a result of breakdown of fat and protein. Vital sign instability can be severe and can include orthostatic hypotension; the pulse becomes irregular, and the rate decreases markedly. Bradycardia and hypothermia can result in cardiac arrest (see Critical Thinking Exercise).

The team responsible for the management of young people with AN arranges a carefully structured environment. First, there must be consistency. The team decides on an approach and adheres to it. The plan is structured with reality testing regarding caloric intake and body-image perception as an essential component. The team members provide a unified front to avoid any possibility of manipulation or inconsistency. Second, all team members are involved; responsibility for the program cannot be left to one person. The role and boundaries of each member are clearly spelled out. Third, continuity of team members is important; it is helpful to have the same team members all the time.

Fourth, communication among team members is essential. Communication with the patient regarding what is expected is also important. Sometimes the limit setting may seem unreasonable; if the adolescent does not understand the rationale for the limits, he or she may sabotage the entire program.

CRITICAL THINKING EXERCISE

Anorexia Nervosa

Jane is a 13-year-old whose grades have been excellent and whom the teachers describe as a "model student." Recently, Jane's teacher told the nurse practitioner that Jane's parents were in the middle of a "messy divorce." In addition, several of Jane's friends told the nurse practitioner that they are concerned about Jane because she runs every day at lunchtime and seldom eats lunch with them. Jane told her friends that she gained weight over the winter months and that she is running because she wants to qualify for the track team this spring. At the time of her routine health interview and sports physical, the nurse practitioner notes that Jane's oral temperature is 36° C (96.8° F) and that she weighs 34 kg (75 pounds). Jane has lost 9 kg (20 pounds) since her last sports physical. Jane tells the nurse practitioner that she has not had her menstrual period for 3 months.

QUESTIONS
1. Evidence—Is there sufficient evidence to draw any conclusions about Jane's behavior?
2. Assumptions—Describe some underlying assumptions about the following:
   a. Personality characteristics of individuals with anorexia nervosa
   b. Factors influencing the development of anorexia nervosa
   c. Clinical manifestations of anorexia nervosa
   d. Treatment of anorexia nervosa
3. What priorities for nursing care should be established for Jane at this time?
4. Does the evidence support your conclusion?
5. Are there alternative perspectives that you should consider?

It is also important to communicate with the family. Fifth, the plan must provide for support of the adolescent, the family, and team members. The adolescent's efforts should be supported, and positive feedback should be provided for accomplishments made in normalizing eating habits. Meetings are held to discuss the feelings and concerns of the patient, immediate caregivers, and team members.

A **behavioral contract,** an agreement that the adolescent makes with others to change a maladaptive behavior, has proved to be effective in some cases. The written contract is constructed by the therapeutic team and approved and signed by the adolescent. Unless the adolescent agrees to its terms, the contract can become the source of a power struggle. However, it can be an effective tool that places the responsibility for weight gain or other behavioral change on the adolescent.

Nursing care of the adolescent with BN is similar to care of the patient with AN. Acute care involves careful monitoring of fluid and electrolyte alterations and observation for signs of cardiac complications. Nutritional consultation and follow-up care are essential. The nurse should encourage the adolescent and family members to structure the environment to reduce the binging behavior. Getting rid of binge foods; restricting eating to one room of the house; not engaging in other activities while eating; and substituting exercise, crafts, visualization, and relaxation techniques for binging are helpful interventions.

Health professionals, patients, and families can find assistance and information from several organizations. The National Association of Anorexia Nervosa and Associated Disor-

ders, Inc.,* and the National Eating Disorders Association† provide counseling, referrals, and self-help programs.

DISORDERS WITH BEHAVIORAL COMPONENTS

ATTENTION DEFICIT HYPERACTIVITY DISORDER AND LEARNING DISABILITY

Attention deficit hyperactivity disorder (ADHD) refers to developmentally inappropriate degrees of inattention, impulsiveness, and hyperactivity. To be diagnosed as ADHD, the symptoms must have been present before age 7 years and must be present in at least two settings. In addition, the persistence of developmentally inappropriate and marked inattention must not be a symptom of another disorder (American Psychiatric Association, 2000). A **learning disability (LD)** refers to a heterogeneous group of disorders manifested by significant difficulties in the acquisition and use of listening, speaking, reading, writing, reasoning, or mathematic skills.

ADHD and LDs affect every aspect of the child's life but are most obvious in the classroom. Early identification of affected children is important because the characteristics of these disorders significantly interfere with the normal course of emotional and psychologic development. Many children develop maladaptive behavior patterns that impede psychosocial adjustment while they try to cope with cognitive dysfunction. Their behavior evokes negative responses from others, and repeated exposure to negative feedback adversely affects their self-concept. The characteristics of ADHD affect the child's written and adaptive skills, social status, and self-esteem (Myers, Eisenhauer, and Ryan, 2003).

Diagnostic Evaluation

The behaviors exhibited by the child with ADHD are not unusual. The difference lies in the quality of motor activity and developmentally inappropriate inattention, impulsivity, and hyperactivity that the child displays. The manifestations may be numerous or few, mild or severe, and vary with the child's developmental level. Any given child will not have every symptom of the condition. The basic characteristics of ADHD are outlined in Box 17-7.

A comprehensive battery of tests is needed to confirm an LD. These include intelligence tests (many children have normal or above-average intelligence quotients [IQs]); hand-eye coordination tests; and measurements of auditory and visual perception, spatial organization, comprehension, and memory. Often there is a wide gap between verbal and performance scores on IQ tests.

Behavioral checklists and adaptive scales are also helpful in measuring school adaptive functioning in children with ADHD. Psychiatric disorders, medical problems, and traumatic experiences are ruled out, including lead poisoning, seizures, partial hearing loss, psychosis, and witnessing of sexual activity or violence.

Therapeutic Management

Management of the child with ADHD usually involves multiple approaches that include family education and counseling, medication, proper classroom placement, environmental

*PO Box 7, Highland Park, IL 60035; (847) 831-3438; e-mail: info@anad.org; http://www.anad.org.
†603 Stewart St., Suite 803, Seattle, WA 98101; (800) 931-2237; http://www.nationaleatingdisorders.org.

BOX 17-7

Diagnostic Criteria for Attention Deficit Hyperactivity Disorder

A. Either (1) or (2):
  (1) Six (or more) of the following symptoms of **inattention** have persisted for at least 6 months to a degree that is maladaptive and inconsistent with developmental level:
  Inattention
  (a) Often fails to give close attention to details or makes careless mistakes in schoolwork, work, or other activities
  (b) Often has difficulty sustaining attention in tasks or play activities
  (c) Often does not seem to listen when spoken to directly
  (d) Often does not follow through on instructions and fails to finish schoolwork, chores, or duties in the workplace (not because of oppositional behavior or failure to understand instructions)
  (e) Often has difficulty organizing tasks and activities
  (f) Often avoids, dislikes, or is reluctant to engage in tasks that require sustained mental effort (such as schoolwork or homework)
  (g) Often loses things necessary for tasks or activities (e.g., toys, school assignments, pencils, books, or tools)
  (h) Is often easily distracted by extraneous stimuli
  (i) Is often forgetful in daily activities
  (2) Six (or more) of the following symptoms of hyperactivity-impulsivity have persisted for at least 6 months to a degree that is maladaptive and inconsistent with developmental level:
  Hyperactivity
  (a) Often fidgets with hands or feet or squirms in seat
  (b) Often leaves seat in classroom or in other situations in which remaining seated is expected
  (c) Often runs about or climbs excessively in situations in which it is inappropriate (in adolescents or adults, may be limited to subjective feelings of restlessness)
  (d) Often has difficulty playing or engaging in leisure activities quietly
  (e) Is often "on the go" or often acts as if "driven by a motor"
  (f) Often talks excessively
  Impulsivity
  (g) Often blurts out answers before questions have been completed
  (h) Often has difficulty awaiting turn
  (i) Often interrupts or intrudes on others (e.g., butts into conversations or games)
B. Some hyperactive-impulsive or inattentive symptoms that caused impairment were present before age 7 years.
C. Some impairment from the symptoms is present in two or more settings (e.g., at school [or work] and at home).
D. There must be clear evidence of clinically significant impairment in social, academic, or occupational functioning.
E. The symptoms do not occur exclusively during the course of a pervasive developmental disorder, schizophrenia, or other psychotic disorder and are not better accounted for by another mental disorder (e.g., mood disorder, anxiety disorder, dissociative disorder, or personality disorder).

American Psychiatric Association: *Diagnostic and statistical manual of mental disorders*, ed 4 (text rev) (DSM-IV TR), Washington, DC, 2000, The Association.

manipulation, and behavioral therapy or psychotherapy for the child. Interventions for children with LD are primarily educational.

Pharmacologic Therapy. Stimulant medications or behavioral therapy are appropriate for the school-age child with ADHD (American Academy of Pediatrics, 2001c). The most frequently prescribed medications are the psychostimulants methylphenidate hydrochloride (Ritalin) and dextroamphetamine sulfate (Dexedrine). These medications increase dopamine and norepinephrine levels that lead to simulation of the inhibitory system of the central nervous system. The tricyclic antidepressants imipramine, desipramine, and nortriptyline are also used; these antidepressants block norepinephrine and serotonin at the nerve endings and increase the action of these substances in nerve cells. Clonidine, used occasionally in the treatment of ADHD, has been recommended primarily for children with ADHD and coexisting conditions such as sleep disturbances (American Academy of Pediatrics, 2001c). Atomoxetine (Strattera), a presynaptic norepinephrine transport inhibitor (nonstimulant), is now available for use in children and adolescents and has proved effective in the treatment of adolescents with ADHD (Michelson, Faries, Wernicke, and others, 2001; Spencer, Wilens, Biederman, and others, 2006).

Regularly scheduled evaluations of the child are essential with all these medications. Children taking stimulant medication may have side effects that include nervousness, tics, insomnia, increased blood pressure, and decreased appetite with subsequent weight loss (see Critical Thinking Exercise). Long-term use of dextroamphetamine may result in suppression of growth.

Behavioral Therapy. Behavioral therapy focuses on the prevention of undesired behavior. Families are helped to identify new appropriate contingencies and reward systems to meet the child's developing needs. They may also receive instruction in effective parenting skills, such as delivering positive reinforcement, rewarding small increments of desired behaviors, and providing age-appropriate consequences (e.g., time-out, response cost). Use of organizational charts for completing self-care activities and use of a word processor instead of manually writing out assignments are emphasized. Through collaborative teamwork, parents learn techniques to help the child become more successful at home and in school.

Environmental Manipulation. Families are encouraged to learn how to modify the environment to allow the child to be more successful. Consistency is especially important for children with ADHD. Consistency between families and teachers in terms of reinforcing the same goals is essential. Fostering improved organizational skills requires a more highly structured environment than most children need. The child should be encouraged to make more appropriate choices and to take responsibility for his or her actions.

Other helpful interventions include teaching parents how to make organizational charts (e.g., listing all activities that must be performed before leaving for school) and decrease distractions in the environment while the child is completing homework (e.g., turning the television off, having a consistent study area equipped with needed supplies) and helping parents to understand ways to model positive behaviors and problem solving. The focus is on strategies to help the child succeed and cope with deficits while emphasizing strengths.

??? CRITICAL THINKING EXERCISE

Attention Deficit Hyperactivity Disorder

Johnnie, age 8 years, is a third-grader who was recently diagnosed with attention deficit hyperactivity disorder (ADHD). He has been taking the drug methylphenidate (Ritalin) for about a month. In the short time that Johnnie has been on this medication, his math teacher has noticed an improvement in his performance in math class. He is receiving a grade of B instead of his previous grades of D on most math quizzes. The math teacher has also noted that Johnnie is socializing more with his classmates and that he now has a "best friend" in math class. Johnnie usually receives his methylphenidate from the school nurse before lunch. Yesterday Johnnie's mother told the school nurse that he has not eaten his lunch for the past week and that he is not hungry.

What important issues regarding Johnnie's medication should the nurse consider in her discussions with Johnnie's mother?

QUESTIONS

1. Evidence—Is there sufficient evidence to draw conclusions about Johnnie's medication from his behavior?
2. Assumptions—Describe some underlying assumptions about the following:
   a. Pharmacologic action of methylphenidate in ADHD
   b. Side effects of methylphenidate
   c. Management of side effects
3. What implications for nursing care can be drawn at this time?
4. Does the evidence objectively support your conclusion?
5. Are there alternative perspectives to your arguments?

Appropriate Classroom Placement. Children with ADHD need an orderly, predictable, and consistent classroom environment with clear and consistent rules. Homework and classroom assignments may need to be reduced, and more time may need to be allotted for tests to allow the child to complete the task. Verbal instructions should be accompanied by visual references such as written instructions on the blackboard. Schedules may need to be arranged so that academic subjects are taught in the morning when the child is experiencing the effects of the morning dose of medication. Low-interest and high-interest classroom activities should be intermingled to maintain the child's attention and interest. Regular and frequent breaks in activity are helpful because sitting in one place for an extended time may be difficult. Computers are helpful for children who have difficulty with writing (dysgraphia) and fine motor skills; in such children handwriting will *not* improve. They need to find alternatives to physical competition that requires coordination of movement (Selekman and Snyder, 2000).

If the child has an LD, special training activities may be accomplished in self-contained classes limited to six to eight children, in special resource rooms with equipment and teaching teams, by mobile consultants who move from room to room to provide assistance to teachers and children, and in special first-grade programs in which high-risk children receive special attention to prevent or reduce the need for services as they progress. The purpose of programs for children with LDs is to assist them toward more successful achievement, personal adjustment, and retention in the regular classroom.

👥 FAMILY FOCUS

A Child's Perception of Taking Ritalin at School

I feel embarrassed by having to leave class early to go take my medication. The other kids always ask where I'm going and why. It would be better if we could leave class at the same time as everyone else, go take the medication, and then just be a little late to the next class. Students don't ask why people are late for class, only why they leave early. It also bothers me when kids tell other kids, "Go take a pill," and other mean things just because someone is acting up.

What could nurses and teachers do to help? Most kids do not understand why other kids have to take medication. I think it would help if a nurse or teacher talked with the other kids and explained why some children take the medication and how ADHD affects people. That way there would be more understanding among all the kids.

—*Marissa White, age 16*

Prognosis. With appropriate intervention ADHD is relatively stable through early adolescence for most children. Some children experience decreased symptoms during late adolescence and adulthood, but a significant number of these children carry their symptoms into adulthood. The goal for children with LDs is to help them identify their areas of weakness and learn to compensate for them.

Nursing Care Management

Nurses are active participants in all aspects of management of the child with ADHD or LD. Nurses in the community work with families and school personnel on a long-term basis to help plan and implement therapeutic regimens and to evaluate the effectiveness of therapy. They coordinate services and serve as a liaison between health and education professionals directly involved in the child's therapy program. School nurses understand the child's special needs and work with teachers (see Family Focus box). Nurses in any setting (community, school, hospital, practitioner's office) provide support and guidance to children and families during the difficult period of the child's growing up with a disabling condition.

Management begins with an explanation to the parents and the child about the diagnosis, including the nature of the problem and the practitioner's concept of the underlying central nervous system basis for the disorder. Most parents are confused and feel some measure of guilt. To some parents, a diagnosis of ADHD is confirmation of the fear that their child has some irreversible, serious disease; to others it is a relief. All need the opportunity to vent their feelings and suspicions.

Parents need information about the prognosis and an understanding of the treatment plan. The greater their understanding of the disorder and its effects, the more likely they will be to carry out the recommended program of therapy. It is important that they understand that the therapy is not necessarily a panacea and that it will extend over a long period. This has particular significance for changes they need to make in environmental management. Reading material to help the child and family can be obtained from a variety of sources.

POSTTRAUMATIC STRESS DISORDER

Posttraumatic stress disorder (PTSD) refers to the development of characteristic symptoms after exposure to an extremely traumatic experience or catastrophic event. The traumatic experience is typically life-threatening to self or a significant other and may involve grotesque mutilation or death, serious injury, or physical coercion (e.g., an assault, a natural disaster, sexual abuse, witnessing violence). It is important to note that PTSD is not limited to children who have lived in "war-torn" countries. Events such as automobile, school, or recreational accidents and bullying have been identified as causes of PTSD (Sundelin-Wahlsten, Ahmad, and von Knorring, 2001). The characteristic symptoms are persistent reexperiencing of the traumatic event, avoidance of stimuli associated with the event or trauma, numbing of general responsiveness, and increased arousal.

The response to the event takes place in three stages. The **initial response** involves intense arousal, which usually lasts for a few minutes to 1 or 2 hours. The stress hormones are at the maximum as the individual prepares for "fight or flight." A prolonged arousal phase may indicate psychosis.

The **second phase,** which lasts approximately 2 weeks, is one in which defense mechanisms are mobilized. It is a period of quiescence in which the event appears to have produced no impression. The child feels numb, and stress hormone secretion is absent. Defense mechanisms are less adaptive to specific situations and may not be what the situation demands. Denial that anything is wrong is a frequently observed defense mechanism.

The **third phase** is one of coping and consciously directed inquiry, which normally extends over 2 to 3 months. The victims want to know what happened and appear to be getting worse, when actually they are getting better. Numerous psychologic symptoms, such as depression, phobia, anxiety, and conversion reactions, may be present. Children frequently display repetitive actions. They play out the situation over and over again in an attempt to come to terms with their fear. Flashbacks are common. This phase can be self-perpetuating, and a prolonged reaction can develop into an obsession with the traumatic event. Some traumatic effects remain indefinitely.

Nursing Care Management

Children need to deal with any traumatic event. Their reactions depend heavily on their social environment and the way in which their caretaking adults react to the event. In the second phase of PTSD, the appropriateness of the defense mechanism must be assessed, and children must be assisted in application of their defense. If children do not engage in some catharsis or if their defense phase is prolonged, they need referral for special psychologic help.

Coping is a learned response, and children in the third phase can be helped to deal with their fear. Children usually are willing to accept reasoning. Those who are assisted in their catharsis and allowed expression will survive without serious lasting effects. They should be encouraged to play out the stress and to discuss their feelings about the event. If they are unable to do this, they may become obsessed with the traumatic event and require professional help. Conversion reactions are common obsessive behaviors in children suffering from PTSD.

Children need professional help if any of the phases of PTSD are prolonged. Boys tend to have a prolonged defense phase more often than girls. Occasionally the event will be unrecognized, and the affected child will engage in what is considered to be unusual behavior. Children exhibiting any sudden change in behavior need to be assessed for a traumatic event. When the change in behavior is traced to a traumatic event, treatment can be implemented.

SCHOOL PHOBIA

Children, other than beginning students, who resist going to school or who demonstrate extreme reluctance to attend school for a sustained period as a result of severe anxiety or fear of school-related experiences are said to have school phobia. The terms **school refusal** and **school avoidance** are also used to describe this behavior. School avoidance behaviors occur in both boys and girls and in children from all socioeconomic levels.

Physical symptoms are prominent and may affect any part of the body (e.g., anorexia, nausea, vomiting, diarrhea, dizziness, headache, leg pains, abdominal pains, even a low-grade fever). A striking feature of school phobia is the prompt subsiding of symptoms when it is evident that the child can remain home. Another significant observation is absence of symptoms on weekends and holidays unless they are related to other places such as Sunday school or parties. Occasional mild reluctance is not uncommon among school children, but if the fear continues for longer than a few days, it must be considered a serious problem.

Nursing Care Management

Treatment for school phobia depends on the cause. The primary goal is *to return the child to school.* The longer a child is permitted to stay out of school, the more difficult it is for the child to reenter. Parents must be convinced gently but firmly that immediate return is essential and that it is their responsibility to insist on school attendance.

A school reentry protocol may be necessary for the child with severe symptoms. In reentry programs, the child role-plays routines involved in getting ready for school and that occur at school. Relaxation techniques are also used. The child usually goes to school initially for a half-day and then progresses to a full day. Often the school nurse is asked to provide support to the parents and the teacher during the reentry process. If the problem persists, professional help is recommended.

RECURRENT ABDOMINAL PAIN

Recurrent abdominal pain (RAP) is a complaint that is often attributed to psychogenic factors, although it can be a symptom of either psychosomatic or organic disease. RAP is defined as three or more separate episodes of abdominal pain during a 3-month period that interferes with functioning; the symptoms may be similar to the "spastic" or "irritable" colon syndrome of adulthood. The American Academy of Pediatrics (2005b) recently suggested retiring the term *recurrent abdominal pain* in favor of **functional abdominal pain,** noting that the majority of cases of chronic abdominal pain in children are functional. Functional abdominal pain is categorized as one or a combination of the following: irritable bowel syndrome, functional stomach upset (dyspepsia), or abdominal migraine. In functional abdominal pain, or RAP, there is no demonstrable evidence of a pathologic condition. Children with RAP have real pain that is usually located in the periumbilical or epigastric area. On palpation the pain is likely to be experienced in the epigastric area or in the lower right or left quadrant and is accompanied by vague tenderness without muscle guarding. The pain is irregular in time, duration, and intensity and associated with either loose or pellet-formed stools. Other symptoms that may accompany the pain are headache, pallor, dizziness, dysuria, flushing, vomiting, diarrhea, and fatigue.

Children at risk for RAP tend to be high achievers who have extensive personal goals or whose parents have unusually high expectations. They are described as sensitive and overly concerned about what others think of them. They are uncomfortable with expressions of anger or argument, especially with persons who are significant in their life. School attendance is adversely affected, and these children may exhibit poor learning performance. It is not uncommon for symptoms to be aggravated during school days.

Treatment involves providing reassurance and reducing or eliminating the symptoms. Hospitalization may be necessary, and the child frequently shows improvement in the hospital. Initial efforts are directed toward ruling out organic causes of the pain, relieving discomfort, and attempting to determine the situations that precipitate attacks. A high-fiber diet, psyllium bulk agents, lubricants such as mineral oil, and bowel training are emphasized for pain associated with bowel patterns. Treatment may also include acid-reduction therapy for pain associated with dyspepsia, antispasmodic agents, smooth muscle relaxants, or low doses of psychotropic agents. Other treatments include cognitive-behavioral therapy and biofeedback.

Nursing Care Management

Once the diagnosis has been established, the parents and the child need an explanation of the pain, which can be compared to a skeletal muscle cramp, "charley horse," or headache for easier comprehension. Reassurance that the symptoms are not unique to their child and that the pain is rarely associated with a severe disease can be helpful in relieving parental fears and anxieties.

The simple measure of having the child rest in a peaceful, quiet environment and providing comfort will often relieve the symptoms in a short time. A heating pad may also help ease the discomfort (see Nonpharmacologic Management, Chapter 7). When pain is not relieved by these simple measures, the parents are taught how to administer antispasmodics, if prescribed. For example, if pain is precipitated by meals, having the child take the medication 20 to 30 minutes before mealtime may prevent an episode.

The most valuable assistance that the nurse can provide is support and reassurance to the family. When open communication is established and families appreciate the relationship between stress-provoking situations and the child's symptoms, the chance for remedial action is enhanced. Follow-up care and continued support are essential because the symptoms tend to remit and exacerbate. The availability of a supportive health professional is a source of comfort to the child and family.

CONVERSION REACTION

Conversion reaction, also known as **hysteria, hysterical conversion reaction,** and **childhood hysteria,** is a psychophysiologic disorder with a sudden onset that can usually be traced to a precipitating environmental event. In childhood the disorder is observed with equal frequency in both sexes, but girls outnumber boys during adolescence.

The manifestations involve primarily the voluntary musculature and special senses. Symptoms include abdominal pain, fainting, pseudoseizures, paralysis, headaches, and visual field restriction. The most common symptom is seizure activity, which can be differentiated from symptoms of neurogenic origin by formal tests. A normal electroencephalogram indicates that the origin is not neurogenic. Many children with a conversion reaction have experienced a major family crisis (such as the loss of a parent or other significant person through death, divorce, or moving) before the onset of symptoms.

Nursing Care Management

Nursing care is similar to that for the child with RAP. If significant personality problems are evident, psychiatric consultation is indicated.

CHILDHOOD DEPRESSION

Depression in childhood is often difficult to detect because children may be unable to express their feelings and tend to act out their problems and concerns. Some states of depression are temporary, such as acute depression precipitated by a traumatic event. The event might include a period of hospitalization; loss of a parent through death or separation; or loss of a significant relationship with something (a pet), a person (a friend, significant other, or family member), or a place (move from a familiar home, neighborhood, or city). Children with depression may demonstrate a variety of behaviors (Box 17-8). Most responses in children are not sustained and can be modified with social and family support.

More serious and less common are the depressive responses to chronic stress and loss; these are frequently observed in children with chronic illness or disability when other family

---

BOX 17-8

Characteristics of Children with Depression

BEHAVIOR

Predominantly sad facial expression with absence or diminished range of affective response

Solitary play or work; tendency to be alone; disinterest in play

Withdrawal from previously enjoyed activities and relationships

Lowered grades in school; lack of interest in doing homework or achieving in school

Diminished motor activity; tiredness

Tearfulness or crying

Dependent and clinging or aggressive and disruptive

INTERNAL STATES

Utterance of statements reflecting lowered self-esteem, sense of hopelessness, or guilt

Suicidal ideations

PHYSIOLOGY

Constipation

Nonspecific complaints of not feeling well

Change in appetite resulting in weight loss or gain

Alterations in sleeping pattern, sleeplessness, or hypersomnia members have denial depression. There is no apparent precipitating event, but there is often a history of frequent disruptions in important relationships. Often, there is also a history of depressive illness in one or both parents. Manifestations in the child are similar to those observed in acute depression, but they occur more frequently and extend over a longer period.

Nursing Care Management

Depressed children are managed by a health team especially prepared in the care of children with mental disorders. Treatment is highly individualized and undertaken in the least restrictive environment. Suicidal children are admitted to the hospital for protection if the family is unable to provide constant monitoring. Pharmacotherapy may involve tricyclic antidepressants or SSRIs such as fluoxetine (Prozac), trazodone (Desyrel), sertraline (Zoloft), paroxetine (Paxil), bupropion (Wellbutrin), and venlafaxine (Effexor).

Nurses should be aware that depression is a problem that can be easily overlooked in the child and one that can interrupt normal growth and development. Recognizing depression and suicidal tendencies in depressed adolescents and making appropriate referrals are important nursing functions. Identification of the depressed child requires a careful history (health, growth and development, social and family health); interviews with the child; and observations by the nurse, parents, and teachers (see also Suicide, p. 568). Some antidepressant medications may cause increased suicidal thinking and behaviors in pediatric patients. This has prompted the U.S. Food and Drug Administration (FDA) to recommend black box drug warnings detailing potential suicide-related risks for pediatric patients (Jick, Kaye, and Jick, 2004; US Food and Drug Administration, 2004). In 2007 the FDA expanded the black box warning, noting that the risk of suicide was highest among adolescents and young adults ages 18 to 24 years, yet added that there is risk in not administering antidepressants. Some data suggest that the suicide rate among adolescents on therapeutic doses of SSRIs was lower than among those who were not being treated with antidepressant medication (Gibbons, Hur, Bhaumik, and others, 2006). However, the issue remains controversial, and further studies are needed.

CHILDHOOD SCHIZOPHRENIA

Childhood schizophrenia is a term that refers to severe deviations in ego functioning and is generally reserved for psychotic disorders that appear in children younger than 15 years of age. Childhood schizophrenia is a rare illness among children in the general population; among children with mental illness, only about two in every 1000 have childhood schizophrenia.

Childhood schizophrenia is characterized by symptoms that last for at least 6 months and that seriously interfere with the child's functioning in school, at home, or in other social situations. The basic disturbance is a lack of contact with reality and the subsequent development of a world of the child's own. Other areas of development that may be impaired include cognition, perception, emotion, language, and physical motor control. The most common manifestations involve language disturbances, impaired interpersonal relationships, and inappropriate affect (outward expression of emotion). Treatment involves management of the symptoms, prevention of relapse, and social and occupational rehabilitation of the

young person. Antipsychotic drugs that may be used include haloperidol, clozapine, chlorpromazine, olanzapine, quetiapine fumarate, and risperidone. Family interventions and family therapy often result in improvements in psychotic symptoms, thought disorders, and social functioning among children with schizophrenia.

Nursing Care Management

Nursing of psychotic children is a highly specialized area. However, nurses should be alert to the possibility that schizophrenia can occur in children and refer children who consistently demonstrate abnormal behavior to a psychiatrist for evaluation. In addition, nurses will need to teach family members of children taking antipsychotic drugs to observe for possible side effects. Common side effects of these drugs include dizziness; drowsiness; tachycardia; hypotension; and extrapyramidal effects, such as abnormal movements and seizures.

SERIOUS HEALTH PROBLEMS OF LATER CHILDHOOD AND ADOLESCENCE

SUBSTANCE ABUSE

Although experimentation with drugs during childhood and adolescence is widespread, most children and teens do not become high-risk users. National and statewide surveys indicate that despite a steady increase in the incidence of adolescents using tobacco, alcohol, and marijuana between the ages of 12 and 18, experimentation is limited to one adolescent in eight for stimulants and inhalants and to less than one adolescent in 10 for "hard" drugs such as hallucinogens, sedatives, and crack cocaine. It has been reported that as many as 51% of American youth have tried an illegal drug by the time of high school graduation (American Academy of Pediatrics, 2005c). Although surveys demonstrate a modest decrease in the use of certain substances among youth (marijuana, amphetamines, barbiturates, and tranquilizers), abuse of other drugs (cocaine, steroids, heroine, flunitrazepam) has remained steady (American Academy of Pediatrics, 2005c; Centers for Disease Control and Prevention, 2006b).

Drug abuse, misuse, and **addiction** are culturally defined and are voluntary behaviors. **Drug tolerance** and **physical dependence** are involuntary physiologic responses to the pharmacologic characteristics of the drugs, such as opioids and alcohol. Consequently, an individual can be addicted to a narcotic with or without being physically dependent. A person can also be physically dependent on a narcotic without being addicted (e.g., patients who use opioids to control pain).

Motivation

Most drug use begins with experimentation. The drug may be used only once, may be used occasionally, or may become part of a drug-centered lifestyle. Children and adolescents initiate drug use out of curiosity. Adolescents who use drugs may fall into one of two broad categories—experimenters and compulsive users—or they may fall into a third category somewhere on the continuum between these extremes, referred to as recreational users, principally of drugs such as marijuana, cocaine, alcohol, and prescription drugs. For many the goal is peer acceptance; these users fit more closely with the experimenting, intermittent users. For others the goal is intoxication or the sustained intense effects from using a particular drug; these users resemble the compulsive users. These users may engage in periodic heavy use, or binges. The groups of greatest concern to health care workers are those whose patterns of use involve high doses or mixed drugs with the danger of overdose, and those compulsive users with the threat of dependence, withdrawal syndromes, and altered lifestyle.

Types of Drugs Abused

Any drug can be abused, and most are potentially harmful to adolescents still going through formative life experiences. Although rarely considered drugs by society, the chemically active substances frequently abused are the xanthines and theobromines contained in chocolate, tea, coffee, and colas. Ethyl alcohol and nicotine are other drugs that are legal and socially sanctioned. Any of these substances can produce mild to moderate euphoric or stimulant effects and can lead to physical and psychologic dependence.

Drugs with mind-altering abilities that are available on the "street" and are of medical and legal concern are the hallucinogenic, narcotic, hypnotic, and stimulant drugs. In addition, health professionals are concerned about the use of alcohol and volatile substances that are inhaled to achieve altered sensation (such as gasoline, antifreeze, plastic model airplane cement, typewriter correction fluid, and organic solvents). Recently, abuse of prescription and synthetic drugs such as oxycodone, alprazolam (Xanax), and amphetamine-dextroamphetamine (Adderall) has become a concern for professionals who work with children and adolescents. Many of the prescription drugs are available at a decreased cost in comparison to the more exotic drugs of abuse and are often found in the medicine cabinet at home. Internet websites also promote the "safe use" of some psychoactive drugs and supply information on new "designer" drugs that are not detectable on a standard urine drug screening test.

Tobacco. Cigarette smoking has continued to decline since the late 1990s, in part due to increased costs, changes in community attitudes about smoking among adults, decreased advertising of cigarettes to children, and increased antismoking advertising as a result of the government lawsuits against tobacco companies (Johnston, O'Malley, Bachman, and others, 2005). From 2001 to 2002, 13.3% of children in middle school and 28.2% of high school students reported tobacco use of some type (Centers for Disease Control and Prevention, 2006c). In another survey cigar smoking ranked second for form of tobacco used among those surveyed, and smokeless tobacco reportedly was third (Centers for Disease Control and Prevention, 2006b).

Although the number of adult and adolescent smokers has declined in recent years, cigarette smoking is still considered the chief avoidable cause of death. The hazards of smoking at any age are undisputed; however, a preventive approach to teenage smoking is especially important. Because of its addictive nature, smoking begun in childhood and adolescence can result in a lifetime habit, with increased morbidity and early mortality. Smoking in adolescence has also been related to other risk behaviors: approximately three times as many adolescents who smoke report carrying weapons and drinking alcohol compared with adolescents who do not smoke; other associated risks in Caucasians include use of smokeless tobacco, marijuana use, multiple sexual partners, not using bicycle helmets, and binge drinking. Research also indicates an association between current use of tobacco and the development of depression (Goodman and Capitman, 2000) and

COMMUNITY FOCUS

Early Sexual Maturation, Alcohol, and Cigarettes

Smoking cigarettes and drinking alcohol among adolescents are complex behaviors that are not explained by any one cause or factor. Some theorists and investigators believe there is a relationship between biologic maturation and these risk-taking behaviors. For example, young girls who are sexually mature at an earlier age than their peers are often attracted to older girls and boys who may engage in risk-taking behaviors. If older teens smoke, drink, and drive while under the influence of alcohol with no adverse consequences (e.g., no motor vehicle accidents), young girls may believe that they, too, will be safe while smoking, drinking, or riding in an automobile with friends who are drinking.

Although parents and nurses cannot influence the time of biologic maturation, they can identify young girls who are at risk for the initiation of risk-taking behaviors because of early puberty. Parents need to understand that an early-maturing daughter might be uncomfortable with her body, and they should take advantage of opportunities to build her self-esteem. Parental sensitivity to the importance of peer-group acceptance and parental support of a teenage daughter who feels left out or different are crucial. School nurses can provide anticipatory guidance to these girls and help them to role-play coping strategies for situations that involve offers to smoke and drink. In addition, school nurses can provide information about physical development during puberty and emphasize the fact that not all teenagers mature at the same time or rate.

Teachers, coaches, and church leaders can provide opportunities for these girls to "fit in" with their same-age peers through activities that stress mutual goals. For example, an early-maturing girl is typically taller than her age-mates and can be an asset in sports such as basketball and track-and-field events.

sleep problems (Patten, Choi, Gillin, and others, 2000) in adolescence. Cigarettes are considered to be a gateway drug, and teenagers who smoke are 11.4 times more likely to use illicit drugs (Gordon, 2000).

The effects of second-hand smoke exposure are also well known and include increased incidence of low birth weight and subsequent illness, increased incidence of sudden infant death syndrome (if mother smoked during pregnancy), increased incidence of acute lower respiratory tract infections, and exacerbation of asthma symptoms (wheezing, cough, phlegm, breathlessness) in asthmatic children (US Department of Health and Human Services, 2006).

Etiology. Teenagers begin smoking for a variety of reasons, including imitation of adult behavior; peer pressure; a desire to imitate behaviors and lifestyles portrayed in movies and advertisements; and a desire to control weight, especially among females. Teenagers who do not smoke usually have family members and friends who do not smoke or who oppose smoking. Most teens who refrain from smoking have a desire to succeed in academics or athletics (particularly high-performance sports, such as basketball, swimming, and track) and plans to go to college (see Community Focus box). Although smoking among college students has increased in recent years, rates of smoking are highest among adolescents who do not complete high school.

Case Study—Teen Smoking

Smokeless Tobacco. The term *smokeless tobacco* refers to tobacco products that are placed in the mouth but not ignited (e.g., snuff and chewing tobacco). This substitute for cigarettes continues to pose a hazard to adolescents, although use has declined by about 50% since the peak prevalence in 1995; in 2004 only 16.7% of teens tried smokeless tobacco by the twelfth grade (Johnston, O'Malley, Bachman, and others, 2005). Many children and adolescents believe that smokeless tobacco is a safe alternative to cigarette smoking and is not addictive, and they believe they can stop using it at any time. However, the number of adolescents who identify it as a health risk has increased since the mid-1990s, with nearly half now agreeing it has health risks (Johnston, O'Malley, Bachman, and others, 2005). These products have also been proved to be carcinogenic, and regular use can cause dental problems, foul-smelling breath, and tooth erosion or loss.

Nursing Care Management. Prevention of regular smoking in teenagers is the most effective way to reduce the overall incidence of smoking. A variety of methods have been employed. Posters, charts, displays, statistics, and the use of examples of actual damaged lungs to communicate the hazards of smoking all have their supporters and doubters. Some schools also use films and demonstrations in science classes.

For the most part, smoking-prevention programs that focus on the negative, long-term effects of smoking on health have been ineffective. Youth-to-youth programs and those emphasizing the immediate effects are more effective but primarily in improving teenagers' attitudes toward not smoking. Because smoking and smoking-related behaviors are social symbols, antismoking campaigns must address the norms of potential smokers. Anything that ridicules or threatens the social norms of the peer group can be unproductive or counterproductive. Investigators have found that teaching resistance to peer pressure to smoke is effective in early adolescence. Although the effects of these programs may decrease with time, the effects can be enhanced in older adolescents by presenting information in class instead of simply handing out written material to the students (Adelman, Duggan, Hauptman, and others, 2001).

Two areas of focus for antismoking programs are peer-led programs and use of media in smoking prevention (e.g., CDs, videotapes, and films). Peer-led programs emphasizing the social consequences of smoking have proved most successful. If a significant number of influential peers can "sell" their classmates on the idea that the habit is not popular, the followers will imitate their behavior. Such programs emphasize short-term rather than long-term consequences (e.g., the effects of smoking on personal appearance, such as unattractive stains on teeth and hands and unpleasant odor of breath and clothing).

The impact of school-based antismoking programs can be strengthened by expanding these programs to include parents, mass media, youth groups, and community organizations. For example, mass media efforts that involve antismoking radio campaigns have been identified as the most cost-effective mass media intervention.

Smoking bans in schools also accomplish several goals: (1) they discourage students from starting to smoke, (2) they reinforce knowledge of the health hazards of cigarette smoking and exposure to environmental tobacco smoke, and (3) they promote a smoke-free environment as the norm (see Community Focus box).

COMMUNITY FOCUS

Nonsmoking Strategies

Nurses who work in schools, hospitals, and community agencies can take advantage of all opportunities to provide education about the dangers of smoking, to discourage smoking initiation by children and adolescents, to encourage smoking cessation, and to promote smoke-free environments. In particular, school nurses must be alert to the vulnerability of young preteens when they enter junior high school. These nurses are in an ideal position to assess stress, personal conflict, weight concerns, peer pressures, and other factors that place preteens at risk for smoking initiation. Nurses should serve as counselors to student, teacher, and parent groups and as advocates for antismoking legislative efforts. Several additional strategies are recommended*:

- Provide only brief information about long-term health consequences (e.g., cardiovascular, cancer risks).
- Discuss immediate physiologic consequences (e.g., changes in heart rate, blood pressure, respiratory symptoms, blood carbon monoxide concentrations).
- Mention alternatives to smoking that also establish a self-image that appears independent, mature, or sophisticated (e.g., weightlifting; running; dancing; joining a boys or girls club; volunteering for a hospital or political, religious, or community group).
- Mention the negative effects in detail (e.g., earlier wrinkling of skin; yellow stains on teeth and fingers; tobacco odor on breath, hair, and clothing).
- Mention the increasing ostracism of smokers by nonsmokers, both legal and informal, in the workplace and in public places.
- Mention the increasing evidence that second-hand smoke is injurious to the health of nonsmokers who are regularly exposed, especially small children.
- Acknowledge that many adults who were enticed to start smoking as teenagers because of its social benefits now wish they could stop smoking.
- Give cooperative adolescents effective arguments to deal with peer pressure (e.g., by not smoking, a teenager demonstrates independence and nonconformity, traits normally prized by youth).
- Request posters or pamphlets from local agencies (e.g., American Cancer Society, American Heart Association, American Lung Association) to display in prominent places at school.

*The Centers for Disease Control and Prevention has information on the effects of tobacco, smoking cessation, and tobacco control programs: 1600 Clifton Rd, Atlanta, GA 30333; (800) 232-4636; email: tobaccoinfo@cdc.gov; http://www.cdc.gov/tobacco.

Alcohol. Acute or chronic abuse of alcohol (ethanol) is responsible for many acts of violence, suicide, accidental injury, and death. Alcohol drinking is likely to begin in the middle school years and increases with age. By 18 years of age, 80% to 90% of adolescents have tried alcohol. Ethanol is a depressant that reduces inhibitions against aggressive and sexual acting out. Severe physical and psychologic symptoms accompany abrupt withdrawal, and long-term use leads to slow tissue destruction, especially of the brain and liver cells. The most noticeable effects of alcohol occur within the central nervous system and include changes in cognitive and autonomic functions such as judgment, memory, learning ability, and other intellectual capacities. Young alcoholics often drink alone and cannot control their use of alcohol. They often rely on the substance as a defense against depression, anxiety, fear, or anger. Not all of these characteristics are observed in the adolescent who is abusing alcohol, but if several signs are evident, the child or adolescent should be considered at risk. Referral to a health care professional and detoxification therapy may be necessary. Information about alcohol and answers to questions are available through the Alcohol Hotline.* Other groups that provide support and counseling for families are Al-Anon, Ala-Teen, Ala-Tot, and Alcoholics Anonymous (an organization that has listings in all local telephone directories).

Cocaine. Although cocaine is not pharmacologically considered a narcotic, it is legally categorized as such. Cocaine is available in two forms: water-soluble cocaine hydrochloride, which is administered by "snorting" or intravenous injection, and nonsoluble alkaloid (freebase) cocaine, which is used primarily for smoking. Crack, or "rock," is a purer, more menacing form of the drug. It can be produced cheaply and smoked in either water pipes or mentholated cigarettes. The use of cocaine has increased in recent years because of its availability and affordability, its association with persons in glamorous occupations, peer pressure, and its reputation as a sexually enhancing drug.

Cocaine creates a sense of euphoria, or an indefinable high. Withdrawal does not produce the dramatic symptoms observed in withdrawal from other substances. The effects are those commonly seen in depression, including lack of energy and motivation, irritability, appetite changes, psychomotor retardation, and irregular sleep patterns. More serious symptoms include cardiovascular manifestations and seizures. Physical withdrawal should not be confused with the so-called crash after a cocaine high, which consists of a long period of sleep. Answers to questions about the risks of using cocaine are available at the National Cocaine Hotline,† which also provides referrals to support groups and treatment centers.

Narcotics. Narcotic drugs include opiates such as heroin and morphine, and opioids (opiate-like drugs), such as hydromorphone (Dilaudid), hydrocodone, fentanyl, meperidine (Demerol), and codeine. These drugs produce a state of euphoria by removing painful feelings and creating a pleasurable experience and a sense of success accompanied by clouding of the consciousness and a dreamlike state. Physical signs of narcotic abuse include constricted pupils, respiratory depression, and, often, cyanosis. Needle marks may be visible on the arms or legs in chronic users. Physical withdrawal from opiates is extremely unpleasant unless controlled with supervised tapering doses of the opioid or substitution of methadone.

As important as the physical effects are the indirect consequences related to the illegal status of narcotic use and the problems associated with securing the drug (e.g., the time-consuming searches to obtain the drug and the often illegal methods used to meet the high cost of purchasing it). Health problems also result from self-neglect of physical needs (nutrition, cleanliness, dental care); overdose; contamination; and infection, including HIV and hepatitis B and C infection.

Central Nervous System Depressants. Central nervous system depressants include a variety of hypnotic drugs that produce physical dependence and withdrawal symptoms on abrupt discontinuation. They create a feeling of relaxation and sleepiness but impair general functioning. Drugs in this category include barbiturates, nonbarbiturates, and alcohol. Barbiturates combined with alcohol produce a profound depressant effect. Flunitrazepam (Rohypnol), known as the

"date rape drug," is a recent hypnotic drug abused by adolescents. Many women and men report being raped after unknowingly being given Rohypnol in a drink. Rohypnol is 10 times more powerful than diazepam (Valium). It produces prolonged sedation, a feeling of well-being, and short-term memory loss.

Central Nervous System Stimulants. Amphetamines and cocaine do not produce strong physical dependence and can be withdrawn without much danger. However, psychologic dependence is strong, and acute intoxication can lead to violent aggressive behavior or psychotic episodes characterized by paranoia, uncontrollable agitation, and restlessness. When combined with barbiturates, the euphoric effects are particularly addictive.

Methamphetamine can be snorted, injected, swallowed, or smoked and produces a burst of energy in its users, along with intense, alternating attacks of boldness and paranoia. It provokes excitement far more intense than that caused by cocaine. The drug, with the street names *crank, meth,* and *crystal,* is inexpensive and has a longer period of action than cocaine. Instead of a short (few minutes) high, as achieved with cocaine, a user can remain "up" for hours on a similar dose of crank.

Health care professionals are concerned about the use of various volatile substances, or **inhalants** such as gasoline, model airplane cement, and organic solvents; these substances are inhaled by the user to achieve an altered sensation, and the most recent surveillance has indicated a modest increase in use, after nearly a decade of decline. Adolescents breathe or place these substances into paper or plastic bags or soda cans from which they rebreathe the fumes to produce a feeling of euphoria and altered consciousness. These substances contain chemical solvents and are extremely hazardous. Dusters contain Freon, a substance that can cause fatal cardiac arrhythmias. The use of inhalants is increasing, and inhalants are becoming a gateway drug for young children and preteens, who often progress to other harder drugs such as marijuana, heroin, and cocaine. Many young children are unaware of the dangers of "sniffing" or "huffing." In addition to rapid loss of consciousness and respiratory arrest, these substances may cause visual scanning problems, language deficiencies, motor instability, memory deficits, and attention and concentration problems.

Mind-Altering Drugs. Hallucinogens (psychedelics, psychotomimetics, psychotropics, or illusionogenics) are drugs that produce vivid hallucinations and euphoria. These drugs do not produce physical dependence, and they can be abruptly withdrawn without ill effect. However, the acute and long-term effects are variable, and in some individuals the dissociative behavior may be prolonged. Cannabis (marijuana, hashish) and lysergic acid diethylamide (LSD) are also included in this category of drugs.

Nursing Care Management Related to Therapeutic Management

Nurses who have contact with children and adolescents are in an excellent position to provide information about substance abuse and to serve as patient advocates. The nurse most often encounters young drug abusers when they are (1) experiencing overdose or withdrawal symptoms, (2) manifesting bizarre behavior or confusion secondary to drug ingestion, (3) worried that they are or will become addicted, or (4) worried about a friend or family member who is addicted.

---

*800-ALCOHOL.
†800-COCAINE.

In particular, nurses who care for hospitalized adolescents need to know if these youths use drugs compulsively. Drug withdrawal can seriously complicate other illnesses. Nurses should be alert for any physical or behavioral clues that indicate the onset of withdrawal or the effects of drugs. School nurses and nurses who work in the community play an essential role in identifying children, adolescents, and families with substance abuse problems. The school nurse may be the first to identify a child or adolescent who has ingested a particular drug by the child's erratic behavior in class or on the school grounds. Early identification of those at risk for substance abuse problems is an essential aspect of prevention. Pediatric health care professionals also prevent substance abuse by creating trusting relationships so that children and adolescents feel comfortable asking questions about drugs and health professionals can alert them to websites and other aspects of society that encourage experimentation with drugs.

Acute Care. Adolescents experiencing toxic drug effects or withdrawal symptoms are usually seen initially in the emergency department. Experienced emergency department personnel are familiar with the management of acute drug toxicity and the signs, symptoms, and behavioral characteristics associated with a variety of substances. When the drug is questionable or unknown, knowledge of these factors facilitates management and treatment. Often, observation or description of the child's or adolescent's behavior is more valuable than reports by patients or their friends

The treatment for drug toxicity or withdrawal varies according to the drug and the method used. Every effort is made to determine the type, the time of ingestion, the amount of drug taken, the mode of administration, and the factors related to the onset of presenting symptoms. It is helpful to know the individual's pattern of use. For example, if two types of drugs are involved, they may require different treatments. Gastric lavage may be employed when the drug has been ingested recently and the cough reflex is intact, but it is of little value when the drug has been administered by the intravenous ("mainlined") or intranasal ("sniffed") route. Because the actual content of most street drugs is highly questionable, other pharmaceutical agents are administered with caution, except perhaps the narcotic antagonists in cases of suspected opiate overdoses. It is also necessary to assess for possible trauma sustained while the patient was under the influence of the drug.

Long-Term Management. A major factor in the treatment and rehabilitation of young drug users is careful assessment in the nonacute stage to determine the function that the drug plays in the adolescent's life. The motivation phase is directed toward exploring the factors that influence drug use. It also involves establishing a feeling of self-worth and a commitment to self-help in the teen.

Rehabilitation begins when adolescents decide that they can and are willing to change. **Rehabilitation** involves fostering healthy interdependent relationships with caring and supportive adults and exploring alternate mechanisms for problem solving while simultaneously reducing or eliminating drug use. Persons working with troubled youth must be prepared for **recidivism,** or the tendency to relapse, and maintain a plan for reentry into the treatment process.

Family Support. Most treatment programs for substance abusers are based on adult 12-step models such as Al-coholics Anonymous. Research is needed to determine whether these adult models are effective for adolescents. Tough Love* is one program that is based on the conviction that parents have the right and responsibility to be the policymakers in the family, to set limits on the behavior of their children, and to take control of the household from out-of-control adolescents. The premise is that allowing teenagers to experience the negative consequences of their behavior will bring them closer to accepting help or changing their behavior. Another group that provides support and counseling for families experiencing substance abuse and seeking strategies to cope with their children is Parents Anonymous.† Another source of information is the Substance Abuse and Mental Health Services Administration's National Clearinghouse for Alcohol and Drug Information.‡

Prevention. Nurses play an important role in education efforts, as well as in individual observation, assessment, and therapy related to substance abuse. In recent years a variety of educational programs have been applied with promising results. The most effective prevention strategies are those that are part of a broader, more general effort to promote overall health and success. Health-compromising behaviors are often interconnected and have common antecedents. Prevention efforts that focus on changing only one behavior (e.g., alcohol, other drug use) are less likely to be successful. Successful programs are those that have promoted parenting skills, social skills among distractible children, academic achievement, and skills to resist peer pressure.

Peer pressure is a powerful tool and can be used effectively in substance abuse prevention. A group that has had some success in reducing injury from drunk driving is Students Against Destructive Decisions (SADD).§ Techniques used by this group include peer counseling, parental guidelines for teenage parties, and community awareness. Nurses should encourage the formation of SADD chapters in the high schools in their communities.

SUICIDE

Suicide is defined as the deliberate act of self-injury with the intent that the injury results in death. Most experts distinguish between suicidal ideation, suicide attempt (or parasuicide), and suicide.

Suicidal ideation involves a preoccupation with thoughts about committing suicide and may be a precursor to suicide. Although it is not uncommon for adolescents to experience occasional suicidal thoughts, expressions of preoccupation with suicide should be taken seriously, and an assessment should be conducted for appropriate referral. A **suicide attempt** is intended to cause injury or death. The term **parasuicide** is used to refer to behaviors ranging from gestures to serious attempts to kill oneself. *Parasuicide* is a preferred term because it makes no reference to intent and because a person's motive may be too difficult or complex to determine. However, all parasuicidal activity should be taken seriously.

---

*http://www.toughlove.com.
†675 W. Foothill Blvd., Suite 220, Claremont, CA 91711; (909) 621-6184; http://www.parentsanonymous.org.
‡PO Box 2345, Rockville, MD 20847; (800) 729-6686; e-mail: info@health. org; http://ncadi.samhsa.gov.
§255 Main St., Marlborough, MA 01752; (877) SADD-INC; http://www.sadd. org.

NURSING ALERT

A history of a previous suicide attempt is a serious indicator for possible suicide completion in the future. Studies of adolescent suicides have found that as many as half of the adolescents had made previous attempts.

Recent results from the Youth Risk Behavior Surveillance, 2005, indicated that 8.4% of students nationwide had attempted suicide at least once during the 12 months preceding the survey; the range of suicide attempts by adolescents across the states varied from 6.2% to 13.1% (Centers for Disease Control and Prevention, 2006b). The overall incidence of youth suicide has decreased since 1992, yet the Centers for Disease Control and Prevention notes the incidence is still too high. Approximately 13% of the students in this survey reported that they had made a specific plan to attempt suicide in the 12 months preceding the survey. Suicide is currently the third leading cause of death during the teenage years, surpassed only by death from motor vehicle crash and homicide (see Chapter 1).

Etiology

Individual, family, and social or environmental factors have all been implicated in suicide. The single most important individual factor is the presence of an active psychiatric disorder (depression, bipolar disorder, psychosis, substance abuse, or conduct disorder). Comorbidity of an affective disorder and substance abuse also increases the risk for suicide. Alcohol use has been associated with more than 50% of suicides (American Academy of Pediatrics, 2000). Gay and lesbian adolescents are at particularly high risk for suicide completion, especially if raised in an environment in which they are denied support systems (see Community Focus box). Family factors influencing suicide include parental loss; family disruption; a family history of suicide, depression, substance abuse, or emotional disturbance; child abuse or neglect; unavailable parents; poor communication and isolation within the family; family conflict; and unrealistically high parental expectations or parental indifference with low expectations. Social or environmental factors include incarceration, isolation, acute loss of a boyfriend or girlfriend, lack of future options, and availability of firearms in the home.

Methods

Firearms are by far the most commonly used instruments in completed suicides among males and females (American Academy of Pediatrics, 2000). For adolescent males, the second and third most common means of suicide are hanging and overdose, respectively; for females the second and third most common means are overdose and strangulation, respectively.

The most common method of suicide attempt is overdose or ingestion of a potentially toxic substance, such as drugs. The second most common method of suicide attempt is self-inflicted laceration.

NURSING ALERT

Given what is known about youth suicide, nurses should ask parents, especially those with at-risk teenagers, if firearms are available in the house and, if so, recommend their removal. Parents must ensure that their children—especially those who are depressed, have poor problem-solving skills, or use drugs or alcohol—do not have access to firearms. Parents must also be educated on the warning signs of suicide (Box 17-9).

COMMUNITY FOCUS

Suicide, Sexual Identity, and Sexual Orientation

A significant number of teenage suicides occur among homosexual youths. Gay or lesbian adolescents who live in families or communities that do not accept homosexuality are likely to suffer low self-esteem, self-loathing, depression, and hopelessness. Such internalization, without treatment and support, can lead to substance abuse and, eventually, suicide. Youths most at risk are those who struggle with gender identity issues such as gay identity formation at a young age, intrapersonal conflict regarding sexuality, and nondisclosure of orientation to others.

Supportive parents, friends, or relationships serve as protective factors against suicide. However, many gay, lesbian, and bisexual adolescents do not feel supported, understood, or accepted by their friends, parents, and families. Nurses who interact with adolescents must be aware of the association between suicide and adolescent homosexuality and gender nonconformity. School nurses may be the first individuals to discuss issues of sexual identity and orientation with adolescents or their families. In their professional capacity, nurses can also serve as support persons for these adolescents. Nurses can provide guidance and resources to families so that they know and understand how best to nurture and support their child.

Nurses must also capitalize on opportunities or experiences that promote the healthy development of self-esteem in youths who choose nontraditional sexual orientation. Educational programs to raise the level of consciousness about the risk factors for and warning signs of suicide are one example. Another possibility could be programs conducted in or outside of school that are designed to foster peer relationships and competency in social skills among high-risk adolescents and young adults, such as support groups and social organizations for these young people.

BOX 17-9

Warning Signs of Suicide

- Preoccupation with themes of death—focuses on morbid thoughts
- Wants to give away cherished possessions
- Talks of own death, desire to die
- Loss of energy—loss of interest, listlessness
- Exhaustion without obvious cause
- Changes in sleep patterns—too much or too little
- Increased irritability, argumentativeness, or stubbornness
- Physical complaints—recurrent stomachaches, headaches
- Repeated visits to physician, nurse practitioner, or emergency department for treatment of injuries
- Reckless behavior
- Antisocial behavior—engages in drinking, uses drugs, fights, commits acts of vandalism, runs away from home, becomes sexually promiscuous
- Sudden change in school performance—lowered grades, cutting classes, dropping out of activities
- Resists or refuses to go to school
- Remains distant, sad, remote—flat affect, frozen facial expression
- Describes self as worthless
- Sudden cheerfulness following deep depression
- Social withdrawal from friends, activities, interests that were previously enjoyed
- Impaired concentration
- Dramatic change in appetite

Motivation

Suicidal ideation is not uncommon in adolescents. It represents numerous fantasies, such as relief from suffering, a means of gaining comfort and sympathy, or a means of revenge against those who have hurt them. Adolescents have the erroneous perception that the act of suicide will evoke remorse and pity and that they will be able to return and witness the grief. Angry children who are unable to directly punish those who have injured or insulted them may take revenge on those who love them through self-destruction ("They'll be sorry when they find me dead"; "They'll be sorry they were mean to me").

For adolescents who are severely depressed, suicide seems to be the only release from their despair. These adolescents rarely provide evidence of their intent and frequently conceal their suicidal thoughts. Many adolescents, however, tell their peers of their suicidal thoughts or plans but avoid telling adults. Social isolation is a significant factor in distinguishing adolescents who will kill themselves from those who will not. It is also more characteristic of those who complete suicide than of those who make attempts or threats.

The frequency of **contagion,** or **copycat suicides** (i.e., an increase in youth suicide that occurs after the suicide of one teenager is publicized) is disturbing and may indicate that teenagers perceive suicide as glamorous. In addition, young people may not realize the finality of suicide because they have become desensitized from constantly viewing violence and death on television.

Diagnostic Evaluation

Depression is common among adolescents who attempt suicide. Depression is characterized by both subjective symptoms and objective signs that reflect the adolescent's sadness and despair. Adolescents describe feelings of sadness, despair, helplessness, hopelessness, boredom, loss of interest, and isolation. They may also feel self-reproach, self-deprecation, and guilt. Subjective symptoms of depression or specific changes in behavior place an adolescent at risk for suicide.

Therapeutic Management

Threats of suicide should always be taken seriously. There has been a tendency to dismiss a suicide attempt as an impulsive act resulting from a temporary crisis or depression. If a suicide attempt fails to draw attention to their problems or makes them worse, the child or adolescent may conclude that suicide is the only answer. Children and adolescents need to know that someone cares and must be provided with swift and efficient crisis intervention. Although ordinary practitioners can manage an acute depressive reaction without difficulty, the adolescent who has made a serious attempt or has a specific plan for suicide should receive immediate attention and competent psychiatric care.

> **NURSINGALERT**
>
> Adolescents who express suicidal feelings and have a specific plan should be monitored at all times. They should not have access to firearms, prescription or over-the-counter drugs, belts, scarves, shoestrings, sharp objects, matches, or lighters. If they are intoxicated, they must be restrained or placed in a protective environment until a psychiatrist or psychologist can assess them.

Nursing Care Management

Nurses play a pivotal role in reducing adolescent suicide. Nurses have the opportunity to provide anticipatory guidance to parents and adolescents. They can teach parents to be supportive and to develop positive communication patterns that help teens feel connected with and loved by their families. To foster healthy development, parents can be encouraged to provide teens with creative outlets and to assist young people in accepting strong emotions—pain, anger, and frustration—as a normal part of the human experience.

Care of the suicidal adolescent includes early recognition, management, and prevention. The most important aspect of management is the recognition of warning signs that indicate an adolescent is troubled and might attempt suicide. Health professionals must be alert to the signs of depression, and anyone who exhibits such behavior should be referred for thorough psychologic assessment. Depression is manifested differently in children and adolescents than in adults. In teens it may be masked by impulsive aggressive behaviors. Defiance, disobedience, behavior problems, and psychosomatic disturbances can indicate underlying depression, suicidal ideation, and impending suicide attempts.

> **NURSINGALERT**
>
> No threat of suicide should be ignored or challenged. Threats are a symptom that must be taken seriously. Too often, suicidal threats or minor attempts are confused with bids for attention. It is also a mistake to be lulled into a false sense of security when the adolescent's depression is apparently relieved. The improvement in attitude may mean that the adolescent has made the decision and found the means to carry out the threat.

Peers or other confidants are valuable observers and excellent sources of information about potential suicide attempts. They may not be able to diagnose depression, but they are able to sense when a friend has undergone a marked personality change. It is important to emphasize that the peer who detects any changes in a friend is a potential rescuer and should not remain silent about the observations. Friendship does not imply collusion. A peer who believes that a friend may be suicidal should alert someone who can help (e.g., a parent, teacher, guidance counselor, school nurse).

Routine health assessments of adolescents should include questions that assess the presence of suicidal ideation or intent. The following questions can be asked (Greydanus and Pratt, 1995):

- Do you consider yourself more a happy person, an unhappy person, or somewhere in the middle?
- Have you ever been so unhappy or upset that you felt like being dead?
- Have you ever thought about hurting yourself?
- Have you ever developed a plan to hurt yourself or kill yourself?
- Have you ever attempted to kill yourself?

If children or adolescents express suicidal intent, nurses make a contract, asking them to sign an agreement that they will not attempt suicide during an agreed-on period and that they will call the 24-hour crisis line immediately if they feel that they cannot keep to their contract. The amount of time an adolescent feels comfortable contracting is usually an indication of his or her risk and stability.

Because a suicide attempt is frequently an outgrowth of family distress, it is essential to intervene with the family. It is important to assess family interactions and to recognize disturbed relationships. The most effective approach is recognition of susceptible adolescents during the early stages of family distress so that family counseling can be started. Prevention must be directed toward improving childrearing practices through support and education of parents and changing societal conditions that generate defeat, despair, and maladaptive behavior.

Although confidentiality is an essential part of adolescent counseling, in the case of self-destructive behaviors confidentiality cannot be honored. Suicidal behavior is reported to the family and other professionals, and adolescents are informed that this will be done. Such action conveys an important message to the youth: that the professionals understand and care.

Many schools have instituted suicide prevention programs. These programs include services such as drop-in counseling and a peer-counseling telephone line. Information can also be obtained from the American Association of Suicidology.*

---

*5221 Wisconsin Ave. NW, Washington, DC 20015; (202) 237-2280; http://www.suicidology.org.

KEY POINTS

- Participation in sports predisposes children and adolescents to both acute injuries and overuse syndromes.
- Alterations in growth and maturation may be manifested as short or tall stature, precocious puberty, or delayed sexual development.
- The most frequent health problems related to the female reproductive system involve menstrual dysfunction.
- Health problems related to sexuality include pregnancy, sexual assault, and STDs; prevention includes sex education and contraceptive counseling.
- Eating disorders observed in middle and late childhood include obesity, AN, and BN.
- Behavior problems in middle childhood can result from ADHD, enuresis, encopresis, school phobia, recurrent abdominal pain, childhood depression, conversion reaction, and childhood schizophrenia.
- Signs of depression in children and adolescents are often subtle and require astute observation by parents and health professionals.
- The substances abused by children and adolescents include alcohol, marijuana, narcotics, opiates, central nervous system depressants or stimulants, inhalants, and mind-altering drugs.
- Tobacco smoking is a significant problem among teenagers; reasons for smoking include social pressures, mass media influence, and a need to develop a self-concept.
- Suicide, the deliberate act of self-injury with the intent to kill, is often associated with depression, substance abuse, difficulties in coping with stress, an affective disorder, or a disturbed family environment.

answers to CRITICAL THINKING EXERCISES

TESTICULAR SELF-EXAMINATION

1. Yes. Although testicular cancer is not common in adolescence, when it does occur, it is generally malignant. Testicular cancer is very curable if detected early.

2. a. The best way to detect testicular tumors is by performing TSE every month.
   b. The usual presenting symptom for testicular cancer is a heavy, hard painless mass (either smooth or nodular) that is palpated on the testis.
   c. Adolescent boys are self-conscious about their genital anatomy. However, as a pediatric nurse practitioner at the school-based clinic, Paul is in an excellent position to teach young men how to perform this examination. It is highly probable that he has already won their trust and confidence through his routine daily nursing activities, such as providing sports physicals and treating their episodic illnesses. Paul will be able to present the class in a manner that is respectful of the young boys, while allaying their anxieties and providing them with an important health skill.
   d. The class should be presented in a matter-of-fact way, with an explanation of both the characteristics of the normal testicle as well as a description of abnormal findings.

3. The first priority is to make certain that all adolescent boys with health problems feel comfortable visiting the health suite and sharing their concerns with the nurse practitioner. The ultimate goal is to be certain that no adolescent boy with a potential testicular tumor fails to get an immediate assessment and referral for treatment.

4. Yes, the information about testicular cancer and the importance of detecting it early provides a definite rationale for the class.

5. If it is difficult to find the time for the class in the regular school health curriculum, Paul should suggest other options. Perhaps Paul could provide the information on TSE as part of an extra class that students volunteer to attend, or he could develop a self-learning packet that male students could complete when they visit the health suite.

ANOREXIA NERVOSA

1. Using the clinical manifestations of anorexia nervosa (AN) (see Box 17-4) and the diagnostic criteria for anorexia nervosa (see Box 17-5), there is sufficient evidence to support the conclusion that Jane has AN.

2. a. Young adolescent girls with AN are often high achievers or excellent students. They have an abundance of energy, a distorted body image, and a fear of gaining weight.
   b. A family crisis can influence AN. Jane's parents are currently in the middle of a divorce, and, in this type of situation, some teens feel they have no control over events in their life. Consequently, some adolescents take control by refusing to eat and developing AN.
   c. Jane is engaging in increased physical activity and is skipping lunch several days each week. On physical examination, she has a decreased body temperature (36° C [96.8° F]), and she has lost 9 kg (20 pounds) in the past year (she is at <85% of her expected weight). She also told the nurse practitioner that she has not had her menstrual period for 3 months. These manifestations are all congruent with AN.
   d. AN is treated by a team of health professionals who address the abnormal eating patterns and altered body image of the patient and the dysfunctional family dynamics that accompany this disorder.

3. Jane should be referred to a specialist who deals with adolescents with AN.

4. Yes, the evidence supports the conclusion.

5. Because Jane has not had her menstrual period for 3 months, there is a possibility that Jane is pregnant. The nurse practitioner should obtain a pregnancy test to rule out this possibility.

ATTENTION DEFICIT HYPERACTIVITY DISORDER

1. Yes, there are sufficient data to arrive at a possible conclusion.
2. a. Methylphenidate is a stimulant that increases dopamine and norepinephrine levels that lead to stimulation of the inhibitory system of the central nervous system.
   b. Common side effects of methylphenidate include nausea, anorexia, decreased appetite, and insomnia.
   c. Although the absorption rate of methylphenidate is increased when the drug is taken with meals, side effects such as decreased appetite may become more pronounced with this schedule of administration. Side effects can be alleviated by changing the times that the drug is administered or by switching to a sustained time-release form of the drug that is taken once per day in the morning.
3. Although Johnnie seems to have responded favorably to his medication and has demonstrated several positive effects of methylphenidate (improvement in math class and increasing self-confidence in social skills), the nurse should be concerned about the fact that Johnnie has not eaten his lunch for the past week and that he is not hungry. Decreased appetite is a negative side effect of methylphenidate.
4. Yes, the data indicate that Johnnie is currently experiencing a decrease in his appetite. Because decreased appetite is a common side effect of methylphenidate, there is a high probability that this symptom is related to Johnnie's medication. However, adjusting or changing the times the medication is administered can often alleviate this side effect. Another option is to ask Johnnie's physician to switch his medication to a sustained time-release form of methylphenidate that can be given once per day in the morning.
5. It is possible that Johnnie's decreased appetite is due to some other factor and is not related to his medication. Therefore the nurse should encourage the mother to communicate information about this side effect to Johnnie's primary care physician so that a more complete evaluation can be made.

REFERENCES

Adelman WP, Duggan AK, Hauptman P, and others: Effectiveness of a high school smoking cessation program, *Pediatrics* 107(4):e50, 2001.

America Academy of Pediatrics, Committee on Infectious Diseases: *Red book: 2006 report of the Committee on Infectious Diseases,* ed 27, Elk Grove Village, Ill, 2006, The Academy.

American Academy of Pediatrics, Committee on Adolescence: Adolescent pregnancy: current trends and issues, *Pediatrics* 116(1):281-286, 2005a.

American Academy of Pediatrics, Subcommittee on Chronic Abdominal Pain: Chronic abdominal pain in children, *Pediatrics* 115(3):812-815, 2005b.

American Academy of Pediatrics: Tobacco, alcohol, and other drugs: the role of the pediatrician in prevention, maintenance, and identification of substance abuse, *Pediatrics* 115(3):816-821, 2005c.

American Academy of Pediatrics, Committee on Adolescence: Identifying and treating eating disorders, *Pediatrics* 111(1):204-211, 2003.

American Academy of Pediatrics, Committee on Adolescence: Care of the adolescent sexual assault victim, *Pediatrics* 107(6):1476-1479, 2001a.

American Academy of Pediatrics, Committee on Public Education: Children, adolescents, and television, *Pediatrics* 107(2):423-426, 2001b.

American Academy of Pediatrics: Treatment of the school-aged child with attention-deficit/hyperactivity disorder, *Pediatrics* 108(4):1033-1044, 2001c.

American Academy of Pediatrics, Committee on Adolescence: Suicide and suicide attempts in adolescents, *Pediatrics* 105(4):871-874, 2000.

American Academy of Pediatrics, American College of Obstetricians and Gynecologists: Menstruation in girls and adolescents: using the menstrual cycle as a vital sign, *Pediatrics* 118(5):2245-2250, 2006.

American Dietetic Association: Position of the American Dietetic Association: Nutrition intervention in the treatment of anorexia nervosa, bulimia nervosa, and other eating disorders, *J Am Diet Assoc* 106(12):2073-2082, 2006.

American Psychiatric Association: *Diagnostic and statistical manual of mental disorders,* ed 4 (text rev) (DSM-IV TR), Washington, DC, 2000, The Association.

Anderson JE, Santelli JS, Morrow B: Trends in adolescent contraceptive use, unprotected and poorly protected sex, 1991-2003, *J Adolesc Health* 38(6):734-739, 2006.

Angulo P: Nonalcoholic fatty liver disease, *N Engl J Med* 346(16):1221-1231, 2002.

Baker S, Barlow S, Cochran W, and others: Overweight children and adolescents: a clinical report of the North American Society for Pediatric Gastroenterology, Hepatology and Nutrition, *J Pediatr Gastroenterol Nutr* 40:533-543, 2005.

Berkowitz RI, Fujioka K, Daniels SR, and others: Effects of sibutramine treatment in obese adolescents, *Ann Intern Med* 145(2):81-90, 2006.

Berry AK: Helping children with nocturnal enuresis: the wait-and-see approach may not be in everyone's interest, *Am J Nurs* 106(8):56-63, 2006.

Centers for Disease Control and Prevention: Sexually transmitted diseases treatment guidelines, 2006, *MMWR* 55(RR-11):1-94, 2006a.

Centers for Disease Control and Prevention: Youth risk behavior surveillance—United States, 2005, *MMWR* 55(SS-5):1-64, 2006b.

Centers for Disease Control and Prevention: Youth tobacco surveillance—United States, 2001-2002, *MMWR* 55(SS03):1-56, 2006c.

Clements PT, Speck PM, Crane PA, and others: Issues and dynamics of sexually assaulted adolescents and their families, *Int J Mental Health Neurosurg* 13:267-274, 2004.

Coughlin EC: Assessment and management of pediatric constipation in primary care, *Pediatr Nurs* 29(4):296-301, 2003.

Dennehy CE: The use of herbs and dietary supplements in gynecology: an evidence-based review, *J Midwifery Womens Health* 51(6):402-409, 2006.

Ehtisham S, Barrett TG, Shaw NJ: Type 2 diabetes mellitus in UK children—an emerging problem, *Diabetes Med* 17(12):867-871, 2000.

Feldman M, Friedman LS, Sleisenger MH: Obesity: a historical perspective and disease prevalence estimates. In Feldman M, Friedman LS, Sleisenger MH, editors: *Sleisenger and Fordtran's gastrointestinal and liver disease,* ed 7, Philadelphia, 2002, Saunders.

Forman SF: Eating disorders: epidemiology, pathogenesis, and clinical features, *UpToDate,* 2007, retrieved July 31, 2007, from http://www.uptodate.com.

Gibbons RD, Hur K, Bhaumik DK, and others: The relationship between antidepressant prescription rates and rate of early adolescent suicide, *Am J Psychiatry* 163(11):1898-1904, 2006.

Goodman E, Capitman J: Depressive symptoms and cigarette smoking among teens, *Pediatrics* 106(4):748-755, 2000.

Gordon SM: *Adolescent drug use: trends in abuse, treatment and prevention,* Wernersville, Penn, 2000, Caron Foundation.

Greaser J, Whyte JJ: Childhood obesity: is there effective treatment? *Consult Pediatr* 4(10):474-478, 2004.

Greydanus DE, Pratt HD: Emotional and behavioral disorders of adolescence, part 2, *Adolesc Health Update* 8(1):1-8, 1995.

Hamilton BE, Martin JA, Ventura SJ: Births: preliminary data for 2005, *Natl Vital Stat Rep* 55(11):1-18, 2006.

Hardy LR, Harrell JS, Bell RA: Overweight in children: definitions, measurements, confounding factors, and health consequences, *J Pediatr Nurs* 19(6):376-383, 2004.

Hedley AA, Ogden CL, Johnson CL, and others: Prevalence of overweight and obesity among US children, adolescents, and adults, 1999-2002, *JAMA* 291(3):2847-2850, 2004.

Hill JO, Wyatt HR, Reed GW, and others: Obesity and the environment: where do we go from here? *Science* 299(5608):853-855, 2003.

Jick H, Kaye JA, Jick SS: Antidepressants and the risk of suicidal behaviors, *JAMA* 292(3):338-343, 2004.

Johnston LD, O'Malley PM, Bachman JG, and others: *Monitoring the future national results on adolescent drug use: overview of key findings, 2004,* NIH Pub No 05-5726, Bethesda, Md, 2005, National Institute on Drug Abuse.

Kandakai TL, Smith LC: Denormalizing a historical problem: teen pregnancy, policy and public health action. *Am J Health Behav* 31(2):170-180, 2007.

Kiess W, Galler A, Reich A, and others: Clinical aspects of obesity in childhood and adolescence, *Obesity Rev* 1:29-36, 2001.

Koeppen-Schomerus G, Wardle J, Plomin R: A genetic analysis of weight and overweight in 4-year-old twin pairs, *Int J Obes Relat Metab Dis* 25(6):838-844, 2001.

Lord J, Winell JJ: Overuse injuries in pediatric athletes, *Curr Opin Pediatr* 16(1):47-50, 2004.

MacKenzie NR: Childhood obesity: strategies for prevention, *Pediatr Nurs* 26(5):527-530, 2000.

Master-Hunter T, Heiman DL: Amenorrhea: evaluation and treatment, *Am Fam Physician* 73(8):1374-1382, 2006.

Mehler PS: Diagnosis and care of patients with anorexia nervosa in primary care settings, *Ann Intern Med* 134:1048-1059, 2001.

Michelson D, Faries, D, Wernicke J, and others: Atomoxetine in the treatment of children and adolescents with attention-deficit/hyperactivity disorder: a randomized, placebo-controlled, dose-response study, *Pediatrics* 108:E83, 2001.

Moran R: Breaking the cycle of childhood obesity, *Clin Advisor* 6(2):62-67, 2003.

Mosher WD, Chandra A, Jones J: Sexual behavior and selected health measures: men and women 15-44 years of age, United States, 2002, *Adv Data,* Sep 15(362):1-55, 2005.

Myers SM, Eisenhauer NJ, Ryan ME: ADHD: it is real, and it can be treated, *Clin Advisor* 6(3):15-25, 2003.

National Institute for Health Care Management Foundation: *Childhood obesity: advancing effective prevention and treatment: an overview for health professionals,* prepared for National Institute for Health Care Management Foundation Forum, Washington, DC, April 9, 2003.

Neinstein LS: *Adolescent health care: a practical guide,* ed 4, Philadelphia, 2002, Lippincott Williams & Wilkins.

Patel M, Minshall L: Management of sexual assault, *Emerg Clin North Am* 19(3):817-831, 2001.

Patten CA, Choi WS, Gillin JC, and others: Depressive symptoms and cigarette smoking predict development and persistence of sleep problems in US adolescents, *Pediatrics* 106(2):E23, 2000.

Rideout VJ, Foehr UG, Roberts DF, and others: *Kids and media @ new millennium,* New York, 1999, Kaiser Family Foundation.

Rimsza ME, Kirk GM: Common medical problems of the college student, *Pediatr Clin North Am* 52(1):9-24, vii, 2005.

Robinson TN: Television viewing and childhood obesity, *Pediatr Clin North Am* 48:1017-1025, 2001.

Rome ES, Ammerman S, Rosen DS, and others: Children and adolescents with eating disorders: the state of the art, *Pediatrics* 111(1):e98-e108, 2003.

Schwartz RH, Milteer R, LeBeau MA: Drug facilitated sexual assault ("date rape"), *South Med J* 93(6):558-561, 2000.

Schwimmer JB: Managing overweight in older children and adolescents, *Pediatr Ann* 33(1):39-44, 2004.

Selekman J, Snyder M: Learning disabilities and/or attention deficit disorder. In Jackson P, Vessey JA, editors: *Primary care of children with chronic conditions,* ed 3, St Louis, 2000, Mosby.

Sethi S, Bhargava S, Shipra PM: Nocturnal enuresis: a review, *J Pediatr Neurol* 3(1):11-18, 2005.

Shrier LA: Sexually transmitted diseases in adolescents: biologic, cognitive, psychologic, behavioral, and social issues, *Adolesc Med Clin* 15(2):215-234, 2004.

Shulman ST: The overweight epidemic, *Pediatr Ann* 33(1):6, 2004.

Sjöberg RL, Nilsson KW, Leppert J: Obesity, shame, and depression in school-aged children: a population-based study, *Pediatrics* 116(3):e389-e393, 2005.

Sondike S, Copperman N, Jacobson MS: Effects of a low-carbohydrate diet on weight loss and cardiovascular risk factors in overweight adolescents, *J Pediatr* 142(3):253-258, 2003.

Spencer TJ, Wilens TE, Biederman J, and others: Efficacy and safety of mixed amphetamine salts extended release (Adderall XR) in the management of attention-deficit hyperactivity disorder in adolescent patients: a 4-week, randomized, double-blind, placebo-controlled, parallel-group study, *Clin Ther* 28(2):266-279, 2006.

Sugerman HJ, Sugerman EL, DeMaria EJ, and others: Bariatric surgery for severely obese adolescents, *J Gastrointest Surg* 7(1):102-107, 2003.

Sundelin-Wahlsten V, Ahmad A, von Knorring A-L: Traumatic experiences and post-traumatic stress reactions in children from Kurdistan and Sweden, *Acta Paediatr* 90:563-568, 2001.

Taylor ED, Theim KR, Mirch MC, and others: Orthopedic complications of overweight in children and adolescents, *Pediatrics* 117(6):2167-2173, 2006.

Tsai WS, Inge TH, Burd RS: Bariatric surgery in adolescents: recent national trends in use and in-hospital outcomes, *Arch Pediatr Adolesc Med* 161(3):217-221, 2007.

US Department of Health and Human Services: *The health consequences of involuntary exposure to tobacco smoke: a report of the surgeon general,* Washington, DC, 2006, US Department of Health and Human Services.

US Food and Drug Administration: *Antidepressant use in children, adolescents, and adults,* March 22, 2004 (updated July 12, 2005), retrieved Jan 22, 2008, from http://www.fda.gov/cder/drug/antidepressants/default.htm.

Weiss R, Dziura J, Burgert TS, and others: Obesity and the metabolic syndrome in children and adolescents, *N Engl J Med* 350(23):2362-2374, 2004.

Yanovski SZ, Yanovski JA: Obesity, *N Engl J Med* 346(8):591-602, 2002.

18

Chronic Illness, Disability, or End-of-Life Care for the Child and Family

ANGELA M. ETHIER

CHAPTER OUTLINE

PERSPECTIVES ON THE CARE OF CHILDREN WITH SPECIAL NEEDS, 575
Scope of the Problem, 575
Trends in Care, 575
  Developmental Focus, 575
  Family-Centered Care, 576
  Family–Health Care Provider
    Communication, 576
  Establishing Therapeutic Relationships, 576
  The Role of Culture in Family-Centered
    Care, 577
  Shared Decision Making, 577
  Normalization, 577
  Managed Care, 578
**THE FAMILY OF THE CHILD WITH
SPECIAL NEEDS, 578**
Impact of the Child's Chronic Illness
  or Disability, 578
  Parents, 579
  Siblings, 580
Coping with Ongoing Stress and Periodic
  Crises, 581
  Concurrent Stresses Within the Family, 581
  Coping Mechanisms, 581
  Parental Empowerment, 581
Assisting Family Members in Managing
  Their Feelings, 581
  Shock and Denial, 582
  Adjustment, 582
  Reintegration and Acknowledgment, 582
Establishing a Support System, 583

THE CHILD WITH SPECIAL NEEDS, 583
Developmental Aspects, 583
Coping Mechanisms, 584
  Hopefulness, 584
  Health Education and Self-Care, 584
Responses to Parental Behavior, 585
Type of Illness or Disability, 585
**NURSING CARE OF THE FAMILY
AND CHILD WITH SPECIAL NEEDS, 585**
Assessment, 585
Provide Support at the Time
  of Diagnosis, 586
Support Family's Coping Methods, 587
  Parents, 587
  Parent-to-Parent Support, 589
  Advocate for Empowerment, 589
  The Child, 589
  Siblings, 590
Educate About the Disorder and General
  Health Care, 590
  Activities of Daily Living, 590
  Safe Transportation, 591
  Primary Health Care, 591
Promote Normal Development, 591
  Early Childhood, 591
  School Age, 593
  Adolescence, 594
Establish Realistic Future Goals, 594
**PERSPECTIVES ON THE CARE OF
CHILDREN AT THE END OF LIFE, 595**
Principles of Palliative Care, 595

Decision Making at the End of Life, 595
  Ethical Considerations in End-of-Life
    Decision Making, 595
  Physician–Health Care Team Decision
    Making, 596
  Parental Decision Making, 597
  The Dying Child, 597
  Treatment Options for Terminally Ill
    Children, 599
**NURSING CARE OF THE CHILD AND
FAMILY AT THE END OF LIFE, 600**
Nursing Care Plan: The Child Who Is
  Terminally Ill or Dying, 600
Fear of Pain and Suffering, 600
  Pain and Symptom Management, 602
  Parents' and Siblings' Need for Education
    and Support, 603
Fear of Dying Alone or of Not Being
  Present When the Child Dies, 603
Fear of Actual Death, 603
  Home Deaths, 603
  Hospital Deaths, 604
Organ or Tissue Donation and
  Autopsy, 605
Grief and Mourning, 605
  Parental Grief, 606
  Sibling Grief, 606
Nurses' Reactions to Caring for Dying
  Children, 607

LEARNING OBJECTIVES

On completion of this chapter the reader will be able to:

- Identify the scope of and changing trends in care of children with special needs.
- Identify the major reactions of and effects on the family of a child with a special need.

- Define the stages of adjustment to the diagnosis of a chronic condition.
- Recognize the impact of the illness or disability on the developmental stages of childhood.

- Outline nursing interventions that promote the family's optimal adjustment to the child's chronic disorder.
- Outline nursing interventions that support the family at the time of death.
- Define the usual symptoms of normal grief.

RELATED TOPICS and ADDITIONAL RESOURCES

 IN TEXT

Childhood Morbidity, *Ch. 1*
Communicating with Families, *Ch. 6*
Compliance, *Ch. 22*
Cultural and Religious Influences on Health Care, *Ch. 4*
Developmental Assessment, *Ch. 5*
Discharge Planning and Home Care: High-Risk Newborn and Family, *Ch. 9*
Family Assessment, *Ch. 6*
Family-Centered Care, *Ch. 1*

Family-Centered Care of the Child During Illness and Hospitalization, *Ch. 21*
Family-Centered Home Care, *Ch. 20*
Health Promotion: Infant, *Ch. 10;* Toddler, *Ch. 12;* Preschooler, *Ch. 13;* School-Age Child, *Ch. 15;* Adolescent, *Ch. 16*
Mortality, *Ch. 1*
Nursing Care of the High-Risk Newborn and Family, *Ch. 9*
Pain Management, *Ch. 7*
School Phobia, *Ch. 17*

 COMPANION CD

Critical Thinking Exercise—Neonatal Loss
Case Study—The Dying Child
NCLEX Review Questions

evolve

evolve.elsevier.com/Wong/essentials/

NCLEX Review Questions
Nursing Care Plan—The Child Who Is Terminally Ill or Dying
WebLinks

PERSPECTIVES ON THE CARE OF CHILDREN WITH SPECIAL NEEDS

SCOPE OF THE PROBLEM

A number of terms and defining characteristics have been used to describe chronic illness and disability in children (Box 18-1). In recent years there have been continuing efforts to develop a definition that better identifies the numbers of children living with chronic conditions, as well as the impact on health and social services (Jackson, 2000; van Dyck, Kogan, Heppel, and others, 2004). Currently children with special health care needs are defined as children who have or are at increased risk for a chronic physical, developmental, behavioral, or emotional condition and who also require health and related services of a type or amount beyond that generally required by children (Msall, Avery, Tremont, and others, 2003; Newacheck, Strickland, Shonkoff, and others, 1998).

Ongoing progress in medical and technologic disease management has contributed to the growing number of children with special health care needs (Palfrey, Tonniges, Green, and others, 2005). The number of U.S. children with acquired immunodeficiency syndrome (AIDS) diagnosed each year declined by 75% from 1992 to 2000 (Yogev and Chadwick, 2004). Technologic advances have substantially increased the survival of extremely low– and very low–birth-weight infants (Jackson, 2000). Children with disabilities are more likely to be in poor health than children without disabilities (Newacheck and Halfon, 1998). The result of such progress is that an estimated 15% to 18% of the children in the United States live with a chronic illness or disability and require specialized health care

of a type or amount beyond that generally required by children (Perrin, 2004).

The most commonly occurring conditions causing disability are diseases of the respiratory tract and impairments of speech, special senses, and intelligence. Mental and nervous system disorders account for about one sixth of all childhood disability (Newacheck and Halfon, 1998).

The impact of chronic illness and disability in children is wide ranging. Chronic conditions in children present most families with additional tasks, responsibilities, and concerns (Ray, 2002). A child's activity level and developmental opportunities can be affected. Days can be lost from school. Children with chronic illness or disability may be at increased risk for behavior or emotional problems. Parents may lose days from work, experience financial strain, and be challenged both emotionally and physically as they cope with care of the child.

Siblings are also affected by having a "different" brother or sister and may simultaneously feel guilt and anger or jealousy toward their ill sibling. Additionally, secondary losses such as the ability to participate in extracurricular activities or social events occur because of routines imposed by the affected child's chronic condition.

TRENDS IN CARE

Developmental Focus

Focusing on the child's **developmental level** rather than chronologic age or diagnosis emphasizes the child's abilities and strengths rather than disabilities. Attention is directed to normalizing experiences, adapting the environment, and pro-

Common Terms Regarding Children with Special Needs

Chronic illness—A condition that interferes with daily functioning for more than 3 months in a year, causes hospitalization of more than 1 month in a year, or (at time of diagnosis) is likely to do either of these

Congenital disability—A disability that has existed since birth but is not necessarily hereditary

Developmental delay—A maturational lag; an abnormal, slower rate of development in which a child demonstrates a functioning level below that observed in normal children of the same age

Developmental disability—Any mental or physical disability that is manifested before age 22 years and is likely to continue indefinitely

Disability—A functional limitation that interferes with a person's ability, for example, to walk, lift, hear, or learn

Handicap—A condition or barrier imposed by society, the environment, or one's own self; not a synonym for disability

Impairment—A loss or abnormality of structure or function

Life-limiting illness—Any illness or condition developed in childhood whereby the child is likely to die before adulthood or with a limited expectation of life thereafter.

Technology-dependent child—A child between the ages of birth and 21 years with a chronic disability that requires the routine use of a medical device to compensate for the loss of a life-sustaining body function; requires daily ongoing care or monitoring by trained personnel

Data from Westbrook LE, Silver EJ, Stein RE: Implications for estimates of disability in children: a comparison of definitional components, *Pediatrics* 101(6):1025-1030, 1998; Newacheck PW, Halfon N: Prevalence and impact of disabling chronic conditions in childhood, *Am J Public Health* 88(4):610-617, 1998; Danvers L, Freshwater D, Cheater F, and others: Providing seamless service for children with life-limiting illness: experiences and recommendations of professional staff at the Diana Princess of Wales Children's Community Service, *J Clin Nurs* 12(3):351-359, 2003.

moting coping skills. Nurses often are in vital positions to redirect attention from the pathologic model with its focus on weaknesses and problems to the developmental model to meet the unique needs of the child and family.

A developmental focus also considers family development. The life cycle of the family unit reflects changing ages and needs of family members, as well as changing external demands. A family member's serious illness or disability can cause significant stress or crisis at any stage of the family life cycle. Just as with individual development, family development may be interrupted or even regress to an earlier level of functioning. Nurses can use the concept of family development to plan meaningful interventions and evaluate care (see Developmental Theory, Chapter 3).

Family-Centered Care

Children's physical and emotional health, as well as cognitive and social functioning, is strongly influenced by how well their families function (Schor, 2003). The importance of family-centered care—a philosophy that considers the family as the constant in the child's life—is especially evident in the care of children with special needs (see also Family-Centered Care, Chapter 1). As parents learn about the youngster's health care needs, they often become experts in delivering care. Health care providers, including nurses, are adjuncts to the child's care and need to form partnerships with parents. Effective communication and negotiation be-

tween parents and nurses are essential to forming trusting and effective partnerships and finding the best ways to meet the needs of the child and family (Corlett and Twycross, 2006). Collaborative relationships are characterized by communication, dialogue, active listening, awareness, and acceptance of differences (Schor, 2003).

Family–Health Care Provider Communication

The disclosure of a serious acute or chronic illness of a child is one of the most stressful aspects of communication between families and health care professionals. Often, parents have suspected for some time that something is wrong with their child and believe that their concerns were minimized or ignored by health care professionals (Whitehead and Gosling, 2003; Thomlinson, 2002; Cohen, 1995). After a diagnosis is made, numerous studies have shown that parents are not always satisfied with the way in which information is given. Factors that influence parent dissatisfaction with communication include unsympathetic and brief diagnostic interviews, lack of privacy during diagnostic discussions, and lack of opportunity to ask questions. Conversely, parents report satisfaction when they perceive the health care providers giving information in an open and honest manner with respect for the parents' need for privacy and time to express emotions and ask questions (Davies, Davis, and Seibert, 2003). Similar factors are important in communication of changes in the child's condition throughout the course of the illness.

Providing information to families with a chronically ill child should be a process of repeated discussions to allow the family to process the information and their reactions to that information, and allow them to ask for clarification and further information. Nurses play an important role in ensuring that families' needs are met during discussions related to the child's diagnosis, condition, and treatment. This requires assessment regarding how much information the family is comfortable with, what they understand of the information already given to them, and how they are coping with the information both cognitively and emotionally. Nurses should ensure that the appropriate health care professionals address any concerns or further questions that families may have.

Establishing Therapeutic Relationships

Another important aspect of family-centered care of chronically ill children is establishing a therapeutic relationship with the child and family, which has been shown to predict improved health-related outcomes (Denboba, McPherson, Kenney, and others, 2006). Families, most often the mother, take on enormous responsibility in providing technical care and symptom management of their child's condition outside the health care institution (O'Brien and Wegner, 2002; Raina, O'Donnell, Rosenbaum, and others, 2005; Swallow and Jacoby, 2001). To build successful therapeutic relationships with families, it is necessary for nurses to recognize parents' expertise with regard to their child's condition and needs. Care conferences, especially multidisciplinary meetings that include the family and key health professionals, provide an opportunity for sharing ideas and expressing feelings or concerns.

Individual discussions, especially with the case manager, primary nurse, clinical nurse specialist, or nurse practitioner, help establish a consistent and flexible care plan that can prevent conflicts or deal with these conflicts before they disrupt care. In family-centered care, the goal is to maintain the integrity of the leadership role and support the family during times of crisis or stress.

The Role of Culture in Family-Centered Care

Issues of culture, ethnicity, and race affect access to services, utilization, and follow-through with referrals and recommendations (van Dyck, Kogan, McPherson, and others, 2004; Wise, Wampler, Chavkin, and others, 2002; Wood, Smith, Romero, and others, 2002; Zuvekas and Taliaferro, 2003). For some ethnic and minority populations, cultural understandings of illness and disability, the structure of family life, social roles for individuals who are disabled, and other factors related to the perception of children may differ from those of mainstream American culture. These factors may affect family needs and family choices regarding the care of their child with special needs.

Although culture cannot completely explain how an individual will think and act, understanding cultural perspectives can help the nurse anticipate and understand why families may make certain decisions. Cultural attributes such as values and beliefs regarding illness or disability and its causation, social roles for the ill or disabled, family structure, the role of children, childrearing practices, self vs group orientation, spirituality, and time orientation also affect a family's response to illness or disability in a child (Carnevale, Alexander, Davis, and others, 2006; Carter, 2002; Marshall, Olsen, Mandleco, and others, 2003; Rehm, 1999; Sterling and Peterson, 2003).

When parents are informed of their child's chronic illness, interpreters familiar with both culture and language should be used. Children, family members, and friends of the family should not be used as translators because their presence may prevent parents from openly discussing the issues. When working with people of cultural backgrounds different from their own, nurses must listen carefully with an initial goal of understanding and articulating the family's perspective. The ability to interpret the mainstream medical culture to the family is also important. Furthermore, every effort is made to incorporate traditional cultural beliefs of a family into treatment plans. Developing a care plan in conjunction with the family, considering their preferences and priorities, is an important first step in formulating a plan that best meets the family's needs, no matter what their cultural background (Ahmann, 1994; Ochieng, 2003).

Shared Decision Making

Shared decision making among the child, family, and health care team can result from open, honest, culturally sensitive communication and the establishment of a therapeutic relationship between the family and health care providers. In a shared decision-making model the health care professionals provide honest, clear information regarding diagnosis, prognosis, treatment options, and risk/benefit assessment. The patient and/or family then shares information with the health care team regarding important family values, acceptable levels of discomfort or inconvenience, and the ability to comply with treatments being recommended (Charles, Gafni, and Whelan, 1997). This process allows them to discuss all options in terms of the risks and benefits to the child and family, the prognosis or expected course of the illness, and the impact on the family's resources (Box 18-2).

BOX 18-2
Facilitating Shared Decision Making

- Continually assess the impact of the child's illness and treatment on the family.
- Provide honest, accurate information regarding the trajectory of the disease, anticipated complications, and prognostic information.
- Discuss what the family desires for the child's quality of life.
- Avoid personal opinion or judgment of the family's questions and decisions.

Normalization

Normalization refers to behaviors and intentions of the disabled to integrate into society by living life as persons without a disability would (Morse, Wilson, and Penrod, 2000). For the chronically ill or disabled child, such behaviors could include attending school, pursuing hobbies and recreational interests, and achieving employment and a level of independence. For their families, it may entail adapting the family routine to accommodate the ill or disabled child's health and physical needs (McDougal, 2002).

Children with chronic illness and disability and their families face numerous challenges in achieving normalization. Families move between the "normal" of living with the experience of chronic childhood illness and the "normal" of the healthy outside world; they often redefine "normal" based on their particular experiences, needs, and circumstances (Nelson, 2002; Deatrick, Knafl, and Murphy-Moore, 1999).

Nurses can assist families in normalizing their lives by assessing the family's everyday life, social support systems, coping strategies, family cohesiveness, and family and community resources. Interventions could include encouraging families to reduce stress through delegation of care and family tasks, identifying ways to incorporate care into current routines, structuring the home environment to encourage the child's engagement in age-appropriate activities, and ensuring families have access to appropriate community support services (Jokinen, 2004; Shepard and Mahon, 2000). Being supportive of the child's illness and treatment and actively including the family in all aspects of care will improve their self-esteem and promote further development (Shepard and Mahon, 2000).

Home care represents the return to a system and set of priorities in which family values are as important in the care of a child with a chronic health problem as they are in the care of other children. Home care seeks to achieve goals that are consistent with the developmental model (Stein, 1985):

Goals for Home Care
- Normalize the life of a child with special needs, including those with technologically complex care, in a family and community context and setting.
- Minimize the disruptive impact of the child's condition on the family.
- Foster the child's maximum growth and development.

With appropriate training and support, families provide complex procedures and treatments in the home. Parents are challenged to retain a homelike setting among monitors, ventilators, and other sophisticated equipment. Throughout the text, home care is discussed as appropriate for specific conditions. The process of transition from hospital to home is elaborated on in Chapters 20 and 21.

Paralleling normalization and home care is the process of **mainstreaming,** or integrating children with special needs into regular classrooms. Just as the home is the natural environment for children, so school must also be included as an essential component of the children's overall physical, intellectual, and social development. Children who attend school have the advantages of learning and socializing with a wide group of peers. There is an increased focus on individualization as plans are made to meet the academic needs of these children along with those of the rest of the students.

A variety of supplemental programs have been designed in the school system to accommodate special needs, both at school age and younger, through **early intervention,** which consists of any sustained and systematic effort to assist children from birth to age 3 years who are disabled and developmentally vulnerable. This change and increasing opportunities for normalization for children with special needs in large part have resulted from the passage of (1) the Education for All Handicapped Children Act of 1975 (Public Law 94-142) and its 1990 amendments (Public Law 101-476), which changed the name of the act to the Individuals with Disabilities Education Act (IDEA); (2) the Education of the Handicapped Act Amendments of 1986 (Public Law 99-457), which directs states to develop and implement statewide comprehensive, coordinated, multidisciplinary interagency programs of early intervention services for infants and toddlers with disabilities, as well as support services for their families; and (4) the Americans with Disabilities Act of 1990. Nurses can provide parents with information about these laws and in some cases may participate in the development of individualized educational programs (IEPs) or individualized family service plans (IFSPs) for children with special needs.

Managed Care

Managed care programs have become the major form of health care provision in the United States (Jackson, 2000). The transition to this model of care presents both opportunities and challenges with respect to the care of children with special health care needs. Managed care may promote continuity and coordination of care. Children rely on adults for access to health care and follow-up with treatment regimens, making it necessary to manage the child's care in the context of the family (McPherson, Weissman, Strickland, and others, 2004; van Dyck, Kogan, McPherson, and others, 2004).

THE FAMILY OF THE CHILD WITH SPECIAL NEEDS

A major goal in working with the family of a child with special needs is to support the family's coping and promote their optimal functioning throughout the child's life. Long-term, comprehensive, family-centered approaches extend beyond supporting the child and family during the critical periods of diagnosis and hospitalization. Rather, comprehensive care involves forming parent-professional partnerships that can support a family's adaptation to the many changes that may be necessary in day-to-day life, determine expectations of and for the child, and provide a long-term perspective (Box 18-3).

BOX 18-3

Adaptive Tasks of Parents Having Children with Chronic Conditions

1. Accept the child's condition.
2. Manage the child's condition on a day-to-day basis.
3. Meet the child's normal developmental needs.
4. Meet the developmental needs of other family members.
5. Cope with ongoing stress and periodic crises.
6. Assist family members to manage their feelings.
7. Educate others about the child's condition.
8. Establish a support system.

From Canam C: Common adaptive tasks facing parents of children with chronic conditions, *J Adv Nurs* 18:46-53, 1993.

The impact of a child's medical or developmental condition is often experienced over time, initially as a crisis at the time of diagnosis, which may occur at birth, after a long period of physical or psychologic testing, or immediately after a tragic injury. The impact may also be felt before the diagnosis is made, when parents are aware that something is wrong with their child but before medical confirmation (Whitehead and Gosling, 2003; Thomlinson, 2002; Cohen, 1995).

The diagnosis and initial discharge home are critical times for parents (Coffey, 2006). Several factors can make it particularly difficult, including a long duration of uncertainty in the diagnostic process, negative perceptions of chronic illness or disability, insufficient information, and lack of mutual trust between parents and their child's health care team (Cohen, 1995; Garwick, Patterson, Bennett, and others, 1995; Nuutila and Salanterä, 2006). Parental feelings of shock, helplessness, isolation, fear, and depression are common (Coffey, 2006; Nuutila and Salanterä, 2006). Throughout the first year, parents struggle to accept the child's diagnosis, care, and uncertainty of the future (Coffey, 2006). Providing explicit and uncomplicated information to parents in an empathic way (Nuutila and Salanterä, 2006); assessing the family's daily routine, living conditions, background knowledge, skills and abilities, and coping behaviors; and evaluating the family's understanding of the information can encourage optimal support at the time of diagnosis and initial discharge home. It is also necessary to reassess parental needs for information and support on a routine basis (Nuutila and Salanterä, 2006).

Other critical times include the exacerbation of the child's physical symptoms, which increases parental care; significant milestones for the child and his or her peers, particularly toddlerhood, entering kindergarten, and turning 18 years old, which increases parental stress; and advocating for the child during these times. Supporting parents, respecting their stress and emotions, and acknowledging their role as team members in the care of their child are important aspects of nursing care (Coffey, 2006; Nuutila and Salanterä, 2006).

IMPACT OF THE CHILD'S CHRONIC ILLNESS OR DISABILITY

Each member of a family who has a child with special needs is affected by the experience (Sullivan-Bolyai, Sadler, Knafl, and others, 2003). The effects on the parents and their responses

BOX 18-4
Anticipated Parental Stress Points

Diagnosis of the condition—Parents require considerable education while dealing with an emotional response.

Developmental milestones—Times that children normally achieve walking, talking, and self-care are delayed or impossible for the child.

Start of schooling—Particularly stressful are situations in which appropriate schooling will not be in a regular class placement.

Reaching the ultimate attainment—Parents must handle situations such as realizing that ambulation will be impossible or that the child will not learn to read.

Adolescence—Issues such as sexuality and independence become prominent.

Future placement—Decisions about placement must be made when the child becomes an adult or when the parents can no longer care for the child.

Death of the child

are so critical that they directly influence the other members' reactions and the child's own coping.

Parents

In addition to the stress of grieving for the loss of a perfect child, parents are affected by whether or not they receive positive feedback from transactions with their child. Many parents feel satisfaction and fulfillment from the parenting role. For others, parenting may be a series of unrewarding experiences that contribute to feelings of inadequacy and failure (Box 18-4). These responses may be most evident in parents who are responsible for the child's care. For example, parents may become preoccupied with their ability to carry out certain procedures, overlooking the child's personal comfort and satisfaction or failing to offer praise for anything less than perfect cooperation or performance. They may pursue a frustrating activity until they achieve "success"—long after the child has become irritable and uncooperative. As a result, parents can become caught in a pattern of interaction that is mutually unrewarding and minimally productive. For these parents, several strategies may be helpful: education regarding what can reasonably be expected of their child, assistance in identifying the child's strengths, praise for a parental job well done, and respite care so that parents can renew their energies.

Parental Roles. Parenting a child with a chronic illness or disability requires much more than raising a typical child. In addition to attending to the routine aspects of parenting, parents of chronically ill children take on the added responsibility of performing complex technical care and symptom management, advocating for their child, and seeking and coordinating health and social services for their ill or disabled child. These added responsibilities must then be balanced with the needs of other family members, extended family and friends, and personal health and obligations to minimize consequences to the overall functioning of the family (Coffey, 2006; Ray, 2002).

Enormous demands may be placed on parental time, energy, and financial resources.

Often one partner remains at home to manage existing family responsibilities while the other remains with the ill child. The partner who is not included in the caregiving activities may feel neglected because all of the attention is directed toward the child and resentful that he or she is not sufficiently informed to be competent in the care. Without active participation in the child's care, the parent has little appreciation of the time and energy involved in performing those activities. When this partner does attempt to participate, the other parent may criticize the less skillful efforts. As a result, communication and support for each other may be adversely affected.

The nurse can assist parents in avoiding role conflicts by providing anticipatory guidance early on. Teaching should address stressors often identified as having an impact on the marriage: (1) the burden of care at home assumed by primarily one parent, (2) the financial burden, (3) the fear of the child dying, (4) pressure from relatives, (5) the hereditary nature of the disease (if applicable), and (6) fear of pregnancy. Other causes of tension may center on the inconveniences associated with care, such as long waits for an appointment, lack of parking near care facilities, or lack of overnight accommodations. Certainly, these last stressors are within health professionals' domain to minimize, if not eliminate.

Mother-Father Differences. Mothers and fathers in the same family often adjust and cope differently as parents of a child with special needs. Some mothers experience a peaks-and-valleys periodic crisis pattern, whereas most fathers tend to experience a steady, gradual recovery. Some research suggests that mothers of children with certain conditions may be more susceptible to psychologic distress and fatigue than fathers (Tong, Kandala, Haig, and others, 2002). Mothers are most often the primary caregiver and are more likely than fathers to give up their job to care for their child, often resulting in social isolation (Coffey, 2006). Mothers often have greater needs for social support and positive appraisal of the situation, whereas fathers are more likely to use self-controlling behaviors to cope (Goldbeck, 2001; Mastroyannopoulou, Stallard, Lewis, and others, 1997).

The father of a child with special needs struggles with issues that may be distinct from those of the mother. He may think that his role of protector is challenged because he does not know how to help and cannot protect the family from the seemingly overwhelming recurring problems. With today's increased emphasis on fathers' involvement in the lives of their children, this loss is felt more profoundly than in the past. The extensive stresses in the family can leave the father feeling depressed, weak, guilty, powerless, isolated, embarrassed, and angry. Fearful that he will lose control or be viewed as weak or ineffectual, however, the father often hides his feelings and displays an outward confidence that may lead others to believe that everything is fine. Fathers worry about what the future holds for their children, their ability to manage the increasing financial burden, and the daily disruptions of the entire family (Davies, Gudmundsdottir, Worden, and others, 2004). Some fathers escape in their work as a means of dulling the pain. Common coping strategies are problem oriented and include praying, getting information, looking at options, and weighing choices, in addition to withdrawal (Mastroyannopoulou, Stallard, Lewis, and others, 1997).

Single-Parent Families. Single-parent families are of special concern. The absence of a parent may result from divorce or death, or the parents may never have married. As the only parent of a child who may require extensive, sophisticated, and lifelong care, the single parent may feel an enormous burden. Available financial and emotional resources may already be stretched to the limit. A special effort should be made to assist the single parent in finding financial and support services that can ease the burden of care. Nurses can also assist the single parent in identifying helping roles that may be acceptable to relatives and friends.

Siblings

Results of studies on how siblings, almost exclusively European Americans, are affected by having a brother or sister with special needs are unclear (Barlow and Ellard, 2006). Generally, there is evidence that there is a negative effect on siblings of children with a chronic illness when compared with siblings of healthy children. This effect appears, however, to be decreasing in significance in recent years—most likely because of changes in public attitudes toward the ill and disabled (Sharpe and Rossiter, 2002). Siblings of children with chronic illness or disability report depression and anxiety more often than their peers (Rossiter and Sharpe, 2001). However, most investigators do agree that brothers and sisters of children with special needs are no more at risk for *severe* psychiatric problems than are siblings of children without chronic or disabling conditions. A number of factors increase the risk of negative effects for siblings of ill children. Responsibility for caregiving, differential treatment by parents, and limitations in family resources and recreational time are often the experience of siblings of ill or disabled children (Lobato and Kao, 2002) (Box 18-5).

An important factor in sibling adjustment and coping is information and knowledge regarding their brother's or sister's illness or disability. What siblings piece together or overhear is often much worse than the truth. Often they imagine gruesome things regarding the experiences related to the illness, treatment, and hospitalization (Shepard and Mahon, 2000). Latino siblings have reported less accurate information about their sibling's condition than non-Latino siblings (Lobato, Kao, and Plante, 2005). Parents are usually in the best position to impart information, although they are often overwhelmed

 FAMILY FOCUS

Reflection of an Older Brother

My youngest sister, Kerry, was on an apnea monitor 3 years ago, when I was 15. I was never embarrassed about Kerry being on the monitor, except for the time it went off in church and everyone turned around to look at us.

Joey Bellino
Oldest sibling of an infant on an apnea monitor
Washington, DC

BOX 18-5

Supporting Siblings of Children with Special Needs

PROMOTE HEALTHY SIBLING RELATIONSHIPS

Value each child individually and avoid comparisons. Remind each child of his or her positive qualities and contribution to other family members.

Help siblings see the differences and similarities between themselves and a child with special needs. Create a climate in which children can achieve successes without feeling guilty.

Teach siblings ways to interact with the child.

Seek to be fair in terms of discipline, attention, and resources; require the affected child to do as much for himself or herself as possible.

Let siblings settle their own differences; intervene only to prevent siblings from hurting one another.

Legitimize reasonable anger. Even children with special needs behave badly sometimes.

Respect a sibling's reluctance to be with or to include the child with special needs in activities.

HELP SIBLINGS COPE

Listen to siblings to let them know that their thoughts and suggestions are valued.

Praise siblings when they have been patient, have sacrificed, or have been particularly helpful. Do not expect siblings to always act in this manner.

Acknowledge the personal strengths siblings have and their ability to cope with stress successfully.

Provide age-appropriate information about the child's condition, and update when appropriate.

Let teachers know what is happening so they can be understanding and helpful.

Recognize special stress times for siblings and plan to minimize negative effects.

Schedule special time with siblings; have a friend or family member substitute when parent is unavailable.

Encourage siblings to join or help establish a sibling support group.

Use the services of professionals when needed. If parent feels that such a service is necessary, it should be provided in as vigorous a manner as a service for the child with special needs.

INVOLVE SIBLINGS

Seek out ways to realistically include siblings in the care and treatment of the child with special needs.

Limit caregiving responsibilities and give recognition when siblings perform them.

Develop a library of children's books on special needs.

Invite siblings to attend meetings to develop plans for the child with special needs (e.g., individualized educational program, individualized family service plan).

Discuss future plans with them.

Solicit their ideas on treatment and service needs.

Have them visit professionals who work with the child.

Help them develop competencies to teach the child new skills.

Provide opportunities for siblings to advocate for the child.

Allow siblings to set their own pace for learning and involvement.

Data from Powell T, Ogle P: *Brothers and sisters—a special part of exceptional families*, Baltimore, 1985, Paul H Brooks; Spokane Washington Deaconess Medical Center, Pediatric Oncology Unit: Tips for dealing with siblings, *Candlelighters Childhood Cancer Found Q Newslett* 11(3,4):7, 1987; and Carlson J, Leviton A, Mueller M: Services to siblings: an important component of family-centered practice, *ACCH Advocate* 1(1):53-56, 1993.

with the medical crisis at hand (Fleitas, 2000). Nurses can encourage parents to talk with the siblings about how they perceive their sick brother or sister and to be accepting of the siblings' feelings. Nurses can be ideal educators and counselors of siblings during the course of their brother's or sister's illness (Shepard and Mahon, 2000).

COPING WITH ONGOING STRESS AND PERIODIC CRISES

Professionals can help families cope with stress by providing anticipatory guidance, providing emotional support, assisting the family in assessing and identifying specific stressors, aiding the family in developing coping mechanisms and problem-solving strategies, and working collaboratively with parents so that they become empowered in the process.

Concurrent Stresses Within the Family

The ability to deal with the overwhelming stress of a lifelong disability or illness is challenged further when additional stresses are present. Stressors may be situational or developmental. They may be related to marital difficulties, sibling needs, homelessness, or social isolation. Some families may simultaneously be struggling with a family member's alcohol or other drug problem. Even relatively minor stressors, such as arranging care for siblings, managing the home, and traveling to distant treatment centers, can challenge a family's ability to cope successfully.

Most families, regardless of their income or insurance coverage, have financial concerns. The costs of caring for a child with special needs can be overwhelming. Nurses and social workers can help a family review various options for financial assistance, including insurance, managed care, or health maintenance organization policies; Medicaid; Supplemental Security Income; Women, Infants, and Children program (WIC); the state Program for Children with Special Health Needs; disease-related associations; and local philanthropic organizations.

Coping Mechanisms

Coping mechanisms are behaviors aimed at reducing the tension caused by a crisis. **Approach behaviors** are coping mechanisms that result in movement toward adjustment and resolution of the crisis. **Avoidance behaviors** result in movement away from adjustment and represent maladaptation to the crisis. Several approach and avoidance behaviors used in coping with a chronic illness or disability are listed in the Nursing Care Guidelines box. None of the indexes can be used singly to assess the possible success or failure in resolving the crisis. Each behavior must be viewed in the context of all of the variables affecting the family. For example, the observation of several avoidance behaviors in an emotionally healthy family may denote significantly less risk to the successful resolution of the crisis than an equal number of avoidance behaviors in an individual who has few available supports.

Parental Empowerment

Empowerment can be seen as a process of recognizing, promoting, and enhancing competence. For parents of children with chronic conditions, empowerment may occur gradually as strength and capabilities are drawn on to master the child's care, manage family life, and plan for the future. Advocating

for the child and developing parent-professional partnerships are part of taking charge (Ray, 2002).

ASSISTING FAMILY MEMBERS IN MANAGING THEIR FEELINGS

Although some previous research has postulated stages of adaptation to a chronic illness or disability, there is a great deal of individual variation in responses to the diagnosis, adjustments made, and time frames for coming to terms with a diagnosis. It is important that professionals recognize and respect a wide range of reactions and coping mechanisms. In fact, members of the family of a child with a chronic illness or disability may experience a number of difficult emotions, including fear, guilt, anger, resentment, and anxiety. Learning to manage these

---

nursingcareguidelines

Assessing Coping Behaviors
APPROACH BEHAVIORS
Asks for information regarding diagnosis and child's present condition
Seeks help and support from others
Anticipates future problems; actively seeks guidance and answers
Endows the illness or disability with meaning
Shares burden of disorder with others
Plans realistically for the future
Acknowledges and accepts child's awareness of diagnosis and prognosis
Expresses feelings such as sorrow, depression, and anger and realizes reason for the emotional reaction
Realistically perceives child's condition; adjusts to changes
Recognizes own growth through passage of time, such as earlier denial and nonacceptance of diagnosis
Verbalizes possible loss of child

AVOIDANCE BEHAVIORS
Fails to recognize seriousness of child's condition despite physical evidence
Refuses to agree to treatment
Intellectualizes about the illness, but in areas unrelated to child's condition
Is angry and hostile to members of the staff, regardless of their attitude or behavior
Avoids staff, family members, or child
Entertains unrealistic future plans for child, with little emphasis on the present
Is unable to adjust to or accept a change in progression of disease
Continually looks for new cures with no perspective toward possible benefit
Refuses to acknowledge child's understanding of disease and prognosis
Uses magical thinking and fantasy; may seek "occult" help
Places complete faith in religion to point of relinquishing own responsibility
Withdraws from outside world; refuses help
Punishes self because of guilt and blame
Makes no change in lifestyle to meet needs of other family members
Resorts to excessive use of alcohol or drugs to avoid problems
Verbalizes suicidal intents
Is unable to discuss possible loss of child or previous experiences with death

emotions promotes adaptive coping (see Nursing Care Guidelines box). Support from professionals, other family members, and friends can assist family members in managing their feelings. The following discussion examines some common phases of adjustment and emotional reactions.

Shock and Denial

The initial diagnosis of a chronic illness or disability is often met with intense emotion and is characterized by shock, disbelief, and sometimes denial, especially if the disorder is not obvious, as in chronic illness. Denial as a defense mechanism is a necessary cushion to prevent disintegration and is a normal response to grieving for any type of loss. Probably all family members experience various degrees of adaptive denial as they learn of the impact that the diagnosis has on their lives.

Shock and denial can last from days to months, sometimes even longer. Examples of denial that may be exhibited at the time of diagnosis include:

- Physician shopping
- Attributing the symptoms of the actual illness to a minor condition
- Refusing to believe the diagnostic tests
- Delaying consent for treatment
- Acting happy and optimistic despite the revealed diagnosis
- Refusing to tell or talk to anyone about the condition
- Insisting that no one is telling the truth, regardless of others' attempts to do so
- Denying the reason for admission
- Asking no questions about the diagnosis, treatment, or prognosis

Generally, these mechanisms should be respected as short-term responses that allow individuals to distance themselves from the tremendous emotional impact and to collect and mobilize their energies toward goal-directed, problem-solving behaviors.

In children, the importance of denial has repeatedly been demonstrated as a factor in their positive coping with the diagnosis. Denial allows the child to maintain hope in the face of overwhelming odds and to function adaptively and productively. Like hope, denial may be an adaptive mechanism for dealing with loss that persists until a family or patient is ready or needs other responses.

Denial is probably the least understood and most poorly dealt-with reaction. Health professionals typically label denial as maladaptive and act inappropriately by attempting to strip it away by repeated and sometimes blunt explanations of the prognosis. However, denial becomes maladaptive only when it prevents recognition of treatment or rehabilitative goals necessary for the child's optimal survival or development.

Adjustment

For most families, adjustment gradually follows shock and is usually characterized by an open admission that the condition exists. This stage may be accompanied by several responses, which are normal parts of the adaptation process. Probably the most universal of these feelings are **guilt** and **self-accusation.** Guilt is often greatest when the cause of the disorder is directly traceable to the parent, as in genetic diseases or accidental injury. However, it can occur even without any scientific or realistic basis for parental responsibility. Frequently the guilt stems from a false assumption that the disability is a result of personal failure or wrongdoing, such as

not doing something correctly during pregnancy or the birth. Guilt may also be associated with cultural or religious beliefs. Some parents are convinced that they are being punished for some previous misdeed. Others may see the disorder as a trial sent by God to test their religious strength and faith. With correct information, support, and time, most parents master guilt and self-accusation. The ability to master resentful and self-accusatory feelings of having "caused" the child's disorder is a crucial factor in determining the parents' acceptance of their child.

Children, too, may interpret their serious illness as retribution for past misbehavior. The nurse should be particularly sensitive to the child who passively accepts all painful procedures. This child may believe that such acts are inflicted as deserved punishment. It is vital that parents and health care professionals reassure children that their illness is not their fault.

Other common and normal reactions to a diagnosis are **bitterness** and **anger.** Anger directed inward may be evident as self-reproaching or punitive behavior, such as neglecting one's health and verbally degrading oneself. Anger directed outward may be manifested in either open arguments or withdrawal from communication and may be evident in the person's relationship with any number of individuals, such as the spouse, the child, and siblings. Passive anger toward the ill child may be evident in decreased visiting, refusal to believe how sick the child is, or inability to provide comfort. Among the most common targets for parental anger are members of the staff. Parents may complain about the nursing care, the insufficient time physicians spend with them, or the lack of skill of those who draw blood or start intravenous infusions.

Children are apt to respond with anger as well, and this includes the affected child and the well siblings. Children are aware of the loss engendered by their illness or disability and may react angrily to the restrictions imposed or the feelings of being different. Siblings may also feel anger and resentment toward the ill child and parents for the loss of routine and parental attention. It is difficult for older children and almost impossible for younger children to comprehend the plight of the affected child. Their perception is of a brother or sister who has the undivided attention of their parents, is showered with cards and gifts, and is the focus of everyone's concern.

During the period of adjustment, four types of parental reactions to the child influence the child's eventual response to the disorder:

Overprotection, in which the parents fear letting the child achieve any new skill, avoid all discipline, and cater to every desire to prevent frustration (Box 18-6)

Rejection, in which the parents detach themselves emotionally from the child but usually provide adequate physical care or constantly nag and scold the child

Denial, in which parents act is if the disorder does not exist or attempt to have the child overcompensate for it

Gradual acceptance, in which parents place necessary and realistic restrictions on the child, encourage self-care activities, and promote reasonable physical and social abilities

Reintegration and Acknowledgment

For many families the adjustment process culminates in the development of realistic expectations for the child and reintegration of family life with the illness or disability in a manageable perspective. Because a large portion of this phase is one

BOX 18-6

Characteristics of Parental Overprotection

- Sacrifices self and rest of family for the child
- Continually helps the child, even when the child is capable
- Is inconsistent with regard to discipline or employs no discipline; frequently applies different rules to the siblings
- Is dictatorial and arbitrary, making decisions without considering the child's wishes, such as keeping the child from attending school
- Hovers and offers suggestions; calls attention to every activity, overdoes praise
- Protects the child from every possible discomfort
- Restricts play, often because of fear that the child will be injured
- Denies the child opportunities for growing up and assuming responsibility, such as learning to give own medications or perform treatments
- Does not understand the child's capabilities and sets goals too high or too low
- Monopolizes the child's time, such as sleeping with the child, permitting few friends, or refusing participation in social or educational activities

BOX 18-7

Concept of Functional Burden

IMPACT OF THE CHILD WITH SPECIAL NEEDS
The child's need for medical and nursing care
The child's fixed deficits
The child's age-appropriate dependency in activities of daily living
The disruptions in the family routine caused by the care
The psychologic burden of the prognosis on the family

FAMILY RESOURCES AND ABILITY TO COPE
The family's physical resources
The family's emotional resources
The family's educational resources
The family's social supports and available help
The competing demands for family members' time and energy

Data from Stein REK: Home care: a challenging opportunity, *Child Health Care* 14(2):90-95, 1985.

of grief for a loss, total resolution is not possible until the child dies or leaves home as an independent adult. Therefore one can regard adjustment as "increased comfort" with everyday living rather than a complete resolution.

This adjustment phase also involves social reintegration in which the family broadens its activities to include relationships outside of the home, with the child as an acceptable and participating member of the group. This last criterion often differentiates the reaction of gradual acceptance during the adjustment period from total acceptance, or perhaps is more descriptive of the acknowledgment process.

Many parents of children with chronic illnesses experience **chronic sorrow,** feelings of sorrow and loss that recur in waves over time. As the child's condition progresses, parents experience repeated losses that represent further declines and new caregiving demands. Consequently, families must be assessed on an ongoing basis and offered appropriate support and resources as their needs change over time (Gravelle, 1997).

ESTABLISHING A SUPPORT SYSTEM

The diagnosis of a child with a serious health problem or disability is a major situational crisis that affects the entire family system. However, families can experience positive outcomes as they successfully deal with the many challenges that accompany a child with chronic illness or disability.

One nursing goal is to assess which families are at greater or lesser risk for succumbing to the effects of the crisis. Several variables—available support system, perception of the event, coping mechanisms, reactions to the child, available resources, and concurrent stresses within the family—influence the resolution of a crisis. Although most families cope well, the needs of families at risk are great. If they receive emotional support and guidance early, there is an increased likelihood that they will also cope successfully.

Although it is easy to assume that families of children with the most severe illnesses or disabilities would have the poorest adjustment, the severity of the condition reflects only one part

of the overall picture. The level of adjustment is significantly influenced by the **functional burden** on the individual family (Stein, 1985). This concept considers the issues related to caring for and living with the child in relation to the family's resources and ability to cope (Box 18-7). The family of a child with multiple disabilities demanding complex care, yet having many resources and coping skills, may adjust more successfully to the child's situation than the family of a child with a less serious condition and few resources to counterbalance.

Intrafamilial resources, social support from friends and relatives, parent-to-parent support, parent-professional partnerships, and community resources interweave to provide a flexible web of support for the family of a child with a chronic condition.

THE CHILD WITH SPECIAL NEEDS

The child's reaction to chronic illness or disability depends to a great extent on his or her developmental level, temperament, and available coping mechanisms; on the reactions of family members or significant others; and, to a lesser extent, on the condition itself. A child's conceptual understanding of his or her own illness is based not only on age and developmental level, but also on the duration and type of experience accumulated with the disease. Knowledge of these variables is essential in providing the kind of information and support needed by these children to cope with a sometimes overwhelming situation.

DEVELOPMENTAL ASPECTS

The impact of a chronic illness or disability is influenced by the age at onset. Chronic illness affects children of all ages, but the developmental aspects of each age-group dictate particular stresses and risks for the child. The nurse must also recognize that children need to redefine their condition and its implications as they develop and grow. For example, appearance, skills, and abilities are highly valued by peers (Fig. 18-1); a teenager who is limited in any of these qualities is subject to rejection. This is especially marked when a physical disability interferes with sexual attractiveness.

Children's developmental concepts of illness are discussed in Chapter 21. An understanding of these developmental fac-

FIG. 18-1 ■ Children with any type of impairment should have the opportunity to develop their skills. (Courtesy Poyo/Hinton Photography.)

FIG. 18-2 ■ Periods of sadness and anger are appropriate in the child's adjustment to a chronic illness or disability, especially during exacerbations of the disorder.

BOX 18-8

Coping Patterns Used by Children with Special Needs

Develops competence and optimism—Accentuates the positive aspects of the situation and concentrates more on what he or she has or can do than on what is missing or on what he or she cannot do; is as independent as possible

Feels different and withdraws—Sees self as being different from other children because of the chronic health condition; views being different as negative; sees self as less worthy than others; focuses on things he or she cannot do and sometimes overrestricts activities needlessly

Is irritable, is moody, and acts out—Uses proactive and self-initiated coping behaviors, although usually counterproductive in that the behaviors are not ego enhancing or socially responsible and do not result in desired outcomes; acts out irritability, which may or may not be associated with condition's symptoms

Complies with treatment—Takes necessary medications, treatments; adheres to activity restrictions; also uses behaviors that indicate developing independence (e.g., assumes responsibility for taking medication)

Seeks support—Talks with adults, children, physicians, and nurses; develops plans to handle problems as they occur; uses downward comparison (i.e., realizes that others have it worse)

Modified from Austin J, Patterson J, Huberty T: Development of the Coping Health Inventory for children, *J Pediatr Nurs* 6(3):166-174, 1991.

---

tors facilitates planning care to support the child and minimize the risks. Developmental aspects of chronic illness or disability on children are described in Table 18-2.

COPING MECHANISMS

Children with chronic conditions tend to use five distinct patterns of coping (Box 18-8). Children with more positive and accepting attitudes about their chronic illness use a more adaptive coping style characterized by optimism, competence, and compliance. They show fewer behavior problems at home and at school. The two maladaptive coping patterns—"Feels different and withdraws" and "Is irritable, is moody, and acts out"—are associated with poorer adaptation; children using these strategies have poorer self-concepts, more negative attitudes about their conditions, and more behavior problems at home and at school.

Well-adapted children gradually learn to accept their physical limitations and find achievement in a variety of compensatory motor and intellectual pursuits. They function well at home, at school, and with peers. They have an understanding of their disorder that allows them to accept their limitations, assume responsibility for care, and assist in treatment and rehabilitation regimens. They express appropriate emotions, such as sadness, anxiety, and anger, at times of exacerbations but confidence and guarded optimism during periods of clinical stability (Fig. 18-2). They are able to identify with other similarly affected individuals, promoting positive self-images and displaying pride and self-confidence in their ability to master a productive, successful life despite the disability.

Hopefulness

Children, particularly adolescents, are sensitive to the presence or absence of hope. Hopefulness is an internal quality that mobilizes humans into goal-directed action that may be satisfying and life sustaining. A sense of hopefulness can produce increased participation in health-seeking behaviors and an improved sense of well-being (Ritchie, 2001).

Health Education and Self-Care

Health education is an intervention that promotes coping. Children need information about their condition, the therapeutic plan, and how the disease or the therapy might affect their particular situation. Children nearing puberty also need to understand the maturation process and how their disability may alter this event. For example, a youngster with Crohn disease should understand that this disorder is associated with growth failure and delayed puberty; a child with diabetes needs to know that hormonal changes and increased growth needs will alter food and insulin requirements at this time; and a sexually active girl with sickle cell anemia or systemic lupus erythematosus needs to be aware of the risks of preg-

nursingprocess | The Child with Special Needs

ASSESSMENT

Knowledge of the family's available support system is essential and may include the marital relationship, nonmarital partners, extended family, colleagues and coworkers, friends, and professionals. The family's perception of the illness or disability is also an area that influences family adjustment. Assessment questions should focus on members' general knowledge of the condition even before the child's diagnosis was made, the influence of culture and religion on their thinking, imagined causes of the condition, and the effects of the child's disorder on the family.

DIAGNOSIS (PROBLEM IDENTIFICATION)

After a thorough assessment, several nursing diagnoses are evident:
- Ineffective Coping
- Compromised Family Coping
- Interrupted Family Processes

PLANNING

Expected patient outcomes for the child with special needs include:
- Child and family will accept support at the time of diagnosis.
- Family's emotional reactions will be accepted.
- Child and family will cope with stresses of the situation.
- Child and family will receive appropriate information about the condition.
- Family will establish an environment of normalization for the child.
- Family will establish realistic future goals.

IMPLEMENTATION

Numerous intervention strategies are discussed on pp. 586-590.

EVALUATION

The effectiveness of nursing interventions is determined by continual reassessment and evaluation of nursing care based on the following observational guidelines:
- Assess how parents verbalize feelings and concerns regarding the disease or disability.
- Observe parents' attitudes, acceptance, and adjustment.
- Determine how family demonstrates understanding of the disease and treatment options.
- Assess family members' goals for themselves and the child.
- Observe whether family demonstrates positive, growth-promoting behaviors for the child and other family members.

nancy. The information should not be given all at once but should be timed appropriately to meet the changing needs of the youngsters, and it should be described and repeated as often as the situation demands.

RESPONSES TO PARENTAL BEHAVIOR

Parental behavior towards the child is one of the most important factors influencing the child's adjustment. Children's perceptions of their mothers' support and maternal perceptions of psychosocial impact of the child's chronic illness on the family were shown to be two of the greatest predictors of children's psychologic adjustment (Immelt, 2006). In addition, family organization and illness-related support and involvement of parents influence children's adjustment to chronic illness (Schor, 2003). They often display pride and confidence in their ability to cope successfully with the challenges imposed by their disorder. Anticipatory guidance by the nurse and encouragement of normalizing practices may assist parents in facilitating positive adjustment in their children.

TYPE OF ILLNESS OR DISABILITY

The type of illness or disability also influences the child's emotional response. Interestingly, children with *more* severe disorders often cope better than those with milder conditions. However, the presence of multiple conditions may place a child at risk for more behavioral problems (Newacheck and Halfon, 1998). Considering children's cognitive ability and their delay in achieving abstract thinking until adolescence, it is likely that an obvious condition is easier to accept because its limitations are concrete. For example, children who are blind or physically disabled are constantly reminded of their

inability to run. However, children with cardiac defects not only live by rules they do not understand, but also only vaguely and occasionally sense their illness, such as when they try to run and experience dyspnea and fatigue. Therefore some chronic illnesses pose special threats to children.

The onset of a disabling condition may generate a state of confusion for children, who may have trouble differentiating between actual bodily functions and their image of their bodies. They may also experience problems in identifying themselves and those extensions of self (e.g., wheelchairs, braces, crutches, other mechanical or prosthetic devices) and may have difficulty in accepting functional aids.

NURSING CARE OF THE FAMILY AND CHILD WITH SPECIAL NEEDS

ASSESSMENT

Because the nurse may meet a family during any phase of the adjustment process, several assessment areas are important (see Nursing Process box). The family's ability to cope with previous stresses influences the current situation, and answers to questions about their usual coping skills are enlightening. Knowledge of concurrent stresses, such as financial, marital or nonmarital, and career or unemployment, helps identify families who may have fewer resources to cope with the child's needs.

Finally, awareness of the family members' reactions to the child and the illness or disability is important. Sample questions that the nurse and family can use to evaluate the support system, perception of the illness, coping mechanisms, resources, and concurrent stresses are listed in Table 18-1. Because factors affecting the family's response may change at any

TABLE 18-1

Assessment of Factors Affecting Family Adjustment

FACTORS AFFECTING ADJUSTMENT	ASSESSMENT QUESTIONS
AVAILABLE SUPPORT SYSTEM	
Status of marital relationship	To whom do you talk when you have something on your mind? (If answer is not the spouse, ask for the reason.)
Alternate support systems	When something is worrying you, what do you do?
	What helps you most when you are upset?
Ability to communicate	Does talking seem to help when you feel upset?
PERCEPTION OF THE ILLNESS OR DISABILITY	
Previous knowledge of disorder	Have you ever heard the word (name of diagnosis) before? Tell me about it (if answer is yes).
Imagined cause of disorder	What are your thoughts about the causes of the disorder?
Effects of illness or disability on family	How has your child's illness or disability affected you and your family?
	How has your lifestyle changed?
COPING MECHANISMS	
Reactions to previous crises	Tell me one time you've had another crisis (problem, bad time) in your family. How did you solve that problem?
Reactions to the child	Do you find yourself being a little more cautious with this child than with your other children?
Childrearing practices	Do you feel as comfortable disciplining this child compared as your other children?
Influence of religion	Has your religion or faith been of help to you? Tell me how (if answer is yes).
Attitudes	How is this child different from the siblings or other children of similar age?
	Describe your child's personality. Is it easy, difficult, or in between?
	When you think of your child's future, what thoughts come to mind?
AVAILABLE RESOURCES	
	What parts of your child's care are causing the most difficulty for you or your family?
	What services are available to help?
	What services do you need that currently are not available?
CONCURRENT STRESSES	
	What other problems are you facing now? (Be specific; ask about financial, marital, sibling, and extended family or friends concerns.)

point during the illness, assessment must be a continuous process.

Special challenges exist in assessing the child's feelings about having a disability. Chapter 6 presents several approaches to encourage a child to discuss feelings about the condition. The nurse should use a variety of communication techniques, such as drawing and play, as assessment tools rather than relying solely on parental reports. Often, children are neglected partners in their care, and their unique needs are not identified (Young, Dixon-Woods, Windridge, and others, 2003; Dixon-Woods, Young, and Henry, 1999).

The needs of working parents and siblings also should be assessed, a goal that requires flexibility in scheduling appointments to include these important family members. When working parents know that their input is valuable, they will often change their work schedule to meet with a health professional. Because siblings can be of any age, the use of appropriate communication strategies for assessment must be considered. Nonverbal techniques such as those discussed in Chapter 6 should be considered for these children.

The main objective in working with the family is to help them cope effectively with those stresses imposed by the child's special needs. To achieve this goal, the entire family

 FAMILY FOCUS

Identifying Family Needs

To ensure an effective care plan, attention to family-identified needs and priorities is essential. For example, a family may have difficulty focusing on treatment issues if their current priority is obtaining enough food to feed their children.

should be considered in every aspect of the implementation process (see Family Focus box).

PROVIDE SUPPORT AT THE TIME OF DIAGNOSIS

The diagnosis is a critical time for parents and can influence how they perceive their health care providers throughout care. Although they may not hear or remember all that is said to them, they frequently sense a certain attitude of acceptance, rejection, hope, or despair that may influence their ability to absorb the shock and begin adapting to the family's altered future.

Parents may be encouraged to be together when they are informed of their child's condition, thus avoiding the problem

FIG. 18-3 ■ Informing session should take place in a private, comfortable setting free of distractions and interruptions.

of one parent having to interpret complex findings and deal with the initial emotional reaction of the other. The informing session should take place in a private, comfortable setting free of distractions and interruptions, in an atmosphere in which the parents feel free to express their emotions (Fig. 18-3). Their emotional needs are acknowledged by showing acceptance of such expressions as crying, sadness, anger, and disappointment. Emotional support is offered by having tissues available if a family member cries and demonstrating through facial and body language that indeed this is a difficult and painful period. Although touching is a powerful expression of empathy, it must be used wisely. For example, it can prematurely terminate free expression of feelings, especially when combined with statements such as "Everything will be all right." Nurses should also be aware of cultural issues regarding touching (see Chapter 4).

Parents should receive the kind of information they desire. This can be assessed by asking questions such as, "Do you prefer to hear detailed information?" Parents or other family members may have different preferences regarding the amount of information they wish to hear. Most parents want a clear, simple explanation of the diagnosis; a prediction of possible futures for the child; advice on what to do next; an opportunity to ask questions; a warm, sympathetic listener; and, most important, time. Understanding of explanations is elicited with such questions as "Do you see what I mean?" or "Is this clear to you?" Technical terms are used with simple definitions. If the parents are unaware of the term, they are given written literature or at least a written summary of the diagnosis.

> **NURSING TIP**
>
> Develop a glossary of commonly used terms, acronyms, and abbreviations to distribute to parents. The list can stand alone or become a part of patient or parent handbooks.

Finally, the informing conference does not end with the presentation of devastating news. Instead, the child's strengths, appealing behaviors, and potential for development are

stressed, as are available rehabilitation efforts or treatment. Parents can be encouraged to view their experiences as a series of challenges that they are capable of handling, particularly with available professional feedback. The parents are assured that the nurse will be available to answer questions and to provide further assistance as needed.

The preceding discussion relates primarily to the initial informing interview. However, because of the need for long-term follow-up, it is only one in a series of continuing discussions. In all interactions the family's input is solicited and incorporated into the care plan. Some situations require consideration of special problems (see Nursing Care Guidelines box).

SUPPORT FAMILY'S COPING METHODS

For the family to meet the stresses of optimally adjusting to the child's condition, each member must be individually supported so that the family system is strong. Although the family can indefinitely support a member who is in need of assistance, its greatest strength lies in every member supporting each other. The nurse should bear in mind that the family member in greatest need is not necessarily the affected child but may be a parent or sibling who is dealing with stresses that require intervention.

Parents

The nurse can provide support by being attentive to families' responses to their children. Mothers and fathers need to experience success, joy, and pride in their children to give the support they need. Children, too, require support for their interactions, adjustments, and efforts. They must be reinforced for attempts to get to know their care providers and to communicate their needs to them.

It is important for nurses to examine their attitudes to determine their ability to engage in parent-professional partnerships. An essential characteristic is the belief that parents are equal to professionals and are experts regarding their child (see Nursing Care Guidelines box).

Communication among all family members is encouraged. Parent group sessions can help parents verbalize thoughts and feelings to each other but often do not take into account siblings' or the child's viewpoint. Therefore the nurse may need to set up a family session, such as during a home or clinic visit. Although the ideal situation is to have all the members present at one time, often this is not possible. Inviting members to participate at various visits is an appropriate alternative.

Parents can be encouraged to discuss their feelings toward the child, the impact of this event on their marriage, and associated stresses such as financial burdens. For most families, regardless of their income or insurance coverage, financial concerns exist. The costs of caring for a child with special needs can be overwhelming. In addition, the family wage earner may have to sacrifice job opportunities to remain close to a medical facility or to avoid losing insurance benefits.*

The nurse regards fathers as able, effective parents, competent and capable of coping with the challenges they face. Every effort is made to include the father in visits, such as to the

*Information regarding financial issues is available from the Federation for Children with Special Needs, 1135 Tremont St., Suite 420, Boston, MA 02120; (617) 236-7210; http://www.fcsn.org.

nursingcareguidelines

Situations Requiring Special Consideration

CONGENITAL ANOMALY

Tension in the delivery room conveys the sense that something is seriously wrong. Communication is often delayed while the physician is involved with the mother's care. The manner in which the infant is presented may well set the tone for the early parent-child relationship.

- Clarify role with physician in regard to revealing information to enable immediate parental support.
- Explain to parents briefly in simple language what the defect is and something concerning the immediate prognosis before showing them the infant, when they are more ready to "hear" what is said.
- Be aware of nonverbal communication. Parents watch facial expressions of others for signs of revulsion or rejection.
- Present infant as something precious.
- Emphasize well-formed aspects of infant's body.
- Allow time and opportunity for parents to express their initial response.
- Encourage parents to ask questions, and provide honest, straightforward answers without undue optimism or pessimism.

COGNITIVE IMPAIRMENT

Unless cognitive impairment (or mental retardation) is associated with other physical problems, it is often easy for parents to miss clues to its presence or to make defensive excuses regarding the diagnosis.

- Plan situations that help parents become aware of the problem.
- Encourage parents to discuss their observations of child, but withhold diagnostic opinions.
- Focus on what the child can do and appropriate interventions to promote progress (e.g., infant stimulation programs) to involve parents in their child's care while helping them gain an awareness of the child's disability.

PHYSICAL DISABILITY

If loss of motor or sensory ability occurs during childhood, the diagnosis is readily apparent. The challenge lies in helping the child and parents over the period of shock and grief and toward the phase of acceptance and reintegration.

- Institute early rehabilitation (e.g., using a prosthetic limb, learning to read braille, learning to read lips).
- Be aware that physical rehabilitation usually precedes psychologic adjustment.
- When the cause of the disability is accidental, avoid implying that parents or child was responsible for the injury, yet allow them the opportunity to discuss feelings of blame.
- Encourage expression of feelings (see Communication Techniques, Chapter 6).

CHRONIC ILLNESS

Realization of the true impact may take months or years. Conflict over parent's vs child's concerns may result in serious problems. When condition is inherited, parents may blame themselves or child may blame parents.

- Help each family member gain an appreciation of the other's concerns.
- Discuss hereditary aspect of condition with parents at time of diagnosis to lessen guilt and accusatory feelings.
- Encourage child to express feelings by using third-person technique (e.g., "Sometimes when a person has an illness that was passed on by the parents, that person feels angry or bitter toward them").

MULTIPLE DISABILITIES

The child or parent may require additional time for the shock phase and may be able to attend to only one diagnosis before hearing significant information regarding other disorders.

- Acknowledge parents' understanding and acceptance of all diagnoses, especially when an obvious and more hidden disability coexists.
- Appreciate the devastating consequences of more than one disability for a child, especially if they interfere with expressive-receptive abilities.

TERMINAL ILLNESS

Parents require much support to deal with their own feelings and guidance in how to tell the child the diagnosis. They may want to conceal the diagnosis from the child. They may believe that the child is too young to know, will not be able to cope with the information, or will lose hope and the will to live.

- Approach the subject of disclosure in a positive way by asking, "How will you tell your child about the diagnosis?"
- Help parents understand the disadvantages of not telling children (e.g., deprives them of the opportunity to discuss their feelings openly and ask questions, incurs the risk of them learning the truth from outside and sometimes less tactful sources, may lessen children's trust and confidence in their parents after they learn the truth).
- Guide parents to see the potential problems involved in fostering a conspiracy.
- Offer parents guidelines for how and what to tell children about their disease or the possibility of death. Explanations should be tailored to child's cognitive ability, be based on knowledge child already has, and be honest. Honesty must be tempered with concern for child's feelings.
- Assure parents that telling a child the name of the illness and the reason for treatment instills hope, provides support from others, and serves as a foundation for explaining and understanding subsequent events.
- Acknowledge that being honest is not always easy because the truth may prompt children to ask other distressing questions, such as "Am I going to die?" However, even this difficult question must be answered.

nursingcareguidelines

Developing Successful Parent-Professional Partnerships

- Promote primary nursing; in nonhospital settings designate a case manager.
- Acknowledge parents' overall competence and their unique expertise with their child.
- Respect parents' time as having value equal to that of other members of child's health care team.
- Explain or define any medical, technical, or discipline-specific terms.
- Tell families, "I am not sure" or "I don't know," when appropriate.
- Facilitate family's effectiveness in team meetings (e.g., provide parents with same information as other participants).

nursingcareguidelines

Encouraging Expression of Emotion

Describe the behavior—"You seem angry at everyone."
Give evidence of understanding—"Being angry is only natural."
Give evidence of caring—"It must be difficult to endure so many painful procedures."
Help focus on feelings—"Maybe you wonder why this happened to your child."

nursery, clinic, special school, and stimulation programs. The father is included in the assessment process, with specific emphasis on having him describe the child's strengths and difficulties. It is not unusual to find two parents who have differing views of the child's abilities, especially in the area of developmental disabilities.

Numerous volunteer and community resources are available that provide assistance, rehabilitation, equipment, and funding for a variety of health problems.* National and local disease-oriented organizations may provide needed assistance and support to families that qualify. Many of these are discussed elsewhere in the text under the specific diagnosis. State and federal departments of health, mental health, social service, and labor may be able to help locate appropriate regional resources. For example, state programs for Children with Special Health Needs (formerly Crippled Children's Services) provide financial assistance for children with many disabling conditions. Local and national sources of respite care and medical day care may be useful to families. Nurses should become acquainted with those in their communities and with vocational programs for special groups.

---

*General sources of information are the Clearinghouse on Disability Information, 550 12th St. SW, Room 5133, Washington, DC 20202-2550; (202) 245-7307; http://www.ed.gov; National Dissemination Center for Children with Disabilities, PO Box 1492, Washington, DC 20013; (202) 884-8411 or (800) 695-0285; http://www.nichcy.org. A comprehensive list of books and pamphlets for parents and teachers is available from the Easter Seals, 230 W. Monroe St., Suite 1800, Chicago, IL 60606; (312) 726-6200; http://www.easterseals.com. In Canada: Council of Canadians with Disabilities, 926-294 Portage Ave., Winnipeg, Manitoba R3C 0B9; (204) 947-0303; http://www.ccdonline.ca.

Parent-to-Parent Support

Just being with another parent who has shared similar experiences is helpful. It may not need to be a parent of a child with the same diagnosis, since parents in the process of adjusting to a child with special needs—or finding respite services, educational or rehabilitative services, special equipment vendors, and financial counseling—tread a common path. If the agency does not have a parent staff position, the nurse can contact parent groups that will often send a representative. Another strategy is to ask another parent to talk to the parents. The nurse should seek out a parent who is a good listener, has a nonjudgmental approach to differences in families, and possesses good advocacy and problem-solving skills.

The parent self-help group is another way to promote parent-to-parent support.* Group members feel less alone and have the opportunity to observe both coping and mastery role modeling from other members. Parents' groups are rich resources for information. Even if parents are unable to attend meetings, they can still benefit from group newsletters and other literature that often accompany membership. The nurse can foster parent participation in self-help groups by serving as a referral agent, a group advisory board member, a resource person, a group member, or an assistant in founding a group. Sometimes all that is required in starting a group is identifying one or two parents as leaders; sharing with them the names, telephone numbers, and addresses of other families who have expressed both an interest and a willingness to release their phone number and address; and guiding them in how to initiate a first meeting.

Advocate for Empowerment

Nurses can advocate for methods that foster opportunities for parent empowerment. For example, nurses can suggest reimbursement for travel and child care, plus stipends to enable parents' voices to be heard at meetings and conferences. They can encourage parent membership on staff, committees, and boards. They can keep parents informed of pending legislation on child health issues or take action when parents inform them.

The Child

Through ongoing contacts with the child, the nurse (1) observes the child's responses to the disorder, ability to function, and adaptive behaviors within the environment and with significant others; (2) explores the child's own understanding of his or her illness or condition; and (3) provides support while the child learns to cope with his or her feelings. Children are encouraged to express their concerns rather than allowing others to express them for them, since open discussions may reduce anxiety.

One of the most important interventions is alleviating the child's feeling of being different and normalizing his or her life as much as possible (see Nursing Care Guidelines box). Whenever possible, the nurse assists the family in assessing the child's daily routine for indications of a need for normalizing practices. For example, the child who remains in a bedroom all day requires a restructured daily routine to provide activi-

---

*Information about self-help groups and books and pamphlets are available from the National Self-Help Clearinghouse, 365 Fifth Ave., Suite 3300, New York, NY 10016; (217) 817-1822; http://www.selfhelpweb.org.

Promoting Normalization

Preparation—Prepare child in advance for changes that may occur from the illness or disability.

Example—Tell the child in advance the possible side effects of drug therapy.

Participation—Include child in as many decisions as possible, especially those relating to his or her care regimen.

Example—The child is responsible for taking medications or scheduling home treatments.

Sharing—Allow both family members and child's peers to be a part of the care regimen whenever possible.

Examples—Give the child his or her medication when the other siblings receive their vitamins.

The parent cooks the same menu for the whole family.

If the child is invited to another's home, the parent advises the family of the child's dietary restrictions.

Control—Identify areas where child can be in control so that feelings of uncertainty, passivity, and helplessness are decreased.

Example—The child identifies activities that are appropriate to his or her energy level and chooses to rest when fatigued.

Expectation—Apply the same family rules to the child with a chronic illness or disability as to the well siblings or peers.

Example—The child is disciplined, is expected to fulfill household responsibilities, and attends school in accordance with abilities.

ties in different parts of the house, such as eating in the kitchen or dining room with the family. Such children may also be deprived of social, recreational, and academic activities that can be better accommodated by applying normalization practices. For example, home and out-of-home health-related treatments should be planned at times that least interfere with normal daily activities.

Children who are concerned that their condition detracts from their physical attractiveness need attention focused on the normal aspects of appearance and capabilities. Health professionals help strengthen and consolidate the self-image by emphasizing the normal, while allowing children to express anger, isolation, fear of rejection, feelings of sadness, and loneliness. The children need positive reinforcement for compliance and any evidence of improvement. Anything that might improve attractiveness and contribute to a positive self-image is employed, such as makeup for a teenager with a scar, clothing that disguises a prosthesis, or a hairstyle or wig to cover a deformity or lost hair.

Siblings

The presence of a child with special needs in a family may result in parents paying less attention to the other children. Siblings may respond by developing negative attitudes toward the child or by expressing anger in different forms. The nurse can help by using anticipatory guidance, questioning the parents about what they believe is the best way to have siblings respond to the child and guiding them through ways to meet their other children's needs for attention. This questioning should take place before serious negative effects occur.

Siblings may also experience embarrassment associated with having a brother or sister with an illness or disability.

Parents are then faced with the difficulty of responding to this embarrassment in an understanding and appropriate manner without punishing the siblings for how they feel. Parents are encouraged to talk with the siblings about how they view their affected sibling. For example, siblings of a child who is retarded may express fears about their ability to bear normal children. Adolescents in particular may not be able to discuss these vital issues with their parents and may prefer to consult with the nurse. Many siblings benefit from sharing their concerns with other young people who are experiencing a similar situation. Support groups for siblings can help decrease isolation, promote expression of feelings, and provide examples of effective coping skills.

Many parents express concern about when and how to inform the other children in the family about a sibling's disability. The answer depends on each child's level of sophistication and understanding. However, it is usually best to inform the siblings before a neighbor or other nonfamily member does so. Uninformed siblings may fantasize or develop apprehensions that are out of proportion to the child's actual condition. Furthermore, if parents choose to be silent or deceptive about the issue, they are setting a negative precedent for the siblings to follow, rather than encouraging the siblings to cope with the experience in a healthy and nurturing way.

The nurse is sensitive to the reactions of siblings and whenever possible intervenes to promote more positive adjustment. For example, siblings often mention that they are expected to take on additional responsibilities to help the parents care for the child. It is not unusual for them to express a positive reaction to assuming the extra duties but a negative response to feeling unappreciated for doing so. Such feelings can often be minimized by encouraging siblings to discuss this with the parents and by suggesting to parents ways of showing gratitude, such as an increase in allowance, special privileges, and, most significantly, verbal praise.

EDUCATE ABOUT THE DISORDER AND GENERAL HEALTH CARE

Educating the family about the disorder is actually an extension of revealing the diagnosis. Education involves not only supplying technical information, but also discussing how the condition will affect the child. Parents may be able to digest only so much information at a time. It may be helpful to provide essential information and then follow by asking, "What else would you like to know about your child's condition?" Responding to parents' questions and concerns ensures that their information needs are met.

Activities of Daily Living

Parents also need guidance in how the condition may interfere with or alter activities of daily living, such as eating, dressing, sleeping, and toileting. One area frequently affected is nutrition. Common problems are undernutrition resulting from food being inappropriately restricted or loss of appetite, vomiting, or motor deficits that interfere with feeding; overnutrition may also occur, usually because of a caloric intake in excess of energy expenditure or boredom and lack of stimulation in other areas. Although the child requires the same basic nutrients as other children, the daily requirements may differ. Special nutritional considerations are discussed as appropriate throughout the text.

Safe Transportation

Modifications may also be needed regarding car safety. Children with conditions such as low birth weight (see Discharge Planning and Home Care, Chapter 9) or orthopedic, neuromuscular, or respiratory problems often cannot safely use conventional car restraints. For example, children with hip spica casts cannot sit properly in child safety seats (see Developmental Dysplasia of the Hip, Chapter 31). Modifications can be made to some commercial models, and for older children a special vest is available that secures the child to the back seat in a lying-down position.*

If a child requires a wheelchair, the family should consult the wheelchair manufacturer for specific instructions regarding safe car transportation. Considerations for wheelchairs used with vehicle transportation must address securing both the wheelchair and the occupant in the wheelchair. Wheelchairs should be secured facing forward with tie downs at four points. The tie-down system should be dynamically crash tested, as should the occupant securement system that secures the child in the wheelchair. For example, use of trays would not be recommended for transportation. With children who must travel with additional medical equipment, this equipment (e.g., oxygen, monitors, or ventilators) should be anchored to the floor or underneath the vehicle seat or wheelchair. Soft padding should be added around the equipment to reduce movement. A second adult should be present to monitor the condition of a medically fragile child while traveling.

Primary Health Care

Children with special needs require all the usual health care recommended for any child. Attention to injury prevention, immunizations, dental health, and regular physical examinations is essential. Nurses can play an important role in reminding parents of these aspects of care that are so often neglected when the concern is focused on the child's illness or disability. Specific discussions of nutrition, sleep and activity, dental health, and injury prevention are presented in the chapters on health promotion for specific age-groups. Immunizations are discussed in Chapter 10.

Parents also need to be aware of the importance of communicating the child's condition in the event of a medical emergency. Young children are unable to give information about their disorder, and although older children may be reliable sources, after an accident they may be physically unable to speak. Therefore all children with any type of chronic condition that may affect medical care should wear some type of identification, such as a MedicAlert bracelet,† or carry a card in their wallet that lists the medical condition and a phone number for emergency medical records and other personal information.

PROMOTE NORMAL DEVELOPMENT

Aside from knowledge of the condition and its effect on the child's abilities, the family must be guided toward fostering appropriate development in their child. Although each stage may take longer to achieve, parents are guided toward helping the child fully realize his or her potential in preparation for the next developmental stage. Table 18-2 outlines developmental aspects of chronic illness or disability and supportive interventions. With appropriate planning and knowledge of strategies to improve the child's functional abilities, most children can live fulfilling and productive lives.

One important aspect of promoting normal development is to encourage the child's self-care abilities in both activities of daily living and the medical regimen. An assessment of the child's age and physical, emotional, and mental capacities, as well as the support and structure provided by the family, should be considered in determining the appropriate level of self-care in the medical regimen. Even toddlers can be involved in their own care by holding supplies for the parent during a procedure. Over time, children should be encouraged toward greater autonomy in the self-care arena.

Early Childhood

During infancy the child is achieving basic **trust** through a satisfying, intimate, consistent relationship with his or her parents. However, the affected child's early existence may be stressful, chaotic, and unsatisfying. Consequently, he or she may need more parental support and expressions of affection to achieve trust. Likewise, the parents require assistance in finding ways to meet the infant's needs, such as how to hold a rigid or flaccid infant, how to feed a child with tongue thrust or episodes of dyspnea, and how to stimulate a child who seems incapable of achieving any skills. If hospitalizations are frequent or prolonged, every effort is made to preserve the parent-child relationship (see also Chapter 21). Hospital policies should promote visitation by and involvement of families.

During early childhood the goal is to achieve **separation** from parents, **autonomy,** and **initiative.** However, the natural parental response to having a sick child is overprotection. Parents need help in realizing the importance of brief separations of the child from them and from others involved in the child's care and of providing social experiences outside the home whenever possible. Respite care, which provides temporary relief for family members, can be essential in allowing caregivers time away from the daily burdens.

Young children also need the opportunity to develop **independence.** Frequently the child is able to learn self-help skills, such as holding the bottle, finger feeding, and removing simple articles of clothing, but the parent continues to perform the act. The nurse can guide parents to the usual milestones expected from the child. When a child is unable to perform a skill independently, functional aids should be used. With innovation, many adaptations can be implemented in children's environments to increase their mobility and independence and allow them to play like other children their age. For example, with slight modifications, a child with physical limitations may be able to ride a tricycle (Fig. 18-4).

Another critical component for normal child development is **discipline.** Discipline and guidance serve several purposes, such as providing children with boundaries on which to test out their behavior and teaching them socially acceptable behavior. Resentment and hostility can arise among siblings if different standards are applied to each child. The nurse's responsibility is to help parents learn successful methods of managing a child's behaviors before they become problems (see Limit Setting and Discipline, Chapter 3).

---

*Information on car safety restraints for children with special needs is available from the Automotive Safety Program, 575 West Drive, Room 004, Indianapolis, IN 46202; (800) 543-6227 or (317) 274-2997; http://www.preventinjury.org.

†MedicAlert Foundation International, 2323 Colorado Ave., Turlock, CA 95382; (888) 633-4298; http://www.medicalert.org.

TABLE 18-2

Developmental Effects of Chronic Illness or Disability on Children

DEVELOPMENTAL TASKS	POTENTIAL EFFECTS OF CHRONIC ILLNESS OR DISABILITY	SUPPORTIVE INTERVENTIONS
INFANCY		
Develop a sense of trust	Multiple caregivers and frequent separations, especially if hospitalized	Encourage consistent caregivers in hospital or other care settings.
	Deprived of consistent nurturing	Encourage parental presence, "rooming in" during hospitalization, and participation in care.
Bond, or attach, to parent	Delayed because of separation; parental grief for loss of "dream" child; parental inability to accept the condition, especially a visible defect	Emphasize healthy, perfect qualities of infant. Help parents learn special care needs of infant for them to feel competent.
Learn through sensorimotor experiences	More exposure to painful experiences than pleasurable ones	Expose infant to pleasurable experiences through all senses (touch, hearing, sight, taste, movement).
	Limited contact with environment from restricted movement or confinement	Encourage age-appropriate developmental skills (e.g., holding bottle, finger feeding, crawling).
Begin to develop a sense of separateness from parent	Increased dependency on parent for care	Encourage all family members to participate in care to prevent overinvolvement of one member.
	Overinvolvement of parent in care	Encourage periodic respite from demands of care responsibilities.
TODDLERHOOD		
Develop autonomy	Increased dependency on parent	Encourage independence in as many areas as possible (e.g., toileting, dressing, feeding).
Master locomotor and language skills	Limited opportunity to test own abilities and limits	Provide gross motor skill activity and modification of toys or equipment, such as modified swing or rocking horse.
Learn through sensorimotor experience; beginning preoperational thought	Increased exposure to painful experiences	Give choices to allow simple feeling of control (e.g., choice of what book to look at, what kind of sandwich to eat).
		Institute age-appropriate discipline and limit setting.
		Recognize that negative and ritualistic behaviors are normal.
		Provide sensory experiences (e.g., water play, sandbox play, finger painting).
PRESCHOOL		
Develop initiative and purpose	Limited opportunities for success in accomplishing simple tasks or mastering self-care skills	Encourage mastery of self-help skills.
Master self-care skills		Provide devices that make task easier (e.g., self-dressing).
Begin to develop peer relationships	Limited opportunities for socialization with peers; may appear "like a baby" to age-mates	Encourage socialization (e.g., inviting friends to play, day care experience, trips to park).
	Protection within tolerant and secure family causing child to fear criticism and withdraw	Provide age-appropriate play, especially associative play opportunities.
		Emphasize child's abilities; dress appropriately to enhance desirable appearance.
Develop sense of body image and sexual identification	Awareness of body centering on pain, anxiety, and failure	Encourage relationships with same-sex and opposite-sex peers and adults.
	Sex-role identification focused primarily on mothering skills	
Learn through preoperational thought (magical thinking)	Guilt (thinking he or she caused the illness/disability or is being punished for wrongdoing)	Help child deal with criticisms; realize that too much protection prevents child from realities of world.
		Clarify that cause of child's illness or disability is not his or her fault or a punishment.
SCHOOL AGE		
Develop a sense of accomplishment	Limited opportunities to achieve and compete (e.g., many school absences, inability to join regular athletic activities)	Encourage school attendance; schedule medical visits at times other than school; encourage child to make up missed work.
Form peer relationships	Limited opportunities for socialization	Educate teachers and classmates about child's condition, abilities, and special needs.
		Encourage sports activities (e.g., Special Olympics).
		Encourage socialization (e.g., Girl Scouts, Campfire, Boy Scouts, 4-H Club; having a best friend or club membership).
Learn through concrete operations	Incomplete comprehension of the imposed physical limitations or treatment of the disorder	Provide child with information about his or her condition.
		Encourage creative activities (e.g., VSA Arts).

TABLE 18-2		
Developmental Effects of Chronic Illness or Disability on Children—cont'd		
DEVELOPMENTAL TASKS	**POTENTIAL EFFECTS OF CHRONIC ILLNESS OR DISABILITY**	**SUPPORTIVE INTERVENTIONS**
ADOLESCENCE		
Develop personal and sexual identity	Increased sense of feeling different from peers and reduced ability to compete with peers in appearance, abilities, special skills	Help child realize that many of the difficulties the teenager is experiencing are part of normal adolescence (rebelliousness, risk taking, lack of cooperation, hostility toward authority).
Achieve independence from family	Increased dependency on family; limited job or career opportunities	Provide instruction on interpersonal and coping skills. Encourage increased responsibility for care and management of the disease or condition (e.g., assuming responsibility for making and keeping appointment [ideally alone], sharing assessment and planning stages of health care delivery, contacting resources). Discuss planning for future and how condition can affect choices.
Form heterosexual relationships	Limited opportunities for heterosexual friendships; less opportunity to discuss sexual concerns with peers. Increased concern with issues such as why did he or she get the disorder, can he or she marry and have a family	Encourage socialization with peers, including peers with special needs and those without special needs. Encourage activities appropriate for age (e.g., attending mixed-sex parties, sports activities, driving a car). Be alert to cues that signal readiness for information regarding implications of condition on sexuality and reproduction. Emphasize good appearance and wearing stylish clothes, use of makeup. Understand that adolescent has same sexual needs and concerns as any other teenager.
Learn through abstract thinking	Decreased opportunity for earlier stages of cognition impeding achievement of level of abstract thinking	Provide instruction on decision making, assertiveness, and other skills necessary to manage personal plans.

School Age

For school-age children the major tasks are entry into school and achieving a sense of **industry.** Although the importance of school in the life of all children is well known, school absences are significantly higher among children with chronic illness than among their healthy peers. The more school absences the child experiences, the more difficult it is to resume attendance, and school phobia may result. The child should return to school as soon as possible after diagnosis or treatments.

Preparation for entry into or resumption of school is best accomplished through a team approach with the parents, child, teacher, school nurse, and primary nurse in the hospital. Ideally, this planning should begin before hospital discharge, provided that the child is well enough to resume usual activities. A structured plan should be developed, with attention to those aspects of care that must be continued during school hours, such as administration of medication or other treatments.

Children also need preparation before entering or resuming school. Having a tutor in the hospital or home as soon as children are physically able helps them realize that school will continue and gives them time to consider this prospect (Fig. 18-5). They need to investigate possible answers to the many questions others will ask. One method of anticipatory preparation is to role-play, with the child as the "returned pupil"

FIG. 18-4 ■ A modified tricycle with block pedals, self-adhesive straps for support, and modified seat and handle bars can help a child with disabilities gain mobility.

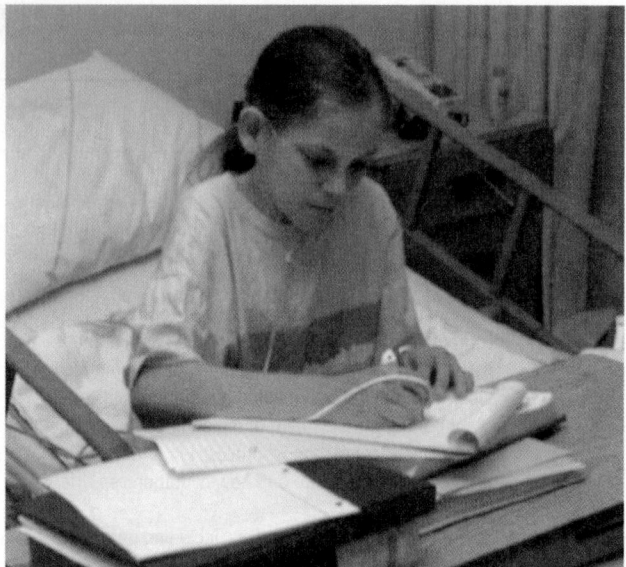

FIG. 18-5 ■ Children with special needs should continue their schooling as soon as their condition permits.

and the nurse or parent as "other schoolmates." If the child returns to school with some obvious physical change, such as hair loss, amputation, or visible scar, the nurse might also ask questions about these alterations to prompt preparatory responses from the child.

Classroom peers also need preparation, and a joint plan of the teacher, nurse, and child is best. At a minimum, classmates should be given a description of the child's condition, prepared for any visible changes in the child, and allowed an opportunity to ask questions. The child should have the option of attending this session. As the child's condition changes, particularly if the illness is potentially fatal, school personnel, including the students, need periodic apprisal of the child's status and preparation for what to expect.

Children with special needs are encouraged to maintain or reestablish relationships with peers and to participate according to their capabilities in any age-appropriate activities. Alternative activities may be substituted for those that are impossible or that place a strain on the child's condition. Programs such as the Special Olympics* offer children an opportunity to compete with their peers and to achieve athletic skill. Summer camps† allow children to associate with peers and develop a wide variety of skills. Children with special needs can derive enormous benefits from expressive activities, such as art, music, poetry, dance, and drama. With adaptive equipment and imagination, children can participate in a va-

riety of activities. Organizations such as VSA Arts allow children to celebrate and share their accomplishments.* Children need the opportunity to interact with healthy peers and to engage in activities with groups or clubs composed of similarly affected age-mates. Such organizations as ostomy clubs, diabetes clubs, and cerebral palsy groups share information and provide support related to the special problems the members face.

Adolescence

Adolescence can be a particularly difficult period for the teenager and family. All of the needs discussed previously apply to this age-group as well. Developing **independence** or **autonomy,** however, is a major task for the adolescent as planning for the future becomes a prominent concern. Although the emphasis in the past has been on achieving independence from physical assistance, recent developments in the fields of special education, adolescent development, and family systems suggest redefining autonomy in terms of individuals' capacities to take responsibility for their own behavior, to make decisions regarding their own lives, and to maintain supportive social relationships. Given this understanding, even individuals with severe impairment can be viewed as autonomous if they perceive their own needs and take responsibility for meeting them, either directly or by engaging the assistance of others. As adolescents become more autonomous, the nurse can help them articulate needs, participate in developing their own care plan, and discover and express how others can be of greatest assistance.

Physical symptoms are high on the teenager's list of health-related concerns. Because adolescence is a time of enormous physical and emotional changes, it is important for the nurse to distinguish between body changes that are related to disability and those that are a result of normal body development. It can be a great comfort for teenagers with disabling conditions to know that many of the changes they experience are normal developmental outcomes.

A sense of feeling different from peers can lead to loneliness, isolation, and depression. Participation in groups of teenagers with chronic conditions or disabilities can alleviate feelings of isolation and smooth the transition to a meaningful relationship with one person in adulthood.

ESTABLISH REALISTIC FUTURE GOALS

One of the most difficult adjustments is setting realistic future goals for the child and for those involved in his or her continued care. Sometimes the impact of this decision does not surface until the child finishes school or the parents approach retirement, when a crisis can arise because of disruption of all of the family roles and relationships that maintained stability.

Planning for the future should be a gradual process. All along, the parents should cultivate realistic vocations for the child. For example, if children have physical disabilities, they are directed to intellectual, artistic, or musical pursuits. Children with developmental disabilities are taught manual skills.

---

*1133 19th St. NW, Washington, DC 20036; (202) 628-3630; http://www.specialolympics.org. Several pamphlets on sports and recreation for children with disabilities are available from Easter Seals (see footnote, p. 589) and American Alliance for Health, Physical Education, Recreation and Dance, 1900 Association Drive, Reston, VA 20191; (703) 476-3400 or (800) 213-7193; http://www.aahperd.org.
†A directory of private/paying camps for children with a variety of chronic illnesses or general physical disabilities is available from the American Camp Association, 5000 State Road 67 North, Martinsville, IN 46151-7902; (765) 342-8456; http://www.acacamps.org.

---

*VSA Arts has affiliate chapters in all 50 states and in selected sites internationally; yearly festivals are held throughout the world. Information is available from VSA Arts, 818 Connecticut Avenue NW, Suite 600, Washington, DC 20006; (202) 628-2800 or (800) 933-8721; http://www.vsarts.org.

In this way, the child's development proceeds in the direction of self-support through gainful employment.

With prolonged survival, young people with chronic illnesses must deal with new decisions and problems, such as marriage, employment, and insurance coverage. With appropriate guidance, individuals with disabilities can attain gainful employment, marriage, and a family. For those whose conditions are genetic, counseling is needed regarding future offspring. Prospective spouses often benefit from an opportunity to discuss their feelings regarding marriage to an individual with continued health needs and possibly a limited life span. Health insurance coverage is a critical issue because some private carriers may no longer insure a young person who leaves home or may be unwilling to reinsure the person who is independent. Life insurance is another dilemma, especially when children have serious defects, such as congenital heart anomalies.

PERSPECTIVES ON THE CARE OF CHILDREN AT THE END OF LIFE

Although most childhood illnesses and many injuries and other trauma respond favorably to treatment, some do not. When a child and family face a prolonged and possibly terminal illness, health professionals must confront the challenge of providing the best possible care to meet the physical, psychologic, spiritual, and emotional needs of the child and family during the uncertain course of the illness and at the time of death. When death is sudden and unexpected, nurses are challenged to respond to grief and shock in families and provide comfort and support in the absence of a prior relationship.

Many factors affect the causes of death that nurses are likely to encounter in children: developmental factors, medical advances and technology, and changing social patterns. In infants the leading causes of death are congenital anomalies, respiratory distress syndrome, disorders related to short gestation and low birth weight, and sudden infant death syndrome (Arias, MacDorman, Strobino, and others, 2003) (see Chapter 1). The leading causes of death in children 5 to 9 years of age include injuries (accidents), malignant neoplasms, congenital anomalies, assault (homicide), and heart disease. In children 10 to 14 years of age, suicide is the third leading cause of death, after injuries (accidents) and malignant neoplasms. In youths 15 to 19 years of age, assault (homicide), suicide, malignant neoplasms, and heart disease follow accidents as the most prevalent causes of death (Anderson and Smith, 2005).

A child who is diagnosed with a life-threatening illness or who is suffering serious, life-threatening trauma needs medical diagnosis and intervention, as well as nursing assessment and care—sometimes for a short time and sometimes over a lengthy period. When cure is no longer possible and life-prolonging measures result in pain and distress to the child, parents need information about care options that are available to assist them in deciding how they want the remaining time with their child to be managed by the health care team. It is important that families are reassured that although their child cannot be cured, active care will continue to be provided to maintain the child's comfort. Support is provided to assist the child and family during the dying process. As a result, nurses may care for children and families who are making the difficult transition from curative or restorative treatments to palliative care.

PRINCIPLES OF PALLIATIVE CARE

Palliative care involves a multidisciplinary approach to the management of a terminal illness or the dying process that focuses on symptom control and support rather than on cure or life prolongation in the absence of the possibility of a cure (Field and Behrman, 2004). The World Health Organization (1996) defines **palliative care** as the "active total care of patients whose disease is not responsive to curative treatment. Control of pain, of other symptoms, and of psychological, social and spiritual problems is paramount. The goal of palliative care is the achievement of the best possible quality of life for patients and their families."

Palliative care interventions do not serve to hasten death; rather, they provide pain and symptom management, attention to issues faced by the child and family with regard to death and dying, and promotion of optimal functioning and quality of life during the time the child has remaining. The implementation of neonatal and pediatric palliative care consulting services within hospitals has led to enhanced quality of life and end-of-life care for children and their families and support for their care providers (Jennings, 2005; Pierucci, Kirby, and Leuthner, 2001). Several principles are hallmarks of palliative care.

The child and family are considered the unit of care. The death of a child is an extremely stressful event for a family because it is out of the natural order of things. Children represent health and hope, and their death calls into question the understanding of life. A multidisciplinary team of health care professionals consisting of social workers, chaplains, nurses, personal care aides, and physicians skilled in caring for dying patients assist the family by focusing care on the complex interactions between physical, emotional, social, and spiritual issues.

Palliative care seeks to create a therapeutic environment, as homelike as possible, if not in the child's own home. Through education and support of family members, an atmosphere of open communication is provided regarding the child's dying process and its impact on all members of the family (see Evidence-Based Practice box).

DECISION MAKING AT THE END OF LIFE

Discussions concerning the possibility that a child's illness or condition is not curable and that death is an inevitable outcome cause everyone involved a great deal of stress. Physicians, other members of the health care team, and families must consider all information regarding the child's situation and make decisions that all parties agree to and that will have a profound impact on the child and family.

Ethical Considerations in End-of-Life Decision Making

A number of ethical concerns arise when parents and health care professionals are deciding on the best course of care for the dying child. Many parents and health care providers are concerned that not offering treatment that would cause potential pain and suffering, but might extend life, would be considered euthanasia or assisted suicide. To eliminate such concerns, it is necessary to understand the various terms. **Euthanasia** involves an action carried out by a person other than the patient to end the life of the patient suffering from a terminal condition. The intent of this action is based on the be-

Pediatric Pain and Symptom Management at the End of Life

ASK THE QUESTION	In children, what is the pain and symptom experience at the end of life?

SEARCH FOR EVIDENCE
Search Strategies Published studies from 2000 to 2005 using the subject terms *child, palliative care, pain,* and *symptoms* were identified and examined. Retrospective descriptive studies dominated the findings describing infants and children's end-of-life experiences through the use of medical record reviews and provider and parental surveys.
Databases Used PubMed, CINAHL

CRITICALLY ANALYZE THE EVIDENCE
Children experienced an average of 11 symptoms during their last week of life (Drake, Frost, and Collins, 2003). Pain, dyspnea, and fatigue were the most frequently documented symptoms, experienced by most children at the end of life (Bradshaw, Hinds, Lensing, and others, 2005; Carter, Howenstein, Gilmer, and others, 2004; Drake, Frost, and Collins, 2003; Hongo, Chieko, Okada, and others, 2003). Children and their parents report high distress with pain and symptoms at the end of life. Parents reported pain and suffering as one of the most important factors in deciding to withhold or withdraw life support from their child in the pediatric intensive care unit (Meert, Thurston, and Sarnaik, 2000).

Documentation was scarce related to symptom management. Morphine was the most commonly prescribed pain medication (Drake, Frost, and Collins, 2003; Hongo, Chieko, Okada, and others, 2003). Parents reported their children as experiencing high levels of pain near the end of life (Contro, Larson, Scofield, and others, 2002). Physicians were more likely than nurses or parents to report that a child's pain and symptoms were well managed at the end of life, whereas the majority of both provider groups believed the child's physical management was difficult (Andresen, Seecharan, and Toce, 2004; Wolfe, Grier, Klar, and others, 2000).

Barriers to the adequate provision of pediatric palliative care include developmental issues specific to infants and children; symptoms, their causes, how they are related, and effective treatment strategies; lack of education; and reimbursement issues (Harris, 2004). Physicians report reliance on trial and error as they learn to care for children at the end of life and the need for specialty consults with palliative care service providers (Hilden, Emanuel, Fairclough, and others, 2001).

APPLY THE EVIDENCE: NURSING IMPLICATIONS
Although the philosophy of palliative care encompasses pain and symptom management for infants and children who may not outlive their disease, the provision of that care to ease suffering and provide comfort to those who will die continues to lag. Studies show that children experience significant pain and other distressing symptoms at the end of life that are not well managed. Discrepancies in perceptions of infant and child pain and suffering continue to exist between providers and parents. Barriers to the provision of pediatric palliative care exist. Improvements are needed in the management of pain and symptoms at the end of life for infants and children.

References
Andresen EM, Seecharan GA, Toce SS: Provider perceptions of child deaths, *Arch Pediatr Adolesc Med* 158:430-435, 2004.
Bradshaw G, Hinds PS, Lensing S, and others: Cancer-related deaths in children and adolescents, *J Palliat Med* 8(1):86-95, 2005.
Carter BS, Howenstein BS, Gilmer MJ, and others: Circumstances surrounding the deaths of hospitalized children: opportunities for pediatric palliative care, *Pediatrics* 114(3):361-366, 2004.
Contro N, Larson J, Scofield S, and others: Family perspectives on the quality of pediatric palliative care, *Arch Pediatr Adolesc Med* 156:1-29, 2002.
Drake R, Frost J, Collins JJ: The symptoms of dying children, *J Pain Symptom Manage* 26(1):594-603, 2003.
Harris B: Palliative care in children with cancer: which child and when? *J Natl Cancer Institute Mono* 32:144-149, 2004.
Hilden JM, Emanuel EJ, Fairclough DL, and others: Attitudes and practices among pediatric oncologists regarding end-of-life care: results of the 1998 American Society of Clinical Oncology Survey, *J Clin Oncol* 19(1):205-212, 2001.
Hongo T, Chieko W, Okada S, and others: Analysis of the circumstances at the end of life in children with cancer: symptoms, suffering and acceptance, *Pediatr Int* 45:60-64, 2003.
Meert KL, Thurston CS, Sarnaik AP: End-of-life decision-making and satisfaction with care: parental perspectives, *Pediatr Crit Care Med* 1(2):179-185, 2000.
Wolfe J, Grier HE, Klar N, and others: Symptoms and suffering at the end of life in children with cancer, *N Engl J Med* 342(5):326-333, 2000.

lief that the act is "putting the person out of his or her misery"; this action has also been called **mercy killing. Assisted suicide** occurs when someone provides the patient with the means to end his or her life and the patient uses that means to do so. The important distinction between these two actions involves who is actually acting to end the person's life.

The American Nurses Association *Code of Ethics for Nurses* (2001) does not support the active intent on the part of a nurse to end a person's life. However, it does permit the nurse to provide interventions to relieve symptoms in the dying patient even when the interventions involve substantial risks of hastening death. When the prognosis for a patient is poor and death is the expected outcome, it is ethically acceptable to withhold or withdraw treatments that may cause pain and suffering and provide interventions that promote comfort and quality of life. Therefore providing palliative care for patients is the ethically correct choice in such a circumstance.

Physician–Health Care Team Decision Making
Decisions by physicians regarding care are often made on the basis of the progression of the disease or amount of trauma, the availability of treatment options that would provide cure from disease or restoration of health, the impact of such treatments on the child, and the child's overall prognosis (Davis and Eng, 1998). Often the main determinants prompting physicians to discuss end-of-life issues and options for children with critical illnesses include the child's age, premorbid cognitive condition and functional status, pain or discomfort, probability of survival, and quality of life (Masri, Farrell, Lacroix, and others, 2000). When the physician discusses this informa-

tion openly with families, a shared decision-making process can occur regarding **do-not-resuscitate (DNR) orders** and care that is focused on the comfort of the child and family during the dying process.

Unfortunately, many families are not given the option of terminating treatment and pursuing care that is focused on comfort and quality of life when cure is unlikely, and staff may be reluctant to raise the question of DNR orders. This occurs for a number of reasons, including the belief that not being able to "save" a child is a "failure." Also, the physician and other members of the health care team may lack knowledge of and experience with the principles of palliative care (Field and Behrman, 2004; Sumner, 2003; Sahler, Frager, Levetown, and others, 2000).

Parental Decision Making

Rarely are families prepared to cope with the numerous decisions that must be made when a child is dying. When the death is unexpected, as in the case of an accident or trauma, the confusion of emergency services and possibly an intensive care setting presents challenges to parents as they are asked to make difficult choices. If the child has either experienced a life-threatening illness such as cancer or lived with a chronic illness that has now reached its terminal phase, parents are often unprepared for the reality of their child's impending death (see Family Focus box). Numerous studies have found that families facing the impending death of a child depend on information provided to them by the health care team, particularly an honest appraisal of the child's prognosis, to make difficult decisions regarding care options for their child (Wolfe, Friebert, and Hilden, 2002; Hinds, Oakes, Furman, and others, 2001; James and Johnson, 1997).

As the group of health professionals who are most involved with families, nurses are in an excellent position to ensure that families are presented with the options available to them. The nurse's first responsibility is to explore the family's wishes. This is best done in concert with the physician, but at times may need to be initiated by the nurse. Statements such as "Tell me about your thoughts for the type of care you want your child to receive when he is dying" or "Have you considered the types of interventions you would like us to use when your child is near death?" can begin discussion of this sensitive but critical aspect of terminal care.

The Dying Child

Children need honest and accurate information about their illness, treatments, and prognosis; this information needs to be given in clear, simple language. In most situations this best occurs as a gradual process over time, characterized by increasingly open dialogue between parents, professionals, and the child (Young, Dixon-Woods, Windridge, and others, 2003). Providing an atmosphere of open communication early in the course of an illness facilitates answering difficult questions as the child's condition worsens. Providing appropriate literature about the disease, as well as the experience of illness and possible death, is also helpful. Exactly how and when to involve children in decisions regarding care during their dying process and death is an individual matter. The child's age or developmental level is an important consideration in the process (Table 18-3). In general, parents should be asked how they would like their child to be told of their prognosis, and they should be included in his or her care. Some parents may request that their

FAMILY FOCUS

Family of the Dying Child

No matter whether you have a PhD or many children, when your child dies, it is a new experience and nothing can prepare you for it. Like so many things in life, experience is the best teacher.

Three of our children have died, and by the time the third was dying, we handled many things differently. We learned a lot about dignity and the rights of the child and family. For example, at first, we didn't know that we had a right to have our child die at home. We also didn't understand pain medications and that if children are taking these medicines and are still in agony, they have not overdosed on the medication.

We learned a lot about case management. With our first two children, lots of different people were making decisions and disagreeing about what was best and what should be done. No one had primary authority. With our third child, one doctor took a primary role. Any questions and problems were handled by one person. I could call him 24 hours a day. It made a lot of difference, and I felt our concerns and needs were better heard and respected.

The nurses caring for our third child at home enabled me to step back and just be his mommy. When I could do this, I realized that we were fighting so hard for his life that we weren't really letting him die. His nurses had worked with him for a long time and really loved him. It was hard for them when we decided to let him die. In his last several days we wanted a lot of family time with our son, and I think the nurses felt left out. Something about their reaction to our increased time with him in the last few days made us feel guilty. If we had all been able to communicate a little more openly, I would have understood that they needed more time with him at the end, too. Everyone's needs could have been met.

Jeni Stepanek
Mother
Upper Marlboro, Maryland

child not be told that he or she is dying, even if the child asks. This often places health care providers in a difficult situation. Children, even at a young age, are perceptive. Even if they are not told outright that they are dying, they realize that something is seriously wrong and that it involves them. Often, helping parents understand that honesty and shared decision making between them and their child are important to the child's and family's emotional health will encourage parents to allow discussion of dying with their child. Parents may require professional support and guidance in this process from a nurse, social worker, or child life specialist who has a good relationship with the child and family.

If given the opportunity, children will tell others how much they want to know. Asking questions such as "If the disease came back, would you want to know?" "Do you want others to tell you everything, even if the news isn't good?" or "If someone were not getting better [or more directly, "were dying"], do you think he would want to know?" helps children set the limits of how much truth they can accept and cope with. Children need time to process many feelings and much information so that they can assimilate and ideally accept the inevitable fact of mortality.

Care of the dying adolescent requires the nurse to become knowledgeable about any possible delays or alterations in normal growth and development. Legal and ethical issues also come to the forefront with respect to the age at which an ado-

TABLE 18-3

Children's Understanding of and Reactions to Death

CONCEPTS OF DEATH	REACTIONS TO DEATH	NURSING CARE MANAGEMENT
INFANTS AND TODDLERS		
Death has least significance to children <6 months of age. After parent-child attachment and trust are established, the loss, even if temporary, of the significant person is profound. Prolonged separation during the first several years is thought to be more significant in terms of future physical, social, and emotional growth than at any subsequent age. Toddlers are egocentric and can only think about events in terms of their own frame of reference—living. Their egocentricity and vague separation of fact and fantasy make it impossible for them to comprehend absence of life. Instead of understanding death, this age-group is affected more by any change in lifestyle.	With the death of someone else, they may continue to act as though the person is alive. As children grow older, they will be increasingly able and willing to let go of the dead person. Ritualism is important; a change in lifestyle could be anxiety producing. This age-group reacts more to the pain and discomfort of a serious illness than to the probable fatal prognosis. This age-group also reacts to parental anxiety and sadness.	Help parents deal with their feelings, allowing them greater emotional reserves to meet the needs of their children. Encourage parents to remain as near to child as possible, yet be sensitive to parents' needs. Maintain as normal an environment as possible to retain ritualism. If a parent has died, encourage having consistent caregiver for child. Promote primary nursing.
PRESCHOOL CHILDREN		
Preschoolers believe their thoughts are sufficient to cause death; the consequence is the burden of guilt, shame, and punishment. Their egocentricity implies a tremendous sense of self-power and omnipotence. They usually have some understanding of the meaning of death. Death is seen as a departure, a kind of sleep. They may recognize the fact of physical death but do not separate it from living abilities. Death is seen as temporary and gradual; life and death can change places with one another. They have no understanding of the universality and inevitability of death.	If they become seriously ill, they conceive of the illness as a punishment for their thoughts or actions. They may feel guilty and responsible for the death of a sibling. Greatest fear concerning death is separation from parents. They may engage in activities that seem strange or abnormal to adults. Because they have fewer defense mechanisms to deal with loss, young children may react to a less significant loss with more outward grief than to the loss of a very significant person. The loss is so deep, painful, and threatening that the child must deny it for a time to survive its overwhelming impact. Behavior reactions such as giggling, joking, attracting attention, or regressing to earlier developmental skills indicate children's need to distance themselves from tremendous loss.	Help parents deal with their feelings, allowing them greater emotional reserves to meet the needs of their children. Help parents understand behavioral reactions of their children. Encourage parents to remain near the child as much as possible, to minimize the child's great fear of separation from parents. If a parent has died, encourage having a consistent caregiver for child. Promote primary nursing.
SCHOOL-AGE CHILDREN		
The children still associate misdeeds or bad thoughts with causing death and feel intense guilt and responsibility for the event. Because of their higher cognitive abilities, they respond well to logical explanations and comprehend the figurative meaning of words. They have a deeper understanding of death in a concrete sense. They particularly fear the mutilation and punishment they associate with death. They personify death as the devil, a monster, or the bogeyman. They may have naturalistic or physiologic explanations of death. By age 9 or 10, children have an adult concept of death, realizing that it is inevitable, universal, and irreversible.	Because of their increased ability to comprehend, they may have more fears, for example: The reason for the illness Communicability of the disease to themselves or others Consequences of the disease The process of dying and death itself Their fear of the unknown is greater than their fear of the known. The realization of impending death is a tremendous threat to their sense of security and ego strength. They are likely to exhibit fear through verbal uncooperativeness rather than actual physical aggression. They are interested in postdeath services. They may be inquisitive about what happens to the body.	Help parents deal with their feelings, allowing them greater emotional reserves to meet the needs of their children. Encourage parents to remain near child as much as possible, yet be sensitive to parents' needs. Because of children's fear of the unknown, anticipatory preparation is important. Because the developmental task of this age is industry, interventions of helping children maintain control over their bodies and increasing their understanding allow them to achieve independence, self-worth, and self-esteem and avoid a sense of inferiority. Encourage children to talk about their feelings and provide aggressive outlets. Encourage parents to honestly answer questions about dying rather than avoiding the subject or fabricating euphemisms. Encourage parents to share their moments of sorrow with their children. Provide preparation for postdeath services.

TABLE 18-3		
Children's Understanding of and Reactions to Death—cont'd		
CONCEPTS OF DEATH	REACTIONS TO DEATH	NURSING CARE MANAGEMENT
ADOLESCENTS		
Adolescents have a mature understanding of death. They are still influenced by remnants of magical thinking and are subject to guilt and shame. They are likely to see deviations from accepted behavior as reasons for their illness.	Adolescents straddle transition from childhood to adulthood. They have the most difficulty in coping with death. They are least likely to accept cessation of life, particularly if it is their own. Concern is for the present much more than for the past or the future. They may consider themselves alienated from their peers and unable to communicate with their parents for emotional support, feeling alone in their struggle. Adolescents' orientation to the present compels them to worry about physical changes even more than the prognosis. Because of their idealistic view of the world, they may criticize funeral rites as barbaric, money making, and unnecessary.	Help parents deal with their feelings, allowing them greater emotional reserves to meet the needs of their children. Avoid alliances with either parent or child. Structure hospital admission to allow for maximum self-control and independence. Answer adolescents' questions honestly, treating them as mature individuals and respecting their needs for privacy, solitude, and personal expressions of emotions. Help parents understand their child's reactions to death and dying, especially that concern for present crises, such as loss of hair, may be much greater than for future ones, including possible death.

lescent should have autonomy in decision making with regard to care and treatment. Effective communication between the patient, family, and health care team is an important part of optimal care for the dying adolescent (Freyer, 2004).

Treatment Options for Terminally Ill Children

Based on the child's and family's decision regarding their wishes for terminal care, they have several options from which to choose.

Hospital. Families may choose to remain in the hospital to receive care if the child's illness or condition is unstable and home care is not an option or the family is uncomfortable with providing care at home. If a family chooses to remain at the hospital for terminal care, the setting should be made as homelike as possible. Families are encouraged to bring familiar items from the child's room at home. In addition, there should be a consistent and coordinated care plan for the child's and family's comfort.

Home Care. Some families prefer to take their child home and receive services from a home care agency. Generally, these services entail periodic nursing visits to administer a treatment or provide medications, equipment, or supplies. The child's care continues to be directed by the primary physician. Home care is often the option chosen by physicians and families because of the traditional view that a child must be considered to have a life expectancy of less than 6 months to be referred to hospice care. Fortunately, a number of hospice organizations are expanding their services to children based on the presence of a life-limiting disease process for which cure is not possible, rather than on the sole criteria of a limited time-projected prognosis.

Hospice Care. Parents should be offered the option of caring for their child at home during the final phases of an illness with the assistance of a hospice organization. **Hospice** is a community health care organization that specializes in the care of dying patients by combining the hospice philosophy

with the principles of palliative care. **Hospice philosophy** regards dying as a natural process and care of dying patients as including management of the physical, psychologic, social, and spiritual needs of the patient and family. Care is provided by a multidisciplinary group of professionals in the patient's home or an inpatient facility that employs the hospice philosophy. Hospice care for children was introduced in the 1970s, and a number of community hospice organizations now accept children into their care (Davies, Davis, and Sibert, 2003; Forrester, 2003; Winkler and Mardegian, 2001; Faulkner and Armstrong-Dailey, 1997). Collaboration between the child's primary treatment team and the hospice care team is essential to the success of hospice care. Families may continue to see their primary care physicians as they choose.*

Hospice care is based on a number of important concepts that significantly set it apart from hospital care:

- Family members are usually the principal caregivers and are supported by a team of professional and volunteer staff.
- The priority of care is comfort. The child's physical, psychologic, social, and spiritual needs are considered. Pain and symptom control are primary concerns, and no extraordinary efforts are used to attempt a cure or prolong life.
- The family's needs are considered to be as important as those of the patient.
- Hospice is concerned with the family's postdeath adjustment, and care may continue for a year or more.

The goal of hospice care is for children to live life to the fullest without pain, with choices and dignity, in the familiar environment of their home, and with the support of their family. Hospice care is covered under state Medicaid programs and by most

---

*For more information, contact National Hospice and Palliative Care Organization, 1700 Diagonal Road, Suite 625, Alexandria, VA 22314; (703) 837-1500; fax: (703) 837-1233; http://www.nho.org; and Children's Hospice International, 1101 King St., Suite 360, Alexandria, VA 22314; (703) 684-0330 or (800) 24-CHILD; http://www.chionline.org.

insurance plans. The service provides home visits from nurses, social workers, chaplains, and, in some cases, physicians. Medications, medical equipment, and any necessary medical supplies are all provided by the hospice organization providing care.

With children, the home has been the more common environment for implementing the hospice concept; it benefits the family in a variety of ways. Children who are dying are allowed to remain with those they love and with whom they feel secure. Many children who were thought to be in imminent danger of death have gone home and lived longer than expected. Siblings can feel more involved in the care and often have more positive perceptions of the death. Parental adaptation is often more favorable, demonstrated by their perceptions of how the experience at home affected their marriage, social reorientation, religious beliefs, and views on the meaning of life and death.

If the home is chosen for hospice care, the child may or may not die in the home. Reasons for final admission to a hospital vary but may be related to the parents' or siblings' wish to have the child die outside the home; exhaustion on the part of the caregivers; and physical problems such as sudden, acute pain or respiratory distress.

NURSING CARE OF THE CHILD AND FAMILY AT THE END OF LIFE

Regardless of where the child is cared for during the terminal stage of illness, both the child and the family usually experience fear of (1) pain and suffering, (2) dying alone (child) or not being present when the child dies (parent), and (3) actual death. Nurses can help families by lessening their fears through attention to the care needs of the child and family (see Nursing Care Plan).

FEAR OF PAIN AND SUFFERING

The presence of unrelieved pain in a terminally ill child can have detrimental effects on the quality of life experienced by the child and family. Parents feel that having their child in pain is unendurable and results in feelings of helplessness and a sense that they must be present and vigilant to get the necessary pain medications. Persistent pain also has an impact on the family as a whole. Nurses can alleviate the fear of pain and suffering by providing interventions aimed at treating the pain and symptoms associated with the terminal process in children.

---

nursingcareplan   The Child Who Is Terminally Ill or Dying

Nursing Diagnosis	Patient Outcomes	Nursing Interventions	Rationale
Anxiety related to fear or worry about dying	Child and family will receive appropriate emotional support during the terminal phase of the child's illness.	Encourage the family to remain near child as much as possible.	To provide support through the presence of a loved one
Child's/Family's Defining Characteristics *(Subjective and Objective Data)*	Child will express fears and anxiety related to dying.	Encourage child to talk about feelings; help the family as they encourage child to express feelings.	To provide a sense of closeness and understanding among family members
Unstable emotions	Family will support the child's ability to express fears and anxiety.	Provide safe, acceptable outlets for aggression or for grieving.	To establish that anger and sadness are normal reactions
Aggressive behavior	Child and family will be informed of symptoms to expect as child nears the end of life.	Answer questions as honestly as possible while maintaining a positive, hopeful approach.	To promote trust as a major strength for therapeutic relationships
Withdrawn behavior			
Depression	Child and family will be informed of procedures and therapies necessary to promote comfort.	Explain progression of physical symptoms as child nears the end of life.	To promote trust and decrease anxiety
	Child and family will be able to cope with the dying process.	Explain all procedures and therapies, especially physical effects child will experience.	To decrease fear of the unknown, which may be more of a concern than the actual procedure or therapy
	The Following NOC Concepts Apply to These Outcomes	Help child distinguish between consequences of treatment and manifestations of the disease.	To focus on interventions that can minimize discomfort
	Anxiety Self-Control	Structure hospital or home environment to allow for maximum self-control and independence within the limitations imposed by child's developmental level and physical condition.	To minimize fear and loss of control
	Coping		
	Fear Self-Control		
		The Following NIC Concepts Apply to These Interventions	
		Active Listening	
		Coping Enhancement	
		Simple Relaxation	
		Touch	

nursingcareplan | The Child Who Is Terminally Ill or Dying—cont'd

Nursing Diagnosis	Patient Outcomes	Nursing Interventions	Rationale
Chronic Pain related to disease process **Child's/Family's Defining Characteristics** *(Subjective and Objective Data)* Crying Withdrawal Aggression Fear of touch Fear of movement	Child will exhibit minimal or no evidence of physical discomfort. Family will be able to participate in the child's care without causing discomfort. Family will be able to provide comfort measures for child. **The Following NOC Concepts Apply to These Outcomes** Comfort Level Pain Control	Assess child's level of comfort. Provide pain management around the clock. Assess child for symptoms associated with pain or its treatment. Provide stool softener, laxative, or diphenhydramine as needed. Provide nonpharmacologic interventions child prefers. Administer anticholinergic drugs as needed. Encourage family to provide comfort measures the child prefers. Provide soothing surroundings for child. Avoid excessive noise or light. Ensure pleasant smell, touch, temperature. Place all commodities within easy reach for the child. Use gentle touch when required to perform physical procedures. Avoid pressure on painful areas. Avoid pressure on bony prominences or painful sites. Use pillows or other supports to prop child in a comfortable position. Place absorbent pads under hips if the child is incontinent. Limit care to essential needs. **The Following NIC Concepts Apply to These Outcomes** Analgesic Administration Patient-Controlled Analgesia Positioning Simple Massage Sleep Enhancement Simple Relaxation Therapy	To ensure child is treated for changes in pain To prevent the recurrence or escalation of pain To ensure child is treated for symptoms accompanying pain or its management To prevent or treat symptoms related to pain or its management To aid pharmacologic management of pain, helping to prevent recurrence or escalation of pain and accompanying symptoms To reduce secretions and lessen "death rattle," which can be distressing to family To provide comfort To minimize irritation and maximize comfort To minimize discomfort from movement To minimize pain when possible To make it easier for the child to breathe To prevent skin breakdown To minimize fatigue
Anticipatory Grieving related to impending loss of child **Child's/Family's Defining Characteristics** *(Subjective and Objective Data)* Parents' feelings and physical responses of loss and depression Parents' feelings of loss of control and uncertainty Child's or sibling's feelings and physical responses of loss and depression Child's or sibling's feelings of loss of control and uncertainty	Family will express fears, concerns, and any special desires for terminal care. Family will demonstrate an understanding of their children's needs. Family members will be actively involved in their child's care. Family members will seek resources needed to assist them during the grieving process. **The Following NOC Concept Applies to These Outcomes** Family Coping	Discuss the grieving process and differences in grieving among men, women, and children with the family and child. Provide opportunities for family members to express emotions independently or together as desired. Facilitate child's or sibling's expression of emotions through art or play activities. Help parents and siblings deal with their feelings about the child's death. Encourage parents to remain as near the child as possible.	To facilitate understanding of what family members are feeling and experiencing To provide an outlet for their emotions To facilitate expression of their emotions To provide support To allow parents to feel they are doing something for their child

Continued

nursingcareplan | The Child Who Is Terminally Ill or Dying—cont'd

Nursing Diagnosis	Patient Outcomes	Nursing Interventions	Rationale
Anticipatory Grieving related to impending loss of child—cont'd		Provide family with information regarding the child's status.	To promote understanding and communication
		Provide family with information on common behavioral reactions.	To promote understanding of their children's behaviors
		Encourage family's assistance with child's care.	To assist with coping and minimize loss of control
		Provide information to family on how to maintain own health care needs.	To give families the approval to take care of themselves
		Provide as much privacy as possible without isolating family from nurse's care.	To provide dignity for the grieving process
		Assist family in assessing their needs for referral services.	To facilitate support for families
		Encourage parents to honestly answer children's questions about dying.	To decrease children's fear and anxiety
		Provide resources for family to facilitate discussions with children about dying.	To provide support and facilitate parents' discussion
		Encourage parents to share their moments of sorrow with their children.	To promote grief expression of children
		Assist family and child with memory-making opportunities.	To facilitate emotions and sharing between family and child
		Assist child as needed to complete any unfinished business.	To facilitate support of child
		Discuss with parents appropriate involvement of siblings.	To prevent siblings from feeling excluded
		Identify family's religious and cultural beliefs related to death.	To provide support and spiritual care
		Provide preparation for postdeath services.	To provide support and guidance
		Discuss with parents the frequent need of children to be given permission to die.	To provide support and guidance
		Discuss with family their preferences for care if death is imminent.	To allow families to be in control
		Facilitate appropriate spiritual care in accordance with family's beliefs or affiliations.	To provide support
		Provide support for families who choose home care for their child.	To allow families to choose where the child is to die and provide guidance for this to occur

The Following NIC Concepts Apply to These Outcomes

Anticipatory Guidance
Anxiety Reduction
Caregiver Support
Counseling
Family Support Family Therapy

Pain and Symptom Management

Pain control for children in the terminal stages of illness or injury must be given the highest priority. Despite ongoing efforts to educate physicians and nurses on pain management strategies in children, studies have reported that children continue to be undermedicated for their pain (Wolfe, Grier, Klar, and others, 2000). Nearly all children experience some amount of pain in the terminal phase of their illness. The current standard for treating children's pain follows the World Health Organization's analgesic stepladder (1996), which promotes tailoring the pain interventions to the child's level of reported pain. Children's pain should be assessed frequently, and medications adjusted as necessary. Pain medications should be given on a regular schedule, and extra doses for breakthrough pain should be available to maintain comfort. Opioid drugs such as morphine should be given for severe pain, and the dose should be increased as necessary to maintain optimal pain relief. Techniques such as distraction, relaxation tech-

BOX 18-9
Ethical Principle of Double Effect

An action that has one good (intended) and one bad (unintended but foreseeable) effect is permissible if the following conditions are met:
- The action itself must be good or indifferent. Only the good consequences of the action must be sincerely intended.
- The good effect must not be produced by the bad effect.
- There must be a compelling or proportionate reason for permitting the foreseeable bad effect to occur.

niques, and guided imagery (Lambert, 1999) should be combined with drug therapy to provide the child and family strategies to control pain (see Chapter 7 for further discussion of pain management strategies).

In addition to pain, children experience a variety of symptoms during their terminal course as a result of their disease process or as a side effect of medicines used to manage pain or other symptoms. These symptoms include fatigue, nausea and vomiting, constipation, anorexia, dyspnea, congestion, seizures, anxiety, depression, restlessness, agitation, and confusion (Wolfe, Friebert, and Hilden, 2002; Hellsten, Hockenberry, Lamb, and others, 2000). Each of these symptoms should be aggressively managed with appropriate medications or treatments and with interventions such as repositioning, relaxation, massage, and other measures to maintain the child's comfort and quality of life.

Occasionally, children require very high doses of opioids to control pain. This may occur for several reasons. The child on long-term opioid pain management can become **tolerant** of the drug, meaning that it is necessary to give more drugs to maintain the same level of pain relief. This should not be confused with **addiction,** which is a psychologic dependence on the side effects of opioids. Addiction is not a factor in managing terminal pain in children. Other obvious reasons for requiring increased doses of opioids include progression of disease and other physiologic experiences of pain. It is important to understand that there is no maximum dose that can be given to control pain. However, nurses often express concern that administering doses of opioids that exceed what they are familiar with will hasten the child's death. The **principle of double effect** (Box 18-9) addresses such concerns. It provides an ethical standard that supports the use of interventions intended to relieve pain and suffering even though there is a foreseeable possibility that death may be hastened (Rousseau, 2001). In cases in which the child is terminally ill and in severe pain, using large doses of opioids and sedatives to manage pain is justified when no other treatment options are available that would relieve the pain but make the risk of death less likely (Hawryluck and Harvey, 2000). See Chapter 7 for an extensive discussion of pain assessment and management.

Parents' and Siblings' Need for Education and Support

Parents are the primary caregivers when the child is at home, and nurses providing care to the child and family need to teach the family about the medications being given to the child, how to administer medications, and the use of nonpharmacologic techniques. Parents are kept informed of all medications and treatments given to a child in the hospital,

and they are encouraged to participate in the child's care to the extent that they desire. This empowers parents and provides a sense of control over the child's comfort and well-being, reducing their fear that their child will be in pain or suffering as he or she is dying. Additionally, better bereavement outcomes (e.g., adaptive coping; family cohesion; less anxiety, stress, and depression) have been reported by parents who were actively involved in the care of their child (Goodenough, Drew, Higgins, and others, 2004; Lauer, Mulhern, Schell, and others, 1989). The grief work of fathers in particular seems to be facilitated when their child dies in the home setting. This finding may be related to the increased opportunity of working fathers to provide care to and spend time with their child at home vs the hospital setting.

Siblings may feel isolated and displaced during the time that their brother or sister is dying. Parents devote the majority of their time to the care and comfort of the dying child, causing siblings to feel left out of the parent–sick child relationship. Siblings may become resentful of their sick sibling and begin to feel guilty or ashamed about such feelings (Murray, 1999). Nurses can assist the family by helping the parents identify ways to involve siblings in the caring process, perhaps by bringing some supplies or favorite toy, game, or food item. Parents should also be encouraged to schedule time to spend with the other children where their focus is on them. Helping parents identify a trusted friend or family member who can sit with the ill child for a short period will allow them to attend to their own needs or those of their other children.

FEAR OF DYING ALONE OR OF NOT BEING PRESENT WHEN THE CHILD DIES

When a child is being cared for at home, the burden of care on parents and family members can be great. Often, as the child's condition declines, family members begin the "death vigil." Rarely is a child left alone for any length of time. This can be exhausting for family members, and nurses can assist the family by helping them arrange shifts so that friends or family members can be present with the child and allow others to rest. If the family has limited resources, community organizations such as hospice or churches often have volunteers who are willing to visit and sit with children. It is important that whoever is sitting with the child be aware of when the parent(s) would like to be notified to return to the child's bedside (Fig. 18-6).

When a child is dying in the hospital, parents should be given full access to the child at all times. If parents need to leave, they should be provided with a pager or other means of immediate communication and alerted if staff members note any change in the child that may indicate imminent death. Nurses advocate for parents' presence in intensive care and emergency departments and attend to the parents' needs for food, drinks, comfortable chairs, blankets, and pillows.

FEAR OF ACTUAL DEATH
Home Deaths

The majority of children receiving hospice care die at home, often in their own room with family, pets, and other loved possessions around them. The physical process of dying can be distressing to parents because often the child slowly become less alert in the days before the actual death. The nurse can assist the family by providing them with information about what changes will occur as the child progresses through

FIG. 18-6 ■ For the dying child there is no greater comfort than the security and closeness of a parent.

BOX 18-10

Physical Signs of Approaching Death

Loss of sensation and movement in the lower extremities, progressing toward the upper body
Sensation of heat, although body feels cool
Loss of senses:
- Tactile sensation decreasing
- Sensitivity to light
- Hearing the last sense to fail

Confusion, loss of consciousness, slurred speech
Muscle weakness
Loss of bowel and bladder control
Decreased appetite and thirst
Difficulty swallowing
Change in respiratory pattern:
- Cheyne-Stokes respirations (waxing and waning of depth of breathing with regular periods of apnea)
- "Death rattle" (noisy chest sounds from accumulation of pulmonary and pharyngeal secretions)

Weak, slow pulse; decreased blood pressure

---

the dying process (Box 18-10). During this time, nursing visits often become more frequent and longer in duration to provide the family with additional support as the death nears. The most distressing change for parents to observe is the change in the respiratory pattern. In the final hours of life, the dying patient's respirations may become labored, with deep breaths and long periods of apnea, referred to as Cheyne-Stokes respirations. Families are reassured that this is not distressing to the child and that it is a normal part of the dying process. However, the use of opioids can slow the respirations to make the child breathe more easily, and scopolamine, usu-

ally applied as a topical patch, can help reduce noisy respirations known as the "death rattle." Noisy respirations are more likely to occur if the child is overhydrated.

All families have the option of admitting their child to the hospital if they feel unable to deal with the death. The child who dies at home must be pronounced dead; hospice programs typically have provisions so that this proceeds smoothly. In some circumstances the police may be notified, with an explanation of the circumstances to prevent unnecessary concern regarding abuse. Providing the police with the number of the responsible practitioner is usually all that is necessary to confirm the cause of death.

Hospital Deaths

Children dying in the hospital of terminal illnesses who are receiving supportive care interventions will experience a similar process. Again, increased nursing presence and attendance to the child's and family's needs provide comfort and support for many families.

Death resulting from accident or trauma or acute illness in settings such as the emergency department or intensive care unit often requires the active withdrawal of some form of life-supporting intervention, such as a ventilator or bypass machine. These situations often raise difficult ethical issues (Sine, Sumner, Gracy, and others, 2001), and parents are often less prepared for the actual moment of death. Nurses can assist these parents by providing detailed information about what will happen as supportive equipment is withdrawn, ensuring that appropriate pain medications are administered to prevent pain during the dying process, and allowing the parents time before the start of the withdrawal to be with and speak to their child. It is important that the nurse attempt to control the environment around the family at this time by providing privacy, asking if they would like to play music, softening lights and monitor noises, and arranging for any religious or cultural rituals that the family may want performed.

After the child's death, the family should be allowed to remain with the body and hold or rock the child if they desire. After the nurse has removed all tubes and equipment from the body, parents should be given the option of assisting with the preparation of the body, such as bathing and dressing. It is important for the nurse to determine whether the family has any specific needs, since many cultures have adopted specific methods for coping with and mourning death and impeding these practices may interfere with the grieving process (Clements, Vigil, Manno, and others, 2003).

At some point the nurse discusses whether the family has made preparations for the burial service and whether the staff can help in any way. Parents often have concerns about the funeral, such as siblings' involvement in the death rituals. Although no absolute answers exist regarding the question of siblings attending the funeral or burial services, the consensus is that the surviving children benefit from being involved in these events. However, children need preparation for postdeath services. They should be told what to expect, particularly how the deceased person will look if the coffin is open; allowed their private time to say good-bye; and permitted to stay as long as they wish. Ideally, the parents should prepare the siblings. If the parents' grief prevents this communication, a significant family member or friend should substitute (see Family Focus box).

FAMILY FOCUS

Children Need to Say Good-Bye

As a nurse and grief counselor, I conduct grief workshops with children who have experienced the death of someone special. Children often communicate their feelings of being excluded through drawings. They may draw a picture of the dying person in a hospital bed that is raised too high for them to see the person's face clearly. Sometimes children reveal that they did not get to say good-bye because a family member told them, for example, "You don't want to see your grandma this way. She is too sick for you to visit." If the special person died at home, the children had to stay in their room when the funeral home staff took away the body.

I have learned never to underestimate the importance of allowing children to be involved with the dying person and the significance of a child's loss. Once, when I asked a 6-year-old girl to draw a picture with the theme "This is what I was doing when my _____ died," she drew a picture and completed the sentence with "when my home died." Her grandmother had been like her mother; to the child, her home was gone. We need to give children the choice of being included in the family's activities of saying good-bye.

Barbara Bilderback, MS, MA, RN
Bereavement Supervisor, Saint Francis Hospice
Tulsa, Oklahoma

ORGAN OR TISSUE DONATION AND AUTOPSY

For some families organ or tissue donation may be a meaningful act—one that benefits another human being despite the loss of their child. Unfortunately, initiating a discussion about tissue donation is often stressful for staff, and there may be confusion regarding whose responsibility this is. In centers in which transplants are performed, a full-time transplant coordinator is usually available to inform the family about organ donation and to take care of details. If such services are not available, the staff needs to determine which members should discuss this topic with the family. Ideally, the person who knows the family best, knows when the death is expected, or has the opportunity to spend time with the family when the death is unexpected takes the role. Often nurses are in an optimal position to suggest tissue donation after consultation with the attending physician. When possible, the topic should be raised before death occurs. The request should be made in a private and quiet area of the hospital and should be simple and direct, with questions such as "Are you a donor family?" or "Have you ever considered organ donation?"

Many states have legislated a mandatory request for organ or tissue donation when a child dies, especially if the patient is brain dead. Written consent from the family is required before donation can proceed. When requests for organ donation are made, health care practitioners must address common misunderstandings families have about brain death and organ donation (Franz, DeJong, Wolfe, and others, 1997). Training health care professionals on sensitive approaches to requests for organ donation has been shown to increase families' willingness to consent to organ donation (American Academy of Pediatrics, 2002; Evanisko, Beasley, Brigham, and others, 1998). The option to donate organs should always be separate from the communication of impending or actual death.

Nurses need to be aware of common questions about organ donation to help families make an informed decision. Healthy children who die unexpectedly are excellent candidates for organ donation. Children with cancer, chronic disease, or infection or those who have suffered prolonged cardiac arrest may not be suitable candidates, although this is individually determined. The nurse should ask whether organ donation was discussed with the child or whether the child ever expressed such a wish. Any number of body tissues or organs can be donated (skin, corneas, bone, kidney, heart, liver, pancreas), and their removal does not mutilate or desecrate the body or cause any suffering. The family may have an open casket, and there is no delay in the funeral. There is no cost to the donor family, but organ donation does not eliminate funeral or cremation responsibilities. Most religions permit organ donation as long as the recipient benefits from the transplant, although Orthodox Judaism forbids it.

In cases of unexplained death, violent death, or suspected suicide, autopsy is required by law. In other instances it may be optional, and parents should be informed of this choice. The procedure, as well as forms that require signing, should be explained. The family should know that the child can be in an open casket after an autopsy.

GRIEF AND MOURNING

Grief is a process, not an event, of experiencing physiologic, psychologic, behavioral, social, and spiritual reactions to the loss of a child. Grief is highly individualized, encompassing a broad range of manifestations from person to person. It is a natural and expected reaction to loss. It is neither orderly nor predictable. Grieving in any form is necessary for healing to occur. When death is the expected or a possible outcome of a disorder, the child and family members may experience **anticipatory grief.** Anticipatory grief may be manifested in varying behaviors and intensities and may include denial, anger, depression, and other psychologic and physical symptoms.

Anticipatory guidance may assist grieving family members. Health care professionals should emphasize that grief reactions such as hearing the dead person's voice, feeling distant from others, or seeking reassurance that they did everything possible for the lost person are normal, necessary, and expected. They in no way signify poor coping, insanity, or an approaching mental breakdown. On the contrary, such behaviors signify that the survivor is working through the acute grief. They are a necessary part of grief work. Anticipatory guidance regarding the mourning process may help families recognize the normalcy of their experiences.

It is important to recognize that some family members may experience complicated grief. **Complicated grief reactions** (more than a year after the loss) include such symptoms as intense intrusive thoughts, pangs of severe emotion, distressing yearnings, feelings of excessive loneliness and emptiness, unusual sleep disturbance, and maladaptive levels of loss of interest in personal activities (Horowitz, Siegel, Holen, and others, 1997). Bereaved persons experiencing such prolonged and complicated grief should be referred to an expert in grief and bereavement counseling.

Another important aspect of grief is the individual nature of the grief experience. Each member of the family will experience the grief of the child's death in his or her own way based on the particular relationship with that child. This can create potential conflict for families, since each family member has expectations that the other family members should feel and grieve as they do. Nurses caring for families experiencing grief should be aware of the different grieving styles and help the family learn to recognize and support the uniqueness of each other's grief.

Parental Grief

Parental grief after the death of a child has been found to be the most intense, complex, long-lasting, and fluctuating grief experience when compared with that of other bereaved individuals. Although parents experience the primary loss of their child, many secondary losses are felt such as the loss of part of one's self, hopes and dreams for the child's future, the family unit, prior social and emotional community supports, and often spousal support. It is common for parents of the same child to experience different grief reactions.

Studies with bereaved parents have shown that grieving does not end with the severing of the bond with the deceased child, but rather involves a continuing bond between the parent and the deceased child (Klass, 2001). Parental resolution of grief is a process of integrating the dead child into daily life where the pain of losing a child is never completely gone, but lessens. There are occasions of brief relapse, but not to the degree experienced when the loss initially occurred. Thus parental grief work is never completed and is a timeless process of accommodating the new reality of being without a child, as it changes over time (Davies, 2004). A child's death can also challenge the marital relationship in several ways. Maternal and paternal reactions often differ (Birenbaum, Stewart, and Phillips, 1996; Moriarty, Carroll, and Cotroneo, 1996; Vance, Najman, Thearle, and others, 1995). Different grieving styles between the couple may hinder communication and support for each other. Differing needs and expectations can place a strain on the marriage.

Sibling Grief

Each child grieves in his or her own way and on his or her own timeline. Children, even adolescents, grieve differently than adults. Adults and children differ more widely in their reactions to death than in their reactions to any other phenomenon. Children of all ages grieve the loss of a loved one, and their understanding and reactions to death depend on their age and developmental level. Children grieve for a longer duration, revisiting their grief as they grow and develop new understandings of death. However, they do not grieve 100% of the time. They grieve in spurts and can be emotional and sad in one instance and then, just as quickly, off and playing. Children express their grief though play and behavior. Children can be exquisitely attuned to their parents' grief and will try to protect them by not asking questions or by trying not to upset them. This can set the stage for the sibling to try to become the "perfect child." Children exhibit many of the grief reactions of adults, including physical sensations and illnesses, anger, guilt, sadness, loneliness, withdrawal, acting out, seep disturbances, isolation, and search for meaning. Again, nurses should be attentive for signs that siblings are struggling with their grief and provide guidance to parents when possible.

At times family members may need assistance in their grieving (see Nursing Care Guidelines box). Communication with the bereaved family is essential, but often nurses do not know what to say and feel helpless in offering words of comfort. The most supportive approach is to avoid judging the

---

nursingcareguidelines

Supporting Grieving Families*

GENERAL

Stay with the family; sit quietly if they prefer not to talk; cry with them if desired.

Accept the family's grief reactions; avoid judgmental statements (e.g., "You should be feeling better by now").

Avoid offering rationalizations for the child's death (e.g., "Your child isn't suffering anymore").

Avoid artificial consolation (e.g., "I know how you feel," or "You are still young enough to have another baby").

Deal openly with feelings such as guilt, anger, and loss of self-esteem.

Focus on feelings by using a feeling word in the statement (e.g., "You're still feeling all the pain of losing a child").

Refer the family to an appropriate self-help group or for professional help if needed.

AT THE TIME OF DEATH

Reassure the family that everything possible is being done for the child, if they want lifesaving interventions.

Do everything possible to ensure the child's comfort, especially relieving pain.

Provide the child and family with the opportunity to review special experiences or memories in their lives.

Express personal feelings of loss or frustrations (e.g., "We will miss him so much," "We tried everything; we feel so sorry that we couldn't save her").

Provide information that the family requests and be honest.

Respect the emotional needs of family members, such as siblings, who may need brief respites from the dying child.

Make every effort to arrange for family members, especially parents, to be with the child at the moment of death, if they want to be present.

Allow the family to stay with the dead child for as long as they wish and to rock, hold, or bathe the child.

Provide practical help when possible, such as collecting the child's belongings.

Arrange for spiritual support, based on the family's religious beliefs; pray with the family if no one else can stay with them.

POSTDEATH

Attend the funeral or visitation if there was a special closeness with the family.

Initiate and maintain contact (e.g., sending cards, telephoning, inviting them back to the unit, making a home visit).

Refer to the dead child by name; discuss shared memories with the family.

Discourage the use of drugs or alcohol as a method of escaping grief.

Encourage all family members to communicate their feelings rather than remaining silent to avoid upsetting another member.

Emphasize that grieving is a painful process that often takes years to resolve.

*"Family" refers to all significant persons involved in the child's life, such as the parents, siblings, grandparents, or other close relatives or friends.

family's reactions or offering advice or rationalizations and to focus on feelings. Perhaps the most valuable supportive measure the nurse can perform for families is to listen. Families understand that no words will relieve their pain; all they want is acceptance, understanding, and respect for their grief.

It is important for families to understand that mourning takes a long time. Whereas acute grief may last only weeks or months, resolving the loss is measured in years. Holidays and anniversaries can be particularly difficult, and people who previously had been supportive may now expect the family to have "adjusted." Consequently, prolonged mourning is often silent and lonely.

Many families never receive the support and guidance that could help them resolve the loss. A plan for regular follow-up with bereaved families can be beneficial. At minimum, one follow-up phone call or meeting with the family should be arranged. Families can also be referred to self-help groups. When such groups are not available, nurses can be instrumental in bringing families together or facilitating parent and sibling groups. Formal bereavement programs or bereavement counseling can be helpful as well.

For more information on end-of-life care, visit these websites:

Americans for Better Care of the Dying—http://www.abcd-caring.org
End-of-Life/Palliative Education Resource Center—http://www.eperc.mcw.edu
Growth House—http://www.growthhouse.org
Robert Wood Johnson Foundation—http://www.rwjf.org

NURSES' REACTIONS TO CARING FOR DYING CHILDREN

The death of a patient is one of the most stressful aspects of critical care or oncology nursing (see Family Focus box).* Nurses experience reactions to a fatal illness that are very

---

*Other sources of publications on life-threatening illness and death are the Compassionate Friends, PO Box 3696, Oak Brook, IL 60522-3696; (630) 990-0010 or (877) 969-0010; http://www.compassionatefriends.org; Centering Corporation, 7230 Maple St., Omaha, NE 68134; (866) 218-0101; http://www.centering.org; Children's Hospice International, 1104 King St., Suite 360, Alexandria, VA 22314; (800) 24-CHILD or (703) 684-0330; e-mail: info@chionline.org; http://www.chionline.org; and National Cancer Institute, Cancer Information Service, Building 21, Room 10A29, Bethesda, MD 20892-2580; (800) 422-6237; http://www.cancer.gov.

FAMILY FOCUS

A Dying Child: A Nurse's Perspective

Claire was unresponsive with slow, gasping breathing. Her mother asked me what I thought was happening. I replied honestly, "Your baby is dying because of her brain tumor." The mother put her arms around me and cried. We arranged for Claire to be baptized.

Honesty. As painful as the loss of a child is, my job is to assist the family through this experience. Although I usually wait until a private moment, such as driving home, I found tears streaming down my face as family and friends gathered for Claire's baptism. I went into the kitchen to compose myself, only to find several of my colleagues crying as well. Saying goodbye to a dying child will always be a difficult but shared experience.

Jeanne O'Connor Egan, RN, MSN
Pediatric Clinical Specialist, Children's Hospital
Washington, DC

---

similar to the responses of family members, including denial, anger, depression, guilt, and ambivalent feelings.

Strategies that can assist the nurse in maintaining the ability to work effectively in these settings include maintaining good general health, developing well-rounded interests, using distancing techniques such as taking time off when needed, developing and using professional and personal support systems, cultivating the capacity for empathy, focusing on the positive aspects of the caregiver role, and basing nursing interventions on sound theory and empiric observations. Attending shared-remembrance rituals assists some nurses in resolving grief (Davis and Eng, 1998). Similarly, attending the funeral services can be a supportive act for both the family and the nurse and in no way detracts from the professionalism of care.

KEY POINTS

■ Trends in the treatment of children with chronic illness or disability have focused on developmental age, the child's strengths and uniqueness, family-centered care, normalization, early discharge, home care, mainstreaming, and early intervention.

■ In response to the child with chronic illness or disability, parents may be affected by feelings of inadequacy and failure; excessive demands on time, energy, and financial resources; and strain on the marital relationship.

■ Families' reactions to disability or chronic illness are manifested in the following stages: shock and denial, adjustment, reintegration, and acknowledgment.

■ The child's reaction to illness or disability depends on the child's developmental level, coping mechanisms, others' reactions, and the illness itself.

■ Assessment of the family's adjustment to a child's chronic illness, disability, or death includes the availability of a support system, their perception of the event, their coping mechanisms, concurrent stressors, and their response to the child.

■ To help parents cope with their child's chronic illness or disability, nurses must offer attentiveness, humanistic support, solicitation of suggestions for care, facilitation of communication, verbalization of feelings, and referral to volunteer and community agencies.

■ Supporting the child involves encouraging self-expression, alleviating feelings of being different, and strengthening the child's self-image.

■ Children's concept of death is determined by their cognitive ability and their experience with life-threatening illness.

■ Young children see death as temporary and reversible and mainly fear separation.

■ School-age children view death as irreversible but not necessarily inevitable and may fear mutilation.

■ Children beyond 9 to 10 years of age realize that death is irreversible, universal, and inevitable but may resist the thought of their own death.

■ Siblings have special needs, including the need for information, reassurance about their own health status, assurance that they are not responsible for the illness or death, and support for their own grieving process.

■ Special needs of the family facing the unexpected death of a child include support while awaiting news of the child's status; a sensitive pronouncement of death; acknowledgment of feelings of denial, guilt, and anger; an opportunity to view the body; and referrals for support.

■ Special decisions at the time of dying and death may involve hospital or hospice care, visualization of the body, tissue donation and autopsy, and siblings' attendance at the funeral.

■ Acute grief is a syndrome with intense and distressing psychologic and somatic symptoms that appear at the time of death.

■ In dealing with stress related to the dying patient, the nurse can cope successfully through self-awareness, consciousness raising, knowledge and practice, an available support system, and maintenance of general good health, and by focusing on the positive rewards of involvement with dying children and their families.

REFERENCES

Ahmann E: "Chunky stew": appreciating cultural diversity while providing health care for children, *Pediatr Nurs* 20(3):320-324, 1994.

American Academy of Pediatrics: Committee on Hospital Care and Section on Surgery: Pediatric organ donation and transplantation, *Pediatrics* 109(5):982-984, 2002.

American Nurses Association: *Code of ethics for nurses with interpretive statements,* Washington, DC, 2001, ANA Publishing.

Anderson RN, Smith BL: Deaths: leading causes, *Natl Vital Stat Rep* 53(17):1-89, 2005.

Arias E, MacDorman MF, Strobino DM, and others: Annual summary of vital statistics—2002, *Pediatrics* 112(6):1215-1230, 2003.

Barlow JH, Ellard DR: The psychosocial well-being of children with chronic disease, their parents and siblings: an overview of the research evidence base, *Child Care Health Dev* 32(1):19-31, 2006.

Birenbaum LK, Stewart BJ, Phillips DS: Health status of bereaved parents, *Nurs Res* 45(2):105-109, 1996.

Carnevale FA, Alexander E, Davis M, and others: Daily living with distress and enrichment: the moral experience of families with ventilator-assisted children at home, *Pediatrics* 117(1):e48-60, 2006.

Carter B: Chronic pain in childhood and the medical encounter: professional ventriloquism and hidden voices, *Qual Health Res* 12:28-41, 2002.

Charles C, Gafni A, Whelan T: Shared decision making in the medical encounter: what does it mean? *Soc Sci Med* 44:681-692, 1997.

Clements PT, Vigil GJ, Manno MS, and others: Cultural perspectives of death, grief, and bereavement, *J Psychosoc Nurs Ment Health Serv* 41(7):18-26, 2003.

Coffey JS: Parenting a child with chronic illness: a metasynthesis, *Pediatr Nurs* 32(1):51-59, 2006.

Cohen MH: The stages of the prediagnostic period in chronic life-threatening childhood illness: a process analysis, *Res Nurs Health* 18(1):39-48, 1995.

Corlett J, Twycross A: Negotiation of parental roles within family-centered care: a review of the research, *J Clin Nurs* 15(10):1308-1316, 2006.

Davies B, Gudmundsdottir M, Worden B, and others: "Living in the dragon's shadow": fathers' experiences of a child's life-limiting illness, *Death Studies* 28(2):111-135, 2004.

Davies R: New understandings of parental grief: literature review, *J Adv Nurs* 46(5):506-513, 2004.

Davies R, Davis B, Sibert J: Parents' stories of sensitive and insensitive care by paediatricians in the time leading up to and including diagnostic disclosure of a life-limiting condition in their child, *Child Care Health Dev* 29(1):77-82, 2003.

Davis B, Eng B: Special issues in bereavement and staff support. In Doyle D, Hanks GWC, MacDonald N, editors: *Oxford textbook of palliative medicine,* ed 2, Oxford University Press, 1998, Oxford.

Deatrick JA, Knafl KA, Murphy-Moore C: Clarifying the concept of normalization, *Image J Nurs Sch* 31:209-214, 1999.

Denboba D, McPherson MG, Kenney MK, and others: Achieving family and provider partnerships for children with special health care needs, *Pediatrics* 118(4):1607-1615, 2006.

Dixon-Woods M, Young B, Henry D: Partnerships with children, *Br J Med* 319:778-780, 1999.

Evanisko MJ, Beasley CL, Brigham LE, and others: Readiness of critical care physicians and nurses to handle requests for organ donation, *Am J Crit Care* 7(1):4-12, 1998.

Faulkner KW, Armstrong-Dailey A: Care of the dying child. In Pizzo PA, Poplack DG, editors: *Principles and practice of pediatric oncology,* Philadelphia, 1997, Lippincott-Raven.

Field MJ, Behrman RE, editors: *When children die: improving palliative and end-of-life care for children and their families,* Washington, DC, 2004, National Academies Press.

Fleitas J: When Jack fell down . . . Jill came tumbling after: siblings in the web of illness and disability, *MCN* 25:267-273, 2000.

Forrester L: One to one care in children's hospice, *Nurs Times* 99(16):44-45, 2003.

Franz HG, DeJong W, Wolfe SM, and others: Explaining brain death: a critical feature of the donation process, *J Transplant Coord* 7(1):14-21, 1997.

Freyer DR: Care of the dying adolescent: special considerations, *Pediatrics* 113(2):381-388, 2004.

Garwick AW, Patterson J, Bennett FC, and others: Breaking the news: how families first learn about their child's chronic condition, *Arch Pediatr Adolesc Med* 149(9):991-997, 1995.

Goldbeck L: Parental coping with the diagnosis of childhood cancer: gender effects, dissimilarity within couples, and quality of life, *Psychooncology* 10:325-335, 2001.

Goodenough B, Drew D, Higgins S, and others: Bereavement outcomes for parents who lose a child to cancer: are place of death and sex of parent associated with differences in psychological functioning? *Psycho-Oncology* 13(11):779-791, 2004.

Gravelle AM: Caring for a child with a progressive illness during the complex chronic phase: parents' experience of facing adversity, *J Adv Nurs* 25:738-745, 1997.

Hawryluck LA, Harvey WR: Analgesia, virtue, and the principle of double effect, *J Palliative Care* 16(Suppl):S24-S30, 2000.

Hellsten MB, Hockenberry M, Lamb D, and others: *End-of-life care for children,* Austin, Tex, 2000, Texas Cancer Council.

Hinds PS, Oakes L, Furman W, and others: End-of-life decision making by adolescents, parents, and healthcare providers in pediatric oncology: research to evidence-based practice guidelines, *Cancer Nurs* 24:122-134, 2001.

Horowitz MJ, Siegel B, Holen A, and others: Diagnostic criteria for complicated grief disorder, *Am J Psychiatry* 154(7):904-910, 1997.

Immelt S: Psychological adjustment in young children with chronic medical conditions, *J Pediatr Nurs* 21(5):362-377, 2006.

Jackson PL: The primary care provider and children with chronic conditions. In Jackson PL, Vessey PA, editors: *Primary care of the child with a chronic condition,* ed 3, St Louis, 2000, Mosby.

James L, Johnson B: The needs of parents of pediatric oncology patients during the palliative care phase, *J Pediatr Oncol Nurs* 14(2):83-95, 1997.

Jennings PD: Providing pediatric palliative care through a pediatric supportive care team, *Pediatr Nurs* 31(3):195-200, 2005.

Jokinen P: The family life-path theory: a tool for nurses working in partnership with families, *J Child Health Care* 8(2):124-133, 2004.

Klass D: The inner representation of the dead child in the psychic and social narratives of bereaved parents. In Neimeyer RA, editor: *Meaning reconstruction and the experience of loss,* Washington, DC, 2001, American Psychological Association.

Lambert S: Distraction, imagery, and hypnosis techniques for management of children's pain, *J Child Fam Nurs* 2(1):5-15, 1999.

Lauer ME, Mulhern RK, Schell MJ, and others: Long-term follow-up of parental adjustment following a child's death at home or hospital, *Cancer* 63(5):988-994, 1989.

Lobato DJ, Kao BT: Integrated sibling-parent group intervention to improve sibling knowledge and adjustment to chronic illness and disability, *J Pediatr Psychol* 27:711-716, 2002.

Lobato DJ, Kao BT, Plante W: Latino sibling knowledge and adjustment to chronic illness, *J Fam Psychol* 19(4):625-632, 2005.

Marshall ES, Olsen SF, Mandleco BL, and others: "This is a spiritual experience": perspectives of Latter-Day Saint families living with a child with disabilities, *Qual Health Res* 13:57-76, 2003.

Masri C, Farrell CA, Lacroix J, and others: Decision making and end-of-life care in critically ill children, *J Palliative Care* 16(Suppl):S45-S52, 2000.

Mastroyannopoulou K, Stallard P, Lewis M, and others: The impact of childhood non-malignant life threatening illness on parents: gender differences and predictors of parental adjustment, *J Child Psychol Psychiatry* 38(7):823-829, 1997.

McDougal J: Promoting normalization in families with preschool children with type 1 diabetes, *J Specialty Pediatr Nurs* 7(3):113-120, 2002.

McPherson M, Weissman G, Strickland BB, and others: Implementing community-based systems of services for child and youths with special health care needs: how well are we doing? *Pediatrics* 113(5):1538-1544, 2004.

Moriarty H, Carroll R, Cotroneo M: Differences in bereavement reactions within couples following the death of a child, *Res Nurs Health* 19:461-469, 1996.

Morse JM, Wilson S, Penrod J: Mothers and their disabled children: refining the concept of normalization, *Health Care Woman Int* 21(8):659-676, 2000.

Msall ME, Avery RC, Tremont MR, and others: Functional disability and school activity limitations in 41,300 school-age children: relationship to medical impairments, *Pediatrics* 111:548-553, 2003.

Murray JS: Siblings of children with cancer: a review of the literature, *J Pediatr Oncol Nurs* 16(1):25-34, 1999.

Nelson AM: A metasynthesis: mothering other-than-normal children, *Qual Health Res* 12:515-530, 2002.

Newacheck PW, Halfon N: Prevalence and impact of disabling chronic conditions in childhood, *Am J Public Health* 88(4):610-617, 1998.

Newacheck PW, Strickland B, Shonkoff JP, and others: An epidemiologic profile of children with special health care needs, *Pediatrics* 102(1):117-123, 1998.

Nuutila L, Salanterä S: Children with a long-term illness: parents' experiences of care, *J Pediatr Nurs* 21(2):153-160, 2006.

O'Brien ME, Wegner CB: Rearing the child who is technology dependent: perceptions of parents and home care nurses, *J Spec Pediatr Nurs* 7:7-15, 2002.

Ochieng BM: Minority ethnic families and family-centered care, *J Child Health Care* 7(2):123-132, 2003.

Palfrey JS, Tonniges TF, Green M, and others: Introduction: addressing the millennial morbidity—the context of community pediatrics, *Pediatrics* 115(4 Suppl):1121-1123, 2005.

Perrin JM: Chronic illness in childhood. In Behrman RE, Kleigman RM, Jensen HB, editors: *Nelson textbook of pediatrics*, ed 17, Philadelphia, 2004, Saunders.

Pierucci RL, Kirby RS, Leuthner SR: End-of-life for neonates and infants: the experience and effects of a palliative care consultation service, *Pediatrics* 108(3):653-660, 2001.

Raina P, O'Donnell M, Rosenbaum P, and others: The health and well-being of caregivers of children with cerebral palsy, *Pediatrics* 115(6):e626-e636, 2005.

Ray LD: Parenting and childhood chronicity: making visible the invisible work, *J Pediatr Nurs* 17(6):424-438, 2002.

Rehm RS: Religious faith in Mexican-American families dealing with chronic childhood illness, *Image J Nurs Sch* 31:33-38, 1999.

Ritchie MA: Self-esteem and hopefulness in adolescents with cancer, *J Pediatr Nurs* 16:35-42, 2001.

Rossiter L, Sharpe D: The siblings of individuals with mental retardation: a quantitative integration of the literature, *J Child Fam Studies* 10(1):65-84, 2001.

Rousseau P: Ethical and legal issues in palliative care, *Prim Care* 28:391-400, 2001.

Sahler O, Frager G, Levetown M, and others: Medical education about end-of-life care in the pediatric setting: principles, challenges, and opportunities, *Pediatrics* 105:575-584, 2000.

Schor EL: Family pediatrics: report of the Task Force on the Family, *Pediatrics* 111:1541-1571, 2003.

Sharpe D, Rossiter L: Siblings of children with a chronic illness: a meta-analysis, *J Pediatr Psychol* 27:699-710, 2002.

Shepard MP, Mahon MM: Chronic conditions and the family. In Jackson PL, Vessey JA, editors: *Primary care of the child with a chronic condition*, ed 3, St Louis, 2000, Mosby.

Sine D, Sumner L, Gracy D, and others: Pediatric extubation: "pulling the tube," *J Palliative Med* 4:519-524, 2001.

Stein REK: Home care: a challenging opportunity, *Child Health Care* 14(2):90-95, 1985.

Sterling YM, Peterson JW: Characteristics of African American women caregivers of children with asthma, *MCN* 28:32-38, 2003.

Sullivan-Bolyai S, Sadler L, Knafl KA, and others: Great expectations: a position description for parents as caregivers, part I, *Pediatr Nurs* 29(6):52-56, 2003.

Sumner LH: Lighting the way: improving the way children die in America, *Caring* 22:14-18, 2003.

Swallow VM, Jacoby A: Mothers' evolving relationships with doctors and nurses during the chronic childhood illness trajectory, *J Adv Nurs* 36:755-764, 2001.

Thomlinson EH: The lived experience of families of children who are failing to thrive, *J Adv Nurs* 39:537-545, 2002.

Tong H, Kandala G, Haig AJ, and others: Physical functioning in female caregivers of children with physical disabilities compared with female caregivers of children with a chronic medical condition, *Arch Pediatr Adolesc Med* 156:1138-1142, 2002.

Vance JC, Najman JM, Thearle MJ, and others: Psychological changes in parents eight months after the loss of an infant from stillbirth, neonatal death, or sudden infant death syndrome—a longitudinal study, *Pediatrics* 96(5):933-938, 1995.

Van Dyck P, Kogan MD, Heppel D, and others: The national survey of children's health: a new data resource, *Matern Child Health J* 8(3):183-188, 2004.

Van Dyck PC, Kogan MD, McPherson MG, and others: Prevalence and characteristics of children with special health care needs, *Arch Pediatr Adolesc Med* 158(9):884-890, 2004.

Whitehead LC, Gosling V: Parent's perceptions of interactions with health professionals in the pathway to gaining a diagnosis of tuberous sclerosis (TS) and beyond, *Res Dev Disabil* 24:109-119, 2003.

Winkler WD, Mardegian CA: Completing the continuum of care: the growth of a pediatric hospice program, *Caring* 20:22-25, 2001.

Wise PH, Wampler NS, Chavkin W, and others: Chronic illness among poor children enrolled in the temporary assistance for needy families program, *Am J Public Health* 92:1458-1461, 2002.

Wolfe J, Friebert S, Hilden J: Caring for children with advanced cancer integrating palliative care, *Pediatr Clin North Am* 49(5):1043-1062, 2002.

Wolfe J, Grier HE, Klar N, and others: Symptoms and suffering at the end of life in children with cancer, *N Engl J Med* 342(5):326-333, 2000.

Wood PR, Smith LA, Romero D, and others: Relationships between welfare status, health insurance status, and health and medical care among children with asthma, *Am J Public Health* 92:1446-1452, 2002.

World Health Organization: *Cancer pain relief and palliative care*, Geneva, 1996, The Organization.

Yogev R, Chadwick EG: Acquired immunodeficiency syndrome. In Behrman RE, Kleigman RM, Jensen HB, editors: *Nelson textbook of pediatrics*, ed 17, Philadelphia, 2004, Saunders.

Young B, Dixon-Woods M, Windridge KC, and others: Managing communication with young people who have a potentially life threatening chronic illness: qualitative study of patients and parents, *BJM* 326(7384):305, 2003.

Zuvekas SH, Taliaferro GS: Pathways to access: health, insurance, the health care delivery system and racial/ethnic disparities, 1996-1999, *Health Affairs* 22(2):139-153, 2003.

19

Impact of Cognitive or Sensory Impairment on the Child and Family

ROSALIND BRYANT

CHAPTER OUTLINE

COGNITIVE IMPAIRMENT, 611
General Concepts, 611
Nursing Care of Children with Impaired Cognitive Function, 612
Nursing Care Plan: The Child with Impaired Cognitive Function, 614

Down Syndrome, 619
Fragile X Syndrome, 622
SENSORY IMPAIRMENT, 623
Hearing Impairment, 623
Visual Impairment, 628

Deaf-Blind Children, 633
Retinoblastoma, 633
Autism Spectrum Disorders, 635

LEARNING OBJECTIVES

On completion of this chapter the reader will be able to:
- Define the classifications of intellectual disability.
- Define developmental delay.
- Outline nursing interventions for the child with cognitive impairment that promote optimal development, including during hospitalization.
- Identify the major biologic and cognitive characteristics of the child with Down syndrome.

- Outline nursing interventions for the child with Down syndrome.
- Identify the major characteristics associated with fragile X syndrome.
- List the general classifications of hearing impairment and the effect on speech.
- Outline nursing interventions for the child with hearing impairment, including during hospitalization.

- List the common types of visual disorders in children.
- Outline nursing interventions for the child with visual impairment, including during hospitalization.
- Outline nursing interventions for the child with retinoblastoma.
- Outline nursing interventions for the child with an autism spectrum disorder.

RELATED TOPICS and ADDITIONAL RESOURCES

 IN TEXT

Auditory Testing, *Ch. 6*
Defects Caused by Chemical Agents, *Ch. 9*
Dental Health: Toddler, *Ch. 12;* School-Age
    Child, *Ch. 15*
Developmental Assessment, *Ch. 6*
Family-Centered Home Care, *Ch. 20*
Chronic Illness, Disability, or End-of-Life
    Care for the Child and Family, *Ch. 18*
Limit Setting and Discipline, *Ch. 3*
Optic, Otic, and Nasal Administration (of
    Medication), *Ch. 22*
Otitis Media, *Ch. 23*

Play: Infant, *Ch. 10;* Toddler, *Ch. 12;*
    Preschooler, *Ch. 13;* School-Age Child,
    Ch. 15
Preparation for Hospitalization, *Ch. 21*
Toilet Training, *Ch. 12*
Toy Safety, *Ch. 5*
Vision Testing, *Ch. 6*

COMPANION CD

Case Study—Down Syndrome
Critical Thinking Exercises—Diagnosis of
    Down Syndrome in the Neonate; Down
    Syndrome; Fragile X Syndrome
NCLEX Review Questions

evolve.elsevier.com/Wong/essentials/

NCLEX Review Questions
Nursing Care Plan—The Child with
    Impaired Cognitive Function
WebLinks

**WONG'S CLINICAL MANUAL
OF PEDIATRIC NURSING, 7th Ed**

Patient and Family Education—Suctioning
    the Nose and Mouth, *p. 566;* Giving Eye
    Medications, *p. 539*

COGNITIVE IMPAIRMENT

GENERAL CONCEPTS

Cognitive impairment (**CI**) is a general term that encompasses any type of mental difficulty or deficiency. In this chapter the term is used synonymously with intellectual disability (**mental retardation**). Although the needs and concerns of the family are a primary focus throughout the chapter, the reader is encouraged to review Chapter 18, which details the family's adjustment to disabilities in general.

The definition of intellectual disability in children consists of three components: intellectual functioning, functional strengths and weaknesses, and age younger than 18 years at time of diagnosis. Intellectual functioning is measured by the intelligence quotient (IQ) of 70 to 75 or below. The child with an intellectual disability must demonstrate functional impairment in at least two of 10 different adaptive skill areas: communication, self-care, home living, social skills, leisure, health and safety, self-direction, functional academics, community use, and work (American Psychiatric Association, 2000). The classification system by the American Association on Intellectual and Developmental Disabilities allows for identification of the individual's specific needs in four established dimensions of care (Box 19-1). Careful evaluation to identify the needs of individuals with CI is focused on promoting habilitation for each person. It is anticipated that the functional capabilities of children with CI will improve over time when support is provided.

Diagnosis and Classification

The diagnosis of CI is usually made after a period of suspicion, by professionals or the family, that the child's developmental progress is delayed. In some cases it is confirmed at birth because of recognition of distinct syndromes, such as Down syndrome and fetal alcohol syndrome. At the other extreme, the diagnosis is made when problems such as speech delays arouse concern. In all cases a high index of suspicion for developmental delay and behavioral signs (Box 19-2) is necessary for early diagnosis; routine developmental screening can assist in early identification (see Chapter 5). Delays are

---

BOX 19-1

Dimensions of Care for the Intellectually Disabled

Dimension I—Intellectual functioning and adaptive skills
Dimension II—Psychologic and emotional considerations
Dimension III—Physical, health, and etiology considerations
Dimension IV—Environmental considerations

BOX 19-2

Early Behavioral Signs Suggestive of Cognitive Impairment

- Dysmorphic features (e.g., Down syndrome, fragile X syndrome)
- Irritability or unresponsiveness to contact
- Abnormal eye contact during feeding
- Gross motor delay
- Decreased alertness to voice or movement
- Language difficulties or delay
- Feeding difficulties

From Crocker A, Nelson R: Mental retardation. In Levine M, Carey WB, Crocker AC, editors: *Developmental-behavioral pediatrics,* ed 3, Philadelphia, 1999, Saunders; and Shapiro B, Batshaw M: Mental retardation. In Behrman RE, Kliegman RM, Jenson HB, editors: *Nelson textbook of pediatrics,* ed 17, Philadelphia, 2004, Saunders.

---

typically seen in gross and fine motor and speech development, although the latter is most predictive. **Developmental delay** can be described as any significant lag in a child's physical, cognitive, behavioral, emotional, or social development, when compared against developmental norms. CI is a permanent impairment encompassing cognitive ability and adaptive behavior that are functioning significantly below average (see Box 19-2). In the absence of clear-cut evidence of CI, it is more appropriate to use a diagnosis of developmental delay (Biasini, Grupe, Huffman, and others, 1999).

Results of standardized tests are used in making the diagnosis of intellectual disability (mental retardation) based on

TABLE 19-1			
Classification of Cognitive Impairment			
LEVEL (IQ)*	PRESCHOOL (BIRTH–5 YEARS)—MATURATION AND DEVELOPMENT	SCHOOL AGE (6-21 YEARS)—TRAINING AND EDUCATION	ADULT (21 YEARS AND OLDER)—SOCIAL AND VOCATIONAL ADEQUACY
Mild—50-55 to approximately 70-75	Often not noticed as delayed by casual observer but is slower to walk, feed self, and talk than most children; follows same sequence in development as normal children	Can acquire practical skills and useful reading and arithmetic to a third- to sixth-grade level with special education; can be guided toward social conformity; achieves mental age of 8-12 years	Can usually achieve social and vocational skills adequate to self-maintenance; may need occasional guidance and support when under unusual social or economic stress; can adjust to marriage but not childrearing
Moderate—35-40 to 50-55	Noticeable delays in motor development, especially in speech; responds to training in various self-help activities	Can learn simple communication, elementary health and safety habits, and simple manual skills; does not progress in functional reading or arithmetic; achieves mental age of 3-7 years	Can perform simple tasks under sheltered conditions; participates in simple recreation; travels alone in familiar places; usually incapable of self-maintenance
Severe—20-25 to 35-40	Marked delay in motor development; little or no communication skills; may respond to training in elementary self-care (e.g., self-feeding)	Usually walks, barring specific disability; has some understanding of speech and some response; can profit from systematic habit training; achieves mental age of toddler	Can conform to daily routines and repetitive activities; needs continuing direction and supervision in protective environment
Profound—below 20-25	Gross delay; minimum capacity for functioning in sensorimotor areas; needs total care	Obvious delays in all areas of development; shows basic emotional responses; may respond to skillful training in use of legs, hands, and jaws; needs close supervision; achieves mental age of young infant	May walk; needs complete custodial care; has primitive speech; usually benefits from regular physical activity

IQ, Intelligence quotient.

*Data from American Psychiatric Association: *Diagnostic and statistical manual of mental disorders*, ed 4 (text rev) (DSM-IV TR), Washington, DC, 2000, The Association; and Rittey CD: Learning difficulties: what the neurologist needs to know, *J Neurol Neurosurg Psychiatry* 74(Suppl 1):30-36, 2005.

cognitive deficits. Tests for assessing adaptive behaviors include the Vineland Social Maturity Scale and the AAMR Adaptive Behavior Scale. Informal appraisal of adaptive behavior may be made by those fully acquainted with the child (e.g., teachers, parents, other care providers). Frequently these observations lead parents to seek evaluation of the child's development.

A more useful approach for clinical application is classification based on educational potential or symptom severity. For educational purposes the term **educable mentally retarded (EMR)** corresponds to the mildly impaired group, which constitutes about 85% of all people with CI. **Trainable mentally retarded (TMR)** generally applies to children with moderate levels of CI and accounts for about 10% of the intellectually disabled population (American Psychiatric Association, 2000; Walker and Johnson, 2006) (Table 19-1). Although nurses may be familiar with the approximate range of IQ for classifying severity, they should refrain from using numbers as the criterion for assessing or evaluating the child's abilities, since numbers are of little value in counseling parents or training these children.

Etiology

The causes of severe CI are primarily genetic, biochemical, and infectious. Although the etiology is unknown in the majority of cases, familial, social, environmental, and organic causes may predominate. Among individuals with CI, a sizable proportion of the cases are linked to Down syndrome, fragile X syndrome, or fetal alcohol syndrome. General categories of events that may lead to CI include (Walker and Johnson, 2006; Kabra and Gulati, 2003):

■ Infection and intoxication, such as congenital rubella, syphilis, maternal drug consumption (e.g., fetal alcohol syndrome), chronic lead ingestion, or kernicterus
■ Trauma or physical agent (i.e., injury to the brain suffered during the prenatal, perinatal, or postnatal period)
■ Inadequate nutrition and metabolic disorders, such as phenylketonuria or congenital hypothyroidism
■ Gross postnatal brain disease, such as neurofibromatosis and tuberous sclerosis
■ Unknown prenatal influence, including cerebral and cranial malformations, such as microcephaly and hydrocephalus
■ Chromosomal abnormalities resulting from radiation; viruses; chemicals; parental age; and genetic mutations, such as Down syndrome and fragile X syndrome
■ Gestational disorders, including prematurity, low birth weight, and postmaturity
■ Psychiatric disorders that have their onset during the child's developmental period up to age 18 years, such as autism spectrum disorders
■ Environmental influences, including evidence of a deprived environment associated with a history of intellectual disability among parents and siblings

NURSING CARE OF CHILDREN WITH IMPAIRED COGNITIVE FUNCTION

Nurses play a major role in identifying children with CI. In the newborn and early infancy periods, few signs are present, with the exception of Down syndrome (p. 619). After this age, however, delayed developmental milestones are the major clues to CI. In addition, nurses must have a high index of suspicion for early behavior patterns that may suggest CI (see Box 19-2). Parental concerns, such as delayed development compared with siblings, need to be taken seriously. All children should receive regular developmental assessment, and the nurse is often the person responsible for performing such assessments (see Chapter 5). When delays are found, the nurse must use sensitivity and discretion in revealing this finding to parents (see Nursing Care Plan).

Educate Child and Family. To teach children with CI, it is necessary to investigate their learning abilities and deficits. This is important for the nurse who may be involved in a home care program or who may be caring for the child in a health care setting. The nurse who understands how these children learn can effectively teach them basic skills or prepare them for various health-related procedures.

Children with CI have a marked deficit in their ability to discriminate between two or more stimuli because of difficulty in recognizing the relevance of specific cues. However, these children can learn to discriminate if the cues are presented in an exaggerated, concrete form and if all extraneous stimuli are eliminated. For example, the use of colors to emphasize visual cues or the use of singing or rhymes to stress auditory cues can help them learn. Their deficit in discrimination also implies that concrete ideas are learned much more effectively than abstract ideas. Therefore demonstration is preferable to verbal explanation, and learning should be directed toward mastering a skill rather than understanding the scientific principles underlying a procedure.

Another cognitive deficit is in short-term memory. Whereas children of average intelligence can remember several words, numbers, or directions at one time, children with CI are less able to do so. Therefore they need simple, one-step directions. Learning through a step-by-step process requires a **task analysis,** in which each task is separated into its necessary components and each step is taught completely before proceeding to the next activity.

One critical area of learning that has had a tremendous impact on education for cognitively impaired individuals is **motivation.** Programs based on the motivational principles of behavior modification, employing positive reinforcement for specific tasks or behaviors, have demonstrated marked improvement in children's ability to learn. Advances in technology have greatly aided in providing reinforcement, especially in children who are severely disabled and who may have physical disabilities that limit their range of capabilities. For example, with the use of specially designed switches, children are given control of some event in the environment, such as turning on the television (Fig. 19-1). The television picture becomes reinforcement for activating the switch. Repetitive use of these switches provides an early, simplistic association with a technical device that may progress to increasingly complex aids.

Early intervention program is a systematic program of therapy, exercises, and activities designed to address developmental delays in disabled children to help achieve their full potentials (American Academy of Pediatrics, 2001; National Down Syndrome Society, 2006). There is considerable evidence that these programs are valuable for cognitively impaired children. Nurses working with these families need to be aware of the types of programs in their community. Under the Individuals with Disabilities Education Act (IDEA) of 1990 (Public Law 101-476), states are encouraged to provide full early intervention services and are required to provide educational opportunities for all children with disabilities from birth to 21 years of age. Services may be provided under state

FIG. 19-1 ■ A push panel allows a child with cognitive impairment to turn a computer on and off.

Programs for Children with Special Health Needs or Head Start, or by private organizations such as National Down Syndrome Society,* Easter Seals,† or the Arc of the United States.‡ Parents should inquire about these programs by contacting the appropriate agencies. The child's education should begin as soon as possible. As children grow older, their education should be directed toward vocational training that prepares them for as independent a lifestyle as possible within their scope of abilities.

Teach Child Self-Care Skills. When a child with CI is born, parents need assistance in promoting normal developmental skills that are almost automatically learned by other children. These include self-care skills such as feeding, toileting, dressing, and grooming. Teaching these skills requires a basic knowledge of the developmental sequence in learning the skills demonstrated by children of average intelligence. For example, children with subaverage intelligence would not be expected to dress themselves as early as unaffected youngsters.

Teaching self-care skills also necessitates a working knowledge of the individual steps needed to master a skill. For example, before beginning a self-feeding program, the nurse performs a task analysis. After a task analysis, the child is observed in a particular situation, such as eating, to determine what skills are possessed and the child's developmental readiness to learn the task. Family members are included in this process because their "readiness" is as important as the child's. Numerous self-help aids are available to facilitate independence and can help eliminate some of the difficulties of learning, such as using a plate with suction cups to prevent accidental spills.§

---

*Information on early intervention programs in each state is available from the National Down Syndrome Society, 666 Broadway, New York, NY 10012-2317; (800) 221-4602; fax: (212) 979-2873; http://www.ndss.org.
†230 W. Monroe St., Suite 1800, Chicago, IL 60606-4802; (800) 221-6827; TTY: (312) 726-4258; fax: (312) 726-1494; http://www.easterseals.com.
‡1010 Wayne Ave., Suite 650, Silver Spring, MD 20910; (301) 565-3842 or (800) 433-5255; fax: (301) 565-5342; http://www.thearc.org.
§A resource for a variety of self-help equipment is Sammons Preston, PO Box 5071, Bolingbrook, IL 60440-5071; (800) 323-5547; fax: (800) 547-4333; http://www.sammonspreston.com. In Canada: (800) 665-9200.

Nursing Diagnosis	Patient Outcomes	Nursing Interventions	Rationale
Delayed Growth and Development related to impaired cognitive functioning	Child will achieve optimum growth and development potential. Child will achieve optimum socialization.	Perform a physical and developmental assessment. Assist with diagnostic tests (e.g., chromosome analysis, metabolic dysfunction, radiography, tomography, electroencephalography).	To further evaluate cognitive impairment
Child's/Family's Defining Characteristics *(Subjective and Objective Data)*	**The Following NOC Concepts Apply to These Outcomes**		
Deprived environment	Cognitive Orientation	Involve child and family in an early infant stimulation program.	To maximize child's development
Psychiatric disorders	Communication: Receptive		
Infections, especially those involving the brain (e.g., meningitis, encephalitis, measles) or a high body temperature	Social Interaction Skills Growth Role Performance Self-Care: Activities of Daily Living (ADL)	Assess child's developmental progress at regular intervals; keep detailed records to distinguish subtle changes in functioning.	To revise the care plan as needed
Chromosomal abnormality		Help family determine child's readiness to learn specific tasks.	To screen for readiness, since it may not be easily recognized
Unresponsiveness to contact		Help family set realistic goals for child.	To encourage successful attainment of goals and to support self-esteem
Poor eye contact during feeding			
Diminished spontaneous activity			
Decreased alertness to voice or movement		Employ positive reinforcement for specific tasks or behaviors.	To improve motivation and learning
Irritability		Encourage learning of self-care skills as soon as child is ready.	To encourage independence
Slow feeding		Reinforce self-care activities.	To facilitate optimum development
		Encourage family to investigate special daycare programs and educational classes as soon as possible.	To promote development
		Emphasize that child has same needs as other children (e.g., play, discipline, social interaction).	To optimize development
		Before adolescence, counsel child and parents regarding physical maturation, sexual behavior, marriage, and childrearing.	To promote the child's potential
		Encourage optimum vocational training	
		Encourage family to teach child socially acceptable behavior (e.g., saying "hello" and "thank you," manners, appropriate touch).	To encourage socialization
		Encourage grooming and age-appropriate dress.	To encourage acceptance by others and support self-esteem
		Recommend programs that provide peer relationships and experiences (e.g., mainstreaming, Boy Scouts, Girl Scouts, Special Olympics).	To promote optimum socialization
		Provide adolescent with practical sexual information and a well-defined, concrete code of conduct.	To decrease risk because of child's easy persuasion and lack of judgment
		Perform or assist with intelligence tests: ▪ Bayley Scales of Infant Development ▪ Mullen Scales of Early Learning ▪ Wechsler Preschool and Primary Scale of Intelligence (WPPSI-R) (preschoolers) ▪ Wechsler Intelligence Scale for Children (WISC III) (school-age children) ▪ Differential Ability Scales ▪ Stanford-Binet Intelligence Scale, ed 4 ▪ Kaufman Assessment Battery for Children	To establish level of cognitive impairment

nursingcareplan | The Child with Impaired Cognitive Function—cont'd

Nursing Diagnosis	Patient Outcomes	Nursing Interventions	Rationale
Delayed Growth and Development related to impaired cognitive functioning—cont'd		Perform or assist with testing of adaptive behaviors: ■ Vineland Social Maturity Scale ■ AAMR Adaptive Behavior Scale ■ Vineland Social Maturity Scale ■ AAMR Adaptive Behavior Scale **The Following NIC Concepts Apply to These Outcomes** Learning Readiness Enhancement Environmental Management Self-Esteem Enhancement Active Listening Developmental Enhancement: Child Family Involvement Promotion Behavior Modification: Social Skills Parent Education: Adolescent Attachment Promotion Parent Education: Infant Sibling Support Caregiver Support Self-Care Assistance Behavior Modification	

Nursing Diagnosis	Patient Outcomes	Nursing Interventions	Rationale
Interrupted Family Processes related to having a child with cognitive impairment **Child's/Family's Defining Characteristics** *(Subjective and Objective Data)* Family history of intellectual disability or hereditary disorders with cognitive impairment Prenatal, perinatal, or postnatal trauma or physical injury Prenatal maternal infection (e.g., rubella), alcoholism, drug consumption Lack of disease understanding Inability to understand plan of treatment Lack of family support	Family will receive adequate information and support. Family will be prepared for long-term care of child. **The Following NOC Concepts Apply to These Outcomes** Family Resiliency Social Support Family Coping Family Functioning Parenting Performance Caregiver Lifestyle Disruption	Inform family at or as soon as possible after birth. Have both parents present at informing conference. Give family, when possible, written information about the condition (e.g., a specific syndrome or disease). Discuss with family members the pros and cons of home care and other placement options; allow them opportunities to investigate all residential alternatives before making a decision. Encourage family to meet other families that have a child with a similar diagnosis. Refrain from giving definitive answers about the degree of impairment; stress the potential learning abilities of each child, especially with early intervention. Demonstrate acceptance of child through own behavior. Emphasize normal characteristics of child. Encourage family members to express their feelings and concerns. Discuss with parents alternatives to home care, especially as child grows older and as parents near retirement or old age.	To prevent fears and concerns and provide immediate support To avoid problem of one parent having to relay complex information to the other parent and deal with the reaction To inform parent of disorder and provide basic education To increase understanding and facilitate decision making To provide additional support To foster hope To demonstrate caring attitude of the professional To help family see child as an individual with strengths and weaknesses To promote adaptation process and effective collaboration To optimize appropriate long-term care that can be provided

Continued

nursingcareplan | **The Child with Impaired Cognitive Function—cont'd**

Nursing Diagnosis	Patient Outcomes	Nursing Interventions	Rationale
Interrupted Family Processes related to having a child with cognitive impairment—cont'd		Encourage family to consider respite care as needed.	To facilitate family's ability to cope with child's long-term care
		Help family investigate residential settings.	To provide the child's optimum care
		Encourage family to include affected member in planning and to continue meaningful relationships after placement.	To promote family development
		Refer to agencies that provide support and assistance.	To promote support

The Following NIC Concepts Apply to These Outcomes

Counseling
Caregiver Support
Family Therapy
Family Involvement Promotion
Parenting Promotion
Referral
Coping Enhancement
Insurance Authorization
Anticipatory Guidance
Support Group
Decision-Making Support

Promote Child's Optimal Development. Optimal development involves more than achieving independence. It requires appropriate guidance for establishing acceptable social behavior and personal feelings of self-esteem, worth, and security. These attributes are not simply learned through a stimulation program. Rather, they must arise from the genuine love and caring that exist among family members. However, families need guidance in providing an environment that fosters optimal development. Often it is the nurse who can provide assistance in these areas of childrearing.

Another important area for promoting optimal development and self-esteem is ensuring the child's physical well-being. Any congenital defects, such as cardiac, gastrointestinal, or orthopedic anomalies, should be repaired. Plastic surgery may be considered when the child's appearance can be substantially improved. Dental health is significant, and orthodontic and restorative procedures can improve facial appearance immensely.

Encourage Play and Exercise. Children who are cognitively impaired have the same needs for recreation and exercise as other children. However, because of the children's slower development, parents may be less aware of the need to provide such activities. Therefore the nurse guides parents toward selection of suitable play and exercise activities. Because play has been discussed for children in each age-group in earlier chapters, only the exceptions are presented here (Fig. 19-2).

The type of play is based on the child's developmental age, although the need for sensorimotor play may be prolonged for several years. Parents should use every opportunity to expose the child to as many different sounds, sights, and sensations as possible. Appropriate play includes musical mobiles, stuffed toys, water play, floating toys, a rocking chair or horse,

FIG. 19-2 ■ Placing an attractive object outside the child's reach encourages crawling movements. (Courtesy James DeLeon, Texas Children's Hospital, Houston.)

a swing, bells, and rattles. The child should be taken on outings, such as trips to the grocery store or shopping center; other people should be encouraged to visit in the home; and the child should be related to directly, such as by cuddling, holding, rocking, talking to the child in the en face (face-to-face) position, and giving "rides" on the parents' shoulders.

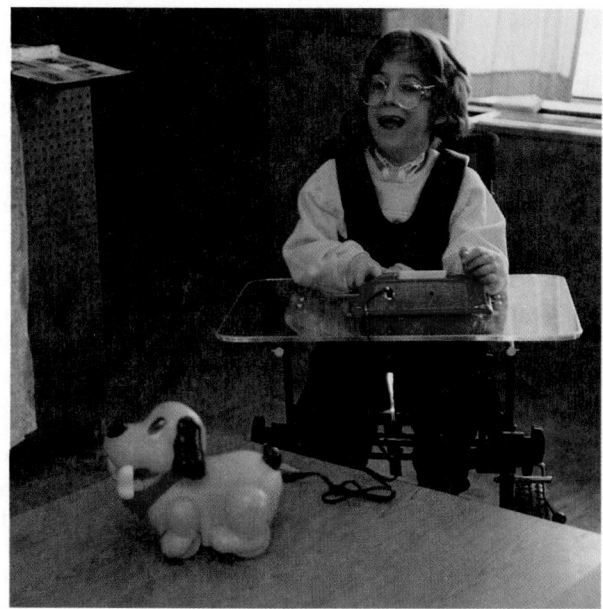

FIG. 19-3 ■ A manual switch allows a child with cognitive impairment to play with a battery-operated toy.

FIG. 19-5 ■ A child with cognitive and physical impairments can activate electronic/communication equipment by moving a device near her head.

FIG. 19-4 ■ A favorite toy provides stimulation for a young child.

Toys are selected for their recreational and educational value. For example, a large inflatable beach ball is a good water toy; it encourages interactive play and can be used to learn motor skills, such as balance, rocking, kicking, and throwing. A doll with removable clothes and different types of closures can help the child learn dressing skills. Musical toys that mimic animal sounds or respond with social phrases are excellent ways of encouraging speech. Toys should be simple in design so that the child can learn to manipulate them without help. For children with severe cognitive and physical impairment, electronic switches can be used to allow them to operate toys (Fig. 19-3).

Suitable activities for physical activity are based on the child's size, coordination, physical fitness and maturity, motivation, and health (Fig. 19-4). Some children may have physical problems that prevent participation in certain sports, such as atlantoaxial instability in children with Down syndrome (p. 619). These children often have greater success in individual and dual sports than in team sports and enjoy themselves most with children of the same developmental level. The Special Olympics* provides these children with a unique competitive opportunity.

Safety is a major consideration in selecting recreational and exercise activities. For example, toys that may be appropriate developmentally may present dangers to a child who is strong enough to break them or use them incorrectly.

Provide Means of Communication. Verbal skills are typically delayed more than other physical skills. Speech requires hearing and interpretation (**receptive skills**) and facial muscle coordination (**expressive skills**). Because both types of skills may be impaired, these children need frequent audiometric testing and should be fitted with hearing aids if indicated. In addition, they may need help in learning to control their facial muscles. For example, some children may need tongue exercises to correct the tongue thrust or gentle reminders to keep the lips closed.

Nonverbal communication may be appropriate for some of these children, and various devices are available. For the child without associated physical disabilities, a talking picture board is helpful. For children with physical limitations, several adaptations or types of communication devices are available to facilitate selection of the appropriate picture or word (Fig. 19-5). Some children may be taught sign language or **Blissymbols**—a highly stylized system of graphic symbols that represent words, ideas, and concepts. Although the symbols require education to learn their meaning, no reading

---

*1133 19th St. NW, Washington, DC 20036; (800) 700-8585 or (202) 628-3630; fax: (202) 824-0200; http://www.specialolympics.org. (Website includes listing of state offices.) In Canada: Special Olympics Canada, 60 St. Clair Ave. E, Suite 700, Toronto, Ontario M4T 1N5; (416) 927-9050; fax: (416) 927-8475; http://www.specialolympics.ca.

skill is needed. The symbols are usually arranged on a board, and the person points or uses some type of selector to convey a message.

Establish Discipline. Discipline must begin early. Limit-setting measures need to be simple, consistently applied, and appropriate for the child's mental age. Control measures are based primarily on teaching a specific behavior rather than on understanding the reasons behind it. Stressing moral lessons is of little value to a child who lacks the cognitive skills to learn from self-criticism or from a lesson based on previous wrong-doing. Behavior modification, especially reinforcement of desired actions, and time-out are appropriate forms of behavior control.

Encourage Socialization. Acquiring social skills is a complex task, as is learning self-care procedures. Active re-hearsal with role-playing and practice sessions and positive reinforcement for desired behavior have been the most successful approaches. Parents should be encouraged early to teach their child socially acceptable behavior: waving good-bye, saying "hello" and "thank you," responding to his or her name, greeting visitors, and sitting modestly. The teaching of socially acceptable sexual behavior is especially important to minimize sexual exploitation. Parents also need to expose the child to strangers so that he or she can practice manners, since there is no automatic transfer of learning from one situation to another.

Dressing and grooming are also important aspects of so-cialization. A child who is dressed in age-appropriate clothing and is well groomed is much more likely to be accepted and to develop good self-esteem. Clothes should be clean, up-to-date, and well fitted. Many attractive outfits can be adapted with self-adhering fasteners and elastic openings to facilitate self-dressing.

As soon as possible, parents should enroll the child in appropriate preschool programs. Not only do these programs provide education and training, but they also offer an opportunity for social experiences among the children. As children grow older, they should have peer experiences similar to those of other children, including group outings, sports, and organized activities such as scouts and Special Olympics. Nurses can assess the child's abilities and encourage others (e.g., parents, teachers) to promote developmentally appropriate peer interaction (Johnson and Walker, 2006; Rehm and Bradley, 2006).

Provide Information on Sexuality. Adolescence may be a particularly difficult time for the family, especially in terms of the child's sexual behavior, possibility of pregnancy, future plans to marry, and ability to be independent. Frequently, little anticipatory guidance has been offered parents to prepare the child for physical and sexual maturation. The nurse can help in this area by providing parents with information about sexuality education that is geared to the child's developmental level. For example, the adolescent girl needs a *simple* explanation of menstruation and instructions on personal hygiene during the menstrual cycle.

These adolescents also need practical sexual information regarding anatomy, physical development, and conception.* Because of their easy persuasion and lack of judgment, they

need a well-defined, concrete code of conduct. The subtleties of social sexual behavior are less beneficial than specific instructions for handling certain situations. For example, an adolescent should be firmly told never to go alone anywhere with any person she does not know well. To protect him or her from abusive sexual activities, parents must closely observe their teenager's activities and associates. The question of contraceptive protection for these adolescents is often a parental concern.

Parents of these adolescents are often concerned about the advisability of marriage between two individuals with an intellectual disability. There is no conclusive answer; each situation must be judged individually. In some instances marriage is possible, but parenthood may not be desirable because of the complexity of childrearing and the potential problem of perpetuating mental deficiency. The nurse should discuss this topic with parents and with the prospective couple, stressing suitable living accommodations and contraceptive methods to prevent pregnancy. If children are conceived, these parents require specialized assistance in learning to meet the needs of their offspring (Johnson and Walker, 2006).

Help Family Adjust to Future Care. Not all families are able to cope with home care of their affected child, especially one who is severely or profoundly impaired or has multiple disabilities. Older parents may not be able to assume care responsibilities after they reach retirement or older age. For these parents, the decision regarding residential placement is a difficult one, and the availability of such facilities varies widely. The nurse working with a family should help them investigate and evaluate various programs, in addition to assisting them in adjusting to the decision for placement.

Care for Child During Hospitalization. Caring for the child during hospitalization can be a special challenge. Frequently, nurses are unfamiliar with children who are cognitively impaired, and they may cope with their feelings of insecurity and fear by ignoring or isolating the child. Not only is this approach nonsupportive, but it may also be destructive for the child's sense of self-esteem and optimal development, and it may hamper the parents' ability to cope with the stress of the experience. One method that successfully avoids this nontherapeutic approach is the use of the mutual participation model in planning the child's care. Parents are encouraged to stay with their child but should not be made to feel as if the responsibility is totally theirs.

When the child is admitted, a detailed history is taken (see Chapter 21), especially in terms of all self-care activity. During the interview the child's developmental age is assessed. It is best to avoid asking directly about IQ levels, since this may make the parents uncomfortable and often tells little about the child's actual abilities. Questions are approached positively. For example, rather than asking, "Is your child toilet trained yet?" the nurse may state, "Tell me about your child's toileting habits." The assessment should also focus on any special devices the child uses, effective measures of limit setting, unusual or favorite routines, and any behaviors that may require intervention. If the parent states that the child engages in self-injurious activities (such as head banging or self-biting), the nurse should inquire about events that precipitate them and techniques that the parents use to manage them (Bosch and Ringdahl, 2001; Walker and Johnson, 2006).

The nurse also assesses the child's functional level of eating and playing; ability to express needs verbally; progress in toilet

---

*Sources of information on sexuality and conception are the Arc of the United States (see footnote, p. 613) and Planned Parenthood Federation of America, 434 W. 33rd St., New York, NY 10001; (212) 541-7800 or (800) 230-7526; fax: (212) 245-1845; http://www.plannedparenthood.org.

training; and relationship with objects, toys, and other children. The child is encouraged to be as independent as possible in the hospital.

Realizing that the child may be lonely in the hospital, the nurse makes certain that toys and other activities are provided. The child is placed in a room with other children of approximately the same developmental age, preferably a room with only two beds to avoid overstimulation. The nurse discusses with the other parents the child's abilities and introduces the parents and children to each other. By the nurse's example of treating the child with dignity and respect, others who may be fearful of what they do not understand are encouraged to accept the child.

Procedures are explained to the child through methods of communication that are at the appropriate cognitive level. Generally, explanations should be simple, short, and concrete, emphasizing what the child will experience *physically.* Demonstration either through actual practice or with visual aids is always preferable to verbal explanation. The nurse repeats instructions often and evaluates the child's understanding by asking questions such as "What will it feel like?" "Show me how you must lie," or "Where will the dressing be?" Parents are included in preprocedural teaching for their own learning and to help the nurse learn effective methods of communicating with the child.

During hospitalization the nurse should also focus on growth-promoting experiences for the child. For example, hospitalization may be an excellent opportunity to emphasize to parents abilities that the child does have but has not had the opportunity to practice, such as self-dressing. It may also be an opportunity for social experiences with peers, group play, or new educational and recreational activities. For example, one child who had the habit of screaming and kicking demonstrated a definite decrease in those behaviors after he learned to pound pegs and use a punching bag. Through social services the parents may become aware of specialized programs for the child. Hospitalization may also offer parents a respite from everyday care responsibilities and an opportunity to discuss their feelings with a concerned professional.

Assist in Measures to Prevent Cognitive Impairment. Besides having a responsibility to families with a child with CI, nurses also need to be involved in programs aimed at preventing CI. Many of the familial, social, and environmental factors known to cause mild impairment are preventable. Counseling and education can reduce or eliminate such factors (e.g., poor nutrition, cigarette smoking, chemical abuse), which increase the risk of prematurity and intrauterine growth restriction. Interventions are directed toward improving maternal health by educating women regarding the dangers of chemicals, including prenatal alcohol exposure, which affects organogenesis, craniofacial development, and cognitive ability (Wilton and Plane, 2006). Other preventive strategies that play an important role include adequate prenatal care; optimal medical care of high-risk newborns; rubella immunization; genetic counseling and prenatal screening, especially in terms of Down or fragile X syndrome; use of folic acid supplements to prevent neural tube defects during pregnancy and during the childbearing years; newborn screening for treatable inborn errors of metabolism, such as congenital hypothyroidism, phenylketonuria, and galactosemia; and early appropriate therapies and rehabilitation services for children with developmental disabilities.

DOWN SYNDROME

Down syndrome is the most common chromosomal abnormality of a generalized syndrome, occurring in one in every 800 to 1000 live births (National Down Syndrome Society, 2006; Skotko, 2005). It occurs slightly more often in Caucasians than in African-Americans, although the incidence is unchanged in various socioeconomic classes.

Etiology

The cause of Down syndrome is not known, but evidence from cytogenetic and epidemiologic studies supports the concept of multiple causality. Approximately 95% of all cases of Down syndrome are attributable to an extra chromosome 21 (group G), thus the name **nonfamilial trisomy 21** (National Down Syndrome Society, 2006; Walker and Johnson, 2006). Although children with trisomy 21 are born to parents of all ages, there is a statistically greater risk in older women, particularly those older than 35 years of age. For example, in women 35 years of age the chance of conceiving a child with Down syndrome is about one in 400 live births, but in women age 40 it is about one in 110. However, the majority (about 80%) of infants with Down syndrome are born to women younger than age 35. About 3% to 4% of the cases may be caused by **translocation** of chromosomes 15 and 21 or 22. This type of genetic aberration is usually hereditary and is not associated with advanced parental age. From 1% to 2% of affected persons demonstrate **mosaicism,** which refers to mixture of normal and abnormal cell types. The degree of cognitive and physical impairment is related to the percentage of cells with the abnormal chromosome makeup.

Diagnostic Evaluation

Down syndrome can usually be diagnosed by the clinical manifestations alone (Box 19-3 and Fig. 19-6), but a chromosome analysis should be done to confirm the genetic abnormality.

Several physical problems are associated with Down syndrome. Many of these children have congenital heart malformations, the most common being septal defects. Respiratory tract infections are prevalent and, when combined with cardiac anomalies, are the chief causes of death, particularly dur-

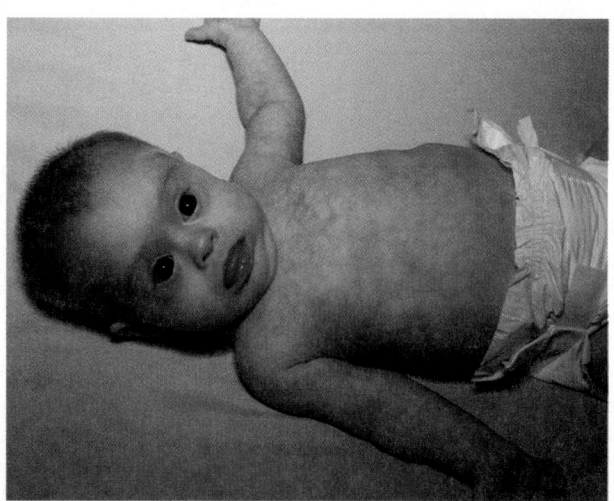

FIG. 19-6 ■ Down syndrome in an infant. Note small, square head with upward slant to eyes, flat nasal bridge, protruding tongue, mottled skin, and hypotonia.

Case Study—Down Syndrome

Critical Thinking Exercise—Down Syndrome

BOX 19-3
Clinical Manifestations of Down Syndrome

HEAD AND EYES
*Separated sagittal suture
Brachycephaly
Rounded and small skull
Flat occiput
Enlarged anterior fontanel
*Oblique palpebral fissures (upward, outward slant)
Inner epicanthal folds
Speckling of iris (Brushfield spots)

NOSE AND EARS
*Small nose
*Depressed nasal bridge (saddle nose)
Small ears and narrow canals
Short pinna (vertical ear length)
Overlapping upper helices
Conductive hearing loss

MOUTH AND NECK
*High, arched, narrow palate
Protruding tongue
Hypoplastic mandible
Delayed teeth eruption and microdontia
Alignment teeth abnormalities common
Periodontal disease
*Neck skin excess and laxity
Short and broad neck

CHEST AND HEART
Shortened rib cage
Twelfth rib anomalies
Pectus excavatum or carinatum
Congenital heart defects common (e.g., atrial septal defect, ventricular septal defect)

ABDOMEN AND GENITALIA
Protruding, lax, and flabby abdominal muscles
Diastasis recti abdominis
Umbilical hernia
Small penis
Cryptorchidism
Bulbous vulva

HANDS AND FEET
Broad, short hands and stubby fingers
Incurved little finger (clinodactyly)
Transverse palmar crease
*Wide space between big and second toes
*Plantar crease between big and second toes
Broad, short feet and stubby toes

MUSCULOSKELETON AND SKIN
Short stature
*Hyperflexibility and muscle weakness
Hypotonia
Atlantoaxial instability
Dry, cracked, and frequent fissuring
Cutis marmorata (mottling)

OTHER
Reduced birth weight
Learning difficulty (average intelligence quotient of 50)
Hypothyroidism common
Impaired immune function
Increased risk of leukemia
Early-onset dementia (in one third)

*Most common findings in modified chart (Pueschel, 1999).

ing the first year of life. Hypotonicity of chest and abdominal muscles and dysfunction of the immune system probably predispose the child to the development of respiratory tract infection. Other physical problems include thyroid dysfunction, especially congenital hypothyroidism, and an increased incidence of leukemia.

Therapeutic Management

Although no cure exists for Down syndrome, a number of therapies are advocated, such as surgery to correct serious congenital anomalies (e.g., heart defects, strabismus). These children also benefit from an evaluative echocardiogram soon after birth and regular medical care. Evaluation of sight and hearing is essential, and treatment of otitis media is required

to prevent auditory loss, which can influence cognitive function. Periodic testing of thyroid function is recommended, especially if growth is severely delayed. Children participating in sports that may involve stress on the head and neck, such as gymnastics, diving, butterfly stroke in swimming, high jump, and soccer, should be evaluated radiologically for **atlantoaxial instability.** Symptoms of the disorder include neck pain, weakness, and torticollis. Affected children are at risk for spinal cord compression.

NURSINGALERT
Report immediately any child with the following signs of spinal cord compression:
- Persistent neck pain
- Loss of established motor skills and bladder or bowel control
- Changes in sensation

Prognosis. Life expectancy for those with Down syndrome has improved in recent years but remains lower than for the general population. More than 80% survive to age 55 years and beyond. As the prognosis continues to improve for these individuals, it will be important to provide for their long-term health care, social, and leisure needs (National Down Syndrome Society, 2006; Van Riper, 2003). (See Ethical Case Study.)

Nursing Care Management
Support Family at Time of Diagnosis. Because of the unique physical characteristics, the infant with Down syndrome is usually diagnosed at birth, and parents should be informed of the diagnosis at this time. Parents usually prefer that both of them be present during the informing interview so that they can support one another emotionally. They appreciate receiving reading material about the syndrome* and being referred to others for help or advice, such as parent groups or professional counseling.

After parents are aware of the diagnosis, they are confronted with the crisis of losing their perfect or dream child and grieving for and accepting their reality child. Consequently, the parents' responses to the child may greatly influence decisions regarding future care. Whereas some families willingly take the child home, others consider immediate residential placement. The nurse must carefully answer questions regarding developmental potential. Institutionalization is no longer an option. For families unable or unready to choose taking the newborn home, specialized foster care or adoption are other options (see Critical Thinking Exercise).

Assist Family in Preventing Physical Problems. Many of the physical characteristics of Down syndrome present nursing problems. The hypotonicity of muscles and hyperextensibility of joints complicate positioning. The limp, flaccid extremities resemble the posture of a rag doll; as a result, holding the infant is difficult and cumbersome. Sometimes parents perceive this lack of molding to their bodies as evidence of inadequate parenting. The extended

*Sources of information include the Arc of the United States (see footnote, p. 613); the American Association on Intellectual and Developmental Disabilities, 444 N. Capitol Street NW, Suite 846, Washington, DC 20001-1512; (800) 424-3688; fax: (202) 387-2193; http://www.aamr.org the National Down Syndrome Society (see footnote, p. 613); and the National Down Syndrome Congress, 1370 Center Drive, Suite 102, Atlanta, GA 30338; (800) 232-6372 or (770) 604-9500; http://www.ndsccenter.org.

ETHICAL CASE STUDY   Child with Down Syndrome

ETHICAL DECISION MAKING MODEL	Elena is a 3-month-old girl with Down syndrome who has an atrioventricular septal defect (AVSD). Elena and her family recently came to the United States from Romania. The cardiologist treating Elena in Romania had not recommended surgery to repair the AVSD. Since arriving in the United States, Elena has been experiencing increased symptoms of heart failure. The child's new pediatrician discussed surgical repair of the AVSD. Elena's parents expressed surprise that reparative surgery was an option, indicating that the cardiologist in Romania believed surgery would be of no benefit to a child with Down syndrome. In addition, they were told that Elena would not live past 1 year of age and thus had not anticipated raising a child with Down syndrome. The father expressed concern about being able to pay for such an expensive operation, stating that, in Romania, surgery would not be considered in a child with Down syndrome. During the discussion with the pediatrician, the mother sat quietly crying while holding the infant.
Evaluate the Issue	There has been discussion in the literature of refusals to perform interventions on individuals with learning disabilities (Bittles and Glasson, 2004; Coats, 2001). This has prompted concern that individuals with disabilities may not receive equal access to health care. Although the life expectancy of children with Down syndrome has increased dramatically in recent decades from 25 years in 1983 to 56 years today (National Down Syndrome Society, 2006; Day, Strauss, Shavelle, and others, 2005; Glasson, Sullivan, Hussain, and others, 2002), there is continued discussion in the literature regarding the restrictions of socialized medicine in industrialized countries and the inadequacies of medical care in less-developed countries. These difficult choices, because of resource-limited medical care, are often not made in the best interest of the child and family.

A second major concern often raised is whether there are increased risks associated with surgery for infants with Down syndrome. Recent studies show no differences in survival after major surgery in children with Down syndrome compared with children with a normal genotype (Formigari, Di Donato, Garguilo, and others, 2004; Al-Hay, MacNeil, Yacoub, and others, 2003). |
Treat All Involved with Respect	Of major importance in this case is listening to the concerns raised by the family. It is important to understand that the parents realize for the first time since the birth of their child that surgery could be of benefit. Nonjudgmental support is essential. The parents need time to evaluate the situation. It is important to consider the mother's feelings as well as those of the father, although culture may determine that the father is the primary decision maker in relation to such matters. Cultural values related to quality of life for a child with Down syndrome must be explored with both parents and extended family.
Hear All Sides	Differences in health care practices in other countries may contribute to the dilemma in ethical cases such as Elena. This case brought renewed concern that a decreased state of health could be accepted for children with Down syndrome and other disabilities. Nurses must critically evaluate their beliefs regarding what is considered quality of life to be of support to all families who seek care and advice regarding the future of a child with a disability such as Down syndrome.
Initiate Action	The first step in this case is to educate the family on the risks and benefits of surgery for an AVSD repair in a child with Down syndrome. Discussions with the family should be coordinated by the health care team. Consideration of the family's support network in the United States is important. Assessment of the family's resources and ability to provide financial support for the surgery must be considered in light of restrictions placed on many hospitals. The implications for the child's life without surgical intervention must be discussed with the family. The family should be given time to ask questions and to consult with other family members and friends. The family needs support for the realization that Elena has a good chance of surviving to an adult age.
Consider the Outcome	The family has been told since Elena's birth that she will not survive past the first year of life. The recent news that Elena has a chance of surviving if she receives surgical intervention is a shock to the family. They have no previous experience with Western medicine and need time to realize that their child has a greater chance of surviving. Surgery to repair the AVSD can change the outcome for this child. The family's awareness that children with Down syndrome have access to modern surgical interventions in the United States is an important ethical issue that the health care team must discuss.

??? CRITICAL THINKING EXERCISE

Diagnosis of Down Syndrome

The parents of Melissa, a newborn diagnosed as having Down syndrome, ask the nurse, "What are we supposed to do with her?" They further state that they already have three other children at home.

QUESTIONS

1. Evidence—Is there sufficient evidence to draw conclusions about the parents' concerns regarding their newborn daughter?

2. Assumptions—Describe an underlying assumption about each of the following:
   a. Newborn diagnosed with Down syndrome
   b. Parental care of a newborn with Down syndrome
   c. Newborn with Down syndrome and older siblings
3. What priorities for the nursing response should be established?
4. Does the evidence support your nursing intervention?
5. What alternative perspectives might you have?

Critical Thinking Exercise—Fragile X Syndrome

body position promotes heat loss because more surface area is exposed to the environment. Parents are encouraged to swaddle or wrap the infant tightly in a blanket before picking up the child to provide security and warmth. The nurse also discusses with parents their feelings concerning attachment to the child, emphasizing that the child's lack of clinging or molding is a physical characteristic, not a sign of detachment or rejection.

Decreased muscle tone compromises respiratory expansion. In addition, the underdeveloped nasal bone causes a chronic problem of inadequate drainage of mucus. The constant stuffy nose forces the child to breathe by mouth, which dries the oropharyngeal membranes, increasing the susceptibility to upper respiratory tract infections. Measures to lessen these problems include clearing the nose with a bulb-type syringe, rinsing the mouth with water after feedings, increasing fluid intake, and using a cool-mist vaporizer to keep the mucous membranes moist and the secretions liquefied. Other helpful measures include changing the child's position frequently, performing postural drainage with percussion if necessary, practicing good hand washing, and properly disposing of soiled articles such as tissues. If antibiotics are ordered, the nurse stresses the importance of completing the full course of therapy for successful eradication of the infection and prevention of growth of resistant organisms.

Inadequate drainage resulting in pooling of mucus in the nose also interferes with feeding. Because the child breathes by mouth, sucking for any length of time is difficult. When eating solids, the child may gag on the food because of mucus in the oropharynx. Parents are advised to clear the nose before each feeding; give small, frequent feedings; and allow opportunities for rest during mealtime.

The protruding tongue also interferes with feeding, especially of solid foods. Parents need to know that the tongue thrust is not an indication of refusal to feed, but a physiologic response. Parents are advised to use a small but long, straight-handled spoon to push the food toward the back and side of the mouth. If food is thrust out, it should be refed.

Dietary intake needs supervision. Decreased muscle tone affects gastric motility, predisposing the child to constipation. Dietary measures such as increased fiber and fluid promote evacuation. The child's eating habits may need careful scrutiny to prevent obesity. Height and weight measurements should be obtained on a serial basis, especially during infancy. Because these children grow more slowly than the general pediatric population's trends, special growth charts developed for these children should be used (American Academy of Pediatrics, 2001).

During infancy the child's skin is pliable and soft. However, it gradually becomes rough and dry and is prone to cracking and infection. Skin care involves the use of minimum soap and application of lubricants. Lip balm is applied to the lips, especially when the child is outdoors, to prevent excessive chapping.

Assist in Prenatal Diagnosis and Genetic Counseling. Prenatal diagnosis of Down syndrome is possible through chorionic villus sampling and amniocentesis, since chromosome analysis of fetal cells can detect the presence of trisomy or translocation. However, analysis will not identify sporadic cases in young women when there is no indication for prenatal testing. Testing for low maternal serum α-fetoprotein, high chorionic gonadotropin, low unconjugated estriol levels, and maternal serum fetal cell markers may

identify an affected fetus in women, who can then undergo amniocentesis (National Down Syndrome Society, 2006; Peterson, 2006; Hall, 2004).

Prenatal testing and genetic counseling should be offered to women of advanced maternal age or those who have a family history of the disorder. If prenatal testing indicates the fetus is affected, the nurse must allow the parents to express their feelings concerning elective abortion and support their decision to terminate or proceed with the pregnancy.

FRAGILE X SYNDROME

Fragile X syndrome is the most common inherited cause of CI and the second most common genetic cause of CI after Down syndrome. It has been described in all ethnic groups and races; the incidence of affected males is one in 3600; the incidence of affected females is one in 4000 to 6000; and the incidence of carrier females is one in 100 to 260 and the incidence of carrier males is one in 250 to 800 worldwide (National Fragile X Foundation, 2006; Phalen, 2005; Crawford, 2001).

The syndrome is caused by an abnormal gene on the lower end of the long arm of the X chromosome. Chromosome analysis may demonstrate a **fragile site** (a region that fails to condense during mitosis and is characterized by a nonstaining gap or narrowing) in the cells of affected males and females and in carrier females. This fragile site has been determined to be caused by a gene mutation that results in excessive repeats of nucleotide in a specific deoxyribonucleic acid (DNA) segment of the X chromosome. The number of repeats in a normal individual is between six and 50. An individual with 50 to 200 base-pair repeats is said to have a **permutation** and is therefore a carrier. When passed from a parent to a child, these base-pair repeats can expand from 200 or more, which is termed a **full mutation.** This expansion occurs only when a carrier mother passes the mutation to her offspring; it does not occur when a carrier father passes the mutation to his daughters.

The inheritance pattern has been termed **X-linked dominant with reduced penetrance.** This is in distinct contrast to the classic X-linked recessive pattern in which all carrier females are normal, all affected males have symptoms of the disorder, and no males are carriers. Consequently, genetic counseling of affected families is more complex than that for families with a classic X-linked disorder, such as hemophilia. Prenatal diagnosis of the fragile X gene mutation is now possible with direct DNA testing in a family with an established history, using amniocentesis or chorionic villus sampling (Centers for Disease Control and Prevention, 2002; Crawford, 2001). Both affected sexes are fertile and therefore capable of transmitting the fragile X disorder.

Clinical Manifestations

The classic trend of physical findings in adult men with fragile X syndrome consists of a long face with a prominent jaw (prognathism); large, protruding ears; and large testes (macroorchidism). In prepubertal children, however, these features may be less obvious, and behavioral manifestations may initially suggest the diagnosis (Box 19-4). In carrier females the clinical manifestations are extremely varied.

Therapeutic Management

No cure exists for fragile X syndrome. Medical treatment may include the use of serotonin agents such as carbamazepine (Tegretol) or fluoxetine (Prozac) to control violent temper

BOX 19-4
Clinical Manifestations of Fragile X Syndrome

PHYSICAL FEATURES
Increased head circumference
Long, wide, and/or protruding ears
Long, narrow face with prominent jaw
Strabismus
Mitral valve prolapse, aortic root dilation
Hypotonia
Enlarged testicles (especially postpubertally)

BEHAVIORAL FEATURES
Mild to severe cognitive impairment
Speech delay; may have rapid speech with stuttering, word repetition
Short attention span, hyperactivity
Hypersensitivity to taste, sounds, touch
Intolerance to change in routine
Autistic-like behaviors

outbursts and the use of central nervous system stimulants or clonidine (Catapres) to improve attention span and decrease hyperactivity. Protein replacement and gene therapy are treatment options that are being investigated (Phalen, 2005).

All affected children require referral to early intervention program (speech and language therapy, occupational therapy, and special education assistance) and multidisciplinary assessment, including cardiology (i.e., mitral valve prolapse), neurology (i.e., seizures), and orthopedic anomalies (Alanay, Unal, Turanh, and others, 2007).

Prognosis. Individuals with fragile X syndrome are expected to live a normal life span. Their CI may be improved by behavioral and educational interventions.

Nursing Care Management

Because CI is a fairly consistent finding in individuals with fragile X syndrome, the care given to these families is the same as for any child with CI. Because the disorder is hereditary, genetic counseling is necessary to inform parents and siblings of the risks of transmission. In addition, any male or female with unexplained or nonspecific mental impairment should be referred for genetic testing and, if needed, counseling. Families with a member affected by the disorder should be referred to the National Fragile X Foundation.*

SENSORY IMPAIRMENT
HEARING IMPAIRMENT

Hearing impairment is one of the most common disabilities in the United States. An estimated three in 1000 well infants have hearing loss of varying degrees (Gregg, Wiorek, and Arvedson, 2004). For infants admitted to the neonatal intensive care unit, the incidence rises sharply to approximately two to four per 100 neonates (Cunningham, Cox, and Committee on Practice and Ambulatory Medicine and the Section on Otolaryngology and Bronchoesophagology, 2003; American Academy of Pediatrics, 1999). In the United States there are

*PO Box 37, Walnut Creek, CA 94597; (800) 688-8765 or (925) 938-9300; fax: (925) 938-9315; http://www.fragilex.org.

about 1 million children with hearing impairment ranging in age from birth to 21 years, and almost a third of these children have other disabilities, such as visual or cognitive deficits.

Definition and Classification

Hearing impairment is a general term indicating disability that may range in severity from mild to profound and includes the subsets of deaf and hard-of-hearing. **Deaf** refers to a person whose hearing disability precludes successful processing of linguistic information through audition, with or without a hearing aid. **Hard-of-hearing** refers to a person who, generally with the use of a hearing aid, has residual hearing sufficient to enable successful processing of linguistic information through audition. Other terms, such as *deaf and dumb, mute,* or *deaf-mute,* are unacceptable. Hearing-impaired persons are not dumb and, if mute, have no physical speech defect other than that caused by the inability to hear.

Hearing defects may be classified according to etiology, pathology, or symptom severity. Each is important in terms of treatment, possible prevention, and rehabilitation.

Etiology. Hearing loss may be caused by a number of prenatal and postnatal conditions. These include a family history of childhood hearing impairment, anatomic malformations of the head or neck, low birth weight, severe perinatal asphyxia, perinatal infection (cytomegalovirus, rubella, herpes, syphilis, toxoplasmosis, bacterial meningitis), chronic ear infection, cerebral palsy, Down syndrome, or administration of ototoxic drugs (Smith, Bale, and White, 2005; Gregg, Wiorek, and Arvedson, 2004).

In addition, high-risk neonates who survive formerly fatal prenatal or perinatal conditions may be susceptible to hearing loss from the disorder or its treatment. For example, sensorineural hearing loss may be a result of continuous humming noises or high noise levels associated with incubators, oxygen hoods, or intensive care units, especially when combined with the use of potentially ototoxic antibiotics.

Environmental noise is a special concern. Sounds loud enough to damage sensitive hair cells of the inner ear can produce irreversible hearing loss. Very loud, brief noise, such as gunfire, can cause immediate, severe, and permanent loss of hearing. Longer exposure to less intense but still hazardous sounds, such as loud persistent music via headphones, sound systems, concerts, or industrial noises, can also produce hearing loss (Daniel, 2007; Kenna, 2004; Segal, Eviatar, Lapinsky, and others, 2003). Loud noises combined with the toxic substances of smoking produces a synergistic effect on hearing that causes hearing loss (Mizoue, Miyamoto, and Shimizu, 2003).

Pathology. Disorders of hearing are divided according to the location of the defect. **Conductive** or **middle-ear hearing loss** results from interference of transmission of sound to the middle ear. It is the most common of all types of hearing loss and most frequently a result of recurrent serous otitis media. Conductive hearing impairment involves mainly interference with loudness of sound.

Sensorineural hearing loss, also called **perceptive** or **nerve deafness,** involves damage to the inner ear structures or the auditory nerve. The most common causes are congenital defects of inner ear structures or consequences of acquired conditions, such as kernicterus, infection, administration of ototoxic drugs, or exposure to excessive noise. Sensorineural hearing loss results in distortion of sound and problems in discrimination. Although the child hears some of everything

TABLE 19-2

Intensity of Sounds Expressed in Decibels

DECIBELS	REPRESENTATIVE SOUND
0	Softest sound normal ear can hear
10	Heartbeat, rustling of leaves
20	Whisper at 1.5 m (5 feet)
30-45	Normal conversation
60	Noise in average restaurant
70-80	Street noises
80	Loud radio in home
90-100	Train
120	Thunder, loud music (e.g., rock concerts)
140	Jet plane during departure
>140	Pain threshold

TABLE 19-3

Classification of Hearing Loss Based on Symptom Severity

HEARING LEVEL (dB)	EFFECT
Slight—16-25	Has difficulty hearing faint or distant speech
	Usually is unaware of hearing difficulty
	Likely to achieve in school but may have problems
	No speech defects
Mild to moderate— 26-55	May have speech difficulties
	Understands face-to-face conversational speech at 0.9-1.5 m (3-5 feet)
Moderately severe— 56-70 (hard of hearing)	Unable to understand conversational speech unless loud
	Considerable difficulty with group or class-room discussion
	Requires special speech training
Severe—71-90 (deaf)	May hear a loud voice if nearby
	May be able to identify loud environmental noises
	Can distinguish vowels but not most consonants
	Requires speech training
Profound—91 (deaf)	May hear only loud sounds
	Requires extensive speech training

going on around him or her, the sounds are distorted, severely affecting discrimination and comprehension.

Mixed conductive-sensorineural hearing loss results from interference with transmission of sound in the middle ear and along neural pathways. It frequently results from recurrent otitis media and its complications.

Central auditory imperception includes all hearing losses that are not linked to defects in the conductive or sensorineural structures. They are usually divided into organic or functional losses. In the **organic** type of central auditory imperception, the defect involves the reception of auditory stimuli along the central pathways and the expression of the message into meaningful communication. Examples are **aphasia,** the inability to express ideas in any form, either written or verbal; **agnosia,** the inability to interpret sound correctly; and **dysacusis,** difficulty in processing details or discriminating among sounds. In the **functional** type of hearing loss, no organic lesion exists to explain a central auditory loss. Examples of functional hearing loss are conversion hysteria (an unconscious withdrawal from hearing to block remembrance of a traumatic event), infantile autism, and childhood schizophrenia.

Symptom Severity. Hearing impairment is expressed in terms of a **decibel (dB),** a unit of loudness (Table 19-2); hearing is measured at various frequencies, such as 500, 1000, and 2000 cycles/sec, the critical listening speech range. Hearing impairment can be classified according to **hearing threshold level** (the measurement of an individual's hearing threshold by means of an audiometer) and the degree of symptom severity as it affects speech (Table 19-3). These classifications offer only general guidelines regarding the effect of the impairment on any individual child, since children differ greatly in their ability to use residual hearing.

Therapeutic Management

Conductive Hearing Loss. Treatment of hearing loss depends on the cause and type of hearing impairment. Many conductive hearing defects respond to medical or surgical treatment, such as antibiotic therapy for acute otitis media or insertion of tympanostomy tubes for chronic otitis media. When the conductive loss is permanent, hearing can be improved with the use of a hearing aid to amplify sound.

The nurse should be familiar with the types, basic care, and handling of hearing aids, especially when the child is hospitalized.* Types of aids include those worn in or behind the ear, models incorporated into an eyeglass frame, or types worn on the body with a wire connection to the ear (Fig. 19-7). One of the most common problems with a hearing aid is **acoustic feedback,** an annoying whistling sound usually caused by improper fit of the ear mold. Sometimes the whistling may be at a frequency that the child cannot hear but that is annoying to others. In this case, if children are old enough, they are told of the noise and asked to readjust the aid.

NURSINGTIP
To reduce or eliminate whistling from a hearing aid, try reinserting the aid, making certain that no hair is caught between the ear mold and the canal, cleaning the ear mold or ear, or lowering the volume of the aid.

As children grow older, they may be self-conscious about the device. Every effort is made to make the aid inconspicuous, such as an appropriate hairstyle to cover behind-the-ear or in-the-ear models; attractive frames for glasses; and placement of the on-the-body type where it is not seen, such as under a blouse or sweater. Children are given responsibility for the care of the device as soon as they are able, since fostering independence is a primary goal of rehabilitation.

---

*Information about hearing aids is available from the International Hearing Society, 16880 Middlebelt Road, Suite 4, Livonia, MI 48154; (800) 521-5247 or (734) 522-7200; fax: (734) 522-0200; http://ihsinfo.org.

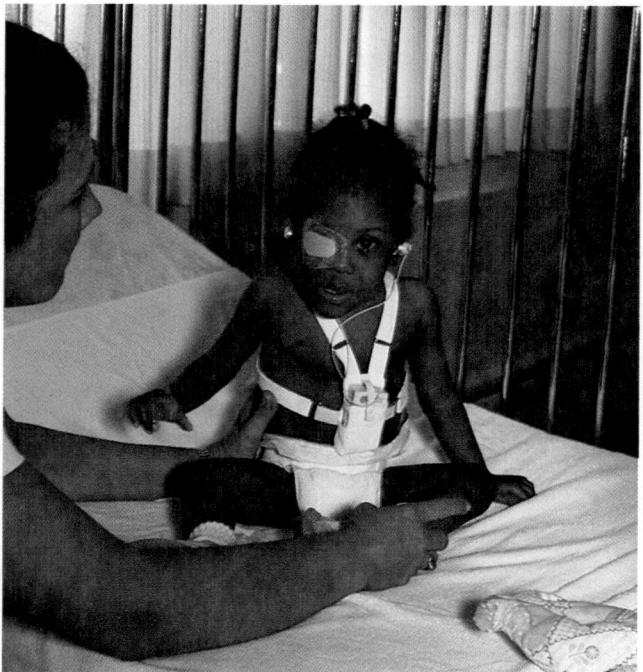

FIG. 19-7 ■ On-the-body hearing aids are convenient for young children, such as this child with severe bilateral hearing loss. Note eye patching for strabismus.

BOX 19-5
Clinical Manifestations of Hearing Impairment

INFANTS

Lack of startle or blink reflex to a loud sound
Failure to be awakened by loud environmental noises
Failure to localize a source of sound by 6 months of age
Absence of babble or voice inflections by age 7 months
Lack of response to the spoken word; failure to follow verbal directions
Response to loud noises as opposed to the voice

CHILDREN

Use of gestures rather than verbalization to express desires
Failure to develop intelligible speech by age 24 months
Monotone and unintelligible speech; lessened laughter
Vocal play, head banging, or foot stamping for vibratory sensation
Yelling or screeching to express pleasure, needs, or annoyance (tantrum)
Asking to have statements repeated or answering them incorrectly
Greater response to facial expression and gestures than to verbal explanation
Avoidance of social interaction; prefer to play alone
Inquiring, sometimes confused facial expression
Suspicious alertness alternating with cooperation
Frequently stubbornness because of lack of comprehension
Irritability at not making themselves understood
Shy, timid, and withdrawn behavior
Often appear "dreamy," "in a world of their own," or exhibit inattentiveness

---

NURSING ALERT

When parents express concern about their child's hearing and speech development, refer the child for a hearing evaluation. Absence of well-formed syllables (*da, na, yaya*) by 11 months of age should result in immediate referral.

Sensorineural Hearing Loss. Treatment for sensorineural hearing loss is much less satisfactory. Because the defect is not one of intensity of sound, hearing aids are of less value in this type of defect. The use of **cochlear implants*** (a surgically implanted prosthetic device) provides a sensation of hearing for individuals who have severe or profound hearing loss (Zeng and Liu, 2006; Downs and Buchman, 2005). Children with sensorineural hearing loss have lost or damaged some or all of their hair cells or auditory nerve fibers. Often these children cannot benefit from conventional hearing aids because they only amplify sound that cannot be processed by a damaged inner ear. A cochlear implant bypasses the hair cells to directly stimulate surviving auditory nerve fibers so that they can send signals to the brain. These signals can be interpreted by the brain to produce sound and sensations (Zeng and Liu, 2006; Gregg, Wiorek, and Arvedson, 2004).

Multichanneled implants are now available. This more sophisticated device stimulates the auditory nerve at a number of locations with differently processed signals. This type of stimulation allows a person to use the pitch information present in speech signals, leading to better understanding of

---

speech. The trend is toward early use of cochlear implants, usually by 18 months of age, to give the child maximum opportunity to develop listening, language, and speaking skills.

Nursing Care Management

Assessment of children for hearing impairment is a critical nursing responsibility. Early detection of hearing loss, preferably within the first 3 to 6 months of life, is essential to improve the language and educational outcomes of those with hearing impairments (Gregg, Wiorek, and Arvedson, 2004; Kenna, 2004). To accomplish this goal, the current recommendation is universal newborn hearing screening before discharge from the newborn nursery (Gregg, Wiorek, and Arvedson, 2004; Cunningham, Cox, and Committee on Practice and Ambulatory Medicine and the Section on Otolaryngology and Bronchoesophagology, 2003; American Academy of Pediatrics, 1999). This discussion focuses on developmental and behavioral indexes associated with hearing impairment. Auditory testing is presented in Chapter 6.

Infancy. At birth the nurse can observe the neonate's response to auditory stimuli, as evidenced by the startle reflex, head turning, eye blinking, and cessation of body movement. The infant may vary in the intensity of the response, depending on the state of alertness. However, a consistent absence of a reaction should lead to suspicion of hearing loss. Box 19-5 summarizes other clinical manifestations of hearing impairment in the infant.

Childhood. The child who is profoundly deaf is much more likely to be diagnosed during infancy than the less severely affected one. If the defect is not detected during early

---

*Hearing Enrichment Language Program of the Hough Ear Institute, 3434 N.W. 56th St., Oklahoma City, OK 73112; (405) 945-7186; fax: (405) 947-6266; http://www.integris-health.com/INTEGRIS/en-US/Specialties/EarInstitute/ HELP.

childhood, it likely will become evident during entry into school, when the child has difficulty learning. Unfortunately, some of these children are mistakenly placed in special classes for students with learning disabilities or CI. Therefore it is essential that the nurse suspect a hearing impairment in any child who demonstrates the behaviors listed in Box 19-5.

Of primary importance is the effect of hearing impairment on speech development.* A child with a mild conductive hearing loss may speak fairly clearly but in a loud, monotone voice. A child with a sensorineural defect usually has difficulty in articulation. For example, inability to hear higher frequencies may result in the word *spoon* being pronounced "poon." Children with articulation problems need to have their hearing tested.

NURSINGALERT

Stress to parents the importance of storing batteries for hearing aids in a safe location and teaching children or supervising young children not to remove the battery from the hearing aid. Ingestion of batteries is most often of those from hearing aids, including the child's own aid.

Lipreading. Even though the child may become an expert at lipreading, only about 40% of the spoken word is understood, and less if the speaker has an accent, mustache, or beard. Exaggerating pronunciation or speaking in an altered rhythm further reduces comprehension. Parents can help the child understand the spoken word by using the suggestions in the Nursing Care Guidelines box. The child learns to supplement the spoken word with sensitivity to visual cues, primarily body language and facial expression (e.g., tightening the lips, muscle tension, eye contact).

Cued Speech. This method of communication is an adjunct to straight lipreading. It uses hand signals to help the child with a hearing impairment distinguish between words that look alike when formed by the lips (e.g., mat, bat). It is most often used by children with hearing impairments who are using speech rather than those who are nonverbal.

Sign Language. Sign language, such as **American Sign Language (ASL)** or **British Sign Language (BSL),** is a visual gestural language that uses hand signals that roughly correspond to specific words and concepts in the English language. Family members are encouraged to learn signing because using or watching hands requires much less concentration than lipreading or talking. Also, a symbol method enables some children to learn more and to learn faster.

Speech Language Therapy. The most formidable task in the education of a child who is profoundly hearing impaired is learning to speak. Speech is learned through a multisensory approach, using visual, tactile, kinesthetic, and auditory stimulation. Parents are encouraged to participate fully in the learning process.

Additional Aids. Everyday activities present problems for older children with hearing impairment. For example, they may not be able to hear the telephone, doorbell, or alarm clock. Several commercial devices are available to help them

nursingcareguidelines

Facilitating Lipreading

- Attract child's attention before speaking; use light touch to signal speaker's presence.
- Stand close to child.
- Face child directly or move to a 45-degree angle.
- Stand still; do not walk back and forth or turn away to point or look elsewhere.
- Establish eye contact and show interest.
- Speak at eye level and with good lighting on speaker's face.
- Be certain nothing interferes with speech patterns, such as chewing food or gum.
- Speak clearly and at a slow and even rate.
- Use facial expression to assist in conveying messages.
- Keep sentences short.
- Rephrase message if child does not understand the words.

adjust to these dilemmas. Flashing lights can be attached to a telephone or doorbell to signal its ringing. Trained hearing ear dogs can provide great assistance because they alert the person to sounds, such as someone approaching, a moving car, a signal to wake up, or a child's cry. Special **teletypewriters** or **telecommunications devices for the deaf** (TDD or TTY) help people with impaired hearing communicate with each other over the telephone; the typed message is conveyed via the telephone lines and displayed on a small screen.*

Any audiovisual medium presents dilemmas for these children, who can see the picture but cannot hear the message. However, with **closed captioning** a special decoding device is attached to the television, and the audio portion of a program is translated into subtitles that appear on the screen.†

Socialization. As children learn to compensate for their lack of hearing, they become extremely perceptive to visual and vibratory changes. Children often know when another person wants to talk to them because the person will walk close by but not pass. They learn to be alert to other people approaching them by seeing their shadows or feeling the vibrations of their footsteps. They are acutely aware of facial expressions and may comprehend unspoken messages more quickly than the spoken word.

Because socialization is extremely important to the child's development, the nurse discusses with the family methods of fostering social contact. If children attend a special school for the deaf, they are able to socialize with peers in that setting. Classmates become a potential source of close friendships because they communicate more easily among themselves. Parents are encouraged to promote these relationships whenever possible.

Children with a hearing impairment may need special help with school or social activities. For children wearing hearing aids, background noise should be kept to a minimum. Because

---

*Other sources of information on several aspects of hearing loss and on the International Parents' Organization are the Alexander Graham Bell Association for the Deaf and Hard of Hearing, 3417 Volta Place NW, Washington, DC 20007; voice: (202) 337-5220; TTY: (202) 337-5221; fax: (202) 337-8314; http://www.agbell.org; and Canadian Hearing Society, 271 Spadina Road, Toronto, Ontario M5R 2V3; voice: (416) 928-2500; TTY: (416) 964-0023; fax: (416) 928-2506; http://www.chs.ca.

*Directory listings stating "TDD or TTY only" before a phone number indicate that regular telephone use is not possible; "TDD or TTY and voice" indicates that both TDD/TTY users and speaking, hearing people can use the telephone number.
†Additional information is available from the National Captioning Institute, 1900 Gallows Road, Suite 3000, Vienna, VA 22182; (703) 917-7600; fax: (703) 917-9878; http://www.ncicap.org.

many of these children are able to attend regular classes, the teacher may need assistance in adapting methods of teaching for the child's benefit. The school nurse is often in an optimal position to emphasize methods of facilitated communication, such as lipreading (see Nursing Care Guidelines box, p. 626). Because group projects and audiovisual teaching aids may hinder the child's learning, these educational methods should be carefully evaluated.

In a group setting it is helpful for the other members to sit in a semicircle in front of the child. Because one of the difficulties in following a group discussion is that the child is unaware of who will speak next, someone should point out each speaker. Speakers can also be given numbers, or their names can be written down as each person talks. If one person writes down the main topic of the discussion, the child is able to follow lipreading more closely. Such suggestions can increase the child's ability to participate in sports, organizations such as Boy Scouts or Girl Scouts, and group projects.

Support Child and Family. After the diagnosis of hearing impairment is made, parents need extensive support to adjust to the shock of learning about their child's disability and an opportunity to realize the extent of the hearing loss. If the hearing loss occurs during childhood, the child also requires sensitive, supportive care during the long and often difficult adjustment to this sensory loss. Early rehabilitation is one of the best strategies for fostering adjustment. However, progress in learning communication may not always coincide with emotional adjustment. Depression or anger is common, and such feelings are a normal part of the grieving process. (See also Chapter 18 for an extensive discussion of the emotional support of the child and family.)

Care for Child During Hospitalization. The needs of the hospitalized child with impaired hearing are the same as those of any other child, but the disability presents special challenges to the nurse (see Critical Thinking Exercise). For example, verbal explanations must be supplemented by tactile and visual aids, such as books or actual demonstration and practice. Children's understanding of the explanation needs to be constantly reassessed. If their verbal skills are poorly developed, they can answer questions through drawing, writing, or gesturing. For example, if the nurse is attempting to clarify where a spinal tap is done, the child is asked to point to where the procedure will be done on the body. Because these children often need more time to grasp the full meaning of an explanation, the nurse needs to be patient, allowing ample time for understanding.

When communicating with the child, the nurse should use the same principles as those outlined for facilitating lipreading. Ideally, nurses without foreign accents should be assigned to the child. The child's hearing aid is checked to ensure that it is working properly. If it is necessary to awaken the child at night, the nurse gently shakes the child or turns on the hearing aid before arousing the child. The nurse always makes certain that the child can see him or her before any procedures, even routine ones such as changing a diaper or regulating an infusion. It is important to remember that the child may not be aware of one's presence until alerted through visual or tactile cues.

Ideally, parents are encouraged to room with the child. However, it must be conveyed to them that this is not to serve as a convenience to the nurse but as a benefit to the child. Although the parents' aid can be enlisted in familiarizing the child with the hospital and explaining procedures, the nurse

also talks directly to the youngster, encouraging expression of feelings about the experience. If the child's speech is difficult to understand, the nurse makes an effort to become familiar with his or her pronunciation of words. Parents often can be helpful by explaining the child's usual speech habits. Nonverbal communication devices that employ pictures or words that the child can point to are also available. Such boards can also be made by drawing pictures or writing the words of common needs on cardboard, such as *parent, food, water,* or *toilet.*

The nurse has a special role as child advocate and is in a strategic position to alert other health team members and other patients to the child's special needs regarding communication. For example, the nurse should accompany other practitioners on visits to the child's room to ensure that they speak to the child and that the child understands what is said. Caregivers sometimes forget that the child has the abilities to perceive and learn despite a hearing loss, and consequently they communicate only with the parents. As a result, the child's needs and feelings remain unrecognized and unmet.

Because children with impaired hearing may have difficulty forming social relationships with other children, the child is introduced to roommates and encouraged to engage in play activities. The hospital setting can provide growth-promoting opportunities for social relationships. With the assistance of a child life specialist, the child can learn new recreational activities, experiment with group games, and engage in therapeutic play. The use of puppets, dollhouses, role-playing with dress-up clothes, building with a hammer and nails, finger painting, and water play can help the child express feelings that previously were suppressed.

Assist in Measures to Prevent Hearing Impairment. A primary nursing role is prevention of hearing loss. Because the most common cause of impaired hearing is chronic otitis media, it is essential that appropriate measures be instituted to treat existing infections and prevent recurrences (see Chapter 23). Children with a history of ear or respiratory infections or any other condition known to increase the risk of hearing impairment should receive periodic auditory testing.

To prevent the causes of hearing loss that begin prenatally and perinatally, pregnant women need counseling regarding the necessity of early prenatal care, including genetic counseling for known familial disorders; avoidance of all ototoxic drugs, especially during the first trimester; tests to rule out syphilis, rubella, or blood incompatibility; medical management of maternal diabetes; strict control of alcohol intake; adequate dietary intake; and avoidance of smoke exposure. The necessity of routine immunization during childhood to eliminate the possibility of acquired sensorineural hearing loss from rubella, mumps, or measles (encephalitis) is stressed.

Excessive noise pollution with or without smoke exposure causes sensorineural hearing loss (Daniel, 2007). The nurse should routinely assess the possibility of environmental pollution (e.g., loud noise and smoking) and advise children and parents of the potential danger of hearing loss. When individuals engage in activities associated with high-intensity noise, such as flying model airplanes, target shooting, or snowmobiling, they should wear ear protection such as earmuffs or earplugs. Even common household equipment, such as lawn mowers, vacuum cleaners, and cordless telephones, may cause noise-induced hearing loss.

> **NURSINGALERT**
>
> Suspect hazardous noise if the listener experiences (1) difficulty in communication while hearing the sound, (2) ringing in the ears (tinnitus) after exposure to the sound, or (3) muffled hearing after leaving the sound.

VISUAL IMPAIRMENT

Visual impairment is a common problem during childhood. In the United States the prevalence of blindness and serious visual impairment in the pediatric population is estimated at 30 to 64 children per 100,000 population. Vision problems occur in 5% to 10% of all preschoolers and include refractive error, strabismus, and amblyopia (Tingley, 2007). The nurse's role is clearly one of early assessment and detection, prevention, referral, and, in some instances, rehabilitation.

Definition and Classification

Visual impairment is a general term that refers to visual loss that cannot be corrected with regular prescription lenses. However, more useful definitions for classifying visual impairments exist. **School vision** (also known as *partially sighted*) refers to visual acuity between 20/70 and 20/200. The child should be able to obtain an education in the usual public school system with the use of normal-sized print. Near vision is almost always better than distance vision. **Legal blindness,** visual acuity of 20/200 or less and/or a visual field of 20 degrees or less in the better eye, is useful only as a legal definition, not as a medical diagnosis. It allows special considerations with regard to taxes, entrance into special schools, eligibility for aid, and other benefits.

Etiology

Visual impairment can be caused by a number of genetic and prenatal or postnatal conditions. These include perinatal infections (herpes, chlamydia, gonococci, rubella, syphilis, toxoplasmosis); retinopathy of prematurity; trauma; postnatal infections (meningitis); and disorders such as sickle cell disease, juvenile rheumatoid arthritis, Tay-Sachs disease, albinism, and retinoblastoma. In many instances, such as with refractive errors, the cause of the defect is unknown.

Refractive errors are the most common types of visual disorders in children. The term **refraction** means bending and refers to the bending of light rays as they pass through the lens of the eye. Normally, light rays enter the lens and fall directly on the retina. However, in refractive disorders the light rays either fall in front of the retina (**myopia**) or beyond it (**hyperopia**). Other eye problems, such as strabismus, may or may not include refractive errors, but they are important because, if untreated, they result in blindness from amblyopia. These, along with other less frequent visual disorders, are summarized in Box 19-6. In addition to these disorders, other visual problems can be a result of infection or trauma.

BOX 19-6

Types of Visual Impairment

REFRACTIVE ERRORS

Myopia

Nearsightedness—Ability to see objects clearly at close range but not at a distance

Pathophysiology
Results from eyeball that is too long, causing image to fall in front of retina

Clinical Manifestations
Excessive eye rubbing
Head tilt or forward head thrusts
Difficulty in reading or doing other close work
Headaches
Dizziness
Clumsiness; walking into objects
Blinking more than usual or irritability when doing close work

Inability to see objects clearly
Poor school performance, especially in subjects that require demonstration, such as arithmetic

Treatment
Corrected with biconcave lenses that focus rays on retina
May be corrected with laser surgery

Hyperopia

Farsightedness—Ability to see objects at a distance

Pathophysiology
Results from eyeball that is too short, causing image to focus beyond retina

Clinical Manifestations
Because of accommodative ability, child can usually see objects at all ranges
Most children normally hyperopic until about 7 years of age

BOX 19-6

Types of Visual Impairment—cont'd

Hyperopia—cont'd
Treatment
When required, corrected with convex lenses that focus rays on retina
May be corrected with laser surgery

Astigmatism
Unequal curvatures in refractive apparatus

Pathophysiology
Results from unequal curvatures in cornea or lens that cause light rays to bend in different directions

Clinical Manifestations
Depend on severity of refractive error in each eye
Possible clinical manifestations of myopia

Treatment
Corrected with special lenses that compensate for refractive errors
May be corrected with laser surgery

Anisometropia
Different refractive strength in each eye

Pathophysiology
May develop amblyopia as weaker eye is used less

Clinical Manifestations
Depend on severity of refractive error in each eye
Possible clinical manifestations of myopia

Treatment
Treated with corrective lenses, preferably contact lenses, to improve vision in each eye so they work as a unit
May be corrected with laser surgery

AMBLYOPIA
Lazy eye—Reduced visual acuity in one eye

Pathophysiology
Results when one eye does not receive sufficient stimulation
Each retina receives different images, resulting in diplopia (double vision)
Brain accommodates by suppressing less intense image
Visual cortex eventually does not respond to visual stimulation, with resultant loss of vision in that eye

Clinical Manifestations
Poor vision in affected eye

Treatment
Preventable if treatment of primary visual defect, such as anisometropia or strabismus, begins before 6 years of age

STRABISMUS
"Squint" or cross-eye—Malalignment of eyes
Esotropia—Inward deviation of eye
Exotropia—Outward deviation of eye

Pathophysiology
May result from muscle imbalance or paralysis, poor vision, or congenital defect
Because visual axes are not parallel, brain receives two images, and amblyopia can result

Clinical Manifestations
Squints eyelids together or frowns
Has difficulty focusing from one distance to another
Inaccurate judgment in picking up objects
Unable to see print or moving objects clearly
Closes one eye to see
Tilts head to one side
If combined with refractive errors, may see any of the manifestations listed for refractive errors
Diplopia
Photophobia
Dizziness
Headaches
Crossed eyes

Treatment
Depends on cause of strabismus
May involve occlusion therapy (patching stronger eye) or surgery to increase visual stimulation to weaker eye
Early diagnosis essential to prevent vision loss

CATARACTS
Opacity of crystalline lens

Pathophysiology
Prevents light rays from entering eye and refracting on retina

Clinical Manifestations
Gradual decrease in ability to see objects clearly
Possible loss of peripheral vision
Nystagmus (with complete blindness)
Gray opacities of lens
Strabismus
Absence of red reflex

Treatment
Requires surgery to remove cloudy lens and replace lens (with intraocular lens implant, removable contact lens, prescription glasses)
Must be treated early to prevent blindness from amblyopia

GLAUCOMA
Increased intraocular pressure

Pathophysiology
Congenital type results from defective development of some component related to flow of aqueous humor
Increased pressure on optic nerve causes eventual atrophy and blindness

Clinical Manifestations
Loss of peripheral vision—mostly seen in acquired types
Possible bumping into objects
Perception of halos around objects
Possible complaint of pain or discomfort (pain, nausea, or vomiting if sudden rise in pressure)
Eye redness
Excessive tearing (epiphora)
Photophobia
Spasmodic winking (blepharospasm)
Corneal haziness
Enlargement of eyeball (buphthalmos)

Treatment
Requires surgical treatment (goniotomy) to open outflow tracts
May require more than one procedure

Trauma. Trauma is a common cause of blindness in children. Injuries to the eyeball and adnexa (supporting or accessory structures, such as eyelids, conjunctiva, or lacrimal glands) can be classified as penetrating or nonpenetrating. **Penetrating wounds** are most often a result of sharp instruments, such as sticks, knives, or scissors; propulsive objects, such as firecrackers, guns, arrows, or slingshots; or a powerful contusion by a blunt object, which may occur during a fight or from a serious car accident. **Nonpenetrating injuries** may be a result of foreign objects in the eyes, lacerations, a blow from a blunt object such as a ball (baseball, softball, basketball, racquet sports) or fist, or thermal or chemical burns.

Treatment is aimed at preventing further ocular damage and is primarily the responsibility of the ophthalmologist. It involves adequate examination of the injured eye (with the child sedated or anesthetized in severe injuries); appropriate immediate intervention, such as removal of the foreign body or suturing of the laceration; and prevention of complications, such as administration of antibiotics or steroids and complete bed rest to allow the eye to heal and blood to reabsorb (see Emergency Treatment box). The prognosis varies according to the type of injury. It is usually guarded in all cases of penetrating wounds because of the high risk of serious complications.

Infections. Infections of the adnexa and structures of the eyeball or globe may occur in children. The most common eye infection is **conjunctivitis** (see Chapter 14). Treatment is usually with ophthalmic antibiotics. Severe infections may require systemic antibiotic therapy. Steroids are used cautiously because they exacerbate viral infections such as herpes simplex, increasing the risk of damage to the involved structures.

Nursing Care Management

Assessment of children for visual impairment is a critical nursing responsibility. Discovery of a visual impairment as early as possible is essential to prevent social, physical, and psychologic damage to the child. Assessment involves (1) identifying those children who by virtue of their history are at risk, (2) observing for behaviors that indicate a vision loss, and (3) screening all children for visual acuity and signs of other ocular disorders such as strabismus. This discussion focuses on clinical manifestations of various types of visual problems (see Box 19-6). Vision testing is discussed in Chapter 6.

Infancy. At birth the nurse should observe the neonate's response to visual stimuli, such as following a light or object and cessation of body movement. The infant may vary in the intensity of the response, depending on the state of alertness.

Of special importance in detecting visual impairment during infancy are the parents' concerns regarding visual responsiveness in their child. Their concerns, such as lack of eye contact from the infant, must be taken seriously. During infancy the child should be tested for strabismus. Lack of binocularity after 4 months of age is considered abnormal and must be treated to prevent amblyopia.

> **NURSINGALERT**
>
> Suspect blindness if the infant does not react to light or if parents of a child at any age express concern.

Childhood. Because the most common visual impairment during childhood is refractive errors, testing for visual acuity is essential. The school nurse usually assumes major responsibility for vision testing in schoolchildren. Besides refractive errors, the nurse should be aware of signs and symptoms that indicate other ocular problems. If a referral is made to the family requesting further eye testing, the nurse is responsible for follow-up concerning the recommendation.

The shock of learning that their child is blind or partially sighted is an immense crisis for families. The family is encouraged to investigate appropriate stimulation and educational programs for their child as soon as possible. Sources of infor-

---

emergencytreatment

Eye Injuries

FOREIGN OBJECT

Examine eye for presence of a foreign body (evert upper lid to examine upper eye).

Remove a freely movable object with pointed corner of gauze pad lightly moistened with water.

Do not irrigate eye or attempt to remove a penetrating object (see following section).

Caution child against rubbing eye.

CHEMICAL BURNS

Irrigate eye copiously with tap water for 20 minutes.

Evert upper lid to flush thoroughly.

Hold child's head with eye under tap of running lukewarm water.

Take to emergency department.

Have child rest with eyes closed.

Keep room darkened.

ULTRAVIOLET BURNS

If skin is burned, patch both eyes (make certain lids are completely closed); secure dressing with Kling bandages wrapped around head rather than tape.

Have child rest with eyes closed.

Refer to an ophthalmologist.

HEMATOMA ("BLACK EYE")

Use a flashlight to check for gross **hyphema** (hemorrhage into anterior chamber; visible fluid meniscus across iris; more easily seen in light-colored than in brown eyes).

Apply ice for first 24 hours to reduce swelling if no hyphema is present.

Refer to an ophthalmologist immediately if hyphema is present.

Have child rest with eyes closed.

PENETRATING INJURIES

Take child to emergency department.

Never remove an object that has penetrated eye.

Follow strict aseptic technique in examining eye.

Observe for:

- Aqueous or vitreous leaks (fluid leaking from point of penetration)
- Hyphema
- Shape and equality of pupils, reaction to light, prolapsed iris (not perfectly circular)

Apply a Fox shield if available (not a regular eye patch) and apply patch over unaffected eye to prevent bilateral movement.

Maintain bed rest with child in 30-degree Fowler position.

Caution child against rubbing eye.

Refer to ophthalmologist.

mation include state commissions for the blind, local schools for the blind, American Foundation for the Blind,* National Federation of the Blind,† National Association for Parents of Children with Visual Impairments,‡ National Association for Visually Handicapped,§ American Council of the Blind,‖ and CNIB.¶

Promote Parent-Child Attachment. A crucial time in the life of blind infants is when they and their parents are getting acquainted with each other. Pleasurable patterns of interaction between the infant and parents may be lacking if there is not enough reciprocity. For example, if the parent gazes fondly at the infant's face and seeks eye contact but the infant fails to respond because he or she cannot see the parent, a troubled cycle of responses may occur. The nurse can help parents learn to look for other cues that indicate the infant is responding to them, such as whether the eyelids blink; whether the activity level accelerates or slows; whether respiratory patterns change, such as faster or slower breathing, when the parents come near; and whether the infant makes throaty sounds when they speak to the infant. In time parents learn that the infant has unique ways of relating to them. They are encouraged to show affection using nonvisual methods, such as talking or reading, cuddling, and walking the child.

Promote Child's Optimal Development. Promoting the child's optimum development requires rehabilitation in a number of important areas. These include learning self-help skills and appropriate communication techniques to become independent. Although nurses may not be directly involved in such programs, they can provide direction and guidance to families regarding the availability of programs and the need to promote these activities in their child.

Development and Independence. Motor development depends on sight almost as much as verbal communication depends on hearing. From earliest infancy, parents are encouraged to expose the infant to as many visual-motor experiences as possible, such as sitting supported in an infant seat or swing and being given opportunities for holding up the head, sitting unsupported, reaching for objects, and crawling.

Despite visual impairment, the child can become independent in all aspects of self-care. The same principles used for promoting independence in sighted children apply, with additional emphasis on nonvisual cues. For example, the child may need help in dressing, such as special arrangement of clothing for style coordination and braille tags to distinguish colors and prints.

The blind child also must learn to become independent in navigational skills. The two main techniques are the **tapping method** (use of a cane to survey the environment for direction and to avoid obstacles) and **guides,** such as a sighted human guide or a dog guide, such as a Seeing Eye dog. Chil-

dren who are partially sighted may benefit from ocular aids, such as a monocular telescope.

Play and Socialization. Blind children do not learn to play automatically. Because they cannot imitate others or actively explore the environment as sighted children do, they depend much more on others to stimulate and teach them how to play. Parents need help in selecting appropriate play material, especially those that encourage fine and gross motor development and stimulate the senses of hearing, touch, and smell. Toys with educational value are especially useful, such as dolls with various clothing closures.

Blind children have the same needs for socialization as sighted children. Because they have little difficulty in learning verbal skills, they are able to communicate with age-mates and participate in suitable activities. The nurse discusses with parents opportunities for socialization outside the home, especially regular preschools. The trend is to include these children with sighted children to help them adjust to the outside world for eventual independence.

To compensate for inadequate stimulation, these children may develop **blindisms** (self-stimulatory activities, such as body rocking, finger flicking, or arm twirling). Such habits restrict the child's social acceptance and are discouraged. Behavior modification is often successful in reducing or eliminating blindisms.

Education. The main obstacle to learning is the child's total dependence on nonvisual cues. Although the child can learn via verbal lecturing, he or she is unable to read the written word or to write without special education. Therefore the child must rely on **braille,** a system that uses raised dots to represent letters and numbers. The child can then read the braille with the fingers and can write a message using a braille writer. However, unless others read braille, this system is not useful for communicating with others. A more portable system for written communication is the use of a braille slate and stylus or a microcassette tape recorder. A recorder is especially helpful for leaving messages for others and taking notes during classroom lectures. For mathematic calculations, portable calculators with voice synthesizers are available.*

Records and tapes are significant sources of reading material other than braille books, which are large and cumbersome. The Library of Congress† has talking books, braille books, and a special records program, which are available at many local and state libraries and directly from the Library of Congress. The talking book machine and tape player are provided at no cost to families, and there is no postage fee for returning the materials. Recording for the Blind and Dyslexic‡ also provides texts and tapes of books, which are helpful for secondary and college students who are blind.

Learning to use a regular typewriter is another form of writing but has the disadvantage of the blind person's being

*11 Penn Plaza, Suite 300, New York, NY 10001; (800) 232-5463 or (212) 502-7600; fax: (212) 502-7777; http://www.afb.org.

†1800 Johnson St., Baltimore, MD 21230; (410) 659-9314; fax: (410) 685-5653; http://www.nfb.org.

‡PO Box 317, Watertown, MA 02471; (800) 562-6265; fax: (617) 972-7444; http://www.napvi.org.

§22 W. 21st St., 6th Floor, New York, NY 10010; (212) 889-3141; fax: (212) 727-2931; http://www.navh.org.

‖1155 15th St. NW, Suite 1004, Washington, DC 20005; (800) 424-8666; fax: (202) 467-5085; http://www.acb.org.

¶1929 Bayview Ave., Toronto, Ontario M4G 3E8; (800) 563-2642; fax: (416) 480-7700; http://www.cnib.ca.

*A catalog of numerous products for people with vision problems is available from American Foundation for the Blind (see previous footnote) and from Lighthouse International, 111 E. 59th St., New York, NY 10022-1202; (212) 821-9200 or (800) 829-0500; http://www.lighthouse.org.

†National Library Service for the Blind and Physically Handicapped, (888) 657-7323; TTD: (202) 707-0744; fax: (202) 707-0712; http://www.loc.gov/nls. (A state-by-state listing of libraries for blind and physically handicapped readers, as well as other reference circulars, is available from this office.)

‡20 Roszel Road, Princeton, NJ 08540; (800) 221-4792 or (866) RFBD-585; http://www.rfbd.org.

unable to check what he or she has written. Computers eliminate this drawback; a home computer with a voice synthesizer can be adapted to speak each letter or word that has been typed.

The child with partial sight benefits from specialized visual aids that produce a magnified retinal image. The basic devices are accommodation (e.g., bringing the object closer), special plus lenses, handheld and stand magnifiers, telescopes, video projection systems, and large print. Special equipment is available to enlarge print. Information about services for the partially sighted is available from the National Association for Visually Handicapped and American Foundation for the Blind. Children with diminished vision often prefer to do close work without their glasses and compensate by bringing the object very near to their eyes. This should be allowed. The exception is the child with vision in only one eye, who should always wear glasses for protection.

Care for the Child During Hospitalization. Because nurses are more likely to care for children who are hospitalized for procedures that involve temporary loss of vision than for children who are blind, the following discussion concentrates primarily on the needs of such children. The nursing care objectives in either situation are to (1) reassure the child and family throughout every phase of treatment, (2) orient the child to the surroundings, (3) provide a safe environment, and (4) encourage independence. Whenever possible, the same nurse should care for the child to ensure consistency in the approach.

When sighted children temporarily lose their vision, almost every aspect of the environment becomes bewildering and frightening. They are forced to rely on nonvisual senses for help in adjusting to the blindness without the benefit of any special training. Nurses have a major role in minimizing the effects of temporary loss of vision. They need to talk to the child about everything that is occurring, emphasizing aspects of procedures that are felt or heard. They should approach the child by always identifying themselves as soon as they enter the room. Because unfamiliar sounds are especially frightening, these are explained. Parents are encouraged to room with their child and participate in the care. Familiar objects, such as a teddy bear or doll, should be brought from home to help lessen the strangeness of the hospital. As soon as the child is able to be out of bed, he or she is oriented to the immediate surroundings. If the child is able to see on admission, this opportunity is taken to point out significant aspects of the room. The child is encouraged to practice ambulating with the eyes closed to become accustomed to this experience.

The room is arranged with safety in mind. For example, a stool or chair is placed next to the bed to help the child climb in and out of bed. The furniture is always placed in the same position to prevent collisions. Cleaning personnel are reminded of the need to keep the room in order. If the child has difficulty navigating by feeling the walls, a rope can be attached from the bed to the point of destination, such as the bathroom. Attention to details such as well-fitting slippers or robes that do not drag on the floor is important in preventing tripping. Unlike the child who is blind, these children are not familiar with navigating with a cane.

The child is encouraged to be independent in self-care activities, especially if the visual loss may be prolonged or potentially permanent. For example, during bathing the nurse sets up all the equipment and encourages the child to participate.

At mealtime the nurse explains where each food item is on the tray, opens any special containers, prepares cereal or toast, and encourages the child in self-feeding. Favorite finger foods, such as sandwiches, hamburgers, hot dogs, or pizza, may be good selections. The child is praised for efforts at being cooperative and independent. Any improvements made in self-care, no matter how small, are stressed.

Appropriate recreational activities are provided, and if a child life specialist is available, such planning is done jointly. Because children with temporary blindness have a wide variety of play experiences to draw on, they are encouraged to select activities. For example, if they like to read, they may enjoy being read to. If they prefer manual activity, they may appreciate playing with clay or building blocks or feeling different textures and naming them. If they need an outlet for aggression, activities such as pounding or banging on a drum can be helpful. Simple board and card games can be played with a "seeing partner" or an opponent who helps with the game. They should have familiar toys from home to play with, since familiar items are more easily manipulated than new ones. If parents want to bring presents, they should be objects that stimulate hearing and touch, such as a radio, music box, or stuffed animal.

Occasionally, children who are blind come to the hospital for procedures to restore their vision. Although this is an extremely happy time, it also requires intervention to help them adjust to sight. They need an opportunity to take in all that they see. They should not be bombarded with visual stimuli. They may need to concentrate on people's faces or their own to become accustomed to this experience. They often need to talk about what they see and to compare the visual images with their mental ones. The children may also go through a period of depression, which must be respected and supported. The nurse or parents should refrain from statements such as "How can you be so sad when you can see again?" Instead the children should be encouraged to discuss how it feels to see, especially in terms of seeing themselves.

Newly sighted children also need time to adjust to the ability to engage in activities that were impossible before. For example, they may prefer to use braille to read, rather than learning a new "visual approach," because of familiarity with the touch system. Eventually, as they learn to recognize letters and numbers, they will integrate these new skills into reading and writing. However, parents and teachers must be careful not to push them before they are ready. This applies to social relationships and physical activities as well as learning situations.

Assist in Measures to Prevent Visual Impairment. An essential nursing goal is to prevent visual impairment. This involves many of the same interventions discussed under hearing impairments:

- Prenatal screening for pregnant women at risk, such as those with rubella or syphilis infection and family histories of genetic disorders associated with visual loss
- Adequate prenatal and perinatal care to prevent prematurity
- Periodic screening of all children, especially newborns through preschoolers, for congenital blindness and visual impairments caused by refractive errors, strabismus, and other disorders
- Rubella immunization of all children
- Safety counseling regarding the common causes of ocular trauma and safe practices when working with, playing with, or carrying objects such as scissors, knives, and balls

After detection of eye problems, the nurse has a responsibility to prevent further ocular damage by ensuring that corrective treatment is used. For the child with strabismus, this often necessitates occlusion patching of the stronger eye. Compliance with the procedure is greatest during the early preschool years. It is more difficult to encourage school-age children to wear the occlusive patch because the poor visual acuity of the uncovered weaker eye interferes with school work and the patch sets them apart from their peers. In school they benefit from being positioned favorably (closer to the chalkboard or other visual media) and allowed extra time to read or complete an assignment. If treatment of the eye disorder requires instillation of ophthalmic medication, the family is taught the correct procedure (see Chapter 22).

For the child with refractive errors, the nurse helps the child adjust to wearing **glasses.** Young children who often pull glasses off benefit from temporal pieces that wrap around the ears or an elastic strap attached to the frames and around the back of the head to hold the glasses on securely. After children appreciate the value of clear vision, they are more likely to wear the corrective lenses.

Glasses should not interfere with any activity. Special protective guards are available during contact sports to prevent accidental injury, and all corrective lenses should be made from safety glass, which is shatterproof. Often, corrective lenses improve visual acuity so dramatically that children are able to compete more effectively in sports. This in itself is a tremendous inducement to continue wearing glasses.

Contact lenses are a popular alternative, especially for adolescents. Several types are available, such as hard lenses, including gas-permeable ones, and soft lenses, which may be designed for daily or extended wear. Contact lenses offer several advantages over glasses, such as greater visual acuity, total corrected field of vision, convenience (especially with the extended-wear type), and optimal cosmetic benefit. Unfortunately, they are usually more expensive and require much more care than glasses, including considerable practice to learn techniques for insertion and removal. If they are prescribed, the nurse can be helpful in teaching parents or older children how to care for the lenses.

Because trauma is the leading cause of blindness, the nurse has the major responsibility of preventing further eye injury until specific treatment is instituted. The major principles to follow when caring for an eye injury are outlined in the Emergency Treatment box on p. 630. Because patients with a serious eye injury fear blindness, the nurse should stay with the child and family to provide support and reassurance.

DEAF-BLIND CHILDREN

The most traumatic sensory impairment is loss of sight and hearing. Obviously, auditory and visual disabilities have profound effects on the child's development. They interfere with the normal sequence of physical, intellectual, and psychosocial growth. Although such children often achieve the usual motor milestones, their rate of development is slower. These children learn communication only with specialized training. **Finger spelling** is one desirable method often taught to these children. Some deaf-blind children, especially those with residual hearing or sight, can learn to speak. Whenever possible, speech is encouraged because it allows communication with other individuals.

The future prospects for deaf-blind children are, at best, unpredictable. Congenital blindness or deafness may be accompanied by other physical or neurologic problems, which further diminish the child's learning potential. The most favorable prognosis is for children who have acquired deafness and blindness and have few, if any, associated disabilities. Their learning capacity is greatly potentiated by their developmental progress before the sensory impairments. Although total independence, including gainful vocational training, is the goal, some deaf-blind children are unable to develop to this level. They may require lifelong parental or residential care. The nurse working with such families helps them deal with future goals for the child, including possible alternatives to home care during the parents' advancing years.

RETINOBLASTOMA

Retinoblastoma, which arises from the retina, is the most common congenital malignant intraocular tumor of childhood. Approximately 11 cases per million occur annually, primarily in children younger than 5 years of age. Retinoblastoma is caused by a mutation in a gene and may occur sporadically or be inherited (Hurwitz, Shields, Shields, and others, 2006). Retinoblastoma develops when the mutated gene is unable to produce the natural signals to stop the growth of retinal cells. Of all cases, the majority are nonhereditary and unilateral, with the remainder divided between hereditary and unilateral, and hereditary and bilateral. Hereditary retinoblastomas are transmitted as an autosomal dominant trait with a 90% penetrance (Hurwitz, Shields, Shields, and others, 2006).

Diagnostic Evaluation

Retinoblastoma has few grossly obvious signs (Box 19-7). Typically the most common sign is observed by the parent as a whitish "glow" in the pupil, known as the white reflex or **leukokoria.** Leukokoria represents visualization of the tumor as the light momentarily falls on the mass (Fig. 19-8). The second most common sign of retinoblastoma is acquired strabismus (Hurwitz, Shields, Shields, and others, 2006).

The first step in diagnosis is carefully listening to and recognizing the significance of reports from family members regarding suspected abnormalities within the eye. Eye abnormalities, including white reflex, strabismus, decreased vision, and persistent painful erythematous eyes, are referred to an ophthalmologist. Definitive diagnosis is usually based on ophthalmoscopic examination with the patient under general anesthesia. Imaging studies, including ultrasonography and computed tomography of the orbit, are done to determine the extent of the disease.

BOX 19-7

Clinical Manifestations of Retinoblastoma

- White eye reflex (most common sign)
- Strabismus (second most common sign)
- Red, painful eye, often with glaucoma
- Blindness (late sign)

FIG. 19-8 ■ White reflex. Whitish appearance of lens is produced as light falls on tumor mass in left eye.

FIG. 19-9 ■ The same infant with left prosthetic eye.

Therapeutic Management

The aim of therapy is to preserve useful vision and eradicate the tumor. Treatment of retinoblastoma depends chiefly on the stage of the tumor at the time of diagnosis. Some of the common focal therapies are (1) plaque brachytherapy (surgical radioactive implant on the sclera until maximum dose has been delivered to the tumor), (2) laser photocoagulation (laser beam to coagulate blood supply to the tumor), (3) cryotherapy (freezing the tumor by destroying the microcirculation to the tumor through microcrystal formation, and (4) thermotherapy (using microwaves or infrared radiation to deliver heat to the tumor) (Melamud, Palekar, and Singh, 2006; De Potter, 2002; Schouten–van Meeteren, Moll, Imhof, and others, 2002).

Chemotherapy is being used in the early RE groups in an attempt to reduce tumor size to facilitate focal intraocular treatment (chemoreduction). Chemotherapy has been used for several years to prevent metastatic disease in the RE groups IV and V and relapsed patients (chemoprevention or chemoprophylaxis). Chemoreduction and chemoprevention minimize the use of external beam radiation treatment and therefore reduce the risk of radiation-induced malignancies and facial disfigurement.

With advanced tumor growth into the optic nerve, choroid, orbit, and anterior chamber or no hope for useful vision, **enucleation** (removal) of the affected eye is the treatment of choice. After enucleation, an orbital implant is placed to provide a more natural cosmetic appearance, minimize sinking of the prosthesis, and enable motility of the prosthesis. With bilateral disease, every attempt is made to preserve useful vision in both eyes. Chemotherapy, external beam, radiotherapy, and other treatments (i.e., cryotherapy, laser, plaque brachytherapy, thermotherapy) to both eyes may prevent the need for enucleation.

Prognosis. The overall prognosis for retinoblastoma is favorable, with a survival rate of nearly 90% for both unilateral and bilateral tumors. Retinoblastoma is one of the tumors that may spontaneously regress. Of major concern in long-term survivors is the development of decreased visual acuity, facial disfiguration, and secondary tumors—especially osteo-

genic sarcoma, other sarcomas, and melanoma. Children with bilateral disease (hereditary form) are more likely to develop secondary cancers than are children with unilateral disease. It is thought that these individuals are predisposed to developing cancer and that radiation increases their risk.

Nursing Care Management

One of the most important nursing goals is to have a high index of suspicion for this rare malignancy. If parents report noticing a strange light in the eye or expression, these concerns must be taken seriously. Families with a history of retinoblastoma require follow-up, and the nurse can be instrumental in reminding parents of appointments.

Because the tumor is usually diagnosed in infants or very young children, most of the preparation for diagnostic tests and treatment involves parents. After indirect ophthalmoscopy, the child may not see clearly, or the eyes may be sensitive to light because of pupillary dilation. Parents are made aware of these normal reactions before the procedure. Screening tests, such as bone surveys and bone marrow aspiration, are rarely performed unless metastatic disease is suspected.

The treatment plan may include focal intraocular therapy with or without chemotherapy, external beam radiation, and, if necessary, enucleation. Enucleation is the treatment of choice if there is extensive disease threatening metastasis or no chance for useful vision. The enucleation procedure and the positive benefits of a prosthesis are explained to the parents. Showing them pictures of another child with an artificial eye may help them adjust to the thought of disfigurement (Fig. 19-9).

After surgery the parents are prepared for the child's facial appearance. An eye patch is in place, and the child's face may be edematous or ecchymotic. Parents often fear seeing the surgical site because they imagine a cavity in the skull. A surgically implanted sphere maintains the shape of the eyeball, and the implant is covered with conjunctiva. When the lids are open, the exposed area resembles the mucosal lining of the mouth. After the child is fitted for a prosthesis, usually within 3 weeks, the facial appearance returns to normal. Initial instructions for care of the prosthesis are given by the ocularist who fits and manufactures the device.

Care of the socket is minimal and easily accomplished. The wound itself is clean and has little or no drainage. If an antibiotic ointment is prescribed, it is applied in a thin line on the surface of the tissues of the socket. To cleanse the site, an irrigating solution may be ordered and is instilled daily or more frequently, *before* application of the antibiotic ointment. The dressing, consisting of an eye pad taped over the surgical site, is changed daily. After the socket has healed completely, a dressing is no longer necessary, although it is a preventive measure against infection.

AUTISM SPECTRUM DISORDERS

Autism spectrum disorders (ASDs) are complex neurodevelopmental disorders of brain function accompanied by intellectual and social behavioral deficits. ASDs include autistic disorder, Asperger syndrome, and pervasive developmental disorder not otherwise specified, which are impairments ranging from mild to severe (Croen, Najjar, Ray, and others, 2006). ASD is typically noticed during early childhood, primarily from 24 to 48 months of age. It occurs in one in 166 children; is about four times more common in males than in females (although females are more severely affected); and is not related to socioeconomic level, race, or parenting style (Courtney-Manning, 2007; Schaefer and Lutz, 2006; Fombonne, 2003).

Etiology

ASD is now recognized as a genetic disorder of prenatal and postnatal brain development (Bloom-DiCicco, Lord, Zwaigenbaum, and others, 2006). Immune and environmental factors (e.g., viral infections) may interact with the genetic susceptibility to increase the incidence of ASD (Bloom-DiCicco, Lord, Zwaigenbaum, and others, 2006). Individuals with ASD may have abnormal electroencephalograms, epileptic seizures, delayed development of hand dominance, persistence of primitive reflexes, metabolic abnormalities (elevated blood serotonin), cerebellar vermal hypoplasia (part of the brain involved in regulating motion and some aspects of memory), and infantile abnormal head enlargement (Dawson, 2007; Bloom-DiCicco, Lord, Zwaigenbaum, and others, 2006).

The strong evidence for a genetic basis in twins is consistent with an autosomal recessive pattern of inheritance. Twin studies demonstrate a high concordance (60% to 96%) for monozygotic (identical) twins and less than 5% concordance for dizygotic (nonidentical) twins. In addition, between 5% and 16% of males with ASD are positive for the fragile X chromosome.

There is a relatively high risk of recurrence of ASD in families with one affected child (Schaefer and Lutz, 2006; Muhle, Trentacoste, and Rapin, 2004). Although several genes have been suggested as possible causative factors in ASD, no specific gene for the disorder has been identified (Dawson, 2007; Kolevzon, Gross, and Reichenberg, 2007; Schanen, 2006).

Contrary to previous reports, autism does not appear to be caused by the measles-mumps-rubella (MMR) and thimerosal-containing vaccines (D'Souza, Fombonne, and Ward, 2006; DeStefano, Bhasin, Thompson, and others, 2004; Muhle, Trentacoste, and Rapin, 2004) (see Evidence-Based Practice box). ASD has been reported in association with a number of conditions such as fragile X syndrome, tuberous sclerosis, metabolic disorders, fetal rubella syndrome, *Haemophilus influenzae* meningitis, and structural brain anomalies (Dawson, 2007; Muhle, Trentacoste, and Rapin, 2004). Recent reports have retrospectively tied ASD to prenatal and perinatal events such as maternal and paternal ages over 40 years (for fathers, one in 116 births; for mothers, one in 123 births), uterine bleeding during pregnancy, low Apgar score, fetal distress, and neonatal hyperbilirubinemia (Croen, Najjar, Fireman, and others, 2007; Kolevzon, Gross, and Reichenberg, 2007; Muhle, Trentacoste, and Rapin, 2004). These same researchers, however, urge caution in interpreting these findings.

Clinical Manifestations and Diagnostic Evaluation

Children with ASD demonstrate several peculiar and often seemingly bizarre characteristics, primarily in social interactions, communication, and behavior. One hallmark characteristic is the inability to maintain eye contact with another person. Parents of autistic children have noted their infants had difficulties with eye contact, avoidance of body contact, and language delay at a very early age (Belschner, 2007; Dawson, 2007). Children with ASD also display limited functional play and may interact with toys in an unusual or odd manner (Belschner, 2007). ASD children may have significant gastrointestinal symptoms. Constipation is a common symptom and can be associated with acquired megarectum in children with ASD (Afzal, Murch, Thirrupathy, and others, 2003). Other clinical manifestations typically seen in children with autism are described in Box 19-8.

Children with autism do not always have the same manifestations, from mild forms requiring minimal supervision, to severe forms in which self-abusive behavior is common. The majority (50% to 70%) of children with autism have some degree of cognitive impairment, with scores typically in the moderate to severe range. More females than males tend to have very low intelligence scores. Despite their relatively moderate to severe disability, some children with autism (known as **savants**) excel in particular areas, such as art, music, memory, mathematics, or perceptual skills such as puzzle building.

> **NURSING TIP**
>
> Claims of beneficial results from the use of secretin, a peptide hormone that stimulates pancreatic secretion, have not been substantiated by scientific study (Dalton, Forman, and Boris, 2004).*

Speech and language delays are also common in ASD children. Any child who does not display such language skills as babbling or gesturing by 12 months, single words by 16 months, and two-word phrases by 24 months is recommended for immediate hearing and language evaluation (Grizzle and Simms, 2005). A sudden deterioration in extant expressive speech is also a red-flag event for further evaluation.

Early recognition, referral, diagnosis, and intensive early intervention tend to improve outcomes for children with ASD (Belschner, 2007; Courtney-Manning, 2007). Unfortunately, diagnosis is often not made until 2 to 3 years after symptoms are first recognized. The American Academy of Neurology report has a comprehensive set of suggested diagnostic criteria to be used to either rule out or establish the diagnosis of childhood ASD (Belschner, 2007; Filipek, Accardo, Ashwal, and others, 2000) (see Box 19-8).

*Additional information on secretin may be found at http://www.autism.org/secretin.html and by contacting the Autism Society of America, 7910 Woodmont Ave., Suite 300, Bethesda, MD 20814-3067; (800) 3AUTISM or (301) 657-0881; http://www.autism-society.org.

Thimerosal-Containing Vaccines and Autism Spectrum Disorders

ASK THE QUESTION Is the incidence of autism spectrum disorders (ASDs) or other neurodevelopmental disorders increased in children receiving vaccines containing thimerosal?

SEARCH FOR EVIDENCE
Search Strategies Search selection criteria included English language, publication within the past 15 years, research-based articles (level 3 or lower), and child populations.
Databases Used PubMed, Cochrane Collaboration, MD Consult, Vaccine Adverse Events Reporting System (VAERS) database, American Academy of Pediatrics, Autism Research Institute

CRITICALLY ANALYZE THE EVIDENCE

■ A two-phased retrospective study used computerized health maintenance organization (HMO) databases to assess the possible toxicity of thimerosal-containing vaccines among infants. Phase I screened for associations between neurodevelopmental disorders and thimerosal exposure in 124,170 infants born from 1992 to 1999. Phase II screened for the most common disorders found during phase I in 16,717 children born from 1991 to 1997 in another HMO database. In the analyses of the data, no significant associations were found between receipt of thimerosal-containing vaccines and neurodevelopmental outcomes (Verstraeten, Davis, DeStefano, and others, 2003).

■ A cohort study of 467,450 children in Denmark compared the incidence of ASDs in children vaccinated with thimerosal-containing vaccines with that in children vaccinated with a thimerosal-free formulation of the same vaccine. Results found no relationship between childhood vaccination with thimerosal-containing vaccines and the development of ASDs (Hviid, Stellfeld, Wohlfahrt, and others, 2003).

■ A retrospective cohort study involved 109,863 children in the United Kingdom from 1988 to 1997. This study was designed to investigate the relationship between the amount of thimerosal in a diphtheria-pertussis-tetanus (DTP) or diphtheria-tetanus (DT) vaccination administered at a young age and the subsequent occurrence of neurodevelopmental disorders. The study found no evidence that thimerosal exposure from DTP or DT vaccines causes neurodevelopmental disorders, except for tics (Andrews, Miller, Path, and others, 2004).

■ A longitudinal study evaluated over 14,000 children in the United Kingdom. The mercury exposure from thimerosal-containing vaccines was recorded and calculated at age 3, 4, and 6 months and compared to cognitive and behavioral-developmental assessments performed from 6 to 91 months of age. Researchers found no evidence that early exposure to thimerosal had any deleterious effect on neurologic or psychologic outcome (Heron, Golding, and the ALSPAC study team, 2004).

■ Between 1985 and 1989 and again during the late 1990s, Stehr-Green, Tull, Stellfeld, and others (2003) compared the incidence and prevalence of autism-like disorders in California, Sweden, and Denmark. Findings indicated that the incidence and prevalence of autism-like disorders began to rise from 1985 to 1989 and increased in incidence until the early 1990s. In the United States the thimerosal level in vaccines increased throughout the 1990s, whereas in Sweden and Denmark the already low thimerosal level in the vaccines steadily decreased in the 1980s and was virtually eliminated from all vaccines in the early 1990s. This study concludes that an increased exposure to thimerosal-containing vaccines does not correlate with the increased rates of autism in young children observed in Sweden and Denmark.

■ Madsen, Lauritsen, Pedersen, and others (2003) studied 956 children diagnosed with autism from 1971 to 2000 and showed that the incidence was stable until 1990 with increased rates thereafter, in spite of the decreased amount of thimerosal used from 1970 to 1992. The rise in the incidence of autism continued even in children born after discontinuation of thimerosal-containing vaccines in Denmark in 1992.

■ In 2004 the Institute of Medicine (IOM) completed an update to the review of the evidence and concluded that the epidemiological evidence supports the rejection of a causal relationship between thimerosal exposure from childhood vaccines and the onset of autism. The IOM supported the effort to remove thimerosal from vaccines to reduce any mercury exposure to infants and children.

APPLY THE EVIDENCE: NURSING IMPLICATIONS

Decisions about the total elimination of thimerosal (even traces) from vaccines must balance the potential benefit of no exposure to mercury against the risks of decreased vaccine coverage because of higher cost of the thimerosal-free vaccine, the risks of sepsis due to the potential bacterial contamination of the preservative-free formulations, and the risk of exposure to alternative preservatives that might replace the thimerosal preservative.

Thimerosal as a preservative has been removed or reduced to trace amounts in all vaccines routinely administered to children except influenza vaccine. The maximum total exposure during the first 6 months of life is less than 3 mcg of mercury. Based on guidelines established by the U.S. Food and Drug Administration (2007) and other government monitoring agencies, no children will be exposed to excessive mercury from childhood vaccines.

References

Andrews N, Miller E, Path FRC, and others: Thimerosal exposure in infants and developmental disorders: a retrospective cohort study in the United Kingdom does not support a causal association, *Pediatrics* 114(3):584-591, 2004.
Heron J, Golding J, ALSPAC study team: Thimerosal exposure in infants and developmental disorders: a prospective cohort study in the United Kingdom does not support a causal association, *Pediatrics* 114(3):577-583, 2004.
Hviid A, Stellfeld M, Wohlfahrt J, and others: Association between thimerosal-containing vaccine and autism, *JAMA* 290(13):1763-1766, 2003.
Institute of Medicine: *Immunization safety review: vaccines and autism,* Washington, DC, 2004, National Academy Press.
Madsen KM, Lauritsen MB, Pedersen CB, and others: Thimerosal and the occurrence of autism: negative ecological evidence from Danish population-based data, *Pediatrics* 112(3):604-606, 2003.
Stehr-Green P, Tull P, Stellfeld M, and others: Autism and thimerosal-containing vaccines: lack of consistent evidence for an association, *Am J Prev Med* 25(2):101-106, 2003.
US Food and Drug Administration: *Thimerosal in vaccines,* 2007, retrieved March 7, 2008, from http://www.fda.gov/cber/vaccine/thimerosal.htm.
Verstraeten T, Davis RL, DeStefano F, and others: Safety of thimerosal-containing vaccines: a two-phased study of computerized health maintenance organization databases, *Pediatrics* 112(5):1039-1048, 2003.

BOX 19-8

Diagnostic Criteria for Autistic Disorder

A. A total of six (or more) items from (1), (2), and (3), with at least two from (1), and one each from (2) and (3):

(1) Qualitative impairment in social interaction, as manifested by at least two of the following:

(a) Marked impairment in the use of multiple nonverbal behaviors such as eye-to-eye gaze, facial expression, body postures, and gestures to regulate social interaction

(b) Failure to develop peer relationships appropriate to developmental level

(c) A lack of spontaneous seeking to share enjoyment, interests, or achievements with other people (e.g., by a lack of showing, bringing, pointing out objects of interest)

(d) Lack of social or emotional reciprocity

(2) Qualitative impairments in communication as manifested by at least one of the following:

(a) Delay in, or total lack of, the development of spoken language (not accompanied by an attempt to compensate through alternative modes of communication such as gestures or mime)

(b) In individuals with adequate speech, marked impairment in the ability to initiate or sustain a conversation with others

(c) Stereotyped and repetitive use of language or idiosyncratic language

(d) Lack of varied, spontaneous make-believe play or social imitative play appropriate to developmental level

(3) Restricted repetitive and stereotyped patterns of behavior, interests, and activities, as manifested by at least one of the following:

(a) Encompassing preoccupation with one or more stereotyped and restricted patterns of interest that is abnormal either in intensity or focus

(b) Apparently inflexible adherence to specific, nonfunctional routines or rituals

(c) Stereotyped and repetitive motor mannerisms (e.g., hand or finger flapping or twisting, complex whole-body movements)

B. Delays or abnormal functioning in at least one of the following areas, with onset before age 3 years: (1) social interaction, (2) language as used in social communication, or (3) symbolic or imaginative play.

C. The disturbance is not better accounted for by Rett's disorder or childhood disintegrative disorder.

From American Psychiatric Association: *Diagnostic and statistical manual of mental disorders,* ed 4, rev trans (DSM-IV TR), Washington, DC, 2000, The Association.

Prognosis

ASD is usually a severely disabling condition. However, some children improve with acquisition of language skills and communication with others (Bloom-DiCicco, Lord, Zwaigenbaum, and others, 2006). Some ultimately achieve independence, but most require lifelong adult supervision. Aggravation of psychiatric symptoms occurs in about half of the children during adolescence, with girls having a tendency for continued deterioration.

Early recognition of behaviors associated with ASD is critical to implement appropriate interventions and family involvement. The prognosis is most favorable for children with communicative speech development by age 6 years and an IQ above 50 at the time of diagnosis.

Nursing Care Management

Therapeutic intervention for the child with ASD is a specialized area involving professionals with advanced training. Although there is no cure for ASD, numerous therapies have been used. The most promising results have been through highly structured and intensive behavior modification programs. In general, the objective in treatment is to promote positive reinforcement, increase social awareness of others, teach verbal communication skills, and decrease unacceptable behavior. Providing a structured routine for the child to follow is a key in the management of ASD.

When these children are hospitalized, the parents are essential to planning care and ideally should stay with the child as much as possible. Nurses should recognize that not all children with ASD are the same and will require individual assessment and treatment. Decreasing stimulation by using a private room, avoiding extraneous auditory and visual distractions, and encouraging the parents to bring in possessions the child is attached to may lessen the disruptiveness of hospitalization. Because physical contact often upsets these children, minimum holding and eye contact may be necessary to avoid behavioral outbursts. Care must be taken when performing procedures on, administering medicine to, or feeding these children, since they may be either fussy eaters who willfully starve themselves or gag to prevent eating or indiscriminate hoarders, swallowing any available edible or inedible items, such as a thermometer. Eating habits of ASD children may be particularly problematic for families and may involve food refusal, mouthing objects, eating nonedibles, and smelling and throwing food (Belschner, 2007; Caronna, Augustyn, and Zuckerman, 2007).

Children with ASD need to be introduced slowly to new situations, with visits with staff caregivers kept short whenever possible. Because these children have difficulty organizing their behavior and redirecting their energy, they need to be told directly what to do. Communication should be at the child's developmental level, brief, and concrete.

Family Support. ASD, as with so may other chronic conditions, involves the entire family and often becomes "a family disease." Nurses can help alleviate the guilt and shame often associated with this disorder by stressing what is known from a biologic standpoint and provide family support. It is imperative to help parents understand that they are not the cause of the child's condition.

Parents need expert counseling early in the course of the disorder and should be referred to the Autism Society of America.* The society provides information about education, treatment programs and techniques, and facilities such as camps and group homes. Other helpful resources for parents of children with ASD are the local and state departments of mental health and developmental disabilities; these organizations provide important programs for ASD children and in-school programs throughout the United States.

As much as possible, the family is encouraged to care for the child in the home. With the help of family support programs in many states, families are often able to provide home care and assist with the educational services the child needs. As the child approaches adulthood and parents become older, the family may require assistance in locating a long-term placement facility.

*See footnote on p. 635.

KEY POINTS

- The American Association on Intellectual and Developmental Disabilities defines intellectual disability as significantly subaverage general intellectual functioning existing concurrently with deficits in adaptive behavior and manifested during the developmental period.
- Causes of severe CI are primarily genetic, biochemical, and infectious. Mild CI is associated primarily with familial, social, and environmental causes, whereas severe CI is more likely to be associated with specific syndromes.
- Education of children with CI emphasizes sensory and verbal discrimination, improvement of short-term memory, motivation, and technologic support.
- Optimal development may be promoted through family guidance regarding play, communication, discipline, socialization, and sexuality.
- Prevention of CI focuses on support for the preterm neonate and other high-risk newborns, rubella immunization, genetic counseling, and maternal education regarding the risks of chemical use (e.g., alcohol ingestion) and the importance of adequate nutrition.
- Down syndrome, a chromosomal abnormality, is characterized by mild to moderate range of CI (most often), physical characteristics, slowed language development, congenital anomalies, sensory problems, and diminished growth and sexual development.
- Fragile X syndrome is characterized by CI and phenotypic findings in affected males. It is considered the most common hereditary cause and the second leading chromosomal cause of CI after Down syndrome.
- Hearing disorders may be classified according to the location of the defect: conductive, sensorineural, mixed conductive-sensorineural, and central auditory imperception.
- Rehabilitation for hearing loss involves parent education and support, hearing aids, lipreading, sign language, speech therapy, and promotion of socialization.
- Prevention of hearing loss includes treatment of infection, universal newborn screening and child auditory testing, immunization, pregnancy and genetic counseling, and reduction of noise pollution.
- Common visual impairments in childhood include refractive errors, amblyopia, strabismus, cataracts, glaucoma, trauma, and infections.
- Prevention of visual impairment focuses on prenatal screening, prenatal and perinatal care, periodic vision screening, immunization, and safety counseling.
- Nursing goals in visual rehabilitation include helping the family and child adjust to the child's visual impairment, promoting parent-child attachment, fostering optimal development and independence, providing for play and socialization, and being aware of educational facilities.
- For the child undergoing ocular surgery, nursing care is aimed at reassuring the child and family throughout treatment, orienting the child to the surroundings, providing a safe environment, and encouraging independence.
- Retinoblastoma is a rare congenital malignant tumor; its most common clinical manifestations are white pupil reflex and strabismus.
- ASDs are a complex neurodevelopmental disorder of brain function accompanied by a broad range and severity of intellectual and behavioral deficits.

answers to CRITICAL THINKING EXERCISES

DIAGNOSIS OF DOWN SYNDROME

1. Yes. Shocked parents with three children are notified their newborn has Down syndrome.
2. a. Melissa is a developmentally delayed newborn who requires time-consuming care.
   b. Melissa will develop a variety of medical problems, causing a huge financial expense.
   c. Melissa will always require parent and sibling supervision and care.
3. The first priority is to allow the parents to express their feelings of grief, anger, sadness, and guilt regarding the birth of a mentally intellectually disabled child.
   - The nurse should not take anything for granted or give definite suggestions regarding disabled children.
   - The nurse should demonstrate acceptance of the child because parents are sensitive to the professional's attitude.
4. Yes. The parents' response suggests unexpressed feelings of anger, loss, sadness, and confusion.
5. The nurse should guide the parents toward appropriate resources when asked, such as written information and organizations.
   - The nurse may ask the pediatrician and the social worker to talk with the parents.
   - Emphasize normal characteristics of the child to help the parents see the child as an individual.
   - Encourage parents to meet other families with a similarly affected child for additional support.

HEARING IMPAIRMENT

1. Yes. Jason is severely hearing impaired and awakening in an unfamiliar environment after a surgical procedure. Jason recovers in an unfamiliar environment with monitors, an intravenous line, and other equipment that may create fear, anxiety, and agitation.
2. a. Jason's inability to hear and communicate promotes frustration and fear.
   b. Jason's increasing agitation may be due to not having his hearing aids.
   c. Jason, who is recovering from regional block for herniorrhaphy, is unable to clearly verbalize or use sign language to express needs.
3. The first priority is to establish communication with Jason by directly facing him to facilitate lip reading, touching him to get his attention, and correctly placing his hearing aids if available.
   - Determine his usual means of communicating and encourage expression of feelings and questions regarding environment, equipment, and procedures.
   - Explain procedures before performing them, using gestures, objects, or pictures; speak slowly and clearly.
   - Allow ample time for child to show understanding of explanations.
   - Decrease environmental noise.
   - Listen closely as the child speaks, and focus on his pronunciation of words.
4. Yes. Jason's behavior does not suggest the transitory confusion associated with the initial emergence from anesthesia. Rather, it suggests that he became increasingly frustrated as he became aware of his environment with the inability to communicate his desires and feelings. Although pain is a possibility and needs to be evaluated, regional blocks are typically given during surgery to keep children comfortable until after they are discharged.

5. It would be appropriate to make a referral to the child life therapist during the hospitalization. The child life therapist would encourage Jason to express his feelings, fears, and anxieties regarding surgery, the hospital environment, equipment, and procedures through therapeutic play.

REFERENCES

Afzal N, Murch S, Thirrupathy K, and others: Constipation with acquired megarectum in children with autism, *Pediatrics* 112(4):939-942, 2003.

Alanay Y, Unal F, Turanh G, and others: Multidisciplinary approach to the management of individuals with fragile X syndrome, *J Intellect Disabil Res* 51:151-161, 2007.

Al-Hay AA, MacNeil SJ, Yacoub M, and others: Complete atrioventricular septal defect, Down syndrome, and surgical outcome: risk factors, *Ann Thorac Surg* 75(2):412-421, 2003.

American Academy of Pediatrics, Committee on Genetics: Health supervision for children with Down syndrome, *Pediatrics* 107(2):442-449, 2001.

American Academy of Pediatrics, Task Force on Newborn and Infant Hearing: Newborn and infant hearing loss: detection and intervention, *Pediatrics* 103(2):527-530, 1999.

American Psychiatric Association: *Diagnostic and statistical manual of mental disorders,* ed 4 (text rev) (DSM-IV TR), Washington, DC, 2000, The Association.

Belschner RA: Stop, assess and motivate: the SAM approach to autism spectrum disorder, *Am J Nurse Pract* 11(4):43-50, 2007.

Biasini FJ, Grupe L, Huffman L, and others: Mental retardation: a symptom and a syndrome. In Netherton SD, Holmes D, Walker E, editors: *Child and adolescent psychological disorders: a comprehensive textbook,* vol 4, New York, 1999, Oxford University Press.

Bittles AH, Glasson EJ: Clinical, social, and ethical implications of changing life expectancy in Down syndrome, *Dev Med Child Neurol* 46(4):282-286, 2004.

Bloom-DiCicco E, Lord C, Zwaigenbaum L, and others: The development neurobiology of autism spectrum disorder, *J Neurosci* 26(26):6897-6906, 2006.

Bosch JJ, Ringdahl J: Functional analysis of problem behavior in children with mental retardation: what is it, and why should pediatric nurses care? *MCN* 26(6):307-311, 2001.

Caronna EB, Augustyn M, Zuckerman B: Revisiting parental concerns in the age of autism spectrum disorders, *Arch Pediatr Adolesc Med* 161:406-407, 2007.

Centers for Disease Control and Prevention: Delayed diagnosis of fragile X syndrome—United States, 1990-1999, *MMWR* 51(33):740-742, 2002.

Coats AJ: Making choices in cardiology: difficulties of rationing and equality of access, *Int J Cardiol* 78(3):209-212, 2001.

Courtney-Manning P: Addressing the crisis in access to autism treatment using health care improvement science, *Arch Pediatr Adolesc Med* 161:414-415, 2007.

Crawford DC: FMR1 and the fragile X syndrome, *CDC Fact Sheet,* 2001, retrieved Feb 28, 2008, from http://www.cdc.gov/genomics/hugenet/factsheets/FS_FragileX.htm.

Croen LA, Najjar DV, Fireman B, and others: Maternal and paternal age and the risk of autism spectrum disorders, *Arch Pediatr Adolesc Med* 161:334-340, 2007.

Croen, LA, Najjar DV, Ray T, and others: A comparison of health care utilization and costs of children with and without autism spectrum disorders in a large group-model health plan, *Pediatrics* 118(4):1203-1211, 2006.

Cunningham M, Cox EO, Committee on Practice and Ambulatory Medicine and the Section on Otolaryngology and Bronchoesophagology: Hearing assessment in infants and children: recommendations beyond neonatal screening, *Pediatrics* 111(2):436-440, 2003.

Dalton R, Forman MA, Boris NW: Pervasive development disorders and childhood psychosis. In Behrman RE, Kliegman RM, Jenson HB, editors: *Nelson textbook of pediatrics,* ed 17, Philadelphia, 2004, Saunders.

Daniel E: Noise and hearing loss: a review, *J School Health* 77(5):225-231, 2007.

Dawson G: Despite major challenges, autism research continues to offer hope, *Arch Pediatr Adolesc Med* 161:411-412, 2007.

Day SM, Strauss DJ, Shavelle RM, and others: Mortality and causes of death in persons with Down syndrome in California, *Dev Med Child Neurol* 47(3):171-176, 2005.

De Potter P: Current treatment of retinoblastoma, *Curr Opin Ophthalmol* 13(5):331-336, 2002.

DeStefano F, Bhasin TK, Thompson WW, and others: Age at first measles-mumps-rubella vaccination in children with autism and school-matched control subjects: a population-based study in metropolitan Atlanta, *Pediatrics* 113(2):259-266, 2004.

Downs BW, Buchman CA: External auditory canal translocation for cochlear implantation, *Laryngoscope* 115:555-556, 2005.

D'Souza Y, Fombonne E, Ward BJ: No evidence of persisting measles virus in blood mononuclear cells from children with autism spectrum disorder, *Pediatrics* 118:1664-1675, 2006.

Filipek P, Accardo PJ, Ashwal S, and others: Practice parameter: screening and diagnosis of autism: report of the Quality Standards Subcommittee of the American Academy of Neurology and the Child Neurology Society, *Neurology* 55(2 of 2):468-479, 2000.

Fombonne E: The prevalence of autism, *JAMA* 289:87-89, 2003.

Formigari R, Di Donato RM, Garguilo G, and others: Better surgical prognosis for patients with complete atrioventricular septal defect and Down's syndrome, *Ann Thorac Surg* 78(2):666-672, 2004.

Glasson EJ, Sullivan SG, Hussain R, and others: The changing survival profile of people with Down's syndrome: implications for genetic counseling, *Clin Genet* 62(5):390-393, 2002.

Gregg RB, Wiorek MA, Arvedson JC: Pediatric audiology: a review, *Pediatr Rev* 25(7):224-234, 2004.

Grizzle KL, Simms MD: Early language development and language learning disabilities, *Pediatr Rev* 26(8):274-283, 2005.

Hall JG: Chromosomal clinical abnormalities. In Behrman RE, Kliegman RM, Jenson HB, editors: *Nelson textbook of pediatrics,* ed 17, Philadelphia, 2004, Saunders.

Hurwitz RL, Shields CL, Shields JA, and others: Retinoblastoma. In Pizzo PA, Poplack DG, editors: *Principle and practice of pediatric oncology,* ed 5, Philadelphia, 2006, Lippincott.

Johnson CP, Walker WO: Mental retardation: management and prognosis, *Pediatr Rev* 27(7):249-256, 2006.

Kabra M, Gulati S: Mental retardation, *Indian J Pediatr* 70(2):153-158, 2003.

Kenna MA: Medical management of childhood hearing loss, *Pediatr Ann* 33(12):822-832, 2004.

Kolevzon A, Gross R, Reichenberg A: Prenatal and perinatal risk factors for autism: a review and integration of findings, *Arch Pediatr Adolesc Med* 161:326-333, 2007.

Melamud A, Palekar R, Singh A: Retinoblastoma, *Am Fam Physician* 73(6):1041-1044, 2006.

Mizoue T, Miyamoto R, Shimizu T: Combined effect of smoking and occupational exposure to noise on hearing loss in steel factory workers, *J Occup Environ Med* 60(10):56-59, 2003.

Muhle E, Trentacoste SV, Rapin I: The genetics of autism, *Pediatrics* 113(5):e472-486, 2004.

National Down Syndrome Society: *About Down syndrome,* 2006, retrieved March 7, 2008, from http://www.ndss.org.

National Fragile X Foundation: *Prevalence of fragile X syndrome,* 2006, retrieved Jan 21, 2007, from http://www.fragilex.org/html/prevalence.htm.

Peterson CC: A review of biochemical and ultrasound markers in detection of Down syndrome, *J Perinatal Educ* 15(1):19-25, 2006.

Phalen JA: Fragile X syndrome, *Pediatr Rev* 26(5):181-182, 2005.

Pueschel SM: The child with Down syndrome. In Levine MD, Carey WB, Crocker AC, editors: *Developmental-behavioral pediatrics,* ed 3, Philadelphia, 1999, Saunders.

Rehm RS, Bradley JF: Social interactions at school of children who are medically fragile and developmentally delayed, *J Pediatr Nurs* 21(4):299-307, 2006.

Schaefer GB, Lutz RE: Diagnostic yield in the clinical genetic evaluation of autism spectrum disorders, *Genet Med* 8(9):549-556, 2006.

Schanen NC: Epigenetics of autism spectrum disorders, *Hum Molec Genet* 15(R1-2):R138-R150, 2006.

Schouten–van Meeteren AYN, Moll AC, Imhof SM, and others: Overview chemotherapy for retinoblastoma: an expanding area of clinical research, *Med Pediatr Oncol* 38:428-438, 2002.

Segal S, Eviatar E, Lapinsky J, and others: Inner ear damage in children due to noise exposure from toy cap pistols and firecrackers: a retrospective review of 53 cases, *Noise Health* 5(18):13-18, 2003.

Skotko B: Mothers of children with Down syndrome reflect on their postnatal support, *Pediatrics* 115(1):64-77, 2005.

Smith RJH, Bale JF, White KR: Sensorineural hearing loss in children, *Lancet* 365:879-890, 2005.

Tingley DH: Vision screening essentials: screening today for eye disorders in the pediatric patient, *Pediatr Rev* 28(2):54-61, 2007.

Van Riper M: A change of plans: the birth of a child with Down syndrome doesn't have to be a negative experience, *Am J Nurs* 103(6):71-74, 2003.

Walker WO, Johnson CP: Mental retardation: overview and diagnosis, *Pediatr Rev* 27(6):204-212, 2006.

Wilton G, Plane MB: The family empowerment network: a service model to address the needs of children and families affected by fetal alcohol spectrum disorders, *Pediatr Nurs* 32(4):299-305, 2006.

Zeng FG, Liu S: Speech perception in individuals with auditory neuropathy, *J Speech Lang Hearing Res* 49:367-380, 2006.

20

Family-Centered Home Care

MARILYN J. HOCKENBERRY

CHAPTER OUTLINE

GENERAL CONCEPTS OF HOME CARE, 642
Home Care Trends, 642
Effective Home Care, 643
Discharge Planning and Selection of a Home Care Agency, 644

Care Coordination (Case Management), 646
Role of the Nurse, Training, and Standards of Care, 647
FAMILY-CENTERED HOME CARE, 648
Diversity in Home Care, 648

Parent-Professional Collaboration, 649
The Nursing Process, 650
Promotion of Optimum Development, Self-Care, and Education, 651
Safety Issues in the Home, 653
Family-to-Family Support, 654

LEARNING OBJECTIVES

On completion of this chapter the reader will be able to:
- Differentiate home care from hospice care.
- List at least three factors contributing to the increasing emphasis on home care services.

- Describe case management/care coordination and its importance in home care.
- List general principles of a family-centered assessment and planning process.

- Identify five key characteristics of collaborative relationships.
- Describe approaches to promoting optimal development, self-care, and education in home care.
- Outline six areas in need of attention for promoting safety in home care.

RELATED TOPICS and ADDITIONAL RESOURCES

 IN TEXT

Communicating with Families, *Ch. 6*
Family-Centered Care (Children with Chronic Illness or Disability), *Ch. 18*
Family-Centered Care of the Child During Illness and Hospitalization, *Ch. 21*
Family Influences on Child Health Promotion, *Ch. 3*

Pediatric Variations of Nursing Interventions, *Ch. 22*
Social, Cultural, and Religious Influences on Child Health Promotion, *Ch. 4*

 COMPANION CD

Case Study—Home Care
NCLEX Review Questions

evolve
evolve.elsevier.com/Wong/essentials/
NCLEX Review Questions
WebLinks

 WONG'S CLINICAL MANUAL OF PEDIATRIC NURSING, 7th Ed

Unit 5—Patient and Family Education: Care in the Home and Community, *pp. 503-589*

GENERAL CONCEPTS OF HOME CARE

Home care nursing has become a routine option for the pediatric patient in today's health care environment. Advances in medical technology have produced a large population of children with a variety of health care needs. The growing demand for home care services came in part as the result of increasing health costs of institutionalized care. More important, home-based health care recognizes the family's valuable contribution to the child's overall health in his or her natural environment. Although there is limited evidence on the ability of home care to reduce hospital admissions and emergency department visits, home care programs lead to greater parent satisfaction, improved quality of life, and a reduction in length of hospital stay (Cooper, Wheeler, Woolfenden, and others, 2006).

Home care is not a new concept in pediatrics. Over time the term has referred to parents caring for mildly ill children at home, nursing home visits after children are discharged from the hospital, hospice care, and care at home for children with more serious chronic illness and dependence on medical technology. As discussed in this chapter, **home care** refers to care provided for children with simple or complex health care needs and their families in their places of residence for the purpose of promoting, maintaining, or restoring health or for maximizing the level of independence while minimizing the effects of disability and illness, including terminal illness.

Home care differs from **hospice care**—a program of palliative and supportive care services that provides physical, psychologic, social, and spiritual care for dying persons, their families, and other loved ones. Hospice services are available both in the home and in inpatient settings (Carlin, 1999) and are discussed more fully in Chapter 18. **End-of-life care** and planning should be considered for any child with a terminal diagnosis. Some patients may receive end-of-life home care services before being ready for admission to hospice services. Many hospice programs have admission criteria that do not permit therapies such as intravenous antibiotics, total parenteral nutrition, or enteral feedings that the family may wish to continue. It is therefore important to discuss the type of care the family wishes for the child early in discharge planning to clarify expectations for home care.

HOME CARE TRENDS

The shift toward home-based health care is propelled by numerous factors. Providing high-quality home health care for children generally requires parental desire and ability, professional assistance, and community preparedness. A natural family environment optimizes growth and development when stress is minimum and support is maximized.

Advances in medical technology have resulted in increased survival for children with congenital and acquired illnesses. Preterm infants or children who are ventilator dependent were once cared for indefinitely in an intensive care unit or long-term care facility. These children are now able to live with their families in their own home (Feudtner, Villareale, Morray, and others, 2005).

Children with cancer, kidney disorders, cystic fibrosis, spina bifida, cardiac anomalies, gastrointestinal disorders, neurodegenerative diseases, and human immunodeficiency virus infection may have ongoing health care needs as a result of the disease, its treatment, or side effects of treatment (Magrabi, Lovell, Henry, and others, 2005; Nazer, Abdulhamid, Thomas,

and others, 2006; Stevens, McKeever, Law, and others, 2006). Parents frequently have ongoing stressors after a child's hospitalization for diagnosis and treatment. Subsequent needs may include reinforcing teachings about the disease process, addressing the child's physical care needs, providing emotional support during this change in parental role, and teaching in a low-stress environment. Home-based nutrition programs are useful, safe, and well tolerated in children. There is sufficient evidence that these programs provide a better quality of life, decrease cost of therapy, and improve survival (Daveluy, Guimber, Uhlen, and others, 2006).

Improving the quality of life for both the child and the family is one of the driving forces in the efforts to move technology-dependent children from the hospital to the home setting. The concept of **normalization** describes the process whereby families of children with chronic illness over time begin to perceive the child and their family life as normal (Knafl and Deatrick, 2002). This has important implications for pediatric home care nurses in relation to assessing family function and understanding family dynamics. The normalized family tends to be more flexible with treatments and incorporates the child with a disability or illness into the routines of daily living (Knafl and Deatrick, 2002).

The **cost of care** is an important factor in the health care delivery system today. Shorter inpatient stays are due in part to the overwhelming cost of lengthy hospitalizations. Children either are not admitted to the hospital at all or are returned home as soon as possible after their illness. Home-based nursing care has decreased the length of hospital stay (Cooper, Wheeler, Woolfenden, and others, 2006). Likewise, a portion of the financial burden is shifted to the family. The family may be forced to absorb the costs of certain medications, supplies, transportation, shelter, utilities, food, laundry, housekeeping, and a portion of the nursing care. Over time chronically ill children can cause a financial burden to the family (see Evidence-Based Practice box).

Home health care of children, however, is not restricted to children with chronic health care needs. Several short-term intermittent therapies such as phototherapy, apnea monitoring, and intravenous antibiotic administration may be successfully provided in a home setting rather than in an acute care setting. A recent study found that home health nurses providing asthma education to families of children hospitalized for an asthma exacerbation increased the family's and caregiver's knowledge about asthma symptoms, triggers, and management (Navaie-Waliser, Misener, Mersman, and others, 2004). A number of strategies can be implemented in the home setting to reduce the triggers that cause acute asthma exacerbations and often result in hospitalization (see Asthma, Chapter 23).

With the increased demand for nurses in home health and continued pervasive short supply, increasing attention has focused on the role of the **family caregiver** in providing home care. A recent survey by the National Alliance for Caregiving (2005) revealed that 21% of U.S. households have a person being cared for by another family member; this represents care above and beyond the daily routine care of the family household.

Sullivan-Bolyai, Sadler, Knafl, and others (2003) explored the literature on adult and pediatric family caregivers' responsibilities in the care of a family member who has a chronic illness. Their review of the literature revealed four family-

EVIDENCE-BASED PRACTICE

Home Care Decreases Length of Hospital Stay

ASK THE QUESTION   In children does the availability of home care services decrease hospital length of stay?

SEARCH FOR EVIDENCE
Search Strategies   Searched the literature to obtain clinical research studies related to this issue. Selection criteria included English, publications within past 10 years, research-based articles, infant and child populations.
Databases Used   PubMed, CINAHL, Cochrane Collaboration, AHRQ

CRITICALLY ANALYZE THE EVIDENCE
In a Cochrane Review on home-based nursing services for children with acute and chronic illnesses, three randomized controlled trials were found evaluating the impact of available home health care services on a child's length of stay. Length of stay was evaluated using bed days, inpatient stay, and use of hospital-based services. The length of hospital stay was significantly reduced when children received home-based care (Cooper, 2007; Daveluy, Guimber, Uhlen, and others, 2006; Bagust, Haycox, Sartain, and others, 2002; Dougherty, Schiffrin, White, and others, 1999; Dougherty, Soderstrom, and Schiffrin, 1998; Strawczynski, Stachewitsch, Morgenstern, and others, 1973).

APPLY THE EVIDENCE: NURSING IMPLICATIONS
Access to home care services contributes to reduction in hospital length of stay.

References
Bagust A, Haycox A, Sartain SA, and others: Economic evaluation of an acute paediatric hospital at home clinical trial, *Arch Dis Child* 87:489-492, 2002.
Cooper C: *Specialist home-based nursing services for children with acute and chronic illnesses* (review), The Cochrane Collaboration, London, 2007, Wiley & Sons.
Daveluy W, Guimber D, Uhlen S, and others: Dramatic changes in home-based enteral nutrition practices in children during an 11-year period, *J Pediatr Gastroenterol Nutr* 43(2):240-244, 2006.
Dougherty G, Schiffrin A, White D, and others: Home-based management can achieve intensification cost-effectively in type I diabetes, *Pediatrics* 103(1):122-128, 1999.
Dougherty GE, Soderstrom L, Schiffrin A: An economic evaluation of home care for children with newly diagnosed diabetes: results from a randomized controlled trial, *Medical Care* 36(4):586-598, 1998.
Strawczynski H, Stachewitsch A, Morgenstern G, and others: Delivery of care to hemophilic children: home care versus hospitalization, *Pediatrics* 51(6):986-991, 1973.

related caregiving responsibilities adapted from the adult literature that may be applied to children's caregivers as well:

Managing the illness—providing daily hands-on care, monitoring the child's medical condition, and educating others to care for the child

Identifying, accessing, and coordinating resources—locating appropriate resources in the community to meet the needs of the child and of the family as the child's caregiver

Maintaining the family unit—continuing to nurture the family unit: siblings' needs, husband-wife relationships, and maintaining the household

Maintaining self—grieving the loss of the healthy child; balancing caregiver responsibilities with own physical, emotional, mental, and personal needs; recognizing stressors and potential caregiver burnout

The researchers developed a multifaceted list of parent caregiving management responsibilities and associated activities that the home health nurse may use to facilitate discussions with parents and families regarding caregiving in the home and its unique requirements (Sullivan-Bolyai, Knafl, Sadler, and others, 2004). Nurses can use the results of this research to better understand the magnitude of responsibilities facing the caregiving family and assist in finding resources to provide the family some respite from caring for the child to care for each other and maintain self and family integrity.

The American Academy of Pediatrics supports the philosophy of **permanency planning,** wherein children with special health care needs obtain permanent family placement and ongoing relationship with caring adults (Johnson, Kastner, and American Academy of Pediatrics Committee on Children with Disabilities, 2005). Within this framework, the home environment with the child's family is perceived as the best place for

the child to be reared. Should the family be unable to support the child as a result of poor resources or family structure, options include extended family members, birth family plus an unrelated family sharing parental responsibilities, or two unrelated families sharing parental responsibilities. In addition, adoptive families may participate in care of the child with special health care needs. The American Academy of Pediatrics further stresses the importance of providing the child's family with adequate resources and support to promote family well-being (Johnson, Kastner, and American Academy of Pediatrics Committee on Children with Disabilities, 2005). In addition, primary care physicians play a vital role in the process of care coordination in collaboration with the family and nursing home care team (American Academy of Pediatrics, 2005).

Respite care for caregivers of children with special care needs has been slow in its development and availability, although respite care centers are now common for adults. Such care for ventilator-dependent children and those with skilled technologic care requirements is lacking throughout the United States (Parra, 2003). Respite care provides temporary relief to parents and allows for a break from the responsibilities of caring for the child on a daily basis (Parra, 2003). Nurses can play an important role in advocating for the provision of high-quality respite care so families and caregivers can maintain appropriate family function, care for themselves, and continue to provide for the care of the child as necessary (Parra, 2003).

EFFECTIVE HOME CARE

Providing home-based care for children gives the nurse an opportunity to assess and interact with the family in its environment. This assessment can provide the health care team with valuable information about safety, support systems, nu-

BOX 20-1
Intermittent Skilled Nursing

HEALTH CARE NEED

Child at risk—parental substance abuse, failure to thrive, social or family situation potentially detrimental to child's well-being

Chronically ill, but medically stable child with multiple care needs

Education and competency validation of caregiver skills

Skilled procedures—regularly scheduled injections or infusions, dressing changes, phototherapy

Reinforcement of home care teaching; evaluation of caregiver's skills

Technology-dependent child (e.g., ventilator or tracheostomy, home total parenteral nutrition, or enteral feedings by pump)

Chronically ill child with multiple skilled nursing needs

INTERVENTION

Regularly scheduled visits to assess patient status, evaluate home environment, teach care provider skills, determine status of growth and development, set goals with family for positive health outcomes

As-needed home visits during illness exacerbation to assess physical status and determine appropriate intervention

Assistance with transportation of child to ambulatory center or practitioner's office for evaluation and diagnostic services

Regular visits of limited duration to perform skilled nursing intervention, assess parental ability and desire to perform procedure, teach procedure technique, supervise parental performance of procedure

Assessment of patient status; evaluation of safety of home environment; teaching, evaluation, and reinforcement of caregivers' skills; determination of status of growth and development; goal setting with family for positive health outcomes

BOX 20-2
Services Necessary to Support Effective Home Care

- Adequate family training and preparation
- Primary care physician willing to oversee medical aspects of home care
- Professional caregivers trained in relevant nursing and communication skills
- Developmental interventions (e.g., physical, occupational, and speech therapy; early intervention)
- Appropriately designed and well-maintained equipment
- Supportive therapies (e.g., respiratory therapy, parenteral therapy, nutritional support)
- Adequate social and psychologic support services
- High-quality respite care
- Appropriate home renovation
- Telephone service in the home
- Appropriate transportation
- Appropriate locally available emergency facilities
- Competent case management services
- Safe home environment (electricity, refrigeration, cleanliness)

trition, parental ability, and actual health care practices. This information will inform future decisions for individualized care and realistic outcomes (Thompson, 2000).

There are two distinct areas of implementation of care for the pediatric home care nurse. Nurses who perform **intermittent skilled nursing visits** may see many different types and numbers of patients each day. These nurses typically have a caseload assigned to them and accept responsibility for implementing the care plan. This mode of nursing care is the most commonly used today as a result of personnel shortages and decreased reimbursement. Most home visits now focus on helping the patient and caregiver achieve independence with care in the home (including home care by therapists, home infusion teaching by nurses, and care management), rather than direct provision of physical care.

Nurses who perform **private-duty nursing** or block nursing are usually assigned individual patients, and they remain in the home for a predetermined amount of time (e.g., 8- or 12-hour blocks). The care plan is implemented over the course of the time in the home. Required nursing skills are determined by patient need, parental ability, family structure, and the home environment. In both types of home care, the pediatric nurse is responsible for patient and family assessment, evaluating the appropriateness of the care plan (Petit de Mange, 1998) (Box 20-1).

A major issue in providing home care in this era is the **nursing shortage.** Agencies and families are facing much more difficulty in staffing required home care services; thus more and more of the home care must be carried out by family members or other caregivers. According to Page (2001), the

lack of pediatric training in some nursing programs, increased acuity of home care patients, and increased pay for nurses working in acute care settings have contributed to a greater than ever nursing shortage in pediatric home health care. An increasing trend resulting from the nursing shortage and limitations in reimbursement is to have patients receive short-term treatment in non–hospital ambulatory settings (such as ambulatory infusion centers).

Consideration of the caregiver's willingness, ability, and limitations are of utmost importance when assessing the appropriateness of the care plan (Box 20-2). It is vital to ensure that patients and families have adequate back-up support and access to resources such as social services. An increasing concern in pediatric home health care is obtaining a managing practitioner. Declining reimbursement and short hospital stays have increased patients' rapid movement through the continuum of care; a patient may be seen in the emergency department or neonatal intensive care unit, then discharged to home health without ever seeing a primary care physician. It is therefore imperative that the provision of care for home patients involve multidisciplinary cooperation and communication among health care workers.

DISCHARGE PLANNING AND SELECTION OF A HOME CARE AGENCY

Identifying appropriate local community resources is critical to a successful transfer to home care (Box 20-3). The ultimate goal of discharge planning is for the family to become familiar with the child's needs and to be competent in providing that care. A discharge plan should include emergency management and provision of social and emotional support. The American Academy of Pediatrics (Johnson, Kastner, and American Academy of Pediatrics Committee on Children with Disabilities, 2005) emphasizes that the goal for a home health care program for infants, children, or adolescents with chronic conditions or disabilities is the provision of community-based, culturally effective, comprehensive, and cost-effective health care within a nurturing home environment that maximizes

BOX 20-3

Characteristics of a High-Quality Pediatric Home Care Agency

- Fully trained pediatric staff to provide for all aspects of care (nursing, rehabilitation therapies, pharmacy, dietitian, social work, home medical equipment)
- Prompt, responsive staff with 24-hour availability
- Family-centered care
- Comprehensive continuing education programs
- Certification of local, state, and federal regulatory agencies
- Accreditation by Joint Commission or Community Health Accreditation Program

Data from Dittbrenner H: Pediatric home care as a viable new service, *Caring* 18(2):12-15, 1999; and Lovejoy D: *Making the transition to home health nursing: a practical guide*, New York, 1997, Springer.

the capabilities of the individual and minimizes the effects of the disabilities.

NURSINGTIP

If home care equipment is different from hospital equipment, have the portable equipment delivered to the hospital to allow family use before discharge.

Much of the success of home care, particularly for the child who is dependent on medical technology or who has complex medical problems, depends on careful planning and preparation. General principles of discharge planning and the transition to home care are presented in Chapter 26. Discharge planning must begin early; should be based on criteria of child and family readiness; must be a multidisciplinary process, including representatives from acute care facilities, home care, and community settings; and must involve the family. Predischarge assessment (Box 20-4) and planning should include the following areas:

- The child's medical, nursing, educational, and other therapeutic needs
- Family members' (including siblings') education and training, coping skills, and adjustment needs
- Community readiness in areas such as availability of equipment, appropriate nursing and other personnel, educational and developmental services, respite care, and emergency plans
- Financial arrangements

Creative financial planning, including negotiating arrangements with the insurance company, health maintenance or managed care organization, and public programs, may be required.

Early involvement of the home care agency in the discharge planning process promotes continuity of care and a smooth transition from hospital to home (Box 20-5). Before discharge, a general plan, sometimes called an **individualized home care plan,** should be developed with multidisciplinary input. This care plan should address the range of needs identified as part of the comprehensive predischarge assessment.

NURSINGTIP

An excellent method of providing home care instructions is with video recordings. Once the family masters the procedures, consider video recording their performance. Visual learning is most helpful for people who cannot read or who are not fluent in English.

BOX 20-4

Assessment for Technology-Dependent Home Care

FAMILY CARE PROVIDERS
Identification and training of primary care providers
Identification and training of care providers for respite and emergency care
Parent employment status while caring for child at home
Family financial status, especially if one parent must stop working
Sibling understanding
Availability of psychosocial support services

PRIMARY CARE PROVIDER
Identification of local primary provider or pediatrician who is able to assume direct care responsibility
Inclusion of local provider in discharge planning
Information needs of local provider before child's discharge

HOME CARE SUPPORT
Home care agency's availability and pediatric experience
Home care agency's coordination of services with local health care providers
Twenty-four–hour availability and coverage for unexpected situations
Adequacy of number of personnel to meet needs
Additional training of staff, if needed
Twenty-four–hour availability of ambulance services

HOME PHYSICAL ENVIRONMENT
Adequacy of space for equipment and supplies
Room for heavy equipment (e.g., ventilator, oxygen tanks, compressor)
Layout of home (e.g., number of floors, stairways, room accessibility, room sizes)
If in an apartment, elevator and fire escape access
Telephone access
Type of transportation used by family
Ability to modify living space to minimize technology invasiveness without isolating child
Adequacy of heating and cooling systems
Adequacy of electrical system to accommodate equipment

EMERGENCY PREPAREDNESS
Written implementation plan: who, what, where, when, how (include telephone numbers)
Notification of utility companies for priority repairs and maintenance
Notification of emergency medical unit (911)
Emergency drill

Adapted from Bakewell-Sachs S, Porth S: Discharge planning and home care of the technology-dependent infant, *J Obstet Gynecol Neonatal Nurs* 24(1):77-83, 1995.

The plans for transition from hospital to home should include family members (ideally two persons) both learning and demonstrating all aspects of the child's care in the hospital. An in-hospital trial period, during which parents provide total care for the child, is generally beneficial. After a successful trial, the family may benefit from taking the child home on a brief pass before making final discharge plans. (Although this arrangement is ideal, most insurance companies will not approve payment for such a visit.) The home care nurse plays an

FIG. 20-1 ■ An essential aspect of preparation for home care is the arrangement of equipment and supplies.

BOX 20-5

Critical Home Care Referral Information

- Scheduled medications
- Durable medical equipment
- Medical supplies
- Transportation needs
- Adaptive equipment
- Rehabilitation therapies (occupational, physical, and speech therapy)
- Psychologic counseling
- Social work referral
- Nursing care
- Respite plans
- Key family members
- Demographic information
- Reimbursement information

Modified from Townsend JL: Assessment of the child and family. In Votroubek WL, Townsend JL, editors: *Pediatric home care*, ed 2, Gaithersburg, Md, 1997, Aspen.

---

important role in assessing this experience with the family. Whether or not the child is taken home on a pass, a predischarge home visit allows the home care nurse to meet the family, help them assess their preparedness and the preparedness of the home environment, discuss plans for arranging the child's equipment at home (Fig. 20-1), reinforce prior discharge teaching, and implement any additional teaching that may be necessary (Bakewell-Sachs, Carlino, Ash, and others, 2000). A comprehensive discharge plan includes the care plan, specific written instructions to facilitate continuity, and detailed information about home care outcomes.

CARE COORDINATION (CASE MANAGEMENT)

Traditional definitions of **case management** generally focus on cost control, attainment of desired clinical outcomes, and the monitoring and evaluation of care provided. However, for optimum home care of the child who is technology dependent, case management (or care coordination) should be viewed more broadly.

Changes in health care over the past two decades not only have improved survival and decreased morbidity among children with special health care needs, but also have heralded higher costs for health care and services provided. As a result, insurance companies have focused on reducing services to contain costs. The advent of managed care and fee-for-service reimbursement has changed the outlook for families desiring to have the child in the home. Often services are provided by multiple organizations and multiple vendors with different missions and a consistent lack of single systems linking home health care. In addition, eligibility criteria to determine the availability of funding and services are complex and vary from one state to another. As a result, coordination of home care can be challenging, frustrating, and complicated for the family (American Academy of Pediatrics, 2005).

The concept of **care coordination** is to link children with special home health care needs (and their families) to services and resources in a coordinated effort to provide the child with optimum care (American Academy of Pediatrics, 2005). Care coordination has several purposes. Its primary goal is ensuring continuity for the child and family across hospital, home, educational, therapeutic, and other settings. Other goals involve facilitating timely access to services and enhancing child and family well-being (Lindeke, Leonard, Presler, and others, 2002). Care should be coordinated among multiple providers to reduce the complexity of care for the child, reduce fragmentation of care, prevent duplication of services, and decrease the burden of care for the family. Case managers from a number of agencies may be involved in the patient's care, which may add to the parents' confusion; the home care nurse should try to coordinate meetings between all case managers and the family to minimize confusion and prevent duplication. Lindeke, Leonard, Presler, and others (2002) proposed that the ideal situation is when the family serves as lead care coordinator within the context of family-centered care. Care coordination should ensure that the child's medical, nursing, and health maintenance needs, as well as financial issues, psychosocial concerns, and educational needs of the child and family, are addressed (American Academy of Pediatrics, 2005; Dittbrenner, 1999).

Care coordination is most effective if a single person works with the family to accomplish the many tasks and responsibilities involved (Box 20-6). The nurse case coordinator should have a minimum of a baccalaureate degree in nursing and 3 years' experience (American Nurses Association, 1998). The nurse case manager should be knowledgeable about community resources, including primary, secondary, and tertiary health care services; speech, language, hearing, and vision resources; respite care services; financial assistance programs; parent groups; advocacy groups; local, state, and federal public officials; transportation services; and private-sector individuals with an interest in children with disabilities (Thompson, 2000). With a greater focus on outcomes of care in home health care, the nurse case manager is challenged to be resourceful and skilled in communication at a number of levels (Rice, 2001).

A valuable tool for nurse case managers is the **care path,** which is a multidisciplinary care plan aimed at measuring the quality of patient care outcomes derived from standardized patient outcomes; the care path evaluates the quality of patient care with respect to cost-effectiveness and timeliness. (For samples of home care clinical care paths, see Rice, 2001.) Care paths may also be used to help nurses and other health care workers learn home care and should be shared with the family members involved in patient care to provide direction and help the family see the eventual goals of care (Rice, 2001).

BOX 20-6

Care Coordination for Children with Special Health Care Needs

- Facilitate timely access to services and resources.
- Promote continuity of care.
- Ensure high-quality care is performed in the home.
- Provide family support and enhance family well-being.
- Improve health, developmental, educational, vocational, psychosocial, and functional outcomes.
- Maximize efficient, effective use of resources.

Modified from Presler B: Care coordination for children with special health care needs, *Orthop Nurs* 17(25 Suppl):45-51, 1998.

FIG. 20-2 ■ The nurse in the home care setting requires expertise to care for a child who is technology dependent.

BOX 20-7

Qualities of a Pediatric Home Care Nurse

- Competent in skills and case management
- Demonstrates expertise in pediatrics
- Recognizes that the nurse is a guest in the home
- Respects family culture and adapts appropriately
- Works as an interdisciplinary team member
- Demonstrates expertise in pediatric care (assessment and technical skills)
- Possesses and uses effective communication skills

Although professionals must always see part of their role as ensuring that integrated, coordinated care is provided, care coordination should promote the family's role as primary decision maker and enhance the family's capability to meet the special needs of the child and the family unit. Families may choose to be involved to varying degrees in coordinating their child's care. Many parents take on increasing responsibility for care coordination over time; they should be encouraged and supported in this role. Home care nurses and case managers should be aware that the termination of private-duty or home care nursing can be a difficult transition for which families may need preparation. A gradual reduction in services provided allows patients and families to adjust favorably to the changes.

ROLE OF THE NURSE, TRAINING, AND STANDARDS OF CARE

The home care nurse must share a level of technical expertise with the critical care nurse while being able to adapt equipment, procedures, and the nursing process to the home setting. The need for technical expertise must be matched by knowledge of child development and the ability to work creatively with the child who is challenged by chronic illness and technology dependence (Fig. 20-2). When practicing in the home, the nurse must be comfortable making independent nursing judgments and solving problems with no immediate assistance. At the same time the nurse must have excellent interpersonal skills, an ability to work with other professionals and the family, and, most important, respect for family autonomy. Patient outcomes are more readily achieved with a balance of nursing skills that demonstrate clinical excellence; adaptability; accountability; and the ability to develop positive relationships with patients, families, and practitioners (Box 20-7).

When working with a home care agency, nurses should expect to receive patient placements appropriate to their expertise. They should also expect to receive orientation to the skills and knowledge base of the home health care nursing specialty and subsequent continuing education to develop as expert practitioners. The minimum initial orientation should include the individual patient's care plan and equipment needs; the agency's policies and procedures, including procedures for addressing any problems that may occur when care is provided in the home; legal liability issues; and documentation procedures. Stronger emphasis should be placed on issues specific to home care.

Supervision of practice, including occasional site visits by a nursing supervisor, should be provided. Mentoring or precepting is ideal. Because of the unique practice environment of home health nurses, it is important for an agency to facilitate sharing among peers to decrease work-related stress, increase job satisfaction, and support high-quality patient care.

Nurses in pediatric home health face increasing demands for providing high-quality care with fewer resources to achieve positive patient outcomes. In doing so, nurses often must rely on **delegation** skills to ensure the patient and family receive the necessary care. Delegation often involves assigning nursing tasks to other health care professionals (Timm, 2003).

Public or private home care agencies that participate in the Medicare or Medicaid programs must be certified by a federally designated state certification body and abide by federal and state regulations. Additionally, the American Nurses Association has developed standards of nursing practice for both (community) public health and home health nurses (American Nurses Association, 1999b, 1999c). Generalist and clinical specialist certification in both home health and community health is offered by the American Nurses Credentialing Center,* a subsidiary of American Nurses Association. The Hospice Nurses Association offers certification in hospice nursing. Despite important differences between pediatric and adult care in the home, as of this writing no national standards specific to pediatric home care practice have been developed. Nursing practice in pediatric home care should be guided by

---

*8515 Georgia Ave., Suite 400, Silver Spring, MD 20910-3492; (800) 284-2378; http://www.nursecredentialing.org.

BOX 20-8

Selected Resources for Home Care

American Academy of Pediatrics
141 Northwest Point Blvd.
Elk Grove Village, IL 60007
(847) 434-4000
Fax: (847) 434-8000
http://www.aap.org

Association of Maternal and Child Health Programs
1220 19th St. NW, Suite 801
Washington, DC 20036
(202) 775-0436
Fax: (202) 775-0061
http://www.amchp.org

Children's Hospice International
1101 King St., Suite 360
Alexandria, VA 22314
(800) 2-4-CHILD or (703) 684-0330
http://www.chionline.org

Father's Network
Kindering Center
16120 N.E. Eighth St.
Bellevue, WA 98008-3937
(425) 653-4286
http:// www.fathersnetwork.org

National Association for Home Care and Hospice
228 Seventh St. SE
Washington, DC 20003
(202) 547-7424
Fax: (202) 547-3540
http://www.nahc.org

National Dissemination Center for Children with Disabilities
PO Box 1492
Washington, DC 20013-1492
(800) 695-0285 (voice/TTY)
Fax: (202) 884-8441
http://www.nichcy.org

Pediatric Home Care Association of America
An affiliate of the National Association for Home Care and Hospice (see contact information above)
Special feature on website is peds@home, an electronic newsletter

PediatricNursing.com
Health Resources for Parents
http://www.pediatricnursing.com/parents

---

published guidelines, textbooks, peer-reviewed articles, and written standards of care for pediatric patients. In addition, professional organizations have published standards of care that apply to pediatric home health nursing practice and are found in Box 20-8.

A **quality improvement program** is an important component of an effective home care agency. **Evidence-based practice** is rapidly becoming an important aspect of home health care, as is **benchmarking,** in which the product or practice (in this case, patient outcome) is compared with other agencies' outcomes and practices to determine best practice; this allows agencies to see how they measure in comparison to other similar agencies (Wilson, 2003; Yoder-Wise, 2003). The **OASIS (Outcome and Assessment Information Set),** as part of Medicare, has been established for adults in home health care; however, as of this writing no such data exist for children younger than age 18 years. As a part of OASIS, home health care quality measures have been established to measure patient care outcomes for Medicare reimbursement purposes. Other certification and licensing organizations that may oversee and regulate practice in home health include The Joint Commission, Centers for Medicare and Medicaid Services (formerly the Health Care Financing Administration), Occupational Safety and Health Administration, and Community Health Accreditation Program. The Health Insurance Portability and Accountability Act of 1996 guidelines affect the manner in which patient records are handled in home health care to ensure patient confidentiality (Wilson, 2004).

FAMILY-CENTERED HOME CARE

Technology dependence, chronic illness, and complex care requirements cross social, cultural, spiritual, and economic boundaries. Regardless of a family's background, family values must be respected in the provision of home care services. *The home is the family's domain,* and the child is at home because the family's central role is to nurture and raise the child. The ultimate responsibility for managing the child's health, developmental, and emotional needs lies with the family. Roush and Cox (2000) developed a framework for helping the home health care nurse understand the significance of the home to the family. The three central concepts of the model are:

Home as familiar—the environment where one is comfortable and at ease because of the familiarity with living arrangements and routines of home
Home as center—the location of everyday experiences related to time, space, and one's social life
Home as protector—the preservation of privacy, safety, and identity in the environment of the home

The nurse must respect and encourage the family's central role in care of the child and must work in collaboration with the family in efforts to care for the child. Family-centered nursing practice is essential in the home setting. Family-centered care has become acknowledged as the standard of care for children with special health care needs (Johnson, 2000).

The philosophic basis for family-centered practice is the recognition that the family is the constant in the child's life, whereas the service systems and personnel within those systems fluctuate. Professionals working with families of children with complex chronic problems must respect the family's central, caring role; their knowledge; and their particular and unique expertise. Families have the most intimate knowledge of the child's strengths and abilities, the challenges of providing care, and the abilities and needs of other family members (Newton, 2000). Believing that no one knows the child better than the family is critical to the success of any health care plan.

DIVERSITY IN HOME CARE

Respect for varied family structures and for racial, ethnic, cultural, and socioeconomic diversity among families is essential in home care. Home care nurses work in close relationship with family members throughout the course of illness (see Family Focus box). The nurse must assess and respect the

FAMILY FOCUS

Developing Relationships with Culturally Diverse Families

I work in the inner city, and my home care patients come from a variety of racial and ethnic backgrounds. I am Caucasian, from Australia. Often, when I first visit a family, there is an initial coolness or apprehension toward me. This is understandable because I am a stranger, and perhaps families think I'll judge them in one way or another. By the end of the first visit, however, there is usually a smile as I leave; by the second visit they often greet me with a smile at the door; and by the third visit we usually have a friendship, trust, and an ease of communication.

If I'm working on a case for an extended time, I use a holistic nursing approach. This involves being aware of how the illness of the child affects the entire family. As I listen over many weeks to their fears and questions, and often as I share faith perspectives, a bond begins to form. I find it a privilege to share in their joys and their pain, and I feel rewarded by the trust that they invest in me.

Julie Edgerton, RN
Home Care Nurse
Children's National Medical Center
Washington, DC

family's background and lifestyle choices. Particular attention is given to communication. The meaning of the words used and the way in which they are said may affect various cultural groups in different ways. Volume of speech and language style must be taken into consideration as part of a family cultural assessment. The home health care nurse must pay particular attention to nonverbal communication. Body language, eye contact, and degree of physical contact have different meanings within a particular culture.

NURSINGTIP

One should not assume that everyone who speaks English can read the language. Color-coded medication bottles, written schedules, and pillboxes or oral syringes may aid compliance with prescription administration. Pictures or special symbols may be helpful when providing instructions for procedures and medication administration.

Families may also differ in their cultural view of children, health care, childrearing practices, illness, and its causes and meaning. The family's health care practices and beliefs may influence the level of investment a family will make in the child's care. The family's religion or spirituality is another factor that can have a major influence on a family's response to the child's special health care needs. Some families look for spiritual meaning and purpose for the illness. Other families may choose to reject past religious ties. In some cultures, religion and beliefs about health care and illness are closely intertwined (McEvoy, 2003); thus it is important that home care nurses assess the relationship between culture, religion, and the family's beliefs about the child's illness.

A variety of cultural assessment tools are available (Giger and Davidhizar, 2002; Spector, 2000). The home care nurse, aware that personal values drive behavior, needs to learn about the family's culture, ask questions without implying judgment, interpret the mainstream medical culture for the family, and help families design interventions that meet their

preferences. When possible, culture-specific teaching materials should be used. In the United States increased emphasis has been placed on health care workers becoming culturally competent to better understand and effectively deliver holistic care to the patient populations they serve (National Center for Cultural Competence, 2002).

Respect for family diversity and an awareness of family developmental stages and the stages of a family's adjustment to a child's illness will assist the home care nurse in recognizing and promoting family strengths and in respecting various coping mechanisms. Labels such as *dysfunctional, difficult,* and *noncompliant* can reinforce negative expectations and shape the behaviors of both parents and professionals (Hostler, 1999). On the other hand, identifying, emphasizing, and building on family strengths and coping mechanisms are strategies that promote a central goal in nursing care of the child and family: family empowerment.

PARENT-PROFESSIONAL COLLABORATION

Family-centered nursing practice is built on a foundation of parent-professional collaboration, which represents a shift from the traditional unidirectional relationships between health care providers and families. The Collaborative Family Healthcare Association* has developed core competencies for professionals collaborating with families.

Collaborative caring allows the nurse and family to work together and share outcomes in a deep and meaningful way. This approach, essential in the home care setting, is characterized by (Kellett and Mannion, 1999):

- Encouraging activities to develop self-confidence and self-esteem
- Displaying increased awareness of and respect for family caregivers
- Recognizing that families vary in defining their role
- Demonstrating an understanding of the family's approach to caregiving
- Sharing perspectives, not just tasks and functions
- Supporting family in their primary, irreplaceable role as caregiver
- Exchanging expertise in providing care to the child
- Assisting family in recognizing their contributions as worthwhile
- Identifying strengths and resources of child and family
- Negotiating options, priorities, and preferences
- Assisting with coping by allowing family to find meaning in caring for the child at home

Communication with the family should not be intrusive. There is no need to collect information from the family that can be obtained from the child's records. The nurse should explain to families the reason for questions, particularly those they may perceive as intrusive, and should tell families who will have access to the information (see Critical Thinking Exercise). The nurse must also assure families that they have a right to expect confidentiality in regard to the data collected. When working in the home, the nurse must respect the privacy of family communications that may be overheard.

Communication with family members should include sharing with the family, in a supportive manner, complete and unbiased information about all aspects of the child's

*PO Box 23980, Rochester, NY 14692-3980; (585) 482-8210; fax: (585) 482-2901; http://www.cfha.net.

CRITICAL THINKING EXERCISE

Family-Centered Home Care and Conflicts

A family wants to begin oral feeding with a tracheostomy of their 3-year-old daughter, Sarah, who is ventilator dependent and is being tube fed through a skin-level gastrostomy feeding tube (MIC-KEY). The mother, who has assumed the role of Sarah's primary caretaker, is adamant about starting oral feedings so Sarah can be more like other children her age. One day the mother asks you, the nurse case manager overseeing the child's home care, to feed Sarah baby food by mouth to see how she tolerates the feeding. The child is alert and sociable yet cannot communicate her wishes except through crying and whining. She has a seizure disorder and has had several episodes of aspiration pneumonia since birth. Sarah appears to have a considerable amount of tongue thrusting and copious amounts of oral mucus that must be suctioned frequently to prevent aspiration; her cough reflex is compromised and usually elicited only with tracheal suctioning.

QUESTIONS

1. Evidence—Is there sufficient evidence to draw any conclusions about the issue of feeding Sarah at this time?
2. Assumptions—Describe some underlying assumptions about the following:
   a. Sarah's readiness for oral feedings
   b. Sarah's ability to tolerate oral feedings
   c. The mother's request for Sarah to start oral feedings
3. What implications and priorities for nursing care may be drawn at this time?
4. Does the evidence objectively support your argument (conclusion)?
5. Are there alternative perspectives to your arguments? What are they?

FAMILY FOCUS

Knowledgeable Parents

It is not unusual for parents, particularly those whose children have chronic illnesses or complex care regimens, to be more knowledgeable about their child's condition than a nurse who is assigned to the child's care. This can be disconcerting for both the parents and the nurse. It is important to remember and reinforce that, regardless of the condition, parents will always know more about their child than the professional caring for the child. The nurse and parents can set goals for care in an atmosphere of mutual respect. If the parents' goal is respite from prolonged caregiving, they are less likely to want to give long explanations about the child's care, and it may be more appropriate for the nurse to seek assistance from an experienced peer. If the parents wish to maintain maximum participation in care delivery, the nurse and the parents can negotiate the collaboration.

When teaching parents to perform complex chronic care regimens at home, include teaching them to expect to know more about their child's care than professionals who may come to assist them, whether that be home health, hospital, or outpatient personnel. At the same time, assure them that various professionals, experienced in working with a multitude of families, will have a scientific knowledge base and a wealth of options for addressing and solving care problems.

Teresa L. Hall, MS, RN
Hathaway Children's Services
Sylmar, California

---

condition and care. Parents often feel overwhelming frustration related to obtaining accurate information about their child's illness and its management. Parents want information given slowly and repeated as necessary over time; they want explanations in terms they can understand; and they want the opportunity to ask questions, which should be answered in a straightforward manner. Stating "I don't know" or "I'll find out" is better than pretending to know or giving excuses. Unfortunately, the home health care nurse may become a source of added stress on the caregiver or family when the nurse displays unprofessional attitudes or fails to show proper respect for the family's knowledge of the child's needs and care (Harrigan, Ratliffe, Patrinos, and others, 2002).

A plan can be made with the parents to gather relevant information when necessary (Hanson and Randall, 1999; Newton, 2000). Information should be shared with families in a way that has meaning in their cultural context (Davidhizar, Havnes, and Bechtel, 1999). Many parents report a preference for interactions with professionals who communicate empathy and concern (Harrigan, Ratliffe, Patrinos, and others, 2002). Families vary in the amount and delivery of information they can tolerate regarding their child's status.

NURSING ALERT

Home care nurses should restrict their communications with other professionals involved in the case to clinically relevant information about the family.

On occasion, disagreements may arise between parents and nurses over proper procedures for the child's care. Nurses should respect parental preferences in any situation that does not pose danger or risk for the child (see Family Focus box). If parents wish to alter a treatment plan that is part of medical orders, the nurse should ask that they negotiate the change with the practitioner because the nurse must follow the written medical orders. If disagreements cannot be resolved, a home care supervisor or case manager (care coordinator) should be contacted to assist with problem solving. Increasingly, home care agencies are developing ethics committees and policies for managing difficult situations such as treatment refusal (see Critical Thinking Exercise).

A tool that might be helpful to the pediatric home care nurse is the Caregiver Strain Index, a 13-item assessment designed to ascertain caregiver stress and subsequently develop appropriate strategies for individual and family coping (Sullivan, 2003).

THE NURSING PROCESS

In the home the family is a partner in each step of the nursing process. Assessment should address family strengths and resources (Box 20-9).* The principles of communication discussed previously guide data collection.

All information gathered as part of the assessment process is shared with the family. The nurse should recognize that the family's perception of their most important need will gener-

---

*Self-report instruments to help families identify concerns, priorities, resources, and sources of support include Family Needs Survey, which is available from FPG Child Development Institute, CB 8180, Chapel Hill, NC 27599; (919) 966-0857; or can be downloaded from http://www.fpg.unc.edu.

BOX 20-9

Sample Family Assessment Questions

- What are the child's and family's experiences and expectations of disease or illness?
- How does that affect the current situation?
- Is the current coping status a reflection of a new condition, the same chronic condition, or a new phase in a chronic condition?
- How can the nurse address family needs and promote health among all family members?
- What specific nursing interventions will facilitate a healthy response to child and family limitations caused by the illness?

Modified from Gedaly-Duff V, Heims ML: Family child health nursing. In Hanson SMH, Boyd ST, editors: *Family health care nursing*, Philadelphia, 1996, Davis.

FAMILY FOCUS

What I Learned About Home Care

I learned many things as a result of having home care for four children over a period of 8 years. Two of the major areas I learned about were communication and families' rights. It took a long time to learn some of these things.

Initially I tried hard to be sensitive to the professionals and often put my own feelings and needs aside. It took a while to learn that I could stand up for myself and my family and that my child could continue to receive good care. One area important to me was to have nurses withhold judgment on our parenting style, even if they might have parented differently.

Communication needs to be open and two way. Families and nurses ought to tell each other what is going well. For example, "Thanks for keeping the room so neat while you're here" can help a nurse see a family's appreciation. There was so little I could do as just "Mommy" that it really meant a lot to me when nurses would say, "That's such a cute outfit you picked out for him today." Communicating about little things, even inconsequential topics such as favorite television shows, makes it easier to communicate about more important things and about problems. Communication has to be open about problems, too.

Jeni Stepanek
Mother
Upper Marlboro, Maryland

ally guide their behavior and consume their attention and energy. Both short- and long-term goals should be outlined and agreed on by the child, family, and professionals involved. The care plan should integrate various disciplines that may be involved with the child to eliminate duplication and coordinate and consolidate care requirements. Cross-training of professionals and a transdisciplinary mode of treatment can also be useful when a child has multiple and complex care requirements (Rothkopf and Rothkopf, 1997). For example, certain physical or occupational therapy routines may be incorporated into the child's morning nursing procedures, or speech therapy interventions may be conducted by the parent or nurse around eating times so that the entire day is not occupied by procedures. A written schedule of daily routines should be developed and followed by all caregivers.

NURSING TIP

At each visit physically handle and look at all medications. Check them against the medical orders and read the labels. There may be discrepancies, duplications, or changes between hospitalizations or follow-up visits. Clarify medication purpose, effect, and dosages for the family.

Goals of care and achievement of established outcomes are supported by intervention strategies that reflect normalization (see Chapter 18) and the interests and abilities of the child and family. Nurses can help the family explore a range of alternative strategies, services, and resources so that the family can choose the best match for their situation.

Families can participate in evaluating a home care plan on several levels. Families and care providers should regularly review the goals of care and update the care plan as required. The nurse can ask the family open-ended questions at regular intervals to assess their opinions on the effectiveness of care. As part of the evaluation process, families should be acknowledged for their successes and accomplishments. Finally, families should be given an opportunity to evaluate individual home care nurses, the home care agency, and other service providers periodically. The evaluation should address the nurse's knowledge, skills, and respect for the family's choices. The agency should use the evaluations to improve quality of care (see Family Focus box).

In addition to maintaining a sense of control over their child's care, families need to control their home and personal lives. For this reason, nurses should discuss "house rules" with the family and address issues such as the physical environment, private areas in the home, responsibility for maintain-

ing the child's environment, and interactions with siblings (see Nursing Care Guidelines box). Home care nursing encourages a close and rewarding relationship with the family. One of the most important aspects of this relationship is maintaining professional boundaries and a therapeutic role that is supportive but not intrusive (McKlindon and Barsteiner, 1999) (see Critical Thinking Exercise).

Technologic trends that influence the nursing process in home care include the use of **laptop computers** (notebooks) to document the home visit; **personal data assistants,** or small hand-held computers that store large amounts of data, including addresses, appointments, patient tracking systems, textbooks, and pharmacologic databases (Lewis and Sommers, 2003); **Internet and e-mail** services, which increase patient-practitioner accessibility and communication; and **telemedicine or telehealth,** which has various features, including electronic systems that can transmit physiologic data directly to the practitioner via the telephone. The American Nurses Association (1999a) has established a list of competencies for nurses involved in telehealth technology. **Telephone triage** has become standard in many health care institutions. Concerns with the increasing use of technology in health care are cost, governmental regulations and patient care standards, liability and malpractice issues, ethics, and confidentiality matters (Rice, 2001). In addition, concerns regarding the nurse-patient relationship (high tech–low touch) and the nurse's role are raised with the use of any technology.

PROMOTION OF OPTIMUM DEVELOPMENT, SELF-CARE, AND EDUCATION

There is little question that living at home offers most children with complex medical problems great social and emotional advantages over living in the hospital or other institutional

nursingcareguidelines

Negotiating "House Rules" for Home Care

HOUSE RULES

Parking—Specify where the nurse should park and any community regulations.

Access—Specify where the nurse enters the home. Is knocking preferred or ringing the bell?

Personal belongings—Where does the nurse store own coat, boots, etc.? Does the family prefer slippers to shoes in the home?

Meals—Where can the nurse store own food? NOTE: This is important given cultural diversity of families.

Radio and television—Identify preferences regarding usage. Remember, this may help nurses remain awake at night.

Patient room—The nurse is responsible for the child's immediate environment. Maintaining a clean working area and cleaning up the room at the end of the shift is the nurse's responsibility.

Telephone—Agency policy may dictate that all personal calls be limited to brief periods and be charged to the nurse making them. NOTE: Many nurses do need to check in with home at some time during the evening.

Visitors—Identify who may enter the home when the parents are away (e.g., child's friends or grandparents). A list of names should be available.

Privacy—Describe what parts of the home are off limits to the nurse and at what times.

CHILD

Routine—Specify times for playtime, bath time, and bedtime. To what extent does the parent want to participate in these routines?

Mealtime—Specify where the family wants the child fed; if tube fed, specify a preference as to how and where it is done.

Clothing—Identify who picks out the child's clothes. Identify where the laundry is and who is responsible for washing the sick child's clothing.

Discipline—Discuss specific guidelines for discipline.

Homework—Discuss when it should be done and who is responsible for it being completed.

SIBLINGS

Discipline—Establish guidelines regarding how parents should be informed of siblings' conflicts and how discipline should be handled. NOTE: Parents or another caregiver must be in the home when siblings are home.

Patient care—Be specific regarding how children can help with the child's care. Discuss any concerns regarding behavior that may compromise the child's or siblings' safety.

NURSING

Parental notification—Specify what information the family wishes to be aware of immediately and what can wait until they are home.

Limits of responsibility—Specify duties the nurse may not perform, such as transportation of the child to care facilities, baby-sitting the child or siblings not under the nurse's care.

Environment—Discuss the need to have adequate lighting and a comfortable working area.

Modified from Klug R: Clarifying roles and expectations in home care, *Pediatr Nurs* 19(4):375, 1993.

??? CRITICAL THINKING EXERCISE

Maintaining Therapeutic Boundaries

As the home care nurse who has been working with a 4-year-old ventilator-dependent child, Derek, weekly for about 5 months, you are aware that the parents have become increasingly argumentative with each other. Most of the arguments are about whether Mr. Jones helps enough with the child's care and the house cleaning. Mr. Jones works full time at one job, then supplements the family income by working at a part-time job every weekend. Ms. Jones approaches you to complain about her husband's lack of involvement with the child and his care. Derek requires constant care, and the family has many expenses related to his physical care; the child is severely developmentally impaired and is not expected to improve significantly despite numerous medical interventions. He is the only child, although Ms. Jones stated at one time they wanted to have many children.

QUESTIONS
1. Evidence—Is there sufficient evidence to draw any conclusions about the family situation at this time?
2. Assumptions—Describe some underlying assumptions about the following:
   a. Home care of the child with a chronic, terminal condition (see p. 642)
   b. Impact of the chronic condition, child's prognosis, and required care on the parents
   c. Status of the marriage relationship between Mr. and Ms. Jones
3. What implications and priorities for nursing care may be drawn at this time?
4. Does the evidence objectively support your argument (conclusion)?
5. Are there alternative perspectives to your arguments? What are they?

setting (see Evidence-Based Practice box, p. 643). However, in infancy and throughout the developmental stages, a child's medical condition and dependence on medical technology can place constraints on and pose challenges to **normal development.** For example, the child may have lengthy and repeated hospitalizations; developmental regression can occur in response to stress; fatigue may result from an underlying pathologic condition, the exacerbation of an illness, or medication side effects; and equipment requirements may impede mobility, exploration, and independence. The challenge of providing support for normal development in a child who is chronically ill and technology dependent requires optimizing opportunities for developmentally appropriate experiences within the constraints posed by the medical condition and the equipment requirements.

Home care plans are designed to promote optimum child development through assessment, planning, and referrals and through interventions that address normalization issues and self-care (Box 20-10). General principles for a family-centered assessment and planning process are addressed earlier in this chapter and are also applied in developmental assessment and planning.

Some parents may not pursue early developmental intervention because they do not believe their child needs the services. In this case professionals need to explain the child's developmental needs to parents in ways that are meaningful

---

BOX 20-10

Incorporating Developmental Support into the Home Care Plan

Example: 6-month-old infant with a history of 24-week prematurity; currently using cardiorespiratory monitor, oxygen via nasal cannula, and nasogastric feeding tube

OUTCOME CRITERIA

Age-appropriate growth—developmental activities promoted with normal parameters achieved

Absence of growth and development deficits for age within limits imposed by illness

INTERVENTION

Assess growth and development with the Denver II Developmental Assessment (see Appendix A).

Reassess growth and development every 4 weeks.

Provide consistent caregiver.

Instruct parents in normal growth and development for child's age, reasons for delay, and anticipated outcomes.

Inform parents of age-related play and other activities that enhance growth and development and provide stimulation.

Consult with physical, occupational, and speech therapists to incorporate recommendations in daily routines.

Provide visual, auditory, and tactile stimulation, including mobiles with or without color, music, toys, books, television.

Hold, rock, pat, and talk to child.

Data from Klijanowicz AS: Care of high-risk infant. In Votroubek WL, Townsend JL, editors: *Pediatric home care*, ed 2, Gaithersburg, Md, 1997, Aspen; Jaffe M: *Pediatric nursing care plans*, ed 2, Englewood, Col, 1998, Skidmore-Roth; and Luxner K, Jaffe M: *Delmar's pediatric nursing care plans*, ed 3, Clifton Park, NY, 2004, Thomson Delmar Learning.

from the parents' own cultural and socioeconomic perspectives. Only then can parents make truly informed decisions. Once parents have been fully informed of the child's condition, likely developmental sequelae, and the expected benefits of intervention, developmental goals outlined by the child and family should guide planning and intervention.

The impact of chronic illness on development is discussed in Chapter 18. Behaviors that may be observed in children receiving home care that need to be addressed by the nurse include:

Infants—crying, withdrawal, detachment, inability to achieve developmental milestones

Toddlers—inactivity; sadness; screaming; regressive behavior; delays in motor, speech, social skills

Preschoolers—temper tantrums, refusal to comply with routines, refusal to eat or participate in self-care

School-age children—expression of loneliness, boredom, isolation, depression, and worry about school absences; altered physical growth

Adolescents—dependency, uncooperativeness, withdrawal, fear of loss of peer status or acceptance at school, altered image

Promoting coping and capability can buffer stress and contribute to mental health and self-esteem in a child with a chronic illness. The extent to which a child is involved in his or her own care depends on many factors, including parental comfort and support and the child's developmental age, level

of interest, and physical ability. Self-care, both in activities of daily living and in regard to the medical condition, is important. The goal for self-care in activities of daily living should be attainment of age-appropriate competence. Some modifications in the environment, the medical equipment, or the techniques for daily activities may be required to promote and support self-care. Effective teaching for self-care is focused at the child's own level of conceptual understanding and may be augmented by the use of dolls, other models and diagrams, simple explanations, and repetition.

Educational planning is important for the child who has a chronic medical condition. Federal laws ensure that all children receive a public education. Before age 3 years, children with developmental delays are eligible for an early intervention program. The child can receive rehabilitation therapies as appropriate (physical, occupational, or speech therapy). After age 3 years, the local school system is responsible for providing this education. Some children may be eligible for special education preschools. The home care nurse should refer the family to local educational programs.

Each family is entitled to an individual family service plan (IFSP), or individualized care plan, to help ensure early intervention. All states in the United States provide agencies that develop IFSPs; each state's plan can easily be accessed via the Internet by entering the term *individual family service plan* in an Internet search engine such as Yahoo or Google. The IFSP provides the child with a disability, from birth to age 3 years, with a plan for integrating early intervention and rehabilitation, based on the child's and family's needs.

When a child requiring special medical care is to be placed in an educational setting, the parents, child, school health coordinator, educational evaluation team, and education and administrative staff should meet to determine safe and appropriate placement and the necessary services and personnel to enable the child to attend school in the least restrictive environment. Training of education staff and caregivers is essential to ensuring the child's safety in the educational setting.* Special assistance can also be beneficial in reintegrating previously schooled children, such as those with cancer, into the school setting. The home care nurse may need to assist parents in developing the skills to advocate effectively for their child in the educational system.

SAFETY ISSUES IN THE HOME

Safety is an important consideration in pediatric home care and should be addressed in the home care plan.

NURSINGTIP

If the family does not have a telephone, arrangements can be made with the telephone company to supply service. Alternatively, one or two nearby neighbors may agree to let the family use their services. In rural areas a local pharmacy or police or ranger station may be willing to receive messages and relay them to the family. A cellular phone may be used in place of a local telephone, but it is advisable to check with the local emergency facilities regarding policies for cell phone use and emergency 911 calls.

---

*A thorough discussion of training issues, content, and guidelines for care in the school is provided in Porter S, Bierle T, Haynie M, and others, editors: *Children and youth assisted by medical technology in educational settings: guidelines for care*, ed 2, Baltimore, 1997, Paul H. Brookes.

The telephone and electric companies (if the use of medical equipment requires electricity) must be notified that the family needs to be placed on a priority service list. In this way the family will learn of any anticipated interruptions in service and will receive priority in reinstatement of interrupted services. Prior contact with rescue squad and local emergency facility personnel can help ensure prompt and appropriate interventions if required. This is especially important if the family lives in a rural location that may not be familiar to local emergency responders. It is recommended that local authorities be given a map marked with key landmarks and intersections for rapid access to the home.

Before hospital discharge, emergency protocols are developed and reviewed with the parents and professional caregivers. Cardiopulmonary resuscitation guidelines, if appropriate, should be posted near the child's bedside or in another accessible location. A list of emergency telephone numbers can be placed near each home phone and should include those of the rescue squad, emergency department, managing physician(s), nursing agency, and equipment vendor(s) or providers. Additional issues to consider are advance directives and out-of-hospital do-not-resuscitate (OHDNR) orders (may vary by state), as indicated. If the patient and family desire enforcement of an **advance directive,** they must follow specific guidelines, which could prevent undesired lifesaving measures for children with terminal illnesses.

Another aspect of safety relates to the provision of care by appropriately trained individuals. Family members should receive thorough training in the child's care requirements and have the opportunity to demonstrate knowledge and confidence before hospital discharge. Children with complex medical care needs are often admitted to an acute care center for nonmedical reasons, including lack of parent training and parents' inability to care for a child with complex medical needs (Schanwald, 2005). Professional staff caring for the child should have the appropriate background and training for the child's particular care needs. Because of the child's body size, special skill and caution are required in the performance of procedures (e.g., gastrostomy feedings, suctioning) and in monitoring the use of equipment (e.g., ventilator settings, intravenous flow rates, and total fluid volumes) (see Chapters 22, 23, 25).

The activity level and curiosity of young children raise additional safety considerations in the provision of home care. All medications, needles, syringes, and contaminated materials must be securely stored well out of the reach of curious hands. Arrangements for the disposal of sharp items or contaminated materials can be made with the home health agency. Special attention is given to childproofing the control panels on ventilators, pumps, monitors, and other equipment. The use of clear plastic tape, covers, or panels to cover control knobs or buttons reduces the risk of accidental changes in settings. Much of the medical equipment now in use has special lock-out capabilities that may be used to prevent accidentally altering settings. Electrical cords are kept short and out of reach, and safety covers are used on any open outlets. Equipment is unplugged when not in use, and any wires (e.g., lead wires for an apnea monitor) are stored out of reach. (See Chapter 11 for use of apnea monitors in the home.)

Care at night poses other safety concerns. Parents or other caregivers need to be able to clearly hear monitor, ventilator, or pump alarms at night; an inexpensive intercom system or baby monitor can be used. Steps must be taken to prevent accidental strangulation by apnea, oximeter, or cardiac monitor wires or lengthy intravenous tubing during sleep.

> **NURSING TIP**
>
> Coiling extra tubing and taping it at the exit site, as well as running wires or tubes out the bottoms of pajamas, are precautions against strangulation.

Safe transportation is a vital concern. Wheelchairs and other medical equipment must be properly secured to the vehicle, including vans and buses. Appropriate child restraints must be used. If necessary, an extra adult should be present to monitor the child while in transit. Information on car seat safety and transportation for children with special needs is available from the American Academy of Pediatrics (1999) reference for guidelines for wheelchairs in cars, supine car seats, and equipment transportation.

FAMILY-TO-FAMILY SUPPORT

Family-to-family support networks can be an important source of emotional and instrumental support and empowerment for families of children with chronic health problems. Family-to-family support does not replace professional sources of support but rather is a unique resource that promotes family strengths through shared experience.

Families will most likely experience increased emotional stress as the result of living with and caring for a child with special needs. Other issues that are likely to arise as a result of the child's illness and the constant attention required include labeling the child as being vulnerable, or **vulnerable child syndrome,** wherein parents may spend too much time preoccupied with the child's welfare while ignoring other family members' needs (Bennett, 2002). As the child with special health care needs develops and grows, parents should impose the same disciplinary rules on the child receiving home care as on siblings to avoid further conflict within the family.

Identifying meaningful sources of support can make a difference in coping abilities. Montagnino and Mauricio (2004) surveyed a group of mothers caring for children in the home who had a tracheostomy and gastrostomy. The researchers found that the mothers experienced significant anxiety, and social interaction within and outside the family was disrupted as a result of the child's condition. The authors recommended that families of children with special health care needs network with other parents in similar conditions through online and local support groups to prevent social disruption and maintain a sense of family normalcy despite the child's condition.

Baum (2004) surveyed caregivers of children with special health care needs about the value of an Internet parent support group; the researcher used stress and coping theory as a guide for measuring perceived satisfaction and a number of other characteristics. The survey indicated that parents were satisfied with the information obtained through the Internet support group, and improved caregiver-child relationship was the strongest outcome factor. The author suggests that undesirable results may also be obtained via such an Internet group and that the quality of such support groups should be carefully evaluated by those involved.

The nurse can assist the family in increasing their involvement in community social networks. For example, a referral to a parent support group may meet an individual family's needs. The nurse should inform the parents of the group's goals so that they can determine whether they might benefit from this connection. In addition, informal support networks can be extremely beneficial. A link to a family in the same or a similar situation allows the sharing of common experiences. This in itself may decrease the sense of isolation and provide a connection with someone who can really identify with family struggles. Positive outcomes can include understanding, empathizing, problem solving, or just talking to someone who will listen.

The nurse should remember that each family member's needs differ. The care plan should acknowledge the needs of each family member (mother, father, siblings, grandparents). Peer support for school-age children and adolescents with complex care needs may be beneficial. These connections can be expanded to include letter writing, e-mails, telephone calls, or specialty camping programs (Johnson, Ravert, and Everton, 2001). Most school-age children and adolescents just want to be accepted by their peers and fit in as a part of the group. Same-age peers may at first be standoffish to children with disabilities, but this is likely out of fear and lack of understanding; helping others see that they have the same dreams, desires, goals, and interests promotes group cohesiveness and understanding.

KEY POINTS

- Effective home care depends on many factors, including the child's medical stability; the family's willingness, training, and ability to accommodate the child's care requirements; and professional, financial, and community support.
- Comprehensive, multidisciplinary discharge planning should begin early and should include the family and a home care coordinator in addition to hospital personnel.
- Thorough education and training of the family or primary caregiver can ease the transition to home.
- Care coordination ensures continuity of care, prevents duplication of services, and reduces fragmentation of services. The family may assume responsibility for varying degrees of care coordination over time.
- The home care nurse must possess a high level of technical expertise while being able to adapt equipment, procedures, and the nursing process to the home setting.
- Federal standards apply to agencies that participate in Medicare or Medicaid; standards of practice by the American Nurses Association and other professional nursing organizations can guide nurses in the home setting.
- Family-centered nursing practice is applied in the home setting; diversity in family structures, cultural backgrounds, strengths, and coping mechanisms is respected.
- Collaborative relationships between parents and home care providers are characterized by communication, dialog, active listening, awareness and acceptance of differences, and negotiation.
- The nursing process is adapted to involve the family in each step and to preserve the family's central role in decision making.
- House rules agreed on by the nurse, child, and family allow the family to maintain a feeling of control over their own environment when professionals are present.
- Individualized home care plans are designed to promote optimum development of the child and to focus on normalization, the impact of the child's medical condition and technologic requirements on development, self-care, and educational needs.

- Safety in the provision of home care services involves emergency preparations and protocols, appropriate training of family and home care personnel, and the safe use and childproofing of medical equipment.
- Family-to-family support networks can provide emotional and instrumental support and encourage family empowerment.

answers to CRITICAL THINKING EXERCISES

FAMILY-CENTERED HOME CARE AND CONFLICTS

1. Yes, there is sufficient evidence to arrive at some possible conclusions (see pp. 648-650).
2. a. Sarah demonstrates tongue thrusting, which is common in healthy children from birth to 4 or 5 months. The extrusion reflex is common in children who have little experience with oral feedings and oral stimulation (see Feeding Resistance, Chapter 9).
   b. Given Sarah's history and assessment data, there are risks involved in starting oral feedings, primarily choking and aspiration.
   c. The mother's request is not unusual. Parents want the best for their children despite handicaps that often set them apart from other peers. Although it may seem complicated to engage in communication, negotiation, and consultation over the seemingly simple issue of giving baby food to a 3-year-old, many issues must be considered.

   The family appears to have legitimate reasons for wanting their daughter started on baby foods. The nurse should further explore reasons for wanting the child to be fed orally. The parents may believe that health care providers have overlooked this aspect of normal development. The implications may be that the family is attempting to assist their daughter in achieving age-appropriate skills and may also want their daughter to participate in family mealtimes. These are legitimate, commendable goals, and the family should be supported in making such choices for their child.
3. A child who is 3 years old and has not been fed orally will benefit from an oral-motor assessment by an occupational therapist/speech language pathologist (OT/SLP) to explore the possibility of starting minimum oral feedings. Specific plans with incremental steps to reduce oral-motor defensiveness and improve the ability to accept foods orally should precede feeding. Nutritional consultation may also be important as feeding plans shift from gastrostomy to oral feedings. The nurse and family should continue to discuss the issue, plan for consultations and evaluations related to the child's oral-motor progress, and thereby arrange to meet the family's goals of oral feeding in safer incremental steps. Communication between the nurse and the family may also lead to other approaches to normalizing mealtimes for Sarah and her family. After the OT/SLP has completed the assessment, specific short- and long-term goals for modified oral feedings may be developed, involving the family in such discussions. In addition, the family should be made aware of potential problems with oral feedings, including aspiration pneumonia or airway obstruction with further respiratory compromise.
4. Yes, the evidence supports implementing this care plan. The nurse should not dismiss the parents' request for oral feedings, yet should not acquiesce to their request without assessing the situation, developing conclusions based on the assessment, and implementing an appropriate care plan that may be evaluated by the outcomes. It would not be appropriate to begin oral feedings without first consulting an OT/SLP regarding Sarah's oral-motor abilities.

5. Assessment of the child's status may reveal deficiencies that could preclude attempts at oral feedings. In this case it would be important to involve other health care workers in a discussion with the parents regarding the issue of oral feedings. The home health care nurse must remember, however, that the child is the parents' responsibility and the ultimate decision about oral feedings rests with them. Home care issues that produce conflict about what constitutes the best care for the child between the primary caretaker or parents and the health care team must be handled with utmost care because the parents are ultimately responsible for the child. Such conflicts may lead to mistrust and further alienation if not handled properly. Each case should be handled on an individual basis and all available resources used to make the best care possible available to the child.

MAINTAINING THERAPEUTIC BOUNDARIES

1. Yes, there is sufficient evidence to arrive at some conclusions regarding the situation.
2. a. Home care of any person, especially a child with a chronic debilitating condition, is stressful on any family regardless of its stability and resources. The seeming lack of coping skills and decreased financial resources make the stress worse. It is not unusual for stress and conflict to surround the child's care, especially if one parent seems to be less involved in the daily care. The needs of the primary caretaker, Ms. Jones in this instance, are not being met, and she is expressing that frustration to the nurse, who perhaps is perceived as an ally in the situation.
   b. The impact of a chronic condition on parents can be devastating and lead to misunderstandings, competition over the child's care, and neglect of the feelings of one's partner. Because the child's prognosis is poor, this can exacerbate feelings of frustration, anger, helplessness, fatigue, and conflict among parents. Parents may feel guilty about their feelings toward the child. On one hand, they may love and care for the child; on the other hand, the presence of a child with a chronic condition with poor prognosis who requires constant physical care may engender a desire to see an end to the situation with the child's death. These ambivalent feelings are not unusual in parents, and there may also be gender differences in how they express feelings over such conditions. Unmet expectations are a source of conflict among parents with a child who is sick; expectations of each other's role in the family setting may have suffered with the loss of the "perfect" child. These feelings may last for months or even years without an appropriate resolution if adequate resources for resolution are not provided.

c. The status of the marriage appears to be strained at this time; however, there is not sufficient evidence to draw a simple conclusion without further exploration (assessment). This may be the way each parent deals with crisis situations—the mother fusses and complains, and the father withdraws by going to work and being less involved. Some anticipatory grieving may be occurring, but this needs to be explored by health care persons who can be objective and properly evaluate the marriage status.

3. The concept of therapeutic boundaries supports the idea that they are not rigid and fixed. The home care nurse must be responsive to the relationship preferred by the family and the style with which the family operates. Individual roles change according to the expectations that person has about her or his role and the context within which that person is living the role. In this situation it would be appropriate for the nurse to mention that home care can be stressful for a family, indicate that referrals for counseling may be provided if desired by the parents, and listen and reflect with Ms. Jones about her feelings. Exploring issues such as an additional home care aide to help take care of Derek might be appropriate; this would enable Ms. Jones to take a break from his care and have time to herself. Additional financial aid may be explored by a qualified case manager or social worker so Mr. Jones would not have to work as much away from home. It is important to explore the couple's feelings regarding Derek's condition and care and their role in providing for him, as well as their relationship to each other. It is not unusual for families in crisis to become so involved in the care of the child that they forget what their marriage and relationship are about. If one or both parties do not desire counseling by another professional, perhaps they could explore other options such as family support groups. For any conclusion you may reach, it would be inappropriate to agree with Ms. Jones that her husband is not helping enough with the child's care. Such an action implies a judgment that is not within the nurse's role to make and undermines rather than supports the family system. Families in crisis often require professional assistance in the form of counseling to explore coping skills and help involve appropriate community resources.

4. Some preliminary evidence supports the argument that professional help is warranted in this situation. In addition, as the feelings of Mr. and Ms. Jones are explored, additional evidence may arise that alters the course of action proposed.

5. Alternative perspectives may arise as more data are obtained during a family interview. It would not be appropriate for the home health care nurse to take sides with Ms. Jones or with Mr. Jones to avoid the main issues, which involve Ms. Jones's sense of isolation in the care of her child.

REFERENCES

American Academy of Pediatrics: Care coordination in the Medical Home: integrating health and related systems of care for children with special health care needs, *Pediatrics* 116(5):1238-1244, 2005.

American Academy of Pediatrics: Transporting children with special health care needs, *Pediatrics* 104(4):988-992, 1999.

American Nurses Association: *Competencies for telehealth technologies in nursing*, Washington, DC, 1999a, The Association.

American Nurses Association: *Standards of home health nursing practice*, Washington, DC, 1999b, The Association.

American Nurses Association: *Standards of public health nursing practice*, Washington, DC, 1999c, The Association.

American Nurses Association: *Nursing case management*, Washington, DC, 1998, The Association.

Bakewell-Sachs S, Carlino H, Ash L, and others: Home care considerations for chronic and vulnerable populations, *Nurse Pract Forum* 11(1):65-72, 2000.

Baum LS: Internet parent support groups for primary caregivers of a child with special health care needs, *Pediatr Nurs* 30(5):381-388, 401, 2004.

Bennett AD: Home apnea monitoring for infants: a discussion of primary care issues, *Adv Nurs Pract* 10(3):48-53, 2002.

Carlin MC: Hospice nursing: more than a job, *Caring* 18(1):8-9, 1999.

Cooper C, Wheeler DM, Woolfenden SR, and others: Specialist home-based nursing services for children with acute and chronic illnesses, *Cochrane Database Sys Rev* 18(4):CD004383, 2006.

Daveluy W, Guimber D, Uhlen S, and others: Dramatic changes in home-based enteral nutrition practices in children during an 11-year period, *J Pediatr Gastroeneterol Nutr* 43(2):240-244, 2006.

Davidhizar R, Havnes R, Bechtel G: Assessing culturally diverse pediatric clients, *Pediatr Nurs* 25(4):371-376, 1999.

Dittbrenner H: Pediatric home care as a viable new service, *Caring* 18(2):12-15, 1999.

Feudtner C, Villareale NL, Morray B, and others: Technology-dependence among patients discharged from a children's hospital: a retrospective cohort study, *BMC Pediatrics* 5(8):1-8, 2005.

Giger JN, Davidhizar R: The Giger and Davidhizar Transcultural Assessment Model, *J Transcult Nurs* 13(3):185-188, 2002.

Hanson JL, Randall VF: Evaluating and improving the practice of family-centered care, *Pediatr Nurs* 25(4):445-449, 1999.

Harrigan RC, Ratliffe C, Patrinos ME, and others: Medically fragile children: an integrative review of the literature and recommendations for future research, *Issues Compr Pediatr Nurs* 25(1):1-20, 2002.

Hostler SL: Pediatric family-centered rehabilitation, *J Head Trauma Rehabil* 14(4):384-393, 1999.

Johnson BH: Family-centered care: facing the new millennium: interview by Elizabeth Ahmann, *Pediatr Nurs* 26(1):87-90, 2000.

Johnson CP, Kastner TA, American Academy of Pediatrics Committee on Children with Disabilities: Helping families raise children with special health care needs at home, *Pediatrics* 115(2):507-511, 2005.

Johnson KB, Ravert RD, Everton A: Hopkins Teen Central: assessment of an internet-based support system for children with cystic fibrosis, *Pediatrics* 107(2):e24, 2001.

Kellett UM, Mannion J: Meaning in caring: reconceptualizing the nurse–family carer relationship in community practice, *J Adv Nurs* 29(3):697-703, 1999.

Knafl KA, Deatrick JA: The challenges of normalization for families of children with chronic conditions, *Pediatr Nurs* 28(1):49-53, 56, 2002.

Lewis JA, Sommers CO: Personal data assistants: using new technology to enhance nursing practice, *MCN* 28(2):66-71, 2003.

Lindeke LL, Leonard BJ, Presler B, and others: Family-centered care coordination for children with special needs across multiple settings, *J Pediatr Health Care* 16(6):290-297, 2002.

Magrabi F, Lovell NH, Henry RL, and others: Designing home telecare: a case study in monitoring cystic fibrosis, *Telemed J E Health* 11(6):707-719, 2005.

McEvoy M: Culture and spirituality as an integrated concept in pediatric care, *MCN* 28(1):39-43, 2003.

McKlindon D, Barsteiner JH: Therapeutic relationships, *MCN* 24(5):237-243, 1999.

Montagnino BA, Mauricio RV: The child with a tracheostomy and gastrostomy: parental stress and coping in the home—a pilot study, *Pediatr Nurs* 30(5):373-380, 401, 2004.

National Alliance for Caregiving: *Family caregiving in the U.S.: findings from a national survey*, 2005, The Alliance, retrieved March 13, 2006, from http://www.caregiving.org.

National Center for Cultural Competence: Developing cultural competence in health care settings, *Pediatr Nurs* 28(2):133-137, 2002.

Navaie-Waliser M, Misener M, Mersman C, and others: Evaluating the needs of children with asthma in home care: the vital role of nurses as caregivers and educators, *Pub Health Nurs* 21(4):306-315, 2004.

Nazer D, Abdulhamid I, Thomas R, and others: Home versus hospital intravenous antibiotic therapy for acute pulmonary exacerbations in children with cystic fibrosis, *Pediatr Pulmonol* 41(8):744-749, 2006.

Newton MS: Family-centered care: current realities in parent participation, *Pediatr Nurs* 26(2):164-168, 2000.

Page DR: Pediatric home care: nursing the shortage, *Caring* 20(6):46-47, 2001.

Parra MM: Nursing and respite care services for ventilator-assisted children, *Caring* 22(5):6-9, 2003.

Petit de Mange EA: Pediatric considerations in homecare, *Crit Care Nurs Clin North Am* 10(3):339-346, 1998.

Rice R: Case management and leadership strategies for home care nurses. In Rice R, editor: *Home care nursing practice: concepts and application*, ed 3, St Louis, 2001, Mosby.

Rothkopf MM, Rothkopf GS: The home care team. In Rothkopf MM, editor: *Standards and practice of homecare therapeutics*, ed 2, Baltimore, 1997, Williams & Wilkins.

Roush CV, Cox JE: The meaning of home: how it shapes the practice of home and hospice care, *Home Healthcare Nurs* 18(6):388-394, 2000.

Schanwald PR: Gaps in pediatric care, *Caring* 25(9):20-25, 2005.

Spector RE: *Cultural diversity in health and illness*, ed 5, Upper Saddle River, NJ, 2000, Prentice-Hall Health.

Stevens B, McKeever P, Law MP, and others. Children receiving chemotherapy at home: perceptions of children and parents, *J Pediatr Oncol Nurs* 23(5):276-285, 2006.

Sullivan T: Caregiver Strain Index, *Home Healthcare Nurse* 21(3):197-198, 2003.

Sullivan-Bolyai S, Knafl K, Sadler L, and others: Great expectations: a position description for parents as caregivers, part II, *Pediatr Nurs* 30(1):52-56, 2004.

Sullivan-Bolyai S, Sadler L, Knafl K, and others: Great expectations: a position description for parents as caregivers, part I, *Pediatr Nurs* 29(6):457-460, 2003.

Thompson J: Pediatric assessment in the home, *Home Health Nurs* 18(10):639-646, 2000.

Timm S: Effectively delegating nursing activities in home care, *Home Healthcare Nurse* 21(4):260-265, 2003.

Wilson A: Understanding benchmarks, *Home Healthcare Nurse* 21(2):102-107, 2003.

Wilson H: HIPAA: the big picture for home care and hospice, *Home Health Care Manage Pract* 16(2):127-137, 2004.

Yoder-Wise P: *Leading and managing in nursing*, ed 3, St Louis, 2003, Mosby.

http://evolve.elsevier.com/Wong/essentials/

21

Family-Centered Care of the Child During Illness and Hospitalization

JENNIFER SANDERS

CHAPTER OUTLINE

STRESSORS OF HOSPITALIZATION AND CHILDREN'S REACTIONS, 659
Separation Anxiety, 659
  Early Childhood, 661
  Later Childhood and Adolescence, 661
Loss of Control, 661
  Infants, 661
  Toddlers, 662
  Preschoolers, 662
  School-Age Children, 662
  Adolescents, 662
Effects of Hospitalization on the Child, 663
  Individual Risk Factors, 663
  Beneficial Effects of Hospitalization, 664

STRESSORS AND REACTIONS OF THE FAMILY OF THE CHILD WHO IS HOSPITALIZED, 664
Parental Reactions, 664
Sibling Reactions, 664
Altered Family Roles, 664
NURSING CARE OF THE CHILD WHO IS HOSPITALIZED, 664
Preparation for Hospitalization, 664
  Admission Assessment, 665
  Preparing Child for Admission, 665
Nursing Interventions, 668
  Preventing or Minimizing Separation, 668
  Minimizing Loss of Control, 670
  Preventing or Minimizing Fear of Bodily Injury, 672
  Providing Developmentally Appropriate Activities, 672

Providing Opportunities for Play and Expressive Activities, 673
Maximizing Potential Benefits of Hospitalization, 675
NURSING CARE OF THE FAMILY, 676
Supporting Family Members, 676
Providing Information, 677
Encouraging Parent Participation, 677
Preparing for Discharge and Home Care, 678
CARE OF THE CHILD AND FAMILY IN SPECIAL HOSPITAL SITUATIONS, 679
Ambulatory or Outpatient Setting, 679
Isolation, 680
Emergency Admission, 680
Intensive Care Unit, 681

LEARNING OBJECTIVES

On completion of this chapter the reader will be able to:
- Identify the stressors of illness and hospitalization for children during each developmental stage.
- List essential priorities of nursing care for a child on admission to the hospital.

- Outline nursing interventions that prevent or minimize the stress of separation during hospitalization.
- Outline nursing interventions that minimize the stress of loss of control during hospitalization.
- Outline nursing interventions that minimize the fear of bodily injury during hospitalization.

- Outline nursing interventions that support parents, siblings, and family during a child's illness and hospitalization.
- Describe nursing interventions needed when children are admitted to special units such as the emergency department.

RELATED TOPICS and ADDITIONAL RESOURCES

 IN TEXT

Administration of Medication, *Ch. 22*
Compliance, *Ch. 22*
Cultural and Religious Influences on Health
    Care, *Ch. 4*
Developmental Assessment, *Ch. 5*
Family-Centered Care, *Ch. 18*
Family-Centered Home Care, *Ch. 20*
Impact of the Child's Chronic Illness
    or Disability, *Ch. 18*
Neonatal Pain, *Ch. 9*
Normalization, *Ch. 18*
Nursing Diagnosis, *Ch. 1*

Pain Assessment and Management in
    Children, *Ch. 7*
Physical Examination, *Ch. 6*
Preparation for Diagnostic and Therapeutic
    Procedures, *Ch. 22*
Surgical Procedures, *Ch. 22*

 COMPANION CD

Critical Thinking Exercise—Discharge
    Planning
NCLEX Review Questions

evolve.elsevier.com/Wong/essentials/

NCLEX Review Questions
Nursing Care Plan—The Child Undergoing
    Surgery
Skills—Admitting a Child to the Health
    Care System; Therapeutic Play; Preparing
    the Child for Surgery
WebLinks

**WONG'S CLINICAL MANUAL
OF PEDIATRIC NURSING, 7th Ed**

Patient and Family Education—Measuring
    your Child's Temperature, *p. 508;*
    Applying a Topical Anesthetic, *p. 546;*
    Giving Oral Medications, *p. 523;* Giving
    Intramuscular (IM) Injections, *p. 525*

STRESSORS OF HOSPITALIZATION AND CHILDREN'S REACTIONS

Often, illness and hospitalization are the first crises children must face. Especially during the early years, children are particularly vulnerable to the crises of illness and hospitalization because (1) stress represents a change from the usual state of health and environmental routine and (2) children have a limited number of coping mechanisms to resolve **stressors** (those events that produce stress). Major stressors of hospitalization include separation, loss of control, bodily injury, and pain. Children's reactions to these crises are influenced by their developmental age; their previous experience with ill-

ness, separation, or hospitalization; their innate and acquired coping skills; the seriousness of the diagnosis; and the support system available.

SEPARATION ANXIETY

The major stress from middle infancy throughout the preschool years, especially for children ages 6 to 30 months, is separation anxiety, also called **anaclitic depression.** The principal behavioral responses to this stressor during early childhood are summarized in Box 21-1. During the phase of **protest,** children react aggressively to the separation from the parent. They cry and scream for their parents, refuse the atten-

---

| BOX 21-1

Manifestations of Separation Anxiety in Young Children

PHASE OF PROTEST
Behaviors observed during later infancy include:
- Cries
- Screams
- Searches for parent with eyes
- Clings to parent
- Avoids and rejects contact with strangers

Additional behaviors observed during toddlerhood include:
- Verbally attacks strangers (e.g., "Go away")
- Physically attacks strangers (e.g., kicks, bites, hits, pinches)
- Attempts to escape to find parent
- Attempts to physically force parent to stay

Behaviors may last from hours to days.
Protest, such as crying, may be continuous, ceasing only with physical exhaustion.
Approach of stranger may precipitate increased protest.

PHASE OF DESPAIR
Observed behaviors include:
- Is inactive
- Withdraws from others

- Is depressed, sad
- Lacks interest in environment
- Is uncommunicative
- Regresses to earlier behavior (e.g., thumb sucking, bed-wetting, use of pacifier, use of bottle)

Behaviors may last for variable length of time.
Child's physical condition may deteriorate from refusal to eat, drink, or move.

PHASE OF DETACHMENT
Observed behaviors include:
- Shows increased interest in surroundings
- Interacts with strangers or familiar caregivers
- Forms new but superficial relationships
- Appears happy

Detachment usually occurs after prolonged separation from parent; it is rarely seen in hospitalized children.
Behaviors represent a superficial adjustment to loss.

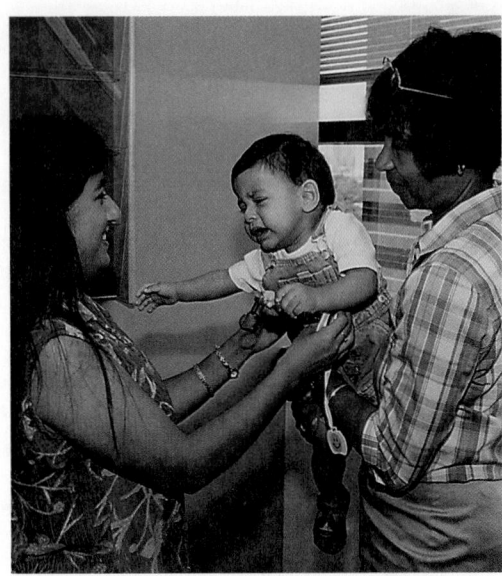

FIG. 21-1 ■ In the protest phase of separation anxiety, children cry loudly and are inconsolable in their grief for the parent. (Courtesy James DeLeon, Texas Children's Hospital, Houston.)

FIG. 21-3 ■ Young children may appear withdrawn and sad even in the presence of a parent. (Courtesy E. Jacob, Texas Children's Hospital, Houston.)

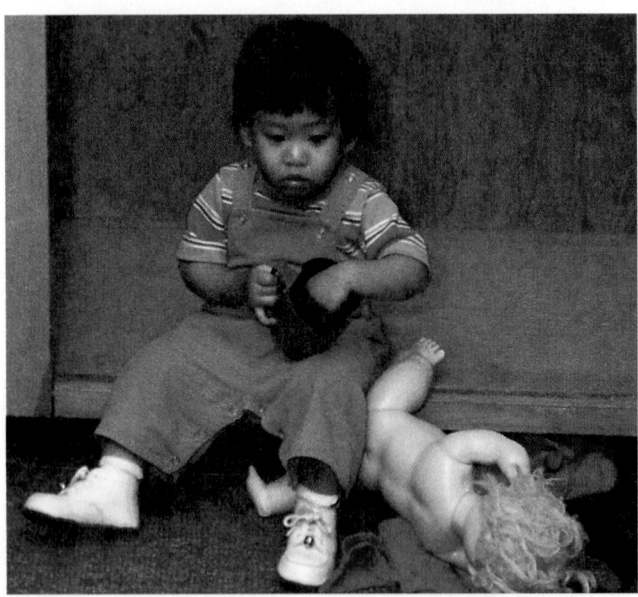

FIG. 21-2 ■ During the despair phase of separation anxiety, children are sad, lonely, and uninterested in food and play.

tion of anyone else, and are inconsolable in their grief (Fig. 21-1). During the phase of **despair,** the crying stops and depression is evident. The child is much less active, is uninterested in play or food, and withdraws from others (Fig. 21-2).

The third stage is **detachment,** also called **denial.** Superficially it appears that the child has finally adjusted to the loss. The child becomes more interested in the surroundings, plays with others, and seems to form new relationships. However, this behavior is the result of resignation and is not a sign of contentment. The child detaches from the parent in an effort

to escape the emotional pain of desiring the parent's presence and copes by forming shallow relationships with others, becoming increasingly self-centered, and attaching primary importance to material objects. This is the most serious stage in that reversal of the potential adverse effects is less likely to occur after detachment is established. However, in most situations, the temporary separations imposed by hospitalization do not cause such prolonged parental absences that the child enters into detachment. In addition, considerable evidence suggests that even with stressors such as separation, children are remarkably adaptable and permanent ill effects are rare.

Although progression to the stage of detachment is uncommon, the initial stages are frequently observed even with brief separations from either parent. Unless health team members understand the meaning of each stage of behavior, they may erroneously label the behaviors as positive or negative. For example, they may see the loud crying of the protest phase as "bad" behavior. Because the protests increase when a stranger approaches the child, they may interpret that reaction as meaning they should stay away. During the quiet, withdrawn phase of despair, health team members may think that the child is finally "settling in" to the new surroundings, and they may see the detachment behaviors as proof of a "good adjustment." The faster this stage is reached, the more likely it is that the child will be regarded as the "ideal patient."

Because children seem to react "negatively" to visits by their parents, uninformed observers feel justified in restricting parental visiting privileges. For example, during the protest stage, children outwardly do not appear happy to see their parents (Fig. 21-3). In fact, they may even cry louder. If they are depressed, they may reject their parents or begin to protest again. Often they cling to their parents in an effort to ensure their continued presence. Consequently, such reactions may be regarded as "disturbing" the child's adjustment to the new surroundings. If the separation has progressed to the phase of detachment, children will respond no differently to their parents than they would to any other person.

Such reactions are distressing to parents, who are unaware of their meaning. If parents are regarded as intruders, they will see their absence as "beneficial" to the child's adjustment and recovery. They may respond to the child's behavior by staying for only short periods, visiting less frequently, or deceiving the child when it is time to leave. The result is a destructive cycle of misunderstanding and unmet needs.

Early Childhood

Separation anxiety is the greatest stress imposed by hospitalization during early childhood. If separation is avoided, young children have a tremendous capacity to withstand any other stress. During this age period, the typical reactions just described are seen. However, children in the toddler stage demonstrate more goal-directed behaviors. For example, they may plead with the parents to stay and physically try to keep the parents with them or try to find parents who have left. They may demonstrate displeasure on the parents' return or departure by having temper tantrums; refusing to comply with the usual routines of mealtime, bedtime, or toileting; or regressing to more primitive levels of development. However, temper tantrums, bed-wetting, or other behaviors may also be expressions of anger, a physiologic response to stress, or symptoms of illness.

Because preschoolers are more secure interpersonally than toddlers, they can tolerate brief periods of separation from their parents and are more inclined to develop substitute trust in other significant adults. However, the stress of illness usually renders preschoolers less able to cope with separation; as a result, they manifest many of the stage behaviors of separation anxiety, although in general the protest behaviors are more subtle and passive than those seen in younger children. Preschoolers may demonstrate separation anxiety by refusing to eat, experiencing difficulty in sleeping, crying quietly for their parents, continually asking when the parents will visit, or withdrawing from others. They may express anger indirectly by breaking their toys, hitting other children, or refusing to cooperate during usual self-care activities. Nurses need to be sensitive to these less obvious signs of separation anxiety in order to intervene appropriately.

Later Childhood and Adolescence

Previous research, usually based on adult recollections, indicated that the family does not play as important a role for school-age children as it does during the toddler and preschool years. However, in a recent study that asked children about their fears when hospitalized, children listed their greatest fears regarding hospitalization as being separated from family and friends, being in an unfamiliar environment, receiving investigations or treatments, and losing self-determination or choices (Coyne, 2006).

Although school-age children are better able to cope with separation in general, the stress and often accompanying regression imposed by illness or hospitalization may increase their need for parental security and guidance. This is particularly true for young school-age children who have only recently left the safety of the home and are struggling with the crisis of school adjustment. Middle and late school-age children may react more to the separation from their usual ac-

tivities and peers than to the absence of their parents. These children have a high level of physical and mental activity that frequently finds no suitable outlets in the hospital environment, and even when they dislike school, they admit to missing its routine and worry that they will not be able to compete or "fit in" with their classmates when they return. Feelings of loneliness, boredom, isolation, and depression are common. Such reactions may occur more as a result of separation than of concern over the illness, treatment, or hospital setting.

School-age children may need and desire parental guidance or support from other adult figures but may be unable or unwilling to ask for it. Because the goal of attaining independence is so important to them, they are reluctant to seek help directly, fearing that they will appear weak, childish, or dependent. Cultural expectations to "act like a man" or to "be brave and strong" weigh heavily on these children, especially boys, who tend to react to stress with stoicism, withdrawal, or passive acceptance. Often the need to express hostile, angry, or other negative feelings finds outlets in alternate ways, such as irritability and aggression toward parents, withdrawal from hospital personnel, inability to relate to peers, rejection of siblings, or subsequent behavioral problems in school.

For adolescents, separation from home and parents may produce varied emotions, ranging from difficulty coping to welcoming the event. However, loss of peer-group contact may pose a severe emotional threat because of loss of group status, inability to exert group control or leadership, and loss of group acceptance. Deviations within peer groups are poorly tolerated, and although group members may express concern for the adolescent's illness or need for hospitalization, they continue their group activities, quickly filling the gap of the absent member. During the temporary separation from their usual group, ill adolescents may benefit from group associations with other hospitalized teens.

LOSS OF CONTROL

One of the factors influencing the amount of stress imposed by hospitalization is the amount of control that persons perceive themselves as having. Lack of control increases the perception of threat and can affect children's coping skills. Many hospital situations decrease the amount of control a child feels. Although the usual sensory stimulations are lacking, the additional hospital stimuli of sight, sound, and smell may be overwhelming. Without an insight into the type of environment conducive to children's optimal growth, the hospital experience can at best temporarily slow development and at worst permanently restrict it. Because children's needs vary greatly depending on their age, the major areas of loss of control in terms of physical restriction, altered routine or rituals, and dependency are discussed for each age-group.

Infants

Infants are developing the most important attribute of a healthy personality—trust. Trust is established through consistent, loving care by a nurturing person. Infants attempt to control their environment through emotional expressions, such as crying or smiling. In the hospital setting, cues may be missed or misinterpreted, and routines may be established to meet the hospital staff's needs instead of the infant's needs. Inconsistent care and deviations from the infant's daily routine may lead to mistrust and a decreased sense of control.

Toddlers

Toddlers are striving for autonomy, and this goal is evident in most of their behaviors: motor skills, play, interpersonal relationships, activities of daily living, and communication. When their egocentric pleasures meet with obstacles, toddlers react with negativism, especially temper tantrums. Any restriction or limitation of movement, such as the simple act of making toddlers lie down, can cause forceful resistance and noncompliance.

Loss of control also results from altered routines and rituals. Toddlers rely on the consistency and familiarity of daily rituals to provide a measure of stability and control in their complex world of growing and developing. The experience of hospitalization or illness severely limits their sense of expectation and predictability, since practically every detail of the hospital environment differs from that of the home.

Toddlers' main areas for rituals include eating, sleeping, bathing, toileting, and play. When the routines are disrupted, difficulties can occur in any or all of these areas. The principal reaction to such change is regression. For example, when mealtime and food choices differ from those at home, toddlers often refuse to eat, demand a bottle, or ask others to feed them. Although regression to earlier forms of behavior may seem to increase toddlers' security and comfort, in reality it is threatening for them to relinquish their most recently acquired achievements.

Enforced dependency is a chief characteristic of the sick role and accounts for the numerous instances of toddler negativism. For example, rigid schedules, different clothes, altered caregiving activities, unfamiliar surroundings, separation from parents, and medical procedures usurp toddlers' control over their world. Although most toddlers initially react negatively and aggressively to such dependency, prolonged loss of autonomy may result in passive withdrawal from interpersonal relationships and regression in all areas of development. Therefore the effects of the sick role are most severe in instances of chronic, long-term illnesses or in those families who foster the sick role despite the child's improved state of health.

Preschoolers

Preschoolers also suffer from loss of control caused by physical restriction, altered routines, and enforced dependency. However, their specific cognitive abilities, which make them feel all-powerful, also make them feel out of control. This loss of control in the context of their sense of self-power is a critical influencing factor in their perception of and reaction to separation, pain, illness, and hospitalization.

Preschoolers' egocentric and magical thinking limits their ability to understand events because they view all experiences from their own self-referenced (egocentric) perspective. Without adequate preparation for unfamiliar settings or experiences, preschoolers' fantasy explanations for such events are usually more exaggerated, bizarre, and frightening than the facts. One typical fantasy to explain the illness or hospitalization is that it represents punishment for real or imagined misdeeds. In response to such thinking the child usually feels shame, guilt, and fear.

Preschoolers' preoperational thinking means that they understand explanations only in terms of real events. Purely verbal instructions are often inadequate for them because they are unable to abstract and synthesize beyond what their senses tell them. When combined with their egocentric and magical thinking, this characteristic may lead them to interpret messages according to their particular past experiences. Even with the best preparation for a procedure, they may misconstrue the details.

Transductive reasoning implies that preschoolers deduct from the particular to the particular, rather than from the specific to the general, or vice versa. For example, if preschoolers' concept of nurses is that they inflict pain, preschoolers will think that every nurse, or everyone wearing a similar uniform, will also inflict pain.

School-Age Children

Because of their striving for independence and productivity, school-age children are particularly vulnerable to events that may lessen their feeling of control and power. In particular, altered family roles; physical disability; fears of death, abandonment, or permanent injury; loss of peer acceptance; lack of productivity; and inability to cope with stress according to perceived cultural expectation may result in loss of control.

Because of the nature of the patient role, many routine hospital activities usurp individual power and identity. For school-age children, dependent activities such as enforced bed rest, use of a bedpan, inability to choose a menu, lack of privacy, help with a bed bath, or transport by a wheelchair or stretcher can be a direct threat to their security. Although all these procedures seem routine and inconsequential, they allow no freedom of choice to children who want to "act grown-up." However, when children are allowed to exert a measure of control, regardless of how limited it may be, they generally respond well to any procedure. For example, some of the most cooperative, satisfied, and contented patients are school-age children who help make their beds, choose their schedule of activities, and assist in their own care. An increased sense of control usually results from a feeling of usefulness and productivity.

In addition to the hospital environment, illness may also cause a feeling of loss of control. One of the most significant problems of children in this age-group is boredom. When physical or enforced limitations curtail their usual ability to care for themselves or to engage in favorite activities, school-age children generally respond with depression, hostility, or frustration. Keeping a normally active child on bed rest is difficult. However, emphasizing areas of control and capitalizing on quiet activities, particularly hobbies such as building models or playing age-appropriate video or board games, promotes their adjustment to physical restriction.

Adolescents

Adolescents' struggle for independence, self-assertion, and liberation centers on the quest for personal identity. Anything that interferes with this poses a threat to their sense of identity and results in a loss of control. Illness, which limits one's physical abilities, and hospitalization, which separates one from one's usual support systems, constitute major situational crises.

The patient role fosters dependency and depersonalization. Adolescents may react to dependency with rejection, uncooperativeness, or withdrawal. They may respond to depersonalization with self-assertion, anger, or frustration. Regardless of the response elicited, hospital personnel often regard them as difficult, unmanageable patients. Parents may not be a source of help because these behaviors serve to isolate them further from understanding the adolescent. Although peers may visit, they may not be able to offer the kind of support and guidance needed. Sick adolescents often voluntarily isolate themselves from age-mates until they feel they can compete on an equal basis and meet group expectations. As a result, ill adolescents may be left with virtually no support system.

Loss of control also occurs for many of the reasons discussed for school-age children. However, adolescents are more sensitive to potential instances of loss of control and dependency than are younger children. For example, both groups seek information about their physical status and rely heavily on anticipatory preparation to decrease fear and anxiety. However, adolescents react not only to the kinds of information supplied them, but also to the means by which it is conveyed. They may feel threatened by others who convey facts in a condescending manner. Adolescents want to know that others can relate to them on their own level. This necessitates a careful assessment of their intellectual abilities, previous knowledge, and present needs. It may also require the nurse's willingness to learn the adolescent's language.

EFFECTS OF HOSPITALIZATION ON THE CHILD

Children may react to the stresses of hospitalization before admission, during hospitalization, and after discharge. A child's concept of illness is even more important than age and intellectual maturity in predicting the level of anxiety before hospitalization (Clatworthy, Simon, and Tiedeman, 1999). This may or may not be affected by the duration of the condition or prior hospitalizations; therefore nurses should avoid overestimating the illness concepts of children with prior medical experience (Box 21-2).

Individual Risk Factors

A number of risk factors make certain children more vulnerable than others to the stresses of hospitalization (Box 21-3). Rural children may exhibit significantly greater degrees of psychologic upset than urban children, possibly because urban children have opportunities to become familiar with a local hospital. Because separation is such an important issue surrounding hospitalization for young children, children who are active and strong willed tend to fare better when hospitalized than youngsters who are passive. Consequently, nurses should be alert to children who passively accept all changes and requests; these children may need more support than the "oppositional" child.

The stressors of hospitalization may cause young children to experience short- and long-term negative outcomes. Adverse outcomes may be related to the length and number of admissions, multiple invasive procedures, and the parents' anxiety. Common responses include regression, separation anxiety, apathy, fears, and sleeping disturbances, especially for children younger than 7 years of age (Melnyk, 2000). Supportive practices, such as family-centered care and frequent family visiting, may lessen the detrimental effects of such admissions. Research also indicates that a child's pain experience determines how the overall hospitalization is experienced (Woodgate and Kristjanson, 1996). Consequently, nurses should attempt to identify children at risk for poor coping strategies (Small, 2002).

Changes in the Pediatric Population. The pediatric population in hospitals has changed dramatically over the past two decades. With a growing trend toward shortened

---

BOX 21-2

Posthospital Behaviors in Children

YOUNG CHILDREN

They show initial aloofness toward parents; this may last from a few minutes (most common) to a few days.

This is frequently followed by dependency behaviors:

- Tendency to cling to parents
- Demands for parents' attention
- Vigorous opposition to any separation (e.g., staying at preschool or with a baby-sitter)

Other negative behaviors include:

- New fears (e.g., nightmares)
- Resistance to going to bed, night waking
- Withdrawal and shyness
- Hyperactivity
- Temper tantrums
- Food finickiness
- Attachment to blanket or toy
- Regression in newly learned skills (e.g., self-toileting)

OLDER CHILDREN

Negative behaviors include:

- Emotional coldness, followed by intense, demanding dependence on parents
- Anger toward parents
- Jealousy toward others (e.g., siblings)

BOX 21-3

Risk Factors That Increase Children's Vulnerability to the Stresses of Hospitalization

- "Difficult" temperament
- Lack of fit between child and parent
- Age (especially between 6 months and 5 years)
- Male gender
- Below-average intelligence
- Multiple and continuing stresses (e.g., frequent hospitalizations)

---

hospital stays and outpatient surgery, a greater percentage of the children hospitalized today have more serious and complex problems than those hospitalized in the past. Many of these children are fragile newborns and children with severe injuries or disabilities who have survived because of major technologic advances, yet have been left with chronic or disabling conditions that require often frequent and lengthy hospital stays. The nature of their conditions increases the likelihood that they will experience more invasive and traumatic procedures while they are hospitalized. These factors make them more vulnerable to the emotional consequences of hospitalization and result in their needs being significantly different from those of the short-term patients of the past (see Chapter 18 for further discussion on children with special needs). The majority of these children are infants and toddlers, the age-group most vulnerable to the effects of hospitalization.

Concern in recent years has focused on the increasing length of hospitalization because of complex medical and nursing care, elusive diagnoses, and complicated psychosocial issues. Without special attention devoted to meeting the child's psychosocial and developmental needs in the hospital environment, the detrimental consequences of prolonged hospitalization may be severe.

Beneficial Effects of Hospitalization

Although hospitalization can be and usually is stressful for children, it can also be beneficial. The most obvious benefit is the recovery from illness, but hospitalization also can present an opportunity for children to master stress and feel competent in their coping abilities. The hospital environment can provide children with new socialization experiences that can broaden their interpersonal relationships. The psychologic benefits need to be considered and maximized during hospitalization. Appropriate nursing strategies to achieve this goal are presented on p. 668.

STRESSORS AND REACTIONS OF THE FAMILY OF THE CHILD WHO IS HOSPITALIZED

PARENTAL REACTIONS

The crisis of childhood illness and hospitalization affects every member of the family. Parents' reactions to illness in their child depend on a variety of factors. Although one cannot predict which factors are most likely to influence their response, a number of variables have been identified (Box 21-4). (See also Chapter 18.)

Recent research has identified common themes among parents whose children were hospitalized, including feeling an overall sense of helplessness, questioning the skills of staff, accepting the reality of hospitalization, needing to have information explained in simple language, dealing with fear, coping with uncertainty, and seeking reassurance from caregivers. This reassurance involves staff being compassionate, expressing concern for the child, and attending to detail in the child's care (Stranton, 2004).

SIBLING REACTIONS

Siblings' reactions to a sister's or brother's illness or hospitalization are discussed in Chapter 18 and differ little when a child becomes temporarily ill. Siblings experience loneliness, fear, and worry, as well as anger, resentment, jealousy, and guilt. Various factors have been identified that influence the effects of the child's hospitalization on siblings. Although these factors are similar to those seen when a child has a

chronic illness, Craft (1993) reported that the following factors regarding siblings are related specifically to the hospital experience and increase the effects on the sibling:

- Being younger and experiencing many changes
- Being cared for outside the home by care providers who are not relatives
- Receiving little information about their ill brother or sister
- Perceiving that their parents treat them differently compared with before their sibling's hospitalization

Parents are often unaware of the number of effects that siblings experience during the sick child's hospitalization and the benefit of simple interventions to minimize such effects, such as explicit explanations about the illness and provisions for the siblings to remain at home. Sibling visitation is usually beneficial to the patient, sibling, and parent but should be evaluated on an individual basis. Siblings should be prepared for the visit with developmentally appropriate information and be given the opportunity to ask questions.

ALTERED FAMILY ROLES

In addition to the effects of separation on family roles, loss of parenting, sibling, and offspring roles may affect each family member differently. One of the most common reactions of parents is specialized and intensified attention toward the sick child. The other siblings may regard this as unfair and interpret the parents' attitude toward them as rejection. Although such responses are usually unconscious and unintended, they place unique burdens on ill children. For example, the ill child may feel obligated to play the sick role to meet parents' expectations, especially those children who have had limited physical ability and regain normal health status, such as after corrective heart surgery. Parents may be unable to perceive the child's recovery and therefore continue the pattern of overprotection and indulgent attention.

Ill children may also feel jealousy and resentment from other siblings. Because of their singular position in the family, they may be denied the companionship of their brothers and sisters. Rivalry between siblings tends to be greatest for the sibling who is nearest in age to the ill child. Without an understanding of the interpersonal dynamics between siblings, parents are likely to blame the well children for antisocial behavior. Illness may also result in children's loss of status within either their family or social group. For example, illness in the oldest child may temporarily terminate special privileges as "big" brother or sister.

NURSING CARE OF THE CHILD WHO IS HOSPITALIZED

PREPARATION FOR HOSPITALIZATION

Children and families require individualized care to minimize the potential negative effects of hospitalization. One method that can decrease negative feelings and fear in children is preparation for hospitalization. The rationale for preparing children for the hospital experience and related procedures is based on the principle that fear of the unknown (fantasy) exceeds fear of the known. When children do not have paralyzing fear to cope with, they are able to direct their energies toward dealing with the other, unavoidable stresses of hospitalization.

Although preparation for hospitalization is a common practice, there is no universal standard or program for all

---

BOX 21-4
Factors Affecting Parents' Reactions to Their Child's Illness
■ Seriousness of the threat to the child
■ Previous experience with illness or hospitalization
■ Medical procedures involved in diagnosis and treatment
■ Available support systems
■ Personal ego strengths
■ Previous coping abilities
■ Additional stresses on the family system
■ Cultural and religious beliefs
■ Communication patterns among family members

settings. The preparation process may be elaborate with tours, puppet shows, and playtime with miniature hospital equipment; it may involve the use of books, videos, or films; or it may be limited to a brief description of the major aspects of any hospital stay (Stewart, Algren, and Arnold, 1994). No consensus exists on the timing of preparation. Some authorities recommend preparing children 4 to 7 years of age about 1 week in advance so that they can assimilate the information and ask questions. For older children the time may be longer. However, for young children, who may begin to fantasize about what they observed, 1 or 2 days before admission is sufficient time for anticipatory preparation. The length of the session should be tailored to the children's attention span—the younger the child, the shorter the program. The optimal approach is one that is individualized for each child and family.

Regardless of the specific type of program, all children, even those who have been hospitalized before, benefit from an introduction to the environment and routine of the unit. Sometimes it is not possible to prepare children and families for hospitalization, such as in the event of sudden, acute illness. However, care should be taken to orient the child and family to hospital routines, establish expectations, and allow for questions.

> ### FYI
>
> In many hospitals, child life specialists—health care professionals with extensive knowledge of child growth and development and of the special psychosocial needs of children who are hospitalized and their families—help prepare children for hospitalization, surgery, and procedures. A collaborative effort between the nurse, child life specialist, and other members of the child's health care team helps ensure the best possible hospital experience for the child and family.

Admission Assessment

The nursing admission history refers to a systematic collection of data about the child and family that allows the nurse to plan individualized care. The nursing admission history presented in Box 21-5 is organized according to the Functional Health Patterns outlined by Gordon (1994, 2002) (see Nursing Diagnosis, Chapter 1). This assessment framework is a guideline for formulating nursing diagnoses. One of the main purposes of the history is to assess the child's usual health habits at home to promote a more normal environment in the hospital. Therefore questions related to activities of daily living in the nutritional-metabolic, elimination, sleep-rest, and activity-exercise patterns are a major part of the assessment. The questions found under the health perception–health management pattern are directed toward evaluation of the child's preparation for hospitalization and are key factors in determining whether additional preparation is needed. The questions included in the self-perception–self-concept and role-relationship patterns offer insight into the child's potential reaction to hospitalization, especially in terms of separation.

The nurse should also inquire about the use of any medications at home, including complementary medicine practices (Box 21-6). In a study of children with cancer, 42% had used alternative or complementary therapies simultaneously with or after conventional treatments (Fernandez, Pyesmany, and Stutzer, 1999). It is important that the use of any herbal or complementary therapy be noted in a preoperative assessment because of possible anesthesia or surgical complications re-

lated to herbal products (Flanagan, 2001) (see Critical Thinking Exercise).

After collecting the admission data, the nurse must apply the information to the nursing process and communicate it to other staff. Information gathered in the nursing admission assessment can offer insight into family dynamics, assist in normalization of the hospital environment, and aid staff members in meeting the child's and family's needs. Asking questions and seeking information directly from the child in an age-appropriate manner can yield a wealth of information regarding understanding of their illness and hospitalization.

Besides completing the nursing admission history, nurses should also perform a physical assessment (see Chapter 6) before planning care. At the very least, the nurse's physical assessment of the child should include observation of the body for any bruises, rashes, signs of neglect, deformities, or physical limitations. The nurse should also listen to the heart and lungs to assess overall physical status. For example, it is impossible to evaluate improvement in respiratory function in a child admitted with pulmonary disease unless there are baseline data with which to compare subsequent findings.

Preparing Child for Admission

The preparation that children require on the day of admission depends on the kind of prehospital counseling they have received. If they have been prepared in a formalized program, they will usually know what to expect in terms of initial medical procedures, inpatient facilities, and nursing staff. However, prehospital counseling does not preclude the need for support during procedures such as obtaining blood specimens, x-ray tests, or physical examination. For example, undressing young

> ### ??? CRITICAL THINKING EXERCISE
>
> #### Complementary and Alternative Medicine
>
> Maria, a 10-year-old Hispanic girl, has had severe nosebleeds. She is admitted to the hospital for a complete workup in an attempt to determine the cause. Her parents and grandparents have gathered around her bed. When you enter her room to begin admitting procedures, you notice an unusual scent. Maria's mother is rubbing the contents from an unfamiliar bottle of liquid on Maria. Meanwhile, the grandmother is rubbing Maria's head. She is startled at your entry and drops something on the floor near your feet. You bend over to pick it up and discover that it is a penny.
>
> #### QUESTIONS
> 1. Evidence—Is there sufficient evidence to draw any conclusions?
> 2. Assumptions—What are some underlying assumptions that may be drawn from the data about the following:
>   a. Complementary or alternative medical remedies
>   b. The role of ethnic or folk remedies in modern health care practice
>   c. The nurse's role in cases where alternative medicine is practiced (vs traditional medicine)
> 3. What implications and priorities for nursing care can be drawn at this time?
> 4. Does the evidence objectively support your argument (conclusion)?
> 5. Are there alternative perspectives to your arguments? If so, what are they?

BOX 21-5

Nursing Admission History According to Functional Health Patterns*

HEALTH PERCEPTION–HEALTH MANAGEMENT PATTERN

Why has your child been admitted?

How has your child's general health been?

What does your child know about this hospitalization?

- Ask the child why he or she came to the hospital.
- If the answer is "For an operation or for tests," ask the child to tell you about what will happen before, during, and after the operation or tests.

Has your child ever been in the hospital before?

- How was that hospital experience?
- What things were important to you and your child during that hospitalization? How can we be most helpful now?

What medications does your child take at home?

- Why are they given?
- When are they given?
- How are they given (if a liquid, with a spoon; if a tablet, swallowed with water; or other)?
- Does your child have any trouble taking medication? If so, what helps?
- Is your child allergic to any medications?

What, if any, forms of complementary medicine practices are being used?

NUTRITION-METABOLIC PATTERN

What are the family's usual mealtimes?

Do family members eat together or at separate times?

What are your child's favorite foods, beverages, and snacks?

- Average amounts consumed or usual size of portions
- Special cultural practices, such as family eats only ethnic food

What foods and beverages does your child dislike?

What are your child's feeding habits (bottle, cup, spoon, eats by self, needs assistance, any special devices)?

How does your child like the food served (warmed, cold, one item at a time)?

How would you describe your child's usual appetite (hearty eater, picky eater)?

- Has being sick affected your child's appetite? In what ways?

Are there any known or suspected food allergies?

Is your child on a special diet?

Are there any feeding problems (excessive fussiness, spitting up, colic); any dental or gum problems that affect feeding?

- What do you do for these problems?

ELIMINATION PATTERN

What are your child's toilet habits (diaper, toilet trained—day only or day and night, use of word to communicate urination or defecation, potty chair, regular toilet, other routines)?

What is your child's usual pattern of elimination (bowel movements)?

Do you have any concerns about elimination (bed-wetting, constipation, diarrhea)?

- What do you do for these problems?

Have you ever noticed that your child sweats a lot?

SLEEP-REST PATTERN

What is your child's usual hour of sleep and awakening?

What is your child's schedule for naps; length of naps?

Is there a special routine before sleeping (bottle, drink of water, bedtime story, night-light, favorite blanket or toy, prayers)?

Is there a special routine during sleep time, such as waking to go to the bathroom?

What type of bed does your child sleep in?

Does your child have a separate room or share a room; if shares, with whom?

Does your child sleep with someone or alone (e.g., sibling, parent, other person)?

What is your child's favorite sleeping position?

Are there any sleeping problems (falling asleep, waking during night, nightmares, sleep walking)?

Are there any problems in awakening and getting ready in the morning?

- What do you do for these problems?

ACTIVITY-EXERCISE PATTERN

What is your child's schedule during the day (preschool, daycare center, regular school, extracurricular activities)?

What are your child's favorite activities or toys (both active and quiet interests)?

What is your child's usual television-viewing schedule at home?

What are your child's favorite programs?

Are there any television restrictions?

Does your child have any illness or disabilities that limit activity? If so, how?

What are your child's usual habits and schedule for bathing (bath in tub or shower, sponge bath, shampoo)?

What are your child's dental habits (brushing, flossing, fluoride supplements or rinses, favorite toothpaste); schedule of daily dental care?

Does your child need help with dressing or grooming, such as hair combing?

Are there any problems with these patterns (dislike of or refusal to bathe, shampoo hair, or brush teeth)?

- What do you do for these problems?

Are there special devices that your child requires help in managing (eyeglasses, contact lenses, hearing aid, orthodontic appliances, artificial elimination appliances, orthopedic devices)?

NOTE: Use the following code to assess functional self-care level for feeding, bathing/hygiene, dressing/grooming, toileting:

- 0—Full self-care
- I—Requires use of equipment or device
- II—Requires assistance or supervision from another person
- III—Requires assistance or supervision from another person and equipment or device
- IV—Is totally dependent and does not participate

COGNITIVE-PERCEPTUAL PATTERN

Does your child have any hearing difficulty?

- Does the child use a hearing aid?
- Have "tubes" been placed in your child's ears?

Does your child have any vision problems?

- Does the child wear glasses or contact lenses?

Does your child have any learning difficulties?

What is the child's grade in school?

For information on pain, see Chapter 7.

SELF-PERCEPTION–SELF-CONCEPT PATTERN

How would you describe your child (e.g., takes time to adjust, settles in easily, shy, friendly, quiet, talkative, serious, playful, stubborn, easygoing)?

What makes your child angry, annoyed, anxious, or sad? What helps?

How does your child act when annoyed or upset?

*The focus of the admission history is the child's psychosocial environment. Most of the questions are worded in terms of parental responses. Depending on the child's age, they should be addressed directly to the child when appropriate.

BOX 21-5

Nursing Admission History According to Functional Health Patterns—cont'd

SELF-PERCEPTION–SELF-CONCEPT PATTERN—cont'd

What have been your child's experiences with and reactions to temporary separation from you (parent)?

Does your child have any fears (places, objects, animals, people, situations)?

■ How do you handle them?

Do you think your child's illness has changed the way he or she thinks about self (e.g., more shy, embarrassed about appearance, less competitive with friends, stays at home more)?

ROLE-RELATIONSHIP PATTERN

Does your child have a favorite nickname?

What are the names of other family members or others who live in the home (relatives, friends, pets)?

Who usually takes care of your child during the day/night (especially if other than parent, such as baby-sitter, relative)?

What are the parents' occupations and work schedules?

Are there any special family considerations (adoption, foster child, stepparent, divorce, single parent)?

Have any major changes in the family occurred lately (death, divorce, separation, birth of a sibling, loss of a job, financial strain, mother beginning a career, other)? Describe child's reaction.

Who are your child's play companions or social groups (peers, younger or older children, adults, prefers to be alone)?

Do things generally go well for your child in school or with friends?

Does your child have "security" objects at home (pacifier, bottle, blanket, stuffed animal or doll)? Did you bring any of these to the hospital?

How do you handle discipline problems at home? Are these methods always effective?

Does your child have any condition that interferes with communication? If so, what are your suggestions for communicating with your child?

Will your child's hospitalization affect the family's financial support or care of other family members (e.g., other children)?

What concerns do you have about your child's illness and hospitalization?

Who will be staying with your child while hospitalized?

How can we contact you or another close family member outside of the hospital?

SEXUALITY-REPRODUCTIVE PATTERN

(Answer questions that apply to your child's age-group.)

Has your child begun puberty (developing physical sexual characteristics, menstruation)? Have you or your child had any concerns?

Does your daughter know how to do breast self-examination?

Does your son know how to do testicular self-examination?

How have you approached topics of sexuality with your child?

Do you think you might need some help with some topics?

Has your child's illness affected the way he or she feels about being a boy or a girl? If so, how?

Do you have any concerns with behaviors in your child, such as masturbation, asking many questions or talking about sex, not respecting others' privacy, or wanting too much privacy?

Initiate a conversation about an adolescent's sexual concerns with open-ended to more direct questions and using the terms "friends" or "partners" rather than "girlfriend" or "boyfriend":

■ Tell me about your social life.

■ Who are your closest friends? (If one friend is identified, could ask more about that relationship, such as how much time they spend together, how serious they are about each other, if the relationship is going the way the teenager hoped.)

■ Might ask about dating and sexual issues, such as the teenager's views on sexuality education, "going steady," "living together," or premarital sex.

■ Which friends would you like to have visit in the hospital?

COPING-STRESS TOLERANCE PATTERN

(Answer questions that apply to your child's age-group.)

What does your child do when tired or upset?

■ If upset, does your child want a special person or object?

■ If so, explain.

If your child has temper tantrums, what causes them and how do you handle them?

Whom does your child talk to when worried about something?

How does your child usually handle problems or disappointments?

Have there been any big changes or problems in your family recently? If so, how have you handled them?

Has your child ever had a problem with drugs or alcohol or tried to commit suicide?

Do you think your child is "accident prone"? If so, explain.

VALUE-BELIEF PATTERN

What is your religion?

How is religion or faith important in your child's life?

What religious practices would you like continued in the hospital (e.g., prayers before meals or bedtime; visit by minister, priest, or rabbi; prayer group)?

BOX 21-6

Complementary Medicine Practices and Examples

Nutrition, diet, and lifestyle or behavioral health changes—Macrobiotics, megavitamins, diets, lifestyle modification, health risk reduction and health education, wellness

Mind-body control therapies—Biofeedback, relaxation, prayer therapy, guided imagery, hypnotherapy, music or sound therapy, massage, aromatherapy, education therapy

Traditional and ethnomedicine therapies—Acupuncture, ayurvedic medicine, herbal medicine, homeopathic medicine, Native American medicine, natural products, traditional Asian medicine

Structural manipulation and energetic therapies—Acupressure, chiropractic medicine, massage, reflexology, rolfing, therapeutic touch, Qi Gong

Pharmacologic and biologic therapies—Antioxidants, cell treatment, chelation therapy, metabolic therapy, oxidizing agents

Bioelectromagnetic therapies—Diagnostic and therapeutic application of electromagnetic fields (e.g., transcranial electrostimulation, neuromagnetic stimulation, electroacupuncture)

FIG. 21-4 ■ The initial admission procedures give the nurse an opportunity to get to know the child and to assess the child's understanding of the hospital experience.

Guidelines for Admission

PREADMISSION

Assign a room based on developmental age, seriousness of diagnosis, communicability of illness, and projected length of stay.

Prepare roommate(s) for the arrival of a new patient; when children are too young to benefit from this consideration, prepare parents.

Prepare room for child and family, with admission forms and equipment nearby to eliminate need to leave child.

ADMISSION

Introduce primary nurse to child and family.

Orient child and family to inpatient facilities, especially to assigned room and unit; emphasize positive areas of pediatric unit.
  Room—Explain call light, bed controls, television, bathroom, telephone, etc.
  Unit—Direct to playroom, desk, dining area, or other areas.

Introduce family to roommate and his or her parents.

Apply identification band to child's wrist, ankle, or both (if not already done).

Explain hospital regulations and schedules (e.g., visiting hours, mealtimes, bedtime, limitations [give written information if available]).

Perform nursing admission history (see Box 21-5).

Take vital signs, blood pressure, height, and weight.

Obtain specimens as needed and order needed laboratory work.

Support child and assist practitioner with physical examination (for purposes of nursing assessment).

children before they feel comfortable in their new surroundings can be upsetting. Causing needless anxiety and fear during admission may adversely affect the nurse's establishment of trust with these children. Therefore nursing assistance during the admission procedure is vital, regardless of how well prepared any child is for the experience of hospitalization. In addition, spending this time with the child gives the nurse an opportunity to evaluate the child's understanding of subsequent procedures (Fig. 21-4). Ideally, a primary nurse is assigned whenever possible to allow for individualized care and to provide a substitute support person for the child.

When a child is admitted, nurses follow several fairly universal admission procedures (Box 21-7). One particularly important decision is room assignment. The minimum considerations for room assignment are age, sex, and nature of the illness. No absolute rules govern room selection, but in general, placing children of the same age-group and with similar types of illness in the same room is both psychologically and medically advantageous. However, there are many exceptions. For example, a child in traction may be therapeutic for another child confined to bed because of a serious illness. A child who is independent despite physical disabilities may help another child with similar or different limitations, and the parents of the child with disabilities may achieve deeper insight and acceptance of their child's disorder.

Age-grouping is especially important for adolescents. Many hospitals make an effort to place teenagers on their own unit or in a separate, designated section of the pediatric or general unit whenever possible.

NURSING INTERVENTIONS
Preventing or Minimizing Separation

A primary nursing goal is to prevent separation, particularly in children younger than 5 years of age. Changes in hospitals' policies over recent years reflect a changed attitude toward parents; many hospitals no longer consider parents "visitors" and welcome their presence at all times throughout the child's hospitalization. Many hospitals have developed a system of **family-centered care.** This philosophy of care recognizes the integral role of the family in a child's life and acknowledges the family as an essential part of the child's care and illness experience. The family is considered to be partners in the care of the child (Smith and Conant Rees, 2000) (see Chapter 1). Family-centered care also supports the family by establishing priorities based on the needs and values of the family unit (Lewandowski and Tesler, 2003).

At the very least, most hospitals welcome parents at any time. Many provide facilities such as a chair or bed for at least one person per child, unit kitchen privileges, and other amenities that create a welcoming atmosphere for parents. However, not all hospitals provide such amenities, and parents' own schedules may prevent rooming-in (see Ethical Case Study). In such instances, strategies to minimize the effects of separation must be implemented.

Nurses must have an appreciation of the child's separation behaviors. As discussed earlier, the phases of protest and despair are normal. The child is allowed to cry. Even if the child rejects strangers, the nurse provides support through physical presence. **Presence** is defined as spending time being physi-

ETHICAL CASE STUDY | Maternal Absence During Infant Hospitalization

ETHICAL DECISION MAKING MODEL	Carrie is a 3-month-old infant who has been admitted to the hospital for bronchiolitis and respiratory syncytial virus (RSV). She also is diagnosed with failure to thrive. Carrie's mother is 18 years of age and has a history of substance abuse. On arrival at the hospital, Carrie's mother informs the nurse that she cannot stay with Carrie because she has to go to work. She leaves shortly after the nurse completes the admission history and has not returned to the hospital for 2 days. No other family members are listed in the chart, and no one has visited Carrie since her mother left.
Evaluate the Issue	The first priority is Carrie's recovery from bronchiolitis and RSV. The hospital policies for supervision of a young infant without family presence should be followed. Social services should be involved, and an investigation of the mother should occur before Carrie's discharge. A review of any past hospital or emergency department visits could be helpful in trying to locate a family member and obtain additional information on Carrie's health.
Treat All Involved with Respect	It is difficult for nursing staff not to judge a mother who has left her young child in a hospital for 2 days without visiting. Nurses who realize the difficulties facing this mother with a history of substance abuse can provide support and serve as resources for helping the mother receive care and improve parenting skills.
Hear All Sides	Assumptions are easily made in this case because the mother is young and has a history of substance abuse. It is important for the nursing staff to remember to be objective during the investigation of the mother and to provide professional support for needed referrals for counseling and guidance.
Initiate Action	Carrie's situation warrants immediate action to begin plans for her care outside the hospital. If the mother cannot be found, social services must begin working with outside resources to place Carrie in a foster home. While investigation of Carrie's mother continues, comfort and support for Carrie should be provided by child life specialists, volunteers, and the nursing staff.
Consider the Outcome	There are a number of outcomes to consider that could positively affect Carrie's well-being. One is that the mother would receive the appropriate counseling needed to cope with her problems without depending on substances or drugs that could affect her and her daughter. If the mother demonstrates the capacity to adequately care for Carrie at home, it would be best for the child to remain in the home setting with her mother. Carrie's failure to thrive must be adequately addressed before such actions take place. The second scenario would entail Carrie recovering from the bronchiolitis and RSV and going into a temporary foster home while her mother receives appropriate assistance for substance abuse. Carrie needs a constant, stable primary caretaker and home environment to be able to grow and develop appropriately. The issue of her failure to thrive must be investigated to ensure that organic problems are not contributing factors. If the lack of an appropriate and consistent home environment is the cause of her failure to thrive, this must be addressed by the nursing staff and social services.

cally close to the child while using a quiet tone of voice, appropriate choice of words, eye contact, and touch in ways that establish rapport and communicate empathy. If behaviors of detachment are evident, the nurse maintains the child's contact with the parents by frequently talking about them; encouraging the child to remember them; and stressing the significance of their visits, telephone calls, or letters. The use of cellular phones can increase the contact between the hospitalized child and parents or other significant family members and friends. However, many cell phone signals are not compatible with medical equipment, and use may be restricted in certain areas within the hospital.

Separation may be equally difficult for parents, especially when they do not understand the behaviors of separation anxiety. To avoid the immediate protest, parents may sneak out or lie to the child about leaving. As a result, instead of learning that absence is associated with a guaranteed return, the child learns that absence means loss of parents. Helping parents recognize that separation behaviors are normal and expected can decrease the parents' anxiety and may ease

their fears about leaving their child. Explaining to parents how the child reacts after they leave may also be helpful. Many parents imagine that the child cries for hours after they leave, whereas in reality the child may cry for a few minutes but settle down when comforted by someone else.

Toddlers and preschoolers have a limited concept of time. Time is measured in associations, such as eating dinner "when Daddy comes home." Therefore, when helping parents with children's fears of separation, nurses need to suggest ways of explaining leaving and returning. For example, if parents must leave to go to work or to make meals for the other family members, they should tell the child the reason for leaving. They also need to convey the expected time of return in terms of anticipated events. For example, if the parents will return in the morning, they can say to the child, "We'll see you after the sun comes up" or "We'll come back when [a favorite program] is on television."

The young child's ability to tolerate parental absence is limited. Therefore parental visits should be frequent (e.g., visiting three times a day for short periods rather than once a

FIG. 21-5 ■ When parents cannot visit, other significant persons can provide comfort to the hospitalized child.

FIG. 21-6 ■ For extended hospitalizations children enjoy having projects with other patients to occupy time.

day for an extended time). This may necessitate that each parent visit at different times to lessen the length of separation. When parents cannot visit, the presence of other significant people can be most comforting for the child (Fig. 21-5).

If parents leave after the child is asleep, they still need to communicate their absence. The parents of a 5-year-old boy solved this problem by devising a sign; on one side they drew a picture of a telephone, and on the other they drew a hamburger. Before they left, they turned the sign to the appropriate side to tell the child when he awoke that they were out using the telephone or eating.

Older children who know how to tell time may find it helpful to have a clock or watch. However, these children have the same need for honesty from their parents regarding visiting schedules. Because their peer groups are important, adolescents often appreciate planning visiting hours with their parents to ensure that the patient has some private time for friends.

Familiar surroundings also increase the child's adjustment to separation. If parents cannot stay with the child, they should leave favorite articles from home with the child, such as a blanket, toy, bottle, feeding utensil, or article of clothing. Because young children associate such inanimate objects with significant people, they gain comfort and reassurance from these possessions. They make the association that if the parents left this, the parents will surely return. Placing an identification band on the toy lessens the chances of its being misplaced and provides a symbol that the toy is experiencing the same needs as the child. Other mementos of home include photographs and audiotape or videocassette recordings of family members reading a story, singing a song, saying prayers before bedtime, relating events at home, or taking a "talking walk" through the home. The tapes can be played at lonely times, such as on awakening or before sleeping. Some units allow pets to visit, which can have therapeutic benefits

for a child. Animals should be carefully screened for medical or behavioral problems, and patients should be screened for allergies.

Older children also appreciate familiar articles from home, particularly photographs, a radio, a favorite toy or game, and their own pajamas. Often the importance of treasured objects to school-age children is overlooked or criticized. However, many school-age children have a special object to which they formed an attachment in early childhood. Therefore such treasured or transitional objects can help even older children feel more comfortable in a strange environment.

The strange sights, smells, and sounds in the hospital that are commonplace for the nurse can be frightening and confusing for children. It is important for the nurse to try to evaluate stimuli in the environment from the child's point of view (considering also what the child may see or hear happening to other patients) and to make every effort to protect the child from frightening and unfamiliar sights, sounds, and equipment. The nurse should offer explanations or prepare the child for those experiences that are unavoidable. Combining familiar or comforting sights with the unfamiliar can relieve much of the harshness of medical equipment.

Helping children maintain their usual contacts also minimizes the effects of separation imposed by hospitalization. This includes continuing school lessons during the illness and confinement, visiting with friends either directly or through letter writing or telephone calls, and participating in stimulating projects whenever possible (Fig. 21-6). For extended hospitalizations, youngsters enjoy personalizing the hospital room to make it "home" by decorating the walls with posters and cards, rearranging the furniture (when possible), and displaying a collection or hobby.

Minimizing Loss of Control

Feelings of loss of control result from separation, physical restriction, changed routines, enforced dependency, and magical thinking. Although some of these cannot be prevented, most can be minimized through individualized planning of nursing care.

Promoting Freedom of Movement. Younger children react most strenuously to any type of physical restriction or immobilization. Although temporary immobilization may be necessary for some interventions such as maintaining an intravenous line, most physical restriction can be prevented if the nurse gains the child's cooperation.

For young children, particularly infants and toddlers, preserving parent-child contact is the best means of decreasing the need for or stress of restraint. For example, almost the entire physical examination can be done in a parent's lap, with the parent hugging the child for procedures such as otoscopy. For painful procedures, the nurse should assess the parents' preferences for assisting, observing, or waiting outside the room.

Environmental factors may also restrict movement. Keeping children in cribs or playpens may not represent immobilization in a concrete sense, but it certainly limits sensory stimulation. Increasing mobility by transporting children in carriages, wheelchairs, carts, or wagons provides them with a sense of freedom.

In some cases, physical restraint or isolation is necessary due to the child's medical diagnosis. In these cases, the environment can be altered to increase sensory freedom (e.g., moving the bed toward the window; opening window shades; providing musical, visual, or tactile activities).

Maintaining Child's Routine. Altered daily schedules and loss of rituals are particularly stressful for toddlers and early preschoolers and may increase the stress of separation. The nursing admission history provides a baseline for planning care around the child's usual home activities. A frequently neglected aspect of altered routines is the change in the child's daily activities. A nonhospitalized child's day, especially during the school years, is structured with specific times for eating, dressing, going to school, playing, and sleeping. However, this time structure vanishes when the child is hospitalized. Although nurses have a set schedule, the child is frequently unaware of it, and the new schedules that are imposed may be rigid. For example, some units have uniform nap times and bedtimes for all children, whereas others allow children to stay up late at night. Many children obtain significantly less sleep in the hospital than at home; the primary causes are delay in sleep onset and early termination of sleep because of hospital routines. Not only are hours of sleep disrupted, but waking hours are spent in passive activities. For example, few institutions impose any limits on the amount of time the child spends watching television. This may lead to the child being less "tired" at bedtime and delay the onset of sleep.

One technique that can minimize the disruption in the child's routine is establishing a daily schedule. This approach is most suitable for the non–critically ill school-age or adolescent child who has mastered the concept of time. It involves scheduling the child's day to include all those activities that are important to the child and nurse, such as treatment procedures, schoolwork, exercise, television, playroom, and hobbies. Together, the nurse, parent, and child then plan a daily schedule with times and activities written down (Fig. 21-7). This is left in the child's room, and a clock or watch is available for the child's use. Whenever possible, a calendar is also constructed with special events marked, such as favorite television programs, visits by friends or relatives, events in the playroom, and holidays or birthdays. If specific changes in treatment are

Eric's Daily Schedule			
7:30 AM	– Breakfast, morning bath	3:00 PM	– Tutor (M, W, F) – Study time (T, Th)
9:00	– Medications, – dressing change	4:00	– Physical therapy
		5:30	– Dinner
11:00	– Physical therapy	9:00	– Medications, dressing change
12:00 PM	– Lunch	9:15	– Bedtime

FIG. 21-7 ■ Time structuring is an effective strategy for normalizing the hospital environment and increasing the child's sense of control.

expected (e.g., "beginning physical therapy in 2 days"), these are added.

Ask the young child to select or draw pictures or symbols to represent daily or weekly fun activities (e.g., favorite television programs, family visits, playroom times). Draw a clock face with the hands of the clock depicting the time each event will occur next to the child's representation. Have the child compare the clock on the schedule with a clock or watch in the room. When the two match, the child knows it is time for a favorite activity.

Encouraging Independence. The dependent role of the hospitalized patient imposes tremendous feelings of loss on older children. Principal interventions should focus on respect for individuality and the opportunity for decision making. Although these sound simple, their efficacy lies with nurses who are flexible and tolerant. It is also important for the nurse to empower the patient while not feeling threatened by a sense of lessened control.

Enabling children's control involves helping them maintain independence and promoting the concept of self-care. **Self-care** refers to the practice of activities that individuals personally initiate and perform on their own behalf in maintaining life, health, and well-being (Orem, 2001). Although self-care is limited by the child's age and physical condition, most children beyond infancy can perform some activities with little or no help. Whenever possible, these activities are encouraged in the hospital. Other approaches include jointly planning care, time structuring, wearing street clothes, making choices in food selections and bedtime, continuing school activities, and rooming with an appropriate age-mate.

Promoting Understanding. Loss of control can occur from feelings of having too little influence on one's destiny or from sensing overwhelming control or power over fate. Although preschoolers' cognitive abilities predispose them most to magical thinking and delusions of power, all children are vulnerable to misinterpreting causes for stresses such as illness and hospitalization.

Most children feel more in control when they know what to expect, since the element of fear is reduced. Anticipatory preparation and provision of information help to lessen stress and increase understanding (see Preparation for Diagnostic and Therapeutic Procedures, Chapter 22).

Informing children of their rights while hospitalized fosters greater understanding and may relieve some of the feel-

BOX 21-8

Bill of Rights for Children and Teens

In this hospital you and your family have the right to:

- Respect and personal dignity
- Care that supports you and your family
- Information you can understand
- Quality health care
- Emotional support
- Care that respects your need to grow, play, and learn
- Make choices and decisions

From Association for the Care of Children's Health: *A pediatric bill of rights*, Bethesda, Md, 1991, The Association.

ings of powerlessness they typically experience. Hospitals providing services to children should have a hospital-wide policy on the rights and responsibilities of these patients and of their parents or guardians (The Joint Commission, 2004). An increasing number of hospitals and organizations have developed a patient "bill of rights" that is prominently displayed throughout the hospital or is presented to children and their families on admission (Box 21-8).

Preventing or Minimizing Fear of Bodily Injury

Beyond early infancy all children fear bodily injury from mutilation, bodily intrusion, body-image change, disability, or death. In general, preparation of children for painful procedures decreases their fears and increases cooperation. Manipulating procedural techniques for children in each age-group also minimizes fear of bodily injury. For example, because toddlers and young preschoolers are traumatized by insertion of a rectal thermometer, axillary temperatures or temperatures taken with electronic or tympanic membrane devices can effectively be substituted. Whenever procedures are performed on young children, the most supportive intervention is to do the procedure as quickly as possible while maintaining parent-child contact.

Because of toddler and preschool children's poorly defined body boundaries, the use of bandages may be particularly helpful. For example, telling children that the bleeding will stop after the needle is removed does little to relieve their fears, whereas applying a small Band-Aid usually reassures them. The size of bandages is also significant to children in this age-group; the larger the bandage, the more importance is attached to the wound. Watching their surgical dressings become successively smaller is one way young children can measure healing and improvement. Prematurely removing a dressing may cause these children considerable concern for their well-being. Specific pain management strategies are discussed in Chapter 7.

For children who fear mutilation of body parts, it is essential that the nurse repeatedly stress the reason for a procedure and evaluate the child's understanding. For example, explaining cast removal to preschoolers may seem simple enough, but children's comprehension of the details may vary considerably from the explanation. Asking them to draw a picture of what they think will happen presents substantial evidence of how they perceive events.

Children may fear bodily injury from a great variety of sources. Imaging machines, strange equipment used for ex-

amination, unfamiliar rooms, or awkward positions can be perceived as potentially hazardous. In addition, thoughts and actions can be imagined sources of bodily damage. Therefore it is important to investigate imagined reasons, particularly of a sexual nature, for illness. Because children may fear revealing such thoughts, using techniques such as drawing or doll play may elicit previously undisclosed misconceptions.

Older children fear bodily injury of both internal and external origins. For example, school-age children are aware of the significance of the heart and may fear the actual operation as much as the pain, the stitches, and the possible scar. Adolescents may express concern about the actual procedure but be much more anxious over the resulting scar.

Children can grasp information only if it is presented on or close to their level of cognitive development. This necessitates an awareness of the words used to describe events or processes. For example, young children told that they are going to have a CAT (i.e., CT, computed tomography) scan may wonder, "Will there be cats? Or something that scratches?" It is clearer to describe the procedure in simple terms and explain what the letters of the common name stand for. Therefore, to prevent or alleviate fears, nurses must be keenly aware of the medical terminology and vocabulary that they use every day.

When children are upset about their illness, their perception can be changed by (1) providing a somewhat different and less negative account of the disease or (2) offering an explanation that is characteristic of the next stage of cognitive development. An example of the first strategy is reassuring a preschooler who fears that after a tonsillectomy, another sore throat means a second operation. Explaining that after tonsils are "fixed" they do not need fixing again can help relieve the fear. An example of the latter strategy is to explain that germs made the tonsils sick and even though germs can cause another sore throat, they cannot cause the tonsils to ever be sick again. This higher-level explanation is based on the school-age child's concept of germs as a cause of disease.

Providing Developmentally Appropriate Activities

A primary goal of nursing care for the child who is hospitalized is to minimize threats to the child's development. Many strategies (e.g., minimizing separation) have been discussed and may be all that the short-term patient requires. However, children who experience prolonged or repeated hospitalization are at greater risk for developmental delays or regression. The nurse who provides opportunities for the child to participate in developmentally appropriate activities further normalizes the child's environment and helps reduce interference with the child's ongoing development (see Normalization, Chapter 18).

Interference with normal development may have long-term implications for the developing infant and toddler. The nurse plays a primary role in identifying children at risk and helping to plan, implement, and evaluate developmental intervention (see Chapters 10 and 12).

School is an integral part of the school-age child's and adolescent's development. Accreditation standards for hospitals serving children consider access to appropriate educational services a key factor in the accreditation decision process when a child's treatment requires a significant absence from school (The Joint Commission, 2004). The nurse can encourage children to resume schoolwork as quickly as their condition permits, help them schedule and protect a selected time for studies, and help the family coordinate hospital educational services with their children's schools. Children should have the opportunity to continue art and music classes, as well as their academic subjects.

To meet the unique developmental needs of adolescents, special units may be developed that provide privacy, increased socialization, and appropriate activities for these young people. Typically these units can be set apart from the general pediatric facility so that the teenagers do not share space with younger children, who are often perceived as a threat to their maturity.

In caring for the adolescent patient, it is essential to provide flexible routines and activities, such as more group activity, wearing of street clothes, and access to the items so critical to adolescents—telephones, compact disc players, DVD players, videocassette recorders, computers, e-mail, video games, and televisions. Because adolescents' food habits are rarely limited to the three traditional meals a day, a ready supply of snacks should be available. However, the most important benefit of these units is increased socialization with peers. In addition, staff members usually enjoy working with this age-group and are able to establish the trust so essential for communication.

NURSING TIP
When adolescents must share a common activity room with younger patients, referring to the area as the "activity" room rather than the "playroom" may entice them to visit the room and participate in activities.

Although regression is expected and normal for all age-groups, nurses have the responsibility for fostering the child's growth and development. Hospitalization can become a significant opportunity for learning and advancing. Extended hospitalizations for long-term chronic illness or situations of failure to thrive, abuse, or neglect represent instances in which regression must be seen as an adjustment period, to be followed by plans for promoting appropriate developmental skills.

Providing Opportunities for Play and Expressive Activities

Play is one of the most important aspects of a child's life and one of the most effective tools for managing stress. Because illness and hospitalization constitute crises in a child's life and often involve overwhelming stresses, children need to act out their fears and anxieties as a means of coping with these stresses. Play is essential to children's mental, emotional, and social well-being. As with their other developmental needs, play does not stop when children are ill or in the hospital. On the contrary, play in the hospital serves many functions (Box 21-9). Of all hospital facilities, no room probably alleviates the stressors of hospitalization more than the playroom (or activity room). In the playroom, children temporarily distance themselves from their illness, hospitalization, and the associated stressors. This room should be a safe haven for children, free from medical or nursing procedures (including medication administration), strange faces, and probing questions. The playroom then becomes a sanctuary in an otherwise frightening environment.

Engaging in play activities gives children a sense of control. In the hospital environment, most decisions are made for the

FIG. 21-8 ■ Play materials for children in the hospital need to be appropriate for their age, interests, and limitations.

BOX 21-9
Functions of Play in the Hospital

- Provides diversion and brings about relaxation
- Helps the child feel more secure in a strange environment
- Lessens the stress of separation and the feeling of homesickness
- Provides a means for release of tension and expression of feelings
- Encourages interaction and development of positive attitudes toward others
- Provides an expressive outlet for creative ideas and interests
- Provides a means for accomplishing therapeutic goals (see Use of Play in Procedures, Chapter 22)
- Places child in active role and provides opportunity to make choices and be in control

child; play and other expressive activities offer the child much-needed opportunities to make choices for themselves. Even if a child chooses not to participate in a particular activity, the nurse has offered the child a choice, perhaps one of only a few real choices the child has had that day.

The hospitalized child typically has lower energy levels than healthy children of the same age. Therefore children may not appear engaged and enthusiastic about an activity, even though they are enjoying the experience. Activities may need to be adjusted or limited based on the child's age, endurance, and any special needs.

Diversional Activities. Almost any form of play can be used for diversion and recreation, but the activity should be selected on the basis of the child's age, interests, and limitations (Fig. 21-8). Children do not necessarily need special direction for using play materials. All they require is the raw materials with which to work and adult approval and supervision to help keep their natural enthusiasm or expression of feelings from getting out of control. Small children enjoy a variety of small, colorful toys that they can play with in bed or in their room, or more elaborate play equipment, such as playhouses, sandboxes, rhythm instruments, or large boxes and blocks, that may be a part of the hospital playroom.

Games that can be played alone or with another child or an adult are popular with older children, as are puzzles; reading material; quiet, individual activities, such as sewing, stringing beads, and weaving; and Lego blocks and other building materials. Assembling models is an excellent pastime, but one should make certain that all pieces and necessary materials are included in the package so that the child is not disappointed and frustrated.

Well-selected books are of infinite value to the child. Children never tire of stories; having someone read aloud gives them endless hours of pleasure and is of special value to the child who has limited energy to expend in play. A radio, DVD player, electronic games, and television, included among most hospital room equipment, are useful tools for entertaining a child. Computers with access to the Internet can provide diversion, educational opportunities, and online support groups.

When supervising play for ill or convalescent children, it is best to select activities that are simpler than would normally be chosen for the child's specific developmental level. These children usually do not have the energy to cope with more challenging activities. Other limitations also influence the type of activities. Special consideration must be given to the child who is confined in terms of movement, has a restricted extremity, or is isolated. Toys for isolated children must be disposable or need to be disinfected after every use. Therefore toys that are not able to be disinfected (e.g., stuffed animals) cannot be used as community toys.

Toys. Parents of hospitalized children often ask nurses about the types of toys that would be best to bring for their child. Although parents often want to buy new toys for the hospitalized child to offer cheer and comfort, it is often better to wait to bring new things, especially in the case of younger children. Small children need the comfort and reassurance of familiar things, such as the stuffed animal the child hugs for comfort and takes to bed at night. These familiar items are a link with home and the world outside the hospital. All toys brought into the hospital should be assessed for safety.

Large numbers of toys often confuse and frustrate a small child. A few small, well-chosen toys are usually preferred to one large, expensive one. Children who are hospitalized for an extended time benefit from changes. Rather than a confusing accumulation of toys, older toys should be replaced periodically as interest wanes.

> **NURSING TIP**
>
> Have parents provide the child with a shoe box, a child's small suitcase, or a backpack to attach to the bed for an easy storage receptacle to prevent small items from becoming lost in the sheets or under the bed.

A highly successful diversion for a child who is hospitalized for a length of time and whose parents are unable to visit frequently is having the parents bring a box with several small, inexpensive, brightly wrapped items with a different day of the week printed on the outside of each package. The child will eagerly anticipate the time for opening each one. If the parents know when their next visit will be, they can provide the number of packages that corresponds to the time between visits. In this way the child knows that the diminishing packages also represent the anticipated visit from the parent.

Expressive Activities. Play and other expressive activities provide one of the best opportunities for encouraging emotional expression, including the safe release of anger and hostility. Nondirective play that allows children freedom for expression can be tremendously therapeutic. Therapeutic play, however, should not be confused with **play therapy,** a psycho-

FIG. 21-9 ■ Drawing and painting are excellent media for expression.

logic technique reserved for use by trained and qualified therapists as an interpretative method with emotionally disturbed children. **Therapeutic play,** on the other hand, is an effective, nondirective modality for helping children deal with their concerns and fears, and at the same time it often helps the nurse gain insights into children's needs and feelings.

Tension release can be facilitated through almost any activity; with younger ambulatory children, large-muscle activity such as use of tricycles and wagons is especially beneficial. Much aggression can be safely directed into pounding and throwing games or activities. Beanbags are often thrown at a target or open receptacle with surprising vigor and hostility. A pounding board is employed with enthusiasm by young children; clay and Play-Doh are beneficial for use at any age.

Creative Expression. Although all children derive physical, social, emotional, and cognitive benefits from engaging in art or other creative activities, children's need for such activities is intensified when they are hospitalized. Drawing and painting are excellent media for expression. Children are more at ease expressing their thoughts and feelings through art, since humans think first in images and later learn to translate these images into words. The child needs only to be supplied with the raw materials, such as crayons and paper; large brushes and an ample supply of newsprint supported on easels; or materials for finger painting (Fig. 21-9). Children can work individually or work together on a group project, such as a mural painted on a long piece of paper.

Although interpretation of children's drawings requires special training, observing changes in a series of the child's drawings over time can be helpful in assessing psychosocial adjustment and coping. The nurse can use children's drawings, stories, poetry, and other products of creative expression as a springboard for discussion of thoughts, fears, and understanding of concepts or events (see Communication Techniques, Chapter 6). A child's drawing before surgery, for example, may reveal unvoiced concerns about mutilation, body changes, and loss of self-control.

Nurses can incorporate opportunities for musical expression into routine nursing care. For example, simple musical instruments, such as bracelets with bells, can be placed on infants' legs for them to shake to accompany mealtime music or dressing changes. Dance and movement suggestions may encourage a child to ambulate.

Holidays provide stimulus and direction for unlimited creative projects. Children can participate in decorating the pediatric unit; making pictures and decorations for their rooms gives the children a sense of pride and accomplishment. This is especially beneficial for children who are immobilized and isolated. Making gifts for someone at home helps to maintain interpersonal ties.

Dramatic Play. Dramatic play is a well-recognized technique for emotional release, allowing children to reenact frightening or puzzling hospital experiences. Through use of puppets, replicas of hospital equipment, or some actual hospital equipment, children can act out the situations that are a part of their hospital experience. Dramatic play enables children to learn about procedures and events that concern them and to assume the roles of the adults in the hospital environment.

Puppets are universally effective for communicating with children. Most children see them as peers and readily communicate with them. Children will tell the puppet feelings that they hesitate to express to adults. Puppets can share children's own experiences and help them to find solutions to their problems. Puppets dressed to represent figures in the child's environment—for example, a physician, nurse, child patient, therapist, and members of the child's own family—are especially useful. Small, appropriately attired dolls are equally effective in encouraging the child to play out situations, although puppets are usually best for direct conversation.

NURSINGTIP

Make a simple puppet using a large handkerchief. Place some cotton balls in the center of the cloth and wrap a rubber band over the handkerchief and cotton balls to form a "head." Place the head over the index finger so that the rubber band secures it to the finger. Let the cloth drape over the front and back of the hand. The cloth forms four parts of the puppet: the index finger is the head, the thumb and other fingers are the arms, and the draped cloth is the body. Decorate the head by drawing features on it.

Play must consider medical needs, but at times a procedure can be postponed briefly to allow the child to complete a special activity (see Critical Thinking Exercise). Play must consider any limitations imposed by the child's condition. For example, small children may eat paste and other creative media; therefore a child who is allergic to wheat should not be given finger paint made from wallpaper paste or modeling dough made with flour. A child on a restricted salt intake should not play with modeling dough because salt is one of its major constituents. At home the play program can be planned around the therapy regimen. However, play can be satisfactorily incorporated into the child's care if the nurse and others involved allow some flexibility and use creativity in planning for play.

Maximizing Potential Benefits of Hospitalization

Although hospitalization generally represents a stressful time for children and families, it also represents an opportunity for facilitating positive change within the child and among family members. For some families the stress of a child's illness, hos-

---

??? CRITICAL THINKING EXERCISE

Playroom and Hospital Procedures

Hannah, a 7-year-old with cystic fibrosis, has been hospitalized numerous times with complications from the condition. She is playing Candyland with her brother, sister, and several other children in the playroom on the pediatric unit. A pediatric phlebotomist enters the playroom and says, "Hannah, I need to take some blood. I can see that you are playing a game, so I'll just do it while you play. It will just take a minute." Hannah nods her head indicating that she agrees to let the phlebotomist draw the blood at this time. The playroom is usually off-limits for invasive procedures. As Hannah's nurse, you are aware that Dr. Lung wants the results of the laboratory studies as soon as possible to make a decision about her course of therapy.

QUESTIONS
1. Evidence—Is there sufficient evidence to draw any conclusions about this situation at this time?
2. Assumptions—What are some underlying assumptions about the following:
   a. Children and painful procedures such as venipunctures
   b. The function of play in a hospitalized child
   c. The priority in performing the procedure
   d. Implications of performing the procedure in the playroom
3. What implications and priorities for nursing care can be drawn at this time (i.e., what will you do)?
4. Does the evidence objectively support your argument (conclusion)?
5. Are there alternative perspectives to your conclusions? If so, what are they?

---

pitalization, or both can lead to strengthening of family coping behaviors and the emergence of new coping strategies.

Fostering Parent-Child Relationships. The crisis of illness or hospitalization can mobilize parents into more acute awareness of their child's needs. For example, hospitalization provides opportunities for parents to learn more about their children's growth and development. When parents are helped to understand children's usual reactions to stress, such as regression or aggression, they are not only better able to support the child through the hospital experience, but also may extend their insights into childrearing practices after discharge.

Difficulties in parent-child relationships that existed before hospitalization that are characterized by feeding problems, negative behavior, and sleep disturbances may decrease during hospitalization. The temporary cessation of such problems sometimes alerts parents to the role they may be playing in propagating the negative behavior. With assistance from health professionals, parents can restructure ways of relating to their children to foster more positive behavior.

Hospitalization may also represent a temporary reprieve or refuge from a disturbed home. Typically, abused or neglected children's dramatic physical and social improvement during hospitalization is proof of the benefits and potential growth that can occur during hospitalization. These children temporarily are able to seek support, reassurance, and security from new relationships, particularly with nurses and hospitalized peers.

Providing Educational Opportunities. Illness and hospitalization represent excellent opportunities for children and other family members to learn more about their bodies, each other, and the health professions. For example, during a hospital admission for a diabetic crisis, the child may learn about the disease; the parents may learn about the child's needs for independence, normalcy, and appropriate limits; and each of them may find a new support system in the hospital staff.

Illness or hospitalization can also help older children in choosing a career. Frequently, children have impressions of physicians or nurses that are disproportionately positive or negative. Actual experience with different health professionals can influence their attitude about health professionals and even a decision regarding a career in healthcare.

Promoting Self-Mastery. The experience of facing a crisis such as illness or hospitalization, coping successfully with it, and maturing as a result of it constitutes an opportunity for self-mastery. Younger children have the chance to test fantasy vs reality fears. They realize that they were not abandoned, mutilated, or punished. In fact, they were loved, cared for, and treated with respect for their individual concerns. It is not unusual for children who have undergone hospitalization or surgery to tell others that "it was nothing" or to display proudly their scars or bandages. For older children, hospitalization may represent an opportunity for decision making, independence, and self-reliance. They are proud of having survived the experience and may feel a genuine self-respect for their achievements. Nurses can facilitate such feelings of self-mastery by emphasizing aspects of personal competence in the child and not focusing on uncooperative or negative behavior.

Providing Socialization. Hospitalization may offer children a special opportunity for social acceptance. Lonely, asocial, and even delinquent children find a sympathetic environment in the hospital. Children who have a physical handicap or are in some other way "different" from their age-mates may find an accepting social peer group (Fig. 21-10). Although this does not always spontaneously occur, nurses can structure the environment to foster a supportive child group. For example, selection of a compatible roommate can help children gain a new friend and learn more about themselves. Forming relationships with significant members of the health care team, such as the physician, nurse, child life specialist, or social worker, can greatly enhance children's adjustment in many areas of life.

Parents may also encounter a new social group in other parents who have similar problems. The waiting room or hallway "self-help" groups are inherent to every institution. Parents meet while in the hospital or clinic and discuss their children's illnesses and treatments. Nurses can capitalize on this informal gathering by encouraging parents to discuss collectively their concerns and feelings. Nurses can also refer parents to organized parent groups or can use the help and support of parents of recovered hospitalized patients. It is important that nurses emphasize to families that each child responds differently to disease, treatments, and care. Any questions raised during group discussions should be clarified with a nurse or physician.

NURSING CARE OF THE FAMILY

Although it is not possible to predict exactly which factors are most likely to have an effect on the family's reactions, important variables are (1) the seriousness of the child's illness, (2) the family's previous experience with hospitalization, and (3)

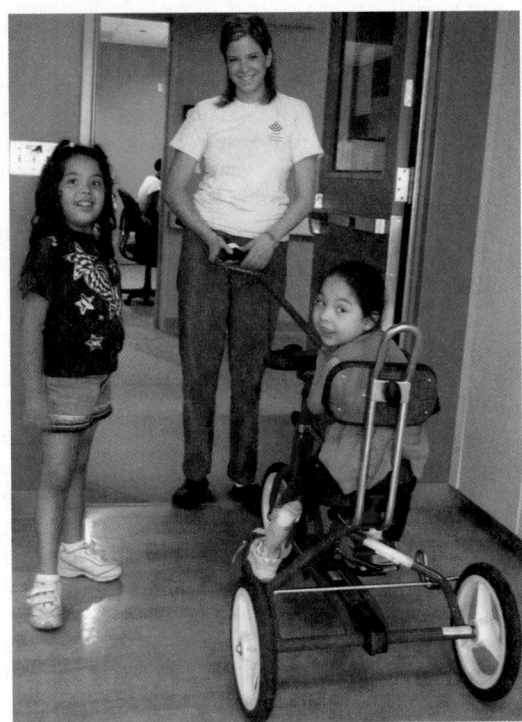

FIG. 21-10 ■ Placing children of the same age-group with similar illnesses near each other on the unit is both psychologically and medically supportive. (Courtesy E. Jacob, Texas Children's Hospital, Houston.)

the medical procedures involved in the diagnosis and treatment. Important information is also obtained in the nursing admission history (see Box 21-5).

SUPPORTING FAMILY MEMBERS

Support involves the willingness to stay and listen to parents' verbal and nonverbal messages. Sometimes the nurse does not give this support directly. For example, the nurse may offer to stay with the child to allow the parents time alone or may discuss with other family members the parents' need for extra relief. Often relatives and friends want to help but do not know how. Suggesting ways, such as baby-sitting, preparing meals, doing laundry, or transporting the siblings to school, can prompt others to help reduce the responsibilities that burden parents. An ongoing parent support group held on the pediatric unit during the children's traditional nap time has also proved effective in helping parents share emotions and concerns related to hospitalization (Bracht, Ardal, Bot, and others, 1998).

Support may also be provided through the clergy. Parents with deep religious beliefs may appreciate the counsel of a clergy member, but because of their stress they may not have sufficient energy to initiate the contact. Nurses can be supportive by arranging for clergy to visit, upholding parents' religious beliefs, and respecting the individual meaning and significance of those beliefs (Feudtner, Haney, and Dimmers, 2003).

Support involves accepting cultural, socioeconomic, and ethnic values. For example, health and illness are defined differently by various ethnic groups. For some, a disorder that has few outward manifestations of illness, such as diabetes,

FAMILY-CENTERED CARE

Supporting Siblings During Hospitalization

Trade off staying at the hospital with spouse or have a surrogate who knows the siblings well stay in the home.

Offer information about the child's condition to young siblings as well as older siblings; respect the sibling who avoids information as a means of coping with the situation.

Arrange for children to visit their brother or sister in the hospital if possible.

Encourage phone visits and mail between brothers and sisters; provide children with phone numbers, writing supplies, and stamps.

Help each sibling identify an extended family member or friend to be their support person and provide extra attention during parental absence.

Make or buy inexpensive toys or trinkets for siblings, one gift for each day the child will be hospitalized.

- Wrap each gift separately and place in a basket, box, or other container at each child's bedside.
- Instruct siblings to open one gift each night at bedtime and to remember that he or she is in the parent's thoughts.

If the child's condition is stable and distance is not prohibitive, plan a special time at home with the siblings or have spouse or another relative or friend bring the children to meet parent(s) at a restaurant or other location near the hospital.

- Have extended family members or friends schedule a visit to the child in the hospital during parental absence.
- Arrange a pass for the child to leave the hospital to join the family if the child's condition permits.

Modified from Craft M, Craft J: Perceived changes in siblings of hospitalized children: a comparison of sibling and parent reports, *Child Health Care* 18(1):42-48, 1989; Rollins J: *Brothers and sisters: a discussion guide for families,* Landover, Md, 1992, Epilepsy Foundation of America.

hypertension, or cardiac problems, is not a sickness. Consequently, following a prescribed treatment may be seen as unnecessary. Nurses who appreciate the influences of culture are more likely to intervene therapeutically. (See also Cultural and Religious Influences on Healthcare, Chapter 4.)

Parents need help in accepting their own feelings toward the ill child. If given the opportunity, parents often disclose their feelings of loss of control, anger, and guilt. They often resist admitting to such feelings because they expect others to disapprove of behavior that is less than perfect. Unfortunately, health personnel, including nurses, sometimes do exercise little tolerance for deviation from the norm. This only increases the psychologic impact of a child's illness on family members. Helping parents identify the specific reason for such feelings and emphasizing that each is a normal, expected, and healthy response to stress may reduce the parents' emotional burden.

Family-centered care also addresses the needs of siblings. Support may involve preparing siblings for hospital visits, assessing their adjustment, and providing appropriate interventions or referrals when needed. The Family-Centered Care box suggests ways that parents can support siblings during hospitalization.

PROVIDING INFORMATION

One of the most important nursing interventions is providing information about (1) the disease, its treatment, prognosis, and home care; (2) the child's emotional and physical reac-

tions to illness and hospitalization; and (3) the probable emotional reactions of family members to the crisis.

For many families the child's illness is the first contact they have with the hospital experience. Often parents are not prepared for the child's behavioral reactions to hospitalization, such as separation behaviors, regression, aggression, and hostility. Providing the parents with information about these normal and expected behavioral responses can lessen the parents' anxiety during the hospital admission. The family is equally unfamiliar with hospital rules, which often compounds their confusion and anxiety. Therefore the family needs clear explanations about what to expect and what is expected of them.

Parents also need to be aware of the effects of illness on the family and strategies that prevent negative changes. Specifically, parents should keep the family well informed and communicate with everyone as much as possible. They should treat all the children equally and as normally as before the illness occurred. Discipline, which initially may be lessened for the ill child, should be continued to provide a measure of security and predictability. When ill children know that their parents expect certain standards of conduct from them, they feel certain that they will recover. Conversely, when all limits are removed, they fear that something catastrophic will happen.

Helping parents understand the meaning of posthospitalization behaviors in the sick child is necessary for them to tolerate and support such behaviors. In addition, parents should be forewarned of the common reactions following discharge (see Box 21-2). Parents who do not expect such reactions may misinterpret them as evidence of the child's "being spoiled" and demand perfect behavior at a time when the child is still reacting to the stress of illness and hospitalization. If the behaviors, especially the demand for attention, are dealt with in a supportive manner, most children are able to relinquish them and assume precrisis levels of functioning.

Nurses should also prepare parents for the reactions of siblings—particularly anger, jealousy, and resentment. Older siblings may deny such reactions because they provoke feelings of guilt. However, everyone needs outlets for emotions, and the repressed feelings may surface as problems in school or with age-mates, as psychosomatic illnesses, or in delinquent behavior.

Probably one of the most neglected areas of communication involves giving information to siblings. Frequently, age becomes the only factor that leads to an awareness of this problem, since older children may begin to ask questions or request explanations. Even in this situation, however, the information may be seriously inadequate. Children in every age-group deserve some explanation of the sibling's illness or hospitalization. Although the exact wording may differ, the explanation should focus on the following concerns: (1) "Will I get sick and have to go to the hospital?" (2) "Did I cause the illness?" (for actual or imagined reasons), and (3) "Will my parents abandon me if my brother or sister doesn't recover?" If parents or nurses address these three questions, the siblings' own fears of illness, guilt, and abandonment are minimized (Melnyk and Alpert-Gillis, 1998).

ENCOURAGING PARENT PARTICIPATION

Preventing or minimizing separation is a key nursing goal with the child who is hospitalized, but maintaining parent-child contact is also beneficial for the family. One of the best approaches is encouraging parents to stay with their child and to participate in the care whenever possible. Although some health facilities provide special accommodations for parents, the concept of rooming in can be instituted anywhere. The first requirement is the staff's positive attitude toward parents. A negative attitude toward parent participation can create barriers to collaborative working relationships.

When hospital staff genuinely appreciate the importance of continued parent-child attachment, they foster an environment that encourages parents to stay. When parents are included in the care planning and understand that they are a contributing factor to the child's recovery, they are more inclined to remain with their child and have more emotional reserves to support themselves and the child through the crisis. An empowerment model of helping allows the nurse to focus on parents' strengths and seek ways to promote growth and family functioning so that the parents become empowered in caring for their child.

Because the mother tends to be the usual family caregiver, she usually spends more time in the hospital than the father. However, not all mothers (or fathers) feel equally comfortable assuming responsibility for their child's care. Some may be under such great emotional stress that they need a temporary reprieve from total participation in caregiving activities (see Ethical Case Study). Others may feel insecure in participating in specialized areas of care, such as bathing the child after surgery. On the other hand, some mothers may feel a great need to control their child's care. This seems particularly true of young mothers, who have recently established their role as a parent; mothers of children too young to verbalize their needs; and ethnic minority mothers when the hospital setting is predominantly staffed by nonminority personnel. Individual assessment of each parent's preferred involvement is necessary to prevent the effects of separation while supporting parents in their needs as well.

With lifestyles and gender roles changing, fathers may assume all or some of the usual "mothering" roles in the household. In this case it may be the father-child relationship that requires preservation. Fathers need to be included in the care plan and respected for their parental role. For some fathers the child's hospitalization may represent an opportunity to alter their usual caregiving role and increase their involvement. In single-parent families the caregiver may not be a parent but an extended family member, such as a grandparent or aunt.

One of the potential problems with continuous parent involvement is neglect of the parent's need for sleep, nutrition, and relaxation. Often the sleeping accommodations are limited to a chair, and sleep is disrupted by nursing procedures. Encouraging the parents to leave for brief periods, arranging for sleeping quarters on the unit but outside the child's room, and planning a schedule of alternating visits with another family member can minimize the stresses for the parent.

All too often, nurses respond to parent participation by abandoning their patient responsibilities. Nurses need to restructure their roles to complement and augment the caregiving functions of parents. Even in units structured to provide care by parents, parents frequently feel anxiety in their caregiving responsibilities; those more involved in direct care may feel more anxiety than those less involved in direct care. Therefore 24-hour responsibility may be too much for some parents. Assistance and relief by nursing personnel should always be available to these families, and nurses may need to

work diligently to establish the strong bond of trust some parents need to take advantage of these opportunities.

PREPARING FOR DISCHARGE AND HOME CARE

Most hospitalizations necessitate some type of discharge preparation. Often this involves education of the family for continued care and follow-up in the home. Depending on the diagnosis, this may be relatively simple or highly complex. Preparing the family for home care demands a high degree of competence in planning and implementing discharge instructions. This usually is best accomplished using an **interdisciplinary team approach,** which requires a shift from the **multidisciplinary team approach** used during an acute phase of a child's illness (Hornick, 1996).

Nurses are often key individuals in initiating and carrying out the discharge process. They collaborate with others in the planning and implementation phases to ensure appropriate care after hospitalization. Throughout the hospitalization the nurse should be aware of the need for discharge planning and those assessment factors that affect the family's ability to provide home care. A thorough assessment of the family and home environment should be performed to ensure that the family's emotional and physical resources are sufficient to manage the tasks of home care. (For a discussion of family and home assessment strategies, see Chapter 6.) In addition to adequate family resources, an investigation of community services, including respite care, is needed to ensure that appropriate support agencies are available, such as emergency facilities, home health agencies, and equipment vendors. Financial resources are also a consideration. To coordinate the immense task of assessment and to plan implementation, a care coordinator or manager should be appointed early in the discharge process.

The preparation for hospital discharge and home care begins during the admission assessment. Short- and long-term goals are established to meet the child's physical and psychosocial needs. For children with complex care needs, discharge planning focuses on obtaining appropriate equipment and healthcare personnel for the home. Discharge planning is also concerned with those treatments that parents or children are expected to continue at home. In planning appropriate teaching, nurses need to assess (1) the actual and perceived complexity of the skill, (2) the parents' or child's ability to learn the skill, and (3) the parents' or child's previous or present experience with such procedures.

The teaching plan incorporates levels of learning, such as observing, participating with assistance, and finally, acting without help or guidance. The skill is divided into discrete steps, and each step is taught to the family member until it is learned. Return demonstration of the skill is requested before new skills are introduced. A record of teaching and performance provides an efficient checklist for evaluation. All families need to receive detailed *written* instructions about home care, with telephone numbers for assistance, before they leave the hospital. Communication between the nurse performing discharge planning and home health care is essential for ensuring a smooth transition for the child and family.

After the family is competent in performing the skill, they are given responsibility for the care. When possible, the family should have a transition or trial period to assume care with minimal health care supervision. This may be arranged on the unit; during a home pass; or in a facility, such as a motel, near the hospital. Such transitions provide a safe practice period for the family, with assistance readily available when needed, and are especially valuable when the family lives far from the hospital.

In many instances parents need only simple instructions and understanding of follow-up care. However, the often overwhelming care assumed by some families, coupled with other stressors they may be experiencing, necessitates continued professional support after discharge. A follow-up home visit or telephone call gives the nurse an opportunity to individualize care and provide information in perhaps a less stressful learning environment than the hospital. Appropriate referrals and resources may include visiting nurse or home health agencies, private nurse services, the school system, a physical therapist, a mental health counselor, a social worker, and any number of community agencies. Sharing the important issues surrounding the child's and family's needs is essential. Referral summaries should be concise, specific, and factual. When numerous support services are required, periodic collaboration among the professionals involved and the family is an excellent strategy to ensure efficient usage and comprehensive delivery of services.

CARE OF THE CHILD AND FAMILY IN SPECIAL HOSPITAL SITUATIONS

In addition to a general pediatric unit, children may be admitted to special facilities such as an ambulatory or outpatient setting, an isolation room, or intensive care.

AMBULATORY OR OUTPATIENT SETTING

The ambulatory or outpatient setting provides needed medical services for the child while eliminating the necessity of overnight admission. Among the benefits of ambulatory care are (1) minimization of the stressors of hospitalization, especially separation from the family; (2) reduced chance of infection; and (3) cost savings. Admission to the ambulatory or outpatient hospital setting usually is for surgical or diagnostic procedures, such as insertion of tympanostomy tubes, hernia repair, adenoidectomy, tonsillectomy, cystoscopy, or bronchoscopy.

In the ambulatory or outpatient setting, adequate preparation is particularly challenging. Ideally, the child and parents should receive preadmission preparation, including a tour of the facility and a review of the day's events (Brewer and Lambert, 1997). Parents need information in advance to help prepare the child and themselves for surgery and enable them to care for the child at home after the procedure. Parents also appreciate suggestions for items to bring to the hospital, such as blankets or stuffed animals. When preadmission preparation is not possible, time should be allowed on the day of the procedure for children to become acquainted with their surroundings and for nurses to assess, plan, and implement appropriate teaching.

Waiting is usually inevitable in ambulatory settings. Families frequently report waiting to be the most stressful part of the experience. Providing a pager is one way to allow the family (and at times the child) to leave the area and then be paged to return when needed (Ashenberg, Lambert, Maier, and others, 1996).

Explicit discharge instructions are important after outpatient surgery (see Family-Centered Care box and Preparing for Discharge and Home Care, p. 678). Parents need guide-

FAMILY-CENTERED CARE

Discharge from Ambulatory Settings

Before beginning, explain that all instructions will also be presented in writing for the family to refer to later.

Provide an overview of the typical trajectory (expected pattern) of recovery.

Discuss expected progression of the child's activity level during the postdischarge period (e.g., "Mary will probably sleep for the rest of the day, feel kind of tired most of tomorrow, but be back to her usual activities the next day").

Explain which activities the child is allowed and what is not permitted (e.g., bed rest, bathing).

Discuss dietary restrictions, being very specific and giving examples of "clear fluids" or what is meant by a "full liquid diet."

Discuss nausea and vomiting, if applicable, explaining how much is "normal" and what to do if more occurs (e.g., "Juan may be sick to his stomach and vomit. This is normal. However, if he vomits more than three times, please call us at this number right away.").

Discuss fever and appropriate comfort measures, explaining how much fever is considered "normal," and specifically what to do if the child goes beyond the range.

Explain the amount, location, and kind of pain or discomfort the child may experience.

Give any prescribed medication before leaving the facility.

Send a pain scale home with the family.

Explain how much pain and discomfort is "normal" and what to do if the child surpasses that level or if pain management interventions are unsuccessful.

Discuss pain management, including dosage for pain medications and details on how to administer them.

Describe appropriate nonpharmacologic comfort measures, such as holding, rocking, or swaddling.

Provide information about each medication that the child will be taking at home.
- Review the details, including dose and route.
- Demonstrate how to administer medications, if necessary (e.g., how to take wrapping off suppositories, how to insert).

Discuss guidelines for requesting other medications.

Request that all prescriptions be filled and given to the family before discharge.

Make certain the family has all of the equipment and supplies (e.g., gauze and tape for dressing changes) they will need at home.

Discuss complications that may occur and the steps to take if they do.

Ensure that appropriate measures are in place for safe transport home.
- Remind family to use a seat belt or car seat for the child.
- Determine if there will be one person whose sole responsibility is helping ensure the child's safety and comfort during transport.
- Discuss measures the driver may need to take if this is impossible (e.g., be certain a basin is within the child's reach should vomiting occur; take a route that permits slower traffic and has places along the roadside to stop if necessary).
- Determine the availability of a blanket, pillow, and cup with a lid and straw for the child's use in the car.
- Provide a basin or plastic bag in case of vomiting.

Provide emergency phone numbers for the family to call with any concerns.

Explain that the family will be contacted (give an approximate time) to follow up on the child but that they should not hesitate to call if concerns arise before then.

Ask the family and child, if appropriate, if they have any questions, and problem solve with family members to meet their unique needs.

lines on when to call their practitioner regarding a change in the child's condition. A follow-up telephone call system allows for nurses to check on the child's progress within 48 to 72 hours after discharge. It also provides an opportunity for the nurse to review discharge information and answer questions.

NURSINGTIP

Help the family prepare for the transportation home by offering these suggestions:

■ Have a blanket and pillow in the car. (Always use the car safety restraint system.)
■ Take a basin or plastic bag in case of vomiting.
■ Use a cup with a cap and straw for the child to drink fluids (except in cases of orofacial surgery where a straw may be contraindicated).
■ Give any prescribed pain medication before leaving facility.
■ Provide parents verbal and written information regarding potential side effects of pain medication for which they should be vigilant after discharge.

ISOLATION

Admission to an isolation room increases all of the stressors typically associated with hospitalization. There is further separation from familiar persons; additional loss of control; and added environmental changes, such as sensory deprivation and the strange appearance of visitors. Orientation to time and place is affected. These stressors are compounded by children's limited understanding of isolation. Preschool children have difficulty understanding the rationale for isolation because they cannot comprehend the cause-and-effect relationship between germs and illness. They are likely to view isolation as punishment. Older children understand the causality better but still require information to decrease fantasizing or misinterpretation.

When a child is placed in isolation, preparation is essential for the child to feel in control. With young children the best approach is a simple explanation, such as "You need to be in this room to help you get better. This is a special place to make all the germs go away. The germs made you sick, and you could not help that."

All children, but especially younger ones, need preparation in terms of what they will see, hear, or feel in isolation. Therefore they are shown the mask, gloves, and gown and are encouraged to "dress up" in them. Playing with the strange apparel lessens the fear of seeing "ghostlike" people walk into the room. Before entering the room, nurses and other health personnel should introduce themselves and let the child see their face before donning a mask. In this way the child associates them with significant experiences and gains a sense of familiarity in an otherwise strange and lonely environment.

When the child's condition improves, appropriate play activities are provided to minimize boredom, stimulate the senses, provide a real or perceived sense of movement, orient the child to time and place, provide social interaction, and reduce depersonalization. For example, the environment can be manipulated to increase sensory freedom by moving the bed toward the door or window. Opening window shades; providing musical, visual, or tactile toys; and increasing interpersonal contact can substitute mental mobility for the limitations of physical movement. Rather than dwelling on the negative aspects of isolation, the child can be encouraged to view this experience as challenging and positive. For example,

the nurse can help the child look at isolation as a method of keeping others out and letting only special people in. Children often think of intriguing signs for their doors, such as "Enter at your own risk." These signs also encourage people "on the outside" to talk with the child about the ominous greeting.

NURSINGTIP

Have the child select a place he or she would like to visit. Help the child decorate the bed and equipment to suit the theme (e.g., truck, circus tent, spaceship, sky). At a set time each day pretend to go with the child to the special place. Consider including props such as a suitcase or picnic basket.

EMERGENCY ADMISSION

One of the most traumatic hospital experiences for the child and parents is an emergency admission. The sudden onset of an illness or the occurrence of an injury leaves little time for preparation and explanation. Sometimes the emergency admission is compounded by admission to an intensive care unit (ICU) or the need for immediate surgery. However, even in those instances requiring only outpatient treatment, the child is exposed to a strange, frightening environment and to experiences that may elicit fear or cause pain.

There is a wide discrepancy between what constitutes a medically defined emergency and a client-defined emergency. A growing concern is the use of major emergency departments for routine primary care health visits. To offset overcrowding in emergency departments, many facilities have minor emergency units or pediatric minor emergency units for after-hours health care. Telephone triage for minor illnesses for patients is also emerging as a health care delivery mode to differentiate illnesses such as a common cold from true life-threatening conditions that require immediate practitioner attention and intervention. Other factors contributing to the overuse of emergency departments (as opposed to the primary practitioner's office) include the increasing number of uninsured persons and households where both parents work full time and cannot afford to take off during the daytime to take the sick child to a practitioner.

In pediatric populations most visits to an emergency department are for respiratory infections, with skin conditions, gastrointestinal disorders, and trauma such as poisoning accounting for the remainder of cases. The most common reason parents give for bringing the child to the emergency department is concern about the illness worsening. However, practitioners may not think that the progressive symptoms necessitate immediate or emergency care. One of the nurse's primary goals is to assess the parents' perception of the event and their reasons for considering it serious or life threatening.

Lengthy preparatory admission procedures are often inappropriate for emergency situations. In such instances, nurses must focus their nursing interventions on the essential components of admission counseling (Box 21-10) and complete the process as soon as the child's condition has stabilized.

Unless an emergency is life threatening, children need to participate in their care to maintain a sense of control. Because emergency departments are frequently hectic, there is a tendency to rush through procedures to save time. However, the extra few minutes needed to allow children to participate may save many more minutes of useless resistance and unco-

BOX 21-10

Guidelines for Special Hospital Admission*

EMERGENCY ADMISSION

Lengthy preparatory admission procedures are often impossible and inappropriate for emergency situations.

Focus assessment on airway, breathing, and circulation; weigh child whenever possible for calculation of drug dosages.

Unless an emergency is life threatening, children need to participate in their care to maintain a sense of control.

Focus on essential components of admission counseling, including:

- Appropriate introduction to the family
- Use of child's name, not terms such as "honey" or "dear"
- Determination of child's age and some judgment about developmental age (If the child is of school age, asking about the grade level will offer some evidence of intellectual ability.)
- Information about child's general state of health, any problems that may interfere with medical treatment (e.g., allergies), and previous experience with hospital facilities
- Information about the chief complaint from both the parents and the child

ADMISSION TO INTENSIVE CARE UNIT (ICU)

Prepare child and parents for elective ICU admission, such as for postoperative care after cardiac surgery.

Prepare child and parents for unanticipated ICU admission by focusing primarily on the sensory aspects of the experience and on usual family concerns (e.g., persons in charge of child's care, schedule for visiting, area where family can stay).

Prepare parents regarding child's appearance and behavior when they first visit child in ICU.

Accompany family to bedside to provide emotional support and answer questions.

Prepare siblings for their visit; plan length of time for sibling visitation; monitor siblings' reactions during visit to prevent them from becoming overwhelmed.

Encourage parents to stay with their child:

- If visiting hours are limited, allow flexibility in schedule to accommodate parental needs.
- Give family members a written schedule of visiting times.
- If visiting hours are liberal, be aware of family members' needs and suggest periodic respites.
- Assure family they can call the unit at any time.

Prepare parents for expected role changes and identify ways for parents to participate in child's care without overwhelming them with responsibilities:

- Help with bath or feeding.
- Touch and talk to child.
- Help with procedures.

Provide information about child's condition in understandable language:

- Repeat information often.
- Seek clarification of understanding.
- During bedside conferences, interpret information for family members and child or, if appropriate, conduct report outside room.

Prepare child for procedures, even if this involves explanation while procedure is performed.

Assess and manage pain; recognize that a child who cannot talk, such as an infant or child in a coma or on mechanical ventilation, can be in pain.

Establish a routine that maintains some similarity to daily events in child's life whenever possible:

- Organize care during normal waking hours.
- Keep regular bedtime schedules, including quiet times when television or radio is lowered or turned off.
- Provide uninterrupted sleep cycles (60 minutes for infant, 90 minutes for older child).
- Close and open drapes and dim lights to allow for day/night.
- Place curtain around bed for privacy.
- Orient child to day and time; have clocks or calendars in easy view for older children.

Schedule a time when child is left undisturbed (e.g., during naps, visit with family, playtime, or favorite program).

Provide opportunities for play.

Reduce stimulation in environment:

- Refrain from loud talking or laughing.
- Keep equipment noise to a minimum:
  —Turn alarms as low as safely possible.
  —Perform treatments requiring equipment at one time.
  —Turn off bedside equipment that is not in use, such as suction and oxygen.
- Avoid loud, abrupt noises.

*See also Box 21-7.

---

operativeness during subsequent procedures. Other supportive measures include ensuring privacy, accepting various emotional responses to fear or pain, preserving parent-child contact, explaining all events before or as they occur, and personally remaining calm. Pain management strategies are discussed in Chapter 7.

At times, because of the child's physical condition, little or no preparatory counseling for emergency hospitalization can be done. In such situations the implementation of **postvention,** or counseling subsequent to the event, has therapeutic value. The process of postvention involves evaluating children's thoughts regarding admission and related procedures. It is similar to precounseling techniques; however, instead of supplying information, the nurse listens to the explanations offered by the child. Projective techniques such as drawing, doll play, or storytelling are especially effective. The nurse

then bases additional information on what has already been understood.

INTENSIVE CARE UNIT

Admission to an ICU can be traumatic for both the child and parents (Fig. 21-11). The nature and severity of the illness and the circumstances surrounding the admission are major factors, especially for parents. Parents experience significantly more stress when the admission is unexpected rather than expected. One study found that parental anxiety reached near panic levels initially (Huckabay and Tilem-Kessler, 1999). Stressors for the child and parent are described in Box 21-11. Although several studies have described what parents perceive as most stressful, the most effective strategy may be to simply ask parents what is stressful and implement interventions that will enhance their ability to cope (Board and Ryan-Wenger,

FIG. 21-11 ■ Parental presence during hospitalization provides emotional support for the child and increases the parent's sense of empowerment in the caregiver role. (Courtesy E. Jacob, Texas Children's Hospital, Houston.)

BOX 21-11

Neonatal or Pediatric Intensive Care Unit Stressors for the Child and Family

PHYSICAL STRESSORS

Pain and discomfort (e.g., injections, intubation, suctioning, dressing changes, other invasive procedures)
Immobility (e.g., use of restraints, bed rest)
Sleep deprivation
Inability to eat or drink
Changes in elimination habits

ENVIRONMENTAL STRESSORS

Unfamiliar surroundings (e.g., crowding)
Unfamiliar sounds

- Equipment noise (e.g., monitors, telephone, suctioning, computer printout)
- Human sounds (e.g., talking, laughing, crying, coughing, moaning, retching, walking)

Unfamiliar people (e.g., health care professionals, patients, visitors)
Unfamiliar and unpleasant smells (e.g., alcohol, adhesive remover, body odors)
Constant lights (disturb day/night rhythms)
Activity related to other patients
Sense of urgency among staff
Unkind or thoughtless comments from staff

PSYCHOLOGIC STRESSORS

Lack of privacy
Inability to communicate (if intubated)
Inadequate knowledge and understanding of situation
Severity of illness
Parental behavior (expression of concern)

SOCIAL STRESSORS

Disrupted relationships (especially with family and friends)
Concern with missing school or work
Play deprivation

Data primarily from Tichy AM, Braam CM, Meyer TA, and others: Stressors in pediatric intensive care units, *Pediatr Nurs* 14(1):40-42, 1988.

 FAMILY FOCUS

Artists as Partners in Care

A teenage boy with a rare genetic disorder, having made steady progress after awakening from a coma, relapsed and seemed very depressed. When told that a musician was visiting the pediatric intensive care unit, he immediately perked up and asked to have his room lights turned on. He whispered endless song requests to the musician. Family members and staff were treated to some of his first smiles in days; his biggest came when the musician held his hand and guided it across the guitar strings while they sang "Born to Be Wild" together at the boy's request. His dad was misty eyed as he thanked the musician for the visit.

A few weeks later the boy's condition worsened and he again lapsed into a coma. There was nothing more to be done. His parents began the necessary preparations to take their son home to die.

We continued to visit our friend and his family, offering a song, a story, or a simple hello. I hold a vivid picture of our final visit. We stood around the boy's bed with his parents singing together songs they remembered from their youth, from more carefree times. Song and laughter filled the boy's room.

Perhaps the boy heard his parents' laughter and knew then that they would be okay. He died a few days later on the morning he was to have been discharged.

Judy Rollins, MS, RN
Washington, DC

Modified from Rollins J: *Placed in our keeping,* 1995, Unpublished.

2003; Melnyk and Alpert-Gillis, 1998). Assessment should be repeated periodically to account for changes in perceptions over time.

The family's emotional needs are paramount when a child is admitted to an ICU. Although the same interventions discussed earlier for the stressors of separation and loss of control apply here, additional interventions may also benefit the family and child (see Box 21-11 and Family Focus box). In a qualitative study of 19 parents of 10 children in an ICU, parents reported that they simply wanted nurses to nurture the child in the same way the family would (Harbaugh, Tomlinson, and Kirschbaum, 2004). Nurse behaviors that exemplified caring and affection were perceived as helpful in decreasing stress. Behaviors perceived as not helpful included separating the child from the parents and communicating poorly with parents. Therefore even critical care must be centered on the family. It is important that visiting hours be liberal and flexible enough to accommodate parental needs and involvement (Hazinski, 1999).

Critically ill children become the focus of the parents' lives, and parents' most pressing need is for information (Scott, 1998). They want to know if their child will live and, if so, whether the child will be the same as before. They need to know why various interventions are being done for the child, that the child is being treated for pain or is comfortable, and that the child may be able to hear them even though not awake. When parents first visit the child in the ICU, they need preparation regarding the child's appearance. Ideally, the nurse should accompany the parents to the bedside to provide emotional support and answer any questions.

Despite the stresses normally associated with ICU admission, a special security develops from being carefully monitored and receiving individualized care. Therefore planning for transition to the regular unit is essential and should include:

- Assignment of a primary nurse on the regular unit
- Continued visits by the ICU staff to assess the child's and parents' adjustment and to act as a temporary liaison with the nursing staff
- Explanation of the differences between the two units and the rationale for the change to less intense monitoring of the child's physical condition
- Selection of an appropriate room, such as one that is close to the nursing station, and a compatible roommate

KEY POINTS

- Children are particularly vulnerable to the stressors of illness and hospitalization because stress represents a change from the usual state of health and routine and because they possess limited coping mechanisms.
- The three phases of separation anxiety are protest, despair, and detachment.
- Feelings of loss of control are caused by unfamiliar environmental stimuli, physical restriction, altered routine, and dependency.
- Fear of bodily pain may be manifested in the following ways: infants—facial expressions, body movements; toddlers—intense emotional upset, physical resistance; preschoolers—aggression, verbal expression, dependency; school-age children—precise verbalization of pain, passive requests for support or help, procrastination technique; adolescents—self-control, limited movement.
- Because of their separation from significant people, children who are hospitalized may lack the opportunity to form new attachments in the strange environment of the hospital and exhibit negative behaviors after discharge.
- Nursing care of the child in the hospital is aimed at preventing or minimizing separation, decreasing loss of control, minimizing fear of bodily injury, using play or expressive activities to lessen stress, and maximizing the potential benefits of hospitalization.
- The nurse can maximize potential benefits of hospitalization by fostering parent-child relations, providing educational opportunities, promoting self-mastery, and encouraging socialization.
- Family reactions are influenced by the seriousness of the illness, experience with illness or hospitalization and diagnostic or therapeutic procedures, available support systems, personal ego strengths, coping abilities, presence of additional stressors, cultural and religious beliefs, and family communication patterns.
- Fear of contracting illness, their younger age, a close relationship with the ill sibling, substitute child care, minimal explanation of the illness, and perceived changes in parenting all increase the deleterious effects of a brother's or sister's illness and hospitalization on siblings.
- Nursing care of the family involves listening to parents' verbal and nonverbal messages; providing clergy support; accepting cultural, socioeconomic, and ethnic values; giving information to families and siblings; and preparing for discharge and home care.
- Admission to an outpatient setting, emergency department, isolation room, or ICU requires additional intervention strategies to meet the child's and family's needs.

answers to CRITICAL THINKING EXERCISES

COMPLEMENTARY AND ALTERNATIVE MEDICINE

1. There is limited evidence to draw certain conclusions without obtaining more data from the parents. It would be appropriate to gather more information before jumping to any major conclusions at this time.

2. Assumptions:
   a. Complementary and alternative medicine (CAM) is more common in U.S. households than previously reported. Much of the concern surrounding complementary therapies, especially in children, is the lack of sufficient data regarding their effectiveness, benefit, and the potential harm that may occur as a result of such treatments. In some cases CAM therapies may counteract certain medications or the effects of prescribed therapies. It has become more common for practitioners in emergency medicine to encounter patients who are taking CAM therapy in addition to prescription medications or treatments for conditions such as eczema, asthma, colds, and upper respiratory tract problems.
   b. Folk remedies are common among certain ethnic groups and subgroups within the United States. Many are based on traditional family remedies that have been proven neither to be effective or entirely harmful in most cases. However, a few remedies could be potentially harmful, especially to children, if these remedies counteract the effects of prescribed treatments that are known to be effective.
   c. The nurse's role in such cases is to gather sufficient data from the family about the practice, discuss the treatment (CAM) in a nonjudgmental manner, and be cognizant of the effects of the treatment on the child's current health status and potential effects on other medical treatment regimens.

3. Give the family their penny and open a dialog about the traditional practice they are using. Additional information should be gathered in a nonjudgmental manner, and the discussion should center on the family's traditional beliefs regarding the practices, the prescribed medical regimen, and whether there is conflict or potential for harm. There is no need to stop the treatment unless potential harm to the child may occur. A discussion with the primary practitioner regarding the use of CAM for Maria should ensue, followed by a discussion with the entire family, if necessary. The contents of the bottle will more than likely be revealed during the discussion with the family. It is important to respect the family's wishes regarding traditional folk or CAM rituals, yet remain mindful of potential harmful effects on the child. It is not likely that telling the family to stop the ritual will be successful because these beliefs are deeply ingrained into cultural, religious, and medical practice; the family is more likely to continue the ritual at home on discharge and further disregard other instructions for care should a confrontational approach be adopted by the nursing and medical staff. The important concept for the staff and family to focus on is the ultimate well-being of the child. What you have probably observed is Santeria, the African-Caribbean religion that was brought to the New World by slaves from West Africa. It is common among immigrants from Cuba, Puerto Rico, Brazil, and Santo Domingo, and it is believed that a majority of Latin American immigrants will have contact with Santeria sometime in their lives.

4. As yet, there is insufficient evidence to indicate that harm is being done by the CAM ritual. Further data need to be gathered, and then a decision about further discussion of the CAM practice may occur.

5. There are no alternative views.

PLAYROOM AND HOSPITAL PROCEDURES

1. There is sufficient evidence regarding this incident to draw some conclusions.

2. a. Regardless of how minor a procedure such as a venipuncture may seem to an adult health care worker, it represents a major threat to a child. One must consider the child's age, illness, developmental level, and previous experiences with venipunctures.

   b. Play is an important function of childhood whether the child is sick or well. Through play children may act out fears, concerns, anger, and other behaviors they may not feel comfortable expressing to adults in a confrontational manner. Play is an important part of the hospitalized child's life, and it is a vehicle for promoting optimal development.

   c. It is important to have the blood drawn so Dr. Lung may plan a therapeutic regimen; however, one must consider another issue: there appears to have been no advance preparation of the child's skin to minimize or prevent pain from the procedure. Regardless of the phlebotomist's skill in performing the procedure, it is also important to consider the fact that the negative repercussions for performing the procedure at this point may outweigh the positive benefits.

   d. All staff on the pediatric floor must be in agreement about respecting the child's personal space in the playroom and about adhering to unit policies or rules so that respect is maintained. Failure to respect the child's space may engender fear in other children who perceive that the playroom is not a safe place after all. The fear of having other procedures performed in the playroom may prevent children from going there to participate in therapeutic and interactive play.

3. It is important to maintain a fair balance between what constitutes therapeutic management of illness and childhood recreation. It would be appropriate in this situation to intervene and ask the phlebotomist to return in 30 minutes to an hour and indicate that the child will be ready for the venipuncture in the treatment room at that time. It is important to stress that the playroom is off-limits for procedures. It would be appropriate to discuss this plan with Hannah, indicating that the procedure will be performed at the designated

time. It is also important to explore pain management issues with Hannah—does she usually use EMLA (an eutectic mix of local anesthetics) or other topical remedy to prevent pain at the site? If so, it will be necessary to make such arrangements in advance, possibly now, so her pain is managed appropriately. As the nurse, it is appropriate to discuss a delay in obtaining the laboratory results with Dr. Lung and the reasons for the delay. As workers on the pediatric floor, it is important for medical and nursing staff to communicate effectively. Should this arrangement not suit Dr. Lung's time frame for accomplishing certain tasks, one might suggest a trade-off. The nurse may draw the blood in the treatment room after preparations are made and Hannah agrees on a time. Remember, however, that school-age children are prone to "bargain" for more time to delay or prevent the event because it is painful. One must be gently firm about the agreed-on time of the procedure and not allow further delays to accommodate the child who just does not want the procedure performed—ever, in most cases.

Even if one accepts the conclusion that it is okay with Hannah, it is important to consider the possible negative implications for the other children in the room, who may be confused about even a simple procedure (e.g., checking blood pressure) or the sanctuary status of the playroom for themselves. Drawing blood in the playroom would violate the child's trust in what adult health care workers say regarding the purpose of the playroom as a sanctuary from painful procedures. Such action would likely result in less cooperation from the children who are present and may also make other parents present (or who learn about the incident) wonder about the staff's sincerity. Interrupting the children's game is not necessary because this does not represent a life-threatening condition at this time.

4. Yes, there is sufficient evidence to support these decisions and the plan of action.

5. An exception is sometimes made when all the children present are older and the procedure is a quick, painless one (e.g., checking blood pressure, giving oral medication) that all the children present have experienced. In such cases the patient and the other children are asked if it is okay and give permission before the procedure is undertaken.

REFERENCES

Ashenberg MD, Lambert SA, Maier NP, and others: Easing the wait: development of a pager program for families, *Pediatr Nurs* 22(2):103-107, 1996.

Board R, Ryan-Wenger N: Stressors and symptoms of mothers with children in the PICU, *J Pediatr Nurs* 18(3):195-201, 2003.

Bracht M, Ardal F, Bot A, and others: Initiation and maintenance of a hospital-based parent group for parents of premature infants: key factors for success, *Neonatal Netw* 17(3):33-37, 1998.

Brewer S, Lambert C: Preparing children for same day surgery: innovative approaches, *J Pediatr Nurs* 12(4):257-259, 1997.

Clatworthy S, Simon K, Tiedeman ME: Child drawing: hospital—an instrument designed to measure the emotional status of hospitalized school-aged children, *J Pediatr Nurs* 14(1):2-9, 1999.

Coyne I: Children's experiences of hospitalization, *J Child Health Care* 10(4):326-336, 2006.

Craft MJ: Siblings of hospitalized children: assessment and intervention, *J Pediatr Nurs* 8(5):289-297, 1993.

Fernandez C, Pyesmany A, Stutzer C: Alternative therapies in childhood cancer, *N Engl J Med* 340(7):569-570, 1999.

Feudtner HJ, Haney J, Dimmers MA: Spiritual care needs of hospitalized children and their families: a national survey of pastoral care providers' perceptions, *Pediatrics* 111(1):e67-e72, 2003.

Flanagan K: Preoperative assessment: safety considerations for patients taking herbal products, *J Perianesth Nurs* 16(1):19-26, 2001.

Gordon M: *Manual of nursing diagnosis*, ed 10, St Louis, 2002, Mosby.

Gordon M: *Nursing diagnosis: process and application*, ed 3, St Louis, 1994, Mosby.

Harbaugh BL, Tomlinson PS, Kirschbaum M: Parents' perceptions of nurses' caregiving behaviors in the pediatric intensive care unit, *Issues Compr Pediatr Nurs* 27(3):163-178, 2004.

Hazinski MF: *Manual of pediatric critical care*, St Louis, 1999, Mosby.

Hornick R: Discharge teams. In Gunter K, Manago R, editors: *Beyond discharge: interdisciplinary per-

spectives for transitioning children with complex medical needs from hospital to home*, Bethesda, Md, 1996, Association for the Care of Children's Health.

Huckabay LMD, Tilem-Kessler D: Patterns of parental stress in PICU emergency admission, *Dimens Crit Care Nurs* 18(2):36-42, 1999.

Lewandowski LA, Tesler MD: *Family centered care: putting it into action*, Washington, DC, 2003, American Nurses Association.

Melnyk BM: Intervention studies involving parents of hospitalized young children: an analysis of the past and future recommendations, *J Pediatr Nurs* 15(1):4-13, 2000.

Melnyk B, Alpert-Gillis L: The COPE Program: a strategy to improve outcomes of critically ill young children and their parents, *Pediatr Nurs* 24(6):521-527, 1998.

Orem D: *Nursing: concepts of practice*, ed 5, New York, 2001, Mosby.

Scott LD: Perceived needs of parents of critically ill children, *J Soc Pediatr Nurs* 3(1):4-12, 1998.

Small L: Early predictors of poor coping outcomes in children following intensive care hospitalization and stressful medical encounters, *Pediatr Nurs* 28(4):393-401, 2002.

Smith T, Conant Rees HL: Making family-centered care a reality, *Semin Nurs Manage* 8(3):136-142, 2000.

Stewart E, Algren C, Arnold S: Preparing children for a surgical experience, *Today's OR Nurse* 16(2):9-14, 1994.

Stranton KM: Parents' experiences of their child's care during hospitalization, *J Cult Divers* 11(1):4-11, 2004.

The Joint Commission on Accreditation of Healthcare Organizations: *AMH92 accreditation manual for hospitals,* Chicago, 2004, The Commission.

Woodgate R, Kristjanson L: "Getting better from my hurts": toward a model of the young child's pain experience, *J Pediatr Nurs* 11(4):233-242, 1996.

22

Pediatric Variations of Nursing Interventions

TERRI L. BROWN

CHAPTER OUTLINE

GENERAL CONCEPTS RELATED TO PEDIATRIC PROCEDURES, 687
Informed Consent, 687
  Requirements for Obtaining Informed Consent, 687
  Eligibility for Giving Informed Consent, 689
Preparation for Diagnostic and Therapeutic Procedures, 689
  Psychologic Preparation, 689
  Performance of the Procedure, 693
  Postprocedural Support, 694
  Use of Play in Procedures, 694
Surgical Procedures, 694
  Preoperative Care, 694
  Postoperative Care, 697
Compliance, 698
  Compliance Strategies, 699
GENERAL HYGIENE AND CARE, 700
Maintaining Healthy Skin, 700
Bathing, 701
Oral Hygiene, 701
Hair Care, 702
Feeding the Sick Child, 702
Controlling Elevated Temperatures, 702
  Fever, 703
  Hyperthermia, 704
Family Teaching and Home Care, 704
SAFETY, 705
Environmental Factors, 705
  Toy Safety, 705
  Preventing Falls, 706
Infection Control, 706
Transporting Infants and Children, 708
Restraining Methods and Therapeutic Holding, 708
  Jacket Restraint, 709
  Mummy Restraint or Swaddle, 709

Arm and Leg Restraints, 709
Elbow Restraint, 710
Positioning for Procedures, 710
  Femoral Venipuncture, 710
  Extremity Venipuncture, 710
  Lumbar Puncture, 710
  Bone Marrow Aspiration or Biopsy, 711
COLLECTION OF SPECIMENS, 711
Urine Specimens, 711
  Clean-Catch Specimens, 712
  Twenty-Four-Hour Collection, 712
  Bladder Catheterization and Other Techniques, 713
Stool Specimens, 715
Blood Specimens, 715
Respiratory Secretion Specimens, 717
ADMINISTRATION OF MEDICATION, 717
Determination of Drug Dosage, 717
  Checking Dosage, 718
  Identification, 718
Oral Administration, 718
  Preparation, 718
  Administration, 719
Intramuscular Administration, 719
  Selecting the Syringe and Needle, 719
  Determining the Site, 720
  Administration, 720
Subcutaneous and Intradermal Administration, 723
Intravenous Administration, 725
  Peripheral Intermittent Infusion Device, 725
  Central Venous Access Device, 725
Nasogastric, Orogastric, or Gastrostomy Administration, 730
Rectal Administration, 730
Optic, Otic, and Nasal Administration, 730
Family Teaching and Home Care, 731

MAINTAINING FLUID BALANCE, 732
Measurement of Intake and Output, 732
  Special Needs When the Child Is NPO, 732
Parenteral Fluid Therapy, 733
  Site and Equipment, 733
  Safety Catheters and Needleless Systems, 734
  Infusion Pumps, 735
  Securement of a Peripheral Intravenous Line, 735
  Removal of a Peripheral Intravenous Line, 737
  Complications, 738
PROCEDURES FOR MAINTAINING RESPIRATORY FUNCTION, 738
Inhalation Therapy, 738
  Oxygen Therapy, 738
  Monitoring Oxygen Therapy, 739
  Aerosol Therapy, 740
Bronchial (Postural) Drainage, 741
Chest Physical Therapy, 741
Artificial Ventilation, 741
  Artificial Airways, 741
  Tracheostomy, 741
PROCEDURES RELATED TO ALTERNATIVE FEEDING TECHNIQUES, 745
Gavage Feeding, 745
Gastrostomy Feeding, 746
Nasoduodenal and Nasojejunal Tubes, 749
Total Parenteral Nutrition, 749
Family Teaching and Home Care, 750
PROCEDURES RELATED TO ELIMINATION, 750
Enema, 750
Ostomies, 750
Family Teaching and Home Care, 751

LEARNING OBJECTIVES

On completion of this chapter the reader will be able to:

- Identify those instances in which informed consent is required and in which minors may be considered emancipated.
- Formulate general guidelines for preparing children for procedures, including surgery.
- Implement play in therapeutic procedures.
- List general strategies for enhancing compliance in children and families.

- Outline general hygiene and care procedures for hospitalized children.
- Implement feeding techniques that encourage food and fluid intake.
- Describe methods of reducing temperature of child with fever or hyperthermia.
- Describe systems that can be used for infection control.
- Describe safe methods of administering oral, parenteral, rectal, optic, otic, and nasal medications to children.

- Identify nursing responsibilities in maintaining fluid balance.
- Demonstrate correct procedures for postural drainage and tracheostomy care.
- Describe the procedures involved in providing nutrition via gavage, gastrostomy, and parenteral routes.
- Describe the procedures involved in administering an enema and ostomy care to children.

RELATED TOPICS and ADDITIONAL RESOURCES

 IN TEXT

Communicating with Families, *Ch. 6*
Dental Health: Infant, *Ch. 10;* Toddler, *Ch. 12;* Preschooler, *Ch. 13;* School-Age Child, *Ch. 15;* Adolescent, *Ch. 16*
Family-Centered Home Care, *Ch. 20*
Febrile Seizures, *Ch. 28*
Feeding Resistance, *Ch. 9*
Injury Prevention: Infant, *Ch. 10;* Toddler, *Ch. 12;* Preschooler, *Ch. 13;* School-Age Child, *Ch. 15;* Adolescent, *Ch. 16*
Limit Setting and Discipline, *Ch. 3*
Nutritional Assessment, *Ch. 6*
Pain Assessment and Management in Children, *Ch. 7*
Preparation for Hospitalization, *Ch. 21*
Providing Opportunities for Play and Expressive Activities, *Ch. 21*
Spina Bifida (Myelomeningocele), *Ch. 32*
Temperature (Measurement), *Ch. 6*
Wounds, *Ch. 30*

 COMPANION CD

Animations—Central Venous Access via Femoral Vein; Central Venous Access via Jugular Vein; Foley Catheter Insertion; IV Line Placement; Lumbar Puncture, Infant; PICC Line Placement
Case Study—Pediatric Procedures
Critical Thinking Exercise—Central Venous Access Device
NCLEX Review Questions

evolve
evolve.elsevier.com/Wong/essentials/
NCLEX Review Questions
Nursing Care Plans—The Child Undergoing Surgery; The Child with Elevated Body Temperature
Skills—Preparing the Child for Procedures; Administering Oral Medications; Urine Specimen Collection; Measuring Oxygen Saturation
WebLinks

 WONG'S CLINICAL MANUAL OF PEDIATRIC NURSING, 7th Ed

Patient and Family Education—Measuring Your Child's Temperature, *p. 508;* Giving Medications to Children, *p. 522;* Obtaining a Urine Sample, *p. 514;* Giving Subcutaneous (Sub Q) Injections, *p. 527;* Giving Intramuscular (IM) Injections, *p. 525;* Caring for an Intermittent Infusion Device, *p. 531;* Caring for a Central Venous Catheter, *p. 533;* Performing Postural Drainage, *p. 567;* Giving an Enema, *p. 558;* Giving Gastrostomy Feedings, *p. 551;* Caring for the Child with a Colostomy, *p. 557;* Caring for the Child with a Tracheostomy, *p. 570;* Child Cardiopulmonary Resuscitation for the Layperson, *p. 578*

GENERAL CONCEPTS RELATED TO PEDIATRIC PROCEDURES

INFORMED CONSENT

Before undergoing any invasive procedure, the patient or the patient's legal surrogate must receive sufficient information on which to make an informed health care decision. **Informed consent** should include the expected care or treatment, potential risks, benefits, alternatives, and what might happen if the patient chooses not to consent. To obtain valid informed consent, the following three conditions must be met:

1. The person must be capable of giving consent; he or she must be over the age of majority (usually age 18) and must be considered competent (i.e., possessing the mental capacity to make choices and understand their consequences).

2. The person must receive the information needed to make an intelligent decision.
3. The person must act voluntarily when exercising freedom of choice without force, fraud, deceit, duress, or other forms of constraint or coercion.

The patient has the right to accept or refuse any health care. If the patient is treated without consent, the hospital or health care provider may be charged with assault and held liable for damages.

Requirements for Obtaining Informed Consent

Written informed consent of the parent or legal guardian is usually required for medical or surgical treatment, including many diagnostic procedures. One universal consent is not sufficient. Separate informed permissions must be obtained for each surgical or diagnostic procedure, including major or minor surgery, diagnostic tests with an element of risk (e.g., bronchoscopy), and medical treatments with an element of risk (e.g., blood transfusion, radiotherapy).

Other situations that require parental consent include:

■ Photographs for medical, educational, or public use
■ Removal of the child from the health care institution against medical advice
■ Postmortem examinations, except in unexplained deaths, such as sudden infant death, violent death, or suicide
■ Release of medical information

Decision making involving the care of older children and adolescents should include, to the extent feasible, the patient's **assent** as well as that of the parents (see Evidence-Based Practice box). Assent means the child or adolescent has been informed about what will happen during the treatment or procedure and is willing to permit a health care provider to perform it. Assent should include the following elements:

■ Helping the patient achieve a developmentally appropriate awareness of the nature of his or her condition
■ Telling the patient what he or she can expect
■ Making a clinical assessment of the patient's understanding
■ Soliciting an expression of the patient's willingness to accept the proposed procedure of care

EVIDENCE-BASED PRACTICE

Informed Consent and Assent in Children
Janet DeJean

ASK THE QUESTION	At what age should children be able to participate in the informed consent or assent process?

SEARCH FOR EVIDENCE

Search Strategies	Search selection criteria included English-language publications within the past 10 years and research-based articles on informed consent and assent in children receiving medical treatment.
Databases Used	Cochrane Collaboration, Joanna Briggs Institute, PubMed, MD Consult

CRITICALLY ANALYZE THE EVIDENCE

There are numerous opinions on when and how a child should be involved in the medical decision-making process. The determining factor is the child's developmental readiness and the medical procedure involved.

The American Academy of Pediatrics' (1995) position is that patients should participate in decision making commensurate with their development. No specific minimum age for a child is identified.

The Children's Oncology Group (2005) states that in clinical research trials for cancer treatment, a child needs to be at least 9 years of age before he or she would have the ability to understand research-related information.

Two research studies evaluated the understanding of assent. Each recommended a different age of understanding:

1. Ondrusek, Abramovitch, Pencharz, and others (1998) found that in subjects younger than 9 years, understanding of most aspects of a clinical nutrition study involving a nontherapeutic blood sample was poor to nonexistent.
2. Tait, Voepel-Lewis, and Malviya (2003) found children ages 11 years and older had significantly greater understanding of the study protocol, benefits, and freedom to withdraw from a clinical anesthesia or surgical study.

Wendler (2006) suggests that children are capable of assent when they become able to understand the research in question at approximately 14 years of age. Assent is not required when the prospect of direct benefit of treatment is available only within the context of research. Sustained dissent should be respected in all cases.

Two research studies were found examining institutional review board (IRB) practices of determining when assent should be attained. All of the IRBs in these two studies support obtaining assent for children before clinical trials.

1. Kimberly, Hoehn, Feudtner, and others (2006) compared 55 different IRBs across the United States. The majority of the IRBs (83%) included methods for documenting assent, whereas only 45% identified specific age ranges for obtaining assent. The ages ranged from 7 to 18 years.

2. Whittle, Shah, Wilfond, and others (2004) interviewed 188 chairpersons of IRBs nationwide. Half the IRBs had a method, most commonly an age cutoff, they required investigators to follow in determining which children are capable of assent.

APPLY THE EVIDENCE: NURSING IMPLICATIONS

■ Children should be assessed for understanding and ability to participate in the assent process.
■ The age for assent ranged from 7 to 14 years in numerous published articles on obtaining assent in children.
■ The complex nature of some research studies and interventions may preclude children younger than 7, 9, 11, or 14 years of age from complete understanding.
■ Assent should not be sought when the prospect of direct treatment benefit is available only within the context of research.
■ Sustained dissent should be respected.
■ Consent should be obtained at the age of 18 years.

References

American Academy of Pediatrics Committee on Bioethics: Informed consent, parental permission, and assent in pediatric practice, *Pediatrics* 95(2):314-317, 1995.
Children's Oncology Group: *Guidelines for involving children in decision-making about research participation*, 2005, retrieved Aug 21, 2006, from http://www.childrensoncologygroup.org.
Kimberly M, Hoehn K, Feudtner C, and others: Variation in standards of research compensation and child assent practices: a comparison of 69 institutional review board–approved informed permission and assent forms for three multicenter pediatric clinical trials, *Pediatrics* 117:1706-1711, 2006.
Ondrusek N, Abramovitch R, Pencharz P, and others: Empirical examination of the ability of children to consent to clinical research, *J Med Ethics* 24(3):158-165, 1998.
Tait A, Voepel-Lewis T, Malviya S: Do they understand? part II, Assent of children participating in clinical anesthesia and surgery research, *Anesthesiology* 98(3):609-614, 2003.
Wendler D: Assent in paediatric research: theoretical and practical considerations, *J Med Ethics* 32(4):229-234, 2006.
Whittle A, Shah S, Wilfond B, and others: Institutional review board practices regarding assent in pediatric research, *Pediatrics* 113(6):1747-1752, 2004.

Multiple methods should be used to provide information, including age-appropriate methods (e.g., videotapes, peer discussion, diagrams, and written materials). An assent form should be provided to each child to sign, and the child should keep a copy (Broome, 1999). By including children in the decision-making process and gaining their acceptance, staff members demonstrate respect for the child. Assent is not a legal requirement but an ethical one to protect the rights of children.

Eligibility for Giving Informed Consent

Informed Consent of Parents or Legal Guardians. Parents have full responsibility for the care and rearing of their minor children, including legal control over them. As long as children are minors, their parents or legal guardians are required to give informed consent before medical treatment is rendered or any procedure is performed. If parents are married to each other, consent from only one parent is required for nonurgent pediatric care. If the parents are divorced, consent usually rests with the parent who has legal custody (Berger and AAP Committee on Medical Liability, 2003). Parents also have a right to withdraw consent at any time.

Evidence of Consent. Obtaining informed consent varies from state to state, and policies differ at each health care facility. It is the physician's responsibility to explain the procedure, risks, benefits, and alternatives. The nurse witnesses the patient's, parent's, or legal guardian's signature on the consent form and may reinforce what the patient has been told. A signed consent form is the legal document that signifies that the process of informed consent has occurred. If parents are unavailable to sign consent forms, verbal consent may be obtained via the telephone in the presence of two witnesses. Both witnesses record that informed consent was given and by whom. Their signatures indicate that they witnessed the verbal consent.

Informed Consent of Mature and Emancipated Minors. State laws differ with regard to the so-called **age of majority,** the age at which a person is considered to have all the legal rights and responsibilities of an adult. In most states, 18 is the age of majority. Competent adults can give informed consent on their own behalf. An **emancipated minor** is one who is legally under the age of majority but is recognized as having the legal capacity of an adult under circumstances prescribed by state law, such as pregnancy, marriage, high school graduation, living independently, or military service.

Treatment Without Parental Consent. Exceptions to requiring parental consent before treating minor children occur when children need urgent medical or surgical treatment and a parent is not readily available or refuses to give consent. For example, a child may be brought to an emergency department accompanied by a grandparent, child care provider, teacher, or others. In the absence of parents or legal guardians, persons in charge of the child may be given permission by the parents to give informed consent by proxy. In emergencies, including danger to life or the possibility of permanent injury, appropriate care should not be withheld or delayed because of problems obtaining consent (Berger and AAP Committee on Medical Liability, 2003; American Academy of Pediatrics, 2003). Efforts made to obtain consent should be documented.

Refusal to give consent can occur when the treatment, such as blood transfusions, conflicts with the parents' religious beliefs. All states recognize such exceptions and have statutory procedures to permit treatment if the life or health of such a minor is in jeopardy or if delayed treatment would create a risk to the minor's health. In most states evaluation for child abuse or neglect can occur without parental consent and without notification of the state prior to evaluation.

Adolescents, Consent, and Confidentiality. The Health Insurance Portability and Accountability Act of 1996 (HIPAA) was passed to help protect and safeguard the security and confidentiality of a person's health information. Because adolescents are not yet adults, parents have the right to make most decisions on their behalf and receive information. Adolescents, however, are more likely to seek care in a setting in which they believe their privacy will be maintained. All 50 states have enacted legislation that entitles adolescents to consent to treatment without their parents' knowledge for one or more "medically emancipated" conditions, such as sexually transmitted infections, alcohol and drug abuse, and need for contraceptive advice (Anderson, Schaechter, and Brosco, 2005; Tillett, 2005). Consent to abortion is controversial, and statutes vary widely by state. State law preempts HIPAA regardless of whether that law prohibits, mandates, or allows discretion about a disclosure.

Informed Consent and Parental Right to the Child's Medical Chart. Some state statutes give parents the unrestricted right to a copy of children's medical records. In states without statutes, the best practice is to allow parents to review or have a copy of minors' charts under reasonable circumstances. Practitioners should avoid restrictive requirements such as review permitted only in the presence of a clinician. Rather, an appropriate practitioner should be available to answer any questions that parents may have during reviews.

PREPARATION FOR DIAGNOSTIC AND THERAPEUTIC PROCEDURES

Technologic advances and changes in health care have resulted in more pediatric procedures being performed in a variety of settings. Many procedures are both stressful and painful experiences. For most procedures the focus of care is psychologic preparation of the child and family. However, some procedures require the administration of sedatives or analgesics.

Psychologic Preparation

Preparing children for procedures decreases their anxiety, promotes their cooperation, supports their coping skills and may teach them new ones, and facilitates a feeling of mastery in experiencing a potentially stressful event. Many institutions have developed preadmission teaching programs designed to educate the pediatric patient and family by offering hands-on experience with hospital equipment, information about the procedure to be performed, and an overview of departments they may visit (Algren, Ireland, and Stewart, 1998). Preparatory methods may be formal, such as group preparation for hospitalization. Most preparation strategies used by nurses are informal, focus on providing information about the experience, and are directed at stressful or painful procedures. The most effective preparation includes providing sensory-procedural information and helping the child develop coping skills, such as imagery, distraction, or relaxation (Broome, Rehwaldt, and Fogg, 1998).

General guidelines for preparing children for procedures are described in Box 22-1, and age-specific guidelines that consider children's developmental needs and cognitive abili-

BOX 22-1
General Guidelines for Preparing Children for Procedures

- Determine details of exact procedure to be performed.
- Review parents' and child's present understanding.
- Base teaching on developmental age and existing knowledge.
- Incorporate parents in the teaching if they desire, especially if they plan to participate in care.
- Inform parents of their supportive role during procedure, such as standing near child's head or in child's line of vision and talking softly to child.
- Allow for ample discussion to prevent information overload and ensure adequate feedback.
- Use concrete, not abstract, terms and visual aids to describe procedure. For example, use a simple line drawing of a boy or girl and mark the body part that will be involved in the procedure. Use nonthreatening but realistic models.*
- Emphasize that no other body part will be involved.
- If the body part is associated with a specific function, stress the change in or noninvolvement of that ability (e.g., after tonsillectomy, child can still speak).

- Use words appropriate to child's level of understanding.
- Avoid words and phrases with dual meanings (see Nursing Care Guidelines box, p. 693) unless child understands such words.
- Clarify all unfamiliar words (e.g., "Anesthesia is a *special* sleep").
- Emphasize sensory aspects of procedure—what child will feel, see, hear, smell, and touch and what child can do during procedure (e.g., lie still, count out loud, squeeze a hand, hug a doll).
- Allow child to practice procedures that require cooperation (e.g., turning, deep breathing, incentive spirometry).
- Introduce anxiety-laden information last (e.g., starting an intravenous line).
- Be honest with child about unpleasant aspects of a procedure but avoid creating undue concern. When discussing that a procedure may be uncomfortable, state that it feels differently to different people.
- Emphasize end of procedure and any pleasurable events afterward (e.g., going home, seeing parents).
- Stress positive benefits of procedure (e.g., "After your tonsils are fixed, you won't have as many sore throats").

*Soft-sculptured dolls and customized adapters and overlays for preparing children and families about procedures and as teaching models for technical care are available from Legacy Products, Inc., 508 Green St., Cambridge City, IN 47327; (800) 238-7951; e-mail: info@legacyproductsinc.com; http://www.legacyproductsinc.com.

ties are presented in Box 22-2. In addition to these suggestions, nurses should consider the child's temperament, existing coping strategies, and previous experiences. Children who are distractible and highly active, as well as those who are "slow to warm up," may need individualized sessions that are shorter for the active child but more slowly paced for the shy child. Youngsters who tend to cope well may need more emphasis on using their present skills, whereas those who appear to cope less adequately can benefit from more time devoted to simple coping strategies, such as relaxing, breathing, counting, squeezing a hand, or singing.

NURSINGTIP

Prepare a basket, toy chest, or cart to keep near the treatment area. Items ideal for the basket include a Slinky; a sparkling "magic" wand (sealed acrylic tube partially filled with liquid and suspended metallic confetti); a soft foam ball; bubble solution; party blowers; pop-up books with foldout, three-dimensional scenes; real medical equipment, such as a syringe, adhesive bandages, and alcohol packets; toy medical supplies or a toy medical kit; marking pens; a notepad; and stickers. Have the child choose an item to help distract and relax during a procedure. After the procedure, allow the child to choose a small gift, such as a sticker, or to play with items, such as medical equipment.

Children differ in their "information-seeking dimension." Some actively solicit information about the intended procedure, whereas others avoid information. Parents can often guide nurses in deciding how much information is enough, since parents know whether the child is typically inquisitive or satisfied with short answers. Asking older children their preferences about the amount of explanation is also important. Drawings may also be helpful in preparing children for procedures.

The exact timing of the preparation for a procedure varies with the child's age and type of procedure. No exact guidelines govern timing, but in general the younger the child, the closer the explanation should be to the actual procedure to prevent undue fantasizing and worrying. With complex procedures, more time may be needed for assimilation of information, especially with older children. For example, the explanation for an injection can immediately precede the procedure for all ages, whereas preparation for surgery may begin the day before for young children and a few days before for older children (although older children's preferences should be elicited).

Establish Trust and Provide Support. The nurse who has spent time with and established a positive relationship with a child will usually find it easier to gain cooperation. If the relationship is based on trust, the child will associate the nurse with caregiving activities that give comfort and pleasure most of the time rather than discomfort and stress. If the nurse does not know the child, it is best to be introduced by another staff person whom the child trusts. The first visit with the child should not include any painful procedure and ideally should focus on the child first, then on the explanation of the procedure.

Parental Presence and Support. Children need support during procedures, and for young children the greatest source of support is the parents. They represent security, safety, and comfort. Controversy exists regarding the role parents should assume during the procedure, especially if discomfort is involved. Parental presence is preferable, however, since it can reduce patient and parent anxiety and decrease the need for sedation (Nelson, 1999). The nurse should assess the parents' preferences for assisting, observing, or waiting outside the room, as well as the child's preference for parental presence. The child's and parents' choice should be respected. Parents who wish to stay should be given appropriate explanation about the procedure and coached about what to do, where to sit or stand, and what to say to help the child through the procedure. Simple instructions such as clarifying where parents can stand or sit in the room and positioning them

BOX 22-2

Age-Specific Preparation of Children for Procedures Based on Developmental Characteristics

INFANT: DEVELOPING A SENSE OF TRUST AND SENSORIMOTOR THOUGHT

Attachment to Parent
Involve parent in procedure if desired.*
Keep parent in infant's line of vision.
If parent is unable to be with infant, place familiar object with infant (e.g., stuffed toy).

Stranger Anxiety
Have usual caregivers perform or assist with procedure.*
Make advances slowly and in nonthreatening manner.
Limit number of strangers entering room during procedure.*

Sensorimotor Phase of Learning
During procedure use sensory soothing measures (e.g., stroking skin, talking softly, giving pacifier).
Use analgesics (e.g., topical anesthetic, intravenous opioid) to control discomfort.*
Cuddle and hug infant after stressful procedure; encourage parent to comfort infant.

Increased Muscle Control
Expect older infant to resist.
Immobilize adequately.
Keep harmful objects out of reach.

Memory for Past Experiences
Realize that older infants may associate objects, places, or persons with prior painful experiences and will cry and resist at the sight of them.
Keep frightening objects out of view.*
Perform painful procedures in a separate room, not in crib (or bed).*
Use nonintrusive procedures whenever possible (e.g., axillary temperatures, oral medications).*

Imitation of Gestures
Model desired behavior (e.g., opening mouth).

TODDLER: DEVELOPING A SENSE OF AUTONOMY AND SENSORIMOTOR TO PREOPERATIONAL THOUGHT
Use same approaches as for infant plus the following.

Egocentric Thought
Explain procedure in relation to what child will see, hear, taste, smell, and feel.
Emphasize those aspects of procedure that require cooperation (e.g., lying still).
Tell child it is okay to cry, yell, or use other means to express discomfort verbally.

Negative Behavior
Expect treatments to be resisted; child may try to run away.
Use firm, direct approach.
Ignore temper tantrums.
Use distraction techniques (e.g., singing a song *with* a child).
Restrain adequately.

Animism
Keep frightening objects out of view (young children believe objects have lifelike qualities and can harm them).

Limited Language Skills
Communicate using behaviors.
Use a few, simple terms familiar to child.
Give one direction at a time (e.g., "Lie down," then "Hold my hand").
Use small replicas of equipment; allow child to handle equipment.
Use play; demonstrate on doll but avoid child's favorite doll, since child may think doll is really "feeling" procedure.
Prepare parents separately to avoid child's misinterpreting words.

Limited Concept of Time
Prepare child shortly or immediately before procedure.
Keep teaching sessions short (about 5 to 10 minutes).
Have preparations completed before involving child in procedure.
Have extra equipment nearby (e.g., alcohol swabs, new needle, adhesive bandages) to avoid delays.
Tell child when procedure is completed.

Striving for Independence
Allow choices whenever possible; child may still be resistant and negative.
Allow child to participate in care and to help whenever possible (e.g., drink medicine from a cup, hold a dressing).

PRESCHOOLER: DEVELOPING INITIATIVE AND PREOPERATIONAL THOUGHT

Egocentric
Explain procedure in simple terms and in relation to how it affects child (as with toddler, stress sensory aspects).
Demonstrate use of equipment.
Allow child to play with miniature or actual equipment.
Encourage "playing out" experience on a doll both before and after procedure to clarify misconceptions.
Use neutral words to describe the procedure (see Nursing Care Guidelines box, p. 693).

Increased Language Skills
Use verbal explanation; avoid overestimating comprehension.
Encourage child to verbalize ideas and feelings.

Limited Concept of Time and Frustration Tolerance
Implement same approaches as for toddler but may plan longer teaching session (10 to 15 minutes); may divide information into more than one session.

Illness and Hospitalization Viewed as Punishment
Clarify why each procedure is performed; a child will find it difficult to understand how medicine can make him or her feel better and can taste bad at the same time.
Ask child thoughts regarding why a procedure is performed.
State directly that procedures are never a form of punishment.

*Applies to any age.

Continued

BOX 22-2

Age-Specific Preparation of Children for Procedures Based on Developmental Characteristics—cont'd

PRESCHOOLER: DEVELOPING INITIATIVE AND PREOPERATIONAL THOUGHT—cont'd

Animism
Keep equipment out of sight, except when shown to or used on child.

Fears of Bodily Harm, Intrusion, and Castration
Point out on drawing, doll, or child where procedure is performed.
Emphasize that no other body part will be involved.
Use nonintrusive procedures whenever possible (e.g., axillary temperature, oral medication).
Apply an adhesive bandage over puncture site.
Encourage parental presence.
Realize that procedures involving genitalia provoke anxiety.
Allow child to wear underpants with gown.
Explain unfamiliar situations, especially noises or lights.

Striving for Initiative
Involve child in care whenever possible (e.g., hold equipment, remove dressing).
Give choices whenever possible but avoid excessive delays.
Praise child for helping and attempting to cooperate; never shame child for lack of cooperation.

SCHOOL-AGE CHILD: DEVELOPING INDUSTRY AND CONCRETE THOUGHT

Increased Language Skills; Interest in Acquiring Knowledge
Explain procedures using correct scientific or medical terminology.
Explain reason for procedure using simple diagrams.
Explain function and operation of equipment in concrete terms.
Allow child to manipulate equipment; use doll or another person as model to practice using equipment whenever possible (doll play may be considered childish by older school-age child).
Allow time before and after procedure for questions and discussion.

Improved Concept of Time
Plan for longer teaching sessions (about 20 minutes).
Prepare before procedure.

Increased Self-Control
Gain child's cooperation.
Tell child what is expected.
Suggest ways of maintaining control (e.g., deep breathing, relaxation, counting).

Striving for Industry
Allow responsibility for simple tasks (e.g., collecting specimens).
Include child in decision making (e.g., time of day to perform procedure, preferred site).
Encourage active participation (e.g., removing dressings, handling equipment, opening packages).

Developing Relationships with Peers
Prepare two or more children for same procedure or encourage one peer to help prepare another.
Provide privacy from peers during procedure to maintain self-esteem.

ADOLESCENT: DEVELOPING IDENTITY AND ABSTRACT THOUGHT

Increasing Abstract Thought and Reasoning
Supplement explanations with reasons why procedure is necessary or beneficial.
Explain long-term consequences of procedures.
Realize adolescent may fear death, disability, or other risks.
Encourage questioning regarding fears, options, and alternatives.

Conscious of Appearance
Provide privacy.
Discuss how procedure may affect appearance (e.g., scar) and what can be done to minimize it.
Emphasize any physical benefits of procedure.

Concerned More with Present Than with Future
Realize that immediate effects of procedure are more significant than future benefits.

Striving for Independence
Involve in decision making and planning (e.g., time, place, individuals present during procedure, clothing).
Impose as few restrictions as possible.
Suggest methods of maintaining control.
Accept regression to more childish methods of coping.
Realize that adolescent may have difficulty accepting new authority figures and may resist complying with procedures.

Developing Peer Relationships and Group Identity
Same as for school-age child but assumes greater significance.
Allow adolescents to talk with other adolescents who have had same procedure.

---

where they have eye contact with the child provide support and lessen anxiety. Parents who do not want to be present or participate are supported in their decision and encouraged to remain close by so that they can be available to console the child immediately after the procedure. Parents should also know that someone will be with their child to provide support. Ideally, this person should inform the parents after the procedure about how the child did.

Provide an Explanation. Age-appropriate explanations are one of the most widely used interventions for reducing anxiety in children undergoing procedures. Before performing a procedure, explain what is to be done and what is expected of the child. The explanation should be short, simple, and appropriate to the child's level of comprehension. Long

explanations may increase anxiety in a young child. When explaining the procedure to parents with the child present, the nurse uses language appropriate to the child because unfamiliar words can be misunderstood (see Nursing Care Guidelines box). If the parents need additional preparation, this is done in an area away from the child. Teaching sessions are planned at times most conducive to the child's learning (e.g., after a rest period) and for the usual span of attention.

Special equipment is not necessary for preparing a child, but for young children who cannot yet think in concepts, using objects to supplement verbal explanation is important. Allowing children to handle actual items that will be used in their care, such as a stethoscope, sphygmomanometer, or oxygen mask, helps them develop familiarity with these

nursingcareguidelines

Selecting Nonthreatening Words or Phrases

Words and Phrases to Avoid	Suggested Substitutions
Shot, bee sting, stick	Medicine under the skin
Organ	Special place in body
Test	See how (specify body part) is working
Incision	Special opening
Edema	Puffiness
Stretcher, gurney	Rolling bed
Stool	Child's usual term
Dye	Special medicine
Pain	Hurt, discomfort, "owie," "boo-boo"
Deaden	Numb, make sleepy
Cut, fix	Make better
Take, as in "take your temperature"	See how warm you are
Take, as in "take your arm blood pressure"	Check your pressure; hug your arm
Put to sleep, anesthesia	Special sleep
Catheter	Tube
Monitor	Television screen
Electrodes	Stickers, ticklers
Specimen	Sample

items and reduces the threat often associated with their use. Miniature versions of hospital items such as gurneys and x-ray and intravenous (IV) equipment can be used to explain what the children can expect and permit them to safely experience situations that are unfamiliar and potentially frightening. Written and illustrated materials are also valuable aids to preparation.*

> **NURSINGTIP**
>
> Use photographs of children in different areas of the hospital (e.g., radiology department, operating room) to give children a more realistic idea of equipment they may encounter.

Physical Preparation. One area of special concern is the administration of sedation and analgesia before stressful procedures. Refer to Chapter 7 for information on sedating children.

Performance of the Procedure

Supportive care continues during the procedure and can be a major factor in a child's ability to cooperate. Ideally, the same nurse who explains the procedure should perform or assist with the procedure. Before beginning, all equipment is assembled and the room is readied to prevent unnecessary delays and interruptions that increase the child's anxiety.

*Preparatory materials include *Going to the Hospital* and *Going to the Doctor*, available from Family Communications, Inc., 4802 Fifth Ave., Pittsburgh, PA 15213; (412) 687-2990; http://www.fci.org; *Hospital Friends*, available from the Centering Corporation, 7230 Maple St., Omaha, NE 68134; (866) 218-0101. Other resources include *Berenstein Bears Go to the Doctor* and *Berenstein Bears Visit the Dentist* (New York, Random House), available in most bookstores.

> **NURSINGTIP**
>
> To avoid a delay during a procedure, have extra supplies handy. For example, have tape, bandages, alcohol swabs, and an extra needle when performing an injection or venipuncture.

If possible, procedures should be performed in a special treatment room rather than the child's hospital room. Traumatic procedures should never be performed in "safe" areas, such as the playroom. If the procedure is lengthy, avoid conversation that could be misinterpreted by the child. As the procedure is nearing completion, inform the child that it is almost over in language the child understands.

Expect Success. Nurses who approach children with confidence and who convey the impression that they expect to be successful are less likely to encounter difficulty. It is best to approach a child as though cooperation is expected. Children sense anxiety and uncertainty in an adult and respond by striking out or actively resisting. Although it is not possible to eliminate such behavior in every child, a firm approach with a positive attitude tends to convey a feeling of security to most children.

Involve the Child. Involving children helps to gain their cooperation. Permitting choices gives them some measure of control. However, a choice is given only in situations in which one is available. Asking children, "Do you want to take your medicine now?" leads them to believe they have an option and provides them with the opportunity to legitimately refuse or delay the medication. This places the nurse in an awkward, if not impossible, position. It is much better to state firmly, "It's time to drink your medicine now." Children usually like to make choices, but the choice must be one that they do indeed have (e.g., "It's time for your medicine. Do you want to drink it plain or with a little water?").

Many children respond to tactics that appeal to their maturity or courage. This also gives them a sense of participation and achievement. For example, preschool children will be proud that they can hold the dressing during the procedure or remove the tape. The same is true for the school-age child, who often cooperates with minimal resistance.

Provide Distraction. Distraction is a powerful coping strategy during painful procedures (Algren and Algren, 1997). It is accomplished by focusing the child's attention on something other than the procedure. Singing favorite songs, listening to music, counting aloud, or blowing bubbles to "blow the hurt away" are effective techniques.

> **NURSINGTIP**
>
> Help the child select and practice a coping technique before the procedure. Consider having the parent or some other supportive person, such as a child life specialist, "coach" the child in learning and using the coping skill.

For other nonpharmacologic interventions that may lessen discomfort, see Pain Management, Chapter 7.

Allow Expression of Feelings. The child should be allowed to express feelings of anger, anxiety, fear, frustration, or any other emotion. It is natural for children to strike out in frustration or to try to avoid stress-provoking situations. The child needs to know that it is all right to cry. Behavior is children's primary means of communication and coping and

FIG. 22-1 ■ Playing with hospital equipment provides children with the opportunity to play out fears and concerns.

should be permitted unless it inflicts harm on them or those caring for them.

Postprocedural Support

After the procedure, the child continues to need reassurance that he or she performed well and is accepted and loved. If the parents did not participate, the child is united with them as soon as possible so that they can provide comfort.

Encourage Expression of Feelings. Planned activity after the procedure is helpful in encouraging constructive expression of feelings. For verbal children, reviewing the details of the procedure can clarify misconceptions and garner feedback for improving the nurse's preparatory strategies. Play is an excellent activity for all children. Infants and young children are given the opportunity for gross motor movement. Older children are able to vent their anger and frustration in acceptable pounding or throwing activities. Play-Doh is a remarkably versatile medium for pounding and shaping. Dramatic play provides an outlet for anger and places the child in a position of control, in contrast to the position of helplessness in the real situation. Puppets can also allow the child to communicate feelings in a nonthreatening way. One of the most effective interventions is **therapeutic play,** which includes well-supervised activities such as permitting the child to give an injection to a doll or stuffed toy to reduce the stress of injections (Fig. 22-1).

Provide Positive Reinforcement. Children need to hear from adults that they know the youngsters did the best they could in the situation, no matter how they behaved. It is important for children to know that their worth is not being judged on the basis of their behavior in a stressful situation. Reward systems, such as earning stars, stickers, or a badge of courage, are appealing to children.

Returning to the child a short while after the procedure helps the nurse strengthen a supportive relationship. Relating with the child in a relaxed and nonstressful period allows him or her to see the nurse not only as someone associated with stressful situations but as someone with whom to share pleasurable experiences.

Use of Play in Procedures

The use of play is an integral part of relationships with children. As such, its value in specific situations is discussed throughout this book, such as in Chapter 21, in relation to hospitalization. Many institutions have elaborate and well-organized play areas and programs under the direction of child life specialists; other institutions have limited facilities. No matter what the institution provides for children, nurses can include play activities as part of nursing care. Play can be used to teach, express feelings, or achieve a therapeutic goal. Consequently, it should be included in preparing children for and encouraging their cooperation during procedures. Play sessions after procedures can be structured, such as directed toward needle play, or general, with a wide variety of equipment available for children to play with. Routine procedures such as measuring blood pressure and oral administration of medication may be of concern to children. Box 22-3 offers suggestions for incorporating play into nursing procedures and activities for the hospitalized child that facilitate learning and adjustment to a new situation.

> **NURSINGTIP**
>
> Play can also be spontaneous at the bedside and does not always require many supplies or much nursing time. Small items such as finger puppets or a small bottle of bubbles can be kept in the nurse's pocket for immediate use.

SURGICAL PROCEDURES
Preoperative Care

Children experiencing surgical procedures require both psychologic and physical preparation. In general, psychologic preparation is similar to that previously discussed for any procedure and employs many of the same techniques used in preparing a child for hospitalization, such as films, books, brochures, play, and tours. However, some important differences exist. Even though children are asleep for the actual surgical intervention, they are subjected to numerous preoperative and postoperative procedures. Stress points before and after surgery include the admission process, blood tests, injection of preoperative medication (if prescribed), transport to the operating room, and the stay in the postanesthesia care unit (PACU).

Psychologic intervention consisting of systematic preparation, rehearsal of the forthcoming events, and supportive care at each of these points has been shown to be more effective than a single-session preparation or consistent supportive care without systematic preparation and rehearsal. Play is always an effective strategy in preparing children, and increased familiarity with medical procedures decreases anxiety.

Surprisingly little research has been conducted on children's perception of the surgical experience and their fears of the event. Although fear of anesthesia is thought to be a major concern among children, little evidence exists. School-age children report few remembered events and even fewer fears. Those events recalled most often were riding to and arriving in the operating room, receiving the preoperative or induction injection, waking up in pain, and not being allowed to eat or drink. The most feared events were the preoperative injection and the mask on the face.

Parental presence during induction of anesthesia is allowed in some institutions (Fig. 22-2). Potential benefits include

BOX 22-3
Play Activities for Specific Procedures

FLUID INTAKE
Make ice pops using child's favorite juice.
Cut gelatin into fun shapes.
Make a game out of taking a sip when turning page of a book or in games such as Simon Says.
Use small medicine cups; decorate the cups.
Color water with food coloring or powdered drink mix.
Have a tea party; pour at a small table.
Let child fill a syringe and squirt into mouth or use to fill small cups.
Cut straws in half and place in a small container (much easier for child to suck liquid).
Use a "crazy" straw.
Make a "progress poster"; give rewards for drinking a predetermined quantity.

DEEP BREATHING
Blow bubbles with a bubble blower.
Blow bubbles with a straw (no soap).
Blow on a pinwheel, feather, whistle, harmonica, balloon, horn, party blower.
Practice band instruments.
Have blowing contest using balloons,* boats, cotton balls, feathers, marbles, Ping-Pong balls, pieces of paper; blow objects on a table top over a goal line, over water, through an obstacle course, into the air, against an opponent, or up and down a string.
Suck paper or cloth from one container to another using a straw.
Use blow bottles with colored water to transfer water from one side to the other.
Dramatize stories such as "I'll huff and puff and blow your house down" from the Three Little Pigs.
Do straw-blowing painting.
Take a deep breath and "blow out the candles" on a birthday cake.
Use a little paint brush to "paint" nails with water and blow nails dry.

RANGE OF MOTION AND USE OF EXTREMITIES
Throw beanbags at a fixed or movable target or throw wadded-up paper into a wastebasket.
Touch or kick Mylar balloons held or hung in different positions (if child is in traction, hang balloon from a trapeze).
Play "tickle toes"; wiggle them on request.
Play Twister game or Simon Says.
Play pretend and guessing games (e.g., imitate a bird, butterfly, horse).
Have tricycle or wheelchair races in safe area.
Play kickball or throw ball with a soft foam ball in a safe area.
Position bed so that child must turn to view television or doorway.
Climb wall like a "spider."
Pretend to teach "aerobic" dancing or exercises; encourage parents to participate.

Encourage swimming if feasible.
Play video games or pinball (fine motor movement).
Play "hide and seek": hide toy somewhere in bed (or room if ambulatory) and have child find it using specified hand or foot.
Provide clay to mold with fingers.
Paint or draw on large sheets of paper placed on floor or wall.
Encourage combing own hair; play "beauty shop" with "customer" in different positions.

SOAKS
Play with small toys or objects* (cups, syringes, soap dishes) in water.
Wash dolls or toys.
Pick up marbles or pennies* from bottom of bath container.
Make designs with coins* on bottom of container.
Pretend a boat is a submarine by keeping it immersed.
During soaks, read to child; sing with child; or play game, such as cards, checkers, or other board game (if both hands are immersed, move board pieces for child).
During a sitz bath, give child something to listen to (music, stories) or look at (View-Master, book).
Punch holes in bottom of plastic cup, fill with water, and let it "rain" on child.

INJECTIONS
Let child handle syringe, vial, and alcohol swab, and give an injection to doll or stuffed animal.
Use syringes to decorate cookies with frosting, squirt paint, or target shoot into a container.
Draw a "magic circle" on area before injection; draw smiling face in circle after injection, but avoid drawing on puncture site.
Allow child to have a "collection" of syringes (without needles); make "wild" creative objects with syringes.
If child has multiple injections or venipunctures, make a "progress poster"; give rewards for predetermined number of injections.
Have child count to 10 or 15 during injection.

AMBULATION
Give child something to push.
Toddler—push-pull toy
School-age child—wagon or a doll in a stroller or wheelchair
Adolescent—decorated IV stand
Have a parade; make hats, drums, etc.

EXTENDING ENVIRONMENT (e.g., FOR PATIENTS IN TRACTION)
Make bed into a pirate ship or airplane with decorations.
Put up mirrors so patient can see around room.
Move bed frequently to playroom, hallway, or outside.

*Small objects such as marbles or coins, as well as gloves or balloons, are unsafe for young children because of possible aspiration. Latex products also carry the risk of an allergic reaction.

minimizing the need for premedication and reducing the struggle that often occurs during separation (Kain, Caldwell-Andrews, and Wang, 2002). Other benefits are controversial but may include decreasing the child's anxiety during induction (e.g., breath holding and laryngospasm) and decreasing long-term behavioral effects of surgery (Romino, Keatley, Secrest, and others, 2005). Although few institutions endorse the policy, reports from parents who attend the induction are favorable (Kain, Caldwell-Andrews, Krivutza, and others, 2004). Even though some parents may become anxious, most control their anxiety, do not disrupt the induction, and support the child (Hall, Payne, Stack, and others, 1995; LaRosa-Nash and Murphy, 1997; Munro and D'Errico, 2000). Clinical observations show parental presence decreases anxiety in the child and reduces the need for heavy doses of preoperative sedation (Fennell, 1999).

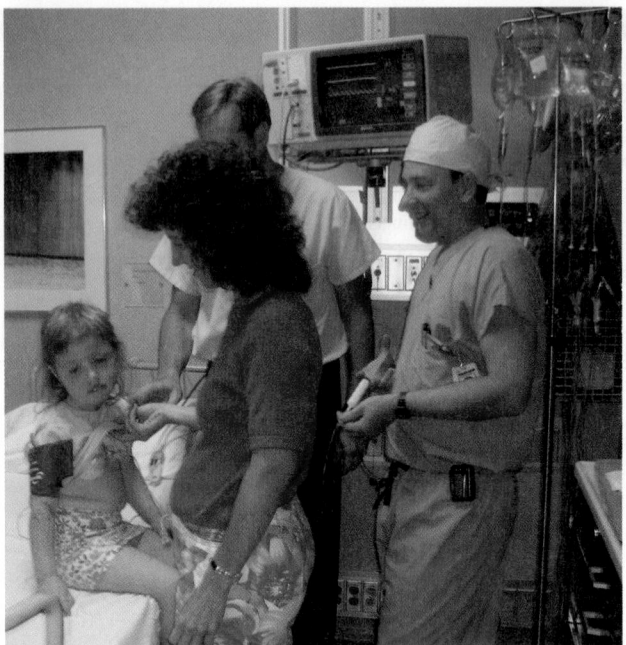

FIG. 22-2 ■ Parental presence during induction of anesthesia can minimize child's and parents' anxiety during the preoperative period.

	TABLE 22-1

Fasting Recommendations to Reduce the Risk of Pulmonary Aspiration*

INGESTED MATERIAL	MINIMUM FASTING PERIOD (hours)†
Clear liquids‡	2
Breast milk	4
Infant formula	6
Nonhuman milk§	6
Light meal‖	6

From American Society of Anesthesiologists: Practice guidelines for preoperative fasting and the use of pharmacologic agents to reduce the risk of pulmonary aspiration: application to healthy patients undergoing elective procedures, *Anesthesiology* 90(3):896-905, 1999; retrieved from http://www.asahq.org/publicationsAndServices/NPO.pdf.
*These recommendations apply to healthy patients who are undergoing elective procedures. They are not intended for women in labor. Following the guidelines does not guarantee a complete gastric emptying has occurred.
†Fasting periods noted in chart apply to all ages.
‡Examples of clear liquids include water, fruit juices without pulp, carbonated beverages, clear tea, and black coffee.
§Because nonhuman milk is similar to solids in gastric emptying time, the amount ingested must be considered when determining appropriate fasting period.
‖A light meal typically consists of toast and clear liquids. Meals that include fried or fatty foods or meat may prolong gastric emptying time. Both the amount and type of foods ingested must be considered when determining appropriate fasting period.

Some concern exists regarding the appropriateness of this practice for all parents. Some parents may become upset by the rapid succession of induction events, by observing their child becoming limp, and by leaving the child in the care of strangers. Parents who are anxious before surgery tend to become even more anxious after the induction, whereas the reverse is true of parents with little anxiety.

However, based on the parents' favorable response to the practice and most children's desire to have parents with them during any stressful procedure, parents should have the option of attending the induction. Appropriate education is essential to help parents understand the stages of anesthesia, what to expect, and how to support their child (Fennell, 1999), combined with a program that prepares them for what to expect and what is expected of them. When parents choose not to or are not allowed to attend this induction, leaving a favorite possession with the child and uniting the child and parents as soon as possible after surgery (preferably in the PACU) are important interventions. During surgery the family should have a designated place to wait and should be kept informed of the child's progress. They also should know where and when they can visit the child after surgery.

Aside from possibly being separated from the parents before and after surgery, children may be cared for by a number of unfamiliar practitioners, which promotes fear and uncertainty. Although the same supportive nurse should remain with the child through as many of the procedures as possible, the child may have other nurses, especially if the patient returns to a special care unit postoperatively. Many hospitals have surgical tours for children and parents to familiarize them with the strange environment and to introduce them to other individuals who will be involved in their care.

An important concern is restriction of food and fluids before surgery to avoid aspiration during anesthesia. Infants require special attention to fluid needs. They should not be

without oral fluids for an extended period preoperatively to avoid glycogen depletion and dehydration. Current preoperative fasting guidelines are found in Table 22-1.

Although most preoperative care procedures are routine, nurses should keep in mind that they can be anxiety provoking for children and parents. For example, wearing a hospital gown without the security of underpants or pajama bottoms can be traumatic. Therefore these articles of clothing should be allowed to be worn into the operating room and removed after induction of anesthesia.

Preoperative Sedation. Historically the most upsetting event for children has been the preoperative injection. Significant increases have recently occurred in the number of anesthesiologists who use preoperative sedatives, usually midazolam (Versed), and parental presence for children undergoing surgery (Kain, Caldwell-Andrews, Krivutza, and others, 2004). When drugs are administered, they should be delivered atraumatically via oral or IV routes. Numerous preanesthetic drug regimens are used with children, and no consensus exists on the optimal method. The goals for using preoperative medications include (1) anxiety reduction, (2) amnesia, (3) sedation, (4) antiemetic effect, and (5) reduction of secretions (Landsman and Cook, 1998; Manworren and Fledderman, 2000). Midazolam provides excellent preoperative anxiety reduction, amnesia, and sedation. It is popular because of its short duration, predictable onset, and rare occurrence of respiratory depression. Oral transmucosal fentanyl (OTFC, or Oralet) is available as a sweetened lozenge on a plastic stick. When first approved, this appeared to be an excellent, atraumatic route of administration. However, associated nausea and vomiting, respiratory depression, and the need for more intensive monitoring and observation than with other oral sedatives have limited its popularity (Klein, Diekema, Paris, and others, 2002). If children have no preoperative pain, are well prepared psychologically for surgery, and have their parents nearby, preoperative medication may be unnecessary.

Anesthesia induction of the pediatric patient is commonly accomplished by administering inhalation agents in combination with nitrous oxide and oxygen by mask. Children may fear induction of anesthesia by mask. Practices that can minimize anxiety related to inhalation anesthesia are (1) disguising the unpleasant odor of anesthetic gases by applying a pleasant-smelling substance on the mask; (2) using a transparent plastic mask rather than an opaque black mask and gradually bringing it toward the face; (3) directing a stream of gas toward the child's face from the bare tube until the child becomes drowsy, then using the mask; (4) allowing the child to sit up rather than lie down for anesthesia induction; and (5) allowing preoperative play with a mask and a doll or manikin.

Postoperative Care

Various psychologic and physical interventions and observations are required to prevent or minimize possible untoward effects from anesthesia and the surgical procedure (see Nursing Care Guidelines box). Although the incidence of serious postoperative complications in healthy children undergoing surgery is less than 1% (Maxwell and Yaster, 2000), continuous monitoring of cardiopulmonary status is essential during the immediate postoperative period. Postanesthesia complications such as airway obstruction, postextubation croup, laryngospasm, and bronchospasm make maintaining a patent airway and maximum ventilation critical.

Monitoring oxygen saturation and providing supplemental oxygen as needed, maintaining body temperature, and promoting fluid and electrolyte balance are important aspects of immediate postoperative care. Vital signs are continuously monitored, and each vital sign is evaluated in terms of side effects from anesthesia, shock, or respiratory compromise (Table 22-2).

A change in vital signs that demands immediate attention in the perioperative period is caused by **malignant hyperthermia** (MH), a potentially fatal genetic myopathy. In susceptible children, anesthetics such as succinylcholine and halothane trigger the disorder, producing hypermetabolism, muscle rigidity, and an elevated temperature. Early symptoms of MH include tachycardia and tachyarrhythmias, tachypnea, hypercarbia, and metabolic and respiratory acidosis. An elevated temperature is considered by many to be a late sign of the disorder (Redmond, 2001). A family or previous history of sudden high fever associated with a surgical procedure and certain neuromuscular disorders increase risk for MH; children who have successfully undergone prior surgery without adverse effects may still be considered susceptible. Treatment includes immediate discontinuation of the triggering agent and surgical procedure, hyperventilation with 100% oxygen, and IV dantrolene sodium. Infusions of cool saline, cooling blankets, gastric or peritoneal lavage, packed ice bags in the axillae and groin, and, possibly, cardiopulmonary bypass reduce core temperature (Redmond, 2001). The patient should be transferred to an intensive care unit and closely monitored for stabilization of vital signs, metabolic state, and possible recurrence of symptoms.

Managing pain is a major nursing responsibility after surgery (see Chapter 7). The nurse should assess pain frequently and administer analgesics to provide comfort and facilitate cooperation with postoperative care such as ambulation and deep breathing. Opioids are the most commonly used analgesics. Routinely scheduled IV analgesics, patient-controlled

---

nursingcareguidelines

Postoperative Care

Ensure that preparations are made to receive child:
- Bed or crib is ready.
- Intravenous pumps and poles, suction apparatus, and oxygen flow meter are at bedside.

Obtain baseline information:
- Take vital signs, including blood pressure; keep blood pressure cuff in place and deflated to lessen amount of disturbance to child.
- Take and record vital signs more frequently if any value fluctuates.
- Inspect operative area.
- Check dressing if present:
  —Outline any bleeding area on dressing or cast with pen.
  —Reinforce, but do not remove, loose dressing.
  —Observe areas below surgical site for blood that may have drained toward bed.
  —Assess for bleeding and other symptoms in areas not covered with a dressing, such as throat after tonsillectomy.
- Assess skin color and characteristics.
- Assess level of consciousness and activity.

Notify physician of any irregularities in child's condition.

Assess for evidence of pain (see Pain Assessment, Chapter 7).

Review surgeon's orders after completing initial assessment, and check that any preoperative orders, such as seizure or cardiac medications, have been reordered and can be given by available routes (oral preparations may be contraindicated).

Monitor vital signs as ordered and more often if indicated.

Check dressings for bleeding or other abnormalities.

Check bowel sounds.

Observe for signs of shock, abdominal distention, and bleeding.

Assess for bladder distention.

Observe for signs of dehydration.

Detect presence of infection:
- Take vital signs every 2 to 4 hours, as ordered.
- Collect or request needed specimens.
- Inspect wound for signs of infection—redness, swelling, heat, pain, and purulent drainage.

---

analgesia, and epidural infusions, rather than as needed (PRN) orders, provide excellent analgesia in postoperative pediatric patients.

Because respiratory infections are a potential complication, every effort is taken to aerate the lungs and remove secretions. The lungs are auscultated regularly to identify abnormal sounds or any areas of diminished or absent breath sounds. To prevent hypostatic pneumonia, respiratory movement can be encouraged with incentive spirometers or other motivating activities (see Box 22-3). If these measures are presented as games, the child is more likely to comply. The child's position is changed every 2 hours, and deep breathing is encouraged.

NURSINGTIP

Because deep breathing is usually painful after surgery, be certain the child has received analgesics. Have the child splint the operative site (depending on its location) by hugging a small pillow or a favorite stuffed animal.

TABLE 22-2

Potential Causes of Postoperative Vital Sign Alterations in Children

ALTERATION	POTENTIAL CAUSE	COMMENTS
HEART RATE		
Increase	Decreased perfusion (shock)	Heart rate may increase to maintain cardiac output.
	Elevated temperature	
	Pain	
	Respiratory distress (early)	
	Medications (atropine, morphine, epinephrine)	
Decrease	Hypoxia	Bradycardia is of more concern in the young child
	Vagal stimulation	than tachycardia.
	Increased intracranial pressure	
	Respiratory distress (late)	
	Medications	
RESPIRATORY RATE		
Increase	Respiratory distress	Body responds to respiratory distress primarily by
	Fluid volume excess	increasing rate.
	Hypothermia	
	Elevated temperature	
	Pain	
Decrease	Anesthetics, opioids	Decreased respiratory rate from opioids may be com-
	Pain	pensated for by increase depth of respiration.
BLOOD PRESSURE		
Increase	Excess intravascular volume	This is serious in preterm infants because it increases
	Increased intracranial pressure	risk of intraventricular hemorrhage.
	Carbon dioxide retention	
	Pain	
	Medication (ketamine, epinephrine)	
Decrease	Vasodilating anesthetic agents (halothane, isoflurane, enflurane)	Decreased blood pressure is late sign of shock
	Opioids (morphine)	because of elasticity and constriction of vessels to maintain cardiac output.
TEMPERATURE		
Increase	Shock (late sign)	Fever associated with infection usually occurs later
	Infection	than fever of noninfectious origin.
	Environmental causes (warm room, excess coverings)	Absence of fever does not rule out infection,
	Malignant hyperthermia	especially in infants.
Decrease	Vasodilating anesthetic agents (halothane, isoflurane, enflurane)	Malignant hyperthermia requires immediate
	Muscle relaxants	treatment.
	Environmental causes (cool room)	Neonates are especially susceptible to hypothermia,
	Infusion of cool fluids or blood	with serious or fatal consequences.

From Smith DP: *Comprehensive child and family nursing skills*, St Louis, 1991, Mosby.

During the recovery period, some time should be spent with children to assess their perception of surgery. Play, drawing, and storytelling are excellent methods of discovering their thoughts. With such information the nurse can support or correct their perceptions and boost children's self-esteem for having endured a stressful procedure.

COMPLIANCE

Compliance, also termed **adherence,** refers to the extent to which the patient's behavior coincides with the prescribed regimen in terms of taking medication, following diets, or executing other lifestyle changes. In developing strategies to promote compliance, the nurse must first assess level of compliance. Because many children are too young to assume par-

tial or total responsibility for their care, parents are usually primarily responsible for home management.

Factors relating to the care setting are important in ensuring compliance and should be considered in planning strategies to improve compliance. Basically, any aspect of the health care environment that increases the family's satisfaction with the physical setting and the relationship with the practitioner positively influences adherence to the treatment regimen. However, the more complex, expensive, inconvenient, and disruptive the treatment protocol, the less likely the family is to comply. During long-term conditions that involve multiple treatments and considerable rearrangement of lifestyle, compliance is severely affected.

Although it is helpful to know those factors that influence compliance, assessment must include more direct measurement techniques. A number of methods exist, each with advantages and disadvantages. The most successful approach includes a combination of at least two of the following methods:

Clinical judgment—This is subject to bias and inaccuracy unless the nurse carefully evaluates the criteria used in assessment.

Self-reporting—Most people overestimate compliance by about 20% even when they admit to lapses.

Direct observation—This is difficult to employ outside the health care setting, and awareness of being observed frequently affects performance.

Monitoring appointments—Keeping appointments indirectly indicates compliance with the prescribed care.

Monitoring therapeutic response—Few treatments yield directly measurable results (e.g., decreased blood pressure, weight loss); record on a graph or chart.

Pill counts—The nurse counts the number of pills remaining in the original container and compares the number missing with the number of times the medication should have been taken. Families may forget to bring the container or deliberately alter the number of pills to avoid detection. This method is also poorly suited to liquid medication. Another technique is the use of pill container caps that record every opening as a presumptive dose.

Chemical assay—For certain drugs, such as digoxin and phenytoin, measurement of plasma drug levels provides information on the amount of drug recently ingested. However, this method is expensive, indicates only short-term compliance, and requires precise timing of the assay for accurate results.

Compliance Strategies

Strategies to improve compliance are composed of interventions that encourage families to follow the prescribed treatment regimen. Some evidence suggests that higher levels of self-esteem and increased autonomy favorably affect adolescent compliance (KyngAs, Kroll, and Duffy, 2000). However, family factors are important, and characteristics associated with good compliance include family support, family reminders, good communication, and expectations for successful completion of the therapeutic regimen (KyngAs, Kroll, and Duffy, 2000). No one approach is always successful, and the best results occur when at least two strategies are used.

Organizational strategies involve the care setting and the therapeutic plan. They include manipulating the factors listed in Box 22-4 that positively affect compliance. This may involve increasing the frequency of appointments, designating a primary practitioner, reducing the cost of medication by prescribing generic brands, reducing the treatment's disruption of the family's lifestyle, and using cues to minimize forgetting. Numerous devices are available commercially or can be improvised for cueing, such as pill dispensers; watches with alarms; charts to record completed therapy; messages on the refrigerator or morning coffee pot; and treatment schedules that incorporate the treatment plan into the daily routine, such as physical therapy after the evening bath.

Educational strategies instruct the family about the treatment plan. Although education is an important factor in enhancing compliance and patients who are more knowledgeable about their condition are more likely to comply, education alone does not ensure compliant behavior. The nurse should incorporate teaching principles known to enhance understanding and retention of material (see Nursing Care Guidelines box). Written materials are essential, especially in any

---

BOX 22-4

Factors That Positively Influence Compliance

INDIVIDUAL AND FAMILY FACTORS
High self-esteem
Positive body image
High degree of autonomy (increased locus of control)
Supportive and well-adjusted family
Effective family communication
Family expectation for successful completion of therapy

CARE SETTING FACTORS
Perceived satisfaction with care
Positive interactions with practitioners
Continuity of care
Individualized care
Minimum waiting time for appointments
Convenient care setting

TREATMENT FACTORS
Simple regimen
Minimum disruption in usual lifestyle
Short duration
Inexpensive
Visible benefits
Tolerable side effects

---

nursingcareguidelines

Effective Teaching of Family Members

- Establish rapport; reduce anxiety and fear.
- Assess what family members know and expect to learn and address their concerns before beginning teaching.
- Assess learning style; ask if they prefer to have everything explained in detail or if they prefer knowing only the major facts.
- Use a variety of teaching materials (lecture, demonstration, video, written material).
- Be specific when giving information.
- Divide the information into small steps.
- Keep information short, simple, and concrete.
- Introduce most important information first.
- Use "verbal" headings to organize information, such as "There are two things you need to learn: how to give the medicine and what side effects to look for. First, how to give. . . . Second, what side effects. . . ."
- Stress how important the instructions are and the expected benefits; explain the detrimental effects of inadequate treatment, but avoid fear tactics.
- Evaluate the teaching by eliciting feedback to ensure that family members understand the information.
- Repeat information as needed.
- Reward family for learning through verbal praise.
- Use "teachable moments"—times when family members are most likely to accept new information (e.g., when a member asks a question or when symptoms are present).
- Use hands-on demonstration and return demonstration to encourage mastery of skills and retention of information.

regimen requiring multiple or complex treatments, and they need to be understandable to the average individual, who reads at about the fourth-grade level. Involvement of the immediate and extended family (e.g., grandparents) in education sessions may enhance compliance.

Treatment strategies relate to the child's refusal or inability to take the prescribed medication. The family may also have difficulty following a prescribed treatment regimen. They may remember and understand the instructions but may not be able to give the medicine as prescribed. Assess the reason for refusal. For example, the child may not be able to swallow pills. In this case, perhaps pills can be crushed or a liquid medication substituted (always review medication to ensure that crushing is acceptable before giving this instruction).

Assess the treatment and medication schedule to determine if it is reasonable for a home situation. Although an every-6-hour or every-8-hour schedule is reasonable for hospitals, a parent would have difficulty getting up once or twice nightly; instead a medication could be given during the day at times that would be easy to remember.

Behavioral strategies are designed to modify behavior directly. Several strategies encouraging the desired behavior are effective with children. Ideally, positive reinforcement should be employed to strengthen the behavior and may consist of earning stars or tokens, which gains the child a special privilege or gift. At times, however, disciplinary techniques such as time-out for young children or withholding privileges for older children may be needed to improve compliance (see Limit Setting and Discipline, Chapter 3). **Contracting,** a formal process in which exact elements of desired behavior are explicitly outlined along with rewards or negative consequences, is an effective method with older children.

> **NURSINGTIP**
>
> To encourage a child to perform a treatment (e.g., soaking a foot) for a certain time frame, ask the child to soak during a favorite television show, including commercials. This technique also helps evaluate compliance by asking the child what show was watched.

GENERAL HYGIENE AND CARE
MAINTAINING HEALTHY SKIN*

Maintaining an IV line, removing a dressing, positioning a child in bed, changing a diaper, using electrodes, and using restraints have the potential to contribute to skin injury. Skin care must go beyond the daily bath and become a part of each nursing intervention (see Nursing Care Guidelines box). Specific guidelines for skin care of neonates are provided in Skin Care, Chapter 9.

Assessment of the skin is most easily accomplished during the bath. Examine for early signs of injury. Risk factors include impaired mobility, protein malnutrition, edema, incontinence, sensory loss, anemia, infection, failure to turn the patient, and intubation. Critically ill children often are at higher risk of pressure ulcers and skin breakdown, since they often have several risk factors combined. Identification of risk factors helps to determine those children who need a more thorough skin assessment. Assessment should occur within 24 hours of admission so that pressure ulcers and

*This section was revised by Shannon McCord, MSN, RN, CPNP.

---

nursingcareguidelines

Skin Care

- Cleanse skin with mild nonalkaline soap or soap-free cleaning agents for routine bathing.
- Provide daily cleansing of eyes, oral and diaper or perineal areas, and any areas of skin breakdown.
- Apply moisturizing agents during or immediately after bathing; cleanse skin of old cream before adding a new layer.
- Use minimum tape and adhesives. On very sensitive skin, use a protective, pectin-based or hydrocolloid skin barrier between skin and tape or adhesives.
- Use water or adhesive remover (if skin is not fragile) when removing tape or adhesives.
- Place pectin-based or hydrocolloid skin barriers directly over excoriated skin. Leave barrier undisturbed until it begins to peel off, or for 5 to 7 days. With wet, oozing excoriations, place a small amount of stoma powder on site, remove excess powder, and apply skin barrier. Hold barrier in place for several minutes to allow barrier to soften and mold to skin surface.
- Alternate electrode placement and thoroughly assess skin underneath electrodes at least every 24 hours. Alcohol-free skin sealant under leads protects skin from epidermal stripping.
- Be certain fingers or toes are visible whenever extremity is used for intravenous (IV) or arterial line.
- Keep skin dry (may apply absorbent powder, e.g., cornstarch) and use soft, smooth bed linen and clothes.
- Use a draw sheet to move a child in bed or onto a gurney; do not drag the child from under the arms.
- Identify children at risk for skin breakdown before it occurs. Employ measures such as pressure-reducing or pressure-relieving devices (e.g., mattress overlay, low–air-loss bed, gel pillows).
- Do not massage reddened bony prominences, since this can cause deep tissue damage; provide pressure relief to those areas instead.
- Keep skin free of excess moisture (e.g., urine or fecal incontinence, wound drainage, excessive perspiration).
- Routinely assess the child's nutritional status. A child who is NPO (nothing by mouth) for several days and is receiving only IV fluid is nutritionally at risk, which can also affect the skin's ability to maintain its integrity. Consider parenteral nutrition.

---

wounds that occurred before admission can be identified (Ratliff and Rodheaver, 1999; Quigley and Curley, 1996).

When capillary blood flow is interrupted by pressure, the blood flows back into the tissue when the pressure is relieved. As the body attempts to reoxygenate the area, a bright red flush appears. This **reactive hyperemia,** or flush, is the earliest sign of tissue compromise and pressure-related ischemia. If pressure is prolonged, reactive hyperemia will not be sufficient to revitalize ischemic tissue (Calianno, 1999).

Staging of pressure ulcers is used to classify the amount of tissue damage.* Necrotic tissue must be removed so that the tissue depth can accurately be assessed. Accurate documentation of redness or obvious skin breakdown is essential. Color, size (diameter and depth), location, presence of sinus tracts, odor, exudate, and response to treatment are observed and recorded at least daily. (For treatment of wounds, see Chapter 30.)

*Staging of pressure ulcers and guidelines for prevention and management of pressure ulcers can be found at http://wocn.org.

Pressure ulcers can develop when the pressure on the skin and underlying tissues is greater than the capillary closing pressure, causing capillary occlusion. If the pressure remains unrelieved, vessels can collapse, resulting in tissue anoxia and cellular death. Pressure ulcers most often occur over bony prominences and are usually very deep, extending into subcutaneous tissue or even deeper into muscle, tendon, or bone. A **pressure-reduction device** reduces pressure but does not prevent pressure from causing capillary closure; therefore turning and repositioning are always included when using these devices. Most of these items are overlays that are placed on top of the regular mattress. A **pressure-relief device** maintains pressure below that which would cause capillary closure. These devices are usually high-technology beds that are used for patients who have multiple problems and cannot be turned effectively.

Friction and shear contribute to pressure ulcers. **Friction** occurs when the surface of the skin rubs against another surface, such as the bed sheets. Skin damage most often occurs over the elbows, heels, or occiput; is usually limited to the epidermal and upper layers; and may have the appearance of an abrasion. Prevention of friction injury includes the use of protective sheepskin over the elbows or heels; gel pillows under the head of infants and toddlers; moisturizing agents; transparent dressings over susceptible areas; and soft, smooth bed linen and clothing. **Shear** is the result of the force of gravity pushing down on the body and friction of the body against a surface, such as the bed or chair. For example, when a patient is in the semi-Fowler position and begins to slide to the foot of the bed, the skin over the sacral area remains in the same place because of the resistance of the bed surface. The blood vessels in the area are stretched and may cause small-vessel thrombosis and tissue death (Bryant and Doughty, 2000). Prevention of shear injury includes using *lift sheets* when repositioning a patient, elevating the bed no more than 30 degrees for short periods, and using the knee gatch to interrupt the pull of gravity on the body toward the foot of the bed.

Epidermal stripping results when the epidermis is unintentionally removed with tape removal. These lesions are usually shallow and irregularly shaped and may blister or weep. Babies are at increased risk for epidermal injury. Prevention includes using no tape when possible, securing dressings with laced binders (Montgomery straps) or stretchy netting (Spandage or stockinette). Using porous or low-tack tapes (e.g., Medipore, paper, hydrogel), using alcohol-free skin sealants (No Sting Barrier Film), or picture framing wounds with hydrocolloid or wafer barriers (e.g., DuoDERM, Coloplast, Stomahesive) and then taping on top of the barrier also will reduce epidermal stripping.

Tape is placed so that there is no tension, traction, or wrinkles on the skin. To remove tape, slowly peel the tape away while stabilizing the underlying skin. Adhesive remover may be used to break the adhesive bond but may be drying to the skin; adhesive removers should be avoided in preterm neonates, since absorption rates vary and toxicity may occur. The adhesive is removed with water to prevent absorption and irritation. Wetting the tape with water or alcohol-based foam hand cleansers may facilitate removal.

Chemical factors can also lead to skin damage. Fecal incontinence, especially when mixed with urine; wound drainage; or gastric drainage around gastrostomy tubes can erode epidermis. The skin can quickly progress from redness to de-

nudement if exposure continues. Moisture barriers, gentle cleansing as soon after exposure as possible, and skin barriers can be used to prevent damage caused by chemical factors (see also Diaper Dermatitis, Chapter 30). In addition, foam dressings that wick moisture away from the skin are helpful around gastrostomy tubes and tracheostomy sites.

BATHING

Most infants and children can be bathed in a basin at the bedside, on the bed, or in a standard bathtub or shower. For infants and young children confined to bed, the towel method can be used. Two towels are immersed in a diluted soap solution and wrung damp. With the child lying supine on a dry towel, one damp towel is placed on top of the child and used to gently clean the body. This towel is discarded, and the child is dried and turned prone. The procedure is repeated using the second damp towel. Commercially available bath cloths may also be used.

Infants and small children are *never* left unattended in a bathtub, and infants who are unable to sit alone are securely held with one hand during the bath. The nurse should securely support the infant's head with one hand, or grasp the farther arm firmly while the head rests comfortably on the nurse's arm. Children who are able to sit without assistance need only close supervision and a pad placed in the bottom of the tub to prevent slipping and loss of balance.

School-age children and adolescents may shower or bathe. Nurses need to use judgment regarding the amount of supervision the child requires. Some can assume this responsibility unaided, whereas others will need someone in constant attendance. Children with cognitive impairments, physical limitations, or suicidal or psychotic problems (who may commit bodily harm) require close supervision.

Areas that require special attention are ears, between skinfolds, neck, back, and genital area. The genital area should be carefully cleansed and dried with particular care given to skinfolds, and in uncircumcised boys, usually those older than 3 years of age, the foreskin should be gently retracted, the exposed surfaces cleansed, and the foreskin then replaced. If the condition of the glans indicates inadequate cleaning, such as accumulated smegma, inflammation, phimosis, or foreskin adhesions, teaching proper hygiene is indicated. In the Vietnamese and Cambodian cultures the foreskin is traditionally not retracted until adulthood. Older children have the tendency to avoid cleaning the genitalia; therefore they may need a gentle reminder.

Children who are ill or debilitated need more extensive assistance with bathing, but should be encouraged to perform as much as they can without overtaxing their energies. Expect increasing involvement with improved strength and endurance.

ORAL HYGIENE

Mouth care is an integral part of daily hygiene and should be continued in the hospital. Infants and debilitated children require the nurse or a family member to perform mouth care. Although young children can manage a toothbrush and are encouraged to use it, most need assistance to perform satisfactorily. Older children, although capable of brushing and flossing without assistance, sometimes need to be reminded. (See Dental Health, Chapters 10 and 12, for specific oral hygiene techniques; mouth care of children with mucosal ulcers is discussed under nursing care of the child with leukemia in Chapter 26.)

HAIR CARE

Children should have their hair brushed and combed at least once daily. The hair is styled for comfort and in a manner pleasing to the child and parents. The hair should not be cut without parental permission, although clipping hair to provide access to a scalp vein for IV insertion may be necessary.

If children are hospitalized for more than a few days, the hair may need shampooing. With infants the hair may be washed during the daily bath or less frequently. For most children, washing the hair and scalp once or twice weekly is sufficient unless there is an indication for more frequent washing, such as following a high fever and profuse sweating. Adolescents normally have increased oily sebaceous secretions that require frequent hair care and more frequent shampoos.

Almost any child can be transported to an accessible sink for shampooing. Those who are unable to be transported can receive a shampoo in their beds with adequate protection, specially adapted equipment or positioning, or dry shampoo caps. When necessary, a shampoo basin may be used or the child may be positioned near the edge of the bed, towels placed under the shoulders, a large plastic garbage bag draped at the edge of the bed with one open end under the shoulders, and the hair placed inside the opening. The other end is opened and placed in a collection container. Water can be transported in a basin.

> **NURSING TIP**
>
> For a convenient source of water, fill an empty enema bag with warm water, hang the bag from an IV pole, and use the clamp on the bag's tubing to adjust the flow of water.

African-American children require special hair care. For the child with curly hair, most standard combs are inadequate and may cause hair breakage and discomfort. Use a special comb with widely spaced teeth. It is also much easier to comb the hair after shampooing when it is wet. Use a special hair dressing or pomade, which usually has a coconut oil base. The preparation is rubbed on the hands and then transferred to the hair to make it more pliable and manageable. Consult the parents regarding the preparation to use on their child's hair and ask if they can provide some for use during the hospitalization. Petroleum jelly should *not* be used. If braiding or plaiting the hair, the nurse should weave it loosely while the hair is damp. The hair tightens as it dries, which could result in tension folliculitis.

FEEDING THE SICK CHILD

Loss of appetite is a symptom common to most childhood illnesses. Because an acute illness is usually short, the nutritional state is seldom compromised. Urging foods on the sick child may precipitate nausea and vomiting, and in most cases children can be permitted to determine their own need for food.

Refusing to eat may also be one way children can exert power and control in an otherwise helpless situation. For young children, loss of appetite may be related to the depression caused by separation from their parents. Parents' concern with eating can intensify the problem. Forcing a child to eat meets with rebellion and reinforces the behavior as a control mechanism. Parents are encouraged to relax any pressure during an acute illness. Although it is best to encourage high-quality nutritious foods, the child may desire foods and liquids that contain mostly empty or nonnutritional calories. Some well-tolerated foods include gelatin, diluted clear soups, carbonated drinks, flavored ice pops, dry toast, and crackers. Even though these substances are not nutritious, they can provide necessary fluid and calories.

Dehydration is always a hazard when children are febrile or anorexic, especially when accompanied by vomiting or diarrhea. Offer small amounts of favored fluids at frequent intervals and provide salty foods (which increase thirst) if allowed. If diarrhea is present, avoid high-carbohydrate liquids (e.g., carbonated beverages, gelatin, flavored ice pops) because they may aggravate the diarrhea by an osmotic effect. Replacing abnormal losses with plain water or undiluted broth may worsen the electrolyte imbalance. Fluids should not be forced, and the child is not awakened to take fluids. Forcing fluids may create the same difficulties as urging unwanted food. Gentle persuasion with preferred beverages will usually meet with success. Using play techniques can also be very effective (see Nursing Care Guidelines box).

Once the child is feeling better, appetite usually begins to improve. It is best to take advantage of any hungry period by serving high-quality foods and snacks. If the child still refuses to eat, nutritious fluids, such as prepared breakfast drinks, should be encouraged. Parents can help by bringing in food items from home, especially if the family's cultural eating habits differ from the hospital food. A clinical dietitian may also be consulted for alternative food choices.

When children are placed on special diets, such as clear liquids after surgery or during episodes of diarrhea, assessment of their intake and readiness to advance to more complex foods is essential. Regardless of the type of diet, charting of the amount consumed is an important nursing responsibility. Descriptions need to be detailed and accurate, such as "4 ounces of orange juice, one pancake, and 8 ounces of milk." Comments such as "ate well" or "ate poorly" are inadequate. Charting the percentage of the meal eaten is also inadequate unless food is measured before serving.

If parents are involved in the child's care, they are encouraged to keep a list of everything eaten. Using a premeasured cup for fluids ensures a more accurate estimate of intake. A comparison of the intake at each meal can isolate food deficiencies, such as insufficient intake of meat or vegetables. Behaviors associated with mealtime also may point to possible factors influencing appetite. For example, the observation that "child eats well when with other children but plays with food if left alone in room" helps the nurse plan mealtime activities that stimulate the appetite.

CONTROLLING ELEVATED TEMPERATURES

An elevated temperature, most frequently from fever but occasionally caused by hyperthermia, is one of the most common symptoms of illness in children. This manifestation is of great concern to parents. To facilitate an understanding of fever, the following terms are defined:

Set point—The temperature around which body temperature is regulated by a thermostat-like mechanism in the hypothalamus

Fever (hyperpyrexia)—An elevation in set point such that body temperature is regulated at a higher level; may be arbitrarily defined as temperature above 38° C (100.4° F)

nursingcareguidelines

Feeding the Sick Child

Take a dietary history (see Chapter 6) and use information to make eating time as much like home as possible.

Encourage parents or other family members to feed child or to be present at mealtimes.

Make mealtimes pleasant; avoid any procedures immediately before or after eating; make certain child is rested and pain free.

Serve small, frequent meals rather than three large meals or serve three meals and nutritious between-meal snacks.

Provide finger foods for young children.

Involve children in food selection and preparation whenever possible.

Serve small portions, and serve each course separately, such as soup first; followed by meat, potatoes, and vegetables; and ending with dessert.
- With young children, camouflage size of food by cutting meat thicker so that less appears on plate or by folding a cheese slice in half.
- Offer second helpings.

Ensure a variety of foods, textures, and colors.

Provide food selections that are favorites of most children, such as peanut butter and jelly sandwiches, hot dogs, hamburgers, macaroni and cheese, pizza, spaghetti, tacos, fried chicken, corn, and fruit yogurt.

Avoid foods that are highly seasoned, have strong odors, or are all mixed together, unless typical of cultural practices.

Provide fluid selections that are favorites of most children, such as fruit punch, cola, ginger ale, sweetened tea, flavored ice pops, sherbet, ice cream, milk, milkshakes, eggnog, pudding, gelatin, clear broth, or creamed soups.

Offer nutritious snacks, such as frozen yogurt or pudding, ice cream, oatmeal or peanut butter cookies, hot cocoa, cheese slices, pieces of raw vegetable or fruit, and dried fruit or cereal.

Make food attractive and different; for example:
- Serve a "picnic lunch" in a paper bag.
- Pack food in a Chinese take-out container; decorate container.
- Put a "face" or a "flower" on a hamburger or sandwich with pieces of vegetable.
- Use a cookie cutter to shape a sandwich.
- Serve pudding, yogurt, or juice frozen as an ice pop.
- Make Slurpies or snow cones by pouring flavored syrup on crushed ice.
- Add food coloring to water or milk.
- Serve fluids through brightly colored or unusually shaped straws.
- Make "bowtie" sandwiches by cutting them in triangles and placing two points together.
- Slice sandwiches into "fingers."
- Grate mounds of cheese.
- Cut apples horizontally to make circles.
- Put a banana on a hot dog bun and spread with peanut butter.
- Break uncooked spaghetti into toothpick lengths and skewer cheese, cold meat, vegetables, or fruit chunks.

Praise children for what they do eat.

Do not punish children for not eating by removing their dessert or putting them to bed

---

Hyperthermia—Body temperature exceeding the set point, which usually results from the body or external conditions creating more heat than the body can eliminate, such as in heatstroke, aspirin toxicity, seizures, or hyperthyroidism

Body temperature is regulated by a thermostat-like mechanism in the hypothalamus. This mechanism receives input from centrally and peripherally located receptors. When temperature changes occur, these receptors relay the information to the thermostat, which either increases or decreases heat production to maintain a constant set point temperature. However, during an infection, pyrogenic substances cause an increase in the body's normal set point, a process that is mediated by prostaglandins. Consequently, the hypothalamus increases heat production until the core temperature reaches the new set point.

Most fevers in children are of brief duration with limited consequences and are viral in origin. When fever is caused by bacteria, endotoxins are produced that activate the inflammatory process and produce fever (Rote, Huether, and McCance, 2000). Contrary to popular belief, neither the rise in temperature nor its response to antipyretics indicates the severity or etiology of infection, which casts doubt on the value of using fever as a diagnostic or prognostic indicator.

Therapeutic management of elevated temperature depends on whether it is due to a fever or hyperthermia. Because the set point is normal in hyperthermia but increased in fever, different approaches must be used to lower body temperature successfully.

Fever

The principal reason for treating fever is the relief of discomfort. Relief measures include pharmacologic or environmental intervention. The most effective intervention is the use of antipyretics to lower the set point.

Antipyretic drugs include acetaminophen, aspirin, and nonsteroidal antiinflammatory drugs (NSAIDs). Acetaminophen is the preferred drug; aspirin should *not* be given to children because of the association between aspirin use in children and influenza virus or chickenpox and Reye syndrome. One nonprescription NSAID, ibuprofen, is approved for fever reduction in children as young as 6 months of age. Dosage is based on the initial temperature level: 5 mg/kg of body weight for temperatures less than 39.2° C (102.6° F) or 10 mg/kg for temperatures greater than 39.2° C. The recommended dosage for pain is 10 mg/kg every 6 to 8 hours, and the recommended maximum daily dose for pain and fever is 40 mg/kg. The duration of fever reduction is generally 6 to 8 hours and is longer with the higher dose (see Chapter 6). It may be given every 4 hours but no more than five times in 24 hours. Because body temperature normally decreases at night, three or four doses in 24 hours will control most fevers. The nurse should retake the temperature 30 minutes after the antipyretic is given to assess its effect, but temperature should not be repeatedly measured; the child's level of discomfort is the best indication for continued treatment.

Environmental measures to reduce fever may be used if tolerated by the child and if they do not induce shivering. Shivering is the body's way of maintaining the elevated set point by producing heat. Compensatory shivering greatly increases metabolic requirements above those already caused by the fever.

Traditional cooling measures, such as wearing minimum clothing, exposing the skin to the air, reducing room temperature, increasing air circulation, and applying cool, moist compresses to the skin (e.g., the forehead), are effective if employed approximately 1 hour *after* an antipyretic is given so that the set point is lowered. Cooling procedures such as sponging or tepid baths are ineffective in treating febrile children (these measures are effective for hyperthermia) either when used alone or in combination with antipyretics, and they cause considerable discomfort (Sharber, 1997).

Seizures associated with a fever occur in 3% to 4% of all children, usually those 3 months to 5 years of age. Although most children never have febrile seizures after the first occurrence, a younger age at onset and a family history of febrile seizures are associated with recurring episodes (Berg, Shinnar, Levy, and others, 1999; Shinnar, Pellock, Berg, and others, 2001). There is little evidence to support the use of antipyretic drugs to prevent febrile seizures; nursing interventions should focus on ways to provide care and comfort during a febrile illness (Purssell, 2000).

Hyperthermia

Unlike fever, antipyretics are of no value in hyperthermia because the set point is already normal. Consequently, cooling measures are used. Cool applications to the skin help reduce the core temperature. Cooled blood from the skin surface is conducted to inner organs and tissues, and warm blood is circulated to the surface, where it is cooled and recirculated. The surface blood vessels dilate as the body attempts to dissipate heat to the environment and facilitate the cooling process.

Commercial cooling devices, such as cooling blankets or mattresses, are available to reduce body temperature. Place on the bed and cover with a sheet or lightweight blanket. Frequent temperature monitoring is essential to prevent excessive cooling of the body.

Traditionally, cool compresses have been used to decrease high temperature. For tepid tub baths it is usually best to start with warm water and gradually add cool water until the desired water temperature of 37° C (98.6° F) is reached to accustom the child to the lower water temperature. Generally, the temperature of the water only has to be 1° C or 2° F less than the child's temperature to be effective. The child is placed directly in the tub of tepid water for 15 to 20 minutes while water is gently squeezed from a washcloth over the back and chest or gently sprayed over the body from a sprayer. In the bed or crib, cool washcloths or towels are used, exposing only one area of the body at a time. The sponging is continued for approximately 20 minutes. After the tub or sponge bath, the child is dried and dressed in lightweight pajamas, a nightgown, or a diaper and placed in a dry bed. The child is dried by gently rubbing the skin surface with a towel to stimulate circulation. The temperature is retaken 30 minutes after the tub bath or sponge bath. The tub or sponge bath should not be continued or restarted until the skin surface is warm or if the child feels chilled. Chilling causes vasoconstriction, which defeats the purpose of the cool applications. In this condition, little blood is carried to the skin surface; the blood remains primarily in the viscera to become heated.

Whether a temperature elevation in the critically ill child is caused by fever or hyperthermia, it should be treated aggressively. The metabolic rate increases 10% for every 1° C increase in temperature and three to five times during shivering, thus increasing oxygen, fluid, and caloric requirements. If the child's cardiovascular or neurologic system is already compromised, these increased needs are especially hazardous. In all children with elevated temperature, attention to adequate hydration is essential. Most children's needs can be met through additional oral fluids.

FAMILY TEACHING AND HOME CARE

Although most children have learned self-care and hygiene in the home or at school, many have not. For some young children, this is their first introduction to the use of a toothbrush. Much health teaching can be accomplished even when the child is hospitalized for only a short time. The daily bath, hand washing before meals and after bowel and bladder evacuation, and conscientious dental hygiene are taught during routine care. Clean hair, nails, and clothing and good grooming are emphasized as being essential to a pleasing appearance. Positive reinforcement of good hygiene practices helps create a positive body image, enhances self-esteem, and prevents health problems (e.g., teaching girls to wipe the genital area from front to back after toileting).

Although sick children's appetites may be poor and not characteristic of their home eating habits, the hospital stay provides numerous opportunities for nurses to assess the family's knowledge of good nutrition and to implement teaching as needed to improve nutritional intake.

Fever is one of the most common problems for which parents seek health care. Parental anxiety increases with temperature elevation and its management (Liebman and Barnsteiner, 2001). Parents need to know that sponging is indicated for elevated temperatures from hyperthermia rather than fever and that ice water and alcohol are inappropriate, potentially dangerous solutions (Axelrod, 2000). Parents should know how to take the child's temperature and read the thermometer

FAMILY-CENTERED CARE

The Child with Fever
CALL THE OFFICE IMMEDIATELY IF:
Your child is younger than 2 months old.
The fever is over 40.6° C (105° F).
Your child looks or acts very sick: stiff neck, persistent vomiting, purplish spots on skin, confusion, trouble breathing after you have cleaned his nose, or inability to be comforted.

CALL WITHIN 24 HOURS IF:
The fever is between 40° and 40.6° C (104° and 105° F), especially if your child is younger than 2 years old.
Your child has:
■ Had a fever for more than 24 hours without an obvious cause or location of infection
■ Had a fever for more than 3 days
■ Burning or pain with urination
■ A history of febrile seizures
The fever went away for more than 24 hours and then returned.
You have other concerns or questions.

Modified from Schmitt BD: *Instructions for pediatric patients*, ed 2, Philadelphia, 1999, Saunders.

accurately and should have guidelines for seeking professional care (see Family-Centered Care box). Some of the newer temperature-measuring devices, such as plastic strips or digital thermometers, may be better suited for home use than hospital use (see Temperature, Chapter 6). If the use of acetaminophen or ibuprofen is indicated, the parents need instruction in administering the drug. Emphasize accuracy in both the amount of drug given and the time intervals at which the drug is administered.

SAFETY

Safety is an essential component of any patient's care, but children have special characteristics that require an even greater concern for safety. Because small children in the hospital are separated from their usual environment and do not possess the capacity for abstract thinking and reasoning, it is the responsibility of everyone who comes in contact with them to maintain protective measures throughout their hospital stay. Nurses need to understand the age level at which each child is operating and plan for safety accordingly.

Identification bands are particularly important for children. Infants and unconscious patients are unable to tell or respond to their names. Toddlers may answer to any name or to a nickname only. Older children may exchange places, give an erroneous name, or choose not to respond to their own names as a form of joke, unaware of the hazards of such practices.

ENVIRONMENTAL FACTORS

All of the environmental safety measures for the protection of adults apply to children, including good illumination, floors clear of fluid or objects that might contribute to falls, and nonskid surfaces in showers and tubs. All staff members should be familiar with the area-specific fire plan. Elevators and stairways should be made safe

All windows should be secured. Blind and curtain cords should be out of reach, with split cords to prevent strangulation.

Electrical equipment is maintained in good working order, is operated only by personnel familiar with its use, and is not in contact with moisture or situated near tubs. Electrical outlets should be provided with covers to prevent burns in small children, whose exploratory activities may extend to inserting objects into the small openings.

Staff members should practice proper care and disposal of small objects such as syringe caps, needle covers, and temperature probe covers (Fig. 22-3).

Bathwater is carefully checked before placing the child in it, and children must never be left alone in a bathtub. Infants are helpless in water, and small children (and some older ones) may turn on the hot water faucet and be severely burned.

Furniture is safest when it is scaled to the child's proportions, is sturdy, and is well balanced to prevent its being easily tipped over. A special hazard for children is the danger of entrapment under an electronically controlled bed when it is activated to descend. Infants and small children must be securely strapped into infant seats, feeding chairs, and strollers. Baby walkers should not be used because they provide access to hazards and can cause injuries by tipping over. Infants; young children; and those who are weak, paralyzed, agitated, confused, sedated, or cognitively impaired are never left unattended on treatment tables, on scales, or in treatment areas. Even preterm infants are capable of surprising mobility; therefore portholes in incubators must be securely fastened when not in use. Beds of ambulatory patients should remain locked in place and at a height that allows easy access to the floor.

Crib sides are kept up and fastened securely unless an adult is at the bedside. It is safer to leave crib sides up, regardless of the child's ability to get out and even when the crib is unoccupied, to remove the child's temptation to climb in. Anyone attending an infant or small child in a crib with the sides down should never turn away without maintaining hand contact with the child; that is, one hand should be kept on the child's back or abdomen to prevent the child from rolling, crawling, or jumping from the open crib (Fig. 22-4). A child who is apt to or has demonstrated the inclination to climb over the sides of the crib is safest when placed in a specially constructed crib with a cover.

Toy Safety

Toys play a vital role in the everyday life of children, and they are no less important in the hospital setting. Nurses are responsible for assessing the safety of toys brought to the hospital by well-meaning parents and friends. Toys should be appropriate to the child's age, condition, and treatment. For example, if

FIG. 22-3 ■ To prevent needlestick injuries, used needles (and other sharp instruments) are not capped or broken and are disposed of in a rigid, puncture-resistant container located near the site of use. Note placement of the container to prevent children's access to the contents.

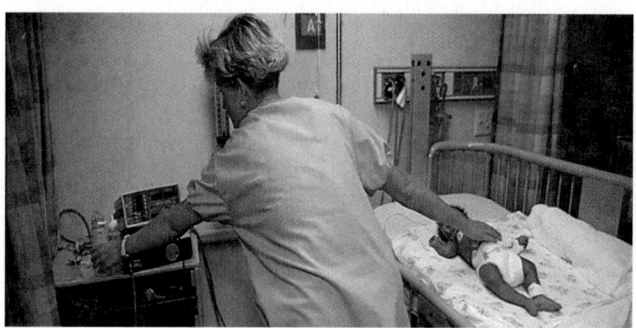

FIG. 22-4 ■ Nurse maintains hand contact when back is turned.

the child is receiving oxygen, electrical or friction toys are not safe, since sparks can cause oxygen to ignite. Inspect toys to ensure they are nonallergenic, washable, and unbreakable and have no small, removable parts that can be aspirated or swallowed or in other ways injure a child. All objects within reach of children younger than 3 years should pass the choke tube test. A toilet paper roll is a handy guide. If a toy or object fits into the cylinder (items less than 1¼ inches across or balls smaller than 1¾ inches), it is a potential choking danger to the child. Latex balloons pose a serious threat to children of all ages. If the balloon breaks, a child may put a piece of the latex in his or her mouth. If it is aspirated or swallowed, the latex piece is difficult to remove, resulting in choking. Latex balloons should *never* be permitted in the hospital setting.

Preventing Falls

Multiple interventions are needed to minimize pediatric patients' risk of falling. Once individual children are identified as at risk for falling, visual identification and communication of the risk among all health care providers is essential. Reduce the risk of falling through patient, family, and staff education.

1. Identify children at risk of falling. Perform a fall risk assessment on patients on admission and throughout hospitalization to identify patients at high risk for falls. Risk factors for hospitalized children include:
   - Medication effects—postanesthesia or sedation; analgesics or narcotics, especially in those who have never had narcotics in the past and in whom effects are unknown
   - Altered mental status—secondary to seizures, brain tumors, or medications
   - Altered or limited mobility—reduced skill at ambulation secondary to developmental age, disease process, tubes, drains, casts, splints, or other appliances; new to ambulation with assistive devices such as walkers or crutches
   - Postoperative children—risk of hypotension or syncope secondary to large blood loss, a heart condition, or extended bed rest
   - History of falls
   - Infants or toddlers in cribs with side rails down or on the daybed with family members
2. Visually identify patients at risk with one or more of the following:
   - Post signs on the door and at the bedside.
   - Apply a special colored armband labeled "Fall Precautions."
   - Label the chart with a sticker.
   - Document information on the chart.
3. Alter the environment:
   - Keep bed in lowest position, breaks locked, and side rails up.
   - Place call bell within reach.
   - Ensure that all necessary and desired items are within reach (e.g., water, glasses, tissues, snacks).
   - Offer toileting on a regular basis, especially if patient is taking diuretics or laxatives.
   - Keep lights on at all times, including dim lights while sleeping.
   - Lock wheelchairs before transferring patients.
   - Ensure that patient has appropriate size gown and nonskid footwear. Do not allow gowns or ties to drag on the floor when ambulating.
   - Keep floor clean and free of clutter. Post "wet floor" sign if floor is wet.
   - Ensure that patient has glasses on if he or she normally wears them.
4. Educate patients (as age appropriate):
   - Assist with ambulation even though the child may have ambulated well before hospitalization.
   - Patients who have been lying in bed will need to get up slowly, sitting on the side of the bed before standing.
5. Educate family members:
   - Call the nursing staff for assistance, and do not allow patients to get up independently.
   - Keep the side rails of the crib or bed up whenever patient is in the crib or bed.
   - Do not leave infants on the daybed; put them in the crib with the side rails up.
   - When all family members need to leave the bedside, notify staff and ensure the patient is in the bed or crib with side rails up and call bell within reach (if appropriate).

INFECTION CONTROL

According to the Centers for Disease Control and Prevention, approximately 2 million patients each year develop nosocomial (hospital-acquired) infections. These infections occur when there is interaction among patients, health care personnel, equipment, and bacteria (Quality, equipment hold keys to infection control, 2006). Nosocomial infections are preventable if caregivers practice meticulous cleaning and disposal techniques. **Standard precautions** synthesize the major features of universal (blood and body fluid) precautions (designed to reduce the risk of transmission of blood-borne pathogens) and body substance isolation (designed to reduce the risk of transmission of pathogens from moist body substances). Standard precautions involve the use of **barrier protection,** such as gloves, goggles, gown, or mask, to prevent contamination from (1) blood; (2) all body fluids, secretions, and excretions *except sweat,* regardless of whether they contain visible blood; (3) nonintact skin; and (4) mucous membranes. Standard precautions are designed for the care of all patients to reduce the risk of transmission of microorganisms from both recognized and unrecognized sources of infection.

Transmission-based precautions are designed for patients with documented or suspected infection or colonization (presence of microorganism in or on patient but without clinical signs and symptoms of infection) with highly transmissible or epidemiologically important pathogens for which additional precautions beyond standard precautions are needed to interrupt transmission in hospitals. There are three types of transmission-based precautions: airborne precautions, droplet precautions, and contact precautions. They may be combined for diseases that have multiple routes of transmission (Box 22-5). They are to be used in addition to standard precautions.

Airborne precautions reduce the risk of airborne transmission of infectious agents. Airborne transmission occurs by dissemination of either airborne droplet nuclei (small-particle residue [5 μm or smaller in size] of evaporated droplets that may remain suspended in the air for long periods) or dust particles containing the infectious agent. Microorganisms carried in this manner can be dispersed widely by air currents and may become inhaled by or deposited on a susceptible host within the same room or over a longer distance from the source patient, depending on environmental factors. Special air handling and ventilation are required to prevent airborne transmission. Airborne precautions apply to patients with

BOX 22-5

Types of Precautions and Patients Requiring Them

STANDARD PRECAUTIONS
Use standard precautions for the care of all patients.

AIRBORNE PRECAUTIONS
In addition to standard precautions, use airborne precautions for patients known or suspected to have serious illnesses transmitted by airborne droplet nuclei. Examples of such illnesses include measles, varicella (including disseminated zoster), and tuberculosis.

DROPLET PRECAUTIONS
In addition to standard precautions, use droplet precautions for patients known or suspected to have serious illnesses transmitted by large-particle droplets. Examples of such illnesses include:

- Invasive *Haemophilus influenzae* type b, including meningitis, pneumonia, epiglottitis, and sepsis
- Invasive *Neisseria meningitidis*, including meningitis, pneumonia, and sepsis
- Other serious bacterial respiratory infections spread by droplet transmission, including diphtheria (pharyngeal), mycoplasmal pneumonia, pertussis, pneumonic plague, streptococcal pharyngitis, pneumonia, or scarlet fever in infants and young children
- Serious viral infections spread by droplet transmission, including adenovirus, influenza, mumps, parvovirus B19, rubella

CONTACT PRECAUTIONS
In addition to standard precautions, use contact precautions for patients known or suspected to have serious illnesses easily transmitted by direct patient contact or by contact with items in the patient's environment. Examples of such illnesses include:

- Gastrointestinal, respiratory, skin, or wound infections or colonization with multidrug-resistant bacteria judged by the infection control program, based on current state, regional, or national recommendations, to be of special clinical and epidemiologic significance
- Enteric infections with a low infectious dose or prolonged environmental survival, including *Clostridium difficile;* for diapered or incontinent patients: enterohemorrhagic *Escherichia coli* O157:H7, *Shigella* sp., hepatitis A, or rotavirus
- Respiratory syncytial virus, parainfluenza virus, or enteroviral infections in infants and young children
- Skin infections that are highly contagious or that may occur on dry skin, including diphtheria (cutaneous), herpes simplex virus (neonatal or mucocutaneous), impetigo, major (noncontained) abscesses, cellulitis or decubiti, pediculosis, scabies, staphylococcal furunculosis in infants and young children, zoster (disseminated or in the immunocompromised host)
- Viral or hemorrhagic conjunctivitis
- Viral hemorrhagic infections (Ebola, Lassa, or Marburg)

From Garner JS: Guidelines for isolation precautions in hospitals, *Infect Control Hosp Epidemiol* 17(1):66, 1996.

known or suspected infection with pathogens transmitted by the airborne route such as measles, varicella, and tuberculosis.

Droplet precautions reduce the risk of droplet transmission of infectious agents. Droplet transmission involves contact of the conjunctivae or the mucous membranes of the nose or mouth of a susceptible person with large-particle droplets (larger than 5 μm in size) containing microorganisms generated from a person who has a clinical disease or who is a carrier of the microorganism. Droplets are generated from the source person primarily during coughing, sneezing, or talking and during procedures such as suctioning and bronchoscopy. Transmission requires close contact between source and recipient persons, since droplets do not remain suspended in the air and generally travel only short distances, usually 3 feet or less, through the air. Because droplets do not remain suspended in the air, special air handling and ventilation are not required to prevent droplet transmission. Droplet precautions apply to any patient with known or suspected infection with pathogens that can be transmitted by infectious droplets (see Box 22-5).

Contact precautions reduce the risk of transmission of microorganisms by direct or indirect contact. Direct-contact transmission involves a skin-to-skin contact and physical transfer of microorganisms to a susceptible host from an infected or colonized person, such as occurs when turning or bathing patients. Direct-contact transmission also can occur between two patients (e.g., by hand contact). Indirect-contact transmission involves contact of a susceptible host with a contaminated intermediate object, usually inanimate, in the patient's environment. Contact precautions apply to specified patients known or suspected to be infected or colonized with microorganisms that can be transmitted by direct or indirect contact.

> **NURSINGALERT**
> The most common piece of medical equipment, the stethoscope, can be a potent source of harmful microorganisms and nosocomial infections. One study found that 80% of 200 stethoscopes were contaminated with at least one microbe (Eckler, 1997).

Nurses caring for young children are frequently in contact with body substances, especially urine, feces, and vomitus. They should exercise judgment concerning those situations when gloves, gowns, or masks are necessary. For example, gloves and possibly gowns should be worn for changing diapers when there are loose or explosive stools. Otherwise, the plastic lining of disposable diapers provides a sufficient barrier between the hands and body substances. The type of diaper may be an important aspect of infection control. Super absorbent disposable diapers with elastic legs contain urine and feces better than cloth diapers.

Antimicrobial-resistant organisms are causing increasing numbers of nosocomial infections. Nearly 70% of nosocomial infections can be attributed to seven pathogens: the gram-positive organisms *Staphylococcus aureus*, coagulase-negative staphylococci, and enterococci; and the gram-negative organisms *Escherichia coli, Pseudomonas aeruginosa, Enterobacter* organisms, and *Klebsiella pneumoniae*. In hospitals, patients are the most significant sources of methicillin-resistant *S. aureus* (MRSA), and the main mode of transmission is patient to patient via the hands of a health care provider (Eaton, 2005; Quality, equipment hold keys to infection control, 2006).

> **NURSINGALERT**
> Hand washing is the most critical infection-control practice.

During feedings, gowns should be worn if the child is likely to vomit or spit up, which often occurs during burping. When gloves are worn, wash hands thoroughly after removing the gloves, since gloves fail to provide complete protection. The absence of visible leakage does not indicate gloves are intact.

Another essential practice of infection control is that all needles (uncapped and unbroken) are disposed of in a rigid, puncture-resistant container located near the site of use. Consequently, these containers are installed in patients' rooms. Since children are naturally curious, extra attention is needed in selecting a suitable type of container and a location that prevents access to disposed needles (see Fig. 22-3). The use of needleless systems allows secure syringe or IV tubing attachment to vascular access devices without the risk of needlestick injury to the child or nurse.

TRANSPORTING INFANTS AND CHILDREN

Infants and children usually need to be transported within the unit and to areas outside the pediatric unit. Infants and small children can be carried for short distances within the unit, but for more extended trips the child should be securely transported in a suitable conveyance.

Small infants can be held or carried in the horizontal position with the back supported and the thigh grasped firmly by the carrying arm (Fig. 22-5, *A*). In the football hold, the infant is carried on the nurse's arm with the head supported by the hand and the body held securely between the nurse's body and elbow (Fig. 22-5, *B*). Both of these holds leave the nurse's other arm free for activity. The infant also can be held in the upright position with the buttocks on the nurse's forearm and the front of the body resting against the nurse's chest. The infant's head and shoulders are supported by the nurse's other arm in case the infant moves suddenly (Fig. 22-5, *C*). Older infants are able to hold their heads erect but are still subject to sudden movements.

Infants can be transported to other areas, such as the radiology department, in their bassinet or crib. Strollers and wheeled feeding chairs or tables are also convenient transporters in some situations, such as trips to the playroom or nurse's station.

The method of transporting children is determined by their age, condition, and destination. Older children are safe in wheelchairs or on stretchers. Younger children can be transported in a crib, on a stretcher, in a wagon with raised sides, or in a wheelchair with a safety belt. Stretchers should be equipped with high sides and a safety belt, both of which are secured during transport.

RESTRAINING METHODS AND THERAPEUTIC HOLDING

The Joint Commission on Accreditation of Healthcare Organizations (now known as The Joint Commission) (2001) defines restraint as "any method, physical or mechanical, which restricts a person's movement, physical activity, or normal access to his or her body." Before initiating restraints, the nurse completes a comprehensive assessment of the patient to determine whether the need for a restraint outweighs the risk of not using one. Restraints can result in loss of dignity, violation of patient rights, psychologic harm, physical harm, and even death. Alternative methods should first be considered and documented in the patient's record. The nurse is responsible for selecting the least restrictive type of restraint. Using less restrictive restraints is often possible by gaining the cooperation of the child and parents.

The two types of restraints used with children are classified as medical-surgical and behavioral restraints. When a standard or protocol states that immobilization is required 100% of the time as a part of the procedure or postprocedural care process, the restraint device is considered a part of routine care. For example, the postoperative use of elbow restraints after a cleft lip repair, if written in the protocol or standard of care and used for 100% of patients, would not fall under The Joint Commission or Centers for Medicare and Medicaid Services mandates for restraints.

Medical-surgical restraints are used for children with an artificial airway or airway adjunct for delivery of oxygen, indwelling catheters, tubes, drains, lines, pacemaker wires, or suture sites. The medical-surgical restraint is used to ensure that safe care is given to the patient. The potential risks of the restraint are offset by the potential benefit of providing safer

FIG. 22-5 ■ Transporting infants. **A,** Infant's thigh firmly grasped in nurse's hand. **B,** Football hold. **C,** Back supported.

care. Medical-surgical restraints may be instituted for any of the following reasons:

- Risk for interruption of therapy used to maintain oxygenation or airway patency
- Risk of harm if indwelling catheter, tube, drain, line, pacemaker wire, or sutures are removed, dislodged, or ruptured
- Patient confusion, agitation, unconsciousness, or developmental inability to understand direct requests or instructions

Medical-surgical restraints can be initiated by an individual order or by protocol; the use of the protocol must be authorized by an individual order. Continued use of restraints must be renewed each day. Patients are monitored at least every 2 hours.

Behavioral restraints are limited to situations with a significant risk of patients physically harming themselves or others because of behavioral reasons and when nonphysical interventions are not effective. Before initiating a behavioral restraint, the nurse should assess the patient's mental, behavioral, and physical status to determine the cause for the child's behavior that may be harmful to the patient or others. If behavioral restraints are indicated, a collaborative approach involving the patient, if appropriate, the family, and the health care team should be used. An order must be obtained as soon as possible, but no longer than 1 hour after the initiation of behavioral restraints. Behavioral restraints for children must be reordered every 1 to 2 hours, based on age. A licensed independent practitioner must conduct an in-person evaluation within 1 hour and again every 4 hours until restraints are discontinued. Children in behavioral restraints must be *continuously* observed and assessed every 15 minutes. Assessment components include signs of injury associated with applying restraint, nutrition and hydration, circulation and range-of-motion of extremities, vital signs, hygiene and elimination, physical and psychologic status and comfort, and readiness for discontinuation of restraint. The nurse must use clinical judgment in setting a schedule for when each of these parameters needs to be evaluated because every parameter must be assessed during each 15-minute physical assessment.

Restraints with ties must be secured to the bed or crib frame, not the side rails. Suggestions for increasing safety and comfort while the child is in a restraint include leaving one finger breadth between skin and the device; tying knots that allow for quick release; ensuring the restraint does not tighten as the child moves; decreasing wrinkles or bulges in the restraint; placing jacket restraints over an article of clothing; placing limb restraints below waist level, below knee level, or distal to the IV; and tucking in dangling straps (Selekman and Snyder, 1997).

An alternative approach for temporary restraint is therapeutic holding. **Therapeutic holding** is the use of a secure, comfortable, temporary holding position that provides close physical contact with the parent or caregiver for 30 minutes or less (Fig. 22-6).

The use of restraints can often be avoided with adequate preparation of the child; parental or staff supervision of the child; or adequate protection of a vulnerable site, such as an infusion device. The nurse needs to assess the child's development, mental status, potential to hurt others or self, and safety. The nurse should carefully consider alternatives to using restraints. Some examples of alternative measures include bringing a child to the nurses' station for continuous observation, providing diversional activities such as music, or encouraging the participation of the parents.

Jacket Restraint

A jacket restraint is sometimes used to keep the child safe in various chairs. The jacket is put on the child with the ties in back so that the child is unable to manipulate them. The long tapes, secured to the understructure of the chair, keep the child inside the chair. The jacket restraint is also useful as a means of maintaining the child in a desired horizontal position.

Mummy Restraint or Swaddle

When an infant or small child requires short-term restraint for examination or treatment that involves the head and neck, such as venipuncture, throat examination, and gavage feeding, a papoose board with straps or a mummy wrap effectively controls the child's movements. A blanket or sheet is opened on the bed or crib with one corner folded to the center. The infant is placed on the blanket with shoulders at the fold and feet toward the opposite corner. With the infant's right arm straight down against the body, the right side of the blanket is pulled firmly across the infant's right shoulder and chest and secured beneath the left side of the body (Fig. 22-7, *A*). The left arm is placed straight against the infant's side, and the left side of the blanket is brought across the shoulder and chest and locked beneath the body on the right side. The lower corner is folded and brought over the body and tucked or fastened securely with safety pins. Safety pins can be used to fasten the blanket in place at any step in the process.

To modify the mummy restraint for chest examination, the folded edge of the blanket is brought over each arm and under the back, after which the loose edge is folded over and secured at a point below the chest to allow visualization of and access to the chest (Fig. 22-7, *B*).

Arm and Leg Restraints

Occasionally, one or more extremities must be restrained or limited in motion. Several commercial restraining devices are available, including disposable wrist and ankle restraints. The restraints must be appropriate to the child's size and padded to prevent undue pressure, constriction, or tissue injury; and the extremity must be observed frequently for signs of irrita-

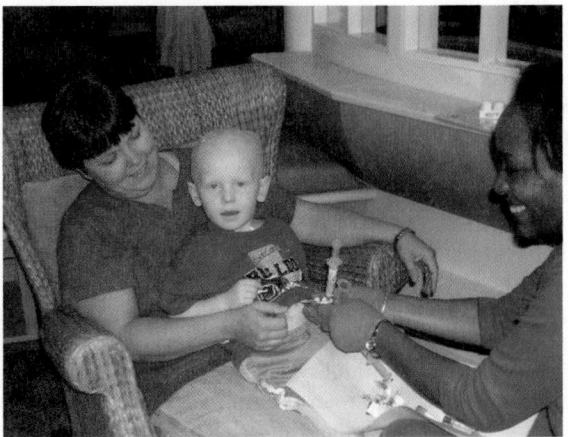

FIG. 22-6 ■ Therapeutic holding of child for extremity venipuncture with parental assistance.

FIG. 22-7 ■ Application of mummy restraint. **A,** Infant placed on folded corner of blanket and one corner of blanket brought across body and secured beneath body. **B,** Second corner brought across body and secured, and lower corner folded and tucked or pinned in place; modified mummy restraint with chest uncovered.

FIG. 22-8 ■ Restraining infant for femoral venipuncture.

tion or impairment of circulation. The ends of the restraints are never tied to the side rails, since lowering the rail will disturb the extremity, frequently with a jerk that may hurt or injure the child.

Elbow Restraint

Sometimes it is important to prevent the child from reaching the head or face (e.g., after lip surgery, when a scalp vein infusion is in place, or to prevent scratching in skin disorders). Elbow restraints fashioned from a variety of materials function well. Commercial elbow restraints are available. An improvised form of elbow restraint consists of a piece of muslin long enough to reach comfortably from just below the axilla to the wrist with a number of vertical pockets into which tongue depressors are inserted. The restraint is wrapped around the arm and secured with tape or pins. It may be necessary to pin the top of the restraint to the undershirt sleeve to prevent the restraint from slipping.

POSITIONING FOR PROCEDURES

Infants and small children are unable to cooperate for many procedures; therefore the nurse is responsible for minimizing their movement and discomfort with proper positioning. Older children usually need only minimal, if any, restraint. Careful explanation and preparation beforehand and support and simple guidance during the procedure are usually sufficient. For painful procedures the child should receive adequate analgesia and sedation to minimize pain and the need for excessive restraint. For local anesthesia, use buffered lidocaine to reduce the stinging sensation or a topical anesthetic (see Pain Management, Chapter 7).

Femoral Venipuncture

The nurse places the child supine with the legs in a frog position to provide extensive exposure of the groin area. The infant's legs can be effectively controlled by the nurse's forearms and hands (Fig. 22-8). Only the side used for the venipuncture

is uncovered, so the practitioner is protected should the infant urinate during the procedure. Apply pressure to the site to prevent oozing from the site.

Extremity Venipuncture

The most common sites of venipuncture are the veins of the extremities, especially the arm and hand. A convenient position is to place the child in the parent's (or assistant's) lap, with the child facing the parent and in the straddle position. Next, place the child's arm for venipuncture on a firm surface, such as a treatment table. The child's outstretched arm is partially stabilized by the technician drawing the blood. Then have the parent hug the child's upper body, preventing movement, and use an arm to immobilize the venipuncture site. This type of restraint also comforts the child because of the close body contact and allows each person to maintain eye contact (see Fig. 22-6).

Lumbar Puncture

Pediatric lumbar puncture (LP) sets contain smaller spinal needles, but sometimes the practitioner will specify a different size or type of needle. The technique for LP in infants and children is similar to that in the adult, although modifications are suggested in neonates, who have less distress in a side-lying position with modified neck extension than in flexion or a sitting position.

Children are usually controlled best in the side-lying position, with the head flexed and the knees drawn up toward the chest. Even cooperative children need to be held gently to prevent possible trauma from unexpected, involuntary movement. They can be reassured that, although they are trusted, the holding will serve as a reminder to maintain the desired position. It also provides a measure of support and reassurance to them.

The child is placed on the side with the back close to the edge of the examining table on the side from which the practitioner is working. Maintain the child's spine in a flexed position by holding the child with one arm behind the neck and the other behind the thighs (Fig. 22-9). The flexed position enlarges the spaces between the lumbar vertebrae, which facilitates access to the spinal fluid space. It is helpful to wrap the legs before positioning to decrease leg movement (see Atraumatic Care box).

FIG. 22-9 ■ Child in side-lying position for lumbar puncture.

Lumbar Puncture and Bone Marrow Test

Apply EMLA (an eutectic mixture of lidocaine and prilocaine) to the puncture site at least 60 minutes or LMX cream (lidocaine) at least 30 minutes before the procedure. To identify the lumbar puncture site, draw an imaginary line from the posterior iliac crest across the spine to the opposite iliac crest. The puncture site is intersected by the line at approximately L4. For additional anesthesia, buffered lidocaine with a 30-gauge needle can be used. **Sedation** with agents such as propofol (Diprivan) or ketamine is recommended for bone marrow biopsy and aspiration.

An alternate position used with small infants and some older children is the sitting position. The child is placed with the buttocks at the edge of the table and with the neck flexed so that the chin rests on the child's chest or the nurse's arm. The infant's arms and legs are immobilized by the nurse's hands.

> **NURSINGALERT**
>
> The sitting position may interfere with chest expansion and diaphragm excursion, and in infants the soft, pliable trachea may collapse. Therefore observe the child for difficulty with breathing.

Specimens and spinal fluid pressure are obtained, measured, and sent for analysis in the same manner as for the adult patient. Vital signs are taken as ordered, and the child is observed for any changes in level of consciousness, motor activity, or other neurologic signs. Post-LP headache may occur and is related to postural changes; this is less severe when the child lies flat. Headache is seen much less frequently in young children than in adolescents.

Bone Marrow Aspiration or Biopsy

The position for a bone marrow aspiration or biopsy depends on the chosen site. In children the posterior or anterior iliac crest is most frequently used, although in infants the tibia may be selected because of easy access to the site and holding of the child. The sternum, which is the most frequent site in adults,

is generally avoided in children because the bone is more fragile and adjacent to vital organs.

If the posterior iliac crest is used, the child is positioned prone. Sometimes a small pillow or folded blanket is placed under the hips to facilitate obtaining the bone marrow specimen. Children should receive adequate analgesia or anesthesia to relieve pain. If the child may awaken, holding may be needed and is best done with two people—one person to immobilize the upper body and a second person to immobilize the lower extremities (see Atraumatic Care box).

COLLECTION OF SPECIMENS
URINE SPECIMENS

Older children and adolescents can use a bedpan or urinal or can be trusted to follow directions for collection in the bathroom. However, they may have special needs. School-age children are cooperative but curious. They are concerned about the reasons behind things and are likely to ask questions regarding the disposition of their specimen and what one expects to discover from it. Self-conscious adolescents may be reluctant to carry a specimen through a hallway or waiting room and appreciate a paper bag or other means for disguising the container. The presence of menses may be an embarrassment or a concern to teenage girls; therefore it is a good idea to ask if they are menstruating and to make adjustments as necessary. The specimen can be delayed or a notation made on the laboratory slip to explain the presence of red blood cells.

Preschoolers and toddlers are usually unable to void on request. It is often best to offer them water or other liquids that they enjoy and wait about 30 minutes until they are ready to void voluntarily.

> **NURSINGTIP**
>
> Wipe the abdomen with an alcohol pad and fan it dry; the cooling effect often causes voiding within 2 minutes. Apply pressure over the suprapubic area or stroke the paraspinal muscles (along the spine) to elicit the Perez reflex; in infants 4 to 6 months of age, this reflex causes crying, extension of the back, flexion of the extremities, and urination.

Children will better understand what is expected if the nurse uses familiar terms, such as "pee-pee," "wee-wee," "tee-tee," or "tinkle." Some will have difficulty voiding in an unfamiliar receptacle. Potty chairs or a potty hat placed on the toilet is usually satisfactory. Toddlers who have recently acquired bladder control may be especially reluctant, since they undoubtedly have been admonished for "going" in places other than those approved by parents. A useful approach is to enlist the help of parents; they are likely to be successful.

For infants and toddlers who are not toilet trained, special urine collection bags with self-adhering material round the opening at the point of attachment are used. To prepare the infant, the genitalia, perineum, and surrounding skin are washed and dried thoroughly because the adhesive will not stick to a moist, powdered, or oily skin surface. The collection bag is easiest to apply if attached first to the perineum, progressing to the symphysis pubis (Fig. 22-10). With girls, the perineum is stretched taut during application to that area to ensure a leak-proof fit. With boys the penis and sometimes the scrotum are placed inside the bag. The adhesive portion of the bag must be firmly applied to the skin all around the genital area to avoid leakage. For low-birth-weight infants, small bags

FIG. 22-10 ■ Application of urine collection bag. **A,** On female infants, adhesive portion is applied to exposed and dried perineum first. **B,** Bag adheres firmly around perineal area to prevent urine leakage.

with adhesive that is gentle to the skin are available.* Anatomically correct urine collection bags are also available.† The diaper is carefully replaced. The bag is checked frequently and removed as soon as the specimen is available, since the moist bag may become loosened on an active child. When urine is collected for culture, the bag is removed immediately. For some types of urine testing, such as specific gravity, ketones, glucose, and protein, urine can be aspirated directly from the diaper. If the urine is not tested within 30 minutes, the specimen is refrigerated or placed in a sterile container with a preservative.

> **FYI**
>
> Urine obtained from disposable diapers can be tested accurately for glucose, ketones, protein, blood, and urea. In one study, urine obtained from a disposable diaper provided a valid sample for diagnosing urinary tract infections (Cohen, Woloch, Linder, and others, 1997). Superabsorbent disposable diapers may produce a false crystalluria. Specific gravity measurements are accurate for up to 4 hours provided that the disposable diapers are kept folded. Urine samples collected by the cotton ball method were accurate for pH and specific gravity and were atraumatic to the skin of newborns (Burke, 1995).

> **NURSING TIP**
>
> ■ When using a urine collection bag, cut a small slit in the diaper and pull the bag through to allow room for urine to collect and to facilitate checking on the contents.
> ■ To obtain small amounts of urine, use a syringe without a needle to aspirate urine directly from the diaper; if diapers with absorbent gelling material that trap urine are used, place a small gauze dressing, some cotton balls, or a urine collection device‡ inside the diaper to collect urine and aspirate the urine with a syringe.

At times parents may be asked to bring a urine sample to a health care facility for examination, especially when infants are unable to void during an outpatient visit. In this instance parents need instruction on applying the collection device and storing the specimen. Ideally, the specimen should be

brought to the designated place as soon as possible; if there is a delay, the sample is refrigerated and the lapsed time reported to the examiner.

Clean-Catch Specimens

Clean-catch specimens traditionally refer to a urine sample obtained for culture after the urethral meatus is cleaned and the first few milliliters of urine are voided before the urine is collected (**midstream specimen**). In girls, the perineum is wiped with an antiseptic-soaked cotton ball or pad from front to back at least three times, using a new cotton ball or pad each time. In boys, the tip of the penis is cleansed. The area may be wiped with sterile water to prevent accidental contamination of the urine with a solution that may destroy pathogens.

> **FYI**
>
> Although this traditional cleansing procedure is often practiced, it does not significantly reduce contamination rates in infants, circumcised or uncircumcised males, or toilet-trained prepubertal children.

Twenty-Four-Hour Collection

Collection bags are required to collect specimens from infants and small children. Older children require special instruction about notifying someone when they need to void or have a bowel movement so that urine can be collected separately and not discarded. Some older school-age children and adolescents can take responsibility for collection of their own 24-hour specimens and can keep output records and transfer each voiding to the 24-hour collection container.

The collection period always starts and ends with an empty bladder. At the time the collection begins, the child is instructed to void and the specimen is discarded. All urine voided in the subsequent 24 hours is saved in a container with a preservative or is placed on ice. Twenty-four hours from the time the precollection specimen was discarded, the child is again instructed to void, the specimen is added to the container, and the entire collection is taken to the laboratory.

Infants and small children who are bagged for a 24-hour urine collection require a special collection bag. Frequent removal and replacement of adhesive collection devices can produce skin irritation. A thin coating of sealant, such as Skin-Prep, applied to the skin helps to protect it and aids adhesion, unless its use is contraindicated, such as in a preterm infant or

*Available from Hollister, Inc., 2000 Hollister Drive, Libertyville, IL 60048; (800) 323-4060; http://www.hollister.com.
†Available from ConvaTec, PO Box 5254, Princeton, NJ 08543-5254; (800) 422-8811; http://www.convatec.com.
‡The Bard Sure Catch is available from Bard Urological Division, C.R. Bard, Inc., 13183 Harland Drive, Covington, GA 30014; (888) 367-2273; http://www.crbard.com.

a child with irritated skin. Plastic collection bags with collection tubes attached are ideal when the container must be left in place for a time. These can be connected to a collecting device or emptied periodically by aspiration with a syringe. When such devices are not available, a regular bag with a feeding tube inserted through a puncture hole at the top of the bag serves as a satisfactory substitute. However, care is taken to empty the bag as soon as the infant urinates to prevent leakage and loss of contents. An indwelling catheter may also be placed for the collection period.

Bladder Catheterization and Other Techniques

Bladder catheterization or suprapubic aspiration is employed when a specimen is urgently needed or when the child is unable to void or otherwise provide an adequate specimen. Catheterization is used to obtain a sterile urine specimen and when urethral obstruction or anuria caused by renal failure is believed to be the cause of the child's failure to void. The American Academy of Pediatrics recommends that urine collected by the bag can be used to determine whether it is necessary to obtain a catheterized urine specimen for culture (Wald, 2005). Suprapubic aspiration is useful in clarifying the diagnosis of suspected urinary tract infection in acutely ill infants.

Preparation for catheterization includes instruction on pelvic muscle relaxation. The toddler, preschooler, or younger child is taught to blow a pinwheel and to press the hips against the bed or procedure table during catheterization to relax the pelvic and periurethral muscles. The location and function of the pelvic muscles are described briefly to the older child or adolescent. The patient is then taught to contract and relax the pelvic muscles, and the relaxation procedure is repeated during catheter insertion. If the patient vigorously contracts the pelvic muscles when the catheter reaches the striated sphincter (proximal urethra in boys and midurethra in girls), catheter insertion is temporarily stopped. The catheter is neither removed nor advanced; instead, the child is helped to press the hips against the bed or examining table and relax the pelvic muscles. The catheter is then gently advanced into the bladder (Gray, 1996).

Children and adolescents experience some discomfort and anxiety during this procedure. Assistance and gentle holding may be necessary, especially for the younger child. Most children prefer to have the parents remain with them during the procedure. Encourage the parent to talk softly and hold the child's hand as the catheter is inserted. Using distractions such as reading a book, singing a song, or playing with small toys may decrease the child's anxiety. Older children and adolescents may wish to listen to music with headphones. Adolescents should be asked if they would like a parent to remain with them during the procedure. The decision should be made before the perineum is exposed and the sterile field is prepared.

Catheterization is a sterile procedure, and standard precautions for body substance protection should be followed. When placing a catheter to obtain a sterile urine specimen or to check for residual urine, the nurse may use a sterile feeding tube if a catheter is unavailable. If the catheter is to remain in place, a Foley catheter is used. Table 22-3 gives guidelines for choosing the appropriately sized catheter and length of insertion. The supplies needed for this procedure include sterile gloves, sterile lubricant anesthetic, an appropriately sized

TABLE 22-3
Straight Catheter or Foley Catheter*

	SIZE (LENGTH OF INSERTION [cm]) FOR GIRLS	SIZE (LENGTH OF INSERTION [cm]) FOR BOYS
Term neonate	5-6 (5)	5-6 (6)
Infant–3 years	5-8 (5)	5-8 (6)
4-8 years	8 (5-6)	8 (6-9)
8 years–prepubertal	10-12 (6-8)	8-10 (10-15)
Pubertal	12-14 (6-8)	12-14 (13-18)

*Foley catheters are approximately 1 French size larger because of the circumference of the balloon. Example: 10 French Foley = approximately 12 French calibration.

catheter, povidone-iodine (Betadine) swabs or an alternative cleansing agent and 4 × 4 inch gauze squares, a sterile drape, and a syringe with sterile water if a Foley catheter is used. Test the balloon of the Foley catheter by injecting sterile water before catheter insertion.

NURSING ALERT

Identify patients who have allergies to povidone-iodine or latex before using these items in catheterization.

Adolescent boys and children with a history of urethral surgery may be catheterized using a coudé-tipped catheter. The child with myelodysplasia or one who has been identified as being sensitive or allergic to latex is catheterized with a catheter manufactured from an alternative material. When an indwelling catheter is indicated for urinary drainage, a lubricious-coated or silicone catheter is selected because these materials produce less irritation of the urethral mucosa when compared with a Silastic or latex catheter when the catheter is left in place for more than 72 hours.

A 2% lidocaine lubricant with applicator is assembled according to the manufacturer's instructions,* and several drops of the lubricant are placed at the meatus. Advise the child that the lubricant is used to reduce discomfort associated with inserting the catheter and that introduction of the lubricant and catheter into the urethra will produce a sensation of pressure and a desire to urinate (Gray, 1996) (see Evidence-Based Practice box).

In male patients, grasp the penis with the nondominant hand and retract the foreskin. In uncircumcised newborns and infants, the foreskin may be adhered to the shaft; use care when retracting. If the penis is pendulous, place a sterile drape under the penis. Using the sterile hand, swab the glans and meatus three times with povidone-iodine. Gently introduce the tip of the lidocaine jelly applicator into the urethra 1 to 2 cm (0.4 to 0.8 inch) so that the lubricant flows only into the urethra; insert 5 to 10 ml 2% lidocaine lubricant into the urethra and hold in place for 2 to 3 minutes by gently squeezing the distal penis. Lubricate the catheter and insert into the urethra while gently stretching the penis and lifting it to a 90-degree angle to the body. Resistance may occur when the catheter meets the

*Lidocaine hydrochloride 2% jelly is available from International Medication Systems, Ltd., 1886 Santa Anita Ave., South El Monte, CA 91733; (800) 423-4136; http://www.ims-limited.com; and from AstraZeneca, 1800 Concord Pike, Wilmington, DE 19801; (800) 842-992; http://www.astrazeneca-us.com.

EVIDENCE-BASED PRACTICE

Use of Lidocaine Lubricant for Urethral Catheterization
Marilyn J. Hockenberry

ASK THE QUESTION   In children, does a lidocaine lubricant decrease the pain associated with urethral catheterization?

SEARCH FOR EVIDENCE
Search Strategies   Search selection criteria included English-language publications within the past 10 years, and research-based and review articles on use of the lidocaine lubricant before urethral catheterization.
Databases Used   Cochrane Collaboration, PubMed, MD Consult, BestBETS, American Academy of Pediatrics

CRITICALLY ANALYZE THE EVIDENCE

Smith and Adams (1998) surveyed 46 children's hospitals to determine the existence of standardized practice guidelines for urethral catheter insertion in children. Only 54% of the institutions had a written policy providing guidelines for the procedure, and the hospitals' recommendations lacked consistency.

Grey (1996) published a review of strategies to minimize distress associated with urethral catheterization in children and supported the use of a local anesthetic that contains 2% lidocaine before insertion.

One prospective, double-blind, placebo-controlled trial evaluated the use of lidocaine lubricant for discomfort in 20 children before urethral catheterization. Findings revealed that lidocaine lubricant significantly reduced pain with pediatric urethral catheterization (Gerard, Cooper, Duethman, and others, 2003).

APPLY THE EVIDENCE: NURSING IMPLICATIONS

- Although only one research study was found to support the use of a topical anesthetic before urethral catheterization, the study found significant reductions in procedural pain. Several publications support its effectiveness in clinical practice.
- A topical anesthetic before urethral catheterization may be helpful, but further evidence is needed.

References

Gerard LL, Cooper CS, Duethman KS, and others: Effectiveness of lidocaine lubricant for discomfort during pediatric urethral catheterization, *J Urol* 170:564-567, 2003.
Grey M: Atraumatic urethral catheterization of children, *Pediatr Nurs* 22(4):306-310, 1996.
Smith AB, Adams LL: Insertion of indwelling urethral catheters in infants and children: a survey of current nursing practice, *Pediatr Nurs* 24(3):229-234, 1998.

---

urethral sphincter. Ask the patient to inhale deeply and advance the catheter. Do not force a catheter that does not easily enter the meatus, particularly if the child has had corrective surgery. For indwelling catheters, once urine is obtained, advance the catheter to the hub, inflate the balloon with sterile water, pull it back gently to test inflation, and connect it to the closed drainage system. Cleanse the glans and meatus and replace retracted foreskin. If blood is seen at any time during the procedure, discontinue the procedure and notify the practitioner.

In female patients, place a sterile drape under the buttocks. Use the nondominant hand to gently separate and pull up the labia minora to visualize the meatus. Swab the meatus from front to back three times, using a different povidone-iodine swab each time. Place 1 to 2 ml 2% lidocaine lubricant on the periurethral mucosa, and insert 1 to 2 ml into the urethral meatus. Delay catheterization for 2 to 3 minutes to maximize absorption of the anesthetic into the periurethral and intraurethral mucosa. Add lubricant to the catheter, and gently insert into the urethra until urine returns then advance the catheter an additional 2.5 to 5 cm (1 to 2 inches). When using a Foley catheter, inflate the balloon with sterile water and gently pull back, then connect to a closed drainage system. Cleanse the meatus and labia (see Cultural Awareness box). Because the use of lidocaine jelly can increase the volume of intraurethral lubricant, urine return may not be as rapid as when minimal lubrication is used.

Suprapubic aspiration is mainly used when the bladder cannot be accessed through the urethra (such as with some congenital urologic birth defects) or to reduce the risk of contamination that may be present when passing a catheter. With

CULTURAL AWARENESS

Bladder Catheterization

Parents may be upset when their child is catheterized. Aside from the trauma the child experiences, some parents may fear that the procedure affects the daughter's virginity. To correct this misconception, the family may benefit from a detailed explanation of the genitourinary anatomy, preferably with a model that shows the separate vaginal and urethral openings. The nurse can also indicate that catheterization has no effect on virginity.

the advent of small catheters (5 and 6 French), the need for suprapubic aspiration has decreased. Access to the bladder via the urethra has a much higher success rate than suprapubic aspiration, where success depends on the practitioner's skill at assessing the location of the bladder and the amount of urine in the bladder. Suprapubic aspiration involves aspirating bladder contents by inserting a 20- or 21-gauge needle in the midline approximately 1 cm (0.4 inch) above the symphysis pubis and directed vertically downward. The skin is prepared as for any needle insertion, and the bladder should contain an adequate volume of urine. This can be assumed if the infant has not voided for at least 1 hour or the bladder can be palpated above the symphysis pubis. This technique is useful for obtaining sterile specimens from young infants, since the bladder is an abdominal organ and is easily accessed. Suprapubic aspiration is painful, and therefore pain management during the procedure is important.

STOOL SPECIMENS

Stool specimens are frequently collected in children to identify parasites and other organisms that cause diarrhea, to assess gastrointestinal function, and to check for occult (hidden) blood. Ideally, stool should be collected without contamination with urine, but in children wearing diapers this is difficult unless a urine bag is applied. Children who are toilet trained should urinate first, flush the toilet, then defecate in the toilet, a bedpan (preferably one that is placed on the toilet to avoid embarrassment), or a commercial potty hat.

> **NURSINGTIP**
>
> To obtain a stool specimen, place plastic wrap over the toilet bowl to collect the stool. Use a tongue depressor or disposable spoon or knife to collect the stool.

Stool specimens should be large enough to obtain an ample sampling, not merely a fecal fragment. Specimens are placed in an appropriate container, which is covered and labeled. If several specimens are needed, the containers are marked with the date and time and kept in a specimen refrigerator. Care is exercised in handling the specimen because of the risk of contamination.

BLOOD SPECIMENS

Whether the specimen is collected by the nurse or others, the nurse is responsible for making certain that specimens, such as serial examinations and fasting specimens, are collected on time and the proper equipment is available. Collecting, transporting, and storing specimens can have a major impact on laboratory results.

Venous blood samples can be obtained by venipuncture or by aspiration from a peripheral or central access device (see Evidence-Based Practice box). Withdrawing blood specimens through peripheral lock devices in small peripheral veins has met with varying degrees of success. Although it avoids an additional venipuncture for the child, attempting to aspirate blood from the peripheral lock may shorten the life of the device. When using an IV infusion site for specimen collection, consider the type of fluid being infused. For example, a specimen collected for glucose level would be inaccurate if removed from a catheter through which glucose-containing solution was being administered.

> **NURSINGTIP**
>
> ■ To obtain a blood specimen from a peripheral lock when the infusion solution may interfere with tests results, first aspirate a quantity of blood equal to the volume of fluid in the catheter and discard; then aspirate the blood sample.
> ■ For a blood culture, use the first sample of blood, since organisms are most likely to collect within the catheter itself.

> **NURSINGALERT**
>
> On small or anemic children, keep track of the amount drawn and discarded over time. Frequent taking of blood specimens can rapidly decrease a child's blood volume. Coordinate blood samples and ask the laboratory to save as much blood as possible to reduce the frequency.

Arterial blood samples are sometimes needed for blood gas measurement, although noninvasive techniques, such as trans-cutaneous oxygen monitoring and pulse oximetry, are used frequently. Arterial samples may be obtained by arterial puncture using the radial, brachial, or femoral arteries; by deep heel puncture; or from indwelling arterial catheters. Adequate circulation should be assessed before arterial puncture by observing capillary refill or performing the **Allen test,** a procedure that assesses the circulation of the radial, ulnar, or brachial arteries. Because unclotted blood is required, only heparinized collection tubes are used. In addition, no air bubbles should enter the tube, since they can alter blood gas concentration. Crying, fear, and agitation also affect blood gas values; therefore every effort is made to comfort the child. The nurse should pack the sample in ice to reduce blood cell metabolism and take it to the laboratory for immediate analysis.

Capillary blood samples are taken from children by a finger stick. A common method for taking peripheral blood samples from infants younger than 6 months of age is by a heel stick. Before the blood sample is taken, the heel is warmed for 3 minutes. The area is cleansed with alcohol, the infant's foot firmly restrained with the free hand, and the heel punctured with an automatic lancet device (Clinical and Laboratory Standards Institute, 2006). An automatic device delivers a more precise puncture depth and is less painful than using a lance (Vertanen, Fellman, Brommels, and others, 2001). A surgical blade of any kind is contraindicated. An example of a safe device is the BD Quickheel Safety Lancet. The Tenderfoot Preemie device was compared with the Monolet lancet and was found to be safer than the lancet and required fewer heel punctures, less collection time, and lower recollection rates (Kellam, Sacks, Wailer, and others, 2001). Shepherd, Glenesk, Niven, and others (2006) reported the Tenderfoot device was more effective and safer than a lancet for newborn screening tests. Although obtaining capillary blood gases is a common practice, these measures may not accurately reflect arterial values.

The most serious complications of infant heel puncture are necrotizing osteochondritis from lancet penetration of the underlying calcaneus bone, infection, or abscess (Meehan, 1998). To avoid osteochondritis, the puncture should be no deeper than 2 mm and should be made at the outer aspect of the heel. The boundaries of the calcaneus can be marked by an imaginary line extending posteriorly from a point between the fourth and fifth toes and running parallel to the lateral aspect of the heel and another line extending posteriorly from the middle of the great toe and running parallel to the medial aspect of the heel (Fig. 22-11). Repeated trauma to the walking surface of the heel can cause fibrosis and scarring that may interfere with locomotion.

The specimens are quickly collected, and pressure is applied to the puncture site with dry gauze until bleeding stops. The arm is kept extended, not flexed, while pressure is applied for a few minutes after venipuncture in the antecubital fossa to reduce bruising. The site is covered with an adhesive bandage. In young children, adhesive bandages pose an aspiration hazard; they should be avoided or removed as soon as the bleeding stops. Applying warm compresses to ecchymotic areas increases circulation, helps remove extravasated blood, and decreases pain.

No matter how or by whom the specimen is collected, children, even some older ones, fear the loss of their blood. This is particularly true for children whose condition requires frequent blood specimens. They mistakenly believe that blood

Obtaining Blood Specimens from Central Venous Catheters in Children
Joy Hesselgrave

ASK THE QUESTION	In children, do blood specimens obtained from central venous catheters using the discard, reinfusion, or push-pull method yield more accurate samples?

SEARCH FOR EVIDENCE

Search Strategies	Search selection criteria included English-language research-based publications within the past 15 years on pediatric blood specimen collection from central venous access.
Databases Used	National Guideline Clearinghouse (AHRQ), Cochrane Collaboration, Joanna Briggs Institute, PubMed, TRIP Database Plus, MD Consult, PedsCCM, BestBETs

CRITICALLY ANALYZE THE EVIDENCE

Limited scientific research exists that describes the optimal method for drawing blood samples from central venous access devices (VAD) in the pediatric patient.

A convenience sample of paired specimens compared blood drawn from central lines via push-pull method and discard method on 28 pediatric patients 6 months to 12 years of age. Of the 438 pairs of measurements that were compared, 420, or 95.9%, were within limits of agreement for hemograms, electrolytes, and glucose. The push-pull method eliminates loss of blood and decreases the amount of times the central line is accessed (Barton, Chase, Latham, and others, 2004).

Forty-two nonneutropenic pediatric patients ages 2 to 20 years were randomly assigned to one of two syringe-handling methods for blood sampling. The discard specimen, routinely reinfused, was collected using the usual clean procedure and an exaggerated unclean alternative procedure. Neither the sterile specimens nor the unclean specimens grew organisms, thus suggesting that the reinfusion of the blood specimen would be safe. This study did not evaluate for clots in the discard specimen (Hinds, Wentz, Hughes, and others, 1991).

Thirty bone marrow transplant units were surveyed to evaluate how blood samples were drawn from central VADs. The average patient age was 5 to 16 years. Seventy-five percent of the units used the discard method, with the volume of discard ranging from 0.5 to 10 ml and an average of 4 to 6 ml. Fourteen percent used the reinfusion method, and 11% used the push-pull or mixing method (Keller, 1994).

The Infusion Nurses Society (2006) recommends that the discard method be used when drawing blood samples from central VADs. The discard volume should be 1.5 to 2 times the fill volume of the central VAD.

Frey (2003) summarizes evidence for the practice of all three blood sampling methods. The discard method is most widely reported, with disadvantages including blood loss, blood exposure risk for clinicians, and the potential to confuse the discard specimen for the blood sample. The reinfusion method does not deplete blood volume but risks blood exposure for clinician and potential to reinfuse a contaminated specimen or clots in the discard volume. The push-pull or mixing method demonstrates accuracy for studies other than coagulation and drug levels and reduces blood loss and clinician exposure risk.

APPLY THE EVIDENCE: NURSING IMPLICATIONS

- There is limited pediatric research that clearly supports any particular central line blood sampling method as being superior. All three methods yield accurate results and appear safe. The discard method is the most frequently reported in the literature and benchmarking. However, if there is a concern about blood volume, the push-pull or reinfusion method should be considered.
- If the catheter has multiple lumens, use the distal lumen for laboratory specimen collection.
- Infusions should be stopped and lumens clamped before blood sampling.
- Cleanse the injection cap with antiseptic agent and allow to dry before drawing laboratory specimens.

References

Barton S, Chase T, Latham B, and others: Comparing two methods to obtain blood specimens from pediatric central venous catheters, *J Pediatr Oncol Nurs* 21(6):320-326, 2004.

Frey M: Drawing blood samples from vascular access devices, *J Infus Nurs* 26(5):285-293, 2003.

Hinds PS, Wentz T, Hughes W, and others: An investigation of the safety of the blood reinfusion step used with tunneled venous access devices in children with cancer, *J Pediatr Oncol Nurs* 8(4):59-64, 1991.

Infusion Nurses Society: *Policies and procedures for infusion nursing,* ed 3, South Norwood, Mass, 2006, The Society.

Keller CA: Methods of drawing blood samples through central venous catheters in pediatric patients undergoing bone marrow transplant: results of a national survey, *Oncol Nurs Forum* 21(5):879-884, 1994.

FIG. 22-11 ■ Puncture site *(colored stippled area)* on sole of infant's foot.

removed from their bodies is a threat to their lives. Explaining to them that their body is continuously producing blood provides them with a measure of reassurance. When the blood is drawn, a comment such as "Just look how red it is. You're really making a lot of nice red blood," confirms this information and affords them an opportunity to express their concern. An adhesive bandage gives them added reassurance that the vital fluids will not leak out.

Children also dislike the discomfort associated with venous, arterial, or capillary punctures. Children have identified these procedures as the ones most frequently causing pain during hospitalization and arterial punctures as being one of the most painful of all procedures experienced (Van Cleve, Johnson, and Pothier, 1996). The ones most distressed by venipunctures are toddlers, followed by school-age children and

ATRAUMATIC CARE

Guidelines for Skin and Vessel Punctures

FOR REDUCTION OF PAIN ASSOCIATED WITH HEEL, FINGER, VENOUS, OR ARTERIAL PUNCTURES

Apply EMLA (an eutectic mixture of lidocaine and prilocaine) topically over the site if time permits (at least 60 minutes). LMX (lidocaine) cream also may be used and requires a shorter application time (30 minutes).

To remove the Tegaderm dressing atraumatically, grasp opposite sides of the film and pull the sides away from each other to stretch and loosen the film. After the film begins to loosen, grasp the other two sides of the film and pull.

Use iontophoresis (Numby Stuff) over the site if time permits (8 to 20 minutes, depending on the amount of current), a vapocoolant spray, or buffered lidocaine (injected intradermally near the vein with a 30-gauge needle) to numb the skin.

Use nonpharmacologic methods of pain and anxiety control (e.g., ask child to take a deep breath when the needle is inserted and again when the needle is withdrawn; exhale a large breath or blow bubbles to "blow hurt away"; count slowly and then faster and louder if pain is felt).

Keep all equipment out of sight until used.

Enlist parents' presence or assistance if they wish.

Restrain child *only as needed* to perform the procedure safely; use therapeutic holding (p. 708).

Allow the skin preparation to dry completely before penetrating the skin.

Use the smallest-gauge needle (e.g., 25 gauge) that permits free flow of blood; a 27-gauge needle can be used for obtaining 1 to 1.5 ml blood and for prominent veins (needle length is only ½ inch).

Emphasize that blood entering the syringe or tube does not hurt, and reassure young children that you did not "take their blood" away and that they have a lot more inside.

Place a small bandage over the puncture site to make removal easy and less painful and to reassure young children that their blood will not "leak out."

Have a "two-try" only policy to reduce excessive insertion attempts—two operators each have two insertion attempts; if insertion is not successful after four punctures, consider alternative venous access, such as a peripherally inserted central catheter (PICC); have a policy for identifying children with difficult access and appropriate interventions (e.g., most experienced operator for the first attempt).

FOR MULTIPLE BLOOD SAMPLES

Use an intermittent infusion device (saline lock) to collect additional samples; consider PICC lines early, not as a last resort.

Coordinate care to allow several tests to be performed on one blood sample using micromethods of testing.

Anticipate tests (e.g., drug levels, chemistry, immunoglobulin levels) and ask the laboratory to save blood for additional testing.

FOR HEEL LANCING IN NEWBORNS

Heel lancing has been shown to be more painful than venipuncture (Larsson, Tannfeldt, Lagercrantz, and others, 1998); consider venipuncture when the amount of blood from the heel would require much squeezing (e.g., genetic screening tests).

The effectiveness of EMLA is controversial, although application of 0.5 g for 30 minutes four times a day in preterm infants was found to be safe (Essink-Tebbes, Wuis, Liem, and others, 1999).

Place diapered newborn against mother's bare chest in skin-to-skin contact 10 to 15 minutes before and during heel lance (Gray, Watt, and Blass, 2000).

During the procedure, allow newborn to suck a pacifier coated with a slurry of sucrose. When commercially manufactured 24% sucrose solution is unavailable, add 1 teaspoon of table sugar to 4 teaspoons of sterile water. Use this solution to coat the pacifier, or administer 2 ml to the tongue 2 minutes before the procedure (Blass and Watt, 1999).

---

then adolescents. Consequently nurses need to institute pain reduction techniques to lessen the discomfort of these procedures (see Atraumatic Care box).

RESPIRATORY SECRETION SPECIMENS

Collection of sputum or nasal discharge is sometimes required for diagnosis of respiratory infections, especially tuberculosis and respiratory syncytial virus (RSV). Older children and adolescents are able to cough and supply sputum specimens when given proper directions. It must be made clear to them that a coughed specimen, not mucus that is cleared from the throat, is needed. It is helpful to demonstrate a deep cough. Infants and small children are unable to follow directions to cough and will swallow any sputum produced; therefore gastric washings (lavage) may be used to collect a sputum specimen. Sometimes a satisfactory specimen can be obtained using a suction device such as a mucus trap if the catheter is inserted into the trachea and the cough reflex is elicited. A catheter inserted into the back of the throat is not sufficient. For children with a tracheostomy, a specimen is easily aspirated from the trachea or major bronchi by attaching a collecting device to the suction apparatus.

Nasal washings are usually obtained to diagnose an infection of RSV. The child is placed supine, and 1 to 3 ml sterile normal saline is instilled with a sterile syringe (without needle) into one nostril. The contents are aspirated using a small, sterile bulb syringe and are placed in a sterile container. Another method uses a syringe with 5 cm (2 inches) of 18- to 20-gauge tubing. The saline is quickly instilled and then aspirated to recover the nasal specimen. To prevent additional discomfort, all of the equipment should be ready before beginning the procedure.

Other respiratory secretion collection methods include nasopharyngeal swabs to diagnose *Bordetella pertussis* and throat cultures. The nurse swabs both the tonsils and the posterior pharynx when obtaining a throat culture. The swab stick is inserted into the culture tube. Some culture kits require squeezing an ampule to release the culture medium.

ADMINISTRATION OF MEDICATION
DETERMINATION OF DRUG DOSAGE

Nurses must have an understanding of the safe dosage of medications they administer to children, as well as the expected action, possible side effects, and signs of toxicity

(Kennedy, 1996). Unlike with adult medications, there are few standardized pediatric dosage ranges, and with a few exceptions, drugs are prepared and packaged in average adult-dosage strengths.

Factors related to growth and maturation significantly alter an individual's capacity to metabolize and excrete drugs. Immaturity or defects in any of the important processes of absorption, distribution, biotransformation, or excretion can significantly alter the effects of a drug. Newborn and preterm infants with immature enzyme systems in the liver (where most drugs are broken down and detoxified), lower plasma concentrations of protein for binding with drugs, and immaturely functioning kidneys (where most drugs are excreted) are particularly vulnerable to the harmful effects of drugs. Beyond the newborn period, many drugs are metabolized more rapidly by the liver, necessitating larger doses or more frequent administration. This is particularly important in pain control, since the dosage of analgesics may need to be increased or the interval between doses decreased.

Various formulas involving age, weight, and body surface area as the basis for calculations have been devised to determine children's drug dosage. Because the administration of medication is a nursing responsibility, nurses need knowledge of not only drug action and patient responses, but also some resources for estimating safe dosages for children. The method most often used to determine children's dosage is based on a specific dose per kilogram of body weight, such as 0.1 mg/kg.

The most reliable method for determining children's dosage is to calculate the proportional amount of **body surface area (BSA)** to body weight. The ratio of BSA to weight varies inversely with length; therefore the infant who is shorter and weighs less than an older child or adult has relatively more surface area than would be expected from the weight. The usual determination of BSA requires the use of the **West nomogram** or an electronic calculator (widely available on the internet). The BSA is estimated from the height and weight of the child.

Checking Dosage

Administering the correct dosage of a drug is a shared responsibility between the practitioner who orders the drug and the nurse who carries out that order. Children react with unexpected severity to some drugs, and ill children are especially sensitive to drugs. When a dose is ordered that is outside the usual range or when there is some question regarding the preparation or the route of administration, the nurse should always check with the prescribing practitioner before proceeding with the administration, since the nurse is legally liable for any drug administered.

Even when it has been determined that the dosage is correct for a particular child, many drugs are potentially hazardous or lethal. Most facilities have regulations requiring specified drugs to be double-checked by another nurse before they are given to the child. Among drugs that require such safeguards are antiarrhythmics, anticoagulants, chemotherapeutic agents, electrolytes, and insulin. Others frequently included are epinephrine, opioids, and sedatives. Even if this precaution is not mandatory, nurses are wise to take such precautions. Errors in decimal point placement may occur and result in a tenfold or greater dosage error.

Identification

Before the administration of any medication, the child must be correctly identified. Two identifiers (e.g., name and medical record number or birth date) are required before medication administration.

ORAL ADMINISTRATION

The oral route is preferred for administering medications to children because of the ease of administration. Most are dissolved or suspended in liquid preparations. Although some children are able to swallow or chew solid medications at an early age, solid preparations are not recommended for young children because of the danger of aspiration.

Most pediatric medications come in palatable and colorful preparations for ease of administration. Some have a slightly unpleasant aftertaste, but most children will swallow these liquids with little if any resistance. The nurse can taste a minute amount of an oral preparation to ascertain whether it is palatable or bitter. Complaints of dislike from the child can be accepted and the taste camouflaged whenever possible. Most pediatric units have preparations available for this purpose (see Atraumatic Care box).

Preparation

The devices available to measure medicines are not always sufficiently accurate for measuring the small amounts needed in pediatric nursing practice. Although molded plastic calibrated cups offer reasonable accuracy in measuring moderate doses of liquids, paper cups are likely to have irregular shapes or crumpled bottoms. Considerable amounts of thick medica-

ATRAUMATIC CARE

Encouraging a Child's Acceptance of Oral Medication

- Give child a flavored ice pop or small ice cube to suck to numb the tongue before giving the drug.
- Mix the drug with a small amount (about 1 teaspoon) of sweet-tasting substance, such as honey (except in infants because of the risk of botulism), flavored syrups, jam, fruit purees, sherbet, or ice cream; avoid essential food items, since the child may later refuse to eat them.
- Give a "chaser" of water, juice, soft drink, ice pop, or frozen juice bar after the drug.
- If nausea is a problem, give a carbonated beverage poured over finely crushed ice before or immediately after the medication.
- When medication has an unpleasant taste, have child pinch the nose and drink the medicine through a straw. Much of what we taste is associated with smell.
- Flavorings such as apple, banana, and bubble gum can be added at many pharmacies (e.g., FLAVORx) at nominal additional cost. An alternative is to have the pharmacist prepare the drug in a flavored, chewable troche or lozenge.*
- Infants will suck medicine from a needleless syringe or dropper in small increments (0.25 to 0.5 ml) at a time. Use a nipple or special pacifier with a reservoir for the drug.

*For information about compounding drugs, contact Technical Staff, Professional Compounding Centers of America (PCCA), 9901 S. Wilcrest Drive, Houston, TX 77099; (800) 331-2498; http://www.pccarx.com.

tion may remain in the cup. Measures of less than a teaspoon are impossible to determine accurately with a cup.

The teaspoon is an inaccurate measuring device and is subject to error. Teaspoons vary greatly in capacity, and different persons using the same spoon will pour different amounts. Therefore a drug ordered in teaspoons should be measured in milliliters; the established standard is 5 ml per teaspoon. A convenient hollow-handled medicine spoon is available to accurately measure and administer the drug. Household *measuring* spoons can also be used when other devices are not available. A device called the Medibottle has been shown to be more effective in delivering oral medication to infants than the oral syringe (Kraus, Stohlmeyer, Hannon, and others, 2001).

Another unreliable device for measuring liquids is the dropper, which varies to a greater extent than the teaspoon or measuring cup. Droppers are available in numerous sizes, but even with the standard USP dropper, the volume of a drop will vary according to the viscosity (thickness) of the liquid measured; viscous fluids produce much larger drops than thin liquids. Many medications are supplied with caps or droppers designed for measuring each specific preparation. These are accurate when used to measure that specific medication but are not reliable for measuring other liquids. Emptying dropper contents into a medicine cup invites additional error. Because some of the liquid clings to the sides of the cup, a significant amount of the drug can be lost.

The most accurate means for measuring small amounts of medication is the plastic disposable syringe, especially the tuberculin syringe for volumes less than 1 ml. Not only does the syringe provide a reliable measure, but it also serves as a convenient means for transporting and administering the medication. The medication can be placed directly into the child's mouth from the syringe.

Young children and some older children have difficulty swallowing tablets or pills. Because a number of drugs are not available in pediatric preparations, the tablet needs to be crushed before it can be given to these children. Commercial devices* are available, or simple methods can be employed for crushing tablets. Not all drugs can be crushed (e.g., medication with an enteric or protective coating or formulated for slow release).

Children who must take oral medication for an extended period can be taught to swallow tablets or capsules. Training sessions include using verbal instruction, demonstration, reinforcement for swallowing progressively larger candy or capsules, no attention for inappropriate behavior, and gradual withdrawal of guidance once children can swallow their medication.

Because pediatric doses often require dividing adult preparations of medication, the nurse may be faced with the dilemma of accurate dosage. With tablets, only those that are scored can be halved or quartered accurately. If the medication is soluble, the tablet or contents of a capsule can be mixed in a small, premeasured amount of liquid and the appropriate portion given. For example, if half a dose is re-

---

*Trademark Medical manufactures a pill crusher and has compiled a list of more than 190 medications that should not be crushed or chewed. Both are available from Trademark Medical, 449 Sovereign Court, St. Louis, MO 63011; (800) 325-9044; http://www.trademarkmedical.com.

quired, the tablet is dissolved in 5 ml water or flavored liquid and 2.5 ml is given.

Administration

Although administering liquids to infants is relatively easy, the nurse must be careful to prevent aspiration. With the infant held in a semireclining position, the medication is placed in the mouth from a spoon, plastic cup, dropper, or syringe (without needle). The dropper or syringe is best placed along the side of the infant's tongue, and the liquid is administered slowly in small amounts, allowing the child to swallow between deposits.

> **NURSINGTIP**
>
> In infants up to 11 months of age and children with neurologic impairments, blowing a small puff of air in the face frequently elicits a swallow reflex.

Medicine cups can be used effectively for older infants who are able to drink from a cup. Because of the natural outward tongue thrust in infancy, medications may need to be retrieved from the lips or chin and refed. Allowing the infant to suck medication that has been placed in an empty nipple or inserting the syringe or dropper into the side of the mouth, parallel to the nipple, while the infant nurses are other convenient methods for giving liquid medications to infants. Medication is not added to the infant's formula feeding because the child may subsequently refuse the formula. Dispose of any plastic covers that may be on the ends of syringes. These covers are small enough to be aspirated by young children.

The young child who refuses to cooperate or resists consistently despite explanation and encouragement may require mild physical coercion. If so, it is carried out quickly and carefully. Every effort is made to determine why the child resists, and the reasons for the coercion are explained to the child in such a way that the child will know that it is being carried out for his or her well-being and is not a form of punishment. There is always a risk in using even mild forceful techniques. A crying child can aspirate a medication, particularly when lying on the back. If the nurse holds the child in the lap with the child's right arm behind the nurse, the left hand firmly grasped by the nurse's left hand, and the head securely restrained between the nurse's arm and body, the medication can be slowly poured into the mouth (Fig. 22-12).

INTRAMUSCULAR ADMINISTRATION
Selecting the Syringe and Needle

The volume of medication prescribed for small children and the small amount of tissue available for injection require that a syringe be selected that can measure small amounts of solution. For volumes of less than 1 ml, the tuberculin syringe, calibrated in one-hundredth-milliliter increments, is appropriate. Minute doses may require the use of a 0.5-ml, low-dose syringe. These syringes, along with specially constructed needles, minimize the possibility of inadvertently administering incorrect amounts of a drug because of **dead space,** which allows fluid to remain in the syringe and needle after the plunger is pushed completely forward. A minimum of 0.2 ml solution remains in a standard needle hub; therefore, when

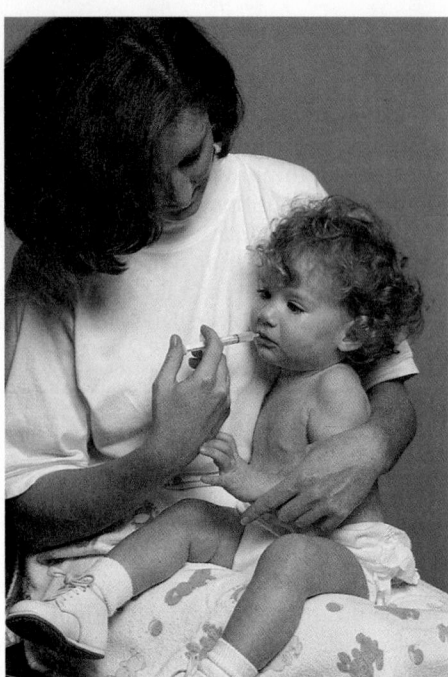

FIG. 22-12 ■ Nurse partially restrains child for easy and comfortable administration of oral medication.

very small amounts of two drugs are combined in the syringe, such as mixtures of insulin, the ratio of the two drugs can be altered significantly. Measures that minimize the effect of dead space are:

- When two drugs are combined in the syringe, always draw them up in the same order to maintain a consistent ratio between the drugs.
- Use the same brand of syringe (dead space may vary between brands).
- Use one-piece syringe units (needle permanently attached to the syringe).

Dead space is also an important factor to consider when injecting medication, since flushing the syringe with an air bubble adds an additional amount of medication to the prescribed dose. This can be hazardous when very small amounts of a drug are given. Consequently, flushing is not advisable, especially when less than 1 ml of medication is given. Syringes are calibrated to deliver a prescribed drug dose, and the amount of medication left in the hub and needle is not part of the syringe barrel calibrations. Certain drugs such as iron dextran and diphtheria and tetanus toxoid may cause irritation when tracked into the subcutaneous tissue. The Z-track method is recommended for use in infants and children rather than an air bubble. Changing the needle after withdrawing the fluid from the vial is another technique to minimize tracking.

The **needle length** must be sufficient to penetrate the subcutaneous tissue and deposit the medication into the body of the muscle. The needle gauge should be as small as possible to deliver fluid safely. Smaller-diameter (25- to 30-gauge) needles cause the least discomfort, but larger diameters are needed for viscous medication and prevention of accidental bending of longer needles (Table 22-4).

Determining the Site

Older children and adolescents usually pose few problems in selecting a suitable site for IM injections, but infants, with their small and underdeveloped muscles, have fewer available sites. It is sometimes difficult to assess the amount of fluid that can be safely injected into a single site. Usually 1 ml is the maximum volume that should be administered in a single site to small children and older infants. The muscles of small infants may not tolerate more than 0.5 ml. As the child approaches adult size, volumes approaching those given to adults may be used. However, the larger the amount of solution, the larger the muscle must be into which it is injected.

Major nerves and blood vessels must be avoided. The preferred site for infants is the vastus lateralis (the rectus femoris is not an acceptable site). The ventrogluteal site is relatively free of major nerves and blood vessels, is a relatively large muscle with less subcutaneous tissue than the dorsal site, has well-defined landmarks for safe site location, is less painful than the vastus lateralis, and is easily accessible in several positions. Cook and Murtagh's (2006) research into IM injection sites in children indicates that the ventrogluteal site has not been associated with complications and is the preferred site in children of all ages (see Table 22-4). In clinical practice, this site has been safely used in children as young as newborns. The deltoid muscle, a small muscle near the axillary and radial nerves, can be used for small volumes of fluid in children as young as 18 months of age. Its advantages are less pain and fewer side effects from the injectate (as observed with immunizations), compared with the vastus lateralis (Ipp, Gold, Goldback, and others, 1989). Table 22-4 summarizes the three major injection sites and illustrates the location of the preferred IM injection sites for children.

Administration

Although injections that are executed with care seldom cause trauma to the child, there have been reports of serious disability related to IM injections in children. Repeated use of a single site has been associated with fibrosis of the muscle with subsequent muscle contracture. Injections close to large nerves, such as the sciatic nerve, have been responsible for permanent disability, especially when potentially neurotoxic drugs are administered. There are several reports of tissue damage from penicillin. One of the difficulties in administering the opaque preparations, such as penicillin G (Bicillin), is that aspirated blood cannot be detected at the bottom of the syringe, thus increasing the risk of injecting into a blood vessel. When such drugs are injected, great care must be used in locating the correct site. When aspirating, the nurse should look for blood at the *top* of the syringe near the plunger, since blood may be drawn up through the column of penicillin. One study of IM injection techniques revealed that the straighter the path of needle insertion (e.g., 90-degree angle), the less displacement and shear to tissue, causing less discomfort (Katsma and Smith, 1997).

A reported potential hazard with medication in glass ampules is the presence of glass particles in the ampule after the container is broken. When the medication is withdrawn into the syringe, the glass particles may also be withdrawn and subsequently injected into the patient. As a precaution, medication from glass ampules should be drawn up only through a needle with a filter or injected intravenously through a site in the tubing that is distal to an IV filter.

TABLE 22-4
Intramuscular Injection Sites in Children

SITE	DISCUSSION
VASTUS LATERALIS 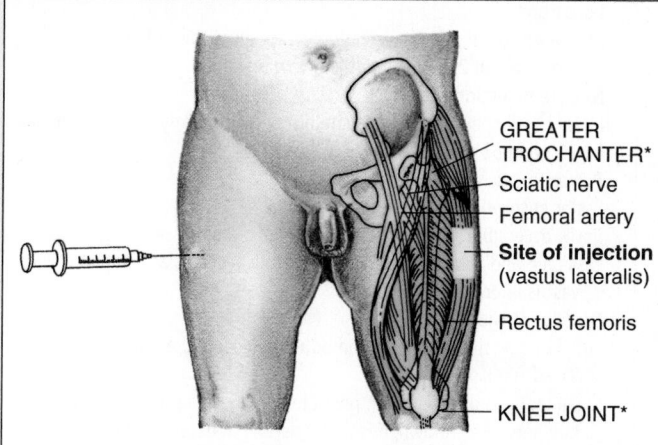 GREATER TROCHANTER* / Sciatic nerve / Femoral artery / **Site of injection** (vastus lateralis) / Rectus femoris / KNEE JOINT*	**Location*** Palpate to find greater trochanter and knee joints; divide vertical distance between these two landmarks into thirds; inject into middle third. **Needle insertion and size** Insert needle perpendicular to knee in infants and young children or perpendicular to thigh or slightly angled toward anterior thigh. 22-25 gauge, ⅝-1 inch† **Advantages** Large, well-developed muscle that can tolerate larger quantities of fluid (0.5 ml [infant] to 2.0 ml [child]) Easily accessible if child is supine, side-lying, or sitting **Disadvantages** Thrombosis of femoral artery from injection in midthigh area Sciatic nerve damage from long needle injected posteriorly and medially into small extremity More painful than deltoid or gluteal sites
VENTROGLUTEAL 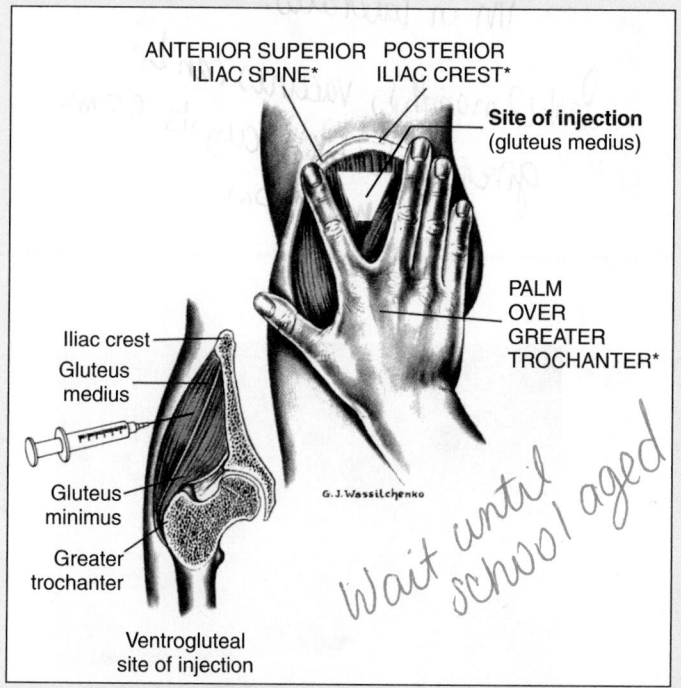 ANTERIOR SUPERIOR ILIAC SPINE* / POSTERIOR ILIAC CREST* / **Site of injection** (gluteus medius) / PALM OVER GREATER TROCHANTER* / Iliac crest / Gluteus medius / Gluteus minimus / Greater trochanter / Ventrogluteal site of injection / G.J.Wassilchenko / *Wait until school aged*	**Location*** Palpate to locate greater trochanter, anterior superior iliac tubercle (found by flexing thigh at hip and measuring up to 1-2 cm above crease formed in groin), and posterior iliac crest; place palm of hand over greater trochanter, index finger over anterior superior iliac tubercle, and middle finger along crest of ileum posteriorly as far as possible; inject into center of V formed by fingers. **Needle insertion and size** Insert needle perpendicular to site but angled slightly toward iliac crest. 22-25 gauge, ½-1 inch† **Advantages** Free of important nerves and vascular structures Easily identified by prominent bony landmarks Thinner layer of subcutaneous tissue than in dorsogluteal site, thus less chance of depositing drug subcutaneously rather than intramuscularly Can accommodate larger quantities of fluid (0.5 ml [infant] to 2.0 ml [child]) Easily accessible if child is supine, prone, or side-lying Less painful than vastus lateralis **Disadvantages** Health professionals' unfamiliarity with site

*Locations are indicated by asterisks on illustrations.
†Research has shown that a 1-inch needle is needed for adequate muscle penetration in infants 4 months old and possibly in infants as young as 2 months (Cook and Murtagh, 2002).

Continued

TABLE 22-4
Intramuscular Injection Sites in Children—cont'd

SITE	DISCUSSION

DELTOID

Clavicle
ACROMION PROCESS*
Site of injection (deltoid)
Axilla
Brachial artery
Humerus
Radial nerve

G.J. Wassilchenko

Location*
Locate acromion process; inject only into upper third of muscle that begins about 2 fingerbreadths below acromion.
Needle insertion and size
Insert needle perpendicular to site but angled slightly toward shoulder. 22-25 gauge, ½-1 inch
Advantages
Faster absorption rates than gluteal sites
Easily accessible with minimal removal of clothing
Less pain and fewer local side effects from vaccines as compared with vastus lateralis
Disadvantages
Small muscle mass; can accommodate only limited amounts of drug (0.5-1.0 ml)
Small margins of safety with possible damage to radial nerve and axillary nerve (not shown, lies under deltoid at head of humerus)

[handwritten] less than 12 mos, always give IM in lateralis.

Past 12 months, vaccines can be given in deltoid cuz its 0.5mL max is 1.0mL

*Locations are indicated by asterisks on illustrations.

Most children are unpredictable and few are totally cooperative when receiving an injection. Even children who appear to be relaxed and constrained can lose control under the stress of the procedure. It is advisable to have someone available to help hold the child if needed. Because children often jerk or pull away unexpectedly, the nurse should carry an extra needle to exchange for a contaminated one so that the delay is minimal. The child, even a small one, is told that he or she is receiving an injection (preferably using a phrase such as "putting medicine under the skin"), and then the procedure is carried out as quickly and skillfully as possible to avoid prolonging the stressful experience. Invasive procedures such as injections are especially anxiety provoking in young children, who may associate any assault to the "behind" area with punishment. Because injections are painful, the nurse should employ excellent injection technique and effective pain reduction measures to reduce discomfort (see Nursing Care Guidelines box).

Small infants offer little resistance to injections. Although they squirm and may be difficult to hold in position, they can usually be restrained without assistance. The body of a larger infant can be securely held between the nurse's arm and body (Fig. 22-13). To inject into the body of the muscle, the nurse firmly grasps the muscle mass between the thumb and fingers to isolate and stabilize the site. In obese children, however, it is preferable to first spread the skin with the thumb and index finger to displace subcutaneous tissue and then grasp the muscle deeply on each side.

FIG. 22-13 ■ Holding small child for intramuscular injection. Note how nurse isolates and stabilizes muscle.

If the medication is given around the clock, the nurse must wake the child. Although it may seem to be easier to surprise the sleeping child and do it quickly, this can cause the child to fear going back to sleep. When awakened first, children know that nothing will be done unless they are forewarned. See Nursing Care Guidelines box for techniques that maximize safety and minimize discomfort.

nursingcareguidelines

Intramuscular Administration of Medication

Use safety precautions in administering medication (e.g., check child's identification).

Apply EMLA (an eutectic mix of lidocaine and prilocaine) topically over site if time permits (at least 60 minutes, preferably 2 to 2½ hours for (intramuscular [IM] injection). LMX (lidocaine) cream may be applied for a shorter interval (see Pain Management, Chapter 7).

Prepare medication.
- Select needle and syringe appropriate to the following:
  —Amount of fluid to be administered (syringe size)
  —Viscosity of fluid to be administered (needle gauge)
  —Amount of tissue to be penetrated (needle length)
- Maximum volume to be administered in a single site is 1 ml for older infants and small children.

Determine site of injection (see Table 22-4), making certain that muscle is large enough to accommodate volume and type of medication.
- Acceptable sites for infants and small or debilitated children are the vastus lateralis muscle and the ventrogluteal muscle.
- The dorsogluteal muscle is insufficiently developed to be a safe site for infants and small children.

Administer medication.
- Obtain sufficient help in restraining child; children are often uncooperative, and their behavior is usually unpredictable.
- Explain briefly what is to be done and, if appropriate, what child can do to help.
- Expose injection area for unobstructed view of landmarks.
- Select a site where skin is free of irritation and danger of infection; palpate for and avoid sensitive or hardened areas. With multiple injections, rotate sites.
- Place child in a lying or sitting position; child is not allowed to stand because:
  —Landmarks are more difficult to assess.
  —Restraint is more difficult.
  —Child may faint and fall.
- Use a new, sharp needle with smallest diameter that permits free flow of the medication.
- Grasp muscle firmly between thumb and fingers to isolate and stabilize muscle for deposition of drug in its deepest part; in obese children, spread skin with thumb and index finger to displace subcutaneous tissue and grasp muscle deeply on each side.
- Allow skin preparation to dry completely before skin is penetrated.
- Have medication at room temperature.

Decrease perception of pain.
- Distract child with conversation.
- Give child something on which to concentrate (e.g., squeezing a hand or side rail, pinching own nose, humming, counting, yelling "Ouch!").
- Spray vapocoolant (e.g., ethyl chloride or fluorimethane) on site 11 to 15 seconds before injection or place a cold compress or wrapped ice cube on site about a minute before injection, or apply cold to contralateral site.
- Say to child, "If you feel this, tell me to take it out, please."
- Have child hold a small adhesive bandage and place it on puncture site after IM injection is given.

Insert needle quickly, using a dartlike motion at a 90-degree angle unless contraindicated.
- Use new needle, not one that has pierced rubber stopper on vial.

Avoid tracking any medication through superficial tissues:
- Replace needle after withdrawing medication, or wipe medication from needle with sterile gauze.
- If withdrawing medication from an ampule, use a needle equipped with a filter that removes glass particles; then use a new, nonfilter needle for injection.
- Use the Z-track or air-bubble technique as indicated.
- Avoid depressing the plunger during insertion of the needle.

Aspirate for blood.
- If blood is found, remove syringe from site, change needle, and reinsert into new location.
- If no blood is found, inject into a relaxed muscle:
  Ventrogluteal—Place child on side with upper leg flexed and placed in front of lower leg.
  Vastus lateralis—Child can be supine, lying on the side, or sitting.

Inject medication slowly.

Remove needle quickly; hold gauze sponge firmly against skin near needle when removing it to avoid pulling on tissue.

Apply firm pressure to site after injection; massage site to hasten absorption unless contraindicated, as with irritating drugs.

Place a small adhesive bandage on puncture site; with young children decorate it by drawing a smiling face or other symbol of acceptance.

Hold and cuddle young child and encourage parents to comfort child; praise older child.

Allow expression of feelings.

Discard syringe and uncapped, uncut needle in puncture-resistant container located near site of use.

Record time of injection, drug, dose, and injection site.

A needless injection system delivers IM or subcutaneous injections without the use of a needle and eliminates the risk of accidental needle puncture. This needle-free injection system involves a carbon dioxide cartridge that provides the power to deliver the medication through the skin. Although it is not painless, it may reduce pain and also the anxiety of seeing the needle (Polillio and Killy, 1997).

SUBCUTANEOUS AND INTRADERMAL ADMINISTRATION

Subcutaneous and intradermal injections are frequently administered to children, but the technique differs little from the method used with adults. Examples of **subcutaneous injections** include insulin, hormone replacement, allergy desensitization, and some vaccines. Tuberculin testing, local anesthesia, and allergy testing are examples of frequently administered **intradermal injections** (see Evidence-Based Practice box).

Techniques to minimize the pain associated with these injections include changing the needle if it pierced a rubber stopper on a vial, using 26- to 30-gauge needles (only to inject the solution), and injecting small volumes (up to 0.5 ml). The angle of the needle for the subcutaneous injection is typically 90 degrees. In children with little subcutaneous tissue, some practitioners insert the needle at a 45-degree angle. However, the benefit of using the 45-degree angle rather than the 90-degree angle remains controversial.

Although subcutaneous injections can be given anywhere there is subcutaneous tissue, common sites include the center

EVIDENCE-BASED PRACTICE

Medication Safety and Insulin Therapy
Shelly Nalbone

ASK THE QUESTION   In children, what practices decrease the number of errors in patients receiving insulin therapy?

SEARCH FOR EVIDENCE

Search Strategies   Search selection criteria included English-language publications within the past 10 years, research-based studies, and pediatric populations.

Databases Used   National Guideline Clearinghouse (AHRQ), Cochrane Collaboration, PubMed, CINAHL, University of Michigan Evidence-Based Pediatrics, Micromedex, EMBASE, ProQuest, TRIP Database, Medscape, RxMed, STAT!Ref, RxKinetics

CRITICALLY ANALYZE THE EVIDENCE

The American Society of Health-System Pharmacists (2006) conducted a review of all relevant literature and evidence-based reviews surrounding insulin therapy focusing on safety and patient outcomes in the hospital setting. Practice recommendations included preprinted order sets or computerized order entry and ongoing and annual training.

A quality improvement project to reduce medication errors and assess a standardized protocol for supplemental sliding scale insulin (SSI) in nonintensive care units was described by Donihi, DeVita, and Korytkowski (2006). Before implementation, more than 20 different types of SSI were used. The number of prescribing errors found on chart review 1 year after implementation was reduced from 10.3 to 1.2 per 100 SSI days. Authors recommend preprinted standardized SSI protocols and intense, ongoing education for direct patient care providers.

Ragone and Lando (2002) evaluated sources of errors and stated that, with the advent of new insulin analogs and premixed insulin combinations, the potential for errors in insulin therapy has increased. Errors have occurred when health care workers have mistaken rapid-acting insulin (Humalog) for glargine at bedtime. Inappropriate use of the proper insulin syringe has also led to errors. Excessive heat, inappropriate labeling of vials after opening, and improper handling of insulin pens can affect the efficacy of insulin. Staff education leads to decreased errors and improved patient outcomes.

Heatlie (2003) found in a qualitative study that long delays existed in the dosing of insulin after blood glucose was obtained. Recommendations included preprinted insulin order forms, increased nursing education surrounding diabetes management, and implementation of a 1-hour time limit from blood glucose specimen to insulin administration.

Davis, Harwood, Midgett, and others (2005) described the safety and efficacy of insulin therapy in intermediate care units. They reviewed staffing patterns, order trends, and past errors. Intense educational offerings were developed and implemented. Three months of data collection revealed 275 correct insulin drip rate calculations out of a possible 276. Audit results indicated that insulin therapy could be safely managed with a 1:5 to 1:6 nurse/patient ratio with proper nursing education.

Cohen, Robinson, and Mandrack (2003) identified methods to increase the safety of medication administration, including preprinted medication orders, the use of "smart pumps" for medication administration, and routine double checking by two licensed nurses when administering high-alert medications such as insulin.

APPLY THE EVIDENCE: NURSING IMPLICATIONS

- Preprinted order sets or computerized order entry for insulin therapy should be used in hospital settings.
- SSI should have a set of standardized protocols for hospitals, and use should be minimized.
- Staff education should be ongoing.
- Direct care provider education should be performed annually and be readily available for just-in-time training.
- Processes should be implemented to include annual education and competency validation for all involved staff.
- Patients receiving insulin therapy should be limited to designated areas of the hospital where staff have received appropriate training and development.
- Well-defined policies should be in place to support appropriate patient placement, safe and effective medication administration, strict insulin management, and judicious documentation.

References

American Society of Health-System Pharmacists: *Professional practice recommendations for safe use of insulin in hospitals*, Bethesda, Md, 2006, Inpatient Care Practitioners.

Cohen H, Robinson E, Mandrack M: Getting to the root of medication errors, *Nursing* 33(9):36-46, 2003.

Davis E, Harwood K, Midgett L, and others: Implementation of a new intravenous insulin method in intermediate-care units in hospitalized patients, *Diabetes Educ* 31(6):818-823, 2005.

Donihi A, DeVita M, Korytkowski M: Use of a standardized protocol to decrease medication errors and adverse events related to sliding scale insulin, *Qual Saf Health Care* 15:89-91, 2006.

Heatlie J: Reducing insulin medication errors: evaluation of a quality improvement initiative, *J Nurs Staff Dev* 19(2):92-98, 2003.

Ragone M, Lando H: Errors of insulin commission? *Clin Diabetes* 20(4):221-222, 2002.

third of the lateral aspect of the upper arm, the abdomen, and the center third of the anterior thigh. Some practitioners believe it is not necessary to aspirate before injecting subcutaneously; for example, this is an accepted practice in the administration of insulin. Automatic injector devices do not aspirate before injecting.

When giving an intradermal injection into the volar surface of the forearm, the nurse should avoid the medial side of the arm, where the skin is more sensitive.

NURSINGTIP

Families often need to learn subcutaneous injection techniques to administer medications, such as insulin, at home. Begin teaching as early as possible to allow the family the maximum amount of practice time possible.

INTRAVENOUS ADMINISTRATION

The IV route for administering medications is frequently used in pediatric therapy. For some drugs it is the only effective route. This method is used for giving drugs to children who have poor absorption as a result of diarrhea, dehydration, or peripheral vascular collapse; who need a high serum concentration of a drug; who have resistant infections that require parenteral medication over an extended time; who need continuous pain relief; and who require emergency treatment.

Insertion sites and observation of the IV infusion are discussed on p. 733. Several factors need to be considered in relation to IV medication. When a drug is administered intravenously, the effect is almost instantaneous and further control is limited. Most drugs for IV administration require a specified minimum dilution and/or rate of flow, and many are highly irritating or toxic to tissues outside the vascular system. In addition to the precautions and nursing observations related to IV therapy, factors to consider when preparing and administering drugs to infants and children by the IV route include:

- Amount of drug to be administered
- Minimum dilution of drug and whether child is fluid restricted
- Type of solution in which drug can be diluted
- Length of time over which drug can be safely administered
- Rate of infusion that child and vessels can tolerate safely
- IV tubing volume capacity
- Time that this or another drug is to be administered
- Compatibility of all drugs that child is receiving intravenously
- Compatibility with infusion fluids

Before any IV infusion, the site of insertion is checked for patency. Medications are never administered with blood products. Only one antibiotic should be administered at a time.

IV infusion is suitable for children who can tolerate the necessary infusion rate and the extra fluid needed to administer the medication. For the very small infant or fluid-restricted child who is not able to tolerate the increased rate of fluids, special delivery systems, such as syringe pumps, are used. Regardless of the technique, the nurse must know the minimum dilutions for safe administration of IV medications to infants and children.

Peripheral Intermittent Infusion Device

The **peripheral lock,** also known as an **intermittent infusion device** or **saline** or **heparin lock,** is an alternative to a keep-open infusion when extended access to a vein is required without the need for continuous fluid. It is most frequently employed for intermittent infusion of medication into a peripheral venous route. A short, flexible catheter is used as the lock device, and a site is selected where there will be minimal movement, such as the forearm. The catheter is inserted and secured in the same manner as for any IV infusion device, but the hub is occluded with a stopper or injection cap.

The type of device used may vary, and the care and use of the peripheral lock are carried out according to the protocol of the institution or unit. However, the general concept is the same. The catheter remains in place and is flushed with saline after infusion of the medication. See the Evidence-Based Practice box on flushing with normal saline or heparin.

Children may be discharged with a peripheral lock in place to continue receiving medications without hospitalization; this is usually reserved for children who require medications on a short-term basis and are referred to a home-based infusion company. Those with chronic illnesses who require repeated blood sampling or medications, long-term chemotherapy, or frequent hyperalimentation or antibiotic therapy are best managed with a central venous catheter.

Central Venous Access Device

Central venous access devices (VADs) have several different characteristics. Factors that can influence the type of VAD include the reason for placement of the catheter (diagnosis), length of therapy, risk to the patient in placement of the catheter, and availability of resources to assist the family in maintaining the catheter.

Short-term or **nontunneled catheters** are used in acute care, emergency, and intensive care units. These catheters are made of polyurethane and are placed in large veins such as the subclavian, femoral, or jugular. Insertion is by surgical incision or large percutaneous threading. A chest x-ray film should be taken to verify placement of the catheter tip before administration of fluids or medications.

Peripherally inserted central catheters (PICCs) can be used for short-term to moderate-length therapy. These catheters consist of silicone or polymer material and are placed by specially trained nurses, physicians, or interventional radiologists (Gamulka, Mendoza, and Connolly, 2005). The most common insertion site is above the antecubital area using the median, cephalic, or basilic vein. The catheter is threaded either with or without a guidewire into the superior vena cava. PICCs can be trimmed before insertion, and the decision can be made to insert the catheter midline, which is considered between the insertion site and the axilla. The midline has a dwell time of 2 to 4 weeks. If the catheter is threaded midline, total parenteral nutrition (TPN) or any other drug known to irritate a peripheral vein (e.g., chemotherapy drugs) should not be administered. The high concentration of glucose in TPN makes it irritating to the vessel; it should be infused through a central catheter.

The decision to insert a PICC needs to be made *before* several attempts at IV insertion are done. Once the antecubital veins have been punctured repeatedly, they are not considered candidates for this type of catheter. Because this catheter is the least costly and has less chance of complications than other central VADs, it is an excellent choice for many pediatric patients.

> **NURSING ALERT**
>
> Most PICC lines are not sutured into place, so care is needed when changing the dressing.

Long-term central VADs include tunneled catheters and implanted infusion ports (Table 22-5 and Fig. 22-14). They may have single, double, or triple lumens. Several lumens (multilumen) catheters allow more than one therapy to be administered at the same time. Reasons to use multilumen catheters include repeated blood sampling, TPN, administration of blood products or infusion of large quantities and/or concentrations of fluids, administration of incompatible drugs or fluids at the same time (through different lumens), and central venous pressure monitoring.

With any of the central venous catheters, medication is easily instilled through the injection cap. Maintenance of the

Critical Thinking Exercise—Central Venous Access Device

Animation—PICC Line Placement

EVIDENCE-BASED PRACTICE

Normal Saline or Heparinized Saline Flush Solution in Pediatric Intravenous Lines
David Wilson

ASK THE QUESTION   Is there a significant difference in the longevity of intravenous (IV) intermittent infusion locks in children when normal saline (NS) is used instead of a heparinized saline (HS) solution as a flush?

SEARCH FOR EVIDENCE

Search Strategies   Selection criteria included English-language publications within the past 15 years with the following terms: *saline vs heparin intermittent flush, children's heparin lock flush, heparin lock patency,* and *peripheral venous catheter in children.*

Databases Used   CINAHL, PubMed

CRITICALLY ANALYZE THE EVIDENCE

- A Cochrane systematic review by Shah and Sinha (2002) revealed eight studies that were randomized or quasirandomized trials of HS administration vs NS, placebo, or no treatment in neonates. The authors of the review concluded that, because of the studies' heterogeneity and variability in methodologic quality, clinical details, and reporting outcomes, they provided no strong evidence regarding the effectiveness and safety of heparin to prolong catheter life in neonates.

- No significant statistical difference was found between HS and NS flushes for maintaining catheter patency in children (Hanrahan, Kleiber, and Fagan, 1994; Kotter, 1996; Schultz, Drew, and Hewitt, 2002; Hanrahan, Kleiber, and Berends, 2000; Heilskov, Kleiber, Johnson, and others, 1998).

- Several studies reported increased incidence of pain or erythema with HS flushing of infusion devices (Hanrahan, Kleiber, and Fagan, 1994; Robertson, 1994; Nelson and Graves, 1998; McMullen, Fioravanti, Pollack, and others, 1993).

- Several studies found increased patency and/or longer dwell times with HS solutions vs NS in 24-gauge catheters (Mudge, Forcier, and Slattery, 1998; Danek and Noris, 1992; Beecroft, Bossert, Chung, and others, 1997; Gyr, Burroughs, Smith, and others, 1995; Hanrahan, Kleiber, and Berends, 2000).

- Younger children and lower gestational age in preterm neonates were associated with shorter patency of IV catheters (Paisley, Stamper, Brown, and others, 1997; Robertson, 1994; McMullen, Fioravanti, Pollack, and others, 1993).

- Infusion devices flushed with NS lasted longer than those flushed with HS (Nelson and Graves, 1998; Le Duc, 1997; Goldberg, Sankaran, Givelichian, and others, 1999).

- When measured and reported, length of time between flushing peripheral devices affected dwell time (Crews, Gnann, Rice, and others, 1997; Gyr, Burroughs, Smith, and others, 1995).

- None of the studies cited anticoagulation-associated complications with HS, which is a concern in preterm neonates who are at higher risk for development of clotting problems as a result of heparin (Klenner, Fusch, Rakow, and others, 2003).

APPLY THE EVIDENCE: NURSING IMPLICATIONS

- Further research is needed with larger samples of children, especially preterm neonates, using small-gauge catheters (24 gauge) and other gauge catheters, flushed with NS and HS as intermittent infusion devices only (no continuous infusions).

- NS is a safe alternative to HS flush in infants and children with intermittent IV locks larger than 24 gauge; smaller neonates may benefit from HS flush (longer dwell time), but the evidence is inconclusive for all weight ranges and gestational ages.

References

Beecroft PC, Bossert E, Chung K, and others: Intravenous lock patency in children: dilute heparin versus saline, *J Pediatr Pharmacol Practice* 2(4):211-223, 1997.

Crews BE, Gnann KK, Rice MH, and others: Effects of varying intervals between heparin flushes on pediatric catheter longevity, *Pediatr Nurs* 23(1):87-91, 1997.

Danek GD, Noris EM: Pediatric IV catheters: efficacy of saline flush, *Pediatr Nurs* 18(2):111-113, 1992.

Goldberg M, Sankaran R, Givelichian L, and others: Maintaining patency of peripheral intermittent infusion devices with heparinized saline and saline: a randomized double blind controlled trial in neonatal intensive care and a review of literature, *Neonatal Intensive Care* 12(1):18-22, 1999.

Gyr P, Burroughs T, Smith K, and others: Double blind comparison of heparin and saline flush solutions in maintenance of peripheral infusion devices, *Pediatr Nurs* 21(4):383-389, 1995.

Hanrahan KS, Kleiber C, Berends S: Saline for peripheral intravenous locks in neonates: evaluating a change in practice, *Neonatal Netw* 19(2):19-24, 2000.

Hanrahan KS, Kleiber C, Fagan C: Evaluation of saline for IV locks in children, *Pediatr Nurs* 20(6):549-552, 1994.

Heilskov J, Kleiber C, Johnson K, and others: A randomized trial of heparin and saline for maintaining intravenous locks in neonates, *J Soc Pediatr Nurs* 3(3):111-116, 1998.

Klenner AF, Fusch C, Rakow A, and others: Benefit and risk of heparin for maintaining peripheral venous catheters in neonates: a placebo-controlled trial, *J Pediatr* 143(6):741-745, 2003.

Kotter RW: Heparin vs. saline for intermittent intravenous device maintenance in neonates, *Neonatal Netw* 15(6):43-47, 1996.

Le Duc K: Efficacy of normal saline solution versus heparin solution for maintaining patency of peripheral intravenous catheters in children, *J Emerg Nurs* 23(4):306-309, 1997.

McMullen A, Fioravanti ID, Pollack D, and others: Heparinized saline or normal saline as a flush solution in intermittent intravenous lines in infants and children, *MCN* 18(2):78-85, 1993.

Mudge B, Forcier D, Slattery MJ: Patency of 24-gauge peripheral intermittent infusion devices: a comparison of heparin and saline flush solutions, *Pediatr Nurs* 24(2):142-149, 1998.

Nelson TJ, Graves SM: 0.9% Sodium chloride injection with and without heparin for maintaining peripheral indwelling intermittent infusion devices in infants, *Am J Health Syst Pharm* 55:570-573, 1998.

Paisley MK, Stamper M, Brown T, and others: The use of heparin and normal saline flushes in neonatal intravenous catheters, *J Pediatr Nurs* 23(5):521-527, 1997.

Robertson J: Intermittent intravenous therapy: a comparison of two flushing solutions, *Contemp Nurs* 3(4):174-179, 1994.

Schultz AA, Drew D, Hewitt H: Comparison of normal saline and heparinized saline for patency of IV locks in neonates, *Appl Nurs Res* 15(1):28-34, 2002.

Shah PS, Sinha AK: Heparin for prolonging peripheral intravenous catheter use in neonates, *Cochrane Database Syst Rev* (2):1-26, 2002.

TABLE 22-5

Comparison of Long-Term Central Venous Access Devices

DESCRIPTION	BENEFITS	CARE CONSIDERATIONS
TUNNELED CATHETER (e.g., HICKMAN OR BROVIAC CATHETER)		
Silicone, radiopaque, flexible catheter with open ends One or two Dacron cuffs or VitaCuffs (biosynthetic material impregnated with silver ions) on catheter(s) enhances tissue ingrowth May have more than one lumen	Reduced risk of bacterial migration after tissue adheres to cuff Easy to use for self-administered infusions Removal requires pulling catheter from site (nonsurgical procedure)	Requires daily heparin flushes Must be clamped or have clamp nearby at all times Must keep exit site dry Heavy activity restricted until tissue adheres to cuff Water sports may be restricted (risk of infection) Risk of infection still present Protrudes outside body; susceptible to damage from sharp instruments and may be pulled out; may affect body image More difficult to repair Patient or family must learn catheter care
GROSHONG CATHETER		
Clear, flexible, silicone, radiopaque catheter with closed tip and two-way valve at proximal end Dacron cuff or VitaCuff on catheter enhances tissue ingrowth May have more than one lumen	Reduced time and cost for maintenance care; no heparin flushes needed Reduced catheter damage; no clamping needed because of two-way valve Increased patient safety because of minimal potential for blood backflow or air embolism Reduced risk of bacterial migration after tissue adheres to Dacron cuff or VitaCuff Easily repaired Easy to use for self-administered intravenous infusions	Requires weekly irrigation with normal saline Must keep exit site dry Heavy activity restricted until tissue adheres to cuff Water sports may be restricted (risk of infection) Risk of infection still present Protrudes outside body; susceptible to damage from sharp instruments and may be pulled out; can affect body image Patient or family must learn catheter care
IMPLANTED PORTS (e.g., PORT-A-CATH, INFUS-A-PORT, MEDIPORT, NORPORT, GROSHONG PORT)		
Totally implantable metal or plastic device that consists of self-sealing injection port with top or side access with preconnected or attachable silicone catheter that is placed in large blood vessel	Reduced risk of infection Placed completely under the skin; therefore much less likely to be pulled out or damaged No maintenance care and reduced cost for family Heparinized monthly and after each infusion to maintain patency (only Groshong port requires saline) No limitations on regular physical activity, including swimming Dressing needed only when port accessed with Huber needle that is not removed No or only slight change in body appearance (slight bulge on chest)	Must pierce skin for access; pain with insertion of needle; can use local anesthetic (EMLA, LMX) or intradermal buffered lidocaine before accessing port Special noncoring needle (Huber) with straight or angled design must be used to inject into port Skin preparation needed before injection Difficult to manipulate for self-administered infusions Catheter may dislodge from port, especially if child "plays" with port site (twiddler syndrome) Vigorous contact sports generally not allowed Removal requires surgical procedure

catheter includes dressing changes, flushing to maintain patency, and prevention of occlusion or dislodgment.

NURSING ALERT

When working with tunneled catheters, PICCs, and peripheral intravenous lines (PIVs), avoid the use of any scissors around the tubing or dressing. Removal is best accomplished using fingers and much patience. In the event that a tunneled catheter is cut, use a padded clamp to clamp the catheter proximal to the exit site to avoid blood loss. Repair kits are available, which may save the catheter and avoid surgery to replace a cut catheter.

With the implanted device the port must be palpated for placement and stabilized, the overlying skin cleansed, and only special noncoring Huber needles used to pierce the port's diaphragm on the top or side, depending on the style. To avoid repeated skin punctures, a special infusion set with a Huber needle and extension tubing with a Luer connection can be used (see Fig. 22-14). With this attached, the injection procedure is the same as for an intermittent infusion device or a central venous catheter. To prevent infection, meticulous aseptic technique must be used any time the devices are entered, including instillation of heparin or saline to prevent clotting (Harris and Maguire, 1999). There should be a protocol stating that the Huber needle needs to be changed at established intervals, usually 5 to 7 days.

The children and parents are taught the procedure for care of the VAD before discharge from the hospital, including preparation and injection of the prescribed medication, the flush, and dressing changes. A protective device may be rec-

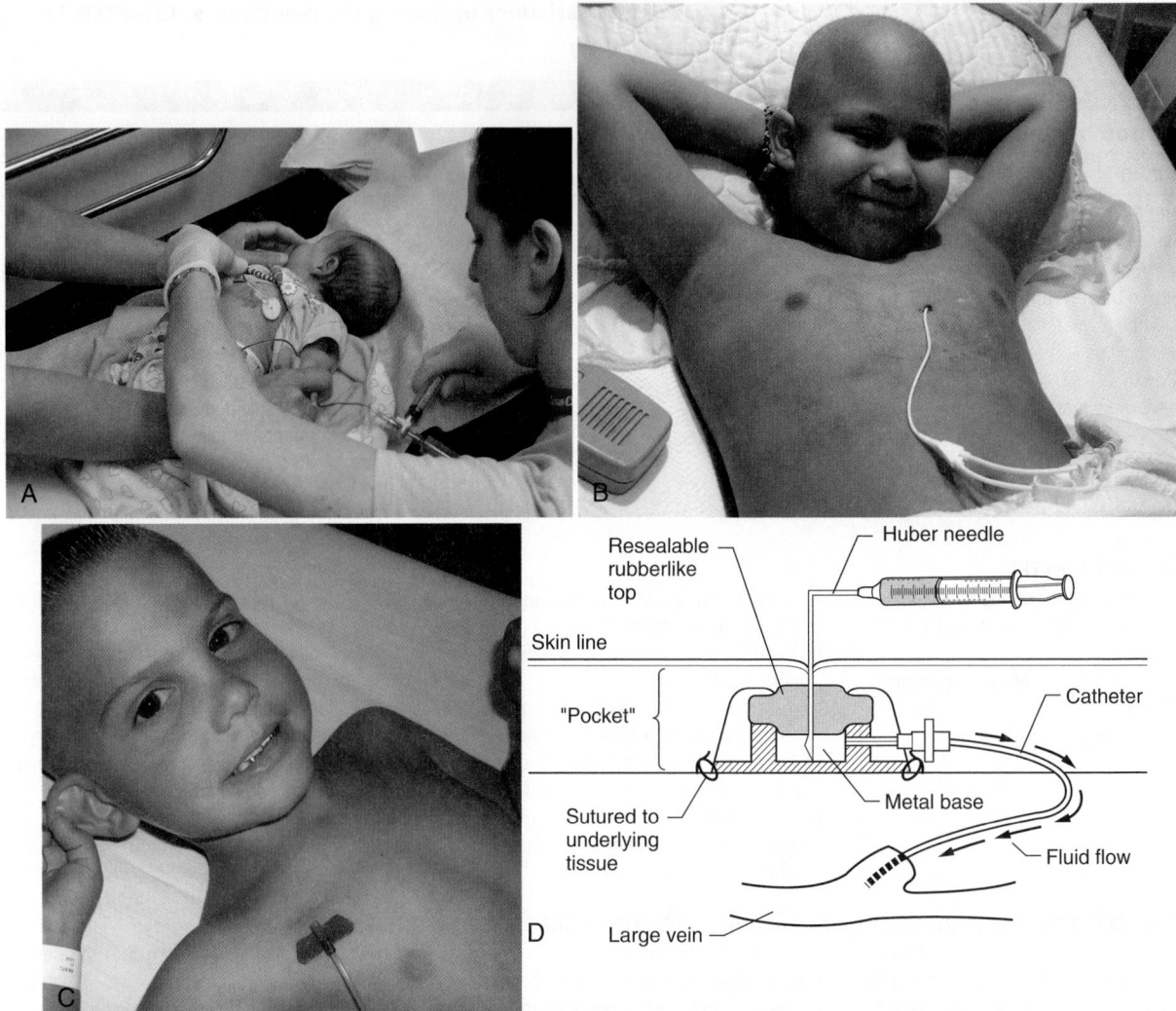

FIG. 22-14 ■ Venous access devices. **A,** Blood being drawn from a central venous catheter. **B,** Child with external central venous catheter. **C,** Child with implanted port with Huber needle in place. **D,** Side view of implanted port.

Labels in figure D:
- Resealable rubberlike top
- Huber needle
- Skin line
- "Pocket"
- Catheter
- Sutured to underlying tissue
- Metal base
- Fluid flow
- Large vein

TABLE 22-6

Flush Guidelines

CHILDREN

Peripheral lines (Heplock)	**≤24-g catheter**	**>24-g catheter**
	10 units/ml 2 ml heparin after meds or every 8 hours	5 ml normal saline after meds or every 8 hours
Midline	10 units/ml 3 ml heparin in a 10-ml syringe after meds or every 8 hours	
External central line (nonimplanted, tunneled, or PICC)	10 units/ml 3 ml heparin in a 10-ml syringe after meds or daily	
Implanted port	**Intermittent**	**Dormant**
	10 units/ml 5 ml heparin after meds	100 units/ml 5 ml heparin every month*
Arterial and central venous pressure continuous monitored lines	1 unit/ml heparin in 55-ml syringes run at 1 ml/hr	

NEONATES AND INFANTS

Peripheral lines (Heplock)	**≤24-g catheter**
	1 unit/ml 2 ml heparin after meds or every 8 hours
Percutaneous central catheter	1 unit/ml heparin in 20-ml syringe run at 0.2 ml/hr
Surgically placed central venous catheter (CVC) ≤5 French	1 unit/ml 2 ml heparin to check for line patency and between meds or TPN known to be compatible or every 8 hours
Surgically placed CVC >5 French	1 unit/ml 3 ml heparin to check for line patency and between meds or TPN known to be compatible or every 8 hours

Modified from Texas Children's Hospital, Houston.
PICC, Peripherally inserted central catheter; *TPN,* total parenteral nutrition.
*Patients <6 months of age: 10 units/ml 5 ml every month or 10 units/ml 5 ml every day if accessed.

EVIDENCE-BASED PRACTICE

Central Venous Catheter Site Care

Terry Jean Brandt, Jessica Hilburn, Anh Mac, Theresa E. Reed, and Brandi Horvath

ASK THE QUESTIONS (1) In children with central venous catheters (CVC), is chlorhexidine gluconate (CHG) a more effective antiseptic solution than povidone-iodine (PI) in preventing CVC-related site infections and bacteremia? (2) In pediatrics, what is the best antiseptic protocol—PI, CHG, or isopropyl alcohol—to use before accessing a CVC?

SEARCH FOR EVIDENCE

Search Strategies Search selection criteria included English-language publications within the past 16 years, research-based articles, for CVC site care in infants, children, and adults.

Databases Used Cochrane Collaboration, Joanna Briggs Institute, CINAHL, PubMed, National Guideline Clearinghouse (AHRQ), Institute for Healthcare Improvement, Centers for Disease Control and Prevention (CDC), Infusion Nurses Society, Oncology Nurses Society, MD Consult, BestBETs, TRIP Database Plus, Children's Health Care Association

CRITICALLY ANALYZE THE EVIDENCE

Dressing Protocol. A Cochrane systematic review and CDC Healthcare Infection Control Practices Advisory Committee found no evidence to demonstrate any difference in the incidence of the catheter-related bloodstream infections between gauze and tape vs transparent dressings (Gillies, O'Riordan, Carr, and others, 2003; O'Grady, Alexander, Dellinger, and others, 2002).

Although data regarding the use of the chlorhexidine-impregnated CVC dressing (Biopatch) in children are limited, one randomized, controlled study involving 705 neonates reported a substantial decrease in colonized catheter tips in infants when the Biopatch was used compared with a group using the standard dressing. Biopatch was associated with localized contact dermatitis in infants of very low birth weight (Garland, Alex, Mueller, and others, 2001). Levy, Katz, Solter, and others (2005) found pediatric patients with Biopatch had a significantly reduced risk of CVC colonization compared with patients with transparent dressing alone. There is clear evidence that CHG sponge dressings should not be used in neonates less than 7 days of age, 26 weeks' gestational age, or 1000 g (O'Grady, Alexander, Dellinger, and others, 2002). Routine application of antibiotic ointment is not recommended because of the risk of fungal infections and antimicrobial resistance (Camp-Sorrell, 2004; O'Grady, Alexander, Dellinger, and others, 2002).

Skin Antisepsis. The Oncology Nursing Society (Camp-Sorrell, 2004) finds chlorhexidine for catheter site care superior to alcohol and PI. Three evidence-based systematic reviews were found regarding CVC site care. Carson (2004) found most studies supported CHG as superior to PI for preventing microbial colonization of the CVC insertion site and catheter tip and for decreasing the risk of local site infection. However, there is still conflicting evidence regarding the efficacy of CHG vs PI for preventing CVC-related bacteremia. A meta-analysis of eight studies by Chaiyakunapruk, Veenstra, Lipsky, and others (2002) found CHG reduced the risk of catheter-related bloodstream infections by 49% compared with PI. Chaiyakunapruk, Veenstra, Lipsky, and others (2003) found the use of

CHG rather than PI for site care led to a cost savings of $113 for each catheter used. In a systematic review focused on bone marrow transplant recipients, CHG was the recommended antisepsis for prevention of catheter-related infection (Zitella, 2003).

APPLY THE EVIDENCE: NURSING IMPLICATIONS

- Weekly dressing changes are advised, using a clear dressing or tape and gauze with a Biopatch.
- Two percent chlorhexidine should be used for catheter site antisepsis; use with caution in preterm and low-birth-weight infants. Biopatch should be used around the catheter site except in low-birth-weight infants in the first 2 weeks of life.

References

Camp-Sorrell D, editor: *Access device guidelines: recommendations for nursing practice and education*, ed 2, Pittsburgh, 2004, Oncology Nursing Society.

Carson S: Chlorhexidine versus povidone-iodine for central venous catheter site care in children, *J Pediatr Nurs* 19(1):74-80, 2004.

Chaiyakunapruk N, Veenstra D, Lipsky B, and others: Vascular catheter site care: the clinical and economic benefits of chlorhexidine gluconate compared with povidone iodine, *Clin Infect Dis* 37(6):764-771, 2003.

Chaiyakunapruk N, Veenstra D, Lipsky B, and others: Chlorhexidine compared with povidone-iodine solution for vascular catheter-site care: a meta-analysis, *Ann Intern Med* 136:792-801, 2002.

Garland JS, Alex CP, Mueller CD, and others: A randomized trial comparing povidone-iodine to a chlorhexidine gluconate impregnated dressing for prevention of central venous catheter infections in neonates, *Pediatrics* 107:1431-1436, 2001.

Gillies D, O'Riordan L, Carr D, and others: Comparison of gauze and tape or transparent polyurethane dressings for central venous catheters, *Cochrane Database Syst Rev* (4): CD003827, 2003.

Levy I, Katz J, Solter E, and others: Chlorhexidine-impregnated dressing for prevention of colonization of central venous catheters in infants and children: a randomized controlled study, *Pediatr Infect Dis J* 24(8):676-679, 2005.

O'Grady N, Alexander M, Dellinger EP, and others: Guidelines for the prevention of intravascular catheter-related infections, *MMWR* 51(RR-10):1-29, 2002.

Zitella L: Central venous catheter site care for blood and marrow transplant recipients, *Clin J Oncol Nurs* 7(3):289-298, 2003.

ommended for some active children to prevent their accidentally dislodging the needle. Many children take responsibility for preparing and administering medications. Both verbal and written step-by-step instructions are provided for the learners (Table 22-6). See the Evidence-Based Practice box for VAD site care.

NURSING TIP

A pocket sewn on the inside of a T-shirt provides a place in which to coil the catheter line while the child is at play if a dressing is not used.

Infection and catheter occlusion are two of the most common complications of central venous catheters. They require treatment with antibiotics for infection and a fibrinolytic agent, such as alteplase, for clots (Fisher, Deffenbaugh, Poole, and others, 2004; Shen, Li, Murdock, and others, 2003). Uncapping can be prevented by taping the cap securely to the catheter and the clamped line to the dressing. Leaks can be prevented by using a smooth-edged clamp only. Parents are cautioned to keep scissors away from the child to prevent accidental cutting of the catheter. If the catheter leaks, they are instructed to tape it above the leak and then clamp the catheter at the taped site. The child should be taken to the practitioner as soon as possible to prevent infection or clotting after a catheter leak.

> ### NURSINGALERT
> If a central venous catheter is accidentally removed, apply pressure to the entry site to the vein, not the exit site on the skin.

NASOGASTRIC, OROGASTRIC, OR GASTROSTOMY ADMINISTRATION

When a child has an indwelling feeding tube or a gastrostomy, oral medications are usually given via that route. An advantage of this method is the ability to administer oral medications around the clock without disturbing the child. A disadvantage is the risk of occluding or clogging the tube, especially when giving viscous solutions through small-bore feeding tubes. The most important preventive measure is adequate flushing after the medication is instilled (see Nursing Care Guidelines box).

RECTAL ADMINISTRATION

The rectal route for administration is less reliable but is sometimes used when the oral route is difficult or contraindicated. It is also used when oral preparations are unsuitable to control vomiting. Some of the drugs available in suppository form are acetaminophen, sedatives, analgesics (morphine), and antiemetics. The difficulty in using the rectal route is that, unless the rectum is empty at the time of insertion, the absorption of the drug may be delayed, diminished, or prevented by the presence of feces. Sometimes the drug is later evacuated, securely surrounded by stool.

The wrapping on the suppository is removed and the suppository lubricated with water-soluble jelly or warm water. Rectal suppositories are traditionally inserted with the apex (pointed end) foremost. Reverse contractions or the pressure gradient of the anal canal may help the suppository slip higher into the canal. Using a glove or finger cot, quickly but gently insert the suppository into the rectum, beyond both of the rectal sphincters. The buttocks are then held together firmly to relieve pressure on the anal sphincter until the urge to expel the suppository has passed—5 to 10 minutes. Sometimes the amount of drug ordered is less than the dosage available. The irregular shape of most suppositories makes the process of dividing them into a desired dose difficult if not dangerous. If the suppository must be halved, it should be cut lengthwise. However, there is no guarantee that the drug is evenly dispersed throughout the petrolatum base.

If medication is administered via a retention enema, the same procedure is used. Drugs given by enema are diluted in the smallest amount of solution possible to minimize the likelihood of being evacuated.

OPTIC, OTIC, AND NASAL ADMINISTRATION

There are few differences between administering eye, ear, and nose medication to children and to adults. The major difficulty is in gaining children's cooperation. Older children need only explanation and direction. Although the administration of optic, otic, and nasal medication is not painful, these drugs can cause unpleasant sensations that can be eliminated with various techniques.

> ### nursingcareguidelines
>
> ## Nasogastric, Orogastric, or Gastrostomy Medication Administration in Children
>
> Use elixir or suspension (rather than tablet) preparations of medication whenever possible.
>
> Dilute viscous medication or syrup with a small amount of water if possible.
>
> If administering tablets, crush tablet to a fine powder and dissolve drug in a small amount of warm water.
>
> Never crush enteric-coated or sustained-release tablets or capsules.
>
> Avoid oily medications because they tend to cling to side of tube.
>
> Do not mix medication with enteral formula unless fluid is restricted. If adding a drug:
> - Check with pharmacist for compatibility.
> - Shake formula well and observe for any physical reaction (e.g., separation, precipitation).
> - Label formula container with name of medication, dosage, date, and time infusion started.
>
> Have medication at room temperature.
>
> Measure medication in a calibrated cup or syringe.
>
> Check for correct placement of nasogastric or orogastric tube (see Nursing Care Guidelines box, p. 747).
>
> Attach syringe (with adaptable tip but without plunger) to tube.
>
> Pour medication into syringe.
>
> Unclamp tube and allow medication to flow by gravity.
>
> Adjust height of container to achieve desired flow rate (e.g., increase height for faster flow).
>
> As soon as syringe is empty, pour in water to flush tubing.
>
> Amount of water depends on length and gauge of tubing.
>
> Determine amount before administering any medication by using a syringe to fill completely an unused nasogastric or orogastric tube with water. Amount of flush solution is usually 1.5 times this volume.
>
> With certain drug preparations (e.g., suspensions) more fluid may be needed.
>
> If administering more than one drug at the same time, flush tube between each medication with clear water.
>
> Clamp tube after flushing, unless tube is left open.

> ### NURSINGTIP
> To reduce unpleasant sensations, when administering medications:
> **Eye**—Apply finger pressure to the lacrimal punctum at the inner aspect of the lid for 1 minute to prevent drainage of medication to the nasopharynx and the unpleasant "tasting" of the drug.
> **Ear**—Allow medications stored in the refrigerator to warm to room temperature before instillation.
> **Nose**—Position the child with the head hyperextended to prevent strangling sensations caused by medication trickling into the throat rather than up into the nasal passages.

To instill eye medication, the child is placed supine or sitting with the head extended, and the child is asked to look up. One hand is used to pull the lower lid downward; the hand that holds the dropper rests on the head so that it may move synchronously with the child's head, thus reducing the possibility of trauma to a struggling child or of dropping medication on the face (Fig. 22-15). As the lower lid is pulled down, a small conjunctival sac is formed; the solution or ointment is applied to this area, never directly on the eyeball. Another effective tech-

FIG. 22-15 ■ Administering eye drops.

FIG. 22-16 ■ Proper position for instilling nose drops.

nique is to pull the lower lid down and out to form a cup effect, into which the medication is dropped. The lids are gently closed to prevent expression of the medication, and the child is asked to look in all directions to enhance even distribution of the preparation. Excess medication is wiped from the inner canthus outward to prevent contamination to the contralateral eye.

Instilling eye drops in infants can be difficult, since they often clench the lids tightly closed. One approach is to place the drops in the nasal corner where the lids meet. The medication pools in this area, and when the infant opens the lids, the medication flows onto the conjunctiva. For young children, playing a game can be helpful, such as instructing the child to keep the eyes closed until the count of 3 and then open them, at which time the drops are quickly instilled. Ointment can be applied by gently pulling down the lower lid and placing the ointment in the lower conjunctival sac.

NURSINGALERT

If both eye ointment and drops are ordered, give drops first, wait 3 minutes, and then apply the ointment to allow each drug to work. When possible, administer eye ointments before bedtime or naptime, since the child's vision will be blurred temporarily.

Ear drops are instilled with the child in the prone or supine position and the head turned to the appropriate side. For children younger than 3 years of age, the external auditory canal is straightened by gently pulling the pinna downward and straight back. The pinna is pulled upward and back in children older than 3 years of age. To place the drops deep in the ear canal without contaminating the tip of the dropper, place a disposable ear speculum in the canal and administer the drops through the speculum. After instillation, the child should remain lying on the unaffected side for a few minutes. Gentle massage of the area immediately anterior to the ear facilitates the entry of drops into the ear canal. The use of cotton pledgets prevents medication from flowing out of the external canal. However, the pledgets should be loose enough to allow any discharge to exit from the ear. Premoistening the

cotton with a few drops of medication prevents the wicking action from absorbing the medication instilled in the ear.

Nose drops are instilled in the same manner as in the adult patient. Unpleasant sensations associated with medicated nose drops are minimized when care is taken to position the child with the head extended well over the edge of the bed or a pillow (Fig. 22-16). Depending on size, the infant can be positioned in the football hold (see Fig. 22-5, *B*); in the nurse's arm with the head extended and stabilized between the nurse's body and elbow, and the arms and hands immobilized with the nurse's hands; or as shown in Fig. 22-16. After instillation of the drops, the child should remain in position for 1 minute to allow the drops to come in contact with the nasal surfaces.

Nasal spray dispensers are inserted into the naris vertically and then angled nasally to avoid trauma to the septum and to direct medication toward the inferior turbinate.

FAMILY TEACHING AND HOME CARE

The nurse usually assumes the responsibility for preparing families to administer medications at home. The family should understand why the child is receiving the medication and the effects that might be expected, as well as the amount, frequency, and length of time the drug is to be administered. Instruction should be carried out in an unhurried, relaxed manner, preferably in an area away from a busy ward or office, following the same guidelines for teaching as outlined in the Nursing Care Guidelines box (p. 699).

The caregiver is carefully instructed regarding the correct dosage. Some persons have difficulty understanding medical terminology from the pharmacy; just because they nod or otherwise indicate an understanding, it cannot be assumed that the message is clear. It is important to ascertain their interpretation of a teaspoon, for example, and to be certain they have acceptable devices for measuring the drug. If the drug is packaged with a dropper, syringe, or plastic cup, the nurse should show or mark the point on the device that indicates the prescribed dose and demonstrate how the dose is drawn up into a dropper or syringe, measured, and the bubbles eliminated. If the nurse has any doubts about the parent's ability to administer the correct dose, the parent should be asked to give a return demonstration. This is essential when the drug has potentially serious consequences from incorrect dosage, such as insulin or digoxin, or when more complex administration is required, such as parenteral injections. When teaching a parent to give an injection, the nurse must allot adequate time for instruction and practice.

Home modifications are often necessary because the availability of equipment or assistance can differ from the hospital setting. For example, the parent may need guidance in devising methods that allow for one person to hold the child and safely give the drug.

NURSINGTIP

To administer oral, nasal, or optic medication when only one person is available to hold the child, use the following procedure:
- Place child supine on flat surface (bed, couch, floor).
- Sit facing child so that child's head is between operator's thighs and child's arms are under operator's legs.
- Place lower legs over child's legs to restrain lower body, if necessary.
- To administer oral medication, place small pillow under child's head to reduce risk of aspiration.
- To administer nasal medication, place small pillow under child's shoulders to aid flow of liquid through nasal passages.

The time that the drug is to be administered is clarified with the parent. For instance, when a drug is prescribed in association with meals, the number of meals that the family is accustomed to eating influences the amount of drug the child receives. Does the child have meals twice a day or five times a day? When a drug is to be given several times during the day, together the nurse and parents can work out a schedule that accommodates the family's routine. This is particularly significant if the drug must be given at equal intervals throughout a 24-hour period. For example, telling parents that the child needs 1 teaspoon of medicine four times a day is subject to misinterpretation, since parents may routinely schedule the doses at incorrect times. Instead, a preplanned schedule based on 6-hour intervals should be set up with the number of days required for therapeutic dosage listed. Modification should also be made to accommodate sleep schedules. Written instruction should accompany all drug prescriptions.

NURSINGTIP

If parents have difficulty reading or understanding English, use colors to convey instructions. For example, mark each drug with a color and place the appropriate color on a calendar chart or on a drawing of a clock to identify when the drug needs to be given. If a liquid medication and syringe are used, also mark the syringe with color-coded tape at the place the plunger needs to be.

MAINTAINING FLUID BALANCE

MEASUREMENT OF INTAKE AND OUTPUT

Accurate measurements of fluid intake and output (I&O) are essential to the assessment of fluid balance. Measurements from all sources—including gastrointestinal and parenteral I&O from urine, stools, vomitus, fistulas, nasogastric suction, sweat, and drainage from wounds—must be taken and considered. Although the practitioner usually indicates when I&O measurements are to be recorded, it is a nursing responsibility

to keep an accurate I&O record on certain children, including those:

- Receiving IV therapy
- Who underwent major surgery
- Receiving diuretic or corticosteroid therapy
- With severe thermal burns or injuries
- With renal disease or damage
- With congestive heart failure
- With dehydration
- With diabetes mellitus
- With oliguria
- In respiratory distress
- With chronic lung disease

Infants or small children who are unable to use a bedpan or those who have bowel movements with every voiding require the application of a collecting device (p. 711). If collecting bags are not used, wet diapers or pads are carefully weighed to ascertain the amount of fluid lost. This includes liquid stool, vomitus, and other losses. The volume of fluid in milliliters is equivalent to the weight of the fluid measured in grams. The specific gravity as a measure of osmolality is determined with a refractometer or urine dipsticks and assists in assessing the degree of hydration (see FYI, p. 712).

NURSINGTIP

1 g of wet diaper weight = 1 ml urine
In infants with diapers, weigh all dry diapers to be used and note in an indelible marker the dry weight of the diaper; when there is fluid (urine or liquid stool) in the diaper, the amount of output can be approximated by subtracting the weight of the dry diaper from the weighed amount of the wet diaper.

Disadvantages of the weighed-diaper method of fluid measurement include (1) inability to differentiate one type of loss from another because of admixture, (2) loss of urine or liquid stool from leakage or evaporation (especially if the infant is under a radiant warmer), and (3) additional fluid in the diaper (superabsorbent disposable type) from absorption of atmospheric moisture (in high-humidity incubators).

Special Needs When the Child Is NPO

Infants or children who are unable or not permitted to take fluids by mouth (NPO) have special needs. To ensure that they do not receive fluids, a sign can be placed in some obvious place, such as over their beds or on their shirts, to alert others to the NPO status. To prevent the temptation to drink, fluids should not be left at the bedside.

Oral hygiene, a part of routine hygienic care, is especially important when fluids are restricted or withheld (p. 701). For the young child who cannot brush the teeth or rinse the mouth without swallowing fluid, the mouth and teeth can be cleaned and kept moist by swabbing with saline-moistened gauze.

NURSINGTIP

To keep the mouth feeling moist when the child is NPO, give ice chips (if this is permitted by the practitioner) or spray the mouth from an atomizer. To meet the need to suck, the infant is provided with a safe commercial pacifier.

The child who is fluid restricted presents an equal challenge. Limiting fluids is often more difficult for the child than being NPO, especially when IV fluids are also eliminated. To make certain the child does not drink the entire amount allowed early in the day, the daily allotment is calculated to provide fluids at periodic intervals throughout the child's waking hours. Serving the fluids in small containers gives the illusion of larger servings. No extra liquid is left at the bedside.

PARENTERAL FLUID THERAPY

Site and Equipment

The site selected for PIV infusion depends on accessibility and convenience. Although it is possible to use any accessible vein in older children, the child's developmental, cognitive, and mobility needs must be considered when selecting a site. Ideally in older children, the superficial veins of the forearm should be used, leaving the hands free. An older child can help select the site and thereby maintain some measure of control. For veins in the extremities it is best to start with the most distal site and avoid the child's favored hand to reduce the disability related to the procedure. Restrict the child's movements as little as possible—avoid a site over a joint in an extremity, such as the antecubital space. In small infants a superficial vein of the hand, wrist, forearm, foot, or ankle is usually most convenient and most easily stabilized (Fig. 22-17). Foot veins should be avoided in children learning to walk and in children already walking. Superficial veins of the scalp have no valves, insertion is easy, and they can be used in infants up to about 9 months of age, but they should be used only when other site attempts have failed. A transilluminator (Fig. 22-18) can aid in finding and evaluating veins for access (see Evidence-Based Practice box).

Selection of a scalp vein may require clipping the area around the site to better visualize the vein and provide a smoother surface on which to tape the catheter hub and tubing. Clipping a portion of the infant's hair is upsetting to parents; therefore they should be told what to expect and reassured that the hair will grow in again rapidly (save the hair because parents often wish to keep it). Remove as little as possible, directly over the insertion site and taping surface. A rubber band slipped onto the head from brow to occiput will usually suffice as a tourniquet, although if the vessel is visible, a tourniquet may not be necessary.

> **NURSINGTIP**
>
> A tab of tape should be placed on the rubber band to help grasp it when removing it from the infant's head. The rubber band should be cut to avoid accidentally dislodging the catheter when moving the rubber band over the IV insertion site. The tape tab will lift the rubber band and allow it to be cut. Hold the rubber band in two places and cut between these areas to prevent the rubber band from snapping on the head.

Situations may occur in which rapid establishment of systemic access is vital, and venous access may be hampered by peripheral circulatory collapse, hypovolemic shock (secondary to vomiting or diarrhea, burns, or trauma), cardiopulmonary arrest, or other conditions (Dubick and Holcomb, 2000). **Intraosseous infusion** provides a rapid, safe, and lifesaving alternate route for administration of fluids and medications until intravascular access can be attained, especially in children who are 6 years of age and younger.

A large-bore needle, such as a bone marrow aspiration needle (e.g., Jamshidi) or an intraosseous needle (e.g., Cook), is inserted into the medullary cavity of a long bone, most often the proximal tibia. This procedure is usually reserved for children who are unconscious or for those who are receiving anal-

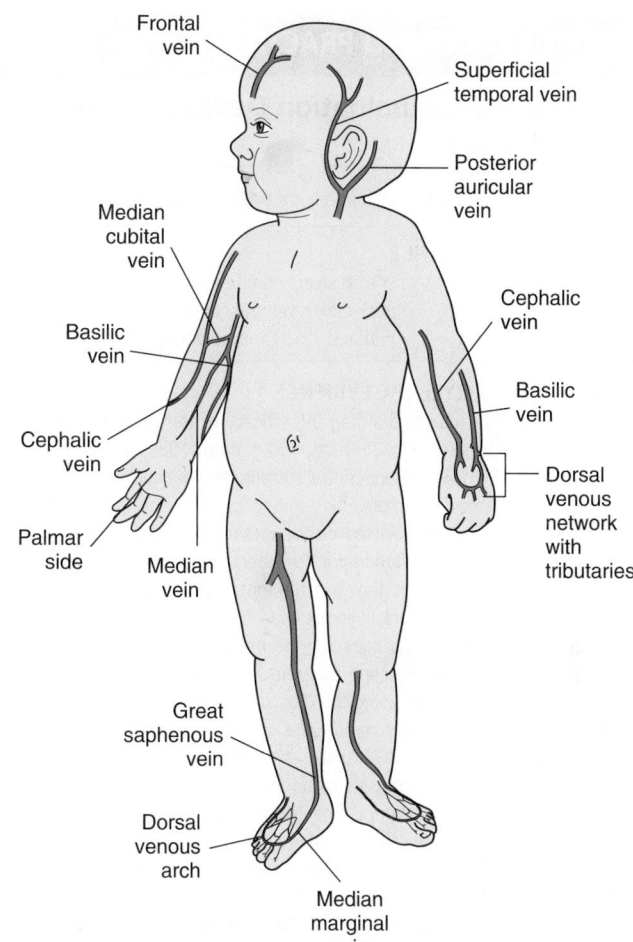

FIG. 22-17 ■ Preferred sites for venous access in infants.

FIG. 22-18 ■ Transilluminator: low-heat light-emitting diode (LED) light placed on the skin to illuminate veins; an opening allows cannulation of vein. (Professor Mark Waltzman, Children's Hospital, Boston.)

gesia, since the procedure is painful. Local anesthesia should be used for a semiconscious patient. Observe the dependent tissue closely for swelling, since extravasation may be hidden under the leg and compartment syndrome may result.

For most IV infusions in children, a 22- to 24-gauge catheter may be used if therapy is expected to last less than 5 days.

EVIDENCE-BASED PRACTICE

Use of Transillumination Devices in Obtaining Vascular Access
Jennifer Sanders

ASK THE QUESTION   In children, do transillumination devices decrease the number of attempts needed to obtain vascular access?

SEARCH FOR EVIDENCE

Search Strategies   Search selection criteria included English-language publications within the past 30 years, research-based articles on children undergoing venipuncture.

Databases Used   PubMed, Cochrane Collaboration, MD Consult, BestBETs

CRITICALLY ANALYZE THE EVIDENCE

Five articles were found regarding the efficacy of transillumination; two were published more than 25 years ago (Curran 1980; Kuhns, Martin, Gildersleeve, 1975). All concluded that transillumination aids in decreasing the number of access attempts.

A letter to the editor focused on the method of using two fiberoptic lights as a venous transilluminator. Peripheral intravenous (PIV) access was usually successful on the first attempt because of the increased visualization of the superficial venous anatomy (Dinner, 1992).

A sample of 100 infants ages 2 to 36 months was evaluated for PIV access using a simple otoscope for transillumination. In 40 of the 100 infants, a vein was visible using the otoscope for transillumination. In 23 of these children, transillumination was used after a vein could not be visualized or palpated. In 17 others, one previous attempt to gain PIV access had failed. With transillumination, 39 of 40 PIV attempts were successful on the first attempt. One patient required a second attempt (Goren, Laufer, Yativ, and others, 2001).

A sample of 240 patients was randomized to receive PIV access either with or without transillumination with the Veinlite. Patients were either less than 3 years old and required elective insertion of an IV, or were 3 to 21 years of age with a chronic illness who were previously identified as having difficult access. Those patients in the Veinlite group were significantly more likely to have a successful IV insertion on the first or second attempt (Katsogridakis, Seshadri, Sullivan, and others, 2005).

APPLY THE EVIDENCE: NURSING IMPLICATIONS

- Transillumination should be used before PIV access to decrease the number of attempts needed to successfully obtain access.
- Education and practice in this technique are needed for success. Since the veins stand out so clearly with transillumination, they appear more superficial than they are.
- An assistant may be needed to hold the device when using the transilluminator to obtain PIV access.
- The heat and temperature of the transilluminator should be monitored to prevent injury to the patient's skin.
- Appropriate equipment should be used to increase the likelihood of visualization of the vasculature.

References

Curran JS: A restraint and transillumination device for neonatal arterial/venipuncture: efficacy and thermal safety, *Pediatrics* 66(1):128-130, 1980.

Dinner M: Transillumination to facilitate venipuncture in children (letter to editor), *Anesthesiol Analg* 74:467-477, 1992.

Goren A, Laufer J, Yativ N, and others: Transillumination of the palm for venipuncture in infants, *Pediatr Emerg Care* 17(2):130-131, 2001.

Katsogridakis Y, Seshadri R, Sullivan C, and others: *Veinlite transillumination in the pediatric emergency department: a therapeutic interventional trial*, retrieved August 2005 from http://www.veinlite.com/public.html.

Kuhns LR, Martin AJ, Gildersleeve RT, and others: Intense transillumination for infant venipuncture, *Radiology* 116:734-735, 1975.

The smallest-gauge and shortest-length catheter that will accommodate the prescribed therapy should be chosen. The length of the catheter may be directly related to infection and/or embolus formation—the shorter the catheter, the fewer the complications (Maki, 1994). The gauge of the catheter should maintain adequate flow of the infusate into the cannulated vein while allowing adequate blood flow around the catheter walls to promote proper hemodilution of the infusate.

Determining the best catheter for the patient early in the therapy provides the best chance of avoiding catheter-related complications (Moureau, 1999). As the length of therapy increases, decisions regarding the type of infusion device (short peripheral, midline, peripherally inserted central catheter, or central venous catheter) should be explored. Guidelines such as flow charts or algorithms are available to help in these decisions (Catudal, 1999).

Safety Catheters and Needleless Systems

Over-the-needle IV catheters with hollow-bore needles carry a high risk for transmission of blood-borne pathogens from needlestick injuries. Safety catheters prevent accidental needlesticks with the use of over-the-needle IV catheters.

Needleless IV systems are designed to prevent needlestick injuries during administration of IV push medications and IV piggyback medications. Some needleless devices can be used with any tubing, whereas others require use of the entire IV delivery system for compatibility. Needleless IV systems rely on prepierced septa that are accessed by blunted plastic cannulas or systems that use valves that open and close a fluid path when activated by insertion of a syringe.

Blunt plastic cannulas and preslit injection port sites (Fig. 22-19) eliminate the need for steel needles and conventional injection port sites but remain accessible via hypodermic needles, a drawback except in emergent situations. Systems that do not permit needled access enhance safety by preventing health care workers from attempting to use needles. A syringe with a blue spike is available to access a single-dose vial (Fig. 22-19, *A*). The preslit injection port sites are identified by a white ring surrounding the port; this ring alerts users that the system is needleless (Fig. 22-19, *B*). Syringes are available with the blunt plastic cannula for accessing these sites (Fig. 22-19, *C*). A lever lock (Fig. 22-19, *D*) or threaded lock cannula (Fig. 22-19, *E*) attaches to an IV line, IV Y site, or peripheral intermittent infusion device. A preslit universal vial adapter (not pictured) provides access to standard multiple-dose vials, and syringe cannulas are then used to access the adapter. Valve technology allows syringes and IV tubing to connect directly in-line without the use of an adapter.

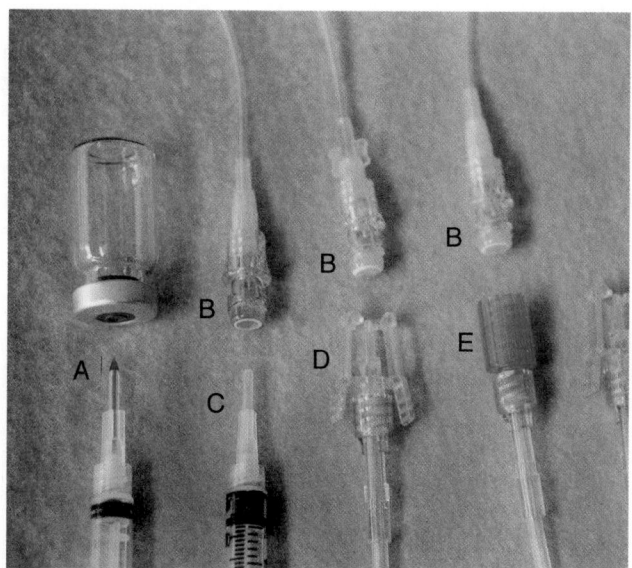

FIG. 22-19 ■ Interlink intravenous access systems. **A,** Blue spike syringe. **B,** Preslit injection port (needleless). **C,** Blunt plastic cannula syringe. **D,** Lever lock cannula. **E,** Threaded lock cannula.

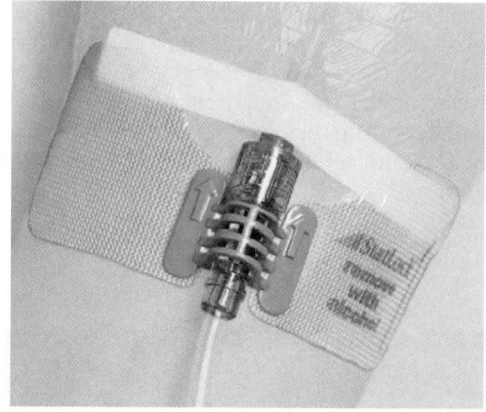

FIG. 22-20 ■ StatLock securement devices enhance peripheral intravenous line dwell time and decrease phlebitis.

NURSINGALERT

Misconnections of tubing have occurred, resulting in patient deaths. Many needleless IV systems allow other types of tubing such as blood pressure and oxygen tubing to connect and instill air directly into the IV line. Before tubing is connected or reconnected to a patient, trace it completely from the patient to the point of origin for verification (Institute for Safe Medication Practices, 2004).

Infusion Pumps

A variety of infusion pumps are available and used in nearly all pediatric infusions to accurately administer medication and minimize the possibility of overloading the circulation. It is important to calculate the amount to be infused in a given length of time, set the infusion rate, and monitor the apparatus frequently (at least every 1 to 2 hours) to make certain that the desired rate is maintained, the integrity of the system remains intact, the site remains intact (free of redness, edema, infiltration, or irritation), and the infusion does not stop. Continuous infusion pumps, although convenient and efficient, are not without risks. Overreliance on the accuracy of the machine can cause either too much or too little fluid to be infused; therefore its use does not eliminate careful periodic assessment by the nurse. Excess pressure can build up if the machine is set at a rate faster than the vein is able to accommodate (or continues to pump when the needle is out of the lumen).

Securement of a Peripheral Intravenous Line

To maintain the integrity of the IV line, adequate protection of the site is required. The catheter hub is firmly secured at the puncture site with a transparent dressing and commercial securement device (e.g., StatLock) (Fig. 22-20) or clear, nonallergenic tape. Transparent dressings are ideal because the insertion site is easily observed. Minimal tape should be used at the puncture site and on about 1 to 2 inches of skin beyond the site to avoid obscuring the insertion site for early detection of infiltration.

FIG. 22-21 ■ I.V. House used to protect intravenous site.

A protective cover is applied directly over the catheter insertion site to protect the infusion site. Easy access to the IV site for frequent (1- to 2-hour) assessments must be considered. Improvised plastic cups that are cut in half with the ridged edges covered with tape should not be used, since they have injured patients. A commercial site protector, I.V. House, is available in different sizes (Fig. 22-21). Its ventilation holes prevent moisture from accumulating under the dome (Lee and Vallino, 1996). This device is designed to protect the IV site; allow for visibility of the site; minimize use of padded boards, splints, or other restraints and tape; and maintain skin integrity. The connector tubing or extension tubing can be looped to make it small enough to fit under the protective cover to prevent accidental snagging of the catheter. It is important to safely secure the IV tubing to prevent infants and children from becoming entangled in the tubing or from accidentally pulling the catheter or needle out. Securing the tubing in this manner also eliminates movement of the catheter hub at the insertion site (mechanical manipulation). A colorful and interesting sticker can be applied to the protecting device to add a positive note to the procedure.

Finger or toe areas are left unoccluded by dressings or tape to allow for assessment of circulation. The thumb is never immobilized because of the danger of contractures with limited movement later on. An extremity should never be encircled with tape. The use of roll gauze, self-adhering stretch bandages (Coban), and Ace bandages can cause the same constriction and hide signs of infiltration (Infusion Nurses Society, 2000a).

> **NURSINGALERT**
>
> Opaque covering should be avoided; however, if any type of opaque covering is used to secure the IV line, the insertion site and extremity distal to the site should be visible to detect an infiltration. If these sites are not visible, they must be checked frequently to detect problems early.

EVIDENCE-BASED PRACTICE

Peripheral Intravenous Site Care
Joy Hesselgrave

ASK THE QUESTION   In children, what site preparation, dressing, and stabilization measures for peripheral intravenous catheters (PIVs) are optimum for preventing complications and extending dwell time?

SEARCH FOR EVIDENCE

Search Strategies   Search selection criteria included English-language and research-based publications within the past 20 years on PIV site care.

Databases Used   National Guideline Clearinghouse (AHRQ), Cochrane Collaboration, Joanna Briggs Institute, PubMed, TRIP Database Plus, MD Consult, PedsCCM, BestBETs

CRITICALLY ANALYZE THE EVIDENCE

Site Preparation. Centers for Disease Control and Prevention recommendations by O'Grady, Alexander, Dellinger, and others (2002) indicate that the skin should be disinfected with an appropriate antiseptic before PIV catheter insertion. A 2% chlorhexidine-based preparation is preferred, but tincture of iodine, an iodophor, or 70% alcohol can be used. The Infusion Nurses Society (2006) recommends cleansing the skin with a preparation that combines alcohol with either chlorhexidine gluconate or povidone-iodine before PIV insertion. There is insufficient evidence to recommend a single product for all neonates; chlorhexidine or povidone-iodine without alcohol may be used, but the disinfectant should be promptly removed with sterile water or normal saline to prevent absorption (Association of Women's Health, Obstetric and Neonatal Nurses, 2007).

Site Dressing. Multiple studies indicate that either gauze dressings changed every 48 hours or clear semipermeable dressings changed as needed are acceptable for PIV sites (Infusion Nurses Society, 2006). Neonatal guidelines recommend a transparent adhesive dressing or clear tape at the PIV site (Callaghan, Copnell, and Johnson, 2002; Tripepi-Bova, Woods, and Loach, 1997; Hoffmann, Wester, Kaiser, and others, 1988).

Stabilization or Securement Devices. A prospective study of 105 PIV placements compared a control group using traditional transparent dressing (Tegaderm) and tape with a study group that used transparent dressings and a catheter securement device (StatLock) (Wood, 1997). The control group had a 65% complication rate (dislodgments, infiltration, and phlebitis) vs a 20% complication rate in the study group, indicating a 45% reduction in overall PIV therapy complications in the study group. When comparing tape, StatLock, and HubGuard for a 96-hour PIV protocol change for adults, researchers found that PIVs with StatLock produced a statistically significant improved survival rate (52%) compared with tape (8%) or HubGuard (9%) (Smith, 2006). Securement devices extend the life of a PIV.

A product trial at 83 hospitals throughout the United States was initiated by Venetec International comparing StatLock with tape, the standard hospital PIV securement for adults and children. The product trial included 10,164 patients, 18 months of age and older, requiring a PIV for more than 24 hours. More than 70% of the PIVs initially placed and secured with tape required a PIV restart within a 72-hour treatment period; only 16.6% of PIVs secured with StatLock stabilization required restarts, representing a 76% overall reduction in the rate of restarts with StatLock (Schears, 2006).

APPLY THE EVIDENCE: NURSING IMPLICATIONS

- PIV sites may be dressed with either gauze or clear dressings, with the advantage of clear dressings allowing continuous site visualization. Commercial securement or protection devices extend the life of the PIV in the pediatric patient.
- For children older than 2 months, chlorhexidine is the preferred skin cleanser. For younger infants, nonalcohol-based cleansers are preferred and should be removed with sterile water or sterile normal saline to prevent absorption.
- Apply a clear semipermeable dressing or gauze dressing and tape. If the child is mobile, consider using a securement or protection device (e.g., StatLock, HubGuard, Ray-Marshall Shield, I.V. House, IV Shield, IV Pro).

References

Association of Women's Health, Obstetric and Neonatal Nurses: *Neonatal skin care: evidence-based clinical practice guideline*, ed 2, Washington, DC, 2007, The Association.

Callaghan S, Copnell B, Johnson L: Comparison of two methods of peripheral intravenous cannula securement in the pediatric setting, *J Infus Nurs* 25(4):256-264, 2002.

Hoffmann K, Wester S, Kaiser D, and others: Bacterial colonization and phlebitis-associated risk with transparent polyurethane film for peripheral intravenous site dressings, *Am J Infect Control* 16(3):101-106, 1988.

Infusion Nurses Society: *Policies and procedures for infusion nursing*, ed 3, South Norwood, Mass, 2006, The Society.

O'Grady N, Alexander M, Dellinger E, and others: Guidelines for the prevention of intravascular catheter–related infections, *MMWR* 51(RR10):1-26, 2002.

Schears G: Summary of product trials for 10,164 patients: comparing an intravenous stabilizing device to tape, *J Infus Nurs* 29(4):225-230, 2006.

Smith B: Peripheral intravenous catheter dwell times: a comparison of three securement methods for implementation of a 96-hour scheduled change protocol, *J Infus Nurs* 29(1):14-17, 2006.

Tripepi-Bova K, Woods K, Loach M: A comparison of transparent polyurethane and dry gauze dressings for peripheral IV catheter sites rates of phlebitis, infiltration and dislodgement by patients, *Am J Crit Care* 6(5):377-381, 1997.

Wood D: A comparative study of two securement techniques for short peripheral intravenous catheters, *J Intraven Nurs* 20(6):280-285, 1997.

Traditionally, padded boards or splints have been used to partially immobilize the IV site. Padded boards or splints and restraints were appropriate when metal needles were inserted into the vein to prevent the sharp end from puncturing the vessel, especially at a joint. With the more recent use of soft, pliable catheters, arm or leg boards may not be necessary and have several disadvantages. They obscure the IV site, can constrict the extremity, may excoriate the underlying tissue and promote infection, can cause a contracture of a joint, restrict useful movement of the extremity, and are uncomfortable. Unfortunately, no research has been conducted to demonstrate their proposed benefit of increasing dwell time (patency of the IV line). Adequate securement should eliminate the need for padded boards in most circumstances. Older children who are alert and cooperative can usually be trusted to protect the IV site (see Evidence-Based Practice boxes).

Removal of a Peripheral Intravenous Line

When it comes time to discontinue an IV infusion, many children are distressed by the thought of catheter removal. Therefore they need a careful explanation of the process and suggestions for helping. Encouraging children to remove or help remove the tape from the site provides them with a measure of control and often fosters their cooperation. The procedure consists of turning off any pump apparatus, occluding the IV tubing, removing the tape, pulling the catheter out of the vessel in the opposite direction of insertion, and exerting firm pressure at the site. A dry dressing (adhesive bandage strip) is placed over the puncture site. The use of adhesive-removal pads can decrease the pain of tape removal, but the skin should be washed after use to avoid irritation. To remove transparent dressings (e.g., OpSite, Tegaderm), pull the opposing edges parallel to the skin to loosen the bond. Inspect

---

EVIDENCE-BASED PRACTICE

Frequency of Changing Intravenous Administration Sets
Brandi Horvath

ASK THE QUESTION	In children, should intravenous (IV) administration sets be changed at 24, 48, 72, or 96 hours to safely prevent patient infection while containing costs?

SEARCH FOR EVIDENCE

Search Strategies	Search selection criteria included English-language publications within the past 10 years and research-based articles on frequency of changing IV administration sets.
Databases Used	National Guideline Clearinghouse (AHRQ), Cochrane Collaboration, Joanna Briggs Institute, PubMed, Infusion Nurses Society, Oncology Nurses Society, MD Consult, BestBETs, TRIP Database Plus, PedsCCM

CRITICALLY ANALYZE THE EVIDENCE

A Cochrane systematic review by Gillies, O'Riordan, Wallen, and others (2005) identified the optimum interval for the routine replacement of IV administration sets when infusate or parenteral nutrition solutions are administered. Data results from 13 randomized or quasirandomized controlled trials were pooled to compare different time intervals of administration set changes: every 24 hours vs 48 hours or greater, 48 hours vs at least 72 hours, and 72 hours vs 96 hours. Findings revealed no evidence that changing IV administration sets more often than every 96 hours reduces the incidence of bloodstream infection. There were no differences in results between patients with central and peripheral catheters and those who did or did not receive parenteral nutrition. For IV administration sets including blood or blood products and lipids, the researchers recommending changing the sets every 24 hours.

The Centers for Disease Control and Prevention (O'Grady, Alexander, Dellinger, and others, 2002) recommends changing IV administration sets for crystalloids at no more than 72-hour intervals. Rates of phlebitis were not substantially different for administration sets left in place 96 hours compared with 72 hours. For tubing used to administer blood and blood products or lipid emulsions, replace tubing within 24 hours of starting the infusion.

The Infusion Nurses Society (2006) and Alexander (2006) recommend replacing continuously infusing IV administration sets no more frequently than every 72 hours. Administration sets used intermittently should be changed every 24 hours. Secondary piggyback sets may be changed no more frequently than every 72 hours when attached to a continuously infusing line; once detached from the primary set, they should be changed at 24 hours. Exceptions include sets used with lipids (change at 24 hours

if continuous or after each unit if intermittently infused) and blood or blood components (change at the end of 4 hours if continuous or after each intermittent component). All sets should be changed immediately if contamination is suspected.

The Oncology Nursing Society (Camp-Sorreli, 2004) recommends replacing IV administration sets every 96 hours or with catheter change, except for fluids that enhance microbial growth. Tubing used to administer blood, blood products, lipids, or total parenteral nutrition should be replaced 24 hours after initiation of therapy.

APPLY THE EVIDENCE: NURSING IMPLICATIONS

- Replace IV administration sets every 96 hours.
- Replace tubing used for lipid emulsions, blood, and blood products every 24 hours.
- Replace blood tubing with in-line filters after 2 units or 4 hours, whichever comes first.

References

Alexander M, editor: Infusion nursing standards of practice, *J Infus Nurs* 29(1S):S48-S50, 2006.

Camp-Sorreli D, editor: *Access device guidelines: recommendations for nursing practice and education*, ed 2, Pittsburgh, 2004, Oncology Nursing Society.

Gillies D, O'Riordan L, Wallen M, and others: Optimal timing for intravenous administration set replacement, *Cochrane Database Syst Rev* (4):CD003588.pub2; DOI: 10.1002/14651858.CD003588.pub2, 2005.

Infusion Nurses Society: *Policies and procedures for infusion nursing*, ed 3, South Norwood, Mass, 2006, The Society.

O'Grady N, Alexander M, Dellinger E, and others: Guidelines for the prevention of intravascular catheter-related infections, *MMWR* 51(RR-10):1-29, 2002.

the catheter tip to ensure the catheter is intact and that no portion remains in the vein.

> **NURSINGALERT**
>
> Consider the child's age, development, and neurologic status, as well as the predictability of the child (how the child responds to painful treatments), when determining the need for assistance to maintain safety. Manual removal of tape is the preferred method. Only if absolutely necessary should a small cut be made in the tape, using bandage scissors, to facilitate its removal. Before cutting the tape:
> - Ensure that all digits are visible.
> - Remove any barrier that hinders visibility, such as a protective covering.
> - Protect the child's skin and digits by sliding own finger(s) between the tape and the child's skin so that the scissors do not touch the patient.
> - Place a cut on the tape located on the medial aspect (thumb side) of the extremity.

Complications

The same precautions regarding maintenance of asepsis, prevention of infection, and observation for infiltration are carried out with patients of any age. However, infiltration is more difficult to detect in infants and small children than in adults. The increased amount of subcutaneous fat and the amount of tape used to secure the catheter often obscure the early signs of infiltration. When the fluid appears to be infusing too slowly or ceases, the usual assessment for obstruction within the apparatus—kinks, screw clamps, shutoff valve, and positioning interference (e.g., a bent elbow)—often locates the difficulty. When these actions fail to detect the problem, it may be necessary to carefully remove some of the dressing to obtain a clear view of the venipuncture site. Dependent areas, such as the palm and undersides of the extremity or the occiput and behind the ears, are examined.

Whenever possible, the IV infusion should be placed in an extremity to which the identification band (or bracelet) is not attached. Serious circulatory impairment can result from infiltrated solution distal to the band, which acts as a tourniquet, preventing adequate venous return. To check for return blood flow through the catheter, the tubing is removed from the infusion pump, and the bag is lowered below the level of the infusion site. Resistance during flushing or aspiration for blood return also indicates that the IV infusion may have infiltrated surrounding tissue. A good blood return, or lack thereof, is not always an indicator of infiltration in small infants. Flushing the catheter and observing for edema, redness, or streaking along the vein are appropriate for assessment of the IV.

IV therapy in pediatrics tends to be difficult to maintain because of mechanical factors such as vascular trauma resulting from the catheter, the insertion site, vessel size, vessel fragility, pump pressure, the patient's activity level, operator skill and insertion technique, forceful administration of boluses of fluid, and infusion of irritants or vesicants through a small vessel (Pettit and Hughes, 1999). These factors cause infiltration and extravasation injuries. **Infiltration** is defined as inadvertent administration of a nonvesicant solution or medication into surrounding tissue. **Extravasation** is defined as inadvertent administration of vesicant solution or medication into surrounding tissue (Infusion Nurses Society, 2000a, 2000b). A **vesicant** or **sclerosing agent** causes varying degrees

of cellular damage when even minute amounts escape into surrounding tissue. Guidelines are available for determining the severity of tissue injury by staging characteristics, such as the amount of redness, blanching, the amount of swelling, pain, the quality of pulses below infiltration, capillary refill, and warmth or coolness of the area (Infusion Nurses Society, 2000a, 2000b; Montgomery, Hanrahan, Korrman, and others, 1999).*

Treatment of infiltration or extravasation varies according to the type of vesicant. Guidelines are available outlining the sequence of interventions and specific treatment of infiltration or extravasation with antidotes (Oncology Nursing Society, 1998; Montgomery, Hanrahan, Korrman, and others, 1999).†

> **NURSINGALERT**
>
> When infiltration or extravasation is observed (signs include erythema, pain, edema, blanching, streaking on the skin along the vein, and darkened area at the insertion site), immediately stop the infusion, elevate the extremity, notify the practitioner, and initiate the ordered treatment as soon as possible. Remove the IV line when it is no longer needed (e.g., after infusing an antidote).

PIV catheters are the most commonly used intravascular device. Heavy cutaneous colonization of the insertion site is the single most important predictor of catheter-related infection with all types of short-term, percutaneously inserted catheters. Phlebitis, largely a mechanical rather than infectious process, remains the most important complication associated with the use of peripheral venous catheters.‡

> **NURSINGALERT**
>
> The most effective ways to prevent infection of an IV site are to cleanse hands between each patient, wear gloves when inserting a catheter, and closely inspect the insertion site and physical condition of the dressing. Proper education of the patient and family regarding signs and symptoms of an infected site can help prevent infections from going unnoticed.

PROCEDURES FOR MAINTAINING RESPIRATORY FUNCTION

INHALATION THERAPY
Oxygen Therapy

Oxygen is administered for hypoxemia and may be delivered by mask, nasal cannula, tent, hood, face mask, or ventilator. Oxygen therapy is frequently administered in the hospital, although increasing numbers of children are receiving oxygen in the home. Oxygen delivered to infants is well tolerated by using a **plastic hood** (Fig. 22-22). The humidified oxygen should not be blown directly into the infant's face. Older, cooperative infants and children can use a **nasal cannula** or **prongs,** which can supply a concentration of oxygen of about 50%. A **mask** is not well tolerated by children.

---

*Guidelines for determining tissue injury severity are available from the Infusion Nurses Society, 315 Norwood Park South, Norwood, MA 02062; (781) 440-9408; fax: (781) 440-9409; http://www.ins1.org.
†Guidelines on interventions for infiltration and extravasation are available from the Oncology Nursing Society, 125 Enterprise Drive, Pittsburgh, PA 15275; (412) 859-6100; fax: (412) 859-6162; http://www.ons.org.
‡Guidelines for prevention of intravascular device–related infections are available from the Centers for Disease Control and Prevention, 1600 Clifton Road, Atlanta, GA 30333; (404) 639-1515; http://www.cdc.gov/ncidod/dhqp/gl_intravascular.html.

FIG. 22-22 ■ Oxygen administered to infant by means of a plastic hood. Note oxygen analyzer (*blue machine*).

FIG. 22-23 ■ The tent provides a comfortable method for oxygen administration. (From Wilson SF, Thompson JM: *Respiratory disorders*, St Louis, 1990, Mosby.)

For children beyond early infancy, the **oxygen tent** is a satisfactory means for administration of oxygen (Fig. 22-23). A tent does not require any device to come into direct contact with the face, but the concentration of oxygen within the tent is difficult to control and to maintain above 30% to 50%. A major difficulty with the use of the tent is keeping the tent closed so that the oxygen concentration is maintained.

To reduce oxygen loss, nursing care is planned carefully so that the tent is opened as little as possible. Because oxygen is heavier than air, loss will be greater at the bottom of the tent; therefore the tent is tucked in snugly without open edges. The bottom of the tent should be examined more often when the child is restless and fussy and liable to pull the covers loose. Some tents are even open at the top. Because of the rapidly diffusing qualities of carbon dioxide, the levels of the gas do not build up within these enclosures.

After the tent has been opened for an extended period, it is flushed with oxygen by increasing the flow meter for a few minutes to quickly raise the oxygen and mist concentration.

The flow meter is then reset to the prescribed number of liters per minute.

The enclosed tent becomes warm; therefore some type of cooling mechanism is provided. The temperature inside the tent must be checked periodically to be certain that it is maintained at the desired level. Although the cool environment can reduce fever and airway inflammation, it can also produce hypothermia and cold stress. It is important to make certain that the child is kept warm and dry. Because oxygen is drying to the tissues, the gas is humidified, which causes moisture to condense on the tent walls.

NURSINGALERT

Keep the child warm and dry by checking the temperature inside the tent and the child's bedding and clothing frequently. Adjust the temperature and change clothing as often as needed.

NURSINGALERT

Inspect all toys for safety and suitability (e.g., vinyl or plastic, not stuffed items that absorb moisture and are difficult to keep dry). The high-level oxygen environment makes any source of sparks (e.g., mechanical or electrical toys) a potential fire hazard.

In some instances the child can be removed from the oxygen tent for activities such as feeding and bathing, whereas in other cases the child is placed in the tent only during periods of rest. Still other children may require oxygen continuously and can be removed from the tent or incubator only if an oxygen source is held close to the child's face. Any change in color, increased respiratory effort, or restlessness is an indication to return the child to the oxygen tent.

Oxygen Toxicity. Prolonged exposure to high oxygen tensions can damage some body tissues and functions. The organs most vulnerable to the adverse effects of excessive oxygenation are the retina of the extremely preterm infant and the lungs of persons at any age.

Oxygen-induced carbon dioxide narcosis is a physiologic hazard of oxygen therapy that may occur in persons with chronic pulmonary disease, such as cystic fibrosis. In these patients the respiratory center has adapted to the continuously higher arterial carbon dioxide tension ($Paco_2$) levels, and therefore hypoxia becomes the more powerful stimulus for respiration. When the arterial oxygen tension (Pao_2) level is elevated during oxygen administration, the hypoxic drive is removed, causing progressive hypoventilation and increased $Paco_2$ levels, and the child rapidly becomes unconscious. Carbon dioxide narcosis can also be induced by the administration of sedation in these patients.

Monitoring Oxygen Therapy

Pulse oximetry is a continuous, noninvasive method of determining oxygen saturation (Sao_2) to guide oxygen therapy. A sensor composed of a light-emitting diode (LED) and a photodetector is placed in opposition around a foot, hand, finger, toe, or earlobe, with the LED placed on top of the nail when digits are used (Fig. 22-24). The diode emits red and infrared lights that pass through the skin to the photodetector. The photodetector measures the amount of each type of light absorbed by functional hemoglobins. Hemoglobin saturated with oxygen (oxyhemoglobin) absorbs more infrared light than does hemoglobin not saturated with oxygen (deoxyhe-

FIG. 22-24 ■ Oximeter sensor on great toe. Note that sensor is positioned with light-emitting diode opposite photodetector. Cord is secured to foot to minimize movement of sensor.

moglobin). Pulsatile blood flow is the primary physiologic factor that influences accuracy of the pulse oximeter. In infants, reposition the probe at least every 3 to 4 hours to prevent pressure necrosis; poor perfusion and very sensitive skin may necessitate more frequent repositioning.

Another noninvasive method is **transcutaneous monitoring (TCM),** which provides continuous monitoring of transcutaneous partial pressure of oxygen in arterial blood (tcPao$_2$) and, with some devices, of carbon dioxide in arterial blood (tcPaco$_2$). An electrode is attached to the warmed skin to facilitate arterialization of cutaneous capillaries. The site of the electrode must be changed every 3 to 4 hours to avoid burning the skin, and the machine must be calibrated with every site change. TCM is used frequently in neonatal intensive care units, but it may not reflect Pao$_2$ in infants with impaired local circulation or in older infants whose skin is thicker.

Oximetry is insensitive to hyperoxia because hemoglobin approaches 100% saturation for all Pao$_2$ readings greater than approximately 100 mm Hg, which is a dangerous situation for the preterm infant at risk for developing retinopathy of prematurity (see Chapter 9). Therefore the preterm infant being monitored with oximetry should have upper limits identified, such as 90% to 95%, and a protocol established for decreasing oxygen when saturations are high.

Oximetry offers several advantages over TCM. Oximetry (1) does not require heating the skin, thus reducing the risk of burns; (2) eliminates a delay period for transducer equilibration; and (3) maintains an accurate measurement regardless of the patient's age or skin characteristics or the presence of lung disease.

Applying the sensor correctly is essential for accurate Sao$_2$ measurements. Because the sensor must identify every pulse beat to calculate the Sao$_2$, movement can interfere with sens-

ing. Some devices synchronize the Sao$_2$ reading with the heartbeat, thereby reducing the interference caused by motion. Sensors are not placed on extremities used for blood pressure monitoring or with indwelling arterial catheters, since pulsatile blood flow may be affected.

Ambient light from ceiling lights and phototherapy, as well as high-intensity heat and light from radiant warmers, can interfere with readings. Therefore the sensor should be covered to block these light sources. IV dyes; green, purple, or black nail polish; nonopaque synthetic nails; and possibly ink used for footprinting can also cause inaccurate Sao$_2$ measurements. The dyes should be removed or, in the case of porcelain nails, a different area used for the sensor. Skin color, thickness, and edema do not affect the readings.

Aerosol Therapy

Aerosol therapy can be effective in depositing medication directly into the airway. The value of aerosolized water, or "mist therapy," is controversial. This route of administration can be useful in avoiding the systemic side effects of certain drugs and in reducing the amount of drug necessary to achieve the desired effect. Bronchodilators, steroids, and antibiotics, suspended in particulate form, can be inhaled so that the medication reaches the small airways. Aerosol therapy is particularly challenging in children who are too young to cooperate with controlling the rate and depth of breathing. Administration of this therapy requires skill, patience, and creativity.

Medications can be aerosolized or nebulized with air or with oxygen-enriched gas. **Handheld nebulizers** are the most frequently used equipment. The medicated mist is discharged into a small plastic mask, which the child holds over the nose and mouth. To avoid particle deposition in the nose and pharynx, the child is instructed to take slow, deep breaths through an open mouth during the treatment. For home use an air compressor is necessary to force air through the liquid medication to form the aerosol. Compact, portable units can be obtained from health equipment companies. The **metered-dose inhaler (MDI)** is a self-contained, handheld device that allows for intermittent delivery of a specified amount of medication. Many bronchodilators are available in this form and are successfully used by children with asthma. For children under the age of 5 or 6 years, a **spacer device** attached to the MDI can help with coordination of breathing and aerosol delivery. It allows the aerosolized particles to remain in suspension longer. (See also Asthma, Chapter 23.)

Assessment of breath sounds and work of breathing should be done before and after treatments. Young children who become upset by having a mask held close to the face may become fatigued with fighting the procedure and may actually appear worse during and immediately after the therapy. It may be necessary to spend a few minutes calming the child after the procedure and allowing the vital signs to return to baseline to accurately assess changes in breath sounds and work of breathing.

BRONCHIAL (POSTURAL) DRAINAGE

Bronchial drainage is indicated whenever excessive fluid or mucus in the bronchi is not being removed by normal ciliary activity and cough. Positioning the child to take maximum advantage of gravity facilitates removal of secretions. Postural drainage can be effective in children with chronic lung disease characterized by thick mucus, such as cystic fibrosis.

Postural drainage is carried out three or four times daily and is more effective when it follows other respiratory therapy, such as bronchodilator or nebulization medication. Bronchial drainage is generally performed before meals (or 1 to 1½ hours after meals) to minimize the chance of vomiting and is repeated at bedtime. The duration of treatment depends on the child's condition and tolerance; it usually lasts 20 to 30 minutes. Several positions facilitate drainage from all major lung segments (Fig. 22-25); all positions are not employed at each session. Children will usually cooperate for four to six positions. Older children can tolerate longer periods.

In the hospital an older child can be positioned over an elevated knee rest. Small children and infants can be positioned with pillows or on the therapist's lap and legs. Infants should not be placed in the Trendelenburg position because they do not have an autonomic regulation of blood flow to the head. Special modifications of the techniques are required in children whose conditions contraindicate the standard positioning, such as head injuries, some types of surgical incisions or burns, and casts.

CHEST PHYSICAL THERAPY

Chest physical therapy (CPT) usually refers to the use of postural drainage in combination with adjunctive techniques that are thought to enhance the clearance of mucus from the airway. These techniques include manual percussion, vibration, and squeezing of the chest; cough; forceful expiration; and breathing exercises. Special mechanical devices are also currently used to perform CPT (e.g., ThAIRapy Vest). Postural drainage in combination with forced expiration has been shown to be beneficial. Noninvasive inspiratory nasal pressure–support ventilation (PSV) during CPT has demonstrated a significant improvement in respiratory muscle performance and a reduction in oxygen desaturation (Fauroux, Boule, Lofaso, and others, 1999).

The most common technique used in association with postural drainage is manual percussion of the chest wall. The patient is dressed in a lightweight shirt and placed in a postural drainage position. The nurse then gently but firmly strikes the chest wall with a cupped hand (Fig. 22-26, *A*). For infants, special devices are available for percussing small areas (Fig. 22-26, *B*). A "popping," hollow sound should be the result, not a slapping sound. The procedure should be done over the rib cage only and should be painless. Percussion can be performed with a soft circular mask (adapted to maintain air trapping) or a percussion cup marketed especially for the purpose of aiding in loosening secretions.

CPT is contraindicated when patients have pulmonary hemorrhage, pulmonary embolism, end-stage renal disease, increased intracranial pressure, osteogenesis imperfecta, or minimal cardiac reserves.

ARTIFICIAL VENTILATION
Artificial Airways

An artificial airway is usually used in association with mechanical ventilation and in children with upper airway obstruction. Endotracheal intubation can be accomplished by the nasal (nasotracheal), oral (orotracheal), or direct tracheal (tracheostomy) routes. Although it is more difficult to place, nasotracheal intubation is preferred to orotracheal intubation because it facilitates oral hygiene and provides more stable fixation, which reduces the complication of tracheal erosion and the danger of accidental extubation. Only uncuffed endotracheal tubes should be used in children younger than 8 years of age (Curley and Moloney-Harmon, 2001). Air or gas delivered directly to the trachea must be humidified.

Tracheostomy

A tracheostomy is a surgical opening in the trachea; the procedure may be done on an emergency basis or may be an elective one, and it may be combined with mechanical ventilation. Pediatric tracheostomy tubes are usually made of plastic or Silastic (Fig. 22-27). The most common types are the Hollinger, Jackson, Aberdeen, and Shiley tubes. These tubes are constructed with a more acute angle than adult tubes, and they soften at body temperature, conforming to the contours of the trachea. Because these materials resist the formation of crusted respiratory secretions, they are made without an inner cannula.

Children who have undergone a tracheostomy must be closely monitored for complications such as hemorrhage, edema, aspiration, accidental decannulation, tube obstruction, and the entrance of free air into the pleural cavity. The focus of nursing care is maintaining a patent airway, facilitating the removal of pulmonary secretions, providing humidified air or oxygen, cleansing the stoma, monitoring the child's ability to swallow, and teaching while simultaneously preventing complications.

Because the child may be unable to signal for help, direct observation and use of respiratory and cardiac monitors are essential. Respiratory assessments include breath sounds and work of breathing, vital signs, tightness of the tracheostomy ties, and the type and amount of secretions. Large amounts of bloody secretions are uncommon and should be considered a sign of hemorrhage. The practitioner should be notified immediately if this occurs.

The child is positioned with the head of the bed raised or in the position most comfortable to the child, with the call light easily available. Suction catheters, suction source, gloves, sterile saline, sterile gauze for wiping away secretions, scissors, an extra tracheostomy tube of the same size with ties already attached, another tracheostomy tube one size smaller, and the obturator are kept at the bedside. A source of humidification is provided because the normal humidification and filtering functions of the airway have been bypassed. IV fluids ensure adequate hydration until the child is able to swallow sufficient amounts of fluids.

Suctioning. The airway must remain patent and requires frequent suctioning during the first few hours after a tracheostomy to remove mucous plugs and excessive secretions. Proper vacuum pressure and suction catheter size are important to prevent atelectasis and decrease hypoxia from the suctioning procedure. Vacuum pressure should range from 60

FIG. 22-25 ■ Bronchial drainage positions for all major segments of child. For each position, model of tracheobronchial tree is projected beside child to show segmental bronchus *(red)* being drained and pathway of secretions out of bronchus. Drainage platform is horizontal unless otherwise noted. Red area on child's chest indicates area to be cupped or vibrated by therapist. **A,** Apical segment of right upper lobe and apical subsegment of apical-posterior segment of left upper lobe. **B,** Posterior segment of right upper lobe and posterior subsegment of apical-posterior segment of left upper lobe. **C,** Anterior segments of both upper lobes. Child should be rotated slightly away from side being drained. **D,** Superior segments of both lower lobes. **E,** Posterior basal segments of both lower lobes. **F,** Lateral basal segments of right lower lobe. Left lateral basal segment would be drained by mirror image of this position (right side down). **G,** Anterior basal segment of left lower lobe. Right anterior basal segment would be drained by mirror image of this position (left side down). **H,** Medial and lateral segments of right middle lobe. **I,** Lingular segments (superior and inferior) of left upper lobe (homologue of right middle lobe). (From Chernick V, editor: *Kendig's disorders of the respiratory tract of children,* ed 6, Philadelphia, 1998, Saunders.)

FIG. 22-26 ■ **A,** Cupped hand position for percussion. **B,** Device for infant percussion.

FIG. 22-27 ■ Silastic pediatric tracheostomy tube and obturator.

to 100 mm Hg for infants and children and from 40 to 60 mm Hg for preterm infants. Unless secretions are thick and tenacious, the lower range of negative pressure is recommended. Tracheal suction catheters are available in a variety of sizes. The catheter selected should have a diameter one-half the diameter of the tracheostomy tube. If the catheter is too large, it can block the airway. The catheter is constructed with a side port so that the catheter is introduced without suction and removed while simultaneous intermittent suction is applied by covering the port with the thumb (Fig. 22-28). The catheter is inserted to 0.5 cm beyond or just to the end of the tracheostomy tube. The practice of instilling sterile saline in the tracheostomy tube before suctioning is not supported by research and is no longer recommended (see Evidence-Based Practice box).

FIG. 22-28 ■ Tracheostomy suctioning. **A,** Insertion, port open. **B,** Withdrawal, port occluded. Note that catheter is inserted just slightly beyond end of tracheostomy tube.

> **NURSINGALERT**
>
> Suctioning should require no more than 5 seconds. Counting one one-thousand, two one-thousand, three one-thousand, and so on while suctioning is a simple means for monitoring the time. Without a safeguard, the airway may be obstructed for too long. Hyperventilating the child with 100% oxygen before and after suctioning (using a bag-valve-mask or increasing the fraction of inspired oxygen concentration [Fio$_2$] ventilator setting) may be performed to prevent hypoxia. Closed tracheal suctioning systems that allow for uninterrupted oxygen delivery may also be used.

> **FYI**
>
> In a closed suction system, a suction catheter is directly attached to the ventilator tubing. This system has several advantages. First, there is no need to disconnect the patient from the ventilator, which allows for better oxygenation. Second, the suction catheter is enclosed in a plastic sheath, which reduces the risk of the nurse being exposed to the patient's secretions (Carroll, 1998).

The child is allowed to rest for 30 to 60 seconds after each aspiration to allow oxygen saturation to return to normal; then the process is repeated until the trachea is clear. Suctioning should be limited to about three aspirations in one period. Oximetry is used to monitor suctioning and prevent hypoxia.

> **NURSINGALERT**
>
> Suctioning is carried out only as often as needed to keep the tube patent. Signs of mucus partially occluding the airway include an increased heart rate, a rise in respiratory effort, a drop in Sao$_2$, cyanosis, and an increase in the positive inspiratory pressure on the ventilator.

In the acute care setting, aseptic technique is used during care of the tracheostomy. Secondary infection is a major concern, since the air entering the lower airway bypasses the natu-

Normal Saline Instillation Before Suctioning—Helpful or Harmful?
Marilyn J. Hockenberry

ASK THE QUESTION   In intubated children and those with tracheostomy, is normal saline instillation before suctioning helpful or harmful?

SEARCH FOR EVIDENCE

Search Strategies   Search selection criteria included English-language publications within the past 20 years and research-based articles on suctioning intubated children and those with a tracheostomy.

Databases Used   PubMed, Cochrane Collaboration, MD Consult, BestBETs, PedsCCM

CRITICALLY ANALYZE THE EVIDENCE

■ Instillation of normal saline before endotracheal (ET) tube suctioning has been used for years as a method to loosen and dilute secretions, lubricate the suction catheter, and promote cough. In recent years the possible adverse effects of this procedure have been explored. Adult studies have found decreased oxygen saturation, increased frequency of nosocomial pneumonia, and increased intracranial pressure after instillation of normal saline before suctioning (O'Neal, Grap, Thompson, and others, 2001; Kinlock, 1999; Hagler and Traver, 1994; Reynolds, Hoffman, Schlichtig, and others, 1990; Ackerman, 1993; Ackerman and Gugerty, 1990; Bostick and Wendelgass, 1987).

■ Two of the first research studies evaluating the effect of normal saline instillation before suctioning in neonates found no deleterious effects. Shorten, Byrne, and Jones (1991) found no significant differences in oxygenation, heart rate, or blood pressure before or after suctioning in a group of 27 intubated neonates. In a second study of nine neonates acting as their own controls, no adverse effects on lung mechanics were found after normal saline instillation and suctioning (Beeram and Dhanireddy, 1992).

■ A recent study evaluating the effects of normal saline instillation before suctioning in children found results similar to those in the previously published adult studies. Ridling, Martin, and Bratton (2003) evaluated the effects of normal saline instillation before suctioning in a group of 24 critically ill children, ages 10 weeks to 14 years. A total of 104 suctioning episodes were analyzed. Children experienced significantly greater oxygen desaturation after suctioning if normal saline was instilled.

■ The American Thoracic Society's (2005) official position statement on the care of children with tracheostomies now states that normal saline should not be instilled before suctioning.

APPLY THE EVIDENCE: NURSING IMPLICATIONS

Studies support that the adverse effects of normal saline instillation before suctioning in children are similar to those found for adults. This technique causes a significant reduction in oxygen saturation that can last up to 2 minutes after suctioning. The evidence does not support the use of normal saline instillation before ET suctioning in children.

References

Ackerman MH: The effect of saline lavage prior to suctioning, *Am J Crit Care* 2(4):326-330, 1993.

Ackerman MH, Gugerty B: The effect of normal saline bolus instillation in artificial airways, *The Journal* Spring:14-17, 1990.

American Thoracic Society: *Care of the child with a chronic tracheostomy*, 2005, retrieved April 17, 2006, from http://www.thoracic.org/sections/publications/statements/pages/respiratory-disease-pediatric/childtrach1-12.html.

Beeram MR, Dhanireddy R: Effects of saline instillation during tracheal suction on lung mechanics in newborn infants, *J Perinatol* 12(2):120-123, 1992.

Bostick J, Wendelgass ST: Normal saline instillation as part of the suctioning procedure: effects of Pao₂ and amount of secretions, *Heart Lung* 16(5):532-537, 1987.

Hagler DA, Traver GA: Endotracheal saline and suction catheters: sources of lower airway contamination, *Am J Crit Care* 3(6):444-447, 1994.

Kinlock D: Instillation of normal saline during endotracheal suctioning: effects on mixed venous oxygen saturation, *Am J Crit Care* 8(4):231-240, 1999.

O'Neal PV, Grap MJ, Thompson C, and others: Level of dyspnoea experienced in mechanically ventilated adults with and without saline instillation prior to endotracheal suctioning, *Intensive Crit Care Nurs* 17(6):356-363, 2001.

Reynolds P, Hoffman LA, Schlichtig R, and others: Effects of normal saline instillation on secretion volume, dynamic compliance, and oxygen saturation (abstract), *Am Rev Respir Dis* 141:A574, 1990.

Ridling DA, Martin LD, Bratton SL: Endotracheal suctioning with or without instillation of isotonic sodium chloride in critically ill children, *Am J Crit Care* 12(3):212-219, 2003.

Shorten DR, Byrne PJ, Jones RL: Infant responses to saline instillations and endotracheal suctioning, *J Obstet Gynecol Neonatal Nurs* 20(6):464-469, 1991.

ral defenses of the upper airway. Gloves are worn during the aspiration procedure, although a sterile glove is needed only on the hand touching the catheter. A new tube, gloves, and sterile saline solution are used each time.

Routine Care. The tracheostomy stoma requires daily care. Assessments of the stoma area include observations for signs of infection and breakdown of the skin. The skin is kept clean and dry, and crusted secretions around the stoma may be gently removed with half-strength hydrogen peroxide. Hydrogen peroxide should not be used with sterling silver tracheostomy tubes because it tends to pit and stain the silver surface. The nurse should be aware of wet tracheostomy dressings, which can predispose the peristomal area to skin breakdown. Several products are available to prevent or treat excoriation. The Allevyn tracheostomy dressing is a hydrophilic sponge with a polyurethane back that is highly absorptive. Other possible barriers to help maintain skin integrity include the use of hydrocolloid wafers (e.g., DuoDERM CGF, Hollister Restore) under the tracheostomy flanges, as well as extrathin hydrocolloid wafers under the chin.

The tracheostomy tube is held in place with tracheostomy ties made of a durable, nonfraying material. The ties are changed daily and when soiled. New ties are looped through the flanges and tied snugly in a triple knot at the side of the neck *before* the soiled ties are cut and removed. Some nurses have found that threading the ties through a piece of 0.25-inch surgical tubing cushions the ties; others have found the tubing to be irritating to the skin. The ties should be tight enough to allow just a fingertip to be inserted between the ties and the neck (Fig. 22-29). It is easier to ensure a snug fit if the child's head is flexed rather than extended while the ties are being secured. Ties fastened with self-adhering closures are also available. These devices, such as the Dale tracheostomy tube holder, are made of a soft, cushioning, and slightly

FIG. 22-29 ■ Tracheostomy ties are snug but allow one finger to be inserted.

stretchy material that is very comfortable. They are becoming increasingly popular because of their ease of use and ability to maintain better skin integrity. However, nurses and family members must consider the safety factor and use them only on a child who will not pull and undo the fastener.

Routine tracheostomy tube changes are usually carried out weekly after a tract has been formed to minimize the formation of granulation tissue. The first change is usually performed by the surgeon; subsequent changes are performed by the nurse and, if the child is discharged home with the tracheostomy, by either a parent or a visiting nurse. Ideally, two caregivers participate in the procedure to assist with positioning the child.

Changing the tracheostomy tube is accomplished using sterile technique. Tube changes should occur before meals or 2 hours after the last meal. Continuous feedings should be turned off at least an hour before a tube change. The new, sterile tube is prepared by inserting the obturator and attaching new ties. The child is suctioned before the procedure to minimize secretions, then restrained and positioned with the neck slightly extended. One caregiver cuts the old ties and removes the tube from the stoma. The new tube is inserted gently into the stoma (using a downward and forward motion that follows the curve of the trachea), the obturator is removed, and the ties are secured. The adequacy of ventilation must be assessed after a tube change because the tube can be inserted into the soft tissue surrounding the trachea; therefore breath sounds and respiratory effort are carefully monitored.

Supplemental oxygen is always delivered with a humidification system to prevent drying of the respiratory mucosa. Humidification of room air for an established tracheostomy can be intermittent if secretions remain thin enough to be coughed or suctioned from the tracheostomy. Direct humidification via a tracheostomy mask can be provided during naps and at night so that the child is able to be up and around unencumbered during much of the day. Room humidifiers are also used successfully.

The inner cannula, if used, should be removed with each suctioning, cleaned with sterile saline and pipe cleaners to remove crusted material, dried thoroughly, and reinserted.

Emergency Care: Tube Occlusion and Accidental Decannulation. Occlusion of the tracheostomy tube is life threatening, and infants and children are at greater risk than adults because of the smaller diameter of the tube. Maintain-

ing patency of the tube is accomplished with suctioning and routine tube changes to prevent the formation of crusts that can occlude the tube.

> **NURSINGALERT**
> Life-threatening occlusion is apparent when the child displays signs of respiratory distress and a suction catheter cannot be passed to the end of the tube despite several attempts and instillation of saline. This situation requires an immediate tube change.

Accidental decannulation also requires immediate tube replacement. Some children have a fairly rigid trachea, so the airway remains partially open when the tube is removed. However, others have malformed or flexible tracheal cartilage, which causes the airway to collapse when the tube is removed or dislodged. Because many infants and children with upper airway problems have little airway reserve, if replacement of the dislodged tube is impossible, a smaller-sized tube should be inserted. If the stoma cannot be cannulated with another tracheostomy tube, oral intubation should be performed.

PROCEDURES RELATED TO ALTERNATIVE FEEDING TECHNIQUES

Some children are unable to take nourishment by mouth because of anomalies of the throat, esophagus, or bowel; impaired swallowing capacity; severe debilitation; respiratory distress; or unconsciousness. These children are frequently fed by way of a tube inserted orally or nasally into the stomach (**orogastric** or **nasogastric gavage**) or duodenum-jejunum (**enteral gavage**), or by a tube inserted directly into the stomach (**gastrostomy**) or jejunum (**jejunostomy**). Such feedings may be intermittent or by continuous drip.

Feeding resistance, a problem that may result from any long-term feeding method that bypasses the mouth, is discussed in Chapter 9. During gavage or gastrostomy feedings, infants are given a pacifier. Nonnutritive sucking has several advantages, such as increased weight gain and decreased crying. However, to prevent the possibility of aspiration, only pacifiers with a safe design may be used. Using improvised pacifiers made from bottle nipples is not a safe practice.

> **NURSINGALERT**
> When a child is concurrently receiving continuous-drip gastric or enteral feedings and parenteral (IV) therapy, the potential exists for inadvertent administration of the enteral formula through the circulatory system, especially when the parenteral solution is a fat emulsion, which looks milky. Safeguards to prevent this potentially serious error include:
> - Use a separate, specifically designed enteral feeding pump mounted on a separate pole for continuous-feeding solutions.
> - Label all tubing for continuous enteral feeding with brightly colored tape or labels.
> - Use specifically designed continuous-feeding bags to contain the solutions instead of parenteral equipment, such as a burette.

GAVAGE FEEDING

Infants and children can be fed simply and safely by a tube passed into the stomach through either the nares or the mouth. The tube can be left in place or inserted and removed with each feeding. In older children it is usually less traumatic to tape the tube securely in place between feedings. When this alternative is used, the tube should be removed and replaced with a new tube according to hospital policy, specific orders,

ATRAUMATIC CARE

Reducing the Distress of Nasogastric Tube Insertion

Numerous strategies can be used to decrease discomfort during nasogastric (NG) tube insertion. Most important, the nurse performing the procedure should be competent in NG tube placement. The nurse should discuss the procedure with the child in a developmentally appropriate way and give family members the details of what to expect during the procedure. Administration of sedation and analgesia should be considered before NG insertion. The use of topical lidocaine and phenylephrine for the nose and tetracaine and benzocaine spray for the throat before NG insertion has been found to reduce pain and discomfort in a group of adult patients (Singer and Konia, 1999). A smaller-caliber, soft, flexible tube should be used. To prevent the trauma of reinsertion, make certain the NG tube is well secured after placement.

Data from Maglinte C: Strategies for reducing the pain and discomfort of nasogastric intubation, *Acad Emerg Med* 6(3):166-168, 1999.

and the type of tube used. Meticulous hand washing is practiced during the procedure to prevent bacterial contamination of the feeding, especially during continuous-drip feedings (see Atraumatic Care box).

Not all feeding tubes are the same. Polyethylene and polyvinylchloride types lose their flexibility and need to be replaced frequently, usually every 3 or 4 days. The polyurethane and silicone tubes are indwelling and remain flexible; so that they can remain in place longer and afford more patient comfort. Use of these small-bore tubes for continuous feeding has reduced the incidence of complications such as pharyngitis, otitis media, and incompetence of the lower esophageal sphincter. Although the increased softness and flexibility of the tubes are advantages, they also have disadvantages such as difficult insertion (may require a stylet or metal guidewire), collapse of the tube during aspiration of gastric contents to test for correct placement, dislodgment during forceful coughing, and unsuitability for thick feedings. Traditional methods for verifying placement are less reliable with the small-bore tubes.

Infants will be easier to control if they are first wrapped in a mummy restraint (see Fig. 22-7). Even tiny infants with random movements can grasp and dislodge the tube. Preterm infants do not ordinarily require restraint, but if they do, a small blanket folded across the chest and secured beneath the shoulders is usually sufficient. Care must be taken so that breathing is not compromised.

Whenever possible, the infant should be held and provided a means of nonnutritive sucking during the procedure to associate the comfort of physical contact with the feeding. When this is not possible, gavage feeding is carried out with the infant or child on the back or toward the right side and the head and chest elevated. Feeding the child in a sitting position helps maintain the placement of the tube in the lowest position, thus increasing the likelihood of correct placement in the stomach (see Nursing Care Guidelines box).

Two standard methods of measuring tube length for insertion are (1) measuring from the nose to the bottom of the earlobe and then to the end of the xiphoid process or (2) measuring from the nose to the earlobe and then to a point midway between the xiphoid process and the umbilicus (Fig. 22-30, *A*). For very low–birth-weight infants, weight can be used to pre-

FIG. 22-30 ■ Gavage feeding. **A,** Measuring tube for orogastric feeding from tip of nose to earlobe and to midpoint between end of xiphoid process and umbilicus. **B,** Inserting tube.

| TABLE 22-7 |

Recommended Minimum Insertion Lengths for Orogastric Tubes in Very Low–Birth-Weight Infants

	DAILY WEIGHT (g)			
	<750	750-999	1000-1249	1250-1499
Insertion length (cm)	13	15	16	17

From Gallaher KJ, Cashwell S, Hall V, and others: Orogastric tube insertion length in very-low-birth-weight infants (<1500 grams), *J Perinatol* 13(2):128-131, 1993.

dict insertion length (Table 22-7). See Evidence-Based Practice box for placement verification techniques.

NURSINGALERT

Nurses need to take precautions when assessing tube placement. One study reported that out of 39 children, 43.5% had nasogastric tube placement errors as viewed by radiography (Ellett and Beckstrand, 1999).

GASTROSTOMY FEEDING

Feeding by way of a gastrostomy tube is a variation of tube feeding that is often used for children in whom passage of a tube through the mouth, pharynx, esophagus, and cardiac sphincter of the stomach is contraindicated or impossible. It

nursingcareguidelines

Nasogastric Tube Feedings in Children

Place child supine with head slightly hyperflexed or in a sniffing position (nose pointed toward ceiling).

Measure the tube for approximate length of insertion, and mark the point with a small piece of tape.

Insert a tube that has been lubricated with sterile water or water-soluble lubricant through either the mouth or one of the nares to the predetermined mark. Because most young infants are obligatory nose breathers, insertion through the mouth causes less distress and helps to stimulate sucking. In older infants and children the tube is passed through the nose and alternated between nostrils. An indwelling tube is almost always placed through the nose.

- When using the nose, slip the tube along the base of the nose and direct it straight back toward the occiput.
- When entering through the mouth, direct the tube toward the back of the throat (Fig. 22-30, B).
- If the child is able to swallow on command, synchronize passing the tube with swallowing.
- Confirm placement by x-ray examination, if available. Document pH and color of aspirate (see Evidence-Based Practice box, p. 748).

Stabilize the tube by holding or taping it to the cheek, not to the forehead, because of possible damage to the nostril. To maintain correct placement, measure and record the amount of tubing extending from the nose or mouth to the distal port when the tube is first positioned. Recheck this measurement before each feeding.

Warm the formula to room temperature. Do not microwave! Document pH and color of aspirate before each feeding to confirm tube placement. Pour formula into the barrel of the syringe attached to the feeding tube. To start the flow, give a gentle push with the plunger, but then remove the plunger and allow the fluid to flow into the stomach by gravity. The rate of flow should not exceed 5 ml every 5 to 10 minutes in preterm and very small infants and 10 ml/min in older infants and children to prevent nausea and regurgitation. The rate is determined by the diameter of the tubing and the height of the reservoir containing the feeding and is regulated by adjusting the height of the syringe. A usual feeding may take from 15 to 30 minutes to complete.

Flush the tube with sterile water (1 or 2 ml for small tubes to 5 to 15 ml or more for large ones), or see discussion of flushing for administering medication through nasogastric tubes in the Nursing Care Guidelines box (p. 730) to clear it of formula.

Cap or clamp indwelling tubes to prevent loss of feeding. If the tube is to be removed, first pinch it firmly to prevent escape of fluid as the tube is withdrawn. Withdraw the tube quickly.

Position the child with the head elevated about 30 degrees and on the right side or abdomen for at least 1 hour in the same manner as after any infant feeding to minimize the possibility of regurgitation and aspiration. If the child's condition permits, bubble the youngster after the feeding.

Record the feeding, including the type and amount of residual, the type and amount of formula, and how it was tolerated.

For most infant feedings, any amount of residual fluid aspirated from the stomach is refed to prevent electrolyte imbalance, and the amount is subtracted from the prescribed amount of feeding. For example, if the infant is to receive 30 ml and 10 ml is aspirated from the stomach before the feeding, the 10 ml of aspirated stomach contents is refed along with 20 ml of feeding. Another method can be used in children. If residual fluid is more than one fourth of the last feeding, return the aspirate and recheck in 30 to 60 minutes. When residual fluid is less than one fourth of the last feeding, give the scheduled feeding. If large amounts of aspirated fluid persist and the child is due for another feeding, notify the practitioner.

is also used to avoid the constant irritation of a gastric tube in children who require tube feeding over an extended period. Placement of a gastrostomy tube may be performed with the patient under general anesthesia or percutaneously using an endoscope with the patient sedated and under local anesthesia (percutaneous endoscopic gastrostomy [PEG]). The tube is inserted through the abdominal wall into the stomach about midway along the greater curvature and, when surgically placed, is secured by a purse-string suture. The stomach is anchored to the peritoneum at the operative site. The tube used can be a Foley, wing-tip, or mushroom catheter. Immediately after surgery the catheter is left open and attached to gravity drainage for 24 hours or more.

Postoperative care of the wound site is directed toward prevention of infection and irritation. The area is cleansed at least daily or as often as needed to keep the area free of drainage. After healing takes place, meticulous care is needed to keep the area surrounding the tube clean and dry to prevent excoriation and infection. Daily applications of antibiotic ointment or other preparations may be prescribed to aid in healing and prevention of irritation. Care is exercised to prevent excessive pull on the catheter that might cause widening of the opening and subsequent leakage of highly irritating gastric juices. The tube is securely taped to the abdomen, leaving a small loop of tubing at the exit site to prevent tension on the site.

Granulation tissue may grow around a gastrostomy site (Fig. 22-31). This moist, beefy red tissue is not a sign of infection. However, if it continues to grow, the excess moisture can irritate the surrounding skin.

For children receiving long-term gastrostomy feeding, a **skin-level device** (e.g., MIC-KEY, Bard Button) offers several advantages. The small, flexible silicone device protrudes slightly from the abdomen, is cosmetically pleasing in appearance, affords increased comfort and mobility to the child, is easy to care for, and is fully immersible in water. The one-way valve at the proximal end minimizes reflux and eliminates the need for clamping. However, the button requires a well-established gastrostomy site and is more expensive than the conventional tube. In addition, the valve may become clogged. When functioning, the valve prevents air from escaping; therefore the child may require frequent bubbling. With some devices, during feedings the child must remain fairly still because the tubing easily disconnects from the opening if the child moves. With other devices, extension tubing can be securely attached to the opening (Fig. 22-32). The feeding is instilled at the other end of the tubing in a manner similar to that for a regular gastrostomy. The extension tubing may also have a separate medication port. Both the feeding and the medication ports have plugs attached. Some skin-level devices require a special tube to decompress the stomach (to check residual or release air).

EVIDENCE-BASED PRACTICE

Assessing Correct Placement of Nasogastric or Orogastric Tubes in Children
Marilyn J. Hockenberry

ASK THE QUESTION   In children, how do we assess for correct placement of nasogastric or orogastric tubes?

SEARCH FOR EVIDENCE

Search Strategies   Search selection criteria included English-language publications within the past 10 years, research-based articles (level 3 or lower), children or adult populations, comparisons to gold standard (x-ray examination).

Databases Used   PubMed, Cochrane Collaboration, MD Consult, Joanna Briggs Institute, National Guideline Clearinghouse (AHRQ), TRIP Database Plus, PedsCCM, BestBETs

CRITICALLY ANALYZE THE EVIDENCE

Studies compared various methods used to evaluate placement of the tube with the gold standard, x-ray examination. Nine articles were found, five adult and four child sample populations.

- pH-assisted feeding tubes, child (Krafte-Jacobs, Persinger, Carver, and others, 1996)
- Bilirubin, adult and child (Westhus, 2004; Metheny, Stewart, Smith, and others, 1999; Metheny, Smith, and Stewart, 2000)
- Enzyme tests, child and adult (Westhus, 2004; Metheny, Stewart, Smith, and others, 1997)
- Bedside sonography for tube placement, adult (Hernandez-Socorro, Marin, Ruiz-Santana, and others, 1996)
- Aspiration of insufflated air for tube placement, adult (Neumann, Meyer, Dutton, and others, 1995; Harrison, Clay, Grant, and others, 1997)

Most reliable tests for determining tube placement in the nine published studies (other than the gold standard of x-ray examination) were the combination of:

- pH testing (Huffman, Jarczyk, O'Brien, and others, 2004; Metheny, Stewart, Smith, and others, 1999; Westhus, 2004; Gharpure, Meert, Sarnaik, and others, 2000)
- Visual inspection of aspirate
- Bilirubin and enzyme tests

Bilirubin and enzyme measures are not currently available at the bedside. Sensitivity and specificity of the bedside tests for children need further evaluation. Auscultation is an unreliable method to confirm tube placement because of the similarity of sounds produced by air in the bronchus, esophagus, or pleural space.

APPLY THE EVIDENCE: NURSING IMPLICATIONS

- Use x-ray to confirm initial placement. Document pH and color of aspirate with initial placement.
- A pH of 5 or less supports the conclusion that the tip of the tube is in a gastric location.
- A pH greater than 5 does not reliably predict the correct distal tip location. It may indicate respiratory or esophageal placement, or presence of medications to suppress acid secretion.
- If pH is greater than 5, use other measures to evaluate tube placement. If bilirubin and enzyme testing is not available, check color of aspirate. Gastric contents are clear, off-white, or tan; they may be brown tinged if blood is present. Respiratory secretions may look the same. Intestinal contents are often bile stained, light to dark yellow, or greenish brown. It may also be necessary to obtain an x-ray.

- A change in pH may indicate tube dislodgment. Check external markings and tube length to ensure tube has not moved. If uncertain about placement, obtain an x-ray.
- pH and color of aspirate can be checked before medication or feeding. For continuous feedings, it is recommended that tube placement be checked every 4 hours.
- A *Visual Bilirubin Scale*, effective in determining bilirubin content in feeding tube aspirates, has been published (Metheny, Smith, and Stewart, 2000). Evaluation of the accuracy of the scale is needed with children.
- Risk factors for improper tube placement are comatose or semicomatose state, swallowing problems, and recurrent retching or vomiting.
- Experience of the individual inserting the tube is always important.

References

Gharpure V, Meert KL, Sarnaik AP, and others: Indicators of postpyloric feeding tube placement in children, *Crit Care Med* 28(8):2962-2966, 2000.

Harrison AM, Clay B, Grant MJ, and others: Nonradiographic assessment of enteral feeding tube position, *Crit Care Med* 25(12):2055-2059, 1997.

Hernandez-Socorro CR, Marin J, Ruiz-Santana S, and others: Bedside sonographic-guided versus blind nasoenteric feeding tube placement in critically ill patients, *Crit Care Med* 24(10):1690-1694, 1996.

Huffman S, Jarczyk KS, O'Brien E, and others: Methods to confirm feeding tube placement: application of research in practice, *Pediatr Nurs* 30(1):10-13, 2004.

Krafte-Jacobs B, Persinger M, Carver J, and others: Rapid placement of transpyloric feeding tubes: a comparison of pH-assisted and standard insertion techniques in children, *Pediatrics* 98(2 Pt 1):242-248, 1996.

Metheny NA, Smith L, Stewart BJ: Development of a reliable and valid bedside test for bilirubin and its utility for improving prediction of feeding tube location, *Nurs Res* 49(6):302-309, 2000.

Metheny NA, Stewart BJ, Smith L, and others: pH and concentration of bilirubin in feeding tube aspirates as predictors of tube placement, *Nurs Res* 48(4):189-197, 1999.

Metheny NA, Stewart BJ, Smith L, and others: pH and concentrations of pepsin and trypsin in feeding tube aspirates as predictors of tube placement, *JPEN* 21:279-285, 1997.

Neumann MJ, Meyer CT, Dutton JL, and others: Hold that x-ray: aspirate pH and auscultation prove tube placement, *J Clin Gastroenterol* 20(4):293-295, 1995.

Westhus N: Methods to test feeding tube placement in children, *MCN Am J Maternal/Child Nurs* 29(5):282-291, 2004.

FIG. 22-31 ■ Appearance of healthy granulation tissue around stoma.

FIG. 22-32 ■ Child with skin-level gastrostomy device (MIC-KEY), which provides for secure attachment of extension tubing to gastrostomy opening.

Feeding of water, formula, or pureed foods is carried out in the same manner and rate as in gavage feeding. A mechanical pump may be used to regulate the volume and rate of feeding. After feedings, the infant or child is positioned on the right side or in the Fowler position, and the tube may be clamped or left open and suspended between feedings, depending on the child's condition. A clamped tube allows more mobility but is appropriate only if the child can tolerate intermittent feedings without vomiting or prolonged backup of feeding into the tube. Sometimes a Y tube is used to allow for simultaneous decompression during feeding. If a Foley catheter is used as the gastrostomy tube, very slight tension is applied. The tube is securely taped to maintain the balloon at the gastrostomy opening to prevent leakage of gastric contents and to prevent the tube's progression toward the pyloric sphincter, where it may occlude the stomach outlet. As a precaution, the length of the tube should be measured postoperatively and then remeasured each shift to be certain it has not slipped. A mark can be made above the skin level to further ensure its placement. When the gastrostomy tube is no longer needed, it is removed; the skin opening usually closes spontaneously by contracture.

NASODUODENAL AND NASOJEJUNAL TUBES

Children at high risk for regurgitation or aspiration such as those with gastroparesis, mechanical ventilation, or brain injuries may require placement of a postpyloric feeding tube. Insertion of a nasoduodenal or nasojejunal tube is done by a trained practitioner because of the risk of misplacement and potential for perforation in tubes requiring a stylet. Accurate placement is verified by radiography. Small-bore tubes may easily clog. Flush tube when feeding is interrupted, before and after medication administration, and routinely every 4 hours or as directed by institutional policy. Tube replacement should be considered monthly to ensure optimal tube patency. Continuous feedings are delivered by mechanical pump to regulate volume and rate. Bolus feeds are contraindicated. Tube displacement is suspected in the child showing signs of feeding intolerance such as vomiting. Stop feedings and notify the practitioner.

TOTAL PARENTERAL NUTRITION

TPN provides for the total nutritional needs of infants or children when feeding by the gastrointestinal tract is impossible, inadequate, or hazardous. Some common conditions include chronic intestinal obstruction, inadequate intestinal length, and prophylactically after surgery or during critical illness.

TPN therapy involves IV infusion of highly concentrated solutions of carbohydrates, lipids, amino acids, vitamins, minerals, water, trace elements and other additives in a single container (Teitelbaum, Guenter, Howell, and others, 2005). The highly concentrated solutions require infusion into a vessel with sufficient volume and turbulence to allow for rapid dilution. The wide-diameter vessels selected are the superior vena cava and innominate or intrathoracic subclavian veins approached by way of the external or internal jugular veins. The highly irritating nature of concentrated glucose precludes the use of the small peripheral veins in most instances. However, dilute glucose-protein hydrolysates that are appropriate for infusing into peripheral veins are being used with increasing frequency. When peripheral veins are used, intralipid becomes the major calorie source. For long-term alimentation, VADs are commonly used (see p. 725).

The major nursing responsibilities are the same as for any IV therapy: control of sepsis, monitoring of the infusion rate, and assessment of the patient's tolerance of the solution. The TPN solution must be prepared under sterile conditions. The infusion is maintained at a constant rate by an infusion pump. The TPN infusion rate should not be increased or decreased without the practitioner being informed, since alterations can cause hyperglycemia or hypoglycemia.

General assessments, such as vital signs, I&O measurements, and laboratory tests, facilitate early detection of infection or fluid and electrolyte imbalance. Additional amounts of potassium and sodium chloride are often required in hyperalimentation; therefore observation for signs of potassium or sodium deficit or excess is part of nursing care. This is rarely a problem except in children with reduced renal function or metabolic defects. Hyperglycemia may occur during the first day or two as the child adapts to the high-glucose load of the hyperalimentation solution. Although hyperglycemia occurs infrequently, insulin may be required to assist the body's adjustment. To prevent hypoglycemia at the time the hyperalimentation is disconnected, the rate of the infusion and the amount of insulin are decreased gradually.

In addition to children's physical needs, their developmental needs must also be considered during the often long-term use of TPN. Development should be regularly assessed to monitor the child's progress, and appropriate interventions should be instituted to encourage expected milestones. Delays in the areas of gross motor and language skills are found most often; therefore special attention should be directed to these areas.

FAMILY TEACHING AND HOME CARE

When alternative feedings are needed for an extended period, the family may need to learn how to feed the child with a nasogastric, gastrostomy, or TPN feeding regimen. The same principles discussed earlier in this chapter for compliance, especially in terms of education (p. 698), and in Chapter 21 for discharge planning and home care are applied. Because of the numerous skills the family must learn for home TPN, ample time must be allowed for the family to learn and perform the procedures under supervision before assuming full responsibility for the child's care.

The family may be referred to community agencies that provide support and practical assistance. The Oley Foundation* is a nonprofit research and education organization that assists persons receiving enteral nutrition and home TPN.

PROCEDURES RELATED TO ELIMINATION

ENEMA

The procedure for giving an enema to an infant or child does not differ essentially from that for an adult, except for the type and amount of fluid administered and the distance for inserting the tube into the rectum. Depending on the volume, a syringe with rubber tubing, an enema bottle, or an enema bag should be used (see Nursing Care Guidelines box).

An isotonic solution is used in children. Plain water is not used because, being hypotonic, it can cause rapid fluid shift and fluid overload. The Fleet enema (pediatric or adult sized) is not advised for children because of the harsh action of its ingredients (sodium biphosphate and sodium phosphate). Commercial enemas can be dangerous to patients with megacolon and to dehydrated or azotemic children. The osmotic effect of the Fleet enema may produce diarrhea, which can lead to metabolic acidosis. Other potential complications are extreme hyperphosphatemia, hypernatremia, and hypocalcemia, which may lead to neuromuscular irritability and coma (Walton, Thomas, Aly, and others, 2000).

> **NURSINGTIP**
> If prepared saline is not available, it can be made by adding 1 teaspoon of table salt to 500 ml (1 pint) of tap water.

Because infants and young children are unable to retain the solution after it is administered, the buttocks must be held together for a short time to retain the fluid. The enema is administered and expelled while the child is lying with the buttocks over the bedpan and with the head and back supported by pillows. Older children are usually able to hold the solution if they understand what to do and if they are not expected to hold it for too long. The nurse should have the bedpan handy or, for the ambulatory child, ensure that the bathroom is available before beginning the procedure. An enema is an intrusive procedure and thus threatening to the preschool child; there-

---

*214 Hun Memorial, MC-28, Albany Medical Center, Albany, NY 12208; (800) 776-OLEY; http://www.oley.org.

nursingcareguidelines

Administration of Enemas to Children

Age	Amount (ml)	Insertion Distance
Infant	120-240	2.5 cm (1 inch)
2-4 years	240-360	5 cm (2 inches)
4-10 years	360-480	7.5 cm (3 inches)
11 years	480-720	10 cm (4 inches)

fore a careful explanation is especially important to ease possible fear.

A preoperative bowel preparation solution given orally or through a nasogastric tube is increasingly being used instead of an enema. The polyethylene glycol–electrolyte lavage solution (GoLYTELY) mechanically flushes the bowel without significant absorption, thereby avoiding potential fluid and electrolyte imbalance. Another effective oral cathartic is magnesium citrate solution.

> **FYI**
> NuLYTELY, a modification of GoLYTELY, has been found to have the same therapeutic advantage as GoLYTELY and was developed to improve on the taste (Diab and Marshall, 1996).

OSTOMIES

Children may require stomas for various health problems. The most frequent causes in the infant are necrotizing enterocolitis and imperforate anus (less often, Hirschsprung disease). In the older child the most frequent causes are inflammatory bowel disease, especially Crohn disease (regional enteritis), and ureterostomies for distal ureter or bladder defects.

Care and management of ostomies in the older child differ little from the care of ostomies in the adult patient. The major emphasis in pediatric care is preparing the child for the procedure and teaching care of the ostomy to the child and family. The basic principles of preparation are the same as for any procedure (see p. 689). Simple, straightforward language is most effective, together with the use of illustrations and a replica model (e.g., drawing a picture of a child with a stoma on the abdomen and explaining it as "another opening where bowel movements [or any other term the child uses] will come out"). At another time the nurse can draw a pouch over the opening to demonstrate how the contents are collected. Using a doll to demonstrate the process is an excellent teaching strategy, and special books are available.*

Ostomy equipment consists of a one- or two-piece system with a hypoallergenic skin barrier to maintain peristomal skin integrity. The pouch should be large enough to contain a moderate amount of stool and flatus but not so large as to overwhelm the infant or child. A backing helps minimize the

---

*Children with ileostomies are fitted immediately after surgery with an appliance to protect the skin from the proteolytic enzymes in the liquid stool. Infants may not be fitted with a pouch in the immediate postoperative period. When stomal drainage is minimal, a gauze dressing will suffice. Parents are usually given a choice of caring for the colostomy with or without an appliance. Pediatric appliances are available in a variety of sizes to ensure an adequate fit. Parents may find the following pamphlets helpful: *A Parent's Guide to Necrotizing Enterocolitis* or *Parent's Guide to Ostomy Care for Children*, available from ConvaTec.

risk of skin breakdown from moisture trapped between the skin and pouch. Small clips or rubber bands should be avoided to prevent choking in the young child. Granulation tissue may grow around an ostomy site (see Fig. 22-31). This moist, beefy red tissue is not a sign of infection. However, if it continues to grow, the excess moisture can cause irritation of the surrounding skin.

Protection of the peristomal skin is a major aspect of stoma care. Well-fitting appliances are important to prevent leakage of contents. Before the appliance is applied, the skin is prepared with a skin sealant that is allowed to dry. Then stoma paste is applied around the base of the stoma or the back of the wafer. The sealant and paste work together to prevent peristomal breakdown.

In infants with a colostomy left unpouched, skin care is similar to that of any diapered infant. However, the peristomal skin is protected with a wafer barrier, such as a hydrocolloid dressing (e.g., DuoDERM) or a barrier substance (e.g., zinc oxide ointment [Desitin], or a mixture of the zinc oxide ointment and stoma [Stomahesive] powder). A gauze dressing may be applied over the stoma and wafer to absorb stomal drainage. If the skin becomes inflamed, denuded, or infected, the care is similar to the interventions used for diaper dermatitis (see Chapter 30). A product that helps protect healthy skin, heal excoriated skin, and minimize pain associated with skin breakdown is Proshield Plus. The skin protectant adheres to denuded weeping skin. Proshield Plus can be applied over topical antifungal and antibacterial agents if infection is present. "No-sting" barrier film is a skin sealant that has no alcohol base and can be used on open skin without stinging.

With young children, protection of the pouch from being pulled off is also an important consideration. One-piece outfits keep exploring hands from reaching the pouch, and the loose waist prevents any pressure on the appliance. Keeping the child occupied with toys during the pouch change is also helpful. As children mature, their participation in ostomy care is encouraged. Even preschoolers can assist by holding supplies, pulling paper backings from the appliance, and helping clean the stoma area. Toilet training for bladder control needs to begin at the appropriate time as for any other child.

Older children and adolescents should eventually have total responsibility for ostomy care just as they would for usual bowel function. During adolescence, concerns for body image and the ostomy's impact on intimacy and sexuality emerge. The nurse should stress to teenagers that the presence of a stoma need not interfere with their activities. These youngsters can choose which ostomy equipment is best suited to their needs. Attractively designed and decorated pouch covers are well liked by teenagers.

An enterostomal therapy nurse specialist is an important member of the health care team and will have additional suggestions and skin care information and ostomy pouching options. Further information may be obtained by contacting the Wound, Ostomy and Continence Nurses Society.*

FAMILY TEACHING AND HOME CARE

Because these children are almost always discharged with a functioning colostomy, preparation of the family should begin as early as possible in the hospital. The family is instructed in the application of the device (if used), care of the skin, and

---

*(888) 224-9626; http://www.wocn.org.

appropriate action in case skin problems develop. Early evidence of skin breakdown or stomal complications, such as ribbonlike stools, excessive diarrhea, bleeding, prolapse, or failure to pass flatus or stool, is brought to the attention of the physician, the nurse, or the stoma specialist. The same principles are applied as discussed earlier in this chapter for compliance, especially in terms of education (p. 699), and in Chapter 21 for discharge planning and home care.

KEY POINTS

- Informed consent is valid when the person is capable of giving consent (is over the age of majority and is competent), is supplied with information needed to make an intelligent decision, and acts voluntarily when exercising freedom of choice.
- Informed consent is needed for major surgery, minor surgery, and diagnostic tests and medical treatments with an element of risk.
- The major principles in psychologic preparation of the child for procedures are to establish trust, provide support, and give an explanation in easy-to-understand terms.
- Preparation for procedures should be based on developmental characteristics of the child and family, emphasizing the importance of the parents' role.
- Most parents and children want to be together during stressful procedures and should be offered this opportunity, with guidance on how the parent can comfort the child.
- In the performance of a procedure the nurse should expect success, involve the child when possible in the procedure, provide distraction, and allow for expression of feelings.
- Proper positioning of infants and small children for procedures is essential to minimize movement and discomfort.
- In giving postprocedural support, encourage children to express feelings and praise for completion of the procedure.
- Stressful times before and after surgery that produce anxiety in children are admission, blood tests, injection of preoperative medication (if used), transportation to the operating room, and return from the PACU.
- Assessment of compliance entails measuring factors that affect compliance through clinical judgment, self-reporting, direct observation, monitoring of appointments and therapeutic response, pill counts, and chemical assays.
- Compliance strategies may be classified as organizational, educational, and behavioral.
- Knowledge of the ill child's eating habits and favorite foods can help in maintaining adequate nutrition.
- Skin care is an essential to prevent skin breakdown.
- Control of fever may be accomplished by administration of antipyretics; hyperthermia is controlled by environmental means (minimum clothing, increased air circulation, hypothermia mattress, or cool compresses).
- Infection control is based on two systems. Standard precautions provide protection when the infected person is undiagnosed. Transmission-based precautions add extra interventions for patients diagnosed with or suspected of having an infection.
- Ensuring safety in the hospital setting is a major concern and can be achieved through environmental measures, limit setting, infection control, and safe transportation.
- Restraints are used cautiously and require a medical order. Therapeutic holding can avoid the use of restraints.

- Factors that affect drug dosage determination are growth and maturation, difficulty in evaluating drug response, and BSA.
- Family teaching regarding medication administration includes telling parents why the child is receiving the drug; its possible effects; and the amount, frequency, and length of time the drug is to be administered.
- The preferred sites for intramuscular injection in children are the vastus lateralis and ventrogluteal areas.
- Intermittent venous access is accomplished by a peripheral intermittent infusion device, a peripherally inserted central catheter, a central venous catheter, or an implanted port.
- Several safety catheters and needleless device systems are available to reduce the risk of needlestick injuries in patients and caregivers.

- Nursing assessment of fluid and electrolyte disturbances entails observation of general appearance, vital signs, and measurement of I&O.
- Oxygen can be administered by hood, mask, nasal cannula, incubator, or oxygen tent.
- Tracheostomy suctioning involves premeasured insertion of the catheter, application of suction for 5 seconds when withdrawing the catheter, and supplemental oxygen before and after suctioning.
- Alternative forms of feeding include gavage feeding, gastrostomy feeding, and TPN.
- In the care of children with ostomies, nurses play an important role in family support and instruction in care of the stoma site.

REFERENCES

Algren C, Algren J: Pediatric sedation essentials for the preoperative nurse, *Nurs Clin North Am* 32(1):17-30, 1997.

Algren C, Ireland D, Stewart E: Perioperative and perianesthesia care of the child. In Albers AC, Schwartz P, editors: *Comprehensive care of the pediatric patient: prehospital through rehabilitation*, Park Ridge, Ill, 1998, Emergency Nurses Association.

American Academy of Pediatrics: Consent for emergency medical services for children and adolescents, *Pediatrics* 111(3):703-705, 2003.

American Academy of Pediatrics: Informed consent, parental permission, and assent in pediatric practice, *Pediatrics* 95(2):314-317, 1995.

Anderson SL, Schaechter J, Brosco JP: Adolescent patients and their confidentiality: staying within legal bounds, *Contemp Pediatr* 22(7):54, 2005.

Axelrod P: External cooling in the management of fever, *Clin Infect Dis* 31(Suppl 5):S224-S229, 2000.

Berg AT, Shinnar S, Levy SR, and others: Childhood-onset epilepsy with and without preceding febrile seizures, *Neurology* 53(8):1742-1748, 1999.

Berger JE, AAP Committee on Medical Liability: Consent by proxy for nonurgent pediatric care, *Pediatrics* 112(5):1186-1195, 2003.

Blass EM, Watt L: Suckling- and sucrose-induced analgesia in human newborns, *Pain* 83(3):611-623, 1999.

Broome M: Consent (assent) for research with pediatric patients, *Semin Oncol Nurs* 15(2):96-103, 1999.

Broome M, Rehwaldt M, Fogg L: Relationship between cognitive behavioral techniques, temperament, observed distress, and pain reports in children and adolescents during lumbar puncture, *J Pediatr Nurs* 13(1):48-54, 1998.

Bryant RA, Doughty D, editors: *Acute and chronic wounds: nursing management*, ed 2, St Louis, 2000, Mosby.

Burke N: Alternative methods for newborn urine sample collection, *Pediatr Nurs* 21(6):546-549, 1995.

Calianno C: Patient hygiene, part II, Skin care: keeping the outside healthy, *Nursing* 29(12 Suppl):1-11, 1999.

Carroll P: Closing in on safer suctioning, *RN* 61(5):22-27, 1998.

Catudal R: Pediatric IV therapy: actual practice, *J Vasc Access Devices* 4(2):27-29, 1999.

Clinical and Laboratory Standards Institute: *Blood collection via capillary puncture in infants*, retrieved March 31, 2006, from http://www.phlebotomypages.com/phleb_infants.htm.

Cohen HA, Woloch B, Linder N, and others: Urine samples from disposable diapers: an accurate method for urine cultures, *J Fam Pract* 44(3):290-292, 1997.

Cook IF, Murtagh J: Ventroluteal area: a suitable site for intramuscular vaccination of infants and toddlers, *Vaccine* 24(13):2403-2408, 2006.

Cook IF, Murtagh J: Needle length required for intramuscular vaccination of infants and toddlers. An ultrasonographic study, *Aust Fam Physician* 31(3):295-297, 2002.

Curley MAQ, Moloney-Harmon PA: *Critical care nursing of infants and children*, ed 2, Philadelphia, 2001, Saunders.

Diab FH, Marshall JB: The palatability of five colonic lavage solutions, *Aliment Pharmacol Ther* 20(5):815-819, 1996.

Dubick MA, Holcomb JB: A review of intraosseous vascular access: current status and military application, *Mil Med* 165(7):552-559, 2000.

Eaton L: Hand washing is more important than cleaner wards in controlling MRSA, *BMJ* 330(7497):922, 2005.

Eckler J: Combating infection, *Nursing* 27(10):20, 1997.

Ellett ML, Beckstrand J: Examination of gavage tube placement in children, *J Soc Pediatr Nurs* 4(2):51-60, 1999.

Essink-Tebbes CM, Wuis EW, Liem KD, and others: Safety of lidocaine-prilocaine cream application four times a day in premature neonates: a pilot study, *Eur J Pediatr* 158(5):421-423, 1999.

Fauroux B, Boule M, Lofaso F, and others: Chest physiotherapy in cystic fibrosis: improved tolerance with nasal pressure support ventilation, *Pediatrics* 103(3):E32, 1999.

Fennell ME: Parents in the OR? You bet! *RN* 62(12):38-40, 1999.

Fisher AA, Deffenbaugh C, Poole RL, and others: The use of alteplase for restoring patency to occluded central venous access devices in infants and children, *J Infus Nurs* 27(3):171-174, 2004.

Gamulka B, Mendoza C, Connolly B: Evaluation of a unique, nurse-inserted, peripherally inserted central catheter program, *Pediatrics* 6(115):1602-1606, 2005.

Gray L, Watt L, Blass EM: Skin-to-skin contact is analgesic in healthy newborns, *Pediatrics* 105(1):110-111, 2000, retrieved July 7, 2007, from http://www.pediatrics.org/cgi/content/full/105/1/E14.

Gray M: Atraumatic urethral catheterization of children, *Pediatr Nurs* 22(4):306-310, 1996.

Hall PA, Payne JF, Stack CG, and others: Parents in the recovery room: survey of parental and staff attitudes, *BMJ* 310(6973):163-164, 1995.

Harris J, Maguire D: Developing a protocol to prevent and treat pediatric central venous catheter occlusions, *J Intraven Nurs* 22(4):194-198, 1999.

Institute for Safe Medication Practices: Problems persist with life-threatening tubing misconnections, *ISMP Medication Safety Alert* June 17, 2004.

Infusion Nurses Society: *Policies and procedures for infusion nursing*, Norwood, Mass, 2000a, The Society.

Infusion Nurses Society: Revised infusion nursing standards of practice, *J Intraven Nurs* 23(6 Suppl): S17, S39, S41, S45, S49-50, S60, 2000b.

Ipp MM, Gold R, Goldback M, and others: Adverse reactions to diphtheria, tetanus, pertussis–polio vaccination at 18 months of age: effect of injection site and needle length, *Pediatrics* 83(5):679-682, 1989.

Joint Commission on Accreditation of Healthcare Organizations: Care of the patient: restraint and seclusion standards, *Comprehensive accreditation manual for hospitals*, Naperville, Ill, 2001, Joint Commission Resources, TX.7.1-TX.7.5.5.

Kain ZN, Caldwell-Andrews AA, Krivutza DM, and others: Trends in the practice of parental presence during induction of anesthesia and the use of preoperative sedative premedication in the United States, 1995-2002: results of a follow-up national survey, *Anesth Analg* 98(5):1252-1259, 2004.

Kain Z, Caldwell-Andrews A, Wang S: Psychological preparation of the parent and pediatric surgical patient, *Anesthesia Clin North Am* 20(1):29-44, 2002.

Katsma D, Smith G: Analysis of needle path during intramuscular injection, *Nurs Res* 46(5):288-292, 1997.

Kellam B, Sacks LM, Wailer JL, and others: Tenderfoot Preemie vs a manual lancet: a clinical evaluation, *Neonatal Netw* 20(7):31-36, 2001.

Kennedy D: Medication "safety checks" in pediatric acute care, *J Intraven Nurs* 19(6):295-302, 1996.

Klein EJ, Diekema DS, Paris CA, and others: A randomized, clinical trial of oral midazolam plus placebo versus oral midazolam plus oral transmucosal fentanyl for sedation during laceration repair, *Pediatrics* 109(5):894-897, 2002.

Kraus D, Stohlmeyer LA, Hannon DR, and others: Effectiveness and infant acceptance of the Rx Medibottle versus the oral syringe, *Pharmacotherapy* 21(4):416-423, 2001.

KyngAs H, Kroll T, Duffy M: Compliance in adolescents with chronic diseases: a review, *J Adolesc Health* 26:379-388, 2000.

Landsman IS, Cook DR: Pediatric anesthesia. In O'Neill J, Rowe MI, Grosfeld JL, and others, editors: *Pediatric surgery*, St Louis, 1998, Mosby.

LaRosa-Nash PA, Murphy JM: An approach to pediatric perioperative care: parent-present induction, *Nurs Clin North Am* 32(1):183-199, 1997.

Larsson BA, Tannfeldt G, Lagercrantz H, and others: Alleviation of the pain of venipuncture in neonates, *Acta Paediatr* 87(7):774-779, 1998.

Lee WE, Vallino LM: Intravenous insertion site protection: moisture accumulation in intravenous site protectors, *J Intraven Nurs* 29(4):194-197, 1996.

Liebman M, Barnsteiner J: Fever education: does it reduce parent fever anxiety? *Pediatr Emerg Care* 17(1):47-51, 2001.

Maki DG: Infections caused by intravascular devices used for infusion therapy: pathogenesis, prevention, and management. In Bisno AL, Waldvogel FA, editors: *Infections associated with indwelling medical devices*, ed 2, Washington, DC, 1994, American Society for Microbiology.

Manworren R, Fledderman M: Preparation of the child and family for surgery. In Wise BV, McKenna C, Garvin G, and others, editors: *Nursing care of the general pediatric surgical patient*, Gaithersburg, Md, 2000, Aspen.

Maxwell LG, Yaster M: Perioperative management issues in pediatric patients, *Anesthesiol Clin North Am* 18(3):601-632, 2000.

Meehan RM: Heelsticks in neonates for capillary blood sampling, *Neonatal Netw* 17(1):17-24, 1998.

Montgomery LA, Hanrahan K, Korrman K, and others: Guidelines for IV infiltrations in pediatric patients, *Pediatr Nurs* 25(2):167-180, 1999.

Moureau N: Practical access, a back-to-basics review of intravenous therapy, *J Vasc Access Devices* 4(2 Suppl):1-4, 1999.

Munro H, D'Errico FC: Parental involvement in perioperative anesthetic management, *J Perianesth Nurs* 15(6):397-400, 2000.

Nelson D: Procedural sedation in the emergency department. In Krauss B, Brustowicz RM, editors: *Pediatric procedural sedation and analgesia*, Philadelphia, 1999, Lippincott Williams & Wilkins.

Oncology Nursing Society: *Cancer chemotherapy guidelines and recommendations for practice*, ed 2, Pittsburgh, 1998, Oncology Nursing Press.

Pettit J, Hughes K: Neonatal intravenous therapy practices, *J Vasc Access Devices* 4:7-16, 1999.

Polillio AM, Killy J: Does a needleless injection system reduce anxiety in children receiving intramuscular injections? *Pediatr Nurs* 23(1):46-49, 1997.

Purssell E: The use of antipyretic medications in the prevention of febrile convulsions in children, *J Pediatr Nurs* 9(4):473-480, 2000.

Quality, equipment hold keys to infection control, *ED Manage* 18(2):19-21, 2006.

Quigley SM, Curley MAQ: Skin integrity in the pediatric population: preventing and managing pressure ulcers, *J Soc Pediatr Nurses* 1(1):7, 1996.

Ratliff CR, Rodheaver GT: Pressure ulcer assessment and management, *Lippincott's Primary Care Pract* 3:242-258, 1999.

Redmond MC: Malignant hyperthermia: perianesthesia recognition, treatment, and care, *J Perianesth Nurs* 16(4):259-270, 2001.

Romino SL, Keatley VM, Secrest J, and others: Parental presence during anesthesia induction in children, *AORN J* 81(4):780-792, 2005.

Rote N, Huether S, McCance K: Hypersensitivities, infection, and immunodeficiencies. In Huether S, McCance K, editors: *Understanding pathophysiology*, ed 2, St Louis, 2000, Mosby.

Selekman J, Snyder B: Institutional policies on the use of physical restraints on children, *Pediatr Nurs* 23(5):531-537, 1997.

Sharber J: The efficacy of tepid sponge bathing to reduce fever in young children, *Am J Emerg Med* 15(2):188-192, 1997.

Shen V, Li X, Murdock M, and others: Recombinant tissue plasminogen activator (alteplase) for restoration of function to occluded central venous catheters in pediatric patients, *J Pediatr Hematol Oncol* 25(1):38-45, 2003.

Shepherd AJ, Glenesk A, Niven CA, and others: A Scottish study of heel-prick blood sampling in newborn babies, *Midwifery* 22(2):158-168, 2006.

Shinnar S, Pellock JM, Berg AT, and others: Short-term outcomes of children with febrile status epilepticus, *Epilepsia* 42(1):47-53, 2001.

Singer AJ, Konia N: Comparison of topical anesthetics and vasoconstrictors vs lubricants prior to nasogastric intubation: a randomized, controlled trial, *Acad Emerg Med* 6(3):184-190, 1999.

Teitelbaum D, Guenter P, Howell WH, and others: Definition of terms, style, and conventions used in A.S.P.E.N. guidelines and standards, *Nutr Clin Pract* 20(2):281-285, 2005.

Tillett J: Adolescents and informed consent: ethical and legal issues, *J Perinatal Neonatal Nurs* 19(2):112-121, 2005.

Van Cleve L, Johnson L, Pothier P: Pain responses of hospitalized infants and children to venipuncture and intravenous cannulation, *J Pediatr Nurs* 11:169-174, 1996.

Vertanen H, Fellman V, Brommels M, and others: An automatic incision device for obtaining blood samples from the heels of the preterm infants causes less damage than a conventional manual lancet, *Arch Dis Child Fetal Neonatal Ed* 84:F53-F55, 200l.

Wald ER: To bag or not to bag, *J Pediatrics* 174(4):418-419, 2005.

Walton DM, Thomas DC, Aly HZ, and others: Morbid hypocalcemia associated with phosphate enema in a six-week-old infant, *Pediatrics* 106(3):e37, 2000.

23

The Child with Respiratory Dysfunction

DAVID WILSON

CHAPTER OUTLINE

RESPIRATORY INFECTION, 755
Nursing Care Plan: The Child with Acute
   Respiratory Tract Infection, 759
**UPPER RESPIRATORY TRACT
INFECTIONS, 759**
Nasopharyngitis, 759
Pharyngitis, 762
Tonsillitis, 763
Influenza, 764
Otitis Media, 765
Infectious Mononucleosis, 768
CROUP SYNDROMES, 769
Acute Epiglottitis, 769
Acute Laryngitis, 770
Acute Laryngotracheobronchitis, 770
Acute Spasmodic Laryngitis, 771
Bacterial Tracheitis, 772
**INFECTIONS OF THE LOWER
AIRWAYS, 772**
Bronchitis, 773

Respiratory Syncytial Virus and
   Bronchiolitis, 773
Pneumonias, 774
   Viral Pneumonia, 775
   Primary Atypical Pneumonia, 775
   Severe Acute Respiratory Syndrome, 775
   Avian Influenza Virus, 775
   Bacterial Pneumonia, 776
**OTHER INFECTIONS OF THE
RESPIRATORY TRACT, 777**
Pertussis (Whooping Cough), 777
Tuberculosis, 777
**PULMONARY DYSFUNCTION CAUSED
BY NONINFECTIOUS IRRITANTS, 780**
Foreign Body Aspiration, 780
Aspiration Pneumonia, 781
Acute Respiratory Distress Syndrome/
   Acute Lung Injury, 781

Smoke Inhalation Injury, 782
Environmental Tobacco Smoke
   Exposure, 783
**LONG-TERM RESPIRATORY
DYSFUNCTION, 783**
Asthma, 783
Nursing Care Plan: The Child with
   Asthma, 792
Cystic Fibrosis, 795
Obstructive Sleep-Disordered
   Breathing, 803
RESPIRATORY EMERGENCY, 803
Respiratory Failure, 803
Cardiopulmonary Resuscitation, 804
   Resuscitation Procedure, 805
Airway Obstruction, 809
   Infants, 809
   Children, 809

LEARNING OBJECTIVES

**On completion of this chapter the
reader will be able to:**
- Identify the factors leading to respiratory
  tract infection in the infant or young child.
- Contrast the effects of various respiratory
  infections observed in infants and
  children.
- Describe the postoperative nursing care of
  the child with a tonsillectomy.
- Outline a nursing care plan for a child
  with croup.

- Describe priorities of nursing care for the
  child with acute otitis media.
- Identify priorities of nursing care for the
  infant with respiratory syncytial virus
  bronchiolitis.
- Describe the various therapeutic measures
  to relieve the symptoms of asthma.
- Outline a plan for teaching home care
  management of the child with asthma.

- Describe the physiologic effects of cystic
  fibrosis on the gastrointestinal and
  pulmonary systems.
- Outline a care plan for the child with
  cystic fibrosis.
- List the major signs of respiratory distress
  in infants and children.
- Describe emergent procedures for the
  relief of foreign body obstruction in an
  infant or child.

RELATED TOPICS and ADDITIONAL RESOURCES

 IN TEXT

Administration of Medication, *Ch. 22*
Apnea and Apparent Life-Threatening Event,
    Ch. 11
Compliance, *Ch. 22*
Controlling Elevated Temperatures, *Ch. 22*
Family-Centered Care of the Child During
    Illness and Hospitalization, *Ch. 21*
Feeding the Sick Child, *Ch. 22*
Hearing Impairment, *Ch. 19*
Immunizations, *Ch. 10*
Impact of Chronic Illness or Disability on the
    Child, *Ch. 18*
Infection Control, *Ch. 22*
Pain Assessment; Pain Management, *Ch. 7*
Physical Examination: Ears, Nose, Mouth
    and Throat, Chest, Lungs, *Ch. 6*
Procedures for Maintaining Respiratory
    Function, *Ch. 22*
Respiratory Complications, *Ch. 9*

Respiratory Secretion and Throat Specimens,
    Ch. 22
Surgical Procedures, *Ch. 22*
Tobacco, *Ch. 17*

 COMPANION CD

Anatomy Reviews—Location of Retractions;
    Location of Tonsillar Masses
Animations—Asthma; Bag Ventilation;
    Bronchi and Bronchioles; Intubation;
    Intubation in Infant; Intubation, Incorrect
    Placement; Lung Sounds; Respiratory
    Failure, Infant
Case Studies—Acute Epiglottitis; Asthma;
    Bronchiolitis; Cystic Fibrosis (2);
    Mononucleosis; Tonsillitis
Critical Thinking Exercises—Cystic Fibrosis
    Inheritance Risks; Ingestion of a Foreign
    Body
NCLEX Review Questions

 evolve
evolve.elsevier.com/Wong/essentials/

Critical Thinking Case Study—Asthma
NCLEX Review Questions
Nursing Care Plans—The Child with Acute
    Respiratory Infection; The Child with
    Asthma; The Child with Respiratory
    Failure; The Infant with Bronchiolitis and
    Respiratory Syncytial Virus (RSV) Infection
WebLinks

**WONG'S CLINICAL MANUAL
OF PEDIATRIC NURSING, 7th Ed**

Nursing Care Plans—The Child with Cystic
    Fibrosis, *p. 420;* The Child with
    Tonsillectomy or Myringotomy, *p. 438*
Patient and Family Education—Giving Nose
    Drops, *p. 541;* Measuring Your Child's
    Temperature, *p. 508;* Giving Medications
    to Children, *p. 522;* Child Cardiopulmonary
    Resuscitation for the Layperson, *p. 578*

RESPIRATORY INFECTION

Infections of the respiratory tract are described according to the anatomic area of involvement. The **upper respiratory tract,** or **upper airway,** consists of the oronasopharynx, the pharynx, the larynx, and the upper part of the trachea. The **lower respiratory tract** consists of the lower trachea, mainstem bronchi, segmental bronchi, subsegmental bronchioles, terminal bronchioles, and alveoli. In this discussion, the trachea is considered with lower tract disorders, and infections of the epiglottis and larynx are categorized as croup syndromes. However, respiratory infections seldom fall into discrete anatomic areas. Infections often spread from one structure to another because of the contiguous nature of the mucous membrane lining the entire tract. Consequently, respiratory tract infections involve several areas rather than a single structure, although the effect on one area may predominate in any given illness.

Etiology and Characteristics

Respiratory tract infections account for the majority of acute illnesses in children. The etiology and course of these infections are influenced by the age of the child, the season, living conditions, and preexisting medical problems.

Infectious Agents. The respiratory tract is subject to a wide variety of infective organisms. Most infections are caused by viruses, particularly respiratory syncytial virus (RSV), nonpolio enteroviruses (coxsackieviruses A and B), adenoviruses, parainfluenza viruses, and human metapneumoviruses. Other agents involved in primary or secondary invasion include group A β-hemolytic streptococci (GABHS), staphylococci, *Haemophilus influenzae, Chlamydia trachomatis, Mycoplasma* organisms, and pneumococci.

Age. Healthy full-term infants under age 3 months are presumed to have a lower infection rate than older infants because of the protective function of maternal antibodies; however, infants may be susceptible to specific respiratory

tract infections, namely pertussis, during this period. The infection rate increases from 3 to 6 months of age, the time between the disappearance of maternal antibodies and the infant's own antibody production. The viral infection rate remains high during the toddler and preschool years. By 5 years of age, viral respiratory tract infections are less frequent, but the incidence of *Mycoplasma pneumoniae* and GABHS infections increases. The amount of lymphoid tissue increases throughout middle childhood, and repeated exposure to organisms confers increasing immunity as children grow older.

Some viral agents produce a mild illness in older children but severe lower respiratory tract illness or croup in infants. For example, pertussis causes a relatively harmless tracheobronchitis in childhood but is a serious disease in infancy.

Size. Anatomic differences influence the response to respiratory tract infections. The diameter of the airways is smaller in young children and subject to considerable narrowing from edematous mucous membranes and increased production of secretions. The distance between structures within the respiratory tract is also shorter in the young child, and organisms may move rapidly down the respiratory tract, causing more extensive involvement. The relatively short and open eustachian tube in infants and young children allows pathogens easy access to the middle ear.

Resistance. The ability to resist pathogens depends on several factors. Deficiencies of the immune system place the child at risk for infection. Other conditions that decrease resistance are malnutrition, anemia, fatigue, and chilling of the body. Conditions that weaken defenses of the respiratory tract and predispose children to infection also include allergies (e.g., allergic rhinitis), preterm birth, bronchopulmonary dysplasia (BPD), asthma, history of RSV infection, cardiac anomalies that cause pulmonary congestion, and cystic fibrosis (CF). Daycare attendance, especially if the caregivers smoke, increases the likelihood of infection.

Seasonal Variations. The most common respiratory pathogens appear in epidemics during the winter and spring months. Mycoplasmal infections occur more often in autumn and early winter. Infection-related asthma (e.g., bronchitis) occurs more frequently during cold weather, whereas winter and early spring are typically the "RSV season."

Clinical Manifestations

Infants and young children, especially those between 6 months and 3 years of age, react more severely to acute respiratory tract infection than older children. Young children display a number of generalized signs and symptoms, as well as local manifestations (Box 23-1).

Nursing Care Management

Assessment of the respiratory system follows the guidelines described in Chapter 6 (for assessment of the ears, nose, mouth and throat, chest, and lungs). Special attention should

also be given to the components and observations listed in Box 23-2. The nursing process in the care of the child with acute respiratory tract infection is outlined in the Nursing Process box.

Ease Respiratory Efforts. Many acute respiratory tract infections are mild and cause few symptoms. Although children may feel uncomfortable and have a "stuffy" nose and some mucosal swelling, respiratory distress occurs infrequently. Interventions delivered at home are usually sufficient to relieve minor discomfort and ease respiratory efforts. However, in some cases the infant or child may require close observation by health professionals for adequate oxygenation and fluid and electrolyte status.

Warm or cool mist is a common therapeutic measure for symptomatic relief of respiratory discomfort. The moisture soothes inflamed membranes and is beneficial when there is hoarseness or laryngeal involvement. Mist tents are sometimes used in the hospital for humidifying the air and relieving dis-

---

Signs and Symptoms Associated with Respiratory Tract Infections in Infants and Small Children

FEVER
May be absent in newborn infants
Greatest at ages 6 months to 3 years
May reach 39.5° to 40.5° C (103° to 105° F) even with mild infections
Often appears as first sign of infection
May lead to listlessness and irritability, with altered activity pattern (usually decreased)
Tendency to develop high temperatures with infection in certain families
May precipitate febrile seizure (see Chapter 28)

POOR FEEDING AND ANOREXIA
Common in infants during breastfeeding or bottle-feeding
Common with most childhood illnesses
Frequently the initial evidence of illness
Persists to a greater or lesser degree throughout febrile stage of illness; often extends into convalescence

VOMITING
Common in small children with illness
Clue to onset of infection
May precede other signs by several hours
Usually short lived but may persist during the illness

DIARRHEA
Usually mild, transient diarrhea but may become severe
Often accompanies viral respiratory infections
Frequent cause of dehydration

ABDOMINAL PAIN
Common complaint
Sometimes indistinguishable from pain of appendicitis
May be caused by mesenteric lymphadenitis
May be linked to muscle spasms from vomiting, especially in nervous, tense child

NASAL BLOCKAGE
Small nasal passages of infants easily blocked by mucosal swelling and exudation
Can interfere with respiration and feeding in infants
May contribute to the development of otitis media and sinusitis

NASAL DISCHARGE
Frequent occurrence
May be thin and watery (rhinorrhea) or thick and purulent
Depends on the type or stage of infection
Associated with itching
May irritate upper lip and skin surrounding the nose

COUGH
Common feature
May be evident only during acute phase
May persist several months after a disease

RESPIRATORY SOUNDS
Sounds associated with respiratory disease:
  ■ Cough
  ■ Hoarseness
  ■ Grunting
  ■ Stridor
  ■ Wheezing
Auscultation:
  ■ Wheezing
  ■ Crackles
  ■ Absence of breath sounds (movement of air)

SORE THROAT
Frequent complaint of older children
Young children (unable to describe symptoms) may not complain even when highly inflamed
Often accompanied by refusal to take oral fluids or solids

MENINGISMUS
Meningeal signs without infection of the meninges
Occurs with abrupt onset of fever
Accompanied by:
  ■ Headache
  ■ Pain and stiffness in the back and neck
Subsides as body temperature decreases

BOX 23-2

Components for Assessing Respiratory Function

RESPIRATIONS

The pattern of respirations is observed for rate, depth, ease, and rhythm of breathing:

Rate—Rapid **(tachypnea),** normal, or slow for the particular child

Depth—Normal depth, too shallow **(hypopnea),** too deep **(hyperpnea);** usually estimated from the amplitude of thoracic and abdominal excursion

Ease—Effortless; labored **(dyspnea); orthopnea** (difficult breathing except in upright position); associated with intercostal or substernal retractions (inspiratory "sinking in" of soft tissues in relation to the cartilaginous and bony thorax); **pulsus paradoxus** (blood pressure falling with inspiration and rising with expiration); nasal flaring; head bobbing (head of sleeping child with suboccipital area supported on caregiver's forearm bobbing forward in synchrony with each inspiration); grunting; wheezing; or stridor

Labored breathing—Continuous, intermittent, becoming steadily worse, sudden onset, at rest or on exertion, associated with wheezing or grunting, associated with pain

Rhythm—Variation in rate and depth of respirations

OTHER OBSERVATIONS

In addition to respirations, particular attention is addressed to:

Evidence of infection—Check for elevated temperature; enlarged cervical lymph nodes; inflamed mucous membranes; and purulent discharges from the nose, ears, or lungs (sputum).

Cough—Observe the characteristics of the cough (if present), under what circumstances the cough is heard (e.g., night only, on arising), nature of the cough (paroxysmal with or without wheeze, "croupy" or "brassy"), frequency of cough, association with swallowing or other activity, character of the cough (moist and dry), productivity.

Wheeze—Observe character of wheezing: expiratory or inspiratory, high pitched or musical, prolonged, slowly progressive or sudden, association with labored breathing.

Cyanosis—Note distribution (peripheral, perioral, facial, trunk, and face), degree, duration, association with activity.

Chest pain—This may be a complaint of older children. Note location and circumstances: localized or generalized; referral to base of neck or abdomen; dull or sharp; deep or superficial; association with rapid, shallow respirations or grunting.

Nasal mucus—Older children may provide sample by blowing nose or provide sputum sample by coughing, whereas young children may need use of bulb suction, wall suction to DeLee mucus trap, or baby nasal aspirator (attaches to wall suction tubing and fits on small nose) to provide a sample. Note volume, color, viscosity, and odor.

Bad breath (halitosis)—May be associated with some upper airway infections, but is more common in mouth breathers.

nursingprocess | The Child with Acute Respiratory Tract Infection

ASSESSMENT

Assessment of the respiratory system follows the guidelines described in Chapter 6 (for nose, ears, mouth and throat, chest, and lungs). In addition, special attention is given to the observations outlined in Box 23-1 and the components in Box 23-2.

- Assess respiratory effort (respiratory rate, accessory muscle use, retractions, nasal flaring).
- Assess oxygenation (pulse oximetry, color).
- Assess body temperature.
- Assess child's activity level.
- Assess child's level of comfort.

DIAGNOSES (PROBLEM IDENTIFICATION)

After a thorough assessment, several nursing diagnoses are evident. Other nursing diagnoses may be apparent in individual cases.

- Ineffective Breathing Pattern related to inflammatory process
- Ineffective Airway Clearance related to mechanical obstruction, inflammation, increased secretions
- Risk for Infection related to presence of infectious organisms, presence of optimum medium (mucus, sputum) for growth of infectious agents
- Activity Intolerance related to inflammatory process, imbalance between oxygen supply and demand
- Altered Family Processes related to child's illness

PLANNING

Expected patient outcomes include:

- Child will have adequate oxygenation.
- Child will demonstrate effective clearance of secretions.
- Optimum patient comfort will be achieved.
- Child will have effective respirations.
- Child will have adequate fluid and nutrient intake.
- Child will remain euthermic.

IMPLEMENTATION

Numerous intervention strategies are discussed on pp. 756-759.

EVALUATION

The effectiveness of nursing interventions is determined by continual reassessment and evaluation of care based on the following observational guidelines:

- Observe child's respiratory effort and chest movements.
- Observe child's behavior and activity.
- Observe other family members and contacts for evidence of infection.
- Take temperature, respiratory rate, pulse oximetry reading, blood pressure, and heart rate.
- Observe for signs of adequate hydration.
- Assess complications, such as dehydration, weight loss, or spread of infection to other areas of the body.
- Observe family's behavior, and interview members regarding their feelings and concerns.

comfort. The use of steam vaporizers in the home is often discouraged because of the hazards related to their use and limited evidence to support their efficacy. Shallow pans with wide surface areas for evaporation increase humidity, but they should be placed where they do not pose a safety hazard.

A time-honored method (albeit not evidence based!) of producing steam is the shower. Running a shower of hot water into the empty bathtub or open shower stall with the bathroom door closed produces a quick source of steam. Keeping a child in this environment for approximately 10 to 15 minutes offers the same advantages as the mist tent without the fear and restraint often associated with the confines of a tent. A small child can be held on the lap of a parent or other adult. Older children can sit in the bathroom under the supervision of an adult.

Promote Rest. Children who have an acute febrile illness should have limited activity or be placed on bed rest. This is usually not difficult while the temperature is elevated but may become a problem when children begin to feel better. In fact, one of the cardinal signs that the child is feeling better is the increase in activity; this may, however, be temporary if a high fever returns after a few hours of increased activity. Often children will comply with bed rest if they are allowed to lie quietly on a couch where they can watch television, play video games, or participate in a quiet activity. If children protest, allowing them to play quietly serves the purpose of rest better than allowing them to cry in bed.

Promote Comfort. Older children are usually able to manage nasal secretions with little difficulty. Parents are instructed in the correct administration of nose drops. For very young infants, who normally breathe through their noses, an infant nasal aspirator or a bulb syringe is helpful in removing nasal secretions, especially before being put to bed to sleep and before feeding. This practice, preceded by instillation of saline nose drops, may clear nasal passages and promote feeding. Saline nose drops can be prepared at home by dissolving 1 teaspoon of salt in 1 pint of warm water.

For older infants and children who can tolerate decongestants, vasoconstrictive nose drops may be administered 15 to 20 minutes before feeding and at bedtime. Two drops are instilled, and because this shrinks only the anterior mucous membranes, two more drops are instilled 5 to 10 minutes later. Older cooperative children often prefer nasal sprays. They are taught to compress the plastic container at the moment of inspiration. Bottles of nose drops should be used for only for one child and one illness because they are easily contaminated with bacteria. To avoid rebound congestion, nose drops or sprays should not be administered for more than 3 days. To prevent cross-contamination with nose drops, draw about 0.25 ml of nose spray solution into a clean tuberculin syringe. Inject a small amount of the nose spray solution into the child's nostrils using the blunt syringe.

Hot or cold applications sometimes provide relief for children with painful cervical adenitis. An ice bag or heating pad applied to the neck may decrease the discomfort, but safety precautions must be observed to prevent burns. The ice bag or heating device must be covered, and the heating pad should not be set at high ranges.

Prevent Spread of Infection. Children and families are taught to use a tissue or their hand to cover their nose and mouth when they cough or sneeze and to dispose of tissues properly, as well as to wash their hands. Remembering to cover the nose or mouth is often difficult for toddlers; therefore frequent hand washing is encouraged to prevent the spread of infection. Used tissues should be immediately thrown into the wastebasket or a special plastic or paper bag, which can be discarded when full. Children with respiratory tract infections should not share drinking cups, washcloths, or hand or face towels. To avoid contamination with respiratory viruses, wash hands and do not touch (rub) your eyes or nose. Careful handwashing is key in the prevention of childhood respiratory tract infections.

Efforts should be made to separate affected children from contact with other children. Parents should keep affected children out of school and daycare settings to prevent the spread of infection. Ideally, ill children should be isolated in a separate bedroom at the first sign of illness. However, this is a problem in households with more than one child. Well children should be told to stay away from ill children.

Reduce Body Temperature. If the child has a significantly elevated body temperature, controlling the fever is important. Parents should know how to take a child's temperature and read the thermometer accurately. Nurses should not assume that all parents can read a thermometer. Parents who cannot perform this skill should receive instruction.

If the practitioner prescribes acetaminophen or ibuprofen, parents may need help giving the drug. Most parents can read the label and calculate the desired dosage, but some may require detailed instruction. It is important to emphasize accuracy in determining both the amount of drug to be given and the time intervals for administration.

Cool liquids are given to reduce the temperature and minimize the chances of dehydration (see Controlling Elevated Temperatures, Chapter 22).

NURSINGALERT
Parents are cautioned regarding over-the-counter combination "cold" remedies, since these often include acetaminophen. Careful calculation of both the acetaminophen given separately and the acetaminophen in combination medications is necessary to avoid an overdose.

Promote Hydration. Dehydration is a potential complication when children have respiratory tract infections and are febrile or anorexic, especially when vomiting or diarrhea is present. Infants are especially prone to fluid and electrolyte deficits when they have a respiratory illness because a rapid respiratory rate that accompanies such illnesses precludes adequate oral fluid intake. In addition, the presence of fever increases the total body fluid turnover in infants. If the infant has nasal secretions, this further prevents adequate respiratory effort by blocking the narrow nasal passages when the infant reclines to bottle-feed or breastfeed and ceases the compensatory mouth breathing effort, thus causing the child to limit intake of fluids. Adequate fluid intake is encouraged by offering small amounts of favorite fluids (clear liquids if vomiting) at frequent intervals. Oral rehydration solutions, such as Infalyte or Pedialyte, should be considered for infants, and sports drinks, such as Gatorade, should be considered for older children. Fluids with caffeine (tea, coffee) are avoided because these may act as diuretics and promote fluid loss. Breastfeeding infants should continue to be breastfed, since human milk confers some degree of protection from infection (see Chapter 8). Fluids should not be forced, and children should not be awakened to take fluids. Forcing fluids creates the same problem as urging unwanted food. Gentle persuasion with preferred beverages or sugar-free popsicles is usually more successful.

To assess their child's level of hydration (see Chapters 9 and 24), parents are advised to observe the frequency of voiding and to notify the nurse or practitioner if there is insufficient voiding. Counting the number of wet diapers in a 24-hour period is a satisfactory method to assess output in infants and toddlers.

Provide Nutrition. Loss of appetite is characteristic of children with acute infections. In most cases, children can be permitted to determine their own need for food. Many children show no decrease in appetite, and others respond well to foods such as gelatin, popsicles, and soup (see Feeding the Sick Child, Chapter 22). Urging solid foods on children who are sick may precipitate nausea and vomiting and cause an aversion to feeding that may extend into the convalescent period and beyond.

Family Support and Home Care. Young children with respiratory tract infections are irritable and difficult to comfort; therefore the family needs support, encouragement, and practical suggestions concerning comfort measures and administration of medication. In addition to antipyretics and nose drops, the child may require antibiotic therapy. Parents of children receiving oral antibiotics must understand the importance of regular administration and of continuing the drug for the prescribed length of time, regardless of whether the child appears ill. Parents are cautioned against giving their

child any medications that are not approved by the health practitioner and are cautioned to avoid giving antibiotics left over from a previous illness or prescribed for another child. Administering unprescribed antibiotics can produce serious side effects and adverse reactions (see Chapter 22 for administration of medications and teaching parents). See also Nursing Care Plan.

UPPER RESPIRATORY TRACT INFECTIONS
NASOPHARYNGITIS

Acute nasopharyngitis, or the equivalent of the "common cold," is caused by the rhinovirus, RSV, adenovirus, influenza virus, and parainfluenza virus. Symptoms are more severe in infants and children than in adults. Fever is common in young children, and older children have low-grade fevers, which appear early in the course of the illness. Other clinical manifestations are listed in Box 23-3.

Therapeutic Management

Children with nasopharyngitis are managed at home. There is no specific treatment, and effective vaccines are not available. Antipyretics are prescribed for mild fever and discomfort (see Chapter 22 for management of fever). Rest is recommended until the child is free of fever for at least 1 day. The provision of a humidified environment and increasing oral fluids may be beneficial to some children with a cold. Decongestants may be prescribed for children and infants older than 6 months of age to shrink swollen nasal passages. The decongestants that

nursingcareplan | The Child with Acute Respiratory Tract Infection

Nursing Diagnosis	Patient Outcomes	Nursing Interventions	Rationale
Ineffective Breathing Pattern related to inflammatory process	Child's respirations will be nonlabored.	Position child for maximal ventilatory efficiency and airway patency.	To allow increased chest expansion
Child's/Family's Defining Characteristics *(Subjective and Objective Data)*	**The Following NOC Concept Applies to These Outcomes**	Position child to facilitate drainage of secretions.	To maintain patent airway and prevent airway obstruction
Use of accessory muscles to breathe	Respiratory Status: Airway Patency, Ventilation	Provide humidified oxygen as necessary.	To improve oxygenation
Dyspnea		Monitor oxygenation status, including vital signs, for changes in condition.	To determine need for additional interventions
Shortness of breath		Suction airway (nose, trachea) as necessary.	To remove secretions and maintain airway patency
Nasal flaring			
Altered chest excursion		Provide gentle chest percussion and chest physical therapy (CPT) as necessary.	To facilitate secretion removal
Assumption of three-point position (tripod)		Administer bronchodilator medications.	To promote bronchodilation and improve ventilation
Respiratory rate outside normal parameter for child's age (increased or decreased rate)		Administer antiinflammatory medications.	To decrease airway inflammation
		Administer antibiotics (if bacterial).	To decrease inflammatory response

The Following NIC Concepts Apply to These Interventions

Aspiration Precautions
Positioning
Respiratory Monitoring Surveillance
Oxygen Therapy
Airway Suctioning
Vital Signs Monitoring
Cough Enhancement

Continued

Nursing Diagnosis	Patient Outcomes	Nursing Interventions	Rationale
Ineffective Airway Clearance related to inflammation, mechanical obstruction, increased secretions **Child's/Family's Defining Characteristics** *(Subjective and Objective Data)* Dyspnea Difficulty vocalizing Orthopnea Adventitious breath sounds (crackles, wheezing, rhonchi) Cough ineffective or absent Restlessness Changes in respiratory rate and rhythm	Child's airways will remain patent. **The Following NOC Concepts Apply to These Outcomes** Aspiration Control Airway Patency	Position child to facilitate drainage of secretions. Perform CPT. Suction airway as necessary. Provide humidified oxygen. Assist with coughing (as developmentally or age appropriate). Avoid throat examination if epiglottitis is suspected. Assure child (as appropriate) all measures will be taken to ensure adequate airway is maintained. Implement comfort measures such as allowing parental presence, parental holding, favorite blanket or stuffed animal at side; explain all procedures beforehand. **The Following NIC Concepts Apply to These Interventions** Cough Enhancement Positioning Chest Physiotherapy Vital Signs Monitoring Anxiety Reduction	To prevent airway obstruction To loosen and remove secretions To remove secretions To moisten secretions and prevent airway drying To remove secretions To prevent airway compromise To allay anxiety To reduce anxiety and decrease effects of medical therapy, including hospitalization if required

Nursing Diagnosis	Patient Outcomes	Nursing Interventions	Rationale
Risk for Injury related to presence (only as indicated) of infective organisms **Child's/Family's Defining Characteristics** *(Subjective and Objective Data)* Tissue hypoxia Abnormal blood profile People or provider (nosocomial agents) Mode of transport Developmental age	Child will remain free from complications of infection. **The Following NOC Concept Applies to These Outcomes** Risk Control	Maintain aseptic environment using sterile suction equipment and technique. Implement and practice standard precautions. Implement contact and airborne precautions as necessary. Obtain (secretion, tissue, or blood) specimen as indicated. Encourage child and family contacts to practice frequent hand washing and avoid hand-to-eye and hand-to-mouth contact. Teach child (as age appropriate) and family how to decrease spread of organisms through coughing and other secretions (e.g., by covering mouth when coughing; disposing of secretions to avoid cross-contamination). Administer antibiotic or antiviral medications. Administer fever reduction medication(s) as appropriate. Monitor and assess for signs and symptoms of secondary complications: hypoxia, skin breakdown, poor nutrient and fluid intake, increased work of breathing, deteriorating cardiorespiratory status. **The Following NIC Concepts Apply to These Interventions** Risk Identification Environmental Management Infection Control Parent Education	To prevent spread of infectious organisms in child and family To identify infective organism To prevent spread of infection To prevent spread of infection To treat infection source To promote comfort if fever is present To implement therapy for prevention of secondary complications

nursingcareplan | The Child with Acute Respiratory Tract Infection—cont'd

Nursing Diagnosis	Patient Outcomes	Nursing Interventions	Rationale
Interrupted Family Processes related to child's illness, hospitalization, and medical or therapeutic regimen	Family will demonstrate ability to cope with child's illness.	Allow family to remain with child. Promote family-centered care. Explain procedures and therapeutic regimen to family.	To decrease effects of separation To promote family integrity To provide accurate information regarding therapy and child's condition
Child's/Family's Defining Characteristics *(Subjective and Objective Data)*	**The Following NOC Concepts Apply to These Outcomes** Family Functioning Family Normalization Parenting	Keep family informed of child's status. Encourage family involvement in child's care. Provide support and referral for continued support as necessary.	To promote family sense of control and involvement in care
Communication patterns Participation in decision making Availability for emotional support Expressions of conflict within family Patterns and rituals		**The Following NIC Concepts Apply to These Interventions** Caregiver Support Family Support Coping Enhancement Emotional Support Financial Resource Assistance	

BOX 23-3

Clinical Manifestations of Nasopharyngitis and Pharyngitis

NASOPHARYNGITIS

Younger Child
Fever
Irritability, restlessness
Poor feeding and decreased fluid intake
Sneezing
Nasal mucus (abundant) causing mouth breathing
Vomiting or diarrhea

Older Child
Dryness and irritation of nose and throat
Sneezing, chilling
Muscle aches
Cough (sometimes)

Physical Assessment Signs
Edema and vasodilation of mucosa

PHARYNGITIS

Younger Child
Fever
General malaise
Anorexia
Moderate sore throat
Headache

Older Child
Fever (may reach 40° C [104° F])
Headache
Anorexia
Dysphagia
Abdominal pain
Vomiting

Physical Assessment Signs
Younger Child
Mild to moderate hyperemia

Older Child
Mild to bright red, edematous pharynx
Hyperemia of tonsils and pharynx; may extend to soft palate and uvula
Often abundant follicular exudate that spreads and coalesces to form pseudomembrane on tonsils
Cervical glands enlarged and tender

---

exert their effect by vasoconstriction are usually less effective when taken orally than when applied topically as nose drops.

Cough suppressants containing dextromethorphan may be prescribed for a dry, hacking cough in older children. However, cough preparations can cause adverse effects such as confusion, hyperexcitability, and sedation; therefore parents should monitor the child carefully for potential adverse effects.

Antihistamines are largely ineffective in treatment of nasopharyngitis. These drugs have a weak atropine-like effect that dries secretions, but they can cause drowsiness or, paradoxically, have a stimulatory effect on children. There is no support for the usefulness of expectorants, and antibiotics are usually not indicated because most infections are viral.

Prevention. Nasopharyngitis is so widespread in the general population that it is impossible to prevent. Children are more susceptible because they have not yet developed resistance to many viruses. Young infants and those with decreased resistance and pulmonary illness are subject to serious complications such as pneumonia, and attempts should be made to protect them from exposure.

Nursing Care Management

A cold is often the parents' first introduction to an illness in their infant. Most discomfort of nasopharyngitis is related to the nasal obstruction, especially in small infants. Elevating the head of the bed or crib mattress assists with drainage of secretions. Suctioning and vaporization may also provide relief. Saline nose drops and gentle suction with a bulb syringe before feeding and sleep time is useful.

Maintaining adequate fluid intake is essential. Although a child's appetite for solid foods is usually diminished for several days, it is important to offer favorite fluids to prevent dehydration. Fluids can be cool or warm, depending on individual preference.

Because nasopharyngitis is spread from secretions, the best means for prevention is avoiding contact with affected per-

BOX 23-4

Early Evidence of Respiratory Complications

Parents are instructed to notify the health professional if any of the following are noted:

- Evidence of earache (see p. 765)
- Respirations faster than 50 to 60 breaths/min
- Fever over 38.3° C (101° F)
- Listlessness
- Confusion
- Increasing irritability with or without fever
- Persistent cough for 2 days or more
- Wheezing
- Crying
- Refusal to take oral fluids and decreased urination
- Restlessness and poor sleep patterns

Modified from National Association of Pediatric Nurse Practitioners (NAPNAP): *Baby's first cold*, New York, 1989, Winthrop Consumer Products. Copies available from NAPNAP, 20 Brace Road, Suite 200, Cherry Hill, NJ 08034-2634; (856) 857-9700; http://www.napnap.org.

FIG. 23-1 ■ Tonsillitis and pharyngitis. (Courtesy Dr. Edward L. Applebaum, Head, Department of Otolaryngology, University of Illinois Medical Center, Chicago.)

sons. This goal is difficult to accomplish in family settings, classrooms, and daycare centers. Family members with a cold should try to "keep it to themselves" by carefully disposing of tissues; not sharing towels, glasses, or eating utensils; covering the mouth and nose with tissues when coughing or sneezing; and washing the hands thoroughly after nose blowing or sneezing. The most frequent carriers of infection are the human hands, which deposit viruses on doorknobs, faucets, and other everyday objects. Children should be taught to wash their hands thoroughly and avoid touching their eyes, nose, or mouth.

Family Support. Support and reassurance are important elements of care for families of young children with recurrent upper respiratory infections (URIs). Because URIs are frequent in children less than 3 years of age, families may feel they are on an endless roller coaster of illness. They need reassurance that frequent colds are a normal part of childhood and that by 5 years of age, their children will have developed immunity to many viruses. Parents who work outside the home should expect to take time off to care for ill children during the fall and winter months. When children spend time in daycare centers, their infection rate is higher than if they are cared for in the home. Parents should know the signs of respiratory complications and should notify a health professional if complications occur or the child does not improve within 2 or 3 days (Box 23-4).

PHARYNGITIS

Children who experience GABHS infection of the upper airway (**strep throat**) are at risk for **rheumatic fever (RF),** an inflammatory disease of the heart, joints, and central nervous system (see Chapter 25), and **acute glomerulonephritis (AGN),** an acute kidney infection (see Chapter 27). Permanent damage can result from these sequelae, especially RF.

Clinical Manifestations

GABHS infection is generally a relatively brief illness that varies in severity from subclinical (no symptoms) to severe toxicity. The onset is often abrupt and characterized by pharyngitis, headache, fever, and abdominal pain. The ton-

sils and pharynx may be inflamed and covered with exudate (Fig. 23-1), which usually appears by the second day of illness. However, streptococcal infections should be suspected in children older than 2 years of age who have pharyngitis without exudate. The tongue may appear edematous and red (strawberry tongue), and the child may have a characteristic erythematous fine sandpaper rash on the trunk, axillae, elbows, and groin; the uvula is edematous and red. Anterior cervical lymphadenopathy (in about 30% to 50% of cases) usually occurs early, and the nodes are often tender. Pain can be relatively mild to severe enough to make swallowing difficult. Clinical manifestations usually subside in 3 to 5 days unless complicated by sinusitis or parapharyngeal, peritonsillar, or retropharyngeal abscess. Nonsuppurative complications may appear after the onset of GABHS—AGN in about 10 days and RF in an average of 18 days.

Diagnostic Evaluation

Although 80% to 90% of all cases of acute pharyngitis are viral, a throat culture should be performed to rule out GABHS. Most streptococcal infections are short-term illnesses, and antibody responses appear later than symptoms and are useful only for retrospective diagnosis.

Rapid identification of GABHS with diagnostic test kits (rapid antigen detection test) is possible in the office or clinic setting. Because of the high specificity of these rapid tests, a positive test result generally does not require throat culture confirmation. However, the sensitivities of these kits vary considerably, and a confirmatory throat culture is recommended in patients who have a negative test result (American Academy of Pediatrics, 2006b).

Therapeutic Management

If streptococcal sore throat infection is present, oral penicillin is prescribed in a dose sufficient to control the acute local manifestations and to maintain an adequate level for at least 10 days to eliminate any organisms that might remain to initiate RF symptoms. Penicillin does not prevent the development of AGN in susceptible children; however, it may prevent the spread of a nephrogenic strain of GABHS to others in the family. Penicillin usually produces a prompt response within 24 hours. Patients who have a history of RF or who remain symptomatic after a full course of antibiotics may require a follow-up throat swab.

Intramuscular (IM) benzathine penicillin G is an appropriate therapy, but it is painful and is not the first choice for children. Oral erythromycin is indicated for children allergic to penicillin. Other antibiotics used to treat GABHS are azithromycin, clarithromycin, oral cephalosporins, amoxicillin, and amoxicillin with clavulanic acid (American Academy of Pediatrics, 2006b; Gerber, 2005).

Nursing Care Management

The nurse often obtains a throat swab for culture and instructs the parents about administering penicillin and analgesics as prescribed. Cold or warm compresses to the neck may provide relief. In children who can cooperate, warm saline gargles may offer relief of throat discomfort. Acetaminophen and ibuprofen may be effective in decreasing the throat pain; liquid preparations or chewable forms may be preferable because of the pain associated with swallowing. Pain may interfere with oral intake, and children should not be forced to eat, but fluid intake is essential. Cool liquids or ice chips are usually more acceptable than solids.

Special emphasis is placed on correct administration of oral medication and completion of the course of antibiotic therapy (see Administration of Medication, and Compliance, Chapter 22). If an injection is required, it must be administered deep into a large muscle mass (e.g., vastus lateralis or ventrogluteal muscle). To prevent pain, application of a topical anesthetic cream such as EMLA (an eutectic mix of lidocaine and prilocaine) or LMX 4 (4% lidocaine) over the injection site before the injection is helpful (see Administration of Medication: Intramuscular Administration, Chapter 22). Parents also need to be aware of residual tenderness at the injection site, which may cause the child to limp for a day or two. Local applications of heat are helpful in relieving this discomfort.

Children are considered infectious to others at the onset of symptoms and up to 24 hours after initiation of antibiotic therapy, but they should not return to school or daycare until they have been taking antibiotics for a full 24-hour period. Nurses should remind the children to discard their toothbrush and replace it with a new one after they have been taking antibiotics for 24 hours. Parents are cautioned to prevent other household members, especially if immunocompromised, from having close contact with the sick child and avoid sharing drinking or eating items.

If the child continues to have a high fever that does not respond to antipyretics, has an extremely sore throat, refuses liquids, and appears toxic 24 to 48 hours after starting antibiotics, further evaluation by the practitioner is recommended.

TONSILLITIS

The tonsils are masses of lymphoid tissue located in the pharyngeal cavity. They filter and protect the respiratory and alimentary tracts from invasion by pathogenic organisms and play a role in antibody formation. Although their size varies, children generally have much larger tonsils than adolescents or adults. This difference is thought to be a protective mechanism because young children are especially susceptible to URIs.

Pathophysiology

Several pairs of tonsils are part of a mass of lymphoid tissue encircling the nasal and oral pharynx, known as the **Waldeyer tonsillar ring** (Fig. 23-2). The **palatine,** or **faucial, tonsils** are located on either side of the oropharynx, behind and below

FIG. 23-2 ■ Location of various tonsillar masses.

the pillars of the fauces (opening from the mouth). A surface of the palatine tonsils is usually visible during oral examination. The palatine tonsils are those removed during tonsillectomy. The **pharyngeal tonsils,** also known as the **adenoids,** are located above the palatine tonsils on the posterior wall of the nasopharynx. Their proximity to the nares and eustachian tubes causes difficulties in instances of inflammation. The **lingual tonsils** are located at the base of the tongue. The **tubal tonsils,** found near the posterior nasopharyngeal opening of the eustachian tubes, are not part of the Waldeyer tonsillar ring.

Etiology

Tonsillitis often occurs with pharyngitis. The causative agent may be viral or bacterial. Because of the abundant lymphoid tissue and the frequency of URIs, tonsillitis is a common cause of illness in young children.

Clinical Manifestations

The manifestations of tonsillitis are caused by inflammation. As the palatine tonsils enlarge from edema, they may meet in the midline (kissing tonsils), obstructing the passage of air or food. The child has difficulty swallowing and breathing. When enlargement of the adenoids occurs, the space behind the posterior nares becomes blocked, making it difficult or impossible for air to pass from the nose to the throat. As a result, the child breathes through the mouth.

Therapeutic Management

Because tonsillitis is self-limiting, treatment of viral pharyngitis is symptomatic. Throat cultures positive for GABHS infection warrant antibiotic treatment. It is important to differentiate between viral and streptococcal infection in febrile exudative tonsillitis. Because most infections are of viral origin, early rapid tests can eliminate unnecessary antibiotic administration.

Tonsillectomy is the surgical removal of the palatine tonsils. Absolute indications for a tonsillectomy are malignancy, recurrent peritonsillar abscess, and airway obstruction. **Adenoidectomy** (the surgical removal of the adenoids) is recommended for children who have hypertrophied adenoids that obstruct nasal breathing; additional indications for adenoidectomy include recurrent adenoiditis and sinusitis, otitis media (OM) with effusion, airway obstruction and subsequent sleep-disordered breathing, and recurrent rhinorrhea (Benninger and Walner, 2007a). The American Academy of Otolaryngology—Head and Neck Surgery (2000) lists "3 or more infections of the tonsils or adenoids per year despite adequate medical therapy" as an indication for tonsillectomy or **adenotonsillectomy**. However, for some children the effectiveness of tonsillectomy or adenoidectomy is modest and may not justify the risk of surgery (van Staaij, van den Akker, Rover, and others, 2004). In practice, many physicians rely on individualized decision making and do not subscribe to an absolute set of eligibility criteria for these surgical procedures (Paradise, Bluestone, Colborn, and others, 2002). Contraindications to either tonsillectomy or adenoidectomy are (1) cleft palate because tonsils help minimize escape of air during speech, (2) acute infections at the time of surgery because locally inflamed tissues increase the risk of bleeding, and (3) uncontrolled systemic diseases or blood dyscrasias.

Nursing Care Management

Nursing care involves providing comfort and minimizing activities or interventions that precipitate bleeding. A soft to liquid diet is preferred. A cool-mist vaporizer keeps the mucous membranes moist during periods of mouth breathing. Warm salt-water gargles, throat lozenges, and analgesic-antipyretic drugs such as acetaminophen are used to promote comfort. Often opioids are needed to reduce pain for the child to drink. Combination nonopioid and opioid elixirs or tablets such as acetaminophen with codeine or with hydrocodone (Lortab) relieve pain and should be given routinely every 4 hours.

If surgery is required, the child requires the same psychologic preparation and physical care as for any other surgical procedure (see Chapters 21 and 22). Most tonsillectomy and adenoidectomy (T&A) surgeries now take place in outpatient settings; however, the priorities of preoperative and postoperative care remain the same. The following discussion focuses on postoperative nursing care for T&A, although both procedures may not be performed.

Until they are fully awake, children are placed on their abdomen or side to facilitate drainage of secretions. Routine suctioning is avoided, and, when performed, it is done carefully to avoid trauma to the oropharynx. When alert, children may prefer sitting up. They are discouraged from coughing frequently, clearing their throat, blowing their nose, or any other activity that may aggravate the operative site.

Some secretions are common, particularly dried blood from surgery. All secretions and vomitus are inspected for evidence of fresh bleeding (some blood-tinged mucus is expected). Dark brown (old) blood is usually present in the emesis, in the nose, and between the teeth. If parents do not expect this, they often become frightened at a time when they need to be calm and reassuring.

The throat is sore after surgery. An ice collar provides relief, but many children find it bothersome and refuse to use it. Most children experience moderate pain after a T&A and need pain medication for at least the first 24 hours. Analgesics

may be given rectally or intravenously to avoid the oral route. Because pain is continuous, analgesics should be administered at regular intervals. An antiemetic such as ondansetron (Zofran) may be administered postoperatively (see Pain Management, Chapter 7).

Food and fluids are restricted until children are fully alert and there are no signs of hemorrhage. Cool water, crushed ice, flavored ice pops, or diluted fruit juice may be given, but fluids with a red or brown color are avoided to distinguish fresh or old blood in emesis from the ingested liquid. Citrus juice may cause discomfort and is usually poorly tolerated. Soft foods, particularly gelatin, cooked fruits, sherbet, soup, and mashed potatoes, are started on the first or second postoperative day or as the child tolerates feeding. The pain from surgery often inhibits fluid intake, reinforcing the need for adequate pain control. Milk, ice cream, and pudding are usually not offered, since milk products coat the mouth and throat and may cause the child to clear the throat, which can initiate bleeding.

Postoperative hemorrhage is uncommon but can occur. The nurse observes the throat directly for evidence of bleeding, using a good source of light and, if necessary, carefully inserting a tongue depressor. Other signs of hemorrhage are tachycardia, pallor, frequent clearing of the throat or swallowing by a younger child, and vomiting of bright red blood. Restlessness, an indication of hemorrhage, may be difficult to differentiate from general discomfort after surgery. Decreasing blood pressure is a late sign of shock.

Surgery may be required to ligate a bleeding vessel. Airway obstruction may also occur as a result of edema or accumulated secretions and is indicated by signs of respiratory distress, such as stridor, drooling, restlessness, agitation, increasing respiratory rate, and progressive cyanosis. Suction equipment and oxygen should be available after tonsillectomy.

NURSINGALERT

The most obvious early sign of bleeding is the child's continuous swallowing of the trickling blood. While the child is sleeping, note the frequency of swallowing. If continuous bleeding is suspected, notify the surgeon immediately.

Family Support and Home Care. Discharge instructions include (1) avoiding irritating or highly seasoned foods, (2) avoiding gargles or vigorous toothbrushing, (3) avoiding coughing or clearing of the throat or putting objects in the mouth, (4) using analgesics or an ice collar for pain, and (5) limiting activity to decrease the potential for bleeding. Objectionable mouth odor and slight ear pain with a low-grade fever are common for a few days postoperatively. However, persistent severe earache, fever, or cough requires medical evaluation. Most children are ready to resume normal activity within 1 to 2 weeks after the operation.

Hemorrhage may occur up to 10 days after surgery as a result of tissue sloughing from the healing process. Any sign of bleeding warrants immediate medical attention.

INFLUENZA

Influenza, or "flu," is caused by three orthomyxoviruses, which are antigenically distinct: types A and B, which cause epidemic disease, and type C, which is unimportant from an epidemiologic standpoint. Influenza is spread from one individual to another by direct contact (large-droplet infection) or by articles recently contaminated by nasopharyngeal secretions.

There is no predilection for a specific age-group, but attack rates are highest in young children who have had no previous contact with a strain. Influenza is frequently most severe in infants. During epidemics, infection among school-age children is believed to be a major source of transmission in a community. The disease is more common during the winter months and has a 1- to 3-day incubation period. Affected persons are most infectious for 24 hours before and after the onset of symptoms. The virus has a peculiar affinity for epithelial cells of the respiratory tract mucosa, where it destroys ciliated epithelium with metaplastic hyperplasia of the tracheal and bronchial epithelium with associated edema. The alveoli may also become distended with a hyaline-like material. The viruses can be isolated from nasopharyngeal secretions early after the onset of infection, and serologic tests identify the type by complement fixation or the subgroups by hemagglutination inhibition.

Clinical Manifestations

The manifestations of influenza may be subclinical, mild, moderate, or severe. Most patients have a dry throat and nasal mucosa, a dry cough, and a tendency toward hoarseness. A flushed face, photophobia, myalgia, hyperesthesia, and sometimes exhaustion and lack of energy accompany a sudden onset of fever and chills. Subglottal croup is common, especially in infants. The symptoms of influenza last for 4 or 5 days. Complications include severe viral pneumonia (often hemorrhagic); encephalitis; and secondary bacterial infections such as OM, sinusitis, or pneumonia.

Therapeutic Management

Uncomplicated influenza in children usually requires only symptomatic treatment: acetaminophen or ibuprofen for fever and sufficient fluids to maintain hydration. Amantadine hydrochloride (Symmetrel) has been effective in reducing symptoms associated with type A disease if administered within 24 to 48 hours after their onset; the symptoms associated with influenza are reportedly shortened by 24 hours, but the drug does not "cure" the disease. It is ineffective against type B or C influenza or other viral diseases. It should not be given to children under 1 year of age but is recommended for unvaccinated high-risk children.

Zanamivir and rimantadine have been approved for the treatment of flu symptoms in children under 18 years of age. Both medications must also be started within 48 hours of symptom onset. Zanamivir is an inhaled medication effective for type A and B influenza. The drug is taken twice daily for 5 days and is administered by a specially designed oral inhaler (Diskhaler). Zanamivir cannot be used for children less than 5 years of age. A fourth drug, oseltamivir (Tamiflu), is a neuroaminidase inhibitor that may be administered orally for 5 days to children over 1 year (and adults) to decrease the flu symptoms; as with other antiviral drugs, this must be taken within 2 days of the onset of symptoms. It is reported to be effective for types A and B influenza (American Academy of Pediatrics, 2006b). Bronchospasm and a decline in lung function can occur when zanamivir is used in patients with underlying airway disease such as asthma or chronic obstructive pulmonary disease. Rimantadine is effective only for type A virus; this drug is taken orally in tablet or syrup twice daily for 7 days. Rimantadine cannot be used for children less than 1 year of age. Children with influenza (or other similar viruses) should not receive aspirin because of its possible link with Reye syndrome.

Prevention. Two vaccines may be administered to prevent influenza. Inactivated trivalent influenza viral (TIV) vaccines are safe and effective provided the antigens in the vaccine correlate with the circulating influenza viruses (see Immunizations, Chapter 10). The live-attenuated influenza vaccine (LAIV) is a nasal spray flu vaccine approved by the U.S. Food and Drug Administration (FDA) that is licensed for administration in children 2 years of age and older. However, this preparation contains a live virus and should not be used in individuals who are immunocompromised, have anaphylactic reactions to egg protein, have reactive airway disease, are receiving immunosuppressive therapy, have a chronic respiratory condition, or have a history of Guillain-Barré syndrome.

Nursing Care Management

Nursing care is the same as for any child with a URI, including implementing measures to relieve symptoms. The greatest danger to affected children is development of a secondary infection. Prolonged fever or appearance of fever during early convalescence is a sign of secondary bacterial infection and should be reported to the practitioner for antibiotic therapy.

OTITIS MEDIA

OM is one of the most prevalent diseases of early childhood. Its incidence is highest in the winter months. Many cases of bacterial OM are preceded by a viral respiratory infection. The two viruses most likely to precipitate OM are RSV and influenza. Most episodes of acute otitis media (AOM) occur in the first 24 months of life, but the incidence decreases with age, except for a small increase at age 5 or 6 years when children enter school. OM occurs infrequently in children older than 7 years of age. Preschool-age boys are affected more frequently than preschool-age girls. Children who have siblings or parents with a history of chronic OM have a higher incidence of OM. Children living in households with many members (especially smokers) are more likely to have OM than those living with fewer persons. Passive smoking increases the risk of persistent middle ear effusion by enhancing attachment of the pathogens that cause otitis to the respiratory epithelium in the middle ear space, by prolonging the inflammatory response, and by impeding drainage through the eustachian tube (American Academy of Pediatrics, 2004a). Family socioeconomic status and extent of exposure to other children are the two most important identifiable risk factors for the occurrence of OM (American Academy of Pediatrics 2004a; Kershner, 2007).

OM has been defined in a variety of ways. The standard terminology used to define OM is outlined in Box 23-5, and AOM treatment guidelines have been published (American Academy of Pediatrics, 2004a, 2004b).

Etiology

Streptococcus pneumoniae, H. influenzae, and *Moraxella catarrhalis* are the three most common bacteria causing AOM. The etiology of noninfectious OM is unknown, although OM may occur because of blocked eustachian tubes from the edema of URIs, allergic rhinitis, or hypertrophic adenoids. Chronic OM is frequently an extension of an acute episode.

A relationship has been observed between the incidence of OM and infant feeding methods. Infants fed breast milk have

Standard Terminology for Otitis Media

Otitis media (OM)—An inflammation of the middle ear without reference to etiology or pathogenesis

Acute otitis media (AOM)—An inflammation of the middle ear space with a rapid onset of the signs and symptoms of acute infection—namely, fever and otalgia (ear pain)

Otitis media with effusion (OME)—Fluid in the middle ear space without symptoms of acute infection

Clinical Manifestations of Otitis Media

ACUTE OTITIS MEDIA
Follows an upper respiratory tract infection
Otalgia (earache)
Fever—may or may not be present
Purulent discharge (otorrhea)—may or may not be present

Infant or Very Young Child
Crying
Fussiness, restlessness, irritability
Tendency to rub, hold, or pull affected ear
Rolling head from side to side
Difficulty comforting child
Loss of appetite

Older Child
Crying or verbalizing feelings of discomfort
Irritability
Lethargy
Loss of appetite

CHRONIC OTITIS MEDIA
Hearing loss
Difficulty communicating
Feeling of fullness, tinnitus, or vertigo may be present

a lower incidence of OM compared with formula-fed infants. Breastfeeding may protect infants against respiratory viruses and allergy because it contains secretory immunoglobulin A, which limits the exposure of the eustachian tube and middle ear mucosa to microbial pathogens and foreign proteins. Reflux of milk up the eustachian tubes is less likely in breast-fed infants because of the semivertical positioning during breastfeeding compared with bottle-feeding.

Pathophysiology

OM is primarily a result of malfunctioning eustachian tubes. The eustachian tube is part of a contiguous system composed of the nares, nasopharynx, eustachian tube, middle ear, and mastoid antrum and air cells. Eustachian tubes have three functions relative to the middle ear: (1) protection of the middle ear from nasopharyngeal secretions, (2) drainage of secretions produced in the middle ear into the nasopharynx, and (3) ventilation of the middle ear to equalize air pressure within the middle ear and atmospheric pressure in the external ear canal and to replenish oxygen that has been absorbed.

Mechanical or functional obstruction of the eustachian tube causes accumulation of secretions in the middle ear. Intrinsic obstruction can be caused by infection or allergy; extrinsic obstruction is usually a result of enlarged adenoids or nasopharyngeal tumors. Persistent collapse of the tube during swallowing can cause functional obstruction associated with decreased stiffness or an inefficient opening mechanism. Eustachian tube obstruction results in negative middle ear pressure and, if persistent, produces a transudative middle ear effusion. Drainage is inhibited by sustained negative pressure and impaired ciliary transport within the tube. When the passage is not totally obstructed, contamination of the middle ear can take place by reflux, aspiration, or insufflation during crying, sneezing, nose blowing, and swallowing when the nose is obstructed.

Diagnostic Evaluation

Careful assessment of tympanic membrane mobility with a pneumatic otoscope is essential to differentiate AOM from OM with effusion (OME) (American Academy of Pediatrics, 2004b). A diagnosis of AOM is made if visual inspection of the tympanic membrane reveals a purulent discolored effusion and a bulging or full, opacified, or reddened immobile membrane. Some practitioners also consider the presence of acute onset of less than 48 hours of ear pain with the above criteria to be a diagnostic factor in AOM (Powers, 2007). An immobile tympanic membrane or an orange discolored membrane indicates OME. Clinical symptoms of otitis are also helpful in making the diagnosis (Box 23-6). In AOM, symp-

toms such as acute onset of ear pain, fever, and a bulging yellow or red tympanic membrane are usually present. In OME, these symptoms may be absent, and other nonspecific symptoms such as rhinitis, cough, or diarrhea are often present (American Academy of Pediatrics, 2004a, 2004b).

Therapeutic Management

Treatment for AOM is one of the most common reasons for antibiotic use in the ambulatory setting. Recently, however, concerns about drug-resistant *S. pneumoniae* and other drug resistances have led infectious disease authorities to recommend careful and judicious use of antibiotics for treatment of this illness. Current literature indicates that waiting up to 72 hours for spontaneous resolution is safe and appropriate management of AOM in healthy infants over 6 months and children (American Academy of Pediatrics, 2004a; Bhetwal and McConaghy, 2007). Furthermore some reviews of the treatment of AOM reveal no clear evidence that antibiotics improve outcomes in children younger than 2 years of age with uncomplicated AOM. However, the watchful waiting approach is not recommended for children younger than 2 years who have persistent acute symptoms of fever and severe ear pain (Carlson and Scudder, 2004). In addition, all cases of AOM in infants younger than 6 months of age should be treated with antibiotics because of the infant's immature immune system and the potential for infection with bacteria other than the three most common organisms found in older infants and children with AOM.

When antibiotics are warranted, oral amoxicillin in high doses (80 to 90 mg/kg/day, divided twice daily) is the treatment of choice for initial episodes of AOM in children who have not received antibiotics within the past month (American Academy of Pediatrics, 2004a; Bhetwal and McConaghy, 2007; Pichichero and Casey, 2005). The recommendation for the duration of antibiotic therapy is 10 to 14 days; in children 6 years and older with uncomplicated AOM, shorter courses may be sufficient (American Academy of Pediatrics, 2006b).

Second-line antibiotics used to treat OM include amoxicillin-clavulanate; azithromycin; and cephalosporins such as cefdinir, cefuroxime, and cefpodoxime. IM ceftriaxone is used if the causative organism is a highly resistant pneumococcus or if the parents are noncompliant with the therapy. An important consideration with the use of single-dose IM injections is the pain involved in this therapy. One strategy to minimize pain at the injection site is to reconstitute the cephalosporin with 1% lidocaine. The use of steroids, decongestants, and antihistamines to treat AOM is not recommended.

Supportive care or symptomatic treatment of AOM includes treating the fever and pain. For fever or discomfort associated with OM, analgesic-antipyretic drugs such as acetaminophen or ibuprofen may be given. Topical pain relief is recommended by external application of heat or cold, or the practitioner may prescribe topical pain relief drops such as benzocaine drops. Antihistamines and decongestants are not recommended. Antibiotic ear drops have no value in treating AOM.

Myringotomy, a surgical incision of the eardrum, may be necessary to alleviate the severe pain of AOM. A myringotomy is also performed to provide drainage of infected middle ear fluid in the presence of complications (mastoiditis, labyrinthitis, or facial paralysis) or to allow purulent middle ear fluid to drain into the ear canal for culture. A minimally invasive laser-assisted myringotomy procedure may be performed in outpatient settings.

Tympanostomy tube placement and adenoidectomy are surgical procedures that may be done to treat recurrent OM. Tympanostomy tubes are pressure-equalizer (PE) tubes or grommets that facilitate continued drainage of fluid and allow ventilation of the middle ear. Adenoidectomy is not recommended for treatment of AOM and is performed only in children with recurrent AOM or chronic OME with postnasal obstruction, adenoiditis, or chronic sinusitis.

In some children, residual middle ear effusions remain after episodes of AOM. Some children have fluid that persists in the middle ear for weeks or months. Antibiotics are not required for initial treatment of OME, but may be indicated for children with persistent effusion for more than 3 months (American Academy of Pediatrics, 2004a). Placement of tympanostomy tubes is recommended after a total of 4 to 6 months of bilateral effusion with a bilateral hearing deficit (American Academy of Pediatrics, 2004b). This therapy allows for mechanical drainage of the fluid, which promotes healing of the membrane and prevents scar formation and loss of elasticity. Myringotomy with or without insertion of PE tubes should not be performed for initial management of OME but may be recommended for children who have recurrent episodes of OME with a long cumulative duration (American Academy of Pediatrics, 2004b). Tonsillectomy either alone or with adenoidectomy is not considered an effective treatment of OME (American Academy of Pediatrics, 2004b).

OME is frequently associated with mild to moderate impairment of hearing; therefore a hearing test should also be performed 3 months after the acute episode of AOM, if OME persists for 3 months or more, or if there is evidence of language or learning delays. Follow-up examinations of children with chronic OME should be maintained on a 3- to 6-month basis until the OME is resolved, a significant hearing loss is identified, or structural defect of the tympanic membrane or middle ear is identified (American Academy of Pediatrics, 2004a). Children with hearing loss should be referred to an otolaryngologist and should receive a speech and language evaluation as necessary.

Prevention. The pneumococcal conjugate vaccine PCV has decreased the incidence of invasive pneumococcal infections by 80% in children under 2 years of age since the year 2000 (American Academy of Pediatrics, 2006b).

Parents are encouraged to reduce risk factors for AOM by breastfeeding infants for at least the first 6 months of life, avoiding propping the bottle, decreasing or discontinuing pacifier use after 6 months, and preventing exposure to tobacco smoke (American Academy of Pediatrics, 2004a).

Nursing Care Management

Nursing objectives for the child with AOM include (1) relieving pain, (2) facilitating drainage when possible, (3) preventing complications or recurrence, (4) educating the family in care of the child, and (5) providing emotional support to the child and family.

Analgesic drugs such as acetaminophen and ibuprofen are used to treat mild pain. For more severe pain, the American Academy of Pediatrics (2004a) guidelines recommend a stronger analgesic such as codeine.

If the ear is draining, the external canal may be cleaned with sterile cotton swabs or pledgets coupled with topical antibiotic treatment. If ear wicks or lightly rolled sterile gauze packs are placed in the ear after surgical treatment, they should be loose enough to allow accumulated drainage to flow out of the ear; otherwise, infection may be transferred to the mastoid process. The wicks need to stay dry during shampoos or baths. Occasionally, drainage is so profuse that the auricle and the skin surrounding the ear become excoriated from the exudate. This is usually prevented by frequent cleansing and application of various moisture barriers (e.g., Proshield Plus) or petrolatum jelly (e.g., Vaseline).

Tympanostomy tubes may allow water to enter the middle ear, but recommendations for earplugs are inconsistent. Research indicates that swimming without earplugs poses a slight increased risk of infection (Goldstein, Mandel, Kurs-Lasky, and others, 2005). However, lake and river water is potentially contaminated, and wearing earplugs while swimming in a lake prevents total flooding of the external canal. Bathwater and shampoo water should be kept out of the ear, if possible, because soap reduces the surface tension of water and facilitates entry through the tube. Parents should be aware of the appearance of a grommet (usually a tiny, white, plastic spool-shaped tube) so that they can recognize it if it falls out. They are reassured that this is normal and requires no immediate intervention, although they should notify the practitioner.

Prevention of recurrence requires adequate education regarding antibiotic therapy. The symptoms of pain and fever usually subside within 24 to 48 hours, but nurses must emphasize that all of the prescribed medication should be taken. Parents should be aware that potential complications of OM, such as hearing loss, can be prevented with adequate treatment and follow-up care.

Parents also need anticipatory guidance regarding methods to reduce the risks of OM, especially in children under 2 years of age. Reducing the chances of OM is possible with simple measures, such as sitting or holding an infant upright for feedings, maintaining routine childhood immunizations, and exclusively breastfeeding until at least 6 months of age. Propping bottles is discouraged to avoid pooling of milk while the child is in the supine position and to encourage human contact during feeding. Eliminating tobacco smoke and known allergens is also recommended. Early detection of middle ear effusion is essential to prevent complications. Infants and preschool children should be screened for effusion, and all schoolchildren, especially those with learning disabilities, should be tested for middle ear effusion. Frequent audiologic evaluations, medical consultation, and education of parents and children are advised when middle ear effusion is detected.

INFECTIOUS MONONUCLEOSIS

Infectious mononucleosis is an acute, self-limiting infectious disease that is common among adolescents. The illness is characterized by an increase in the mononuclear elements of the blood and by general symptoms of an infectious process. The course is usually mild but occasionally can be severe or, rarely, accompanied by serious complications.

Etiology and Pathophysiology

The herpes-like Epstein-Barr virus (EBV) is the principal cause of infectious mononucleosis. It appears in both sporadic and epidemic forms, but the sporadic cases are more common. The mechanism of spread has not been proved, but it is believed to be transmitted in saliva by direct intimate contact. It is mildly contagious, but the period of communicability is unknown. There is evidence that the virus is spread through sexual contact, especially when multiple partners are involved (Rimsza and Kirk, 2005). The incubation period following exposure is approximately 30 to 50 days (American Academy of Pediatrics, 2006).

Diagnostic Tests

The onset of symptoms may be acute or insidious and may appear anywhere from 10 days to 6 weeks after exposure. The presenting symptoms vary greatly in type, severity, and duration (Box 23-7). The clinical manifestations of infectious mononucleosis are usually less severe (often subclinical or unapparent) and the convalescent phase is shorter in younger children than in older children and young adults. The leukocyte count may be normal or low. Usually lymphocytic leukocytosis develops, and there is an increase in atypical leukocytes in the peripheral blood smear. The heterophil antibody test determines the extent to which the patient's serum will agglutinate sheep red blood cells; the response in this test is primarily to immunoglobulin M, which is present in the first 2 weeks of the illness in adolescents.

The **spot test (Monospot)** is a slide test of venous blood that has high specificity. It is rapid, sensitive, inexpensive, and easy to perform, and has the advantage over the heterophil antibody test that it can detect significant agglutinins at lower levels, thus allowing earlier diagnosis. Blood is usually obtained for the test by finger puncture or venous sampling and is placed on special paper. If the blood agglutinates, forming fragments or clumps, the test is positive for the infection.

Therapeutic Management

No specific treatment exists for infectious mononucleosis. Simple remedies ordinarily relieve the symptoms. A mild analgesic is often sufficient to relieve the headache, fever, and malaise. Rest is encouraged for fatigue but is not imposed for any specific period. Affected persons are instructed to regulate

---

BOX 23-7

Clinical Manifestations of Infectious Mononucleosis

EARLY SIGNS	Common Features
Headache	Splenomegaly (may persist for
Malaise	several months)
Fatigue	Palatine petechiae
Chills	Macular eruption (especially on
Low-grade fever	trunk)
Loss of appetite	Exudative pharyngitis or tonsillitis
Puffy eyes	Hepatic involvement to some
	degree, often associated with
ACUTE DISEASE	jaundice
Cardinal Features	
Fever	
Sore throat	
Cervical adenopathy	

---

activities according to their own tolerance unless complicating factors are present. Contact sports are discouraged in the presence of splenomegaly.

Antibiotics are contraindicated unless β-hemolytic streptococci are present. If sore throat is severe, effective therapies include gargles; hot drinks; anesthetic troches; or analgesics, including opioids. Corticosteroids have been used to treat respiratory distress from significant tonsillar inflammation, hemolytic anemia, thrombocytopenia, and neurologic complications; however, routine use of steroids is not recommended (American Academy of Pediatrics, 2006).

Prognosis. The course of this disease is usually self-limiting and uncomplicated. Acute symptoms often disappear within 7 to 10 days, and persistent fatigue subsides within 2 to 4 weeks. Some adolescents may need to restrict activities for 2 to 3 months, but the disease rarely extends for longer periods. Complications are uncommon, but can be serious and require appropriate management.

Nursing Care Management

Nursing responsibilities are directed toward providing comfort measures to relieve symptoms and helping affected adolescents and their families to determine appropriate activities for the stage of the disease. The child is advised to limit exposure to persons outside the family, especially during the acute phase of illness. Children and adolescents may need diet counseling to select foods that contain sufficient calories to meet growth and energy needs but are easy to swallow. It may be more comfortable to limit intake to liquids during the acute phase; milk shakes are a good alternative to solid foods on a temporary basis. Throat pain may be severe enough to require a mild analgesic such as codeine. Careful nursing assessment of swallowing ability is essential because the edema may cause serious airway compromise in some children.

NURSINGALERT

Advise the family to seek medical evaluation of the child or adolescent if:
- Breathing becomes difficult.
- Severe abdominal pain develops.
- Sore throat pain is so severe that the child is unable drink liquids.
- Respiratory stridor is observed.

TABLE 23-1

Comparison of Croup Syndromes

	ACUTE EPIGLOTTITIS	ACUTE LARYNGOTRACHEOBRONCHITIS (LTB)	ACUTE SPASMODIC LARYNGITIS	ACUTE TRACHEITIS
Age-group affected	2-8 years	Infant or child under 5 years	1-3 years	1 month–6 years
Etiologic agent	Bacterial	Viral	Viral with allergic component	Viral or bacterial with allergic component
Onset	Rapidly progressive	Slowly progressive	Sudden; at night	Moderately progressive
Major symptoms	Dysphagia	URI	URI	URI
	Stridor aggravated when supine	Stridor	Croupy cough	Croupy cough
	Drooling	Brassy cough	Stridor	Purulent secretions
	High fever	Hoarseness	Hoarseness	High fever
	Toxic appearance	Dyspnea	Dyspnea	No response to LTB therapy
	Rapid pulse and respirations	Restlessness	Restlessness	
		Irritability	Symptoms awakening child but disappearing during day	
		Low-grade fever	Tendency to recur	
		Nontoxic appearance		
Treatment	Airway protection	Racemic epinephrine	Cool mist	Antibiotics
	Racemic epinephrine	Corticosteroids		Fluids
	Corticosteroids	Fluids		
	Fluids	Reassurance		
	Antibiotics			
	Reassurance			

URI, Upper respiratory infection.

CROUP SYNDROMES

Croup is a general term applied to a symptom complex characterized by hoarseness, a resonant cough described as "barking" or "brassy" (croupy), varying degrees of inspiratory stridor, and varying degrees of respiratory distress resulting from swelling or obstruction in the region of the larynx. Acute infections of the larynx are important in infants and small children because of their increased incidence in these age-groups and because the small diameter of the airway in infants and children places them at risk for significant narrowing with inflammation.

Croup syndromes can affect the larynx, trachea, and bronchi. However, laryngeal involvement often dominates the clinical picture because of the severe effects on the voice and breathing. Croup syndromes are described according to the primary anatomic area affected (i.e., epiglottitis [or supraglottitis], laryngitis, laryngotracheobronchitis [LTB], and tracheitis). In general, LTB occurs in very young children, and epiglottitis is more common in older children. A comparison of croup syndromes is provided in Table 23-1.

With widespread immunization programs aimed at preventing *H. influenzae* type b, the cause of most cases of croup in the United States is attributed to viruses, namely parainfluenza virus, human metapneumovirus, influenza types A and B, adenovirus, and measles.

ACUTE EPIGLOTTITIS

Acute epiglottitis, or **acute supraglottitis,** is a serious obstructive inflammatory process that occurs predominantly in children 2 to 8 years of age (Rotta and Wiryawan, 2003), but can occur from infancy to adulthood. The disorder requires immediate attention. The obstruction is supraglottic as opposed to the subglottic obstruction of laryngitis. The responsible organism is usually *H. influenzae*. LTB and epiglottitis do not occur together.

Clinical Manifestations

The onset of epiglottitis is abrupt, and it can rapidly progress to severe respiratory distress. The child usually goes to bed asymptomatic to awaken later, complaining of sore throat and pain on swallowing. The child has a fever; appears sicker than clinical findings suggest; and insists on sitting upright and leaning forward, with the chin thrust out, mouth open, and tongue protruding (**tripod position**). Drooling of saliva is common because of the difficulty or pain on swallowing and excessive secretions.

> **NURSINGALERT**
>
> Three clinical observations that are predictive of epiglottitis are absence of spontaneous cough, presence of drooling, and agitation.

The child is irritable and extremely restless and has an anxious, apprehensive, and frightened expression. The voice is thick and muffled, with a froglike croaking sound on inspiration, but the child is not hoarse. Suprasternal and substernal retractions may be evident. The child seldom struggles to breathe, and slow, quiet breathing provides better air exchange. The sallow color of mild hypoxia may progress to frank cyanosis. The throat is red and inflamed, and a distinctive large, cherry red, edematous epiglottis is visible on careful throat inspection.

> **NURSINGALERT**
>
> Throat inspection should be attempted only when immediate endotracheal intubation can be performed if needed.

Therapeutic Management

The course of epiglottitis may be fulminant, with respiratory obstruction appearing suddenly. Progressive obstruction leads to hypoxia, hypercapnia, and acidosis followed by decreased muscular tone; reduced level of consciousness; and, when obstruction becomes more or less complete, a rather sudden death. A presumptive diagnosis of epiglottitis constitutes an emergency.

The child who is suspected of having epiglottitis should be examined in a setting where emergency airway equipment is readily available. Examination of the throat with a tongue depressor is contraindicated until experienced personnel and equipment are available to proceed with immediate intubation or tracheostomy in the event that the examination precipitates further or complete obstruction.

If a lateral neck film is indicated, experienced personnel should accompany the child to the radiology department. For a young child who is likely to become more agitated by the procedure, it is preferable that the child not be transported but remain on the parent's lap in the examination area during portable radiology. Other procedures, such as insertion of an intravenous (IV) line, that are likely to further agitate the child are delayed until adequate airway is maintained.

Nasotracheal intubation or tracheostomy is usually considered for the child with epiglottitis with severe respiratory distress. It is recommended that the intubation or tracheostomy and any invasive procedure, such as starting an IV infusion, be performed in an area where emergency airway maintenance can be easily and quickly accomplished. Humidified oxygen is administered as necessary either via mask in older children or flowby in younger children to avoid further agitation. Whether or not there is an artificial airway, the child requires intensive observation by experienced personnel. The epiglottal swelling usually decreases after 24 hours of antibiotic therapy, and the epiglottis is near normal by the third day. Intubated children are generally extubated at this time. Additional treatment for children with moderate or severe disease includes administration of nebulized epinephrine (racemic epinephrine) or a mixture of helium and oxygen (heliox) to decrease edema. The use of corticosteroids for reducing edema has become a mainstay in the treatment of epiglottitis. Oral corticosteroid is preferred, but other routes of administration include IM, IV, and nebulized (Wright, Rowe, Arent, and others, 2005).

Children with suspected bacterial epiglottitis are given antibiotics intravenously, followed by oral administration to complete a 7- to 10-day course.

Nursing Care Management

Epiglottitis is a serious and frightening disease for the child and family. It is important to act quickly but calmly and to provide support without increasing anxiety. The child is allowed to remain in the position that provides the most comfort and security, and parents are reassured that everything possible is being done to obtain relief for their child.

> **NURSINGALERT**
>
> When epiglottitis is suspected, the nurse should not attempt to visualize the epiglottis directly with a tongue depressor or take a throat culture but should refer the child for medical evaluation immediately (see Critical Thinking Exercise).

Acute care of the child is the same as that described later for the child with LTB. Continuous monitoring of respiratory status, including pulse oximetry (and blood gases if the patient is intubated), is an important part of nursing observa-

CRITICAL THINKING EXERCISE

Croup Syndrome

Kim, a 6-year-old, is admitted to the emergency department in the early evening hours with a sore throat, pain on swallowing, drooling, and a fever of 39° C (102.2° F). She looks ill, her skin is flushed, she is agitated, and she prefers to sit up, leaning on her arms. According to the child's mother, she has not had anything to eat or drink in 2 or 3 days. What nursing interventions should the nurse implement in this situation?

QUESTIONS

1. Evidence—Is there sufficient evidence to draw any conclusions about Kim's condition at this time?
2. Assumptions—Describe some underlying assumptions about each of the following:
   a. Epiglottitis in children
   b. Symptoms of epiglottitis
   c. Precautions to be taken when a child has suspected epiglottitis
   d. Immediate nursing interventions when caring for a child with epiglottitis
3. What priorities for nursing care can be drawn at this time?
4. Does the evidence objectively support your argument (conclusion)?
5. Are there alternative perspectives to your arguments? What are they?

tions, and the IV infusion is maintained as described in Chapter 22.

ACUTE LARYNGITIS

Acute infectious laryngitis is a common illness in older children and adolescents. Infants and smaller children experience more generalized involvement (see the following section on LTB). Viruses are the usual causative agents, and the principal complaint is hoarseness, which may be accompanied by other upper respiratory symptoms (e.g., rhinitis, sore throat, nasal congestion) and systemic manifestations (e.g., fever, headache, myalgia, malaise). Associated complaints vary with the infecting virus. Adenoviruses, human metapneumoviruses, and influenza viruses are responsible for more systemic involvement; parainfluenza viruses, rhinoviruses, and RSV cause milder illness.

Therapeutic Management and Nursing Care Management

The disease is usually self-limited without long-term sequelae. Treatment is symptomatic with fluids and humidified air (see Nursing Care Plan, pp. 759-761).

ACUTE LARYNGOTRACHEOBRONCHITIS

LTB is the most common croup syndrome. It primarily affects children younger than 5 years of age, and the causative organisms are the parainfluenza virus types 2 and 3, human metapneumovirus, RSV, influenza A and B, and *M. pneumoniae*. The disease is usually preceded by a URI, which gradually descends to adjacent structures. It is characterized by gradual onset of low-grade fever, and the parents often report that the child went to bed and later awoke with a barky, brassy cough. Inflammation of the mucosa lining the larynx and trachea causes a narrowing of the airway. When the airway is significantly narrowed, the child struggles to inhale air past the ob-

BOX 23-8
Progression of Symptoms in Laryngotracheobronchitis

STAGE I
Fear
Hoarseness
Croupy cough
Inspiratory stridor when disturbed

STAGE II
Continuous respiratory stridor
Substernal retraction
Suprasternal retraction (retraction of soft tissue of neck)
Use of accessory muscles of respiration
Labored respiration

STAGE III
Signs of anoxia and carbon dioxide retention
Restlessness
Anxiety
Pallor
Sweating
Tachypnea

STAGE IV
Intermittent cyanosis
Permanent cyanosis
Cessation of breathing

From Walter EB, Shurin PA: Acute respiratory infections. In Krugman S, Katz SL, Gershon AA, and others, editors: *Infectious diseases of children*, ed 9, St Louis, 1992, Mosby.

struction and into the lungs, producing the characteristic inspiratory stridor and suprasternal retractions; other classic manifestations include cough and hoarseness. Respiratory distress in infants and toddlers may be manifested by nasal flaring, intercostal retractions, tachypnea, and continuous stridor. The typical child with LTB is a toddler who develops the classic barking or seal-like cough and acute stridor after several days of rhinitis. When the child is unable to inhale a sufficient volume of air, symptoms of hypoxia become evident. Obstruction that is severe enough to prevent adequate ventilation and exhalation of carbon dioxide can cause respiratory acidosis and eventually respiratory failure. The progression of symptoms is outlined in Box 23-8.

Therapeutic Management

The major objective in medical management is maintaining the airway and providing adequate respiratory exchange. Children with mild croup (no stridor at rest) can be managed at home. Parents are taught the signs of respiratory distress and instructed to summon professional help early if needed. Children who progress to stage II respiratory symptoms should receive medical attention (see Box 23-8).

High humidity with cool mist provides relief for most children. A cool-air vaporizer can be used at home. In the hospital, a nebulized mist for older infants and toddlers may be used to provide increased humidity and supplemental oxygen. However, controversy surrounds the use of mist therapy to treat croup. Studies have failed to demonstrate any improvement in subglottic edema with mist therapy (Moore and Little, 2006).

Nebulized epinephrine (racemic epinephrine) is often used in children with severe disease, stridor at rest, retractions, or difficulty breathing. The α-adrenergic effects cause mucosal vasoconstriction and subsequently decrease subglottic edema. The onset of action is rapid, and the peak effect is observed in 2 hours. Children may be discharged home following racemic epinephrine after a 2- to 3-hour period of observation for return of acute symptoms.

Oral steroids have proven effective in the treatment of croup; IM dexamethasone may be given to children who are

unable to tolerate oral dosing. Nebulized budesonide may be administered in conjunction with IM dexamethasone. A single dose of oral corticosteroid has been shown to decrease hospitalizations and the need for multiple racemic epinephrine treatments in children with mild croup.

In severe cases of LTB the administration of heliox may serve to reduce the work of breathing and relieve airway obstruction. Because helium has a lower density than room air, it forms a respirable gas (with oxygen) that reduces airway turbulence.

Nursing Care Management

The most important nursing function in the care of children with LTB is continuous, vigilant observation and accurate assessment of respiratory status. Pulse oximetry is commonly used for monitoring oxygenation status. Changes in therapy are frequently based on the nurses' observations and assessments, the child's response to therapy, and tolerance of procedures. The trend away from early intubation of children with LTB emphasizes the importance of nursing observations and the ability to recognize impending respiratory failure so that intubation can be implemented without delay. Intubation equipment must be readily accessible and taken with the child during transport to other areas (e.g., radiology, operating room).

NURSING ALERT

Early signs of impending airway obstruction include increased pulse and respiratory rate; substernal, suprasternal, and intercostal retractions; flaring nares; and increased restlessness.

Infants or small children find that being enclosed in a tent, coughing, having laryngeal spasms, and needing IV therapy are additional sources of distress. In many acute care facilities the mist tent has been abandoned and the infant is allowed to be held by the parent; if cool mist is used in the treatment, it can be administered through a tube held in front of the patient while the child is held on the parent's lap.

Children with mild croup are allowed to drink beverages they like as long as respiratory status is stable, and parents are encouraged to try whatever comforting measures work best (e.g., holding their child, rocking, singing). If the child is unable to take oral fluids, IV fluids may be required in addition to IV medications (dexamethasone).

The rapid progression of croup, the alarming sound of the cough and stridor, and the child's apprehensive behavior and ill appearance combine to create a frightening experience for the parents. Parents need reassurance regarding their child's progress and an explanation of treatments. The family should be allowed to remain with their child as much as possible.

The nurse should provide the parents with an opportunity to express their feelings and referrals as necessary. Parents need frequent reassurance provided in a calm, quiet manner and education regarding what they can do to make their child more comfortable. Home care includes continued humidity, adequate hydration, and nourishment.

ACUTE SPASMODIC LARYNGITIS

Acute spasmodic laryngitis (**spasmodic croup,** "midnight croup," or "twilight croup") is distinct from laryngitis and LTB and is characterized by paroxysmal attacks of laryngeal obstruction that occur chiefly at night. Signs of inflammation are absent or mild, and there is often a history of previous attacks lasting 2 to 5 days, followed by uneventful recovery. This condition usually affects children ages 1 to 3 years. Some children appear to be predisposed to the condition; allergies may be implicated in some cases.

The child goes to bed feeling well or with mild respiratory symptoms but awakens suddenly with characteristic barking, metallic cough; hoarseness; noisy inspirations; and restlessness. The child appears anxious and frightened. Dyspnea is aggravated by excitement, but there is no fever, the attack subsides in a few hours, and the child appears well the next day.

Therapeutic Management and Nursing Care Management

Spasmodic croup is usually self-limiting, and most children are managed at home. A cool mist humidifier may be recommended for home treatment. Sometimes the spasm is relieved by sudden exposure to cold air (as when the child is taken out into the night air to see the practitioner). Parents are usually advised to have the child sleep in humidified air until the cough has subsided to prevent subsequent episodes. Children with moderately severe symptoms may be hospitalized for observation and therapy with cool mist and racemic epinephrine, as for LTB. Some patients respond to corticosteroid therapy.

BACTERIAL TRACHEITIS

Bacterial tracheitis, an infection of the mucosa of the upper trachea, is a distinct entity with features of both croup and epiglottitis. The disease occurs in children under 3 years of age and may be a serious cause of airway obstruction that is severe enough to cause respiratory arrest. It is believed to be a com-

plication of LTB, and although *Staphylococcus aureus* is the most frequent organism responsible, *M. catarrhalis, S. pneumonia,* and *H. influenzae* have also been implicated.

Many of the manifestations of bacterial tracheitis are similar to those of LTB but are unresponsive to LTB therapy. There is a history of previous URI with croupy cough, stridor unaffected by position, toxicity, absence of drooling, and high fever. A prominent manifestation is the production of thick, purulent tracheal secretions. Respiratory difficulties are secondary to these copious secretions. Children with this condition may develop a life-threatening upper airway obstruction, respiratory failure, acute respiratory distress syndrome (ARDS), and multiple organ dysfunction (Hopkins, Lahiri, Salerno, and others, 2006).

Therapeutic Management and Nursing Care Management

Bacterial tracheitis requires vigorous management with antipyretics and antibiotics. Many children require endotracheal intubation and mechanical ventilation; patients are closely monitored for impending respiratory failure if not intubated. Early recognition to prevent life-threatening airway obstruction is essential.

INFECTIONS OF THE LOWER AIRWAYS

The **reactive portion** of the lower respiratory tract includes the bronchi and bronchioles in children. Cartilaginous support of the large airways is not fully developed until adolescence. Consequently, the smooth muscle in these structures represents a major factor in the constriction of the airway, particularly in the bronchioles, that portion that extends from the bronchi to the alveoli. Table 23-2 compares some of the major features of bronchial and bronchiolar infections.

TABLE 23-2
Comparison of Conditions Affecting the Bronchi

	ASTHMA*	BRONCHITIS	BRONCHIOLITIS
Description	Exaggerated response of bronchi to a trigger such as URI, dander, cold air, exercise. Bronchospasm, exudation, and edema of bronchi	Usually occurs in association with URI. Seldom an isolated entity	Most common infectious disease of lower airways. Maximum obstructive impact at bronchiolar level
Age-group affected	Infancy to adolescence	First 4 years of life	Usually children 2-12 months of age; rare after age 2 years
Etiologic agents	Most often viruses such as RSV in infants, but may be any of a variety of URI pathogens	Usually viral. Other agents (e.g., bacteria, fungi, allergic disorders, airborne irritants) can trigger symptoms	Peak incidence approximately age 6 months. Viruses, predominantly respiratory syncytial viruses; also adenoviruses, parainfluenza viruses, human metapneumovirus, and *Mycoplasma pneumoniae*
Predominant characteristics	Wheezing, cough	Persistent dry, hacking cough (worse at night) becoming productive in 2-3 days	Labored respirations, poor feeding, cough, tachypnea, retractions and flaring nares, emphysema, increased nasal mucus, wheezing, may have fever
Treatment	Inhaled corticosteroids, bronchodilators, leukotriene modifiers, allergen and "triggers" control	Cough suppressants if needed	Supplemental oxygen if saturations ≤90%; bronchodilators (optional). Suctioning nasopharynx. Ensure adequate fluid intake. Maintain adequate oxygenation

*See Asthma, p. 783.
URI, Upper respiratory infection.

BRONCHITIS

Bronchitis (sometimes referred to as **tracheobronchitis**) is inflammation of the large airways (trachea and bronchi), which is frequently associated with a URI. Viral agents are the primary cause of the disease, although *M. pneumoniae* is a common cause in children older than 6 years of age. A dry, hacking, nonproductive cough that worsens at night and becomes productive in 2 or 3 days characterizes this condition.

Bronchitis is a mild, self-limiting disease that requires only symptomatic treatment, including analgesics, antipyretics, and humidity. Cough suppressants may be useful to allow rest but can interfere with clearance of secretions. Most patients recover uneventfully in 5 to 10 days.

RESPIRATORY SYNCYTIAL VIRUS AND BRONCHIOLITIS

Bronchiolitis is an acute viral infection with maximum effect at the bronchiolar level. The infection occurs primarily in winter and early spring. By age 3 years most children have been infected at least once. RSV infection is the most frequent cause of hospitalization in children less than 1 year old. In addition, severe RSV infections in the first year of life represent a significant risk factor for the development of asthma up to age 13 (Chávez-Bueno, Mejías, Jafri, and others, 2005). RSV infection may also occur in children older than 1 year who have a chronic or serious disabling illness. Although most cases of bronchiolitis are caused by RSV, adenoviruses and parainfluenza viruses are also implicated; recently, human metapneumovirus has also been associated with bronchiolitis in children.

Pathophysiology

RSV affects the epithelial cells of the respiratory tract. The ciliated cells swell, protrude into the lumen, and lose their cilia. RSV produces a fusion of the infected cell membrane with cell membranes of adjacent epithelial cells, thus forming a giant cell with multiple nuclei. At the cellular level this fusion results in multinucleated masses of protoplasm, or **syncytia.**

The bronchiolar mucosa swells, and lumina are subsequently filled with mucus and exudate. The walls of the bronchi and bronchioles are infiltrated with inflammatory cells, and peribronchiolar interstitial pneumonitis is usually present. Because luminal epithelial cells are shed into the bronchioles when they die, the lumina are frequently obstructed, particularly on expiration. The varying degrees of obstruction produced in small air passages lead to hyperinflation, obstructive emphysema resulting from partial obstruction, and patchy areas of atelectasis. Dilation of bronchial passages on inspiration allows sufficient space for intake of air, but narrowing of the passages on expiration prevents air from leaving the lungs. Thus air is trapped distal to the obstruction and causes progressive overinflation (emphysema).

Clinical Manifestations

The illness usually begins with a URI after an incubation of about 5 to 8 days. Symptoms such as rhinorrhea and low-grade fever often appear first. OM and conjunctivitis may also be present. In time a cough may develop. If the disease progresses, it becomes a lower respiratory tract infection and manifests typical symptoms (Box 23-9). Infants may have several days of URI symptoms or no symptoms except slight lethargy, poor feeding, or irritability.

Once the lower airway is involved, classic manifestations include signs of altered air exchange, such as wheezing, retractions, crackles, dyspnea, tachypnea, and diminished breath sounds. Apnea may be the first recognized indicator of RSV infection in very young infants.

Diagnostic Evaluation

Identification has been simplified by the development of tests done on nasal or nasopharyngeal secretions, using either a rapid immunofluorescent antibody–direct fluorescent antibody staining (DFA) or an enzyme-linked immunosorbent assay (ELISA) for RSV antigen detection (see Respiratory Secretion and Throat Specimens, Chapter 22).

Therapeutic Management

Bronchiolitis is treated symptomatically with cool humidified oxygen, adequate fluid intake, airway maintenance, and medications. Most children with bronchiolitis can be managed at home. Hospitalization is usually recommended for children with respiratory distress or those who cannot maintain adequate hydration. Other reasons for hospitalization include complicating conditions, such as underlying lung or heart disease or associated debilitated states, or a home environment where adequate management is questionable. The infant who is tachypneic or apneic, has marked retractions, seems listless, or has a history of poor fluid intake should be admitted.

Humidified oxygen is administered in concentrations sufficient to maintain adequate oxygenation (SpO_2) at or above 90% as measured by pulse oximetry. The administration of humidified mist is controversial. Routine chest physical therapy (CPT) is not recommended; infants with abundant nasal secretions benefit from periodic suctioning. Fluids by mouth may be contraindicated because of tachypnea, weakness, and fatigue; therefore IV fluids are preferred until the acute stage of the disease has passed.

Clinical assessments, noninvasive oxygen monitoring, and blood gas values guide therapy. Medical therapy for bronchiolitis is primarily supportive and aimed at decreasing airway hyperresonance and inflammation and promoting adequate fluid intake. Bronchodilators may provide short-term benefits, yet overall significant improvement in the child's condition is not always appreciable. Racemic epinephrine has been shown to produce modest improvement in ventilation status. Corti-

---

BOX 23-9

Signs and Symptoms of Respiratory Syncytial Virus

INITIAL	SEVERE ILLNESS
Rhinorrhea	Tachypnea, greater than
Pharyngitis	70 breaths/min
Coughing, sneezing	Listlessness
Wheezing	Apneic spells
Possible ear or eye drainage	Poor air exchange; poor breath
Intermittent fever	sounds

WITH PROGRESSION OF ILLNESS
Increased coughing and wheezing
Tachypnea and retractions
Cyanosis

costeroids and antihistamines have not been shown to be effective in controlled studies and are not recommended for routine use. Antibiotics are not part of the treatment of RSV unless there is a coexisting bacterial infection such as OM (American Academy of Pediatrics, 2006a). Additional treatment recommendations in the American Academy of Pediatrics (2006a) practice guideline are to encourage breastfeeding; avoid passive tobacco smoke exposure; and promote preventive measures, including hand washing and the administration of palivizumab (Synagis) to high-risk infants.

Ribavirin, an antiviral agent (synthetic nucleoside analog), is the only specific therapy approved for hospitalized children; however, use of this drug is controversial because of concerns about the high cost, aerosol route of administration, potential toxic effects among exposed health care personnel, and conflicting results of efficacy trials (American Academy of Pediatrics, 2006a; Chávez-Bueno, Mejías, Jafri, and others, 2005; Ventre and Randolph, 2007). This drug is aerosolized and delivered via a small-particle aerosol generator. It may be administered by hood, tent, or mask or through ventilator tubing for 12 to 20 hours daily; average duration of therapy is 3 days.

Prevention of RSV Infection

The only product available in the United States for prevention of RSV is palivizumab, a monoclonal antibody, which is given monthly in an IM injection. According to the American Academy of Pediatrics (2006a) practice guideline, candidates for palivizumab include infants born before 32 weeks' gestation who required medical therapy such as supplemental oxygen or mechanical ventilation. Infants and children younger than 2 years of age with BPD who have received medical therapy (supplemental oxygen, bronchodilator, diuretic, or corticosteroid therapy) for BPD within 6 months before the anticipated RSV season may benefit from palivizumab prophylaxis. Children with more severe BPD may benefit from palivizumab prophylaxis for two RSV seasons. Children with severe immunodeficiencies (e.g., severe combined immunodeficiency or acquired immunodeficiency syndrome [AIDS]) may also benefit from prophylaxis. Infants and children younger than 2 years of age with hemodynamically significant congenital heart disease will benefit from 5 monthly IM injections of palivizumab. Prophylaxis for RSV should be initiated at the onset of the RSV season and terminated at the end of the season (November to March). Additional age and condition recommendations are outlined in the American Academy of Pediatrics practice guideline (2006a).

> **NURSINGALERT**
>
> The lyophilized powder form of palivizumab should be administered within 6 hours of being reconstituted with sterile water because it is preservative free.

A second-generation monoclonal antibody, motavizumab, is currently undergoing phase III clinical trials; this drug is reported to be more effective in the prevention of RSV than palivizumab (DeVincenzo, 2008).

Nursing Care Management

Children admitted to the hospital with suspected RSV infection may be assigned separate rooms or grouped with other RSV-infected children. Contact and standard precautions are employed, including hand washing, not touching the nasal mucosa or conjunctiva, and using gloves and gowns when entering the patient's room. Other isolation procedures of potential benefit are those aimed at diminishing the number of hospital personnel, visitors, and uninfected children in contact with the child. Another measure is to make patient assignments so that nurses assigned to children with RSV are not caring for other patients who are considered high risk.

Infants with RSV often have copious nasal secretions, making breathing and nursing or bottle-feeding difficult. This engenders concerns that the child will lose weight or stop breastfeeding altogether. Encourage breastfeeding mothers to continue feeding the infant or, if feedings are contraindicated due to the acuity of the illness, mothers should pump their milk and store appropriately for later use (see Chapter 8). Parents are taught how to instill normal saline drops into the nares and suction the mucus with a bulb syringe before feedings and before bedtime so the child may eat and rest better; unfortunately no medications appropriate for infants can help with these symptoms. To address the issue of decreased fluid intake, parents may offer small amounts of clear fluids, 5 to 10 ml at a time, with a medication syringe every 10 minutes or so to maintain adequate hydration. Infants may cough or vomit as the secretions settle in the stomach and make them prone to emesis of such secretions.

Additional nursing care is aimed at monitoring oxygenation with pulse oximetry, ensuring bronchodilator therapy is optimized by using a small mask for delivery, and providing information for the parent regarding the infant's status. The unpredictability of the infant's individual response to the disease compounds parental anxiety when they hear about children who had serious morbidity or died from RSV. However, for the most part infants recover quickly from the disease and resume normal daily activities, including fluid intake. Such infants are at risk for further episodes of wheezing that may or may not involve an RSV infection; parents, however, may be concerned that the infant has another serious case of RSV.

PNEUMONIAS

Pneumonia, inflammation of the pulmonary parenchyma, is common in childhood but occurs more frequently in infancy and early childhood. Clinically, pneumonia may occur either as a primary disease or as a complication of another illness. The various types of pneumonia include:

Lobar pneumonia—All or a large segment of one or more pulmonary lobes is involved.

Bronchopneumonia—This begins in the terminal bronchioles, which become clogged with mucopurulent exudate to form consolidated patches in nearby lobules; also called **lobular pneumonia.**

Interstitial pneumonia—The inflammatory process is more or less confined within the alveolar walls (interstitium) and the peribronchial and interlobular tissues.

Although the morphologic classification is typically used, the most useful classification of pneumonia is based on the etiologic agent (e.g., viral, bacterial, mycoplasmal, or aspiration of foreign substances) (see Aspiration Pneumonia, p. 781). Histomycosis, coccidioidomycosis, and other fungi also cause pneumonia. Other terms that describe pneumonias are *hemorrhagic, fibrinous,* and *necrotizing.* **Pneumonitis** is a

---

BOX 23-10

General Signs of Pneumonia

Fever—Usually high
Respiratory
- Cough—Unproductive to productive with white sputum
- Tachypnea
- Breath sounds—Crackles, decreased breath sounds, rales
- Dullness with percussion
- Chest pain
- Retractions
- Nasal flaring
- Pallor to cyanosis (depends on severity)

Chest x-ray film—Diffuse or patchy infiltration with peribronchial distribution
Behavior—Irritability, restlessness, malaise, lethargy
Gastrointestinal—Anorexia, vomiting, diarrhea, abdominal pain

---

localized acute inflammation of the lung without the toxemia associated with lobar pneumonia.

The clinical manifestations of pneumonia vary depending on the etiologic agent, the child's age, the child's systemic reaction to the infection, the extent of the lesions, and the degree of bronchial and bronchiolar obstruction. The causative agent is identified from the clinical history, the child's age, the general health history, the physical examination, radiography, and the laboratory examination.

Viral Pneumonia

Viral pneumonias, which occur more frequently than bacterial pneumonias, are seen in children of all ages and are often associated with viral URIs. Viruses that cause pneumonia include RSV in infants and parainfluenza, influenza, human metapneumovirus, and adenovirus in older children. There are few clinical symptoms that are unique to a specific virus, and differentiation among viruses is usually made by clinical features such as child's age, past medical history, season of the year, and radiographic and laboratory examination (Box 23-10).

The prognosis is generally good, although viral infections of the respiratory tract render the affected child more susceptible to secondary bacterial invasion, especially when there is denuded bronchial mucosa. Treatment is symptomatic and includes measures to promote oxygenation and comfort, such as oxygen administration with cool mist, CPT and postural drainage, antipyretics for fever management, fluid intake, and family support. Some authorities recommend antimicrobial therapy in the hopes of reducing or preventing secondary bacterial infection, but this therapy should be reserved for children in whom a bacterial infection is demonstrated by appropriate cultures.

Primary Atypical Pneumonia

Atypical pneumonia refers to pneumonia that is caused by pathogens other than the traditionally most common and readily cultured bacteria (e.g., *S. pneumoniae*). In the category of atypical pneumonias, *M. pneumoniae* and *Chlamydia pneumoniae* are the most common cause of community-acquired pneumonia in children 5 years or older (Rafei and Lichenstein, 2006). It occurs in the fall and winter months and is more

prevalent in crowded living conditions. Most affected persons recover from acute illness in 7 to 10 days with symptomatic treatment, followed by a week of convalescence. Hospitalization is rarely necessary.

Severe Acute Respiratory Syndrome

A severe form of atypical pneumonia identified as severe acute respiratory syndrome (SARS) was first reported in Asia in 2003. SARS is caused by a previously unrecognized coronavirus called SARS-associated coronavirus (SARS Co-V). Additional human coronavirus types have since been identified in Canada, Hong Kong, and the Netherlands. Clinical manifestations of this disorder include a fever greater than 38° C (100.4° F); headache; cough; shortness of breath; difficulty breathing; and, after 2 to 7 days, a dry, nonproductive cough and dyspnea. In some patients the symptoms are severe enough to require intubation and mechanical ventilation. The disease is spread by close contact with a person with SARS. Most cases have involved people who have cared for or lived with someone with SARS or people who have traveled to areas with reported cases of SARS.

In children, two distinct forms of the illness have been observed. Adolescents have malaise, myalgia, chills, and rigor, whereas young children have mainly cough and runny nose. In younger children the clinical course seems to be milder and the disease resolves more quickly than in adolescents or adults (Denison, 2005; Stockman, Massoudi, Helfand, and others, 2007).

Laboratory findings include lymphopenia; leukopenia; thrombocytopenia; and elevated lactate dehydrogenase, aspartate aminotransferase, and creatinine kinase levels. The most reliable laboratory diagnostic test is positive antibodies for the SARS Co-V. Chest radiographs in a substantial number of patients reveal focal interstitial infiltrates that progress to more generalized, patchy interstitial infiltrates.

Treatment of SARS involves predominantly supportive care measures. Other therapies such as antibiotics, antiviral drugs such as ribavirin, and steroids have been used with mixed results (O'Connor, 2003).

Nursing Care Management. The Centers for Disease Control and Prevention recommends that patients with SARS receive the same treatment as any patient with serious community-acquired atypical pneumonia. This includes the use of strict hand washing, contact precautions, and airborne precautions (e.g., an isolation room with negative pressure relative to the surrounding area and the use of an N95 filtering disposable respirator for persons entering the room). Recommendations for stopping the spread of SARS have also been developed. When triaging patients, nurses should place a surgical mask on any patient who has had close contact with someone who has SARS or who has a history of international travel to an area with cases of SARS. Health care workers who have had high-risk, unprotected exposure to SARS should be excluded from duty and remain home from work to monitor their health for 10 days.

Avian Influenza Virus

Several types of influenza were identified in Asian countries that caused mild to severe disease in adults and children. The avian influenza that has resulted in several deaths in Hong Kong, Vietnam, and Thailand has been identified as subtypes H5 and H7 and has as its host chickens and wild ducks, in which the mortality rates range from 90% to 100% (Lee and Krilov, 2005). The virus has also been reported to spread among other animals such as pigs and tigers. In humans the viral manifestations of avian influenza often consist of fever and respiratory symptoms—sore throat, rhinorrhea, and cough—occurring within 3 to 5 days of illness (Chokephaibulkit, 2004). Laboratory findings include leukopenia and thrombocytopenia, and moderately elevated liver transaminases are often identified. Patients may rapidly progress to ARDS with acute lung injury. In some children the virus is manifest only as an eye infection (conjunctivitis).

Treatment is aimed at prompt diagnosis and intervention to reduce the onset of ARDS. The virus may respond to influenza drugs such as amantadine, rimantadine, oseltamivir, and zanamivir, but cases of avian flu in Southeast Asia were resistant to amantadine and rimantadine (Lee and Krilov, 2005). Rimantadine is not indicated for children. At present laboratory testing in the United States is indicated only in the case of a hospitalized patient with a severe respiratory illness without a diagnosis who has traveled to a country with documented avian influenza (Lee and Krilov, 2005). To obtain updated information on the emergence and progress in treatment of these and other respiratory viruses, the reader is encouraged to visit the Centers for Disease Control and Prevention website.*

Bacterial Pneumonia

S. pneumoniae is the most common bacterial pathogen responsible for community-acquired pneumonia in both children and adults (Rafei and Lichenstein, 2006). Other bacteria that cause pneumonia in children are group A streptococcus, *S. aureus, M. catarrhalis, M. pneumoniae,* and *C. pneumoniae.*

Beyond the neonatal period, bacterial pneumonias display distinct clinical patterns that facilitate their differentiation from other forms of pneumonia. The onset of illness is abrupt and generally follows a viral infection that disturbs the natural defense mechanisms of the upper respiratory tract.

The child with bacterial pneumonia usually appears ill. Symptoms include fever, malaise, rapid and shallow respirations, cough, and chest pain. The pain of pneumonia may be referred to the abdomen and confused with appendicitis. Chills and meningeal symptoms (**meningism**) are common.

Most older children with pneumonia can be treated at home if the condition is recognized and treatment is initiated early. Antibiotic therapy, bed rest, liberal oral intake of fluid, and administration of an antipyretic for fever are the principal therapeutic measures. Follow-up examination is recommended for small infants and toddlers. Hospitalization is indicated when pleural effusion or empyema accompanies the disease, in situations where compliance with therapy is estimated to be poor, in infants less than 1 month old, and when there are chronic illnesses such as congenital heart disease or BPD (Rafei and Lichenstein, 2006). IV fluids may be necessary to ensure adequate hydration, and oxygen is required if the child is in respiratory distress; some children may require initial therapy with parenteral antibiotics due to the severity of illness.

Complications. At present the classic features and clinical course of pneumonia are seen infrequently because of early and vigorous antibiotic and supportive therapy. However, some children, especially infants, with staphylococcal

pneumonia develop empyema, pyopneumothorax, or tension pneumothorax. AOM and pleural effusion are common in children with pneumococcal pneumonia.

Continuous closed chest drainage may be instituted when purulent fluid is aspirated. If a large amount of purulent drainage is obtained, an appropriate antibiotic is instilled into the chest cavity, and chest drainage is discontinued for approximately 1 hour after the instillation. Closed drainage is continued until drainage fluid is free of pathogens, which rarely requires more than 5 to 7 days. Sometimes, repeated pleural taps are sufficient to remove fluid; however, if the purulent drainage accumulates rapidly and is highly viscous, continuous drainage is preferred. Thoracotomy with open debridement of the infected lung tissue may be required; if empyema and pneumothorax tend to recur, a partial thoracoscopic lobectomy may be performed.

Prognosis. The prognosis for pneumonia is generally good, with rapid recovery when symptoms are recognized and treated early. Streptococcal infections vary in duration but usually resolve spontaneously. The course of staphylococcal pneumonia is generally prolonged. The prognosis varies with the length of illness before treatment is begun, although early recognition and treatment are usually effective.

Prevention. The use of the heptavalent pneumococcal vaccine (PCV; Prevnar) is recommended for infants and children younger than 23 months of age to be administered at 2, 4, 6, 12, and 15 months of age; studies have demonstrated a decrease in pneumococcal pneumonia in children less than 24 months. The polyvalent pneumococcal vaccine (PPV) provides protection from pneumococcal serotypes in children 24 months old and older (American Academy of Pediatrics, 2006b). (See Immunizations, Chapter 10.)

Nursing Care Management

For the child being cared for at home the nurse educates the parent regarding antibiotic and antipyretic administration, assessment of respiratory status, and oral fluid intake. If the child is ill, solid foods may be rejected; fluid intake is encouraged until the child feels well enough to eat solids. Parents are reassured that the child's appetite will return once the acute phase of the illness has passed. If the cough is disturbing, judicious use of antitussives, especially at bed time, is often helpful. Most sick children are adept at self-regulation of activity and rest; parents are encouraged to allow the child appropriate rest and discourage vigorous activities until the child has been afebrile for 24 hours or more. Return to school or daycare is usually permitted according to the type of pneumonia, severity of illness, and practitioner recommendation. It should be emphasized that the infection may be transmitted to other children with close contact.

Nursing care of the hospitalized child with pneumonia is primarily supportive and symptomatic but necessitates thorough respiratory assessment, antibiotics, and evaluation of hydration status; supplemental oxygen may be required if oxygenation status is compromised. The child's respiratory rate and oxygenation status, as well as vital signs, pain level, and general disposition and level of activity, are frequently assessed. Isolation procedures are implemented according to hospital policy, but standard and contact precautions are recommended initially for all children with a URI until the exact cause is known. To prevent dehydration, fluids are frequently administered intravenously during the acute phase.

FIG. 23-3 ■ Child placed in semierect position is often more comfortable, and this position enhances diaphragmatic expansion.

If needed, supplemental oxygen may be administered by nasal cannula or face mask (or face tent [bucket]); small infants may be given humidified oxygen via a plastic head hood or rarely via a mist tent. Children are usually more comfortable in a semierect position (Fig. 23-3) but should be allowed to determine the position of comfort. Lying on the affected side (if pneumonia is unilateral) splints the chest on that side and reduces the pleural rubbing that often causes discomfort. Fever is controlled by the cool environment and administration of antipyretic drugs.

Children, especially infants, with ineffectual cough or difficulty handling secretions require suctioning to maintain a patent airway. A simple bulb suction syringe is usually sufficient for clearing the nares and nasopharynx of infants, but mechanical suction should be readily available if needed. A noninvasive suction device may be used to suction the infant's nares without the danger of causing nasal trauma; the device may be connected to mechanical suction for best results. Older children can usually handle secretions without assistance. Postural drainage, CPT, and nebulized bronchodilator treatments may be prescribed depending on the child's condition.

The hospitalized child may be apprehensive, and the treatments and tests are frightening and stress producing. It is important to involve the entire family in the care as appropriate and to encourage questions and facilitate effective communication. Allowing the child to be involved in regular activities such as quiet play may help reduce the anxiety of hospitalization and separation from friends and family. Reducing anxiety and apprehension reduces psychologic distress in the child, and when the child is more relaxed, the respiratory efforts are lessened. Easing respiratory efforts makes the child less apprehensive, and encouraging the presence of the caregiver provides the child with a source of comfort and support.

OTHER INFECTIONS OF THE RESPIRATORY TRACT

PERTUSSIS (WHOOPING COUGH)

Pertussis, or whooping cough, is an acute respiratory tract infection caused by *Bordetella pertussis,* which in the past primarily occurred in children younger than 4 years of age who were not immunized. It is highly contagious and is particularly

threatening in young infants, who have a higher morbidity and mortality rate. Infants less than 6 months of age may not come in to the practitioner with the typical cough; in this age-group, apnea is a common presenting manifestation (American Academy of Pediatrics, 2006b). Likewise, older children are known to manifest the disease with a persistent cough and the absence of the characteristic whoop (see Table 14-1 for signs, symptoms, and management of pertussis). The incidence is highest in the spring and summer months, and a single attack confers lifetime immunity. The resurgence of pertussis in the United States, particularly among children 10 years old and older, has prompted concerns of the long-term effects of the pertussis vaccine. Consequently two acellular pertussis booster vaccines have been approved for children: Boostrix (for children ages 10 to 18 years) and Adacel (for persons ages 11 to 64 years). (See also Immunizations, Chapter 10.)

TUBERCULOSIS

Tuberculosis (TB) is the second leading cause of death from an infectious disease. Ten million to 15 million persons in the United States are infected with TB. Case rates of TB for all ages are higher in urban, low-income areas and among non-Caucasian racial and ethnic groups. In recent years, foreign-born children have accounted for more than one fourth of newly diagnosed cases of TB in children 14 years of age or younger in the United States (American Academy of Pediatrics, 2006b).

TB is caused by *Mycobacterium tuberculosis*, an acid-fast bacillus not readily decolorized by acids after staining. Children are susceptible to the human (*M. tuberculosis*) and the bovine (*Mycobacterium bovis*) organisms. In parts of the world where TB in cattle is not controlled or milk is not pasteurized, the bovine type is a common source of infection.

Although the causative agent for TB is the tubercle bacillus, other factors influence the degree to which the organism produces an altered state in the host. These factors include heredity (resistance to the infection may be genetically transmitted), gender (higher rates in adolescent girls), age (lower resistance in infants, higher incidence during adolescence), stress (emotional or physical), nutritional state, and intercurrent infection (especially human immunodeficiency virus [HIV], measles, and pertussis). Children with HIV infection have an increased incidence of TB disease, and all children with TB should be tested for HIV.

The source of TB infection in children is usually an infected member of the household or a frequent visitor to the home such as a baby-sitter or domestic worker. The airway is the usual portal of entry for the organism. In the lungs a proliferation of epithelial cells surrounds and encapsulates the multiplying bacilli in an attempt to wall it off, thus forming the typical tubercle. Extension of the primary lesion at the original site causes progressive tissue destruction as it spreads within the lung, discharges material from foci to other areas of the lungs (e.g., bronchi, pleura), or produces pneumonia. Erosion of blood vessels by the primary lesion can cause widespread dissemination of the tubercle bacillus to near and distant sites (miliary TB). Extrapulmonary TB may be manifested as superior lymphadenitis, meningitis, and osteoarthritis and may appear in the middle ear and mastoid and on the skin (American Academy of Pediatrics, 2006b). With the exception of meningitis, treatment for extrapulmonary TB may be the same drug regimen as for pulmonary TB.

Nasopharyngeal swab, Antimicrobials, O₂ management, IV fluids, ICU, mechanical ventilation? Prevention → DTAP & Tdap

Clinical Manifestations of Tuberculosis

May be asymptomatic or produce a broad range of symptoms:
- Fever
- Malaise
- Anorexia
- Weight loss
- Cough (may or may not be present; progresses slowly over weeks to months)
- Aching pain and tightness in the chest
- Hemoptysis (rare)

With progression:
- Increasing respiratory rate
- Poor expansion of lung on the affected side
- Diminished breath sounds and crackles
- Dullness to percussion
- Persistent fever
- Generalized symptoms
- Pallor, anemia, weakness, and weight loss

Diagnostic Evaluation

Diagnosis is based on information derived from physical examination, history, tuberculin skin testing, radiographic examinations, and cultures of the organism. The clinical manifestations of the disease are extremely variable (Box 23-11).

The **tuberculin skin test (TST)** is the most important indicator of whether a child has been infected with the tubercle bacillus. The standard dose of purified protein derivative (PPD) is 5 tuberculin units, which is administered using a 27-gauge needle and a 1-ml syringe intradermally into the volar aspect of the forearm. Creation of a visible wheal is crucial to accurate testing. A change in TB screening procedures has been recommended by the American Academy of Pediatrics (2006b); universal testing of all children for TB is no longer recommended. Subsequently a targeted testing method is employed wherein only children and adolescents at high risk for contracting the disease, in addition to those patients at risk for progression to TB disease, are screened. A risk factor questionnaire has been developed to facilitate screening pediatric populations at high risk; factors on the questionnaire include a close association with persons having latent or active disease, foreign birth, or foreign travel (Pediatric Tuberculosis Collaborative Group, 2004). The entire questionnaire is available in the Pediatric Tuberculosis Collaborative Group (2004) reference. Recommendations for TST of children are listed in Box 23-12.

A **positive reaction** indicates that the individual has been infected and has developed sensitivity to the tubercle bacillus. It does not, however, confirm the presence of active disease. Once an individual reacts positively, he or she will always react positively. A previously negative reaction that becomes positive indicates that the person has been infected since the last test. Guidelines for interpreting the TST are listed in Box 23-13. Prompt radiographic evaluation of all children with a positive TST reaction is recommended. The American Academy of Pediatrics (2006b) recommends that administration of the TST and interpretation of the results be performed and read by trained health care professionals.

Tuberculin Skin Test (TST) Recommendations for Infants, Children, and Adolescents*

CHILDREN FOR WHOM IMMEDIATE TST IS INDICATED
Contacts of persons with confirmed or suspected contagious tuberculosis (contact investigation).
Children with radiographic or clinical findings suggesting tuberculosis disease.
Children immigrating from endemic countries (e.g., Asia, Middle East, Africa, Latin America).
Children with travel histories to endemic countries or significant contact with indigenous persons from such countries.†

CHILDREN WHO SHOULD HAVE ANNUAL TST‡
Children infected with human immunodeficiency virus (HIV).
Incarcerated adolescents.

CHILDREN WHO SOME EXPERTS RECOMMEND SHOULD BE TESTED EVERY 2 TO 3 YEARS
Children with ongoing exposure to the following people: HIV-infected people, homeless people, residents of nursing homes, institutionalized adolescents or adults, users of illicit drugs, incarcerated adolescents or adults and migrant farm workers; foster children with exposure to adults in the preceding high-risk groups are included.

CHILDREN WHO SOME EXPERTS RECOMMEND SHOULD BE CONSIDERED FOR TST AT 4 TO 6 AND 11 TO 16 YEARS
Children whose parents immigrated (with unknown TST status) from regions of the world with high prevalence of tuberculosis; continued potential exposure by travel to the endemic areas or household contact with persons from the endemic areas (with unknown TST status) should be an indication for repeat TST.

CHILDREN AT INCREASED RISK FOR PROGRESSION OF INFECTION TO DISEASE
Children with other medical risk factors, including diabetes mellitus, chronic renal failure, malnutrition, and congenital or acquired immunodeficiencies, deserve special consideration. Without recent exposure, these people are not at increased risk of acquiring tuberculosis infection. Underlying immune deficiencies associated with these conditions theoretically would enhance the possibility for progression to severe disease. Initial histories of potential exposure to tuberculosis should be included for all of these patients. If these histories or local epidemiologic factors suggest a possibility of exposure, immediate and periodic TST should be considered. **An initial TST should be performed before initiation of immunosuppressive therapy, including prolonged steroid administration, for any child with an underlying condition that necessitates immunosuppressive therapy.**

From American Academy of Pediatrics, Committee on Infectious Diseases, Pickering L, editor: *Red book: 2006 report of the Committee on Infectious Diseases*, ed 27, Elk Grove Village, Ill, 2006, The Academy.
*Bacille Calmette-Guérin (BCG) immunization is not a contraindication to TST.
†If child is well, TST should be delayed for up to 10 weeks after return.
‡Initial tuberculin skin testing is done at the time of diagnosis or circumstance, beginning as early as 3 months of age.

The term **latent tuberculosis infection** (LTBI) is used to indicate infection in a person who has a positive TST, no physical findings of disease, and normal chest radiograph findings. The term **tuberculosis disease** is used when a child has clinical symptoms or radiographic manifestations caused by the *M. tuberculosis* organism. A diagnosis of LTBI or TB

BOX 23-13

Definition of Positive Tuberculin Skin Test (TST) Results in Infants, Children, and Adolescents*

INDURATION ≥5 mm

Children in close contact with known or suspected contagious cases of tuberculosis disease

Children suspected to have tuberculosis disease:
- Findings on chest x-ray film consistent with active or previously active tuberculosis
- Clinical evidence of tuberculosis disease†

Children receiving immunosuppressive therapy‡ or who have immunosuppressive conditions, including human immunodeficiency virus (HIV) infection

INDURATION ≥10 mm

Children at increased risk of disseminated disease:
- Those younger than 4 years of age
- Those with other medical risk conditions, including Hodgkin disease, lymphoma, diabetes mellitus, chronic renal failure, or malnutrition

Children at increased risk of exposure to tuberculosis disease:
- Those born, or whose parents were born, in high-prevalence (TB) regions of the world
- Those frequently exposed to adults who are HIV infected, homeless, users of illicit drugs, residents of nursing homes, incarcerated or institutionalized, or migrant farm workers
- Those who travel to high-prevalence (TB) regions of the world

INDURATION ≥15 mm

Children 4 years of age or older without any risk factors

From American Academy of Pediatrics, Committee on Infectious Diseases, Pickering L, editor: *Red book: 2006 report of the Committee on Infectious Diseases*, ed 27, Elk Grove Village, Ill, 2006, The Academy.

*These definitions apply regardless of previous Bacille Calmette-Guérin (BCG) immunization; erythema at TST site does not indicate a positive test result. TSTs should be read at 48 to 72 hours after placement.

†Evidence by physical examination or laboratory assessment that would include tuberculosis in the working differential diagnosis (e.g., meningitis).

‡Including immunosuppressive doses of corticosteroids.

---

disease in a child is a sentinel event usually representing recent transmission of the *M. tuberculosis* organism.

Therapeutic Management

Medical management of TB disease in children consists of adequate nutrition, pharmacotherapy, general supportive measures, prevention of unnecessary exposure to other infections that further compromise the body's defenses, prevention of reinfection, and sometimes surgical procedures.

The recommended drug regimen for LTBI in children and adolescents includes a daily dose of isoniazid (INH) for 9 months or alternatively 2 or 3 times per week with direct observation of therapy (DOT). DOT means that a health care worker or other responsible, mutually agreed-on individual is present when medications are administered to the patient. Rifampin (daily for 6 months; alternatively DOT twice weekly for 6 months) may be used to treat the child or adolescent who is INH resistant (American Academy of Pediatrics, 2006b).

For the child with clinically active TB, the goal is to achieve sterilization of the tuberculous lesion. Recommended drug therapy for treating TB disease includes combinations of INH, rifampin, and pyrazinamide (PZA). The American Academy of Pediatrics (2006b) recommends a 6-month regimen consisting of INH, rifampin, and PZA given daily for the first 2 months, followed by INH and rifampin given 2 or 3 times a week by DOT for the remaining 4 months. DOT decreases the rates of relapse, treatment failures, and drug resistance and is recommended for treatment of children and adolescents with TB in the United States.

If the child is suspected of having multidrug-resistant TB, a fourth medication such as streptomycin (IM injection only) or ethambutol is added. Optimal therapy for TB in children with HIV infection has not been established, and consultation with a specialist is advised. Therapy should always include at least three drugs initially and be continued for at least 9 months. INH, rifampin, and PZA usually with ethambutol or an aminoglycoside should be given for at least the first 2 months. The three-drug regimen can be used after drug-resistant disease is excluded.

Surgical procedures may be required to remove the source of infection in tissues that are inaccessible to pharmacotherapy or that are destroyed by the disease. Orthopedic procedures may be performed for correction of bone deformities, and bronchoscopy may be done for removal of a tuberculous granulomatous polyp.

Prognosis. Most children recover from primary TB infection and are often unaware of its presence. However, very young children have a higher incidence of disseminated disease. TB is a serious disease during the first 2 years of life, during adolescence, and in children who are HIV positive. Except in cases of tuberculous meningitis, death seldom occurs in treated children. Antibiotic therapy has decreased the death rate and the hematogenous spread from primary lesions.

Prevention. The only definite means to prevent TB is to avoid contact with the tubercle bacillus. Maintaining an optimal state of health with adequate nutrition and avoiding fatigue and debilitating infections promote natural resistance but do not prevent infection. Pasteurization and routine testing of milk and elimination of diseased cattle have reduced the incidence of bovine TB.

Limited immunity can be produced by administration of BCG (bacille Calmette-Guérin), a live vaccine containing bovine bacilli with reduced virulence (attenuated). In most instances, positive tuberculin reactions develop after inoculation with BCG. The distribution of BCG is controlled by local or state health departments, and the vaccine is not used extensively, even in areas with a high prevalence of disease. BCG vaccination is not generally recommended for use in the United States. However, it may be recommended for long-term protection of infants and children with negative TST who are not infected with HIV and who (1) are at high risk for continuing exposure to persons with infectious pulmonary TB or (2) are continuously exposed to persons with TB who have bacilli resistant to both INH and rifampin when the child cannot be removed from the environment or given antituberculosis drug therapy (American Academy of Pediatrics, 2006b).

Nursing Care Management

Children with TB receive their nursing care in ambulatory settings, outpatient departments, schools, and public health settings. Most children are not contagious and require only standard precautions. Children with no cough and negative *peanuts eat lung tissue if aspirated.*

sputum smears can be hospitalized in a regular patient room. However, airborne precautions and a negative-pressure room are required for children who are contagious and hospitalized with active TB disease. Infection control for hospital personnel in contagious cases should include the use of a personally fitted air-purifying N95 or N100 respirator (PAPR) for all patient contacts.

Asymptomatic children with TB can attend school or daycare facilities if they are receiving pharmacotherapy. They can return to regular activities as soon as effective therapy has been instituted, adherence to therapy has been documented, and clinical symptoms have diminished. Children receiving pharmacotherapy for TB can receive measles and other age-appropriate live virus vaccines unless they are receiving high-dose corticosteroids, are severely ill, or have specific contraindications to immunization. Children with TB should also receive optimal nutrition and adequate rest.

Nurses assume several roles in management of the disease, including helping the family understand the rationale for diagnostic procedures, assisting with radiographic examinations, performing and interpreting skin tests, and obtaining specimens for laboratory examination. Skin tests must be carried out correctly to obtain accurate results. The tuberculin is injected intradermally with the bevel of the needle pointing upward. A wheal 6 to 10 mm in diameter should form between the layers of the skin when the solution is injected properly. If the wheal is not formed, the procedure is repeated. The volar or dorsal surface of the forearm is the usual injection site. The reaction to the skin test is determined in 48 to 72 hours; reactions occurring after 72 hours should be measured and considered the result. The size of the transverse diameter of induration, not the erythema, is measured. The diameter transverse to the long axis of the forearm is the only one standardized for measurement purposes (American Academy of Pediatrics, 2006b).

Sputum specimens are difficult or impossible to obtain from an infant or young child because they swallow any mucus coughed from the lower respiratory tract. The best means for obtaining material for smears or culture is by gastric washing (i.e., aspiration of lavaged contents from the fasting stomach). The procedure is carried out and the specimen obtained early in the morning before the customary breakfast time. In some cases an induced sputum specimen may be obtained by administering aerosolized normal saline for 10 to 15 minutes, followed by CPT and suctioning of the nasopharynx for sputum collection.

Because the success of therapy depends on compliance with the drug regimen, parents are instructed about the importance and rationale for DOT. Case finding in the community and follow-up of known contacts—individuals from whom the affected child may have acquired the disease and persons who may have been exposed to the child with the disease—are essential control measures.

PULMONARY DYSFUNCTION CAUSED BY NONINFECTIOUS IRRITANTS

FOREIGN BODY ASPIRATION

Small children characteristically explore matter with their mouths and are prone to aspirate a foreign body (FB). Small children also place objects such as beads, paper clips, small magnets, or food items in the nose, which can easily be aspirated into the trachea. FB aspiration can occur at any age but

is most common in children 1 to 3 years of age. Severity is determined by the location, type of object aspirated, and extent of obstruction. For example, dry vegetable matter, such as a seed, nut, or piece of carrot or popcorn, that does not dissolve and that may swell when wet creates a particularly difficult problem. The high fat content of potato chips and peanuts may cause the added risk of lipoid pneumonia. "Fun foods" are the worst offenders in terms of potential for choking. Offending foods in the order of frequency of choking are hot dog, round candy, peanut or other nut, grape, cookie or biscuit, other meat, carrot, peas, apple, and peanut butter. Other items include plastic or glass beads, button or disc batteries, and coins. Objects such as small lithium or cadmium batteries may cause esophageal or tracheal corrosion.

Raw carrot—big offender

Diagnostic Evaluation

The diagnosis of FB aspiration is suspected on the basis of the history and physical signs. Initially, an FB in the air passages produces choking, gagging, wheezing, or coughing. Laryngotracheal obstruction most commonly causes dyspnea, cough, stridor, and hoarseness because of decreased air entry. Up to half of all children with FB ingestion may be asymptomatic (Uyemura, 2005). Cyanosis may occur if the obstruction becomes worse. Bronchial obstruction usually produces cough (frequently paroxysmal), wheezing, asymmetric breath sounds, decreased airway entry, and dyspnea. When an object is lodged in the larynx, the child is unable to speak or breathe. If the obstruction progresses, the child's face may become livid, and if the obstruction is total, the child can become unconscious and die of asphyxiation. If obstruction is partial, hours, days, or even weeks may pass without symptoms after the initial period. Secondary symptoms are related to the anatomic area in which the object is lodged and are usually caused by a persistent respiratory tract infection distal to the obstruction. FB aspiration should also be suspected in the presence of acute or chronic pulmonary lesions. Often, by the time secondary symptoms appear, the parents have forgotten the initial episode of coughing and gagging.

Radiographic examination reveals opaque FBs but is of limited use in localizing nonradiographic matter. Bronchoscopy is required for a definitive diagnosis of objects in the larynx and trachea. Fluoroscopic examination is valuable in detecting FBs in the bronchi. The mainstay of diagnosis and management of FBs is endoscopy. If there is doubt about the presence of an FB, endoscopy can be diagnostic and therapeutic.

Therapeutic Management

FB aspiration may result in life-threatening airway obstruction, especially in infants because of the small diameters of their airways. Current recommendations for the emergency treatment of the choking child include the use of abdominal thrusts for children older than 1 year of age and back blows and chest thrusts for children younger than 1 year of age (see Airway Obstruction, p. 809).

An FB is rarely coughed up spontaneously. Most frequently, it must be removed instrumentally by endoscopy. Endoscopy and bronchoscopy require sedation with an agent such as IV propofol or midazolam. The procedure is carried out as quickly as possible because the progressive local inflammatory process triggered by the foreign material hampers removal. A chemical pneumonia soon develops, and vegetable matter begins to macerate within a few days, making it even more difficult to remove. After removal of the FB, the child is usually observed for any complications such as laryngeal edema, then discharged home within a matter of hours if vital signs are stable and recovery is satisfactory.

Nursing Care Management

A major role of nurses caring for a child who has aspirated an FB is to recognize the signs of FB aspiration and implement immediate measures to relieve the obstruction. All persons working with children must be prepared to deal effectively with aspiration of an FB. Choking on food or other material should not be fatal. Back blows and chest thrusts in infants and abdominal thrusts in children are simple procedures that can be used by both health professionals and laypersons to save lives. It is the responsibility of nurses to learn these techniques and to teach them to parents and other groups (see Figs. 23-16 and 23-17). To aid a child who is choking, nurses must recognize the signs of distress. Not every child who gags or coughs while eating is truly choking.

> **NURSINGALERT**
>
> The child in severe distress (1) cannot speak, (2) becomes cyanotic, and (3) collapses. These three signs indicate that the child is truly choking and requires immediate action. The child can die within 4 minutes.

Prevention. Nurses are in a position to teach prevention in a variety of settings. They can educate parents singly or in groups about hazards of aspiration in relation to the developmental level of their children and encourage them to teach their children safety. Parents should be cautioned about behaviors that their children might imitate (e.g., holding foreign objects, such as pins, nails, and toothpicks, in their lips or mouth). (Prevention based on the child's age is discussed in Chapters 10 and 12.)

ASPIRATION PNEUMONIA

Aspiration pneumonia occurs when food, secretions, inert materials, volatile compounds, or liquids enter the lung and cause inflammation and a chemical pneumonitis. Aspiration of fluid or foods is a particular hazard in the child who has difficulty with swallowing or is unable to swallow because of paralysis, weakness, debility, congenital anomalies, or absent cough reflex or in the child who is force-fed, especially while crying or breathing rapidly. Clinical signs of the aspiration of oral secretions may not be distinguishable from those of other forms of acute bacterial pneumonia. For example, if vegetable matter has been aspirated, manifestations may not appear for several weeks after the event. Classic symptoms include an increasing cough or fever with foul-smelling sputum, deteriorating chest radiographs, and other signs of lower airway involvement. These deviations may persist for weeks, however, while the child starts to feel better. Rarely, aspiration causes immediate death from asphyxia; more often the irritated mucous membrane becomes a site for secondary bacterial infection. In addition to fluids, food, vomitus, and nasopharyngeal secretions, other substances that may cause pneumonia are hydrocarbons, lipids, powder, and barium.

Nursing Care Management

Care of the child with aspiration pneumonia is the same as that described for the child with pneumonia from other causes. However, the major focus of nursing care is on prevention of aspiration. Proper feeding techniques should be carried out for weak, debilitated, and uncooperative children, and preventive measures should be used to prevent aspiration of any material that might enter the nasopharynx. Nasogastric tubes used for feedings are checked before the initiation of bolus feedings; continuous nasogastric tube feedings are also evaluated periodically for proper tube placement. Children who are at risk for swallowing difficulties as a result of illness, physical debilitation, anesthesia, or sedation are kept NPO (nothing by mouth) until they can properly swallow fluids effectively. The child who is at risk for vomiting and incapable of protecting the airway should be positioned in a side-lying recovery position (see Fig. 23-18).

ACUTE RESPIRATORY DISTRESS SYNDROME/ ACUTE LUNG INJURY

ARDS is recognized in children and adults and has been associated with clinical conditions and injuries such as sepsis, trauma, viral pneumonia, fat emboli, drug overdose, reperfusion injury after lung transplantation, smoke inhalation, and near-drowning. It is characterized by respiratory distress and hypoxemia that occur within 72 hours of a serious injury or surgery in a person with previously normal lungs. Acute lung injury (ALI) is said to involve a spectrum of inflammatory disease responses to a precipitating event (Frye, 2005). Acute pulmonary inflammation with alveolar capillary membrane destruction results in significant hypoxemia, and mechanical ventilation is often required. ARDS is the most severe in the spectrum of illnesses in relation to the degree of hypoxemia. Hypoxemia is expressed as the ratio of partial pressure of oxygen (Pao_2) to fraction of inspired oxygen (Fio_2), or P/F ratio, with the P/F ratio for ALI being 300 or less, whereas the P/F ratio for ARDS is 200 or less. Both ALI and ARDS demonstrate radiographic evidence of bilateral alveolar infiltrates without evidence of left-sided heart failure (Rice and Bernard, 2006).

The hallmark of ARDS is increased permeability of the alveolar-capillary membrane that results in pulmonary edema. During the acute phase of ARDS, the alveolocapillary membrane is damaged, with an increasing pulmonary capillary permeability and resulting interstitial edema. Later stages are characterized by pneumocyte and fibrin infiltration of the alveoli, with the start of either the healing process or fibrosis. When fibrosis occurs, the child may demonstrate respiratory distress and the need for mechanical ventilation. In ARDS the lungs become stiff as a result of surfactant inactivation, gas diffusion is impaired, and eventually bronchiolar mucosal swelling and congestive atelectasis occur. The net effect is decreased functional residual capacity, pulmonary hypertension, and increased intrapulmonary right-to-left shunting of pulmonary blood flow. Surfactant secretion is reduced, and the atelectasis and fluid-filled alveoli provide an excellent medium for bacterial growth.

The criteria for diagnosis of ARDS in children are an acute antecedent illness or injury, acute respiratory distress or failure, no evidence of prior cardiopulmonary disease, and diffuse bilateral infiltrates evidenced on chest radiography. The child with ARDS may first demonstrate only symptoms caused by an injury or infection, but, as the condition deteriorates, hyperventilation, tachypnea, increasing respiratory effort, cyanosis, and decreasing oxygen saturation occur. At times the developing hypoxemia is not responsive to oxygen administration.

Treatment involves supportive measures, such as maintenance of adequate oxygenation and pulmonary perfusion, treatment of infection (or the precipitating cause), maintenance of adequate cardiac output and vascular volume, hydration, adequate nutritional support, comfort measures, prevention of complications such as gastrointestinal ulceration and aspiration, and psychologic support. Prone positioning may be used to improve oxygenation; this requires close communication and coordination among the health care team (Frye, 2005). Definitive therapy is directed toward improvement of oxygenation. The use of endotracheal intubation, positive end-expiratory pressure, and low tidal volume may be required to ensure maximum oxygen delivery by increasing functional residual capacity, reducing intrapulmonary shunting, and reducing pulmonary fluid. Additional supportive strategies in the treatment of ARDS in children include the use of lung-protective ventilator strategies, permissive hypercapnia, inhaled nitric oxide, exogenous surfactant administration, high-frequency ventilation, partial liquid ventilation, and extracorporeal life support (extracorporeal membrane oxygenation, or ECMO). Once the underlying cause is identified, specific treatment (e.g., antibiotics for infection) is initiated.

Prognosis. In spite of advances in understanding and treating ARDS and ALI, mortality in children ranges from 22% (after severe trauma) to 88% (after bone marrow transplant) (Flori, Glidden, Rutherford, and others, 2005; Frankel and DiCarlo, 2004). The precipitating disorder influences the outcome; the worst prognosis is associated with uncontrolled sepsis, bone marrow transplantation, cancer, and multisystem involvement with hepatic failure. Children who recover may have persistent cough and exertional dyspnea.

Nursing Care Management

The child with ARDS is cared for in intensive care during the acute stages of illness. Nursing care involves close monitoring of cardiac output, perfusion, fluid and electrolyte balance, and renal function (urinary output), as well as assessment of oxygenation and respiratory status. Blood gas analysis and pulse oximetry are important evaluation tools. Parenteral and enteral nutritional support are often required because of the length of the acute phase of the illness. Diuretics may be administered to reduce pulmonary fluid, and vasodilators may be administered to decrease pulmonary vascular pressure. Pain management is another important consideration in the management of the child with ARDS. Nursing management also includes monitoring the effects of the numerous parenteral fluids and drugs used to stabilize the child and monitoring for changes in the child's hemodynamic status. Most children with ARDS require invasive monitoring via a central venous line and possibly a pulmonary artery catheter to monitor oxygenation and administer medications. The nursing care of the child with ARDS also involves close observance of skin condition and prevention of breakdown, passive range of motion for prevention of muscle atrophy and contractures, and nutritional support. Respiratory distress is a frightening situation for both the child and the parents, and attention to their psychologic needs is a major element in the care of these children. The child is often sedated during the acute phase of the illness, and weaning from sedation requires close monitoring for anxiety reduction and comfort.

SMOKE INHALATION INJURY

A number of noxious substances that may be inhaled are toxic to humans. They are primarily products of incomplete combustion and cause more deaths from fires than flame injuries. The severity of the injury depends on the nature of the substances generated by the material burned, whether the victim is confined in a closed space, and the duration of contact with the smoke. Smoke inhalation results in three types of injury: heat, chemical, and systemic. Three distinct stages occur in the child suffering from inhalation injury:

- Pulmonary insufficiency, usually during the initial 12 hours
- Pulmonary edema, usually after 6 to 72 hours, with an increase in the lung fluid and interstitial edema
- Bronchopneumonia, usually after 72 hours with a resulting airway obstruction or atelectasis

Heat injury involves thermal injury to the upper airway. Air has low specific heat; therefore the injury goes no farther than the upper airway. Reflex closure of the glottis prevents injury to the lower airway.

Chemical injury involves gases that may be generated during the combustion of materials such as clothing, furniture, and floor coverings. Acids, alkalis, and their precursors in smoke can produce chemical burns. These substances can be carried deep into the respiratory tract, including the lower respiratory tract, in the form of insoluble gases. Soluble gases tend to dissolve in the upper respiratory tract.

Synthetic materials are especially toxic, producing gases such as oxides of sulfur and nitrogen, acetaldehyde, formaldehyde, hydrocyanic acid, and chlorine. Heated plastics are the source of extremely toxic vapors, including chlorine and hydrochloric acid from polyvinylchloride, and hydrocarbons, aldehydes, ketones, and acids from polyethylene. Irritant gases such as nitrous oxide or carbon dioxide combine with water in the lungs to form corrosive acids; aldehydes cause denaturation of proteins, cellular damage, and edema of pulmonary tissues. Chemical burns to the airways are similar to burns on the skin, except they are painless because the tracheobronchial tree is relatively insensitive to pain.

Inhalation of small amounts of noxious irritants produces alveolar and bronchiolar damage that can lead to obstructive bronchiolitis. Severe exposure causes further injury, including alveolocapillary damage with hemorrhage, necrotizing bronchiolitis, inhibited secretion of surfactant, and formation of hyaline membranes—manifestations of ARDS.

Systemic injury occurs from gases that are nontoxic to the airways (e.g., carbon monoxide [CO], hydrogen cyanide). However, these gases cause injury and death by interfering with or inhibiting cellular respiration. CO is responsible for more than half of all fatal inhalation poisonings in the United States. CO is a colorless, odorless gas with an affinity for hemoglobin 230 times greater than that of oxygen. When it enters the bloodstream, CO combines readily with hemoglobin to form carboxyhemoglobin (COHb). Because it is released less readily, tissue hypoxia reaches dangerous levels before oxygen is available to meet tissue needs.

NURSINGALERT

The oxygen saturation (Sao_2) obtained by pulse oximetry will be normal because the device measures only oxygenated and deoxygenated hemoglobin; it does not measure dysfunctional hemoglobin, such as COHb.

Accidental CO poisoning is most often a result of exposure to fumes of heaters or smoke from structural fires, although poorly ventilated recreational vehicles with improperly operated or maintained gas lamps or stoves and cooking in underventilated areas with charcoal grills are also frequent causes. CO is produced by incomplete combustion of carbon or carbonaceous material such as wood or charcoal.

The signs and symptoms of CO poisoning are secondary to tissue hypoxia and vary with the level of COHb. Mild manifestations include headache, visual disturbances, irritability, and nausea, whereas more severe intoxication causes confusion, hallucinations, ataxia, and coma. The bright, cherry red lips and skin often described are less often observed; pallor and cyanosis are seen more frequently.

Therapeutic Management

Treatment of children with smoke inhalation injury is largely symptomatic. The most widely accepted treatment is placing the child on humidified 100% oxygen as quickly as possible and monitoring for signs of respiratory distress and impending failure. Baseline arterial blood gases (ABGs) and COHb levels are obtained. Pao_2 may be within normal limits unless there is marked respiratory depression. If CO poisoning is confirmed, 100% oxygen is continued until COHb levels fall to the nontoxic range of about 10%. If CO poisoning is severe, the patient may benefit from hyperbaric oxygen therapy; however, the benefits and risks of treatment are debatable (Kao and Nañagas, 2004); at this time there are no published clinical practice guidelines for the therapy, especially in children. Hyperbaric oxygen therapy may be useful in the treatment of neurologic complications related to CO poisoning.

Respiratory distress may occur early in the course of smoke inhalation as a result of hypoxia, or patients who are breathing well on admission may suddenly develop respiratory distress. Therefore intubation equipment should be readily available. Transient edema of the airways can occur at any level in the tracheobronchial tree. Assessment and localization of the obstruction should be accomplished before severe swelling of the head, neck, or oropharynx occurs. Intubation is often necessary when (1) severe burns in the area of the nose, mouth, and face increase the likelihood of developing oropharyngeal edema and obstruction; (2) vocal cord edema causes obstruction; (3) the patient has difficulty handling secretions; and (4) progressive respiratory distress requires artificial ventilation. Controversy surrounds tracheostomy, but many prefer this procedure when the obstruction is proximal to the larynx and reserve nasotracheal intubation for lower tract involvement.

Nursing Care Management

Nursing care of the child with inhalation injury is the same as that for any child with respiratory distress. Vital signs and other respiratory assessments are performed frequently, and the pulmonary status is carefully observed and maintained. Pulmonary physical therapy is often part of the therapy, as well as mechanical ventilation if needed. Fluid requirements for children experiencing inhalation injury are greater than for those with surface burns alone; however, one concern is the development of pulmonary edema. Therefore accurate monitoring of intake and output is essential.

In addition to observation and management of the physical aspects of inhalation injury, the nurse also deals with the psychologic needs of a frightened child and distraught parents. As with any accidental injury, the parents may feel overwhelming guilt, even when the injury occurred through no fault of their own. Parents need support, reassurance, and information regarding the child's condition, treatment, and progress.

ENVIRONMENTAL TOBACCO SMOKE EXPOSURE

Numerous investigations indicate that parental smoking is an important cause of morbidity in children. Children exposed to passive or environmental tobacco smoke have an increased number of respiratory illnesses, increased respiratory symptoms (i.e., cough, sputum, and wheezing), and reduced performance on pulmonary function tests. AOM and OME are also increased in children who have smoking parents. Indoor exposure to environmental tobacco smoke has been linked to asthma in children. Among children with asthma, there is an association between parental cigarette smoking and asthma exacerbations, trips to the emergency department, medication use, and impaired recovery after hospitalization for acute asthma. Maternal cigarette smoking is associated with increased respiratory symptoms and illnesses in children; decreased fetal growth; increased deliveries of low-birth-weight, preterm, and stillborn infants; and a greater incidence of sudden infant death syndrome (SIDS). Antenatal maternal smoking has emerged as a significant risk factor for SIDS (American Academy of Pediatrics, 2005). The risk for diagnosis of early-onset asthma in the first 3 years of life is associated with in utero exposure to maternal smoking; grandmaternal smoking was also associated with an increased risk of early-onset asthma in the grandchild even if the mother did not smoke during pregnancy (Li, Langholz, Salam, and others, 2005). Exposure to tobacco smoke during childhood may also contribute to the development of chronic lung disease in the adult.

Nursing Care Management

Nurses must provide information about the hazards of environmental smoke exposure in all their interactions with children and their family members. This information is especially important for children with respiratory and allergic illnesses. In families where smokers refuse to quit, appropriate guidance is provided for reducing smoke in the child's environment (see Family-Centered Care box). Nurses should set an example for children and families and become advocates for "no smoking" ordinances in public places, prohibition of advertising tobacco products in the media, and inclusion of health warnings of sidestream smoke on tobacco products.* Nurses also have an important role in providing parents with affordable smoking cessation education resources, including the appropriate use of smoking cessation pharmacologic aids (Sheahan and Free, 2005).

LONG-TERM RESPIRATORY DYSFUNCTION

ASTHMA

Asthma is a chronic inflammatory disorder of the airways in which many cells (mast cells, eosinophils, and T lymphocytes) play a role. In susceptible children, inflammation causes recurrent episodes of wheezing, breathlessness, chest tightness, and cough, especially at night or in the early morning. These asthma episodes are associated with airflow limitation or ob-

---

*For further information on the effects of second-hand smoke on child health go to http://www.cdc.gov/tobacco/secondhand_smoke/index.htm.

Case Study—Asthma

FAMILY-CENTERED CARE

Decreasing Childhood Exposure to Environmental Tobacco Smoke

- Maintain a smoke-free home.
- Avoid exposing an infant to environmental smoke.
- Use an air-purifying filter in the home where smoking is unavoidable.
- Encourage exclusive breastfeeding for the first 6 months.
- If smoking cessation is in progress by breastfeeding mother, suggest she change upper clothing after smoking and before breastfeeding infant.
- Do not smoke around children.
- Change clothing after smoking and before holding an infant in close proximity.
- Restrict smoking to an isolated area of the house where the children do not play or sleep.
- Do not smoke in motor vehicles with children.
- Do not smoke in rooms children use.
- Do not allow visitors to smoke in the home.

BOX 23-14
Asthma Severity Classification in Children: Ages 0 to 11*

STEP 5 OR 6: SEVERE PERSISTENT ASTHMA
Continual symptoms throughout the day
Frequent nighttime symptoms
Peak expiratory flow (PEF): <60%
Forced expiratory volume in 1 second (FEV_1): <75% of predicted value
Interference with normal activity: extremely limited
Use of short-acting β-agonist for symptom control: several times a day

STEP 3 OR 4: MODERATE PERSISTENT ASTHMA
Daily symptoms
Nighttime symptoms: 3 to 4 times a month (ages 0 to 4), >1 per week but not nightly (ages 5 to 11)
PEF: 60% to 80% of predicted value
FEV_1: 75% to 80%
PEF variability: >30%
Interference with normal activity: some limitation
Use of short-acting β-agonist for symptom control: daily

STEP 2: MILD PERSISTENT ASTHMA
Symptoms >2 times a week, but <1 time a day
Nighttime symptoms: 1 to 2 times a month (ages 0 to 4), 3 to 4 times a month (ages 5 to 11)
PEF or FEV_1: ≥80% of predicted value
PEF variability: 20% to 30%
Interference with normal activity: minor limitation
Use of short-acting β-agonist for symptom control: <2 days a week but not daily

STEP 1: INTERMITTENT ASTHMA
Symptoms <2 days/week
Nighttime symptoms (awakenings): none (ages 0 to 4), >2 times a month (ages 5 to 11)
PEF or FEV_1: ≥80% of predicted value
PEF variability: <20%
Interference with normal activity: none
Use of short-acting β-agonist for symptom control: <2 days/week

From National Asthma Education and Prevention Program: *Guidelines for the diagnosis and management of asthma: summary report 2007,* retrieved March 8, 2008, from http://www.nhlbi.nih.gov/guidelines/asthma/index.htm.
*The presence of one clinical feature of severity is sufficient to place a patient in that category. An individual should be assigned to the most severe grade in which any feature occurs. The characteristics in this table are general and may overlap because asthma is highly variable. An individual's classification may change over time. Risk factors for each category are not presented in this table. See the original table referenced above for additional classification data. Asthma treatment should not be based on this table.

---

struction that is reversible either spontaneously or with treatment. The inflammation also causes an increase in bronchial hyperresponsiveness to a variety of stimuli (National Asthma Education and Prevention Program, 2007). Recognition of the importance of inflammation has made the use of antiinflammatory agents, especially inhaled steroids, a key component in the treatment of asthma.

Asthma is classified into four categories based on the symptom indicators of disease severity. These categories are intermittent, mild persistent, moderate persistent, and severe persistent. The intermittent category has the least number of symptoms; symptoms increase in frequency or intensity until the last category of severe persistent asthma (Box 23-14). These categories provide a stepwise approach to the pharmacologic management, environmental control, and educational interventions needed for each category (National Asthma Education and Prevention Program, 2007). A new component of the asthma severity classification system includes the domains of impairment and risk for each category; these categories emphasize the multifaceted aspect of the disease for consideration of effects on present quality of life and functional capacity and the future risk of adverse events (National Asthma Education and Prevention Program, 2007).

Asthma prevalence, morbidity, and mortality are increasing in the United States, especially among African-Americans (Linzer, 2007). These increases may result from worsening air pollution, poor access to medical care, or underdiagnosis and undertreatment. Asthma is the most common chronic disease of childhood, the primary cause of school absences, and the third leading cause of hospitalizations in children under the age of 15. Although the onset of asthma may occur at any age, 80% to 90% of children have their first symptoms before 4 or 5 years of age. Boys are affected more frequently than girls until adolescence, when the trend reverses.

Etiology

Studies of children with asthma indicate that allergy influences both the persistence and the severity of the disease. In fact, atopy, or the genetic predisposition for the development of an immunoglobulin E (IgE)–mediated response to common aeroallergens, is the strongest identifiable predisposing factor for developing asthma (National Asthma Education and Prevention Program, 2007). Although allergens play an important role in asthma, 20% to 40% of children with asthma have no evidence of allergic disease. In addition to allergens, other substances and conditions can serve as triggers that may exacerbate asthma (Box 23-15). Asthma is a complex disorder involving biochemical, genetic, immunologic, environmental, infectious, endocrine, and psychologic factors. Evidence shows that viral respiratory infections may have a significant role in the development and expression of asthma (National Asthma Education and Prevention Program, 2007).

BOX 23-15

Triggers Tending to Precipitate or Aggravate Asthmatic Exacerbations

- Allergens
  Outdoor—Trees, shrubs, weeds, grasses, molds, pollens, air pollution, spores
  Indoor—Dust or dust mites, mold, cockroach antigen
- Irritants—Tobacco smoke, wood smoke, odors, sprays
- Exposure to occupational chemicals
- Exercise
- Cold air
- Changes in weather or temperature
- Environmental change—Moving to new home, starting new school, etc.
- Colds and infections
- Animals—Cats, dogs, rodents, horses
- Medications—Aspirin, nonsteroidal antiinflammatory drugs, antibiotics, beta blockers
- Strong emotions—Fear, anger, laughing, crying
- Conditions—Gastroesophageal reflux, tracheoesophageal fistula
- Food additives—Sulfite preservatives
- Foods—Nuts, milk or other dairy products
- Endocrine factors—Menses, pregnancy, thyroid disease

Pathophysiology

There is general agreement that inflammation contributes to heightened airway reactivity in asthma. The mechanisms contributing to airway inflammation are multiple and involve a number of different pathways. It is unlikely that asthma is caused by either a single cell or a single inflammatory mediator; rather, it appears that asthma results from complex interactions among inflammatory cells, mediators, and the cells and tissues present in the airways (National Asthma Education and Prevention Program, 2007). However, recognition of the importance of inflammation has made the use of antiinflammatory agents a key component of asthma therapy.

Another important component of asthma is bronchospasm and obstruction. The mechanisms responsible for the obstructive symptoms in asthma include (Fig. 23-4) (1) inflammatory response to stimuli; (2) airway edema and accumulation and secretion of mucus; and (3) spasm of the smooth muscle of the bronchi and bronchioles, which decreases the caliber of the bronchioles.

Bronchial constriction is a normal reaction to foreign stimuli, but in the child with asthma it is abnormally severe, producing impaired respiratory function. The smooth muscle arranged in spiral bundles around the airway causes narrowing and shortening of the airway, which significantly increases airway resistance to airflow. Airflow is determined by the size of the airway lumen, degree of bronchial wall edema, mucus production, smooth muscle contraction, and muscle hypertrophy. Because the bronchi normally dilate and elongate during inspiration and contract and shorten on expiration, the respiratory difficulty is more pronounced during the expiratory phase of respiration.

Increased resistance in the airway causes forced expiration through the narrowed lumen. The volume of air trapped in the lungs increases as airways are functionally closed at a point between the alveoli and the lobar bronchi. This trapping of gas forces the individual to breathe at higher and higher lung volumes. Consequently, the person with asthma fights to inspire sufficient air. This expenditure of effort for breathing causes fatigue, decreased respiratory effectiveness, and increased oxygen consumption. The inspiration occurring at higher lung volumes hyperinflates the alveoli and reduces the effectiveness of the cough. As the severity of obstruction increases, there is a reduced alveolar ventilation with carbon dioxide retention, hypoxemia, respiratory acidosis, and, eventually, respiratory failure.

FIG. 23-4 ■ Mechanisms of obstruction in asthma.

Chronic inflammation may also cause permanent damage (airway remodeling) to airway structures, which cannot be prevented by and is not responsive to current treatments (National Asthma Education and Prevention Program, 2007).

Diagnostic Evaluation

The classic manifestations of asthma are dyspnea, wheezing, and coughing. However, children may experience symptoms that range from acute episodes of shortness of breath, wheezing, and cough followed by a quiet period to a relatively continuous pattern of chronic symptoms that fluctuate in severity (Box 23-16). An attack may develop gradually or appear abruptly and may be preceded by a URI. The age of the child is often a significant factor, since the first attack frequently occurs before the age of 5 years, with some children manifesting clinical signs and symptoms in infancy. In infancy an attack usually follows a respiratory infection. Some children may experience a prodromal itching at the front of the neck or over the upper part of the back just before an attack.

NURSING ALERT

Shortness of breath with air movement in the chest restricted to the point of absent breath sounds accompanied by a sudden rise in respiratory rate is an ominous sign indicating ventilatory failure and imminent respiratory arrest.

The diagnosis is determined primarily on the basis of clinical manifestations, history, physical examination, and, to a lesser extent, laboratory tests. Generally, chronic cough in the absence of infection or diffuse wheezing during the expiratory phase of respiration is sufficient to establish a diagnosis.

Pulmonary function tests (PFTs) provide an objective method of evaluating the presence and degree of lung disease, as well as the response to therapy. Spirometry can generally be

Animation—Asthma

Animation—Bronchi and Bronchioles

BOX 23-16
Clinical Manifestations of Asthma

COUGH

Hacking, paroxysmal, irritative, and nonproductive
Becomes rattling and productive of frothy, clear, gelatinous sputum

RESPIRATORY-RELATED SIGNS

Shortness of breath
Prolonged expiratory phase
Audible wheeze
May have a malar flush and red ears
Lips deep, dark red color
May progress to cyanosis of nail beds or circumoral cyanosis
Restlessness
Apprehension
Prominent sweating as the attack progresses
Older children sitting upright with shoulders in a hunched-over position, hands on the bed or chair, and arms braced (tripod)
Speaking with short, panting, broken phrases

CHEST

Hyperresonance on percussion
Coarse, loud breath sounds
Wheezes throughout the lung fields
Prolonged expiration
Crackles
Generalized inspiratory and expiratory wheezing; increasingly high pitched

WITH REPEATED EPISODES

Barrel chest
Elevated shoulders
Use of accessory muscles of respiration
Facial appearance—flattened malar bones, circles beneath the eyes, narrow nose, prominent upper teeth

nursingcareguidelines

Interpreting Peak Expiratory Flow Rates*

- **Green (80% to 100% of personal best)** signals all clear. Asthma is under reasonably good control. No symptoms are present, and the routine treatment plan for maintaining control can be followed.
- **Yellow (50% to 79% of personal best)** signals caution. Asthma is not well controlled. An acute exacerbation may be present. Maintenance therapy may need to be increased. Call the practitioner if the child stays in this zone.
- **Red (below 50% of personal best)** signals a medical alert. Severe airway narrowing may be occurring. A short-acting bronchodilator should be administered. Notify the practitioner if the peak expiratory flow rate does not return immediately and stay in yellow or green zones.

*These zones are guidelines only. Specific zones and management should be individualized for each child.

performed reliably on children by the age of 5 or 6 years and includes either the traditional and simple mechanical spirometer often used in clinics, offices, and the home or new computerized versions. The National Asthma Education and Prevention Program (2007) recommends that spirometry testing be done at the time of initial assessment of asthma, after treatment is initiated and symptoms have stabilized, and at least every 1 to 2 years to assess the maintenance of airway function.

Another key measurement is the **peak expiratory flow rate (PEFR),** which measures the maximum flow of air that can be forcefully exhaled in 1 second. PEFR is measured in liters per minute using a **peak expiratory flow meter (PEFM).** Three zones of measurement are typically used to interpret PEFR. The zone system is patterned after a traffic light to make the categories easy to understand and remember (see Nursing Care Guidelines box). Each child needs to establish his or her personal best value. A personal best value should be established during a 2- to 3-week period when the child's asthma is stable. During this period, the child records the PEFR at least twice a day. After the personal best value has been established, the child's current PEFR on any occasion can be compared with the personal best value.

Bronchoprovocation testing, direct exposure of the mucous membranes to a suspected antigen in increasing concen-

trations, helps to identify inhaled allergens. Exposure to methacholine, histamine, or cold or dry air may be performed to assess airway responsiveness or reactivity. Exercise challenges may be used to identify children with exercise-induced bronchospasm (Liu, Spahn, and Leung, 2004). Although these tests are highly specific and sensitive, they place the child at risk for an asthmatic episode and should be done under close observation in a qualified laboratory or clinic.

Skin testing is useful in identifying specific allergens, and those obtained by the puncture technique correlate better than intracutaneous tests with symptoms and measurements of specific IgE antibody. The radioallergosorbent test (RAST) helps identify antigens against various foods and is often useful in determining appropriate therapy. It is recommended that all patients with year-round asthma symptoms be tested with skin tests or laboratory blood analysis to determine sensitization to perennial allergens (e.g., house dust mites, cats, dogs, cockroaches, molds, and fungus) (National Asthma Education and Prevention Program, 2007).

In addition to these tests, other important tests include laboratory tests (complete blood count with differential) and chest radiographs. The complete blood count may show a slight elevation in the white blood cell count during acute asthma, but elevations to more than 12,000/mm^3 or an increased percentage of band cells may indicate respiratory tract infection. The presence of eosinophilia of greater than 500/mm^3, on the other hand, tends to suggest an allergic or inflammatory disorder.

Frontal and lateral radiographs show infiltrates and hyperexpansion of the airways, with the anteroposterior diameter on physical examination indicating an increased diameter (suggestive of barrel chest). Additional diagnostic tests for conditions such as gastroesophageal reflux may be carried out to determine whether they may contribute to asthma symptoms. Radiography may assist in ruling out a respiratory tract infection.

Therapeutic Management

The overall goals of asthma management are to maintain normal activity levels, maintain normal pulmonary function, prevent chronic symptoms and recurrent exacerbations, pro-

FAMILY-CENTERED CARE

"Allergy-Proofing" the Home and Community

- Keep humidity between 30% and 50%; use dehumidifier or air conditioner if available; keep air conditioners clean and free of mold; do not use vaporizers or humidifiers.
- Encase pillows in zippered allergen-impermeable covers or wash pillows in hot water (at least 54.4° C [130° F]) every week.
- Encase mattress and box springs in zippered allergen-impermeable cover.
- Use foam rubber mattress and pillows or Dacron pillows and synthetic blankets.
- Wash bed linens every 7 to 10 days in hot water (at least 54.4° C).
- Encase polyester comforters in allergen-impermeable covers or wash in hot water (at least 54.4° C) every week; if possible, do not use comforters and use cotton blankets.
- Do not use a canopy above the bed; children should not sleep on the bottom bunk of a bunk bed.
- Store nothing under the bed; keep clothing in a closet with the door shut.
- Use washable window shades; avoid heavy curtains; if curtains are used, launder them frequently.
- Remove all carpeting if possible; if not possible, vacuum carpet once or twice a week while the child wears a mask; have child remain out of the room while vacuuming occurs and for 30 minutes after vacuuming.
- If possible, use a central vacuum cleaner with a collecting bag outside of the home or use cleaner filters (e.g., high-efficiency particulate air [HEPA] filters).
- Have air and heating ducts cleaned annually; change or clean filters monthly; cover heating vents with filter material (e.g., cheesecloth) to prevent circulation of dust, especially when heat is turned on.
- Remove unnecessary furniture, rugs, stuffed or real animals, toys, books, upholstered furniture, plants, aquariums, and wall hangings from child's room.
- Use wipeable furniture (wood, plastic, vinyl, or leather) in place of upholstered furniture; avoid rattan or wicker furniture.
- Cover walls with washable paint or wallpaper.
- Limit child's exposure to animals (rabbits, gerbils, hamsters) at school; teach child to stay away from zoos, petting farms, and neighbor's pets.
- Change child's clothes after playing outdoors; wash child's hair nightly if child is outside and pollen count is high.
- Keep child indoors while lawn is being mowed, bushes or trees are being trimmed, or pollen count is high.
- Keep windows and doors closed during pollen season; use air conditioner if possible or go to places that are air conditioned, such as libraries and shopping malls, when the weather is hot.
- Wet-mop bare floors weekly; wet-dust and clean child's room weekly; child should not be present during cleaning activities.
- Wash showers and shower curtains with bleach or Lysol at least once a month.
- Limit or prevent child's exposure to tobacco and wood smoke; do not allow cigarette smoking in the house or car; select daycare centers, play areas, and shopping malls that are smoke free.
- Avoid odors or sprays (e.g., perfumes, talcum powder, room deodorizers, chalk dust at school, fresh paint, cleaning solutions).
- Avoid cellar (basement) as a play area if it is damp, and use a dehumidifier in damp basement.
- Cover all food, including pet food, and put food away in cabinets.
- Store garbage in closed containers.
- Use pesticide sprays, roach bait traps, and boric acid powder to kill cockroaches; if living in an apartment or adjacent housing, encourage neighbors to work together to get rid of cockroaches and mice.
- Repair leaking or dripping faucets; seal cracks and crevices in cabinets and pantry areas.

vide optimum drug therapy with minimum or no adverse effects, and assist the child in living as normal and happy a life as possible. This includes facilitating the child's social adjustments in the family, school, and community and normal participation in recreational activities and sports. To accomplish these goals, several treatment principles need to be followed (National Asthma Education and Prevention Program, 2007):

- A continuous care approach with regular visits (at least every 1 to 6 months) to the health care provider is necessary to control symptoms and prevent exacerbations.
- Prevention of exacerbations includes avoiding triggers, avoiding allergens, and using medications as needed.
- Therapy includes efforts to reduce underlying inflammation and to relieve or prevent symptomatic airway narrowing.
- Therapy includes patient education, environmental control, pharmacologic management, and the use of objective measures to monitor the severity of disease and guide the course of therapy.

Allergen Control. Nonpharmacologic therapy is aimed at the prevention and reduction of exposure to airborne allergens and irritants. **House dust mites** and other components of house dust are frequent agents identified in children allergic to inhalants. The **cockroach,** another common household inhabitant, is an important allergen in many locations. Exterminating live cockroaches, carefully cleaning kitchen floors and cabinets, putting food away after eating, and taking trash out in the evening are essential measures to control cockroaches. The mouse allergen is the most recent allergen to be identified in the homes of inner-city children with asthma. The role of cat and dog dander in allergen-induced asthma has also been studied. Sensitized persons should carefully evaluate having such pets in the household; there are inconclusive data on cat dander, but there is some evidence that dog dander either has no effect or may be protective (Sharma, Hansel, Matsui, and others, 2007). Additional sources of pollutants include ozone, particulate matter produced by tobacco smoke, wood-burning stoves, pesticides, lead, mold spores, nitrogen dioxide, and sulfur dioxide; these are believed to contribute to asthma morbidity in children and should be avoided or minimized. Exposure to tobacco smoke is a significant contributing factor in the development of asthma in infants and small children (Sharma, Hansel, Matsui, and others, 2007). Recommendations for controlling allergens are found in the Family-Centered Care box.

Skin testing identifies specific allergens so steps can be taken to eliminate or avoid them. Often, simply removing the offending environmental allergens or irritants (e.g., removing carpeting from the home of a child sensitive to mold and dust particles) will decrease the frequency of asthma episodes. Dehumidifiers or air conditioners control nonspecific factors that trigger an episode, such as extremes of temperature.

Despite the proven association between the incidence of asthma and exposure to these residential hazards, little evidence-based research demonstrates an overall reduction in symptoms even with significant interventions aimed at environmental (housing) modifications such as removal of carpeting, cleaning, and extermination (Sandel, Phelan, Wright, and others, 2004; Sharma, Hansel, Matsui, and others, 2007).

Drug Therapy. Pharmacologic therapy is used to prevent and control asthma symptoms, reduce the frequency and severity of asthma exacerbations, and reverse airflow obstruction. A stepwise approach is recommended based on the severity of the child's asthma. Because inflammation is considered an early and persistent feature of asthma, therapy is directed toward long-term suppression of inflammation.

Asthma medications are categorized into two general classes: **long-term control medications (preventive medications)** to achieve and maintain control of inflammation, and **quick-relief medications (rescue medications)** to treat symptoms and exacerbations (National Asthma Education and Prevention Program, 2007).

Quick-relief and long-term medications are often used in combination. Inhaled corticosteroids, cromolyn sodium and nedocromil, long-acting β_2-agonists, methylxanthines, and leukotriene modifiers are used as long-term control medications. Short-acting β_2-agonists, anticholinergics, and systemic corticosteroids are used as quick-relief or rescue medications. Bronchodilators that relax bronchial smooth muscle and dilate the airways include β_2-agonists, methylxanthines, and anticholinergics that can be used as both quick-relief and long-term medications.

Many asthma medications are given by inhalation with a nebulizer or a **metered-dose inhaler (MDI).** The MDI should always be attached to a spacer when an inhaled corticosteroid is administered to prevent yeast infections in the mouth. Spacers are also important for children who have difficulty coordinating or learning proper inhalation technique (Pongracic, 2003). The spacer and holder can be equipped with a mask or a mouthpiece. Pharmaceutical companies are currently mandated to produce inhalers that do not contain chlorofluorocarbons (CFCs) as the propellant because CFCs have been linked to damage and depletion of the earth's ozone level. An alternative propellant to the CFCs is hydrofluoroalkanes (HFAs); the purported advantages include delivery of more fine particles and less oral deposition (Pongracic, 2003). The FDA mandated December 2008 as the targeted cessation date for MDIs containing CFCs to be produced and sold (US Food and Drug Administration, 2005). Several currently available CFC-free MDI devices use dry powder (and also called dry powder inhalers [DPIs]); these include the Diskus inhaler and the Turbuhaler. These devices are breath activated, and the child needs to inhale as quickly and deeply as possible to use them effectively. The Diskhaler and Aerosolizer are similar, but with the Aerosolizer the medication must be loaded into the inhaler before use. Infants and very young children who have difficulty using MDIs or other inhalers can receive their asthma medications via a **nebulizer.** When this device is used, the medication is mixed with saline (also available in premixed form) and nebulized with compressed air. Children are instructed to breathe normally with the mouth open to provide a direct route to the trachea.

Corticosteroids are antiinflammatory drugs used to treat reversible airflow obstruction and to control symptoms and reduce bronchial hyperresponsiveness in chronic asthma. A major change in the last two revisions of the National Asthma Education and Prevention Program guidelines is the recommendation that inhaled corticosteroids be used as first-line therapy in children over 5 years of age. Clinical studies of corticosteroids have indicated significant improvement of all asthma parameters, including decreases in symptoms, emergency visits, and medication requirements (National Asthma Education and Prevention Program, 2007).

Corticosteroids may be administered parenterally, orally, or by inhalation. Oral medications are metabolized slowly, with an onset of action up to 3 hours after administration and peak effectiveness occurring within 6 to 12 hours. Oral systemic steroids may be given for short periods of time (e.g., 3- or 10-day "bursts") to gain prompt control of inadequately controlled persistent asthma or to manage severe persistent asthma. These drugs should be given in the lowest effective dose. These medications have few side effects (cough, dysphonia, and oral thrush), and there is strong evidence that they improve the long-term outcomes for children of all ages with mild or moderate persistent asthma. Evidence from clinical trials that monitored children for 6 years indicate that the use of inhaled corticosteroids at recommended doses does not have long-term significant effects on growth, bone mineral density, ocular toxicity, or suppression of the adrenal-pituitary axis (National Asthma Education and Prevention Program, 2007). However, primary care providers should frequently monitor (at least every 3 to 6 months) the growth of children and adolescents taking corticosteroids to assess the systemic effects of these drugs and make appropriate reductions in dosages or changes to other types of asthma therapy when necessary. The inhaled corticosteroids include budesonide and fluticasone.

Cromolyn sodium is a nonsteroidal antiinflammatory drug (NSAID) for asthma. It stabilizes mast cell membranes; inhibits activation and release of mediators from eosinophil and epithelial cells; and inhibits the acute airway narrowing after exposure to exercise, cold dry air, and sulfur dioxide. There is no way to reliably predict whether a child will respond to the drug. Cromolyn sodium has minimal side effects (occasional coughing on inhalation of the powder formulation) and may be given via nebulizer or MDI. **Nedocromil sodium** inhibits the bronchoconstrictor response to inhaled antigens and inhibits the activity of and release of histamine, leukotrienes, and prostaglandins from inflammatory cells associated with asthma. The drug has few side effects and is used for maintenance therapy in asthma; it is not effective for reversal of acute exacerbations and is not used in children under 5 years of age

β-Adrenergic agonists (short acting) (primarily albuterol, levalbuterol [Xopenex], and terbutaline) are used for treatment of acute exacerbations and for the prevention of exercise-induced bronchospasm. These drugs bind with the β-receptors on the smooth muscle of airways, where they activate adenylate cyclase and convert adenosine monophosphate (AMP) to cyclic AMP (cAMP). It is believed that the increased cAMP enhances binding of intracellular calcium to the cell membrane, reducing the availability of calcium and thus allowing smooth muscle to relax. Other effects of the drug help stabilize mast cells to prevent release of mediators. Most β-adrenergics used in asthma therapy affect predominantly the β$_2$-receptors, which help eliminate bronchospasm. β$_1$ effects, such as increased heart rate and gastrointestinal disturbances, have been minimized. These drugs can be given via inhalation or as oral or parenteral preparations. The inhaled drug has a more rapid onset of action than the oral form. Inhalation also reduces troublesome systemic side effects: irritability, tremor, nervousness, and insomnia. Levalbuterol reportedly causes fewer side effects; however, its overall effectiveness in childhood asthma is controversial (Linzer, 2007). The 2007 National Asthma Education and Prevention Program guidelines recommend the addition of a long-acting β$_2$-agonist to a low- or medium-dosage inhaled corticosteroid to improve lung function and asthma symptoms and decrease the need for a short-acting β$_2$-agonist. There is some evidence that this combination may actually enable the practitioner to lower the corticosteroid dose and manage asthma symptoms just as effectively (Mintz, 2004). Inhaled β-adrenergic agents should not be taken more than three or four times daily for acute symptoms.

Salmeterol (Serevent) is a long-acting β$_2$-agonist (bronchodilator) that is used twice a day (no more frequently than every 12 hours). This drug is added to antiinflammatory therapy and used for long-term prevention of symptoms, especially nighttime symptoms, and exercise-induced bronchospasm. Salmeterol is not used in children less than 12 years of age, and it is not used to treat acute symptoms or exacerbations.

Theophylline was used for decades to relieve symptoms and prevent asthma attacks; however, it is now used primarily in the emergency department when the child is not responding to maximal therapy (Linzer, 2007). Therapeutic levels should be obtained with this drug, since it has a narrow therapeutic window.

Leukotrienes are mediators of inflammation that cause increases in airway hyperresponsiveness. Leukotriene modifiers (such as zafirlukast [Accolate] and montelukast sodium [Singulair]) block inflammatory and bronchospasm effects. These drugs are not used to treat acute episodes, but are given orally in combination with β-agonists and steroids to provide long-term control and prevent symptoms in mild persistent asthma. Montelukast is approved for children 12 months old and older, whereas zafirkulast is approved for children 7 years and older.

Anticholinergics (atropine and ipratropium [Atrovent]) may also be used for relief of acute bronchospasm. However, these drugs have adverse side effects that include drying of respiratory secretions, blurred vision, and cardiac and central nervous system stimulation. The primary anticholinergic drug used is ipratropium, which does not cross the blood-brain barrier and therefore elicits no central nervous system effects. Ipratropium, when used in combination with albuterol, has been shown to be effective during acute severe asthma in significantly improving lung function and reducing hospitalizations in children coming to the emergency department (Liu, Spahn, and Leung, 2004).

A fairly new asthma drug, omalizumab (Xolair), is a monoclonal antibody that blocks the binding of IgE to mast cells. Blocking this interaction eventually inhibits the inflammation that is associated with asthma. Because many patients with asthma are atopic and possess specific IgE antibodies to allergens responsible for airway inflammation, this drug is a promising adjunct to the treatment of asthma. It has been approved for use in children 12 years and older. The drug is administered once or twice a month by subcutaneous injection. Efficacy of omalizumab is not immediate, and clinical trials report that response to the drug was not evident before 12 weeks (Strunk and Bloomberg, 2006). Clinical trials of the drug indicate that it can be an effective therapy for patients with symptomatic moderate to severe allergic asthma that is poorly controlled with inhaled corticosteroids. The drug is expensive (Courtney, McCarter, and Pollart, 2005), however, and there have been reported cases of severe anaphylactic reactions. In early 2007 the FDA added a "black box warning" to the drug, which highlights the risk of anaphylaxis.

The use of complementary and alternative medicine (CAM) in children with asthma is reported by several sources; most common are the use of herbal products, breathing techniques, homeopathy, and acupuncture (Slader, Reddel, Jenkins, and others, 2006). The use of CAM should be carefully evaluated in conjunction with other therapies in the overall management of asthma.

Exercise. Exercise-induced bronchospasm (EIB) is an acute, reversible, usually self-terminating airway obstruction that develops during or after vigorous activity, reaches its peak 5 to 10 minutes after stopping the activity, and usually stops in another 20 to 30 minutes. Patients with EIB have cough, shortness of breath, chest pain or tightness, wheezing, and endurance problems during exercise, but an exercise challenge test in a laboratory is necessary to make the diagnosis.

The problem is rare in activities that require short bursts of energy (e.g., baseball, sprints, gymnastics, skiing) and more common in those that involve endurance exercise (e.g., soccer, basketball, distance running). Swimming is well tolerated by children with EIB because they are breathing air fully saturated with moisture and because of the type of breathing required in swimming.

Children with asthma are often excluded from exercise by parents, teachers, and practitioners, as well as by the children themselves, since they are reluctant to provoke an attack. However, this practice can seriously hamper peer interaction and physical health. Exercise is advantageous for children with asthma, and most children can participate in activities at school and in sports with minimal difficulty, provided their asthma is under control. Participation should be evaluated on an individual basis. Appropriate prophylactic treatment with β-adrenergic agents or cromolyn sodium before exercise will usually permit full participation in strenuous exertion.

Chest Physical Therapy. CPT includes breathing exercises and physical training. These therapies help produce physical and mental relaxation, improve posture, strengthen respiratory musculature, and develop more efficient patterns of breathing. For the motivated child, breathing exercises and controlled breathing are of value in preventing overinflation and improving efficiency of the cough. However, CPT is not recommended during acute, uncomplicated exacerbations of asthma.

Hyposensitization. The role of hyposensitization in childhood asthma has become controversial. In the past, immunotherapy was used for seasonal allergies and when single substances were identified as the offending allergen. It is not recommended for allergens that can be eliminated, such as foods, drugs, and animal dander.

The National Asthma Education and Prevention Program guidelines (2007) recommend immunotherapy for asthma patients in the following situations:

■ When there is evidence of a relationship between asthma symptoms and unavoidable exposure to an allergen to which the patient is sensitive

■ When symptoms occur all year or at least during a major portion of the year

■ When symptom control is difficult with drug therapy because multiple medications are required, or the patient is not responsive to available drugs, or the patient refuses to take the medications

Injection therapy is usually limited to clinically significant allergens. The initial dose of the offending allergen(s), based on the size of the skin reaction, is injected subcutaneously. The amount is increased at weekly intervals until a maximum tolerance is reached, after which a maintenance dose is given at 4-week intervals. This may be extended to 5- or 6-week intervals during the off-season for seasonal allergens. Successful treatment is continued for a minimum of 3 years and then stopped. If no symptoms appear, acquired immunity is assumed; if symptoms recur, treatment is reinstituted. Hyposensitization injections should be administered only with emergency equipment and medications readily available in the event of an anaphylactic reaction.

Prognosis. The outlook for children with asthma varies widely. Some children's asthma symptoms may improve at puberty, but up to two thirds of children with asthma continue to have symptoms through puberty and into adulthood. The prognosis for control or disappearance of symptoms varies in children from those who have rare and infrequent attacks to those who are constantly wheezing or are subject to status asthmaticus. In general, when symptoms are severe and numerous, when symptoms have been present for a long time, and when there is a family history of allergy, there is a greater likelihood of a poor prognosis. Risk factors that may predict persistence of symptoms into childhood (from infancy) include atopy, male gender, exposure to environmental tobacco, and maternal history of asthma (Ross, Mjaanes, and Lemanske, 2003). Many children who outgrow their exacerbations continue to have airway hyperresponsivenesss and cough as adults. Furthermore, airway hyperresponsiveness in adults appears to be associated with decreased lung function.

Although deaths from asthma have been relatively uncommon, especially in the young age-groups, since the 1980s the rate of death from asthma has increased steadily in the United States and other countries. Data indicate a significant increase in asthma symptoms, emergency department visits, and hospitalization among children ages birth to 4 years of age in 2003 to 2004. Most asthma deaths for the same period were in children ages 11 to 17 years, with significant increases seen in non-Hispanic African-Americans (Linzer, 2007). Mortality and morbidity for asthma are especially high among African-American children, whose hospitalization and death rates are three times higher than those of Caucasian and Hispanic children (Liu, Spahn, and Leung, 2004).

The adolescent age-group appears to be the most vulnerable, with the greatest increase occurring in children 10 to 14 years of age. No reliable data exist to explain this increase. Factors that have been postulated include exposure of atopic persons to more allergens (particularly in large urban centers), change in severity of the disease, abuse of drug therapy (toxicity), failure of families and practitioners to recognize the severity of asthma, and psychologic factors such as denial and refusal to accept the disease.

Risk factors for asthma deaths include early onset, frequent attacks, difficult-to-manage disease, adolescence, history of respiratory failure, psychologic problems (refusal to take medications), dependency on or misuse of asthma drugs (high use), presence of physical stigmata (barrel chest, intercostal retractions), and abnormal PFTs.

Status Asthmaticus. Children who continue to display respiratory distress despite vigorous therapeutic measures, especially the use of sympathomimetics (e.g., albuterol, epinephrine), are considered to be in status asthmaticus. The condition may develop gradually or rapidly, often coincident with complicating conditions, such as pneumonia or a respiratory virus, that can influence the duration and treatment of the exacerbation.

> **NURSINGALERT**
>
> Status asthmaticus is a medical emergency that can result in respiratory failure and death if untreated.

Therapy for status asthmaticus is aimed at improving ventilation, decreasing airway resistance and relieving bronchospasm, correcting dehydration and acidosis, allaying child and parent anxiety related to the severity of the event, and treating any concurrent infection. Humidified oxygen is recommended and should be given to maintain an oxygen saturation greater than 90%. Inhaled aerosolized short-acting β_2-agonists are recommended for all patients. Three treatments of β_2-agonists spaced 20 to 30 minutes apart are usually given as initial therapy, and continuous administration of β_2-agonists may be initiated. A systemic corticosteroid (oral, IV, or IM) may also be given to decrease the effects of inflammation. An anticholinergic such as ipratropium bromide may be added to the aerosolized solution of the β_2-agonist. Anticholinergics have been shown to result in additional bronchodilation in patients with severe airflow obstruction. An IV infusion is often initiated to provide a means for hydration and to administer medications. Correction of dehydration, acidosis, hypoxia, and electrolyte disturbance is guided by frequent determination of arterial pH, blood gases, and serum electrolytes.

Additional therapies in acute asthma attacks include the use of IV magnesium sulfate, a potent muscle relaxant that acts to decrease inflammation and improves pulmonary function and peak flow rate among pediatric patients treated in the emergency department with moderate to severe asthma. Heliox may be administered to decrease airway resistance, and thereby decrease the work of breathing; heliox can be delivered via a nonrebreathing face mask from premixed tanks, which may be blended in a stand-alone unit or within a ventilator. Heliox may be used in acute exacerbations as an adjunct to β_2-agonist and IV corticosteroid therapy to improve pulmonary function until the two latter medications have time to take full effect in decreasing bronchospasm; the effects of heliox are usually seen within 20 minutes of administration, whereas other drugs may take longer to exert the desired effect (Liu, Spahn, and Leung, 2004). Ketamine, a dissociative anesthetic, is believed to cause smooth muscle relaxation and decrease airway resistance caused by severe bronchospasm in acute asthma (Linzer, 2007); it may be administered as an adjunct to other therapies mentioned previously. Inhaled magnesium sulfate used in addition to a β_2-agonist for acute asthma attacks has also been effective in treating acute asthma exacerbation (Blitz, Blitz, Beasley, and others, 2005).

Antibiotics should not be used to treat acute asthma attacks except when a bacterial infection resulting from another condition such as pneumonia or sinusitis is present (National Asthma Education and Prevention Program, 2007).

A child suspected of having status asthmaticus is usually seen in the emergency department and is often admitted to a pediatric intensive care unit for close observation and continuous cardiorespiratory monitoring. A key component in the prevention of morbidity is helping the child, parents, teachers, coaches, and other adults recognize features of deteriorating respiratory status, use the correct rescue drugs effectively, and immediately place the child with deteriorating respiratory status into the care of trained health care professionals instead of waiting to see if the asthma gets better on its own. The child going into early status asthmaticus is no different from the adult who is having a myocardial infarction in terms of needing trained medical assistance before the condition deteriorates to irreversible respiratory failure and possible death. Community education regarding asthma recognition and management is an important component of nursing care.

Nursing Care Management

The nursing care of the child with asthma begins with a review of the child's health history; the home, school, and play environment; parent and child attitudes about the child's condition; and a comprehensive physical assessment with focus on the respiratory system. Nursing care of children with asthma involves both acute and long-term care. Nurses who are involved with children in the home, hospital, school, outpatient clinic, or practitioner's office play an important role in helping children and their families learn to live with the condition. The disease can be managed so that it does not require hospitalization or interfere with family life, physical activity, or school attendance. The nursing process in the care of the child with asthma is outlined in the Nursing Care Plan.

Physical assessment of asthma involves the same observations and techniques described in Chapter 6. In addition, the nurse notes and evaluates physical characteristics of chronic respiratory involvement, including chest configuration (e.g., barrel chest), posturing, and type of breathing. A history of the current and previous episodes and precipitating factors or events provides important information.

Nurses may perform a variety of functions in asthma care. These may include asthma education in the primary care setting and in schools and other community settings, care of the child with asthma in the acute care setting, ambulatory care, and intensive care. Nurses also obtain information on how asthma affects the child's everyday activities and self-concept, the child's and family's adherence to the prescribed therapy, and their personal treatment goals. Every effort is made to build a partnership between the child and family and the health care team. Communication is an essential part of this partnership, and health care providers should routinely assess the effectiveness of patient-provider communication. In particular, the child and family's satisfaction with asthma control and with the quality of care should be assessed. The nurse should also assess their perception of the severity of the disease and their level of social support.

One of the major emphases of nursing care is outpatient management by the family. Parents are taught how to avoid allergens, to recognize and respond to symptoms of bronchospasm, to maintain health and prevent complications, and to promote normal activities. The nurse should determine any cultural or ethnic beliefs or practices that influence self-management and that may necessitate modifications in educational approaches to meet the family's needs.

Avoid Allergens. One goal of asthma management is avoidance of an exacerbation. Parents need to know how to avoid allergens that precipitate asthma episodes. The nurse assists the parent in modifying the environment to reduce contact with the offending allergen(s) (see Family-Centered Care box, p. 787). Parents are cautioned to avoid exposing a sensitive child to excessive cold, wind, or other extremes of weather; smoke; sprays; or other irritants. Foods known to provoke symptoms should be eliminated from the diet.

Approximately 2% to 6% of children with asthma are sensitive to aspirin; therefore nurses should caution parents to use other analgesic-antipyretic drugs for discomfort or fever and to read package labeling. Although aspirin is rarely given to children in the United States, salicylate compounds are in other common medicines such as Pepto-Bismol. Children with aspirin-induced asthma may also be sensitive to NSAIDs and tartrazine (yellow dye number 5, a common food coloring).

> **NURSING ALERT**
>
> Parents are encouraged to avoid administering aspirin to *any* child unless specifically recommended by and under the supervision of a health practitioner. Acetaminophen is safe for children and is the analgesic of choice.

Relieve Bronchospasm. Parents and older children are taught to recognize early signs and symptoms of an impending attack so that it can be controlled before symptoms become distressing. Most children can recognize prodromal symptoms well before an attack (about 6 hours) and implement preventive therapy. Objective signs that parents may observe include rhinorrhea, cough, low-grade fever, irritability, itching (especially in front of the neck and chest), apathy, anxiety, sleep disturbance, abdominal discomfort, and loss of appetite. A variety of easy-to-use, inexpensive PEFMs are available for use in the home and at school to assess changes in pulmonary function (see Family-Centered Care box). In general, children 5 years of age and older are able to use a PEFM successfully. However, young children need to be supervised while they are learning to use their PEFM, and their technique should be checked frequently to ensure it is correct. Children should use the same peak flow meter over time, and they should bring their peak flow meter for use at every follow-up visit. Using the same brand of meter is recommended because different brands can give significantly different values. The use of a PEFM provides objective monitoring regarding the severity of asthma and can decrease asthma episodes, health care visits, and missed school days (Burkhart, Rayens, Revelette, and others, 2007).

Nursing Diagnosis	Patient Outcomes	Nursing Interventions	Rationale
Risk for Suffocation related to interaction between individual and triggering factors (allergens, respiratory tract infection, exercise, irritants, emotions, temperature changes) **Child's/Family's Defining Characteristics** *(Subjective and Objective Data)* Wheezing Dry cough Labored respirations Dyspnea Intercostal retractions Complaints of tightness in chest, shortness of breath Bronchial inflammation and airway constriction	Child will have adequate airway exchange. Family and child will assume responsibility for asthma symptom management. **The Following NOC Concepts Apply to These Outcomes** Asthma Control Anxiety Control Child Development	Assist child and family in recognizing factors such as allergens, irritants, temperature changes, and upper respiratory infections (URIs) that trigger asthma symptoms. Assist child (according to developmental age) and family in recognizing early signs of an asthmatic episode (use peak expiratory flow meter [PEFM]). Educate child and family in the use of inhaled corticosteroids and bronchodilator. Educate child and family regarding proper use of rescue medications in case of disease exacerbation. Educate child and family regarding the proper use of metered-dose inhaler with spacer, aerosolized nebulizer, and PEFM (know child's personal best). **The Following NIC Concepts Apply to These Interventions** Respiratory Monitoring Administering Inhaled Medications Risk Identification Family Integrity Promotion Energy Management Coping Enhancement Environmental Management	To avoid asthma exacerbations To control symptoms with medication To control symptoms and minimize shortness of breath To prevent illness exacerbations and hospitalization; to prevent side effects from improper use of certain asthma drugs To help child and family effectively manage asthma symptoms independently

Nursing Diagnosis	Patient Outcomes	Nursing Interventions	Rationale
Interrupted Family Processes related to child with a chronic illness **Child's/Family's Defining Characteristics** *(Subjective and Objective Data)* Anxiety Disruptive family interactions with child and members Family conflicts Inadequate child support Child's health status ignored Family ignoring other members' needs for those of the child with asthma	Family will cope with effects of the disease. Family will provide child an appropriate protective environment. **The Following NOC Concepts Apply to These Outcomes** Family support Family normalization	Provide family and child (as age appropriate) with explanations about the disease and management. Cooperate with family to develop a written action plan for asthma management. Discuss facilitators and barriers to effective asthma management. Encourage family and child (as age appropriate) to discuss the impact of the illness on the family's lifestyle. Evaluate family resources for asthma management in relation to the following: ■ Access to health care ■ Medication availability in home and school (or daycare, as appropriate) ■ Allergen exposure control and eradication **The Following NIC Concepts Apply to These Interventions** Emotional Support Anticipatory Guidance Family Involvement Promotion Financial Resource Assistance Decision-Making Support Mutual Goal Setting	To provide adequate information To provide realistic expectations To provide family and child sense of control To assist family members in understanding their role as being vital in the management of asthma To provide opportunity to verbalize frustrations and challenges of having a child with a chronic illness To enhance family's ability to cope with child's chronic illness

FIG. 23-5 ■ Child using metered-dose inhaler with spacer and face mask.

FAMILY-CENTERED CARE

Use of a Peak Expiratory Flow Meter

1. Before each use, make certain the sliding marker or arrow on the peak expiratory flow meter (PEFM) points to zero or is at the bottom of the numbered scale.
2. Stand up straight.
3. Remove gum or any food from the mouth.
4. Close your lips tightly around the mouthpiece. Be sure to keep your tongue away from the mouthpiece.
5. Blow out as hard and as quickly as you can, a "fast hard puff." Blow from the diaphragm, not the cheeks.
6. Note the number by the marker on the numbered scale.
7. Repeat entire routine three times; wait 30 seconds between each routine.
8. Record the highest of the three readings, not the average.
9. Measure the peak expiratory flow rate (PEFR) close to the same time and same way each day (e.g., morning and evening; before or 15 minutes after taking medication).
10. Keep a chart of your PEFRs.

Children who use a nebulizer, MDI, Diskus, or Turbuhaler to deliver drugs need to learn how to use the device correctly. A study of school-age children with asthma indicated that only 7% of these children had effective MDI skills (Winkelstein, Huss, Butz, and others, 2000). The MDI device (Fig. 23-5) delivers medication directly to the airways; therefore the child needs to learn to breathe slowly and deeply for better distribution to narrowed airways (see Family-Centered Care box).

Young children and those who are unable to manipulate the MDI or coordinate breathing should use spacers. These devices allow the parent or child to deliver the medication from the MDI into the spacer, from which the child then inhales the medication. Spacers also prevent yeast infections in the mouth when corticosteroids are inhaled via an MDI.

FAMILY-CENTERED CARE

Use of a Metered-Dose Inhaler*
STEPS FOR CHECKING HOW MUCH MEDICINE IS IN THE CANISTER
1. If the canister is new, it is full.
2. If the canister has been used repeatedly, it might be empty. (Check product label to see how many inhalations should be in each canister.)
3. The most accurate way to determine how many doses remain in a metered-dose inhaler (MDI) is to count and record each actuation as it is used.
4. Many dry powder inhalers have a dose-counting device or dose indicator on the canister to let you know when the canister is empty.

STEPS FOR USING THE INHALER
1. Remove the cap and hold inhaler upright.
2. Shake the inhaler.
3. Tilt the head back slightly and breathe out slowly.
4. With the inhaler in an upright position, position the mouthpiece:
   ■ About 3 to 4 cm from the mouth *or*
   ■ Insert into an AeroChamber *or* spacer (this method is recommended for young children and for people using corticosteroids)
5. At the end of a normal expiration, depress the top of the inhaler canister firmly to release the medication (into either the AeroChamber or the mouth), and breathe in slowly (about 3 to 5 seconds). Relax the pressure on the top of the canister.
6. Hold the breath for at least 5 to 10 seconds to allow the aerosol medication to reach deeply into the lungs.
7. Remove the inhaler and breathe out slowly through the nose.
8. Wait 1 minute between puffs (if additional one is needed).

Modified from National Asthma Education and Prevention Program: *Expert Panel report II: guidelines for the diagnosis and management of asthma*, NIH Pub No 97-4051, Bethesda, Md, 1997, National Heart, Lung, and Blood Institute.
*NOTE: Some inhaled dry-powder inhalers require a different inhalation technique. To use these dry-powder inhalers, it is important to close the mouth tightly around the mouthpiece of the inhaler and inhale rapidly and deeply.

The child and parents also need to be cautioned about the adverse effects of prescribed drugs and the dangers of overuse of β_2-agonists. They should know that it is important to use these drugs when needed but not indiscriminately or as a substitute for avoiding the symptom-provoking allergen. Parents are cautioned against purchasing over-the-counter preparations because these medications can place the children at risk for increased dosage of a drug and toxicity.

NURSING ALERT
Long-acting β-adrenergic inhalers (salmeterol) should be used only as directed (usually every 12 hours) and not more frequently. They are not intended to relieve acute asthmatic symptoms.

The family should obtain a PEFM and learn to use this device to monitor the child's asthma. A written asthma action plan that includes the three peak flow meter zones and the child's asthma medications may be obtained from the child's primary care provider. Medications used for asthma exacerbations are also included in the asthma plan. This action plan should be used to make decisions about asthma management at home and at school. The nurse may assist the child and family in preparing the written action plan, emphasizing that the child and family determine the success of the plan, not the health professionals.

Foods known to provoke symptoms should be eliminated from the diet, and parents are advised to read labels on prepared foods and snacks to determine the presence of allergens.

The child should be protected from a respiratory tract infection that can trigger an attack or aggravate the asthmatic state, especially in young children whose airways are mechanically smaller and more reactive. Annual influenza vaccinations are recommended for children with persistent asthma (American Academy of Pediatrics, 2008). Equipment used for the child, such as nebulizers, must be kept absolutely clean to decrease the chances of contamination with bacteria and fungi.

Breathing exercises and controlled breathing are taught and encouraged for motivated children, and the nurse should provide information concerning activities that promote diaphragmatic breathing, side expansion, and improved mobility of the chest wall. Play techniques that can be used for younger children to extend their expiratory time and increase expiratory pressure include blowing cotton balls or a Ping-Pong ball on a table, blowing a pinwheel, blowing bubbles, or preventing a tissue from falling by blowing it against the wall.

Self-care and asthma self-management programs are important in helping the child and family cope with asthma. Most asthma self-management programs for children convey several principles. First, asthma is a common disease that can be controlled with appropriate drug therapy, environmental control, education, and management skills. Second, it is much easier to prevent than to treat an asthma episode; adherence to a therapeutic program is necessary to prevent exacerbations. Third, children with asthma can live full and active lives.

Asthma camps provide an opportunity for children with asthma to engage in physical activity while learning about their disease in a controlled environment with their peers and health professionals. Children who attend asthma camps often demonstrate improved asthma self-management skills.

Self-contained programs and brochures for patient education are available from the Asthma and Allergy Foundation of America* and the American Lung Association.† The National Heart, Lung, and Blood Institute‡ provides educational materials for asthma education in the school setting and also copies of the *Guidelines for the Diagnosis and Management of Asthma* for the practitioner (National Asthma Education and Prevention Program, 2007). Another publication designed for health care practitioners, *Pediatric Asthma: Promoting Best Practice,* can be obtained from the American Academy of Allergy Asthma and Immunology.§

Provide Acute Asthma Care. Children who are admitted to the hospital with acute asthma are ill, anxious, and uncomfortable. The progression or resolution of status asth-

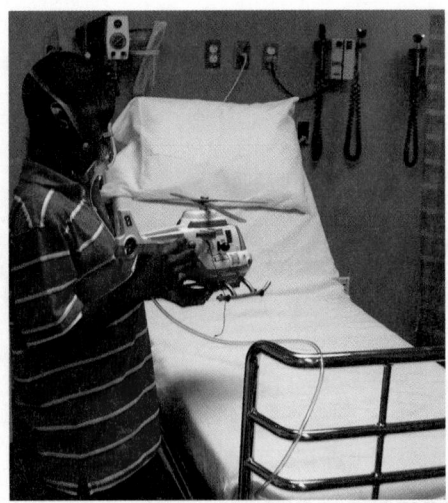

FIG. 23-6 ■ Child with asthma is allowed play activity as tolerated.

maticus is variable. The importance of continual observation and assessment cannot be overemphasized.

When β$_2$-agonists and corticosteroids are given, the child is monitored closely and continuously for relief of respiratory distress and signs of side effects or toxicity. Oral fluid intake may be limited during the acute phase; IV fluid replacement may be required to provide adequate tissue hydration.

Older children may be more comfortable standing (Fig. 23-6), sitting upright, or leaning slightly forward (Fig. 23-7). When possible, the nurse communicates in such a way that a child can reply in a few words to avoid fatigue. Shortness of breath makes talking difficult.

Children with acute asthma are apprehensive and anxious. The calm, efficient presence of a nurse helps reassure them that they are safe and will be cared for during this stressful period. It is important to assure children that they will not be left alone and that their parents are allowed to remain with them.

Parents need reassurance and want to be informed of their child's condition and therapies. They may believe that they have in some way contributed to the child's condition or could have prevented the episode. Reassurance regarding their efforts expended on the child's behalf and their parenting capabilities can help alleviate their stress. Efforts to reduce parental apprehension will also reduce the child's distress. Anxiety is easily communicated to the child from parents and members of the staff.

Support Child or Adolescent and Family. The nurse working with children with asthma can provide support in a number of ways. Many children voice frustration because their exacerbations interfere with their daily activities and social lives. They need education about what to do to prevent an asthma episode. These children also need reassurance from the health team that they can learn to control and cope with their asthma and live a normal life. Be aware of children, especially adolescents, who demonstrate signs of depression and may not comply with therapy as a means of passive suicide.

Children in disruptive family situations (divorce, separation, violence, custodial battles) may disregard daily asthma medication regimen or may be at higher risk as a result of

*1233 20th St., NW, Suite 402, Washington, DC 20036; (800) 7-Asthma; http://www.aafa.org.

†61 Broadway, 6th Floor, New York, NY 10006; (800) 548-8252; national headquarters: (212) 315-8700; http://www.lungusa.org.

‡NHLBI Health Information Center, PO Box 30105, Bethesda, MD 20824-0105; (301) 592-8573; fax: (240) 629-3246; http://www.nhlbi.nih.gov.

§555 E. Wells St., Suite 1100, Milwaukee, WI 53202; (414) 272-6071; http://aaaai.org.

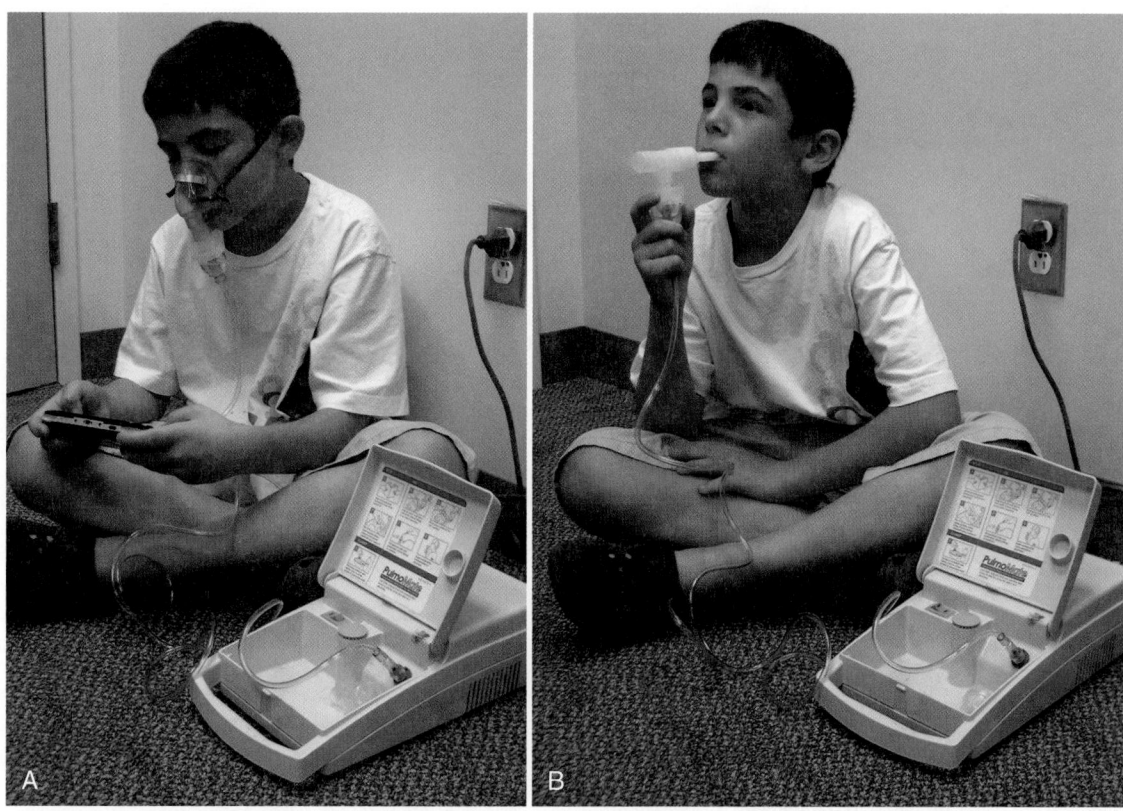

FIG. 23-7 ■ Children with asthma may take a nebulized aerosol treatment with **(A)** a mask or **(B)** mouthpiece. (Courtesy Texas Children's Hospital, Houston.)

neglect by adults who are in charge of their care. Adolescents struggling with a sense of identity and body image often regard asthma as a condition that will "go away," especially if there is a time lapse between symptoms, and may abandon the therapeutic regimen. In some cases adolescents find themselves in charge of other siblings in blended family situations and may ignore their own health needs. Referral for counseling and guidance is appropriate in these situations where the child's or adolescent's life is potentially in harm's way and the therapeutic regimen for asthma is abandoned due to other crises.

The short- and long-term adaptation of children with asthma often depends on the family's acceptance of the disorder. The task of living day-to-day with affected children involves the entire family. There are periodic crises and the ever-present threat of a crisis, requiring parental vigilance; sleepless nights; frequent trips to the physician, emergency department, or hospital; and often overwhelming medical expenses. Throughout these stresses, parents are encouraged to promote as normal a life as possible for their children.

CYSTIC FIBROSIS *inherited*

CF is inherited as an autosomal recessive trait; the affected child inherits the defective gene from both parents, with an overall incidence of 1:4. The mutated gene responsible for CF is located on the long arm of chromosome 7. This gene codes a protein of 1480 amino acids called the **cystic fibrosis transmembrane regulator (CFTR).** The CFTR protein is related to a family of membrane-bound glycoproteins. The glycopro-

teins constitute a cAMP-activated chloride channel and also regulate other chloride and sodium channels at the surfaces of the epithelial cells.

Pathophysiology

CF is characterized by several clinical features: increased viscosity of mucous gland secretions, a striking elevation of sweat electrolytes, an increase in several organic and enzymatic constituents of saliva, and abnormalities in autonomic nervous system function. Although both sodium and chloride are affected, the defect appears to be primarily a result of abnormal chloride movement; the CFTR appears to function as a chloride channel. Children with CF demonstrate decreased pancreatic secretion of bicarbonate and chloride and an increase in sodium and chloride in both saliva and sweat. This characteristic is the basis for the sweat chloride diagnostic test. The sweat electrolyte abnormality is present from birth, continues throughout life, and is unrelated to the severity of the disease or the extent to which other organs are involved.

The primary factor, and the one that is responsible for many of the clinical manifestations of the disease, is mechanical obstruction caused by the increased viscosity of mucous gland secretions (Fig. 23-8). Instead of forming a thin, freely flowing secretion, the mucous glands produce a thick mucoprotein that accumulates and dilates them. Small passages in organs such as the pancreas and bronchioles become obstructed as secretions precipitate or coagulate to form concretions in glands and ducts. The earliest postnatal manifestation of CF is often **meconium ileus** in the newborn, in which the

FIG. 23-8 ■ Various effects of exocrine gland dysfunction in cystic fibrosis.

small intestine is blocked with thick, puttylike, tenacious, mucilaginous meconium.

In the pancreas the thick secretions block the ducts, eventually causing **pancreatic fibrosis.** This blockage prevents essential pancreatic enzymes from reaching the duodenum, which causes marked impairment in the digestion and absorption of nutrients. The disturbed function is reflected in bulky stools that are frothy from undigested fat (**steatorrhea**) and foul smelling from putrefied protein (**azotorrhea**). The endocrine function of the pancreas often remains unchanged because the islets of Langerhans are normal but may decrease in number as pancreatic fibrosis progresses. The incidence of diabetes mellitus (cystic fibrosis–related diabetes [CFRD]) is greater in CF children than in the general population (Balinsky and Zhu, 2004), which may be caused by changes in pancreatic architecture and diminished blood supply over time. Consequently, with increased survival, and primarily in adolescents and adults, type 1 diabetes is becoming a more frequent finding. There is no relationship between the progression of pulmonary disease and the development of diabetes mellitus in CF. In the liver, localized biliary obstruction and fibrosis are common and become more extensive with time.

A common gastrointestinal complication associated with CF is **prolapse of the rectum,** which occurs in infancy and childhood and is related to large, bulky stools; malnutrition; and increased intraabdominal pressure secondary to paroxysmal cough. Affected children of all ages are subject to intestinal obstruction from inspissated or impacted feces. Gumlike masses can obstruct the bowel and produce a partial or complete obstruction, a condition that is referred to as **distal intestinal obstruction syndrome.**

Pulmonary complications are present in almost all children with CF, but the onset and extent of involvement are variable. Symptoms are produced by stagnation of mucus in the airways, with eventual bacterial colonization leading to destruction of lung tissue. The abnormally viscous and tenacious secretions are difficult to expectorate and gradually obstruct the bronchi and bronchioles, causing scattered areas of bronchiectasis, atelectasis, and hyperinflation. The stagnant mucus offers a favorable environment for bacterial growth. The most common pathogens are *Pseudomonas aeruginosa, Burkholderia cepacia, S. aureus, H. influenzae, Escherichia coli,* and *Klebsiella pneumoniae.*

The reproductive systems of both males and females with CF are affected. Females with CF have normal fallopian tubes and ovaries. Fertility can be inhibited by highly viscous cervical secretions, which act as a plug, blocking sperm entry. Women with CF who become pregnant have an increased incidence of premature labor and delivery and low birth weight in the infant. Favorable nutritional status and pulmonary function are positively correlated with favorable pregnancy outcomes. Most adult men (95%) with CF are sterile, which may be caused by blockage of the vas deferens with abnormal secretions or by failure of normal development of the wolffian duct structures (vas deferens, epididymis, and seminal vesicles), resulting in decreased or absent sperm production.

Growth and development are often affected in children with moderate to severe forms of CF. Physical growth may be

BOX 23-17
Clinical Manifestations of Cystic Fibrosis

MECONIUM ILEUS*
Abdominal distention
Vomiting
Failure to pass stools
Rapid development of dehydration

GASTROINTESTINAL MANIFESTATIONS
Large, bulky, loose, frothy, extremely foul-smelling stools
Voracious appetite (early in disease)
Loss of appetite (later in disease)
Weight loss
Marked tissue wasting
Failure to grow
Distended abdomen
Thin extremities
Sallow skin
Evidence of deficiency of fat-soluble vitamins A, D, E, and K
Anemia

PULMONARY MANIFESTATIONS
Initial signs:
- Wheezy respirations
- Dry, nonproductive cough

Eventually:
- Increased dyspnea
- Paroxysmal cough
- Evidence of obstructive emphysema and patchy areas of atelectasis

Progressive involvement:
- Overinflated, barrel-shaped chest
- Cyanosis
- Clubbing of fingers and toes
- Repeated episodes of bronchitis and bronchopneumonia

*In about 10% of cases.

restricted as a result of decreased absorption of nutrients, including vitamins and fat; increased oxygen demands for pulmonary function; and delayed bone growth. The usual pattern is one of growth failure (failure to thrive), with increased weight loss despite an increased appetite, and gradual deterioration of the respiratory system. Clinical manifestations of CF are listed in Box 23-17.

Diagnostic Evaluation

Traditionally the diagnosis of CF was based on a positive sweat chloride test, absence of pancreatic enzymes, radiography, chronic obstructive pulmonary disease, and family history. Newer diagnostic methods make it possible to diagnose CF early in infancy so therapies can be implemented to increase the child's overall survival and quality of life. In addition to the sweat chloride test and factors listed above, diagnosis may be confirmed by any one of the following: newborn screening, deoxyribonucleic acid (DNA) identification of mutant genes, and abnormal nasal potential difference measurement.

Universal newborn screening for CF has been proposed yet remains controversial, since many states lack the resources for such screening programs. Currently 12 states offer some type of CF newborn screening (Wilfond and Gollust, 2005); the

Centers for Disease Control and Prevention (2004) emphatically recommends newborn screening for CF. The newborn screening test consists of an immunoreactive trypsinogen (IRT) analysis performed on a dried spot of blood, which may be followed by direct analysis of DNA for the presence of the ΔF508 mutation or other mutations on the same dried blood spot. Benefits of early screening and detection include earlier nutritional intervention for identified infants (Farrell, Lai, Li, and others, 2007); disadvantages include the parental anxiety false-positive results may generate. Children who were identified and treated early in infancy with aggressive nutritional support had improved height and weight well into adolescence. Although the technology is available to conduct carrier screening for the general population, this issue remains controversial, and widespread implementation of carrier screening programs is not recommended. An in utero diagnosis of CF is also possible, based on detection of two CF mutations in the fetus.

The consistent finding of abnormally high sodium and chloride concentrations in the sweat is a unique characteristic of CF. Parents may report that their infant tastes "salty" when they kiss him or her. The quantitative sweat chloride test (pilocarpine iontophoresis) involves stimulating the production of sweat with a special device (involves stimulation with 3 mA electric current), collecting the sweat on filter paper, and measuring the sweat electrolytes. The quantitative analysis requires a sufficient volume of sweat (>75 mg). Two separate samples are collected to ensure the reliability of the test for any individual. Normally sweat chloride content is less than 40 mEq/L, with a mean of 18 mEq/L. A chloride concentration greater than 60 mEq/L is diagnostic of CF; in infants less than 3 months, a sweat chloride concentration greater than 40 mEq/L is highly suggestive of CF. In some situations DNA testing may be substituted for the sweat test. The presence of a mutation known to cause CF on each CFTR gene predicts with a high degree of certainty that the individual has CF; however, multiple CFTR mutations may also be present and detected with DNA assay.

Chest radiography reveals characteristic patchy atelectasis and obstructive emphysema. PFTs are sensitive indexes of lung function, providing evidence of abnormal small airway function in CF. Other diagnostic tools that may aid in diagnosis include stool fat or enzyme analysis. Stool analysis requires a 72-hour sample with accurate recording of food intake during that time. Radiographs, including barium enema, are used for diagnosis of meconium ileus.

Therapeutic Management

Improved survival among patients with CF during the past two decades is attributable largely to antibiotic therapy and improved nutritional and respiratory management. Goals of CF therapeutic management are to (1) prevent or minimize pulmonary complications, (2) ensure adequate nutrition for growth, (3) encourage appropriate physical activity, and (4) promote a reasonable quality of life for the child and the family. A multidisciplinary approach to treatment is needed to accomplish these goals.

Management of Pulmonary Problems. Management of pulmonary problems is directed toward prevention and treatment of pulmonary infection by improving ventilation, removing mucopurulent secretions, and administering antimicrobial agents. Many children will develop respiratory

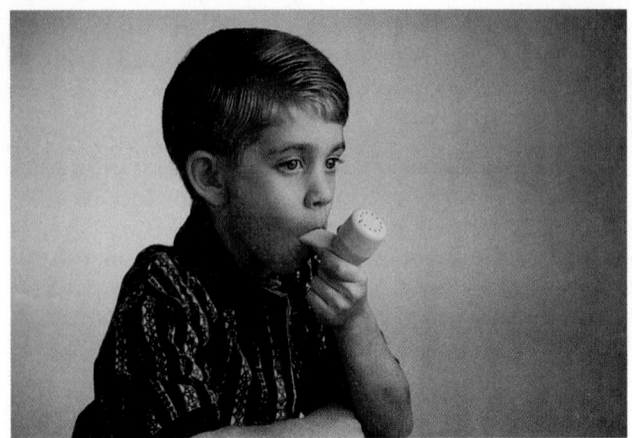

FIG. 23-9 ■ Child using Flutter mucus clearance device. (Courtesy Scandipharm, Inc.)

symptoms by 3 years of age. The large amounts and viscosity of respiratory secretions in children with CF contribute to the likelihood of respiratory tract infections. Recurrent pulmonary infections in the child with CF result in greater the damage to the airways; small airways are destroyed, causing bronchiectasis.

The most common pathogens responsible for pulmonary infections are *P. aeruginosa, B. cepacia, S. aureus, H. influenzae, E. coli,* and *K. pneumoniae. P. aeruginosa* and *B. cepacia* are particularly pathogenic for children with CF, and infections with these organisms are difficult to clear. In addition, children with CF who are chronically colonized with these organisms have poorer survival rates than children who are not colonized. Colonization and infection with methicillin-resistant *S. aureus* (MRSA) has recently emerged as a critical factor in lung infection and pulmonary function in patients with CF. Patients with MRSA required longer hospitalization and multiple antibiotic regimens (Ren, Morgan, Konstan, and others, 2007). Fungal colonization with *Candida* or *Aspergillus* organisms in the respiratory tract is also common in CF patients.

Prevention of infection involves a daily routine of CPT to maintain pulmonary hygiene. CPT is usually performed on average twice daily (on rising and in the evening) and more frequently if needed, especially during pulmonary infection. The **Flutter mucus clearance device** is a small, hand-held plastic pipe with a stainless-steel ball on the inside that facilitates removal of mucus (Fig. 23-9). It has the advantage of increasing sputum expectoration and being used without an assistant. Hand-held percussors may be used to loosen secretions. Another method to clear mucus is high-frequency chest compression, in which the child temporarily wears a mechanical vest device that provides high-frequency chest wall oscillation. Some children and adolescents with an implantable port may experience localized pain with the vest.

Patients with CF have been found to regress when conventional CPT is discontinued. Therefore, although it is time consuming for the child and family, CPT remains the cornerstone of pulmonary therapy. Forced expiration, or "huffing," with the glottis partially closed helps move secretions from the small airways so that subsequent coughing can move secretions forcefully from the large airways. Several studies indicate

that this maneuver enhances the pulmonary function of patients with CF. Autogenic drainage involves a variety of breathing techniques, which the older child can use to force mucus in lower lobes up into the airways so it can be successfully expelled. Another mucus-clearing technique involves use of a positive expiratory pressure mask; this technique involves breathing into a mask attached to a one-way valve, which creates resistance—as the patient exhales, the airway is kept open by the pressure and mucus is forced into the upper airway for expulsion.

Bronchodilator medication delivered in an aerosol opens bronchi for easier expectoration and is administered before CPT when the patient exhibits evidence of reactive airway disease or wheezing. Another aerosolized medication is recombinant human deoxyribonuclease (DNase, known generically as dornase alfa [Pulmozyme]), which decreases the viscosity of mucus. It is well tolerated and has no major adverse effects; minor reactions are voice alterations and laryngitis. This medication, given daily via nebulization, has resulted in improvements in spirometry, PFTs, dyspnea scores, and perceptions of well-being and has reduced the viscosity of sputum.

Physical exercise is an important adjunct to daily CPT. Exercise stimulates mucus excretion and provides a sense of well-being and increased self-esteem. Any aerobic exercise that the patient enjoys should be encouraged. The ultimate aim of exercise is to increase lung vital capacity, remove secretions, increase pulmonary blood flow, and maintain healthy lung tissue for effective ventilation.

Pulmonary infections are treated as soon as they are recognized. In CF patients characteristic signs of pulmonary infection—fever, tachypnea, and chest pain—may be absent; therefore a careful history and physical examination are essential. The presence of anorexia, weight loss, and decreased activity alert the practitioner to pulmonary infection and the need for an antibiotic regimen (Boat and Acton, 2007). Aerosolized antibiotics such as tobramycin, ticarcillin, and gentamicin are beneficial for patients with frequent pulmonary exacerbations. It is not uncommon for the hospitalized child with CF to be placed on as many as two or three antibiotics and one antifungal medication to treat coexisting pulmonary infections.

IV antibiotics may be administered at home as an alternative to hospitalization. The use of peripherally inserted central catheters (PICCs) for the administration of antibiotics in children with CF is a viable option with limited complications and fewer needle punctures to obtain blood specimens and to maintain often lengthy treatment with parenteral antibiotics (Tolomeo and Mackey, 2003). Alternatively, an implanted port offers the advantage of access for blood draws and antibiotic infusion. Patients may receive antibiotic therapy at home and continue daily activities with minimum disruptions. However, when pulmonary function does not improve with outpatient management, hospitalization may be recommended for continued antibiotic therapy and vigorous CPT and postural drainage. Oxygen administration is used for children with acute episodes but must be used cautiously because many children with CF have chronic carbon dioxide retention, and the unsupervised use of oxygen can be harmful (see Oxygen Therapy, Chapter 22). With repeated infection and inflammation, bronchial cysts and emphysema may develop. These cysts may rupture, resulting in a pneumothorax.

Blood streaking of the sputum is usually associated with increased pulmonary infection and often requires no specific treatment. Hemoptysis greater than 250 ml/24 hr for the older child (less for a younger child) indicates a potentially life-threatening event and needs to be treated immediately. Sometimes bleeding can be controlled with bed rest, IV antibiotics, replacement of acute blood loss, IV conjugated estrogens (Premarin) or vasopressin (Pitressin), and correction of any coagulation defects with vitamin K or fresh frozen plasma. If hemoptysis persists, the site of bleeding should be localized via bronchoscopy and cauterized or embolized.

Treatment of nasal polyps includes intranasal corticosteroids, oral antihistamines, and decongestants. If these measures are ineffective, surgical interventions may be necessary.

Because pulmonary damage in patients with CF is believed to be caused by the inflammatory process that occurs with frequent infections, the use of corticosteroids has been studied; however, treatment with corticosteroids for prolonged periods has been associated with linear growth restriction, glucose tolerance abnormalities, and cataract formation. Antiinflammatory medications such as ibuprofen are becoming more important in the treatment of CF, but careful monitoring for adverse effects (gastrointestinal bleeding) is essential.

Management of Gastrointestinal Problems. The principal treatment for pancreatic insufficiency is replacement of pancreatic enzymes, which are administered with meals and snacks to ensure that digestive enzymes are mixed with food in the duodenum. Enteric-coated products prevent the neutralization of enzymes by gastric acids, thus allowing activation to occur in the alkaline environment of the small bowel. The amount of enzymes depends on the severity of the insufficiency, the child's response to enzyme replacement, and the practitioner's philosophy. Usually one to five capsules are administered with a meal, and a smaller amount is taken with snacks. Capsules can be swallowed whole or taken apart and the contents sprinkled on a small amount of food to be taken at the beginning of the meal. The amount of enzyme is adjusted to achieve normal growth and a decrease in the number of stools to one or two per day. Pancreatic enzymes should be taken within 30 minutes of eating. The enteric-coated beads should not be chewed or crushed, since destroying the enteric coating can lead to inactivation of the enzymes and excoriation of oral mucosa. The powder form should be used cautiously because inhalation of the powder may precipitate acute bronchospasm.

Children with CF require a well-balanced, high-protein, high-caloric diet (because of the impaired intestinal absorption). In fact, they often require up to 150% of the recommended daily allowances to meet their needs for growth. Breastfeeding with enzyme supplementation should be continued whenever possible for parents who prefer this method and, when necessary, supplemented with a higher-calorie-per-ounce formula. For formula-fed infants, commercial cow's milk–based formulas are usually adequate, although fre-

quently a partially hydrolysated formula with medium-chain triglycerides (e.g., Pregestimil, Alimentum) may be recommended. Enzymes are mixed into cereal or fruit, such as applesauce. Because the uptake of fat-soluble vitamins is decreased, water-miscible forms of these vitamins (A, D, E, and K) are given, along with multivitamins and the enzymes. When high-fat foods are eaten, the child is encouraged to add extra enzymes. Growth failure despite adequate nutritional support may indicate deterioration of pulmonary status. Patients with CF may experience frequent anorexia as a result of the copious amounts of mucus produced and expectorated, persistent cough, effect of medications, fatigue, and sleep disruption. They may be placed on nighttime supplemental gastrostomy feedings or parenteral alimentation in an effort to build up nutritional reserves if there has been a history of inability to maintain weight.

Meconium ileus and meconium ileus equivalent, or total or partial intestinal obstruction, can occur at any age. Constipation is often the result of a combination of malabsorption (either from inadequate pancreatic enzyme dosage or a failure to take the enzymes), decreased intestinal motility, and abnormally viscous intestinal secretions. These problems usually do not require surgical interventions and may be treated with GoLYTELY or Colyte (osmotic solutions given orally or by nasogastric tubes), other laxatives, stool softeners, or rectal administration of meglumine diatrizoate (Gastrografin).

Rectal prolapse occurs in about 20% to 25% of children with CF (McMullen and Bryson, 2004). The first episode of rectal prolapse is frightening to both parents and child. Its reduction usually requires immediate guidance and intervention, which is managed by simply guiding the rectum back into place with a gloved, lubricated finger. Further management usually involves attempting to decrease the bulk of daily stools through enzyme replacement.

Children with CF often experience transient or chronic gastroesophageal reflux, which should be treated with the appropriate histamine-receptor antagonist and gastrointestinal motility drug, dietary modifications, and an upright position after feedings or meals (McMullen and Bryson, 2004).

Management of Endocrine Problems. The management of CFRD is critical in the therapeutic treatment of the child with CF. CFRD presents a combination of insulin resistance and insulin deficiency, with unstable glucose homeostasis in the presence of acute lung infection and treatment. Children with CFRD require close monitoring of blood glucose, administration of oral glucose-lowering agents or insulin injections, and diet and exercise management; children with CF may be at increased risk for glucose management problems as a result of decreased nutrient absorption, anorexia, and severity of pulmonary illness. The prevalence of CFRD increases with age, and there is increased morbidity and mortality among children with CFRD compared to those without (Strausbaugh and Davis, 2007). Microvascular complications such as retinopathy and nephropathy may occur in children and adolescents with CFRD (Schwarzenberg, Thomas, Olsen, and others, 2007). However, ketoacidosis is reported to be rare in individuals with CFRD (Boat and Acton, 2007).

Bone health is of concern in children and adults with CF. The pancreatic insufficiency of CF and chronic steroid use present potential risks for less than optimum bone growth in such children. Assessment of bone health by history and bone mass density evaluation should be considered in assessing the child's (8 years old and older) health status to detect and prevent osteoporosis or osteopenia (Borowitz, Baker, and Stallings, 2002).

The administration of growth hormone (somatropin [Nutropin]) is being investigated as a nutritional adjunct in children with CF to achieve optimum growth; one small study sample suggests an improvement in CF clinical status (Hardin, Rice, Ahn, and others, 2005).

Prognosis. The median predicted survival age for the CF patient in 2005 was 36.5 years (Cystic Fibrosis Foundation, 2006). Lung, heart, pancreas, and liver transplantation have increased survival rates among some CF patients. Heart-lung and double-lung procedures have been successfully performed in children with advanced pulmonary vascular disease and hypoxia. The obstacles surrounding this technique are availability of donated organs; complications from surgery; pulmonary infections; and recurrence of obstructive bronchiolitis, which decreases transplanted lung function.

Despite considerable progress and a recent surge in new treatment modalities, CF remains a progressive and incurable disease. The pulmonary involvement ultimately determines the patient's outcome because pancreatic enzyme deficiency is less of a problem if adequate nutrition is ensured. With advances in technology, parents and adolescents are challenged to set future goals that may include college, careers, social relationships, and marriage. Concurrently they are faced with increasing morbidity and higher rates of CF complications as they grow older.

Nursing Care Management

Assessment of the child with CF involves both pulmonary and gastrointestinal observations. Pulmonary assessment is the same as that described for asthma, with special attention to lung sounds, observation of cough, and evidence of decreased activity or fatigue. Gastrointestinal assessment primarily involves observing the frequency and nature of the stools and abdominal distention. The observer is also alert to evidence of growth failure (e.g., weight loss, muscle wasting, pallor, anorexia, decreased activity [from baseline norm]). Family members are interviewed to determine the child's eating and eliminating habits and to confirm a history of frequent respiratory tract infections or bowel obstruction in infancy.

The nurse assesses the newborn for feeding and stooling patterns, which may indicate a potential problem such as meconium ileus. The nurse also participates in diagnostic testing such as the initial newborn screening, IRT, DNA analysis, or sweat chloride test.

Parents are often anxious and puzzled about the diagnostic tests and the possible implications of the test results. They need careful explanations of the disease, how it might affect their family, and what they can do to provide the best possible care for their child. It is crucial to involve the parents in the follow-up for early diagnostic testing; the neonate may require several follow-up visits in the first few weeks of life if initial test results are not conclusive.

The uncertainty, fear, and initial shock associated with the diagnosis are overwhelming to parents. They must face the impact of the chronic, life-threatening nature of the disease and the prospect of intensive treatment, for which they must assume a major part of the responsibility and for which they are ill prepared. They often fear that they will be unable to provide the care the child needs. One of the most difficult aspects of the diagnosis is the implications inherent in its etiology (i.e., the recognition that each parent contributed the gene responsible for the defect).

Hospital Care. Most patients with CF require hospitalization only for treatment of pulmonary infection, uncontrolled diabetes, or a coexisting medical problem that cannot be treated on an outpatient basis. Therefore, when patients with CF are hospitalized, standard precautions with meticulous hand washing should be implemented to decrease the nosocomial spread of organisms to the CF patient and between hospitalized CF patients (especially when MRSA is prevalent). Contact precautions may be required for specific infections.

When the child with CF is hospitalized for diagnosis or treatment of pulmonary complications, aerosol therapy, chest percussion therapy, and postural drainage are instituted or continued. Respiratory therapists often initiate, supervise, and provide these treatments; however, it is the nurse's responsibility to monitor the patient's tolerance to the procedure and evaluate the effectiveness of the procedure in relation to treatment goals. The nurse may at times administer aerosol therapy, perform CPT, assist with mucus removal interventions such as the mechanical vest, and teach breathing exercises. CPT should not be performed before or immediately after meals. Planning CPT so that it does not coincide with meals is difficult in the hospital situation, but essential to the effectiveness of this treatment.

Supplemental oxygen therapy is administered to the child with mild or moderate respiratory distress, and the child requires frequent assessment of the tolerance to the procedure. Noninvasive pulse oximetry provides valuable data about the patient's oxygenation status, yet nursing assessments, including observation of respiratory pattern, work of breathing, and lung auscultation, are vital assessments.

One of the nursing challenges in the care of the child with CF is encouraging compliance with the therapeutic medication regimen, which often involves a significant number of medications; pancreatic enzymes; vitamins A, D, E, and K; oral antifungals for *Candida* infection; antihistamines; antiinflammatory agents; and oral antibiotics. This may be overwhelming to the child. Factor in multiple inhaled bronchodilators, CPT and aerosol treatments, blood glucose monitoring and insulin administration, various other medications, and increased mucus production during the acute phase, and it is not uncommon for the child with CF to rebel and be noncompliant with this regimen. Gentle coaxing, positive reinforcement, and frank negotiation may be required to enlist cooperation for effective medication compliance.

The child's sleep is disrupted frequently by hospital routines; therefore nursing care should be flexible enough to allow the child some quiet time without affecting vital care. In some cases a daily schedule of events, including medication administration, CPT, aerosolized therapy, and dressing changes, may need to be mutually developed with the child, nurses, and physician so the child feels he or she has some control of the care.

The diet for the child with CF represents another challenge; careful planning with a pediatric dietitian and the child's input may help decrease the loss of appetite and weight loss that are often part of the condition. Patients with CF, and especially adolescents, enjoy foods brought from home or an occasional fast food of choice (provided these meet therapeutic requirements). Children in the early stages of CF often have a good appetite. With infection and increased lung involvement, their appetite diminishes, and eventually it becomes a challenge to tempt failing appetites. When dietary intake fails to meet the child's needs for growth, enteral feedings or supplements may be considered (Borowitz, Baker, and Stallings, 2002). These feedings may be administered via gastrostomy tube during the night to minimize the disruption of daily activities, including school. A skin-level feeding gastrostomy affords the child few activity restrictions and minimum disruption of body image in comparison to a nasogastric tube or conventional gastrostomy tube. The child and parents are encouraged to not perceive this therapy as a last-ditch effort but as an adjunct therapy to maintain optimum growth and prevent excessive weight loss (Borowitz, Baker, and Stallings, 2002).

The child needs support during the many treatments and tests that are a part of the hospitalization. IV fluids, IV antibiotics and antifungals, and blood tests are almost always a part of the acute care treatment, and the child soon associates hospitalization with these stress-provoking procedures.

Depression, anxiety, and disturbed self-image may occur in children and adolescents with CF; young adults with severe symptoms may be especially prone to depression as a result of the realization of the poor prognosis and the reality of unmet life expectations and goals.

Providing support to both the child and the family is essential. The progressive nature of the disease makes each illness requiring hospitalization a potentially life-threatening event. Skilled nursing care and sympathetic attention to the emotional needs of the child and family help them cope with the stresses associated with repeated respiratory tract infections and hospitalizations.

The care of the child or adolescent who is immobilized as a result of CF requires the same care and attention as the child with immobility from any other chronic or acute illness, including skin care, bowel management, passive range of motion, and positioning.

Home Care. Most children and adolescents with CF can be managed at home. The goals of care include normalization and daily activities, including school and peer involvement. The care plan should be flexible so that family activities are disrupted as little as possible. Parents may initially require assistance finding and contacting durable medical equipment companies that will provide home care equipment. They also need opportunities to learn how to use the equipment and to solve problems they may encounter while delivering therapy at home. The many aspects of home care for the child with CF are similar to those of home care for other children and are discussed in Chapter 20.

Patients and family members need education about the preferred diet of nutritious meals with tolerated fat, increased protein and carbohydrate, and the administration of pancreatic enzymes. For infants and young children, the enzymes can be mixed with pureed fruit, such as applesauce, and fed with a spoon. Capsules are usually suitable for older children. It is important to stress to parents that the enzymes, in the amount regulated to the child's needs, should be administered at the beginning of all meals and snacks.

One of the most important aspects of educating parents for home care is teaching techniques for the removal of mucus

(CPT, vest, forced expiration) and breathing exercises. The success of a therapy program depends on conscientious performance of these treatments regularly as prescribed. The number of times these therapies are performed each day is determined on an individual basis, and often parents readily learn to adjust the number and intensity of the treatments to the child's needs. For pulmonary infection, home IV antibiotics may be prescribed. Home IV care may be preferred for willing and competent families because it reduces tension and usually brings a sense of belonging to the family members; this option, however, depends on a number of factors including availability of an agency with adequate staff to perform multiple daily home antibiotic infusions. With use of the venous access devices, such as PICC lines, and implanted ports, the parents and child can be taught the technique of direct administration into the IV line. Around-the-clock administration may be difficult for families and requires certain adjustments such as waking at least once during the night to give the drug.

Families also need information about medications and possible side effects. Children receiving multiple antibiotics may require serum drug levels to ensure therapeutic dosaging.

Children and adolescents with CF should receive routine primary care with special attention to diet, growth and development, and immunizations. Primary care providers should be alert to any weight loss or flattening in the growth curve associated with loss of appetite, which could indicate a pulmonary exacerbation in children with CF (McMullen and Bryson, 2004). In addition to all the recommended routine immunizations, CF patients should be immunized against influenza starting at age 6 months and followed by a yearly booster (American Academy of Pediatrics, 2006b). Anticipatory guidance concerning issues of discipline, how to incorporate aspects of the treatment regimen into the school environment, and delayed pubertal development are also important considerations for the primary care provider.

Home palliative care for the child or adolescent with CF who is in the terminal stages may be carried out with the assistance of hospice (see Chapter 18).

The nurse can assist the family in contacting resources that provide help to families with affected children. Various special child health services, many local clinics, private agencies, service clubs, and other community groups often offer equipment and medications either free or at reduced rates. The Cystic Fibrosis Foundation* has chapters throughout the United States to provide education and services to families and professionals.

Family Support. The most challenging aspect of providing care for the family of a child or adolescent with CF is meeting the emotional needs of the child and family. The di-

*6931 Arlington Road, Bethesda, MD 20814-3205; (301) 951-4422 or (800) FIGHT CF; http://www.cff.org. In Canada: Canadian Cystic Fibrosis Foundation, 2221 Yonge St., Suite 601, Toronto, Ontario M4S 2B4; http://www.cysticfibrosis.ca. Two excellent publications available from the Cystic Fibrosis Foundation are *What Everyone Should Know About Cystic Fibrosis*, and *Cystic Fibrosis: A Summary of Symptoms, Diagnosis, and Treatment*. For information about specialized medications, especially dornase alfa, and equipment for CF and other pulmonary diseases, contact Cystic Fibrosis Pharmacy, HHCS Health Group, 3901 E. Colonial Drive, Orlando, FL 32803; (800) 741-4427; http://www.cfpharmacy.com.

agnosis, treatment, and prognosis for CF are often associated with many problems and frustrations. The diagnosis can evoke feelings of guilt and self-recrimination in parents.

The long-range problems for an infant, child, or adolescent with CF are those encountered in any chronic illness (see Chapter 18). Both the child and the family must make many adjustments, the success of which depends on their ability to cope and also on the quality and quantity of support they receive from outside sources. Combined efforts of a variety of health professionals are needed to provide the most comprehensive services to families. It is often the nurse who assesses the home situation, organizes and coordinates these services, and collects the data needed to evaluate the effectiveness of the services.

The persistent need for treatment several times a day places tremendous strain on the family. When the child is young, a family member must perform postural drainage and CPT. Children often balk at these treatments, and the parents are placed in the position of insisting on adherence. The stress and anxiety related to this routine may produce feelings of resentment in both the child and the family members. When possible, occasional trusted respite care should be available to allow parents to leave the situation for short periods without undue anxiety about the child's welfare.

The affected child or adolescent may become resentful about the disease, its relentless routine of therapy, and the necessary curtailment it places on activities and relationships. The child's activities are interrupted or built around treatments, medications, and diet. This imposes hardships and influences the child's quality of life. The child should be encouraged to attend school and to join age-appropriate peer groups to foster a life that is as normal and productive as possible. Sports are often an important part of the child and adolescent's life; interaction with peers are valuable life experiences, especially to adolescents. The child or adolescent with CF should be encouraged to participate in sports activities inasmuch as physical and pulmonary health allows. Exercise is encouraged to increase pulmonary vital capacity, promote muscle development, and enhance cardiovascular function.

ETHICAL CASE STUDY   Cystic Fibrosis and End-of-Life Care

ETHICAL DECISION MAKING MODEL	Michael, a 15-year-old boy, has cystic fibrosis. Since age 12 years, Michael's respiratory status has been getting progressively worse, and he has been hospitalized for multiple respiratory exacerbations. Last evening he was admitted to the adolescent unit in acute respiratory distress. Today, he told his favorite nurse: "I am so tired, I can't fight anymore. Can't they just let me go home now and be comfortable?" Michael lives with his father and his paternal grandmother. His mother died 6 years ago in a motor vehicle accident.
Evaluate the Issue	Michael's pulmonary specialist, Dr. A., believes Michael's illness is now in the terminal stage. Michael's paternal grandmother does not want Michael to suffer any more. She tells the nurse that she believes Michael is ready to die and she thinks a do-not-resuscitate (DNR) order and hospice care are best for Michael at this time. Michael's father does not believe Michael's condition has become progressively worse. He wants everything medically possible to be done for his son. He will not discuss a DNR order or hospice care.
Treat All Involved with Respect	Michael's wishes must be heard and acknowledged. He is 15 years old and sufficiently mature to deserve respectful honesty and consideration. By approximately age 14 years, adolescents demonstrate the same kind of reasoning abilities as adults concerning health care decisions. The father's concerns must also be addressed in an empathetic manner.
Hear All Sides	The nurse has an obligation to be an advocate for her patient. However, the nurse should also consider the father's reasons for wanting everything possible to be done. Why is the father denying the seriousness of his son's condition? Does the father need more information, or is he overwhelmed and terrified at the prospect of losing his son and experiencing all the grief and emotions he felt when he lost his wife?
Initiate Action	Which of the following actions is most appropriate for the nurse to take: ■ Talk to Michael's father about Michael's comments. ■ Tell the grandmother to try to get the father to agree to a DNR order and hospice. ■ Discuss Michael's comments with Dr. A.

Consider the Outcome	The ethical dilemma is how to meet the needs of Michael and his father and grandmother.
	    The nurse decided to share Michael's comments with Dr. A. and determine whether he is aware of both Michael's wishes and those of his father.
	    After discussion with Dr. A., the nurse and other health team members believed that Michael's father may need more information about his son's condition and feelings. The following plan was implemented: the family care coordinator will arrange a family conference in which all parties (including Michael) can exchange views and arrive at a decision about future care for Michael. If the family conference does not produce a consensus and Michael still maintains his position, the situation will need to be referred to the hospital ethics committee.

As the disease progresses, however, family stress should be expected, and the patient may become angry and noncompliant. It is important for the nurse to recognize the family's changing needs and the grief they may experience as the CF worsens. Families should be made aware of sources for counseling. Patients need to be guided into activities that enable them to express anger, sorrow, and fear without guilt (see Ethical Case Study).

Transition to Adulthood. As life expectancy continues to rise for children and adolescents with CF, issues related to marriage, sexuality, childbearing, and career choice become more pressing. Males must be informed at some point that they will often be unable to produce offspring. It is important that the distinction be made between sterility and impotence. Normal sexual relationships can be expected. Female patients may be able to bear children but should be informed of the possible deleterious effects on the respiratory system created by the burden of pregnancy. They also need to know that their children will be carriers of the CF gene. Adolescent females may need counseling concerning the use of oral contraceptives and other contraceptive options (McMullen and Bryson, 2004).

Adolescents with CF are encouraged to take personal ownership and management of the illness to maximize their life's potential. Many adolescents and young persons with the illness enroll in college or vocational and technical training school and complete degrees either by distance learning or by attending a local school. Young people are encouraged to set life goals and live normal lives to the extent their illness allows.

Life as an independent adult should be encouraged for children with CF. From the time that children can take partial responsibility for their own care (e.g., CPT and taking enzymes), independence and accountability should be fostered. Although the prognosis for these children has improved, many will need continued support as they cope with the demands of surviving with CF.

Anticipatory grieving and other aspects related to care of a child with a terminal illness are also part of nursing care. For example, it is important to prepare the child and family members for end-of-life decisions and care.

OBSTRUCTIVE SLEEP-DISORDERED BREATHING

Pediatric obstructive sleep-disordered breathing reportedly affects between 10% and 12% of children ages 2 to 8 years; obstructive sleep apnea may occur in as many as 2% of all children (Benninger and Walner, 2007b). Obstructive sleep-disordered breathing is said to form a continuum of sleep-disordered breathing ranging from partial obstruction of the upper airway to continuous episodes of complete upper airway obstruction, with the most severe form being **obstructive sleep apnea syndrome (OSAS)** (Benninger and Walner, 2007b). OSAS is defined by the American Thoracic Society (1996) as a disorder of breathing during sleep with prolonged partial upper airway obstruction and/or complete obstruction that disrupts normal respiration during sleep and normal sleep patterns. Common symptoms include nightly snoring, interrupted or disturbed sleep patterns, enuresis, and daytime neurobehavioral problems (American Academy of Pediatrics, 2002; Chan, Edman, and Koltai, 2004). OSAS is to be distinguished from primary snoring, which is snoring without obstructive apnea, frequent sleep arousals, or abnormalities in gas exchange (American Academy of Pediatrics,

2002). Interestingly, children with OSAS do not exhibit daytime sleepiness as do adults; the exception may be obese children (Chan, Edman, and Koltai, 2004). If left untreated, obstructive sleep-disordered breathing may result in complications such as growth failure, cor pulmonale, pulmonary hypertension, poor learning, behavioral problems, attention deficit hyperactivity disorder, and death.

The diagnosis of obstructive sleep-disordered breathing is made by a sleep study (polysomnography), which provides evidence of sleep disturbance, respiratory pauses, and changes in oxygenation. The six-channel polysomnography can be performed in children of all ages with videotaping or audiotaping, and abbreviated (vs full night sleep study) polysomnography may be useful; however, this latter method does not predict the severity of OSAS (American Academy of Pediatrics, 2002).

A common treatment for sleep-disordered breathing in children is adenotonsillectomy, provided there is evidence of adenotonsillar hypertrophy (Benninger and Walner, 2007b). Complications of these surgical interventions are discussed previously in this chapter. Continuous positive airway pressure (CPAP) and bilevel positive airway pressure (BiPAP) may be helpful in older children with sleep-disordered breathing whose condition persists after surgical intervention. CPAP is a long-term therapy with frequent assessments to evaluate the required amount of pressure and the overall effectiveness of the intervention.

Surgical interventions such as tracheotomy may be required for children with craniofacial syndromes such as Goldenhar, Pierre Robin, Apert, and Crouzon, in which there is partial or complete upper airway obstruction (Chan, Edman, and Koltai, 2004).

Nursing care of the child with sleep-disordered breathing involves early detection by observation of the infant's or child's sleep patterns and active participation in the diagnostic polysomnography. Important nursing roles are inserting the pH probe into the esophagus, ensuring accurate placement by radiography, and monitoring the sleep study and the patient's response to diagnostic therapy. Counseling families of children with sleep-disordered breathing may involve dietary counseling for exercise programs and weight management, use of the CPAP or BiPAP equipment, and direct postoperative care after the surgical intervention of tonsillectomy or adenoidectomy. The nurse can be instrumental in helping the child and family cope with the chronic illness diagnosis should intervention such as CPAP or BiPAP be required.

RESPIRATORY EMERGENCY
RESPIRATORY FAILURE

In general, the term **respiratory insufficiency** is applied to two situations: (1) when there is increased work of breathing but gas exchange function is near normal and (2) when normal blood gas tensions cannot be maintained and hypoxemia and acidosis develop secondary to carbon dioxide retention.

Respiratory failure is defined as the inability of the respiratory apparatus to maintain adequate oxygenation of the blood, with or without carbon dioxide retention. This process involves pulmonary dysfunction that generally results in impaired alveolar gas exchange, which can lead to hypoxemia or hypercapnia. Respiratory failure is the most common cause of cardiopulmonary arrest in children (Rotta and Wiryawan, 2003). **Respiratory arrest** is the cessation of respiration. **Apnea**

is the cessation of breathing for more than 20 seconds or for a shorter period when associated with hypoxemia or bradycardia (Curley and Moloney-Harmon, 2001). Apnea can be (1) central, in which respiratory efforts are absent; (2) obstructive, in which respiratory efforts are present; and (3) mixed, in which both central and obstructive components are present.

Effective pulmonary gas exchange requires clear airways, normal lungs and chest wall, and adequate pulmonary circulation. Anything that affects these functions or their relationships can compromise respiration.

Diagnostic Evaluation

Respiratory dysfunction may have an abrupt or an insidious onset. Respiratory failure can occur as an emergency situation or may be preceded by gradual and progressive deterioration of respiratory function. Most clinical manifestations are nonspecific and are affected by variations among individual patients and differences in the severity and duration of inadequate gas exchange.

The diagnosis of respiratory failure is determined by the combined application of three sources of information:

1. Presence or history of a condition that might predispose the patient to respiratory failure
2. Observation of respiratory failure
3. Measurement of ABGs and pH

Nursing observation and judgment are vital to the recognition and early management of respiratory failure. Nurses must be able to assess a situation and initiate appropriate action within moments. Signs of respiratory failure are listed in Box 23-18.

Therapeutic Management

The interventions used in the management of respiratory failure are often dramatic, requiring special skills and emergency procedures. If respiratory arrest occurs, the primary objectives are to recognize the situation and immediately initiate resuscitative measures, such as airway positioning, administration of oxygen, cardiopulmonary resuscitation (CPR), suctioning, or intubation. When the situation is not an arrest, the suspicion of respiratory failure is confirmed by assessment; the severity may be defined by ABG analysis. Interventions such as administering supplemental oxygen, positioning, stimulation, suctioning, and early intubation may avert an arrest. When severity is established, an attempt is made to determine the underlying cause by thorough evaluation.

Treatment of respiratory dysfunction involves both specific and nonspecific therapy. Specific therapies are directed toward reversal of the causative factors. However, nonspecific measures are needed to maintain adequate oxygenation and enhance carbon dioxide removal until specific methods take effect. The major reasons for implementing nonspecific treatments are (1) unknown etiology, (2) lack of specific treatment for a known cause, (3) lack of time for a specific treatment to take effect, and (4) need for specialized personnel or equipment for specific treatment.

The principles of management are to (1) maintain ventilation and maximize oxygen delivery, (2) correct hypoxemia and hypercapnia, (3) treat the underlying cause, (4) minimize extrapulmonary organ failure, (5) apply specific and nonspecific therapy to control oxygen demands, and (6) anticipate complications. Monitoring the patient's condition is critical.

BOX 23-18
Clinical Manifestations of Respiratory Failure

CARDINAL SIGNS
Restlessness
Tachypnea
Tachycardia
Diaphoresis

EARLY BUT LESS OBVIOUS SIGNS
Mood changes, such as euphoria or depression
Headache
Altered depth and pattern of respirations
Hypertension
Exertional dyspnea
Anorexia
Increased cardiac output and renal output
Central nervous system symptoms (decreased efficiency, impaired judgment, anxiety, confusion, restlessness, irritability, depressed level of consciousness)

Flaring nares
Chest wall retractions
Expiratory grunt
Wheezing or prolonged expiration

SIGNS OF MORE SEVERE HYPOXIA
Hypotension or hypertension
Dimness of vision
Somnolence
Stupor
Coma
Dyspnea
Depressed respirations
Bradycardia
Cyanosis, peripheral or central

Nursing Care Management

For families whose child has a respiratory arrest, support is aimed at keeping the family informed of the child's status and helping them cope with a near-death experience or an actual death (see Chapter 18). Knowing that their child requires CPR is a frightening and often overwhelming experience for parents. Uncertainty regarding the outcome—both mortality and morbidity—is a primary concern. Traditionally, family members are not allowed to be present during resuscitation efforts in the emergency department. However, studies indicate that family presence during emergencies alleviates the family's anger about being separated from the patient during a crisis, reduces their anxiety, eliminates doubts about what was done to help the patient, and facilitates the grieving process when the patient dies (Mangurten, Scott, Guzzetta, and others, 2006).

Regardless of whether an institution permits parental presence during CPR, nurses must consider the needs, fears, and concerns of family members during an arrest situation. If family presence is not permitted, nurses should arrange for someone to remain with the family during the code. After the child's recovery or death, the family will continue to need support and thorough medical information regarding lifesaving measures, the prognosis if the child survives, and the cause of death if the child dies.

CARDIOPULMONARY RESUSCITATION

Cardiac arrest in children is less often of cardiac origin than from prolonged hypoxemia secondary to inadequate oxygenation, ventilation, and circulation (shock). Some causes of cardiac arrest include injuries, suffocation (e.g., FB aspiration), smoke inhalation, or infection. In small infants the small size of the airway may easily be compromised by improper positioning with the chin resting on the chest; this can easily be remedied by positioning the infant with the chin elevated (but not hyperextended) so the airway is open. This is common in infants who are not positioned properly in an infant seat or car restraint seat. Respiratory arrest is associated with a better survival rate than cardiac arrest. After cardiac arrest occurs, the outcome of resuscitative efforts is poor.

Complete apnea signals the need for rapid, vigorous action to prevent cardiac arrest. In such situations, nurses must initiate action immediately. In the hospital, emergency equipment must be available and easily accessible in all patient care areas. The status of emergency equipment must be checked at least once daily. Regardless of the cause of the arrest, basic procedures are carried out and modified somewhat according to the child's size.

Rescuers who have infections that may be transmitted by blood or saliva or who believe they have been exposed to such an infection should not perform mouth-to-mouth resuscitation if a barrier device or mask with a one-way valve is not available. If CPR efforts are anticipated in the workplace or other out-of-hospital settings, rescuers should have access to these devices.

Outside the hospital situation the first action in an emergency is to quickly assess the extent of any injury and determine whether the child is unconscious. A child who is struggling to breathe but conscious should be transported immediately to an **advanced life support (ALS)** facility, with the child maintaining whatever position affords the most comfort. Attempting to transport a child by automobile wastes valuable time in obtaining help. Transportation by an **emergency medical service (EMS)** is recommended. Services in most large communities can institute ALS immediately or en route to a medical facility.

An unconscious child is managed with care to prevent additional trauma if a head or spinal cord injury has been sustained (see Spinal Cord Injury, Chapter 32). The circumstances in which the child is found offer clues to a possible injury. For example, a child who has been thrown from a bicycle or fallen from a tree is more likely to have sustained trauma than a child who is discovered in bed.

Resuscitation Procedure

The American Heart Association (2005) implemented several changes in CPR guidelines that incorporate the use of the automatic external defibrillator (AED) as a part of the treatment of cardiorespiratory arrest in children older than 1 year of age. The 2005 guidelines state that AEDs can be safely and effectively used in children ages 1 to 8 years; however, there are insufficient data to support or refute the use of AED in children less than 1 year old. Appropriate-sized pediatric pads must be used for small children. Health care providers are advised to give children 1 year and older a defibrillatory shock after providing approximately five cycles of CPR (approximately 2 minutes of cycles of 30 compressions and two ventilations by the lone rescuer), provided the AED is sensitive to pediatric rhythms, the device is capable of delivering a pediatric dosage of 2 joules/kg, and a shockable rhythm (usually ventricular fibrillation) is present. In a hospital situation, where weight-based defibrillation dosing is possible, manual defibrillation is the mode of choice instead of AED (Samson, Berg, Bingham, and others, 2003). When using an AED, health care providers

are advised to give adults and children older than 8 years a defibrillatory shock within 5 minutes of collapse outside the hospital and within 3 minutes in the hospital.

Changes in resuscitation procedure for the lay rescuer are discussed in the text. The sequence of CPR steps for the health care provider is discussed in both the text and in Fig. 23-10.

If two rescuers are present, one rescuer should begin CPR while the second rescuer activates the EMS system by calling 9-1-1 and obtaining an AED. Pediatric rescuers provide five cycles of basic life support (approximately 2 minutes) before activating EMS; each cycle consists of 30 chest compressions and two ventilations. Because pediatric arrests are most commonly due to respiratory arrest, maintaining ventilation is primary.

Open the Airway. For effective CPR the victim is placed on the back on a firm, flat surface, employing appropriate precautions. With loss of consciousness, the tongue, which is attached to the lower jaw, relaxes and falls back, obstructing the airway. To open the airway, the head is positioned with a head tilt–chin lift maneuver by the lay rescuer. Health professionals should open the airway using either a head tilt–chin lift or jaw thrust maneuver. A head tilt is accomplished by placing one hand on the victim's forehead and applying firm, backward pressure with the palm to tilt the head back. The fingers of the free hand are placed under the bony portion of the lower jaw near the chin to lift and bring the chin forward (chin lift). This supports the jaw and helps tilt the head back (Fig. 23-11).

The jaw thrust is accomplished by grasping the angles of the victim's lower jaw and lifting with both hands, one on each side, displacing the mandible upward and outward. *The jaw thrust is recommended only for health care workers.* In suspected neck injuries the jaw thrust method should be used while the cervical spine is completely immobilized. After a patent airway has been restored by removal of foreign material and secretions (if indicated), and if the child is not breathing, maintenance of the airway is continued and rescue breathing is initiated.

Give Breaths. To ventilate the lungs in the infant (from birth to 1 year of age), the bag-valve mask (BVM) or operator's mouth is placed in such a way that both the mouth and the nostrils are covered (Fig. 23-12). Children (over 1 year of age) are ventilated through the mouth while the nostrils are firmly pinched for airtight contact.

The volume of air in an infant's lungs is small, and the air passages are considerably smaller, with resistance to flow potentially higher than in adults. The rescuer should deliver small puffs of air and assess the rise of the chest to ensure that overinflation does not occur. A gentle rise of the chest is a sufficient indicator of adequate inflation. If air enters freely and the chest rises, the airway is assumed to be clear. Breaths should be given slowly with sufficient volume to make the chest rise.

Pulse Check. After an initial two breaths, the health care provider palpates the pulse to ascertain the presence of a heartbeat. The carotid is the most central and accessible artery in children over 1 year of age. However, the infant's short and often fat neck makes the carotid pulse difficult to palpate. Therefore in the infant it is preferable to use the brachial pulse, located on the inner side of the upper arm midway between the elbow and the shoulder (Fig. 23-13). Absence of a carotid or brachial pulse is considered sufficient indication to begin external cardiac massage. *Lay rescuers are not taught to check the pulse*

Maneuver	Adult Lay rescuer: ≥8 yr HCP: Adolescent and older	Child Lay rescuer: 1–8 yr HCP: 1 yr to adolescence	Infant <1 yr of age
Activate Emergency response Number (1 rescuer)	Activate when victim found unresponsive. **HCP:** If asphyxial arrest likely, call after 5 cycles (2 min) of CPR.	Activate after performing 5 cycles of CPR. For sudden, witnessed collapse, activate after verifying that victim unresponsive.	
Airway	Head tilt–chin lift (**HCP:** suspected trauma, use jaw thrust)		
Breaths Initial	2 breaths at 1 sec/breath	2 effective breaths at 1 sec/breath	
HCP: Rescue breathing without chest compressions	10-12 breaths/min (approximately 1 breath every 5-6 sec)	12-20 breaths/min (approximately 1 breath every 3-5 sec)	
HCP: Rescue breaths for CPR with advanced airway	8-10 breaths/min (approximately 1 breath every 6-8 sec)		
Foreign-body airway obstruction	Abdominal thrusts		Back slaps and chest thrusts
Circulation **HCP:** Pulse check (≤10 sec)	Carotid (**HCP** can use femoral in child)		Brachial or femoral
Compression landmarks	Center of chest, between nipples		Just below nipple line
Compression method Push hard and fast Allow complete recoil	**2 Hands:** Heel of 1 hand, other hand on top	**2 Hands:** Heel of 1 hand with second on top *or* **1 Hand:** Heel of 1 hand only	**1 Rescuer:** 2 fingers **HCP, 2 rescuers:** 2 thumb-encircling hands
Compression depth	1½-2 inches	Approximately ⅓-½ the depth of the chest	
Compression rate	Approximately 100/min		
Compression-ventilation ratio	30:2 (1 or 2 rescuers)	30:2 (1 rescuer) **HCP:** 15:2 (2 rescuers)	
Defibrillation (AED)	Use adult pads. Do not use child pads/child system. **HCP:** For out-of-hospital response, may provide 5 cycles/2 min of CPR before shock if response >4-5 min and arrest not witnessed.	**HCP:** Use AED as soon as available for sudden collapse and in-hospital. **All:** Use after 5 cycles of CPR (out-of-hospital). If available, use child pads/child system for child 1-8 yr. If pads/system not available, use adult AED pads.	No recommendation for infants <1 yr of age.

FIG. 23-10 ■ Summary of basic life support maneuvers for infants, children, and adults (newborn-neonatal information not included). *CPR,* Cardiopulmonary resuscitation; *HCP,* maneuvers used only by health care provider; *AED,* automated external defibrillator. (From American Heart Association: 2005 American Heart Association guidelines for cardiopulmonary resuscitation and emergency cardiovascular care, *Circulation* 112(24 Suppl 1):IV-166, 2005.)

FIG. 23-11 ■ Open airway using the head tilt–chin lift maneuver and check breathing.

FIG. 23-12 ■ Mouth-to–mouth and nose breathing for infant.

FIG. 23-13 ■ Locating brachial pulse in infant.

FIG. 23-14 ■ Combining chest compressions with breathing in infant.

but are taught to look for signs of circulation (e.g., normal breathing, coughing, or air movement) in response to rescue breaths.

Chest Compression. External chest compression consists of serial, rhythmic compressions of the chest to maintain circulation to vital organs until the child achieves spontaneous vital signs or ALS can be provided. *Chest compressions are always interspersed with ventilation of the lungs.** For optimal compressions, it is essential that the child's spine is supported on a firm surface during compressions of the sternum and that sternal pressure is forceful but not traumatic. For a small infant the hard surface can be the rescuer's hand or forearm, with the palm supporting the infant's back. The child's head is positioned for optimal airway opening using the head tilt–chin lift maneuver. It is essential to prevent overextension of the head of small infants, since this tends to close the flexible trachea.

The placement of the fingers for compression in infants is at a point on the lower sternum just below the intersection of the sternum and an imaginary line drawn between the nipples (Fig. 23-14). Compressions on the child 1 to 8 years of age are applied to the lower half of the sternum (Fig. 23-15). Sternal compression to infants is applied with two fingers on the sternum, exerting a firm downward thrust; for children, pressure is applied with the heel of one hand or two hands, depending on the child's size. Current American Heart Association (2005) guidelines include the addition of the two-thumb technique for chest compressions for infants when two health care providers are present. In the two-thumb technique, one of the two rescuers places both thumbs side by side over the lower half of the infant's sternum; the remaining fingers encircle the infant's chest and support the back. The two-thumb technique is not taught to lay rescuers and is not practical for the health care provider working alone.

---

*The American Heart Association now recommends that laypersons who witness an adult cardiac arrest perform continuous chest compressions without ventilations (Sayre, Berg, Cave, and others, 2008).

FIG. 23-15 ■ Chest compressions in child: one hand for smaller child **(A)** and two hands for larger child **(B)**.

The depth of compression is adapted to the child's size. The location, rate, and depth for children older than 8 years of age are the same as for adults.

Lone-rescuer CPR is continued at the ratio of two breaths to 30 compressions for all ages until signs of recovery appear. These signs include palpable peripheral pulses, return of pupils to normal size, the disappearance of mottling and cyanosis, and possibly return of spontaneous respiration. When two rescuers are present, they should deliver two breaths to each 15 compressions. The lay rescuer is not taught two-rescuer CPR according to the new guidelines (American Heart Association, 2005).

Medications. Medications are an important adjunct to CPR, especially cardiac arrest, and are used during and after resuscitation in children. Medications are used to (1) correct hypoxemia, (2) increase perfusion pressure during chest compression, (3) stimulate spontaneous or more forceful myocardial contraction, (4) accelerate cardiac rate, (5) correct metabolic acidosis, and (6) suppress ventricular ectopy (Table 23-3).

Appropriate fluid therapy is initiated immediately in the hospital or by EMS personnel during transport (see Parenteral Fluid Therapy, Chapter 22, and Shock, Chapter 25). A complete supply of emergency medications is kept and maintained in all EMS vehicles and on all hospital units. The supply is

TABLE 23-3

Drugs for Pediatric Cardiopulmonary Resuscitation

DRUG AND DOSE	ACTION	IMPLICATION
Epinephrine HCl* IV/IO—0.01 mg/kg (1:10,000) Endotracheal tube (ET)—0.1 mg/kg (1:1000) Repeat ET doses—0.1 ml/kg (1:1000)	Adrenergic Acts on both α- and β-receptor sites, especially heart and vascular and other smooth muscle	Most useful drug in cardiac arrest Disappears rapidly from bloodstream after injection; instill 5 ml saline after ET administration May produce renal vessel constriction and decreased urine formation
Sodium bicarbonate IV/IO—1 mEq/kg/dose Newborn—0.5 mEq/ml (4.2%)	Alkalinizer Buffers pH	Infuse slowly and only when ventilation is adequate; flush with saline before and after administration Do not mix with catecholamines or calcium
Atropine sulfate* 0.02 mg/kg/dose Minimum dose—0.1 mg Maximum single dose—infants and children, 0.5 mg; adolescents, 1 mg	Anticholinergic-parasympatholytic Increases cardiac output, heart rate by blocking vagal stimulation in heart	Used to treat bradycardia caused by vagal stimulation Always provide adequate ventilation and monitor oxygen saturation Produces pupillary dilation, which constricts with light
Calcium chloride 10% 20 mg/kg IV 0.2 mg/kg/dose q10min	Electrolyte replacement Needed for maintenance of normal cardiac contractility	Used only for hypocalcemia, calcium blocker overdose, hyperkalemia, or hypermagnesemia Administer slowly; very sclerosing; administer in central vein Incompatible with phosphate solutions
Lidocaine HCl* 1 mg/kg/dose	Antidysrhythmic agent Inhibits nerve impulses from sensory nerves	Used for ventricular arrhythmias only
Amiodarone IV—5 mg/kg over 30 min followed by continuous infusion Starting at 5 mcg/kg/min May increase to maximum 10 mcg/kg/min	Antidysrhythmic agent Inhibits adrenergic stimulation; prolongs action potential and refractory period in myocardial tissues; decreases atrioventricular (AV) conduction and sinus node function	Recommended as first choice for shock-refractory ventricular tachycardia Contraindicated in severe sinus node dysfunction, marked sinus bradycardia, second- and third-degree AV block Monitor ECG and blood pressure
Adenosine 0.1-0.2 mg/kg as a rapid IV bolus Maximum single initial dose—6-12 mg (given over 1-2 sec) May repeat administration—double initial dose (maximum dose = 12 mg) Follow with 5 ml normal saline flush	Antidysrhythmic, for supraventricular tachycardia Causes temporary block through AV node and interrupts reentry circuits	Administer by rapid IV push followed by saline flush May cause transient bradycardia
Naloxone (Narcan)* 0.1 mg/kg/dose† May repeat q2-3min	Reverses respiratory arrest caused by excessive opiate administration	Evaluate level of pain after administration because analgesic effects of opioids are reversed with large doses of naloxone
Magnesium 25-50 mg/kg Maximum—2 g	Inhibits calcium channels and causes smooth muscle relaxation	Given by rapid IV infusion for suspected hypomagnesemia torsades de pointes dysrhythmia Have calcium gluconate (IV) available as antidote
INFUSIONS		
Epinephrine HCl infusion 0.05 mcg/kg/min	Adrenergic See above	Titrated to desired hemodynamic effect
Dopamine HCl infusion 2 mcg/kg/min	Agonist Acts on α-receptors, causing vasoconstriction Increases cardiac output	Titrated to desired hemodynamic response
Dobutamine HCl infusion 2 mcg/kg/min	Adrenergic direct-acting β_2-agonist Increases contractility and heart rate	Titrated to desired hemodynamic response Little vasoconstriction, even at high rates
Lidocaine HCl infusion 20-50 mcg/kg/min	Antidysrhythmic Increases electrical stimulation threshold of ventricle	See above Lower infusion dose used in shock

HCl, Hydrochloride; *IO*, intraosseous; *IV*, intravenous.
*These drugs may be administered via ET tube if IV is not available; absorption rate unknown.
†Dose of naloxone to reverse respiratory depression without reversing analgesia from opioids is 0.5 mcg/kg in children <40 kg (88 pounds) (American Pain Society, 1999).

FIG. 23-16 ■ Relief of foreign body obstruction in infant. **A,** Back blows. **B,** Chest thrusts.

checked on a regular basis (usually once on each 8- or 12-hour shift). When administering drugs during CPR (or a "code"), use a saline flush between medications to prevent drug interactions. Document all drugs, dosages, and the time and route of administration.

AIRWAY OBSTRUCTION

Attempts at clearing the airway should be considered for (1) children in whom aspiration of an FB is witnessed or strongly suspected and (2) unconscious, nonbreathing children whose airways remain obstructed despite the usual maneuvers to open them. When aspiration is strongly suspected, the child is encouraged to continue coughing as long as the cough remains forceful. In a conscious choking child, attempt to relieve the obstruction only if:

- The child is unable to make any sounds.
- The cough becomes ineffective.
- There is increasing respiratory difficulty with stridor.

FIG. 23-17 ■ Abdominal thrusts in standing child for relief of foreign body obstruction.

NURSINGALERT

Blind finger sweeps are avoided in infants and children under 8 years old.

Infants

A combination of **back blows** (over the spine between the shoulder blades) and **chest thrusts** (on the sternum, same location as for chest compressions) is recommended to relieve the FB obstruction in infants (Fig. 23-16). A choking infant is placed face down over the rescuer's arm with the head lower than the trunk and the head supported. For additional support the rescuer should support the arm firmly against the thigh. Up to five quick, sharp, back blows are delivered between the infant's shoulder blades with the heel of the rescuer's hand. Less force is required than would be applied to an adult. After delivery of the back blows, the rescuer's free hand is placed flat on the infant's back so that the infant is "sandwiched" between the two hands, making certain the neck and chin are well supported. While the rescuer maintains support with the infant's head lower than the trunk, the infant is turned and placed supine on the rescuer's thigh, where up to five quick downward chest thrusts are applied in rapid succession in the same location as external

chest compressions described for CPR. Back blows and chest thrusts are continued until the object is removed or the infant becomes unconscious.

Children

A series of **subdiaphragmatic abdominal thrusts (Heimlich maneuver)** is recommended for children older than 1 year of age. The maneuver creates an artificial cough that forces air, and with it the FB, out of the airway. The procedure is carried out with the child in a standing, sitting, or lying position (Fig. 23-17). In the conscious choking child, upward thrusts are delivered to the upper abdomen with the fisted hand at a point just below the rib cage. To prevent damage to the internal organs, the rescuer's hands should not touch the xiphoid process of the sternum or the lower margins of the ribs. Up to five thrusts are repeated in rapid succession until the FB is expelled.

It is neither necessary nor desirable to squeeze or compress the arms during the procedure. It is not a punch or a bear hug. The child may vomit after relief of the obstruction and should be positioned to prevent aspiration. After breathing is restored, the child should receive medical attention and be assessed for complications.

FIG. 23-18 ▪ Recovery position for child after respiratory emergency.

The success of the technique is primarily a result of the obstruction occurring at the end of a maximum respiration. The victim is most likely to choke on food during inspiration; therefore the tidal volume plus expiratory reserve volume is present in the lungs. When pressure is exerted on the diaphragm by the maneuver, the food bolus is ejected with considerable force by this trapped air.

If the victim is breathing or resumes effective breathing after emergency interventions, place in the recovery position: move the head, shoulders, and torso simultaneously and turn onto the side. The leg not in contact with the ground may be bent and the knee moved forward to stabilize the victim (Fig. 23-18). The victim should not be moved in any way if trauma is suspected and should not be placed in the recovery position if rescue breathing or CPR is required.

KEY POINTS

- Acute infection of the respiratory tract is the most common cause of illness in infancy and childhood.
- The incidence and severity of respiratory tract infections are influenced by the infectious agents involved, the child's age, and the child's natural defenses.
- Common respiratory tract infections of childhood include nasopharyngitis, pharyngitis (including tonsillitis), influenza, infectious mononucleosis, and OM.
- Croup syndromes involve acute inflammation and variable degrees of obstruction of the epiglottis, larynx, or trachea.
- The primary goals in the care of children with croup are observation for signs of respiratory distress and relief of laryngeal obstruction.
- Common infections of the lower airways are bacterial tracheitis, bronchitis, and RSV-bronchiolitis.
- Pneumonias are classified according to site (lobar, bronchial, or interstitial) or by etiologic agent (viral, bacterial, mycoplasmal), or are associated with aspiration of foreign material.
- In TB, susceptibility to the bacillus can be influenced by heredity, age, stress, poor nutrition, and intercurrent infection.
- Second-hand smoke exposure is a major environmental pollutant contributing to respiratory illness in children.
- Asthma is the leading cause of chronic illness in children.

- General therapeutic management of asthma includes assessment of asthma severity, allergen control, drug therapy, symptom management, and sometimes hyposensitization.
- Support for the family of the child with asthma includes education about the disease and its therapy and facilitation of self-management.
- CF is the most common inherited disease in children.
- The diagnosis of CF is based on newborn screening finding of elevated IRT, DNA analysis showing a CFTR mutation, and a positive sweat chloride test (increased sweat electrolyte content).
- Choking and respiratory failure are respiratory emergencies that require immediate intervention.
- Abdominal thrusts are used in children in whom FB obstruction is witnessed or strongly suspected. A combination of back blows and chest thrusts is used for infants with FB obstruction.
- In a conscious choking child, attempts to relieve the obstruction are used only if the child is unable to make any sounds, the cough becomes ineffective, or the child has increasing respiratory difficulty with stridor.

answers to CRITICAL THINKING EXERCISE

CROUP SYNDROME

1. Yes, there are sufficient data to arrive at a possible conclusion in this situation.
2. a. Epiglottitis is a serious obstructive inflammatory process that occurs in children 2 to 8 years of age.
   b. Symptoms of epiglottitis include throat pain, restlessness, drooling, and the child usually preferring to sit upright rather than lie down.
   c. Because epiglottitis can quickly progress to severe respiratory distress, the nurse should never examine the child's throat with a tongue depressor or take a throat culture.
   d. Nursing interventions for the child with epiglottitis include monitoring the child's respiratory status, allowing the child to remain in the position that is most comfortable, preparing to administer a racemic epinephrine (nebulized) aerosol treatment, having emergency airway equipment available, and assisting with insertion of an intravenous line and administration of antibiotics.
3. The suspicion of epiglottitis constitutes an emergency. The priority for nursing care at this time is to maintain the child's airway, keep the child comfortable, and reassure the child and parent. An antipyretic may be administered for the fever as per standing practitioner's orders.
4. Yes, the evidence supports the conclusion.
5. Alternative perspectives to this situation are not apparent at this time. However, after Kim's respiratory condition stabilizes and her treatment is begun, it would be worthwhile to determine whether her immunizations are up to date. Recently, the number of cases of epiglottitis has been reduced significantly by administration of the *Haemophilus influenzae* type B conjugate vaccine.

REFERENCES

American Academy of Otolaryngology—Head and Neck Surgery: 2000 Clinical indicators compendium, *Bulletin* 19:6, 2000.

American Academy of Pediatrics, Committee on Infectious Diseases: Recommended immunization schedules for children and adolescents—United States, 2008, *Pediatrics* 121(1):219-220, 2008.

American Academy of Pediatrics: Clinical practice guideline: diagnosis and management of bronchiolitis, *Pediatrics* 118(4):1774-1793, 2006a.

American Academy of Pediatrics, Committee on Infectious Diseases, Pickering L, editor: *Red book: 2006 report of the Committee on Infectious Diseases,* ed 27, Elk Grove Village, Ill, 2006b, The Academy.

American Academy of Pediatrics, Task Force on Sudden Infant Death Syndrome: The changing concept of sudden infant death syndrome: diagnostic coding shifts, controversies regarding the sleeping environment, and new variables to consider in reducing risk, *Pediatrics* 116(5):1245-1255, 2005.

American Academy of Pediatrics: Clinical practice guidelines: diagnosis and management of acute otitis media, *Pediatrics* 113(5):1451-1465, 2004a.

American Academy of Pediatrics: Clinical practice guidelines: otitis media with effusion, *Pediatrics* 113(5):1412-1429, 2004b.

American Academy of Pediatrics: Clinical practice guideline: diagnosis and management of childhood obstructive sleep apnea syndrome, *Pediatrics* 109(4):704-712, 2002.

American Heart Association: 2005 American Heart Association guidelines for cardiopulmonary resuscitation and emergency cardiovascular care, *Circulation* 112(24 Suppl 1):IV-166, 2005.

American Pain Society: *Principles of analgesic use in the treatment of acute pain and chronic cancer pain,* ed 4, Skokie, Ill, 1999, The Society.

American Thoracic Society: Standards and indications for cardiopulmonary sleep studies in children, *Am J Respir Crit Care Med* 153(2):866-878, 1996.

Balinsky W, Zhu CW: Pediatric cystic fibrosis: evaluating costs and genetic testing, *J Pediatr Health Care* 18:30-34, 2004.

Benninger M, Walner D: Coblation: improving outcomes for children following adenotonsillectomy, *Clin Cornerstone* 9(Suppl 1):S13-S23, 2007a.

Benninger M, Walner D: Obstructive sleep-disordered breathing in children, *Clin Cornerstone* 9(Suppl 1):S006-S12, 2007b.

Bhetwal N, McConaghy JR: The evaluation and treatment of children with acute otitis media, *Primary Care* 34(1):59-70, 2007.

Blitz M, Blitz S, Beasley R, and others: Inhaled magnesium sulfate in the treatment of acute asthma, *Cochrane Database Syst Rev* 20(3):CD003898, 2005.

Boat TF, Acton JD: Cystic fibrosis. In Behrman RE, Kliegman RM, Jenson HB, editors: *Nelson textbook of pediatrics,* ed 18, Philadelphia, 2007, Saunders.

Borowitz D, Baker RD, Stallings V: Consensus report on nutrition for pediatric patients with cystic fibrosis, *J Pediatr Gastroenterol Nutr* 35(3):246-259, 2002.

Burkhart PV, Rayens MK, Revelette WR, and others: Improved health outcomes with peak flow monitoring for children with asthma, *J Asthma* 44(2):137-142, 2007.

Carlson L, Scudder L: Controversies in the management of pediatric otitis media: are more definitive answers on the horizon? *Adv Nurse Pract* 12(2):73-77, 2004.

Centers for Disease Control and Prevention: Newborn screening for cystic fibrosis, *MMWR* 53(RR13):1-36, 2004.

Chan J, Edman JC, Koltai PJ: Obstructive sleep apnea in children, *Am Fam Physician* 69(5):1147-1154, 1159-1160, 2004.

Chávez-Bueno S, Mejías A, Jafri H, and others: Respiratory syncytial virus: old challenges and new approaches, *Pediatr Ann* 34(1):62-68, 2005.

Chokephaibulkit K: Q & A: avian influenza virus infection of children in Vietnam and Thailand, *Pediatr Infect Dis J* 23(8):793-794, 2004.

Courtney AU, McCarter DF, Pollart SM: Childhood asthma: treatment update, *Am Fam Physician* 71(10):1959-1968, 2005.

Curley MA, Moloney-Harmon PA: *Critical care nursing of infants and children,* Philadelphia, 2001, Saunders.

Cystic Fibrosis Foundation: *CFF Patient Registry: annual data report 2005,* Bethesda, Md, 2006, The Foundation.

Denison MR: Severe acute respiratory syndrome coronavirus pathogenesis, disease and vaccines: an update, *Pediatr Infect Dis J* 23(11 Suppl):S207-S214, 2005.

Farrell PM, Lai HC, Li Z, and others: Evidence on improved outcomes with early diagnosis of cystic fibrosis through neonatal screening: enough is enough! *J Pediatr* 147(3 Suppl):S30-S36, 2007.

Flori HR, Glidden DV, Rutherford GW, and others: Pediatric acute lung injury, *Am J Respir Crit Care Med* 171(9):995-1001, 2005.

Frankel LR, DiCarlo JV: Acute (adult) respiratory distress syndrome (ARDS). In Behrman RE, Kliegman RM, Jenson HB, editors: *Nelson textbook of pediatrics,* ed 17, Philadelphia, 2004, Saunders.

Frye AD: Acute lung injury and acute respiratory distress syndrome in the pediatric patient, *Crit Care Nurs Clin North Am* 17(4):311-318, 2005.

Gerber MA: Diagnosis and treatment of pharyngitis in children, *Pediatr Clin North Am* 52(3):729-747, 2005.

Goldstein NA, Mandel EM, Kurs-Lasky M, and others: Water precautions and tympanostomy tubes: a randomized, controlled trial, *Laryngoscope* 115(2):324-330, 2005.

Hardin DS, Rice J, Ahn C, and others: Growth hormone treatment enhances nutrition and growth in children with cystic fibrosis receiving enteral nutrition, *J Pediatr* 146(3):324-328, 2005.

Hopkins A, Lahiri T, Salerno R, and others: Changing epidemiology of life-threatening upper airway infections: the reemergence of bacterial tracheitis, *Pediatrics* 118(4):1418-1421, 2006.

Kao LW, Nañagas KA: Carbon monoxide poisoning, *Emerg Med Clin North Am* 22(4):985-1018, 2004.

Kershner JE: Otitis media. In Behrman RE, Kliegman RM, Jenson HB, and others, editors: *Nelson textbook of pediatrics,* ed 18, Philadelphia, 2007, Saunders.

Lee PJ, Krilov LR: When animal viruses attack: SARS and avian influenza, *Pediatr Ann* 34(1):43-52, 2005.

Li YF, Langholz B, Salam MT, and others: Maternal and grandmaternal smoking patterns are associated with early childhood asthma, *Chest* 127(4):1232-1241, 2005.

Linzer JF: Review of asthma: pathophysiology and current treatment options, *Clin Pediatr Emerg Med* 8(2):87-95, 2007.

Liu AH, Spahn JD, Leung DYM: Childhood asthma. In Behrman RE, Kliegman RM, Jenson HB, editors: *Nelson textbook of pediatrics,* ed 17, Philadelphia, 2004, Saunders.

Mangurten J, Scott SH, Guzzetta CE, and others: Effects of family presence during resuscitation and invasive procedures in a pediatric emergency department, *J Emerg Nurs* 32(3):225-233, 2006.

McMullen AH, Bryson EA: Cystic fibrosis. In Jackson PL, Vessey JA, editors: *Primary care of the child with a chronic condition,* ed 4, St Louis, 2004, Mosby.

Mintz M: Asthma update, part II, Medical management, *Am Fam Physician* 70(6):1061-1066, 2004.

Moore M, Little P: Humidified air inhalation for treating croup, *Cochrane Database Syst Rev* 19(3):CD002870, 2006.

National Asthma Education and Prevention Program: *Guidelines for the diagnosis and management of asthma,* August 2007, retrieved March 7, 2008, from http://www.nhlbi.nih.gov/guidelines/asthma/index.htm.

O'Connor BB: SARS—the latest menacing microbe, *Nurs Spectrum* 13(12DC):12-13, April 7, 2003.

Paradise JL, Bluestone CD, Colborn DK, and others: Tonsillectomy and adenotonsillectomy for recurrent throat infection in moderately affected children, *Pediatrics* 110:7-15, 2002.

Pediatric Tuberculosis Collaborative Group: Targeted tuberculin skin testing and treatment of latent tuberculosis infection in children and adolescents, *Pediatrics* 114(4 Suppl):1175-1201, 2004.

Pichichero ME, Casey JR: Acute otitis media: making sense of recent guidelines on antimicrobial treatment, *J Fam Pract* 54(4):313-322, 2005.

Pongracic JA: Asthma delivery devices: age-appropriate use, *Pediatr Ann* 32(1):50-54, 2003.

Powers JH: Diagnosis and treatment of acute otitis media: evaluating the evidence, *Infect Dis Clin North Am* 21(2):409-426, 2007.

Rafei K, Lichenstein R: Airway infectious disease emergencies, *Pediatr Clin North Am* 53(2):215-242, 2006.

Ren CL, Morgan WJ, Konstan KW, and others: Presence of methicillin resistant *Staphylococcus aureus* in respiratory cultures from cystic fibrosis patients is associated with lower lung function, *Pediatr Pulmonol* 42(6):513-518, 2007.

Rice TW, Bernard GR: Acute lung injury and the acute respiratory distress syndrome: challenges in clinical trial testing, *Clin Chest Med* 27(4):733-754, 2006.

Ross MH, Mjaanes CM, Lemanske R: Asthma. In Rudolph CD, Rudolph AM, Hostetter MK, editors: *Rudolph's pediatrics,* ed 21, New York, 2003, McGraw-Hill.

Rotta AT, Wiryawan B: Respiratory emergencies in children, *Respir Care* 48(3):248-260, 2003.

Samson RA, Berg RA, Bingham R, and others: Use of automated external defibrillators for children: an update: advisory statement from the pediatric advanced life support task force, International Liaison Committee on Resuscitation, *Circulation* 107(25):3250-3255, 2003.

Sandel M, Phelan K, Wright R, and others: The effects of housing interventions on child health, *Pediatr Ann* 33(7):475-481, 2004.

Sayre MR, Berg RA, Cave DM, and others: Hands-only (compression-only) cardiopulmonary resuscitation: a call to action for bystander response to adults who experience out-of-hospital sudden cardiac arrest, *Circulation* 117(16):2162-2167, 2008.

Schwarzenberg SJ, Thomas W, Olsen TW, and others: Microvascular complications in cystic fibrosis–related diabetes, *Diabetes Care* 30(5):1056-1061, 2007.

Sharma HP, Hansel NH, Matsui E, and others: Indoor environmental influences on children's asthma, *Pediatr Clin North Am* 54(1):103-120, 2007.

Sheahan SL, Free TA: Counseling parents to quit smoking, *Pediatr Nurs* 31(2):98-108, 2005.

Slader CA, Reddel HK, Jenkins CR, and others: Complementary and alternative medicine use in asthma: who is using what? *Respirology* 11(4):373-387, 2006.

Stockman LJ, Massoudi MS, Helfand R, and others: Severe acute respiratory syndrome in children, *Pediatr Infect Dis J* 26(1):68-74, 2007.

Strausbaugh SD, Davis PB: Cystic fibrosis: a review of epidemiology and pathobiology, *Clin Chest Med* 28(2):279-288, 2007.

Strunk RC, Bloomberg GR: Omalizumab for asthma, *N Engl J Med* 354(25):2689-2695, 2006.

Tolomeo C, Mackey W: Peripherally inserted central catheters (PICCs) in the CF population: one center's experience, *Pediatr Nurs* 29(5):355-359, 2003.

US Food and Drug Administration, Center for Drug Evaluation and Research: *Questions and answers on final rule on albuterol MDI's,* March 2005, retrieved June 2007 from http://www.fda.gov/cder/mdi/mdifaqs.htm.

Uyemura MC: Foreign body ingestion in children, *Am Fam Physician* 72(2):287-291, 2005.

Van Staaij BK, van den Akker EH, Rover MM, and others: Effectiveness of adenotonsillectomy in children with mild symptoms of throat infections of adenotonsillar hypertrophy: open, randomized controlled trial, *BMJ* 329(7467):651, 2004.

Ventre K, Randolph AG: Ribavirin for respiratory syncytial virus infection of the lower respiratory tract in infants and young children, *Cochrane Database Syst Rev* 24(1):CD000181, 2007.

Wilfond BS, Gollust SE: Policy issues for expanding newborn screening programs: the cystic fibrosis newborn screening experience in the United States, *J Pediatr* 146(5):668-674, 2005.

Winkelstein ML, Huss K, Butz A, and others: Factors associated with medication self-administration in children with asthma, *Clin Pediatr* 39(6):337-345, 2000.

Wright RB, Rowe BH, Arent RJ, and others: Current pharmacologic options in the treatment of croup, *Expert Opin Pharmacother* 6(2):255-261, 2005.

24

The Child with Gastrointestinal Dysfunction

MARSHA L. ELLETT

CHAPTER OUTLINE

GASTROINTESTINAL DYSFUNCTION, 814
Dehydration, 814
  Water Balance in Infants, 814
  Types of Dehydration, 815
DISORDERS OF MOTILITY, 817
Diarrhea, 817
Constipation, 823
  Newborn Period, 824
  Infancy, 824
  Childhood, 824
Hirschsprung Disease, 825
Vomiting, 826
Gastroesophageal Reflux, 827
FUNCTIONAL ABDOMINAL PAIN DISORDERS, 829

INFLAMMATORY DISORDERS, 829
Acute Appendicitis, 829
Nursing Care Plan: The Child with
  Appendicitis, 831
Meckel Diverticulum, 831
Inflammatory Bowel Disease, 833
Peptic Ulcer Disease, 836
HEPATIC DISORDERS, 838
Acute Hepatitis, 838
Cirrhosis, 841
Biliary Atresia, 842
STRUCTURAL DEFECTS, 843
Cleft Lip or Cleft Palate, 843

Esophageal Atresia with
  Tracheoesophageal Fistula, 846
Hernias, 849
OBSTRUCTIVE DISORDERS, 849
Hypertrophic Pyloric Stenosis, 849
Intussusception, 852
Malrotation and Volvulus, 853
Anorectal Malformations, 854
MALABSORPTION SYNDROMES, 855
Celiac Disease, 855
Short-Bowel Syndrome, 856

LEARNING OBJECTIVES

On completion of this chapter the reader will be able to:
- Describe the characteristics of infants that affect their ability to adapt to fluid loss or gain.
- Formulate a care plan for the infant with acute diarrhea.
- Compare and contrast the inflammatory diseases of the gastrointestinal tract.
- Describe the nursing care of the child with hepatitis.
- Formulate a plan for teaching parents preoperative and postoperative care of the child with a cleft lip or palate.
- Formulate a care plan for the child with an obstructive disorder.
- Identify nutritional therapies for the child with a malabsorption syndrome.

stomachache — ginger Ale.

RELATED TOPICS and ADDITIONAL RESOURCES

IN TEXT

Collection of Specimens, *Ch. 22*
Cystic Fibrosis, *Ch. 23*
Diaper Dermatitis, *Ch. 30*
Encopresis, *Ch. 17*
Family-Centered Care of the Child During
    Illness and Hospitalization, *Ch. 21*
Genitourinary Tract Disorders and Defects,
    Ch. 27
Infection Control, *Ch. 22*
Intestinal Parasitic Diseases, *Ch. 14*
Nursing Care of the High-Risk Newborn and
    Family, *Ch. 9*
Ostomies, *Ch. 22*
Pain Assessment; Pain Management, *Ch. 7*
Preparation for Diagnostic and Therapeutic
    Procedures, *Ch. 22*
Procedures Related to Alternative Feeding
    Techniques, *Ch. 22*
Procedures Related to Elimination, *Ch. 22*

Recommendations for Routine
    Immunizations: Hepatitis, *Ch. 10*
Shock, *Ch. 25*
Surgical Procedures, *Ch. 22*
Total Parenteral Nutrition, *Ch. 22*

COMPANION CD

Animations—Appendicitis; Digestive Tract,
    Passage of Food; Volvulus, Pediatric
Case Studies—Appendicitis, Cleft Lip and
    Palate; Acute Diarrhea (Gastroenteritis);
    Dehydration and Diarrhea
Critical Thinking Exercises—Abdominal
    Pain; Constipation; Hematemesis; Home
    Care for the Adolescent
NCLEX Review Questions

evolve.elsevier.com/Wong/essentials/

Critical Thinking Case Studies—
    Dehydration; Gastroenteritis;
    Gastrointestinal Problems; Hepatitis
NCLEX Review Questions
Nursing Care Plans—The Child with
    Appendicitis; The Child with Acute
    Diarrhea (Gastroenteritis)
WebLinks

WONG'S CLINICAL MANUAL OF PEDIATRIC NURSING, 7th Ed

Nursing Care Plans—The Infant with
    Gastrointestinal Dysfunction, Obstructive,
    p. 431; The Child with Cleft Lip and/or
    Cleft Palate (CL/CP), *p. 433*
Patient and Family Education—Caring for
    the Child with a Colostomy, *p. 557;*
    Giving Gastrostomy Feedings, *p. 551;*
    Caring for a Central Venous Catheter
    (for TPN), *p. 53*

GASTROINTESTINAL DYSFUNCTION

The extensive surface area of the gastrointestinal (GI) tract and its digestive function represent the major means of exchange between the human organism and the environment. Inflammatory and malabsorptive disorders impair the functional integrity of the GI tract. In addition, the infant's intestine is extremely vulnerable to infection. Acute infectious diarrhea causes significant alterations in fluid and electrolyte balance in both infants and children.

Numerous clinical observations provide clues to specific GI problems (Box 24-1). In any disorder that involves GI losses of large amounts of fluid, dehydration poses a serious threat to life and demands immediate attention.

DEHYDRATION *Tsp pedialyte q 5min*

Dehydration is a common body fluid disturbance in infants and children and occurs whenever the total output of fluid exceeds the total intake, regardless of the cause. Dehydration may result from a number of diseases that cause insensible losses through the skin and respiratory tract, through increased renal excretion, and through the GI tract. Although dehydration can result from lack of oral intake (especially in elevated environmental temperatures), more often it is a result of abnormal losses, such as those that occur in vomiting or diarrhea, when oral intake only partially compensates for the abnormal losses. Other significant causes of dehydration are diabetic ketoacidosis and extensive burns.

Water Balance in Infants

Compared with older children and adults, infants and young children have a greater need for water and are more vulnerable to alterations in fluid and electrolyte balance. Infants have a greater fluid intake and output relative to size. Water and electrolyte disturbances occur more frequently and more rapidly, and infants and children adjust less promptly to these alterations.

The fluid compartments in the infant vary significantly from those in the adult, primarily because of an expanded extracellular compartment. The **extracellular fluid (ECF)** compartment constitutes more than half the total body water at birth and has a greater relative content of extracellular sodium and chloride. The infant loses a large amount of fluid at birth and maintains a larger amount of ECF than the adult until about 2 years of age. This contributes to greater and more rapid water loss during this age period.

Fluid losses create compartment deficits that are reflected throughout the duration of dehydration. In general, approximately 60% of fluid is lost from the ECF, and the remaining 40% comes from the **intracellular fluid (ICF).** The amount of fluid lost from the ECF increases with acute illness and decreases with chronic loss.

Fluid losses vary with age and are divided into insensible, urinary, and fecal losses. Approximately two thirds of **insensible losses** occur through the skin; the remaining one third is lost through the respiratory tract. Heat and humidity, body temperature, and respiratory rate influence insensible fluid loss. Infants and children have a greater tendency to become highly febrile than do adults. Fever increases insensible water loss approximately 7 ml/kg/24 hr for each degree rise in temperature above 37.2° C (99° F). Fever and increased surface area relative to volume are factors that contribute to greater insensible fluid losses in young patients.

Body Surface Area. The infant's relatively greater body surface area (BSA) allows larger quantities of fluid to be lost in

BOX 24-1

Clinical Manifestations of Gastrointestinal Dysfunction in Children

Failure to thrive—Weight consistently below the 3rd percentile or body mass index below the 5th percentile or a decrease from established growth pattern

Spitting up or **regurgitation**—Passive transfer of gastric contents into the esophagus or mouth

Vomiting—Forceful ejection of gastric contents; involves a complex process under central nervous system control that causes salivation, pallor, sweating, and tachycardia; usually accompanied by nausea
Projectile vomiting—Vomiting accompanied by vigorous peristaltic waves and typically associated with pyloric stenosis or pylorospasm

Nausea—Unpleasant sensation vaguely referred to the throat or abdomen with an inclination to vomit

Constipation—Delay or difficulty with the passage of stools that is present for 2 or more weeks; associated with symptoms that may include blood-streaked stools and abdominal discomfort

Encopresis—Involuntary overflow of incontinent stool causing soiling or incontinence secondary to fecal retention or impaction

Diarrhea—Increase in the number of stools with increased water content as a result of alterations of water and electrolyte transport by the gastrointestinal (GI) tract; may be acute or chronic

Hypoactive, hyperactive, or **absent bowel sounds**—Evidence of intestinal motility problems that may be caused by inflammation or obstruction

Abdominal distention—Protuberant contour of the abdomen that may be caused by delayed gastric emptying, accumulation of gas or stool, inflammation, or obstruction

Abdominal pain—Pain associated with the abdomen that may be localized or diffuse, acute or chronic; often caused by inflammation, obstruction, or hemorrhage

Gastrointestinal bleeding—May be from an upper or lower GI source and may be acute or chronic
Hematemesis—Vomiting of bright red blood or denatured blood that results from bleeding in the upper GI tract or from swallowed blood from the nose or oropharynx
Hematochezia—Passage of bright red blood per rectum, usually indicating lower GI tract bleeding
Melena—Passage of dark-colored, "tarry" stools resulting from denatured blood, suggesting upper GI tract bleeding or bleeding from the right colon

Jaundice—Yellow coloration of the skin and sclerae associated with liver dysfunction

Dysphagia—Difficulty swallowing caused by abnormalities in the neuromuscular function of the pharynx or upper esophageal sphincter or by disorders of the esophagus

Dysfunctional swallowing—Impaired swallowing caused by central nervous system defects or structural defects of the oral cavity, pharynx, or esophagus; can cause feeding problems or aspiration

Fever—Common manifestation of illness in children with GI disorders; usually associated with dehydration, infection, or inflammation

---

insensible perspiration through the skin. It is estimated that the BSA of the preterm neonate is five times greater, and that of the newborn is two to three times greater, than that of the older child or adult. The proportionately longer GI tract in infancy is another source of fluid loss, especially from diarrhea.

Basal Metabolic Rate. The rate of metabolism in infancy is significantly higher than in adulthood because of the larger BSA in relation to the mass of active tissue. Consequently, there is a greater production of metabolic wastes that must be excreted by the kidneys. Any condition that increases metabolism causes greater heat production, insensible fluid loss, and an increased need for water for excretion. The basal metabolic rate in infants and children is higher to support growth.

Kidney Function. The kidneys of the infant are functionally immature at birth and are inefficient in excreting waste products of metabolism. Of particular importance for fluid balance is the inability of the infant's kidneys to concentrate or dilute urine, to conserve or excrete sodium, and to acidify urine. The infant is less able to handle large quantities of solute-free water than is the older child, and infants are more likely to become dehydrated when given concentrated formulas or overhydrated when given excessive water or dilute formula.

Fluid Requirements. Infants ingest and excrete a greater amount of fluid per kilogram of body weight than do older children. Because electrolytes are excreted with water and the infant has limited ability for conservation, maintenance requirements include both water and electrolytes. The daily exchange of ECF in the infant is greatly increased over that of

BOX 24-2

Daily Maintenance Fluid Requirements

1. Calculate weight of child in kilograms:

$$\frac{\text{Weight of child (in pounds)}}{\text{Divided by 2.2 lb/kg}} = \text{Weight in kilograms}$$

2. Allow 100 ml/kg for first 10 kg.
3. Allow 50 ml/kg for second 10 kg.
4. Allow 20 ml/kg for remainder of weight in kilograms.
5. Divide total amount by 24 hours to obtain rate in milliliters per hour.

older children, which leaves the infant little fluid volume reserve in dehydrated states. Fluid requirements depend on hydration status, size, environmental factors, and underlying disease. Box 24-2 lists daily maintenance fluid requirements.

Types of Dehydration

The pathophysiology of dehydration is understood by recognizing that the distribution of water between the ECF and ICF spaces depends on active transport of potassium into and sodium out of cells by energy-requiring processes. Sodium is the chief solute in ECF and is the primary determinant of ECF volume. Potassium is primarily intracellular. When ECF volume is reduced in acute dehydration, the total body sodium content is almost always reduced as well, regardless of serum sodium measurements. Replacement of fluid volume should therefore be accompanied by sodium repletion. Sodium depletion in diarrhea occurs in two ways: out of the body in stool and into the ICF compartment to replace potassium to maintain electrical equilibrium.

Dehydration is classified into three categories on the basis of osmolality and depends primarily on the serum sodium concentration: (1) isotonic, (2) hypotonic, and (3) hypertonic.

Isotonic (isosmotic or **isonatremic) dehydration,** the primary form of dehydration in children, occurs in conditions in which electrolyte and water deficits are present in approximately balanced proportions. Water and salt are lost in approximately equal amounts. The observable fluid losses are not necessarily isotonic, since losses from other avenues make adjustments so that the sum of all losses, or the net loss, is isotonic. There is no osmotic force between the ICF and the ECF, so the major loss is sustained from the ECF compartment. This significantly reduces the plasma volume and the circulating blood volume, which affects the skin, muscles, and kidneys. Shock is the greatest threat to life, and the child with isotonic dehydration displays symptoms characteristic of hypovolemic shock. Plasma sodium remains within normal limits, between 130 and 150 mEq/L.

Hypotonic (hyposmotic or **hyponatremic) dehydration** occurs when the electrolyte deficit exceeds the water deficit, leaving the serum hypotonic. Because ICF is more concentrated than ECF in hypotonic dehydration, water moves from the ECF to the ICF to establish osmotic equilibrium. This movement further increases the ECF volume loss, and shock is a frequent finding. Because there is a greater proportional loss of ECF in hypotonic dehydration, the physical signs tend to be more severe with smaller fluid losses than with isotonic or hypertonic dehydration. Serum sodium concentration is less than 130 mEq/L.

Hypertonic (hyperosmotic or **hypernatremic) dehydration** results from water loss in excess of electrolyte loss and is usually caused by a proportionately larger loss of water or a larger intake of electrolytes. This type of dehydration is the

most dangerous and requires more specific fluid therapy. Hypertonic diarrhea may occur in infants who are given fluids by mouth that contain large amounts of solute, or in children who receive high-protein nasogastric (NG) tube feedings that place an excessive solute load on the kidneys. In hypertonic dehydration, fluid shifts from the lesser concentration of the ICF to the ECF. Plasma sodium concentration is greater than 150 mEq/L.

Because the ECF volume is proportionally larger, hypertonic dehydration consists of a greater degree of water loss for the same intensity of physical signs. Shock is less apparent. However, neurologic disturbances, including alterations in consciousness, poor ability to focus attention, lethargy, increased muscle tone with hyperreflexia, and hyperirritability to stimuli, are more likely to occur. Cerebral changes are serious and may result in permanent damage.

Diagnostic Evaluation

Diagnosis of the type and degree of dehydration is necessary to develop an effective plan of therapy. The degree of dehydration has been described as a percentage: 3% to 5% (mild), 6% to 9% (moderate), or more than 10% (severe) (American Academy of Pediatrics, 1996). Water constitutes only 60% to 70% of the infant's weight. However, adipose tissue contains little water and is highly variable in individual infants and children. A more accurate means of describing dehydration is to reflect acute loss (over 48 hours or less) in milliliters per kilogram of body weight. For example, a loss of 50 ml/kg is considered to be a mild fluid loss, whereas a loss of 100 ml/kg produces severe dehydration. Weight is the most important determinant of the percent of total body fluid loss in infants and younger children. However, often the preillness weight is unknown. Other predictors of fluid loss include a changing level of consciousness (irritability to lethargy), response to stimuli, decreased skin elasticity and turgor, prolonged capillary refill, increased heart rate, and sunken eyes and fontanels. Clinical signs provide clues to the extent of dehydration (Table 24-1). Using multiple predictors increases the sensitivity of assessing

---

TABLE 24-1

Evaluating Extent of Dehydration

CLINICAL SIGNS	LEVEL OF DEHYDRATION		
	MILD	MODERATE	SEVERE
Weight loss—infants	3%-5%	6%-9%	≥10%
Weight loss—children	3%-4%	6%-8%	10%
Pulse	Normal	Slightly increased	Very increased
Respiratory rate	Normal	Slight tachypnea (rapid)	Hyperpnea (deep and rapid)
Blood pressure	Normal	Normal to orthostatic (>10 mm Hg change)	Orthostatic to shock
Behavior	Normal	Irritable, more thirsty	Hyperirritable to lethargic
Thirst	Slight	Moderate	Intense
Mucous membranes*	Normal	Dry	Parched
Tears	Present	Decreased	Absent, sunken eyes
Anterior fontanel	Normal	Normal to sunken	Sunken
External jugular vein	Visible when supine	Not visible except with supraclavicular pressure	Not visible even with supraclavicular pressure
Skin*	Capillary refill > 2 seconds	Slowed capillary refill (2-4 seconds [decreased turgor])	Very delayed capillary refill (>4 seconds) and tenting; skin cool, acrocyanotic or mottled
Urine specific gravity	>1.020	>1.020; oliguria	Oliguria or anuria

Data from Jospe N, Forbes G: Fluids and electrolytes—clinical aspects, *Pediatr Rev* 17(11):395-403, 1996; and Steiner MJ, DeWalt DA, Byerley JS: Is this child dehydrated? *JAMA* 291(22):2746-2754, 2004.

*These signs are less prominent in patients who have hypernatremia.

the fluid deficit, and early studies have shown a reasonably high degree of agreement between experienced observers in assessment of the level of dehydration. Objective signs of dehydration are present at a fluid deficit of less than 5%. Any two of the following signs—capillary refill of 2 seconds, absent tears, dry mucous membranes, and an ill general appearance—are predictors of a deficit of at least 5%. Generally, three or more clinical findings are present at a deficit of 5% to 9%, and four or more findings are found with a deficit of 10% or more (Steiner, DeWalt, Byerley, and others, 2004). Shock, tachycardia, and very low blood pressure are common features of severe depletion of ECF volume (see Shock, Chapter 25).

Therapeutic Management

See discussion on therapeutic management of diarrhea, p. 821.

Nursing Care Management

Nursing observation and intervention are essential for detection and therapeutic management of dehydration. A variety of circumstances cause fluid losses in infants, and changes can take place quickly. An important nursing responsibility is observation for signs of dehydration. Nursing assessment should begin with observation of general appearance and proceed to more specific observations. Conditions in which dehydration may develop quickly include diarrhea; vomiting; sweating; fever; disorders such as diabetes, renal disease, and cardiac anomalies; administration of certain drugs (such as diuretics and steroids); and trauma (major surgery, burns, and other extensive injury).

Intake and Output. Accurate measurements of fluid intake and output are vital to the assessment of dehydration. This includes oral and parenteral intake and losses from urine, stools, vomiting, fistulas, NG suction, sweat, and wound drainage:

- **Urine**—Frequency, color, consistency, and volume (when weighing diapers, approximately 1 g wet diaper weight equals 1 ml urine)
- **Stools**—Frequency, volume, and consistency
- **Vomitus**—Volume, frequency, and type
- **Sweating**—Can be only estimated from frequency of clothing and linen changes

In addition to fluid intake and output, the following observations assist in assessment of dehydration:

- **Vital signs**—Temperature (normal, elevated, or lowered depending on degree of dehydration), pulse (tachycardia), respirations (hyperpnea), and blood pressure (hypotension)
- **Skin**—Color, temperature, turgor, presence or absence of edema, and capillary refill
- **Mucous membranes**—Moisture, color, and presence and consistency of secretions
- **Body weight**—Decreased in relation to degree of dehydration
- **Fontanel (infants)**—Sunken, soft, or normal
- **Sensory alterations**—Presence of thirst

For nursing interventions, see discussion under specific disorders.

DISORDERS OF MOTILITY

DIARRHEA

Diarrhea is a symptom that results from disorders involving digestive, absorptive, and secretory functions. Diarrhea is caused by abnormal intestinal water and electrolyte transport. Worldwide, there are an estimated 1.3 billion episodes of diarrhea each year. Approximately 24% of all deaths in children living in developing countries are related to diarrhea and dehydration. Most children living in developed countries who have gastroenteritis have mild forms. However, in the United States, approximately 200,000 children younger than age 5 are hospitalized and approximately 200 children younger than 5 years die of diarrhea and dehydration each year (Malek, Curns, Holman, and others, 2006; Staat, 2006).

Diarrheal disturbances involve the stomach and intestines (gastroenteritis), the small intestine (enteritis), the colon (colitis), or the colon and intestines (enterocolitis). Diarrhea is classified as acute or chronic.

Acute diarrhea, a leading cause of illness in children younger than 5 years of age, is defined as a sudden increase in frequency and a change in consistency of stools, often caused by an infectious agent in the GI tract. It may be associated with upper respiratory or urinary tract infections, antibiotic therapy, or laxative use. Acute diarrhea is usually self-limited (less than 14 days' duration) and subsides without specific treatment if dehydration does not occur. **Acute infectious diarrhea (infectious gastroenteritis)** is caused by a variety of viral, bacterial, and parasitic pathogens (Table 24-2).

Chronic diarrhea is defined as an increase in stool frequency and increased water content with a duration of more than 14 days. It is often caused by chronic conditions such as malabsorption syndromes, inflammatory bowel disease (IBD), immunodeficiency, food allergy, lactose intolerance, or chronic nonspecific diarrhea, or as a result of inadequate management of acute diarrhea.

Intractable diarrhea of infancy is a syndrome that occurs in the first few months of life, persists for longer than 2 weeks with no recognized pathogens, and is refractory to treatment. The most common cause is acute infectious diarrhea that was not managed adequately.

Chronic nonspecific diarrhea (CNSD), also known as irritable colon of childhood and toddlers' diarrhea, is a common cause of chronic diarrhea in children 6 to 54 months of age. These children have loose stools, often with undigested food particles, and diarrhea greater than 2 weeks' duration. Children with CNSD grow normally and have no evidence of malnutrition, no blood in their stool, and no enteric infection. Dietary indiscretions and food sensitivities have been linked to chronic diarrhea. The excessive intake of juices and artificial sweeteners such as sorbitol, a substance found in many commercially prepared beverages and foods, may be a factor.

Etiology

Most pathogens that cause diarrhea are spread by the fecal-oral route through contaminated food or water or are spread from person to person where there is close contact (e.g., day-care centers). Lack of clean water, crowding, poor hygiene, nutritional deficiency, and poor sanitation are major risk factors, especially for bacterial or parasitic pathogens. The increased frequency and severity of diarrheal disease in infants is also related to age-specific alterations in susceptibility to pathogens. For example, the immune system of infants has not been exposed to many pathogens and has not acquired protective antibodies. Worldwide, the most common causes of acute gastroenteritis are infectious agents, viruses, bacteria, and parasites. In developed nations, viruses, primarily rotavirus, cause 70% to 80% of infectious diarrhea.

TABLE 24-2			
Infectious Causes of Acute Diarrhea			
AGENTS	PATHOLOGY	CHARACTERISTICS	COMMENTS
VIRAL			
Rotavirus Incubation—48 hours Diagnosis—enzyme immunoassay (EIA) 7 groups (A-G)—Most group A virus replicates in mature villus epithelial cells of small intestine; leads to (1) imbalance in ratio of intestinal fluid absorption to secretion and (2) malabsorption of complex carbohydrates	Fecal-oral transmission Mild to moderate fever	Vomiting followed by onset of watery stools Fever and vomiting generally abate in approximately 2 days, but diarrhea persists 5-7 days	Most common cause of diarrhea in children <5 years of age; infants 6-12 months most vulnerable; affects all ages; usually milder in children >3 years of age Immunocompromised children at greater risk for complications Peak occurrences in winter months Important cause of nosocomial infections
Norwalk-like organisms Incubation—12-48 hours Also called caliciviruses Diagnosis—EIA	Fecal-oral; contaminated water Pathology similar to that of rotavirus; affects villus epithelial cells of small intestine, leading to (1) imbalance in ratio of intestinal fluid absorption to secretion and (2) malabsorption of complex carbohydrates	Abdominal cramps, nausea, vomiting, malaise, low-grade fever, watery diarrhea without blood; duration 2-3 days; tends to resemble so-called food poisoning symptoms with nausea predominating	Affects all ages Multiple strains often named for the location of outbreak (e.g., Norwalk, Sapporo, Snow Mountain, Montgomery)
BACTERIAL			
Escherichia coli Incubation—3-4 days; variable depending on strain Diagnosis—Sorbitol MacConkey (SMAC) agar positive for blood, but fecal leukocytes absent or rare	*E. coli* strains produce diarrhea as result of enterotoxin production, adherence, or invasion (enterotoxigenic-producing *E coli*, enterohemorrhagic *E. coli*, enteroaggregative *E. coli*)	Watery diarrhea 1-2 days, then severe abdominal cramping and bloody diarrhea Can progress to hemolytic uremic syndrome	Foodborne pathogen Traveler's diarrhea Highest incidence in summer Cause of nursery epidemics Symptomatic treatment Antibiotics may worsen course Avoid antimotility agents and opioids
***Salmonella* groups** (nontyphoidal) Gram-negative rods, nonencapsulated nonsporulating Incubation—6-72 hours Diagnosis—Gram stain, stool culture	Invasion of mucosa in the small and large intestine, edema of the lamina propria, focal acute inflammation with disruption of the mucosa and microabscesses	Nausea, vomiting, colicky abdominal pain, bloody diarrhea, fever; symptoms variable: mild to severe May have headache and cerebral manifestations (e.g., drowsiness confusion, meningismus, seizures) Infants may be afebrile and nontoxic May result in life-threatening septicemia and meningitis Nausea and vomiting typically of short duration; diarrhea may persist as long as 2-3 weeks Typically shed virus for average of 5 weeks; cases reported up to a year	Incidence highest in warm months: July to November; foodborne outbreaks common Usually transmitted person to person but may transmit via undercooked meats or poultry; about half the cases caused by poultry and poultry products In children, related to pets (e.g., dogs, cats, hamsters, turtles) Communicable as long as organisms are excreted Antibiotics not recommended in uncomplicated cases Antimotility agents also not recommended—prolong transit time and carrier state Incidence decreasing over past 10 years
Salmonella typhi Produces enteric fever—systemic syndrome Incubation usually 7-14 days but could be 3-30 days depending on size of inoculum Diagnosis—positive blood cultures; also sometimes positive stool and urine cultures Late stage—positive bone marrow culture	Bloodstream invasion; after ingestion, organism attaches to microvilli of ileal brush borders and bacteria invade the intestinal epithelium via Peyer patches Next, organism is transported to intestinal lymph nodes and enters bloodstream via thoracic ducts, and circulating organism reaches reticuloendothelial cells, causing bacteremia	Manifestations dependent on age Abdominal pain, diarrhea, nausea, vomiting, high fever, lethargy Must be treated with antibiotics	Incidence much lower in developed countries; about 400 cases per year in United States; 65% of US cases acquired via international cases Ingestion of foods and water contaminated with human feces is most common mode of transmission Congenital and intrapartum transmission possible Three vaccines available

CNS, Central nervous system; *ELISA,* enzyme-linked immunosorbent assay; *GI,* gastrointestinal.

TABLE 24-2

Infectious Causes of Acute Diarrhea—cont'd

AGENTS	PATHOLOGY	CHARACTERISTICS	COMMENTS
BACTERIAL—cont'd ***Shigella* groups** Gram-negative nonmotile anaerobic bacilli Incubation—1-7 days Diagnosis—stool culture loaded with polymorphonuclear leukocytes	Enterotoxins—invades the epithelium with superficial mucosal ulcerations	Children appear sick Symptoms begin with fever, fatigue, anorexia Crampy abdominal pain preceding watery or bloody diarrhea Symptoms usually subside in 5-10 days	Most cases in children younger than 9 years, with about a third of cases in children ages 1-4 weeks Antibiotics shorten illness and lower mortality All patients at risk for dehydration Acute symptoms may persist for a week or more Antidiarrheal medications not recommended, since they may predispose patient to toxic megacolon
***Yersinia* enterocolitis** Incubation period—dose dependent, 1-3 weeks Diagnosis—stool culture, ELISA Patients have leukocytosis, elevated sedimentation rate	Pathology poorly understood; possibly due to production of enterotoxin	Mucoid diarrhea, sometimes bloody; abdominal pain suggestive of appendicitis; fever, vomiting	Seen more frequently in the winter months Transmitted by pets and food Antibiotics usually do not alter the clinical course in uncomplicated cases; antibiotics used in complicated infections and compromised hosts
Campylobacter jejuni Microaerophilic, motile, gram-negative bacilli Incubation period—1-7 days Ability to cause illness appears dose related Diagnosis—stool culture, sometimes blood culture Commonly found in GI tract of wild or domestic animals	Not fully understood, possibly (1) adherence to intestinal mucosa by toxin, (2) invasion of the mucosa in the terminal ileum and colon, (3) translocation in which the organisms penetrate the mucosa and replicate in the lamina propria	Fever, abdominal pain, diarrhea that can be bloody, vomiting Watery, profuse, foul-smelling diarrhea Clinically like infection by *Salmonella* or *Shigella* organisms Fecal-oral transmission	Most infections in humans relate to consumption of contaminated foods or water, such as undercooked meats, particularly chicken Also acquired from contaminated household pets (e.g., dogs, cats, hamsters) Bimodal peaks in infants <1 year and again at ages 15-29 years Antibiotics do not prolong the carriage of bacteria and may eliminate organism more quickly Erythromycin is the drug of choice Antimotility agents not recommended because they tend to prolong symptoms
Vibrio cholerae Gram-negative, motile, curved bacillus living in bodies of salt water Incubation—1-3 days Diagnosis—stool culture	Enters via oral route in contaminated food or water; if survives acid stomach environment, travels to the small intestine, adheres to the mucosa, and produces toxin	Onset abrupt; vomiting, watery diarrhea without cramping or tenesmus Dehydration can occur quickly	More prevalent in developing countries Rehydration most important treatment Antibiotics can shorten diarrhea Despite continued efforts, still no vaccine
Clostridium difficile Gram-positive anaerobic bacillus with the ability to produce spores Diagnosis—by detecting *C. difficile* toxin in stool culture	Produces two important toxins (A and B) Toxin binds to the enterocyte surface receptor, resulting in alteration permeability, protein synthesis, and direct cytotoxicity	Mostly mild watery diarrhea lasting a few days Some prolonged diarrhea and illness May cause pseudomembranous colitis Some individuals extremely ill with high fever, leukocytosis, hypoalbuminemia	Associated with alteration of normal intestinal flora by antibiotics Adults tend to have more severe symptoms than children Treatment with antibiotics in mildly to moderately symptomatic patients—metronidazole; nonresponders—vancomycin Resistant strains have developed Relapse common
Clostridium perfringens Incubation period—8-24 hours; anaerobic, gram-positive, spore-producing bacilli	Toxins produced in the intestine after ingestion of organism	Acute onset—watery diarrhea, crampy abdominal pain Fever, nausea, and vomiting are rare Duration of illness usually 24 hours	Transmitted by contaminated food products, most often meats and poultry Usually self-limiting and medical intervention not needed Oral rehydration usually sufficient Antibiotics serve no purpose and should not be used

Continued

TABLE 24-2

Infectious Causes of Acute Diarrhea—cont'd

AGENTS	PATHOLOGY	CHARACTERISTICS	COMMENTS
BACTERIAL—cont'd			
Clostridium botulinum Incubation period—12-26 hours (range, 6 hours–8 days) Gram-positive anaerobic spore-producing bacilli To detect toxin, submit blood and stool culture to special laboratory (usually state health department)	Botulism caused by binding of toxin to the neuromuscular junction	Clinical presentation related to age and the strain of the botulism GI—abdominal pain, cramping, and diarrhea Other strains—respiratory compromise, CNS symptoms	Transmitted in contaminated food products Can be acquired via wound infection Treatment—supportive care and neutralization of the toxin
***Staphylococcus* organisms** Incubation period—generally short, 1-8 hours Gram-positive nonmotile, aerobic or facultative anaerobic bacteria Diagnosis—identify organism in food, blood, pus, aspirate	Direct tissue invasion and production of toxin	Clinical presentation dependent on site of entry In food poisoning, profuse diarrhea, nausea, and vomiting	Transmitted in inadequately cooked or refrigerated foods Self-limiting Symptomatic treatment

No latex balloons due to aspiration.

Rotavirus is the most important cause of serious gastroenteritis among children and a significant nosocomial (hospital-acquired) pathogen, accounting for 55,000 to 70,000 hospitalizations annually (Staat, 2006). Rotavirus disease is most severe in children 3 to 24 months of age. Children younger than 3 months of age have some protection from the disease because of maternally acquired antibodies. Approximately 25% of severe cases of rotavirus occur in older children (Coffin, 2001).

Salmonella, Shigella, and *Campylobacter* organisms are the most frequently isolated bacterial pathogens. *Salmonella* has the highest occurrence in infants; *Giardia* and *Shigella* have the highest incidence among toddlers. *Shigella* infection is uncommon in the United States, accounting for less than 5% of diarrheal illnesses in infants and toddlers. *Campylobacter* infection has a bimodal presentation (highest in children less than 12 months of age with a second rise in incidence at age 15 to 19 years). *Giardia* and *Cryptosporidium* organisms are parasites. *Giardia* infection represents 15% of nondysenteric illness in the United States; *Cryptosporidium* infection is often associated with outbreaks in young children in daycare centers. *Plesiomonas* and *Yersinia* are also parasites that are frequently responsible for causing diarrhea that lasts more than 10 days in a previously healthy adolescent. (See also Intestinal Parasitic Diseases, Chapter 14.)

Antibiotic administration is frequently associated with diarrhea because antibiotics alter the normal intestinal flora, resulting in an overgrowth of other bacteria such as *Clostridium difficile*. National rates of *C. difficile* have more than doubled since 2000 (Richards, 2006). Antibiotic-associated diarrhea can also be caused by *Salmonella* organisms, *Clostridium porringers* type A, and *Staphylococcus aureus* pathogens (Jabbar and Wright, 2003).

Pathophysiology

Invasion of the GI tract by pathogens results in increased intestinal secretion as a result of enterotoxins, cytotoxic mediators, or decreased intestinal absorption secondary to intestinal damage or inflammation. Enteric pathogens attach to the mucosal cells and form a cuplike pedestal on which the bacteria rest. The pathogenesis of the diarrhea depends on whether the organism remains attached to the cell surface, resulting in a secretory toxin (noninvasive, toxin-producing, noninflammatory type diarrhea), or penetrates the mucosa (systemic diarrhea). Noninflammatory diarrhea is the most common diarrheal illness, resulting from the action of enterotoxin that is released after attachment to the mucosa (Ramaswamy and Jacobson, 2001). The most serious and immediate physiologic disturbances associated with severe diarrheal disease are (1) dehydration, (2) acid-base imbalance with acidosis, and (3) shock that occurs when dehydration progresses to the point that circulatory status is seriously impaired.

Diagnostic Evaluation

Evaluation of the child with acute gastroenteritis begins with a careful history that seeks to discover the possible cause of diarrhea, to assess the severity of symptoms and the risk of complications, and to elicit information about current symptoms indicating other treatable illnesses that could be causing the diarrhea. The history should include questions about recent travel, exposure to untreated drinking or washing water sources, contact with animals or birds, daycare center attendance, recent treatment with antibiotics, or recent diet changes. History questions should also explore the presence or absence of other symptoms such as fever and vomiting, frequency and character of stools (e.g., watery, bloody), urinary output, dietary habits, and recent food intake.

Extensive laboratory evaluation is not indicated in children who have uncomplicated diarrhea and no evidence of dehydration, since most diarrheal illnesses are self-limiting. Laboratory tests are indicated for children who are severely dehydrated and receiving intravenous (IV) therapy. Watery, explosive stools suggest glucose intolerance; foul-smelling, greasy, bulky stools suggest fat malabsorption. Diarrhea that develops after the introduction of cow's milk, fruits, or cereal may be related to enzyme deficiency or protein intolerance.

Neutrophils or red blood cells in the stool indicate bacterial gastroenteritis or IBD. The presence of eosinophils suggests protein intolerance or parasitic infection. Stool cultures should be performed only when blood, mucus, or polymorphonuclear leukocytes are present in the stool, when symptoms are severe, when there is a history of travel to a developing country, and when a specific pathogen is suspected. Gross blood or occult blood may indicate pathogens such as *Shigella, Campylobacter,* or hemorrhagic *Escherichia coli* strains. An enzyme-linked immunosorbent assay (ELISA) may be used to confirm the presence of rotavirus or *Giardia* organisms. If there is a history of recent antibiotic use, the stool should be tested for *C. difficile* toxin. When bacterial and viral cultures are negative and when diarrhea persists for more than a few days, stools should be examined for ova and parasites. A stool specimen with a pH of less than 6 and the presence of reducing substances may indicate carbohydrate malabsorption or secondary lactase deficiency. Stool electrolyte measurements may help identify children with secretory diarrhea.

Urine specific gravity should be determined if dehydration is suspected. A complete blood count (CBC), serum electrolytes, creatinine, and blood urea nitrogen (BUN) should be obtained in the child who requires hospitalization. The hemoglobin, hematocrit, creatinine, and BUN levels are usually elevated in acute diarrhea and should normalize with rehydration.

Therapeutic Management

The major goals in the management of acute diarrhea include (1) assessment of fluid and electrolyte imbalance, (2) rehydration, (3) maintenance fluid therapy, and (4) reintroduction of an adequate diet. Infants and children with acute diarrhea and dehydration should be treated first with **oral rehydration therapy (ORT)**. ORT is one of the major worldwide health care advances. It is more effective, safer, less painful, and less costly than IV rehydration. The American Academy of Pediatrics, World Health Organization, and Centers for Disease Control and Prevention all recommend ORT as the treatment of choice for most cases of dehydration caused by diarrhea (American Academy of Pediatrics, 2001). Oral rehydration solutions (ORSs) enhance and promote the reabsorption of sodium and water, and studies indicate that these solutions greatly reduce vomiting, volume loss from diarrhea, and the duration of the illness. ORSs, including reduced osmolarity ORS, are available in the United States as commercially prepared solutions and are successful in treating the majority of infants with dehydration. Guidelines for rehydration recommended by the American Academy of Pediatrics are included in Box 24-3.

After rehydration, ORS may be used during maintenance fluid therapy by alternating the solution with a low-sodium fluid such as water, breast milk, lactose-free formula, or half-strength lactose-containing formula. In older children ORS can be given and a regular diet continued. Ongoing stool losses should be replaced on a 1:1 basis with ORS. If the stool volume is not known, approximately 10 ml/kg (4 to 8 ounces) of ORS should be given for each diarrheal stool.

Solutions for oral hydration are useful in most cases of dehydration, and vomiting is not a contraindication. A child who is vomiting should be given an ORS at frequent intervals and in small amounts. For young children the caregiver may give the fluid with a spoon or small syringe in 5- to 10-ml incre-

---

BOX 24-3

Model for Rehydration

- Rehydration solution should consist of 75 to 90 mEq of sodium (Na⁺) per liter.
- Give 40 to 50 ml/kg of rehydration solution over 4 hours.
- Replacement and maintenance solution should consist of 40 to 60 mEq of Na⁺ per liter.
- Reevaluate the need for further rehydration; initiate maintenance therapy using maintenance formulations, with daily volumes not to exceed 150 ml/kg/day.
- In children with diarrhea without significant dehydration, the maintenance phase may be initiated without the need for rehydration solution (Acra and Ghishan, 1996).
- If additional fluids are needed, use low-salt fluids such as breast milk or water.

Modified from American Academy of Pediatrics, Provisional Committee on Quality Improvement, Subcommittee on Acute Gastroenteritis: Practice parameter: the management of acute gastroenteritis in young children, *Pediatrics* 97(3):424-435, 1996.

---

ments every 1 to 5 minutes. An ORS may also be given via NG or gastrostomy tube infusion. Infants without clinical signs of dehydration do not need ORT. They should, however, receive the same fluids recommended for infants with signs of dehydration in the maintenance phase and for ongoing stool losses. The use of probiotics reduces the risk of antibiotic-associated diarrhea in children by 56% (Szajewska, Ruszcynski, and Radzikowski, 2006).

Prevention

Human-bovine reassortant rotavirus vaccine (RotaTeq) became available in 2006, and live-attenuated human rotavirus vaccine (Rotarix) will be available soon for the prevention of rotavirus. Infants should receive three doses of RotaTeq oral vaccine at 2, 4, and 6 months of age. Two doses of Rotarix will induce protective immunity (Marshall, 2006).

NURSING ALERT

Diarrhea is not managed by encouraging intake of clear fluids by mouth, such as fruit juices, carbonated soft drinks, and gelatin. These fluids usually have a high carbohydrate content, a very low electrolyte content, and a high osmolality. Caffeinated soda is avoided because caffeine is a mild diuretic and may lead to increased loss of water and sodium. Chicken or beef broth is not given because it contains excessive sodium and inadequate carbohydrate. A BRAT diet (bananas, rice, applesauce, and toast or tea) is contraindicated for the child and especially for the infant with acute diarrhea, since this diet has little nutritional value (low in energy and protein), is high in carbohydrates, and is low in electrolytes (American Academy of Pediatrics, 1996).

Early reintroduction of nutrients is desirable and is gaining more widespread acceptance. Continued feeding or early reintroduction of a normal diet has no adverse effects and actually lessens the severity and duration of the illness and improves weight gain when compared with the gradual reintroduction of foods (Zangwill, 2006). Infants who are breastfeeding should continue to do so, and ORS should be used to replace ongoing losses in these infants. Formula-fed infants should resume their formula; if it is not tolerated, a lactose-free formula may be used for a few days. In older children a regular diet, including milk, can generally be offered after rehydration has been achieved. In toddlers there is no contraindication to continuing soft or pureed foods. A diet of easily digestible foods such as cereals, cooked vegetables, and meats is adequate for the older child.

In cases of severe dehydration and shock, IV fluids are initiated whenever the child is unable to ingest sufficient amounts of fluid and electrolytes to (1) meet ongoing daily physiologic losses, (2) replace previous deficits, and (3) replace ongoing abnormal losses. Patients who usually require IV fluids are those with severe dehydration, those with uncontrollable vomiting, those who are unable to drink for any reason (e.g., extreme fatigue, coma), and those with severe gastric distention.

The IV solution is selected on the basis of what is known regarding the probable type and cause of the dehydration—usually a saline solution containing 5% dextrose in water. Sodium bicarbonate may be added, since acidosis is usually associated with severe dehydration. Although the initial phase of fluid replacement is rapid in both isotonic and hypotonic dehydration, rapid fluid replacement is contraindicated in hypertonic dehydration because of the risk of water intoxication, especially in the brain cells.

After the severe effects of dehydration are under control, specific diagnostic and therapeutic measures are begun to detect and treat the cause of the diarrhea. Because of the self-limiting nature of vomiting and its tendency to improve when dehydration is corrected, the use of antiemetic agents is not recommended. The use of antibiotic therapy in children with acute gastroenteritis is controversial. Antibiotics may shorten the course of some diarrheal illnesses (e.g., those caused by *Shigella* organisms). However, most bacterial diarrheas are self-limiting, and the diarrhea often resolves before the causative organism can be determined. Antibiotics may prolong the carrier period for bacteria such as *Salmonella.* Antibiotics may be considered, however, in patients with immunosuppression, severe symptoms, or persistent disease or in patients who have had transplantation (Jabbar and Wright, 2003) (see Intestinal Parasitic Diseases, Chapter 14).

Nursing Care Management

The management of most cases of acute diarrhea takes place in the home with education of the caregiver. Caregivers are taught to monitor for signs of dehydration (especially the number of wet diapers or voidings) and the amount of fluids taken by mouth, and to assess the frequency and amount of stool losses. Education relating to ORT, including the administration of maintenance fluids and replacement of ongoing losses, is important (see Critical Thinking Exercise). ORS should be administered in small quantities at frequent intervals. Vomiting is not a contraindication to ORT unless it is severe. Information concerning the introduction of a normal diet is essential. Parents need to know that a slightly higher stool output initially occurs with continuation of a normal diet and with ongoing replacement of stool losses. The benefits of a better nutritional outcome with fewer complications and a shorter duration of illness outweigh the potential increase in stool frequency. Parents' concerns should be addressed to ensure adherence to the treatment plan.

If the child with acute diarrhea and dehydration is hospitalized, an accurate weight must be obtained, as well as careful monitoring of intake and output. The child may be placed on parenteral fluid therapy with nothing by mouth (NPO) for 12 to 48 hours. Monitoring the IV infusion is an important nursing function. The nurse must ensure that the correct fluid and

---

??? CRITICAL THINKING EXERCISE

Diarrhea

A mother brings her 8-month-old infant, Mary, to the primary care clinic. The mother reports that Mary has had a "cold" for about 2 days, and this morning she began to vomit and has had diarrhea for the past 8 hours. The mother states that Mary is still breastfeeding, but that she is not taking as much fluid as usual, and she is having three times as many stools as usual (the stools are watery in consistency). When the nurse practitioner examines Mary, she notes that her temperature is 38° C (100.4° F), her pulse and blood pressure are in the normal range, her mucous membranes are moist, and she has tears when she cries. The nurse practitioner also notes that Mary's weight has not changed from what it was when she was seen in the clinic 2 weeks ago for her well-child visit. What interventions should the nurse practitioner include in her initial management of Mary?

QUESTIONS
1. Evidence—Is there sufficient evidence for the nurse practitioner to draw any conclusions for her initial plan of management?
2. Assumptions—Describe some underlying assumptions about:
   a. Clinical manifestations of various levels of dehydration
   b. Management of acute diarrhea
   c. Breastfeeding and the management of acute diarrhea
   d. Use of antidiarrheal medications for acute diarrhea
3. What nursing interventions should the nurse practitioner implement at this time?
4. Does the evidence support the nurse practitioner's conclusion?
5. Are there any alternative perspectives that the nurse practitioner should consider?

---

electrolyte concentration is infused, that the flow rate is adjusted to deliver the desired volume in a given time, and that the IV site is maintained.

Accurate measurement of output is essential to determine whether renal blood flow is sufficient to permit the addition of potassium to the IV fluids. The nurse is responsible for examination of stools and collection of specimens for laboratory examination (see Collection of Specimens, Chapter 22). Care should be taken when obtaining and transporting stools to prevent possible spread of infection. A clean tongue depressor can be used to obtain specimens for laboratory examination or as an applicator for transfer to a culture medium. Stool specimens should be transported to the laboratory in appropriate containers and media according to hospital policy.

Diarrheal stools are highly irritating to the skin, and extra care is needed to protect the skin of the diaper region from excoriation (see Diaper Dermatitis, Chapter 30). Rectal temperatures are avoided because they stimulate the bowel, increasing passage of stool.

Support for the child and family involves the same care and consideration given all hospitalized children (see Chapter 21). Parents are kept informed of the child's progress and instructed in the use of frequent and proper hand washing and the disposal of soiled diapers, clothes, and bed linen. Everyone caring for the child must be aware of "clean" areas and "dirty" areas, especially in the hospital, where the sink in the child's room is used for many purposes. Soiled diapers and linen should be discarded in receptacles close to the bedside. To re-

ASSESSMENT

Observe the infant's or child's general appearance and behavior. Assess for dehydration, such as decreased urinary output; decreased weight; dry mucous membranes; poor skin turgor; sunken fontanel; and pale, cool, dry skin. With severe dehydration, increased pulse and respiration, decreased blood pressure, and a prolonged capillary refill time (>2 seconds) may indicate impending shock (see Table 24-1).

A history provides information about probable etiologic agents, such as introduction of a new food, exposure to infectious agents, travel to an area of high susceptibility, contact with foods that might have been contaminated, and contact with pets known to be sources of enteric infections. An allergic, drug, and dietary history may indicate food allergies, use of laxatives or antibiotics, or sources of excess sorbitol and fructose (e.g., apple juice).

DIAGNOSIS (PROBLEM IDENTIFICATION)

After a thorough assessment, several nursing diagnoses are evident:

- Deficient Fluid Volume related to diarrhea (gastrointestinal) losses, inadequate intake
- Risk for Infection related to microorganisms invading GI tract
- Impaired Skin Integrity related to irritation caused by frequent, loose stools

PLANNING

Expected patient outcomes include:

- Infant or child will maintain adequate hydration.
- Infant or child will maintain appropriate nutrition for age.
- Infant or child will not spread infection (if etiologic agent) to others.
- Family will receive appropriate support and education, especially regarding home care.

IMPLEMENTATION

Numerous intervention strategies are discussed on pp. 822-823.

EVALUATION

The effectiveness of nursing interventions for the family and the child with diarrhea is determined by continual assessment and evaluation of care based on the following guidelines:

- Monitor fluid losses with careful intake and output measurements and daily weights.
- Monitor food intake, especially calories.
- Observe for evidence of complications from underlying disease (specify) or therapy.
- Observe and interview family to determine extent and effectiveness of care.

mind caregivers to keep diapers and other soiled articles away from clean areas, place signs identifying "clean" (e.g., bed table) and "dirty" (e.g., sink, bathroom) areas. List the articles that may be stored in each area on these signs.

Prevention. The best intervention for diarrhea is prevention. The fecal-oral route spreads most infections, and parents need information about preventive measures such as personal hygiene, protection of the water supply from contamination, and careful food preparation.

NURSINGALERT

To reduce the risk of bacteria transmitted via food, encourage parents to:

- Quickly freeze or refrigerate all ground meat and other perishable foods.
- Never thaw food on the counter or let it sit out of the refrigerator for more than 2 hours.
- Wash hands, utensils, and work areas with hot, soapy water after contact with raw meat to keep bacteria from spreading.
- Check ground meat with a fork to make certain no pink is showing before taking a bite.
- Cook all dishes made with ground meat until brown or gray inside or to an internal temperature of 71° C (160° F).

Meticulous attention to perianal hygiene, disposal of soiled diapers, proper hand washing, and isolation of infected persons also minimizes the transmission of infection (see Infection Control, Chapter 22).

Parents need information about preventing diarrhea while traveling. They are cautioned against giving their children adult medications that are used to prevent traveler's diarrhea. Until vaccines or other prophylactic measures are proved to be safe for children, the best measure during travel to areas where water may be contaminated is to allow children to drink only bottled water and carbonated beverages (from the container through a straw supplied from home). Tap water, ice, unpas-

teurized dairy products, raw vegetables, unpeeled fruits, meats, and seafood should also be avoided.

The **expected outcomes** are described in the Nursing Process Box.

CONSTIPATION

Constipation is an alteration in the frequency, consistency, or ease of passing stool. Parents often define constipation as passing less than three stools per week. It may also be defined as painful bowel movements, which are often blood streaked, or include the retention of stool, with or without soiling, even with a stool frequency of more than three stools per week (Loening-Baucke and Pashankar, 2006). The frequency of bowel movements, however, is not considered a diagnostic criterion because it varies widely among children. Having extremely long intervals between defecation is termed **obstipation.** Constipation with fecal soiling is referred to as **encopresis.**

Constipation may arise secondary to a variety of organic disorders or in association with a wide range of systemic disorders. Structural disorders of the intestine, such as strictures, ectopic anus, and Hirschsprung disease (HD), may be associated with constipation. Systemic disorders associated with constipation include hypothyroidism, hypercalcemia resulting from hyperparathyroidism or vitamin D excess, and chronic lead poisoning. Constipation may be associated with drugs such as antacids, diuretics, antiepileptics, antihistamines, opioids, and iron supplementation. Spinal cord lesions may be associated with loss of rectal tone and sensation. Affected children are prone to chronic fecal retention and overflow incontinence.

The majority of children have **idiopathic** or **functional constipation,** since no underlying cause can be identified. Chronic constipation may occur as a result of environmental or psychosocial factors, or a combination of both. Transient illness, withholding and avoidance secondary to painful or negative experiences with stooling, and dietary intake with decreased fluid and fiber all play a role in the etiology of constipation.

Newborn Period

Normally the newborn infant passes a first meconium stool within 24 to 36 hours of birth. Any infant who does not do so should be assessed for evidence of intestinal atresia or stenosis, HD, hypothyroidism, meconium plugs, or meconium ileus. **Meconium plugs** are caused by meconium that has reduced water content and are usually evacuated after digital examination but may require irrigations with a hypertonic solution or contrast medium.

Meconium ileus, the initial manifestation of cystic fibrosis, is the luminal obstruction of the distal small intestine by abnormal meconium. Treatment is the same as for a meconium plug; early surgical intervention may be needed to evacuate the small intestine.

Infancy

The onset of constipation frequently occurs during infancy and may result from organic causes such as HD, hypothyroidism, and strictures. It is important to differentiate these conditions from functional constipation. Constipation in infancy is often related to dietary practices. It is less common in breast-fed infants, who have softer stools than bottle-fed infants. Breast-fed infants may also have decreased stools because of more complete use of breast milk with little residue. When constipation occurs with a change from human milk or modified cow's milk to whole cow's milk, simple measures such as adding or increasing the amount of cereal, vegetables, and fruit in the infant's diet usually corrects the problem. When a bottle-fed infant passes a hard stool that results in an anal fissure, stool-withholding behaviors may develop in response to pain on defecation (see Critical Thinking Exercise).

Childhood

Most constipation in early childhood is due to environmental changes or normal development when a child begins to attain control over bodily functions. A child who has experienced discomfort during bowel movements may deliberately try to withhold stool. Over time, the rectum accommodates to the accumulation of stool, and the urge to defecate passes. When the bowel contents are ultimately evacuated, the accumulated feces are passed with pain, thus reinforcing the desire to withhold stool.

Constipation in school-age children may represent an ongoing problem or a first-time event. The onset of constipation at this age is often the result of environmental changes, stresses, and changes in toileting patterns. A common cause of new-onset constipation at school entry is fear of using the school bathrooms, which are noted for their lack of privacy. Early and hurried departure for school immediately after breakfast may also impede bathroom use.

The management of simple constipation consists of a plan to promote regular bowel movements. Often this is as simple as changing the diet to provide more fiber and fluids, eliminating foods known to be constipating, and establishing a bowel routine that allows for regular passage of stool. Stool-softening agents such as docusate or lactulose may also be helpful. Polyethylene glycol (PEG) 3350 without electrolytes (Miralax) is a chemically inert polymer that has been

??? CRITICAL THINKING EXERCISE

Constipation

Harry, an 8-month-old infant, is seen by the pediatric nurse practitioner for his well-child visit. Harry's mother states that he usually has one hard stool every 4 or 5 days, which causes discomfort when the stool is passed. He has also had one episode of diarrhea and two episodes of ribbonlike stools. Abdominal distention and vomiting have not accompanied the constipation, and Harry's growth has been normal. Currently, his diet consists of formula only. Harry's mother reports that the infrequent passage of hard stools began approximately 6 weeks ago when she stopped breastfeeding. Which interventions should the nurse practitioner include in the initial management of Harry's problem?

QUESTIONS

1. Evidence—Is there sufficient evidence for the nurse practitioner to draw any conclusions about the management of Harry's problem?
2. Assumptions—Describe some underlying assumptions about:
   a. Causes of constipation in infants
   b. Factors associated with functional constipation in infants
   c. Management of functional constipation in infants
3. What interventions should the nurse practitioner implement at this time?
4. Does the evidence support these interventions?
5. Are there alternative perspectives that the nurse practitioner should consider? What are they?

introduced as a new laxative in recent years. It is tolerated well by children because it can be mixed in a beverage of choice (Loening-Baucke and Pashankar, 2006). If other symptoms such as vomiting, abdominal distention, or pain and evidence of growth failure are associated with the constipation, the condition should be investigated further.

Nursing Care Management

Constipation tends to be self-perpetuating. A child who has difficulty or discomfort when attempting to evacuate the bowels has a tendency to retain the bowel contents, and this may initiate a vicious circle. Nursing assessment begins with an accurate history of bowel habits; diet; events associated with the onset of constipation; drugs or other substances that the child may be taking; and the consistency, color, frequency, and other characteristics of the stool. If there is no evidence of a pathologic condition, the major task is to educate the parents regarding normal stool patterns and to participate in the education and treatment of the child.

Dietary modifications are essential in preventing constipation. During infancy, simply increasing the carbohydrate (sugar or corn syrup) in the infant's formula will often relieve the problem. During childhood the diet should contain increased amounts of fiber and fluid. Parents benefit from guidance in selecting foods that facilitate bowel movements (Box 24-4). They need reassurance concerning the benign nature of the condition. It is also important to discuss their attitudes and expectations regarding toilet habits.

When constipation persists despite dietary intervention, more aggressive management may be necessary. It is important to differentiate an acute episode of constipation from chronic functional constipation, which can result from chronic

Failure to pass meconium within 24-48 hrs Indicator of Hirschsprung or CF.

BOX 24-4
High-Fiber Foods

BREAD, GRAINS
Whole-grain bread or rolls
Whole-grain cereals
Bran
Pancakes, waffles, and muffins with fruit or bran
Unrefined (brown) rice

VEGETABLES
Raw vegetables, especially broccoli, cabbage, carrots, cauliflower, celery, lettuce, and spinach
Cooked vegetables, such as those listed above, and asparagus, beans, Brussels sprouts, corn, potatoes, rhubarb, squash, string beans, and turnips

FRUITS
Raw fruits, especially those with skins or seeds, other than ripe banana or avocado
Raisins, prunes, or other dried fruits

MISCELLANEOUS
Nuts, seeds, legumes, popcorn
High-fiber snack bars

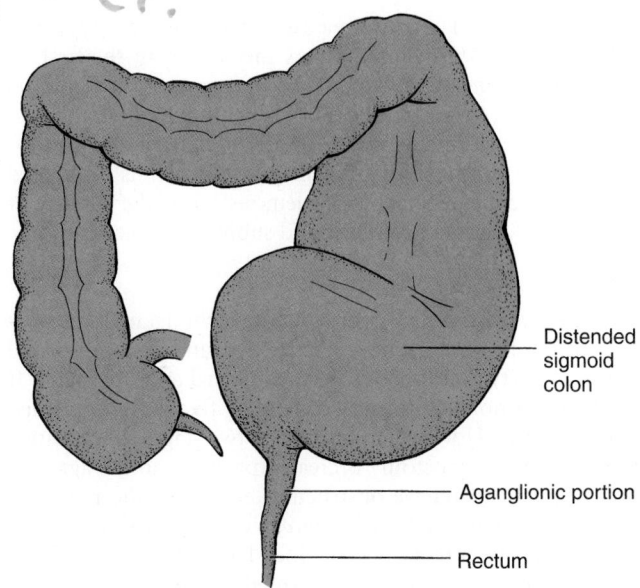

FIG. 24-1 ▪ Hirschsprung disease.

Distended sigmoid colon

Aganglionic portion

Rectum

stool-withholding behavior. As the rectal vault becomes distended over time, further complications such as fecal impaction and encopresis may develop (see Chapter 17).

HIRSCHSPRUNG DISEASE

HD (**congenital aganglionic megacolon**) is a mechanical obstruction caused by inadequate motility of part of the intestine. It accounts for about one fourth of all cases of neonatal obstruction, although it may not be diagnosed until later in infancy or childhood. The incidence is 1 in 5000 live births (Dasgupta and Langer, 2004). It is four times more common in males than in females and may follow a familial pattern in about 10% of cases. HD is usually an isolated birth defect, but it has been associated with other syndromes, including Down syndrome. Mutations in the RET proto-oncogene have been found in 17% to 38% of children with short-segment HD and in 70% to 80% of those with long-segment involvement (Dasgupta and Langer, 2004). Depending on its presentation, it may be an acute, life-threatening, or chronic condition.

Pathophysiology

HD is a developmental disorder of the enteric nervous system that is characterized by the absence of ganglion cells, originating in from the neural crest, in both the Auerbach myenteric and Meissner submucosal plexuses of the distal intestine. The length of the aganglionic distal bowel depends on the timing of the arrest in craniocaudal migration of ganglion cells. The aganglionic bowel is chronically contracted. This results in absent peristalsis in the affected bowel and the development of a functional intestinal obstruction (Fig. 24-1) (Dasgupta and Langer, 2004). Intestinal distention and ischemia may also occur as a result of distention of the bowel wall, which contributes to the development of **enterocolitis** (inflammation of the small bowel and colon). Enterocolitis is characterized by

BOX 24-5
Clinical Manifestations of Hirschsprung Disease

NEWBORN PERIOD
Failure to pass meconium within 24 to 48 hours after birth
Refusal to feed
Bilious vomiting
Abdominal distention

INFANCY
Failure to thrive
Constipation
Abdominal distention
Episodes of diarrhea and vomiting
Signs of enterocolitis
  ▪ Explosive, watery diarrhea
  ▪ Fever
  ▪ Appears significantly ill

CHILDHOOD
Constipation
Ribbonlike, foul-smelling stools
Abdominal distention
Visible peristalsis
Easily palpable fecal mass
Undernourished, anemic appearance

fever, abdominal distention, and diarrhea that may be severe and lead to life-threatening dehydration or sepsis (Dasgupta and Langer, 2004).

Diagnostic Evaluation

Most children with HD are diagnosed in the first few months of life. Clinical manifestations vary according to the age when symptoms are recognized and the presence of complications, such as enterocolitis (Box 24-5). A neonate usually is seen with distended abdomen, feeding intolerance with bilious vomiting, and delay in the passage of meconium. Typically, 95% of normal term infants pass meconium in the first 24 hours of life, whereas less than 10% of infants with HD do so. In older children, a careful history is helpful. Radiographs, an unprepped barium enema, and anorectal manometric examinations assist in the differential diagnosis, which is confirmed by a full-thickness rectal biopsy demonstrating the absence of ganglion cells in the myenteric and submucosal plexuses.

Therapeutic Management

Treatment is primarily surgery to remove the aganglionic portion of the bowel to relieve obstruction and restore normal bowel motility and function of the internal anal sphincter. If the bowel is not significantly distended, this is accomplished in one surgery. However, in most cases two stages are required. First, a temporary ostomy is created proximal to the aganglionic segment to relieve obstruction and allow the normally enervated and dilated bowel to return to its normal size. Complete corrective surgery is performed later. The various surgical procedures that can be performed are the Swenson, Duhamel, Boley, and Soave procedures. The Soave endorectal pull-through procedure, one of the most frequently used procedures, consists of pulling the end of the normal bowel through the muscular sleeve of the rectum, from which the aganglionic mucosa has been removed. The ostomy is usually closed at the time of the pull-through procedure.

Prognosis. Most children with HD require surgery rather than medical therapy. Once the child is stabilized with fluid and electrolyte replacement, if needed, the temporary colostomy is performed and has a high rate of success. After the later pull-through procedure, anal stricture and incontinence are potential complications, requiring further therapy, including dilation or bowel-retraining therapy.

Nursing Care Management

The nursing concerns depend on the child's age and the type of treatment. If the disorder is diagnosed during the neonatal period, the main objectives are (1) to help the parents adjust to a congenital defect in their child, (2) to foster infant-parent bonding, (3) to prepare them for the medical-surgical intervention, and (4) to assist them in colostomy care after discharge.

Preoperative Care. The child's preoperative care depends on the age and clinical condition. A child who is malnourished may not be able to withstand surgery until his or her physical status improves. Often this involves symptomatic treatment with enemas; a low-fiber, high-calorie, and high-protein diet; and in severe situations the use of total parenteral nutrition (TPN).

Physical preoperative preparation includes the same measures that are common to any surgery (see Surgical Procedures, Chapter 22). In the newborn, whose bowel is sterile, no additional preparation is necessary. However, in other children, preparation for the pull-through procedure involves emptying the bowel with repeated saline enemas and decreasing bacterial flora with oral or systemic antibiotics and colonic irrigations using antibiotic solution. Enterocolitis is the most serious complication of HD. Emergency preoperative care includes frequent monitoring of vital signs and blood pressure for signs of shock; monitoring fluid and electrolyte replacements, as well as plasma or other blood derivatives; and observing for symptoms of bowel perforation, such as fever,

increasing abdominal distention, vomiting, increased tenderness, irritability, dyspnea, and cyanosis.

Because progressive distention of the abdomen is a serious sign, the nurse measures abdominal circumference with a paper tape measure, usually at the level of the umbilicus or at the widest part of the abdomen. The point of measurement is marked with a pen to ensure reliability of subsequent measurements. Abdominal measurement can be obtained with the vital sign measurements and is recorded in serial order so that any change is obvious. To reduce stress to the acutely ill child when frequent measurements of abdominal circumference are needed, the tape measure can be left in place beneath the child rather than removed each time.

The child's age dictates the type and extent of psychologic preparation. Because a colostomy is usually performed, the child who is of preschool age is told about the procedure in concrete terms with the use of visual aids (see Chapter 22). It is important to time explanations appropriately to prevent the anxiety and confusion that could result from too much information. It is also important to stress to parents and older children that the colostomy for HD is temporary, unless so much bowel is involved that a permanent ileostomy must be performed. In most instances the extent of bowel resection is known before surgery, although the nurse should be aware of cases when doubt exists concerning repair. The nurse should remember that although a temporary colostomy is favorable in terms of future health and adjustment, it requires additional surgery, which may be stressful to parents and children.

Postoperative Care. Postoperative care is the same as that for any child or infant with abdominal surgery (see Surgical Procedures, Chapter 22). When a colostomy is part of the corrective procedure, stomal care is a major nursing task (see Ostomies, Chapter 22). To prevent contamination of an infant's abdominal wound with urine, the diaper should be pinned below the dressing. Sometimes a Foley catheter is used in the immediate postoperative period to divert the flow of urine away from the abdomen.

Discharge Care. After surgery, parents need instruction concerning colostomy care. Even a preschooler can be included in the care by handing articles to the parent, rolling up the colostomy pouch after it is emptied, or applying barrier preparations to the surrounding skin. Although the diagnosis of HD is less frequent in school-age children or adolescents, children this age can often be involved in colostomy care to the point of total responsibility.

Some institutions and communities have enterostomal therapists who provide expert assistance in planning home care. If families require financial assistance and psychologic support, referral to a social worker, home health care agency, or community health nurse provides continuity of care.

VOMITING

Vomiting is the forceful ejection of gastric contents through the mouth. It is a well-defined, complex, coordinated process that is under central nervous system control and is often accompanied by nausea and retching. Vomiting may be divided into two categories: nonbilious and bilious. Some small intestinal reflux is common in all vomiting. In nonbilious vomiting, the majority of bile drains into the more distal portions of the intestine. If an obstruction is present, nonbilious vomiting suggests a more proximal obstruction. Bilious vomiting implies a disorder of motility or distal physical blockage. Causes of nonbilious vomiting include infectious, inflammatory, metabolic or endocrinologic, neurologic, and psychologic causes and obstructive lesions. Causes of bilious vomiting include intestinal atresia and stenosis, malrotation with or without volvulus, ileus, intussusceptions, intestinal duplication, mass lesions, incarcerated inguinal hernia, and appendicitis. Vomiting may also be associated with other processes, including acute infectious diseases, increased intracranial pressure, toxic ingestions, food intolerances and allergies, mechanical obstruction of the GI tract, metabolic disorders, and psychogenic problems. Vomiting is common in childhood, is usually self-limiting, and requires no specific treatment. However, complications may occur, including dehydration and electrolyte disturbances, malnutrition, aspiration, and Mallory-Weiss syndrome (small tears in the distal esophageal mucosa).

Therapeutic Management

Management is directed toward detection and treatment of the cause of the vomiting and prevention of complications from the loss of fluid. Fluids are administered in the same manner and in a similar electrolyte composition to those administered for diarrhea. Although most children respond to these measures, antiemetic drugs may be needed. Antiemetics such as ondansetron (Zofran) and trimethobenzamide (Tigan) block receptors in the chemoreceptor trigger zone; others such as metoclopramide (Reglan) enhance gastroduodenal peristalsis; still others such as promethazine (Phenergan) compete for H_1-receptor sites. For children who are prone to motion sickness, it is helpful to administer an appropriate dose of dimenhydrinate (Dramamine) before a trip.

Nursing Care Management

The major focus of nursing care is observation and reporting of vomiting behavior and associated symptoms and the implementation of measures to reduce the vomiting. Accurate assessment of the type of vomiting, the appearance of the vomitus, and the child's behavior in association with the vomiting helps to establish a diagnosis.

Nursing interventions are determined by the cause of the vomiting. When the vomiting is a manifestation of improper feeding methods, establishing proper techniques through teaching and example will usually correct the situation. If vomiting is believed to be an indication of obstruction, food is usually withheld or special feeding techniques are implemented. In situations in which vomiting is related to concurrent infection, dietary indiscretion, or emotional factors, efforts are directed toward maintaining hydration or preventing dehydration.

The thirst mechanism is the most sensitive guide to fluid needs, and ad libitum administration of a glucose-electrolyte solution to an alert child will restore water and electrolytes satisfactorily. It is important to include carbohydrate to spare body protein and avoid ketosis resulting from exhaustion of glycogen stores. Small, frequent feedings of fluids or foods are preferred. After vomiting has stopped, more liberal amounts of fluids are offered, followed by gradual resumption of the regular diet.

The vomiting infant or child is positioned on the side or semireclining to prevent aspiration and observed for evidence of dehydration. It is important to emphasize the need for the child to brush the teeth or rinse the mouth after vomiting to dilute hydrochloric acid that comes in contact with the teeth. A flavored mouthwash or tooth brushing will freshen the mouth. Careful monitoring of fluid and electrolyte status is necessary to prevent an electrolyte disturbance.

GASTROESOPHAGEAL REFLUX

Keep HOB upright

Gastroesophageal reflux (GER) is defined as the transfer of gastric contents into the esophagus. This phenomenon is physiologic, occurring throughout the day, most frequently after meals and at night; therefore it is important to differentiate GER from **gastroesophageal reflux disease (GERD)**. GERD represents symptoms or tissue damage that result from GER. Approximately 50% of infants less than 2 months old are reported to have GER (Suwandhi, Ton, and Schwarz, 2006). This "physiologic" GER usually resolves spontaneously by 1 year of age. GER becomes a disease when complications such as failure to thrive, bleeding, or dysphagia develop. GERD is associated with respiratory symptoms, including apnea, bronchospasm, laryngospasm, and pneumonia (Zeiter and Hyams, 1999). Heartburn is also a frequent symptom in children who are able to describe it (Box 24-6). Certain conditions predispose children to a high prevalence of GERD, including neurologic impairment, hiatal hernia, repaired esophageal atresia, and morbid obesity (Suwandhi, Ton, and Schwarz, 2006).

BOX 24-6

Clinical Manifestations and Complications of Gastroesophageal Reflux

SYMPTOMS IN INFANTS
Spitting up, regurgitation, vomiting (may be forceful)
Excessive crying, irritability, arching of the back, stiffening
Weight loss, failure to thrive
Respiratory problems (cough, wheeze, stridor, gagging, choking with feedings)
Hematemesis
Apnea or apparent life-threatening event

SYMPTOMS IN CHILDREN
Heartburn
Abdominal pain
Noncardiac chest pain
Chronic cough
Dysphagia
Nocturnal asthma
Recurrent pneumonia

COMPLICATIONS
Esophagitis
Esophageal stricture
Laryngitis
Recurrent pneumonia
Anemia
Barrett's esophagus

Adapted from Rudolph CD, Mazur LJ, Liptak GS, and others: Guidelines for evaluation and treatment of gastroesophageal reflux in infants and children: recommendations of the North American Society for Pediatric Gastroenterology and Nutrition, *J Pediatr Gastroenterol Nutr* 32(Suppl 2):S1-S31, 2001.

Sandifer syndrome is an uncommon condition, usually occurring in young children, characterized by repetitive stretching and arching of the head and neck that can be mistaken for a seizure. This maneuver likely represents a physiologic neuromuscular response attempting to prevent acid refluxate from reaching the upper portion of the esophagus (Cavataio and Guandalini, 2005).

Pathophysiology

Although the pathogenesis of GER is multifactorial, its primary causative mechanism likely involves inappropriate transient relaxation of the lower esophageal sphincter (LES) (Suwandhi, Ton, and Schwarz, 2006). Factors that increase abdominal pressure such as coughing and sneezing, scoliosis, and overeating may contribute to GERD. Esophageal symptoms are caused by inflammation from the acid in the gastric refluxate, whereas reactive airway disease may result from stimulation of airway reflexes by the acid refluxate.

Diagnostic Evaluation

The history and physical examination are usually sufficiently reliable to establish the diagnosis of GER. However, the upper GI series is helpful in evaluating the presence of anatomic abnormalities (e.g., pyloric stenosis, malrotation, annular pancreas, hiatal hernia, esophageal stricture). The 24-hour intraesophageal pH monitoring study is the gold standard in the diagnosis of GER (Suwandhi, Ton, and Schwarz, 2006). Endoscopy with biopsy may be helpful to assess the presence and severity of esophagitis, strictures, and Barrett esophagus and to exclude other disorders such as Crohn disease. **Scintigraphy** detects radioactive substances in the esophagus after a feeding of the compound and assesses gastric emptying. It can differentiate between aspiration of gastric contents from reflux vs aspiration from poor oropharyngeal muscle coordination.

Therapeutic Management

Therapeutic management of GER depends on its severity. No therapy is needed for the infant who is thriving and has no respiratory complications. Avoidance of certain foods that exacerbate acid reflux (e.g., caffeine, citrus, tomatoes, alcohol, peppermint, spicy or fried foods), lifestyle modifications in children (e.g., weight control if indicated; small, more frequent meals; smoking cessation), and feeding maneuvers in infants (e.g., thickened feedings, upright positioning) can improve mild GER symptoms. Thickened feedings do not improve pH scores on 24-hour intraesophageal monitoring but may decrease the number of vomiting episodes. Feedings thickened with 1 teaspoon to 1 tablespoon of rice cereal per ounce of formula may be recommended. This may benefit infants who are underweight as a result of GERD. Constant NG feedings may be necessary for the infant with severe reflux and failure to thrive until surgery can be performed. Elevating the head of the bed 30 degrees or placing the infant in an infant seat elevated 30 degrees for 1 hour after feedings may decrease GER. Prone positioning of infants also decreases episodes of GER but is recommended only with extreme caution when the risk of GERD complications exceeds the risk of sudden infant death syndrome (Cavataio and Guandalini, 2005). The American Academy of Pediatrics recommends supine positioning for sleep (see Chapter 11). If the prone position is used, parents need to be cautioned to avoid soft bedding.

FIG. 24-2 ■ Nissen fundoplication sutures passing through esophageal musculature. (Redrawn from Campbell A, Ferrara B: Toupet partial fundoplication: correcting, preventing gastroesophageal reflux, *AORN J* 57(3):671-679, 1993.)

Pharmacologic therapy may be used to treat infants and children with GERD. Both H$_2$-receptor antagonists (cimetidine [Tagamet], ranitidine [Zantac], or famotidine [Pepcid]) and proton pump inhibitors (PPIs; esomeprazole [Nexium], lansoprazole [Prevacid], omeprazole [Prilosec], pantoprazole [Protonix], and rabeprazole [Aciphex]) reduce gastric hydrochloric acid secretion and may stimulate some increase in LES tone. Use of available prokinetic drugs (e.g., bethanechol [Urecholine] and metoclopramide) remains controversial. Careful analyses of published data have failed to demonstrate clinical efficacy in modifying the natural history or therapeutic outcomes of GER in childhood (Suwandhi, Ton, and Schwartz, 2006).

Surgical management of GER is reserved for children with severe complications such as recurrent aspiration pneumonia, apnea, severe esophagitis, or failure to thrive, and for children who have failed to respond to medical therapy. The **Nissen fundoplication** (Fig. 24-2) is the most common surgical procedure (Christian and Buyske, 2005). This surgery involves passage of the gastric fundus behind the esophagus to encircle the distal esophagus. The most recent surgical advance is the introduction of the laparoscopic Nissen fundoplication (Jackson, Gleiber, Askar, and others, 2001). Complications following fundoplication include breakdown of the wrap, small bowel obstruction, gas-bloat syndrome, infection, retching, and dumping syndrome (Rudolph, Mazur, Liptak, and others, 2001).

Nursing Care Management

Nursing care is directed at (1) identifying children with symptoms; (2) educating parents regarding home care, including feeding, positioning, and medications; and (3) if appropriate, providing care for the child undergoing surgical repair (see Surgical Procedures, Chapter 22). Early in the treatment program, parents should be reassured that most infants and children outgrow GER and often conservative lifestyle changes are sufficient. Parents need support and reassurance to implement lifestyle changes. Although it is not known if lifestyle changes bring additional benefit to patients receiving pharmacologic interventions, some changes may be helpful. To help parents cope with the inconvenience of dealing with a child who spits up frequently, simple measures such as using bibs and protective cloths during and after feedings are beneficial. Older children and adolescents need to know that caffeine, chocolate, and spicy foods may weaken the LES and aggravate symptoms. Exposure to tobacco and alcohol are also associated with GER. Obesity increases abdominal pressure, and weight management may reduce GER symptoms. When medical management is necessary, parents need information about the medications and their potential side effects. Prokinetic medications must be given before feedings. Medications for acid control must be timed to provide coverage and given regularly and as ordered.

FUNCTIONAL ABDOMINAL PAIN DISORDERS

Functional abdominal pain disorders include **functional abdominal pain (FAP)**, **irritable bowel syndrome (IBS)**, and **abdominal migraine** (Saps and Li, 2006). FAP is defined as nearly continuous abdominal pain in school-aged children or adolescents with only occasional relation of pain to eating, menses, or defecation. This pain may be accompanied by dizziness, headache, nausea, and vomiting. IBS is defined as abdominal pain associated with bowel movements. Patients may experience diarrhea, constipation, mucus in stools, straining, urgency, and/or a sense of incomplete evacuation. As many as 16% of all high school students and 6% of all middle school students report symptoms consistent with IBS (Saps, Sztainberg, DiLorenzo, and others, 2005). Abdominal migraine is characterized by discrete, paroxysmal episodes of severe abdominal pain between which the child is completely normal (Li and Balint, 2000). The child may have an aura and photophobia.

Etiology

There is a higher seasonal prevalence of abdominal pain symptoms during winter months, suggesting that school-related stressors and daylight hours may play a role. Also, an increased prevalence has been found among first-degree relatives.

Pathophysiology

Although the pathogenesis of functional abdominal pain disorders is incompletely understood, most investigators agree on a multifactorial etiology and the presence of an altered brain-gut interaction (Saps and Li, 2006). Children with FAP exhibit generalized visceral hyperanalgesia, whereas those with IBS exhibit rectal hyperanalgesia (DiLorenzo, Youssef, Sigurdsson, and others, 2001). All may have abnormal GI motility.

Diagnostic Evaluation

Exclusion of an organic condition can usually be accomplished through screening diagnostic tests such as CBC; erythrocyte sedimentation rate (ESR); liver transaminases; celiac antibodies; urinalysis; and stool examination for blood, ova, or parasites (Saps and Li, 2006).

Therapeutic Management

Alleviating symptoms is the main goal when treating children with functional abdominal pain disorders because complete eradication of pain often is impossible. Children may experience reduced pain with the use of anticholinergics, tricyclic antidepressants, selective serotonin reuptake inhibitors (SSRIs), or serotonin receptor modulators. Children with FAP may benefit from a smooth muscle relaxant. Children with constipation-dominant IBS may find relief by increasing fiber combined with a laxative as necessary, whereas those with diarrhea-dominant IBS may experience relief by increasing fiber and adding an antidiarrheal medication as necessary. Antimigraine therapy is often used to prevent recurrences of abdominal migraine or to abort attacks.

Nursing Care Management

It is important to validate the child's symptoms by stating that the pain is "real," not just "in the head" (Saps and Li, 2006). In addition to medications, children with functional abdominal pain disorders may benefit from relaxation training. The goals are to return the child to functional status, attending school and extracurricular activities.

INFLAMMATORY DISORDERS

ACUTE APPENDICITIS

Appendicitis, inflammation of the **vermiform appendix** (blind sac at the end of the cecum), is the most common cause of emergency abdominal surgery in childhood. In the United States, 60,000 to 80,000 cases are diagnosed each year. The average age of children with appendicitis is 10 years, with boys and girls equally affected before puberty. Classically, the first symptom of appendicitis is periumbilical pain, followed by nausea, right lower quadrant pain, and later vomiting with fever (Kwok, Kim, and Gorelick, 2004). Perforation of the appendix can occur within approximately 48 hours of the initial complaint of pain. At the time of initial presentation, about one third of all cases involve an already perforated appendix. Complications from appendiceal perforation include major abscess, phlegmon, enterocutaneous fistula, peritonitis, and partial bowel obstruction (Kwok, Kim, and Gorelick, 2004). A **phlegmon** is an acute suppurative inflammation of subcutaneous connective tissue that spreads.

Etiology

The cause of appendicitis is obstruction of the lumen of the appendix, usually by hardened fecal material (fecalith). Swollen lymphoid tissue, frequently occurring after a viral infection, can also obstruct the appendix. Another rare cause of obstruction is a parasite such as *Enterobius vermicularis,* or pinworms, which can obstruct the appendiceal lumen.

Pathophysiology

With acute obstruction, the outflow of mucus secretions is blocked and pressure builds within the lumen, resulting in compression of blood vessels. The resulting ischemia is followed by ulceration of the epithelial lining and bacterial invasion. Subsequent necrosis causes perforation or rupture with fecal and bacterial contamination of the peritoneal cavity. The resulting inflammation spreads rapidly throughout the abdomen **(peritonitis),** especially in young children, who are unable to localize infection. Progressive peritoneal inflammation

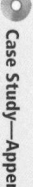

Critical Thinking Exercise—Abdominal Pain

Animation—Appendicitis

Case Study—Appendicitis

results in functional intestinal obstruction of the small bowel (**ileus**) because intense GI reflexes severely inhibit bowel motility. Because the peritoneum represents a major portion of total body surface, the loss of ECF to the peritoneal cavity leads to electrolyte imbalance and hypovolemic shock.

Diagnostic Evaluation

Diagnosis is not always straightforward. Fever, vomiting, abdominal pain, and an elevated white blood count are associated with appendicitis but are also seen in IBD, pelvic inflammatory disease, gastroenteritis, urinary tract infection, right lower lobe pneumonia, mesenteric adenitis, Meckel diverticulum, and intussusception. Prolonged symptoms and delayed diagnosis often occur in younger children, in whom the risk of perforation is greatest because of their inability to verbalize their complaints.

The diagnosis is based primarily on the history and physical examination (Box 24-7). Pain, the cardinal feature, is initially generalized (usually periumbilical); however, it usually descends to the lower right quadrant. The most intense site of pain may be at **McBurney point,** located at a point midway between the anterior superior iliac crest and the umbilicus. Rebound tenderness is not a reliable sign and is extremely painful to the child. Referred pain, elicited by light percussion around the perimeter of the abdomen, indicates peritoneal irritation. Movement, such as riding over bumps in an automobile or gurney, aggravates the pain. In addition to pain, significant clinical manifestations include fever, a change in behavior, anorexia, and vomiting.

Laboratory studies usually include a CBC; urinalysis (to rule out a urinary tract infection); and, in adolescent females, serum human chorionic gonadotropin (to rule out an ectopic pregnancy). A white blood cell (WBC) count greater than 10,000/mm^3 and a C-reactive protein (CRP) are common but are not necessarily specific for appendicitis. An elevated percentage of bands (often referred to as "a shift to the left") may indicate an inflammatory process. CRP is an acute-phase reactant that rises within 12 hours of the onset of infection.

Computed tomography (CT) scan has become the imaging technique of choice, although ultrasound may also be helpful in diagnosing appendicitis. A CT scan is considered positive in the presence of enlarged appendiceal diameter; appendiceal wall thickening; and periappendiceal inflammatory changes,

including fat streaks, phlegmon, fluid collection, and extraluminal gas (Kaiser, Frenchner, and Jorulf, 2002).

> **NURSINGALERT**
>
> Signs of peritonitis, in addition to fever, include sudden relief from pain after perforation, subsequent increase in pain (usually diffuse and accompanied by rigid guarding of the abdomen), progressive abdominal distention, tachycardia, rapid shallow breathing, pallor, chills, and irritability.

Therapeutic Management

Treatment of appendicitis before perforation includes rehydration, antibiotics, and surgical removal of the appendix (**appendectomy**). Laparoscopic surgery is now commonly used to treat nonperforated acute appendicitis (Holcomb, 2001). Recovery is rapid, and, if no complications occur, the hospital stay is short.

Ruptured Appendix. Management of the child diagnosed with peritonitis caused by a ruptured appendix often begins preoperatively with IV administration of fluid and electrolytes, systemic antibiotics, and NG suction. Postoperative management includes IV fluids, continued administration of antibiotics, and NG suction for abdominal decompression until intestinal activity returns. Sometimes surgeons close the wound after irrigation of the peritoneal cavity. Other times, they leave the wound open (delayed closure) to prevent wound infection. A Penrose drain may be used to permit transperitoneal drainage.

Prognosis. Complications are uncommon after a simple appendectomy. The mortality rate for perforating appendicitis has improved from nearly certain death a century ago to 1% or less at present (Strahlman, 2001). Early recognition of the illness is essential to prevent complications.

Nursing Care Management

Because abdominal pain is the most common childhood complaint with appendicitis, it is important to assess the severity of pain (see Pain Assessment, Chapter 7). One of the most reliable estimates is the degree of change in behavior. The younger, nonverbal child will assume a rigid, motionless, side-lying posture with the knees flexed on the abdomen, and there is decreased range of motion of the right hip. Older children may exhibit all of these behaviors while complaining of abdominal pain. They can always indicate a point at which the pain is worse than at any other location.

> **NURSINGALERT**
>
> In any instance when appendicitis is suspected, be aware of the danger of administering laxatives or enemas or applying heat to the area. Such measures stimulate bowel motility and increase the risk of perforation.

Postoperative Care. Postoperative care for the nonperforated appendix is the same as for most abdominal procedures. Care of the child with a ruptured appendix and peritonitis involves more complex care, and the course of recovery is considerably longer (usually 7 to 10 days of hospitalization). The child is maintained on IV fluids, NPO, and the NG tube is kept on low continuous gastric decompression until there is evidence of intestinal activity. Listening for bowel sounds and observing for other signs of bowel activity (e.g., passage of stool) are part of the routine assessment. Management of IV therapy is the same as for any child receiving fluids and par-

---

> ### BOX 24-7
>
> ## Clinical Manifestations of Appendicitis
>
> - Right lower quadrant abdominal pain
> - Fever
> - Rigid abdomen
> - Decreased or absent bowel sounds
> - Vomiting (typically follows onset of pain)
> - Constipation or diarrhea
> - Anorexia
> - Tachycardia, rapid shallow breathing
> - Pallor
> - Lethargy
> - Irritability
> - Stooped posture

enteral antibiotics. A drain is often placed in the wound during surgery, and frequent dressing changes with meticulous skin care are essential to prevent excoriation of the area surrounding the surgical site. Wound care includes irrigation with antibacterial solution.

Management of pain from the incision and repeated dressing changes and irrigations are an essential part of the child's care. Psychologic care of the child and parents is similar to that used in other emergency situations (see Emergency Admission, Chapter 21). Parents and older children need to express their feelings and concerns regarding the events surrounding the illness and hospitalization. The nurse can provide education and psychosocial support to promote adequate coping and alleviate anxiety for both the child and the family (see Nursing Care Plan).

MECKEL DIVERTICULUM

Meckel diverticulum is a remnant of the fetal omphalomesenteric duct that connects the yolk sac with the primitive midgut during fetal life. Normally this structure is obliter-

ated by the fifth to seventh week of gestation, when the placenta replaces the yolk sac as the source of nutrition for the fetus (Sagar, Kumar, and Shah, 2006). Failure of obliteration may result in an **omphalomesenteric fistula,** a fibrous band connecting the small intestine to the umbilicus, known as Meckel diverticulum.

Meckel diverticulum is a true diverticulum because it arises from the antimesenteric border of the small intestine and contains all layers of the intestinal wall with a separate blood supply from the vitelline artery. The diverticulum is usually found within 100 cm (40 inches) of the ileocecal valve and averages 1 to 10 cm (0.4 to 4 inches) in length.

Meckel diverticulum is the most common congenital malformation of the GI tract and is present in 2% to 4% of the population (Sagar, Kumar, and Shah, 2006). Its occurrence in males and females is equal, but the incidence of complications is three to four times greater in males. Most symptomatic cases are seen in childhood. Patients requiring surgery are generally less than 10 years of age, and about 50% are less than 2 years of age (Sagar, Kumar, and Shah, 2006).

nursingcareplan | The Child with Appendicitis

Nursing Diagnosis	Patient Outcomes	Nursing Interventions	Rationale
Acute Pain related to inflamed appendix	The child will have no pain or pain will be reduced to a level acceptable to child	Allow child to choose position most comfortable (usually legs flexed).	To promote the most comfortable position
Child's/Family's Defining Characteristics *(Subjective and Objective Data)*		Provide small pillow for abdomen. Administer analgesia per orders.	To splint the abdomen To provide pain relief
Crying	**The Following NOC Concepts Apply to These Outcomes**	**The Following NIC Concepts Apply to These Interventions**	
Guarding abdomen	Comfort Level		
Limited movement	Pain Control	Analgesic Administration	
Withdrawal	Pain: Disruptive Effects	Positioning	
Refusal to eat or drink		Presence	
Fever		Coping Enhancement	
Increased pulse		Pain Management	

Nursing Diagnosis	Patient Outcomes	Nursing Interventions	Rationale
Risk for Infection related to possibility of rupture	Child will be free of signs and symptoms of peritonitis. Signs of peritonitis will be recognized early.	Provide dietary instructions for foods that reduce excretory demands on kidney and provide sufficient calories and protein for growth.	To support an appropriate diet that can reduce kidney demands
Child's/Family's Defining Characteristics *(Subjective and Objective Data)*		Limit phosphorus, salt, and potassium as prescribed.	To promote nutrition
Abdominal pain	**The Following NOC Concepts Apply to These Outcomes**	Encourage intake of carbohydrates and foods high in calcium.	To provide calories for growth and calcium to prevent bone demineralization
Fever			
Rebound tenderness	Infection Status		
Nausea and vomiting	Wound Healing	Arrange for renal dietitian to meet with family to review allowable foods and assist in dietary planning.	To support the family in understanding the child's dietary needs
Anorexia		Help hemodialysis patient fill out menu requests for meals.	To promote appropriate food choice decisions
Increased white blood cell count			
Fluid around the appendix visualized on ultrasound imaging			
		The Following NIC Concepts Apply to These Interventions	
		Medication Management Laboratory Data Interpretation Vital Signs Monitoring Wound Care Infection Protection	

Continued

nursingcareplan | The Child with Appendicitis—cont'd

Nursing Diagnosis	Patient Outcomes	Nursing Interventions	Rationale
Risk for Deficient Fluid Volume related to decreased intake and losses secondary to loss of appetite, vomiting	Child will receive sufficient fluids to replace losses. Child will exhibit signs of adequate hydration (specify).	Maintain nothing by mouth (NPO) status.	To minimize losses through vomiting and minimize abdominal distention
Child's/Family's Defining Characteristics *(Subjective and Objective Data)*	**The Following NOC Concepts Apply to These Outcomes**	Maintain integrity of infusion site for intravenous (IV) fluids. Administer IV fluids and electrolytes as prescribed.	To infuse fluids and electrolytes To replace losses
Dry mucous membranes Loss of skin turgor Sunken eyes, sunken fontanel Rapid thready pulse, rapid breathing Lethargy	Electrolyte and Acid-Base Balance Fluid Balance	Monitor intake and output. **The Following NIC Concepts Apply to These Interventions** Acid-Base Monitoring Electrolyte Monitoring Fluid Monitoring Fluid Management IV Therapy Laboratory Data Interpretation Vital Signs Monitoring	To assess hydration

Nursing Diagnosis	Patient Outcomes	Nursing Interventions	Rationale
Surgical Recovery, Delayed because of absence of bowel motility	Child will not experience abdominal distention or vomiting caused by delayed bowel mobility.	Maintain NPO status in early postoperative period Maintain nasogastric tube decompression.	To prevent abdominal distention and vomiting To rest bowel until motility returns
Child's/Family's Defining Characteristics *(Subjective and Objective Data)*	**The Following NOC Concept Applies to These Outcomes**	Assess abdomen for distention, tenderness, and presence of bowel sounds.	To assess presence of peristalsis To assess for an indicator of bowel motility
Abdominal distention Nausea and vomiting Absence of bowel sounds Abdominal tenderness No passage of stools	Immobility Consequences: Physiological	Monitor passage of flatus and stool. **The Following NIC Concepts Apply to These Interventions** Bowel Management Flatulence Reduction Positioning	

Pathophysiology

The symptomatic complications of Meckel diverticulum are ulceration, bleeding, intussusception, intestinal obstruction, diverticulitis, and perforation; bleeding is the most common problem in children. Gastric mucosa is the most common ectopic tissue found in Meckel diverticulum. Bleeding is caused by peptic ulceration or perforation because of the un-buffered acidic gastric secretion. Several mechanisms can cause obstruction. Intussusception may be led by the diverticulum. Obstruction may also be caused by entanglement of the small intestine around a fibrous cord, trapping of a loop of intestine under the band, incarceration within a hernia sac, or volvulus of the intestinal segment containing the diverticulum. Diverticulitis occurs when peptic ulceration or obstruction leads to inflammation.

Diagnostic Evaluation

Diagnosis is usually based on the history, physical examination, and a specialized radiographic study. The most common clinical presentation in children includes painless rectal bleeding, abdominal pain, or signs of intestinal obstruction (Box 24-8). Bleeding, which may be mild or profuse, often appears as dark red or "currant jelly" stools; bleeding may be significant enough to cause hypotension. The Meckel scan, a technetium-99m pertechnate scan, detects the presence of gastric mucosa with an overall diagnostic accuracy of 90%. Blood studies are performed to screen for bleeding disorders and anemia.

Therapeutic Management

The standard treatment is surgical removal of the diverticulum. When severe hemorrhage increases the surgical risk, interventions to correct hypovolemic shock, such as blood replacement, IV fluids, and oxygen, may be necessary. Antibiotics may be used preoperatively to control infection. If intestinal obstruction has occurred, appropriate preoperative measures are used to reverse electrolyte imbalances and prevent abdominal distention.

Prognosis. If this condition is diagnosed and treated early, full recovery is likely. The mortality rate of untreated Meckel diverticulum ranges from 2.5% to 15%. Complications of untreated Meckel diverticulum include GI hemorrhage and bowel obstruction.

BOX 24-8
Clinical Manifestations of Meckel Diverticulum

ABDOMINAL PAIN
Similar to appendicitis
May be vague and recurrent

BLOODY STOOLS*
Painless
Bright or dark red with mucus ("currant jelly" stool)
In infants, bleeding sometimes accompanied by pain

SOMETIMES
Severe anemia
Shock

*Often a presenting sign.

TABLE 24-3
Clinical Manifestations of Inflammatory Bowel Diseases

CHARACTERISTICS	ULCERATIVE COLITIS	CROHN DISEASE
Rectal bleeding	Common	Uncommon
Diarrhea	Often severe	Moderate to severe
Pain	Less frequent	Common
Anorexia	Mild or moderate	May be severe
Weight loss	Moderate	May be severe
Growth retardation	Usually mild	May be severe
Anal and perianal lesions	Rare	Common
Fistulas and strictures	Rare	Common
Rashes	Mild	Mild
Joint pain	Mild to moderate	Mild to moderate

Nursing Care Management

Nursing objectives are similar to those for any child undergoing surgery (see Chapter 22). Because the onset of this condition is often rapid, parents require psychologic support. The massive intestinal bleeding that can accompany a Meckel diverticulum is traumatic to both the child and the parents and may significantly affect their emotional reaction to hospitalization and surgery.

Specific preoperative considerations with intestinal bleeding include (1) frequent monitoring of vital signs and blood pressure for shock, (2) keeping the child on bed rest, and (3) recording the approximate amount of blood lost in stools. In the absence of frank hemorrhage, the nurse tests the stools for occult blood. Postoperatively, the child requires IV fluids and an NG tube for the decompression and evacuation of gastric contents.

INFLAMMATORY BOWEL DISEASE

Inflammatory bowel disease (IBD) is a term that is used for two forms of chronic intestinal inflammation: **ulcerative colitis (UC)** and **Crohn disease (CD).** Although UC and CD have similar epidemiologic, immunologic, and clinical features, there are important differences (Table 24-3).

GI symptoms, extraintestinal and systemic inflammatory responses, and exacerbations and remissions without complete resolution characterize these diseases. Growth failure, particularly common in CD, is an important problem unique to the pediatric population. CD is more disabling, has more serious complications, and has less effective medical and surgical treatment than UC. Because UC is confined to the colon, theoretically it may be cured with a colectomy. Over the past 30 years, the incidence of CD has risen, whereas the incidence of UC in children has remained stable (Silbermintz and Markowitz, 2006). The incidence of UC in children has been estimated as 3.5 new cases per 100,000 per year; the incidence of CD is 3.11 per 100,000 per year (Jackson and Grand, 1999).

Etiology

Despite decades of research, the etiology of IBD is not completely understood, and there is no known cure. There is evidence to indicate a multifactorial etiology. Research is focused on theories of defective immunoregulation of the inflammatory response to bacteria or viruses in the GI tract in individuals with a genetic predisposition (Silbermintz and Markowitz, 2006). In CD the chronic immune process is characterized by a T helper 1 cytokine profile, whereas in UC the response is more humoral and mediated by T helper 2 cells (Silbermintz and Markowitz, 2006). An epidemiologic study by Kugathasan, Judd, Hoffman, and others (2003) found an equal distribution of IBD among all racial and ethnic groups, contrasting with earlier studies that suggested IBD typically affects Caucasians (especially Ashkenazi Jews) more than those of Asian or African decent. The Kugathasan study also did not demonstrate a higher risk for developing IBD in urban populations, as had been reported in earlier studies.

There is an influence of genetics in the development of CD. Several CD susceptibility genes have now been identified, including *NOD2/CARD15* on chromosome 16 associated with ileal disease, *IBD5* on chromosome 5, and *IBD6* on chromosome 6 (Kugathasan, Collins, Maresso, and others, 2004; Ahmad, Armuzzi, Bunce, and others, 2002). The influence of genetics in UC appears to be smaller than in CD; however, the *MDRI* gene has been associated with UC (Schwab, Schaeffeler, Marx, and others, 2003). Environmental factors appear to play a role in the development of IBD. Breastfeeding decreases the risk of developing CD, whereas infantile diarrhea seems to increase the risk.

Pathophysiology of Ulcerative Colitis

The inflammation is limited to the colon and rectum, with the distal colon and rectum the most severely affected. Inflammation affects the mucosa and submucosa and involves continuous segments along the length of the bowel with varying degrees of ulceration, bleeding, and edema. The presentation may be mild, moderate, or severe, depending on the extent of mucosal inflammation and systemic symptoms. Children with UC usually are seen with diarrhea, rectal bleeding, and abdominal pain, often associated with tenesmus and urgency (Silbermintz and Markowitz, 2006). Thickening of the bowel wall and fibrosis are unusual, but longstanding disease can result in shortening of the colon and strictures. Extraintestinal manifestations are less common in UC than in CD. Toxic megacolon is the most dangerous form of severe colitis.

Pathophysiology of Crohn Disease

The chronic inflammatory process of CD involves any part of the GI tract from the mouth to the anus but most often affects the terminal ileum. The disease involves all layers of the bowel wall (transmural) in a discontinuous fashion, meaning that between areas of intact mucosa, there are areas of affected mucosa (skip lesions). The most common symptoms are abdominal pain, diarrhea, and decrease in appetite resulting in weight loss. Perianal disease, including skin tags, fistulas, and abscesses, occur in CD. Fever, growth delay, and delayed sexual development are seen commonly (Silbermintz and Markowitz, 2006). Mild GI symptoms, poor growth, and extraintestinal manifestations may be present for several years before overt GI symptoms occur. The inflammation may result in ulcerations; fibrosis; adhesions; stiffening of the bowel wall; stricture formation; and fistulas to other loops of bowel, bladder, vagina, or skin. Extraintestinal manifestations include erythema nodosum, pyoderma gangrenosum, arthralgia and arthritis, uveitis and episcleritis, sclerosing cholangitis, autoimmune hepatitis, nephrolithiasis, and pneumonitis (Silbermintz and Markowitz, 2006).

Diagnostic Evaluation

The diagnosis of UC and CD is derived from the history, physical examination, laboratory evaluation, and other diagnostic procedures. Laboratory tests include a CBC to evaluate anemia and an ESR or CRP to assess the systemic reaction to the inflammatory process. Levels of total protein, albumin, iron, zinc, magnesium, vitamin B_{12}, and fat-soluble vitamins may be low in children with CD. Stools are examined for blood, leukocytes, and infectious organisms. A serologic panel is often used in combination with clinical findings to diagnose IBD and to differentiate between CD and UC. In IBD, autoantibodies called antineutrophil cytoplasmic antibodies (ANCAs) may be detected in the blood. The perinuclear antineutrophil cytoplasmic antibody (pANCA) is associated with UC. Approximately 60% of children with UC and 10% of those with CD are pANCA-positive. Anti–*Saccharomyces cerevisiae* antibodies (ASCA) and anti–outer membrane porin of *E. coli* (anti-OmpC) have been found in up to 60% of children with CD (Ruemmele, Targan, Levy, and others, 1998).

In patients with CD, an upper GI series with small bowel follow-through assists in assessing the existence, location, and extent of disease. Upper endoscopy and colonoscopy with biopsies are an integral part of diagnosing IBD. Endoscopy allows direct visualization of the surface of the GI tract so that the extent of inflammation and narrowing can be evaluated. CT and ultrasound also may be used to identify bowel wall inflammation, intraabdominal abscesses, and fistulas. CD lesions may pierce the walls of the small intestine and colon, creating tracts called fistulas between the intestine and adjacent structures such as the bladder, anus, vagina, or skin.

Therapeutic Management

The goals of therapy are to (1) control the inflammatory process to reduce or eliminate the symptoms, (2) obtain long-term remission, (3) promote normal growth and development, and (4) allow as normal a lifestyle as possible. Treatment is individualized and managed according to the type and the severity of the disease, its location, and the response to therapy.

Medical Treatment. The goal of any treatment regimen is first to induce remission of acute symptoms and then to maintain remission over time. **5-Aminosalicylates** (5-ASAs) are effective in the induction and maintenance of remission in mild to moderate UC. Mesalamine, olsalazine, and balsalazide are now preferred over sulfasalazine because of reduced side effects (headache, nausea, vomiting, neutropenia, and oligospermia). Suppository and enema preparations of mesalamine are used to treat left-sided colitis. These drugs decrease inflammation by inhibiting prostaglandin synthesis. 5-ASAs can be used to induce remission in mild CD. Corticosteroids, such as prednisone and prednisolone, are indicated in induction therapy in children with moderate to severe UC and CD. These drugs inhibit the production of adhesion molecules, cytokines, and leukotrienes. Although these drugs reduce the acute symptoms of IBD, they have side effects that relate to long-term use, including growth suppression (adrenal suppression), weight gain, and decreased bone density (Baron, 2002). High doses of IV corticosteroids may be administered in acute episodes and tapered according to clinical response. Budesonide, a synthetic corticosteroid, is designed for controlled release in the ileum and is indicated for ileal and right-sided colitis; budesonide has fewer side effects than prednisone and prednisolone (Silbermintz and Markowitz, 2006). Rectal steroid therapy (enemas and foam-based preparations) are available for both induction and maintenance therapy in left-sided colitis.

Immunomodulators, such as azathioprine and its metabolite 6-mercaptopurine (6-MP), are used to induce and maintain remission in children with IBD who are steroid resistant or steroid dependent and in treating chronic draining fistulas. They block the synthesis of purine, thus inhibiting the ability of deoxyribonucleic acid (DNA) and ribonucleic acid (RNA) to hinder lymphocyte function, especially that of T cells. Side effects include infection, pancreatitis, hepatitis, bone marrow toxicity, arthralgia, and malignancy. Methotrexate has also been shown to be useful in inducing and maintaining remission in CD patients unresponsive to standard therapies. Cyclosporine and tacrolimus have both been shown to be effective in inducing remission in severe steroid-dependent UC. 6-MP or azathioprine is then used to maintain remission. Patients on immunomodulating medications require regular monitoring of their CBC and differential to assess for changes that reflect suppression of the immune system, since many of the side effects can be prevented or managed by dose reduction or discontinuation of medication.

Antibiotics, such as metronidazole and ciprofloxacin, may be used as an adjunctive therapy to treat complications such as perianal disease or small bowel bacterial overgrowth in CD. Side effects of these drugs are peripheral neuropathy, nausea, and a metallic taste.

Biologic therapies act to regulate inflammatory and antiinflammatory cytokines. Tumor necrosis factor-alpha (TNF-α) is believed to influence active inflammation. Infliximab (Remicade) is a chimeric human-murine monoclonal antibody to TNF-α that is administered intravenously. The U.S. Food and Drug Administration (FDA) has approved it for inducing and maintaining remission in adult CD patients with moderate to severe disease who have not responded sufficiently to conventional therapy. Children appear to respond to infliximab similarly to adults. Infliximab is approved for the treatment of fistulas in CD and for systemic manifestations of IBD such as ankylosing spondylitis, pyoderma gangrenosum, and chronic uveitis. Recently infliximab was approved by the FDA for the treatment of UC unresponsive to steroids. Many patients relapse if treatment is stopped; therefore long-term maintenance therapy with infliximab every 8 weeks may be required. Patients generally require concurrent maintenance with 6-MP or methotrexate to avoid the development of antibodies to infliximab, which are associated with infusion reactions and loss of efficacy. Approximately 5% of patients have acute allergic reactions to infliximab and require premedication with prednisone and diphenhydramine before infusion to prevent reactions. Long intervals between infusions may predispose patients to serum sickness (an immune response causing fever, muscle pain, arthritis, and hives) (Baron, 2002). Severe complications of this drug include lupuslike syndrome or lymphoma. Adalimumab (Humira) was introduced in 2007 for adults with IBD who have lost response or are intolerant to infliximab. Tuberculosis and other opportunistic infections have been observed in patients receiving adalimumab (Abbott Laboratories, 2007).

Nutritional Support. Nutritional support is important in the treatment of IBD. Growth failure is a common serious complication, especially in CD. Growth failure is characterized by weight loss, alteration in body composition, retarded height, and delayed sexual maturation. Malnutrition causes the growth failure, and its etiology is multifactorial. Malnutrition occurs as a result of inadequate dietary intake, excessive GI losses, malabsorption, drug-nutrient interaction, and increased nutritional requirements. Inadequate dietary intake occurs with anorexia and episodes of increased disease activity. Excessive loss of nutrients (protein, blood, electrolytes, and minerals) occurs secondary to intestinal inflammation and diarrhea. Carbohydrate, lactose, fat, vitamin, and mineral malabsorption, as well as vitamin B_{12} and folic acid deficiencies, occur with disease episodes and with drug administration and when the terminal ileum is resected. Finally, nutritional requirements are increased with inflammation, fever, fistulas, and periods of rapid growth (e.g., adolescence).

The goals of nutritional support include (1) correction of nutrient deficits and replacement of ongoing losses, (2) provision of adequate energy and protein for healing, and (3) provision of adequate nutrients to promote normal growth. Nutritional support includes both enteral and parenteral nutrition. A well-balanced, high-protein, high-calorie diet is recommended for children whose symptoms do not prohibit an adequate oral intake. There is little evidence that avoiding specific foods influences the severity of the disease. Supplementation with multivitamins, iron, and folic acid is recommended.

Special enteral formulas, given either by mouth or continuous NG infusion (often at night), may be required. Elemental formulas are completely absorbed in the small intestine with almost no residue. A diet consisting only of elemental formula not only improves nutritional status but also induces disease remission, either without steroids or with a diminished dosage of steroids required. An elemental diet is a safe and potentially effective primary therapy for patients with CD. Unfortunately, remission is not sustained when NG feedings are discontinued unless maintenance medications are added to the treatment regimen.

TPN has also improved nutritional status in patients with IBD. Short-term remissions have been achieved after TPN, although complete bowel rest has not reduced inflammation

or added to the benefits of improved nutrition by TPN. Nutritional support is less likely to induce a remission in UC than in CD. Improvement of nutritional status is important, however, in preventing deterioration of the patient's health status and in preparing the patient for surgery.

Surgical Treatment. Surgery is indicated for UC when medical and nutritional therapies fail to prevent complications. Surgical options include a **subtotal colectomy** and **ileostomy** that leaves a rectal stump as a blind pouch. A reservoir pouch is created in the configuration of a J or S to help improve continence postoperatively. An ileoanal pull-through preserves the normal pathway for defecation. Pouchitis, an inflammation of the surgically created pouch, is the most common late complication of this procedure and had been reported to occur in up to 50% of cases. Metronidazole and ciprofloxacin are effective in treating pouchitis (Alexander, Sarigol, DiFiore, and others, 2003). In many cases UC can be cured with a total colectomy.

Surgery may be required in children with CD when complications cannot be controlled by medical and nutritional therapy. Segmental intestinal resections are performed for small bowel obstructions, strictures, or fistulas. Partial colonic resection is not curative, and the disease often recurs.

Prognosis. IBD is a chronic disease. Relatively long periods of quiescent disease may follow exacerbations. The outcome of the disease is influenced by the regions and severity of involvement, as well as by appropriate therapeutic management. Malnutrition, growth failure, and bleeding are serious complications. The overall prognosis for UC is good.

The development of colorectal cancer (CRC) is a long-term complication of IBD. In UC, the cumulative incidence of CRC is 2.5% after 20 years, increasing to 10.8% after 30 years (Rutter, Saunders, Wilkinson, and others, 2006). Surveillance colonoscopy with multiple biopsies should begin approximately 10 years after diagnosis of UC or Crohn colitis and continue every 1 to 2 years (Rubin and Kavitt, 2006). Removal of the diseased colon prevents development of CRC. In CD, however, surgical removal of the affected colon does not prevent cancer from developing elsewhere in the GI tract.

Nursing Care Management

The nursing considerations in the management of IBD extend beyond the immediate period of hospitalization. These interventions involve continued guidance of families in terms of (1) managing diet; (2) coping with factors that increase stress and emotional lability; (3) adjusting to a disease of remissions and exacerbations; and (4) when indicated, preparing the child and parents for the possibility of diversionary bowel surgery.

Because nutritional support is an essential part of therapy, encouraging the anorectic child to consume sufficient quantities of food is often a challenge. Successful interventions include involving the child in meal planning; encouraging small, frequent meals or snacks rather than three large meals a day; serving meals around medication schedules when diarrhea, mouth pain, and intestinal spasm are controlled; and preparing high-protein, high-calorie foods such as eggnog, milkshakes, cream soups, puddings, or custard (if lactose is tolerated) (see Feeding the Sick Child, Chapter 22). Foods that aggravate the condition are avoided. Using bran or a high-fiber diet for active IBD is questionable. Bran, even in small amounts, has been shown to worsen the patient's condition.

??? CRITICAL THINKING EXERCISE

Inflammatory Bowel Disease

Susan, a 13-year-old girl, was admitted to the hospital because of bloody diarrhea, abdominal pain, and weight loss. After a thorough evaluation, including laboratory tests, radiographic studies, and gastrointestinal endoscopy procedures, the diagnosis of Crohn disease (CD) was made. Medical treatment, including corticosteroid drugs and nutritional support, was implemented during this hospitalization.

Susan has improved considerably and is to be discharged home this week. Enteral formula administered by continuous nighttime nasogastric (NG) tube infusion will be continued at home, and both Susan and her family are eager to learn how to perform these feedings. You are the nurse responsible for Susan's discharge planning. Which interventions relating to these feedings should you include in Susan's preparations for discharge?

QUESTIONS

1. Evidence—Are there sufficient data to formulate any specific interventions for discharge?
2. Assumptions—Describe some underlying assumptions about:
   a. The goals of nutritional support for children with CD
   b. Teaching required by an adolescent or family member who is administering NG tube feedings at home
   c. Psychosocial issues related to CD
3. What are the priorities for discharge planning at this time?
4. Does the evidence support your conclusion?
5. Are there alternative perspectives to your conclusion? What are they?

Occasionally the occurrence of aphthous stomatitis further complicates adherence to dietary management. Mouth care before eating and the selection of bland foods help relieve the discomfort of mouth sores.

When NG feedings or TPN is indicated, nurses play an important role in explaining the purpose and the expected outcomes of this therapy. The nurse should acknowledge the anxieties of the child and family members and give them adequate time to demonstrate the skills necessary to continue the therapy at home if needed (see Critical Thinking Exercise).

The importance of continued drug therapy despite remission of symptoms must be stressed to the child and family members. Failure to adhere to the pharmacologic regimen can result in exacerbation of the disease (see Compliance, Chapter 22). Unfortunately, exacerbation of IBD can occur even if the child and family are compliant with the treatment regimen; this is difficult for the child and family to cope with.

Family Support. The nurse should attend to the emotional components of the disease and assess any sources of stress. Frequently, the nurse can help children adjust to problems of growth retardation, delayed sexual maturation, dietary restrictions, feelings of being "different" or "sickly," inability to compete with peers, and necessary absence from school during exacerbations of the illness (see Impact of Chronic Illness or Disability on the Child, Chapter 18).

If a permanent colectomy-ileostomy is required, the nurse can teach the child and family how to care for the ileostomy. The nurse can also emphasize the positive aspects of the surgery, particularly accelerated growth and sexual development,

permanent recovery, and the eliminated risk of colonic cancer in UC, as well as the normality of life despite bowel diversion. Introducing the child and parents to other ostomy patients, especially those who are the same age, can be effective in fostering eventual acceptance. Whenever possible, continent ostomies should be offered as options to the child, although they are not performed in all centers in the United States.

Because of the chronic and often lifelong nature of the disease, families benefit from the educational services provided by organizations such as the Crohn's and Colitis Foundation of America (CCFA).* If diversionary bowel surgery is indicated, United Ostomy Associations of America† and the Wound, Ostomy and Continence Nurses Society‡ are available to assist with ileostomy care and provide important psychologic support through their self-help groups. Adolescents often benefit by participating in peer-support groups, which are sponsored by the CCFA.

PEPTIC ULCER DISEASE

Peptic ulcers may be classified as acute or chronic, and peptic ulcer disease (PUD) is a chronic condition that affects the stomach or duodenum. Ulcers are described as gastric or duodenal and as primary or secondary. A **gastric ulcer** involves the mucosa of the stomach; a **duodenal ulcer** involves the pylorus or duodenum. Most **primary ulcers** occur in the absence of a predisposing factor and tend to be chronic, occurring more frequently in the duodenum. **Stress ulcers** result from the stress of a severe underlying disease or injury (e.g., severe burns, sepsis, increased intracranial pressure, severe trauma, multisystem organ failure) and are more frequently acute and gastric.

About 1.7% of children in general pediatric practices have PUD, and the disease represents about 3.4% per 10,000 of pediatric hospital admissions. Primary ulcers are more common in children older than 6 years, and stress ulcers are more common in infants younger than 6 months. Except for very young children, the incidence is two to three times greater in boys than in girls.

Etiology

The exact cause is unknown, although infectious, genetic, and environmental factors are important. There is an increased familial incidence, and the disease is increased in persons with blood group O.

There is a significant relationship between the bacterium *Helicobacter pylori* (*H. pylori*) and ulcers. *H. pylori* is a microaerophilic, gram-negative, slow-growing, spiral-shaped, and flagellated bacterium known to colonize the gastric mucosa in about half of the population of the world (Cover and Blaser, 1996). It has been identified in 90% to 100% of adult patients with PUD. *H. pylori* synthesizes the enzyme urease, which hydrolyses urea to form ammonia and carbon dioxide. Ammonia then absorbs acid to form ammonium, thus raising

*386 Park Ave. South, 17th Floor, New York, NY 10016; (800) 932-2423; http://www.ccfa.org. In Canada: Crohn's and Colitis Foundation of Canada, http://www.ccfc.ca.

†UOAA, PO Box 66, Fairview, TN 37062-0066; (800) 826-0826; http://www.uoaa.org. In Canada: United Ostomy Association of Canada, PO Box 825-50, Charles St. East, Toronto, Ontario M4Y 2N7; (416) 595-5452; fax: (416) 595-9924; http://www.ostomycanada.ca.

‡1500 Commerce Pkwy., Suite C, Mt. Laurel, NJ; (888) 224-9626; http://www.wocn.org.

the gastric pH. Also, its flagella allow the bacterium to swim across the viscous gastric mucus and reach the more neutral gastric pH below the mucus (Sgouros and Bergele, 2006). *H. pylori* may cause ulcers by weakening the gastric mucosal barrier and allowing acid to damage the mucosa. It is believed that it is acquired via the fecal-oral route, and this hypothesis is supported by finding viable *H. pylori* in feces.

In addition to ulcerogenic drugs, both alcohol and smoking contribute to ulcer formation. There is no conclusive evidence to implicate particular foods, such as caffeine-containing beverages or spicy foods, but polyunsaturated fats and fiber may play a role in ulcer formation. Psychologic factors may play a role in the development of PUD, and stressful life events, dependency, passiveness, and hostility have all been implicated as contributing factors.

Pathophysiology

Most likely, the pathology is due to an imbalance between the destructive (cytotoxic) factors and defensive (cytoprotective) factors in the GI tract. The toxic mechanisms include acid, pepsin, medications such as aspirin and nonsteroidal antiinflammatory drugs (NSAIDs), bile acids, and infection with *H. pylori*. The defensive factors include the mucus layer, local bicarbonate secretion, epithelial cell renewal, and mucosal blood flow. Prostaglandins play a role in mucosal defense because they stimulate both mucus and alkali secretion. The primary mechanism that prevents the development of peptic ulcer is the secretion of mucus by the epithelial and mucus glands throughout the stomach. The thick mucus layer acts to diffuse acid from the lumen to the gastric mucosal surface, thus protecting the gastric epithelium. The stomach and the duodenum produce bicarbonate, decreasing acidity on the epithelial cells and thereby minimizing the effects of the low pH (Chelimsky and Czinn, 2001). When abnormalities in the protective barrier exist, the mucosa is vulnerable to damage by acid and pepsin. Exogenous factors, such as aspirin and NSAIDs, cause gastric ulcers by inhibition of prostaglandin synthesis.

Zollinger-Ellison syndrome may occur in children who have multiple, large, or recurrent ulcers. This syndrome is characterized by hypersecretion of gastric acid, intractable ulcer disease, and intestinal malabsorption caused by a gastrin-secreting tumor of the pancreas.

Diagnostic Evaluation

Diagnosis is based on the history of symptoms, physical examination, and diagnostic testing. The focus is on symptoms such as epigastric abdominal pain, nocturnal pain, oral regurgitation, heartburn, weight loss, hematemesis, and melena (Box 24-9). History should include questions relating to the use of potentially causative substances such as NSAIDs, corticosteroids, alcohol, and tobacco. Laboratory studies may include a CBC to detect anemia, stool analysis for occult blood, liver function tests (LFTs), sedimentation rate, or CRP to evaluate IBD; amylase and lipase to evaluate pancreatitis; and gastric acid measurements to identify hypersecretion. A lactose breath test may be performed to detect lactose intolerance.

Radiographic studies such as an upper GI series may be performed to evaluate obstruction or malrotation. An upper endoscopy is the most reliable procedure to diagnose PUD. A biopsy is taken to determine the presence of *H. pylori*. It can also be diagnosed by a blood test that identifies the presence

---

BOX 24-9

Characteristics of Peptic Ulcers

NEONATES
Usually gastric and secondary ulcers
Commonly a history of prematurity, respiratory distress, sepsis, hypoglycemia, or an intraventricular hemorrhage
Perforation may lead to massive bleeding

INFANTS TO 3-YEAR-OLD CHILDREN
Most likely to have a secondary ulcer located equally in the stomach or duodenum
Primary ulcers less common and usually located in stomach
Likely to be noticed in relation to illness, surgery, or trauma
Hematemesis, melena, or perforation

2- TO 6-YEAR-OLD CHILDREN
Primary or secondary ulcers
Located equally in stomach and duodenum
Perforation more likely in secondary ulcers
Periumbilical pain, poor eating, vomiting, irritability, nighttime wakening, hematemesis, melena

CHILDREN 6 YEARS AND OLDER
Usually primary and most often duodenal ulcers
More typical of adult type
Chance of recurrence greater
Often associated with *Helicobacter pylori*
Epigastric pain or vague abdominal pain
Nighttime wakening, hematemesis, melena, and anemia possible

---

of the antigen to this organism. The C-urea breath test measures bacterial colonization in the gastric mucosa. This test is used to screen for *H. pylori* in adults and children. Polyclonal and monoclonal stool antigen tests are an accurate noninvasive method both for the initial diagnosis of *H. pylori* and for the confirmation of its eradication after treatment (Gisbert, de la Morena, and Abraira, 2006).

Therapeutic Management

The major goals of therapy for children with PUD are to relieve discomfort, promote healing, prevent complications, and prevent recurrence. Management is primarily medical and consists of administration of medications to treat the infection and to reduce or neutralize gastric acid secretion.

Antacids are beneficial medications to neutralize gastric acid.

Histamine (H₂) receptor antagonists (antisecretory drugs) act to suppress gastric acid production. Cimetidine (Tagamet), ranitidine (Zantac), and famotidine (Pepcid) are examples of these medications. These medications have few side effects.

PPIs, such as omeprazole and lansoprazole, act to inhibit the hydrogen ion pump in the parietal cells, thus blocking the production of acid. Controlled studies of these drugs have been done in adults, and these drugs are now commonly used to treat ulcers in children. They appear to be well tolerated and to have infrequent side effects (e.g., headache, diarrhea, nausea and vomiting).

Mucosal protective agents, such as sucralfate and bismuth-containing preparations, may be prescribed for PUD. Sucralfate is an aluminum-containing agent that forms a protective barrier over ulcerated mucosa to protect against acid and pepsin. Sucralfate is available in both pill and liquid forms. Because sucralfate blocks the absorption of other medications, it should be given separately from other medications.

Bismuth compounds are sometimes prescribed for the relief of ulcers, but they are used less frequently than PPIs. Although these compounds inhibit the growth of microorganisms, the mechanism of their activity is poorly understood. In combination with antibiotics, bismuth is effective against *H. pylori*. Although concern has been expressed about the use of bismuth salts in children because of potential side effects, none of these side effects has been reported when these compounds have been used in the treatment of *H. pylori* infection.

Triple drug therapy is the recommended treatment regimen for *H. pylori* (Ford, Delaney, Forman, and others, 2004). Combination therapy has demonstrated 90% effectiveness in eradication of *H. pylori* when compared with antibiotic monotherapy. Examples of drug combinations used in triple therapy are (1) bismuth, clarithromycin, and metronidazole; (2) lansoprazole, amoxicillin, and clarithromycin; and (3) metronidazole, clarithromycin, and omeprazole. Common side effects of medications include diarrhea, nausea, and vomiting. The yearly relapse rate of 80% for duodenal ulcer and 60% for gastric ulcer can be reduced to less than 5% after successful *H. pylori* eradication (Ford, Delaney, Forman, and others, 2004).

In addition to medications, the child with PUD should be given a nutritious diet and advised to avoid caffeine. Adolescents are warned about gastric irritation associated with alcohol use and smoking.

Children with an acute ulcer who have developed complications, such as massive hemorrhage, require emergency care. The administration of IV fluids, blood, or plasma depends on the amount of blood loss. Replacement with whole blood or packed cells may be necessary for significant loss.

Surgical intervention may be required for complications such as hemorrhage, perforation, or gastric outlet obstruction. Ligation of the source of bleeding or closure of a perforation is performed. A vagotomy and pyloroplasty may be indicated in children with recurring ulcers despite aggressive medical treatment.

Prognosis. The long-term prognosis for PUD is variable. Many ulcers are successfully treated with medical therapy; however, primary duodenal peptic ulcers often recur. Complications such as GI bleeding can occur and extend into adult life. The effect of maintenance drug therapy on long-term morbidity remains to be established with further studies.

Nursing Care Management

The primary nursing goal is to promote healing of the ulcer through compliance with the medication regimen. If an analgesic-antipyretic is needed, acetaminophen, not aspirin or NSAIDs, is used. Critically ill neonates, infants, and children in intensive care units should receive H_2 blockers to prevent stress ulcers. Critically ill children receiving IV H_2 blockers should have their gastric pH values checked at frequent intervals.

The role of stress in ulcer formation should be considered for nonhospitalized children with chronic illnesses. In children, many ulcers occur secondary to other conditions, and the nurse should be aware of family and environmental conditions that may aggravate or precipitate ulcers. Children may benefit from psychologic counseling and from learning how to cope constructively with stress.

HEPATIC DISORDERS

ACUTE HEPATITIS
Etiology

Hepatitis is an acute or chronic inflammation of the liver that can result from several different causes (e.g., virus, chemical or drug reaction, or other diseases). Nonviral causes of hepatitis include autoimmune hepatitis, Wilson disease, α_1-antitrypsin deficiency, and steatohepatitis. The following six viruses cause 90% of cases of viral hepatitis (Table 24-4):

1. Hepatitis A virus (HAV)
2. Hepatitis B virus (HBV)
3. Hepatitis C virus (HCV)
4. Hepatitis D virus (HDV)
5. Hepatitis E virus (HEV)
6. Hepatitis G virus (HGV)

Hepatitis A. HAV is the most common form of acute viral hepatitis in most parts of the world. It is a member of the picornavirus family. The virus produces a contagious disease transmitted primarily in contaminated stool spread via the fecal-oral route from person to person. HAV has been associated with miniepidemics in areas of poor hygiene and high population density. There is no chronic or carrier state. HAV infection affects individuals of all ages, but the highest incidence occurs among preschool- or school-age children younger than 15 years. Children may serve as the source of HAV infection in adults, such as in childcare center exposures. Usually HAV disease in children is mild. It is frequently anicteric and often subclinical. Infected children who show no symptoms may still spread the virus to others. HAV can be severe in children with immunodeficiency disorders. The incubation period is approximately 3 weeks. Although some cases may be prolonged, the prognosis is excellent. A highly effective vaccine for HAV was introduced in 1997; in 1999 the Advisory Committee on Immunization Practices recommended vaccination for all children over 24 months old living in the 11 states with the highest incidence of HAV (Amon, Darling, Fiore, and others, 2003; Balistreri, Chang, Ciocca, and others, 2002).

Hepatitis B. HBV infection can occur as an acute or chronic infection and may range from being asymptomatic and limited to causing fatal fulminant (rapid and severe) hepatitis. HBV varies greatly throughout the world. High-prevalence areas have been identified in Africa and Asia; the United States is considered a low-prevalence area. Transmission is usually via the parenteral route through the exchange of blood or any bodily secretion or fluid. Infections from blood transfusion have been reduced as a result of blood product–screening procedures. Transplantation of organs, intimate physical contact, transmission from mother to infant, and the splashing of contaminated fluids into the mouth or eyes are other sources of infection. Adults whose occupations are associated with exposure to blood or blood products (such as health care workers) are at increased risk for infection and should receive HBV vaccination.

Most HBV infection in children is acquired perinatally. Newborns are at risk for hepatitis if the mother is infected with HBV or was a carrier of HBV during pregnancy. Possible routes of maternal-fetal or maternal-infant transmission include (1) leakage of virus across the placenta late in pregnancy or during labor and (2) ingestion of amniotic fluid or maternal blood. Infants who have HBV infection are more than

TABLE 24-4

Comparison of Types A, B, and C Hepatitis

CHARACTERISTICS	TYPE A	TYPE B	TYPE C
Incubation period	15-50 days, average 25-30 days	30-180 days, average 50 days	2 weeks–6 months, average 6-7 weeks
Period of communicability	Believed to be later half of incubation period to the first week after the onset of clinical illness	Variable Virus in blood or other body fluids during late incubation period and acute stage of disease; may persist in carrier state for years to lifetime	Begins before onset of symptoms May persist in carrier state for years
Mode of transmission	Principal route—fecal-oral Rarely—parenteral	Principal route—parenteral Less frequent route—oral, sexual, any body fluid Perinatal transfer—transplacental blood (last trimester), at delivery, or during breastfeeding, especially if mother has cracked nipples	Principal route—parenteral Nonparenteral spread possible
Clinical features			
Onset	Usually rapid, acute	More insidious	Usually insidious
Fever	Common and early	Less frequent	Less frequent
Anorexia	Common	Mild to moderate	Mild to moderate
Nausea and vomiting	Common	Sometimes present	Mild to moderate
Rash	Rare	Common	Sometimes present
Arthralgia	Rare	Common	Rare
Pruritus	Rare	Sometimes present	Sometimes present
Jaundice	Present (many cases anicteric)	Present	Present
Immunity	Present after one attack; no crossover to type B or C	Present after one attack; no crossover to type A or C	Present after one attack; no crossover to type A or B
Carrier state	No	Yes	Yes
Chronic infection	No	Yes	Yes
Prophylaxis			
Immune globulin (IG)	Passive immunity Successful, especially in early incubation period and preexposure prophylaxis	Passive immunity Inconsistent benefits; probably of no use	Not currently recommended by Centers for Disease Control and Prevention
HAV vaccine	Two inactivated vaccines approved for children ages 2-18 years: Havrix and Vaqta; given in a 2-dose schedule (6-12 months between doses)		
HBV immune globulin (HBIG)	No benefit	Passive immunity	No benefit
HBV vaccine	No benefit	Postexposure protection possible if given immediately after definite exposure Provides active immunity Universal vaccination recommended for all newborns	No benefit
Mortality	0.1%-0.2%	0.5%-2.0% in uncomplicated cases; may be higher in complicated cases	1%-2% in uncomplicated cases; may be higher in complicated cases

90% likely to become chronic carriers (Broderick and Jonas, 2003). The incubation period of HBV infection varies from 45 to 160 days.

HBV infection occurs in children and adolescents in the following high-risk groups:

- Individuals with hemophilia and others who have received multiple transfusions
- Children and adolescents involved in IV drug abuse
- Institutionalized children and adolescents
- Preschool-age children in endemic areas
- Individuals engaged in heterosexual or homosexual activity with infected partners

Hepatitis C. Approximately 1 in 50 people in the general population is positive for HCV antibodies (Centers for Disease Control and Prevention, 2001). About 0.2% to 0.4% of children younger than 12 years of age are infected with HCV.

It is estimated that 4 million people in the United States are anti–HCV-positive. Approximately 7% of HCV-infected mothers transmit HCV to their newborns (Balistreri, Chang, Ciocca, and others, 2002). Another common route of infection is by percutaneous exposure, which occurs through transfusion of blood or blood products, transplantation of organs or tissues, or sharing of used needles. Transfusion-associated HCV infection is low, but a common cause of infection is injection drug use. The American Academy of Pediatrics (1998) suggests screening the following groups:

- All infants born to HCV-infected women
- Individuals who received blood products before 1992
- Individuals involved in injection drug use
- Individuals who receive hemodialysis

The clinical course of HCV infection is variable. Incubation averages 6 to 7 weeks, with a range of 2 weeks to 6 months. Both acute and chronic HCV infection often produces only mild nonspecific symptoms or no symptoms at all (Bonkovsky and Mehta, 2001).

The length of time that maternal antibody is present in infants born to HCV-infected women must be considered, and screening should be done after the infant is 12 months old. However, a routine screening program, such as that for HBV, is not recommended. Current recommendations are to evaluate HCV-infected children at regular intervals to monitor for chronic hepatitis. Most children will be asymptomatic with evidence of chronic hepatitis on liver biopsy. Liver enzyme levels may fluctuate between periods of normal and elevated values.

Hepatitis D. HDV is an important cause of acute and chronic liver disease. HDV is a defective RNA virus that requires the presence of HBV. HDV infection occurs primarily in hemophiliac patients and IV drug abusers. The incubation period is 2 to 8 weeks. Both acute and chronic forms are more severe than HBV infection and can lead to cirrhosis. Testing for HDV infection is recommended in children with chronic HBV infection or severe liver disease and in children with acute exacerbation of a previously stable liver disease.

Hepatitis E. HEV infection is enterally transmitted. Transmission may occur through the fecal-oral route or from contaminated water. The incubation period is 2 to 9 weeks. This illness is uncommon in children, does not cause chronic liver disease, is not a chronic condition, and has no carrier state. The mortality rate resulting from submassive hepatic necrosis is low except in pregnant women in their third trimester, in whom mortality reaches 20%.

Hepatitis G. HGV is a blood-borne virus that may also be transmitted by organ transplantation. High-risk groups include transfusion recipients, IV drug users, and individuals infected with HCV. Individuals with the virus are often asymptomatic, and most infections are chronic. The incubation period is unknown.

Diagnostic Evaluation

Diagnosis is based on the history (especially regarding possible exposure to a hepatitis virus); physical examination; and serologic markers (antibodies or antigens) indicating the presence of active infection with hepatitis A, B, or C or previous infection. Because the liver has a large functional reserve, abnormal laboratory tests may be the only indication of hepatitis. However, LFTs are not specific for the diagnosis of viral

hepatitis. Although serum aspartate and alanine aminotransferase (AST and ALT) levels are markedly elevated in viral hepatitis, other diseases or conditions may cause their elevation. Serum bilirubin levels peak 5 to 10 days after clinical jaundice appears. When hepatitis is severe, albumin levels are depressed and prothrombin times are increased.

Diagnosis of viral hepatitis is based on the presence of specific viral markers. Diagnosis of acute HAV infection is based on the presence of anti-HAV immunoglobulin (immunoglobulin M [IgM]) antibody in the serum. HBV diagnosis depends on the presence of hepatitis B surface antigen (HBsAg) or anti-HBV core (anti-HBc) IgM antibody. Chronic HBV infection is associated with the persistence of HBsAg and HBV DNA markers. The diagnosis of HCV is based on the detection of anti-HCV antibodies and confirmation by polymerase chain reaction for hepatitis C RNA.

An abdominal ultrasound provides measurement of liver size, detection of cystic lesions and stones, and imaging of the gallbladder. Cholescintigraphy radionuclide imaging detects abnormalities in liver uptake, concentration, and excretory function. Finally, a liver biopsy aids in assessing the severity of the disease.

Pathophysiology

Pathologic changes occur primarily in the parenchymal cells of the liver and result in varying degrees of swelling, infiltration of liver cells by mononuclear cells, subsequent degeneration, necrosis, and fibrosis.

Hepatitis can be self-limited, and complete regeneration of liver cells without scarring may occur. However, some forms of hepatitis do not result in complete return of liver function. These include **fulminant hepatitis,** which is characterized by a severe, acute course and massive destruction of the liver, resulting in liver failure and death in 1 to 2 weeks. **Subacute** or **chronic active hepatitis** is characterized by progressive liver destruction, uncertain regeneration, scarring, and potential cirrhosis.

The initial **anicteric** (absence of jaundice) **phase** usually lasts 5 to 7 days and is often mistaken for influenza. Symptoms include nausea, vomiting, extreme anorexia, malaise, easy fatigability, arthralgia, skin rashes, slight to moderate fever, and epigastric or upper right quadrant abdominal pain. Dark urine is a symptom of the **icteric** (jaundice) **phase.** Pruritus may accompany jaundice and can be bothersome, but many children with acute viral hepatitis do not develop jaundice.

Therapeutic Management

Treatment options for viral hepatitis are limited. The goals of management include early detection, recognition of chronic liver disease, support and monitoring, and prevention of spread of the disease.

HAV infection is an acute disease that resolves with support and management of symptoms. HBV and HCV treatment is directed at managing the viral load to prevent further destruction of the liver. Currently, HBV and HCV are treated with interferons, naturally occurring proteins that exert antiviral, antiproliferative, and immunomodulatory effects. A recent interferon formulation, pegylated interferon, can be administered once a week and has been found to sustain plasma levels and enhance viral suppression (Karnam and Reddy, 2003). Lamivudine and adefovir are two other interferon analogs that suppress the replication of HBV (Yuen and Lai,

2001). A combination of α-interferon and ribavirin has resulted in a sustained response in only 50% of patients with HBV and HCV (Waters and Nelson, 2006).

Another important aspect of the therapeutic management of hepatitis involves hospitalization. Hospitalization is necessary if coagulopathy or fulminant hepatitis is present.

Prevention. Proper hand washing and standard isolation precautions can prevent the spread of hepatitis. Prophylactic use of standard immune globulin (Ig) is effective in preventing HAV infection in situations of preexposure (e.g., anticipated travel to areas where HAV is prevalent) or in situations of postexposure during the early part of the incubation period. Hepatitis B immune globulin (HBIg) is effective in preventing HBV infection after exposure. Ig and HBIg must be administered less than 2 weeks after exposure.

Vaccines have been developed to prevent HAV and HBV infection. HBV vaccination is recommended for all newborns and for high-risk groups. HAV is also recommended for high-risk groups (see Immunizations, Chapter 10). Active immunizations are not available against HCV. It is possible to prevent HDV infection by preventing HBV infection.

Prognosis. The prognosis for children with hepatitis is variable and depends on the type of virus. HAV usually causes a mild and brief illness with no carrier state. HBV causes a wide spectrum of acute and chronic illness. Approximately 5% of individuals develop chronic hepatitis B each year, and about half of these develop fulminant liver failure, leading to death in the absence of liver transplantation (Kim, Gores, Benson, and others, 2005). Hepatocellular carcinoma is a potentially fatal complication of HBV infection. HCV causes acute hepatitis that progresses to chronic disease in more than 85% of affected individuals, with approximately 15% to 20% developing cirrhosis or hepatocellular carcinoma (Centers for Disease Control and Prevention, 2001; Richmond, Dunning, and Desmond, 2004). Chronic HCV infection is the leading indication for liver transplantation in adults in the United States (Regev and Schiff, 2000).

Nursing Care Management

Nursing objectives depend on the severity of the hepatitis, the medical management, and factors influencing the control and transmission of the disease. Children with benign viral hepatitis are frequently cared for at home, and the clinic or office nurse must explain the medical therapy and control measures. If further assistance is needed for parents to comply with therapy, a public health nursing referral may be necessary.

A well-balanced diet and a realistic schedule of rest and activity adjusted to the child's condition are encouraged. HAV is not infectious within a week after the onset of jaundice, and children may feel well enough to resume school. Parents are cautioned about administering any medication to the child, since normal dosages of many drugs may become dangerous because of the liver's inability to detoxify and excrete them. Hand washing is the single most critical measure in reducing risk of transmission. The nurse should explain to parents and children the ways in which HAV (oral-fecal route) and HBV (parenteral route) are spread.

Nurses caring for young people with HBV infection and a known or suspected history of illicit drug use should help these teens realize the dangers of drug abuse. Nurses should stress the parenteral mode of transmission of hepatitis and encourage them to seek counseling through a drug program.

HBV and HCV are chronic diseases that require frequent monitoring and management. Many communities have multidisciplinary clinics dedicated to the management of these diseases.

CIRRHOSIS

Cirrhosis occurs at the end stage of many chronic liver diseases, including biliary atresia (BA) and chronic hepatitis. Cirrhosis can also result from infectious, autoimmune, or toxic factors and from chronic diseases such as hemophilia and cystic fibrosis. A cirrhotic liver is irreversibly damaged.

Clinical manifestations in children are similar to those seen with all chronic liver disorders. Children exhibit jaundice, poor growth, anorexia, muscle weakness, and lethargy. Ascites, edema, GI bleeding, anemia, and abdominal pain may be present with impaired intrahepatic blood flow. Pulmonary function may be impaired because of pressure against the diaphragm from hepatosplenomegaly and ascites. Dyspnea and cyanosis may occur, especially on exertion. Intrapulmonary arteriovenous shunts may develop and cause hypoxemia. Spider angiomas and prominent blood vessels are often present on the upper torso.

Therapeutic Management

Therapy is directed toward (1) frequent assessment of liver status with physical examination and LFTs and (2) management of specific complications. The only successful treatment for end-stage liver disease and liver failure may be **liver transplantation,** which has improved the prognosis substantially for many children with cirrhosis. Currently, the 1-year survival rate for liver transplantation is 85%. Increasing numbers of recipients are reaching their second decade after transplant. The increasing life span after transplantation is related to advances in surgical techniques and improved preoperative, intraoperative, and postoperative care (Atkison, Ross, Williams, and others, 2002).

Prognosis. Liver transplantation has revolutionized the approach to liver cirrhosis. Liver failure and cirrhosis are indications for transplantation. Liver transplantation reflects the failure of other medical and surgical measures to prevent or treat cirrhosis. Careful monitoring of the child's condition and quality of life is necessary to evaluate the need for and timing of transplantation (see Family Focus box).

FAMILY FOCUS

End-Stage Liver Disease

In many cases the child and family must cope with an uncertain progression of the disease. The only hope for long-term survival may be liver transplantation. Transplantation can be successful, but the waiting period may be long, and there are many more children in need of organs than there are donors. The procedure is expensive and is performed only at designated medical centers, which are often far from the family's home. The nurse should recognize the unique stresses of coping with end-stage liver disease and waiting for transplantation and assist the family in coping with these stressors. The assistance of social workers and support from other parents can be beneficial.

Nursing Care Management

Nursing care of the child with cirrhosis is determined by the cause of the cirrhosis, the severity of complications, and the prognosis. The prognosis for life is poor unless successful liver transplantation occurs. Nursing care of this child is similar to that for any child with a life-threatening illness (see Chapter 18). Hospitalization is usually required when complications occur.

BILIARY ATRESIA

BA is a destructive, idiopathic, inflammatory process that leads to fibrosis and obliteration of the biliary tree (Emerick and Whitington, 2006). BA has been detected in 3.7 in 10,000 live births (Chen, Chang, Du, and others, 2006). The disorder is more common in girls and preterm infants. In the United States, the incidence is twice as high in African-Americans as in Caucasian infants, and more common in Chinese than in either Japanese or Caucasian populations.

Etiology and Pathophysiology

The exact cause of BA is unknown. Because BA has two distinct forms, postnatal and fetal-embryonic, different pathogenic mechanisms are suggested. Postnatal BA represents 65% to 90% of cases and is probably the result of infection or an immune-mediated mechanism. Jaundice, manifesting with yellow discoloration of the skin or sclerae, is the most common early symptom of BA. Jaundice, indicating cholestasis (the accumulation of compounds that cannot be excreted because of occlusion or obstruction of the biliary tree), can be visible at a total serum bilirubin concentration as low as 5.0 mg/dl. An abnormal direct bilirubin has been designated as greater than 1.0 mg/dl if the total bilirubin is less than 5 mg/dl or a value of direct bilirubin that represents more than 20% of the total bilirubin if it is greater than 5 mg/dl (Emerick and Whitington, 2006). Direct hyperbilirubinemia first appears after the resolution of physiologic jaundice. Jaundice is often associated with pale stool and dark urine. Histologic study demonstrates bile duct remnants and a progressive inflammatory process. In the fetal embryonic form of BA, which represents 10% to 35% of cases, there is a congenital absence of biliary ductal patency and an absence of bile duct remnants. Many infants have associated congenital anomalies. Varying degrees of cholestasis occur, resulting in retention of irritants and toxins. Injury to the liver occurs as the result of the inflammation caused by the cholestasis.

Diagnostic Evaluation

Early diagnosis is the key to the survival of the child with BA. Infants who undergo surgery in the first 60 days of life have an 80% chance of establishing bile flow. Between 60 to 90 days of life, the chance of reestablishing flow drops to 50%, and after 90 days to 10% (Chen, Chang, Du, and others, 2006). The typical infant is thriving, appears well, and has only very mild jaundice during the first 6 to 8 weeks (Emerick and Whitington, 2006) but will soon begin failing to thrive. Several clinical signs may indicate the presence of BA (Box 24-10). Blood tests should include a CBC, electrolytes, bilirubin, and liver enzymes. Additional laboratory analyses, including α_1-antitrypsin level, TORCH titers (see Maternal Infections, Chapter 9), hepatitis serology, α-fetoprotein, urine cytomegalovirus, and a sweat test, are indicated to rule out other conditions that cause persistent cholestasis and jaundice. Abdominal ultrasonography allows

---

BOX 24-10

Clinical Manifestations of Extrahepatic Biliary Atresia

Jaundice
- Earliest manifestation and most striking feature of disorder
- First observed in sclera
- May be present at birth, but usually not apparent until age 2 to 3 weeks

Urine dark and stains diaper
Stools lighter than expected or white or tan
Hepatomegaly and abdominal distention common
Splenomegaly occurs later
Poor fat metabolism results in:
- Poor weight gain
- Failure to thrive

Pruritus
Irritability; difficulty comforting infant

---

inspection of the liver and biliary system. Hepatobiliary scintigraphy demonstrates biliary patency but does not provide diagnostic certainty. Endoscopic retrograde cholangiopancreatography (ERCP) is performed in very young infants. This procedure, which is done using general anesthesia, has an 80% reported diagnostic accuracy. Percutaneous liver biopsy is highly reliable when the biopsy contains specimens from a number of portal areas. Definitive diagnosis of BA is obtained during surgical laparotomy and an intraoperative cholangiogram.

Therapeutic Management

The primary treatment of BA is **hepatic portoenterostomy (Kasai procedure)**, in which a segment of intestine is anastomosed to the resected porta hepatis to attempt bile drainage. Bile drainage is achieved in approximately 80% to 90% of infants who undergo surgery when younger than 10 weeks of age (Ohi, 2001). However, progressive cirrhosis still occurs in many children, necessitating liver transplantation. Prophylactic antibiotics are given after the Kasai procedure to minimize the risk of ascending cholangitis.

Medical management is primarily supportive. It includes nutritional support with infant formulas that contain medium-chain triglycerides and essential fatty acids. Supplementation is usually required with fat-soluble vitamins; a multivitamin; and minerals, including iron, zinc, and selenium. Aggressive nutritional support with continuous tube feedings or TPN is indicated for moderate to severe failure to thrive. The enteral solution should be low in sodium. Ursodeoxycholic acid is used to treat pruritus and hypercholesterolemia.

Prognosis. Untreated BA results in progressive cirrhosis and death in most children by 2 years of age. The Kasai procedure improves the prognosis but is not a cure. Biliary drainage can often be achieved if the surgery is done before the intrahepatic bile ducts are destroyed. Long-term survival has been reported in children who receive the Kasai procedure; however, even with successful bile drainage, many children ultimately develop liver failure.

Advances in surgical techniques and the use of immunosuppressive and antifungal drugs have improved the success of transplantation. The major obstacle continues to be a shortage of donor livers. Reduced-size, split-liver transplantation, retransplantation, and increased public awareness may improve donor organ availability in the future (see Ethical Case Study).

ETHICAL CASE STUDY | Liver Transplant

ETHICAL DECISION MAKING MODEL	J.T. is a 3-year-old African-American boy diagnosed with biliary atresia at the age of 6 months. Although he underwent a Kasai procedure, no bile ducts were found. His condition has progressively deteriorated until he is in need of a liver transplant. There are not enough donated livers to go around. If J.T. receives a liver, his biliary atresia will be cured, and he can be expected to live a normal life. Should he and other children like him with curable diseases receive preference over adults with diseases that could recur in the new liver (such as those with hepatitis B or C)?
Treat All Involved with Respect	Representatives of all sides of the issue from various racial, ethnic, and socioeconomic groups should be included in the discussion.
Hear All Sides	The voices representing all sides of this issue should be listened to, including pediatric proponents, adult proponents, geriatric proponents, and recovered alcoholics.
Initiate Action	After all sides have had their say, those who set the priorities regarding who gets available livers will decide whether the priorities need to be revised. They might want to consider increasing the pool of available livers by allowing relatively healthy older adults to donate to other adults whose disease is likely to return in the new liver.
Consider the Outcome	If children with curable diseases were to receive preference for available livers over adults whose disease is likely to recur in the new liver, the number of years of productive life posttransplant may be increased. A research study would provide the data.

Nursing Care Management

Nursing interventions for the child with BA include support of the family before, during, and after surgical procedures and education regarding the treatment plan. In the postoperative period of a portoenterostomy, nursing care is similar to that after major abdominal surgery. Family members need education relating to the proper administration of medications and nutritional therapy, including special formulas, vitamin and mineral supplements, tube feedings, or parenteral nutrition. Pruritus can often be relieved by drug therapy or comfort measures such as baths.

Children and their families also need psychosocial support. The uncertain prognosis, discomfort, and waiting for transplantation produce stress, and hospitalizations, pharmacologic therapy, and nutritional therapy impose financial burdens on the family. Families can receive help from the Children's Liver Disease Foundation,* an organization that provides educational materials, programs, and support systems.

STRUCTURAL DEFECTS

CLEFT LIP OR CLEFT PALATE

Clefts of the lip (CL) and palate (CP) are facial malformations that occur during embryonic development and are the most common congenital deformities of the head and neck. They may appear separately or, more often, together. CL results from failure of the maxillary and median nasal processes to fuse; CP is a midline fissure of the palate that results from failure of the two sides to fuse.

CL may vary from a small notch to a complete cleft extending into the base of the nose (Fig. 24-3). Clefts can be unilateral or bilateral. Deformed dental structures are associated

with CL. CP alone occurs in the midline and may involve the soft and hard palates. When associated with CL, the defect may involve the midline and extend into the soft palate on one or both sides.

Cleft lip and palate (CL/P) is more common than CP alone and varies by ethnicity. The occurrence is 1 in 1000 births in Caucasians; 1 in 500 births in Native Americans and Asians, and 1 in 2000 births in African-Americans. CP occurs alone in only 1 in 2500 cases and does not display variation by ethnicity (Wilkins-Haug, 2003). Approximately 60% to 80% of children born with CL/P are male. Females have a higher frequency of isolated clefts of the secondary palate. Unilateral clefts are nine times more common than bilateral clefts and occur twice as frequently on the left side. Isolated bilateral CLs are uncommon; approximately 86% of those with bilateral CL also have palatal clefts. Approximately 68% of those with unilateral CLs have an associated palatal cleft (Kirschner and LaRossa, 2000).

Etiology

Cleft deformities may be an isolated anomaly, or they may occur with a recognized syndrome. CL with or without CP is distinct from isolated CP. Clefts of the secondary palate alone are more likely to be associated with syndromes than is isolated CL or CL with CP.

CL and CP may be caused by exposure to teratogens such as alcohol, anticonvulsants, steroids, and retinoids, but there is little evidence to link isolated clefts to any single teratogenic agent with the exception of phenytoin. Use of phenytoin during pregnancy is associated with a tenfold increase in the incidence of CL. The incidence of CL among mothers who smoke during pregnancy is twice as great as the incidence in mothers who do not (Eppley, van Aalst, Robey, and others, 2005).

*36 Great Charles St., Birmingham, B3 3JY, United Kingdom; (0121) 212-3839; fax: (0121) 212-4300; http://www.childliverdisease.org.

FIG. 24-3 ■ Variations in clefts of lip and palate at birth. **A,** Notch in vermilion border. **B,** Unilateral cleft lip and palate. **C,** Bilateral cleft lip and palate. **D,** Cleft palate.

Pathophysiology

Cleft deformities represent a genetic defect in cell migration that results in a failure of the maxillary and premaxillary processes to come together between the third and twelfth week of embryonic development. Although often appearing together, CL and CP are distinct malformations embryologically, occurring at different times during the developmental process. Merging of the upper lip at the midline is completed between the seventh and eleventh weeks of gestation. Fusion of the secondary palate (hard and soft palate) takes place later, between the seventh and twelfth weeks of gestation. In the process of migrating to a horizontal position, the palates are separated by the tongue for a short time. If there is delay in this movement, or if the tongue fails to descend soon enough, the remainder of development proceeds but the palate never fuses.

Diagnostic Evaluation

CL with or without CP is apparent at birth. The defect elicits severe emotional reactions in parents. CP is less obvious than CL and may not be detected without a thorough assessment of the mouth. CP is identified when the examiner places a gloved finger directly on the palate. Clefts of the hard palate form a continuous opening between the mouth and the nasal cavity. The severity of the CP has an impact on feeding; the infant is unable to generate negative pressure and create suction in the oral cavity. This impairs feeding, even though in most cases the infant's ability to swallow is normal.

Prenatal diagnosis with fetal ultrasound is not reliable until the soft tissues of the fetal face can be visualized at 13 to 14 weeks. The sensitivity of fetal ultrasound for facial clefting is almost 100% when CL/P is associated with other structural anomalies. An intact lip is the most difficult to diagnose prenatally (Wilkins-Haug, 2003).

Therapeutic Management

Treatment of the child with CL is surgical and involves no long-term interventions other than possible scar revision. The management of CP involves the cooperative efforts of a multidisciplinary health care team, including pediatrics, plastic surgery, orthodontics, otolaryngology, speech/language pathology, audiology, nursing, and social work. Management is directed toward closure of the cleft(s), prevention of complications, and facilitation of normal growth and development in the child. Until recently, repair of cleft deformities in the neonate was not considered safe. Surgery is now possible in younger neonates because of advances in pediatric anesthesiology and neonatology. However, the infant must be free of any oral, respiratory, or systemic infections. In deformities of both the lip and palate, the palate is repaired first to avoid disrupting the lip after it has been repaired.

Surgical Correction of Cleft Lip. The two most common procedures for repair of CL are the Tennison-Randall triangular flap (Z-plasty) and the Millard rotational advancement technique. The difference between these two is that the Tennison-Randall procedure crosses the philtral line and the Millard procedure advances a triangle of tissue in the upper third of the lip and does not cross the midline. Surgeons often use a combination of these two techniques to address individual differences. Improved surgical techniques have minimized scar retraction, and in the absence of infection or trauma, healing occurs with little scar formation. Optimal cosmetic results, however, are difficult to obtain in severe defects. Additional revisions may be necessary at a later age.

Surgical Correction of Cleft Palate. CP repair was previously postponed until a later age than the repair of the CL to take advantage of palatal changes that take place with normal growth. With advanced surgical and anesthesia techniques, many surgeons are currently performing palatal repairs in the neonatal period (Sandberg, Magee, and Denk, 2002). The timing of repair remains controversial. Most surgeons prefer to close the cleft before the child develops faulty speech habits.

Prognosis. Even with good anatomic closure, most children with CL/P have some degree of speech impairment that requires speech therapy. Physical problems result from inefficient functioning of the muscles of the soft palate and nasopharynx, improper tooth alignment, and varying degrees of hearing loss. Improper drainage of the middle ear, as a result of inefficient function of the eustachian tube, contributes to recurrent otitis media with scarring of the tympanic membrane, which leads to hearing impairment in many children with CP. Upper respiratory tract infections require immediate and meticulous attention, and extensive orthodontics and prosthodontics may be needed to correct malposition of teeth and maxillary arches.

Long-term problems are related to the child's social adjustment. The better the physical care, the better is the chance for emotional and social adjustment, although the degree of residual disability are not always directly related to a satisfactory adjustment. Physical defects are a threat to the self-image, and abnormal speech quality is an impediment to social expression.

Nursing Care Management

The immediate nursing problems for an infant with CL/P deformities are related to feeding and dealing with the parental reaction to the defect. Facial deformities are particularly disturbing to parents. CL is a visible defect that may produce a strong negative response in parents, which could influence maternal- and paternal-infant attachment. However, a study of infants with CL or CP indicated that maternal-infant attachment was not negatively affected when measured at 1 year of age (Speltz, Endriga, Fisher, and others, 1997). During the initial phase following birth, it is important for the nurse to emphasize not only on the infant's physical needs, but also the parents' emotional needs. The manner of handling the infant should convey to the parents that the infant is a precious human being. (See Chapter 18 for interventions in assisting parents in accepting a birth defect.) Throughout the course of therapy, parents need explanations of the immediate and long-range problems associated with CP. They may be unaware that more is involved than repairing the defect. Whenever possible, they should be referred to a comprehensive CP team.

Feeding. Feeding the infant presents a challenge to nurses and parents. Growth failure in infants with CL or CP has been attributed to preoperative feeding difficulties. After surgical repair, most infants who have isolated CL or CP with no associated syndromes gain weight or achieve adequate weight and height for age.

CL or CP reduces the infant's ability to suck, making bottle-feeding and breastfeeding difficult. In breastfeeding the CL or CP interferes with compression of the areola. Liquid taken into the mouth escapes via the cleft through the nose. Feeding is best accomplished with the infant's head in an upright position, either held in the caregiver's hand or cradled in the arm. Normal nipples are unsuitable for these infants, who are unable to generate the suction required. A variety of special "cleft palate" nipples have been devised and used with some success. However, large, soft nipples with large holes; Nursettes; or long, soft lamb's nipples appear to offer the best means for

nipple feeding. The newer "gravity flow" nipple attached to a squeezable plastic bottle allows formula to be deposited directly into the mouth in the same manner as with a bulb syringe. Success has also been achieved by modification of a standard nipple. A single small slit or crosscut is made in the end of the nipple with a sharp surgical blade or pair of sharp, thin scissors. The enlarged opening, which can be adjusted to the infant's individual needs, allows the infant to swallow the formula easily, bypassing the suction problem.

The ESSR feeding technique also works well with these infants. The steps in ESSR are (1) *E*nlarge the nipple, (2) *S*timulate the suck reflex, (3) *S*wallow fluid appropriately, and (4) *R*est when the infant signals with facial expression. Infants fed with the ESSR method revealed a significantly greater increase in their mean weight before surgery than infants fed with traditional methods (Richard, 1994).

Using special or modified nipples or feeding techniques helps meet the infant's sucking needs. Muscle development is important for later development of speech. During feeding, the nipple is positioned so that it is compressed by the infant's tongue and existing palate. If a single-slit nipple is used, the slit is placed vertically so that the infant will be able to produce and stop a flow of milk by alternately opening and closing the opening. No matter which type of nipple is used, gentle, steady pressure on the base of the bottle reduces the chance of choking or coughing. The person feeding should resist the temptation to remove the nipple because of the noise the infant makes or fear that the infant will choke. These infants swallow excessive amounts of air, and they require frequent burping.

When the infant has trouble with nipple feeding, a rubber-tipped medicine dropper, Asepto syringe, or Breck feeder (a large syringe with soft rubber tubing) provides an efficient, safe feeding device. The rubber extension should be long enough to extend back into the mouth to reduce the likelihood of regurgitation through the nose. The formula is deposited on the back of the tongue, and the flow is controlled by bulb or syringe compression that is adjusted to the infant's needs. With some infants, spoon feeding works best, especially if the formula is slightly thickened with cereal. After feeding, the infant is given water to rinse the mouth.

Many infants with CL/P can breastfeed. The nipple is positioned and stabilized well back in the oral cavity so that tongue action facilitates milk expression. The suction required to stimulate milk may be absent, so a breast pump may be useful before nursing to stimulate the let-down reflex.

Regardless of the feeding method used, the mother should begin feeding the infant as soon as possible, preferably after the initial nursery feeding. When maternal feeding is initiated early, the mother can help to determine the method best suited to her and the infant and can become adept in the technique before discharge from the hospital.

Preoperative Care. In preparation for surgical repair, parents are frequently taught to accustom the infant to the needs of the early postoperative period, especially if surgery is delayed for several months. It is mandatory for the infant to be positioned on the back or side postoperatively. Most infants tolerate these positions well because they are accustomed to being supine for sleeping. It is also helpful to place the infant or child in arm restraints periodically before admission and to feed the infant with a rubber-tipped Asepto syringe or other device that will be used postoperatively.

Postoperative Care for Cleft Lip. The major efforts in the postoperative period are directed toward protecting the operative site. After CL repair (**cheiloplasty**), a metal appliance or adhesive strips are securely taped to the cheeks to relax the surgical site and prevent tension on the suture line caused by crying or other facial movement. Efforts should be made to prevent crying as much as possible to avoid stress on the suture line. Elbow restraints to prevent the infant from rubbing or disturbing the suture line are applied immediately after surgery. It is advisable to pin the cuff of the restraints to the infant's clothing to keep the restraints in place. Older infants who roll over require a jacket restraint in addition to restricting arm movement to prevent rolling on the abdomen and rubbing the face on the sheet, especially if the repair involves the lip. It is important to remove the elbow restraints periodically to exercise the arms, to provide relief from restrictions, to observe the skin for signs of irritation, and to provide an opportunity for cuddling and body contact. Restraints should be released one at a time. Sitting the infant in an infant seat provides a change of position and a different view of the environment. Adequate analgesia is required to relieve postoperative pain and to prevent restlessness.

Clear liquids are offered when the infant has fully recovered from the anesthesia, and feeding is resumed when tolerated. The suture site is carefully cleansed of formula or serosanguineous drainage as needed with a cotton-tipped swab dipped in saline. A thin layer of antibiotic ointment may be prescribed for application to the suture line after cleansing. Meticulous care of the suture line is essential because inflammation or infection will interfere with optimal healing and the ultimate cosmetic effect of the surgical repair. Gentle aspiration of mouth and nasopharyngeal secretions may be necessary to prevent aspiration and respiratory complications. An upright or infant seat position is helpful in the immediate postoperative period (especially for the infant who has difficulty handling secretions).

Postoperative Care of Cleft Palate. The child with CP repair (**palatoplasty**) is allowed to lie on the abdomen immediately postoperatively. The child may resume feeding by bottle, breast, or cup shortly after surgery.

> **NURSINGALERT**
>
> Avoid the use of suction or other objects in the mouth, such as tongue depressors, thermometers, pacifiers, spoons, or straws.

Oral packing may be secured to the palate after palatoplasty; this packing is usually removed after 2 to 3 days. Sometimes the infant will have difficulty breathing after surgery, since it is often necessary to alter an established pattern of breathing and adjust to breathing through the nose. This is frustrating but seldom requires more than positioning and support. The elbows may be restrained to keep the child's hands away from the mouth. Parents are instructed to maintain elbow restraints at home until the palate is healed, usually in 4 to 6 weeks. They are instructed to remove the restraints (one at a time) frequently to allow the child to exercise the arms.

The nurse must assess the infant's or child's level of postoperative pain. Opioids may be prescribed initially, and acetaminophen may be given as needed thereafter. It is important to manage pain to decrease crying in infants with CL repair.

The older infant or child may be discharged on a blenderized or soft diet, and parents are instructed to continue the diet until the surgeon directs them otherwise. Parents are cautioned against allowing the child to eat hard items (such as toast, hard cookies, and potato chips) that can damage the repaired palate. The expected outcomes are described in the Nursing Process box.

Long-Term Care. Children with CL/P often require a variety of services during recovery. Family members need support and encouragement by health professionals and guidance in activities that facilitate a normal outcome for their child. Parents frequently cite financial stress as a difficult issue. With the combined efforts of the family and the health team, most children achieve a satisfactory outcome. Many children with CL/P have surgical correction that creates a near normal–appearing lip and permits good function. Parents need to understand the function of therapy and the purpose and care of all appliances, as well as the importance of establishing good mouth care and proper brushing habits.

Throughout the child's development, an important goal is the development of a healthy personality and self-esteem. Many communities have CP parents' groups that offer help and support to families. Agencies that provide services and information for children with CL/P and their families include the American Cleft Palate–Craniofacial Association, the Cleft Palate Foundation, the Birth Defects Research for Children, the March of Dimes, and various state children's medical services.

ESOPHAGEAL ATRESIA WITH TRACHEOESOPHAGEAL FISTULA

Congenital atresia of the esophagus and tracheoesophageal fistula (TEF) are rare malformations that result from failed separation of the esophagus and trachea by the fourth week of gestation. These defects occur as separate entities or in combination (Fig. 24-4). They have a fatal outcome without early diagnosis and treatment.

Etiology

Esophageal atresia (EA) with or without an associated TEF is the most common esophageal malformation, occurring in approximately 1 in 3500 live births (Shaw-Smith, 2006). There appears to be an equal sex incidence, but the birth weight of most affected infants is significantly lower than average, and incidence of prematurity is unusually high. A history of maternal polyhydramnios is present in approximately 50% of infants with the defects. EA/TEF is often present with the VATER or VACTERL syndromes, acronyms for syndromes involving a combination of Vertebral, Anorectal, Cardiovascular, Tracheoesophageal, Renal, and Limb abnormalities. The cardiac and renal anomalies occur most frequently with EA/TEF.

Pathophysiology

The cause of EA/TEF is unknown. In the most frequently encountered form of EA and TEF (80% to 95% of cases), the proximal esophageal segment terminates in a blind pouch, and the distal segment is connected to the trachea or primary bronchus by a short fistula at or near the bifurcation (see Fig. 24-4, *C*). The second most common variety (5% to 8%) consists of a blind pouch at each end, widely separated and with no communication to the trachea (see Fig. 24-4, *A*). Less frequently, an otherwise normal trachea and esophagus are connected by a common fistula (see Fig. 24-4, *E*). Extremely rare anomalies involve a fistula from the trachea to the upper

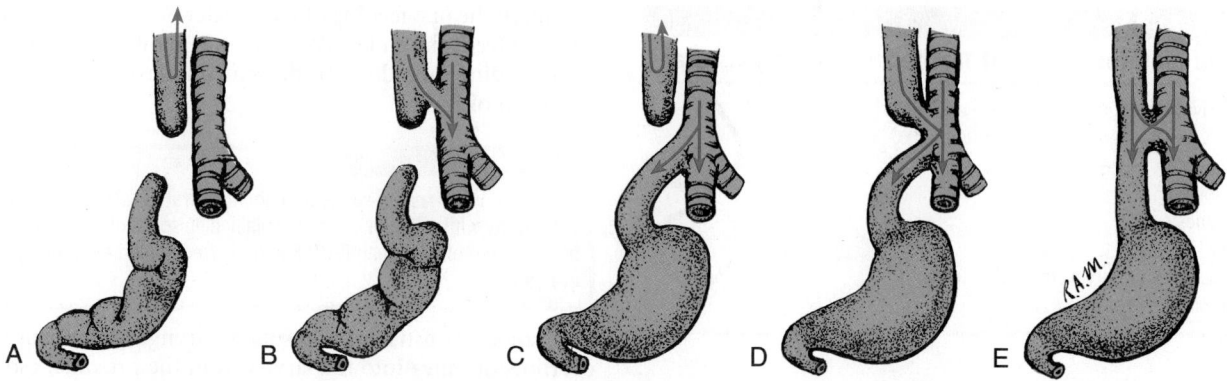

FIG. 24-4 ■ A-E, Five most common types of esophageal atresia and tracheoesophageal fistula.

---

nursingprocess | **The Child with a Cleft Lip or Cleft Palate**

ASSESSMENT
The lip defect is visible at birth, and assessment involves describing the location and extent of the defect; the cleft palate (CP) is estimated by visualization during crying. CP without cleft lip (CL) is detected by palpating the palate with the gloved finger during the newborn assessment. The emotional impact of the birth of a child with a cosmetic and functional disability is especially traumatic to the family. Consequently, nursing assessment is also concerned with the family's emotional reaction.

DIAGNOSIS (PROBLEM IDENTIFICATION)
After a thorough assessment, several nursing diagnoses are evident:
- Altered Nutrition: Less Than Body Requirements related to physical defect
- Risk for Altered Parenting related to infant with a highly visible physical defect
- Risk for Trauma of the surgical site related to surgical procedure, dysfunctional swallowing
- Altered Nutrition: Less Than Body Requirements related to difficulty eating following surgical procedure
- Pain related to surgical procedure
- Altered Family Processes related to child with a physical defect, hospitalization

PLANNING
The goals of care are related to preoperative care, short-term postoperative care, and long-term management. Goals for the infant and family include:
Preoperative care:
- Family will cope with the impact of an infant with a defect.
- Infant will receive optimum nutrition.
- Infant will be prepared for surgery.

Postoperative care:
- Infant will experience no trauma and minimal or no pain.
- Infant will receive optimum nutrition.
- Infant will experience no complications.
- Infant and family will receive adequate support.
- Family will be prepared for care at home and long-term needs of a child with CP.

IMPLEMENTATION
Numerous intervention strategies are discussed on pp. 845-846.

EVALUATION
The effectiveness of nursing interventions for the family and the child who has CP is determined by continual assessment and evaluation of care based on the following guidelines:
Preoperative care:
- Observe and interview family members about their understanding, feelings, and concerns regarding the defect, any anticipated surgery, and their interactions with the infant.
- Observe infant during feeding.
- Complete preoperative checklist.
Postoperative care:
- Inspect operative site, including the protective device, for evidence of infection, bleeding, sloughing, or irritation.
- Observe for behavioral and physiologic indicators of pain and response to analgesics.
- Observe infant during feeding, measure intake and output, and weigh infant daily.
- Observe and interview family regarding their understanding and concerns about the infant, including long-term needs.

---

esophageal segment (see Fig. 24-4, *B*) or to both the upper and the lower segments (see Fig. 24-4, *D*).

Diagnostic Evaluation

The disorder is suspected on the basis of clinical manifestations (Box 24-11). EA should also be suspected in cases of maternal polyhydramnios. Although the diagnosis is established on the basis of clinical signs and symptoms, the exact type of anomaly is determined by radiographic studies. A radiopaque catheter is inserted into the hypopharynx and ad-

vanced until it encounters an obstruction. Chest films are taken to ascertain esophageal patency or the presence and level of a blind pouch. Sometimes fistulas are not patent, which makes them more difficult to diagnose. The presence of gas in the stomach or small bowel is indicative of a coexisting TEF.

Therapeutic Management

EA is a surgical emergency. The treatment includes maintenance of a patent airway, prevention of pneumonia, gastric or blind pouch decompression, and surgical repair of the anom-

---

BOX 24-11

Clinical Manifestations of Tracheoesophageal Fistula

Excessive salivation and drooling
Three Cs of tracheoesophageal fistula:
    Coughing
    Choking
    Cyanosis
Apnea
Increased respiratory distress after feeding
Abdominal distention

---

aly. When EA/TEF is suspected, the infant is immediately taken off oral intake, started on IV fluids, and placed in the position least likely to cause aspiration of either mouth or stomach secretions. Removal of secretions from the mouth and upper pouch requires frequent or continuous suction. Because aspiration pneumonia is almost inevitable and appears early, broad-spectrum antibiotic therapy is often instituted.

Primary surgical correction consists of a thoracotomy with division and ligation of the TEF and an end-to-side anastomosis of the esophagus. This may consist of one operation or be staged with two or more procedures. For infants who are preterm, have multiple anomalies, or are in poor condition, a staged procedure is preferred that involves palliative measures, including gastrostomy, ligation of the TEF, and provision of constant drainage of the esophageal pouch. A delayed esophageal anastomosis is usually attempted after several weeks to months when the upper pouch elongates. Further surgical techniques may be performed later to facilitate esophageal lengthening. If an esophageal anastomosis still cannot be accomplished, a **cervical esophagostomy** (to allow drainage of saliva) and gastrostomy are performed.

A primary anastomosis may be impossible because of insufficient length of the two segments of the esophagus. In these cases, an esophageal replacement procedure using a part of the colon, or gastric tube interposition may be necessary to bridge the missing esophageal segment. Endotracheal intubation may be required, since many infants (10% to 20%) also have **tracheomalacia,** a weakness in the tracheal wall that occurs when a dilated proximal pouch compresses the trachea in early fetal life or when the trachea does not develop normally because of a loss of intratracheal pressure.

Complications of a primary repair include an anastomotic leak, strictures resulting from tension or ischemia, esophageal motility disorders causing dysphagia, and GER.

Prognosis. The prognosis is related to the birth weight, associated congenital anomalies, and time of diagnosis. The survival rate is nearly 100% in full-term infants without severe respiratory distress or other anomalies. In preterm low-birth-weight infants with associated anomalies, the incidence of complications is high.

Nursing Care Management

Nursing responsibility for detection of this malformation begins *immediately* after birth. Ideally, the diagnosis should be made before the initial feeding, but often it is not. If fed, the infant swallows normally but suddenly coughs and struggles, and the fluid is aspirated or returns through the nose and mouth. For this reason, it is customary for the nurse to give the infant the first feeding of plain water or to be present when a parent feeds the child to observe the infant's response. Early breastfeeding should not be prevented unless there is a strong suspicion of EA.

NURSINGALERT

Any infant who has an excessive amount of frothy saliva in the mouth or difficulty with secretions and unexplained episodes of cyanosis should be suspected of having an EA/TEF and referred immediately for medical evaluation.

Cyanosis is usually the result of laryngospasm caused by overflow of saliva into the larynx from the proximal esophageal pouch. It normally clears after removal of the secretions from the oropharynx by suctioning. Any suspicion of TEF is reported immediately. The infant is placed in an incubator or a radiant warmer, and oxygen is administered to help relieve respiratory distress. Intubation and assisted mechanical ventilation may be necessary if the infant is in respiratory distress. When a newborn is suspected of having a TEF, the most desirable position is supine with the head elevated at least 30 degrees. This position minimizes the reflux of gastric secretions up the distal esophagus into the trachea and bronchi.

It is imperative that the source of aspiration be removed at once. Oral fluids are withheld, and the infant's fluid needs are met parenterally or via gastrostomy. Until surgery the blind pouch is kept empty by intermittent or continuous suction through an indwelling nasal catheter that extends to the end of the pouch. The catheter needs attention because it has a tendency to become clogged with mucus. It is usually replaced daily. In the event that a staged repair is performed, a gastrostomy tube is inserted and left open so that air entering the stomach through the fistula can escape, thus minimizing the danger that gastric contents will be regurgitated into the trachea. The tube empties by gravity drainage. Feedings through the gastrostomy tube and irrigations with fluid are contraindicated before surgery in the infant with a distal TEF. Nursing interventions include respiratory assessment, airway management, thermoregulation, fluid and electrolyte management, and possibly nutritional support.

Postoperative Care. Postoperative care is essentially the same as for any high-risk newborn (see Nursing Care of the High-Risk Newborn and Family, Chapter 9). The infant is returned to the radiant heater, and the gastrostomy tube is connected to gravity drainage until the infant can tolerate feedings. At this time the tube is elevated and secured at a point above the level of the stomach. This allows gastric secretions to pass to the duodenum, and swallowed air can escape through the open tube. Tracheal suction should be done only using a premeasured catheter and with extreme caution to avoid injury to the suture line. If tolerated, gastrostomy feedings may be started and continued until the esophageal anastomosis is healed. Before oral feedings are initiated and the chest tube is removed, a contrast study or esophagram is performed to verify the integrity of the esophageal anastomosis.

The initial attempt at oral feeding must be carefully observed to make certain that the infant can swallow without choking. Oral feedings are begun with sterile water, followed by frequent small feedings of formula. Until the infant can take a sufficient amount by mouth, gastrostomy feedings or parenteral nutrition may supplement oral intake. Infants are usually not discharged until they are taking oral fluids well and the gastrostomy tube is removed. However, the infant who has palliative surgery will be discharged with the gastrostomy tube in place. The nurse is responsible for making certain that the caregiver is educated and has practiced the care of the gastrostomy (see Chapter 22).

Special Problems. Upper respiratory tract complications are a threat to life in both the preoperative and postoperative periods. In addition to pneumonia, there is a constant danger of respiratory distress resulting from atelectasis, pneumothorax, and laryngeal edema. Any persistent respiratory difficulty after removal of secretions is reported to the surgeon immediately. The infant is monitored for anastomotic leaks, as evidenced by purulent chest tube drainage, increased WBC count, and temperature instability.

In the infant awaiting esophageal replacement surgery, the catheter is removed and the upper esophageal segment is drained through a cervical esophagostomy. An esophagostomy is difficult to care for because the skin becomes irritated by moisture from the continuous discharge of saliva. Frequent removal of drainage and application of a layer of protective ointment may remedy the problem. A dressing or ostomy appliance may be applied to collect the drainage, and an enterostomal therapist can provide additional guidance to prevent or treat skin breakdown.

For the infant who requires esophageal replacement, nonnutritive sucking is provided by a pacifier. Sometimes small amounts of water or formula are given orally, and although the liquid drains from the esophagostomy, this process allows the infant to develop mature sucking patterns. Other appropriate oral stimulation prevents feeding aversions. Infants who remain NPO for an extended period or who have not received oral stimulation have difficulty eating by mouth after corrective surgery and may develop oral hypersensitivity and food aversion. They require patient, firm guidance to learn how to take food into the mouth and swallow after repair. A referral to a multidisciplinary feeding behavior program is often necessary.

As with any congenital anomaly, parents need support in adjusting to the child's condition (see Chapter 18). One difficulty is the immediate transfer of the sick newborn to the intensive care unit and the length of hospitalization. Encouraging parents to visit the infant, participate in care when appropriate, and express their feelings regarding the infant's condition facilitates the attachment process. The nurse in the intensive care unit should assume responsibility for ensuring that the parents are kept fully informed of the infant's progress.

Preparing parents for discharge involves teaching them skills they will need at home. Parents are taught to observe for behaviors that indicate the need for suctioning and for signs of respiratory distress and constriction of the esophagus (e.g., poor feeding, dysphagia, drooling, regurgitation of undigested food). Discharge planning also includes obtaining the necessary equipment and home nursing services to provide home care.

HERNIAS

A **hernia** is a protrusion of a portion of an organ or organs through an abnormal opening. The danger from herniation arises when the organ protruding through the opening is constricted to the extent that circulation is impaired or when the protruding organs encroach on and impair the function of other structures. A hernia that cannot be reduced easily is called an **incarcerated hernia**. A **strangulated hernia** is one in which the blood supply to the herniated organ is impaired. The herniations of concern are those that protrude through the diaphragm, the abdominal wall, or the inguinal canal (see also Genitourinary Tract Disorders and Defects, Chapter 27). The other hernias of significance to the pediatric age-groups are outlined in Table 24-5.

OBSTRUCTIVE DISORDERS

Obstruction in the GI tract occurs when the passage of nutrients and secretions is impeded by a constricted or occluded lumen or when there is impaired motility (**paralytic ileus**). Obstructions may be congenital or acquired. Many congenital obstructions such as atresia, imperforate anus, meconium plug, and meconium ileus usually appear in the neonatal period. Other obstructions of congenital etiology such as malrotation, HD, volvulus, incarcerated hernia, and Meckel diverticulum appear after the first few weeks of life. Intestinal obstruction from acquired causes such as intussusception, pyloric stenosis, and tumors may occur in infancy or childhood. Intestinal obstructions from any cause are characterized by similar signs and symptoms (Box 24-12).

HYPERTROPHIC PYLORIC STENOSIS

Hypertrophic pyloric stenosis (HPS) occurs when the circumferential muscle of the pyloric sphincter becomes thickened, resulting in elongation and narrowing of the pyloric channel. This produces an outlet obstruction and compensatory dilation, hypertrophy, and hyperperistalsis of the stomach. This condition usually develops in the first 2 to 5 weeks of life, causing projectile nonbilious vomiting, dehydration, metabolic alkalosis, and failure to thrive. The precise etiology is unknown. The reported incidence is 2 to 9 per 1000 live births with a male/female ratio of 6:1. There is a genetic predisposition, and siblings and offspring of affected persons are at increased risk of developing HPS. It is more common in full-term than in preterm infants and is seen less frequently in African-American and Asian infants than in Caucasian infants.

Pathophysiology

The circular muscle of the pylorus thickens as a result of hypertrophy (increased size) and hyperplasia (increased mass). This produces severe narrowing of the pyloric canal between the stomach and the duodenum, causing partial obstruction of the lumen (Fig. 24-5, *A*). Over time, inflammation and edema further reduce the size of the opening, resulting in complete obstruction. The hypertrophied pylorus may be palpable as an olivelike mass in the upper abdomen. Pyloric stenosis is not a congenital disorder. There is now substantial evidence to support decreased expression of neuronal nitric oxide synthase in the nerve fibers of the pyloric circular muscle in infants with HPS (Huang, Tiao, Lee, and others, 2006). In most cases HPS is an isolated lesion; however, it may be associated with intestinal malrotation, esophageal and duodenal atresia, and anorectal anomalies.

Diagnostic Evaluation

The diagnosis of HPS is often made after the history and physical examination. The olivelike mass is easily palpated when the stomach is empty, the infant is quiet, and the abdominal muscles are relaxed. Vomiting usually occurs 30 to

TABLE 24-5

Summary Outline of Hernias

MANIFESTATIONS AND TYPE	DIAGNOSTIC EVALUATION	NURSING CARE MANAGEMENT
DIAPHRAGMATIC Protrusion of abdominal organs through opening in diaphragm	**Symptoms**—Mild to severe respiratory distress within a few hours after birth; tachypnea, cyanosis, dyspnea, absent breath sounds in affected area; impaired cardiac output; possible symptoms of shock, severe acidosis **Diagnosis**—Suspected on basis of symptoms, confirmed by radiographic study; often diagnosed prenatally as early as 25th week of gestation	**Therapeutic:** Provide supportive treatment of respiratory distress and correction of acidosis; possibly use endotracheal intubation, gastrointestinal (GI) decompression, and extracorporeal membrane oxygenation (ECMO). Administer prophylactic antibiotics. Perform surgical reduction of hernia and repair of defect. **Nursing:** *Preoperative:* Reduce stimulation—environmental and care activities. Provide prompt recognition, resuscitation, and stabilization. Maintain suction, oxygen, and intravenous (IV) fluids. Position patient with head up. Administer medications. *Postoperative:* Carry out routine postoperative care and observation. Relieve pain and provide comfort. Support family because this is a critical illness.
HIATAL **Sliding**—Protrusion of an abdominal structure (usually stomach) through esophageal hiatus	**Symptoms**—Dysphagia, failure to thrive, vomiting, neck contortions, frequent unexplained respiratory problems, bleeding; usually associated with gastroesophageal reflux (GER); may cause gastric volvulus and obstruction **Diagnosis**—Made by fluoroscopy	**Therapeutic:** Manage GER symptoms; provide patient positioning, pharmacologic treatment, and dietary management. Surgical treatment is necessary when complications are related to GER despite medical management. **Nursing**—Be alert to significant signs and carry out routine postoperative care.
ABDOMINAL **Umbilical**—Weakness in abdominal wall around umbilicus; incomplete closure of abdominal wall, allowing intestinal contents to protrude through opening	**Symptoms**—Noted by inspection and palpation of the abdomen High incidence in preterm and African-American infants Usually closes spontaneously by 1-2 years of age	**Therapeutic:** No treatment is necessary for small defects. Provide operative repair if persists to age 4-6 years or if defect is >1.5-2.0 cm by age 2 years. Strangulation requires immediate attention. **Nursing:** Discourage use of home remedies (e.g., belly bands, coins). Reassure parents.
Omphalocele—Protrusion of intraabdominal viscera into base of umbilical cord; sac covered with peritoneum without skin **Gastroschisis**—Protrusion of intraabdominal contents through defect in abdominal wall lateral to umbilical ring; there is never a peritoneal sac	**Symptoms**—Obvious on inspection Observe for other malformations	**Therapeutic:** Provide surgical repair of defect. *Preoperative:* For large lesions, provide gradual reduction of abdominal contents. Administer prophylactic antibiotics. **Nursing (preoperative):** Keep sac or viscera moist with saline-soaked pads. Use overhead warming unit. Carry out routine care of IV line. Provide nasogastric suction. Keep patient NPO (nothing by mouth).

60 minutes after feeding and becomes projectile as the obstruction progresses. Emesis is nonbilious, usually consisting of stale milk. Often these infants become dehydrated and lethargic and appear significantly malnourished.

If the diagnosis is inconclusive from the history and physical signs (Box 24-13), ultrasonography will demonstrate an elongated, sausage-shaped mass with an elongated pyloric channel. If ultrasound fails to demonstrate a hypertrophied pylorus, then upper GI radiography should be done to rule out other causes of vomiting. Laboratory findings reflect the metabolic alterations created by severe depletion of both fluid and electrolytes from extensive and prolonged vomiting. There are decreased serum levels of both sodium and potassium, although these may be masked by the hemoconcentra-

BOX 24-12

Clinical Manifestations of Mechanical/Paralytic Intestinal Obstruction

Colicky abdominal pain—From peristalsis attempting to overcome the obstruction

Abdominal distention—As a result of accumulation of gas and fluid above the level of the obstruction

Vomiting—Often the earliest sign of a high obstruction; a later sign of lower obstruction (may be bilious or feculent)

Constipation and obstipation—Early signs of low obstructions; later signs of higher obstructions

Dehydration—From losses of large quantities of fluid and electrolytes into the intestine

Rigid and boardlike abdomen—From increased distention

Bowel sounds—Gradually diminish and cease

Respiratory distress—Occurs as the diaphragm is pushed up into the pleural cavity

Shock—Caused by plasma volume diminishing as fluids and electrolytes are lost from the bloodstream into the intestinal lumen

Sepsis—Caused by bacterial proliferation with invasion into the circulation

FIG. 24-5 ■ Hypertrophic pyloric stenosis. **A,** Enlarged muscular area nearly obliterates pyloric channel. **B,** Longitudinal surgical division of muscle down to submucosa establishes adequate passageway.

tion from ECF depletion. Of greater diagnostic value is a decrease in serum chloride levels and increases in pH and bicarbonate (carbon dioxide content) characteristic of metabolic alkalosis. The BUN level will be elevated as evidence of dehydration.

Therapeutic Management

Surgical relief of the pyloric obstruction by **pyloromyotomy** is the standard treatment for this disorder. The procedure is performed through a right upper quadrant incision (laparotomy) and consists of a longitudinal incision through the circular muscle fibers of the pylorus down to, but not including, the submucosa (see Fig. 24-5, *B*). The procedure has a high success rate when infants receive careful preoperative preparation to correct fluid and electrolyte imbalances.

Feedings are usually begun 4 to 6 hours postoperatively, beginning with small, frequent feedings of glucose water or electrolyte solutions followed by formula or breast milk as tolerated. Another procedure, **laparoscopy,** may be performed for infants with HPS. The use of a small incision for the laparoscope results in shorter surgical time, more rapid postoperative feeding, and quicker discharge.

Prognosis. Most infants recover completely and rapidly after pyloromyotomy. Postoperative complications include persistent pyloric obstruction and wound dehiscence. Some infants also have GER.

Nursing Care Management

The diagnosis of HPS is considered in the very young infant who appears alert but fails to gain weight and has a history of vomiting after meals. Assessment is based on observation of eating behaviors and evidence of other characteristic clinical manifestations.

Preoperative Care. Preoperatively the emphasis is placed on restoring hydration and electrolyte balance. Infants are usually given no oral feedings and receive IV fluids

BOX 24-13

Clinical Manifestations of Hypertrophic Pyloric Stenosis

Projectile vomiting
- May be ejected 3 to 4 feet from the child when in a side-lying position, 1 foot or more when in a back-lying position
- Usually occurs shortly after a feeding, but may not occur for several hours
- May follow each feeding or appear intermittently
- Nonbilious vomitus that may be blood-tinged

Infant hungry, avid nurser; eagerly accepts a second feeding after vomiting episode

No evidence of pain or discomfort except that of chronic hunger

Weight loss

Signs of dehydration

Distended upper abdomen

Readily palpable olive-shaped tumor in the epigastrium just to the right of the umbilicus

Visible gastric peristaltic waves that move from left to right across the epigastrium

with glucose and electrolyte replacement based on laboratory serum electrolyte values. Careful monitoring of the IV infusion and diligent attention to intake, output, and urine specific gravity measurements are important. Vomiting and the number and character of stools are observed and recorded accurately.

Observations also include assessment of vital signs, particularly those that might indicate fluid or electrolyte imbalances. These infants are prone to metabolic alkalosis from loss of hydrogen ions and to potassium, sodium, and chloride depletion. The skin, mucous membranes, and daily weight are assessed for alterations in hydration status and water gain or loss.

If stomach decompression and gastric lavage are used preoperatively, the nurse is responsible for ensuring that the tube is patent and functioning properly and for measuring and recording the type and amount of drainage. The infant is usually fed with the head elevated if an NG tube is in place. Infants who are receiving IV fluids or have an NG tube for continuous drainage must be observed to prevent the needle or tube from becoming dislodged.

General hygienic care, with attention to the skin and mouth in dehydrated infants, is essential. Protection from infection is also important because infants with impaired nutritional status are more susceptible than normal newborns. Parental involvement is encouraged and promoted.

Postoperative Care. Postoperative vomiting may occur, and most infants, even with successful surgery, exhibit some vomiting during the first 24 to 48 hours because of edema resulting from the surgery. IV fluids are administered until the infant can retain adequate amounts by mouth. Observation of physical signs, monitoring of IV fluids, careful observation, and recording of intake and output are maintained. The infant is also observed for evidence of pain, and appropriate analgesics are given. The NG tube may be maintained after surgery for a variable time.

Feedings are usually instituted soon after surgery, beginning with clear liquids containing glucose and electrolytes advancing to formula or breast milk as tolerated. They are offered slowly, in small amounts, and at frequent intervals as ordered by the practitioner. Observation and recording of feedings and the infant's responses to feedings are a vital part of postoperative care. Positioning with the head elevated 30% is usually continued postoperatively. Care of the operative site consists of observation for any drainage or signs of inflammation and care of the incision as directed by the surgeon.

Parents are encouraged to remain with their child and become involved in the child's care. Vomiting of a projectile nature is frightening to parents, and they often believe that they may have done something wrong or that surgery was not successful. Most parents need support and reassurance that the condition is caused by a structural problem and is in no way a reflection on their parenting skills and capacities.

INTUSSUSCEPTION

Intussusception is the most common cause of acute intestinal obstruction in children less than 5 years. The peak age is 3 to 9 months (Huppertz, Soriano-Gaabarro, Grimprel, and others, 2006). Intussusception is more common in boys than in girls and in children with cystic fibrosis. Although specific intestinal lesions can be found in about 3% of these children, the cause is usually not known. More than 90% of intussusceptions do not have a pathologic lead point, such as a polyp, lymphoma, or Meckel diverticulum. The idiopathic cases are most likely a result of hypertrophy of intestinal lymphoid tissue secondary to viral infection. Some cases have been associated with administration of the first licensed rotavirus vaccine, the reassortant rhesus-human tetravalent rotavirus vaccine (RRV-IV; RotaShield), which led to its voluntary with-

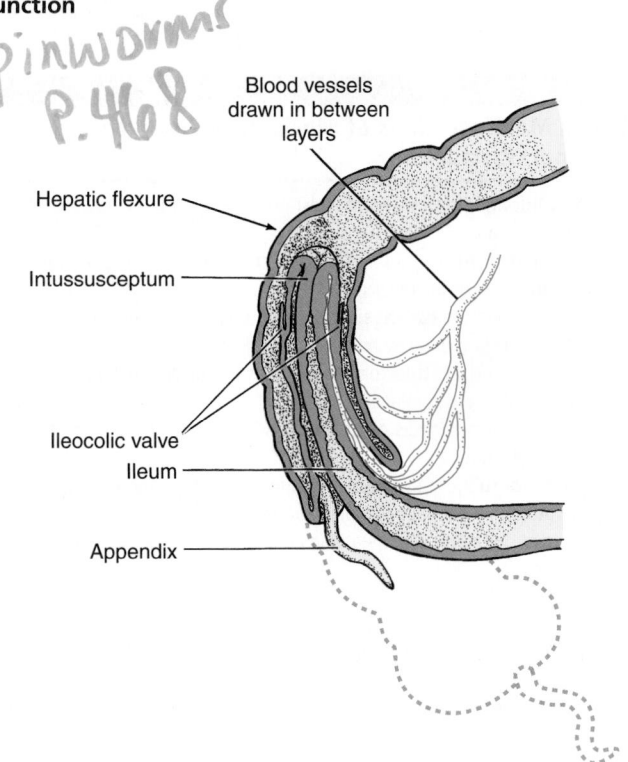

FIG. 24-6 ■ Ileocolic intussusception.

drawal in 1998. No such association has to date been reported from large phase III safety trials with the two new rotavirus vaccines currently being introduced.

Pathophysiology

Intussusception occurs when one portion of bowel invaginates into a more distant portion of the bowel, pulling the mesentery with it. Lymphatic and venous congestion and bowel wall edema can cause obstruction of the intestine, and infarction and perforation of the bowel wall can occur (Huppertz, Soriano-Gaabarro, Grimprel, and others, 2006). Venous engorgement also leads to leaking of blood and mucus into the intestinal lumen, forming the classic currant jelly stools. The most common site is the **ileocecal valve** (ileocolic), where the ileum invaginates into the cecum and colon (Fig. 24-6). Other forms include ileoileal (one part of the ileum invaginates into another section of the ileum) and colocolic (one part of the colon invaginates into another area of the colon, usually in the area of the hepatic or splenic flexure or at some point along the transverse colon).

> **NURSING ALERT**
>
> The classic triad of intussusception symptoms (abdominal pain, abdominal mass, bloody stools) is present in only 29% to 33% of children (Huppertz, Soriano-Gaabarro, Grimprel, and others, 2006). Children might also be initially seen with screaming, irritability, lethargy, vomiting, diarrhea or constipation, fever, dehydration, and shock. Because intussusception is potentially life threatening, the nurse should be aware of alternate presentations, observe these children closely, and refer them for further evaluation.

Diagnostic Evaluation

Frequently subjective findings lead to the diagnosis (Box 24-14), which can be confirmed by ultrasound. Spontaneous reduction occurs in up to 10% of patients.

BOX 24-14
Clinical Manifestations of Intussusception

- Sudden acute abdominal pain
- Child screaming and drawing the knees onto the chest
- Child appearing normal and comfortable between episodes of pain
- Vomiting
- Lethargy
- Passage of red, currant jelly–like stools (stool mixed with blood and mucus)
- Tender, distended abdomen
- Palpable sausage-shaped mass in upper right quadrant
- Empty lower right quadrant (Dance sign)
- Eventual fever, prostration, and other signs of peritonitis

Therapeutic Management

Conservative treatment consists of radiologist-guided pneumoenema (air enema) with or without water-soluble contrast or ultrasound-guided hydrostatic (saline) enema, the advantage of the latter being that no ionizing radiation is needed (Huppertz, Soriano-Gaabarro, Grimprel, and others, 2006). Recurrence of intussusception after conservative treatment occurs in about 1 in 10 patients; no predictable risk factors for recurrence have been identified.

IV fluids, NG decompression, and antibiotic therapy may be used before hydrostatic reduction is attempted. If these procedures are not successful, the child may require surgical intervention. Surgery involves manually reducing the invagination and, when indicated, resecting any nonviable intestine.

Prognosis. Nonoperative reduction is successful in approximately 80% of cases (Huppertz, Soriano-Gaabarro, Grimprel, and others, 2006). Surgery is required for patients in whom the contrast enema is unsuccessful. With early diagnosis and treatment, serious complications and death are uncommon.

Nursing Care Management

The nurse can help establish a diagnosis by listening to the parent's description of the child's physical and behavioral symptoms. It is not unusual for parents to state that they thought something was seriously wrong before others shared their concerns. The description of the child's severe colicky abdominal pain combined with vomiting is a significant sign of intussusception.

As soon as a possible diagnosis of intussusception is made, the nurse prepares the parents for the immediate need for hospitalization, the nonsurgical technique of hydrostatic reduction, and the possibility of surgery. It is important to explain the basic defect of intussusception. A model of the defect is easily demonstrated by pushing the end of a finger on a rubber glove back into itself or using the example of a telescoping rod. The principle of reduction by hydrostatic pressure can be simulated by filling the glove with water, which pushes the "finger" into a fully extended position.

Physical care of the child does not differ from that for any child undergoing abdominal surgery. Even though nonsurgical intervention may be successful, the usual preoperative procedures, such as maintenance of NPO status, routine laboratory testing (CBC and urinalysis), signed parental consent,

and preanesthetic sedation, are performed. For the child with signs of electrolyte imbalance, hemorrhage, or peritonitis, additional preparation, such as replacement fluids, whole blood or plasma, and NG suctioning, may be needed. Before surgery the nurse monitors all stools.

NURSINGALERT
Passage of a normal brown stool usually indicates that the intussusception has reduced itself. This is immediately reported to the practitioner, who may choose to alter the diagnostic and therapeutic care plan.

Postprocedural care includes observations of vital signs, blood pressure, intact sutures and dressing, and the return of bowel sounds. After spontaneous or hydrostatic reduction, the nurse observes for passage of water-soluble contrast material (if used) and the stool patterns, since the intussusception may recur. Children may be admitted to the hospital or monitored on an outpatient basis. A recurrence of intussusception is treated with the conservative reduction techniques described above, but a laparotomy is considered for multiple recurrences.

Because hospitalization may be the child's first separation from the parents, it is important to preserve the parent-child relationship by encouraging rooming-in or extended visiting. It may be the parents' first experience with hospitalization, necessitating their preparation for procedures such as IV therapy, frequent vital sign and blood pressure monitoring, dressings, and NPO. Because of the rapidity of the onset, diagnosis, and treatment, parents may feel stunned or numb. They may ask few questions, or they may constantly make inquiries, sometimes the same ones several times. If the nurse realizes the circumstances surrounding this condition, the parents' reactions are more likely to be understood and accepted.

MALROTATION AND VOLVULUS

Malrotation of the intestine is due to the abnormal rotation of the intestine around the superior mesenteric artery during embryologic development. Malrotation may manifest in utero or may be asymptomatic throughout life. Infants may have intermittent bilious vomiting, recurrent abdominal pain, distention, or lower GI bleeding. Malrotation is the most serious type of intestinal obstruction because, if the intestine undergoes complete volvulus (the intestine twisting around itself), compromise of the blood supply will result in intestinal necrosis, peritonitis, perforation, and death.

Diagnostic Evaluation

It is imperative that malrotation and volvulus be diagnosed promptly and surgical treatment instituted quickly. An upper GI series is the definitive procedure to diagnose this condition.

Therapeutic Management

Surgery is indicated to remove the affected area. Because of the extensive nature of some lesions, short-gut syndrome is a postoperative complication.

Nursing Care Management

Preoperatively the nursing care is the same as that provided to an infant or child with intestinal obstruction. Postoperatively the nursing care is similar to that provided to the infant or child who has undergone abdominal surgery.

ANORECTAL MALFORMATIONS

Anorectal malformations include a number of anomalies of the genitourinary and pelvic organs. These malformations are among the more common congenital malformations caused by abnormal development, with an incidence of 1 in 2000 to 5000 live births (Hendren, 1998). The anus and rectum originate from an embryologic structure called the **cloaca**. Lateral growth of the cloaca forms the urorectal septum that separates the rectum dorsally from the urinary tract ventrally. The rectum and urinary tract separate completely by the seventh week of gestation. Anomalies that occur reflect the stage of development of these processes.

Imperforate anus includes several forms of malformation without an obvious anal opening. Many have a fistula from the distal rectum to the perineum or genitourinary system. Anorectal malformations may occur in isolation or as part of the VACTERL or VATER syndromes.

A **persistent cloaca** is a complex anorectal malformation in which the rectum, vagina, and urethra drain into a common channel that opens onto the perineum via the usual urethral site (Chien, Chen, Tui, and others, 2005). **Cloacal exstrophy** is a rare, severe defect in which there is externalization of the bladder and bowel through the abdominal wall. Often the genitalia are indefinite and chromosome studies are necessary to determine the child's gender, which is almost always female. The exstrophic bladder is separated into two halves by the cecum; other features may include an omphalocele, imperforate anus, and, at times, a neural tube defect. With improved surgical techniques, survival rates for this condition are 88% to 90% (Smith, Woodard, Broecker, and others, 1997).

Anorectal anomalies are classified according to gender and abnormal anatomic features, including genitourinary and associated pelvic anomalies. The level of rectal descent is determined by the relationship of the termination of the bowel to the puborectalis sling of the levator ani musculature. Anorectal malformations are also classified according to the level of the malformation (high, intermediate, and low) (Table 24-6). About 50% of children with anorectal anomalies have a urologic problem.

Diagnostic Evaluation

Checking for patency of the anus and rectum is a routine part of the newborn assessment and should include observations regarding the passage of meconium. Inspection of the perineal area reveals absence of the normal anal opening; however, the appearance of the perineum alone does not accurately predict the level of the lesion. Genitourinary and pelvic anomalies associated with anorectal malformations should be considered.

In the newborn the presence of meconium on the perineum does not always indicate anal patency (particularly in girls), since a fistula may be present and allow evacuation of meconium through the vagina. Fistulas may not be apparent at birth but may become obvious as peristalsis gradually forces the meconium through the fistula. Rectourinary fistulas should be suspected if there is meconium in the urine. Anal stenosis may not be identified until the child is older and comes to the physician with a history of difficult defecation, abdominal distention, and ribbonlike stools.

Abdominal ultrasound is performed to determine the existence of other malformations. An IV pyelogram and voiding cystourethrogram are recommended for an infant with a high malformation to identify anomalies of the urinary tract.

TABLE 24-6

Classification of Anorectal Malformations

LEVEL	MALE	FEMALE
High	Anorectal agenesis	Anorectal agenesis
	With rectoprostatic-urethral fistula	With rectovaginal fistula
	Without fistula	Without fistula
	Rectal atresia	Rectal atresia
Intermediate	Recto-bulbar-urethral fistula	Rectovestibular fistula
		Rectovaginal fistula
Low	Agenesis without fistula	Agenesis without fistula
	Anocutaneous fistula	Anovestibular fistula
	Anal stenosis	Anocutaneous fistula
	Rare malformations	Anal stenosis
		Cloaca
		Rare malformations

From Stephens FD, Smith ED: Classification, identification, and assessment of surgical treatment of anorectal anomalies, *Pediatr Surg Int* 1(4):200-205, 1986.

Further examination is also indicated when there is evidence of urinary tract infection or other symptoms. If a syndrome is suspected, cardiac evaluation and spinal films should be obtained.

Therapeutic Management

Successful treatment for anal stenosis is generally accomplished by manual dilations. The procedure is initiated by a physician and repeated on a regular basis by the nurses in the hospital. Parents are taught to continue the dilations at home. Perineal fistulas are treated by anoplasty during the newborn period. The opening is moved to the center of the external sphincter, and dilations are begun. More extensive defects are usually managed with a colostomy and corrective surgical repair performed later in the first year.

The type of defect, the sacral anatomy, and the quality of muscles influence the long-term prognosis. In general, if the newborn has a deep midline groove, two well-formed buttocks, and an anal dimple, the prognosis for bowel control is better than if the infant has a flat or "rocker" bottom and no midline groove because of associated neurologic problems. A functioning interior anal sphincter is important to achieve continence. In its absence, the child may need a bowel program to achieve socially acceptable bowel continence. Other potential complications after surgical treatment include strictures, recurrent rectourinary fistula, mucosal prolapse, and constipation.

Nursing Care Management

The first nursing responsibility is identification of undetected anorectal malformations. A poorly developed anal dimple, a genitourinary fistula, or vertebral abnormalities suggest a high lesion. A newborn who does not pass a stool within 24 hours of birth requires further assessment. In addition, meconium that appears at an inappropriate orifice is reported. Preoperative care includes diagnostic evaluation, GI decompression, and IV fluids.

Nursing care after an anorectoplasty is directed toward healing the surgical site without infection or complications. Care involves keeping the anal area as clean as possible with scrupulous perineal care. A temporary dressing and drain may be placed initially to manage the continuous passage of stool.

Protective ointments such as zinc oxide and occlusive dressings such as hydrocolloids decrease skin irritation from frequent loose stools. The preferred position is a side-lying prone position with the hips elevated or a supine position with the legs suspended at a 90-degree angle to the trunk to prevent pressure on perineal sutures.

There may be an NG tube for abdominal decompression and IV feedings. The infant is given formula when normal peristalsis is noted. Care of the infant with a colostomy involves frequent dressing changes, meticulous skin care, and correct application of a collection device (see Chapter 22).

Family Support, Discharge Planning, and Home Care. Long-term follow-up is important for children with high malformations. After the definitive pull-through procedure, toilet training is delayed and complete continence is seldom achieved at the usual age of 2 to 3 years. Prevention of constipation is important, and breastfeeding is encouraged postoperatively. If a cow's milk–based formula is used, a laxative may be prescribed. Bowel habit training, diet modification, and administration of stool softeners or fiber are important aspects of bowel management. Optimum bowel function may not be achieved until late childhood or adolescence. Support and reassurance are important during the slow progression to normal function.

Parents are instructed in perineal and wound care or care of the colostomy. Anal dilations may be necessary for some infants. Parents are advised to observe stooling patterns and notify the physician if there are any signs of anal stricture or complications.

MALABSORPTION SYNDROMES

Chronic diarrhea and malabsorption of nutrients characterize malabsorption syndromes. An important complication of malabsorption syndromes in children is failure to thrive. Most cases are classified according to the location of the supposed anatomic or biochemical defect. The term **celiac disease** is often used to describe a symptom complex with four characteristics: (1) steatorrhea (fatty, foul, frothy, bulky stools), (2) general malnutrition, (3) abdominal distention, and (4) secondary vitamin deficiencies.

Digestive defects are conditions in which the enzymes necessary for digestion are diminished or absent, such as (1) cystic fibrosis, in which pancreatic enzymes are absent; (2) biliary or liver disease, in which bile flow is affected; or (3) lactase deficiency, in which there is congenital or secondary lactose intolerance.

Absorptive defects are conditions in which the intestinal mucosal transport system is impaired. This may occur because of a primary defect (e.g., celiac disease) or secondary to inflammatory disease of the bowel that results in impaired absorption because bowel motility is accelerated (e.g., UC). Obstructive disorders (e.g., HD) also cause secondary malabsorption from enterocolitis.

Anatomic defects, such as extensive resection of the bowel or short-bowel syndrome (SBS), affect digestion by decreasing the transit time of substances and affect absorption by severely compromising the absorptive surface.

CELIAC DISEASE

Celiac disease, also known as *gluten-induced enteropathy, gluten-sensitive enteropathy,* and *celiac sprue,* is an immune-mediated enteropathy of the proximal small intestine triggered by inappropriate immune response to ingested gluten and gluten-related proteins found in wheat, rye, and barley. Celiac disease is one of the most common lifelong disorders affecting approximately 1% of the general population. As many as 2 million to 3 million Americans may be affected by celiac disease, but only 70,000 to 80,000 carry the diagnosis. It is second only to cystic fibrosis as a cause of malabsorption in children. The age that this condition first appears and its prevalence have changed over the past 30 to 40 years. Celiac sprue used to be considered a disease of childhood, but adult presentation is becoming more common. It is seen more frequently in Europe than in the United States and is rarely reported in Asians or African-Americans (American Gastroenterological Association Medical Position Statement, 2001). The exact cause of celiac disease is unknown, but there appears to be an inherited predisposition with an influence by environmental factors.

Pathophysiology

Genetic predisposition is an essential factor in the development of celiac disease. Membrane receptors involved in preferential antigen presentation to CD4+ T cells play a crucial role in the immune response characteristic of celiac disease. Genes located on the HLA region of chromosome 6, namely HLA-DQ2 or HLA-DQ8, are found in almost 100% of those affected with celiac disease (Murdock and Johnston, 2005). Once the inflammatory reaction is activated by gluten, CD4+ T cells produce cytokines, which are likely to contribute to the intestinal damage. The damage consists of infiltration of the lamina propria, crypt hyperplasia, and villous atrophy and flattening. With sufficient villous atrophy, malabsorption occurs.

Diagnostic Evaluation

Classic symptoms of celiac disease are GI manifestations usually noted several months after the introduction of gluten-containing grains into the diet, typically between the ages of 6 months and 2 years (Box 24-15). Typically, children are seen with impaired growth, chronic diarrhea, abdominal distention, muscle wasting with hypotonia, poor appetite, and lack of energy. The clinical manifestations are usually insidious and chronic. The first evidence may be failure to thrive and diarrhea. Less typical presentation has been observed in children ages 5 to 7 years, who have abdominal pain; nausea; vomiting; bloating; constipation; or extraintestinal manifestations, including short stature, pubertal delay, iron deficiency, dental enamel defects, and abnormal LFTs. Older children have been found to have osteoporosis. Untreated celiac disease can evolve into celiac crisis, characterized by abdominal distention, explosive watery diarrhea, and dehydration with electrolyte imbalance, leading to hypotensive shock and lethargy.

The diagnosis of celiac disease is based on a biopsy of the small intestine demonstrating the characteristic changes of mucosal inflammation, crypt hyperplasia, and villous atrophy (Dieterich, Esslinger, and Schuppan, 2003). Within a day or two of instituting the diet, most children with celiac disease demonstrate a favorable response, including weight gain and improved appetite. Within a few weeks there is resolution of the diarrhea and steatorrhea.

Commercially available serologic tests for celiac disease include antigliadin antibodies of both the immunoglobulin A and G classes (IgA and IgG); antiendomysium IgA; and anti-tissue transglutaminase IgA and IgG antibodies for screening

Clinical Manifestations of Celiac Disease

IMPAIRED FAT ABSORPTION
Steatorrhea (excessively large, pale, oily, frothy stools)
Exceedingly foul-smelling stools

IMPAIRED NUTRIENT ABSORPTION
Malnutrition
Muscle wasting (especially prominent in legs and buttocks)
Anemia
Anorexia
Abdominal distention

BEHAVIORAL CHANGES
Irritability
Uncooperativeness
Apathy

CELIAC CRISIS*
Acute, severe episodes of profuse watery diarrhea and vomiting
May be precipitated by:
- Infections (especially gastrointestinal)
- Prolonged fluid and electrolyte depletion
- Emotional disturbance

*In very young children.

first-degree relatives of known celiac disease patients and those with known celiac disease–associated disorders such as type 1 diabetes, thyroiditis, arthritis, primary biliary cirrhosis, Down syndrome, Turner syndrome, Williams syndrome, and osteopenia or osteoporosis. False-positive results are likely when only one serologic test is used because patients with these disorders can also test positive for these antibodies. Use of more than one test increases diagnostic accuracy (Gelfond and Fasano, 2006). Ruling out total IgA deficiency is necessary to minimize false-negative results.

Therapeutic Management

Treatment of chronic celiac disease is primarily dietary. Although the diet is called "gluten free," it is actually *low* in gluten, since it is impossible to remove every source of this protein. Because gluten is found primarily in the grains of wheat and rye, but also in smaller quantities in barley and oats, these four foods are eliminated. Corn and rice become substitute grain foods.

Children with untreated celiac disease may have associated lactose intolerance related to intestinal mucosal lesions, which usually improves with gluten withdrawal and intestinal healing. Specific nutritional deficiencies are treated with appropriate supplements, including vitamins, iron, and calories.

Prognosis. Celiac disease is regarded as a chronic disease. The most severe symptoms usually occur in early childhood and again in adult life. Strict dietary avoidance of gluten prevents symptoms and may minimize the risk of developing lymphoma, the most serious complication of the disease.

Nursing Care Management

The main nursing consideration is helping the child adhere to dietary management. Considerable time is involved in explaining to the child and the parents the disease process,

the specific role of gluten in aggravating the condition, and those foods that must be restricted. Also, a lactose-free diet, which necessitates eliminating all milk products, may be needed initially. It is especially difficult to maintain a diet indefinitely when the child has no symptoms and temporary transgressions result in no difficulties. However, evidence indicates that most individuals who relax their diet experience a relapse of their disease and possibly exhibit growth retardation, anemia, or osteomalacia. There is also the risk of developing malignant lymphoma of the small intestine or other GI malignancies.

Although the chief source of gluten is cereal and baked goods, grains are frequently added to processed foods as thickeners or fillers. Gluten is also added to many foods as "hydrolyzed vegetable protein." The nurse must advise parents to read carefully all ingredients on labels to avoid hidden sources of gluten. Many gluten-containing products are easily eliminated from the infant's or young child's diet, but monitoring the diet of a school-age child or adolescent is more difficult. Many "favorite" foods, such as hot dogs, pizza, and spaghetti, are chief offenders. Luncheon preparation away from home is particularly difficult, since bread, luncheon meats, and instant soups are not tolerated.

Generally, management includes a diet high in calories and proteins, with simple carbohydrates, such as fruits and vegetables, but low in fats. Initially the bowel may be inflamed as a result of the pathologic process, so high-fiber foods, such as nuts, raisins, raw vegetables, and raw fruits with skin, are avoided until inflammation has subsided. In a survey of 253 patients with celiac disease in New York State, Lee and Newman (2003) found that 86% experienced difficulties eating out and 82% experienced difficulties traveling because of the constraints of a gluten-free diet.

Several organizations and resources are available to help families cope with this condition. The Celiac Sprue Association/United States of America* provides support, guidance, and educational materials to families concerning a gluten-free diet, food sources, recipes, and travel information. Several published cookbooks contain gluten-free recipes.†

SHORT-BOWEL SYNDROME

SBS is a malabsorptive disorder that occurs when there is decreased mucosal surface area, usually as a result of extensive resection of the small intestine. The most common causes of SBS in children include congenital anomalies (jejunal and ileal atresia, gastroschisis), ischemia (necrotizing enterocolitis), and trauma or vascular injury (volvulus [twisting of bowel on itself]). Other causes include volvulus that results in massive resection, long-segment HD, and omphalocele.

The prognosis for infants and children with SBS has dramatically improved in the past 25 years as a result of advances in parenteral nutrition and enteral feeding. Both the amount and the location of bowel lost are important in determining the severity of the condition. The preservation of the terminal

---

*PO Box 31700, Omaha, NE 68131-0700; (877) CSA-4CSA or (402) 558-0600; http://www.csaceliacs.org. In Canada: Canadian Celiac Association, 5170 Dixie Road, Suite 204, Mississauga, Ontario, L4W 1E3; (905) 507-6208; http://www.celiac.ca.

†A booklet, *Pointers for Parents: Coping with Celiac Sprue,* provides information on shopping, cooking, and living with an affected child and is available from the Clinical Dietetics Department, Children's Memorial Hospital, 2300 Children's Plaza, Chicago, IL 60614; (773) 880-4793.

ileum and ileocecal valve influences fluid and nutrient absorption and may avoid problems of bacterial overgrowth by preventing the entrance of bacteria from the colon into the small intestine.

The small intestine has significant capacity for adaptation after resection. During the **adaptation process,** the villus height increases (villous hyperplasia), and the cell number and absorptive surface area also increase. As villus length and the number of enterocytes available for absorption per centimeter of bowel increase, nutrient absorption increases. Intraluminal enteral feedings stimulate the adaptation process and maintain the structural and functional integrity of the small intestine.

Therapeutic Management

The goals of treatment are (1) to preserve as much length of bowel as possible during surgery; (2) to maintain the child's nutritional status, growth, and development while intestinal adaptation occurs; (3) to stimulate intestinal adaptation with enteral feeding; and (4) to minimize complications related to the disease process and therapy.

Nutritional support is the long-term focus of care. The **initial phase** of therapy includes TPN as the primary source of nutrition. The **second phase** is the introduction of enteral feeding, which usually begins as soon as possible after surgery. Elemental formulas containing glucose, sucrose and glucose polymers, hydrolyzed proteins, and medium-chain triglycerides facilitate absorption. Usually these formulas are given by continuous infusion through an NG or gastrostomy tube. As the enteral feedings are advanced, the TPN solution is decreased in terms of calories, amount of fluid, and total hours of infusion per day. The **final phase** of nutritional support occurs when growth and development are sustained exclusively by enteral feedings. When TPN is discontinued, there is a risk of nutritional deficiency secondary to malabsorption of fat-soluble vitamins (A, D, E, K) and trace minerals (iron, selenium, zinc). Serum vitamin and mineral levels should be obtained, and enteral supplementation of vitamins and minerals may be required. Pharmacologic agents have been used to reduce secretory losses. H_2 blockers, PPIs, and octreotide inhibit gastric or pancreatic secretion. Cholestyramine is often prescribed to improve diarrhea that is associated with bile salt malabsorption. Growth factors have also been used to hasten adaptation and to enhance mucosal growth, but these uses are still experimental.

Numerous complications are associated with SBS and long-term TPN (see Chapter 22). Infectious, metabolic, and technical complications can occur. Catheter sepsis can occur after improper care of the catheter. The GI tract can also be a source of microbial seeding of the catheter. Bowel atrophy may foster increased intestinal permeability of bacteria. A lack of adequate sites for central lines may become a significant problem for the child in need of long-term TPN. Hepatic dysfunction, hepatomegaly with abnormal LFTs, and cholestasis may also occur.

Bacterial overgrowth is likely to occur when the ileocecal valve is absent or when stasis exists as a result of a partial obstruction or a dilated segment of bowel with poor motility. Alternating cycles of broad-spectrum antibiotics are used to reduce bacterial overgrowth. This treatment may also decrease the risk of bacterial translocation and subsequent central venous catheter infections. Other complications of bacterial overgrowth and malabsorption include metabolic acidosis and gastric hypersecretion.

Many surgical interventions, including intestinal valves, tapering enteroplasty or stricturoplasty, intestinal lengthening, and interposed segments, have been used to slow intestinal transit, reduce bacterial overgrowth, or increase mucosal surface area. **Intestinal transplantation** has been performed successfully in children. Only children with a permanent dependence on TPN or severe complications of long-term parenteral nutrition are candidates for transplantation.

Prognosis. The prognosis for infants with SBS has improved with advances in TPN and with the understanding of the importance of intraluminal nutrition. Improved surgical techniques for the management of therapy-related problems and the development of more specific immunosuppressive medications for transplantation have all contributed to improved management. The prognosis depends in part on the length of the residual small intestine. An intact ileocecal valve also improves the prognosis. Infants and children with SBS die from TPN-related problems, such as fulminant sepsis or severe TPN cholestasis.

Nursing Care Management

The most important components of nursing care are administration and monitoring of nutritional therapy. During TPN therapy, care must be taken to minimize the risk of complications related to the central venous access device (i.e., catheter infections, occlusions, dislodgment, or accidental removal). Care of the enteral feeding tubes and monitoring of enteral feeding tolerance are also important nursing responsibilities.

When long-term parenteral nutrition is required, preparing the family for home care is a major nursing responsibility that should be initiated early to prevent a lengthy hospitalization with subsequent problems such as family dysfunction and developmental delays. Many infants and children can be successfully cared for at home with enteral and parenteral nutrition when the family is prepared and provided with adequate support services. Follow-up by a multidisciplinary nutritional support service is essential. The nurse plays an active and important role in the success of a home nutrition program. Home infusion companies provide portable equipment, which enables the child and family to maintain a more normal lifestyle.

When hospitalization is prolonged, the child's developmental and emotional needs must be met. This often requires special planning to promote normal family adjustment and adaptation of the hospital routines. Care of the hospitalized child is discussed in Chapter 21.

KEY POINTS

- Infants are subject to fluid depletion because of their greater surface area relative to body mass, high rate of metabolism, and immature kidney function.
- Dehydration can be classified as isotonic, hypotonic, and hypertonic.
- Vomiting and diarrhea account for significant fluid depletion, especially in infants and small children.
- The amount, frequency, and characteristics of stool and vomitus are important nursing observations.

- Diarrhea can be caused by an inflammatory process of infectious origin, a toxic reaction to ingestion of poisonous substances, dietary indiscretions, or infections outside the alimentary tract. The primary treatment of diarrhea is the use of ORS.
- HD requires surgical removal of aganglionic segments of bowel.
- Postoperative care of the child with abdominal surgery involves assessing the abdomen and providing hydration and nutrition, IV fluids, proper positioning, wound care, and psychologic support.
- Nursing care of GI reflux is aimed at identifying children with suggestive symptoms, helping parents with home care feeding and positioning, and caring for the child undergoing surgical intervention.
- Although the cause of appendicitis is poorly understood, it is typically a result of obstruction of the lumen, usually by a fecalith. Common signs and symptoms are right lower quadrant abdominal pain, tenderness, and fever.
- Meckel diverticulum is a congenital malformation of the GI tract characterized by bloody stools.
- IBD refers to UC and CD. Chronic diarrhea is the most common feature. It is treated by dietary management and medication, although surgery is needed in some cases.
- Peptic ulcers are poorly understood, but contributing factors include interference with the normal protective mechanisms of the mucosal lining and the presence of *H. pylori*.
- Viral hepatitis is caused by six types of virus: HAV, HBV, HCV, HDV, HEV, and HGV.
- HAV is spread by the fecal-oral route, whereas HBV and HCV are transmitted primarily by the parenteral route. The most effective measure in prevention and control of hepatitis in any setting is hand washing.
- Structural disorders of the GI tract include CL, CP, EA with TEF, anorectal malformations, and BA.
- BA is a serious disorder, often causing progressive liver failure, which is an indication for liver transplantation.
- CL/P, the most common facial malformation, may involve nutritional, dental, and speech problems.
- Hernias related to the GI tract can be minor (umbilical) or life-threatening (diaphragmatic, gastroschisis, omphalocele).
- General signs of obstruction include colicky abdominal pain, nausea and vomiting, abdominal distention, and decreased stool output.
- HPS is recognized by characteristic projectile vomiting, malnutrition, dehydration, and a palpable mass in the epigastrium and is relieved by pyloromyotomy.
- Intussusception is one of the most common causes of intestinal obstruction during infancy and is characterized by abdominal pain and blood in stools. Treatment is either nonsurgical hydrostatic reduction or surgical reduction.
- Malabsorption syndromes are disorders associated with some degree of impaired digestion or absorption. They include digestive defects, absorptive defects, and anatomic defects.
- Celiac disease is characterized by an intolerance to gluten. It is thought to be either an inborn error of metabolism or an immunologic response.
- SBS is characterized by a loss of intestine resulting in a diminished ability to absorb a regular diet normally. Specialized enteral and parenteral nutrition is a major element of care for these children.

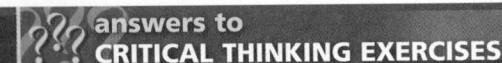

answers to
CRITICAL THINKING EXERCISES

DIARRHEA

1. Yes, there are sufficient data for the nurse practitioner to arrive at some conclusions.
2. a. See Table 24-1, Evaluating Extent of Dehydration, and note the criteria for mild dehydration.
   b. Infants or children with mild dehydration are managed with oral rehydration therapy (ORT) and early reintroduction of an adequate diet. In cases of severe dehydration, or when infants and children have uncontrollable vomiting, intravenous fluids are used in the management of acute diarrhea.
   c. Breastfeeding generally can be continued in mild dehydration.
   d. Antidiarrheal medications are not recommended for the treatment of acute infectious diarrhea. These medications have adverse effects such as slowed motility and can prolong the illness.
3. At present, Mary meets all the criteria for mild dehydration. It is highly probable that she has acute infectious diarrhea because her mother noted that she has had a "cold" for several days, she is vomiting and having diarrhea, and she has an elevated temperature. The priority for nursing care at this time is to provide rehydration via ORT. ORT is an effective, safe, and cost-effective way to treat mild dehydration. The nurse practitioner should provide the mother with instructions to give Mary oral rehydration solution at frequent intervals and in small amounts. The mother should also be instructed to continue with breastfeeding and normal feedings. Early reintroduction of normal nutrients is desirable in cases of mild dehydration; delayed introduction of food may be harmful and can prolong the illness. Mary's mother should also be told to avoid the use of antidiarrheal medications.
4. Yes, the evidence supports this initial plan of management.
5. Mary's mother should be instructed to continue to monitor Mary for signs of improvement (an increase in the number of voidings or the number of wet diapers, and a decrease in vomiting). However, if Mary's condition does not improve, Mary's mother should be instructed to bring Mary back to the clinic or to the local emergency department. Mary's mother should be told to use frequent hand washing when caring for Mary to avoid transferring this infection to other family members.

CONSTIPATION

1. Yes, there are sufficient data to arrive at some conclusions for an initial plan of management.
2. a. Constipation in infancy can be caused by medical conditions such as Hirschsprung disease, hypothyroidism, or strictures, or it can be simple functional constipation.
   b. In infancy, changes in dietary practices such as a change from human milk to formula may precipitate functional constipation.
   c. Functional constipation is usually treated by dietary modifications such as increasing the amount of carbohydrate, fruit, or vegetables in the infant's diet.
3. Initially, the nurse practitioner can tell Harry's mother that functional constipation may occur with changes in the diet (e.g., the change from breastfeeding 6 weeks ago to bottle-formula feeding). The nurse practitioner can recommend that Harry's mother slowly introduce cereal and prune juice into Harry's diet. Cereal and one or two offerings of fruit juice each day may help to prevent further constipation. Often, simple measures such as the introduction of solid foods or other dietary modifications help to remedy functional constipation.

4. The initial data seem to point to the conclusion that Harry has functional constipation. However, the one episode of diarrhea and the two episodes of passage of ribbonlike stools do not usually occur with functional constipation.

5. The nurse practitioner should remember that constipation can be caused by medical conditions such as Hirschsprung disease; therefore a referral to a gastroenterologist for further evaluation is also warranted at this time.

INFLAMMATORY BOWEL DISEASE

1. Yes, there is sufficient evidence to arrive at some conclusions about what to include in Susan's discharge planning.

2. a. The goals of nutritional support for a patient with CD include (1) correction of nutrient deficits and replacement of ongoing losses, (2) provision of adequate energy and protein for healing, and (3) provision of adequate nutrients to support normal growth.
   b. See Gavage Feeding, Chapter 22 (p. 745).
   c. Adolescents who are diagnosed with CD must adjust to the fact that they have a chronic illness that is characterized by remissions and exacerbations. CD may affect their activities of daily living, their social interactions with peers, and their ability to attend school. An important goal of therapy for adolescents with CD is to allow them to have as normal a lifestyle as possible.

3. The most immediate priority for discharge is to teach Susan and her family how to insert the NG tube, how to administer the feedings, how to obtain the supplies needed for the tube feedings at home, and how to observe for any untoward effects of the NG feedings. As Susan's discharge nurse, you should have Susan and another family member insert the NG tube and demonstrate how to check the placement of the NG tube and how to start and stop the feedings while Susan is in the hospital. As Susan's nurse, you will also need to arrange before discharge for the appropriate vendors to deliver the feeding tube supplies and feeding pump to Susan's home so the supplies will be in place when Susan is discharged. While doing all this teaching, you should also be alert to any questions, worries, or anxieties that Susan or her family members may express.

4. Yes, Susan is to receive nighttime NG tube infusions at home, and her family has expressed a desire to perform this procedure at home. Therefore this discharge teaching is needed and required.

5. Now that the acute disease exacerbation is under control, Susan will be able to resume school attendance and activities with her peers. However, some of her activities of daily living have been changed (e.g., the nighttime NG feedings), and she will need to adjust to remissions and exacerbations that characterize CD. To help Susan and her family cope with these changes, you should refer them to the services of the Crohn's and Colitis Foundation of America. Perhaps Susan can become involved in one of the adolescent peer-support groups that are sponsored by this organization.

REFERENCES

Abbott Laboratories: *HUMIRA (adalimumab) for the management of moderate-to-severe Crohn's disease,* Abbott Park, Ill, 2007, The Laboratories.

Acra SA, Ghishan GK: Electrolyte fluxes in the gut and oral rehydration solutions, *Pediatr Clin North Am* 43(2):433-449, 1996.

Ahmad T, Armuzzi A, Bunce M, and others: The molecular classification of the clinical manifestations of Crohn's disease, *Gastroenterology* 122(4):854-866, 2002.

Alexander F, Sarigol S, DiFiore J, and others: Fate of the pouch in 151 pediatric patients after ileal pouch anal anastomosis, *J Pediatr Surg* 38(1):328-332, 2003.

American Academy of Pediatrics: Multicenter, randomized, double-blind clinical trial to evaluate the efficacy and safety of a reduced osmolarity oral rehydration salts solution in children with acute watery diarrhea, *Pediatrics* 107(4):613-619, 2001.

American Academy of Pediatrics, Committee on Infectious Diseases: Hepatitis C virus infection, *Pediatrics* 101(3):481-485, 1998.

American Academy of Pediatrics, Provisional Committee on Quality Improvement, Subcommittee on Acute Gastroenteritis: Practice parameter: the management of acute gastroenteritis in young children, *Pediatrics* 97(3):424-435, 1996.

American Gastroenterological Association Medical Position Statement: Celiac sprue, *Gastroenterology* 120(6):1522-1525, 2001.

Amon JJ, Darling N, Fiore AE, and others: Factors associated with hepatitis A vaccination among children 24-35 months of age: United States, *Pediatrics* 117(1):30-33, 2003.

Atkison PR, Ross BC, Williams S, and others: Long-term results of pediatric liver transplantation in a combined pediatric and adult transplant program, *Can Med Assoc J* 166(13):1663-1671, 2002.

Balistreri WF, Chang MH, Ciocca M, and others: Acute and chronic hepatitis: working group report of the First World Congress of Pediatric Gastroenterology, Hepatology, and Nutrition, *J Pediatr Gastroenterol Nutr* 35(Suppl 2):S62-S73, 2002.

Baron ML: Crohn disease in children: this chronic illness can be painful and isolating, but new treatments may help, *Am J Nurs* 102(10):26-34, 2002.

Bonkovsky HL, Mehta S: Hepatitis C: a review and update, *J Am Acad Dermatol* 44(2):159-182, 2001.

Broderick AL, Jonas MM: Hepatitis B in children, *Semin Liver Dis* 23(1):59-68, 2003.

Cavataio F, Guandalini S: Gastroesophageal reflux. In Guandalini S, editor: *Essential pediatric gastroenterology and nutrition,* New York, 2005, McGraw-Hill.

Centers for Disease Control and Prevention, National Center for HIV/AIDS, Viral Hepatitis, STD, and TB Prevention: *National hepatitis C prevention strategy,* 2001, retrieved April 22, 2007, from http://www.cdc.gov/ncidod/diseases/hepatitis/c/plan/index.htm.

Chelimsky G, Czinn S: Peptic ulcer disease in children, *Pediatr Rev* 22(10):349-355, 2001.

Chen S-M, Chang M-H, Du J-C, and others: Screening for biliary atresia by infant stool color card in Taiwan, *Pediatrics* 117(4):1147-1154, 2006.

Chien JC, Chen SJ, Tui CM, and others: Is urorectal septum malformation sequence a variant of the vertebral defects, anal atresia, tracheo-oesophageal fistula, renal defects and radial dysplasia association? Report of a case and a review of the literature, *Eur J Pediatr* 164(6):350-354, 2005.

Christian DJ, Buyske J: Current status of antireflux surgery, *Surg Clin North Am* 85(5):931-947, 2005.

Coffin SE: Future vaccines: recent advances and future prospects, *Primary Care* 28(4):869-887, 2001.

Cover TL, Blaser MJ: *Helicobacter pylori* infection, a paradigm for chronic mucosal inflammation: pathogenesis and implications for eradication and prevention, *Adv Int Med* 41:85-117, 1996.

Dasgupta R, Langer JC: Hirschsprung disease, *Curr Probl Surg* 41(12):949-988, 2004.

Dieterich W, Esslinger B, Schuppan D: Pathomechanisms in celiac disease, *Int Arch Allergy Immunol* 132(2):98-108, 2003.

DiLorenzo C, Youssef NN, Sigurdsson L, and others: Visceral hyperalgesia in children with functional abdominal pain, *J Pediatr* 139(6):838-843, 2001.

Emerick KM, Whitington PF: Neonatal liver disease, *Pediatr Ann* 35(4):281-286, 2006.

Eppley BL, van Aalst J, Robey A, and others: The spectrum of orofacial clefting, *Plast Reconstr Surg* 115(7):101e-114e, 2005.

Ford AC, Delaney BC, Forman D, and others: Eradication therapy in *Helicobacter pylori* positive peptic ulcer disease: systematic review and economic analysis, *Am J Gastroenterol* 99(9):1833-1855, 2004.

Gelfond D, Fasano A: Celiac disease in the pediatric population, *Pediatr Ann* 35(4):275-279, 2006.

Gisbert JP, de la Morena F, Abraira V: Accuracy of monoclonal stool antigen test for the diagnosis of *H. pylori* infection: a systematic review and meta-analysis, *Am J Gastroenterol* 101(8):1921-1930, 2006.

Hendren WH: Pediatric rectal and perineal problems, *Pediatr Clin North Am* 45(6):1353-1371, 1998.

Holcomb GW: Minimally invasive surgery. In Hoekelman RA, Adam H, Nelson N, and others, editors: *Primary pediatric care,* ed 4, St Louis, 2001, Mosby.

Huang L-T, Tiao M-M, Lee S-Y, and others: Low plasma nitrite in infantile hypertrophic pyloric stenosis patients, *Dig Dis Sci* 51(5):869-872, 2006.

Huppertz H-I, Soriano-Gaabarro M, Grimprel E, and others: Intussusception among young children in Europe, *Pediatr Infect Dis J* 25(1):S22-S29, 2006.

Jabbar A, Wright RA: Gastroenteritis and antibiotic-associated diarrhea, *Primary Care* 30(1):63-80, 2003.

Jackson PG, Gleiber MA, Askar R, and others: Predictors of outcome in 100 consecutive laparoscopic antireflux procedures, *Am J Surg* 181(3):231-235, 2001.

Jackson WD, Grand RJ: Crohn's disease. In McMillan JA, DeAngelis CD, Feigin RD, and others, editors: *Oski's pediatrics: principles and practice*, ed 3, Philadelphia, 1999, Lippincott Williams & Wilkins.

Kaiser S, Frenchner B, Jorulf HK: Suspected appendicitis in children: US and CT—a prospective randomized study, *Radiology* 223(3):633-638, 2002.

Karnam US, Reddy KR: Pegylated interferons, *Clin Liver Dis* 7(1):139-148, 2003.

Kim WR, Gores GJ, Benson JT, and others: Mortality and hospitalization for hepatocellular carcinoma in the United States, *Gastroenterology* 129(2):486-493, 2005.

Kirschner RE, LaRossa D: Cleft lip and palate, *Otolaryngol Clin North Am* 33(6):1191-1215, 2000.

Kugathasan S, Collins N, Maresso K, and others: CARD15 gene mutations and risk for early surgery in pediatric-onset Crohn's disease, *Clin Gastroenterol Hepatol* 2(11):1003-1009, 2004.

Kugathasan S, Judd RH, Hoffman RG, Wisconsin Pediatric Inflammatory Bowel Disease Alliance: Epidemiologic and clinical characteristics of children with newly diagnosed inflammatory bowel disease in Wisconsin: a statewide population-based study, *J Pediatr* 143(4):525-531, 2003.

Kwok MY, Kim MK, Gorelick MH: Evidence-based approach to the diagnosis of appendicitis in children, *Pediatr Emerg Care* 20(10):690-698, 2004.

Lee A, Newman JM: Celiac diet: its impact on quality of life, *J Am Diet Assoc* 103(11):1533-1535, 2003.

Li BU, Balint JP: Cyclic vomiting syndrome: evolution in our understanding of a brain-gut disorder, *Adv Pediatr* 47:117-160, 2000.

Loening-Baucke V, Pashankar DS: A randomized, prospective, comparison study of polyethylene glycole 3350 without electrolytes and milk of magnesia for children with constipation and fecal incontinence, *Pediatrics* 118(2):528-535, 2006.

Malek MA, Curns AT, Holman RC, and others: Diarrhea- and rotavirus-associated hospitalizations among children less than 5 years of age: United States, 1997 and 2000, *Pediatrics* 117(6):1887-1892, 2006.

Marshall GS: Testing new rotavirus vaccines: efficacy and safety. In *The management and prevention of rotavirus*, Thorofare, NJ, 2006, Vindico Medical Education.

Murdock AM, Johnston SD: Diagnostic criteria for coeliac disease: time for change? *Eur J Gastroenterol Hepatol* 17(1):41-43, 2005.

Ohi R: Surgery for biliary atresia, *Liver* 21(3):175-182, 2001.

Ramaswamy K, Jacobson K: Infectious diarrhea in children, *Gastroenterol Clin* 30(3):611-624, 2001.

Regev A, Schiff ER: Viral hepatitis A, B, and C, *Clin Liver Dis* 4(1):47-71, 2000.

Richard ME: Weight comparisons of infants with complete cleft lip and palate, *Pediatr Nurs* 20(20):191-196, 1994.

Richards CA: *C. difficile* epidemic continuing to spread, *Infect Dis Children* 39-41, September, 2006.

Richmond J, Dunning P, Desmond P: Hepatitis C: a medical and social diagnosis, *Austral Nurs J* 12(1):23-25, 2004.

Rubin DT, Kavitt RT: Surveillance for cancer and dysplasia in inflammatory bowel disease, *Gastroenterol Clin North Am* 35(3):581-604, 2006.

Rudolph CD, Mazur LJ, Liptak GS, and others: Guidelines for evaluation and treatment of gastroesophageal reflux in infants and children: recommendations of the North American Society for Pediatric Gastroenterology and Nutrition, *J Pediatr Gastroenterol Nutr* 32(Suppl 2):S1-S31, 2001.

Ruemmele FM, Targan SR, Levy G, and others: Diagnostic accuracy of serological assays in pediatric inflammatory bowel disease, *Gastroenterology* 115(4):822-829, 1998.

Rutter MD, Saunders BP, Wilkinson KH, and others: Thirty-year analysis of colonoscopic surveillance program for neoplasia in ulcerative colitis, *Gastroenterology* 130(4):1030-1038, 2006.

Sagar J, Kumar V, Shah DK: Meckel's diverticulum: a systematic review, *J R Soc Med* 99(10):501-505, 2006.

Sandberg SJ, Magee WP, Denk MJ: Neonatal cleft lip and cleft palate repair, *AORN Online* 75(3):488, 490-499, 501, 503-504, 506-508, 2002.

Saps M, Li BU: Chronic abdominal pain of functional origin in children, *Pediatr Ann* 35(4):246, 249-256, 2006.

Saps M, Sztainberg MO, DiLorenzo C, and others: A prospective community based study of gastroenterological symptoms in school-age children, *Gastroenterology* 128(4 Suppl 2):A169, 2005.

Schwab M, Schaeffeler E, Marx C, and others: Association between the C3435T MDRI gene polymorphism and susceptibility for ulcerative colitis, *Gastroenterology* 124(1):26-33, 2003.

Sgouros SN, Bergele C: Clinical outcome of patients with *Helicobacter pylori* infection: the bug, the host, or the environment? *Postgrad Med J* 82(967):338-342, 2006.

Shaw-Smith C: Oesophageal atresia, tracheo-oesophageal fistula, and the VACTERL association: review of genetics and epidemiology, *J Med Genet* 43(7):545-554, 2006.

Silbermintz A, Markowitz J: Inflammatory bowel diseases, *Pediatr Ann* 35(4):268-274, 2006.

Smith EA, Woodard JR, Broecker BH, and others: Current urologic management of cloacal exstrophy: experience with 11 patients, *J Pediatr Surg* 32(2):256-262, 1997.

Speltz ML, Endriga MC, Fisher PA, and others: Early predictors of attachment in infants with cleft lip and/or palate, *Child Dev* 68(1):12-25, 1997.

Staat MA: What is the disease burden associated with rotavirus? In *The management and prevention of rotavirus*, Thorofare, NJ, 2006, Vindico Medical Education.

Steiner MJ, DeWalt DA, Byerley JS, and others: Is this child dehydrated? *JAMA* 291(22):2746-2754, 2004.

Strahlman RS: Appendicitis. In Hoekelman RA, Adam H, Nelson N, and others, editors: *Primary pediatric care*, ed 4, St Louis, 2001, Mosby.

Suwandhi E, Ton MN, Schwarz SM: Gastroesophageal reflux in infancy and childhood, *Pediatr Ann* 35(4):259-266, 2006.

Szajewska H, Ruszcynski M, Radzikowski A: Probiotics in the prevention of antibiotic-associated diarrhea in children: a meta-analysis of randomized controlled trials, *J Pediatr* 149(3):367-372, 2006.

Waters L, Nelson M: New therapeutic options for hepatitis C, *Curr Opin Infect Dis* 19(6):615-622, 2006.

Wilkins-Haug L: Prenatal diagnosis of orofacial clefts, *Up to Date*, January 7, 2003, retrieved from http://www.uptodate.com.

Yuen MF, Lai CL: Treatment of chronic hepatitis B, *Lancet Infect Dis* 1(4):383-393, 2001.

Zangwill KM: Protecting against rotavirus disease and its complications. In *The management and prevention of rotavirus*, Thorofare, NJ, 2006, Vindico Medical Education.

Zeiter DK, Hyams JS: Gastroesophageal reflux: pathogenesis, diagnosis, and treatment, *Allergy Asthma Proc* 20(1):45-49, 1999.

The Child with Cardiovascular Dysfunction

PATRICIA O'BRIEN AND ANNETTE L. BAKER

CHAPTER OUTLINE

CARDIOVASCULAR DYSFUNCTION, 862
History and Physical Examination, 862
CONGENITAL HEART DISEASE, 865
Circulatory Changes at Birth, 866
Altered Hemodynamics, 866
Classification of Defects, 866
  Defects with Increased Pulmonary Blood
    Flow, 867
  Obstructive Defects, 867
  Defects with Decreased Pulmonary Blood
    Flow, 867
  Mixed Defects, 870
**CLINICAL CONSEQUENCES OF
CONGENITAL HEART DISEASE, 876**
Congestive Heart Failure, 876
Nursing Care Plan: The Child with
  Congestive Heart Failure (CHF), 880
Hypoxemia, 884

**NURSING CARE OF THE FAMILY AND
CHILD WITH CONGENITAL HEART
DISEASE, 886**
Help Family Adjust to the Disorder, 886
Educate Family About the Disorder, 887
Help Families Manage the Illness at
  Home, 887
Prepare Child and Family for Invasive
  Procedures, 888
Provide Postoperative Care, 889
  Observe Vital Signs, 889
  Maintain Respiratory Status, 890
  Monitor Fluids, 890
  Provide Rest and Progressive Activity, 890
  Provide Comfort and Emotional
    Support, 891
Plan for Discharge and Home Care, 891

**ACQUIRED CARDIOVASCULAR
DISORDERS, 891**
Bacterial (Infective) Endocarditis, 891
Rheumatic Fever, 893
Hyperlipidemia (Hypercholesterolemia),
  894
Cardiac Dysrhythmias, 896
Pulmonary Artery Hypertension, 897
Cardiomyopathy, 898
HEART TRANSPLANTATION, 899
VASCULAR DYSFUNCTION, 899
Systemic Hypertension, 899
Kawasaki Disease (Mucocutaneous Lymph
  Node Syndrome), 901
Shock, 902
Anaphylaxis, 904
Septic Shock, 906
Toxic Shock Syndrome, 907

LEARNING OBJECTIVES

On completion of this chapter the reader will be able to:

- Design a plan for assisting a child during a cardiac diagnostic procedure.
- Demonstrate an understanding of the hemodynamics, distinctive manifestations, and therapeutic management of congenital heart disease.
- Outline a care plan for an infant or child with congestive heart failure.
- Describe the care for a child who has hypoxia.
- Describe the care for an infant or a child with a congenital heart defect and its surgical repair.
- Discuss the nurse's role in helping the child and family cope with congenital heart disease.
- Differentiate between rheumatic fever and rheumatic heart disease.
- List the criteria for selected cholesterol screening of children.
- Discuss the assessment and management of hypertension in children and adolescents.
- Outline a care plan for a child with Kawasaki disease.
- Describe the emergency treatment for shock, including anaphylaxis.

RELATED TOPICS and ADDITIONAL RESOURCES

 IN TEXT

Compliance, *Ch. 22*
Controlling Elevated Temperatures, *Ch. 22*
Impact of the Child's Chronic Illness or
     Disability, *Ch. 18*
Latex Allergy, *Ch. 32*
Neonatal Loss, *Ch. 9*
Neonatal Pain, *Ch. 9*
Pain Assessment; Pain Management, *Ch. 7*
Physical Examination: Heart, *Ch. 6*
Physical Examination: Skin, *Ch. 6*
Physiologic Measurements, *Ch. 6*
Preparation for Diagnostic and Therapeutic
     Procedures, *Ch. 22*
Surgical Procedures, *Ch. 22*

 COMPANION CD

Anatomy Reviews—Changes in Circulation
     at Birth; Conduction System of the Heart
Animations—Cardiac Tamponade, Infant;
     Catheter Placement, Umbilical Vein; Heart
     Sounds; Structure of the Heart; Subaortic
     Stenosis
Case Study—Patent Ductus Arteriosus
Critical Thinking Exercises—Patent Ductus
     Arteriosus; Shock; Cardiac
     Catheterization; Digoxin Administration
NCLEX Review Questions
Pediatric Assessment Video Clip

evolve
evolve.elsevier.com/Wong/essentials/
NCLEX Review Questions
Nursing Care Plans—The Child with
     Congestive Heart Failure; The Child in
     Shock (Cardiovascular Failure)
WebLinks

 **WONG'S CLINICAL MANUAL
OF PEDIATRIC NURSING, 7th Ed**

Nursing Care Plans—The Child with
     Congestive Heart Failure (CHF), *p. 439;*
     The Child with Rheumatic Fever (RF),
     p. 441; The Child in Shock
     (Cardiovascular Failure), *p. 443*

Animation—Structure of the Heart

Animation—Heart Sounds

CARDIOVASCULAR DYSFUNCTION

Cardiovascular disorders in children are divided into two major groups: congenital heart disease and acquired heart disorders. **Congenital heart disease (CHD)** includes primarily anatomic abnormalities present at birth that result in abnormal cardiac function. The clinical consequences of congenital heart defects fall into two broad categories: congestive heart failure (CHF) and hypoxemia. **Acquired cardiac disorders** are disease processes or abnormalities that occur after birth and can be seen in the normal heart or in the presence of congenital heart defects. They result from various factors, including infection, autoimmune responses, environmental factors, and familial tendencies.

History and Physical Examination

Taking an accurate health history is an important first step in assessing an infant or child for possible heart disease. Parents may have specific concerns, such as an infant with poor feeding or fast breathing, or a 7-year-old who can no longer keep up with friends on the soccer field. Others may not realize that their child has a medical problem; their baby has always been pale and fussy.

Asking details about the mother's health history, pregnancy, and birth history are important in assessing infants. Mothers with chronic health conditions, such as diabetes or lupus, are more likely to have infants with heart disease. Some medications, such as phenytoin (Dilantin), are teratogenic to the fetus. Maternal alcohol use or illicit drug use increases the risk of congenital heart defects. Exposures to infections, such as rubella, early in pregnancy may result in congenital anomalies. Infants with low birth weight resulting from intrauterine growth restriction are more likely to have congenital anomalies. High-birth-weight infants have an increased incidence of heart disease.

A detailed family history is also important. There is an increased incidence of congenital cardiac defects if either parent or a sibling has a heart defect. Some diseases, such as Marfan syndrome, and some cardiomyopathies are hereditary. A family history of frequent fetal loss, sudden infant death, and sudden death in adults may indicate heart disease. Congenital heart defects are seen in many syndromes such as Down and Turner syndromes.

The physical assessment of suspected cardiac disease begins with observation of general appearance, then proceeds with more specific observations. The following are supplementary to the general assessment techniques described for physical examination of the chest and heart in Chapter 6.

Inspection

Nutritional state—Failure to thrive or poor weight gain is associated with heart disease.

Color—Cyanosis is a common feature of CHD, and pallor is associated with poor perfusion.

Chest deformities—An enlarged heart sometimes distorts the chest configuration.

Unusual pulsations—Visible pulsations of the neck veins are seen in some patients.

Respiratory excursion—This refers to the ease or difficulty of respiration (e.g., tachypnea, dyspnea, expiratory grunt).

Clubbing of fingers—This is associated with cyanosis.

Palpation and Percussion

Chest—These maneuvers help discern heart size and other characteristics (e.g., thrills) associated with heart disease.

Abdomen—Hepatomegaly or splenomegaly may be evident.

Peripheral pulses—Rate, regularity, and amplitude (strength) may reveal discrepancies.

Auscultation

Heart rate and rhythm—Listen for fast heart rates (tachycardia), slow heart rates (bradycardia), or irregular rhythms.

Character of heart sounds—Listen for distinct or muffled sounds, murmurs, and additional heart sounds.

Diagnostic Evaluation

A variety of invasive and noninvasive tests may be used in the diagnosis of heart disease (Table 25-1). Some of the more common diagnostic tools that require nursing assessment and intervention are described here.

TABLE 25-1	
Procedures for Cardiac Diagnosis	
PROCEDURE	**DESCRIPTION**
Chest radiograph (x-ray)	Provides information on heart size and pulmonary blood flow patterns
Electrocardiography (ECG)	Graphic measure of electrical activity of heart
Holter monitor	24-hour continuous ECG recording used to assess dysrhythmias
Echocardiography	Use of high-frequency sound waves obtained by a transducer to produce an image of cardiac structures
Transthoracic	Done with transducer on chest
M-mode	One-dimensional graphic view used to estimate ventricular size and function
Two-dimensional (2-D)	Real-time, cross-sectional views of heart used to identify cardiac structures and cardiac anatomy
Doppler	Identifies blood flow patterns and pressure gradients across structures
Fetal	Imaging fetal heart in utero
Transesophageal (TEE)	Transducer placed in esophagus behind heart to obtain images of posterior heart structures or in patients with poor images from chest approach
Cardiac catheterization	Imaging study using radiopaque catheters placed in a peripheral blood vessel and advanced into heart to measure pressures and oxygen levels in heart chambers and visualize heart structures and blood flow patterns
Hemodynamics	Measures pressures and oxygen saturations in heart chambers
Angiography	Use of contrast material to illuminate heart structures and blood flow patterns
Biopsy	Use of special catheter to remove tiny samples of heart muscle for microscopic evaluation; used in assessing infection, inflammation, or muscle dysfunction disorders; also to evaluate for rejection after heart transplant
Electrophysiology (EPS)	Special catheters with electrodes employed to record electrical activity from within heart; used to diagnose rhythm disturbances
Exercise stress test	Monitoring of heart rate, blood pressure, ECG, and oxygen consumption at rest and during progressive exercise on a treadmill or bicycle
Cardiac magnetic resonance imaging (MRI)	Noninvasive imaging technique; used in evaluation of vascular anatomy outside of heart (e.g., coarctation of the aorta, vascular rings), estimates of ventricular mass and volume; uses for MRI are expanding

Electrocardiogram. Bedside cardiac monitoring with the electrocardiogram (ECG) is commonly used in pediatrics, especially in the care of children with heart disease. The bedside monitor provides valuable information about heart rate and rhythm through a graphic display of the ECG tracing and a digital display. An alarm can be set with parameters for individual patient requirements and will sound if the heart rate is above or below the set parameters. Gelfoam electrodes are commonly used and placed on the right side of the chest (above the level of the heart) and on the left side of the chest, and a ground electrode is placed on the abdomen. Electrodes should be changed every 1 or 2 days because they irritate the skin. Bedside monitors are an adjunct to patient care and should never be substituted for direct assessment and auscultation of heart sounds. The nurse should assess the patient, not the monitor.

NURSINGTIP

Electrodes for cardiac monitoring are often color coded: white for right, green (or red) for ground, and black for left. Always check to ensure that these colors are placed correctly.

Echocardiography. Echocardiography is one of the most frequently used tests for detecting cardiac dysfunction in children. Recent improvements in echocardiographic techniques have made it increasingly possible to confirm the diagnosis without resorting to cardiac catheterization. In more and more cases a prenatal diagnosis of CHD can be made by fetal echocardiography.

Echocardiography involves the use of ultra-high-frequency sound waves to produce an image of the heart's structure. A transducer placed directly on the chest wall delivers repetitive pulses of ultrasound and processes the returned signals (echoes).

Although the test is noninvasive, painless, and associated with no known side effects, it can be stressful for children. The child must lie quietly in the standard echocardiographic positions; crying, nursing, or sitting up often leads to diagnostic errors or omissions. Therefore infants and young children may need a mild sedative; older children benefit from psychologic preparation for the test. The distraction of a video or movie is often helpful.

Cardiac Catheterization. Cardiac catheterization is an invasive diagnostic procedure in which a radiopaque catheter is inserted through a peripheral blood vessel into the heart. The catheter is usually introduced through percutaneous technique, in which the catheter is threaded through a large-bore needle that is inserted into the vein. The catheter is guided through the heart with the aid of fluoroscopy. After the tip of the catheter is within a heart chamber, contrast material is injected, and films are taken of the dilution and circulation of the material (***angiography***). Types of cardiac catheterizations include:

Diagnostic catheterizations—These studies are used to diagnose congenital cardiac defects, particularly in symptomatic infants and before surgical repair. They are divided into right-sided catheterizations, in which the catheter is introduced through a vein (usually the femoral vein) and threaded to the right atrium (most common), and left-sided catheterizations, in which the catheter is threaded through an artery into the aorta and into the heart.

Interventional catheterizations (therapeutic catheterizations)—A balloon catheter or other device is used to alter the cardiac anatomy. Examples include dilating stenotic valves or vessels or closing abnormal connections (Table 25-2).

Animation—Catheter Placement, Umbilical Vein

TABLE 25-2

Current Interventional Cardiac Catheterization Procedures in Children

INTERVENTION	DIAGNOSIS
Balloon atrioseptostomy—Use well established in newborns; may also be done under echocardiographic guidance	Transposition of great arteries Some complex single-ventricle defects

Balloon dilation—Treatment of choice	Valvular pulmonic stenosis
	Branch pulmonary artery stenosis
	Congenital valvular aortic stenosis
	Rheumatic mitral stenosis
	Recurrent coarctation of aorta
	Further follow-up required in:
	    Native coarctation of aorta in patients over 7 months old
	    Congenital mitral stenosis

Coil occlusion—Accepted alternative to surgery	Patent ductus arteriosus (<4 mm)
Transcatheter device closure—Several devices used in clinical trials	Atrial septal defect (ASD)
Amplatzer septal occluder—Approved for ASD closure	ASD
Ventricular septal defect devices—Used in clinical trials	Ventricular septal defects
Stent placement	Pulmonary artery stenosis Coarctation of the aorta in adolescents Use to treat other lesions investigational
Radiofrequency ablation	Some tachydysrhythmias

Data from Allen HD, Beekman RH 3rd, Garson A Jr, and others: Pediatric therapeutic cardiac catheterization: AHA scientific statement, *Circulation* 97:609-625, 1998; updated from Rome J, Kreutzer J: Pediatric interventional catheterization: reasonable expectations and outcomes, *Pediatr Clin North Am* 51:1589-1610, 2004.

Electrophysiology studies—Catheters with tiny electrodes that record the impulses of the heart directly from the conduction system are used to evaluate dysrhythmias and sometimes destroy accessory pathways that cause some tachydysrhythmias.

Nursing Care Management

Cardiac catheterization has become a routine diagnostic procedure and may be done on an outpatient basis. However, it is not without risks, especially in neonates and seriously ill infants and children. Possible complications include acute hemorrhage from the entry site (more likely with interventional procedures because larger catheters are used), low-grade fever, nausea, vomiting, loss of pulse in the catheterized extremity (usually transient, resulting from a clot, hematoma, or intimal tear), and transient dysrhythmias (generally catheter induced) (Uzark, 2001). Rare risks include stroke, seizures, tamponade, and death.

Preprocedural Care. A complete nursing assessment is necessary to ensure a safe procedure with minimum complications. This assessment should include accurate height (essential for correct catheter selection) and weight. Obtaining a history of allergic reactions is important, since some of the contrast agents are iodine based. Specific attention to signs and symptoms of infection is crucial. Severe diaper rash may be a reason to cancel the procedure if femoral access is required. Because assessment of pedal pulses is important after catheterization, the nurse should assess and mark pulses (dorsalis pedis, posterior tibial) before the child goes to the catheterization room. The presence and quality of pulses in both feet are clearly documented. Baseline oxygen saturation using pulse oximetry in children with cyanosis is also recorded.

Preparing the child and family for the procedure is the joint responsibility of the patient care team. School-age children and adolescents benefit from a description of the catheterization laboratory and a chronologic explanation of the procedure, emphasizing what they will see, feel, and hear. Older children and adolescents may bring earphones and favorite music so they can listen during the catheterization procedure. Preparation materials such as picture books, videotapes, or tours of the catheterization laboratory may be helpful. Preparation should be geared to the child's developmental level. The child's caregivers often benefit from the same explanations. Additional information, such as the expected length of the catheterization, description of the child's appearance after catheterization, and usual postprocedure care, should be outlined. (See also Prepare Child and Family for Invasive Procedures, p. 888.)

Methods of sedation vary among institutions and may include oral or intravenous (IV) medications (see Chapter 22). The child's age, heart defect, clinical status, and type of catheterization procedure planned are considered when sedation is determined. General anesthesia may be needed for some interventional procedures. Children are allowed nothing by mouth (NPO) for 4 to 6 hours or more before the procedure according to institutional guidelines. Infants and patients with polycythemia may need IV fluids to prevent dehydration and hypoglycemia.

Postprocedural Care. Patients may recover from the procedure in a recovery unit, their hospital room, or, occasionally, intensive care. Patients are placed on a cardiac monitor and a pulse oximeter for the first few hours of recovery. The most important nursing responsibility is observation of the following for signs of complications:

- Pulses, especially below the catheterization site, for equality and symmetry (Pulse distal to the site may be weaker for the first few hours after catheterization but should gradually increase in strength.)
- Temperature and color of the affected extremity, since coolness or blanching may indicate arterial obstruction

- Vital signs, which are taken as frequently as every 15 minutes, with special emphasis on heart rate, which is counted for 1 full minute for evidence of dysrhythmias or bradycardia
- Blood pressure (BP), especially for hypotension, which may indicate hemorrhage from cardiac perforation or bleeding at the site of initial catheterization
- Dressing, for evidence of bleeding or hematoma formation in the femoral or antecubital area
- Fluid intake, both IV and oral, to ensure adequate hydration (Blood loss in the catheterization laboratory, the child's NPO status, and diuretic actions of dyes used during the procedure put children at risk for hypovolemia and dehydration.)
- Blood glucose levels for hypoglycemia, especially in infants, who should receive dextrose-containing IV fluids

NURSINGALERT

If bleeding occurs, direct continuous pressure is applied 2.5 cm (1 inch) above the percutaneous skin site to localize pressure over the vessel puncture.

Depending on hospital policy, the child may be kept in bed with the affected extremity maintained straight for 4 to 6 hours after venous catheterization and 6 to 8 hours after arterial catheterization to facilitate healing of the cannulated vessel. If younger children have difficulty complying, they can be held in the parent's lap with the leg maintained in the correct position. The child's usual diet can be resumed as soon as tolerated, beginning with sips of clear liquids and advancing as the condition allows. The child is encouraged to void to clear the contrast material from the blood. Generally, there is only slight discomfort at the percutaneous site. To prevent infection, the catheterization area is protected from possible contamination. If the child wears diapers, the dressing can be kept dry by covering it with a piece of plastic film and sealing the edges of the film to the skin with tape. However, the nurse must be careful to continue observing the site for any evidence of bleeding (see Family-Centered Care box and Critical Thinking Exercise).

CONGENITAL HEART DISEASE

The incidence of CHD in children is approximately 5 to 8 per 1000 live births (Park, 2003). About 2 or 3 in 1000 infants will be symptomatic during the first year of life with significant heart disease that will require treatment (Hoffman and Kaplan, 2002). CHD is the major cause of death (other than prematurity) in the first year of life. Although there are more than 35 well-recognized cardiac defects, the most common heart anomaly is ventricular septal defect (VSD).

The exact etiology of most congenital cardiac defects is unknown. Most are thought to be a result of multifactorial inheritance: a complex interaction of genetic and environmental factors. The tremendous amount of information being discovered in molecular biology and the Human Genome Project will likely increase our understanding of the genetic causes of congenital heart defects.

Some risk factors are known to increase the incidence of congenital heart defects. Maternal factors include chronic illnesses such as diabetes or poorly controlled phenylketonuria, alcohol consumption, and exposure to environmental toxins and infections. Family history of a cardiac defect in a parent or sibling increases the likelihood of a cardiac anomaly. The risk of CHD increases if a first-degree relative (parent or sibling) is affected. The familial risk is higher with left-sided obstructive lesions.

FAMILY-CENTERED CARE

After Cardiac Catheterization
- Remove pressure dressing the day after catheterization. Cover site with an adhesive bandage strip for several days.
- Keep site clean and dry. Avoid tub baths for several days; patient may shower.
- Observe site for redness, swelling, drainage, and bleeding. Monitor for fever. Notify practitioner if these occur.
- Avoid strenuous exercise for several days; patient may attend school.
- Resume regular diet without restrictions.
- Use acetaminophen or ibuprofen for pain.
- Keep follow-up appointments per practitioner's instruction.

Modified from Children's Hospital (Boston) Cardiovascular Program, 1996.

??? CRITICAL THINKING EXERCISE

Cardiac Catheterization
Tommy, a 4-year-old with tetralogy of Fallot, has just returned to his hospital room from the cardiac catheterization recovery room. His mother calls you to the bedside to tell you that he is vomiting and bleeding. You arrive to find Tommy anxious, pale, crying, and sitting in a puddle of blood.

QUESTIONS
1. Evidence—Is there sufficient evidence to draw conclusions about Tommy's situation?
2. Assumptions—Describe an underlying assumption about each of the following:
   a. Risks of cardiac catheterization
   b. Association between vomiting and bleeding after cardiac catheterization
   c. Concerns related to acute blood loss
3. What priorities for nursing care should be established for Tommy?
4. Does the evidence support your nursing interventions?
5. What alternative perspectives might you have?

Congenital heart anomalies are often associated with chromosomal abnormalities, syndromes, or congenital defects in other body systems. Down syndrome (trisomy 21) and trisomy 13 and 18 are highly correlated with congenital heart defects.

Recent research in gene mapping has identified deletion of part of chromosome 22 (22q11), which is present in the majority of patients with DiGeorge syndrome, velocardiofacial syndrome, and conotruncal anomaly face syndrome. The features of these syndromes include congenital cardiac defects, soft palate abnormalities, dysmorphic facial features, and speech and developmental delays. Mild immunologic abnormalities of T cells, absence or hypoplasia of the thymus, and parathyroid abnormalities resulting in hypocalcemia are seen with DiGeorge syndrome. Commonly associated cardiac defects are interrupted aortic arch, truncus arteriosus, tetralogy of Fallot, and posterior malaligned VSD (Goldmuntz, Clark, Mitchell, and others, 1998). This syndrome has variable clinical expression, with some patients minimally affected and others having all characteristics.

FIG. 25-1 ■ Changes in circulation at birth. **A,** Prenatal circulation. **B,** Postnatal circulation. *Arrows* indicate direction of blood flow. Although four pulmonary veins enter the LA, for simplicity this diagram shows only two. *RA,* Right atrium; *LA,* left atrium; *RV,* right ventricle; *LV,* left ventricle.

CIRCULATORY CHANGES AT BIRTH

During fetal life, blood carrying oxygen and nutritive materials from the placenta enters the fetal system through the umbilicus via the large umbilical vein. Oxygenated blood enters the heart by way of the inferior vena cava. Because of the higher pressure of blood entering the right atrium, it is directed posteriorly in a straight pathway across the right atrium and through the **foramen ovale** to the left atrium. In this way the better-oxygenated blood enters the left atrium and ventricle to be pumped through the aorta to the head and upper extremities. Blood from the head and upper extremities entering the right atrium from the superior vena cava is directed downward through the tricuspid valve into the right ventricle. From here it is pumped through the pulmonary artery, where the major portion is shunted to the descending aorta via the **ductus arteriosus.** Only a small amount flows to and from the nonfunctioning fetal lungs (Fig. 25-1, *A*).

Before birth the high pulmonary vascular resistance created by the collapsed fetal lung causes greater pressures in the right side of the heart and the pulmonary arteries. At the same time, the free-flowing placental circulation and the ductus arteriosus produce a low vascular resistance in the remainder of the fetal vascular system. With the cessation of placental blood flow from clamping of the umbilical cord and the expansion of the lungs at birth, the hemodynamics of the fetal vascular system undergo pronounced and abrupt changes (Fig. 25-1, *B*).

With the first breath, the lungs are expanded, and increased oxygen causes pulmonary vasodilation. Pulmonary pressures start to fall as systemic pressures, given the removal of the placenta, start to rise. Normally the foramen ovale closes as the pressure in the left atrium exceeds the pressure in the right atrium. The ductus arteriosus starts to close in the presence of increased oxygen concentration in the blood and other factors.

ALTERED HEMODYNAMICS

To appreciate the physiology of heart defects, it is necessary to understand the role of pressure gradients, flow, and resistance within the circulation. As with any fluid, blood flows from an area of high pressure to one of lower pressure and toward the path of least resistance in response to the pumping action of the heart. In general, the higher the pressure gradient, the greater the rate of flow; the higher the resistance, the lesser the rate of flow.

Normally the pressure on the right side of the heart is lower than that on the left side, and the resistance in the pulmonary circulation is less than that in the systemic circulation. Vessels entering or exiting these chambers have corresponding pressures. Therefore, if an abnormal connection exists between the heart chambers (such as a septal defect), blood will necessarily flow from an area of higher pressure (left side) to one of lower pressure (right side). Such a flow of blood is termed a **left-to-right shunt.** Anomalies resulting in cyanosis may result from a change in pressure so that the blood is shunted from the right to the left side of the heart (**right-to-left shunt**) because of either increased pulmonary vascular resistance or obstruction to blood flow through the pulmonic valve and artery. Cyanosis may also result from a defect that allows mixing of oxygenated and deoxygenated blood within the heart chambers or great arteries, such as occurs in truncus arteriosus.

CLASSIFICATION OF DEFECTS

Congenital heart defects have been divided into two categories. Traditionally, cyanosis, a physical characteristic, has been used as the distinguishing feature, dividing the anomalies into **acyanotic defects** and **cyanotic defects.** In clinical practice this system is problematic because children with acyanotic

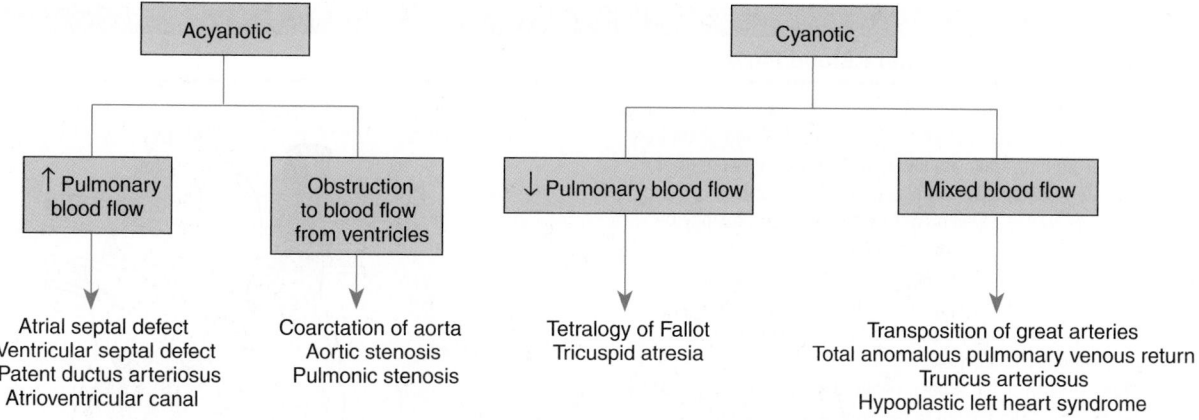

FIG. 25-2 ■ Comparison of acyanotic-cyanotic and hemodynamic classification systems of congenital heart disease.

defects may develop cyanosis. Also, more often, those with cyanotic defects may appear pink and have more clinical signs of CHF.

A more useful classification system is based on hemodynamic characteristics (blood flow patterns within the heart). These blood flow patterns are (1) **increased pulmonary blood flow;** (2) **decreased pulmonary blood flow;** (3) **obstruction to blood flow** out of the heart; and (4) **mixed blood flow,** in which saturated and desaturated blood mix within the heart or great arteries. As a comparison, both classification systems are outlined in Fig. 25-2.

With the hemodynamic classification system, the clinical manifestations of each group are more uniform and predictable. Defects that allow blood flow from the higher pressure left side of the heart to the lower pressure right side (left-to-right shunt) result in increased pulmonary blood flow and cause CHF. Obstructive defects impede blood flow out of the ventricles; obstruction on the left side of the heart results in CHF, whereas severe obstruction on the right side causes cyanosis. Defects that cause decreased pulmonary blood flow result in cyanosis. Mixed lesions present a variable clinical picture based on the degree of mixing and amount of pulmonary blood flow; hypoxemia (with or without cyanosis) and CHF usually occur together. Using this classification system, the clinical presentation and management of the most common defects are outlined in the following sections and Box 25-1.

The outcomes of surgical treatment for patients with moderate to severe disease are variable. Patient risk factors for increased morbidity and mortality include prematurity or low birth weight, a genetic syndrome, multiple cardiac defects, a noncardiac congenital anomaly, and age at time of surgery (neonates are a higher-risk group). For example, aortic stenosis or coarctation manifesting in the first week of life is more severe and carries a higher mortality than if it becomes apparent at 1 year of age. Outcomes for surgical repair of similar congenital heart defects also vary among treatment centers. Most mortality rates are obtained from a large multicenter database maintained by the Society of Thoracic Surgeons (Jacobs, Mavroudis, Jacobs, and others, 2004) to reflect the more likely outcome of present day treatments. Individual center results may be better or worse than the Society of Thoracic Surgeons database. In general, the outcomes of surgical procedures have steadily improved in the past decade, with mortality rates for many severe defects below 10%, and the incidence of complications and length of hospital stay have declined.

Defects with Increased Pulmonary Blood Flow

In this group of cardiac defects, intracardiac communications along the septum or an abnormal connection between the great arteries allows blood to flow from the higher pressure left side of the heart to the lower pressure right side of the heart (Fig. 25-3). Increased blood volume on the right side of the heart increases pulmonary blood flow at the expense of systemic blood flow. Clinically, patients demonstrate signs and symptoms of CHF. Atrial septal defect (ASD), VSD, and patent ductus arteriosus are typical anomalies in this group (Box 25-1).

Obstructive Defects

Obstructive defects are those in which blood exiting the heart meets an area of anatomic narrowing (**stenosis**), causing obstruction to blood flow. The pressure in the ventricle and in the great artery before the obstruction is increased, and the pressure in the area beyond the obstruction is decreased. The location of the narrowing is usually near the valve (Fig. 25-4), as follows:

Valvular—At the site of the valve itself
Subvalvular—Narrowing in the ventricle below the valve (also referred to as the **ventricular outflow tract**)
Supravalvular—Narrowing in the great artery above the valve

Coarctation of the aorta (narrowing of the aortic arch), aortic stenosis, and pulmonic stenosis are typical defects in this group (Box 25-2). Hemodynamically, there is a pressure load on the ventricle and decreased cardiac output. Clinically, infants and children exhibit signs of CHF. Children with mild obstruction may be asymptomatic. Rarely, as in severe pulmonic stenosis, hypoxemia may be seen.

Defects with Decreased Pulmonary Blood Flow

In this group of defects, there is obstruction of pulmonary blood flow and an anatomic defect (ASD or VSD) between the right and left sides of the heart (Fig. 25-5). Because blood has difficulty exiting the right side of the heart via the pulmonary artery, pressure on the right side increases, exceeding left-sided pressure. This allows desaturated blood to shunt right to left, causing desaturation in the left side of the

BOX 25-1
Defects with Increased Pulmonary Blood Flow

ATRIAL SEPTAL DEFECT

Description—Abnormal opening between the atria, allowing blood from the higher-pressure left atrium to flow into the lower-pressure right atrium. There are three types of atrial septal defect (ASD):

Ostium primum (ASD 1)—Opening at lower end of septum; may be associated with mitral valve abnormalities

Ostium secundum (ASD 2)—Opening near center of septum

Sinus venosus defect—Opening near junction of superior vena cava and right atrium; may be associated with partial anomalous pulmonary venous connection

Pathophysiology—Because left atrial pressure slightly exceeds right atrial pressure, blood flows from the left to the right atrium, causing an increased flow of oxygenated blood into the right side of the heart. Despite the low pressure difference, a high rate of flow can still occur because of low pulmonary vascular resistance and the greater distensibility of the right atrium, which further reduces flow resistance. This volume is well tolerated by the right ventricle because it is delivered under much lower pressure than with a ventricular septal defect (VSD). Although there is right atrial and ventricular enlargement, cardiac failure is unusual in an uncomplicated ASD. Pulmonary vascular changes usually occur only after several decades if the defect is left unrepaired.

Clinical manifestations—Patients may be asymptomatic. They may develop congestive heart failure (CHF). There is a characteristic systolic murmur with a fixed split second heart sound. There may also be a diastolic murmur. Patients are at risk for atrial dysrhythmias (probably caused by atrial enlargement and stretching of conduction fibers) and pulmonary vascular obstructive disease and emboli formation later in life from chronically increased pulmonary blood flow.

Surgical treatment—Surgical patch closure (pericardial patch or Dacron patch) is done for moderate to large defects. Open repair with cardiopulmonary bypass is usually performed before school age. In addition, the sinus venosus defect requires patch placement, so the

Atrial septal defect

anomalous right pulmonary venous return is directed to the left atrium with a baffle. The ASD 1 type may require mitral valve repair or, rarely, replacement of the mitral valve.

Nonsurgical treatment—ASD 2 closure with a device during cardiac catheterization is becoming commonplace and can be done as an outpatient procedure. The Amplatzer Septal Occluder is most commonly used. Smaller defects that have a rim around them for attachment of the device can be closed with a device; large, irregular defects without a rim require surgical closure. Successful closure in appropriately selected patients yields results similar to those from surgery but involves shorter hospital stays and fewer complications. Patients receive low-dose aspirin for 6 months (Rome and Kreutzer, 2004).

Prognosis—Operative mortality is very low (<1%).

VENTRICULAR SEPTAL DEFECT

Description—Abnormal opening between the right and left ventricles. May be classified according to location: membranous (accounting for 80%) or muscular. May vary in size from a small pinhole to absence of the septum, which results in a common ventricle. VSDs are frequently associated with other defects, such as pulmonary stenosis, transposition of the great vessels, patent ductus arteriosus (PDA), atrial defects, and coarctation of the aorta. Many VSDs (20% to 60%) will close spontaneously. Spontaneous closure is most likely to occur during the first year of life in children having small or moderate defects. A left-to-right shunt is caused by the flow of blood from the higher-pressure left ventricle to the lower-pressure right ventricle.

Pathophysiology—Because of the higher pressure within the left ventricle and because the systemic arterial circulation offers more resistance than the pulmonary circulation, blood flows through the defect into the pulmonary artery. The increased blood volume is pumped into the lungs, which may eventually result in increased pulmonary vascular resistance. Increased pressure in the right ventricle as a result of left-to-right shunting and pulmonary resistance causes the muscle to hypertrophy. If the right ventricle is unable to accommodate the increased workload, the right atrium may also enlarge as it attempts to overcome the resistance offered by incomplete right ventricular emptying.

Clinical manifestations—CHF is common. There is a characteristic loud holosystolic murmur heard best at the left sternal border. Patients are at risk for bacterial endocarditis and pulmonary vascular obstructive disease.

Ventricular septal defect

Surgical treatment

Palliative—Pulmonary artery banding (placement of a band around the main pulmonary artery to decrease pulmonary blood flow) may be done in infants with multiple muscular VSDs or complex anatomy. Improvements in surgical techniques and postoperative care make complete repair in infancy the preferred approach.

Complete repair (procedure of choice)—Small defects are repaired with sutures. Large defects usually require that a knitted Dacron patch be sewn over the opening. Cardiopulmonary bypass is used for both procedures. The approach for the repair is generally through

BOX 25-1

Defects with Increased Pulmonary Blood Flow—cont'd

VENTRICULAR SEPTAL DEFECT—cont'd

the right atrium and the tricuspid valve. Postoperative complications include residual VSD and conduction disturbances.

Nonsurgical treatment—Device closure during cardiac catheterization is being performed in some centers under investigational protocols. One device has been approved for closure of muscular defects, and another is in clinical trials. Early results are encouraging, with successful defect closure and few complications (Rome and Kreutzer, 2004).

Prognosis—Risks depend on the location of the defect, the number of defects, and the presence of other associated cardiac defects. Single membranous defects are associated with low mortality (<2%); multiple muscular defects can carry a higher risk (Jacobs, Mavroudis, Jacobs, and others, 2004).

ATRIOVENTRICULAR CANAL DEFECT

Description—Incomplete fusion of the endocardial cushions. Consists of a low ASD that is continuous with a high VSD and clefts of the mitral and tricuspid valves, which create a large central atrioventricular (AV) valve that allows blood to flow between all four chambers of the heart. The directions and pathways of flow are determined by pulmonary and systemic resistance, left and right ventricular pressures, and the compliance of each chamber, although flow is generally from left to right. It is the most common cardiac defect in children with Down syndrome.

Pathophysiology—The alterations in hemodynamics depend on the severity of the defect and the child's pulmonary vascular resistance. Immediately after birth, while the newborn's pulmonary vascular resistance is high, there is minimum shunting of blood through the defect. Once this resistance falls, left-to-right shunting occurs and pulmonary blood flow increases. The resultant pulmonary vascular engorgement predisposes the child to development of CHF.

Clinical manifestations—Patients usually have moderate to severe CHF. There is a loud systolic murmur. There may be mild cyanosis that increases with crying. Patients are at high risk for developing pulmonary vascular obstructive disease.

Surgical treatment

Palliative—Pulmonary artery banding is occasionally done in small infants with severe symptoms. Complete repair in infancy is most common.

Atrioventricular canal defect

Complete repair—Surgical repair consists of patch closure of the septal defects and reconstruction of the AV valve tissue (either repair of the mitral valve cleft or fashioning of two AV valves). Postoperative complications include heart block, CHF, mitral regurgitation, dysrhythmias, and pulmonary hypertension.

Prognosis—Operative mortality is less than 5% (Jacobs, Mavroudis, Jacobs, and others, 2004). A potential later problem is mitral regurgitation, which may require valve replacement.

PATENT DUCTUS ARTERIOSUS

Description—Failure of the fetal ductus arteriosus (artery connecting the aorta and pulmonary artery) to close within the first weeks of life. The continued patency of this vessel allows blood to flow from the higher-pressure aorta to the lower-pressure pulmonary artery, which causes a left-to-right shunt.

Pathophysiology—The hemodynamic consequences of PDA depend on the size of the ductus and the pulmonary vascular resistance. At birth the resistance in the pulmonary and systemic circulations is almost identical, so that the resistance in the aorta and pulmonary artery is equalized. As the systemic pressure comes to exceed the pulmonary pressure, blood begins to shunt from the aorta across the duct to the pulmonary artery (left-to-right shunt). The additional blood is recirculated through the lungs and returned to the left atrium and left ventricle. The effect of this altered circulation is increased workload on the left side of the heart, increased pulmonary vascular congestion and possibly resistance, and potentially increased right ventricular pressure and hypertrophy.

Clinical manifestations—Patients may be asymptomatic or show signs of CHF. There is a characteristic machinery-like murmur. A widened pulse pressure and bounding pulses result from runoff of blood from the aorta to the pulmonary artery. Patients are at risk for bacterial endocarditis and pulmonary vascular obstructive disease in later life from chronic excessive pulmonary blood flow.

Patent ductus arteriosus

Medical management—Administration of indomethacin (prostaglandin inhibitor) has proved successful in closing a PDA in preterm infants and some newborns.

Continued

BOX 25-1

Defects with Increased Pulmonary Blood Flow—cont'd

PATENT DUCTUS ARTERIOSUS—cont'd

Surgical treatment—Surgical division or ligation of the patent vessel is performed via a left thoracotomy. In a newer technique, video-assisted thoracoscopic surgery, a thoracoscope and instruments are inserted through three small incisions on the left side of the chest to place a clip on the ductus. The technique is used in some centers and eliminates the need for a thoracotomy, thereby speeding postoperative recovery.

Nonsurgical treatment—Coils to occlude the PDA are placed in the catheterization laboratory in many centers. Preterm or small infants (with small-diameter femoral arteries) and patients with large or unusual PDAs may require surgery.

Prognosis—Both surgical and nonsurgical procedures can be done at low risk with less than 1% mortality. PDA closure in very preterm infants has a higher mortality rate because of the additional significant medical problems.

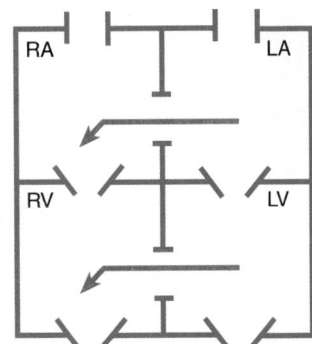

FIG. 25-3 ■ Hemodynamics in defects with increased pulmonary blood flow. See Fig. 25-1 for abbreviations.

FIG. 25-5 ■ Hemodynamic defects with decreased pulmonary blood flow. See Fig. 25-1 for abbreviations.

FIG. 25-4 ■ Obstruction to ventricular ejection can occur at the valvular level (shown), below the valve (subvalvular), or above the valve (supravalvular). Pulmonary stenosis is shown here. *Ao,* Aorta; *PA,* pulmonary artery. See Fig. 25-1 for additional abbreviations.

heart and in the systemic circulation. Clinically, these patients are hypoxemic and usually appear cyanotic. Tetralogy of Fallot and tricuspid atresia are the most common defects in this group (Box 25-3).

Mixed Defects

Many complex cardiac anomalies are classified together in the mixed category (Box 25-4) because survival in the postnatal period depends on mixing of blood from the pulmonary and systemic circulations within the heart chambers. Hemodynamically, fully saturated systemic blood flow mixes with the desaturated pulmonary blood flow, causing a relative desaturation of the systemic blood flow. Pulmonary congestion occurs because the differences in pulmonary artery pressure and aortic pressure favor pulmonary blood flow. Cardiac output decreases because of a volume load on the ventricle. Clinically, these patients have a variable picture that combines some degree of desaturation (although cyanosis is not always visible) and signs of CHF. Some defects, such as transposition of the great arteries, cause severe cyanosis in the first days of life and later cause CHF. Others, such as truncus arteriosus, cause severe CHF in the first weeks of life and mild desaturation.

Text continued on p. 876

BOX 25-2

Obstructive Defects

COARCTATION OF THE AORTA

Description—Localized narrowing near the insertion of the ductus arteriosus, which results in increased pressure proximal to the defect (head and upper extremities) and decreased pressure distal to the obstruction (body and lower extremities).

Pathophysiology—The effect of a narrowing within the aorta is increased pressure proximal to the defect (upper extremities) and decreased pressure distal to it (lower extremities).

Clinical manifestations—The patient may have high blood pressure and bounding pulses in the arms, weak or absent femoral pulses, and cool lower extremities with lower blood pressure. There are signs of congestive heart failure (CHF) in infants. In infants with critical coarctation, the hemodynamic condition may deteriorate rapidly with severe acidosis and hypotension. Mechanical ventilation and inotropic support are often necessary before surgery. Older children may experience dizziness, headaches, fainting, and epistaxis resulting from hypertension. Patients are at risk for hypertension, ruptured aorta, aortic aneurysm, and stroke.

Surgical treatment—Surgical repair is the treatment of choice for infants younger than 6 months of age and for patients with long-segment stenosis or complex anatomy; it may be performed for all patients with coarctation. Repair is by resection of the coarcted portion with an end-to-end anastomosis of the aorta or enlargement of the constricted section using a graft of prosthetic material or a portion of the left subclavian artery. Because this defect is outside the heart and pericardium, cardiopulmonary bypass is not required, and a thoracotomy incision is used. Postoperative hypertension is treated with intravenous sodium nitroprusside, esmolol, or milrinone followed by oral medications, such as angiotensin-converting enzyme inhibitors or beta blockers. Residual permanent hypertension after repair of coarctation of the aorta (COA) seems to be related to age and time of repair. To prevent both hypertension at rest and exercise-provoked

Coarctation of aorta

systemic hypertension after repair, elective surgery for COA is advised within the first 2 years of life. There is a 15% to 30% risk of recurrence in patients who underwent surgical repair as infants (Beekman, 2001). Percutaneous balloon angioplasty techniques have proved to be effective in relieving residual postoperative coarctation gradients.

Nonsurgical treatment—Balloon angioplasty is being performed as a primary intervention for COA in older infants and children. In adolescents, stents may be placed in the aorta to maintain patency. Recent studies have demonstrated that balloon angioplasty is effective in children and that aneurysm formation is rare. The high restenosis rate in young infants limits its application in this group (Rome and Kreutzer, 2004).

Prognosis—Mortality is less than 5% in patients with isolated coarctation; risk is increased in infants with other complex cardiac defects (Jacobs, Mavroudis, Jacobs, and others, 2004).

AORTIC STENOSIS

Description—Narrowing or stricture of the aortic valve, causing resistance to blood flow in the left ventricle, decreased cardiac output, left ventricular hypertrophy, and pulmonary vascular congestion. The prominent anatomic consequence of aortic stenosis (AS) is the hypertrophy of the left ventricular wall, which eventually leads to increased end-diastolic pressure resulting in pulmonary venous and pulmonary arterial hypertension. Left ventricular hypertrophy also interferes with coronary artery perfusion and may result in myocardial infarction or scarring of the papillary muscles of the left ventricle, which causes mitral insufficiency. Valvular stenosis, the most common type, is usually caused by malformed cusps that result in a bicuspid rather than tricuspid valve or fusion of the cusps. Subvalvular stenosis is a stricture caused by a fibrous ring below a normal valve; supravalvular stenosis occurs infrequently. Valvular AS is a serious defect for the following reasons: (1) the obstruction tends to be progressive; (2) sudden episodes of myocardial ischemia, or low cardiac output, can result in sudden death; and (3) surgical repair rarely results in a normal valve. This is one of the rare instances in which strenuous physical activity may be curtailed because of the cardiac condition.

Pathophysiology—A stricture in the aortic outflow tract causes resistance to ejection of blood from the left ventricle. The extra workload on the left ventricle causes hypertrophy. If left ventricular failure develops, left atrial pressure will increase; this causes increased pressure in the pulmonary veins, which results in pulmonary vascular congestion (pulmonary edema).

Clinical manifestations— Newborns with critical AS demonstrate signs of decreased cardiac output with faint pulses, hypotension,

Aortic stenosis

tachycardia, and poor feeding. Children show signs of exercise intolerance, chest pain, and dizziness when standing for a long period. A systolic ejection murmur may or may not be present. Patients are at risk for bacterial endocarditis, coronary insufficiency, and ventricular dysfunction.

Valvular Aortic Stenosis

Surgical treatment—Aortic valvotomy is performed under inflow occlusion. Used rarely since balloon dilation in the catheterization laboratory is the first-line procedure. Newborns with critical AS and small left-sided structures may undergo a stage 1 Norwood procedure (see Hypoplastic Left Heart Syndrome, Box 25-4).

Continued

BOX 25-2

Obstructive Defects—cont'd

AORTIC STENOSIS—cont'd

Valvular Aortic Stenosis—cont'd

Prognosis—Aortic valve replacement offers a good treatment option and may lead to normalization of left ventricular size and function (Arnold, Ley-Zaporozhan, Ley, and others, 2008). Results of aortic valvotomy in older children are very good, with mortality and morbidity close to 0% (Shanmugam, MacArthur, and Pollock, 2005). However, aortic valvotomy remains a palliative procedure, and approximately 25% of patients require additional surgery within 10 years for recurrent stenosis. A valve replacement may be required at the second procedure. An aortic homograft with a valve may also be used (extended aortic root replacement), or the pulmonary valve may be moved to the aortic position and replaced with a homograft valve (Ross procedure).

Nonsurgical treatment—The narrowed valve is dilated using balloon angioplasty in the catheterization laboratory. This procedure is usually the first intervention.

Prognosis—Complications include aortic insufficiency or valvular regurgitation, tearing of the valve leaflets, and loss of pulse in the catheterized limb.

Subvalvular Aortic Stenosis

Surgical treatment—Procedure may involve incising a membrane if one exists or cutting the fibromuscular ring. If the obstruction results from narrowing of the left ventricular outflow tract and a small aortic valve annulus, a patch may be required to enlarge the entire left ventricular outflow tract and annulus and replace the aortic valve; this is known as the Konno procedure.

Prognosis—Mortality from surgical repairs of subvalvular AS is less than 5% in major centers; however, about 20% of these patients develop recurrent subaortic stenosis and require additional surgery (Freed, 2001).

PULMONIC STENOSIS

Description—Narrowing at the entrance to the pulmonary artery. Resistance to blood flow causes right ventricular hypertrophy and decreased pulmonary blood flow. Pulmonary atresia is the extreme form of pulmonic stenosis (PS) in that there is total fusion of the commissures and no blood flows to the lungs. The right ventricle may be hypoplastic.

Pathophysiology—When PS is present, resistance to blood flow causes right ventricular hypertrophy. If right ventricular failure develops, right atrial pressure will increase, and this may result in reopening of the foramen ovale, shunting of unoxygenated blood into the left atrium, and systemic cyanosis. If PS is severe, CHF occurs, and systemic venous engorgement will be noted. An associated defect such as a patent ductus arteriosus partially compensates for the obstruction by shunting blood from the aorta to the pulmonary artery and into the lungs.

Clinical manifestations—Patients may be asymptomatic; some have mild cyanosis or CHF. Progressive narrowing causes increased symptoms. Newborns with severe narrowing will be cyanotic. A loud systolic ejection murmur at the upper left sternal border may be present. However, in severely ill patients the murmur may be much softer due to decreased cardiac output and shunting of blood. Cardiomegaly is evident on chest radiographic films. Patients are at risk for bacterial endocarditis.

Surgical treatment—In infants, transventricular (closed) valvotomy (Brock procedure). In children, pulmonary valvotomy with cardiopulmonary bypass. Need for surgical treatment is rare with widespread use of balloon angioplasty techniques.

Nonsurgical treatment—Balloon angioplasty in the cardiac catheterization laboratory to dilate the valve. A catheter is inserted across the stenotic pulmonic valve into the pulmonary artery, and a balloon at the end of the catheter is inflated and rapidly passed through the narrowed opening (see figure at right). The procedure is associated with few complications and has proved to be highly effective. It is the treatment of choice for discrete PS in most centers and can be done safely in neonates.

Prognosis—Risk is low for both surgical and nonsurgical procedures; mortality is lower than 1%, slightly higher in neonates (Latson, 2001). Both balloon dilation and surgical valvotomy leave the pulmonic valve incompetent because they involve opening the fused valve leaflets; however, these patients are clinically asymptomatic. Long-term problems with restenosis or valve incompetence may occur.

Pulmonic stenosis

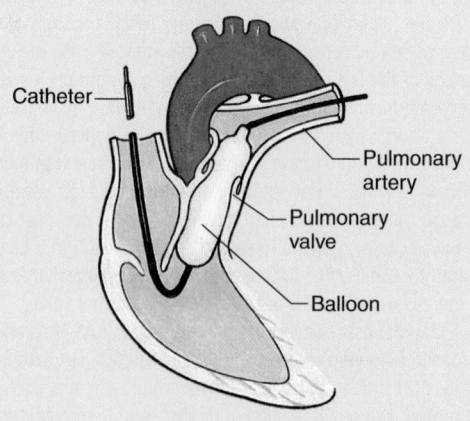

Catheter

Pulmonary artery

Pulmonary valve

Balloon

[handwritten margin notes: "Always will be there will be unless repaired"]

[handwritten margin notes: "Digoxin - 1st dose is double then maintenance dose. Loading dose or digitalizing dose."]

BOX 25-3
Defects with Decreased Pulmonary Blood Flow

TETRALOGY OF FALLOT *[handwritten: Medical emergency.]*

Description—The classic form includes four defects: (1) ventricular septal defect (VSD), (2) pulmonic stenosis (PS), (3) overriding aorta, and (4) right ventricular hypertrophy.

Pathophysiology—The alteration in hemodynamics varies widely, depending primarily on the degree of PS, but also on the size of the VSD and the pulmonary and systemic resistance to flow. Because the VSD is usually large, pressures may be equal in the right and left ventricles. Therefore the shunt direction depends on the difference between pulmonary and systemic vascular resistance. If pulmonary vascular resistance is higher than systemic resistance, the shunt is from right to left. If systemic resistance is higher than pulmonary resistance, the shunt is from left to right. PS decreases blood flow to the lungs and consequently the amount of oxygenated blood that returns to the left side of the heart. Depending on the position of the aorta, blood from both ventricles may be distributed systemically.

Clinical manifestations—Some infants may be acutely cyanotic at birth; others have mild cyanosis that progresses over the first year of life as the PS worsens. There is a characteristic systolic murmur that is often moderate in intensity. There may be acute episodes of cyanosis and hypoxia, called *blue spells* or *tet spells* (see p. 884). Anoxic spells occur when the infant's oxygen requirements exceed the blood supply, usually during crying or after feeding. Patients are at risk for emboli, seizures, and loss of consciousness or sudden death following an anoxic spell.

Surgical treatment

Palliative shunt—In infants who cannot undergo primary repair, a palliative procedure to increase pulmonary blood flow and increase oxygen saturation may be performed. The preferred procedure is a modified Blalock-Taussig shunt operation, which provides blood flow to the pulmonary arteries from the left or right subclavian artery via a tube graft (see Table 25-4). In general, however, shunts are avoided because they may result in pulmonary artery distortion.

[handwritten notes near figure: "Sit upright, nasal cannula, EKG pads, IV fluids."]

[labels on figure: Pulmonic stenosis; Overriding aorta; Ventricular septal defect; Right ventricular hypertrophy]

[handwritten: "Do right away: crunch them back into fetal position. More O2 blood to heart."]

Complete repair—Elective repair is usually performed in the first year of life. Indications for repair include increasing cyanosis and the development of hypercyanotic spells. Complete repair involves closure of the VSD and resection of the infundibular stenosis, with placement of a pericardial patch to enlarge the right ventricular outflow tract. In some repairs, the patch may extend across the pulmonary valve annulus (transannular patch), making the pulmonary valve incompetent. The procedure requires a median sternotomy and the use of cardiopulmonary bypass.

Prognosis—The operative mortality for total correction of tetralogy of Fallot is less than 3% (Jacobs, Mavroudis, Jacobs, and others, 2004). With improved surgical techniques there is a lower incidence of dysrhythmias and sudden death; surgical heart block is rare. Congestive heart failure may occur postoperatively.

TRICUSPID ATRESIA

Description—The tricuspid valve fails to develop; consequently there is no communication from the right atrium to the right ventricle. Blood flows through an atrial septal defect (ASD) or a patent foramen ovale to the left side of the heart and through a VSD to the right ventricle and out to the lungs. The condition is often associated with PS and transposition of the great arteries. There is complete mixing of unoxygenated and oxygenated blood in the left side of the heart, which results in systemic desaturation, and varying amounts of pulmonary obstruction, which causes decreased pulmonary blood flow.

Pathophysiology—At birth the presence of a patent foramen ovale (or other atrial septal opening) is required to permit blood flow across the septum into the left atrium; the patent ductus arteriosus allows blood flow to the pulmonary artery into the lungs for oxygenation. A VSD allows a modest amount of blood to enter the right ventricle and pulmonary artery for oxygenation. Pulmonary blood flow usually is diminished.

[label on figure: Tricuspid atresia]

Clinical manifestations—Cyanosis is usually seen in the newborn period. There may be tachycardia and dyspnea. Older children have signs of chronic hypoxemia with clubbing.

Therapeutic management—For the neonate whose pulmonary blood flow depends on the patency of the ductus arteriosus, a continuous infusion of prostaglandin E_1 is started at 0.1 mcg/kg/min until surgical intervention can be arranged.

Surgical treatment—Palliative treatment is the placement of a shunt (pulmonary–to–systemic artery anastomosis) to increase blood flow to

the lungs. If the ASD is small, an atrial septostomy is performed during cardiac catheterization. Some children have increased pulmonary blood flow and require pulmonary artery banding to lessen the volume of blood to the lungs. A bidirectional Glenn shunt (cavopulmonary anastomosis) may be performed at 4 to 9 months as a second stage.

Modified Fontan procedure—Systemic venous return is directed to the lungs without a ventricular pump through surgical connections between the right atrium and the pulmonary artery. A fenestration (opening) is sometimes made in the right atrial baffle to relieve pressure. The patient must have normal ventricular function and a

Continued

BOX 25-3

Defects with Decreased Pulmonary Blood Flow—cont'd

TRICUSPID ATRESIA—cont'd

low pulmonary vascular resistance for the procedure to be successful. The modified Fontan procedure separates oxygenated and unoxygenated blood inside the heart and eliminates the excess volume load on the ventricle but does not restore normal anatomy or hemodynamics. This operation is also the final stage in the correction of many complex defects with a functional single ventricle, including hypoplastic left heart syndrome.

Prognosis—Surgical mortality is less than 5% (Jacobs, Mavroudis, Jacobs, and others, 2004); the rate increases when the anatomy is more complex and other risk factors are present. Postoperative complications include dysrhythmias, systemic venous hypertension, pleural and pericardial effusions, and ventricular dysfunction. Long-term concerns are the development of protein-losing enteropathy, atrial dysrhythmias, late ventricular dysfunction, and developmental delays.

BOX 25-4

Mixed Defects

TRANSPOSITION OF THE GREAT ARTERIES, OR TRANSPOSITION OF THE GREAT VESSELS

Description—The pulmonary artery leaves the left ventricle, and the aorta exits from the right ventricle, with no communication between the systemic and pulmonary circulations.

Pathophysiology—Associated defects such as septal defects or patent ductus arteriosus must be present to permit blood to enter the systemic circulation or the pulmonary circulation for mixing of saturated and desaturated blood. The most common defect associated with transposition of the great arteries (TGA) is a patent foramen ovale. At birth there is also a patent ductus arteriosus, although in most instances this closes after the neonatal period. Another associated defect may be a ventricular septal defect (VSD). The presence of a VSD increases the risk of congestive heart failure (CHF) because it permits blood to flow from the right to the left ventricle, into the pulmonary artery, and finally to the lungs. However, it also produces high pulmonary blood flow under high pressure, which can result in high pulmonary vascular resistance.

Clinical manifestations—Depend on the type and size of the associated defects. Newborns with minimum communication are severely cyanotic and have depressed function at birth. Those with large septal defects or a patent ductus arteriosus may be less cyanotic but have symptoms of CHF. Heart sounds vary according to the type of defect present. Cardiomegaly is usually evident a few weeks after birth.

Therapeutic management (to provide intracardiac mixing)—The administration of intravenous prostaglandin E_1 may be initiated to keep the ductus arteriosus open to temporarily increase blood mixing and provide an oxygen saturation of 75% or to maintain cardiac output. During cardiac catheterization or under echocardiographic guidance, a balloon atrial septostomy (Rashkind procedure) may also be performed to increase mixing by opening the atrial septum.

Surgical treatment—An arterial switch procedure is the procedure of choice performed in the first weeks of life. It involves transecting the great arteries and anastomosing the main pulmonary artery to the proximal aorta (just above the aortic valve) and anastomosing the ascending aorta to the proximal pulmonary artery. The coronary arteries are switched from the proximal aorta to the proximal pulmonary artery to create a new aorta. Reimplantation of the coronary arteries is critical to the infant's survival, and they must be reattached without torsion or kinking to provide the heart with its supply of oxygen. The advantage of the arterial switch procedure is the reestablishment of normal circulation, with the left ventricle acting as

the systemic pump. Potential complications of the arterial switch include narrowing at the great artery anastomoses and coronary artery insufficiency.

Intraatrial baffle repairs—Intraatrial baffle repairs are rarely performed, although many adolescents and adults survive today with repairs that were done more than 15 years ago. An intraatrial baffle is created to divert venous blood to the mitral valve and pulmonary venous blood to the tricuspid valve using the patient's atrial septum (Senning procedure) or a prosthetic material (Mustard procedure). A disadvantage is the continuing role of the right ventricle as the systemic pump and the late development of right ventricular failure and rhythm disturbances. Other potential postoperative complications include loss of normal sinus rhythm, baffle leaks, and ventricular dysfunction.

Rastelli procedure—This procedure is the operative choice in infants with TGA, VSD, and severe pulmonic stenosis (PS). It involves closure of the VSD with a baffle, so that left ventricular blood is directed through the VSD into the aorta. The pulmonic valve is then closed, and a conduit is placed from the right ventricle to the pulmonary artery to create a physiologically normal circulation. Unfortunately, this procedure requires multiple conduit replacements as the child grows.

Prognosis—Operative mortality is less than 2% (Jacobs, Mavroudis, Jacobs, and others, 2004). Potential long-term problems include suprapulmonic stenosis and neoaortic dilation and regurgitation.

BOX 25-4
Mixed Defects—cont'd

TOTAL ANOMALOUS PULMONARY VENOUS CONNECTION

Description—Rare defect characterized by failure of the pulmonary veins to join the left atrium. Instead, the pulmonary veins are abnormally connected to the systemic venous circuit via the right atrium or various veins draining toward the right atrium, such as the superior vena cava. The abnormal attachment results in mixed blood being returned to the right atrium and shunted from the right to the left through an atrial septal defect (ASD). Total anomalous pulmonary venous connection (TAPVC; also called *total anomalous pulmonary venous return* or *total anomalous pulmonary venous drainage*) is classified according to the pulmonary venous point of attachment as follows:

Supracardiac—Attachment above the diaphragm, such as to the superior vena cava (most common form) (see Fig. 25-9)

Cardiac—Direct attachment to the heart, such as to the right atrium or coronary sinus

Infradiaphragmatic—Attachment below the diaphragm, such as to the inferior vena cava (most severe form)

Pathophysiology—The right atrium receives all the blood that normally would flow into the left atrium. As a result, the right side of the heart hypertrophies, whereas the left side, especially the left atrium, may remain small. An associated ASD or patent foramen ovale allows systemic venous blood to shunt from the higher-pressure right atrium to the left atrium and into the left side of the heart. As a result, the oxygen saturation of the blood in both sides of the heart (and ultimately in the systemic arterial circulation) is the same. If the pulmonary blood flow is large, pulmonary venous return is also large, and the amount of saturated blood is relatively high. However, if there is obstruction to pulmonary venous drainage, pulmonary venous return is impeded, pulmonary venous pressure rises, and pulmonary interstitial edema develops and eventually contributes to CHF. Infradiaphragmatic TAPVC is often associated with obstruction to pulmonary venous drainage and is a surgical emergency.

Clinical manifestations—Most infants develop cyanosis early in life. The degree of cyanosis is inversely related to the amount of pulmonary blood flow—the more pulmonary blood, the less cyanosis. Children with unobstructed TAPVC may be asymptomatic until pulmonary

vascular resistance decreases during infancy, increasing pulmonary blood flow, with resulting signs of CHF. Cyanosis becomes worse with pulmonary vein obstruction; once obstruction occurs, the infant's condition usually deteriorates rapidly. Without intervention, cardiac failure will progress to death.

Surgical treatment—Corrective repair is performed in early infancy. The surgical approach varies with the anatomic defect. In general, however, the common pulmonary vein is anastomosed to the back of the left atrium, the ASD is closed, and the anomalous pulmonary venous connection is ligated. The cardiac type is most easily repaired; the infradiaphragmatic type carries the highest morbidity and mortality because of the higher incidence of pulmonary vein obstruction. Potential postoperative complications include reobstruction; bleeding; dysrhythmias, particularly heart block; pulmonary artery hypertension; and persistent heart failure.

Prognosis—Mortality for all types is less than 10% (Jacobs, Mavroudis, Jacobs, and others, 2004) and is lowest for the cardiac type; morbidity increases with the presence of pulmonary vein obstruction.

TRUNCUS ARTERIOSUS

Description—Failure of normal septation and division of the embryonic bulbar trunk into the pulmonary artery and the aorta, which results in development of a single vessel that overrides both ventricles. Blood from both ventricles mixes in the common great artery, which leads to desaturation and hypoxemia. Blood ejected from the heart flows preferentially to the lower-pressure pulmonary arteries, so that pulmonary blood flow is increased and systemic blood flow is reduced. There are three types:

Type I—A single pulmonary trunk arises near the base of the truncus and divides into the left and right pulmonary arteries.

Type II—The left and right pulmonary arteries arise separately but in close proximity and at the same level from the back of the truncus.

Type III—The pulmonary arteries arise independently from the sides of the truncus.

Pathophysiology—Blood ejected from the left and right ventricles enters the common trunk, so that pulmonary and systemic circulations are mixed. Blood flow is distributed to the pulmonary and systemic circulations according to the relative resistances of each system. The amount of pulmonary blood flow depends on the size of the pulmonary arteries and the pulmonary vascular resistance. Generally, resistance to pulmonary blood flow is less than systemic vascular

resistance, which results in preferential blood flow to the lungs. Pulmonary vascular disease develops at an early age in patients with truncus arteriosus.

Clinical manifestations—Most infants are symptomatic with moderate to severe CHF and variable cyanosis, poor growth, and activity intolerance. There is a holosystolic murmur at the left sternal murmur

Continued

BOX 25-4

Mixed Defects—cont'd

TRUNCUS ARTERIOSUS—cont'd

with a diastolic murmur present if truncal regurgitation is present. Thirty-five percent of patients have 22q11 deletions (Goldmuntz, Clark, Mitchell, and others, 1998).

Surgical treatment—Early repair is performed in the first month of life. It involves closing the VSD so that the truncus arteriosus receives the outflow from the left ventricle, and excising the pulmonary arteries from the aorta and attaching them to the right ventricle by means of a homograft. Currently homografts (segments of cadaver aorta and pulmonary artery that are treated with antibiotics and cryopreserved) are preferred over synthetic conduits to establish continuity between the right ventricle and pulmonary artery. Homografts are more flexible and easier to use during the procedure and appear less prone to obstruction. Postoperative complications include persistent heart failure, bleeding, pulmonary artery hypertension, dysrhythmias, and residual VSD. Because conduits are not living tissue, they will not grow along with the child and may also become narrowed with calcifications. One or more conduit replacements will be needed in childhood.

Prognosis—Mortality is greater than 10%; future operations are required to replace the conduits.

HYPOPLASTIC LEFT HEART SYNDROME

Description—Underdevelopment of the left side of the heart, resulting in a hypoplastic left ventricle and aortic atresia. Most blood from the left atrium flows across the patent foramen ovale to the right atrium, to the right ventricle, and out the pulmonary artery. The descending aorta receives blood from the patent ductus arteriosus supplying systemic blood flow.

Pathophysiology—An ASD or patent foramen ovale allows saturated blood from the left atrium to mix with desaturated blood from the right atrium and to flow through the right ventricle and out into the pulmonary artery. From the pulmonary artery, the blood flows both to the lungs and through the ductus arteriosus into the aorta and out to the body. The amount of blood flow to the pulmonary and systemic circulations depends on the relationship between the pulmonary and systemic vascular resistances. The coronary and cerebral vessels receive blood by retrograde flow through the hypoplastic ascending aorta.

Clinical manifestations—The patient has mild cyanosis and signs of congestive failure until the patent ductus arteriosus closes, then progressive deterioration with cyanosis and decreased cardiac output, leading to cardiovascular collapse. The condition is usually fatal in the first months of life without intervention.

Therapeutic management—Neonates require stabilization with mechanical ventilation and inotropic support preoperatively. A prostaglandin E_1 infusion is needed to maintain ductal patency and ensure adequate systemic blood flow.

Surgical treatment—Multiple-stage approach is used. The first stage is a Norwood procedure, which involves an anastomosis of the main pulmonary artery to the aorta to create a new aorta, shunting to provide pulmonary blood flow (usually with a modified Blalock-Taussig shunt), and creation of a large ASD. Postoperative complications include imbalance of systemic and pulmonary blood flow, bleeding, low cardiac output, and persistent heart failure. A new modification of the first stage repair is the use of a right ventricle–to–pulmonary artery homograft conduit instead of a shunt to supply pulmonary blood flow (Sano procedure). The second stage is often a bidirectional Glenn shunt procedure (see Fig. 25-9) or a hemi-Fontan operation. Both involve anastomosing the superior vena cava to the right pulmonary artery so

Hypoplastic ascending aorta

Hypoplastic left ventricle

superior vena cava flow bypasses the right atrium and flows directly to the lungs. The procedure is usually done at 3 to 6 months of age to relieve cyanosis and reduce the volume load on the right ventricle. The final repair is a modified Fontan procedure (see Tricuspid Atresia, Box 25-3).

Transplantation—Heart transplantation in the newborn period is another option for these infants. Problems include the shortage of newborn organ donors, risk of rejection, long-term problems with chronic immunosuppression, and infection (see Heart Transplantation, p. 899).

Prognosis—For the first-stage repair, survival rates vary widely in different centers. Much progress has been made, and some experienced centers are reporting mortality rates of about 10% (Tweddell, Hoffman, Mussatto, and others, 2002), but a large multicenter series reports a mortality rate of about 30% (Jacobs, Mavroudis, Jacobs, and others, 2004). Long-term problems with repair include worsening ventricular function, tricuspid regurgitation, recurrent aortic arch narrowing, dysrhythmias, and developmental delays. There is a risk of mortality between surgical procedures. The mortality for the later two operations is less than 5%.

CLINICAL CONSEQUENCES OF CONGENITAL HEART DISEASE

CONGESTIVE HEART FAILURE

CHF is the inability of the heart to pump an adequate amount of blood to the systemic circulation at normal filling pressures to meet the body's metabolic demands. In children, CHF most frequently occurs secondary to structural abnormalities (e.g., septal defects) that result in increased blood volume and pressure within the heart. It can also result from myocardial failure in which the contractility of the ventricle is impaired. This can occur with cardiomyopathy, dysrhythmias, or severe electrolyte disturbances. CHF can also occur because of excessive demands on a normal heart muscle, such as sepsis or severe anemia.

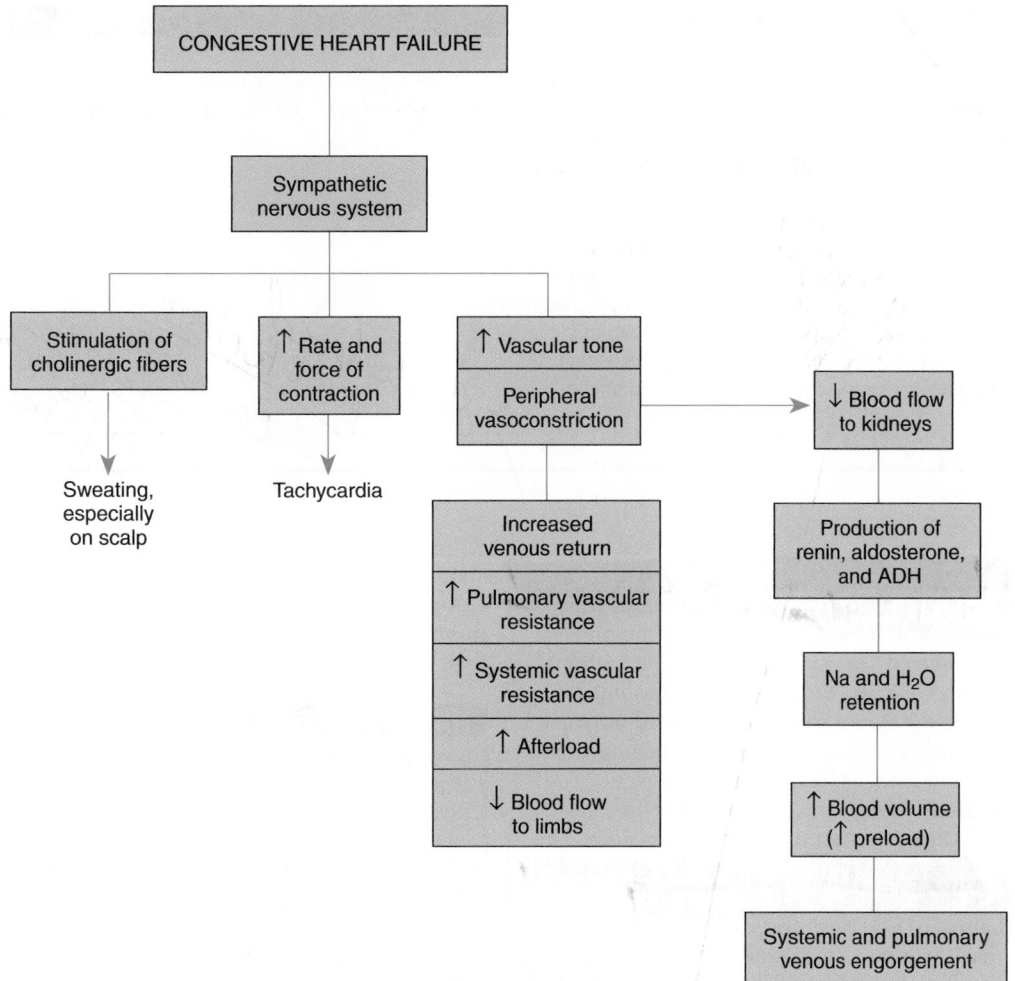

FIG. 25-6 ■ Pathophysiology of congestive heart failure. *ADH*, Antidiuretic hormone.

Pathophysiology

Heart failure is often separated into two categories: right-sided and left-sided failure. In **right-sided failure** the right ventricle is unable to pump blood effectively into the pulmonary artery, resulting in increased pressure in the right atrium and systemic venous circulation. Systemic venous hypertension causes hepatosplenomegaly and occasionally edema. In **left-sided failure** the left ventricle is unable to pump blood into the systemic circulation, resulting in increased pressure in the left atrium and pulmonary veins. The lungs become congested with blood, causing elevated pulmonary pressures and pulmonary edema.

Although each type of heart failure produces different signs and symptoms, clinically it is unusual to observe solely right- or left-sided failure in children. Because each side of the heart depends on adequate function of the other side, failure of one chamber causes a reciprocal change in the opposite chamber.

If the abnormalities precipitating CHF are not corrected, the heart muscle becomes damaged. Despite compensatory mechanisms, the heart is unable to maintain an adequate cardiac output. Decreased blood flow to the kidneys continues to stimulate sodium and water reabsorption, leading to fluid overload, increased workload on the heart, and congestion in the pulmonary and systemic circulations (Fig. 25-6).

The signs and symptoms of CHF can be divided into three groups: (1) impaired myocardial function, (2) pulmonary congestion, and (3) systemic venous congestion (Box 25-5). Because these hemodynamic changes occur from different causes and at differing times, the clinical presentation may vary among children.

Diagnostic Evaluation

Diagnosis is made on the basis of clinical symptoms such as tachypnea and tachycardia at rest, dyspnea, retractions, activity intolerance (especially during feeding in infants), weight gain caused by fluid retention, and hepatomegaly. A chest x-ray film demonstrates cardiomegaly and increased pulmonary blood flow. Ventricular hypertrophy appears on the ECG. An echocardiogram is done to determine the cause of CHF such as a congenital heart defect or poor ventricular function.

Therapeutic Management

The goals of treatment are to (1) improve cardiac function (increase contractility and decrease afterload), (2) remove accumulated fluid and sodium (decrease preload), (3) decrease

---

BOX 25-5

Clinical Manifestations of Congestive Heart Failure

IMPAIRED MYOCARDIAL FUNCTION	PULMONARY CONGESTION	SYSTEMIC VENOUS CONGESTION
Tachycardia	Tachypnea	Weight gain
Sweating (inappropriate)	Dyspnea	Hepatomegaly
Decreased urinary output	Retractions (infants)	Peripheral edema, especially periorbital
Fatigue	Flaring nares	Ascites
Weakness	Exercise intolerance	Neck vein distention (children)
Restlessness	Orthopnea	
Anorexia	Cough, hoarseness	
Pale, cool extremities	Cyanosis	
Weak peripheral pulses	Wheezing	
Decreased blood pressure	Grunting	
Gallop rhythm		
Cardiomegaly		

[handwritten margin notes: "WBN bradycardia, anorexia"; "check apical pulse for 1 min."; "calculate safe dose"; "Infants 90-110 bpm Children <70 bpm"; "toxicity = N V=08"; "2mg/ml"; "Pull the serum potassium level"]

---

cardiac demands, and (4) improve tissue oxygenation and decrease oxygen consumption. For most infants diagnosed with CHF, the cause is CHD. Infants are stabilized on medical therapy and then referred for surgical repair. For children newly diagnosed with CHF, the cause may be worsening ventricular function after a previous cardiac repair, cardiomyopathy, dysrhythmia, or other causes. In addition to management of CHF, the underlying cause is treated if possible.

Improve Cardiac Function. Myocardial efficiency is improved through administration of digitalis glycosides. The beneficial effects are increased cardiac output, decreased heart size, decreased venous pressure, and relief of edema. In pediatrics, **digoxin (Lanoxin)** is used almost exclusively because of its more rapid onset. It is available as an elixir (0.05 mg/ml) for oral administration. For infants the dose is calculated in micrograms (1000 mcg = 1 mg).

Treatment consists of a digitalizing dosage, given orally or intravenously in divided doses over 24 hours to produce optimal cardiac effects, and a maintenance dosage, given orally twice a day to maintain blood levels. During digitalization the child is monitored by means of an ECG to observe for the desired effects (prolonged PR interval and reduced ventricular rate) and detect side effects, especially dysrhythmias.

A newer group of drugs used in the treatment of CHF are the **angiotensin-converting enzyme (ACE) inhibitors.** As their name implies, these drugs inhibit the normal function of the renin-angiotensin system in the kidney. The ACE inhibitors block the conversion of angiotensin I to angiotensin II so that, instead of vasoconstriction, vasodilation occurs. Vasodilation results in decreased pulmonary and systemic vascular resistance, decreased BP, and a reduction in afterload. Common medications used in pediatrics are **captopril (Capoten), enalapril (Vasotec),** and lisinopril. The principal side effects of ACE inhibitors are hypotension, cough, and renal dysfunction.

Carvedilol, a beta blocker, is the newest medication to be added to the treatment of some children with chronic CHF. It blocks the α- and β-adrenergic receptors, causing decreased heart rate, decreased BP, and vasodilation. It has been shown to decrease morbidity and mortality in some adults with heart failure and is being used selectively in children. Side effects included dizziness, headache, and hypotension.

A new and promising therapy for some patients with severe ventricular dysfunction may be biventricular pacing, also called resynchronization therapy. Both ventricles are paced to closely mimic normal ventricular conduction and thereby improve the mechanical function of the heart muscle (Rosenthal, Chrisant, Edens, and others, 2004).

NURSINGALERT

Because ACE inhibitors also block the action of aldosterone, the addition of potassium supplements or spironolactone (Aldactone) to the drug regimen of patients taking diuretics is usually not needed and may cause hyperkalemia.

Remove Accumulated Fluid and Sodium. Treatment consists of diuretics, possible fluid restriction, and possible sodium restriction. Diuretics are the mainstay of therapy to eliminate excess water and salt to prevent reaccumulation. The most frequently used agents are listed in Table 25-3. Because furosemide and the thiazides are potassium-losing diuretics, potassium supplements may be prescribed, and rich sources of the electrolyte are encouraged in the diet.

NURSINGALERT

A fall in the serum potassium level enhances the effects of digitalis, increasing the risk of digoxin toxicity. Therefore serum potassium levels must be carefully monitored.

Fluid restriction may be required in the acute stages of CHF and must be carefully calculated to avoid dehydrating the child, especially if cyanotic CHD and significant polycythemia are present. Infants rarely need fluid restrictions because CHF makes feeding so difficult that they struggle to take maintenance fluids.

Sodium-restricted diets are used less often in children than in adults to control CHF because of their potential negative effects on appetite. If salt intake is restricted, additional table salt and highly salted foods are avoided.

Decrease Cardiac Demands. The workload on the heart is reduced when metabolic needs are kept to a minimum. This is accomplished by limiting physical activity (bed rest), maintaining body temperature, treating any infections, reducing the effort of breathing (semi-Fowler position), and using medication to sedate an irritable child.

Improve Tissue Oxygenation. All of the preceding measures serve to increase tissue oxygenation, either by im-

TABLE 25-3
Diuretics Used in Congestive Heart Failure   *Remove fluid & sodium*

ACTIONS	COMMENTS	NURSING CARE MANAGEMENT
Furosemide (Lasix)—Blocks reabsorption of sodium and water in proximal renal tubule and interferes with reabsorption of sodium *~Top of line "Big Guns"*	Drug of choice in severe congestive heart failure (CHF) Causes excretion of chloride and potassium (hypokalemia may precipitate digitalis toxicity)	Begin to record output as soon as drug is given. Observe for dehydration caused by profound diuresis. Observe for side effects (nausea and vomiting, diarrhea, ototoxicity, hypokalemia, dermatitis, postural hypotension). Encourage foods high in potassium and/or give potassium supplements. Monitor chloride and acid-base balance with long-term therapy. Observe for signs of digoxin toxicity.
Chlorothiazide (Diuril)—Acts directly on distal tubules to decrease sodium, water, potassium, chloride, and bicarbonate absorption	Less frequently used drug Causes hypokalemia, acidosis from large doses	Observe for side effects (nausea, weakness, dizziness, paresthesia, muscle cramps, skin eruptions, hypokalemia, acidosis). Encourage foods high in potassium and/or give potassium supplements.
Spironolactone (Aldactone)—Blocks action of aldosterone, which promotes retention of sodium and excretion of potassium	Weak diuretic Has potassium-sparing effect; frequently used with thiazides, furosemide Poorly absorbed from gastrointestinal tract Takes several days to achieve maximum actions	Observe for side effects (skin rash, drowsiness, ataxia, hyperkalemia). Do not administer potassium supplements.

proving myocardial function or by lessening tissue oxygen demands. In addition, supplemental cool humidified oxygen may be administered to increase the amount of available oxygen during inspiration. Oxygen administration is especially helpful in patients with pulmonary edema, intercurrent respiratory tract infections, and increased pulmonary vascular resistance (oxygen is a vasodilator that decreases pulmonary vascular resistance).

NURSING ALERT
Oxygen is a drug and is administered only with an appropriate order. There are some uncommon circumstances in patients with complex hemodynamics in which oxygen can be detrimental.

An oxygen hood, nasal cannula, or face tent is used to deliver oxygen. Nasal cannulas are ideal for long-term oxygen administration because the child can be ambulatory and can easily eat and drink. Cool humidification is necessary to counteract the drying effect of oxygen. The amount of cool humidity is carefully regulated to prevent chilling.

Nursing Care Management
The infant or child with CHF may be acutely ill, and some may require intensive care until the symptoms improve. Expert nursing care is essential to reduce the cardiac demands that strain the failing heart muscle. During this time the child and family require emotional support. Although the objectives of nursing care are the same, interventions differ depending on the child's age (see Nursing Process box).

Assist in Measures to Improve Cardiac Function. The nurse's responsibility in administering digoxin includes calculating and administering the correct dosage, observing for signs of toxicity, and instituting parental teaching regarding drug administration at home. The child's apical pulse is always checked before administering digoxin. As a general rule,

BOX 25-6
Common Signs of Digoxin Toxicity in Children

GASTROINTESTINAL	CARDIAC
Nausea	Bradycardia
Vomiting	Dysrhythmias
Anorexia	

the drug is not given if the pulse is below 90 to 110 beats/min in infants and young children or below 70 beats/min in older children (the cutoff point for adults is 60 beats/min). However, because the pulse rate varies in children in different age-groups, the written drug order should specify at what heart rate the drug is withheld. The nurse should also use judgment in evaluating the pulse rate. If it is significantly lower than the previous recording, the dose should be withheld until the practitioner is notified.

The apical rate is taken because a pulse deficit (radial pulse rate lower than apical) may be present with decreased cardiac output. It is auscultated for 1 full minute to evaluate alterations in rhythm. If the child is monitored by means of an ECG, a rhythm strip is obtained and attached to the chart for rate and rhythm analysis, such as abnormal lengthening of the PR interval (>50% increase over predigitalization interval) and dysrhythmias.

Digoxin is a potentially dangerous drug because of its narrow margin of safety of therapeutic, toxic, and lethal doses. Many toxic responses are extensions of its therapeutic effects. Therefore the nurse must maintain a high index of suspicion for signs of toxicity when administering digoxin (Box 25-6).

Because digoxin toxicity can occur from accidental overdose, great care must be taken in properly calculating and measuring

nursingprocess | The Child with Congestive Heart Failure

ASSESSMENT

Assess for signs and symptoms of congestive heart failure (CHF) in children with congenital heart defects or suspected defects. (See Box 25-5 and the defining characteristics in the Nursing Care Plan below.)

DIAGNOSIS (PROBLEM IDENTIFICATION)

After a thorough assessment, several nursing diagnoses are evident (see Nursing Care Plan below). Other nursing diagnoses include:

- Fluid Volume Excess related to edema secondary to congestive heart failure
- Risk for Infection related to reduced body defenses, pulmonary congestion
- Imbalanced Nutrition: Less Than Body Requirements related to respiratory distress, feeding difficulties
- Interrupted Family Processes related to the presence of a child with a life-threatening illness
- Activity Intolerance related to respiratory distress, fatigue

PLANNING

Expected patient outcomes include:

- Child will have adequate cardiac output.
- Child will have decreased cardiac demands.
- Child will have improved respiratory function.
- Child will have no evidence of fluid excess.
- Child and family will have adequate support and education.

IMPLEMENTATION

Numerous intervention strategies are discussed on pp. 879-884.

EVALUATION

The effectiveness of nursing interventions for the child with CHF and his or her family is determined by continual assessment and evaluation of care based on the following guidelines:

- Monitor vital signs, child's color and perfusion, and fluid status. Assess activity level and observe for signs of fatigue.
- Observe nutritional intake and feeding behaviors.
- Monitor intake and output and weight.
- Observe the family's behaviors.

nursingcareplan | The Child with Congestive Heart Failure (CHF)

Nursing Diagnosis	Patient Outcomes	Nursing Interventions	Rationale
Decreased Cardiac Output related to structural defect, myocardial dysfunction, altered hemodynamics	Child will have adequate cardiac output as evidenced by: ■ Heart rate within acceptable range (state specific range) ■ Respiratory rate within acceptable range (state specific range) ■ Skin warm to touch ■ Strong and equal peripheral pulses ■ Blood pressure normal for age ■ Brisk capillary refill, within 2 to 3 seconds ■ Lack of distended neck veins ■ Normal sinus rhythm ■ Lack of edema ■ Adequate urinary output (state specific; 1 to 2 ml/kg/hr)	Assess and record heart rate, respiratory rate (RR), blood pressure, and any signs and symptoms of decreased cardiac output (listed under defining characteristics) every 2 to 4 hours and as needed (PRN).	To assess for changes in vital signs and child's physical status that reflect altered cardiac output
Child's/Family's Defining Characteristics *(Subjective and Objective Data)*		Administer cardiac drugs on schedule. Assess for and record any side effects or any signs or symptoms of toxicity. Follow hospital protocol for administration.	To improve heart function by giving drugs on time and to avoid dangers by giving as prescribed and with careful assessment before administration
Tachycardia Tachypnea Ineffective peripheral circulation, cool extremities Hypotension Rapid, weak peripheral pulses Prolonged capillary refill, longer than 2 to 3 seconds Narrow pulse pressure Distended neck veins in older children Cardiomegaly revealed on chest x-ray film Gallop rhythm Edema Rapid weight gain Feeding difficulty Irritability		Keep accurate record of intake and output.	To assess for CHF, which causes decreased urinary output
		Weigh child or infant on same scale at same time of day. Document results and compare with previous weight.	To observe for weight increase that may indicate excess fluid accumulation
		Administer diuretics on schedule. Assess and record effectiveness and any side effects noted.	To prevent fluid retention, which commonly occurs with CHF; to eliminate excess water and salt
	Child will have age-appropriate weight gain on standardized growth curve. Infant will demonstrate successful feeding.	Elevate head of bed at a 30- to 45-degree angle.	To promote maximum chest expansion
		Offer small, frequent feedings to infant's or child's tolerance.	To prevent fatigue during feeding and to ensure adequate nutrition, since metabolic rate is greater because of poor cardiac function
	Child and/or family will be able to state at least four characteristics of congestive heart failure such as: ■ Rapid heart rate ■ Fast breathing ■ Cool extremities ■ Puffiness (edema) ■ Fussiness ■ Decreased appetite	Organize nursing care to allow child or infant uninterrupted rest.	To account for decreased energy level and lower tolerance to activity
		Educate child and family about characteristics of CHF. Assess and record teaching session.	To provide parent education that can promote measures to improve cardiac function and decrease demands

nursingcareplan | The Child with Congestive Heart Failure (CHF)—cont'd

Nursing Diagnosis	Patient Outcomes	Nursing Interventions	Rationale
Decreased Cardiac Output related to structural defect, myocardial dysfunction, altered hemodynamics—cont'd	Child and/or family will be able to state knowledge of care regarding: ■ Medication administration ■ Head elevated positioning ■ Sufficient rest periods ■ Monitoring intake and output ■ When to contact health care provider **The Following NOC Concepts Apply to These Outcomes** Cardiac Pump Effectiveness Knowledge: Illness Care Tissue Perfusion: Cardiac	Educate child and family about care such as medication administration. Assess and record results and family's participation in care. **The Following NIC Concepts Apply to These Interventions** Cardiac Care Fluid Management Medication Administration Positioning Vital Signs Monitoring Respiratory Monitoring	To educate on proper medication administration, promote safety, and minimize medication side effects

Nursing Diagnosis	Patient Outcomes	Nursing Interventions	Rationale
Ineffective Breathing Pattern related to pulmonary congestion, decreased cardiac output **Child's/Family's Defining Characteristics** *(Subjective and Objective Data)* Tachypnea Dyspnea Retractions Crackles Shortness of breath Cyanosis Pallor Mottling Nasal flaring Grunting Head bobbing Cough Use of accessory muscles Activity intolerance	Child will have effective breathing pattern as evidenced by: ■ Respiratory rate within acceptable range (state specific range) ■ Clear and equal breath sounds bilaterally anterior and posterior ■ Pink or tan color ■ Absence of nasal flaring, retractions, cough, and head bobbing ■ Unlabored breath sounds ■ Tolerance of activities appropriate for age Child and/or family will be able to state four characteristics of ineffective breathing pattern such as: ■ Color change from pink or tan to pale, dusky, or blue color ■ Fast breathing ■ Change in amount and/or characteristics of secretions ■ Retractions, head bobbing ■ Ineffective cough ■ Decreased or altered activity level Child and/or family will be able to state knowledge of care regarding: ■ Positioning to facilitate respiratory effort ■ Oxygen administration ■ When to contact health care provider **The Following NOC Concepts Apply to These Outcomes** Activity Tolerance Knowledge: Illness Care Respiratory Status: Gas Exchange Tissue Perfusion: Pulmonary	Assess and record RR, breath sounds, and any signs and symptoms of ineffective pattern (listed under characteristics) every 2 to 4 hours and PRN. Administer humidified oxygen in correct amount and using correct route of delivery. Record percent of oxygen and route of delivery. Assess and record child's response to therapy. Keep head of bed elevated at a 30- to 45-degree angle. Suction if child has ineffective cough or is unable to manage secretions. Assess and record amount and characteristics of secretions. Assess and record oxygen saturation every 2 to 4 hours and PRN. Educate child and family about characteristics of ineffective breathing pattern. Assess and record results. Educate child and family about care. Assess and record results and family participation in care. **The Following NIC Concepts Apply to These Interventions** Airway Management Airway Suctioning Chest Physiotherapy Family Involvement Promotion Health Education	To assess for respiratory changes that can be indicators of worsening CHF To provide oxygen, which can reduce respiratory distress by easing respiratory effort To promote maximum chest expansion To maintain patent airway to promote respiratory expansion To evaluate pulmonary effectiveness To provide parent education that can promote measures to improve breathing effort To promote family support

FAMILY-CENTERED CARE

Administering Digoxin

- Give digoxin at regular intervals, usually every 12 hours, such as at 8 AM and 8 PM.
- Administer the drug carefully by slowly directing it to the side and back of the mouth.
- Do not mix the drug with foods or other fluids, since refusal to consume these results in inaccurate intake of the drug.
- If the child has teeth, give water after administering the drug; whenever possible, brush the teeth to prevent tooth decay from the sweetened liquid.
- If a dose is missed, do not give an extra dose or increase the dose. Stay on the same medication schedule.
- If the child vomits, do not give a second dose.
- If more than two consecutive doses have been missed, notify the physician or other designated practitioner.
- Frequent vomiting, poor feeding, or slow heart rate can be signs of toxicity; if they occur, contact the physician.
- If the child becomes ill, notify the physician or other designated practitioner immediately.
- Keep digoxin in a safe place, preferably in a locked cabinet.
- In case of accidental overdose of digoxin, call the nearest poison control center immediately.

??? CRITICAL THINKING EXERCISE

Digoxin Toxicity

You are visiting a 3-month-old infant at home who began receiving digoxin and furosemide (Lasix) 5 days ago for management of congestive heart failure (CHF). A brief assessment indicates that the infant appears well but is not very active, has a weak suck reflex, and does not exhibit much spontaneous movement during interaction with the mother. The mother mentions that the infant is a good baby and does not cry much except when he is very hungry. She also mentions that he vomited several times yesterday and vomited twice this morning; this was not perceived as unusual because her 3-year-old did the same thing and was diagnosed with gastroesophageal reflux. Further assessment of the infant reveals an irregular heartbeat of 86 to 104 beats/min at rest; the heart rhythm is also noted to be irregular. No murmur or other significant sounds are auscultated.

QUESTIONS

1. Evidence—Is there sufficient evidence to draw conclusions about this infant?
2. Assumptions—Describe an underlying assumption about each of the following:
   a. Side effects of furosemide
   b. Side effects of digoxin
   c. Infants with CHF
3. What priorities for nursing care should be established for this infant?
4. Does the evidence support your nursing interventions?
5. What alternative perspectives might you have?

---

the dosage. When converting milligrams to micrograms to milliliters, the nurse carefully checks the placement of the decimal point, since an error causes a significant change in dosage. For example, 0.1 mg is 10 times the dosage of 0.01 mg.

NURSINGALERT

Infants rarely receive more than 1 ml (50 mcg, or 0.05 mg) in one dose; a higher dose is an immediate warning of a dosage error. To ensure safety, compare the calculation with another staff member's calculation before giving the drug.

These same principles are taught to parents in preparation for discharge, although the correct dose in milliliters is usually specified on the container, thus reducing potential errors in calculation. The nurse watches the parent measure the elixir in the dropper and stresses the level mark as the meniscus of the fluid that is observed at eye level. Other instructions for administering digoxin are listed in the Family-Centered Care box and the Critical Thinking Exercise.

Parents are also advised of the signs of toxicity. According to the practitioner's preference, they may be taught to take the pulse before giving the drug. A return demonstration of the procedure from the parents or another principal caregiver is included as part of the teaching plan. Their level of anxiety in counting the pulse is assessed, since overconcern about the heart rate may result in excessive withholding of the drug.

Monitor Afterload Reduction. For patients receiving ACE inhibitors for afterload reduction, the nurse should carefully monitor BP before and after dose administration, observe for symptoms of hypotension, and notify the practitioner if BP is low. Numerous medications affecting the kidney can potentiate renal dysfunction, so children taking multiple diuretics and an ACE inhibitor require careful assessment of serum electrolytes and renal function.

Decrease Cardiac Demands. The infant requires rest and conservation of energy for feeding. Every effort is made to organize nursing activities to allow for uninterrupted periods of sleep. Whenever possible, parents are encouraged to stay with their infant to provide the holding, rocking, and cuddling that help children sleep more soundly. To minimize disturbing the infant, changing bed linen and complete bathing are done only when necessary. Feeding is planned to accommodate the infant's sleep and wake patterns. The child is fed at the first sign of hunger, such as when sucking on fists, rather than waiting until he or she cries for a bottle, since the stress of crying exhausts the limited energy supply. Because infants with CHF tire easily and may sleep through feedings, smaller feedings every 3 hours may be helpful. Gavage feedings may be instituted to provide adequate nutrition and allow the infant to rest.

Every effort is made to minimize unnecessary stress. Older children need an explanation of what is happening to them to decrease anxiety about their illness and necessary treatments such as cardiac monitoring, oxygen administration, and medications. Outlining a plan for the day, preparing the child for tests and procedures, providing quiet activities, and providing adequate rest periods are all helpful interventions with older children. Some infants and children require sedation during the acute phase of illness to allow them to rest.

Temperature is carefully monitored because hyperthermia or hypothermia increases the need for oxygen. Febrile states are reported to the physician, since infection must be promptly treated. Maintaining body temperature is of special importance in children who are receiving cool, humidified oxygen and in infants, who tend to be diaphoretic and lose heat by way of evaporation.

Skin breakdown from edema is prevented with a change of position every 2 hours (from side to side while in semi-Fowler position) and use of a pressure-relieving mattress or bed. The skin, especially over the sacrum, is checked for evidence of redness from pressure.

Reduce Respiratory Distress. Careful assessment, positioning, and oxygen administration can reduce respiratory distress. Respirations are counted for 1 full minute during a resting state. Any evidence of increased respiratory distress is reported, since this may indicate worsening CHF.

Infants are positioned to encourage maximum chest expansion, with the head of the bed elevated; they should sit up in an infant seat or be held at a 45-degree angle. Children prefer to sleep on several pillows and remain in a semi-Fowler or high-Fowler position during waking hours. Safety restraints, such as those used with infant seats, are applied low on the abdomen and loosely enough to provide both safety and maximum expansion.

The infant or child is often given humidified supplemental oxygen via oxygen hood or tent, nasal cannula, or mask. The child's response to oxygen therapy is carefully evaluated by noting respiratory rate, ease of respiration, color, and especially oxygen saturation as measured by oximetry.

Respiratory tract infections can exacerbate CHF and should be appropriately treated and prevented if possible. The child should be protected from persons with respiratory tract infections and have a noninfectious roommate. With an older child, it is advantageous to choose a roommate who is also confined to bed and relatively quiet to promote a restful environment. Good hand washing is practiced before and after caring for any hospitalized child. Antibiotics may be given to combat respiratory tract infection. The nurse ensures that the drug is given at equally divided times over a 24-hour schedule to maintain high blood levels of the antibiotic.

Maintain Nutritional Status. Meeting the nutritional needs of infants with CHF or serious cardiac defects is a nursing challenge. The metabolic rate of these infants is greater because of poor cardiac function and increased heart and respiratory rates. Their caloric needs are greater than those of the average infant because of their increased metabolic rate, yet their ability to take in adequate calories is hampered by their fatigue. Feeding for a fragile infant with serious CHD is similar to exercising for an adult, and these infants often do not have the energy or cardiac reserve to do extra work. The nurse seeks measures to enable the infant to feed easily without excess fatigue and to increase the caloric density of the formula.

The infant should be well rested before feeding and fed soon after awakening so as not to expend energy on crying. A 3-hour feeding schedule works well for many infants. (Feeding every 2 hours does not provide enough rest between feedings, and a 4-hour schedule requires an increased volume of feeding, which many infants are unable to take.) The feeding schedule should be individualized to the infant's needs. A feeding goal of 150 ml/kg/day and at least 120 kcal/kg/day is common for newborns with significant heart disease (Stetzler, Rudd, and Pick, 2005). A soft preemie nipple or a slit in a regular nipple to enlarge the opening decreases the infant's energy expenditure while sucking. Infants should be well sup-

ported and fed in a semiupright position. The infant may need to rest frequently and may need to have the jaw and cheeks stroked to encourage sucking. Generally, giving an infant about a half hour to complete a feeding is reasonable. Prolonging the feeding time can exhaust the infant and decrease the rest period between feedings.

Infants with feeding difficulties are often gavage fed using a nasogastric tube to supplement their oral intake and ensure adequate calories. If they are very stressed and fatigued, in respiratory distress, or tachypneic to 80 to 100 breaths/min, oral feedings may be withheld and all nutrition given by gavage feedings. Gavage feedings are usually a temporary measure until the infant's medical status improves and nutritional needs can be met through oral feedings. Some infants with severe CHF, neurologic deficits, or significant gastroesophageal reflux may need placement of a gastrostomy tube to allow adequate nutrition.

Caloric density of formulas is frequently increased by concentration and then adding Polycose, medium-chain triglyceride oil, or corn oil. Infant formulas provide 20 kcal/oz, and the use of additives can increase the calories to 30 kcal/oz or more. This allows the infant to obtain more calories despite a smaller volume intake of formula. The caloric density of the formula needs to be increased slowly (by 2 kcal/oz/day) to prevent diarrhea or formula intolerance. Breastfeeding mothers are encouraged to provide the infant with alternating feedings of breast milk and high-calorie formulas. Some lactating mothers prefer to feed the child expressed breast milk that has been fortified with Similac or Enfamil powder, Polycose, or corn oil to increase caloric intake. A supplemental nurser may also be helpful. A diet plan specific to the individual infant's needs is calculated and prescribed by the nutritionist in collaboration with the other health personnel. The nurse needs to reinforce this information with the parents as necessary.

Assist in Measures to Promote Fluid Loss. When diuretics are given, the nurse records fluid intake and output and monitors body weight at the same time each day to evaluate benefit from the drug. Because profound diuresis may cause dehydration and electrolyte imbalance (loss of sodium, potassium, chloride, bicarbonate), the nurse observes for signs indicating either complication, as well as signs and symptoms suggesting reactions to the drugs. Diuretics should be given early in the day to children who are toilet trained to avoid the need to urinate at night. If potassium-losing diuretics are given, the nurse encourages foods high in potassium, such as bananas, oranges, whole grains, legumes, and leafy vegetables, and administers prescribed supplements. Serum potassium levels are checked frequently.

NURSING TIP

Mix the elixir with fruit juice (red punch or grape juice works well) to disguise the bitter taste and to prevent intestinal irritation from a concentrated solution.

Fluid restriction is rarely necessary in infants because of their difficulty in feeding. However, if fluids are restricted, the nurse plans fluid intake schedules for a 24-hour period, allowing for most fluids during waking hours. Toddlers and preschoolers should be given small amounts of liquid in small cups so that the containers appear full. Older children's cooperation is gained by placing them in charge of recording fluid intake.

If salt is limited, the nurse discusses food sources of sodium with the family and discourages their bringing salt-containing treats to the child. At mealtime the child's tray is checked to make sure the appropriate diet is given.

Support Child and Family. CHF is a serious complication of heart disease. Parents and older children are usually acutely aware of the critical nature of the condition. Because stress places additional demands on cardiac function, the nurse should focus on reducing anxiety through anticipatory preparation, frequent communication with the parent regarding the child's progress, and constant reassurance that everything possible is being done.

Home care involves many of the same interventions discussed under Plan for Discharge and Home Care (p. 891). The nurse teaches the family about the medications that need to be administered and alerts them to the signs of worsening CHF that require medical attention, such as increased sweating, decreased urinary output (noted in fewer wet diapers or infrequent use of the toilet), or poor feeding. Every effort is made to improve the family's adherence to the medication schedule by adapting the schedule to their usual home routines, avoiding medications during the night, making it as simple as possible, and using charts or visual aids to remember when to give medications (see Chapter 22). Written instructions regarding correct administration of digoxin are essential (see Family-Centered Care box, p. 882), including an explanation regarding signs of toxicity.

If CHF is the end stage of a severe heart defect, the nurse cares for this child as for any child who is terminally ill, using the principles discussed in Chapter 18.

HYPOXEMIA

Hypoxemia refers to an arterial oxygen tension (or pressure, Pao_2) that is less than normal and can be identified by a decreased arterial saturation or a decreased Pao_2. **Hypoxia** is a reduction in tissue oxygenation that results from low oxygen saturations and Pao_2 and results in impaired cellular processes. **Cyanosis** is a blue discoloration in the mucous membranes, skin, and nail beds of the child with reduced oxygen saturation. It results from the presence of deoxygenated hemoglobin (hemoglobin not bound to oxygen) in a concentration of 5 g/dl of blood. Cyanosis is usually apparent when arterial oxygen saturations are 80% to 85%. Determination of cyanosis is subjective. It can vary depending on skin pigment, quality of light, color of the room, or clothing worn by the child. The presence of cyanosis may not accurately reflect arterial hypoxemia, since both oxygen saturation and the amount of circulating hemoglobin are involved. Children with severe anemia may not be cyanotic despite severe hypoxemia, since the hemoglobin level may be too low to produce the characteristic blue color. Conversely, patients with polycythemia may appear cyanotic despite a near-normal Pao_2. Heart defects that cause hypoxemia and cyanosis result from desaturated venous blood (blue blood) entering the systemic circulation without passing through the lungs.

Clinical Manifestations

Over time, two physiologic changes occur in the body in response to chronic hypoxemia: polycythemia and clubbing. **Polycythemia,** an increased number of red blood cells, increases the oxygen-carrying capacity of the blood. However, anemia may result if iron is not readily available for the for-

FIG. 25-7 ■ Clubbing of the fingers.

mation of hemoglobin. Polycythemia increases the viscosity of the blood and crowds out clotting factors. **Clubbing,** a thickening and flattening of the tips of the fingers and toes, is thought to occur because of chronic tissue hypoxemia and polycythemia (Fig. 25-7). Infants with mild hypoxemia may be asymptomatic except for cyanosis and exhibit near-normal growth and development. Those with more severe hypoxemia may exhibit fatigue with feeding, poor weight gain, tachypnea, and dyspnea. Severe hypoxemia resulting in tissue hypoxia is manifested by clinical deterioration and signs of poor perfusion.

Hypercyanotic spells, also referred to as **blue spells** or **tet spells** because they are often seen in infants with tetralogy of Fallot, may occur in any child whose heart defect includes obstruction to pulmonary blood flow and communication between the ventricles. The infant becomes acutely cyanotic and hyperpneic because sudden infundibular spasm decreases pulmonary blood flow and increases right-to-left shunting (the proposed mechanism in tetralogy of Fallot). Spells, rarely seen before 2 months of age, occur most frequently in the first year of life. They occur more often in the morning and may be preceded by feeding, crying, defecation, or stressful procedures (see Critical Thinking Exercise). Because profound hypoxemia causes cerebral hypoxia, hypercyanotic spells require prompt assessment and treatment to prevent brain damage or possibly death.

Persistent cyanosis as a result of cyanotic heart defects places the child at risk for significant **neurologic complications.** Cerebrovascular accident (CVA, stroke), brain abscess, and developmental delays (especially in motor and cognitive development) may result from chronic hypoxia.

Therapeutic Management

Newborns generally exhibit cyanosis within the first few days of life as the ductus arteriosus, which provided pulmonary blood flow, begins to close. Prostaglandin E_1, which causes vasodilation and smooth muscle relaxation, thus increasing dilation and patency of the ductus arteriosus, is administered intravenously to reestablish pulmonary blood flow. The use of prostaglandins has been lifesaving for infants with ductus-dependent cardiac defects. The increase in oxygenation allows the infant to be stabilized and have a complete diagnostic evaluation performed before further treatment is needed.

Hypercyanotic spells occur suddenly, and prompt recognition and treatment are essential. In the hospital setting, spells are often seen during blood drawing or IV insertion, when the

??? CRITICAL THINKING EXERCISE

Hypercyanotic Spell

A 4-month-old infant known to have tetralogy of Fallot is seen in the emergency department because of a 2-day history of diarrhea, low-grade fever, and poor oral intake. When blood tests are obtained, he becomes acutely cyanotic with rapid shallow respirations.

QUESTIONS

1. Evidence—Is there sufficient evidence to draw conclusions about this infant's condition?
2. Assumptions—Describe an underlying assumption about each of the following:
   a. Symptoms associated with tetralogy of Fallot
   b. Diarrhea, low-grade fever, and poor oral intake in a 4-month-old infant
   c. Acute cyanotic episodes in a 4-month-old infant
3. What priorities for nursing care should be established for this infant?
4. Does the evidence support your nursing interventions?
5. What alternative perspectives might you have?

FIG. 25-8 ■ Infant held in knee-chest position.

nursingcareguidelines

Treating Hypercyanotic Spells

- Place infant in knee-chest position (Fig. 25-8).
- Employ calm, comforting approach.
- Administer 100% oxygen by blow-by.
- Give morphine subcutaneously or through existing intravenous (IV) line.
- Begin IV fluid replacement and volume expansion if needed.
- Repeat morphine administration.

child is highly agitated, or after cardiac catheterization. Treatment of a hypercyanotic spell is outlined in the Nursing Care Guidelines box. Morphine, administered subcutaneously or through an existing IV line, helps reduce infundibular spasm. A spell indicates the need for prompt surgical treatment if possible. In infants with defects not amenable to surgical repair, a shunt may be created surgically to increase blood flow to the lungs. Several commonly used shunt procedures are described in Table 25-4 and Fig. 25-9.

The cyanotic infant and child are well hydrated to keep the hematocrit and blood viscosity within acceptable limits to reduce the risk of CVAs. Fevers are carefully evaluated because bacteremia can result in bacterial endocarditis. The infant is monitored closely for anemia because of the risk of CVAs and the reduced arterial oxygen-carrying capacity that occurs. Iron supplementation and possibly blood transfusion are used as needed.

Respiratory tract infections or reduced pulmonary function from any cause can worsen hypoxemia in the cyanotic child. Aggressive pulmonary hygiene, chest physical therapy, administration of antibiotics, and use of oxygen to improve arterial saturations are important interventions.

Nursing Care Management

The general appearance of infants and children with significant cyanosis poses unique concerns. Blue lips and fingernails are obvious signs of their hidden cardiac defect. Clubbing and small, thin stature in older children further indicate severe heart disease. Adolescents are especially concerned about their body image; children with cyanosis are often teased about their appearance and singled out as different. Many children, when asked what surgery will do, reply, "Make me pink." Their joy and excitement after surgery are evident when they see their pink fingers. Parents are often fearful of their child's bluish color, since cyanosis is usually associated with lack of oxygen and severe illness. They also must deal with comments from relatives, friends, and strangers about their child's ab-

normal color. They need a simple explanation of hypoxemia and cyanosis and reassurance that cyanosis does not imply a lack of oxygen to the brain. Their questions and fears need to be addressed in a calm, supportive manner, and positive aspects of their child's growth and development are emphasized. They are taught the treatment for hypercyanotic spells (see Nursing Care Guidelines box above).

Dehydration must be prevented in hypoxemic children because it potentiates the risk of CVAs. Fluid status is carefully monitored, with accurate intake and output and daily weight measurements. Maintenance fluid therapy is the minimum requirement, supplemental fluids should be readily available, and gavage feeding or IV hydration is given to children unable to take adequate oral fluids. Fever, vomiting, and diarrhea can cause dehydration and require prompt treatment. Parents are instructed in the importance of adequate fluid intake and measures to prevent dehydration. An oral electrolyte solution should be available at home in the event that the infant is unable to tolerate the usual formula. The practitioner should be notified of fever, vomiting, diarrhea, or other problems.

Preventive measures and accurate assessment of respiratory infection are important nursing considerations. Any compromise in pulmonary function will increase the infant's hypoxemia. Good hand washing and protection from individuals with an obvious respiratory tract infection are impor-

TABLE 25-4

Selected Shunt Procedures for Children with Cardiac Defects

SHUNT TYPE	COMMENTS
Modified Blalock-Taussig shunt—Subclavian artery to pulmonary artery using Gore-Tex or Impra tube graft	Shunt flow sometimes excessive, requiring use of diuretics
	Possibility of thrombosis; aspirin usually prescribed postoperatively
	Easy to ligate at time of definitive correction
	Shunt size fixed and may become too small as child grows
Central shunt—Ascending aorta to main pulmonary artery using Gore-Tex graft	Length of shunt acts to restrict blood flow; possibility of symptoms of congestive heart failure; diuretic therapy sometimes required
	Uncommon; used when modified Blalock-Taussig shunt cannot be used
	Easy to insert and remove at time of repair
	Possibility of thrombosis; aspirin usually prescribed postoperatively
Bidirectional Glenn shunt (cavopulmonary anastomosis)—Superior vena cava to side of right pulmonary artery; blood flow to both lungs	Done as a second shunt; often used as a staging step to a Fontan procedure
	Can be incorporated into eventual modified Fontan procedure
	Relieves severe cyanosis and decreases volume overload on ventricle
	Carries risk of embolic events (mixing defect); aspirin often prescribed
	Pulmonary arteriovenous fistulas may occur months or years later, causing desaturation (uncommon finding)

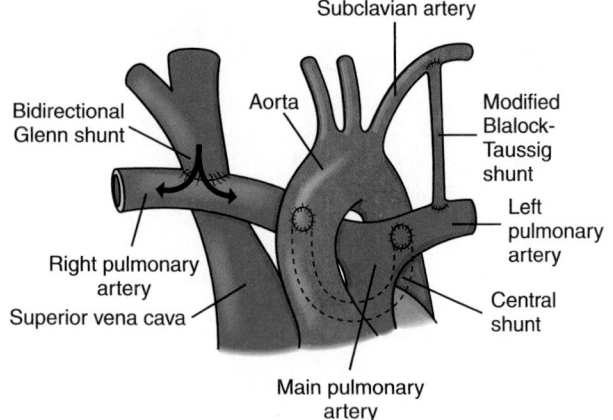

FIG. 25-9 ■ Schematic diagram of cardiac shunts.

tant. Aggressive pulmonary hygiene, treatment with antibiotics or antiviral agents as indicated, and supplemental oxygen to decrease hypoxemia are necessary measures. Infants may need to be gavage fed or given parenteral hydration if respiratory distress prevents oral feeding.

NURSING ALERT

Intracardiac shunting of blood from the right side (desaturated) to the left side of the heart allows air in the venous system to go directly to the brain, resulting in an air embolism. Therefore all IV lines should have filters in place to prevent air from entering the system, the entire tubing should be checked for air, all connections should be taped securely, and any air should be removed.

NURSING CARE OF THE FAMILY AND CHILD WITH CONGENITAL HEART DISEASE

When a child is born with a severe cardiac anomaly, the parents are faced with the immense psychologic and physical tasks of adjusting to the birth of a child with special needs. Family issues and nursing interventions to support the family are similar to those discussed in Chapters 11 and 22. The fol-

lowing discussion is primarily directed (1) toward the family of an infant who has a serious heart defect and requires home care before definitive repair and (2) toward preparation and care of the child and family when invasive procedures (catheterization and surgery) are performed. For nursing care related to the child with hypoxemia and CHF, the reader should refer to earlier discussions of these topics.

Nursing care of the child with a congenital heart defect begins as soon as the diagnosis is suspected. Prenatal diagnosis of congenital heart defects is becoming increasingly frequent. New demands are being placed on nurses to counsel and support families as they prepare for the birth of these infants.

HELP FAMILY ADJUST TO THE DISORDER

Once parents learn of the heart defect, they are initially in a period of shock, followed by high anxiety and fear that the child will die. The family needs time to grieve before they can assimilate the meaning of the defect. Unfortunately, the demands for medical treatment may not allow this, instead necessitating that the parents immediately give informed consent for diagnostic-therapeutic procedures. The nurse can be instrumental in supporting parents in their loss, assessing their level of understanding, supplying information as needed, and helping other members of the health care team understand the parents' reactions (see Family Focus box).

Severely ill newborns usually remain in the hospital. Parent-infant attachment is supported by encouraging parents to hold, touch, and look at their child and providing time and privacy for the parents to spend with their newborn. (See Chapter 10 for suggestions on promoting attachment between parents and their hospitalized newborn.)

The effect of a child with a serious heart defect on the family is complex. No member, regardless of the degree of positive adjustment, is unaffected. Mothers frequently feel inadequate in their mothering ability because of the more complex care infants with congenital heart defects require. They often feel exhausted from the pressures of caring for these children and the other family members. Fathers and siblings may feel neglected and resentful, a reaction similar to the feelings toward family members with other chronic conditions (see Chapter

FAMILY FOCUS

Diagnosis of Heart Disease

Remember, we don't have your experience. We don't see children everyday who have heart disease. We would have been upset finding out our child had to have his tonsils out. How could we ever be prepared for this? Please remember, we only know people who have trivial heart murmurs. How could we ever expect this to happen? And to us, this is the worst problem we've ever heard of.

We still fear most what we don't know and understand. Be honest with us. If you don't know either, tell us. But at least don't leave us wondering about what you know and we don't. Not knowing anything really can be worse than knowing something bad. Be honest, but don't strip us of hope. . . .

Please, remember we are trying to learn complex information in a moment of time. And trying to learn it in a context of great pain and emotional investment. This is our lives you're talking about. Please be thorough, but keep it simple. Tell us again, maybe even again and again, when we can hear better.

From Schrey C, Schrey M: A parent's perspective: our needs and our message, *Crit Care Nurs Clin North Am* 6(1):113-119, 1994.

18). Often, parents do not feel confident leaving the child in another's care. This often sets up a trap for parents, especially mothers, who become locked into the child's care with no relief. Although the fears are justified, they can be minimized by gradually teaching someone (a reliable relative or neighbor) how to care for the child.

The need to maintain discipline and set consistent limits can be difficult for parents. Using behavior modification techniques, in the form of either concrete awards (e.g., a favorite activity) or social reinforcement (e.g., approval), can be effective. However, it is most beneficial if employed *before* the child learns to control the family. To prevent later problems, it is necessary to begin discussions with parents while the child is in infancy regarding the need for discipline as the child gets older.

Another issue that may develop within family relationships is the child's overdependency. This is often the result of parental fear that the child may die. Parents need guidance to recognize the eventual hazards of continuing dependency and protectiveness as the child grows older, and the nurse can assist parents in learning ways to foster optimum development. Unless parents are shown what activities the child can do, they may focus on physical limitations and encourage dependency.

The child also needs opportunities for normal social interaction with peers. These children do not need to be prevented from playing with other children because of concern regarding overexertion. Children usually limit their activities if allowed to set their own pace. A child with CHD may constitute a long-term family crisis. Frequently the continuing unremitting stresses of care—physical exhaustion, financial costs, emotional upset, fear of death, and concern for the child's future—are not fully appreciated by those caring for the family. Even when the child's condition is stabilized or corrected, the family may need to make adjustments in their lifestyle. Introducing them to other families with similarly affected children can help them adjust to the daily stresses.

EDUCATE FAMILY ABOUT THE DISORDER

When parents are ready to hear about the heart condition, they require a clear explanation based on their level of understanding. A review of the basic structure and function of the heart is helpful before describing the defect. A simple diagram, pictures, or a model of the heart can help parents visualize the heart and the congenital defect.* Parents appreciate receiving written information about the specific condition. A glossary of frequently used terms is also helpful. Parents also require information about prognosis and treatment options.

Increasingly, families are using the Internet as a source of information about heart disease in children.† They are also finding support through contacts with other parents and parent groups. It is important for parents to realize that not all websites offer medically accurate information and that information from other parents might not be applicable to their own situation. Some children with rare, complex heart defects require individualized treatment plans, and general information on the Internet or in books may not apply to their child. Parents should use their health care team, in particular their cardiologist, to discuss information they have received from other sources.

Information given to the child must be tailored to the child's developmental age. As the child matures, the level of information is revised to meet the child's new cognitive level. Preschoolers need basic information about what they will experience more than what is actually occurring physiologically. School-age children benefit from a concrete explanation of the defect. Preadolescents and adolescents often appreciate a more detailed description of how the defect affects their heart. Children of all ages need to express their feelings concerning the diagnosis.

HELP FAMILIES MANAGE THE ILLNESS AT HOME

Parents are the child's principal caregivers and need to develop a positive, supportive working relationship with the health care team. Since most children spend the majority of their time at home with episodic trips to the hospital, parents manage their child's illness on a daily basis. They monitor for signs of illness, give medications and treatments, bring their child to appointments, work with a variety of caregivers, and alert the team about problems. Successful relationships are a partnership between parents and caregivers that is built on mutual trust and respect. Good communication among the family, the cardiology specialists, and the primary care practitioner is essential. As children reach adolescence, they begin to take a larger role in managing their illness and making decisions about their care.

Parents should be aware of the symptoms of their child's cardiac condition and signs of worsening clinical status. Parents of children who may develop CHF should be familiar with the symptoms (see Box 25-5) and know when to contact the practitioner. Parents of children with cyanosis should be informed about fluid management and hypercyanotic spells

---

*The booklet *If Your Child Has a Congenital Heart Defect: A Guide for Parents,* as well as other information, is available from the American Heart Association, 7272 Greenville Ave., Dallas, TX 75231; (214) 373-6300 or (800) AHA-USA1; http://www.americanheart.org.

†The Congenital Heart Information Network (TCHIN), First Floor, 600 North 3rd Street, Philadelphia, PA 19123-2902; (215) 627-4034; fax: (215) 627-4036; http://tchin.org.

(see p. 885). Parents should have an information sheet with their child's diagnosis, significant treatments such as surgical procedures, allergies, other health care problems, current medications, and health care providers' contact numbers available in case of emergencies and to share with other caregivers such as teachers, baby-sitters, or daycare providers.

The family also needs to be knowledgeable regarding the therapeutic management of the disorder and the role that surgery, other procedures, medications, and healthy lifestyle play in maintaining good health. Medications play a critical role in managing some cardiac conditions such as dysrhythmias, severe CHF, anticoagulation for artificial valves, and antirejection medications after heart transplantation. Some patients must take multiple medications daily for their lifetime. Many medications can be dangerous if taken incorrectly and require close monitoring. Parents are taught the correct procedure for giving medications and cautioned to keep them in a safe area to prevent accidental ingestion (see Family-Centered Care box, p. 882).

Another area of parental concern is the child's level of physical activity. Most children do not need to restrict activity, and the best approach is to treat the child normally and allow self-limited activity. Exceptions to self-determined activity primarily involve strenuous recreational and competitive sports in children with specific cardiac problems. Activities and exercise restrictions should be discussed with the child's cardiologist. Deliberately attempting to prevent crying should be avoided because it can establish a maladaptive parental pattern of relating to the infant.

Infants and children with CHD require good nutrition. Breastfeeding should be possible for many infants with CHD. Providing adequate nutrition to infants with CHF or complex congenital defects is especially difficult because of their high caloric requirements and inability to suck effectively because of fatigue and tachypnea. Instructing parents in feeding methods that decrease the infant's work and giving high-calorie formula are important interventions (see p. 883 for a discussion on feeding the infant with CHF). Children with severe cardiac defects are often anorexic. Encouraging them to eat can be a tremendous challenge. Consultation with a dietitian is often helpful. The child should be given a choice of available high-nutrient foods.

Infants with heart disease should be immunized according to the current guidelines. Immunization schedules may need to be modified around times of acute illness or surgical procedures (Smith, 2001). Infants and children less than 2 years of age with unrepaired heart defects, cyanotic lesions, pulmonary hypertension, or history of prematurity should receive the vaccine for respiratory syncytial virus (RSV) monthly during RSV season (November to April in North America) (American Academy of Pediatrics, 2006).

Infants and children who have serious heart disease are at risk for developmental delays. Multiple factors can influence neurodevelopmental outcomes, including genetics (chromosomal abnormalities and microdeletions), family background (parental intelligence quotient [IQ] and socioeconomic status), preoperative factors (including prematurity, cyanosis, shock), intraoperative factors (use of cardiopulmonary bypass, deep hypothermic circulatory arrest), and postoperative factors (hemodynamic instability, hypoxia, acidosis, cardiac arrest, stroke, ischemic events). Recent efforts to limit the time of deep hypothermic circulatory arrest and provide better neuroprotection during infant surgery may improve outcomes in the future. Although most children with serious heart disease are within the normal range for IQ, there is a higher incidence of neurodevelopmental deficits in children after heart surgery than in the normal population, specifically in speech and language, fine motor skills, and cognitive processes (Majnemer and Limperopoulos, 1999). Severe neurologic problems such as cerebral palsy, epilepsy, and mental retardation are uncommon.

PREPARE CHILD AND FAMILY FOR INVASIVE PROCEDURES

Chapter 22 provides an extensive discussion of the principles for preparing children for invasive procedures. The American Heart Association published a scientific statement "Recommendations for Preparing Children and Adolescents for Invasive Cardiac Procedures" (LeRoy, Elixson, O'Brien, and others, 2003), which addresses issues specific to the child with heart disease. The following discussion highlights some important aspects of preparation for cardiac catheterization and cardiac surgery.

The expected outcomes for preprocedure preparation include reducing anxiety, improving patient cooperation with procedures, enhancing recovery, developing trust with caregivers, and improving long-term emotional and behavioral adjustments after procedures (LeRoy, Elixson, O'Brien, and others, 2003). Important factors to consider in planning preparation strategies are the child's cognitive development, previous hospital experiences, child's temperament and coping style, timing of preparation, and the involvement of the parents. The most beneficial preparation strategies usually combine information giving and coping skills training such as conscious breathing exercises, distraction techniques, guided imagery, or other behavioral interventions.

Outpatient preoperative and precatheterization workups are common for most elective procedures. Children are then admitted on the morning of the procedure. Preprocedure teaching is often done in the clinic setting or at home and may include a tour of the intensive care unit (ICU) and inpatient facilities. Children of different ages and developmental levels require different amounts of information and different approaches. Young children should be prepared close in time to the event, whereas older children and adolescents may benefit from teaching several weeks in advance. Parents should be included in the preparation session to support their child and learn about upcoming events.

Topics to include in preoperative or precatheterization preparation include information on the environment, equipment, and procedures that the child will encounter during and following the procedure. Many information-giving techniques can be used such as verbal and written information, hospital tours, preoperative classes, picture books, or videos. Information about what the child will see, hear, and feel should be included, especially for older children and adolescents. Some of the sensory experiences of being in an ICU or catheterization laboratory include sights (monitors, many people, lots of equipment), sounds (beeping noises, alarms, voices), and sensations (lines and dressings, tape, discomfort, thirst). Familiar aspects of the environment, like BP cuffs, stethoscopes, or oximeter probes, are reviewed; and new equipment, such as monitors, IV lines, and oxygen masks, are described. Comforting aspects of the environment, such as play areas, chairs for parents, and televisions, are emphasized. Many patients who will be sedated during catheterization or receiving narcotic pain relievers after surgery will have minimal recall of that period and will not need detailed information about the equipment or procedures used. Information should be specific to the planned procedure for each patient.

A discussion of ways the child can cope with the experience should be included. For a young child, bringing a familiar stuffed animal or comfort object will help relieve anxiety, whereas advising an older child to bring headphones and favorite music to the catheterization laboratory will help distract him or her during the procedure. Recovery topics after catheterization include lying still to prevent bleeding at the catheter site, advancing diet, controlling pain, and monitoring. After surgery, the nurse reviews the importance of ambulation, coughing, deep breathing, drinking, and eating and describes pain management and monitoring routines. Simple coping strategies for use during painful procedures should be reviewed; these include distraction techniques such as counting, blowing, singing, or telling stories.

Children and their families should have a choice about an ICU tour. Exposure to the ICU environment can actually increase anxiety in some children, particularly young children, those with previous hospital experiences, and those who are highly anxious (LeRoy, Elixson, O'Brien, and others, 2003). Usually the day before the procedure is ample time to allow the child to ask questions and to prevent undue fantasizing about the experience. The child should be protected from the frightening sights in the unit; equipment not in view postoperatively, such as equipment located behind or below the bed, needs less attention. The child and parents are encouraged to ask questions or to explore further any equipment in the room, but they should not be pushed to assimilate more information than they are able.

Preoperative physical care differs little, if any, from that for any other surgery and is discussed in Chapter 22. The child should be assured that the parents will be there when the child wakes up; they should be allowed to accompany their child as far as possible to the operating suite (see Surgical Procedures, p. 694). After all of the equipment and procedures have been explained, it is important to talk about "getting well" and going home.

PROVIDE POSTOPERATIVE CARE

Immediate postoperative care is usually provided by specially trained nurses in ICUs. Many of the procedures, such as arterial pressure and central venous pressure (CVP) monitoring, and the observations related to vital functions require advanced educational training (the reader should refer to critical care texts for further information). However, nurses caring for the child before surgery and during the convalescent period need to be familiar with the major principles of care. Selected complications that may occur postoperatively are described in Box 25-7.

Observe Vital Signs

Vital signs and BP are recorded frequently until stable. Heart rate and respirations are counted for 1 full minute, compared with the ECG monitor, and recorded with activity. The heart rate is normally increased after surgery. The nurse observes cardiac rhythm and notifies the practitioner of any changes in regularity. Dysrhythmias may occur postoperatively sec-

BOX 25-7
Selected Complications After Cardiac Surgery and Treatment Approaches

CARDIAC
Congestive heart failure—Digoxin, diuretics (p. 876)
Low cardiac output—Intravenous inotropes (Shock, p. 902)
Dysrhythmias—Identification, drug treatment, possible pacing, cardioversion (p. 896)
Tamponade (blood or fluid in the pericardial space constricting the heart)—Prompt removal of fluid by pericardiocentesis

RESPIRATORY
Atelectasis—Chest physical therapy, coughing, deep breathing, ambulation
Pulmonary edema—Diuretics
Pleural effusions—Diuretics, possible chest tube drainage
Pneumothorax—Possible chest tube drainage

NEUROLOGIC
Seizures—Assessment, antiepileptic drugs
Cerebrovascular accident (stroke), cerebral edema, neurologic deficits—Assessment and treatment

INFECTIOUS DISEASE
Infections (especially wound, pneumonia, otitis media, and sepsis)—Antibiotics

HEMATOLOGIC
Anemia—Iron supplementation, possible transfusion
Postoperative bleeding—Initially, clotting factors, blood products; may need repeat surgery to locate and ligate source of bleeding

OTHER
Postpericardiotomy syndrome (syndrome of fever, leukocytosis, friction rub, pericardial and pleural effusions, and lethargy seen about 7 to 21 days after cardiac surgery; possible viral or autoimmune etiologies)—Antipyretics, diuretics, antiinflammatory medications

ondary to anesthetics, acid-base and electrolyte imbalance, hypoxia, surgical intervention, or trauma to conduction pathways (p. 896).

At least hourly, the lungs are auscultated for breath sounds. Diminished or absent sounds may indicate an area of atelectasis or a pleural effusion or pneumothorax, which necessitates further medical assessment. Temperature changes are typical during the early postoperative period. Hypothermia is expected immediately after surgery from hypothermia procedures, effects of anesthesia, and loss of body heat to the cool environment. During this period the child is kept warm to prevent additional heat loss. Infants may be placed under radiant heat warmers. During the next 24 to 48 hours the body temperature may rise to 37.7° C (100° F) or slightly higher as part of the inflammatory response to tissue trauma. After this period an elevated temperature is most likely a sign of infection and warrants immediate investigation for probable cause.

Intraarterial monitoring of BP is commonly done after open-heart surgery. A catheter is passed into the radial artery or other artery, and the other end is attached to an electronic monitoring system, which provides a continuous recording of the BP. The intraarterial line is maintained with a low-rate, constant infusion of heparinized saline to prevent clotting.

Several IV lines are inserted preoperatively: a peripheral IV to give fluids and medications, and a CVP, which is usually inserted in a large vessel in the neck. Additionally, intracardiac monitoring lines are sometimes placed intraoperatively in the right atrium, left atrium, or pulmonary artery. Intracardiac lines allow assessment of pressures inside the cardiac chambers, providing vital information about volume status, cardiac output, and ventricular function. All lines must be cared for using strict aseptic technique, and patients must be carefully assessed for bleeding at the time of line removal.

Maintain Respiratory Status

Infants usually require mechanical ventilation in the immediate postoperative period. Early extubation in the operating room or early postoperative period is becoming more common. Children, especially those who did not require cardiopulmonary bypass, may be extubated in the operating room or in the first few postoperative hours. Suctioning is performed only as needed and performed carefully to avoid vagal stimulation (which can trigger cardiac dysrhythmias) and laryngospasm, especially in infants. Suctioning is intermittent and maintained for no more than 5 seconds at a time to avoid depleting the oxygen supply. Supplemental oxygen is administered with a manual resuscitation bag before and after the procedure to prevent hypoxia. The heart rate is monitored after suctioning to detect changes in rhythm or rate, especially bradycardia. The child should always be positioned facing the nurse to permit assessment of the child's color and tolerance of the procedure.

> **NURSINGALERT**
>
> During suctioning, observe for signs and symptoms of respiratory distress, such as tachypnea, use of accessory muscles for breathing, and restlessness.

When weaning and extubation are completed, humidified oxygen is delivered by mask, hood, or nasal cannula to prevent drying of mucosa. The child is encouraged to turn and deep breathe at least hourly. Measures are employed to enhance ventilation and decrease pain, such as splinting of the operative site and use of analgesics. Chest tubes are inserted into the pleural or mediastinal space during surgery or in the immediate postoperative period to remove secretions and air to allow reexpansion of the lung. Drainage is checked hourly for color and quantity. Immediately after surgery the drainage may be bright red, but afterward it should be serous. The largest volume of drainage occurs in the first 12 to 24 hours and is greater in extensive heart surgery.

> **NURSINGALERT**
>
> Chest tube drainage greater than 3 ml/kg/hr for more than 3 consecutive hours or 5 to 10 ml/kg in any 1 hour is excessive and may indicate postoperative hemorrhage. The surgeon is notified immediately because cardiac tamponade can develop rapidly and is life threatening.

Chest tubes are usually removed on the first to third postoperative day. Removal of chest tubes is a painful, frightening experience. Analgesics such as morphine sulfate, often combined with midazolam (Versed), should be given before the procedure. Older children are forewarned that they will feel a sharp, momentary pain. After the suture is cut, the tubes are quickly pulled out at the end of full inspiration to prevent intake of air into the pleural cavity. A purse-string suture (placed when the tubes were inserted) is pulled tight to close the opening. A petrolatum-covered gauze dressing is immediately applied over the wound and securely taped on all four sides to the skin so that an airtight seal is formed. It is left on for 1 or 2 days. Breath sounds are checked to assess for a pneumothorax.

Monitor Fluids

Intake and output of all fluids must be accurately calculated. Intake is primarily IV fluids; however, a record of fluid used to flush the arterial and CVP lines or to dilute medications is also kept. Output includes hourly recordings of urine (usually a Foley catheter is inserted and attached to a closed collecting device), drainage from chest and nasogastric tubes, and blood drawn for analysis. Urine is analyzed for specific gravity to assess the concentrating ability of the kidneys and to assess approximately the body's degree of hydration. Renal failure is a potential risk from a transient period of low cardiac output.

> **NURSINGALERT**
>
> The signs of renal failure are decreased urinary output (<1 ml/kg/hr) and elevated levels of blood urea nitrogen and serum creatinine.

Fluids are restricted during the immediate postoperative period to prevent hypervolemia, which places additional demands on the myocardium, predisposing the patient to cardiac failure. To monitor fluid retention, the child is weighed daily, and the same scale is used at approximately the same time each day to avoid errors in measurement. The child is usually given nothing by mouth for the first 24 hours. If an endotracheal (ET) tube is inserted, oral fluids are usually withheld until the child is extubated. Fluid restriction may be imposed even when oral fluids are given. The nurse calculates the distribution over a 24-hour period based on the child's preoperative weight and drinking habits. The distribution should allow for most fluid to be given during the child's most wakeful and active periods.

Provide Rest and Progressive Activity

After heart surgery, rest should be provided to decrease the workload of the heart and promote healing. The simplest way to ensure individualized, efficient, high-quality care is to plan at the beginning of the shift the nursing procedures to be done, with periods of rest identified. The schedule should be shared with parents to allow them to visit at the most advantageous times, such as after a rest period when no special treatments are anticipated.

A progressive schedule of ambulation and activity is planned, based on the child's preoperative activity patterns and postoperative cardiovascular and pulmonary function. Ambulation is initiated early, usually by the second postoperative day, when chest tubes, arterial lines, and assisted ventilatory equipment may be removed. Activity progresses from sitting on the edge of the bed and dangling the legs to standing up and sitting in a chair. Heart rate and respirations are carefully monitored to assess the degree of cardiac demand imposed by each activity. Tachycardia, dyspnea, cyanosis, desaturation, progressive fatigue, or dysrhythmias indicate the need to limit further energy expenditure.

Provide Comfort and Emotional Support

Heart surgery is both painful and frightening for children, and comfort is a primary nursing concern. Several incisions may be used for heart surgery. A median sternotomy is most common, following the sternum down the center of the chest. A ministernotomy opens the lower sternum. A thoracotomy incision is most uncomfortable because it goes through muscle tissue. It allows access to the side of the chest through an incision from under the arm around the back to the scapula.

Most patients need IV analgesics for pain control during the immediate postoperative period. Patient-controlled analgesia may be used with children old enough to understand the concept. Nonsteroidal antiinflammatory drugs (NSAIDs) such as ketorolac (Toradol) may be used intravenously. Paralyzing agents may also be used with the analgesics for children who are agitated or hemodynamically unstable.

After extubation and removal of lines and tubes, pain can be satisfactorily controlled with oral medications such as ibuprofen, codeine with acetaminophen (Tylenol No. 3), or oxycodone and acetaminophen (Tylox). Acetaminophen alone provides adequate pain relief for most children at discharge. Sternotomy incisions are usually well tolerated, with some discomfort when walking and coughing. Thoracotomy incisions are usually more painful because the incision is through muscle; a more aggressive pain management plan with around-the-clock medications for several days is often necessary to allow for adequate rest, ambulation, and pulmonary hygiene.

In addition to pharmacologic pain control, every effort is made to minimize the discomfort of procedures, such as using a firm pillow or favorite stuffed animal placed against the chest incision during movement and performing treatments *after* pain medication is given, preferably at a time that coincides with the drug's peak effect. Nonpharmacologic measures are used to lessen the perception of pain, and parents are encouraged to comfort their child as much as possible. (See also Pain Assessment; Pain Management, Chapter 7.)

Children may become depressed after surgery. This is thought to be caused by preoperative anxiety, postoperative psychologic and physiologic stress, and sensory overstimulation. Typically the child's disposition improves on leaving the ICU.

Children may also be angry and uncooperative after surgery as a response to the physical pain and to the loss of control imposed by the surgery and treatments. They need an opportunity to express feelings, either verbally or through activity. Children often regress in their behavior during the stress of surgery and hospitalization. They also may express feelings of anger or rejection toward parents. The nurse can support the parents by being available for information and explaining all the procedures to them. The first few postoperative days are particularly difficult because parents see their child in pain and realize the potential risks from surgery. They often are overwhelmed by the physical environment of the ICU and feel useless because they can do so little for their child. The nurse can minimize such feelings by including parents in caregiving activities and comfort and play activities, by providing information about the child's condition, and by being sensitive to their emotional and physical needs. The importance of their presence in making the child feel more secure is stressed, even if they do not provide physical care.

FAMILY-CENTERED CARE

Topics to Include in Discharge Teaching After Cardiac Surgery
- Medication teaching (for digoxin, see Family-Centered Care box, p. 882)
- Activity restrictions
- Diet and nutrition
- Wound care (including dressings, if any; suture removal; bathing)
- Bacterial endocarditis prophylaxis (see Box 25-9)
- Follow-up appointments (cardiologist, primary care provider)
- Community agencies as needed (visiting nurse service, early developmental intervention)
- When to call practitioner; signs and symptoms of postoperative problems
- Review of cardiac defect and surgical repair

PLAN FOR DISCHARGE AND HOME CARE

Ideally, discharge planning begins on admission for cardiac surgery and includes an assessment of the parents' adjustment to the child's altered state of health. Neonates need additional screening tests (such as newborn metabolic screen and hearing tests) and may need immunizations before discharge (Dodds and Merle, 2005). The family will need both verbal and written instructions on medication, nutrition, activity restrictions, subacute bacterial endocarditis, return to school, wound care, and signs and symptoms of infection or complications (see Family-Centered Care box). Referrals to community agencies may be warranted to assist parents in the transition from hospital to home and to reinforce the teaching.

The parents will also need clear instructions on when to seek medical care for complications and how to contact the health care provider. Follow-up with the cardiologist and primary care provider is also arranged before discharge. Parents should have a summary, including their child's medical condition, medications, and health care providers available for emergencies. Appropriate identification, such as a MedicAlert device, is indicated for children with a pacemaker or a heart transplant and for those receiving anticoagulation therapy or antidysrhythmic medication.

Although surgical correction of heart defects has improved dramatically, it is still not possible to completely repair many of the complex anomalies. For many children, repeat procedures are required to replace conduits or grafts or to manage complications such as restenosis. Consequently, the long-term prognosis is uncertain, and full recovery is not always possible. For these families, medical follow-up and continued emotional support are essential. The nurse can often serve as an important primary health professional and as a resource for referrals when needed.

ACQUIRED CARDIOVASCULAR DISORDERS
BACTERIAL (INFECTIVE) ENDOCARDITIS

Bacterial endocarditis (BE), or infective endocarditis (IE), also referred to as **subacute bacterial endocarditis (SBE),** is an infection of the valves and inner lining of the heart. Although it can occur without underlying heart disease, it is most often a sequela of bacteremia in the child with acquired or congenital anomalies of the heart or great vessels. It especially affects children with valvular abnormalities, prosthetic valves, shunts, recent cardiac surgery with invasive lines, and rheumatic heart disease with valve involvement. The most common causative agent is *Streptococcus viridans;* other causative agents are *Staphylococcus aureus,* gram-negative bacteria, and fungi such as *Candida albicans.*

Pathophysiology

Organisms may enter the bloodstream from any site of localized infection. In the past, endocarditis was believed to be highly associated with invasive procedures; however, endocarditis is most likely to occur from routine exposure to bacteremia associated with usual daily activities, although it can also occur after procedures such as dental work *(S. viridans);* after invasive procedures involving the gastrointestinal-genitourinary tract; after cardiac surgery, especially if synthetic material is used (valves, patches, conduits); or from long-term indwelling catheters. The microorganisms grow on the endocardium, forming vegetations (verrucae), deposits of fibrin, and platelet thrombi. The lesion may invade adjacent tissues, such as aortic and mitral valves, and may break off and embolize elsewhere, especially in the spleen, kidney, and central nervous system.

Diagnostic Evaluation

The diagnosis of IE is suspected on the basis of clinical manifestations (Box 25-8). Several laboratory findings may suggest IE (e.g., ECG changes [prolonged PR interval], radiographic evidence of cardiomegaly, anemia, elevated erythrocyte sedimentation rate, leukocytosis, microscopic hematuria). Vegetations on the valve and abnormal valve function can often be visualized by echocardiography. Definitive diagnosis rests on growth and identification of the causative agent in the blood.

Therapeutic Management

Treatment should be instituted immediately and consists of administration of high doses of appropriate antibiotics intravenously for 2 to 8 weeks. Blood cultures are taken periodically to evaluate response to antibiotic therapy.

Prevention involves administration of prophylactic antibiotic therapy 1 hour before procedures known to increase the risk of entry of organisms in very high–risk patients. New guidelines only require prophylaxis in patients with the highest risk of poor outcome if they develop endocarditis (Box 25-9). Drugs of choice for prophylaxis include amoxicillin, ampicillin, clindamycin, cephalexin, cefadroxil, azithromycin, and clarithromycin.

Nursing Care Management

Ideally, the objective of nursing care is to counsel parents of high-risk children concerning the signs and symptoms of endocarditis and, in certain cases, the need for prophylactic antibiotic therapy before procedures such as dental work. The family's regular dentist should be advised of the child's cardiac diagnosis as an added precaution to ensure preventive treatment. SBE prophylaxis is now reserved for very high–risk patients. Many patients who met criteria established in the past may not require prophylaxis under the new guidelines (Wilson, Taubert, Gewitz, and others, 2007) (see Box 25-9). Parents should be counseled regarding the rationale for discontinuing prophylaxis and should be educated as to the fact

---

BOX 25-8

Clinical Manifestations of Infective Endocarditis

Onset usually insidious
Unexplained fever (low grade and intermittent)
Anorexia
Malaise
Weight loss
Characteristic findings caused by extracardiac emboli formation:
- Splinter hemorrhages (thin black lines) under the nails
- Osler nodes (red, painful intradermal nodes found on pads of phalanges)
- Janeway lesions (painless hemorrhagic areas on palms and soles)
- Petechiae on oral mucous membranes
May be present:
- Congestive heart failure
- Cardiac dysrhythmias
- New murmur or change in previously existing one

BOX 25-9

Cardiac Conditions Associated with the Highest Risk of Adverse Outcome from Endocarditis

Prophylaxis with dental procedures recommended for*:
- Previous episode of infective endocarditis
- Prosthetic cardiac valve
Congenital heart disease (CHD), including only:
- Unrepaired cyanotic CHD, including palliative shunts and conduits
- Completely repaired congenital heart defect with prosthetic material or device, whether placed by surgery or by catheter intervention, during the first 6 months after the procedure
Repaired CHD with residual defects at the site or adjacent to the site of a prosthetic patch or prosthetic device (which inhibit endothelialization)
Cardiac transplantation recipients who develop cardiac valvulopathy

Adapted from Wilson W, Taubert K, Gewitz M, and others: Prevention of infective endocarditis: guidelines from the American Heart Association, *Circulation* 116(15):1736-1754, 2007.
*Except for the conditions listed, antibiotic prophylaxis is no longer recommended for any other form of CHD.

---

that their child is still at risk. It is important that all children with congenital or acquired heart disease maintain the highest level of oral health to reduce the chance of bacteremia from oral infections.

Parents should also have a high index of suspicion regarding potential infections. Without unduly alarming them, the nurse stresses that any unexplained fever, weight loss, or change in behavior (lethargy, malaise, anorexia) must be brought to the practitioner's attention. Such symptoms should not be self-diagnosed as a cold or flu. Early diagnosis and treatment are important in preventing further cardiac damage, embolic complications, and growth of resistant organisms.

Treatment of endocarditis requires long-term parenteral drug therapy. In many cases, IV antibiotics may be administered at home with nursing supervision for part of the treatment course. Nursing goals during this period are (1) preparation of the child for IV infusion, usually with an intermittent-infusion device, and several venipunctures for blood cultures; (2) observation for side effects of antibiotics, especially inflammation along venipuncture sites; (3) observation for complications, including embolism and CHF; and (4) education regarding the importance of follow-up visits for

nursingcareguidelines

Diagnosis of Initial Attack of Rheumatic Fever (Jones Criteria, 1992 Update)*

MAJOR MANIFESTATIONS

Carditis

Tachycardia out of proportion to degree of fever

Cardiomegaly

New murmurs or change in preexisting murmurs

Muffled heart sounds

Pericardial friction rub

Chest pain

Changes in electrocardiogram (especially prolonged PR interval)

Polyarthritis

Swollen, hot, red, painful joint(s)

After 1 to 2 days, different joint(s) affected

Favors large joints—knees, elbows, hips, shoulders, wrists

Erythema Marginatum

Erythematous macules with clear center and wavy, well-demarcated border

Transitory

Nonpruritic

Primarily affects trunk and extremities (inner surfaces)

Chorea (St. Vitus Dance, Sydenham Chorea)

Sudden aimless, irregular movements of extremities

Involuntary facial grimaces

Speech disturbances

Emotional lability

Muscle weakness (can be profound)

Muscle movements exaggerated by anxiety and attempts at fine motor activity; relieved by rest

Subcutaneous Nodes

Nontender swelling

Located over bony prominences

May persist for some time, then gradually resolve

MINOR MANIFESTATIONS

Clinical Findings

Arthralgia

Fever

Laboratory Findings

Elevated acute-phase reactants

- Erythrocyte sedimentation rate
- C-reactive protein

SUPPORTING EVIDENCE OF ANTECEDENT GROUP A STREPTOCOCCAL INFECTION

Positive throat culture or rapid streptococcal antigen test

Elevated or rising streptococcal antibody titer

From Special Writing Group of the Committee on Rheumatic Fever, Endocarditis, and Kawasaki Disease of the Council on Cardiovascular Disease in the Young of the American Heart Association: Guidelines for the diagnosis of rheumatic fever: Jones criteria, 1992 (update), *JAMA* 268:2069-2073, 1992.

*If supported by evidence of preceding group A streptococcal infection, the presence of two major manifestations or of one major and two minor manifestations indicates a high probability of acute rheumatic fever.

cardiac evaluation, echocardiographic monitoring, and blood cultures.

RHEUMATIC FEVER

Rheumatic fever (RF) is a poorly understood inflammatory disease that occurs after infection with group A β-hemolytic streptococcal (GABHS) pharyngitis. It occurs most often in late school-age children or adolescents and is rare in adults. It is a self-limited illness that involves the joints, skin, brain, serous surfaces, and heart. Cardiac valve damage (referred to as **rheumatic heart disease**) is the most significant complication of RF. The mitral valve is most often affected. In developed countries RF and rheumatic heart disease have become uncommon. However, RF remains a devastating problem in developing (Third World) countries and has reappeared in some parts of the United States (Gentles, Colan, Wilson, and others, 2001).

Etiology

Strong evidence supports a relationship between upper respiratory tract infection with GABHS and subsequent development of RF (usually within 2 to 6 weeks). Acute RF is the result of an exaggerated immune response to bacteria in a susceptible host (Carapetis, McDonald, and Wilson, 2005). In almost all cases of RF a previous infection with GABHS can be documented by laboratory evidence of rising antibody titers. Prevention or treatment of GABHS infection prevents RF.

Diagnostic Evaluation

Diagnosis is based on a set of guidelines recommended by the American Heart Association (Newburger, Takahashi, Gerber, and others, 2004). These guidelines, known as **modifications of the Jones criteria,** suggest that the presence of two major manifestations or one major and two minor manifestations, such as fever and arthralgia, with supportive evidence of recent streptococcal infection, indicates a high probability of RF (see Nursing Care Guidelines box).

Children suspected of having RF are tested for streptococcal antibodies. The most reliable and best standardized test is an elevated or rising **antistreptolysin O (ASO or ASLO) titer,** which occurs in 80% of children with RF.

Therapeutic Management

The goals of medical management are (1) eradication of hemolytic streptococci, (2) prevention of permanent cardiac damage, (3) palliation of the other symptoms, and (4) prevention of recurrences of RF. Penicillin is the drug of choice, with erythromycin as a substitute in penicillin-sensitive children. Salicylates are used to control the inflammatory process, especially in the joints, and reduce the fever and discomfort. Bed rest is recommended during the acute febrile phase but need not be strict.

Prophylactic treatment against recurrence of RF is started after the acute therapy and involves monthly intramuscular injections of benzathine penicillin G (1.2 million units), two daily oral doses of penicillin (200,000 units), or one daily dose of sulfadiazine (1 g). The duration of long-term prophylaxis is uncertain, but 5 years since the last episode or age 18, longer with cardiac involvement, is suggested by the World Health Organization (Carapetis, McDonald, and Wilson, 2005).

Children who have had acute RF are susceptible to recurrent RF for the rest of their lives and should be followed medically for at least 5 years. Repeated infections are likely to result in rheumatic heart disease. Children and families must be aware of the need for continuing antibiotic prophylaxis for dental work, infection, and invasive procedures.

Nursing Care Management

The objectives of nursing care for the child with RF are to (1) encourage compliance with drug regimens, (2) facilitate recovery from the illness, (3) provide emotional support, and (4) prevent the disease. Because compliance is a major concern in long-term drug therapy, every effort is made to encourage adherence to the therapeutic plan (see Compliance, Chapter 22). When compliance is poor, monthly injections may be substituted for daily oral administration of antibiotics, and children need preparation for this often-dreaded procedure.

Interventions during home care are primarily concerned with providing rest and adequate nutrition. Usually, after the febrile stage is over, children can resume moderate activity, and their appetite improves. If carditis is present, the family must be aware of any activity restrictions and may need help in choosing less strenuous activities for the child.

One of the most disturbing and frustrating manifestations of the disease is **chorea.** The onset is gradual and may occur weeks to months after the illness; it sometimes even occurs in children who have not been diagnosed with RF. It may be mistaken for nervousness, clumsiness, behavioral changes, inattentiveness, and learning disability. It is usually a source of great frustration to the child because the movements, incoordination, and weakness severely limit physical ability. Of utmost importance is stressing to parents and schoolteachers the involuntary, sudden nature of the movements; that the chorea is transitory; and that all manifestations eventually disappear.

Nurses also have a role in prevention, primarily in screening school-age children for sore throats caused by GABHS. This may involve actively participating in throat culture screening programs or in referring children with a possible streptococcal infection for testing.

HYPERLIPIDEMIA (HYPERCHOLESTEROLEMIA)

Hyperlipidemia is a general term for excessive lipids (fat and fatlike substances); **hypercholesterolemia** refers to excessive cholesterol in the blood. High lipid or cholesterol levels play an important role in producing atherosclerosis (fatty plaque on the arteries), which eventually can lead to coronary artery disease, a primary cause of morbidity and mortality in the adult population. A presymptomatic phase of atherosclerosis can begin in childhood. Preventive cardiology is focusing on the screening and management of lipid levels in childhood. The goal is to identify those children at high risk and intervene early.

Cholesterol is part of the lipoprotein complex in plasma that is essential for cellular metabolism. Triglycerides, natural

---

TABLE 25-5

Classification of Cholesterol Levels in Children from Families with a History of Heart Disease

CATEGORY	TOTAL CHOLESTEROL (mg/dl)	LDL CHOLESTEROL (mg/dl)
Acceptable	<170	<110
Borderline	170-199	110-129
High	≥200	≥130

From National Cholesterol Education Program: Report of the Expert Panel on Blood Cholesterol Levels in Children and Adolescents, *Pediatrics* 89(3 Pt 2):527, 1992.
LDL, Low-density lipoprotein.

---

fats synthesized from carbohydrates, are used for energy. Both are major lipids transported on **lipoproteins,** a combination of lipids and proteins, which include:

Low-density lipoproteins (LDLs)—These contain low concentrations of triglycerides, high levels of cholesterol, and moderate levels of protein. LDL is the major carrier of cholesterol to the cells. Cells use cholesterol for synthesis of membranes and steroid production. Elevated circulating LDL is a strong risk factor in cardiovascular disease.

High-density lipoproteins (HDLs)—These contain very low concentrations of triglycerides, relatively little cholesterol, and high levels of protein. They transport free cholesterol to the liver for excretion in the bile. High levels of HDL are thought to protect against cardiovascular disease.

Diagnostic Evaluation

Hyperlipidemia is diagnosed on the basis of analysis of blood for a full lipid profile, drawn after a 12-hour fast. A screening thyroid-stimulating hormone (TSH) is useful to rule out hypothyroidism as a cause of secondary hypercholesterolemia. In overweight children, a fasting glucose may be obtained to assess for the potential of metabolic syndrome, which is a combination of multiple symptoms that are associated with increased cardiovascular risk in adults. Blood samples should be collected after having the child sit for 5 minutes, and the tourniquet should be applied immediately before the needle puncture, since posture and vascular stasis may affect results. Diagnostic values for acceptable, borderline, and high total cholesterol and LDL cholesterol levels are listed in Table 25-5.

Screening children for hypercholesterolemia is a controversial issue, with some authorities advocating universal screening and others proposing selective screening. Guidelines from the American Academy of Pediatrics' Committee on Nutrition (American Academy of Pediatrics, 1998) recommend a strategy that combines two complementary approaches: (1) a **population approach** that aims to lower the average levels of blood cholesterol among all American children through population-wide changes in nutrient intake and eating patterns, and (2) an **individualized approach** based on selective screening (see Evidence-Based Practice box).

Therapeutic Management

The first step in the treatment of high cholesterol is oriented to lifestyle modification. The American Academy of Pediatrics (1998) guidelines advocate a heart-healthy diet for all children. Children with known elevated cholesterol should have

EVIDENCE-BASED PRACTICE

Cholesterol Screening for Children

ASK THE QUESTION   Should cholesterol screening be performed in children?

SEARCH FOR EVIDENCE
Search Strategies   The literature was searched to locate clinical research studies related to this issue. Selection criteria included English language, publication within the past 10 years, research-based articles (level 3 or lower), infant and child populations.
Databases Used   PubMed, Cochrane Collaboration, MD Consult, Joanna Briggs Institute, National Guidelines Clearinghouse (AHRQ), TRIP Database Plus, PedsCCM, BestBETs

CRITICALLY ANALYZE THE EVIDENCE

The rationale for lipid screening and management in children is evolving now that lipid levels have been monitored from childhood into adulthood. Children who have cholesterol levels in the upper percentiles seem to have an increased risk of remaining in the upper percentiles into adulthood (Nicklas, von Duvillard, and Berenson, 2002). The more severely affected children are generally the ones targeted for dietary and possibly pharmacologic intervention. On the other hand, children in the lower percentiles are unlikely to have high cholesterol levels as adults.

Cholesterol levels in childhood appear to be a major population predictor for adult cholesterol levels (American Academy of Pediatrics, 1998). The precursors of atherosclerosis are present in young people. Findings from autopsy studies from more than 50 years ago of young people who have died of accidents and injuries have shown that the atherosclerotic process begins early in life (Enos, Holmes, and Beyer, 1953; Strong, Malcom, McMahan, and others, 1999). Furthermore, the extent of atherosclerosis is related to the presence and degree of cardiovascular risk factors in adults (Berenson, Srinivasan, Bao, and others, 1998).

Many experts favor selective screening because high blood cholesterol levels aggregate in families as a result of shared genetic and environmental factors (American Academy of Pediatrics, 1998). In addition, the most severely affected children generally come from families in which there is a high incidence of early heart disease.

APPLY THE EVIDENCE: NURSING IMPLICATIONS

Current recommendations include selective screening of children over the age of 2 years who have a sibling, parent, or grandparent with an elevated cholesterol level of 240 mg/dl or higher. In addition, children should be screened if they have a first- or second-degree relative with early atherosclerotic disease (stroke, myocardial infarction, sudden cardiac death, angina, or peripheral vascular disease). Screening should also be done if the child has any individual risk factors such as diabetes, hypertension, obesity, a history of Kawasaki disease, or nephritic syndrome. Lastly, cholesterol screening should be performed if the child's genetic family history is unknown.

References

American Academy of Pediatrics: Cholesterol in childhood, *Pediatrics* 101(1, Pt 1):141-147, 1998.
Berenson GS, Srinivasan SR, Bao W, and others: Association between multiple cardiovascular risk factors and atherosclerosis in children and young adults, *N Engl J Med* 338(23):1650-1656, 1998.
Enos WF, Holmes RH, Beyer J: Coronary disease among United States soldiers killed in action in Korea, *JAMA* 152(12):1090-1093, 1953.
Nicklas TA, von Duvillard SP, Berenson GS: Tracking of serum lipids and lipoproteins from childhood to dyslipidemia in adults: the Bogalusa Heart Study, *Int J Sports Med* 23(Suppl 1):S39-S43, 2002.
Strong JP, Malcom GT, McMahan CA, and others: Prevalence and extent of atherosclerosis in adolescents and young adults: implications for prevention from the Pathobiological Determinants of Atherosclerosis in Youth Study, *JAMA* 281(8):727-735, 1999.

individual nutritional counseling by a nutritionist with expertise in pediatric lipids.

Research continues to support the benefit of diets low in saturated fats (Van Horn, Obarzanek, Friedman, and others, 2005). Current thinking favors a "Mediterranean"-type diet. Whole grains, fruits, and vegetables form the foundation of this diet. In addition, this diet allows the use of monounsaturated fats, such as olive oil and canola oil, which have beneficial effects on HDL-cholesterol values. The use of these fats also makes the diet more realistic. Daily aerobic exercise of at least 60 minutes a day is also recommended for children with high cholesterol. In addition, patients and parents should be counseled regarding the negative effects of smoking (both first hand and second hand).

For children with severe hypercholesterolemia who fail to respond to dietary modifications (after a 6- to 12-month trial), drug therapy may be necessary. Pharmacologic therapy is recommended for children with LDL cholesterol over 190 mg/dl without other risk factors or over 160 mg/dl in patients with two or more other risk factors. In most situations, medication is reserved for boys over 10 years old and for girls once they begin their menses.

In the past, bile acid–binding resins were the only class of drugs recommended for treatment of children. This class of drug acts by binding bile acids in the intestinal lumen. Because they are not absorbed by the intestine, they do not produce systemic toxicity and are safe for children. Cholestyramine (Questran) and colestipol (Colestid) are both powders that are mixed with water or juice just before ingestion. Unfortunately, the vast majority of patients do not get adequate reduction in LDL-cholesterol from bile acid–binding resins. Many cannot tolerate the medication because of the taste; gritty texture; and side effects, the most significant being constipation, abdominal pain, gastrointestinal bloating, flatulence, and nausea. The most recent findings on lipid abnormalities in children recommends treatment with statins if pharmacologic therapy is indicated, using the previously outlined guidelines for treatment (McCrindle, Urbina, Dennison, and others, 2007). Statins are much more effective at lowering LDL cholesterol and triglycerides and raising HDL cholesterol. Statins work by inhibiting the enzyme necessary for cholesterol synthesis. Statins are most effective when taken in the evening and are started at the lowest possible dose in young people. Blood work should be followed closely and should include a fasting lipid profile, liver function tests, and creatinine kinase repeated at 4- and 8-week intervals initially and with dosage changes.

Patients beginning therapy with a statin should be counseled regarding rare but potentially serious side effects such as rhabdomyolysis, elevated transaminases, and elevated creatinine kinase. Patients should discontinue their medication and contact their practitioner if they develop dark urine or new muscle aches. Lastly, statin medications are not safe during pregnancy and therefore sexually active adolescents need to take adequate birth control measures. Very long–term studies are unlikely to be available over decades; however, in the shorter-term studies that have been completed, statins seem to have a similar safety profile for children as they do for adults (McCrindle, Urbina, Dennison, and others, 2007).

Nursing Care Management

Nurses play an important role in the screening, education, and support of children with hyperlipidemia and their families. When a child is referred to a lipid clinic, it is essential that the family be adequately prepared for the first visit. Generally, the parents will be asked to keep a dietary history of the child before this visit. Sometimes they will need to complete a questionnaire regarding the child's normal dietary habits during the preceding year. Families should be instructed to keep their child fasting for at least 12 hours before screening. It is important to schedule the blood test early in the morning and to arrange for nourishment immediately thereafter. At the visit, a full family history should be taken, including the health of both parents and all first-degree relatives. Specific questions should be asked regarding early heart disease, hypertension, strokes (CVAs), sudden death, hyperlipidemia, diabetes, and endocrine abnormalities.

Parents and extended families should be informed about cholesterol and hyperlipidemia. This education should include a brief introduction to the different lipoprotein categories, including cholesterol, HDL, LDL, and triglycerides. Also, behavioral risk factors for heart disease, such as smoking and exercise, should be reviewed. For management to be effective, parents need to understand the rationale for dietary or pharmacologic intervention. The key is prevention of future cardiovascular disease.

Stringent dietary guidelines may become an issue of control and a source of great stress for many families. Children should not be viewed as having a disease. Rather, the positive aspects of healthy eating, regularly exercising, and avoiding smoking should be emphasized. Basic dietary changes should be encouraged for the whole family so that the affected child is not singled out. Cultural differences must be considered and recommendations individualized. Substitution rather than elimination needs to be emphasized. Visual aids (e.g., test tubes depicting the amount of fat in a hot dog) are often helpful, especially for children. Diets should be flexible and individually tailored by a nutritionist experienced in combining recommendations that meet both the nutritional demands of the growing child and the lipid modifications. Parents are encouraged to participate in dietary and educational sessions, ask questions, and share ideas and experiences.

Parents often feel guilty about the hereditary component of hyperlipidemia. Many also believe they have failed if the diet alone is not making a significant difference in their child's lipid profile. They need to be reassured that a dietary approach alone is often not sufficient, especially for children with significantly elevated values.

Parents of children who require pharmacologic therapy need to understand the purpose, dosage, and possible side effects of the various drugs. Medication schedules should remain flexible and should not interfere with the child's daily activities. Follow-up phone calls by the nurse between visits allow parents to discuss their concerns and ask any questions that have arisen.

CARDIAC DYSRHYTHMIAS

Dysrhythmias, or abnormal heart rhythms, can occur in children with structurally normal hearts, as features of some congenital heart defects, and in patients after surgical repair of congenital heart defects. They are also seen in patients with cardiomyopathy and with cardiac tumors. They can occur secondary to metabolic and electrolyte imbalances. They can be classified in several ways, including by heart rate characteristics (bradycardia and tachycardia) and by the origin of the dysrhythmia in the atria or ventricles. Some dysrhythmias are well tolerated and self-limiting. Others may cause decreased cardiac output with associated symptoms. Some dysrhythmias can cause sudden death. Treatment depends on the cause of the dysrhythmia and its severity.

Many advances have been made in the diagnosis and treatment of pediatric dysrhythmias in the past decade. Improvements in technology have allowed better diagnosis, the development of ablation techniques, and the expansion of pacemaker capabilities. New antidysrhythmic medications have proven safe and effective in children. Radiofrequency ablation has offered a cure for some dysrhythmias. Pediatric electrophysiology has become a highly specialized field, and the student should consult more detailed sources for an in-depth discussion. The following sections address diagnostic studies and provide a general discussion of the most common tachycardia (supraventricular tachycardia [SVT]) and the most common bradycardia (complete heart block) that require treatment in the pediatric population.

Diagnostic Evaluation

Nurses must be familiar with the standards of normal heart rate for the particular age-group (see inside back cover). An initial nursing responsibility is recognition of an abnormal heartbeat, either in rate or rhythm. When a dysrhythmia is suspected, the apical rate is counted for a full minute and compared with the radial rate, which may be lower because not all of the apical beats are felt. Consistently high or low heart rates should be regarded as suspicious. The patient should be placed on a cardiac monitor with recording capabilities. A 12-lead ECG yields more information than the monitor recording and should be done as soon as possible.

The basic diagnostic procedure is the ECG, including 24-hour Holter monitoring. **Electrophysiologic cardiac catheterization** allows for identification of the conduction disturbance and immediate investigation of drugs that may control the dysrhythmia. Another procedure that may be employed is **transesophageal recording.** An electrode catheter is passed to the lower esophagus and, when in position at a point proximal to the heart, is used to stimulate and record dysrhythmias.

Dysrhythmias can be classified according to various criteria, such as effect on heart rate and rhythm, as follows:

Bradydysrhythmias—Abnormally slow rate
Tachydysrhythmias—Abnormally rapid rate
Conduction disturbances—Irregular heart rate

Bradydysrhythmias. Sinus bradycardia (slower than normal rate) in children can be due to the influence of the autonomic nervous system, as with hypervagal tone, or in response to hypoxia and hypotension. Sinus bradycardias are also known to develop after some complex cardiac surgical repairs involving extensive atrial suture lines such as atrial baffle repairs (Mustard and Senning repairs) and the Fontan procedure.

Complete atrioventricular block (AV block) is also referred to as **complete heart block.** This can be either congenital (occurring in children with structurally normal hearts) or acquired after surgery to repair cardiac defects. AV blocks are most often related to edema around the conduction system and resolve without treatment. Temporary epicardial wires are placed in most patients at surgery; if a rhythm disturbance occurs, temporary pacing can be employed. Several days after surgery, the health practitioner removes the wires by pulling slowly and deliberately down on them from the site of insertion.

Some children may need a permanent pacemaker. The pacemaker takes over or assists in the heart's conduction function. The implantation of a pacemaker, in the operating room or possibly the catheterization laboratory, is usually a low-risk procedure. The pacemaker is made up of two basic parts: the pulse generator and the lead. The pulse generator is composed of the battery and the electronic circuitry. The lead is an insulated, flexible wire that conducts the electrical impulse from the pulse generator to the heart. Two types of leads are available: transvenous and epicardial. After the lead has been attached to the heart, a small incision is made and a pocket is formed under the muscle to house and protect the generator. Continuous ECG monitoring is necessary during the recovery phase to assess pacemaker function. The nurse should be aware of the programmed rate and expected individual generator variations. The pacemaker insertion site is monitored for signs of infection. Analgesics are given for pain.

Pacemaker functions have become more sophisticated, and some models can adjust heart rate to activity demands or be programmed for overdrive pacing or cardioversion.

Discharge teaching includes information about the signs and symptoms of infection, general wound care, and activity restrictions. Parents, and patients if they are old enough, should be taught to take a pulse and know the settings of the pacemaker. If the patient's low rate is set at 80 beats/min and the heart rate is only 68 beats/min, there is a possible problem with the pacemaker that needs to be investigated. Instructions for telephone transmission of ECG readings are also given. Telephone transmission can be used to transmit ECG strips and also to monitor battery life and pacemaker function. The pacemaker generator will have to be replaced periodically because of battery depletion. Children with pacemakers should wear a medical alert device, and their parents should have a paper identification card with specific pacer data in case of an emergency. Cardiopulmonary resuscitation (CPR) instruction is suggested for parents.

Tachydysrhythmias. **Sinus tachycardia** (abnormally fast heart rate) secondary to fever, anxiety, pain, anemia, dehydration, or any other etiologic factor requiring increased cardiac output should be ruled out before diagnosing an increased heart rate as pathologic. SVT is the most common tachydysrhythmia found in children and refers to a rapid regular heart rate of 200 to 300 beats/min. The onset of SVT is often sudden, the duration is variable, and the rhythm may end abruptly and convert back to a normal sinus rhythm.

Clinical signs in infants and young children are poor feeding, extreme irritability, and pallor. Children may experience palpitations, dizziness, chest pain, and diaphoresis. If SVT is sustained, signs of CHF may be seen.

The treatment of SVT depends on the degree of compromise imposed by the dysrhythmia. In some cases, vagal maneuvers, such as applying ice to the face, massaging the carotid artery (on one side of the neck only), or having an older child perform a Valsalva maneuver (e.g., exhaling against a closed glottis, blowing on a thumb as if it were a trumpet for 30 to 60 seconds), have terminated SVT. If vagal maneuvers fail or the child is hemodynamically unstable, adenosine (a drug that impairs AV conduction) may be used. Adenosine is given by rapid IV push with a saline bolus immediately after the drug because of its very short half-life. If this is unsuccessful or cardiac output is compromised, esophageal overdrive pacing or synchronized cardioversion (delivering an electrical shock to the heart) can be employed in the intensive care setting. Sedation is needed for both procedures. Cardioversion should never be done in a conscious patient. More long-term pharmacologic treatment includes digoxin or possibly propranolol (Inderal) or amiodarone for severe or recurrent SVT.

A primary focus of nursing care is education of the family regarding the symptoms of SVT and its treatment. SVT may occur again despite therapy. Parents should be taught to take a radial pulse for a full minute. If medication is prescribed, instructions regarding accurate dosage and the importance of administering the correct dose at specified intervals are stressed.

Radiofrequency ablation has become first-line therapy for some types of SVT. The procedure is done in the cardiac catheterization laboratory and begins with mapping of the conduction system to identify the dysrhythmia focus. A catheter delivering radiofrequency current is directed at the site, and the area is heated to destroy the tissue in the area. These are lengthy procedures, often 6 to 8 hours, and sedation or general anesthesia is required. Preparation is similar to that for cardiac catheterization.

PULMONARY ARTERY HYPERTENSION

Pulmonary artery hypertension (PAH) describes a group of rare disorders that result in an elevation of pulmonary artery pressure above 25 mm Hg at rest after the neonatal period (Barst, 1999). These disorders are poorly understood, and until recently there was no treatment beyond supportive care. PAH is a progressive, eventually fatal disease for which there is no known cure. It can be difficult to diagnose in the early stages. Often when patients become symptomatic and a diagnosis is made, their disease is rapidly progressing, treatment is unsuccessful, and death occurs within several years. Significant new information about the disease process, genetic links, diagnosis, and treatment has recently been learned that may improve treatments and outcomes for these patients.

PAH affects the small pulmonary arteries and is characterized by vascular narrowing leading to an increase in pulmonary vascular resistance. Why some children develop the disease and others do not is unclear. There are many possible causes of PAH. Cardiac causes occur primarily in patients with a large left-to-right shunt producing increased pulmonary blood flow. If these defects are not repaired early, the high pulmonary flow will cause changes in the pulmonary artery vessels and the vessels will lose their elasticity. Other causes of PAH include hypoxic lung diseases, thromboembolic diseases causing pulmonary vascular obstruction, collagen vascular diseases, and exposure to toxic substances. Many of the patients have no identifiable cause for PAH and have primary or idiopathic PAH.

Clinical Manifestations

The clinical manifestations include dyspnea with exercise, chest pain, and syncope. Dyspnea is the most common symptom and is caused by impaired oxygen delivery. Chest pain is the result of coronary ischemia in the right ventricle from severe hypertrophy. Syncope reflects a limited cardiac output leading to decreased cerebral blood flow. Right-sided heart dysfunction is steadily progressive, and when symptoms of venous congestion and edema are present, prognosis is poor.

Therapeutic Management

Although no cure is known, several therapies have shown promise in slowing the progression of the disease and improving quality of life. In general, situations that may exacerbate the disease and cause hypoxia, such as exercise and high altitudes, are avoided. Supplemental oxygen, especially at night while sleeping, is commonly used to relieve hypoxia. Patients are at risk for thromboembolic events leading to pulmonary emboli, so anticoagulation with warfarin (Coumadin) is often prescribed.

Vasodilator therapy (which relaxes vascular smooth muscle and reduces pulmonary artery pressure) can prolong survival of patients with PAH. Oral calcium channel blockers have been successful in some children. Continuous IV prostacyclin has been used with some success in children who did not respond to oral therapy. Both these therapies, although promising, have been used in only small numbers of patients and are expensive. Lung transplantation may be another treatment option.

CARDIOMYOPATHY

Cardiomyopathy refers to abnormalities of the myocardium in which the cardiac muscles' ability to contract is impaired. Cardiomyopathies are relatively rare in children. Possible etiologic factors include familial or genetic causes, infection, deficiency states, metabolic abnormalities, and collagen vascular diseases. Most cardiomyopathies in children are considered primary or idiopathic, in which the cause is unknown and the cardiac dysfunction is not associated with systemic disease. Some of the known causes of **secondary** cardiomyopathy are anthracycline toxicity (the antineoplastic agents doxorubicin [Adriamycin] and daunomycin), hemochromatosis (from excessive iron storage), Duchenne muscular dystrophy, Kawasaki disease (KD), collagen diseases, and thyroid dysfunction.

Cardiomyopathies can be divided into three broad clinical categories according to the type of abnormal structure and dysfunction present: dilated cardiomyopathy, hypertrophic cardiomyopathy, and restrictive cardiomyopathy.

Dilated cardiomyopathy is characterized by ventricular dilation and greatly decreased contractility resulting in symptoms of CHF. This is the most common type of cardiomyopathy in children. Its cause is often unknown. The clinical findings are of CHF with tachycardia, dyspnea, hepatosplenomegaly, fatigue, and poor growth. Dysrhythmias may be present and may be more difficult to control with worsening heart failure.

Hypertrophic cardiomyopathy is characterized by an increase in heart muscle mass without an increase in cavity size, usually occurring in the left ventricle and associated with abnormal diastolic filling. It is a familial autosomal dominant genetic abnormality in most cases and is probably the most common genetically transmitted cardiovascular disease (Maron, 2001). The expression of clinical disease varies greatly among patients. Clinical symptoms usually appear in school-age period or adolescence and may include anginal chest pain, dysrhythmias, and syncope. Sudden death is possible. Presentation in infancy includes signs of CHF and has a poor prognosis. The ECG demonstrates left ventricular hypertrophy, often with ST-T changes. The echocardiogram is most helpful and demonstrates asymmetric septal hypertrophy and an increase in left ventricular wall thickness, with a small left ventricle cavity.

Restrictive cardiomyopathy, rare in children, describes a restriction to ventricular filling caused by endocardial or myocardial disease or both. It is characterized by diastolic dysfunction and absence of ventricular dilation or hypertrophy. Symptoms are of CHF (see p. 906).

Therapeutic Management

Treatment is directed toward correcting the underlying cause whenever feasible. However, in most affected children this is not possible, and treatment is aimed at managing CHF (p. 906) and dysrhythmias. Digoxin, diuretics, and aggressive use of afterload reduction agents have been found to be helpful in managing symptoms in those with dilated cardiomyopathy. Practice guidelines for the management of heart failure in children have recently been outlined and provide an in-depth review of available therapies (Rosenthal, Chrisant, Edens, and others, 2004). Digoxin and inotropic agents are usually not helpful in the other forms of cardiomyopathy because increasing the force of contraction may exacerbate the muscular obstruction and actually impair ventricular ejection. Beta blockers such as propranolol or calcium channel blockers such as verapamil (Calan) have been used to reduce left ventricular outflow obstruction and improve diastolic filling in those with hypertrophic cardiomyopathy.

Careful monitoring and treatment of dysrhythmias are essential. The placement of an implantable defibrillator (AICD) should be considered for patients at high risk of sudden death due to ventricular dysrhythmias. Anticoagulants may be given to reduce the risk of thromboemboli, a complication of the sluggish circulation through the heart. For worsening heart failure and signs of poor perfusion, IV inotropic or vasodilating drugs may be needed. Severely ill children may require mechanical ventilation, oxygen administration, and IV medications. Heart transplantation may be a treatment option for patients who have worsening symptoms despite maximum medical therapy.

Nursing Care Management

Because of the poor prognosis in many children with cardiomyopathy, nursing care is consistent with that for any child with a life-threatening disorder (see Chapter 18). One of the most difficult adjustments for the child (especially the normally active youngster with hypertrophic cardiomyopathy) may be the realization of failing health and the need for restricted activity. The child should be included in decisions regarding activity and allowed to discuss feelings, particularly if the disease follows a progressively fatal course. After symptoms of CHF or dysrhythmias develop, the same nursing interventions are implemented as discussed on pp. 877-879. If heart transplantation is considered, the needs of the child and family are great in terms of psychologic preparation and postoperative care. The nurse plays an important role in assessing the family's understanding of the procedure and long-term consequences. Children of school age and older should be fully informed to give their assent to the procedure (see Informed Consent, Chapter 22).

HEART TRANSPLANTATION

Heart transplantation has become a treatment option for infants and children with worsening heart failure and a limited life expectancy despite maximum medical and surgical management. Indications for heart transplantation in children are cardiomyopathy and end-stage CHD. It is also an option for patients with some forms of complex congenital cardiac defects, such as hypoplastic left heart syndrome, for whom conventional surgical approaches have a high mortality rate.

The heart transplant procedure may be orthotopic or heterotopic. **Orthotopic heart transplantation** refers to removing the recipient's own heart and implanting a new heart from a donor who has had brain death but a healthy heart. The donor and recipient are matched by weight and blood type. **Heterotopic heart transplantation** refers to leaving the recipient's own heart in place and implanting a new heart to act as an additional pump, or "piggyback" heart; this type of transplant is rarely done in children.

Before transplantation, potential recipients undergo a careful cardiac evaluation to determine if there are any other medical or surgical options to improve the patient's cardiac status. Other organ systems are assessed to identify problems that might increase the risk of or preclude transplantation. A psychosocial evaluation of the patient and family is done to assess family function, support systems, and ability to comply with the complex medical regimen after the transplant. Support services to help the family successfully care for their child are provided when possible. Parents and older adolescents need extensive education about the risks and benefits of transplantation so that they can make an informed decision. Patients are listed on a national computer network organized by the United Network for Organ Sharing to match donors and recipients. (See also Organ or Tissue Donation and Autopsy, Chapter 18.)

The number of heart transplants in pediatric patients has been constant for the past decade at about 400 transplants per year internationally (Boucek, Aurora, Edwards, and others, 2007). This likely reflects a limit in the number of available donors. Infants are the largest group of pediatric transplant recipients and account for about a fourth of all procedures. The International Society for Heart and Lung Transplantation registry data for all pediatric heart transplant recipients from 1982 to 2005 demonstrated a 1-year actuarial survival rate of 85%. Early rejection within the first year posttransplant is associated with increased late mortality. There is an ongoing risk of death with time from transplant. The infant group is associated with higher early mortality and adolescents with higher late mortality. Overall survival was approximately 40% for patients up to 20 years after transplantation (Boucek, Aurora, Edwards, and others, 2007). Surviving pediatric patients have excellent functional recovery with less than 10% reporting activity limitations (Boucek, Aurora, Edwards, and others, 2007). The posttransplant course is complex. Although heart function is greatly improved or normal after transplantation, the risk of rejection is serious. The leading cause of death in the first 3 years after heart transplantation is rejection, with the greatest risk in the first 6 months (Blume, 2003). Rejection of the heart is diagnosed primarily by endomyocardial biopsy in older children. Serial echocardiograms are often used in infants and young children to reduce the need for invasive biopsies. Immunosuppressants must be taken for life and have many systemic side effects. Triple drug therapy for immunosuppression with a calcineurin inhibitor (cyclosporine or tacrolimus), steroids, and azathioprine is most commonly used in pediatric patients, although mycophenolate mofetil is being used more frequently and replacing azathioprine. Steroids are weaned in the first year and may be discontinued in some patients.

Infection is always a risk. Potential long-term problems that may limit survival include chronic rejection, causing coronary artery disease; renal dysfunction and hypertension resulting from cyclosporine administration; lymphoma; and infection. Coronary artery disease is the leading cause of death among late survivors of heart transplantation (Boucek, Aurora, Edwards, and others, 2007). In the short term, after successful transplantation, children are able to return to full participation in age-appropriate activities and appear to adapt well to their new lifestyle. Transplantation is not a cure, since patients must live with the lifetime consequences of chronic immunosuppression.

Nursing Care Management

Successfully caring for a child after a heart transplant requires the expertise and dedication of many members of the health care team. Nurses play vital roles in assessment, coordination of care, psychosocial support, and patient and family education. The heart transplant recipient must be carefully monitored for signs of rejection, infection, and the side effects of the immunosuppressant medications. The patient's and family's psychosocial well-being also needs to be assessed to identify issues such as increased family stress, depression, substance abuse, and school problems. Noncompliance with an intense medication regimen, especially during adolescence, can lead to serious medical problems and can be fatal. Immunosuppressants and nursing implications are discussed in Chapter 27 in relation to renal transplantation. Care of the immunosuppressed child is reviewed in Chapter 26. Psychosocial concerns and appropriate interventions for the child with a life-threatening disorder are presented in Chapter 18.

The first 6 months to 1 year after the transplant are most intense, since the risk of complications is greatest and the patient and family are adjusting to a new lifestyle. Patients are monitored closely by the health care team, with frequent visits and laboratory tests. Care is usually shared between local health care providers and the transplant center. Many patients are able to return to school and other age-appropriate activities within 2 to 3 months after the transplant.

VASCULAR DYSFUNCTION
SYSTEMIC HYPERTENSION

Hypertension is defined as the consistent elevation of BP beyond values considered to be the upper limits of normal. The two major categories are **essential hypertension** (no identifiable cause) and **secondary hypertension** (subsequent to an identifiable cause). In recent years there has been increasing interest in this disorder in adolescents and children. Hypertension in children and adolescents is defined as having a systolic or diastolic BP that consistently falls at or over the 95th percentile. This group is further delineated as follows:

- Stage 1 hypertension includes patients who have BP readings between the 95th and 99th percentiles.
- Stage 2 hypertension describes patients with BP readings over the 99th percentile plus 5 mm Hg.

An additional group includes children and adolescents who have prehypertension (or high-normal BP). This prehypertensive group includes those with BP readings that fall consistently between the 90th and 95th percentiles. *The Fourth Report on the Diagnosis, Evaluation, and Treatment of High Blood Pressure in Children and Adolescents* outlines in detail the identification, testing, and treatment recommendations for young people with high BP (National High Blood Pressure Education Program Working Group on High Blood Pressure in Children and Adolescents, 2004).

Etiology

Most instances of hypertension observed in young children occur secondary to a structural abnormality or an underlying pathologic process, although this is being challenged by screening programs of relatively healthy children. The most common cause of secondary hypertension is renal disease, followed by cardiovascular, endocrine, and some neurologic disorders. As a rule, the younger the child and the more severe the hypertension, the more likely it is to be secondary.

The causes of essential hypertension are undetermined, but evidence indicates that both genetic and environmental factors play a role. The incidence of hypertension has been shown to be higher in children whose parents are hypertensive. African-Americans have a higher incidence of hypertension than Caucasians, and in these persons it develops earlier, is frequently more severe, and results in death at an earlier age. Environmental factors that contribute to the risk of developing hypertension include obesity, salt ingestion, smoking, and stress.

Diagnostic Evaluation

From the increasing numbers of hypertensive or potentially hypertensive children and adolescents being identified, a BP determination should be a routine part of annual assessment in healthy children over 3 years old. BP readings should be done in children less than 3 years old who have high-risk family histories or those with individual risk factors, including CHD, kidney disease, malignancy, transplant, certain neurologic problems, or systemic illnesses known to cause hypertension. Although clinical manifestations associated with hypertension depend largely on the underlying cause, some observations can provide clues to the examiner that an elevated BP may be a factor (Box 25-10). In infants and very young children who cannot communicate symptoms, observation of behavior provides clues, although gross behavioral changes may not be apparent until complications are present.

No definitive cutoff values are used in the diagnosis of hypertension in the pediatric patient. The *Fourth Report on the Diagnosis, Evaluation, and Treatment of High Blood Pressure in Children and Adolescents* (National High Blood Pressure Education Program Working Group on High Blood

---

BOX 25-10

Clinical Manifestations of Hypertension

ADOLESCENTS AND OLDER CHILDREN	INFANTS OR YOUNG CHILDREN
Frequent headaches	Irritability
Dizziness	Head-banging or head-rubbing
Changes in vision	Waking up screaming in the night

Pressure in Children and Adolescents, 2004) provides normative data for children (see inside cover). BP tables now include the 50th, 90th, 95th, and 99th percentiles for BP readings based on age, gender, and height percentiles. These guidelines are based on auscultatory readings, and therefore this is currently the preferred method of assessment. These charts take into account differences in body height. It is therefore important to note that a child who is large for his or her age may normally have a higher BP than a child of average size. Before a diagnosis is made, BP should be measured on at least three separate occasions.

A careful medical history and family history should be obtained to screen for other relatives with hypertension or other cardiovascular risk factors. In children with suspected hypertension, initial laboratory data include a urinalysis, renal function studies such as creatinine and blood urea nitrogen, a lipid profile, complete blood count, and electrolytes. Depending on the severity of hypertension, additional testing may be indicated. Testing may include a renal ultrasound to measure kidney size and Doppler flow to detect the possibility of a renal cause, a cardiac echocardiogram to evaluate the presence of end-organ involvement such as left ventricular hypertrophy, and a retinal examination.

Therapeutic Management

Therapy for secondary hypertension involves diagnosis and treatment of the underlying cause. In cases amenable to surgical repair, the nature of the condition, the type of surgery, and the child's age are all important considerations. Children or adolescents with consistently elevated BP readings from no known cause or those with secondary hypertension not amenable to surgical correction may be treated with a combination of nonpharmacologic and pharmacologic interventions. Dietary practices and lifestyle changes are important in the control of hypertension both for children and for adults. Nonpharmacologic measures, such as weight control in overweight patients, increased exercise, limited salt intake, and avoidance of stress and smoking, carry no risk and should be instituted first, except in severe cases. Because the long-term effects of antihypertensive agents on children are not known, drug treatment of asymptomatic children with mild or borderline hypertension is not recommended.

Drug therapy is instituted with caution in children with significant elevations of BP resistant to nonpharmacologic intervention. The treatment should begin with one drug and should add other drugs only if control is not obtained. The oral antihypertensive drugs used in children include the beta blockers, ACE inhibitors, calcium channel blockers, angiotensin-receptor blockers, and diuretics. The goal is to achieve a normotensive state throughout the day without accompanying drug side effects.

Nursing Care Management

BP measurement should always be a part of the routine assessment of children over 3 years old and patients under 3 years old who are considered to be at high risk for hypertension. To obtain an accurate reading, care is taken to quiet the child or relax the adolescent while the measurement is recorded to avoid false readings caused by excitement. The chief cause of falsely elevated BP readings is the use of improperly fitting, narrow cuffs. Therefore attention to correct measurement technique is essential (see Blood Pressure, Chapter 6).

Nursing counseling and guidance of affected children are challenges. Education aimed at understanding hypertension and its implication over the life span is essential in promoting patient and family compliance with both nonpharmacologic and pharmacologic therapies (see Compliance, Chapter 22).

Home BP measurements can facilitate surveillance in youngsters with chronic hypertension and can document effectiveness of therapy. A family member can be instructed in how to take and record accurate BP measurements, thus decreasing the number of trips to a health care facility. This individual needs to understand when to contact the practitioner regarding elevated values. The school nurse can often be a valuable resource in monitoring BP. The nurse plays an important role in assessing individual families and providing targeted information regarding nonpharmacologic modes of intervention, such as diet, weight loss, smoking cessation, and exercise programs. If extensive dietary counseling is required, the child should be referred to a nutritionist with expertise in working with children and adolescents. Exercise regimens should be individualized. Schoolchildren and young adolescents generally prefer team sports rather than individual training, which they may view as a burden rather than an enjoyable activity. If peers and family members can be encouraged to participate in any of the management strategies, the child's compliance is likely to be greater.

Young hypertensive women should avoid oral contraceptives because of their pressor effects. Other options need to be presented before this form of birth control is discontinued (see Contraception, Chapter 17).

If drug therapy is prescribed, the nurse needs to provide information to the family regarding the reasons for it, how the drug works, and possible side effects. General instructions for antihypertensive drugs include:

- Rise slowly from a horizontal position and avoid sudden position changes.
- Take drug as prescribed.
- Maintain adequate hydration
- Notify practitioner if unpleasant side effects occur, but do not discontinue drug.
- Avoid alcohol and stay on prescribed diet.

The need for follow-up is stressed, especially because antihypertensive therapy can sometimes be safely discontinued if BP remains under control over time.

KAWASAKI DISEASE (MUCOCUTANEOUS LYMPH NODE SYNDROME)

KD is an acute systemic vasculitis of unknown cause. It is seen in every racial group, and about 75% of the cases occur in children younger than the age of 5 years, with peak incidence in the toddler age-group. The acute disease is self-limited. Without treatment, however, approximately 15% to 25% of

---

BOX 25-11

Diagnostic Criteria for Kawasaki Disease

Child must have fever for more than 5 days along with four of five clinical criteria (diagnosis may be made on day 4 by an experienced clinician if child has all the clinical criteria):

1. Changes in the extremities: in the acute phase edema, erythema of the palms and soles; and in the subacute phase, periungual desquamation (peeling) of the hands and feet
2. Bilateral conjunctival injection (inflammation) without exudation
3. Changes in the oral mucous membranes, such as erythema of the lips, oropharyngeal reddening; or "strawberry tongue" (large papillae are exposed)
4. Polymorphous rash
5. Cervical lymphadenopathy (one lymph node >1.5 cm)

NOTE: Kawasaki disease can be diagnosed with fewer clinical criteria when coronary artery changes are noted.

---

children with KD develop coronary artery aneurysms (Belay, Maddox, Holman, and others, 2006). Infants younger than 1 year of age are most seriously affected by KD and are at the greatest risk for heart involvement.

The etiology of KD is unknown. Although it is not spread by person-to-person contact, several factors support infectious etiologic factors. It is often seen in geographic and seasonal outbreaks, with most cases reported in the late winter and early spring (Newburger, Takahashi, Gerber, and others, 2004).

Pathophysiology

The principal area of involvement is the cardiovascular system. During the initial stage of the illness, extensive inflammation of the arterioles, venules, and capillaries occurs. In addition, segmental damage to the medium-sized muscular arteries, mainly the coronary arteries, can occur, causing the formation of coronary artery aneurysms in some children. When death occurs (in <0.05% of cases), it is usually the result of myocardial ischemia from coronary thrombosis or, over time, severe scar formation and stenosis in coronary aneurysms (Wilder, Palinkas, Kao, and others, 2007).

Clinical Manifestations

Because no specific diagnostic test exists for KD, the diagnosis is established on the basis of clinical findings and associated laboratory results (Box 25-11). These criteria should be used as guidelines. It is important to note that many children with KD do not fulfill standard diagnostic criteria, and infants often have an incomplete presentation. It is therefore important to consider KD as a possible diagnosis in any infant or child with prolonged elevated temperature that is unresponsive to antibiotics and is not attributable to another cause.

KD manifests in three phases: acute, subacute, and convalescent. The **acute phase** begins with the abrupt onset of high fever that is unresponsive to antibiotics and antipyretics. The child then develops the remaining diagnostic symptoms. During this stage the child is typically *very* irritable. The **subacute phase** begins with resolution of the fever and lasts until all clinical signs of KD have disappeared. During this phase the child is at greatest risk for the development of coronary artery aneurysms. Echocardiograms are used to monitor myocardial and coronary artery status. A baseline echocardiogram should be obtained at the time of diagnosis for comparison with future studies. Irritability persists during this phase. In the **convalescent phase,** all the clinical signs of KD have resolved, but the laboratory values have not returned to normal. This phase is complete when all blood values are normal (6 to 8 weeks after onset). At the end of this stage the child has regained his or her usual temperament, energy, and appetite.

Cardiac Involvement. Long-term complications of KD include the development of coronary artery aneurysms, disrupting blood flow. In children with aneurysms, there is the potential for myocardial infarction, which can result from thrombotic occlusion of a coronary aneurysm. Over time, as the damaged vessel tries to heal, stenosis of the aneurysm may develop and may lead to myocardial ischemia. Most of the morbidity and mortality occurs in those children affected with the largest aneurysms (giant aneurysms >8 mm). Symptoms of acute myocardial infarction in children may include abdominal pain, vomiting, restlessness, inconsolable crying, pallor, and shock.

Therapeutic Management

The current treatment of KD includes high-dose IV gamma globulin along with salicylate therapy. Gamma globulin has been demonstrated to be effective at reducing the incidence of coronary artery abnormalities when given within the first 10 days of the illness. A single, large infusion of 2 g/kg over 10 to 12 hours is recommended. Retreatment with intravenous gamma globulin is indicated in patients who continue with fever after treatment.

Aspirin is given initially in an antiinflammatory dose (80 to 100 mg/kg/day in divided doses every 6 hours) to control fever and symptoms of inflammation. After fever has subsided, aspirin is continued at an antiplatelet dose (3 to 5 mg/kg/day). Low-dose aspirin is continued in patients without echocardiographic evidence of coronary abnormalities until the platelet count has returned to normal (6 to 8 weeks). If the child develops coronary abnormalities, salicylate therapy is continued indefinitely. Additional anticoagulation (e.g., clopidogrel [Plavix], enoxaparin [Lovenox], or warfarin) may be indicated in children who have medium-sized or giant coronary artery aneurysms.

Prognosis. Most children with KD recover fully after treatment. However, when cardiovascular complications occur, serious morbidity may result. Death occurs rarely but almost always results from coronary thrombosis.

Nursing Care Management

In the initial phase the nurse must monitor the child's cardiac status carefully. Intake and output and daily weight measurements are recorded. Although the child may be reluctant to eat and therefore may be partially dehydrated, fluids need to be administered with care because of the usual finding of myocarditis. The child should be assessed frequently for signs of CHF, including decreased urinary output, gallop rhythm (an additional heart sound), tachycardia, and respiratory distress.

Administration of gamma globulin should follow the same guidelines as for any blood product, with frequent monitoring of vital signs. Patients must be watched for allergic reactions. Cardiac status must be monitored because of the large volume being administered to patients with myocarditis and diminished left ventricular function.

Most nursing care focuses on symptomatic relief. To minimize skin discomfort, cool cloths; unscented lotions; and soft, loose clothing are helpful. During the acute phase, mouth care, including lubricating ointment to the lips, is important for mucosal inflammation. Clear liquids and soft foods can be offered.

Patient irritability is perhaps the most challenging problem. These children need a quiet environment that promotes adequate rest. Their parents need to be supported in their efforts to comfort an often inconsolable child. They may need time away from their child, and nurses can often provide respite care for the family. Parents need to understand that irritability is a hallmark of KD and that they need not feel guilty or embarrassed about their child's behavior.

Discharge Teaching. Parents need accurate information about the progression of KD, including the importance of follow-up monitoring and when they should contact their practitioner. Irritability is likely to persist for up to 2 months after the onset of symptoms. Peeling of the hands and feet is painless and occurs primarily in the second and third weeks. Arthritis, especially of the larger weight-bearing joints, may persist for several weeks. Children are typically most stiff in the mornings, during cold weather, and after naps. Passive range-of-motion exercises in the bathtub are often helpful in increasing flexibility. Any live immunizations (e.g., measles-mumps-rubella, varicella) should be deferred for 11 months after the administration of gamma globulin because the body might not produce the appropriate amount of antibodies (American Academy of Pediatrics, 2006). The decision to give the varicella (chickenpox) vaccine while the child is receiving aspirin therapy is made individually by the practitioner. Temperature should be recorded after discharge until the child has been afebrile for several days.

All parents should understand the unlikely but real possibility of myocardial infarction, as well as the signs and symptoms of cardiac ischemia, in a child. At discharge the ultimate cardiac sequela is generally not known because vessels do not reach their maximum diameter until 4 to 6 weeks after the onset of KD. In addition, the parents of children with known severe coronary artery sequelae may be taught CPR.

SHOCK

Shock, or **circulatory failure,** is a complex clinical syndrome characterized by inadequate tissue perfusion to meet the metabolic demands of the body, resulting in cellular dysfunction and eventual organ failure. Although the causes are different, the physiologic consequences are the same: hypotension, tissue hypoxia, and metabolic acidosis. Circulatory failure in children is a result of hypovolemia, altered peripheral vascular resistance, or pump failure. Types of shock are listed in Box 25-12.

Pathophysiology

A healthy child's circulatory system is able to transport oxygen and metabolic substrates to body tissues, which require a constant source for these essential needs. The cardiac output and distribution to the various body tissues can change rapidly in response to intrinsic (myocardial and intravascular) or extrinsic (neuronal) control mechanisms. In shock states these mechanisms are altered or challenged.

Reduced blood flow, as in hypovolemic shock, causes diminished venous return to the heart, low CVP, low cardiac

BOX 25-12
Types of Shock

HYPOVOLEMIC

Characteristics

Reduction in size of vascular compartment
Falling blood pressure
Poor capillary filling
Low central venous pressure

Most Frequent Causes

Blood loss (hemorrhagic shock)—Trauma, gastrointestinal bleeding, intracranial hemorrhage
Plasma loss—Increased capillary permeability associated with sepsis and acidosis, hypoproteinemia, burns, peritonitis
Extracellular fluid loss—Vomiting, diarrhea, glycosuric diuresis, sunstroke

DISTRIBUTIVE

Characteristics

Reduction in peripheral vascular resistance
Profound inadequacies in tissue perfusion
Increased venous capacity and pooling
Acute reduction in return blood flow to the heart
Diminished cardiac output

Most Frequent Causes

Anaphylaxis (anaphylactic shock)—Extreme allergy or hypersensitivity to a foreign substance
Sepsis (septic shock, bacteremic shock, endotoxic shock)—Overwhelming sepsis and circulating bacterial toxins
Loss of neuronal control (neurogenic shock)—Interruption of neuronal transmission (spinal cord injury)
Myocardial depression and peripheral dilation—Exposure to anesthesia or ingestion of barbiturates, tranquilizers, opioids, antihypertensive agents, or ganglionic blocking agents

CARDIOGENIC

Characteristic

Decreased cardiac output

Most Frequent Causes

After surgery for congenital heart disease
Primary pump failure—Myocarditis, myocardial trauma, biochemical derangements, congestive heart failure
Dysrhythmias—Supraventricular tachycardia, atrioventricular block, and ventricular dysrhythmias; secondary to myocarditis or biochemical abnormalities (occasionally)

BOX 25-13
Clinical Manifestations of Shock

COMPENSATED	DECOMPENSATED
Apprehensiveness	Confusion and somnolence
Irritability	Tachypnea
Unexplained tachycardia	Moderate metabolic acidosis
Normal blood pressure	Oliguria
Narrowing pulse pressure	Cool, pale extremities
Thirst	Decreased skin turgor
Pallor	Poor capillary filling
Diminished urinary output	
Reduced perfusion of extremities	**IRREVERSIBLE**
	Thready, weak pulse
	Hypotension
	Periodic breathing or apnea
	Anuria
	Stupor or coma

As a result of impaired perfusion, oxygen is depleted in the tissue cells, causing them to revert to anaerobic metabolism, producing lactic acidosis. The acidosis places an extra burden on the lungs as they attempt to compensate for the metabolic acidosis by increasing respiratory rate to remove excess carbon dioxide. Prolonged vasoconstriction results in fatigue and atony of the peripheral arterioles, which leads to vessel dilation. Venules, less sensitive to vasodilator substances, remain constricted for a time, causing massive pooling in the capillary and venular beds, which further depletes blood volume.

Complications of shock create further hazards. Central nervous system hypoperfusion may eventually lead to cerebral edema, cortical infarction, or intraventricular hemorrhage. Renal hypoperfusion causes renal ischemia with possible tubular or glomerular necrosis and renal vein thrombosis. Reduced blood flow to the lungs can interfere with surfactant secretion and result in acute respiratory distress syndrome (ARDS), characterized by sudden pulmonary congestion and atelectasis with formation of a hyaline membrane. Gastrointestinal tract bleeding and perforation are always a possibility after splanchnic ischemia and necrosis of intestinal mucosa. Metabolic complications of shock may include hypoglycemia, hypocalcemia, and other electrolyte disturbances.

Diagnostic Evaluation

The etiology of shock can be discerned from the history and the physical examination. The severity of the shock is determined by measurements of vital signs, including CVP and capillary filling (Box 25-13). Shock can be regarded as a form of compensation for circulatory failure. Because of the progressive nature of shock, it can be divided into the following three stages or phases:

1. **Compensated shock**—Vital organ function is maintained by intrinsic compensatory mechanisms; blood flow is usually normal or increased but generally uneven or maldistributed in the microcirculation.
2. **Decompensated shock**—Efficiency of the cardiovascular system gradually diminishes until perfusion in the microcirculation becomes marginal despite compensatory adjustments. The outcomes of circulatory failure that progress beyond the

output, and hypotension. Vasomotor centers in the medulla are signaled, causing a compensatory increase in the force and rate of cardiac contraction and constriction of arterioles and veins, thereby increasing peripheral vascular resistance. Simultaneously the lowered blood volume leads to the release of large amounts of catecholamines, antidiuretic hormone, adrenocorticosteroids, and aldosterone in an effort to conserve body fluids. This causes reduced blood flow to the skin, kidneys, muscles, and viscera to shunt the available blood to the brain and heart. Consequently, the skin feels cold and clammy, there is poor capillary filling, and glomerular filtration rate and urinary output are significantly reduced.

limits of compensation are tissue hypoxia, metabolic acidosis, and eventual dysfunction of all organ systems.

3. **Irreversible, or terminal, shock**—Damage to vital organs, such as the heart or brain, is of such magnitude that the entire organism will be disrupted regardless of therapeutic intervention. Death occurs even if cardiovascular measurements return to normal levels with therapy.

At all stages the principal differentiating signs are observed in the (1) degree of tachycardia and perfusion to extremities, (2) level of consciousness, and (3) BP. Additional signs or modifications of these more universal signs may be present depending on the type and cause of the shock. Initially the child's ability to compensate is effective; therefore early signs are subtle. As the shock state advances, signs are more obvious and indicate early decompensation.

Additional signs may be present, depending on the type and cause of the shock. In early septic shock there are chills, fever, and vasodilation, with increased cardiac output that results in warm, flushed skin (hyperdynamic, or "hot," shock). A later and ominous development is disseminated intravascular coagulation (see Chapter 26), the major hematologic complication of septic shock. Anaphylactic shock is frequently accompanied by urticaria and angioneurotic edema, which is life threatening when it involves the respiratory passages (see Anaphylaxis, below).

Laboratory tests that assist in assessment are blood gas measurements, pH, and sometimes liver function tests. Coagulation tests are evaluated when there is evidence of bleeding, such as oozing from a venipuncture site, bleeding from any orifice, or petechiae. Cultures of blood and other sites are indicated when there is a high suspicion of sepsis. Renal function tests are performed when impaired renal function is evident.

Therapeutic Management

Treatment of shock consists of three major interventions: (1) ventilation, (2) fluid administration, and (3) improvement of the pumping action of the heart (vasopressor support). The first priority is to establish an airway and administer oxygen. After the airway is ensured, circulatory stabilization is the major concern. Establishment of adequate IV access, ideally with multilumen central lines, is essential to deliver fluids and medications.

Ventilatory Support. The lung is the organ most sensitive to shock. Decreased distribution or redistribution of blood flow to respiratory muscles plus the increased work of breathing can rapidly lead to respiratory failure. Critically ill patients are unable to maintain an adequate airway. To place the lung at rest and improve ventilation, tracheal intubation is initiated early with positive-pressure ventilation. Supplemental oxygen is always given as soon as possible. Blood gases and pH are monitored frequently.

Increased extravascular lung water caused by edema contributes to the development of respiratory complications. Therapy is directed toward maintaining normal arterial blood gas measurements, normal acid-base balance, and circulation. Efforts are made to remove fluid and prevent its accumulation with the use of diuretics.

Cardiovascular Support. In most cases, rapid restoration of blood volume is all that is needed for resuscitation of the child in shock. An isotonic crystalloid solution (normal saline or Ringer's lactate) is the fluid of choice; colloids such as albumin are also used. Successful resuscitation is reflected by an increase in BP and a reduction in heart rate; increased cardiac output will result in improved capillary circulation and skin color. CVP measurements of right atrial pressure help guide fluid therapy, and urinary output measurement is an important indicator of adequacy of circulation. Correction of acidosis, hypoxemia, hypoglycemia, hypothermia, and any metabolic derangements is mandatory.

Temporary pharmacologic support may be required to enhance myocardial contractility, to reverse metabolic or respiratory acidosis, and/or to maintain arterial pressure. The principal agents used to improve cardiac output and circulation are catecholamines, such as dopamine (Intropin) or epinephrine (Adrenalin). Vasodilators that are sometimes used include nitroprusside (Nipride) or milrinone.

Nursing Care Management

The child who is in shock requires intensive observation and care. *The initial action is to ensure adequate tissue oxygenation.* The nurse should be prepared to administer oxygen by the appropriate route and to assist with any intubation and ventilatory procedures indicated. Other procedures and activities that require immediate attention are establishing an IV line, weighing the child, obtaining baseline vital signs, placing an indwelling catheter, obtaining blood gases and other measurements, and administering medications as indicated. The child is best positioned flat with the legs elevated.

> **NURSINGALERT**
>
> Early clinical signs of shock include apprehension, irritability, normal BP, narrowing pulse pressure (difference between diastolic and systolic BP), thirst, pallor, diminished urinary output, unexplained mild tachycardia, and decreased perfusion of the hands and feet.

The nurse's responsibilities are to monitor the IV infusion, intake and output, vital signs (including CVP), and general systems assessments on a routine basis. IV medications are titrated according to patient responses, and vital signs are taken every 15 minutes during the critical periods and thereafter as needed. Urinary output is measured hourly; blood gases, hematocrit, pH, and electrolytes are monitored frequently to assess the child's status and the efficacy of therapy. An apnea and cardiac monitor is attached and monitored continuously. In the initial stages of acute shock, more than one nurse is often needed to manage all the necessary activities that must be carried out simultaneously (see Emergency Treatment box).

Throughout the intense activity, support for the family must not be overlooked. Someone should contact family members at frequent intervals to inform them about what is being done and whether there is any progress. Ideally, someone should remain with the parents to serve as liaison between them and the intensive care team. However, this is not always feasible in such a critical situation. As soon as possible, the family should be allowed to see the child. A member of the clergy or a social worker may be called to help provide comfort and support.

ANAPHYLAXIS

Anaphylaxis is the acute clinical syndrome resulting from the interaction of an allergen and a patient who is hypersensitive to that allergen. When the antigen enters the circulatory sys-

Shock

VENTILATION
Establish airway; be prepared for intubation.
Administer oxygen, usually 100% by mask.

FLUID ADMINISTRATION
Obtain vascular access (preferably intravenous [IV]; intraosseous in emergency).
Restore fluid volume as ordered (initial volume resuscitation is 20 ml/kg of isotonic crystalloid [normal saline or Ringer's lactate] over 5 to 20 minutes).

CARDIOVASCULAR SUPPORT
Administer vasopressors, especially IV epinephrine (dose: 0.01 mg/kg = 0.1 ml/kg of 1:10,000 solution).
May repeat this every 3 to 5 minutes for patients in cardiac arrest.

GENERAL SUPPORT
Provide continuous electrocardiographic monitoring.
Monitor pulse oximetry.
Keep child warm and calm.

IN ADDITION:
Septic Shock—Administer broad-spectrum antibiotics IV.
Anaphylaxis—Remove allergen if possible; provide intramuscular epinephrine and corticosteroids as ordered.

---

tem, a generalized reaction rapidly takes place. Vasoactive amines (principally histamine or a histamine-like substance) are released and cause vasodilation, bronchoconstriction, and increased capillary permeability.

Severe reactions are immediate in onset; are often life threatening; and frequently involve multiple systems, primarily the cardiovascular, respiratory, gastrointestinal, and integumentary systems. Exposure to the antigen can be by ingestion, inhalation, skin contact, or injection. Examples of common allergens associated with anaphylaxis include drugs (e.g., antibiotics, chemotherapeutic agents, radiologic contrast media), latex, foods, venom from bees or snakes, and biologic agents (antisera, enzymes, hormones, blood products).

> **NURSINGALERT**
>
> Penicillin allergy is associated with immediate onset (within an hour of administration) or accelerated onset (1 to 72 hours after administration) of skin eruption, especially a urticarial rash, or more serious symptoms such as laryngeal edema or anaphylactic shock.

Clinical Manifestations

The onset of clinical symptoms usually occurs within seconds or minutes of exposure to the antigen, and the rapidity of the reaction is directly related to its intensity: the sooner the onset, the more severe the reaction. The reaction may be preceded by symptoms of uneasiness, restlessness, irritability, severe anxiety, headache, dizziness, paresthesia, and disorientation. The patient may lose consciousness. Cutaneous signs of flushing and urticaria are common early signs, fol-

lowed by angioedema, most notable in the eyelids, lips, tongue, hands, feet, and genitalia.

Bronchiolar constriction may follow, causing narrowing of the airway; pulmonary edema and hemorrhage also may occur. Laryngeal edema with severe acute upper airway obstruction may be life threatening and requires rapid intervention. Shock occurs as a result of mediator-induced vasodilation, which causes capillary permeability and loss of intravascular fluid into the interstitial space. Sudden hypotension and impaired cardiac output with poor perfusion are seen.

Therapeutic Management

Successful outcome of anaphylactic reactions depends on rapid recognition and institution of treatment. The goals of treatment are to provide ventilation, restore adequate circulation, and prevent further exposure by identifying and removing the cause when possible.

A mild reaction with no evidence of respiratory distress or cardiovascular compromise can be managed with subcutaneous administration of antihistamines, such as diphenhydramine (Benadryl) and epinephrine.

Moderate or severe distress presents a potentially life-threatening emergency. Establishing an airway is the first concern, as with all shock states. Epinephrine is given subcutaneously or intravenously as an antihistamine and to support the cardiovascular system and increase BP. Other routes for giving epinephrine are intramuscular and via the airway, either nebulized or injected through an ET tube. In severe anaphylaxis, epinephrine by any route is better than none. Fluids are given to restore blood volume. Additional vasopressors may be given to improve cardiac output.

Prevention of a reaction is preferable. Preventing exposure is more easily accomplished in children known to be at risk, including those with (1) a history of previous allergic reaction to a specific antigen; (2) a history of atopy; (3) a history of severe reactions in immediate family members; and (4) a reaction to a skin test, although skin tests are not available for all allergens. Desensitization may be recommended in certain cases.

Nursing Care Management

When an anaphylactic reaction is suspected, both immediate intervention and preparation for medical therapy are nursing responsibilities. Ventilation is ensured by placing the child in a head-elevated position, unless contraindicated by hypotension, to facilitate breathing and administer oxygen. If the child is not breathing, CPR is initiated and emergency medical services are summoned.

If the cause can be determined, measures are implemented to slow the spread of the offending substance. An IV infusion is established immediately. Emergency medications are given intravenously whenever possible; however, epinephrine may be given subcutaneously (see Emergency Treatment box, above left). Vital signs and urinary output are monitored frequently. Medications are administered as prescribed, with regular assessment to monitor effectiveness and to detect signs of side effects of medication and fluid overload.

To prevent an anaphylactic reaction, parents are always asked about possible allergic responses to foods, latex, medications, and environmental conditions. These are displayed prominently on the patient's chart. The specific allergen is noted, as is the type and severity of the reaction. Parents are excellent historians, especially when the child has displayed a pronounced reaction to a substance. Drugs, including related drugs (e.g., penicillin, nafcillin), and other items, such as latex, that have produced a reaction previously are *never* used. If the child is allergic to insect venom, the family is instructed to purchase an emergency kit to be kept with the child at all times. Both the family and the child, if the child is old enough, are taught how to use the equipment. The patient should carry medical identification at all times.

SEPTIC SHOCK

Sepsis and septic shock are caused by an infectious organism (Maar, 2004). Normally an infection triggers an inflammatory response in a local area, which results in vasodilation, increased capillary permeability, and eventually elimination of the infectious agent. The widespread activation and systemic release of inflammatory mediators is called the **systemic inflammatory response syndrome** (SIRS). Box 25-14 provides the exact definitions for SIRS, infection, sepsis, and severe sepsis. SIRS can occur in response to both infectious and noninfectious (e.g., trauma, burns) causes. When caused by infection, it is called **sepsis.** Septic shock is defined as sepsis with organ dysfunction and hypotension.

Most of the physiologic effects of shock occur because the exaggerated immune response triggers more than 30 different mediators that result in diffuse vasodilation, increased capillary permeability, and maldistribution of blood flow. This impairs oxygen and nutrient delivery to the cells, resulting in cellular dysfunction. If the process continues, multiple organ dysfunction occurs and may result in death. Table 25-6 includes the age-specific vital signs and laboratory values reflective of septic shock in children.

The incidence of septic shock is increasing in adults and children (Arnal and Stein, 2003), possibly as a result of greater numbers of immunosuppressed patients, more widespread use of invasive devices in the seriously ill, increased awareness of the diagnosis, and a growing number of resistant microorganisms.

Three stages have been identified in septic shock. In early septic shock the patient has chills, fever, and vasodilation with increased cardiac output, which results in warm, flushed skin that reflects vascular tone abnormalities and hyperdynamic, warm, or hyperdynamic-compensated responses. BP and urinary output are normal. The patient has the best chance for survival in this stage. The second stage—the normodynamic, cool, or hyperdynamic-decompensated stage—lasts only a few hours. The skin is cool, but pulses and BP are still normal. Urinary output diminishes, and the mental state becomes depressed. With advancing disease, certain signs of circulatory decompensation that deteriorate to signs of circulatory collapse are indistinguishable from late shock of any cause. In the hypodynamic, or cold, stage of shock, cardiovascular function progressively deteriorates, even with aggressive therapy. The patient has hypothermia, cold extremities, weak pulses, hypotension, and oliguria or anuria. Patients are severely lethargic or comatose. Multiorgan failure is common. This is the most dangerous stage of shock.

Management of septic shock involves measures to provide hemodynamic stability and adequate oxygenation to the tissues and the use of antimicrobials to treat the infectious organism. As with other forms of shock, hemodynamic stability is achieved with fluid volume resuscitation and inotropic agents as needed. Providing adequate oxygenation often re-

---

BOX 25-14

Definitions of Systemic Inflammatory Response Syndrome, Infection, Sepsis, and Severe Sepsis

Systemic inflammatory response syndrome (SIRS)—The presence of at least two of the following four criteria, one of which must be abnormal temperature or leukocyte count:
1. Core temperature of more than 38.5° C (101.3° F) or less than 36° C (96.8° F).
2. Tachycardia, defined as a mean heart rate more than 2 SD above normal for age in the absence of external stimulus, chronic drugs, or painful stimuli; or otherwise unexplained persistent elevation over a 0.5- to 4-hour period; or, for children less than 1 year old: bradycardia, defined as a mean heart rate less than the 10th percentile for age in the absence of external vagal stimulus, beta-blocker drugs, or congenital heart disease; or otherwise unexplained persistent depression over a 0.5-hour period.
3. Mean respiratory rate more than 2 SD above normal for age or mechanical ventilation for an acute process not related to underlying neuromuscular disease or the receipt of general anesthesia.
4. Leukocyte count elevated or depressed for age (not secondary to chemotherapy-induced leukopenia) or more than 10% immature neutrophils.

Infection—A suspected or proven (by positive culture, tissue stain, or polymerase chain reaction test) infection caused by any pathogen; or a clinical syndrome associated with a high probability of infection. Evidence of infection includes positive findings on clinical examination, imaging, or laboratory tests (e.g., white blood cells in a normally sterile body fluid, perforated viscus, chest radiograph consistent with pneumonia, petechial or purpuric rash, or purpura fulminans).

Sepsis—SIRS in the presence of or as a result of suspected or proven infection.

Severe sepsis—Sepsis plus cardiovascular organ dysfunction or acute respiratory distress syndrome; or two or more other organ dysfunctions.

From Goldstein B, Giroir B, Randolph A, and others: International Pediatric Sepsis Consensus Conference: definitions for sepsis and organ dysfunction in pediatrics, *Pediatr Crit Care Med* 6(1):2-8, 2005; used with permission.

---

quires intubation and mechanical ventilation, supplemental oxygen, sedation, and paralysis to decrease the work of breathing. Septic shock involves activation of complement proteins that promote clumping of the granulocytes in the lung. The granulocytes can release chemicals that can cause direct lung injury to the pulmonary capillary endothelium. This causes a fluid leak into the alveoli, which causes stiff, noncompliant lungs. Disseminated intravascular coagulation and multiorgan dysfunction may also occur and require prompt assessment and management.

Newer therapies are being developed to modify the host immune response by attempting to block various mediators, thereby interrupting the inflammatory cascade.

Early identification of the symptoms of septic shock is critical to patient survival. A high index of suspicion is required in all critically ill patients who are at greater risk for sepsis because of multiple invasive lines and devices, poor nutrition, and impaired immune function. Subtle alterations in tissue perfusion and unexplained tachypnea and tachycardia often are early warning signs. Identification of the infectious agent and prompt treatment are also critical to patient

TABLE 25-6

Age-Specific Vital Signs and Laboratory Variables in Septic Shock*

AGE-GROUP	HEART RATE (beats/min)		RESPIRATORY RATE (breaths/min)	LEUKOCYTE COUNT (leukocytes × 10³/mm³)	SYSTOLIC BLOOD PRESSURE (mm Hg)
	TACHYCARDIA	BRADYCARDIA			
0 days–1 week	>180	<100	>50	>34	<65
1 week–1 month	>180	<100	>40	>19.5 or <5	<75
1 month–1 year	>180	<90	>34	>17.5 or <5	<100
2-5 years	>140	N/A	>22	>15.5 or <6	<94
6-12 years	>130	N/A	>8	>13.50 or <4.5	<105
13-<18 years	>110	N/A	>4	>11 or <4.5	<117

From Goldstein B, Giroir B, Randolph A, and others: International pediatric sepsis consensus conference: definitions for sepsis and organ dysfunction in pediatrics, *Pediatr Crit Care Med* 6(1):2-8, 2005; used with permission.
N/A, Not applicable.
*Lower values for heart rate, leukocyte count, and systolic blood pressure are for 5th percentile, and upper values for heart rate, respiratory rate, or leukocyte count are for 95th percentile.

survival. Broad-spectrum antibiotics should be given, and the site of infection should be removed if possible (e.g., drain abscesses, remove indwelling lines). Patients should be managed in an intensive care unit, in which continuous monitoring and sophisticated cardiac and respiratory support are available. Multidisciplinary collaboration is essential in managing these critically ill patients.

TOXIC SHOCK SYNDROME

Toxic shock syndrome (TSS) is a relatively rare condition caused by the toxins produced by the *Staphylococcus* bacteria. First described in 1978, TSS can cause acute multisystem organ failure and a clinical picture that resembles septic shock. TSS became well known in 1980 because of the striking relationship between the disease and tampon use (Nakase, 2000). An aggressive health education campaign about the dangers of prolonged tampon use and a change in the chemical composition of tampons has markedly reduced the incidence of TSS in menstruating women. Cases of TSS have also been reported in men, older women, and children.

Diagnostic Evaluation

Diagnosis is established on the basis of the criteria established by the Centers for Disease Control and Prevention's toxic case definition (Box 25-15). A history of tampon use contributes to the diagnosis. Additional laboratory tests include cultures from blood, vagina, cervix, and any discharge. Other laboratory tests are those that facilitate the management of shock.

Therapeutic Management

The management of TSS is the same as management of shock of any cause and may range from supportive care in mild cases to hospitalization and intensive care in severe cases. Appropriate parenteral antibiotics are usually administered after cultures are obtained.

Nursing Care Management

Because the disease is relatively rare, the major efforts of nursing are directed toward prevention. The association between the disease and the use of tampons provides some di-

BOX 25-15

Criteria for Definition of Toxic Shock Syndrome

1. Fever of 38.9° C (102° F) or higher
2. Presence of diffuse macular erythroderma
3. Desquamation, particularly of palms and soles, 1 to 2 weeks after onset of illness
4. Hypotension, defined as a systolic blood pressure of 90 mm Hg or less for adults and below the 5th percentile for children younger than 16 years of age; or an orthostatic drop in diastolic blood pressure of 15 mm Hg or more with a change from lying to sitting; or orthostatic syncope; or orthostatic dizziness
5. Involvement of three or more of the following organ systems: gastrointestinal, muscular, mucous membrane, renal, hepatic, hematologic, or central nervous system

Toxic shock syndrome is probable when four of the five major criteria are fulfilled. In addition, if blood and cerebrospinal fluid cultures are obtained, they must be negative for any organisms other than *Staphylococcus aureus*. Serologic tests for Rocky Mountain spotted fever, leptospirosis, and measles also must be negative.

Modified from American Academy of Pediatrics, Committee on Infectious Diseases, Pickering L, editor: *Red book: 2006 report of the Committee on Infectious Diseases,* ed 27, Elk Grove Village, Ill, 2006, The Academy.

rection for education. Avoiding the use of tampons offers the most certain preventive measure, although this approach is probably unacceptable to most adolescent girls, who prefer the freedom, comfort, and inconspicuousness that tampons afford.

Adolescent girls who use tampons can be taught general hygiene measures, such as good hand washing and careful insertion to avoid vaginal abrasion. It is wise to modify their use, alternating with sanitary napkins—perhaps using the napkins during the night, when at home during the day, and when flow is slight. Young girls are advised not to use superabsorbent tampons and not to leave any tampon in the body for more than 4 to 6 hours.

KEY POINTS

- CHD is the most common form of cardiac disease in children.
- Major categories to investigate in the cardiac history are poor weight gain, poor feeding habits, and fatigue during feeding; frequent respiratory tract infections and difficulties; and evidence of exercise intolerance.
- The most common tests used in assessing cardiac function are radiography, ECG, echocardiography, and cardiac catheterization.
- Cardiac catheterization procedures can be divided into three groups: (1) diagnostic procedures, including angiography, that measure pressures and saturations to establish cardiac diagnosis; (2) interventional procedures, in which catheters or balloon devices are used to correct cardiac defects; and (3) electrophysiology studies, in which catheters with electrodes are used to evaluate dysrhythmias.
- Diagnostic cardiac catheterization provides important information about oxygen saturation of blood within the chambers and great vessels, pressure changes, changes in cardiac output or stroke volume, and anatomic abnormalities.
- Several prenatal factors may predispose children to CHD: maternal rubella during pregnancy, maternal alcoholism, maternal age older than 40 years, and maternal type 1 diabetes.
- Congenital heart defects can be divided into four main groups, as determined by hemodynamic patterns: (1) defects that result in increased pulmonary blood flow, (2) obstructive defects, (3) defects that result in decreased pulmonary blood flow, and (4) mixed defects.
- Clinical consequences of congenital heart defects include CHF and hypoxemia. A child can have both hypoxemia and CHF, although usually they occur independently.
- Clinical manifestations of CHF are impaired myocardial function (tachycardia, cardiomegaly), pulmonary congestion (dyspnea, tachypnea, orthopnea, cyanosis), and systemic congestion (hepatosplenomegaly, edema, distended veins).
- Nursing measures in the care of a child with CHF are to assist in improving cardiac function, decrease cardiac demands, reduce respiratory distress, maintain nutritional status, promote fluid loss, and provide family support.
- Clinical manifestations of hypoxemia are cyanosis, polycythemia, clubbing, and delayed growth and development. The child is at increased risk for hypercyanotic spells, CVAs, brain abscess, and BE.
- Caring for the child with CHD and the family requires helping them to adjust to the disorder and to cope with the effects of the defect, and fostering growth-promoting family relationships.
- Preoperative care of the child with a congenital heart defect involves introducing the child and family to the hospital and preparing them for preoperative and postoperative procedures.
- Providing postoperative care includes observing vital signs and arterial and venous pressures, maintaining respiratory status, allowing maximum rest, providing comfort, monitoring fluids, planning for progressive activities, giving emotional support, observing for complications of surgery, and planning for discharge and home care.
- Acquired cardiovascular disorders include BE, RF, hyperlipidemia (hypercholesterolemia), and cardiac dysrhythmias.
- Prevention of BE in certain children with CHD involves administration of prophylactic antibiotics when specific procedures are performed.
- Acute RF is a systemic inflammatory disease that can damage the cardiac valves and is associated with previous GABHS infection. Its incidence has increased in some areas of the United States.
- Cholesterol screening in children is controversial; currently, children with known risk factors for hyperlipidemia are screened and treated as needed. The influence of childhood cholesterol levels on later development of coronary artery disease is under investigation.
- Common dysrhythmias in children include slow rhythms (bradycardias, heart block) and fast rhythms (sinus tachycardia, SVT).
- Heart transplantation has been extended to infants and children with cardiomyopathy and complex congenital heart defects involving ventricular dysfunction, such as hypoplastic left heart syndrome.
- Education of the child with hypertension and the family focuses on drug therapy, diet control, and appropriate exercise.
- KD is an extensive inflammation of small vessels and capillaries that may progress to involve the coronary arteries, causing aneurysm formation. The administration of gamma globulin is an important aspect of treatment.
- Emergency treatment for shock includes ensuring ventilation; administering vasopressors, fluids, blood, and antibiotics as needed; and providing supportive measures such as correct positioning, warmth, and psychologic reassurance to the child and family.
- Persons at risk for anaphylaxis may be identified by a history of previous allergic reaction, history of atopy, history of severe reactions in family, and positive skin test to the allergen.
- Nursing management of the patient with TSS focuses on prevention primarily through education concerning safe tampon use.

answers to CRITICAL THINKING EXERCISES

CARDIAC CATHETERIZATION

1. Yes. This patient has just undergone an invasive diagnostic procedure. Bleeding is a potential risk after cardiac catheterization.
2. a. Complications after cardiac catheterization can include acute hemorrhage from the catheterization entry site, low-grade fever, nausea and vomiting, loss of pulses in the catheterized extremity, and transient dysrhythmias.
   b. Nausea and vomiting can occur after heart catheterization but are not directly related to acute blood loss. However, if the child had significant vomiting immediately after the procedure and was not able to keep his leg straight, the vomiting might have increased the chance of bleeding at the catheterization entry site.
   c. Significant blood loss can occur in a short time after the use of an artery for cardiac catheterization.
3. The first priority is to prevent bleeding. Pressure is applied above the visible catheterization site where the vessel was accessed. Place the child flat in bed to decrease the effect of gravity on the rate of bleeding. Notify the practitioner immediately. Replacement fluids may need to be administered, and pharmacologic control of emesis is important.
4. This may be an arterial bleed, and Tommy is at risk for losing a large amount of blood in a short time. Your first priority should be to control the bleeding. Appropriate measures are to treat the patient like a shock patient by immediately laying the child flat to help control bleeding.
5. In this case it is essential for the nurse to understand the complications associated with heart catheterization. Observation of acute blood loss at the site of catheter entry does not provide alternative perspectives but supports an immediate need to control bleeding.

DIGOXIN TOXICITY

1. Yes. The infant has been vomiting since yesterday and has an irregular heartbeat.
2. a. Furosemide is a diuretic that is a mainstay of therapy to eliminate excess water and salt to prevent reaccumulation of fluid. Side effects can include nausea and vomiting, diarrhea, ototoxicity, hypokalemia, and postural hypotension.
   b. Digoxin is a potentially dangerous drug because the margin of safety of therapeutic, toxic, and lethal doses is very narrow. Common signs of digoxin toxicity are bradycardia, anorexia, nausea, and vomiting. Dysrhythmias can occur with digoxin toxicity. The dosage of digoxin must be calculated exactly.
   c. The goals of treatment for CHF are to improve cardiac output, remove excess fluid and stabilize the sodium level, decrease cardiac demands and improve tissue oxygenation, and decrease oxygen consumption. Digoxin is used because of its rapid onset and decreased risk of toxicity as a result of a relative short half-life compared with other digitalis preparations.
3. The home health nurse should notify the health care provider of the findings before giving digoxin. The assessment reveals a slow, irregular heartbeat and intermittent vomiting. These are common signs of digoxin toxicity in infants. Because the medication was started only 5 days ago, digoxin toxicity should be a major concern. Because furosemide is a non–potassium-sparing diuretic, a concomitant problem with the vomiting is hypokalemia, which is a common finding in children with CHF, furosemide administration, and vomiting. This should also be further evaluated at this visit.
4. Yes. The implications of the assessment are essential because the margin of safety for digoxin blood levels is narrow. Continuing to give the digoxin can cause a toxic reaction. Further evaluation is important.
5. Vomiting in a young child is a concern, but with a history of congenital heart disease and digoxin therapy, the first priority is to evaluate for digoxin toxicity. As noted above, hypokalemia is also a concern. The vomiting may cause fluid loss above that for which the infant is able to compensate, and the possibility of mild dehydration should be evaluated.

HYPERCYANOTIC SPELL

1. Yes. The patient has a history of tetralogy of Fallot, which is associated with acute episodes of cyanosis and hypoxia. Hypercyanotic episodes occur suddenly and are common with crying.
2. a. Infants with tetralogy of Fallot may be acutely cyanotic at birth; others have mild cyanosis that progresses over the first year of life as pulmonic stenosis worsens.
   b. Symptoms of diarrhea, low-grade fever, and poor oral intake can be indicative of an acute infection in a young child. However, the hypercyanotic spell requires immediate attention.
   c. Acute cyanotic spells, called *blue spells* or *tet spells,* can occur suddenly when the infant's oxygen requirements exceed oxygen availability. This may occur during crying or after feeding.
3. The priorities are to immediately calm the infant, place in the knee-chest position, administer blow-by oxygen, and call for assistance.
4. Yes. The infant is having a hypercyanotic spell, and the first actions should be to calm the infant, place in the knee-chest position, and give supplemental oxygen. A hypercyanotic spell will likely worsen without immediate intervention, so prompt action is needed. If the nurse fails to accept the conclusions, negative implications may result, since a severe hypercyanotic spell may require intravenous medications, hydration, and resuscitative measures to stabilize the infant.
5. An alternative perspective is concern for an infection because of a history of diarrhea and low-grade fever for the past 2 days. However, in the presence of a diagnosis of tetralogy of Fallot, the immediate presentation of a hypercyanotic episode needs immediate attention. There should be a record or notation on the care plan measures that have been effective in calming the child in the past; this information is crucial in the care of such children.

REFERENCES

American Academy of Pediatrics, Committee on Infectious Diseases, Pickering L, editor: *Red book: 2006 report of the Committee on Infectious Diseases,* ed 27, Elk Grove Village, Ill, 2006, The Academy.

American Academy of Pediatrics: Cholesterol in childhood, *Pediatrics* 101(1 Pt 1):141-147, 1998.

Arnal LE, Stein F: Pediatric septic shock: why has mortality decreased? The utility of goal-directed therapy, *Semin Pediatr Infect Dis* 14(2):165-172, 2003.

Arnold R, Ley-Zaporozhan J, Ley S, and others: Outcome after mechanical aortic valve replacement in children and young adults, *Ann Thorac Surg* 85(2):604-610, 2008.

Barst RJ: Recent advances in the treatment of pediatric pulmonary artery hypertension, *Pediatr Clin North Am* 46(2):333-345, 1999.

Beekman RH: Coarctation of the aorta. In Allen HD, Driscoll DJ, Shaddy RE, and others, editors: *Moss and Adams' heart disease in infants, children and adolescents,* ed 6, Philadelphia, 2001, Lippincott Williams & Wilkins.

Belay E, Maddox R, Holman R, and others: Kawasaki syndrome and risk factors for coronary artery abnormalities, *Pediatr Infect Dis* 25(3):245-249, 2006.

Blume ED: Current status of heart transplantation in children: update 2003, *Pediatr Clin North Am* 50:1375-1391, 2003.

Boucek MM, Aurora P, Edwards LB, and others: The Registry of the International Society for Heart and Lung Transplantation: tenth official pediatric heart transplantation report—2007, *J Heart Lung Transplant* 26(8):796-807, 2007.

Carapetis JR, McDonald M, Wilson NJ: Acute rheumatic fever, *Lancet* 366:155-168, 2005.

Dodds KM, Merle C: Discharging neonates with congenital heart disease after cardiac surgery: a practical approach, *Clin Perinatol* 32:1031-1042, 2005.

Freed MD: Aortic stenosis. In Allen HD, Driscoll DJ, Shaddy RE, and others, editors: *Moss and Adams' heart disease in infants, children, and adolescents,* ed 6, Philadelphia, 2001, Lippincott Williams & Wilkins.

Gentles T, Colan SD, Wilson NJ, and others: Left ventricular mechanics during and after acute rheumatic fever: contractile dysfunction is closely related to valve regurgitation, *J Am Coll Cardiol* 37(1):201-207, 2001.

Goldmuntz E, Clark BJ, Mitchell LE, and others: Frequency of 22q11 deletion in patients with conotruncal defects, *J Am Coll Cardiol* 32:492-498, 1998.

Hoffman JIE, Kaplan S: The incidence of congenital heart disease, *J Am Coll Cardiol* 39:1890-1900, 2002.

Jacobs JP, Mavroudis C, Jacobs ML, and others: Lessons learned from the data analysis of the second harvest (1998-2001) of the Society of Thoracic Surgeons (STS) Congenital Heart Surgery Database, *Eur J Cardiothorac Surg* 26(1):18-37, 2004.

Latson LA: Critical pulmonic stenosis, *J Intervent Cardiol* 14(3):345-350, 2001.

LeRoy S, Elixson EM, O'Brien P, and others: Recommendations for preparing children and adolescents for invasive cardiac procedures: AHA Scientific Statement, *Circulation* 108:2550-2564, 2003.

Maar SP: Emergency care in pediatric septic shock, *Pediatr Emerg Care* 20(9):617-624, 2004.

Majnemer A, Limperopoulos C: Developmental progress of children with congenital heart defects requiring open heart surgery, *Semin Pediatr Neurol* 6:12-19, 1999.

Maron BJ: Hypertrophic cardiomyopathy. In Allen HD, Driscoll DJ, Shaddy RE, and others, editors: *Moss and Adams' heart disease in infants, children, and adolescents,* ed 6, Philadelphia, 2001, Lippincott Williams & Wilkins.

McCrindle BW, Urbina EM, Dennison BA, and others: Drug therapy of high-risk lipid abnormalities in children and adolescents: a scientific statement from the American Heart Association Atherosclerosis, Hypertension, and Obesity in Youth Committee, Council of Cardiovascular Disease in the Young, with the Council on Cardiovascular Nursing, *Circulation* 115:1948-1967, 2007.

Nakase J: Update on emerging infections from the Centers for Disease Control and Prevention, *Ann Emerg Med* 36(3):268-270, 2000.

National High Blood Pressure Education Program Working Group on High Blood Pressure in Children and Adolescents: The fourth report on the diagnosis, evaluation, and treatment of high blood pressure in children and adolescents, *Pediatrics* 114(2):555-576, 2004.

Newburger JW, Takahashi M, Gerber MA, and others: Diagnosis, treatment, and long-term management of Kawasaki disease: a statement for health professionals from the Committee on Rheumatic Fever, Endocarditis and Kawasaki Disease, Council on Cardiovascular Disease in the Young, American Heart Association, *Circulation* 110(17):2747-2771, 2004.

Park MK: *Pediatric cardiology handbook,* ed 3, St Louis, 2003, Mosby.

Rome JJ, Kreutzer J: Pediatric interventional catheterization: reasonable expectations and outcomes, *Pediatr Clin North Am* 51:1589-1610, 2004.

Rosenthal D, Chrisant MR, Edens E, and others: International Society for Heart and Lung Transplantation: practice guidelines for management of heart failure in children, *J Heart Lung Transplant* 23(12):1313-1333, 2004.

Shanmugam G, MacArthur K, Pollock J: Mechanical aortic valve replacement: long-term outcomes in children, *J Heart Valve Dis* 14(2):166-171, 2005.

Smith P: Primary care in children with congenital hearth disease, *J Pediatr Nurs* 16(5):308-319, 2001.

Stetzler M, Rudd N, Pick B: Nutrition care for newborns with congenital heart disease, *Clin Perinatol* 32:1017-1030, 2005.

Tweddell JS, Hoffman GM, Mussatto KA, and others: Improved survival of patients undergoing palliation of hypoplastic left heart syndrome: lessons learned from 115 consecutive patients, *Circulation* 106(12 Suppl 1):182-189, 2002.

Uzark K: Therapeutic cardiac catheterization for congenital heart disease: a new era in pediatric care, *J Pediatr Nurs* 16(5):300-307, 2001.

Van Horn L, Obarzanek E, Friedman LA, and others: Children's adaptations to a fat-reduced diet: the dietary intervention study in children, *Pediatrics* 115(60):1723-1733, 2005.

Wilder M, Palinkas L, Kao A, and others: Delayed diagnosis by physicians contributes to the development of coronary artery aneurysms in children with Kawasaki syndrome, *Pediatr Infect Dis* 26(3):256-260, 2007.

Wilson W, Taubert KA, Gewitz M, and others: Prevention of infective endocarditis: guidelines from the American Heart Association, *Circulation* 116(15):1736-1754, 2007.

26

The Child with Hematologic or Immunologic Dysfunction

ROSALIND BRYANT

CHAPTER OUTLINE

HEMATOLOGIC AND IMMUNOLOGIC DYSFUNCTION, 912
RED BLOOD CELL DISORDERS, 912
Anemia, 912
  Classification, 912
  Consequences of Anemia, 912
Iron Deficiency Anemia, 915
Sickle Cell Anemia, 916
β-Thalassemia (Cooley Anemia), 923
Aplastic Anemia, 924
DEFECTS IN HEMOSTASIS, 925
Hemophilia, 925
Idiopathic Thrombocytopenic
  Purpura, 927
Disseminated Intravascular
  Coagulation, 929
Epistaxis (Nosebleeding), 929

NEOPLASTIC DISORDERS, 930
Leukemias, 930
  Prognosis, 931
  Late Effects of Treatment, 932
Nursing Care Plan: The Child with
  Cancer, 932
Lymphomas, 937
Hodgkin Disease, 937
Non-Hodgkin Lymphoma, 939
**IMMUNOLOGIC DEFICIENCY
DISORDERS, 939**
Human Immunodeficiency Virus Infection
  and Acquired Immunodeficiency
  Syndrome, 939

Severe Combined Immunodeficiency
  Disease, 943
Wiskott-Aldrich Syndrome, 943
**TECHNOLOGIC MANAGEMENT OF
HEMATOLOGIC AND IMMUNOLOGIC
DISORDERS, 943**
Blood Transfusion Therapy, 943
Hematopoietic Stem Cell
  Transplantation, 945
Apheresis, 946

LEARNING OBJECTIVES

On completion of this chapter the reader will be able to:
- Distinguish between the various categories of anemia.
- Describe the prevention of and care of the child with iron deficiency anemia.
- Compare sickle cell anemia and β-thalassemia major in relation to pathophysiology and nursing care.

- Describe the mechanisms of inheritance and nursing care of the child with hemophilia.
- Relate the pathophysiology and clinical manifestations of leukemia.
- Demonstrate an understanding of the rationale of therapies for neoplastic disease.

- Outline a care plan for the child with neoplastic disease and the family.
- Contrast the pathophysiology and management of the immunodeficiency disorders.
- List nursing precautions and responsibilities during blood transfusion.
- Describe the types of hematopoietic stem cell transplants.

HEMATOLOGIC AND IMMUNOLOGIC DYSFUNCTION

Several tests can be performed to assess hematologic function, including additional procedures to identify the cause of the dysfunction. The following discussion is limited to a description of the most common and one of the most valuable tests, the **complete blood cell count (CBC).** Other procedures, such as those related to iron, coagulation, and immune status, are discussed throughout the chapter as appropriate. The nurse should be familiar with the significance of the findings from the CBC (Table 26-1) and aware of normal values for age, which are listed in Appendix C.

As with any disorder, the history and physical examination are essential to identify hematologic dysfunction, and the nurse is often the first person to suspect a problem based on information from these sources. Comments by the parent regarding the child's lack of energy, food diary of poor sources of iron, frequent infections, and bleeding that is difficult to control offer clues to the more common disorders affecting the blood. A careful physical appraisal, especially of the skin, can reveal findings (e.g., pallor, petechiae, bruising) that may indicate minor or serious hematologic conditions. Nurses need to be aware of the clinical manifestations of blood diseases to assist in recognizing symptoms and establishing a diagnosis.

FYI

A common term used in describing an abnormal CBC is **shift to the left,** which refers to the presence of immature neutrophils in the peripheral blood from hyperfunction of the bone marrow, as seen during a bacterial infection.

RED BLOOD CELL DISORDERS
ANEMIA

The term **anemia** describes a condition in which the number of red blood cells (RBCs) or the hemoglobin (Hgb or Hb) concentration is reduced below normal values for age. This diminishes the oxygen-carrying capacity of the blood, causing a reduction in the oxygen available to the tissues. Anemia is the most common hematologic disorder of infancy and childhood and is not a disease itself but an indication or manifestation of an underlying pathologic process.

Classification

Anemias are classified in relation to (1) **etiology** or **physiology,** manifested by erythrocyte or Hgb depletion; and (2) **morphology,** the characteristic changes in RBC size, shape, or color (Box 26-1). Although the morphologic classification is more useful in terms of laboratory evaluation of anemia, the etiologic approach provides direction for planning nursing care. For example, anemia with reduced Hgb concentration may be caused by a dietary depletion of iron, and the principal intervention is replenishing iron stores. The classification of anemias is found in Fig. 26-1.

Consequences of Anemia

The basic physiologic defect caused by anemia is a decrease in the oxygen-carrying capacity of blood and consequently a reduction in the amount of oxygen available to the cells. When the anemia has developed slowly, the child usually adapts to the declining Hgb level.

The effects of anemia on the circulatory system can be profound. Because the viscosity of blood depends almost entirely on the concentration of RBCs, the resulting hemodilution of severe anemia decreases peripheral resistance, causing greater quantities of blood to return to the heart. The increased circulation and turbulence within the heart may produce a murmur. Because the cardiac workload is greatly increased, especially during exercise, infection, or emotional stress, cardiac failure may ensue.

Children seem to have a remarkable ability to function well despite low levels of Hgb. **Cyanosis** (the result of the quantity of deoxygenated Hgb in arterial blood) is typically not evident. Growth retardation, resulting from decreased cellular metabolism and coexisting anorexia, is a common finding in chronic severe anemia and is frequently accompanied by delayed sexual maturation in the older child.

TABLE 26-1

Tests Performed as Part of the Complete Blood Cell Count

TEST (AVERAGE VALUE)*	DESCRIPTION AND COMMENTS
Red blood cell (RBC) count (4.5-5.5 million/mm³)	Number of RBCs/mm³ of blood
	Indirectly estimates Hgb content of blood
	Reflects function of bone marrow
Hemoglobin (Hgb) determination (11.5-15.5 g/dl)	Amount of Hgb (g)/dl of whole blood
	Total blood Hgb primarily dependent on number of circulating RBCs but also on amount of Hgb in each cell
Hematocrit (Hct) (35%-45%)	Percent volume of packed RBCs in whole blood
	Indirectly measures Hgb content
	Is approximately three times Hgb content
RBC indexes	
Mean corpuscular volume (MCV) (77-95 fl)	Average or mean volume (size) of a single RBC
	MCV values are expressed as femtoliters (fl) or cubic microns (μm³)
Mean corpuscular hemoglobin (MCH) (25-33 pg/cell)	Average or mean quantity (weight) of Hgb in a single RBC
	MCH values are expressed as picograms (pg) or micromicrograms (μmcg)
	MCV and MCH depend on accurate counts of RBCs, whereas MCHC does not; therefore MCHC is often more reliable
	All indexes depend on average cell measurements and do not show individual RBC variations (anisocytosis)
Mean corpuscular hemoglobin concentration (MCHC) (31%-37% Hgb [g]/dl RBC)	Average concentration of Hgb in a single RBC
	MCHC values are expressed as percent Hgb (g)/cell or Hgb (g)/dl RBC
RBC volume distribution width (RDW) (13.4% ± 1.2%)	Average size of RBCs
	Differentiates some types of anemia
Reticulocyte count (0.5%-1.5% erythrocytes)	Percent reticulocytes in RBCs
	Index of production of mature RBCs by bone marrow
	Decreased count indicates depressed bone marrow function
	Increased count indicates erythrogenesis in response to some stimulus
	When reticulocyte count is extremely high, other forms of immature RBCs (normoblasts, even erythroblasts) may be present
	Indirectly estimates hypochromic anemia
	Usually elevated in patients with chronic hemolytic anemia
White blood cell (WBC) count (4.5-13.5 × 10³ cells/mm³)	Number of WBCs/mm³ of blood
	Total number of WBCs less important than differential count
Differential WBC count	Inspection and quantification of WBC types present in peripheral blood
	Values are expressed as percentages; to obtain absolute number of any type of WBC, multiply its respective percentage by total number of WBCs
Neutrophils (polys) (54%-62%) (3-5.8 × 10³ cells/mm³)	Primary defense in bacterial infection; capable of phagocytizing and killing bacteria
Bands (3%-5%) (0.15-0.4 × 10³ cells/mm³)	Immature neutrophil
	Increased numbers in bacterial infection
	Also capable of phagocytosis and killing
Eosinophils (1%-3%) (0.05-0.25 × 10³ cells/mm³)	Named for their staining characteristics with eosin dye
	Increased in allergic disorders, parasitic diseases, certain neoplasms, and other diseases
Basophils (0.075%) (0.015-0.030 cells/mm³)	Named for their characteristic basophilic stippling
	Contain histamine, heparin, and serotonin; believed to cause increased blood flow to injured tissues while preventing excessive clotting
Lymphocytes (25%-33%) (1.5-3.0 × 10³ cells/mm³)	Involved in development of antibody and delayed hypersensitivity
Monocytes (3%-7%)	Large phagocytic cells that are involved in early stage of inflammatory reaction
Absolute neutrophil count (ANC) (>1000)	Percent neutrophils/bands times WBC count
	Indicates body's capability to handle bacterial infections
Platelet count (150-400 × 10³/mm³)	Number of platelets/mm³ of blood
	Cellular fragments that are necessary for clotting to occur
Stained peripheral blood smear	Visual estimation of amount of Hgb in RBCs and overall size, shape, and structure of RBCs
	Various staining properties of RBC structures may be evidence of immature forms of erythrocytes
	Shows variation in size and shape of RBCs: microcytic, macrocytic, poikilocytic (variable shapes)

*See Appendix C for normal values according to ages.

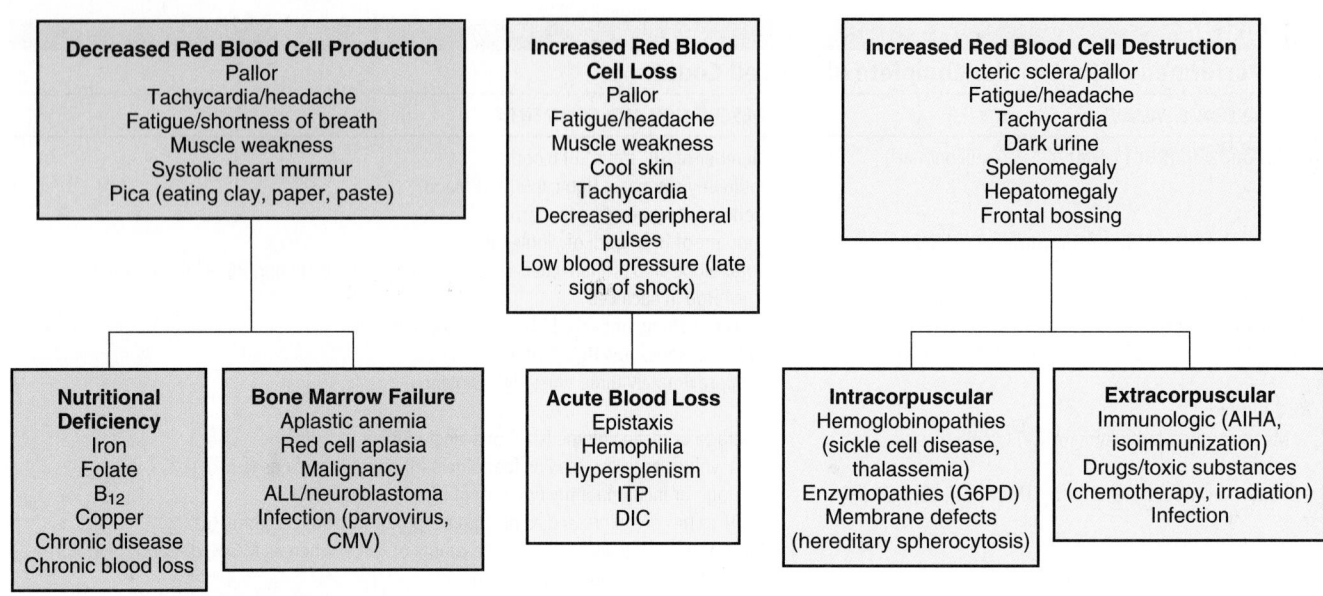

FIG. 26-1 ■ Classifications of anemias. *AIHA,* Autoimmune hemolytic anemia; *ALL,* acute lymphoid leukemia; *CMV,* cytomegalovirus; *DIC,* disseminated intravascular coagulation; *G6PD,* glucose-6-phosphate dehydrogenase; *ITP,* idiopathic thrombocytopenic purpura.

BOX 26-1
Red Blood Cell Morphology

SIZE (CELL SIZE)
Variation in red blood cell (RBC) sizes (anisocytosis)
- Normocytes (normal cell size)
- Microcytes (smaller than normal cell size)
- Macrocytes (larger than normal cell size)

SHAPE (CELL SHAPE)
Variation in RBC shapes (poikilocytosis)
- Spherocytes (globular cells)
- Drepanocytes (sickle-shaped cells)
- Numerous other irregularly shaped cells

COLOR (CELL STAINING CHARACTERISTICS)
Variation in hemoglobin concentration in the RBC
- Normochromic (sufficient or normal amount of hemoglobin per RBC)
- Hypochromic (reduced amount of hemoglobin per RBC)
- Hyperchromic (increased amount of hemoglobin per RBC)

Diagnostic Evaluation

In general, anemia may be suspected based on findings on the history and physical examination, such as lack of energy, easy fatigability, and pallor, but unless the anemia is severe, the first clue to the disorder may be alterations in the CBC, such as decreased RBCs, and decreased Hgb and hematocrit (Hct) levels (see Fig. 26-1). Although anemia is sometimes defined as an Hgb level below 10 or 11 g/dl, this arbitrary cutoff is inappropriate for all children, because Hgb levels normally vary with age (see Table 26-1 and Appendix C).

Other tests specific to a particular type of anemia are employed to determine the underlying cause of anemia. These are discussed in relation to the particular disorder.

Therapeutic Management

The objective of medical management is to reverse the anemia by treating the underlying cause and to make up for any deficiency of blood, blood component, or substance the blood needs for normal functioning. For example, blood or blood cells are replaced after hemorrhage; in nutritional anemias the specific deficiency is replaced.

In patients with severe anemia, supportive medical care may include oxygen therapy, bed rest, and replacement of intravascular volume with intravenous (IV) fluids. The prognosis for anemia depends on the correction of the cause.

Nursing Care Management

The assessment of anemia includes the basic techniques that are applicable to any condition. The age of the infant or child provides some clues regarding the possible etiology of the anemia. For example, iron deficiency anemia occurs more frequently in the toddler between 12 and 36 months of age and during the growth spurt of adolescence.

Racial or ethnic background is significant. For example, the anemias related to abnormal Hgb levels are found in Southeast Asians and persons of African or Mediterranean ancestry. These same groups may be genetically deficient in the enzyme lactase after the period of infancy. Affected individuals are unable to tolerate lactose in the diet, with consequent intestinal irritation and chronic blood loss.

Special emphasis is placed on a careful history to elicit any information that might help identify the cause of the anemia. For example, a statement such as "My child drinks lots of milk" is a frequent finding in toddlers with iron deficiency anemia. An episode of diarrhea may have precipitated temporary lactose intolerance in a young child.

Stool examination for occult (microscopic) blood (Hemoccult test) can identify chronic intestinal bleeding that results from a primary or secondary lactase deficiency. It is also important to understand the significance of various blood tests (see Table 26-1).

Prepare Child and Family for Laboratory Tests. Usually, several blood tests are ordered, but because they are generally done sequentially rather than at one time, the child is subjected to multiple finger or heel punctures or venipunctures. Laboratory technicians frequently are not aware of the trauma that repeated punctures represent to a child. However, these invasive procedures need not be painful (see Blood Specimens, Chapter 22). For example, the topical application of EMLA (an eutectic mix of lidocaine and prilocaine) or 4% lidocaine (Ela-Max) before needle punctures can eliminate pain (see Pain Management, Chapter 7). Therefore the nurse is responsible for preparing the child and family for the tests by:

- Explaining the significance of each test, particularly why the tests are not all done at one time
- Encouraging parents or another supportive person to be with the child during the procedure
- Allowing the child to play with the equipment on a doll or participate in the actual procedure (e.g., by cleansing the finger with an alcohol swab)

Older children may appreciate the opportunity to observe the blood cells under a microscope or in photographs. This experience is especially important if a serious blood disorder, such as leukemia, is suspected, since it serves as a foundation for explaining the pathophysiology of the disorder.

Bone marrow aspiration is not a routine hematologic test but is essential for definitive diagnosis of the leukemias, lymphomas, and certain anemias.

> **NURSING TIP**
>
> The following are suggested explanations for teaching children about blood components:
> **Red blood cells**—Carry the oxygen you breathe from your lungs to all parts of your body
> **White blood cells**—Help keep germs from causing infection
> **Platelets**—Small parts of cells that help make bleeding stop by forming a clot (scab) over the hurt area
> **Plasma**—The liquid portion of blood, which has clotting factors that help make bleeding stop

Decrease Tissue Oxygen Needs. Because the basic pathologic process in anemia is a decrease in oxygen-carrying capacity, an important nursing responsibility is to assess the child's energy level and minimize excess demands. The child's level of tolerance for activities of daily living and play is assessed, and adjustments are made to allow as much self-care as possible without undue exertion. During periods of rest the nurse takes vital signs and observes behavior to establish a baseline of nonexertion energy expenditure. During periods of activity the nurse repeats these measurements and observations to compare them with resting values.

> **NURSING ALERT**
>
> Signs of exertion include tachycardia, palpitations, tachypnea, dyspnea, shortness of breath, hyperpnea, breathlessness, dizziness, lightheadedness, diaphoresis, and change in skin color. The child looks fatigued (sagging, limp posture; slow, strained movements; inability to tolerate additional activity; difficulty sucking in infants).

Prevent Complications. Children who are so severely anemic that they are hospitalized may require oxygen to prevent or reduce tissue hypoxia. Because these children are susceptible to infection, every effort is expended to prevent exposure to infectious agents. All the usual precautions are taken to prevent infection, such as practicing thorough hand washing, selecting an appropriate room in a noninfectious area, restricting visitors or hospital personnel with active infection, and maintaining adequate nutrition. The nurse also observes for signs of infection, particularly temperature elevation and leukocytosis.

IRON DEFICIENCY ANEMIA

Anemia caused by an inadequate supply of dietary iron is the most prevalent nutritional disorder in the United States and the most common mineral disturbance. Children 12 to 36 months of age are at risk for anemia as a result of cow's milk being a major staple of the child's diet (Richardson, 2007; Segel, Hirsh, and Feig, 2002). The prevalence of iron deficiency anemia has decreased, probably in part because of families' participation in the Women, Infants, and Children (WIC) program, which provides iron-fortified formula for the first year of life and routine screening of Hgb levels during early childhood (Bogen, Krause, and Serwint, 2001). Preterm infants are especially at risk because of their reduced fetal iron supply. Adolescents are also at risk because of their rapid growth rate combined with poor eating habits.

Pathophysiology

Iron deficiency anemia can be caused by any number of factors that decrease the supply of iron, impair its absorption, increase the body's need for iron, or affect the synthesis of Hgb. Although the clinical manifestations and diagnostic evaluation are similar regardless of the cause, the therapeutic and nursing care management depend on the specific reason for the iron deficiency. The following discussion is limited to iron deficiency anemia resulting from inadequate iron in the diet.

During the last trimester of pregnancy, iron is transferred from mother to fetus. Most of the iron is stored in the circulating erythrocytes of the fetus, with the remainder stored in the fetal liver, spleen, and bone marrow. These iron stores are usually adequate for the first 5 to 6 months in a full-term infant but for only 2 to 3 months in preterm infants or multiple births. If dietary iron is not supplied to meet the infant's growth demands after the fetal iron stores are depleted, iron deficiency anemia results. Physiologic anemia should not be confused with iron deficiency anemia resulting from nutritional causes.

Although most toddlers with iron deficiency anemia are underweight, many infants are overweight because of excessive milk ingestion (known as **milk babies**). These children become anemic for two reasons: milk, a poor source of iron, is given almost to the exclusion of solid foods, and 50% of iron-deficient infants fed cow's milk have an increased fecal loss of blood.

Therapeutic Management

After the diagnosis of iron deficiency anemia is made, therapeutic management focuses on increasing the amount of supplemental iron the child receives. This is usually done through dietary counseling and the administration of oral iron supplements.

In formula-fed infants the most convenient and best sources of supplemental iron are iron-fortified commercial formula and iron-fortified infant cereal. Iron-fortified for-

constipation

mula provides a relatively constant and predictable amount of iron and is not associated with an increased incidence of gastrointestinal (GI) symptoms, such as colic, diarrhea, or constipation. Infants younger than 12 months of age should *not* be given fresh cow's milk because it may increase the risk of GI blood loss occurring from allergy to the milk protein or from GI mucosal damage resulting from a lack of cytochrome iron (heme protein) (Richardson, 2007; Segel, Hirsh, and Feig, 2002). If GI bleeding is suspected, the child's stool should be guaiac tested on at least four or five occasions to identify any intermittent blood loss.

Dietary addition of iron-rich foods is usually inadequate as the sole treatment of iron deficiency anemia, since the iron is poorly absorbed and thus provides insufficient supplemental quantities of iron. If dietary sources of iron cannot replace body stores, oral iron supplements are prescribed for approximately 3 months. Ferrous iron, more readily absorbed than ferric iron, results in higher Hgb levels. Ascorbic acid (vitamin C) appears to facilitate absorption of iron and may be given as vitamin C–enriched foods and juices with the iron preparation.

If the Hgb level fails to rise after 1 month of oral therapy, it is important to assess for persistent bleeding, iron malabsorption, noncompliance, improper iron administration, or other causes for the anemia. Parenteral (IV or intramuscular [IM]) iron administration is safe and effective, but painful, expensive, and occasionally associated with regional lymphadenopathy or allergic reaction (Andrews, 2003; McKenzie, 2004). Therefore parenteral iron is reserved for children who have iron malabsorption or chronic hemoglobinuria. Transfusions are indicated for the most severe anemia and in cases of serious infection, cardiac dysfunction, or surgical emergency when anesthesia is required. Packed RBCs (2 to 3 ml/kg), not whole blood, are used to minimize the chance of circulatory overload. Supplemental oxygen is administered when tissue hypoxia is severe.

Prognosis. The prognosis for a child with this condition is very good. However, there is some evidence that if the iron deficiency anemia is severe and longstanding, cognitive, behavioral, and motor impairment may result (Burden, Westerlund, Sivan-Armony, and others, 2007; Andrews, 2003).

Nursing Care Management

An essential nursing responsibility is instructing parents in the administration of iron. Oral iron should be given as prescribed in two divided doses between meals, when the presence of free hydrochloric acid is greatest, since more iron is absorbed in the acidic environment of the upper GI tract. A citrus fruit or juice taken with the medication aids in absorption.

> **NURSINGTIP**
>
> Cow's milk contains substances that bind the iron and interfere with absorption. Iron supplements should not be administered with milk or milk products (Carley, 2003).

An adequate dosage of oral iron turns the stools a tarry green color. The nurse advises parents of this normally expected change and inquires about its occurrence on follow-up visits. Absence of the greenish black stool may be a clue to poor administration of iron, either in schedule or in dosage. Vomiting or diarrhea can occur with iron therapy. If the parents report these symptoms, the iron can be given with meals

and the dosage reduced and then gradually increased until tolerated.

Liquid preparations of iron may temporarily stain the teeth. If possible, the medication should be taken through a straw or given through a syringe or medicine dropper placed toward the back of the mouth. Brushing the teeth after administration of the drug lessens the discoloration.

If parenteral iron preparations are prescribed, iron dextran must be injected deeply into a large muscle mass using the Z-track method. The injection site is *not* massaged after injection to minimize skin staining and irritation. Because no more than 1 ml should be given in one site, the IV route should be considered to avoid multiple injections. Careful observation is required because of the risk of adverse reactions, such as anaphylaxis, with IV administration. A test dose is recommended before routine use.

Diet. A primary nursing objective is to prevent nutritional anemia through family education. Because breast milk is a poor iron source after 5 months of lactation, the nurse must reinforce the importance of administering iron supplementation to the exclusively breast-fed infant by 6 months of age (Andrews, 2003; Chandran and Gelfer, 2006; Richardson, 2007). The American Academy of Pediatrics (2005) recommends preterm and low-birth-weight infants or infants with inadequate iron stores at birth receive iron supplements before 6 months of age.

In the formula-fed infant, the nurse discusses with parents the importance of using iron-fortified formula and the introducing solid foods at the appropriate age during the first year of life. Traditionally, cereals are one of the first semisolid foods to be introduced into the infant's diet at approximately 6 months of age (Chandran and Gelfer, 2006; Glader, 2007). The best solid-food source of iron is commercial iron-fortified cereals. It may be difficult at first to teach the infant to accept foods other than milk. The same principles are applied as those for introducing new foods (see Nutrition, Chapter 10), especially feeding the solid food before the milk. Predominantly milk-fed infants rebel against solid foods, and parents are cautioned about this and the need to be firm in not relinquishing control to the child. It may require intense problem solving on the part of both the family and the nurse to overcome the child's resistance.

A difficulty encountered in discouraging the parents from feeding milk to the exclusion of other foods is dispelling the popular myth that milk is a "perfect food." Many parents believe that milk is best for the infant and equate the weight gain with a "healthy child" and "good mothering." The nurse can also stress that overweight is not synonymous with good health.

Diet education of teenagers is especially difficult, especially because teenage girls are particularly prone to following weight-reduction diets. Emphasizing the effect of anemia on appearance (pallor) and energy level (difficulty maintaining popular activities) may be useful. (See Mineral Imbalances, Chapter 11, and Table 11-2 for sources of iron-rich foods.)

SICKLE CELL ANEMIA

Sickle cell anemia (SCA) is one of a group of diseases collectively termed **hemoglobinopathies,** in which normal adult Hgb (Hgb A [HbA]) is partly or completely replaced by abnormal sickle Hgb (HbS). **Sickle cell disease (SCD)** includes all those hereditary disorders whose clinical, hematologic, and pathologic features are related to the presence of HbS. Even though the term *SCD* is sometimes used to refer to SCA, this use is incorrect. Other correct terms for SCA are **SS** and **homozygous SCD.**

The following are the most common forms of SCD in the United States:

SCA, the homozygous form of the disease (HbSS or SS).
Sickle cell–C disease, a heterozygous variant of SCD, including both HbS and HbC (SC).
Sickle cell–hemoglobin E disease, a variant of SCD in which glutamic acid has been substituted for lysine in the number-26 position of the β-chain (SE).
Sickle thalassemia disease, a combination of sickle cell trait and β-thalassemia trait (Sβthal). β⁺ refers to the ability to still produce some normal HbA. β⁰ indicates that there is no ability to produce HbA.

Of the SCDs, SCA is the most common form in African-Americans, followed by sickle cell–C disease and sickle thalassemia. Sickle syndromes exist when the HbS is paired with other mutant globins.

SCA is found primarily in 1 in 375 births of African-Americans, 1 in 1200 births of Hispanics, with lower incidence in the other ethnic groups (Driscoll, 2007). The incidence of the disease varies in different geographic locations. Among African-Americans the incidence of sickle cell trait is about 9%. In West Africa the incidence is reported to be as high as 40% among native Africans. The high incidence of

sickle cell trait in West Africans is believed by some to be the result of selective protection afforded trait carriers against one type of malaria.

The gene that determines the production of HbS is situated on an autosome and, when present, is always detectable and therefore dominant. Heterozygous persons who have both normal HbA and abnormal HbS are said to have **sickle cell trait.** Persons who are homozygous have predominantly HbS and have **sickle cell anemia.** The inheritance pattern is essentially that of an autosomal recessive disorder. Therefore, when both parents have sickle cell trait, there is a 25% chance with each pregnancy of producing an offspring with SCA.

Although the defect is inherited, the sickling phenomenon is usually not apparent until later in infancy because of the presence of fetal Hbg (HbF). As long as the child has predominantly HbF, sickling does not occur because there is less HbS. The newborn with SCA is generally asymptomatic because of the protective effect of HbF (60% to 80% HbF), but this rapidly decreases during the first year, so the child is at risk for sickle cell–related complications (Dover and Platt, 2003; Driscoll, 2007).

Pathophysiology

The clinical features of SCA are primarily the result of (1) **obstruction** caused by the sickled RBCs and (2) increased RBC **destruction** (Fig. 26-2). The abnormal adhesion, entanglement, and enmeshing of rigid sickle-shaped cells with one another

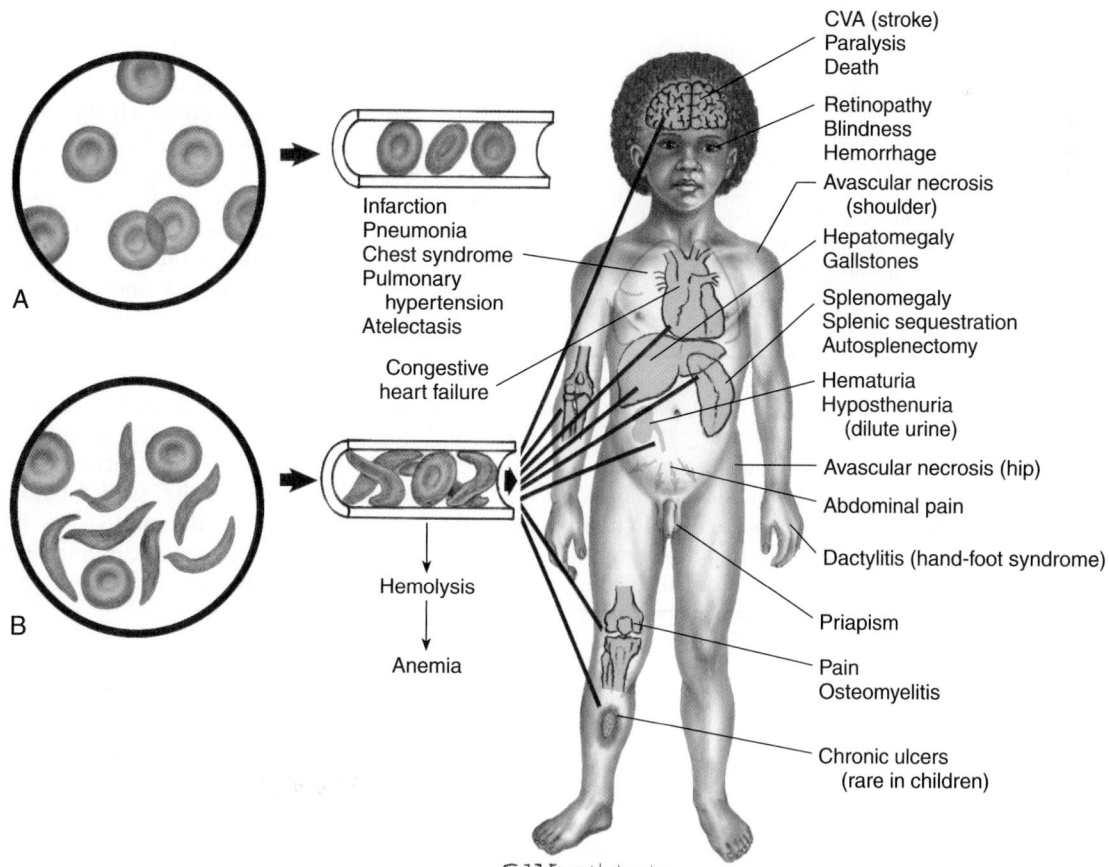

FIG. 26-2 ■ Differences between effects of normal **(A)** and sickled **(B)** red blood cells on circulation with related complications. *CVA,* Cerebrovascular accident.

BOX 26-2

Clinical Manifestations of Sickle Cell Anemia

GENERAL
Possible growth retardation
Chronic anemia (hemoglobin level of 6 to 9 g/dl)
Possible delayed sexual maturation
Marked susceptibility to sepsis

VASOOCCLUSIVE CRISIS
Pain in area(s) of involvement
Manifestations related to ischemia of involved areas
   Extremities—Painful swelling of hands and feet (sickle cell dactylitis, or hand-foot syndrome), painful joints
   Abdomen—Severe pain resembling acute surgical condition
   Cerebrum—Stroke, visual disturbances
   Chest—Symptoms resembling pneumonia, protracted episodes of pulmonary disease
   Liver—Obstructive jaundice, hepatic coma
   Kidney—Hematuria
   Genitalia—Priapism (painful, constant penile erection)

SEQUESTRATION CRISIS
Pooling of large amounts of blood
- Hepatomegaly
- Splenomegaly
- Circulatory collapse

EFFECTS OF CHRONIC VASOOCCLUSIVE PHENOMENA
Heart—Cardiomegaly, systolic murmurs
Lungs—Altered pulmonary function, susceptibility to infections, pulmonary insufficiency
Kidneys—Inability to concentrate urine, enuresis, progressive renal failure
Liver—Hepatomegaly, cirrhosis, intrahepatic cholestasis
Spleen—Splenomegaly, susceptibility to infection, functional reduction in splenic activity progressing to autosplenectomy
Eyes—Intraocular abnormalities with visual disturbances; sometimes progressive retinal detachment and blindness
Extremities—Avascular necrosis of hip or shoulder; skeletal deformities, especially lordosis and kyphosis; chronic leg ulcers; susceptibility to osteomyelitis
Central nervous system—Hemiparesis, seizures

---

intermittently block the microcirculation, causing vasoocclusion. The resultant absence of blood flow to adjacent tissues causes local hypoxia, leading to tissue ischemia and infarction (cellular death). Most of the complications seen in SCA can be traced to this process and its impact on various organs of the body. The effect of sickling and infarction on organ structures occurs in the following sequence (see Box 26-2):

1. Stasis with enlargement
2. Infarction with ischemia and repeated destruction
3. Replacement with fibrous tissue (scarring)

Clinical Manifestations

The clinical manifestations of SCA vary greatly in severity and frequency. The most acute symptoms of the disease occur during periods of exacerbation called **crises.** There are several types of episodic crises: vasoocclusive, acute splenic sequestra-

tion, aplastic, hyperhemolytic, cerebrovascular accident, chest syndrome, and infection. The crises may occur individually or concomitantly with one or more other crises. The episode may be a **vasoocclusive crisis (VOC),** preferably called a "painful episode," characterized by distal ischemia and pain; **sequestration crisis,** a pooling of blood in the liver and spleen with decreased blood volume and shock; **aplastic crisis,** diminished RBC production resulting in profound anemia; or **hyperhemolytic crisis,** an accelerated rate of RBC destruction characterized by anemia, jaundice, and reticulocytosis.

Another serious complication is **acute chest syndrome (ACS),** which is clinically similar to pneumonia. It is the presence of a new pulmonary infiltrate and is associated with chest pain, fever, cough, tachypnea, wheezing, and hypoxia. A **cerebrovascular accident (CVA, stroke)** is a sudden and severe complication, often with no related illnesses. Sickled cells block the major blood vessels in the brain, resulting in cerebral infarction, which causes variable degrees of neurologic impairment. The current treatment for SCD children who have experienced a stroke is chronic transfusion therapy. Repeat CVAs causing progressively greater brain damage occur in approximately 70% of untreated children who have experienced one stroke (Dover and Platt, 2003).

Diagnostic Evaluation

Newborn screening for SCA is mandatory in most of the United States so that infants can be identified before symptoms occur. At birth the infant has up to 80% of HbF, which does not carry the defect. Because levels of HbS are low at birth, Hgb electrophoresis or other tests that measure Hgb concentrations are indicated. Early diagnosis (before 3 months of age) enables initiation of appropriate interventions to minimize complications. The family is taught to administer prophylactic antibiotics and identify early signs of infection to seek medical therapy as soon as possible.

If SCA is not diagnosed in early infancy, it is likely to manifest symptoms during the toddler and preschool years. SCA is occasionally first diagnosed during a crisis that follows an acute respiratory tract or GI infection. Routine hematologic tests are done to evaluate the anemia. Several specific tests detect the presence of the abnormal Hgb in the heterozygote or the homozygote. For **screening** purposes the **sickle-turbidity test (Sickledex)** is frequently used because it can be performed on blood from a fingerstick and yields accurate results in 3 minutes. However, if the test is positive, Hgb electrophoresis is necessary to distinguish between those children with the trait and those with the disease. **Hemoglobin electrophoresis** ("fingerprinting" of the protein) is an accurate, rapid, and specific test for detecting the homozygous and heterozygous forms of the disease, as well as the percentages of the various types of Hgb.

Therapeutic Management

The aims of therapy are (1) to prevent the sickling phenomena, which are responsible for the pathologic sequelae; and (2) to treat the medical emergencies of sickle cell crisis. The successful achievement of the aims depends on prompt nursing interventions, medical therapies, patient and family preventive measures, and use of innovative treatments.

Medical management of a crisis is usually directed toward supportive and symptomatic treatment. The main objectives are to provide (1) rest to minimize energy expenditure and

ETHICAL CASE STUDY	Sickle Cell Disease

ETHICAL DECISION MAKING MODEL	Joey is a 7-year-old with sickle cell disease. His family belongs to a Jehovah's Witnesses congregation, and the parents indicate that they are strong in their faith and beliefs. Joey has had several sickle cell pain crises this past year requiring hospitalization. He has never had a blood transfusion, yet the parents have been informed that a blood transfusion is often required to treat the physical problems associated with sickle cell disease. He arrives in the clinic today looking pale, and his hemoglobin level is 4.9 g/dl (baseline level is 8.0 g/dl), with a reticulocyte count of 1.0%. He has had a cough, fever as high as 37.8° C (100° F), and runny nose for the past week. Physical examination reveals a grade II/VI systolic ejection murmur with gallop at the left lower sternal border. His pulse is 120 beats/min, respirations 20 breaths/min, and blood pressure 102/60 mm Hg. Joey states that he feels tired and has no appetite, and he appears listless.
Evaluate the Issue	The first priority is to evaluate Joey's condition. Children with sickle cell disease are anemic, but when their hemoglobin level drops extremely low, the reticulocyte count should increase as the bone marrow tries to produce new red blood cells. When children with sickle cell disease experience aplastic crisis, the bone marrow does not respond to the decreasing hemoglobin level; this situation is exemplified by Joey's low reticulocyte count. This often occurs after a viral illness, which is indicated in the symptoms experienced by Joey the previous week. The treatment for aplastic crisis in a child with sickle cell disease is blood transfusion, since it can be several weeks before the bone marrow recovers and begins making new red blood cells again. On examination, Joey has clinical symptoms created by the decreasing hemoglobin level.
Treat All Involved with Respect	The physician sits with Joey's parents to discuss the need for a blood transfusion. The physician explains that without a blood transfusion, Joey's condition could become severe and he could die. Joey's mother becomes distraught and states that she cannot give permission to transfuse her son with blood or blood products. The physician listens while the parents discuss their religious beliefs. The controversy in this case is that Joey's family are Jehovah's Witnesses. Individuals of this faith believe that ingesting the blood of any flesh is forbidden and that blood transfusions are equivalent to oral ingestion of blood. Transfusion of whole blood, packed red blood cells, white blood cells, platelets, and plasma (fresh or frozen) is forbidden. If the parents give consent for a blood transfusion, the family will have to leave the congregation, family, friends, and Jehovah's Witnesses community. Refusal of transfusion of blood and blood products is a basic component of the Jehovah's Witnesses faith, and if this precept is broken, the individual loses eternal salvation. Families are often shunned by the Witnesses community, and the child is perceived as an outcast because his future beyond death is affected by the transfusion of blood regardless of its impact on the child's health.
Hear All Sides	Joey's hematology nurse and social worker are asked to spend time with the parents to further explore their concerns regarding the blood transfusion. It becomes evident that the parents cannot give permission for the transfusion. The physician is adamant that the child's best hope for recovery is to receive a blood transfusion.
Initiate Action	For the parents' sake, it is better to obtain a court order for lifesaving transfusion than to ask their permission. This removes the decision from the parents and prevents the parents and child from being ostracized, since the matter was removed from their control. The nurse's role is to be an advocate for the family and a resource to other members of the health care team regarding the family's beliefs.
Consider the Outcome	The eventual outcome if Joey does not receive a blood transfusion is that his hemoglobin level will likely continue to fall as red blood cells are lysed. He will become more ill with ensuing respiratory difficulty, propensity for systemic infections, and eventual cardiac failure and death. If his parents fail to give consent for a blood transfusion, a court order may be obtained and Joey may be given the necessary blood transfusion, which will improve his health status. However, it is possible that Joey will become ill again at some point in the future and will again require a blood transfusion, at which point a court order will again become necessary because the parents will not give consent for such therapy. It is unknown how Joey's parents and Jehovah's Witnesses congregation will react to his receiving a blood transfusion.

oxygen use; (2) hydration through oral and IV therapy; (3) electrolyte replacement, since hypoxia results in metabolic acidosis, which also promotes sickling; (4) analgesics for the severe pain from vasoocclusion; (5) blood replacement to treat anemia and to reduce the viscosity of the sickled blood; and (6) antibiotics to treat any existing infection (see Ethical Case Study).

Administration of pneumococcal and meningococcal vaccines is recommended for these children because of their susceptibility to infection as a result of functional asplenia. In addition to routine immunizations, the child with SCD should

receive a yearly influenza vaccination (see Immunizations, Chapter 10). Oral penicillin prophylaxis is also recommended by 2 months of age to reduce the chance of pneumococcal sepsis (see Evidence-Based Practice box) (American Academy of Pediatrics, 2002; National Institutes of Health, National Heart, Lung, and Blood Institute, 2002; Redding-Lallinger and Knoll, 2006).

Short-term oxygen therapy may be helpful if a child has symptoms of respiratory difficulty. Severe hypoxia must be prevented because this causes massive systemic sickling that can be fatal. Although oxygen may prevent more sickling, it

EVIDENCE-BASED PRACTICE

Sickle Cell Anemia and Penicillin Prophylaxis

ASK THE QUESTION	In children with sickle cell anemia, does prophylaxis with penicillin prevent pneumococcal infection?

SEARCH FOR EVIDENCE

Search Strategies   Search selection criteria included English language, publication within the past 25 years, research-based articles (level 3 or lower), and child populations.

Databases Used   PubMed, Cochrane Collaboration, MD Consult

CRITICALLY ANALYZE THE EVIDENCE

■ Administration of oral prophylactic penicillin was compared with the 14-valent pneumococcal vaccine in preventing pneumococcal infection in 242 children between the ages of 6 months and 3 years with homozygous sickle cell disease. In the first 5 years of the trial, there were 11 pneumococcal infections in the pneumococcal vaccine group and higher infection rates in those given the vaccine before 1 year of age. No pneumococcal isolates were found in the group receiving penicillin, although four pneumococcal isolates were found in this group within 1 year of stopping the penicillin prophylaxis at age 3 years. This study supported the use of penicillin prophylaxis to prevent pneumococcal infection in children younger than 3 years of age (John, Ramlal, Jackson, and others, 1984).

■ In a multicenter, randomized, double-blind, placebo-controlled clinical trial, 105 children received penicillin twice daily; a control group of 110 children received a placebo twice daily. The trial was terminated 8 months early when an 84% reduction in the incidence of pneumococcal infections was observed in the group treated with penicillin compared with the placebo group. There were no deaths in the penicillin group, but three deaths from infection occurred in the placebo group. Researchers stressed the importance of screening children during the neonatal period and prescribing prophylactic penicillin to decrease the morbidity and mortality associated with pneumococcal infection (Gaston, Verter, Woods, and others, 1986).

■ Zarkowsky, Gallagher, Gill, and others (1986) conducted a retrospective analysis of 178 episodes of bacteremia in children with sickle hemoglobinopathies that occurred during 13,771 patient-years of follow-up ($N = 3451$). The predominant pathogen in patients younger than 6 years of age was *Streptococcus pneumoniae* (66%), and gram-negative organisms were responsible for 50% of the bacteremias in patients 6 years and older. The incidence of pneumococcal bacteremia in children with sickle cell anemia younger than 3 years of age was 6.1 events per 100 patient-years. The results of this study supported prophylactic administration of penicillin for prevention of pneumococcal bacteremia in children younger than 3 years of age.

■ A cohort study of 315 patients with homozygous sickle cell disease who lived in Jamaica was conducted between June 1973 and December 1981. The patients were divided into three groups to determine whether interventions such as penicillin prophylaxis, parental education in early diagnosis of acute splenic sequestration, and close monitoring in a sickle cell clinic improved survival. A significant decline in deaths from acute splenic sequestration and pneumococcal septicemia and

meningitis was found. The research indicated that early detection of sickle cell disease and prophylactic measures could significantly reduce deaths associated with homozygous sickle cell disease (Lee, Thomas, Cupidore, and others, 1995).

■ In a retrospective longitudinal study conducted from January 1995 through December 1999, 261 children under 4 years of age with sickle cell disease who did not have adequate health insurance were found to have received inadequate refills for antibiotic prophylaxis that placed them at increased risk of developing pneumococcal infection. Study findings showed that an increased number of outpatient visits for preventive care was associated with improved dispensing of prophylactic antibiotic refills (Sox, Cooper, Koepsell, and others, 2003).

■ Riddington and Owusu-Ofori (2002) conducted a systematic review of randomized controlled trials evaluating the effectiveness of prophylactic antibiotic administration in preventing pneumococcal infection in children with sickle cell disease. The review of published research found that penicillin prophylaxis significantly reduced the risk of pneumococcal infection in children with homozygous sickle cell disease with minimal adverse reactions.

APPLY THE EVIDENCE: NURSING IMPLICATIONS

The evidence demonstrated that penicillin prophylaxis significantly reduces the risk of pneumococcal infection in children with sickle cell anemia. The epidemiologic studies strongly suggest that all children with sickle cell anemia should be started on prophylactic penicillin at 2 months of age. Parents and children with sickle cell anemia should be instructed in the importance of taking the prophylactic penicillin twice daily and seeking medical attention immediately for acute illness, especially if the temperature exceeds 38.3° C (101° F), regardless of the use of prophylaxis.

References

Gaston MH, Verter JI, Woods G, and others: Prophylaxis with oral penicillin in children with sickle cell anemia: a randomized trial, *N Engl J Med* 314(25):1593-1599, 1986.

John AB, Ramlal A, Jackson H, and others: Prevention of pneumococcal infection in children with homozygous sickle cell disease, *BMJ* 288(6430):1567-1570, 1984.

Lee A, Thomas P, Cupidore L, and others: Improved survival in homozygous sickle cell disease: lessons from cohort study, *BMJ* 311(7020):1600-1602, 1995.

Riddington C, Owusu-Ofori S: *Prophylactic antibiotics for preventing pneumococcal infection in children with sickle cell disease*, 2002, retrieved August 19, 2005, from http://www.cochrane.org/reviews/en/ab003427.html.

Sox CM, Cooper WO, Koepsell TD, and others: Provision of pneumococcal prophylaxis for publicly insured children with sickle cell disease, *JAMA* 290(8):1057-1061, 2003.

Zarkowsky HS, Gallagher D, Gill FM, and others: Bacteremia in sickle hemoglobinopathies, *J Pediatr* 109(4):579-585, 1986.

usually is not effective in reversing sickling because the oxygen is unable to reach the enmeshed sickled erythrocytes in clogged vessels (Perkins, 2001; Chiocca, 1996). In addition, prolonged administration can depress bone marrow, further aggravating the anemia (Khoury and Grimsley, 1995: Dover and Platt, 2003).

Exchange transfusion, which reduces the number of circulating sickle cells and slows down the vicious circle of hypoxia, thrombosis, tissue ischemia, and injury, has been successful. The procedure is sometimes advocated as a possible preventive technique. A transcranial Doppler (TCD) test identifies the child with SCD who is at high risk for developing a CVA by monitoring the intracranial vascular flow (American Academy of Pediatrics, 2002; Bulas, 2005; Driscoll, 2007). The TCD is performed yearly on children from 2 to 16 years of age. If the TCD is abnormal, the recommended treatment is chronic transfusion therapy (Driscoll, 2007; Segal, Hirsh, and Feig, 2002). However, multiple transfusions carry the risk of transmission of viral infection, hyperviscosity, transfusion reactions, alloimmunization, and hemosiderosis (Redding-Lallinger and Knoll, 2006; Orkin and Nathan, 2003; Driscoll, 2007). After a CVA, blood transfusions are usually given every 3 to 4 weeks to help prevent a repeat stroke. To reduce iron overload from chronic transfusion therapy, chelation therapy may be started (see p. 924).

In children with recurrent life-threatening splenic sequestration, splenectomy may be a lifesaving measure. However, the spleen usually atrophies on its own through progressive fibrotic changes (**functional asplenia**) by 6 years of age. Prophylactic penicillin postsplenectomy and pneumococcal vaccines have decreased the incidence of pneumococcal sepsis. Packed RBC transfusions are recommended for treatment of splenic sequestration and stroke and preoperatively for most surgical procedures in the child with SCD.

The most frequent problem for patients with SCA is **vasoocclusive pain**. The chronic nature of this pain can greatly affect the child's development. **Priapism (continuous or intermittent)** is defined as painful erection of the penis. As a vasoocclusive crisis, the priapism event is caused by sickling in sinusoids of the corpora cavernosa and is treated with aspiration from the corpora cavernosa only when conventional approaches fail (Redding-Lallinger and Knoll, 2006). A multidisciplinary approach is best for vasoocclusive pain management that includes pharmacologic treatment, hydration, physical therapy, and complementary treatment (e.g., prayer, spiritual healing, massage, herbs, relaxation, acupuncture, and biofeedback) (Redding-Lallinger and Knoll, 2006; Yoon and Black, 2006). When mild to moderate pain is reported, ibuprofen or acetaminophen (Tylenol) is used initially. If these drugs are not effective alone, codeine can be added. The dosages of both drugs are titrated (adjusted) to a therapeutic level. Opioids such as immediate- and sustained-release morphine, oxycodone, hydromorphone (Dilaudid), and methadone are administered intravenously or orally for severe pain and are given around the clock. Patient-controlled analgesia (PCA) has been used successfully for sickle cell–related pain. PCA reinforces the patient's role and responsibility in managing the pain and provides flexibility in dealing with pain, which may vary in severity over time (see Pain Management, Chapter 7).

NURSING ALERT

Meperidine (Demerol) is not recommended. Normeperidine, a metabolite of meperidine, is a central nervous system (CNS) stimulant that produces anxiety, tremors, myoclonus, and generalized seizures when it accumulates with repetitive dosing. Patients with SCD are particularly at risk for normeperidine-induced seizures (Dover and Platt, 2003; National Institutes of Health, National Heart, Lung, and Blood Institute, 2002; American Pain Society, 1999).

Prognosis. The prognosis varies, but most patients live into the fifth decade. Most of the time, children are without symptoms and participate in normal activities without restrictions. The greatest risk is usually in children younger than 5 years of age, and the majority of deaths in these children are caused by overwhelming infection. Consequently, SCA is a chronic illness with a potentially terminal outcome. Physical and sexual maturation are delayed in adolescents with SCA. Although adults achieve normal height, weight, and sexual function, the delay may present problems to the adolescent (Dover and Platt, 2003; Redding-Lallinger and Knoll, 2006).

SCD individuals with higher levels of HbF tend to have a milder disease with fewer complications than those with lower levels (Anderson, 2006; Driscoll, 2007). Hydroxyurea is a U.S. Food and Drug Administration–approved medication that increases the production of HbF, reduces endothelial adhesion of sickle cells, and improves the sickle cell hydration (National Institutes of Health, National Heart, Lung, and Blood Institute, 2002). Long-term follow-up of patients taking hydroxyurea alone revealed a 40% reduction in mortality and decreased frequency of vasoocclusive crisis, ACS, hospital admissions, and need for transfusions, thus making SCD crises milder (Anderson, 2006; Steinberg, Barton, Castro, and others, 2003). Pediatric studies has shown that hydroxyurea can be safely used in children (Miller, Zimmerman, Schultz, and others, 2001; Zimmerman, Schultz, Davis, and others, 2004).

Hematopoietic stem cell transplantation (HSCT) offers the only cure for some children, although the mortality rate is approximately 8% and graft failures after transplantation range from 9% to 14% (Dover and Platt, 2003; Driscoll, 2007) (see p. 945).

Nursing Care Management

Educate Family and Child. Family education begins with an explanation of the disease and its consequences. After this explanation, the most important issues to teach the family are to (1) seek early intervention for problems, such as fever of 38.5° C (101.3° F) or greater; (2) give penicillin as ordered; (3) recognize signs and symptoms of splenic sequestration, as well as respiratory problems that can lead to hypoxia; and (4) treat the child normally. The nurse tells the family that the child is normal but can get sick in ways that other children cannot.

NURSING TIP

One simple yet graphic way to demonstrate the effect of sickling is to roll rounded objects, such as marbles or beads, through a tube to simulate normal circulation and then roll pointed objects, such as screws or jacks, through the tube. The effect of sickling and clumping of the pointed objects is especially noticeable at a bend or slight narrowing of the tube.

The nurse emphasizes the importance of adequate hydration to prevent sickling and to delay the adhesion-stasis-thrombosis-ischemia cycle in a crisis. It is not sufficient to advise parents to "force fluids" or "encourage drinking." They need specific instructions on how many daily glasses or bottles of fluid are required. Many foods are also a source of fluid, particularly soups, flavored ice pops, ice cream, sherbet, gelatin, and puddings.

Increased fluids combined with impaired kidney function result in the problem of **enuresis**. Parents who are unaware of this fact frequently employ the usual measures to discourage bed-wetting, such as limiting fluids at night, and may

FAMILY FOCUS

Fear of Addiction

Although the pain during a sickle cell crisis is usually severe and opioids are needed, many families fear that their child will become addicted to the narcotic. Unfortunately, misinformed health professionals may foster this unfounded fear, which results in needless suffering. Very few children who receive opioids for severe pain become behaviorally addicted to the drug (American Pain Society, 1999; National Institutes of Health, National Heart, Lung, and Blood Institute, 2002). Families and older children, especially adolescents, need to be reassured that opioids are medically indicated, high doses may be needed, and children rarely become addicted.

resort to punishment and shame to force bladder control. Enuresis is treated as a complication of the disease, such as joint pain or some other symptom, to alleviate parental pressure on the child.

Promote Supportive Therapies During Crises. The success of many of the medical therapies relies heavily on nursing implementation. Management of pain is an especially difficult problem and often involves experimenting with various analgesics, including opioids, and schedules before relief is achieved. Unfortunately, these children tend to be undermedicated, resulting in their "clock watching" and demands for additional doses sooner than might be expected. Often this incorrectly raises suspicions of drug addiction, when in fact the problem is one of improper dosage (see Family Focus box). In choosing and scheduling analgesics, the goal should be *prevention* of pain.

NURSING ALERT

Advise parents to be particularly alert to situations in which dehydration may be a possibility, such as hot weather, and to recognize early signs of reduced intake, such as decreased urinary output (e.g., fewer wet diapers) and increased thirst.

Any pain program should be combined with psychologic support to help the child deal with the depression, anxiety, and fear that may accompany the disease. This includes regular visits with the child to discuss any concerns during the hospitalization and positive reinforcement of coping skills, such as successful methods of dealing with the pain and compliance with treatment prescriptions. To reduce the negative connotation associated with the term *crisis*, it is best to say *pain episode.*

Frequently, heat to the affected area is soothing. Cold compresses are not applied to the area because this enhances sickling and vasoconstriction. Bed rest is usually well tolerated during a crisis, although actual rest depends greatly on pain alleviation and organized schedules of nursing care. Some activity, particularly passive range-of-motion exercises, is beneficial to promote circulation. Usually the best course of action is to let children dictate their activity tolerance.

If blood transfusions or exchange transfusions are given, the nurse has the responsibility of observing for signs of transfusion reaction (see Table 26-5). Because hypervolemia from too-rapid transfusion can increase the workload of the heart, the nurse also is alert to signs of cardiac failure.

In splenic sequestration the size of the spleen is gently measured by abdominal palpation (see Abdomen, Chapter 6). The nurse should be aware of spleen size because increasing splenomegaly is an ominous sign. A decreasing spleen size denotes response to therapy. Vital signs and blood pressure are also closely monitored for impending shock. Anemia is typically not a presenting complication in vasoocclusive crises but is a critical problem in other types of crises. The nurse monitors for evidence of increasing anemia and institutes appropriate nursing interventions (see p. 918). Oxygen is not beneficial in vasoocclusive episodes unless hypoxemia is present (Dover and Platt, 2003; Karayalcin, 2000). It does not reverse sickled RBCs, and if used in the nonhypoxic patient, it will decrease erythropoiesis (Khoury and Grimsley, 1995). Because prolonged use of oxygen can aggravate the anemia, signs of lack of therapeutic benefit, such as restlessness, increased pallor, and continued pain, are reported.

Intake, especially of IV fluids, and output are recorded. The child's weight should be taken on admission to serve as a baseline for evaluating hydration. Because diuresis can result in electrolyte loss, the nurse also observes for signs of hypokalemia and should be familiar with normal serum electrolyte values to report changes.

Recognize Other Complications. Nurses also need to be aware of the signs of ACS and CVA, both potentially fatal complications.

NURSING ALERT

Report signs of the following immediately:
ACS:
- Severe chest, back, or abdominal pain
- Fever of 38.5° C (101.3° F) or higher
- Very congested cough
- Dyspnea, tachypnea
- Retractions
- Declining oxygen saturation (oximetry)

CVA:
- Severe, unrelieved headaches
- Severe vomiting
- Jerking or twitching of the face, legs, or arms
- Seizures
- Strange, abnormal behavior
- Inability to move an arm or leg
- Staggering or an unsteady walk
- Stuttering or slurred speech
- Weakness in the hands, feet, or legs
- Changes in vision

Support Family. Families need the opportunity to discuss their feelings regarding transmitting a potentially fatal, chronic illness to their child. Because of the widely publicized prognosis for children with SCA, many parents express their prevalent fear of the child's death. Three manifestations of SCD that may appear in the first 2 years of life (dactylitis, severe anemia, leukocytosis) can be predictors of disease severity (Platt, Brambilla, Roose, and others, 1994; Ohls and Christensen, 2007). However, nursing care for the family should be the same as for any family with a child with a life-threatening illness. Particular emphasis is placed on the siblings' reactions, the stress on the marital relationship, and the childrearing attitudes displayed toward the child (see Chapter 18). Several resources are available to the family with a sickling disorder.*

The nurse advises parents to inform all treating personnel of the child's condition. The use of medical identification, such as a bracelet, is another way of ensuring awareness of the disease.

If family members have the SCD trait or SCA, genetic counseling is necessary. A primary goal is informing parents who carry the trait, in language they can understand, of the 25% chance with each pregnancy resulting in a child with the disease.

β-THALASSEMIA (COOLEY ANEMIA)

The term **thalassemia,** which is derived from the Greek word *thalassa,* meaning "sea," is applied to a variety of inherited blood disorders characterized by deficiencies in the rate of production of specific globin chains in Hgb. The name appropriately refers to descendants of or those people living near the Mediterranean Sea, who have the highest incidence of the disease, namely Italians, Greeks, and Syrians. Evidence suggests that the high incidence of the disorders among these groups is a result of the selective advantage the trait confers in relation to malaria, as is postulated in SCD. However, the disorder has a wide geographic distribution, probably as a result of genetic migration through intermarriage or possibly as a result of spontaneous mutation.

β-Thalassemia is the most common of the thalassemias and occurs in four forms:

- Two heterozygous forms, **thalassemia minor,** an asymptomatic silent carrier, and **thalassemia trait,** which produces a mild microcytic anemia
- **Thalassemia intermedia,** which is manifested as splenomegaly and moderate to severe anemia
- A homozygous form, **thalassemia major** (also known as **Cooley anemia**), which results in a severe anemia that would lead to cardiac failure and death in early childhood without transfusion support

Pathophysiology

Normal postnatal Hgb is composed of two α- and two β-polypeptide chains. In β-thalassemia there is a partial or complete deficiency in the synthesis of the β-chain of the Hgb molecule. Consequently, there is a compensatory increase in the synthesis of α-chains, and γ-chain production remains activated, resulting in defective Hgb formation. This unbalanced polypeptide unit is very unstable; when it disintegrates, it damages RBCs, causing severe anemia.

---

*Sickle Cell Disease Association of America, Inc., 231 E. Baltimore St., Suite 800, Baltimore, MD 21202; (410) 528-1555, (800) 421-8453; fax: (410) 528-1495; e-mail: scdaa@sicklecelldisease.org; http://www.sicklecelldisease.org; Sickle Cell Information Center, PO Box 109, Grady Memorial Hospital, 80 Jesse Hill Jr Drive SE, Atlanta, GA 30303; (404) 616-3572; fax: (404) 616-5998; e-mail: aplatt@emory.edu; http://www.scinfo.org; National Heart, Lung, and Blood Institute, PO Box 30105, Bethesda, MD 20824-0105; (301) 592-8573, fax: (240) 629-3246; http://www.nhlbi.nih.gov. *Sickle Cell Disease in Newborns and Infants: A Guide for Parents,* Pub No AHCPR 93-0564. Available from the AHCPR Publications Clearinghouse, PO Box 8547, Silver Spring, MD 20907-8547; (800) 358-9295; http://www.ahcpr.gov. *Guideline for the Management of Acute and Chronic Pain in Sickle-Cell Disease* is available from the American Pain Society, 4700 W. Lake Ave., Glenview, IL 60025-1485; (847) 375-4715; fax: (877) 734-8758; e-mail: info@ampainsoc.org; http://www.ampainsoc.org.

BOX 26-3

Clinical Manifestations of β-Thalassemia

ANEMIA (BEFORE DIAGNOSIS)
Pallor
Unexplained fever
Poor feeding
Enlarged spleen or liver

PROGRESSIVE ANEMIA
Signs of chronic hypoxia
- Headache
- Precordial and bone pain
- Decreased exercise tolerance
- Listlessness
- Anorexia

OTHER FEATURES
Small stature
Delayed sexual maturation
Bronzed, freckled complexion (if not receiving chelation therapy)

BONE CHANGES (OLDER CHILDREN IF UNTREATED)
Enlarged head
Prominent frontal and parietal bossing
Prominent malar eminences
Flat or depressed bridge of the nose
Enlarged maxilla
Protrusion of the lip and upper central incisors and eventual malocclusion
Generalized osteoporosis

To compensate for the hemolytic process, an overabundance of erythrocytes is formed unless the bone marrow is suppressed by transfusion therapy. Excess iron from hemolysis of supplemental RBCs in transfusions and from the rapid destruction of defective cells is stored in various organs (**hemosiderosis**).

Diagnostic Evaluation

The onset of thalassemia major may be insidious and not recognized until the latter half of infancy. The clinical effects of thalassemia major are primarily attributable to (1) defective synthesis of HbA, (2) structurally impaired RBCs, and (3) shortened life span of erythrocytes (Box 26-3).

Hematologic studies reveal the characteristic changes in RBCs (i.e., microcytosis, hypochromia, anisocytosis, poikilocytosis, target cells, and basophilic stippling of various stages). Low Hgb and Hct levels are seen in severe anemia, although they are typically lower than the reduction in RBC count because of the proliferation of immature erythrocytes. Hgb electrophoresis confirms the diagnosis, and radiographs of involved bones reveal characteristic findings.

Therapeutic Management

The objective of supportive therapy is to maintain sufficient Hgb levels to prevent bone marrow expansion and the resulting bony deformities, and to provide sufficient RBCs to support normal growth and normal physical activity. Transfusions are the foundation of medical management. Recent studies have evaluated the benefits of maintaining the child's Hgb level above 9.5 g/dl, a goal that may require transfusions as often as every 3 to 5 weeks. The advantages of this therapy include (1) improved physical and psychologic well-being because of the ability to participate in normal activities, (2) decreased cardiomegaly and hepatosplenomegaly, (3) fewer bone changes, (4) normal or near-normal growth and development until puberty, and (5) fewer infections.

One of the potential complications of frequent blood transfusions is iron overload. Because the body has no effective means of eliminating the excess iron, the mineral is deposited in body tissues. To minimize the development of hemosiderosis, the new oral iron chelator deferasirox has been shown to be equivalent to **deferoxamine (Desferal),** a parenteral iron-chelating agent, and more tolerable by patients and families (Morris, Singer, and Walters, 2006; Okpala, 2005).

In some children with severe splenomegaly who demonstrate increased transfusion requirements, a splenectomy may be necessary to decrease the disabling effects of abdominal pressure and to increase the life span of supplemental RBCs. Over time, the spleen may accelerate the rate of RBC destruction and thus increase transfusion requirements. After a splenectomy, children generally require fewer transfusions, although the basic defect in Hgb synthesis remains unaffected. A major postsplenectomy complication is severe and overwhelming infection. Therefore these children continue to receive prophylactic antibiotics with close medical supervision for many years and should receive the pneumococcal and meningococcal vaccines in addition to the regularly scheduled immunizations (see Immunizations, Chapter 10).

NURSING ALERT

Ensure that the family and patient understand the need to notify the health professional of all fevers of 38.5° C (101.3° F) or greater because of the risk of sepsis in a child with asplenia.

Prognosis. Most children treated with blood transfusion and early chelation therapy survive well into adulthood. The most common cause of death is iron-induced heart disease, multiple organ failure, postsplenectomy sepsis, liver disease, and malignancy (Paley, 2000). HSCT has the best results in the least symptomatic pediatric patients, with an 85% to 90% rate of complication-free survival (Morris, Singer, and Walters, 2006; Orkin and Nathan, 2003; Richardson, 2007).

Nursing Care Management

The objectives of nursing care are to (1) promote compliance with transfusion and chelation therapy, (2) assist the child in coping with the anxiety-provoking treatments and the effects of the illness, (3) foster the child's and family's adjustment to a chronic illness, and (4) observe for complications of multiple blood transfusions. Basic to each of these goals is explaining to parents and older children the defect responsible for the disorder, its effect on RBCs, and the potential effects of untreated iron overload (such as diabetes and heart disease). Because the prevalence of this condition is high among families of Mediterranean descent, the nurse also inquires about the family's previous knowledge about thalassemia. All families with a child with thalassemia should be tested for the trait and referred for genetic counseling.

As with any chronic illness, the family's needs must be met for optimal adjustment to the stresses imposed by the disorder

(see Chapter 18). Sources of information for the family include the Cooley's Anemia Foundation* and the Northern California Comprehensive Thalassemia Center.† Genetic counseling for the parents and fertile offspring is mandatory, and both prenatal diagnosis using amniocentesis at 20 weeks' gestation or fetal blood sampling at 10 weeks and screening for thalassemia trait are available.

APLASTIC ANEMIA

Aplastic anemia (AA) refers to a bone marrow failure condition in which the formed elements of the blood are simultaneously depressed. The peripheral blood smear demonstrates pancytopenia or the triad of profound anemia, leukopenia, and thrombocytopenia. **Hypoplastic anemia** is characterized by a profound depression of RBCs, but normal or slightly decreased white blood cells (WBCs) and platelets.

Etiology

AA can be **primary** (**congenital,** or present at birth) or **secondary** (**acquired**). The best-known congenital disorder of which AA is an outstanding feature is **Fanconi syndrome,** a rare hereditary disorder characterized by pancytopenia, hypoplasia of the bone marrow, and patchy brown discoloration of the skin resulting from the deposit of melanin and associated with multiple congenital anomalies of the musculoskeletal and genitourinary systems. The syndrome appears to be inherited as an autosomal recessive trait with varying penetrance; therefore affected siblings may demonstrate several different combinations of defects.

Several etiologic factors contribute to the development of acquired hypoplastic anemia; however, most of the cases are considered idiopathic (Box 26-4). Acquired AA is classified as either severe acquired AA or moderate acquired AA. The following discussion focuses on severe acquired AA, which carries a poorer prognosis and follows a more rapidly fatal course than the primary types.

Diagnostic Evaluation

The onset of clinical manifestations, which include anemia, leukopenia, and decreased platelet count, is usually insidious. Definitive diagnosis is determined from bone marrow aspiration, which demonstrates the conversion of red bone marrow to yellow, fatty bone marrow. Severe AA is defined as less than 25% bone marrow cellularity with at least two of the following findings: absolute granulocyte count less than 500/mm^3, platelet count less than 20,000/mm^3, and absolute reticulocyte count less than 40,000/mm^3 (Hord, 2007; Shimamura and Guinan, 2003). Moderate AA is defined as more than 25% bone marrow cellularity with the presence of mild or moderate cytopenia (Shimamura and Guinan, 2003; Shende, 2000).

Therapeutic Management

The objectives of treatment are based on the recognition that the underlying disease process is failure of the bone marrow to carry out its hematopoietic functions. Therefore therapy is directed at restoring function to the marrow and involves two main approaches: (1) immunosuppressive therapy to remove

---

*330 Seventh Ave., No. 900, New York, NY 10001; (800) 522-7222; fax: (212) 279-5999; http://www.cooleysanemia.org.
†747 52nd St., Oakland, CA 94609; (510) 428-3885, ext. 4398; http://www.thalassemia.com.

BOX 26-4
Common Causes of Acquired Aplastic Anemia

- Human parvovirus infection, hepatitis, or overwhelming infection
- Irradiation
- Immune disorders such as eosinophilic fasciitis and hypoimmunoglobulinemia
- Drugs such as certain chemotherapeutic agents, anticonvulsants, and antibiotics
- Industrial and household chemicals, including benzene and its derivatives, which are found in petroleum products, dyes, paint remover, shellac, and lacquers
- Infiltration and replacement of myeloid elements, such as in leukemia or the lymphomas
- Idiopathic (In most cases no identifiable precipitating cause can be found.)

the presumed immunologic functions that prolong aplasia or (2) replacement of the bone marrow through transplantation. Bone marrow transplantation is the treatment of choice for severe AA when a suitable donor exists (see p. 945).

Antilymphocyte globulin (ALG) or **antithymocyte globulin (ATG)** is the principal drug treatment used for AA. The rationale for using ATG is based on the theory that AA may be a result of autoimmunity. ATG and cyclosporine suppress T cell–dependent autoimmune responses but do not cause bone marrow suppression. Cyclosporine is administered orally for several weeks to months. ATG usually is administrated intravenously over 12 to 16 hours for 4 days, after a test dose to check for hypersensitivity. A course may be repeated, depending on the reduction in circulating lymphocytes and the patient's response. Because of the hypersensitivity response associated with ATG (i.e., fever, chills, myalgias), methylprednisolone is given intravenously to prevent these side effects. Colony-stimulating factor (CSF), and granulocyte-macrophage colony-stimulating factor (GM-CSF) given parenterally, may be used to enhance bone marrow production. Androgens may be used with ATG to stimulate erythropoiesis if the AA is unresponsive to initial therapies.

HSCT should be considered early in the course of the disease if a compatible donor can be found. Transplantation is more successful when performed before multiple transfusions have sensitized the child to leukocyte and **human leukocyte antigens (HLA).** HSCT is associated with an 85% survival rate in untransfused patients compared with a 70% survival rate in transfused patients (Marsh, 2005; Shende, 2000).

Nursing Care Management

The care of the child with AA is similar to that of the child with leukemia (see p. 930)—specifically, preparing the child and family for the diagnostic and therapeutic procedures, preventing complications from the severe pancytopenia, and emotionally supporting them in the face of a potentially fatal outcome. Information and support are available from the Aplastic Anemia and MDS International Foundation, Inc.*

Because the aspects of nursing care are discussed in the section on leukemia, only the exceptions are presented here.

*PO Box 310, Churchton, MD 20733 USA; (800) 747-2820, (410) 867-0242; fax: (410) 867-0240; e-mail: help@aamds.org; http://www.aamds.org.

The drug ATG is usually administered by way of a central vein. If not, vigilant care must be directed to the IV infusion to prevent extravasation. Meticulous care of the venous access is essential because of the child's susceptibility to infection. CSFs are usually given by subcutaneous injection over several days. Chemotherapeutic agents have been reported in the treatment of the relapsed patient with AA after ATG and CSF therapy. Many of the side effects associated with chemotherapy such as nausea and vomiting, alopecia, and mucositis are experienced by children receiving treatment for AA. Specialized care is required for children who have HSCT (see p. 945).

DEFECTS IN HEMOSTASIS

Hemostasis is the process that stops bleeding when a blood vessel is injured. Vascular and plasma clotting factors, as well as platelets, are required. A complex system of clotting, anticlotting, and clot breakdown (**fibrinolysis**) mechanisms exists in equilibrium to ensure clot formation only in the presence of blood vessel injury and to limit the clotting process to the site of vessel wall injury. Dysfunction in these systems will lead to bleeding or abnormal clotting. Although the coagulation process is complex, clotting depends on three factors: (1) vascular influence, (2) platelet role, and (3) clotting factors.

HEMOPHILIA

The term **hemophilia** refers to a group of bleeding disorders in which there is a deficiency of one of the factors necessary for coagulation of the blood. Although the symptomatology is similar regardless of which clotting factor is deficient, the identification of specific factor deficiencies allows definitive treatment with replacement agents.

In about 80% of all cases of hemophilia, the inheritance pattern is demonstrated as X-linked recessive. The two most common forms of the disorder are **factor VIII deficiency (hemophilia A,** or **classic hemophilia)** and **factor IX deficiency (hemophilia B,** or **Christmas disease). Von Willebrand disease (vWD)** is another hereditary bleeding disorder characterized by a deficiency, abnormality, or absence of the protein called von Willebrand factor (vWF) and a deficiency of factor VIII. Unlike hemophilia, vWD affects both males and females. The following discussion is primarily concerned with factor VIII deficiency, which accounts for 80% to 85% of all hemophilia cases.

Pathophysiology

The basic defect of hemophilia A is a deficiency of **factor VIII (antihemophilic factor [AHF]).** AHF is produced by the liver and is necessary for the formation of thromboplastin in phase I of blood coagulation. The less AHF found in the blood, the more severe the disease. Individuals with hemophilia have two of the three factors required for coagulation: vascular influence and platelets. Therefore they may bleed for longer periods, but not at a faster rate.

Bleeding into subcutaneous and intramuscular tissue is common. Hemarthrosis, which is bleeding into a joint space, is the most frequent type of internal bleeding. Bony changes and crippling deformities occur after repeated bleeding episodes over several years. Signs of hemarthrosis are swelling, warmth, redness, pain, and loss of movement. Bleeding in the neck, mouth, or thorax is serious because the airway can become obstructed. Intracranial hemorrhage can have fatal consequences and is one of the major causes of death. Hemor-

BOX 26-5
Clinical Manifestations of Hemophilia

- Prolonged bleeding anywhere from or in the body
- Hemorrhage from any trauma—Loss of deciduous teeth, circumcision, cuts, epistaxis, injections
- Excessive bruising, even from a slight injury, such as a fall
- Subcutaneous and intramuscular hemorrhages
- Hemarthrosis (bleeding into the joint cavities), especially the knees, ankles, and elbows
- Hematomas—Pain, swelling, and limited motion
- Spontaneous hematuria

nonactive sports only, mobile riding. Bioaugical risks? (handwritten)

rhage anywhere along the GI tract can lead to anemia, and bleeding into the retroperitoneal cavity is especially hazardous because of the large space for blood to accumulate. Hematomas in the spinal cord can cause paralysis.

Diagnostic Evaluation

Overt, prolonged hemorrhage is readily apparent; bleeding into tissues is less apparent (Box 26-5). The diagnosis is usually made from a history of bleeding episodes, evidence of X-linked inheritance (only one third of the cases are new mutations), and laboratory findings. The tests specific for hemophilia plasma depend on specific factors for a reaction to occur, such as the partial thromboplastin time (PTT). Specific determination of factor deficiencies requires assay procedures normally performed in specialized laboratories. Carrier detection is possible in classic hemophilia using deoxyribonucleic acid (DNA) testing and is an important consideration in families in which female offspring may have inherited the trait.

Therapeutic Management

The primary therapy for hemophilia is replacement of the missing clotting factor. The products available are **factor VIII concentrate** from pooled plasma or a genetically engineered recombinant, to be reconstituted with sterile water immediately before use, and **DDAVP (1-deamino-8-D-arginine vasopressin),** a synthetic form of vasopressin that increases plasma factor VIII and vWF levels and is the treatment of choice in mild hemophilia and vWD if the child shows an appropriate response. DDAVP is not effective in the treatment of severe hemophilia A, severe vWD, or any form of hemophilia B. Vigorous therapy is instituted to prevent chronic crippling effects from joint bleeding.

Other drugs may be included in the therapy plan, depending on the source of the hemorrhage. Corticosteroids are given for hematuria, acute hemarthrosis, and chronic synovitis. Nonsteroidal antiinflammatory drugs (NSAIDs), such as ibuprofen, are effective in relieving pain caused by synovitis; however, they must be used with caution because they inhibit platelet function (Curry, 2004; National Hemophilia Foundation, 2006). Oral administration or local application of ε-aminocaproic acid (Amicar) prevents clot destruction; however, its use is limited to mouth or trauma surgery, and a dose of factor concentrate must be given first.

A regular program of exercise and physical therapy is an important aspect of management. Physical activity within reasonable limits strengthens muscles around joints and may decrease the number of spontaneous bleeding episodes.

Treatment without delay results in more rapid recovery and a decreased likelihood of complications; therefore most children are treated at home. The family is taught the technique of venipuncture and to administer the AHF to children older than 2 to 3 years of age. The child learns the procedure for self-administration at 8 to 12 years of age. Home treatment is highly successful, and the rewards, in addition to the immediacy, are less disruption of family life, fewer school or work days missed, and enhancement of the child's self-esteem and independence.

Primary prophylaxis in hemophilia patients has proved to be effective in preventing bleeding complications by administrating periodic factor replacement. Primary prophylaxis involves the infusion of factor VIII concentrate on a regular basis before the onset of joint damage. Secondary prophylaxis involves the infusion of factor VIII concentrate on a regular basis after the child experiences his or her first joint bleed. The infusions are given three times a week. Aggressive factor replacement may be a cost-effective alternative to primary prophylaxis. This involves the infusion of a high dose of factor VIII concentrate when a joint bleed occurs, followed by 2 days of more standard doses of factor VIII concentrate with consideration of additional treatment every other day for one week (Montgomery, Gill, and Scott, 2003).

Prognosis. Although there is no cure for hemophilia, its symptoms can be controlled and its potentially crippling deformities greatly reduced or even avoided. Today many children with hemophilia function with minimal or no joint damage. They are normal children with an average life expectancy in every respect but one: they have a tendency to bleed, which is a significant inconvenience but not necessarily a life-threatening event.

Gene therapy may prove to be a treatment option in the future. This therapy involves introducing a working copy of the factor VIII gene into a patient who has a flawed copy of the gene. Problems exist with appropriate selection of the vector, identification of the cell for gene expression, and control of side effects (Montgomery, Gill, and Scott, 2003).

Nursing Care Management

The earlier a bleeding episode is recognized, the more effectively it can be treated. Signs that indicate internal bleeding are especially important to recognize. Children are aware of internal bleeding and are reliable in telling the examiner where an internal bleed is. In addition to the manifestations described (see Box 26-5), the nurse maintains a high level of suspicion when a child with hemophilia demonstrates signs such as headache, slurred speech, loss of consciousness (from cerebral bleeding), and black tarry stools (from GI bleeding).

Prevent Bleeding. The goal of prevention of bleeding episodes is directed toward decreasing the risk of injury. Prevention of bleeding episodes is geared mostly toward appropriate exercises to strengthen muscles and joints and to allow age-appropriate activity. During infancy and toddlerhood the normal acquisition of motor skills creates innumerable opportunities for falls, bruises, and minor wounds. Restraining the child from mastering motor development can foster more serious long-term problems than allowing the behavior. However, the environment should be made as safe as possible, with close supervision during playtime to minimize incidental injuries.

Critical Thinking Exercise—Bleeding (sidebar)

@dentist (handwritten)

For older children the family usually needs assistance in preparing for school. A nurse who knows the family can be instrumental in discussing the situation with the school nurse and in jointly planning an appropriate activity schedule. Because almost all persons with hemophilia are boys, the physical limitations in regard to active sports may be a difficult adjustment, and activity restrictions must be tempered with sensitivity to the child's emotional and physical needs. Use of protective equipment, such as padding and helmets, is particularly important, and noncontact sports, especially swimming, walking, jogging, tennis, golf, fishing, and bowling, are encouraged (National Hemophilia Foundation, 2006).

To prevent oral bleeding, some readjustment in terms of dental hygiene may be needed to minimize trauma to the gums, such as use of a water irrigating device, softening the toothbrush in warm water before brushing, or using a sponge-tipped disposable toothbrush. A regular toothbrush should be soft bristled and small.

Because any trauma can lead to a bleeding episode, all persons caring for these children must be aware of their disorder. These children should wear medical identification, and older children should be encouraged to recognize situations in which disclosing their condition is important, such as during dental extraction or injections. Health personnel need to take special precautions to prevent the use of procedures that may cause bleeding, such as IM injections. The subcutaneous route is substituted for IM injections whenever possible. Venipunctures for blood samples are usually preferred for these children. There is usually less bleeding after the venipuncture than after finger or heel punctures. Neither aspirin nor any aspirin-containing compound should be used. Acetaminophen is a suitable aspirin substitute, especially for controlling pain at home.

Recognize and Control Bleeding. As noted, the earlier a bleeding episode is recognized, the more effectively it can be treated. Factor replacement therapy should be instituted according to established medical protocol, and supportive measures may be implemented, such as *RICE,* which stands for *Rest, Ice, Compression,* and *Elevation.* When parents and older children are taught such measures beforehand, they can be prepared to initiate immediate treatment. Plastic bags of ice or cold packs should be kept in the freezer for such emergencies. However, such measures do not take the place of factor replacement.

Prevent Crippling Effects of Bleeding. As a result of repeated episodes of hemarthrosis, incompletely absorbed blood in the joints, and limitation of motion, bone and muscle changes occur that result in flexion contractures and joint fixation. During bleeding episodes the joint is elevated and immobilized. Active range-of-motion exercises are usually instituted after the acute episode. This allows the child to control the degree of exercise and discomfort. If an exercise program is instituted in the home, a physical therapist or public health nurse may need to supervise compliance with the regimen. Rarely, orthopedic intervention, such as casting, application of traction, or aspiration of blood, may be necessary to preserve joint function. Diet is also an important consideration, since excessive body weight can increase the strain on affected joints, especially the knees, and predispose the child to hemarthrosis. Consequently, calories need to be supplied in accordance with energy requirements.

Support Family and Prepare for Home Care. Genetic counseling is essential as soon as possible after diagno-

sis. Unlike many other disorders in which both parents carry the trait, the feeling of responsibility for this condition usually rests with the mother. Without an opportunity to discuss her feelings, the marital relationship can suffer. Technology is now available to identify carriers in approximately 80% of cases and may reduce the anxiety regarding childbearing in women who may be at risk of carrying the defective gene, such as sisters or maternal aunts of an affected male. The discovery of factor concentrates has greatly changed the outlook for these children. Bleeding can be minimized, and the child can live a much more normal, unrestricted life. Children are taught to take responsibility for their disease at an early age. They learn their limitations, other preventive measures, and self-administration of the prophylactic AHF.

The needs of families who have children with hemophilia are best met through a comprehensive team approach of physicians (pediatrician, hematologist, orthopedist), nurse practitioner, nurse, social worker, and physical therapist. Parent-group discussions are beneficial in meeting those needs often best met by similarly affected families. For example, with the improved prognosis for these children, parents and adolescents with hemophilia face vocational and financial problems, in addition to concern over future childbearing. After children reach 21 years of age, many insurance companies will no longer carry them. This can be disastrous in terms of the cost of treatment. The National Hemophilia Foundation* and the Canadian Hemophilia Society† provide numerous services and publications for both health providers and families. Financial support is particularly important. A person with severe hemophilia may require factor replacement therapy and other medical treatments that cost in excess of $70,000 to $90,000 a year.

Children who have become infected with HIV through transfusions and factor replacement products are faced with the consequences of this dreaded disease. Consequently, they need the support of health professionals, especially in the areas of safe sexual practices to avoid disease transmission and public education regarding acquired immunodeficiency syndrome (AIDS) and ways to deal with public reactions to persons who have AIDS (see p. 939).

IDIOPATHIC THROMBOCYTOPENIC PURPURA

Idiopathic thrombocytopenic purpura (ITP) is an acquired hemorrhagic disorder characterized by (1) **thrombocytopenia,** excessive destruction of platelets; (2) **purpura,** a discoloration caused by petechiae beneath the skin; and (3) **normal bone marrow with normal or increased number of immature platelets (megakaryocytes) and eosinophils.** Although the cause is unknown, it is believed to be an autoimmune response to disease-related antigens. It is the most frequently occurring thrombocytopenia of childhood. The greatest frequency of occurrence is between 2 and 10 years of age.

The disease occurs in one of two forms: an acute, self-limiting course or a chronic condition (greater than 6 months' duration). The acute form is most often seen after upper respiratory

*116 W. 32nd St., 11th Floor, New York, NY 10001; (800) 42-HANDI, (212) 328-3700; fax: (212) 328-3777; e-mail: handi@hemophilia.org; http://www.hemophilia.org.
†625 President Kennedy Ave., Suite 505, Montreal, Quebec H3A 1K2; (800) 668-2686, (514) 848-0503; fax: (514) 848-9661; e-mail: chs@hemophilia.ca; http://www.hemophilia.ca.

BOX 26-6

Clinical Manifestations of Idiopathic Thrombocytopenic Purpura

Easy bruising
- Petechiae
- Ecchymoses
- Most often over bony prominences

Bleeding from mucous membranes
- Epistaxis
- Bleeding gums
- Internal hemorrhage evidenced by:
  —Hematuria
  —Hematemesis
  —Melena
  —Hemarthrosis
  —Menorrhagia

Hematomas over lower extremities

BOX 26-7

Criteria for Anti-D Antibody Therapy

- Age between 1 and 19 years; Rh(D)-positive blood type
- Normal white blood count and hemoglobin level for age; platelet count of 20,000/mm^3
- No active mucosal bleeding
- No history of reaction to plasma products
- No known immunoglobulin A deficiency
- No concurrent infection
- Absence of Evans syndrome (characterized by the combination of idiopathic thrombocytopenic purpura and autoimmune hemolytic anemia)
- No suspicion of lupus erythematosus or other collagen-vascular disorder
- No splenectomy

---

tract infections; after the childhood diseases measles, rubella, mumps, and chickenpox; or after infection with parvovirus B19.

Diagnostic Evaluation

The diagnosis is suspected on the basis of clinical manifestations (Box 26-6). In ITP the platelet count is reduced to below 20,000/mm^3; therefore tests that depend on platelet function, such as the tourniquet test, bleeding time, and clot retraction, are abnormal. Although there is no definitive test on which to establish a diagnosis of ITP, several are usually performed to rule out other disorders in which thrombocytopenia is a manifestation, such as systemic lupus erythematosus, lymphoma, or leukemia.

Therapeutic Management

Management of ITP is primarily supportive, since the course of the disease is self-limited in the majority of cases. Activity is restricted at the onset while the platelet count is low and while active bleeding or progression of lesions is occurring. Treatment for acute presentation is symptomatic and has included prednisone, IV immune globulin (IVIG), and anti-D antibody. These are not curative therapies. **Anti-D antibody** is a relatively new therapy for ITP. Infusion of anti-D antibody causes a transient hemolytic anemia in the patient. Along with the clearance of antibody-coated RBCs, there is prolonged survival of platelets resulting from the blockade of the Fc receptors of the reticuloendothelial cells. The platelet count does not increase until 48 hours after an infusion of anti-D antibody; therefore it is not appropriate therapy for patients who are actively bleeding. The benefits of choosing anti-D antibody therapy over prednisone or IVIG is that anti-D antibody can be given in one dose over 5 to 10 minutes and is significantly less expensive than IVIG. Historically, patients who are treated with prednisone may first undergo a bone marrow examination to rule out leukemia. Therefore the use of anti-D antibody alleviates the need for a bone marrow examination. Patients must meet certain criteria before the administration of anti-D antibody (Box 26-7). Premedica-

tion with acetaminophen 5 to 10 minutes before infusion is recommended.

NURSING ALERT

After administration of anti-D antibody, observe the child for a minimum of 1 hour and maintain a patent IV line. Obtain baseline vital signs before the infusion and again 5, 20, and 60 minutes after beginning the infusion. Fever, chills, and headache may occur during or shortly after the infusion. If so, diphenhydramine (Benadryl) and hydrocortisone (Solu-Cortef) should be given and the patient observed for an additional hour.

Splenectomy is reserved for those patients in whom ITP has persisted for 1 year or longer. It is the only treatment associated with long-term remission for 60% to 90% of children. Splenectomy removes the risk of hemorrhage but increases the risk of septicemia (Buchanan, 2005; Scott and Montgomery, 2007). Before splenectomy is considered, waiting until the child is older than 5 years of age is generally recommended because of the increased risk of bacterial infection. Pneumococcal and meningococcal vaccines are recommended before splenectomy (see Immunizations, Chapter 10). The child also receives penicillin prophylaxis after splenectomy. The length of prophylactic therapy is controversial, but in general, a minimum of 3 years is recommended.

Prognosis. The majority of children have a self-limited course without major complications. Some children may develop chronic ITP and require ongoing therapy. A splenectomy may modify the disease process, and the child will be asymptomatic.

Nursing Care Management

Nursing care is largely supportive and should include teaching regarding possible side effects of therapy and limitation in activities while the child's platelet count is 50,000 to 100,000/mm^3. Children with ITP should not participate in *any* contact sports, bike riding, skateboarding, in-line skating, gymnastics, climbing, or running. Parents are encouraged to engage their children in quiet activities and to prevent any injuries to the child's head. The harmful effects of using aspirin and NSAIDs to control pain are critical for these children; therefore salicy-

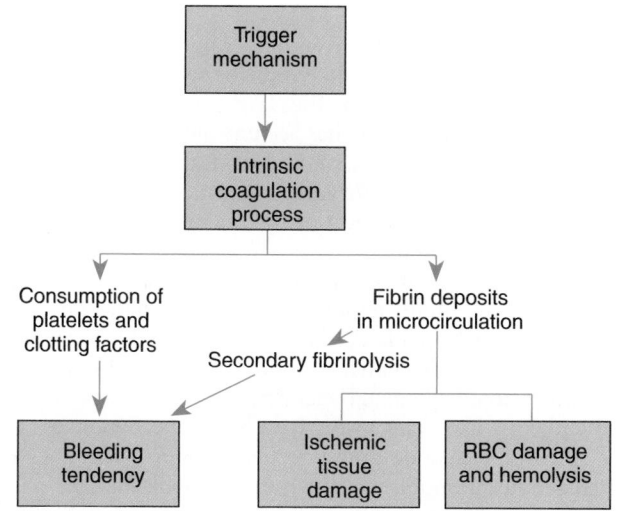

FIG. 26-3 ■ Effects of disseminated intravascular coagulation. *RBC,* Red blood cell.

late substitutes (such as acetaminophen) are always used. As in any condition with an uncertain outcome, the family needs emotional support.

DISSEMINATED INTRAVASCULAR COAGULATION

Disseminated intravascular coagulation (DIC), also known as **consumption coagulopathy,** is characterized by diffuse fibrin deposition in the microvasculature, consumption of coagulation factors, and endogenous generation of thrombin and plasmin. DIC is a secondary disorder of coagulation that occurs as a complication of a number of pathologic processes, such as hypoxia, acidosis, shock, and endothelial damage. It can result from many severe systemic diseases, such as congenital heart disease, necrotizing enterocolitis, gram-negative bacterial sepsis, rickettsial infections, and some severe viral infections.

Pathophysiology

DIC occurs when the first stage of the coagulation process is abnormally stimulated. Although no well-defined sequence of events occurs, two distinct phases can be identified. First, when the clotting mechanism is triggered in the circulation, thrombin is generated in greater amounts than can be neutralized by the body. Consequently, there is rapid conversion of fibrinogen to fibrin, with aggregation and destruction of platelets. If local and widespread fibrin deposition in blood vessels takes place, obstruction and eventual necrosis of tissues occur. Second, the fibrinolytic mechanism is activated, causing extensive destruction of clotting factors. With a deficiency of clotting factors, the child is vulnerable to uncontrollable hemorrhage into vital organs. An additional complication is damage and hemolysis of RBCs (Fig. 26-3).

Diagnostic Evaluation

DIC is suspected when the patient has an increased tendency to bleed (Box 26-8). Hematologic findings include prolonged prothrombin time (PT), PTT, and thrombin time (TT). There is a profoundly depressed platelet count, fragmented RBCs, and depleted fibrinogen.

Therapeutic Management

Treatment of DIC is directed toward control of the underlying or initiating cause, which in most instances stops the coagulation problem spontaneously. Platelets and fresh-frozen plasma may be needed to replace lost plasma components, especially in the child whose underlying disease remains uncontrolled. The extremely ill newborn infant may require exchange transfusion with fresh blood. The IV administration of heparin to inhibit thrombin formation is most often restricted to patients who have not responded to treatment of the underlying disease or replacement of coagulation factors and platelets.

Nursing Care Management

The goals of nursing care are to be aware of the possibility of DIC in the severely ill child and to recognize signs that might indicate its presence. The skills needed to monitor IV infusion and blood transfusions and to administer heparin are the same as for any child receiving these therapies (see p. 943). (See Chapter 18 for care of the child with a life-threatening illness.)

EPISTAXIS (NOSEBLEEDING)

Isolated and transient episodes of epistaxis, or nosebleeding, are common in childhood. The nose, especially the septum, is a highly vascular structure, and bleeding usually results from direct trauma, including blows to the nose, foreign bodies, and nose picking; or from mucosal inflammation associated with allergic rhinitis and upper respiratory tract infections. The bleeding ordinarily stops spontaneously or with minimal pressure and requires no medical evaluation or therapy.

Recurrent epistaxis and severe bleeding may indicate an underlying disease, particularly vascular abnormalities, leukemia, thrombocytopenia, and clotting factor deficiency diseases (e.g., hemophilia, vWD). Nosebleeds are sometimes associated with administration of aspirin, even in normal amounts. Persistent episodes of epistaxis require medical evaluation.

Nursing Care Management

In the event of a nosebleed, an essential intervention is to remain calm. Otherwise, the child will become more agitated, the blood pressure will increase, and the child will not cooperate. Although in most instances a nosebleed is not serious, it can be upsetting to family members as well. They need reassurance that the loss of blood is not serious and that the bleeding usually stops within 10 to 15 minutes.

To control the bleeding, the child is instructed to sit up and lean forward (not to lie down) to avoid aspiration of blood. Most of the nosebleeding originates in the anterior part of the nasal septum and can be controlled by applying pressure to the soft lower portion of the nose with the thumb and forefinger (see Emergency Treatment box). During this time the child breathes through the mouth.

In the event that hemorrhage continues, the child should be evaluated by a practitioner, who may pack the nose with epinephrine-soaked gauze. After a nosebleed, petroleum or water-soluble jelly can be inserted into each nostril to prevent crusting of old blood and to lessen the likelihood of the child's picking at the nose and restarting the hemorrhage. If a child has numerous nosebleeds, factors believed to increase the likelihood of bleeds are eliminated, such as discouraging nose picking or altering the household humidity by placing a cool-mist humidifier in the child's room. Repeated bleeding episodes lasting longer than 30 minutes may be an indication to refer the child for evaluation for the possibility of a bleeding disorder.

NEOPLASTIC DISORDERS

Neoplastic disorders are the leading cause of death from disease in children past infancy, and almost half of all childhood cancers involve the blood or blood-forming organs. Leukemias and lymphomas are discussed here. Malignant solid tumors of childhood are discussed elsewhere in relation to the tissues or organs involved.

Leukemias

Leukemia, cancer of the blood-forming tissues, is the most common form of childhood cancer. The annual incidence is 3 to 4 cases per 100,000 Caucasian children younger than 15 years of age (Margolin, Steuber, and Poplack, 2006; Pearce and Sills, 2005). It is more common in males and Caucasians, with the peak onset between 2 and 5 years of age (Pearce and Sills, 2005; Margolin, Steuber, and Poplack, 2006). It is one of the forms of cancer that has demonstrated dramatic improvements in survival rates. Current long-term disease-free survival for children with acute lymphoid leukemia approaches 80% (Pui, Relling, and Downing, 2004; Pearce and Sills, 2005), whereas acute nonlymphoid leukemia has a nearly 50% survival rate (Pearce and Sills, 2005). (See also Prognosis, p. 931.)

Classification

Leukemia is a broad term given to a group of malignant diseases of the bone marrow and lymphatic system. Research has revealed that it is a complex disease of varying heterogeneity. Consequently, classification has become increasingly complex, sophisticated, and essential, since identification of the subtype of leukemia has therapeutic and prognostic implications. The following is a brief overview of the major classification systems currently being used.

Morphology. Two forms are generally recognized in children: **acute lymphoid leukemia (ALL)** and **acute nonlymphoid (myelogenous) leukemia (ANLL or AML)**. Synonyms for ALL include lymphatic, lymphocytic, lymphoblastic, and lymphoblastoid leukemia. Usually the terms **stem cell** or **blast cell leukemia** also refer to the lymphoid type. Synonyms for the AML type include granulocytic, myelocytic, monocytic, myelogenous, monoblastic, and monomyeloblastic.

- **Cytochemical markers**—Several chemical stains (e.g., terminal deoxynucleotidyl transferase [TdT]) aid in differentiation between ALL and ANLL.
- **Chromosome studies**—Chromosome analysis has become an important tool in the diagnosis of ALL. For example, children with trisomy 21 have 20 times the risk of other children for developing ALL. Children with more than 50 chromosomes on the leukemic cells (hyperdiploid) have the best prognosis (Margolin, Steuber, and Poplack, 2006). Translocations of chromosomes also found on the leukemic cells can denote good prognosis, as in the trisomies 4 and 10, or a poor prognosis, as in the t(9:22) or Philadelphia chromosome.
- **Cell-surface immunologic markers**—Cell-surface antigens have permitted differentiation of ALL into three broad classes: non-T, non-B ALL; B-cell ALL; and T-cell ALL. Children with non-T, non-B ALL have the best prognosis, especially if they have the common ALL antigen, known as CALLA positive (or CD 10+), on their cell surfaces (Margolin, Steuber, and Poplack, 2006).

Pathophysiology

Leukemia is an unrestricted proliferation of immature WBCs in the blood-forming tissues of the body. Although not a "tumor" as such, the leukemic cells demonstrate the same neoplastic properties as solid cancers. Therefore the resulting pathologic condition and clinical manifestations are caused by infiltration and replacement of any tissue of the body with nonfunctional leukemic cells. Highly vascular organs, such as the spleen and liver, are the most severely affected.

To understand the pathophysiology of the leukemic process, it is important to clarify two common misconceptions. First, although leukemia is an overproduction of WBCs, most often in the acute form the leukocyte count is low (thus the term *leukemia*). Second, these immature cells do not deliberately attack and destroy the normal blood cells or vascular tissues. Cellular destruction takes place by infiltration and subsequent competition for metabolic elements (Table 26-2).

In all types of leukemia the proliferating cells depress the production of formed elements of the blood in bone marrow by competing for and depriving the normal cells of the essential nutrients for metabolism. The most frequent presenting signs and symptoms of leukemia are a result of infiltration of the bone marrow. The three main consequences are (1) **anemia** from decreased RBCs, (2) **infection** from neutropenia,

TABLE 26-2

Pathology and Related Clinical Manifestations of Leukemia

ORGAN OR TISSUE	CONSEQUENCES	MANIFESTATIONS
Bone marrow dysfunction	Decreased RBCs—Anemia	Pallor, fatigue
	Neutropenia—Infection	Fever
	Decreased platelets—Bleeding tendencies	Hemorrhage (petechiae)
	Invasion of bone marrow—Bone weakness; invasion of periosteum	Tendency toward fractures
		Pain
Liver	Infiltration, enlargement, eventual fibrosis	Hepatomegaly
Spleen		Splenomegaly
Lymph glands		Lymphadenopathy
Central nervous system—Meninges	Increased intracranial pressure, ventricular enlargement	Severe headache
		Vomiting
		Irritability, lethargy
		Papilledema
	Meningeal irritation	Eventual coma
		Pain
		Stiff neck and back
Hypermetabolism	Cell deprivation of nutrients by invading cells	Muscle wasting
		Weight loss
		Anorexia
		Fatigue

and (3) **bleeding** from decreased platelet production. The invasion of the bone marrow with leukemic cells gradually causes a weakening of the bone and a tendency toward fractures. As leukemic cells invade the periosteum, increasing pressure causes severe pain.

The spleen, liver, and lymph glands demonstrate marked infiltration, enlargement, and eventually fibrosis. Hepatosplenomegaly is typically more common than lymphadenopathy. The next most important site of involvement is the CNS secondary to leukemic infiltration, which may cause increased intracranial pressure (see Box 28-1).

Leukemic cells may also invade the testes, kidneys, prostate, ovaries, GI tract, and lungs. With long-term survivors becoming more common, such sites of leukemia invasion, especially the testes, are becoming more important clinically.

Diagnostic Evaluation

Leukemia is usually suspected based on the history, physical manifestations (see Table 26-2), and a peripheral blood smear that contains immature forms of leukocytes, frequently combined with low blood counts. Definitive diagnosis is based on flow cytometry of the cells obtained in the bone marrow aspiration or biopsy. Flow cytometry identifies the specific type of blast cell. Typically, the bone marrow is hypercellular, with primarily blast cells. After the diagnosis is confirmed, a lumbar puncture is performed to determine whether there is any CNS involvement. A few children will have CNS involvement at diagnosis, although most are asymptomatic.

Therapeutic Management

Treatment of leukemia involves the use of chemotherapeutic agents, with or without cranial irradiation, in four phases: (1) **induction therapy,** which achieves a complete remission or less than 5% leukemic cells in the bone marrow; (2) **CNS**

prophylactic therapy, which prevents leukemic cells from invading the CNS; (3) **intensification therapy** (consolidation), which eradicates residual leukemia cells, followed by delayed intensification, which prevents emergence of resistant leukemic clones; and (4) **maintenance therapy,** which serves to maintain the remission phase. Although the combination of drugs and radiation may vary according to institutions, the prognostic or risk characteristics of the patient, and the type of leukemia being treated.

Hematopoietic Stem Cell Transplantation. HSCT has been used successfully for treating children who have ALL and AML. HSCT is *not* recommended for children with ALL during the first remission because of the excellent results possible with chemotherapy. Because of the poorer prognosis in children with AML, HSCT may be considered during the first remission when a suitable donor is available (Bollard, Krance, and Heslop, 2006).

HSCT may be not only from antigen-matched related donors, but also from matched unrelated donors or mismatched donors. Peripheral blood stem cell transplants are capable of differentiating into specialized cells of the hematologic system and can be obtained from related or unrelated donors or from umbilical cord blood. Regardless of the type of transplant, it is accompanied by significant morbidity and mortality, including graft-vs-host disease (GVHD), overwhelming infection, or severe organ damage.

Prognosis

The most important prognostic factors for determining long-term survival for children with ALL (in addition to treatment) are (1) the initial WBC count, (2) the child's age at the time of diagnosis, (3) the type of cell involved, (4) the sex of the child, and (5) karyotype analysis. Children with a normal or low WBC count and who have non-T, non-B ALL and are CALLA

Critical Thinking Exercise—Bone Marrow Test

Case Study—Acute Lymphoblastic Leukemia

positive have a much better prognosis than those with a high count or other cell types. Children diagnosed between 2 and 9 years of age have consistently demonstrated a better outlook than those diagnosed before 2 or after 10 years of age, and girls appear to have a more favorable prognosis than boys. Children with a DNA index greater than 1.16 (hyperdiploid) and translocation of chromosomes 4 and 10 have a better prognosis (Margolin, Steuber, and Poplack, 2006).

Late Effects of Treatment

Although vigorous treatment of childhood cancers has resulted in dramatically improved survival rates, increasing concern surrounds late effects—adverse changes related to treatment modalities—and recurrence of the disease process. Almost no organ is exempt, and almost every antineoplastic agent, especially irradiation, is responsible for some adverse effect.

The most devastating late effect is development of a second malignancy. Children who received cranial irradiation at age 5 years or younger are most susceptible to developing brain tumors (Silverman and Sallan, 2003; Bhatia, 2004). Treatment with an anthracycline is associated with cardiomyopathy; cranial irradiation and intrathecal chemotherapy are associated with cognitive and neuropsychologic deficits, which are just a few of the long-term sequelae. Consequently, close monitoring for late effects is essential, especially with the advent of additional clinical trials.

Nursing Care Management

Nursing care of the child with leukemia is directly related to the therapeutic regimen. General psychologic interventions during each phase of therapy are discussed in Chapter 18. The Nursing Care Plan for the Child with Cancer appears below.

Prepare Child and Family for Diagnostic and Therapeutic Procedures. From the time before diagnosis to cessation of therapy, children must undergo several tests; the most traumatic are bone marrow aspiration, bone marrow biopsy, and lumbar punctures. Multiple finger sticks and venipunctures for blood analysis and drug infusion are common occurrences. Therefore the child needs an explanation of each procedure and what can be expected. In addition, effective pharmacologic measures, including conscious and unconscious sedation, and nonpharmacologic strategies are used to reduce discomfort associated with these painful procedures.

Relieve Pain. The effective use of analgesia is especially important when the malignant process is uncontrolled and causes acute pain. Dosages of opioids (narcotics) are adjusted, or *titrated,* to the child's needs and administered *around the clock* for optimal pain control. Nonpharmacologic strategies should be implemented as needed but are not substitutes for pharmacologic management. The reader is encouraged to review the principles of pain assessment and management presented in Chapter 7 and Preparation for Diagnostic and

nursingcareplan | The Child with Cancer

Nursing Diagnosis	Expected Patient Outcomes	Nursing Interventions	Rationale
Risk for Injury related to chemotherapy treatment	Child will exhibit no complications of chemotherapy.	Administer chemotherapeutic agents using established guidelines.	To minimize inappropriate administration techniques
Child's/Family's Defining Characteristics	Child will receive prompt, appropriate treatment of complications.	Assist with procedures for administration of chemotherapeutic agents.	To promote safer cancer treatment
(Subjective and Objective Data)	**The Following NOC Concept Applies to These Outcomes**	Administer medications around the clock to prevent nausea and vomiting before chemotherapy.	To minimize side effects of nausea and vomiting
Anaphylaxis—Wheezing, hypotension, urticaria, cyanosis	Risk Control	Administer IV fluid as prescribed.	To maintain hydration
Nausea, vomiting		Encourage frequent intake of fluids in small amounts.	To promote hydration
Intravenous (IV) infiltration—Pain, redness, swelling at IV infusion site		Observe for signs of infiltration of IV site: pain, stinging, swelling redness.	To prevent infiltration when possible
		Institute policies to treat infiltration if it occurs.	To prevent complications
		Observe child for 20 minutes after infusion of drugs that are associated with risk of anaphylaxis.	To prevent anaphylaxis
		Stop infusion of drug and flush IV line with normal saline is reaction if suspected.	To prevent further reaction
		Have emergency equipment and emergency drugs readily available.	To prevent delay in treatment
		The Following NIC Concepts Apply to These Interventions	
		Chemotherapy Management	
		Nausea Management	

Nursing Diagnosis	Expected Patient Outcomes	Nursing Interventions	Rationale
Risk for Infection related to depressed body defenses	Child will not exhibit signs of infection. Child will not come in contact with infected persons.	Use good hand-washing technique.	To minimize exposure to infective organisms
Child's/Family's Defining Characteristics *(Subjective and Objective Data)*	**The Following NOC Concepts Apply to These Outcomes**	Screen all visitors and staff for signs of infection.	To decrease exposure to possible infective organisms
		Use aseptic technique for all invasive procedures.	To decrease chance of infection spread
Fever	Risk Control	Monitor temperature.	To detect possible infection
Altered vital signs	Immune Status	Evaluate child for any potential sites of infection: needle puncture sites, mucosa for ulceration, minor abrasions.	To detect signs of possible infection
Lethargy	Infection Severity		
Change in behavior			
Septic shock			
		Provide nutritionally complete diet.	To support body's natural defenses
		Avoid giving live attenuated virus vaccines.	To prevent overwhelming infection
		Give inactivated virus vaccines.	To prevent specific infections and to avoid placing the child at risk for acquiring the illness
		Administer antibiotics as prescribed.	To treat a specific infection
		Administer granulocyte colony-stimulating factor (G-CSF) as prescribed.	To promote production of infection-fighting cells
		The Following NIC Concepts Apply to These Interventions	
		Infection Protection Infection Control Immunization/Vaccination Management	

Nursing Diagnosis	Expected Patient Outcomes	Nursing Interventions	Rationale
Imbalanced Nutrition: Less Than Body Requirements related to loss of appetite	Child's nutritional intake will be adequate.	Encourage parents to relax pressure placed on child concerning eating.	To educate that loss of appetite is a consequence of chemotherapy
Child's/Family's Defining Characteristics *(Subjective and Objective Data)*	**The Following NOC Concepts Apply to These Outcomes**	Allow child any food tolerated; selections can improve once appetite increases.	To encourage child to eat
	Nutritional Status: Food and Fluid Intake	Explain expected increase in appetite if child will be taking steroids.	To prepare child and family for this change
Weight loss	Nutritional Status: Nutrient Intake	Fortify foods with nutritious supplements.	To maximize quality of intake
Lack of appetite		Allow child to be involved in food preparation and selection.	To encourage eating
Nausea		Make food appealing.	To encourage eating
		Monitor child's weight.	To evaluate for weight change
		The Following NIC Concepts Apply to These Interventions	
		Nutrition Management Nutrition Therapy	

Nursing Diagnosis	Expected Patient Outcomes	Nursing Interventions	Rationale
Pain (Specify: Acute, Chronic) related to diagnosis, treatment, physiologic effects of cancer	Child will experience no pain or reduction of pain to level acceptable to the child.	Use pharmacologic and nonpharmacologic interventions before painful procedures.	To minimize discomfort
Child's/Family's Defining Characteristics *(Subjective and Objective Data)*	**The Following NOC Concepts Apply to These Outcomes**	Assess pain with each vital sign measurement.	To determine level of pain
	Pain Level	Evaluate effectiveness of pain relief.	To determine effectiveness
Crying	Pain: Disruptive Effects	Administer analgesics as prescribed on preventive schedule (around the clock) when needed.	To prevent pain from recurring
Withdrawal	Pain Control		
Fear of procedures			
Reluctance to move		**The Following NIC Concept Applies to These Interventions**	
Change in vital signs		Pain Management	

Continued

nursingcareplan | The Child with Cancer—cont'd

Nursing Diagnosis	Expected Patient Outcomes	Nursing Interventions	Rationale
Fear related to diagnostic tests, procedures, treatment **Child's/Family's Defining Characteristics** *(Subjective and Objective Data)* Worry and anxiety before procedures Withdrawal Lack of control Outbursts, anger Lack of cooperation	Child will have reduced fear related to diagnostic procedures and treatment. **The Following NOC Concepts Apply to These Outcomes** Fear Self-Control Pain Control	Explain procedures carefully at child's level of understanding. Explain what will take place and what child will feel, see, and hear. Listen to special requests of child when possible. Provide child with some means of involvement with procedures (e.g., holding a piece of equipment, helping put on bandage, counting). Implement distraction techniques and pain reduction interventions. **The Following NIC Concept Applies to These Interventions** Pain Management	To reduce fear of unknown To provide sense of control To encourage cooperation To provide sense of control, encourage cooperation, and support child's coping skills To reduce pain

Nursing Diagnosis	Expected Patient Outcomes	Nursing Interventions	Rationale
Body Image Disturbance related to changes caused by cancer and treatment **Child's/Family's Defining Characteristics** *(Subjective and Objective Data)* Sadness Depression Withdrawal Anger	Child will exhibit positive coping skills. **The Following NOC Concepts Apply to These Outcomes** Body Image	Encourage child to decide how he or she will cope with hair loss (e.g., wig, cap, scarf). Provide adequate covering during exposure to sunlight, wind, or cold. Explain that hair begins to regrow in 3 to 6 months and may be a different color and texture. Encourage good hygiene and grooming. Encourage rapid return to peer group and friends. Encourage visits from friends before discharge. **The Following NIC Concepts Apply to These Interventions** Counseling Body Image Enhancement	To promote early adjustment and preparation for hair loss To prevent exposure To prepare child and family for changes in appearance To reduce risk of infection To prepare child for reactions of others To support child

Nursing Diagnosis	Expected Patient Outcomes	Nursing Interventions	Rationale
Altered (Interrupted) Family Processes related to having a child with a life-threatening disease **Child's/Family's Defining Characteristics** *(Subjective and Objective Data)* Lack of understanding of disease and treatment Inability to identify side effects of treatment Inability to understand child's treatment plan Lack of family support	Child and family will demonstrate understanding of the disease and treatment. **The Following NOC Concepts Apply to These Outcomes** Family Functioning Family Coping Family Normalization Knowledge: Illness Care	Teach parents and child about the disease, and explain all procedures. Advise family of expected side effects and toxicities; clarify which demand medical evaluation. Reassure family that reactions are complications of treatment. Prepare family for what to do when side effects occur. Interpret prognostic statistics carefully, realizing family's level of understanding. Schedule time for family to be together without interruptions. Help family plan for future. Encourage family to discuss feelings regarding child's disease. **The Following NIC Concepts Apply to These Interventions** Counseling Family Support	To promote understanding To prevent delay in treatment To provide support To prevent delay in treatment To promote understanding To encourage communication and expression of feelings To promote child's development To promote expression of feelings

Therapeutic Procedures, Chapter 22, when caring for a child with leukemia.

Prevent Complications of Myelosuppression. The leukemic process and most of the chemotherapeutic agents cause myelosuppression. The reduced numbers of blood cells result in secondary problems of infection, bleeding tendencies, and anemia. Supportive care involves both medical and nursing management. Because these are so closely linked, they are discussed together.

Infection. A frequent complication of treatment for childhood cancer is overwhelming infection secondary to neutropenia. The child is most susceptible to overwhelming infection during three phases of the disease: (1) at the time of diagnosis and relapse when the leukemic process has replaced normal leukocytes; (2) during immunosuppressive therapy; and (3) after prolonged antibiotic therapy, which predisposes the child to the growth of resistant organisms. However, the use of granulocyte colony-stimulating factor (GCSF) has reduced the incidence and duration of infection in children receiving treatment for cancer.

The first defense against infection is prevention. When the child is hospitalized, the nurse employs all measures to control transfer of infection. These typically include the use of a private room, restriction of all visitors and health personnel with active infection, and strict hand-washing technique with an antiseptic solution. In some research centers, special germ-free environments are available during complete myelosuppression from intensive chemotherapy or for bone marrow transplant.

> **NURSINGALERT**
>
> Because the usual viral infections of childhood are particularly dangerous, the child is not immunized against these diseases (measles, rubella, mumps, and polio) until the immune system is capable of responding appropriately to the vaccine. If given when the immune system is depressed, the attenuated virus can result in an overwhelming infection. The child can receive the Salk (inactivated) vaccine for poliomyelitis. Children with cancer should not routinely receive the varicella vaccine. Siblings and other family members can receive the varicella vaccine without risk to the child with cancer (American Academy of Pediatrics, 2006; Walsh, Roilides, and Groll, 2006) (see Chapter 10).

The child is evaluated for potential sites of infection (e.g., mucosal ulceration; skin abrasion; skin tear, such as a hangnail) and observed for any elevation in temperature. To identify the source of infection, chest radiographs and blood, stool, urine, and nasopharyngeal cultures are taken. IV antibiotics are administered, and if this therapy is prolonged, a venous access device, such as a peripherally inserted central catheter or intermittent infusion device (saline lock or PRN adaptor), is used to maintain IV access.

Prevention of infection continues to be a priority after discharge from the hospital. Ordinarily, the child is allowed to return to school when the WBC count is at a satisfactory level, usually an absolute neutrophil count (ANC) greater than 500/mm³ (see Nursing Care Guidelines box). At all times, family members are encouraged to practice good hand washing to prevent introducing pathogens into the home. The child may need to be isolated from school contacts in the event of an outbreak of a childhood disease, especially chickenpox.

Nutrition is another important component of infection prevention. An adequate protein-caloric intake provides the

> **nursingcareguidelines**
>
> **Calculating the Absolute Neutrophil Count**
> Determine the total percent of neutrophils (polys, or segs, and bands). Multiply white blood cell (WBC) count by percent of neutrophils.
>
> **EXAMPLE:**
> WBC = 1000; neutrophils = 7%; nonsegmented neutrophils (bands) = 7%
> *Step 1:* 7% + 7% = 14%
> *Step 2:* 0.14 × 1000 = 140 absolute neutrophil count (ANC)

child with better host defenses against infection and increased tolerance to chemotherapy and irradiation. However, providing optimal nutrition during periods of anorexia and vomiting from chemotherapy is a tremendous challenge (see Feeding the Sick Child, Chapter 22).

Hemorrhage. Before the use of transfused platelets, hemorrhage was a leading cause of death in patients with leukemia. Now most bleeding episodes can be prevented or controlled with the administration of platelet concentrates or platelet-rich plasma.

Because infection increases the tendency toward hemorrhage, and because bleeding sites become more easily infected, skin punctures are avoided whenever possible. When finger sticks, venipunctures, IM injections, and bone marrow aspirations are performed, aseptic technique must be employed, along with continued observation for bleeding. Meticulous mouth care is essential, since gingival bleeding with resultant mucositis is a frequent problem. Because the rectal area is prone to ulceration from various drugs, feces and urine are removed immediately, and the perianal area is washed. Using rectal temperatures is avoided to prevent trauma. Children are advised to avoid activities that might cause injury or bleeding, such as riding bicycles or skateboards, climbing trees or playground equipment, and playing contact sports.

Platelet transfusions are generally reserved for active bleeding episodes that do not respond to local treatment and that may occur during induction or relapse therapy. Epistaxis and gingival bleeding are the most common. The nurse teaches parents and older children measures to control nosebleeding (see pp. 929-930). Pressure at the site without disturbing clot formation is the general rule.

During bleeding episodes the parents and child need much emotional support. Often parents will request a platelet transfusion, unaware of the need for trying local measures first. The nurse can be instrumental in allaying anxiety by acknowledging the feelings of the child and family and explaining the reason for delaying a platelet transfusion until absolutely necessary.

Anemia. Initially, anemia may be profound from complete replacement of the bone marrow by leukemic cells. During induction therapy, blood transfusions may be necessary. The usual precautions in caring for the child with anemia are instituted (see p. 914).

Use Precautions in Administering and Handling Chemotherapeutic Agents. In addition to the nurse's many responsibilities in regard to the child and family, nurses must also use safeguards to protect themselves. Handling chemotherapeutic agents may present risks to handlers and to their offspring, although the exact degree of risk is not known. Many chemotherapeutic agents are vesicants (sclerosing agents) that can cause severe cellular damage if even minute amounts of the drug infiltrate surrounding tissue. Only nurses experienced with chemotherapeutic agents should administer vesicants. Guidelines are available* and must be followed exactly to prevent tissue damage to patients. Interventions for extravasation vary, but each nurse should be aware of the institution's policies and implement them at once.

In addition to extravasation, a potentially fatal complication is anaphylaxis, especially from L-asparaginase, teniposide (VM-26), etoposide (VP-16), bleomycin, and cisplatin. Nursing responsibilities include prevention of, recognition of, and preparation for serious reactions. Prevention begins with a careful history for known allergies.

Most children with cancer have a venous access device, which facilitates administration of IV drugs. During treatment and remission, many drugs are taken orally at home. Compliance with the medication schedule is essential, and nurses play an important role in educating the family about the drugs and encouraging adherence to the plan.

> **NURSINGALERT**
>
> Chemotherapeutic drugs must be given through a free-flowing IV line. The infusion is stopped immediately if any sign of infiltration (pain, stinging, swelling, or redness at the cannulation site) occurs.

> **NURSINGALERT**
>
> When chemotherapeutic and immunologic agents are given, the child must be observed for 20 minutes after the infusion for signs of anaphylaxis (cyanosis, hypotension, wheezing, severe urticaria). Emergency equipment (especially blood pressure monitor and bag-valve-mask) and emergency drugs (especially oxygen, epinephrine, antihistamine, aminophylline, corticosteroids, and vasopressors) must be available. If a reaction is suspected, the drug is discontinued, the IV line is flushed with saline, and the child's vital signs and subsequent responses are monitored.

Manage Problems of Drug Toxicity. Chemotherapy presents several nursing challenges. The complexity of the treatment protocols is often overwhelming to families. In addition, each therapy is associated with a number of predictable side effects. Nurses must be aware of these side effects and use judgment in recognizing reactions, as well as toxicities.†

Nausea and Vomiting. The nausea and vomiting that occur shortly after administration of several of the drugs and from cranial or abdominal radiation can be profound. The serotonin-receptor antagonists (e.g., ondansetron, granisetron) are effective in the control of nausea and vomiting occurring after emetogenic chemotherapy and radiotherapy. When combined with dexamethasone, these agents are the treatment of choice in the prevention of delayed emesis (Berde, Billett, and Collins, 2006).

The most beneficial regimen for antiemetic control has been the administration of the antiemetic *before* the chemotherapy begins. The goal is to prevent the child from ever experiencing nausea or vomiting, thus preventing development of anticipatory symptoms (the conditioned response of developing nausea and vomiting before receiving the drug).

Anorexia. Loss of appetite is a direct consequence of the chemotherapy or irradiation. It is a major problem for parents because it is the one area they feel responsible for, particularly when so many other facets of care are outside their control. There are no universally successful techniques for encouraging a sick child to eat. However, the guidelines in Chapter 22 can be helpful during the anorexic period and can prevent additional problems during the remission.

Some children still do not eat despite these approaches. When loss of appetite and weight persist, the nurse should investigate the family situation to determine whether any factors (e.g., conditioned aversion to food, environmental stress related to eating, controlling behavior, anger) might be contributing to the problem. Nasogastric tube feedings or total parenteral nutrition may be implemented for children with significant nutritional problems.

Mucosal Ulceration. One of the most distressing side effects of several drugs is GI mucosal cell damage, which can produce ulcers anywhere along the alimentary tract. Oral ulcers greatly compound anorexia because eating is extremely uncomfortable, but the following interventions may be helpful: (1) provide a bland, moist, soft diet appropriate for the child's age and preferences; (2) use a soft sponge toothbrush (Toothettes) or cotton-tipped applicator; (3) provide frequent mouthwashes with normal saline (using a solution of 1 teaspoon of table salt and 1 pint of water) or sodium bicarbonate mouth rinses (using a solution of 1 teaspoon of baking soda in 1 quart of water); and (4) use local anesthetics (e.g., Chloraseptic lozenges) or nonprescription preparations without alcohol (e.g., hydrocortisone dental paste [Orabase], antiseptic mouth rinse [UlcerEase], diphenhydramine [Benadryl] and aluminum and magnesium hydroxide [Maalox] solution). Although local anesthetics are effective in temporarily relieving the pain, many children dislike the taste and numb feeling they produce.

> **NURSINGALERT**
>
> Viscous lidocaine is not recommended for young children; if applied to the pharynx, it may depress the gag reflex, increasing the risk of aspiration. Seizures have been rarely associated with the use of oral viscous lidocaine (Berde, Billett, and Collins, 2006; Cho, Cheng, and Cheng, 2000).

Other preparations that may be used to prevent or treat mucositis include chlorhexidine gluconate (Peridex) because of its dual effectiveness against candidal and bacterial infections, antifungal troches (lozenges) or mouthwash, and lip balm (e.g., Aquaphor) to keep the lips moist. Agents that should not be used include lemon glycerin swabs (irritate eroded tissue and can decay teeth), hydrogen peroxide (delays healing by breaking down protein), and milk of magnesia (dries mucosa).

Stomatitis may cause such difficulty with eating that the child may require hospitalization for hydration, parenteral nutrition, and pain control (often with IV morphine). The child will usually choose the foods that are best tolerated, and

---

Cancer Chemotherapy Guidelines can be obtained from the Oncology Nursing Society, 125 Enterprise Drive, Pittsburgh, PA 15275; (866) 257-4ONS, (412) 859-6100; fax: (877) 369-5497; e-mail: customer.service@ons.org; http://www.ons.org.

†Detailed chemotherapeutic agents are outlined in Wilson D, Hockenberry MJ: *Wong's clinical manual of pediatric nursing*, ed 7, St Louis, 2008, Mosby, pp 301-307.

the nurse should encourage parents to relax any eating pressures. Because the stomatitis is a temporary condition, the child can resume good food habits after the ulcers heal. Dental hygiene can become a serious problem for children with orthodontic appliances. Sometimes it may be necessary to remove the braces to allow chemotherapy to continue.

Rectal ulcers are managed by meticulous toilet hygiene, warm sitz baths after each bowel movement, and use of an occlusive ointment or dressing applied to the ulcerated area to promote epithelialization. Stool softeners are necessary to prevent further discomfort. Parents are advised to record bowel movements, since the child may voluntarily avoid defecation to prevent discomfort. Rectal thermometers and suppositories are contraindicated because insertion may further traumatize the area.

Neuropathy. Vincristine and, to a lesser extent, vinblastine can cause various neurotoxic effects. Nursing interventions for management of these effects include (1) administering stool softeners or laxatives for severe constipation caused by decreased bowel innervation; (2) maintaining good body alignment and, if patient is on bed rest, using a footboard or high-top shoes to minimize or prevent footdrop; (3) carrying out safety measures during ambulation because of weakness and numbing of the extremities, which may cause difficulty in walking or fine hand movement; and (4) providing a soft or liquid diet for severe jaw pain.

Hemorrhagic Cystitis. Sterile hemorrhagic cystitis, a side effect of chemical irritation to the bladder from cyclophosphamide, can be decreased and often prevented by (1) promoting a liberal fluid intake (at least one and a half times the recommended daily fluid requirement); (2) frequent voiding immediately after feeling the urge, before bed, and after arising; (3) administering the drug early in the day to allow for sufficient oral intake and voiding; and (4) administering mesna (an agent that provides protection to the bladder) as ordered. If oral home administration is prescribed, the family needs *specific* instructions regarding exactly how much fluid the child must have.

> **NURSINGALERT**
>
> If signs of cystitis occur, such as burning or bleeding on urination, prompt medical evaluation is needed.

Alopecia. Hair loss is a common side effect of several chemotherapeutic drugs and cranial irradiation, although not all children lose their hair during drug therapy. It is better to warn children and parents of this side effect than to allow them to think that it is only a remote possibility. A soft cotton cap is the most comfortable head wear for children. Polyester increases perspiration and causes itching. Other options include scarves, hats, or a wig.

> **NURSINGTIP**
>
> If the child chooses to wear a wig, encouraging the child to select one similar to his or her own hairstyle and color before the hair falls out is helpful in fostering later adjustment to hair loss.

The nurse should also inform the family that hair regrows in 3 to 6 months and may be of a different color and texture. Frequently the hair is darker, thicker, and curlier than before. If the child chooses not to wear a wig, attention to some type of head covering, especially in cold climates and during exposure to sun, and scalp hygiene are important. The scalp should be washed like any other body part.

Moon Face. Short-term steroid therapy produces no acute toxicities and produces two beneficial reactions: increased appetite and a sense of well-being. However, it does produce alterations in appearance, which, although not clinically significant, can be extremely distressing to older children. One of these is moon face, in which the child's face becomes rounded and puffy. It is helpful to reassure the child that after cessation of the drug, the facial shape will return to normal. Unlike hair loss, little can be done to camouflage this obvious change. If the child resumes activity early in the course of treatment, the change may be less noticeable to peers than after a long absence.

Mood Changes. Shortly after beginning steroid therapy, children experience a number of mood changes that range from feelings of well-being and euphoria to depression and irritability. If parents are unaware of these drug-induced changes, they may become unduly concerned. The nurse should warn them of the reactions and encourage them to discuss the behavioral changes with each other and the child.

Provide Emotional Support. An important aspect of continued emotional support involves the prognosis. Although leukemia is no longer invariably fatal, it must be remembered that survival statistics are only average estimates and apply to those children treated with the latest protocols since diagnosis. For the low-risk child the chances may be better, but for the high-risk child they may be significantly poorer. Of those who do survive after discontinuing therapy, some will relapse. Therefore, at present, only the passage of time is positive confirmation of the child's being ultimately "cured" of the disease. Remission, even in excess of 5 years, cannot be equated with a cure. With increasing concern regarding late effects of treatment, continued surveillance of the child's health status is needed. The nurse who is working with family members must individualize information regarding the "numbers" and the potential risks. An understanding of each member's emotional needs, as well as competent care of physical ones, is essential to the positive, growth-promoting support of the family. Comprehensive emotional support for the family of the child with a potentially fatal illness is discussed in Chapter 18.

Lymphomas

Pediatric lymphomas are the third most common group of malignancies in children and adolescents. The lymphomas, a group of neoplastic diseases that arise from the lymphoid and hematopoietic systems, are divided into Hodgkin disease and non-Hodgkin lymphoma (NHL). These diseases are further subdivided according to tissue type and extent of disease. NHL is more prevalent in children younger than 14 years of age, whereas Hodgkin disease is prevalent in adolescence and the young adult period, with a striking increase between ages 15 and 19 years.

HODGKIN DISEASE

Hodgkin disease is a neoplastic disease that originates in the lymphoid system and primarily involves the lymph nodes. It predictably metastasizes to nonnodal or extralymphatic sites, especially the spleen, liver, bone marrow, and lungs, although no tissue is exempt from involvement (Fig. 26-4). It is classified according to four histologic types: (1) lymphocytic predomi-

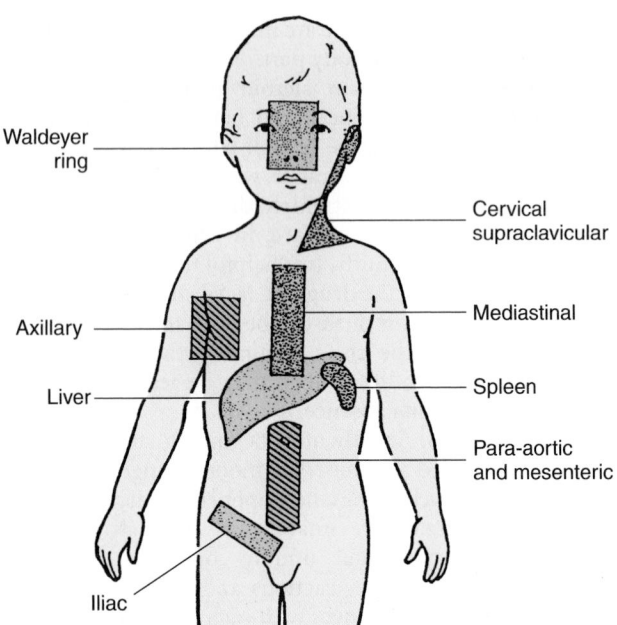

Waldeyer ring

Axillary

Liver

Iliac

Cervical supraclavicular

Mediastinal

Spleen

Para-aortic and mesenteric

FIG. 26-4 ■ Main areas of lymphadenopathy and organ involvement in Hodgkin disease.

nance, (2) nodular sclerosis, (3) mixed cellularity, and (4) lymphocytic depletion. Accurate staging of the extent of disease is the basis for treatment protocols and expected prognoses.

The Ann Arbor staging system assigns a stage based on the number of sites of lymph node involvement, presence of extranodal disease, and history of any symptoms. Patients are classified as A if asymptomatic and as B if they have the following symptoms: temperature of 38° C (100.4° F) or higher for 3 consecutive days, drenching night sweats, or unexplained loss of body weight (10% or more) over the preceding 6 months (Hudson, Onciu, and Donaldson, 2006).

Asymptomatic enlarged cervical or supraclavicular lymphadenopathy is the most common presentation of Hodgkin disease. Other systemic symptoms may be manifested, including fever, weight loss, night sweats, cough, abdominal discomfort, anorexia, nausea, and pruritus. Because multiple organs may be involved, diagnosis is based on several tests and the extent of metastatic disease. Tests include a CBC, erythrocyte sedimentation rate, serum copper, ferritin level, fibrinogen, immunoglobulins, uric acid level, liver function tests, T-cell function studies, and urinalysis. Radiographic tests include computed tomography (CT) scans of the neck, chest, abdomen, and pelvis; a gallium scan (identifies metastatic or recurrent disease); a chest x-ray film; and, if clinically indicated, a bone scan to identify metastatic disease.

Although used rarely, **lymphangiography** may be performed. This is visualization of the lymphatic circulation of the lower extremities, groin, ileopelvic and abdominal-aortic regions, and thoracic duct by way of a radiopaque medium injected in the feet or hands.

A lymph node biopsy is essential to establish histologic diagnosis and staging. The presence of Reed-Sternberg cells is characteristic of Hodgkin disease. These large cells, which are multilobed and nucleated with abundant cytoplasm and a typically halolike clear zone around the nucleolus, are often described as having an "owl's eyes" appearance (Hudson, Onciu, and Donaldson, 2006). A bone marrow aspiration or biopsy is usually performed. With the advent of CT and gallium scans to

identify metastatic disease and multiagent chemotherapy to eradicate metastatic disease, a laparotomy without splenectomy is avoided except in a few selected cases.

Therapeutic Management

The primary modalities of therapy are radiation and chemotherapy. Each may be used alone or in combination based on the clinical staging. Radiation may involve only the involved field (IF), an extended field (EF) (involved areas plus adjacent nodes), or total nodal irradiation (TNI), depending on the extent of involvement.

An effective combination of chemotherapy widely used is MOPP (mechlorethamine, vincristine [Oncovin], procarbazine, prednisone) or ABVD (adriamycin, bleomycin, vinblastine, dacarbazine). However, this therapy combination has caused severe late effects, especially secondary malignancies. Other drug combinations such as COPP (cyclophosphamide, vincristine, prednisone, procarbazine) as a substitute for MOPP have minimized late effects.

Follow-up care of children no longer receiving therapy is essential to identify relapse and secondary cancers. In children with splenectomy resulting from laparotomy or splenic irradiation, prophylactic antibiotics are administered for an indefinite period. Also, immunizations against pneumococci and meningococci are recommended before the splenectomy.

Prognosis. Long-term survival for all stages of Hodgkin disease is excellent. Early-stage disease can have survival rates greater than 90%, with advanced stages having rates between 65% and 75%.

Nursing Care Management

Nursing care involves the same objectives as for patients with other types of cancer, specifically: (1) preparation for diagnostic and operative procedures, (2) explanation of treatment side effects, and (3) child and family support (see Chapter 18). Because this is most often a disease of adolescents and young adults, the nurse must have an appreciation of their psychologic needs and reactions during the diagnostic and treatment phases (see Nursing Care Plan, pp. 932-934).

The most common side effect of irradiation is fatigue. This is particularly difficult for active, outgoing school-age children and adolescents, since it prevents them from keeping up with their peers. Sometimes adolescents will push themselves to the point of physical exhaustion rather than admit and succumb to the decreased activity tolerance. The nurse cautions parents to observe for behavior such as extreme fatigue at the end of the day, falling asleep at the dinner table, inability to concentrate on homework, or an increased susceptibility to infection. A regular bedtime and scheduled rest periods are important for these children, especially during chemotherapy, when myelosuppression increases the risk of infection and debilitation. Before discharge the nurse should discuss a feasible school schedule with the parents and child.

An area of concern for adolescents is the high risk of sterility from irradiation and chemotherapy. Both drugs, particularly procarbazine and alkylating agents, and irradiation to the gonads can lead to infertility. Adolescents should be informed of these side effects early in the course of the diagnosis and treatment. Sperm banking is now offered at many cancer centers before the initiation of treatment in adolescent boys. Sexual function is not altered, although the appearance of secondary sexual characteristics and menstruation may be delayed in the pubescent child. Delayed sexual maturation may be an extremely sensitive and stressful issue for children (see Chapter 17).

NON-HODGKIN LYMPHOMA

NHL occurs more frequently in children than Hodgkin disease. NHL is diagnosed in approximately 750 to 800 children each year in the United States (Link and Weinstein, 2006). Histologic classification of childhood NHL is strikingly different from that of Hodgkin disease, as demonstrated in the following statements:

- The disease is usually diffuse rather than nodular.
- The cell type is either undifferentiated or poorly differentiated.
- Dissemination occurs early, more often, and rapidly.
- Mediastinal involvement and invasion of meninges are common.

NHL exhibits a variety of morphologic, cytochemical, and immunologic features, not unlike the diversity seen in leukemia. Classification is based on the histologic pattern: (1) lymphoblastic, (2) Burkitt or non-Burkitt, or (3) large cell. Immunologically these cells are also classified as T cells; B cells; or non-T, non-B cells (lacking immunologic properties). The clinical staging system used in Hodgkin disease is of little value in NHL, although it has been modified and other systems have been developed.

Diagnostic Evaluation

Because the clinical presentation of most children with NHL is widespread disseminated disease, thorough pathologic staging is unnecessary. Clinical manifestations depend on the anatomic site and extent of involvement. These manifestations include many of those seen in Hodgkin disease and leukemia, as well as organ symptoms related to pressure from enlargement of adjacent lymph nodes, such as intestinal or airway obstruction, cranial nerve palsies, and spinal paralysis.

Recommendations for staging include a surgical biopsy of an enlarged node, histopathologic confirmation of disease with cytochemical and immunologic evaluation, bone marrow examination, radiographic studies (especially tomograms of the lungs and GI organs), and lumbar puncture.

Therapeutic Management

The treatment protocols for NHL include aggressive use of irradiation and chemotherapy. Similar to leukemic therapy, the protocols include induction, consolidation, and maintenance phases, some with intrathecal chemotherapy. Several antineoplastic agents used in the treatment of NHL include vincristine, prednisone, L-asparaginase, methotrexate, 6-mercaptopurine, cytarabine, cyclophosphamide, anthracyclines, and teniposide or etoposide (Link and Donaldson, 2003; Link and Weinstein, 2006).

Prognosis. The prognosis is excellent for children with localized disease, and long-term remissions are possible in many patients, even in those with disseminated disease. Because relapse after 2 years is rare, survival after 24 months is considered a cure.

Nursing Care Management

Nursing care of the child with NHL is similar to that required for children with leukemia. Many of the same drugs are employed, although the schedules differ. Because of the intense chemotherapy, nursing care is primarily directed toward managing the side effects of these agents and providing supportive care to the child and family (see Nursing Care Plan, pp. 932-934).

IMMUNOLOGIC DEFICIENCY DISORDERS

A number of disorders can cause profound, often life-threatening alterations within the body's immune system. The most serious are those conditions that completely depress immunity, such as severe combined immunodeficiency disease (SCID). However, the one disorder that generates the most anxiety, within both the family and the community at large, is HIV infection/AIDS.

Several classifications of immune dysfunction exist. **AIDS,** SCID, and **Wiskott-Aldrich syndrome (WAS)** are syndromes wherein the body is unable to mount an immune response. The immune response can also be misdirected. In **autoimmune disorders,** antibodies, macrophages, and lymphocytes attack healthy cells.

HUMAN IMMUNODEFICIENCY VIRUS INFECTION AND ACQUIRED IMMUNODEFICIENCY SYNDROME

Since the first cases of AIDS were identified in the early 1980s, HIV infection has generated intense medical investigation. Research has led to early diagnosis of and improved medical treatments for HIV infection, changing this disease from a rapidly fatal one to a chronic, but terminal, disease of childhood.

Epidemiology

The first AIDS cases in the pediatric population in the United States were identified in children born to HIV-infected mothers and in children who received blood products. More than 90% of these children acquired the disease perinatally from their mothers. Smaller numbers of children were infected through the transfusion of contaminated blood or blood products before 1985 or were infected through sexual abuse. In contrast, sexual activity and IV drug use are major sources of HIV infection in adolescents.

The estimated number of children with perinatally acquired AIDS peaked in 1992; subsequent years have seen significant declines. This trend is a result of implementation of recommended HIV counseling and voluntary testing practices and the use of highly active antiretroviral therapy (HAART) to prevent perinatal transmission. HAART, typically a combination of two nucleoside analog reverse transcriptase inhibitors and a protease inhibitor, is the current standard in the United States for the treatment of HIV-infected pregnant women, and it has significantly reduced the transmission of HIV (Cibulka, 2006; Perinatal HIV Guidelines Working Group, 2007). Routine HIV screening and voluntary testing for pregnant women are recommended (Centers for Disease Control and Prevention, 2006), and guidelines for the use of antiretroviral drugs in HIV-infected pregnant women to reduce perinatal transmission are available (Perinatal HIV Guidelines Working Group, 2007).

Etiology

HIV is a retrovirus that is transmitted by lymphocytes and monocytes. It is found in the blood, semen, vaginal secretions, and breast milk. It has an incubation period of months to years (Ezekowitz and Stockman, 2003). There are different strains of HIV. HIV-2 is prevalent in Africa, whereas HIV-1 is the dominant strain in the United States and elsewhere. **Horizontal transmission** of HIV occurs through intimate sexual contact or parenteral exposure to blood or body fluids containing visible blood. **Perinatal (vertical) transmission** occurs when an HIV-infected pregnant woman passes the infection to her infant. There is no evidence that *casual* contact between infected and uninfected individuals can spread the virus.

Pathophysiology

The HIV virus primarily infects a specific subset of T lymphocytes, the CD_4^+ T cells. The virus takes over the machinery of the CD_4^+ lymphocyte, using it to replicate itself, rendering the CD_4^+ cell dysfunctional. The CD_4^+ lymphocyte count gradually decreases over time, leading to progressive immunodeficiency. The count eventually reaches a critical level below which there is substantial risk of opportunistic illnesses, followed by death.

Clinical Manifestations

Common clinical manifestations of HIV infection in children are varied (Box 26-9). The diagnosis of AIDS is associated with certain illnesses or conditions. The most common AIDS-defining conditions observed among American children are listed in Box 26-10. Other problems in these children may include short stature, malnutrition, and cardiomyopathy. CNS abnormalities resulting from HIV infection may include neuropsychologic deficits; developmental disabilities; and deficits in motor skills, communication, and behavioral functioning.

Diagnostic Evaluation

For children 18 months of age and older, the HIV enzyme-linked immunosorbent assay (ELISA) and Western blot immunoassay are performed to determine HIV infection. In infants born to HIV-infected mothers, these assays will be positive because of the presence of maternal antibodies derived transplacentally. Maternal antibodies may persist in the infant up to 18 months of age. Therefore other diagnostic tests are employed, most commonly the HIV polymerase chain reaction (PCR) for detection of proviral DNA. With this technique, more than 95% of infected infants can be diagnosed by 1 to 4 months of age (Ezekowitz and Stockman, 2003; Goldschmidt and Fogler, 2006).

The Centers for Disease Control and Prevention (1994) has developed a classification system to describe the spectrum of HIV disease in children (Table 26-3). The system indicates the severity of clinical signs and symptoms and the degree of immunosuppression. Mild signs and symptoms include lymphadenopathy, parotitis, hepatosplenomegaly, and recurrent or persistent sinusitis or otitis media. Moderate signs and symptoms include lymphoid interstitial pneumonitis (LIP) and a variety of organ-specific dysfunctions or infections. Severe signs and symptoms include AIDS-defining illnesses with the exception of LIP. Children with LIP have a better prognosis than those with other AIDS-defining illnesses. In children whose HIV infection is not yet confirmed, the letter *E* (vertically exposed) is placed in front of the classification. The immune categories are based on CD_4^+ lymphocyte counts and percentages. Age adjustment of these numbers is necessary because normal counts, which are relatively high in infants,

BOX 26-9

Common Clinical Manifestations of Human Immunodeficiency Virus Infection in Children

- Lymphadenopathy
- Hepatosplenomegaly
- Oral candidiasis
- Chronic or recurrent diarrhea
- Failure to thrive
- Developmental delay
- Parotitis

BOX 26-10

Common Defining Conditions for Acquired Immunodeficiency Syndrome in Children

- *Pneumocystis carinii* pneumonia
- Lymphoid interstitial pneumonitis
- Recurrent bacterial infections
- Wasting syndrome
- Candidal esophagitis
- Human immunodeficiency virus encephalopathy
- Cytomegalovirus disease
- *Mycobacterium avium-intracellulare* complex infection
- Pulmonary candidiasis
- Herpes simplex disease
- Cryptosporidiosis

decline steadily until 6 years of age, when they reach adult norms (Table 26-4).

Therapeutic Management

The goals of therapy for HIV infection include slowing the growth of the virus, preventing and treating opportunistic infections, and providing nutritional support and symptomatic treatment. **Antiretroviral drugs** work at various stages of the HIV life cycle to prevent reproduction of functional new virus particles. Although not a cure, these drugs can suppress viral replication, preventing further deterioration of the immune system, and thus delay disease progression. Classes of antiretroviral agents include nucleoside reverse transcriptase inhibitors (e.g., zidovudine, didanosine, stavudine, lamivudine, abacavir), nonnucleoside reverse transcriptase inhibitors (e.g., nevirapine, delavirdine, efavirenz), nucleotide reverse transcriptase inhibitors (e.g., adefovir), protease inhibitors (e.g., indinavir, saquinavir, ritonavir, nelfinavir, amprenavir), and adjunctive antiretrovirals (e.g., hydroxyurea). Combinations of these drugs are used to forestall the emergence of drug resistance. Antiretroviral therapy regimens and guidelines are continually evolving. Therapy is lifelong, making adherence difficult. Laboratory markers (CD_4^+ lymphocyte count, viral load) assist in monitoring both disease progression and response to therapy.

Pneumocystis carinii pneumonia (PCP) is the most common opportunistic infection of children infected with HIV. It occurs most frequently between 3 and 6 months of age. All infants born to HIV-infected women should receive prophylaxis during the first year of life, according to guidelines from the Centers for Disease Control and Prevention (1995) and the American Academy of Pediatrics (2000a). Trimethoprim-sulfamethoxazole (TMP-SMZ) is the agent of choice. If ad-

TABLE 26-3

Pediatric HIV Infection Classification*

IMMUNOLOGIC CATEGORY	N: NO SIGNS/ SYMPTOMS	A: MILD SIGNS/ SYMPTOMS	B: MODERATE SIGNS/ SYMPTOMS†	C: SEVERE SIGNS/ SYMPTOMS†
No evidence of suppression	N1	A1	B1	C1
Evidence of moderate suppression	N2	A2	B2	C2
Severe suppression	N3	A3	B3	C3

From Centers for Disease Control and Prevention: 1994 Revised classification system for human immunodeficiency virus infection in children less than 13 years of age, *MMWR Recomm Rep* 43(RR-12):1-10, 1994.
*Children whose human immunodeficiency virus infection status is not confirmed are classified by using the above table with the letter *E* (for perinatally exposed) placed before the appropriate classification code (e.g., EN2).
†Both category C and lymphoid interstitial pneumonitis in category B are reportable to state and local health departments as acquired immunodeficiency syndrome.

TABLE 26-4

Immunologic Categories Based on Age-Specific CD$_4$$^+$ T-Lymphocyte Counts and Percent of Total Lymphocytes

	AGE OF CHILD					
	<12 MONTHS		1-5 YEARS		6-12 YEARS	
IMMUNOLOGIC CATEGORY	μl	(%)	μl	(%)	μl	(%)
No evidence of suppression	≥1500	(≥25)	≥1000	(≥25)	≥500	(≥25)
Evidence of moderate suppression	750-1499	(15-24)	500-999	(15-24)	200-499	(15-24)
Severe suppression	<750	(<15)	<500	(<15)	<200	(<15)

From Centers for Disease Control and Prevention: 1994 Revised classification system for human immunodeficiency virus infection in children less than 13 years of age, *MMWR Recomm Rep* 43(RR-12):1-10, 1994.

verse effects are experienced with TMP-SMZ, dapsone or pentamidine can be used.

Prophylaxis is often employed for other opportunistic infections, such as disseminated *Mycobacterium avium-intracellulare* complex (MAC), candidiasis, or herpes simplex. IVIG has been helpful in preventing recurrent or serious bacterial infections in some HIV-infected children.

Immunization against common childhood illnesses is recommended for all children exposed to and infected with HIV (American Academy of Pediatrics, 2000b). Varicella (chickenpox) vaccine and measles-mumps-rubella (MMR) vaccine can be administered if there is no evidence of severe immunocompromise. Because antibody production to vaccines may be poor or decrease over time, immediate prophylaxis after exposure to several vaccine-preventable diseases (e.g., measles, varicella) is warranted. It should be recognized that children receiving IV gamma globulin prophylaxis may not respond to the MMR vaccine (Centers for Disease Control and Prevention, 2003).

HIV infection often leads to marked failure to thrive and multiple nutritional deficiencies. Nutritional management may be difficult because of recurrent illness, diarrhea, and other physical problems. Intensive nutritional interventions should be instituted when the child's growth begins to slow or weight begins to decrease.

Prognosis. Early recognition and improved medical care have changed HIV disease from a rapidly fatal illness to a chronic disease. After the introduction of combination antiretroviral therapy, the numbers of new AIDS cases and deaths declined substantially. Between 1995 and 1998, the annual number of AIDS cases declined by 38% and deaths declined

by 63% (Centers for Disease Control and Prevention, 2003; 2007). The annual number of AIDS cases has remained stable in children less than 13 years of age since 1998 (Klause and Johnson, 2007).

Nursing Care Management

Education concerning transmission and control of infectious diseases, including HIV infection, is essential for children with HIV infection and anyone involved in their care. The basic tenets of standard precautions should be presented in an age-appropriate manner, with careful consideration of the educational levels of the individuals (see Infection Control, Chapter 22). Safety issues, including appropriate storage of special medications and equipment (e.g., needles and syringes), are emphasized.

Unfortunately, relatives, friends, and others in the general public may be fearful of contracting HIV infection, and criticism and ostracism of the child and family may occur. In an effort to protect the child, the family may limit the child's activities outside the home. Although certain precautions are justified in limiting exposure to sources of infections, they must be tempered with concern for the child's normal developmental needs. Both the family and the community need ongoing education about HIV to dispel many of the myths that have been perpetuated by uninformed persons.*

Prevention is a key component of HIV education. Educating adolescents about HIV is essential in preventing HIV infection in this age-group. Education should include the routes

---

*Additional information is available from the AIDS Hotline: (800) 342-2437 (342-AIDS).

of transmission, the hazards of IV and other recreational drug use, and the value of sexual abstinence and safe sex practices. Such education should be a part of anticipatory guidance provided to all adolescent patients. Nurses can also encourage adolescents at risk to undergo HIV counseling and testing. In addition to identifying infected teenagers and getting them into care, such counseling affords adolescents an opportunity to learn about, and possibly change, their risky behaviors.

The multiple complications associated with HIV disease are potentially painful (Ezekowitz and Stockman, 2003; Sullivan and Woda, 2003). Aggressive pain management is essential for these children to have an acceptable quality of life. Their pain may be due to infections (e.g., otitis media, dental abscess),

encephalopathy (e.g., spasticity), adverse effects of medications (e.g., peripheral neuropathy), or an unknown source (e.g., deep musculoskeletal pain). Sources of pain are related not only to disease processes, but also to various treatments these children often undergo, including venipunctures, lumbar punctures, biopsies, and endoscopies. Ongoing assessment of pain is crucial and is most easily accomplished in older children who are able to communicate. Nonverbal and developmentally delayed children are more difficult to assess. The nurse should be alert for signs of pain such as emotional detachment, lack of interactive play, irritability, and depression. Effective pain management depends on the appropriate use of pharmacologic agents, including EMLA cream, acetaminophen, NSAIDs, muscle relaxants, and opioids. Tolerance to opioids may indicate increased dosing; monitored use ensures safety. Nonpharmacologic interventions (e.g., guided imagery, hypnosis, relaxation, and distraction techniques) are useful adjuncts.

Common psychosocial concerns include disclosing the diagnosis to the child, making custody plans when the parent is infected, and anticipating the loss of a family member. Other stressors may include financial difficulties, HIV-associated stigma, efforts to keep the diagnosis secret, other infected family members, and the multiple losses associated with HIV. Most mothers of these children are single mothers who are also HIV infected. As primary caretakers, they often attend to the needs of their child first, neglecting their own health in the process (see Family Focus box). The nurse can encourage the mother to receive regular health care. Family members are often involved in the care of the child, particularly if the mother has symptomatic illness. After the mother's death, a grandparent or other relative typically assumes responsibility for care of the child. The nurse can provide support and encouragement for the new surrogate parent, particularly during the transition phase. If no family member is available, the

---

FAMILY FOCUS

Caregivers and the Infant with Human Immunodeficiency Virus Infection

Unlike other fatal pediatric diseases, human immunodeficiency virus (HIV) infection is associated with special family alterations. The infant infected in utero faces multiple physical and parental problems. Because the mother is infected, she may be ill or dying and therefore unable to care for the child. If possible, grandparents or other relatives may assume care. Foster care is often difficult to arrange because of the nature of the disease, especially in relation to the social stigma and the child's multiple medical needs. When these children are hospitalized, the importance of consistent caregivers, especially primary nurses, who attend to the youngsters' physical, developmental, and emotional needs, cannot be overemphasized. However, primary nurses may face the risk of overinvolvement and must be aware of the boundaries of a therapeutic relationship.

---

nursingprocess | The Child with Human Immunodeficiency Virus Infection

ASSESSMENT
Assess for signs and symptoms of infection (see Boxes 26-9 and 26-10).

DIAGNOSIS (PROBLEM IDENTIFICATION)
After a thorough assessment, several nursing diagnoses are evident:
- Risk for Infection related to impaired body defenses, presence of infective organisms
- Altered Nutrition: Less Than Body Requirements related to recurrent illness, diarrheal losses, loss of appetite, oral candidiasis
- Impaired Social Interaction related to physical limitations, hospitalizations, social stigma of infection with human immunodeficiency virus (HIV)
- Chronic Pain related to disease process
- Interrupted Family Processes related to having a child with a dreaded and life-threatening disease
- Anticipatory Grieving related to having a child with a potentially fatal illness
- Interrupted Family Processes related to a situational crisis

PLANNING
Expected patient outcomes include the following:
- No infection will be evident.
- Disease will not be spread to others.
- Adequate nutrition will be maintained.
- Child will participate in activities with peer group and family.
- Pain will be controlled or alleviated.
- Child and family will receive appropriate support.

IMPLEMENTATION
Numerous intervention strategies are discussed on pp. 941-943.

EVALUATION
The effectiveness of nursing interventions for the child with HIV infection and his or her family is determined by continual assessment and evaluation of care based on the following guidelines:
- Observe child and family for their ability to cope with the situation and comply with care.
- Observe for and document child's emotional and physical needs, especially assessment of adherence to medications.
- Evaluate for signs of infection and disease progression.
- Observe behaviors of family.
- Educate child and family on importance of disease prevention.
- Interview and observe child and family for evidence of their understanding of the condition.

child may be placed in a foster or group home. Nursing is an integral part of the multidisciplinary team necessary for the successful management of the complex medical and social problems of these families.

Children with HIV infection attend daycare centers and schools. It is well established that the risk of HIV transmission in these settings is minimal. These institutions are required to follow Centers for Disease Control and Prevention and Occupational Safety and Health Administration (OSHA) guidelines for infection control measures. Standard precautions describing proper management of blood and body fluids should also be followed. It is recommended that school personnel receive current HIV information and include it in the health education curriculum for kindergarten through twelfth grade (American Academy of Pediatrics, 2000a, 1999). School nurses play a vital role in educating the school staff, students, and parents. They are also invaluable in monitoring the needs of known affected children.

Confidentiality is a major issue in daycare or school attendance. Parents and legal guardians have the right to decide whether they inform these agencies of their child's HIV diagnosis. Unfortunately, myths about HIV infection continue to exist, and the family often wishes to avoid any potential criticism or ostracism of the child.

SEVERE COMBINED IMMUNODEFICIENCY DISEASE

SCID is a defect characterized by absence of both humoral and cell-mediated immunity. The terms **Swiss-type lymphopenic agammaglobulinemia** (an autosomal recessive form of the disease) and **X-linked lymphopenic agammaglobulinemia** have been used to describe this disorder, which, as the names imply, can follow either mode of inheritance.

Susceptibility to infection occurs early in life, most often in the first month of life. The child suffers from chronic infection, fails to completely recover from an infection, is frequently reinfected, and is infected with unusual agents. Failure to thrive is a consequence of the persistent illnesses.

Diagnosis is usually based on a history of recurrent, severe infections from early infancy; a familial history of the disorder; and specific laboratory findings, which include lymphopenia, lack of lymphocyte response to antigens, and absence of plasma cells in the bone marrow. Documentation of immunoglobulin deficiency is difficult during infancy because of the normally delayed response of infants in producing their own immunoglobulins and material transfer of immunoglobulin G (IgG).

Therapeutic Management

The definitive treatment for SCID is HSCT from a histocompatible donor, a haplo-identical donor (usually a parent), or a matched unrelated donor. IVIG infusions and PCP prophylaxis are used to augment the humoral immunity until the transplant is performed. Several investigators are attempting gene therapy with some success, but there is a potential complication of insertional mutagenesis (Buckley, 2007).

Nursing Care Management

Nursing care focuses on preventing infection and supporting the child and family. The care is consistent with that needed for HSCT for any condition (see p. 945). Because the prognosis for SCID is very poor if a compatible bone marrow donor is not available, nursing care is directed at supporting the family in caring for a child with a life-threatening illness (see Chapter 18). Genetic counseling is essential because of the modes of transmission in either form of the disorder.

WISKOTT-ALDRICH SYNDROME

WAS is an X-linked recessive disorder characterized by a triad of abnormalities: (1) thrombocytopenia, (2) eczema, and (3) immunodeficiency of selective functions of B lymphocytes and T lymphocytes. A defective gene has been identified and designated the WAS protein (Bonilla and Geha, 2003; Fleisher, 2006). At birth the presenting symptoms may be bloody diarrhea as a result of thrombocytopenia. As the child grows older, recurrent infection and eczema become more severe, and the bleeding becomes less frequent.

Eczema is typical of the allergic type and easily becomes superinfected. Chronic infection with herpes simplex is a frequent problem and may lead to chronic keratitis of the eye with loss of vision. Chronic pulmonary disease, sinusitis, and otitis media result from repeated infections. In those children who survive the bleeding episodes and overwhelming infections, malignancy presents an additional risk to survival. Medical treatment involves:

■ Counteracting the bleeding tendencies with platelet transfusions
■ Using IV gamma globulin to provide passive immunity
■ Administering prophylactic antibiotics to prevent and control infection.

The only curative therapy is HSCT from a matched donor (Buckley, 2007).

Nursing Care Management

Because of the poor prognosis for these children, the main nursing consideration is supporting the family in the care of a fatally ill child (see Chapter 18). Physical care is directed at controlling the problems imposed by the disorder. The measures used to control bleeding are similar to those for hemophilia and vWD (see previous discussions). Another major goal is prevention or control of infection. Because eczema is a troublesome problem, nursing measures specific to this condition are especially important (see Chapter 30). The genetic implications of this X-linked recessive disorder differ little from those of any other X-linked disorder.

TECHNOLOGIC MANAGEMENT OF HEMATOLOGIC AND IMMUNOLOGIC DISORDERS

BLOOD TRANSFUSION THERAPY

Technologic advances in blood banking and transfusion medicine enable the administration of only the blood component needed by the child, such as packed RBCs in anemia or platelets for bleeding disorders. However, regardless of the blood component infused, all transfusions have some risks. Therefore nurses need to be aware of the possible complications and the appropriate interventions. Table 26-5 summarizes the major hazards of transfusions, the signs and symptoms typically associated with each, and nursing responsibilities. General guidelines that apply to all transfusions include:

■ Take vital signs, including blood pressure, *before* administering blood to establish baseline data for intratransfusion and posttransfusion comparison, then every 15 minutes for 1 hour while blood is infusing and on completion of transfusion.

TABLE 26-5

Nursing Care of the Child Receiving Blood Transfusions

COMPLICATION	SIGNS AND SYMPTOMS	PRECAUTIONS AND NURSING RESPONSIBILITIES
IMMEDIATE REACTIONS **Hemolytic Reactions** Most severe type, but rare Incompatible blood Incompatibility in multiple transfusions	Sudden severe headache Chills Shaking Fever Pain at needle site and along venous tract Nausea and vomiting Sensation of tightness in chest Red or black urine Flank pain Progressive signs of shock or renal failure	Identify donor and recipient blood types and groups before transfusion is begun; verify with another nurse or practitioner. Transfuse blood slowly for first 15-20 minutes and/or initial 20% of blood volume; remain with patient. Stop transfusion immediately in event signs or symptoms occur, maintain patent intravenous line, and notify practitioner. Save donor blood to recrossmatch with patient's blood. Monitor for evidence of shock. Insert urinary catheter and monitor hourly outputs. Send sample of patient's blood and urine to laboratory for presence of hemoglobin (indicates intravascular hemolysis). Observe for signs of hemorrhage resulting from disseminated intravascular coagulation. Support medical therapies to reverse shock.
Febrile Reactions Leukocyte or platelet antibodies Plasma protein antibodies	Fever Chills	May give acetaminophen for prophylaxis. Leukocyte-poor red blood cells (RBCs) are less likely to cause reaction. Stop transfusion immediately; report to practitioner for evaluation.
Allergic Reactions Recipient reaction to allergens in donor's blood	Urticaria Pruritus Flushing Asthmatic wheezing Laryngeal edema	Give antihistamines for prophylaxis to children with tendency to allergic reactions. Stop transfusion immediately. Administer epinephrine for wheezing or anaphylactic reaction.
Circulatory Overload Too rapid transfusion (even a small quantity) Transfusion of excessive quantity of blood (even slowly)	Precordial pain Dyspnea Rales Cyanosis Dry cough Distended neck veins Hypertension	Transfuse blood slowly. Prevent overload by using packed RBCs or administering divided amounts of blood. Use infusion pump to regulate and maintain flow rate. Stop transfusion immediately if signs of overload. Place child upright with feet in dependent position to increase venous resistance.
Air Emboli May occur when blood is transfused under pressure	Sudden difficulty in breathing Sharp pain in chest Apprehension	Normalize pressure before container is empty when infusing blood under pressure. Clear tubing of air by aspirating air with syringe at nearest Y connector if air is observed in tubing; disconnect tubing and allow blood to flow until air has escaped only if a Y connector is not available.
Hypothermia	Chills Low temperature Irregular heart rate Possible cardiac arrest	Allow blood to warm at room temperature (<1 hour). Use approved mechanical blood warmer or electric warming coil to warm blood rapidly; never use microwave oven. Take temperature if patient complains of chills; if subnormal, stop transfusion.
Electrolyte Disturbances Hyperkalemia (in massive transfusions or in patients with renal problems)	Nausea, diarrhea Muscle weakness Flaccid paralysis Paresthesia of extremities Bradycardia Apprehension Cardiac arrest	Use washed RBCs or fresh blood if patient is at risk.

TABLE 26-5		
Nursing Care of the Child Receiving Blood Transfusions—cont'd		
COMPLICATION	**SIGNS AND SYMPTOMS**	**PRECAUTIONS AND NURSING RESPONSIBILITIES**
DELAYED REACTIONS **Transmission of Infection** Hepatitis Human immunodeficiency virus (HIV) infection Malaria Syphilis Other bacterial or viral infection	Signs of infection (e.g., jaundice) Toxic reaction—High fever, severe headache or substernal pain, hypotension, intense flushing, vomiting or diarrhea	Blood is tested for antibodies to HIV, hepatitis C virus, and hepatitis B core antigen; in addition, blood is tested for hepatitis B surface antigen and alanine aminotransferase, and a serologic test is performed for syphilis; units that test positive are destroyed; individuals at risk for carrying certain viruses are deterred from donation. Report any sign of infection and, if it occurs during transfusion, stop transfusion immediately, send sample for culture and sensitivity testing, and notify practitioner.
Alloimmunization Antibody formation Occurs in patients receiving multiple transfusions	Increased risk of hemolytic, febrile, and allergic reactions	Use limited number of donors. Observe carefully for signs of reactions.
Delayed Hemolytic Reaction	Destruction of RBCs and fever 5-10 days after transfusion	Observe for posttransfusion anemia and decreasing benefit from successive transfusion.

■ Check the identification of the recipient with the donor's blood group and type, regardless of the blood product being used.

■ Administer the first 50 ml of blood or 20% of the volume (whichever is smaller) *slowly* and stay with the child.

■ Administer with normal saline on a piggyback setup or have normal saline available.

■ Administer blood through an appropriate filter to eliminate particles in the blood and prevent the precipitation of formed elements; gently shake the container frequently.

■ Use blood within 30 minutes of its arrival from the blood bank; if it is not used, return to the blood bank—do not store in the regular unit refrigerator.

■ Infuse a unit of blood (or the specified amount) within 4 hours. If the infusion will exceed this time, the blood should be divided into appropriately sized quantities by the blood bank, and the unused portion refrigerated under controlled conditions.

■ If a reaction of any type is suspected, take vital signs, stop the transfusion, maintain a patent IV line with normal saline and new tubing, notify the practitioner, and do not restart the transfusion until the child's condition has been medically evaluated.

Although hemolytic reactions are rare, ABO incompatibility remains the most common cause of death from blood transfusion, and human error is usually responsible (administration of the wrong type to the patient or mislabeling of the blood product) (Norville and Bryant, 2002; Bell, 2007). Hemolysis can also cause the release of large quantities of phospholipids, which are capable of stimulating DIC (see p. 929). Acute kidney shutdown and eventual renal failure are a result of renal vasoconstriction from antigen-antibody complexes derived from the RBC surface.

Blood is usually administered to children by infusion pump; therefore the usual precautions and management related to pumps apply. When the blood is started with a standard transfusion set, the filter chamber is filled to allow the total filter to be used. The drip chamber is partially filled with blood to permit counting of the drops. In adjusting the flow rate, it is important to remember that blood administration sets do not use microdrops (60 drops/ml) but regular drops (usually 10 or 15 drops/ml).

HEMATOPOIETIC STEM CELL TRANSPLANTATION

HSCT is used to establish healthy hematopoiesis in both malignant and nonmalignant disease. Candidates for transplantation are children who have disorders that are unlikely to be cured by other means. Most HSCT patients undergo intensive ablative therapy using high-dose combination chemotherapy with or without total body irradiation (Bollard, Krance, and Heslop, 2006). After the immune system is suppressed to prevent rejection of the transplanted marrow, the stem cells harvested from the bone marrow, peripheral blood, or the umbilical vein of the placenta are given to the patient by IV transfusion. The newly transfused stem cells will begin to repopulate the ablative bone marrow. In essence, a new blood-forming organ will be accepted by the recipient.

The selection process for a suitable donor and the potential complications in transplantation are related to the **HLA system complex.** Some of the major HLA antigens are A, B, C, D, and DR. There is a wide diversity for each of these HLA loci. There are more than 20 different HLA-A antigens that can be inherited and more than 40 different HLA-B antigens.

The genes are inherited as a single unit or **haplotype.** A child inherits one unit from each parent; thus a child and each parent have one identical and one nonidentical haplotype. Because the possible haplotype combinations among siblings follow the laws of mendelian genetics, there is a one-in-four chance that two siblings have two identical haplotypes and are perfectly matched at the HLA loci.

The importance of HLA matching is to prevent the serious complication known as **GVHD.** Because the child's immune system is essentially rendered nonfunctional, there is little difficulty with bone marrow rejection by the recipient. However, the donor's marrow may contain antigens not matched to the recipient's antigens, which begin attacking body cells. The more closely the HLA systems match, the less likely GVHD is to develop. However, it can occur even with a perfect HLA match, since there are as yet unidentified and thus unmatched histocompatibility antigens (Bollard, Krance, and Heslop, 2006).

Different types of HSCT are now performed in children with cancer. **Allogeneic HSCT** involves matching a histocompatible donor with the recipient. However, allogeneic HSCT is limited by the presence of a suitable marrow donor.

Because of the limited numbers of patients having HLA-identical siblings, other types of allogeneic transplants have evolved. **Umbilical cord blood stem cell transplantation** is an established, rich source of hematopoietic stem cells for use in children with cancer. Because stem cells can be found with high frequency in the circulation of newborns, cord blood transplantation has become an alternative for some children. The benefit of using umbilical cord blood is the blood's relative immunodeficiency at birth, allowing for partially matched unrelated cord blood transplants to be successful, with a lower risk of GVHD-related problems (Bollard, Krance, and Heslop, 2006; Ryan, Kristovich, Haugen, and others, 2002).

Autologous HSCTs use the patient's own marrow that was collected from disease-free tissue, frozen, and sometimes treated to remove malignant cells. Children with solid tumors such as neuroblastoma, Hodgkin disease, NHL, rhabdomyosarcoma, Ewing sarcoma, and Wilms tumor have been treated with autologous HSCTs.

Peripheral stem cell transplants (PSCTs) are also used in children with cancer. PSCT, a type of autologous transplant, differs in the way stem cells are collected from the patient. CSF is first given to stimulate the production of many stem cells (Ryan, Kristovich, Haugen, and others, 2002). After the WBC count is high enough, the stem cells are collected by an apheresis machine. This machine filters out peripheral stem cells from whole blood, returning the remainder of the blood cells and plasma to the child. Stem cells have been collected in very small children without problems (Lipton, 2003). The peripheral stem cells are then frozen until the patient is ready for the PSCT.

Nursing Care Management

The care of children undergoing HSCT is similar to that of any child receiving chemotherapy and radiotherapy. The hospitalization is typically 3 to 6 weeks in an isolated environment, during which time the child is subjected to numerous procedures and side effects of therapy. Throughout this long ordeal the family is concerned with successful engraftment and fear of fatal complications (see Family Focus box). Consequently, nurses involved with the child and family need to provide sensitive care and maintain a supportive attitude during the many crises that may arise. If the procedure is not successful, the families need care consistent with that required by the family of any child with a life-threatening disorder (see Chapter 18).

APHERESIS

Apheresis is the removal of blood from an individual, separation of the blood into its components, retention of one or more of these components, and reinfusion of the remainder

of the blood into the individual. Apheresis is most often used to remove large quantities of platelets from healthy adult donors. These transfusion products have greatly prolonged the survival of patients with hematologic and oncologic diseases.

This technique is used to remove peripheral blood stem cells (PBSCs) from children before they receive HSCT or high-dose chemotherapy or radiotherapy, which is severely toxic to the bone marrow. These PBSCs can then be used to restore the child's bone marrow. Apheresis is also used as a therapeutic modality. The blood component that is diseased or toxic is separated from the blood, and the remainder is returned to the individual. Therapeutic apheresis is considered part of standard therapy for many diseases. Plasma is selectively removed from individuals with hyperviscosity, life-threatening complications of myasthenia gravis, Guillain-Barré syndrome, thrombotic thrombocytopenic purpura, and certain drug overdoses. WBCs are removed from individuals with high-WBC-count leukemia.

Nursing Care Management

Difficult venous access and small blood volume can limit the ability to use this therapy in the infant and young child. Education of the family and child includes the purposes of the therapy and the technology.

Specially trained individuals perform the apheresis procedure. Attention focuses on rate of removal, blood component separation, and reinfusion of blood into the child. Vital signs are monitored, and the child is continuously observed for any adverse reactions secondary to the circulatory volume changes and the anticoagulant used.

When apheresis components are infused, nursing measures differ depending on whether the product is autologous (blood component from the child) or allogeneic (blood component from another individual). Autologous components are the child's own blood; therefore a major precaution is proper identification to ensure the correct component. The rate of infusion should be adjusted to the child's tolerance. If the product is allogeneic, all precautions for blood transfusions apply.

KEY POINTS

- Anemia is defined as reduction of RBCs or Hgb concentration to levels below normal for age; disorders are classified either by etiology and physiology or by morphology.
- The nurse's role in treatment of anemia is to assist in establishing a diagnosis, prepare the child for laboratory tests, administer prescribed medications, decrease tissue oxygen needs, implement safety precautions, and observe for complications.
- The main nursing goal in prevention of nutritional anemia is parent education regarding correct feeding practices.
- Sickle cell anemia is a hereditary hemoglobinopathy caused by normal adult Hgb (HbA) being partly or completely replaced by sickle Hgb (HbS).
- Nursing care of the child with sickle cell anemia focuses on teaching the family how to prevent and recognize sickle cell problems; managing pain during crises; and helping the child and parents adjust to a lifelong, chronic disease.
- Nursing care of the child with β-thalassemia includes observing for complications of multiple blood transfusions, assisting the child in coping with the effects of illness, and fostering parent-child adjustment to long-term illness.
- Causes of acquired AA include irradiation, drugs, industrial and household chemicals, infections, and infiltration and replacement of myeloid elements; however, the majority cases are idiopathic.
- Clotting depends on three processes: vascular spasm, platelet aggregation, and coagulation and clot formation.
- Nursing care of the child with hemophilia involves preventing bleeding by decreasing the risk of injury, recognizing and managing bleeding with factor replacement, preventing the crippling effects of joint degeneration, and preparing and supporting the child and family for home care.
- Goals in the care of the child with leukemia are to prepare the family for diagnostic and therapeutic procedures, prevent complications of myelosuppression, manage problems of irradiation and drug toxicity, and provide continued emotional support.
- The lymphomas include Hodgkin lymphoma and NHL and are disorders involving the lymphoid system.
- Immunodeficiency disorders render the affected individual unable to fight infectious organisms.
- HIV infection is primarily acquired in infants during pregnancy or birth from an infected mother and in adolescents from engaging in high-risk behaviors.
- Blood transfusions supply needed blood components.
- HSCT replaces the diseased or malfunctioning bone marrow with viable blood stem cells.
- Apheresis is the selective removal of a blood component. It can be used to supply cellular elements needed for therapy (i.e., platelets or stem cells) or to remove diseased components.

REFERENCES

American Academy of Pediatrics, Committee on Infectious Diseases, Pickering L, editor: *Red book: 2006 report of the Committee on Infectious Diseases*, ed 27, Elk Grove Village, Ill, 2006, The Academy.

American Academy of Pediatrics: Breastfeeding and the use of human milk, *Pediatrics* 115(2):496-506, 2005.

American Academy of Pediatrics, Section on Hematology/Oncology, Committee on Genetics: Health supervision for children with sickle cell disease, *Pediatrics* 109(3):526-536, 2002.

American Academy of Pediatrics, Committee on Pediatric AIDS: Identification and care of HIV-exposed and HIV-infected infants, children, and adolescents in foster care, *Pediatrics* 106(1):149-153, 2000a.

American Academy of Pediatrics, Committee on Pediatric AIDS: Technical report: perinatal human immunodeficiency virus testing and prevention of transmission, *Pediatrics* 106(6):1-12, 2000b.

American Academy of Pediatrics, Committee on Pediatric AIDS and Committee on Infectious Diseases: Issues related to human immunodeficiency virus transmission in schools, child care, medical settings, the home, and community, *Pediatrics* 104(2):318-324, 1999.

American Pain Society: *Guidelines for the management of acute and chronic pain in sickle-cell disease*, Glenview, Ill, 1999, The Society.

Anderson N: Hydroxyurea therapy: improving the lives of patients with sickle cell disease, *Pediatr Nurs* 32(6):541-543, 2006.

Andrews NC: Disorders of iron metabolism and sideroblastic anemia. In Nathan D, Orkin SH,

Ginsburg D, and others, editors: *Nathan and Oski's hematology of infancy and childhood*, ed 6, Philadelphia, 2003, Saunders.

Bell MD: Red blood cell transfusions, *Pediatr Rev* 28(8):299-304, 2007.

Berde CB, Billett AM, Collins JJ: Symptom management in supportive care. In Pizzo PA, Poplack DG, editors: *Principles and practice of pediatric oncology*, ed 5, Philadelphia, 2006, Lippincott.

Bhatia S: Epidemiology. In Wallace WHB, Green DM, editors: *Late effects of childhood cancer*, London, 2004, Arnold.

Bogen DL, Krause JP, Serwint JR: Outcome of children identified as anemic by routine screening in an inner-city clinic, *Arch Pediatr Adolesc Med* 155:366-371, 2001.

Bollard CM, Krance RA, Heslop HE: Hematopoietic stem cell transplantation in pediatric oncology. In Pizzo PA, Poplack DG, editors: *Principles and practice of pediatric oncology*, ed 5, Philadelphia, 2006, Lippincott.

Bonilla FA, Geha RS: Primary immunodeficiency diseases. In Nathan D, Orkin SH, Ginsburg D, and others, editors: *Nathan and Oski's hematology of infancy and childhood*, ed 6, Philadelphia, 2003, Saunders.

Buchanan GR: Thrombocytopenia during childhood: what the pediatrician need to know, *Pediatr Rev* 26(11):401-409, 2005.

Buckley RH: Evaluation of the immune system. In Behrman RE, Kliegman RM, Jenson HTS, and others, editors: *Nelson textbook of pediatrics*, ed 18, Philadelphia, 2007, Saunders.

Bulas D: Screening children for sickle cell vasculopathy: guidelines for transcranial Doppler evaluation, *Pediatr Radiol* 35:235-241, 2005.

Burden MJ, Westerlund AJ, Sivan-Armony R, and others: An event-related potential study of attention and recognition memory in infants with iron-deficiency anemia, *Pediatrics* 120(2):336-345, 2007.

Carley A: Anemia: when is it iron deficiency? *Pediatr Nurs* 29(2):127-133, 2003.

Centers for Disease Control and Prevention: *HIV/AIDS surveillance report, 2005*, Vol 17, revised edition, Atlanta, 2007, The Centers, pp. 1-54; available online at http://www.cdc.gov/hiv/topics/surveillance/resources/reports.

Centers for Disease Control and Prevention: Revised recommendations for HIV testing of adults, adolescents and pregnant women in health-care settings, *MMWR* 55(RR-14):1-13, 2006.

Centers for Disease Control and Prevention: Advancing HIV prevention: new strategies for a changing epidemic—United States, *MMWR* 52(15):329-332, 2003.

Centers for Disease Control and Prevention: 1995 revised guidelines for prophylaxis against *Pneumocystis carinii* pneumonia for children infected with or perinatally exposed to human immunodeficiency virus, *MMWR* 44(RR-4):1-11, 1995.

Centers for Disease Control and Prevention: 1994 revised classified system for human immunodeficiency virus infection in children less than 13 years of age, *MMWR* 43(RR-12):1-10, 1994.

Chandran L, Gelfer P: Breastfeeding: the essential principles, *Pediatr Rev* 27(11):409-417, 2006.

Chiocca EM: Sickle cell crisis: severe pain and potential tissue necrosis are the major concerns, *Am J Nurs* 96(9):49, 1996.

Cho S, Cheng AC, Cheng MCK: Oral care for children with leukemia, *Hong Kong Med J* 6(2):203-208, 2000.

Cibulka NJ: Mother-to-child transmission of HIV in the United States, *AJN* 106(7):56-63, 2006.

Curry H: Bleeding disorder basics, *Pediatr Nurs* 30(5):402-405, 2004.

Dover GJ, Platt OS: Sickle cell disease. In Nathan D, Orkin SH, Ginsburg D, and others, editors: *Nathan and Oski's hematology of infancy and childhood,* ed 6, Philadelphia, 2003, Saunders.

Driscoll MC: Sickle cell disease, *Pediatr Rev* 28(7):259-267, 2007.

Ezekowitz RAB, Stockman III JA: Hematologic manifestations of systemic diseases. In Nathan D, Orkin SH, Ginsburg D, and others, editors: *Nathan and Oski's hematology of infancy and childhood,* ed 6, Philadelphia, 2003, Saunders.

Fleisher TA: Primary immune deficiencies: windows into the immune system, *Pediatr Rev* 27(10):363-373, 2006.

Glader B: Anemias of inadequate production. In Behrman RE, Kliegman RM, Jenson HTS, and others, editors: *Nelson textbook of pediatrics,* ed 18, Philadelphia, 2007, Saunders.

Goldschmidt RH, Fogler JA: Opportunities to prevent HIV transmission to newborns, *Pediatrics* 117(1):208-209, 2006.

Hord JD: The acquired pancytopenia. In Behrman RE, Kliegman RM, Jenson HTS, and others, editors: *Nelson textbook of pediatrics,* ed 18, Philadelphia, 2007, Saunders.

Hudson MM, Onciu M, Donaldson SS: Hodgkin's disease. In Pizzo PA, Poplack DG, editors: *Principles and practice of pediatric oncology,* ed 4, Philadelphia, 2006, Lippincott.

Karayalcin G: Hemolytic anemia (sickle cell anemia). In Lanzkowsky P, editor: *Manual of pediatric hematology and oncology,* ed 3, San Diego, 2000, Academic Press.

Khoury H, Grimsley E: Oxygen inhalation in non-hypoxic sickle cell patients during vaso-occlusive crisis, *Blood* 86(10):3998, 1995.

Klause BD, Johnson M: Paradigm shift: new testing guidelines for HIV, *Adv Nurse Pract* 15(3):59-93, 2007.

Link MP, Donaldson SS: The lymphomas and lymphadenopathy. In Nathan D, Orkin SH, Ginsburg D, and others, editors: *Nathan and Oski's hematology of infancy and childhood,* ed 6, Philadelphia, 2003, Saunders.

Link MP, Weinstein HJ: Malignant non-Hodgkin lymphomas in children. In Pizzo PA, Poplack DG, editors: *Principles and practice of pediatric oncology,* ed 5, Philadelphia, 2006, Lippincott.

Lipton JM: Peripheral blood as a stem cell source for hematopoietic cell transplantation in children: is the effort in vein? *Pediatr Transplant* 7(Suppl 3):65-70, 2003.

Margolin JF, Steuber CP, Poplack DG: Acute lymphoblastic leukemia. In Pizzo PA, Poplack DG, editors: *Principles and practice of pediatric oncology,* ed 4, Philadelphia, 2006, Lippincott.

Marsh JCW: Management of acquired aplastic anemia, *Blood Rev* 19:143-151, 2005.

McKenzie SB: Anemias of disordered iron metabolism and heme synthesis. In McKenzie SB, editor: *Clinical laboratory hematology,* Upper Saddle River, NJ, 2004, Pearson Prentice Hall.

Miller M, Zimmerman S, Schultz W, and others: Hydroxyurea therapy for pediatric patients with hemoglobin SC disease, *J Pediatr Hematol Oncol* 23(5):306-308, 2001.

Montgomery RR, Gill JC, Scott JP: Hemophilia and von Willebrand disease. In Nathan D, Orkin SH, Ginsburg D, and others, editors: *Nathan and Oski's hematology of infancy and childhood,* ed 6, Philadelphia, 2003, Saunders.

Morris CR, Singer ST, Walters MC: Clinical hemoglobinopathies: iron, lungs and new blood, *Curr Opin Hematol* 13:407-418, 2006.

National Hemophilia Foundation, Bleeding Disorders Information Center: *Newly diagnosed: parents FAQ 2006,* retrieved March 25, 2008, from http://www.hemophilia.org/bdi/bdi_newly7c.htm.

National Institutes of Health; National Heart, Lung, and Blood Institute, Division of Blood Disease and Resources: *The management of sickle cell disease,* NIH Pub No 02-2117, Bethesda, Md, 2002, NHLBI Health Information Network.

Norville R, Bryant R: Blood component deficiencies. In Baggott CR, Kelly KP, Fochtman D, and others, editors: *APON nursing care of children and adolescents with cancer,* ed 3, Philadelphia, 2002, Saunders.

Ohls R, Christensen RD: Hemoglobin disorders. In Behrman RE, Kliegman RM, Jenson HTS, and others, editors: *Nelson textbook of pediatrics,* ed 18, Philadelphia, 2007, Saunders.

Okpala I: New therapies for sickle cell disease, *Hematol Oncol Clin North Am* 19:975-987, 2005.

Orkin SH, Nathan DG: The thalassemias. In Nathan D, Orkin SH, Ginsburg D, and others, editors: *Nathan and Oski's hematology of infancy and childhood,* ed 6, Philadelphia, 2003, Saunders.

Paley C: Hemolytic anemia (thalassemias). In Lanzkowsky P, editor: *Manual of pediatric hematology and oncology,* San Diego, 2000, Academic Press.

Pearce JM, Sills RH: Childhood leukemia, *Pediatr Rev* 26(3):96-104, 2005.

Perinatal HIV Guidelines Working Group, Public Health Service Task Force: *Recommendations for use of antiretroviral drugs in pregnant HIV-infected women for maternal health and interventions to reduce perinatal HIV transmission in the United States,* 2007, retrieved March 24, 2008, from http://www.aidsinfo.nih.gov/ContentFiles/PerinatalGL.pdf.

Perkins S: Disorders of hematopoiesis. In Collins RD, Swerdlow SH, editors: *Pediatric hematopathology,* ed 1, Philadelphia, 2001, Churchill Livingstone.

Platt OS, Brambilla DJ, Roose WF, and others: Mortality in sickle cell disease: life expectancy and risk factors for early death, *N Engl J Med* 330:1639-1644, 1994.

Pui CH, Relling MV, Downing JR: Acute lymphoblastic leukemia, *N Engl J Med* 350:1535-1548, 2004.

Redding-Lallinger R, Knoll C: Sickle cell disease—pathophysiology and treatment, *Curr Probl Pediatr Adolesc Health Care* 36(10):346-376, 2006.

Richardson M: Microcytic anemia, *Pediatr Rev* 28(1):5-13, 2007.

Ryan LG, Kristovich KM, Haugen MS, and others: Hematopoietic stem cell transplantation. In Baggott CR, Kelly KP, Fochtman D, and others, editors: *Nursing care of children and adolescents with cancer,* ed 3, Philadelphia, 2002, Saunders.

Scott JP, Montgomery RR: Platelet and blood vessel disorder. In Behrman RE, Kliegman RM, Jenson HTS, and others, editors: *Nelson textbook of pediatrics,* ed 18, Philadelphia, 2007, Saunders.

Segel GB, Hirsch MG, Feig SA: Managing anemia in a pediatric office practice, part I, *Pediatr Rev* 23(3):75-83, 2002.

Shende A: Bone marrow failure. In Lanzkowsky P, editor: *Manual of pediatric hematology and oncology,* ed 3, San Diego, 2000, Academic Press.

Shimamura A, Guinan EC: Acquired aplastic anemia. In Nathan D, Orkin SH, Ginsburg D, and others, editors: *Nathan and Oski's hematology of infancy and childhood,* ed 6, Philadelphia, 2003, Saunders.

Silverman LB, Sallan SE: Acute lymphoblastic leukemia. In Nathan D, Orkin SH, Ginsburg D, and others, editors: *Nathan and Oski's hematology of infancy and childhood,* ed 6, Philadelphia, 2003, Saunders.

Steinberg MH, Barton F, Castro O, and others: Effect of hydroxyurea on mortality and morbidity in adult sickle cell anemia: risks and benefits up to 9 years of treatment, *JAMA* 289(13):1645-1651, 2003.

Sullivan JL, Woda BA: Lymphohistiocytic disorders. In Nathan D, Orkin SH, Ginsburg D, and others, editors: *Nathan and Oski's hematology of infancy and childhood,* ed 6, Philadelphia, 2003, Saunders.

Walsh TJ, Roilides E, Groll AH: Infectious complications in pediatric cancer patients. In Pizzo PA, Poplack DG, editors: *Principles and practice of pediatric oncology,* ed 4, Philadelphia, 2006, Lippincott.

Yoon SL, Black S: Comprehensive, integrative management of pain for patients with sickle-cell disease, *J Altern Complement Med* 12(10):995-1001, 2006.

Zimmerman S, Schultz W, Davis J, and others: Sustained long-term hematologic efficacy of hydroxyurea at maximum tolerated dose in children with sickle cell disease, *Blood* 103(6):2039-2045, 2004.

27

The Child with Genitourinary Dysfunction

BARBARA A. MONTAGNINO AND PATRICIA A. RING

CHAPTER OUTLINE

GENITOURINARY DYSFUNCTION, 950
GENITOURINARY TRACT DISORDERS
AND DEFECTS, 950
Urinary Tract Infection, 950
Obstructive Uropathy, 956
External Defects, 957
    Psychologic Problems Related to Genital
        Surgery, 957

GLOMERULAR DISEASE, 958
Nephrotic Syndrome, 958
Acute Glomerulonephritis, 961
MISCELLANEOUS RENAL
DISORDERS, 962
Hemolytic Uremic Syndrome, 962
Wilms Tumor, 963
RENAL FAILURE, 965

Acute Renal Failure, 965
Nursing Care Plan: The Child with Acute
    Renal Dysfunction, 967
Chronic Renal Failure, 967
TECHNOLOGIC MANAGEMENT
OF RENAL FAILURE, 970
Dialysis, 970
Transplantation, 971

LEARNING OBJECTIVES

On completion of this chapter the reader will be able to:

- Describe the various factors that contribute to urinary tract infections in infants and children.
- Discuss the preoperative preparation of the child and parents when the child has a structural defect of the genitourinary tract.

- Demonstrate an understanding of the causes and mechanisms of edema formation in nephrotic syndrome.
- Outline a nursing care plan for a child with nephrotic syndrome.
- Compare the child with minimal-change nephrotic syndrome and the child with acute glomerulonephritis in terms of clinical manifestations and nursing care.

- Contrast the causes, complications, and management of acute and chronic renal failure.
- List the types of renal dialysis.
- Recognize signs of kidney transplant rejection.

RELATED TOPICS and ADDITIONAL RESOURCES

 IN TEXT

Administration of Medication, *Ch. 22*
Anemia, *Ch. 26*
Collection of Specimens, *Ch. 22*
Impact of Chronic Illness or Disability on the Child, *Ch. 18*
Infection Control, *Ch. 22*
Physical Examination: Genitalia, *Ch. 6*
Preparation for Diagnostic and Therapeutic Procedures, *Ch. 22*

Surgical Procedures, *Ch. 22*
Systemic Hypertension, *Ch. 25*

 COMPANION CD

Animations—Bladder; Kidney Function
NCLEX Review Questions

evolve

evolve.elsevier.com/Wong/essentials/

Critical Thinking Case Studies—Acute Renal Failure; Urinary Tract Infection

NCLEX Review Questions
Nursing Care Plan—The Child with Acute Renal Dysfunction
WebLinks

 WONG'S CLINICAL MANUAL OF PEDIATRIC NURSING, 7th Ed

Patient and Family Education—Giving Medications to Children, *p. 522;*
Obtaining a Urine Sample, *p. 514*

GENITOURINARY DYSFUNCTION

Assessment of kidney and urinary tract integrity and diagnosis of renal or urinary tract disease are based on several evaluative tools. Physical examination, history taking, and observation of symptoms are the initial procedures. In suspected urinary tract diseases or disorders, further assessment by laboratory, radiologic, and other evaluative methods is carried out.

Clinical Manifestations

As in most disorders of childhood, the incidence and type of kidney or urinary tract dysfunction change with the age and maturation of the child. In addition, the presenting complaints and the significance of these complaints vary with maturation. For example, a complaint of enuresis has greater significance at age 8 years than at age 4. In the newborn, urinary tract disorders are associated with a number of obvious malformations of other body systems, including the curious and unexplained but frequent association between malformed or low-set ears and urinary tract anomalies.

Many of the clinical manifestations of renal disease are common to a variety of childhood disorders, but their presence is an indication to obtain further information from the child's history, family history, and laboratory studies as part of a complete physical examination. Suspected renal disease can be further evaluated by means of radiographic studies and renal biopsy (Table 27-1).

Laboratory Tests

Both urine and blood studies contribute vital information for detection of renal problems. The single most important test is probably routine urinalysis. Specific urine and blood tests provide additional information. Because nurses are usually the persons who collect the specimens for examination and who often perform many of the screening tests, they should be familiar with the test, its function, and factors that can alter or distort the results of the test. The major urine and blood tests are outlined in Tables 27-2 and 27-3.

Nursing Care Management

Nursing responsibilities in assessment of genitourinary disorders or diseases begin with observation of the child for any manifestations that might indicate dysfunction. Many conditions have specific characteristics that distinguish them from other disorders. These are discussed as appropriate throughout the chapter.

The nurse is generally the one who is responsible for preparing infants, children, and parents for tests and for collection of urine and (sometimes) blood specimens for observation and laboratory analysis (see Preparation for Diagnostic and Therapeutic Procedures, and Collection of Specimens, Chapter 22). An important nursing responsibility is to maintain careful **intake and output** measurements and **blood pressure** on most children with genitourinary dysfunction and those who might be at risk for developing renal complications (e.g., children in shock, postoperative patients). For example, any significant degree of renal disease can diminish the glomerular filtration rate, a measure of the amount of plasma from which a given substance is totally cleared in 1 minute. A number of substances can be used, but the most useful clinical estimation of glomerular filtration is the clearance of **creatinine,** an end product of protein metabolism in muscle and a substance that is freely filtered by the glomerulus and secreted

by renal tubular cells. The nurse's responsibility in this test is collection of urine, usually a 12- or 24-hour specimen.

GENITOURINARY TRACT DISORDERS AND DEFECTS

URINARY TRACT INFECTION

Infection of the genitourinary tract is one of the most common conditions of childhood. Up to 10% of children will have a febrile urinary tract infection (UTI) during the first 2 years of life (Kanellopoulos, Salakos, Spiliopoulou, and others, 2006). Among febrile males, circumcision status is important in determining risk for UTI. Uncircumcised male infants younger than 3 months of age had the highest prevalence of UTI (20.1%) of any group, male or female (Shaikh, Morone, Bost, and others, 2008). Circumcision status should be assessed in male infants with unexplained fever. UTI may involve the urethra and bladder (lower urinary tract) or the ureters, renal pelvis, calyces, and renal parenchyma (upper urinary tract). Because it is often impossible to localize the infection, the broad designation UTI is applied to the presence of significant numbers of microorganisms anywhere within the urinary tract, except the distal third of the urethra, which is usually colonized with bacteria.

Classification

Infection of the urinary tract may be present with or without clinical symptoms. As a result, the site of infection is often difficult to pinpoint with any degree of accuracy. Various terms used to describe urinary tract disorders include:

Bacteriuria—Presence of bacteria in the urine
Asymptomatic bacteriuria—Significant bacteriuria (usually defined as >100,000 colony-forming units [CFUs]) with no evidence of clinical infection
Symptomatic bacteriuria—Bacteriuria accompanied by physical signs of UTI (dysuria, suprapubic discomfort, hematuria, fever)
Recurrent UTI—Repeated episode of bacteriuria or symptomatic UTI
Persistent UTI—Persistence of bacteriuria despite antibiotic treatment
Febrile UTI—Bacteriuria accompanied by fever and other physical signs of UTI; presence of a fever typically implies a pyelonephritis
Cystitis—Inflammation of the bladder
Urethritis—Inflammation of the urethra
Pyelonephritis—Inflammation of the upper urinary tract and kidneys
Urosepsis—Febrile UTI coexisting with systemic signs of bacterial illness; blood culture reveals presence of urinary pathogen

Etiology

A variety of organisms can be responsible for UTI. *Escherichia coli* (80% of cases) and other gram-negative enteric organisms are most frequently implicated; these organisms are usually found in the anal and perineal region. Other organisms associated with UTI include *Proteus, Pseudomonas, Klebsiella, Staphylococcus aureus, Haemophilus,* and coagulase-negative *Staphylococcus* organisms. Several factors contribute to the development of UTI in childhood.

Anatomic and Physical Factors. The structure of the lower urinary tract is believed to account for the increased incidence of bacteriuria in females (Rosenthal, 2004). The short urethra, which measures about 2 cm (0.75 inch) in young girls and 4 cm (1.6 inches) in mature women, provides

Text continued on p. 954

TABLE 27-1

Radiologic and Other Tests of Urinary System Function

TEST	PROCEDURE	PURPOSE	COMMENTS AND NURSING RESPONSIBILITIES
Urine culture and sensitivity	Collection of sterile specimen	Determines presence of pathogens and the drugs to which they are sensitive	Does not require specific parental permission Send specimen to laboratory immediately after collection Catheterization, clean-catch, or suprapubic specimen
Renal/bladder ultrasound	Transmission of ultrasonic waves through renal parenchyma, along ureteral course, and over bladder	Allows visualization of renal parenchyma and renal pelvis without exposure to external beam radiation or radioactive isotopes Visualization of dilated ureters and bladder wall also possible	Noninvasive procedure
Testicular (scrotal) ultrasound	Transmission of ultrasonic waves through scrotal contents and testis	Allows visualization of scrotal contents, including testis Testicular ultrasound is used to identify masses, and Doppler-enhanced ultrasound is used to differentiate hyperemia of epididymo-orchitis from ischemia or torsion	Noninvasive procedure
Scout film	Flat plate roentgenogram of abdomen and pelvis for kidney, ureters, bladder (KUB)	Detects and establishes renal outlines, presence of calculi, or opaque foreign bodies in bladder	Prepare as for routine x-ray film
Voiding cystourethrography	Contrast medium injected into bladder through urethral catheter until bladder is full; films taken before, during, and after voiding	Visualizes bladder outline and urethra, reveals reflux of urine into ureters, and shows complications of bladder emptying	Prepare child for catheterization
Radionuclide (nuclear) cystogram	Radionuclide-containing fluid injected through urethral catheter until bladder is full; images generated before, during, and after voiding	Alternative to voiding cystourethrography in children with allergy to intravesical contrast material Allows evaluation of reflux, although visualization of anatomic details is relatively poor	Prepare child for catheterization Reassure patient and parents that allergic response to contrast materials is avoided by use of radionuclide
Radioisotope imaging studies	Contrast medium injected intravenously; computer analysis to measure uptake or washout (excretion) for analysis of organ function	DTPA radioisotope used to measure glomerular filtration rate; estimate of differential renal function and renal washout to determine presence and location of upper urinary tract obstruction DMSA radioisotope used to visualize renal scars and differential renal function; does not visualize ureters and bladder MAG3 radioisotope combines features of DTPA (evaluation of upper urinary tract obstruction) with features of DMSA radioisotope (differential renal function)	Insert or assist with insertion of intravenous infusion Monitor intravenous infusion Urethral catheterization may accompany DTPA radioisotope scan; prepare child for catheterization when indicated
Intravenous pyelography (IVP) (intravenous urogram; excretory urogram)	Intravenous injection of a contrast medium Medium secreted and concentrated by tubules X-ray films made 5, 10, and 15 minutes after injection; delayed films (30, 60 minutes, etc.) are obtained if obstruction suspected	Defines urinary tract Provides information about integrity of kidneys, ureters, and bladder Retroperitoneal masses visualized when they shift position of ureters	Preparation for test: *Infants <2 years of age*—no solid food, omit one bottle on morning of examination; perform studies early to avoid withholding of fluids *Children ages 2-14 years of age*—give cathartic evening before examination, nothing orally after midnight, enema (soapsuds) morning of examination

DMSA, Dimercaptosuccinic acid; *DTPA*, diethylenetriamine pentaacetic acid; *MAG3*, mercaptoacetyltriglycine.

Continued

TABLE 27-1

Radiologic and Other Tests of Urinary System Function—cont'd

TEST	PROCEDURE	PURPOSE	COMMENTS AND NURSING RESPONSIBILITIES
Computed tomography (CT)	Narrow-beam x-rays and computer analysis providing precise reconstruction of area	Visualizes vertical or horizontal cross section of kidney Especially valuable to distinguish tumors and cysts	Noncontrast scan is noninvasive Contrast-enhanced CT scan preparation similar to that for IVP
Cystoscopy	Direct visualization of bladder and lower urinary tract through small scope inserted via urethra	Investigation of bladder and lower tract lesions; visualizes ureteral openings, bladder wall, trigone, and urethra	Give nothing orally after midnight Carry out preoperative preparations Prepare the child for cystoscopy
Retrograde pyelography	Contrast medium injected through ureteral catheter	Visualizes pelvic calyces, ureters, and bladder	Give cathartic if ordered Give preoperative medication if ordered Observe for reaction to contrast medium Monitor vital signs after procedure
Renal angiography	Contrast medium injected directly into renal artery via catheter placed in femoral artery (or umbilical artery in newborn) and advanced to renal artery	Visualizes renal vascular system, especially for renal arterial stenosis	Prepare child for insertion of a spinal needle or perfusion catheter in renal pelvis (anesthetic often required)
Whitaker perfusion test	Injection of contrast material through renal pelvis and ureters Measures pressures in renal pelvis and urinary bladder	Determine presence of obstruction causing upper urinary tract dilation	Give nothing orally 4-6 hours before test Premedicate as ordered Prepare setup for procedure Assist with procedure Take vital signs Apply pressure to area with pressure dressing and, if feasible, a sandbag Bed rest for 24 hours Observe for abdominal pain, tenderness Monitor input and output; surgical incision may be required in infants
Renal biopsy	Removal of kidney tissue by open or percutaneous technique for study by light, electron, or immunofluorescent microscopy	Yields histologic and microscopic information about glomeruli and tubules; helps distinguish between types of nephritic syndromes Distinguishes other renal disorders	Prepare child for catheterization Insertion of a rectal tube produces feelings of rectal fullness or pressure Insertion of needles may be required for sphincter electromyography
Urodynamics	Set of tests designed to measure bladder filling, storage, and evacuation functions **Uroflowmetry**—Test to determine efficiency of urination **Cystometrogram**—Graphic comparison of bladder pressure as a function of volume **Voiding pressure study**—Comparison of detrusor contraction pressure, sphincter electromyelogram, and urinary flow	Determine characteristic of voiding dysfunction Used to identify type (cause) of incontinence or urinary retention Especially valuable for voiding dysfunction complicated by urinary infection, urinary retention, or neurogenic bladder dysfunction	Prepare child for urinary catheterization The bladder will be filled with saline solution, and filling pressures will be recorded; the child may experience fullness, coolness from the saline fluid, and urine leakage during the study

TABLE 27-2

Urine Tests of Renal Function

TEST	NORMAL RANGE	DEVIATIONS	SIGNIFICANCE OF DEVIATIONS
PHYSICAL TESTS			
Volume	Age-related	Polyuria	Osmotic factors (urinary glucose level in diabetes mellitus)
	Newborn—30-60 ml	Oliguria	Retention caused by obstructive disease
	Children—Bladder capacity (oz) = Age (years) + 2		Inadequate bladder emptying caused by neurogenic bladder or obstructive disorder
		Anuria	Obstruction of urinary tract; acute renal failure
Specific gravity	With normal fluid intake—1.016-1.022	High	Dehydration
			Presence of protein or glucose
	Newborn—1.001-1.020		Presence of radiopaque contrast medium after radiologic examinations
	Others—1.001-1.030	Low	Excessive fluid intake
			Distal tubular dysfunction
			Insufficient antidiuretic hormone
			Diuresis
Osmolality	Newborn—50-600 mOsm/L	Fixed at 1.010	Chronic glomerular disease
	Thereafter—50-1400 mOsm/L	High or low	Same as for specific gravity
			More sensitive index than specific gravity
Appearance	Clear pale yellow to deep gold	Cloudy	Contains sediment
		Cloudy reddish pink to reddish brown	Blood from trauma or disease
			Myoglobin after severe muscle destruction
		Light	Dilute
		Dark	Concentrated
		Red	Trauma
CHEMICAL TESTS			
pH	Newborn—5-7	Weak acid or neutral	If associated with metabolic acidosis, suggests tubular acidosis
	Thereafter—4.8-7.8		If associated with metabolic alkalosis, suggests potassium deficiency
	Average—6		Urinary infection
		Alkaline	Metabolic alkalosis
Protein level	Absent	Present	Abnormal glomerular permeability (e.g., glomerular disease, changes in blood pressure)
			Most kidney disease
			Orthostatic in some individuals
Glucose level	Absent	Present	Diabetes mellitus
			Infusion of concentrated glucose-containing fluids
			Glomerulonephritis
			Impaired tubular reabsorption
Ketone levels	Absent	Present	Conditions of acute metabolic demand (stress)
			Diabetic ketoacidosis
Leukocyte esterase	Absent	Present	Can identify both lysed and intact white blood cells via enzyme detection
Nitrites	Absent	Present	Most species of bacteria convert nitrates to nitrites in the urine
MICROSCOPIC TESTS			
White blood cell count	<1 or 2	>5 polymorphonuclear leukocytes/field	Urinary tract inflammatory process
		Lymphocytes	Allograft rejection
			Malignancy
Red blood cell count	<1 or 2	4-6/field in centrifuged specimen	Trauma
			Stones
			Glomerular injury
			Infection
			Neoplasms
Presence of bacteria	Absent to a few	More than 100,000 organisms/ml in centrifuged specimen	Urinary tract infection
Presence of casts	Occasional	Granular casts	Tubular or glomerular disorders
			Degenerative process in advanced renal disease
		Cellular casts	Pyelonephritis
		White blood cell	Glomerulonephritis
		Red blood cell	Proteinuria; usually transient
		Hyaline casts	

TABLE 27-3

Blood Tests of Renal Function

TEST	NORMAL RANGE (mg/dl)	DEVIATIONS	SIGNIFICANCE OF DEVIATIONS
Blood urea nitrogen (BUN)	Newborn—4-18 Infant, child—5-18	Elevated	Renal disease—acute or chronic (the higher the BUN, the more severe the disease) Increased protein catabolism Dehydration Hemorrhage High protein intake Corticosteroid therapy
Uric acid	Child—2.0-5.5	Increased	Severe renal disease
Creatinine	Infant—0.2-0.4 Child—0.3-0.7 Adolescent—0.5-1.0	Increased	Severe renal impairment

a ready pathway for invasion of organisms. In addition, the closure of the urethra at the end of micturition may return contaminated bacteria to the bladder. The longer male urethra (as long as 20 cm [8 inches] in an adult) and the antibacterial properties of prostatic secretions inhibit the entry and growth of pathogens.

> **FYI**
>
> Considerable evidence suggests there are fewer UTIs among circumcised male infants than among uncircumcised male infants, but the difference is not significant enough to recommend routine circumcision in newborns (American Academy of Pediatrics, 1999).

The single most important host factor influencing the occurrence of UTI is **urinary stasis.** Ordinarily, urine is sterile, but at 37° C (98.6° F) it provides an excellent culture medium. Under normal conditions the act of completely and repeatedly emptying the bladder flushes away any organisms before they have an opportunity to multiply and invade surrounding tissue. However, urine that remains in the bladder allows bacteria from the urethra to rapidly become established in the rich medium. Incomplete bladder emptying (stasis) may result from **reflux** (see Vesicoureteral Reflux, p. 955), anatomic abnormalities (especially those involving the ureters), dysfunction of the voiding mechanism, or extrinsic ureteral or bladder compression that may be caused by constipation. The key to preventing UTI is to maintain adequate blood supply to the bladder wall by avoidance of overdistention and high bladder pressure.

Altered Urine and Bladder Chemistry. Several mechanical and chemical characteristics of the urine and bladder mucosa help maintain urinary sterility. An increased fluid intake promotes flushing of the normal bladder and lowers the concentration of organisms in the infected bladder. Diuresis also seems to enhance the antibacterial properties of the renal medulla.

Most pathogens favor an alkaline medium. Normally, urine is slightly acidic with a median pH of 6.0. A urine pH of about 5 hampers but does not eliminate bacterial multiplication. Much has been reported about the use of cranberry products to increase urine acidity in an effort to prevent UTI. Studies done in adults offer limited evidence for the value of cran-

berry products in promoting urinary tract health (Jepson, Mihaljevic, and Craig, 2004; Bailey, Dalton, Daugherty, and others, 2007). Further research that controls for type of cranberry product used, dosing regimens, and patient selection based on age and underlying medical condition is required to clarify unanswered questions before recommendations can be made regarding the use of this supplement, especially in the pediatric population.

Diagnostic Evaluation

The clinical manifestations of UTI depend on the child's age (Box 27-1). Diagnosis of UTI is confirmed by detection of bacteriuria in urine culture, but urine collection is often difficult, especially in infants and very small children. Several factors may alter a urine specimen, and contamination of a specimen by organisms from sources other than the urine, such as perineal and perianal flora in bag specimens, is the most frequent cause of false-positive results. Unless the specimen is a first morning sample, a recent high fluid intake may indicate a falsely low organism count. Therefore children should not be encouraged to drink large volumes of water in an attempt to obtain a specimen quickly.

> **NURSINGALERT**
>
> A child who exhibits the following should be evaluated for UTI:
> - Incontinence in a toilet-trained child
> - Strong-smelling urine
> - Frequency or urgency

More accurate estimates of bacterial content are obtained from **suprapubic aspiration** (in children younger than 2 years of age) and properly performed bladder catheterization (as long as the first few milliliters are excluded from collection). The specimen should be taken directly to the laboratory for immediate culture.

Tests to detect bacteriuria are being used with increased frequency in screening for UTI. The dipstick tests for leukocyte esterase or nitrite are quick and inexpensive methods for detecting infection before obtaining final culture results.

Localization of the infection site may involve more specific tests, including percutaneous kidney taps and bladder washout procedures. Other tests such as ultrasonography, voiding

BOX 27-1

Clinical Manifestations of Urinary Tract Disorders or Disease

NEONATAL PERIOD (BIRTH TO 1 MONTH)
Poor feeding
Vomiting
Failure to gain weight
Rapid respiration (acidosis)
Respiratory distress
Spontaneous pneumothorax or pneumomediastinum
Frequent urination
Screaming on urination
Poor urine stream
Jaundice
Seizures
Dehydration
Other anomalies or stigmata
Enlarged kidneys or bladder

INFANCY (1 TO 24 MONTHS)
Poor feeding
Vomiting
Failure to gain weight
Excessive thirst
Frequent urination
Straining or screaming on urination

Foul-smelling urine
Pallor
Fever
Persistent diaper rash
Seizures (with or without fever)
Dehydration
Enlarged kidneys or bladder

CHILDHOOD (2 TO 14 YEARS)
Poor appetite
Vomiting
Growth failure
Excessive thirst
Enuresis, incontinence, frequent urination
Painful urination
Swelling of face
Seizures
Pallor
Fatigue
Blood in urine
Abdominal or back pain
Edema
Hypertension
Tetany

cystourethrogram (VCUG), intravenous pyelogram (IVP), and DMSA (dimercaptosuccinic acid) scan may be performed after the infection subsides to identify anatomic abnormalities contributing to the development of infection and existing kidney changes from recurrent infection.

Therapeutic Management

The objectives of treatment of children with UTI are (1) to eliminate current infection, (2) to identify contributing factors to reduce the risk of recurrence, (3) to prevent systemic spread of the infection, and (4) to preserve renal function. Antibiotic therapy should be initiated on the basis of identification of the pathogen, the child's history of antibiotic use, and the location of the infection. Several antimicrobial drugs are available for treating UTI, but all of them can occasionally be ineffective because of resistance of organisms. Common antiinfective agents used for UTI include the penicillins, sulfonamide (including trimethoprim and sulfisoxazole in combination), the cephalosporins, and nitrofurantoin.

If anatomic defects such as primary reflux or bladder neck obstruction are present, surgical correction of these abnormalities may be necessary to prevent recurrent infection. Follow-up study is an important component of medical management, since the relapse rate is high and infection tends to recur 1 to 2 months after termination of treatment. The aim of therapy and careful follow-up is to reduce the chance of renal scarring. However, recurrent infection of the urinary bladder predisposes the individual to transient episodes of vesicoureteral reflux (VUR).

Vesicoureteral Reflux. VUR refers to the abnormal retrograde flow of bladder urine into the ureters. During voiding, urine is swept up the ureters and then flows back into the empty bladder, where it acts as a reservoir for bacterial growth until the next void. **Primary reflux** results from congenitally abnormal insertion of ureters into the bladder; **secondary reflux** occurs as a result of an acquired condition.

It is not clear that reflux necessarily causes infections. What is clear is that reflux is more likely to be associated with recurring kidney infections rather than simple bladder infections (cystitis). In the presence of reflux, infected urine (bacteria) from the bladder has access to the kidney, resulting in kidney infections (pyelonephritis). These children are usually very symptomatic with high fevers, vomiting, and chills. Reflux, when associated with UTI, is the most common cause of renal scarring in children. Renal scarring may occur with the first episode of febrile UTI. Reflux in the presence of sterile urine does not cause renal damage. Therefore the most important concept in managing VUR is preventing bacteria from reaching the kidneys. VUR is managed conservatively with daily low-dose antibiotic therapy. A urine culture should be done every 2 to 3 months and any time the child has a fever. This method of management requires a motivated, reliable, and cooperative family. Many children will outgrow the reflux over a period of years. An annual VCUG is done to assess the status of the reflux.

For children with mild to moderate reflux, a minimally invasive endoscopic option (subtrigonal injection, or STING) is an alternative to daily antibiotics or open surgical intervention. A bulking agent—dextranomer-hyaluronic acid polymer (Deflux)—is injected into the mucous membrane of the ureter, making retrograde flow of urine more difficult. Overall cure rates relate to degree of reflux and range from 72% to 84% (Kirsch, Perez-Brayfield, and Scherz, 2003; Lavelle, Conlin, and Skoog, 2005).

Indications for open surgical intervention include significant anatomic abnormality at the ureterovesical junction, recurrent UTIs, severe forms of VUR, noncompliance with medical therapy, intolerance to antibiotics, and VUR after puberty in females.

Prognosis. With prompt and adequate treatment at the time of diagnosis, the long-term prognosis for UTI is usually excellent. However, the hazard of progressive renal injury is greatest when infection occurs in young children (especially those younger than 2 years of age) and is associated with congenital renal malformations and reflux. Therefore early diagnosis of children at risk is particularly important.

Nursing Care Management

Nurses should instruct parents to observe regularly for clues suggesting UTI. Unfortunately, the signs of UTI are not as evident as those of upper respiratory tract infection. Therefore many cases go undetected because no one thought to investigate this very common problem.

Because infants and young children often are unable to express their feelings and sensations verbally, it is difficult to detect discomfort they may be experiencing from dysuria. A careful history regarding voiding habits, stooling pattern, and episodes of unexplained irritability may assist in detecting less obvious cases of UTI. Consequently, parents should be cautioned to observe for specific clues of UTI in suspected cases.

When infection is suspected, collecting an appropriate specimen is essential. It is the nurse's responsibility to take every precaution to obtain acceptable clean-voided specimens to avoid the use of other, more invasive collecting procedures except when absolutely indicated. Because of the unreliability of a specimen obtained via a urine collection bag, suprapubic aspiration of urine or sterile catheterization should be done in the infant or young child who is seen with fever.

Frequently, additional tests are performed to detect anatomic defects. Children are prepared for these tests as appropriate for their age. This includes an explanation of the procedure, its purpose, and what the children will experience (see Preparation for Diagnostic and Therapeutic Procedures, Chapter 22). Sometimes a simple description of the urinary system is helpful. Especially for preschool children, the nurse must clarify that the urinary tract is separate from any sexual function and that the test is for a problem that they did not cause. Children may associate blame for perceived wrongdoing (e.g., masturbation) or unacceptable thoughts with the reason for the illness or the tests. For children younger than 3 to 4 years of age, the procedure can be explained on a doll. For those who are older, a simple drawing of the bladder, urethra, ureters, and kidneys makes the procedure more understandable.

Handling actual equipment when feasible can be helpful in allaying anxiety in children of all ages. Anticipatory instruction on distraction techniques such as deep breathing, storytelling, and imagery may help the child relax and be more cooperative during the actual procedures. If surgery is indicated, facts and understanding of the procedure will help decrease the child's fear and anxiety concerning more extensive medical-surgical intervention.

Because antibacterial drugs are indicated in UTI, the nurse advises parents of proper dosage and administration. When antiseptics such as nitrofurantoin are used for prolonged therapy to maintain urine sterility, parents need an explanation of the drug's continued necessity when no signs of infection are present. For all children an adequate or increased fluid intake is encouraged.

Prevention. Prevention is the most important goal in both primary and recurrent infection, and most preventive measures are simple hygienic habits that should be a routine part of daily care (see Nursing Care Guidelines box). For example, parents are taught to cleanse their infant's genital areas from front to back to avoid contaminating the urethral area with fecal organisms. Girls are taught to wipe from front to back after voiding or defecating. Children should void as soon as they feel the urge (see Critical Thinking Exercise).

Sexually active adolescent females are advised to urinate as soon as possible after they have intercourse to flush out bacteria introduced during the activity. Children who have recurrent UTIs or neurogenic bladder are frequently maintained on daily low-dose antibiotics. Giving the dose at bedtime allows the drug to remain in the bladder overnight. The nurse should

reinforce the importance of compliance to parents and older children.

OBSTRUCTIVE UROPATHY
Structural or functional abnormalities of the urinary system that obstruct the normal flow of urine can produce renal disorders. When there is interference with urine flow, the backup of urine above the obstruction causes **hydronephrosis** (dilation of the renal pelvis from distention) with eventual pressure destruction of renal parenchyma, although the dilating ureters form a reservoir that reduces the effect on the kidneys for a long time.

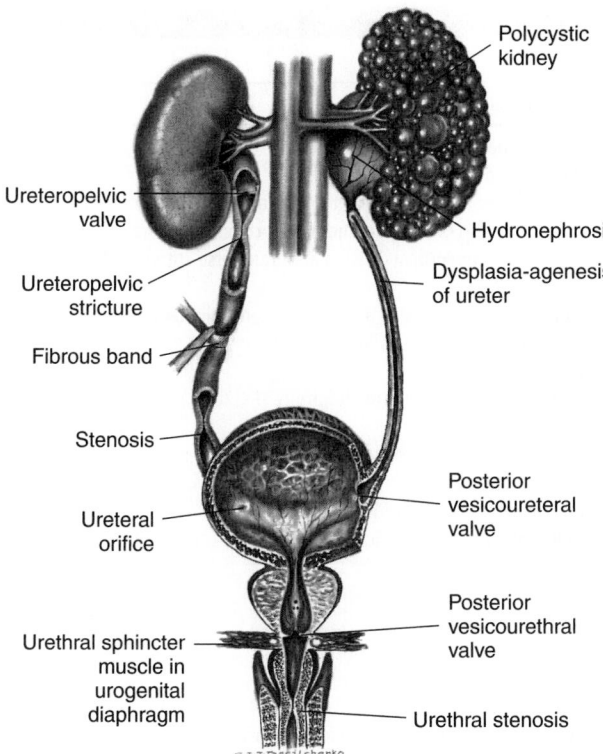

Polycystic kidney

Ureteropelvic valve

Hydronephrosis

Ureteropelvic stricture

Dysplasia-agenesis of ureter

Fibrous band

Stenosis

Ureteral orifice

Posterior vesicoureteral valve

Posterior vesicourethral valve

Urethral sphincter muscle in urogenital diaphragm

Urethral stenosis

FIG. 27-1 ■ Major sites of urinary tract obstruction.

Obstruction may be congenital or acquired, unilateral or bilateral, complete or incomplete, with acute or chronic manifestations. The obstruction can occur at any level of the upper or lower urinary tract (Fig. 27-1). Partial obstruction may not be symptomatic unless there is a water or solute diuresis. Boys are affected more frequently than girls, and malformations should be suspected when patients have some other congenital defects (e.g., prune belly syndrome, chromosomal anomalies, anorectal malformations, defects of the pinna of the ear).

Damage to distal nephrons in chronic uropathy alters the ability to concentrate urine, contributing to increased urine flow and metabolic acidosis occurring from decreased excretion of acid secondary to impaired ability of the distal nephron to secrete hydrogen ions. Partial obstruction results in progressive loss of renal function as a result of irreversible damage to the nephrons. Pooled urine serves as a medium for bacterial growth; therefore UTIs further increase the extent of renal damage.

Early diagnosis and surgical correction or procedures that divert the flow of urine to bypass the obstruction, such as placement of a temporary percutaneous nephrostomy tube or cutaneous ureterostomy, are essential to prevent progressive renal damage. Medical complications of acute or chronic renal failure or infection are managed as described for those disorders.

Nursing Care Management

Nursing goals in urinary tract obstruction include helping to identify cases, assisting with diagnostic procedures, and caring for children with complications (described elsewhere). Preparing parents and children for procedures is a major nursing responsibility. Preparation for urinary diversion procedures is

of special importance (see Preparation for Diagnostic and Therapeutic Procedures, Chapter 22).

Parents and children need emotional support and counseling during the lengthy management of these disorders. Many children are discharged with ureteral drainage systems in place that must be protected from damage, and the danger of infection is a constant concern. Parents are taught to care for the equipment and recognize the signs of possible obstruction or infection within the system. Maintaining adequate urine flow is imperative. Fluids should be encouraged. The tube should be observed frequently for indications of obstruction resulting from sediment, small blood clots, or kinking. The physician should inspect any drainage from around the tube.

Children with external diversional systems need psychologic support and guidance, especially as they reach adolescence and body image concerns assume more prominence. Those with progressive renal deterioration may face the prospect of dialysis or transplantation and the emotions that accompany these procedures.

EXTERNAL DEFECTS

Defects of the external genitourinary tract are serious conditions primarily because of the psychologic impact on the child. Satisfactory surgical repair is successful for the more common disorders and is carried out or initiated as early as possible. The major anomalies of the lower genitourinary tract, their description, and their management are outlined in Table 27-4.

Psychologic Problems Related to Genital Surgery

Surgery involving sexual organs can be particularly disruptive to children, especially preschoolers fearing punishment, retaliation, body mutilation, or castration. Some of the problems of hospitalization, separation, and anxiety can be eased by hospital practices that are sensitive to the child's needs (see Chapter 21).

A child's body image is largely derived as a result of feedback from the primary caregivers, and parental anxiety regarding an acceptable physical appearance and adequate future sexual competency is readily communicated to an affected child. Therefore children with birth defects are at risk for developing a distorted body image that reflects the caregiver's subtly communicated evaluation of their bodies. The trend toward repair of visible genital defects is based in large part on these psychologic variables. The earlier a repair can be achieved, the more likely it is that the child will develop a normal body image.

During the years from 3 to 6, the phallic-oedipal period, children show a strong interest and concern about the genital area, sex differences, and genital normality or its lack. It is also a time when children are frightened of what they perceive to be threats to their body and bodily function. They also view any untoward happening as a punishment for real or imagined wrongdoing or unacceptable sexual feelings, such as masturbation, sex play, or erotic feelings. Surgical repair is recommended before these fears and anxieties develop.

After extensive review of the emotional, cognitive, and body-image problems that may occur in children undergoing surgical reconstruction of a genital deformity, Kass (1996) recommended that surgery be accomplished between the ages

TABLE 27-4

Defects of the Genitourinary Tract

DEFECT	THERAPEUTIC MANAGEMENT
Inguinal hernia—Protrusion of abdominal contents through inguinal canal into scrotum	Detected as painless inguinal swelling of variable size Surgical closure of inguinal defect
Hydrocele—Fluid in scrotum	Surgical repair indicated if spontaneous resolution not accomplished in 1 year
Phimosis—Narrowing or stenosis of preputial opening of foreskin	**Mild cases**—manual retraction of foreskin and proper cleansing of area **Severe cases**—circumcision or vertical division and transverse suturing of foreskin
Hypospadias—Urethral opening located behind glans penis or anywhere along ventral surface of penile shaft	Objectives of surgical correction: Enable child to void in standing position and direct stream voluntarily in usual manner Improve physical appearance of genitalia Produce a sexually adequate organ
Chordee—Ventral curvature of penis, often associated with hypospadias	Surgical release of fibrous band causing the deformity
Epispadias—Meatal opening located on dorsal surface of penis	Surgical correction, usually including penile and urethral lengthening and bladder neck reconstruction (if necessary)
Cryptorchidism—Failure of one or both testes to descend normally through inguinal canal	Detected by inability to palpate testes within scrotum **Medical**—Administration of human chorionic gonadotropin (older child) **Surgical**—Orchiopexy Objectives of therapy: Prevent damage to undescended testicle Decrease incidence of malignant tumor formation Avoid trauma and torsion Close inguinal canal Prevent cosmetic and psychologic disability from empty scrotum
Exstrophy of bladder—Eversion of posterior bladder through anterior bladder wall and lower abdominal wall; associated with open pubic arch (a severe defect)	Potential objectives of surgical correction: Preserve renal function Attain urinary control Provide adequate reconstructive repair Improve sexual function (especially in males)
Ambiguous genitalia Masculinized female (female pseudohermaphrodite)	Assign gender as female; assign gender while avoiding irreversible surgery, realizing some children may change gender later in life; family participation essential
Incompletely masculinized male (male pseudohermaphrodite)	Assign gender while avoiding irreversible surgery, realizing some children may change gender later in life; family participation essential
True hermaphrodite (both ovaries and testes)	Assign gender while avoiding irreversible surgery, realizing some children may change gender later in life; gender assignment depends on predominant characteristics; family participation essential
Mixed gonadal dysgenesis	Assign gender while avoiding irreversible surgery, realizing some children may change gender later in life; gender assignment depends on predominant characteristics; family participation essential

of 6 and 15 months to minimize the psychologic effects of surgery and anesthesia.

Nursing Care Management

Preparing children and their families for diagnostic and surgical procedures (see Preparation for Diagnostic and Therapeutic Procedures, Chapter 22) and for home care is a major nursing function. Most postoperative care involves care of the surgical site. Tub baths are discouraged for 1 week after simple surgeries. The surgical site is kept clean and otherwise protected from infection and is inspected for signs of infection. Dressings, if any, are inspected regularly. More complex surgeries require additional care and observation (e.g., catheter care for urethral reconstruction and care of urinary diversion stomas and collection devices).

Some older children's activities, such as pushing, lifting, playing with straddle toys or in sandboxes, swimming, and rough activities, may be restricted after some types of surgical repairs. Precise restrictions depend on the specific type of surgery. Activities of infants and toddlers are not limited.

In most cases the results of surgery are satisfactory. However, in some of the more severe defects, such as exstrophy and those that require stomas, additional emotional interventions may be needed. A major concern of parents and children is related to surgery affecting the genitalia directly. Concerns about penis size, appearance of the genitalia, potential ability to procreate, and rejection by peers (especially the opposite sex) are potential fears that require psychologic adjustment, particularly during adolescence.

GLOMERULAR DISEASE

NEPHROTIC SYNDROME

Nephrotic syndrome is a clinical state that includes massive proteinuria, hypoalbuminemia, hyperlipidemia, and edema. The disorder can occur as (1) a primary disease known as **idiopathic nephrosis, childhood nephrosis,** or **minimal-**

FIG. 27-2 ■ Sequence of events in nephrotic syndrome. *ADH,* Antidiuretic hormone.

change nephrotic syndrome (MCNS); (2) a secondary disorder that occurs as a clinical manifestation after or in association with glomerular damage that has a known or presumed cause; or (3) a congenital form inherited as an autosomal recessive disorder. The disorder is characterized by increased glomerular permeability to plasma protein, which results in massive urinary protein loss. The glomerulus is responsible for the initial step in the formation of urine, and the filtration rate depends on an intact glomerular membrane. This discussion is devoted to MCNS because it constitutes 80% of nephrotic syndrome cases.

Pathophysiology

The onset of MCNS can occur at any age but predominantly occurs in children between 2 and 7 years of age. It is rare in children younger than 6 months of age, uncommon in infants younger than 1 year of age, and unusual after the age of 8. Patients with MCNS are twice as likely to be male.

The pathogenesis of MCNS is not understood. There may be a metabolic, biochemical, physiochemical, or immune-mediated disturbance that causes the basement membrane of the glomeruli to become increasingly permeable to protein, but the cause and mechanisms are only speculative.

The glomerular membrane, normally impermeable to albumin and other proteins, becomes permeable to proteins, especially albumin, which leak through the membrane and are lost in urine (**hyperalbuminuria**). This reduces the serum

albumin level (**hypoalbuminemia**), decreasing the colloidal osmotic pressure in the capillaries. As a result, the vascular hydrostatic pressure exceeds the pull of the colloidal osmotic pressure, causing fluid to accumulate in the interstitial spaces (**edema**) and body cavities, particularly in the abdominal cavity (**ascites**). The shift of fluid from the plasma to the interstitial spaces reduces the vascular fluid volume (**hypovolemia**), which in turn stimulates the renin-angiotensin system and the secretion of antidiuretic hormone and aldosterone. Tubular reabsorption of sodium and water is increased in an attempt to increase intravascular volume. The elevation of serum lipids is not fully understood. The sequence of events in nephrotic syndrome is diagrammed in Fig. 27-2.

Diagnostic Evaluation

The disease is suspected on the basis of clinical manifestations (Box 27-2), especially when weight gain in a previously well child increases slowly over days or weeks. The generalized edema may develop rapidly or gradually but eventually prompts the family to seek medical attention. Parents usually give a history of the child being well but steadily gaining weight, appearing edematous, and then becoming anorexic, irritable, and less active.

The diagnosis of MCNS is suspected on the basis of the history and clinical manifestations (edema, proteinuria, hypoalbuminemia, and hypercholesterolemia in the absence of hematuria and hypertension) in children between the ages

---

BOX 27-2

Clinical Manifestations of Nephrotic Syndrome

Weight gain
Puffiness of face (facial edema):
- Especially around the eyes
- Apparent on arising in the morning
- Subsides during the day

Abdominal swelling (ascites)
Pleural effusion
Labial or scrotal swelling
Edema of intestinal mucosal, possibly causing:
- Diarrhea
- Anorexia
- Poor intestinal absorption

Ankle or leg swelling
Irritability
Easily fatigued
Lethargic
Blood pressure normal or slightly decreased
Susceptibility to infection
Urine alterations:
- Decreased volume
- Frothy

---

of 2 and 8 years. The hallmark of MCNS is massive proteinuria (higher than 3+ on urine dipstick). Hyaline casts, oval fat bodies, and a few red blood cells can be found in the urine of some affected children, although there is seldom gross hematuria. The glomerular filtration rate is usually normal or high.

Total serum protein concentration is low, with the serum albumin significantly reduced and plasma lipids elevated. Hemoglobin and hematocrit are usually normal or elevated as a result of hemoconcentration. The platelet count may be elevated. Serum sodium concentration may be low. If the patient does not respond to a 4- to 8-week course of steroids, a renal biopsy may be needed to distinguish between other types of nephrotic syndrome. The biopsy results of children with MCNS are remarkable for effacement of the foot processes of the epithelial cells lining the basement membrane, but otherwise the kidney tissue is normal.

Therapeutic Management

Objectives of therapeutic management include (1) reducing excretion of urinary protein, (2) reducing fluid retention in the tissues, (3) preventing infection, and (4) minimizing complications related to therapies. Dietary restrictions include a low-salt diet and, in more severe cases, fluid restriction. If complications of edema develop, diuretic therapy may be initiated to provide temporary relief from edema. Sometimes infusions of 25% albumin are used. Acute infections are treated with appropriate antibiotics.

Corticosteroids are the first line of therapy for MCNS. The starting dosage for prednisone is usually 2 mg/kg body weight/day, in one or more divided doses. In most children this response occurs within 7 to 21 days. The medication is then tapered over a period of several months and eventually stopped if the child remains asymptomatic. About two thirds of children with MCNS have a relapse, heralded first by increased urine protein. Relapses can be diagnosed early if parents are taught routine home monitoring of urine protein by dipstick. Relapses are treated with a repeated course of high-dose steroid therapy. Side effects of the steroids include weight gain, rounding of the face, behavior changes, and increased appetite. Long-term therapy may result in hirsutism, growth retardation, cataracts, hypertension, gastrointestinal bleeding,

bone demineralization, infection, and hyperglycemia. Children who do not respond to steroid therapy, those who have frequent relapses, and those in whom the side effects threaten their growth and general health may be considered for a course of therapy using other immunosuppressant medications (cyclophosphamide, chlorambucil, or cyclosporine).

MCNS episodes, both the first episode and relapse, often happen in conjunction with a viral or bacterial infection. Relapses can also be triggered by allergies and immunizations. Relapses in children with MCNS may continue over many years.

Complications of nephrotic syndrome include infection, circulatory insufficiency secondary to hypovolemia, and thromboembolism. Infections that may be seen in children with nephrotic syndrome include peritonitis, cellulitis, and pneumonia and require prompt recognition and vigorous treatment with appropriate antibiotic therapy.

Prognosis. The prognosis for ultimate recovery in most cases is good. It is a self-limiting disease, and in children who respond to steroid therapy the tendency to relapse decreases with time. With early detection and prompt implementation of therapy to eradicate proteinuria, progressive basement membrane damage is minimized, so that when the tendency to relapse is past, renal function is usually normal or near normal. It is estimated that approximately 80% of affected children have this favorable prognosis.

Nursing Care Management

Continuous monitoring of fluid retention or excretion is an important nursing function. Strict intake and output records are essential but may be difficult to obtain from very young children. Application of collection bags is irritating to edematous skin that is readily subject to breakdown. Applying diapers or weighing wet pads may be necessary.

NURSINGTIP

Another strategy for obtaining a daily urine protein is to place cotton balls in the diaper at night before bedtime and then squeeze them out in the morning.

Other methods of monitoring progress include urine examination for albumin, daily weight, and measurement of abdominal girth. Assessment of edema (e.g., increased or decreased swelling around the eyes and dependent areas), the degree of pitting, and the color and texture of skin are part of nursing care. Vital signs are monitored to detect any early signs of complications such as shock or an infective process.

Infection is a constant source of danger to edematous children and those receiving corticosteroid therapy. These children are particularly vulnerable to upper respiratory tract infection; therefore they must be kept warm and dry, active, and protected from contact with infected individuals (e.g., roommates, visitors, and personnel). Vital signs are monitored to detect any early signs of an infective process.

Loss of appetite accompanying active nephrosis creates a perplexing problem for nurses. During this time the combined efforts of nurse, dietitian, parents, and child are needed to formulate a nutritionally adequate and attractive diet. Salt is usually restricted (but not eliminated) during the edema phase and while the child is on steroid therapy. Fluid restriction (if prescribed) is limited to short-term use during massive edema. Every effort should be made to serve attractive meals with preferred foods and a minimum of fuss, but it usually requires considerable ingenuity to entice the child to eat (see Feeding the Sick Child, Chapter 22).

Children usually adjust activities according to their tolerance level. However, they may require guidance in selecting play activities. Suitable recreational and diversional activities are an important part of their care. Irritability and mood swings that accompany steroid therapy are not unusual in these children and may create an additional challenge for the nurse and family.

Family Support and Home Care. Continuous support of the child and family is one of the major nursing considerations. Many children are treated at home during relapses. Parents are taught to detect signs of relapse and to call for changes in treatment at the earliest indications. Unless the edema and proteinuria are severe or the parents, for some reason, are unable to care for the ill child, *home care is preferred*. Parents are instructed in testing urine for albumin, administering medications, and providing general care. Parents are also instructed regarding avoiding contact with infected playmates, but the child should attend school.

The prolonged course of the relapsing form of nephrotic syndrome is taxing to both the child and the family. The up-and-down course of remissions and exacerbations with periodic disruption of family life by hospitalization places a severe strain on the child and the family, both psychologically and financially. Reassurance regarding this characteristic of the course of the disease, with emphasis on the importance of long-term care, needs to be provided to parents and children to gain their cooperation. A satisfactory response is more likely when relapses are detected and therapy is instituted early, and remissions are prolonged when instructions are carried out faithfully. Continuous support of the child and family is one of the major nursing considerations (see Chapter 18).

ACUTE GLOMERULONEPHRITIS

Acute glomerulonephritis (AGN) may be a primary event or a manifestation of a systemic disorder that can range from minimal to severe. Common features include oliguria, edema, hypertension and circulatory congestion, hematuria, and proteinuria. Most cases are postinfectious and have been associated with pneumococcal, streptococcal, and viral infections. **Acute poststreptococcal glomerulonephritis (APSGN)** is the most common of the postinfectious renal diseases in childhood and the one for which a cause can be established in the majority of cases. APSGN can occur at any age but affects primarily early school-age children, with a peak age of onset of 6 to 7 years. It is uncommon in children younger than 2 years of age, and males outnumber females 2:1.

Etiology

APSGN is an immune-complex disease that occurs after an antecedent streptococcal infection with certain strains of the group A β-hemolytic streptococcus. Most streptococcal infections *do not* cause APSGN. A latent period of 10 to 21 days occurs between the streptococcal infection and the onset of clinical manifestations. Disease secondary to streptococcal pharyngitis is more common in the winter or spring, but when APSGN is associated with pyoderma (principally **impetigo**), it may be more prevalent in later summer or early fall, especially in warmer climates. Second episodes of AGN are rare.

BOX 27-3

Clinical Manifestations of Acute Poststreptococcal Glomerulonephritis

Edema:
- Especially periorbital
- Facial edema more prominent in the morning
- Spreads during the day to involve extremities and abdomen

Anorexia

Urine:
- Cloudy, smoky brown (resembles tea or cola)
- Severely reduced volume

Pallor

Irritability

Lethargy

Child appearing ill

Child seldom expresses specific complaints

Older children complaining of:
- Headaches
- Abdominal discomfort
- Dysuria

Vomiting possible

Mild to moderately elevated blood pressure

Pathophysiology

The pathophysiology of APSGN is still uncertain. Immune complexes are deposited in the glomerular basement membrane. The glomeruli become edematous and infiltrated with polymorphonuclear leukocytes, which occlude the capillary lumen. The resulting decrease in plasma filtration results in an excessive accumulation of water and retention of sodium that expands plasma and interstitial fluid volumes, leading to circulatory congestion and edema. The cause of the hypertension associated with AGN cannot be completely explained by fluid retention. Excess renin may also be produced.

Diagnostic Evaluation

Typically, affected children are in good health until they experience the streptococcal infection. In some instances they have a history of only a mild cold or no previous infection at all. The onset of nephritis appears after an average latency period of about 10 days (Box 27-3). Because the child appears to be well during the latency period, parents do not recognize the association. The edema is relatively moderate and may not be appreciated by someone unfamiliar with the child's normal appearance.

Urinalysis during the acute phase characteristically shows hematuria and proteinuria. Proteinuria generally parallels the hematuria and may be 3+ or 4+ in the presence of gross hematuria. Gross discoloration of the urine reflects red blood cell and hemoglobin content. Microscopic examination of the sediment shows many red blood cells, leukocytes, epithelial cells, and granular and red blood cell casts. Bacteria are not seen.

Azotemia that results from impaired glomerular filtration is reflected in elevated blood urea nitrogen (BUN) and creatinine levels in at least 50% of cases. Occasionally proteinuria is excessive and the patient may have nephrotic syndrome (i.e., hypoproteinemia and hyperlipidemia).

Cultures of the pharynx are rarely positive for streptococci, since the renal disease occurs weeks after the infection.

Some serologic tests are necessary to make the diagnosis of AGN. Circulating serum antibodies to streptococci indicate the presence of a previous infection. The antistreptolysin O (ASO) titer is the most familiar and readily available test for streptococcal infection. Other antibodies that may aid in diagnosis are elevated antihyaluronidase (AHase), antideoxyribonuclease B (ADNase-B), and streptozyme.

All patients with APSGN have reduced serum complement (C3) activity in the early stages of the disease. Rising C3 levels are used as a guide to indicate improvement of the disease and should be normal in almost all patients 8 weeks after the disease onset.

Studies that may be useful include chest x-ray examination, which generally shows cardiac enlargement, pulmonary congestion, or pleural effusion during the edematous phase of acute disease. Renal biopsy for diagnostic purposes is seldom required but may be useful in the diagnosis of atypical cases.

Therapeutic Management

Management consists of general supportive measures and early recognition and treatment of complications. Children who have normal blood pressure and a satisfactory urinary output can generally be treated at home. Those with substantial edema, hypertension, gross hematuria, or significant oliguria should be hospitalized because of the unpredictability of complications.

Dietary restrictions depend on the stage and severity of the disease, especially the extent of edema. Moderate sodium restriction and even fluid restriction may be instituted for children with hypertension and edema. Foods with substantial amounts of potassium are generally restricted during the period of oliguria.

Regular measurement of vital signs, body weight, and intake and output is essential to monitor the progress of the disease and to detect complications that may appear at any time during the course of the disease. *A record of daily weight is the most useful means for assessing fluid balance.* Rarely, children with AGN will develop acute renal failure (ARF) with oliguria that significantly alters the fluid and electrolyte balance (resulting in hyperkalemia, acidosis, hypocalcemia, and/or hyperphosphatemia). These children require careful management. Peritoneal dialysis or hemodialysis is seldom needed.

Acute hypertension must be anticipated and identified early. Blood pressure measurements are taken every 4 to 6 hours. A variety of antihypertensive medications and diuretics are used to control hypertension. Antibiotic therapy is indicated only for those children with evidence of persistent streptococcal infections. It is used to prevent transmission of nephritogenic streptococci to other family members.

Prognosis. Almost all children correctly diagnosed as having APSGN recover completely, and specific immunity is conferred, so that subsequent recurrences are uncommon. Some of these children have been reported to develop chronic disease, but most of these cases are now believed to be different glomerular diseases misdiagnosed as poststreptococcal disease.

Nursing Care Management

Nursing care of the child with glomerulonephritis involves careful assessment of the disease status, with regular monitoring of vital signs (including frequent measurement of blood pressure), fluid balance, and behavior.

Vital signs provide clues to the severity of the disease and early signs of complications. They are carefully measured, and any deviations are reported and recorded. The volume and character of urine are noted, and the child is weighed daily. Children with restricted fluid intake, especially those who are not severely edematous or those who have lost weight, are observed for signs of dehydration.

Assessment of the child's appearance for signs of cerebral complications is an important nursing function, since the severity of the acute phase is variable and unpredictable. The child with edema, hypertension, and gross hematuria may be subject to complications, and anticipatory preparations such as seizure precautions and intravenous (IV) equipment are included in the nursing care plan.

For most children a regular diet is allowed, but it should contain no added salt. Foods high in sodium and salted treats are eliminated, and parents and friends are advised not to bring snacks such as potato chips or pretzels. However, the total amount of salt ingested is usually less than prescribed because of the child's poor appetite. Fluid restriction, if prescribed, is more difficult, and the amount permitted should be evenly divided throughout the waking hours. Meal preparation and service require special attention, since the child is indifferent to meals during the acute phase. Again, collaboration with parents and the dietitian and special consideration for food preferences facilitate meal planning.

During the acute phase children are generally content to lie in bed. As they begin to feel better and their symptoms subside, they will want to be up and about. Activities should be planned to allow for frequent rest periods and avoidance of fatigue. Children who have mild edema and no hypertension, as well as convalescent children who are being treated at home, need follow-up care. Parents are instructed regarding general measures, including diet and prevention of infection.

Health supervision is continued, with weekly, followed by monthly, visits for evaluation and urinalysis. Parent education and support in preparation for discharge and home care include education in home management and the need for follow-up care and health supervision.

MISCELLANEOUS RENAL DISORDERS
HEMOLYTIC UREMIC SYNDROME

Hemolytic uremic syndrome (HUS) is an uncommon, acute renal disease that occurs primarily in infants and small children between the ages of 6 months and 5 years. HUS is one of the most frequent causes of acquired ARF in children (Davis and Avner, 2004). The clinical features of the disease include acquired hemolytic anemia, thrombocytopenia, renal injury, and central nervous system symptoms. The etiology of HUS is thought to be associated with bacterial toxins, chemicals, and viruses. The appearance of the disease has been associated with *Rickettsia* organisms, viruses (especially coxsackievirus, echovirus, and adenovirus), *Escherichia coli,* pneumococci, shigellae, and salmonellae and may represent an unusual response to these infections. Multiple cases of HUS caused by enteric infection of the *E. coli* O157:H7 serotype have been traced to undercooked meat, especially ground beef. Other sources are unpasteurized milk or fruit juice, especially apple; alfalfa sprouts; lettuce; and salami; drinking or swimming in sewage-contaminated water can also cause infection. The clinical presentation is usually a history of a prodromal illness (most often gastroenteritis or an upper respiratory tract infec-

BOX 27-4
Clinical Manifestations of Hemolytic Uremic Syndrome

Vomiting	Oliguria or anuria
Irritability	Central nervous system
Lethargy	involvement:
Marked pallor	■ Seizures
Hemorrhagic manifestations:	■ Stupor or coma
■ Bruising	Signs of acute heart failure
■ Petechiae	(sometimes)
■ Jaundice	
■ Bloody diarrhea	

BOX 27-5
Clinical Manifestations of Wilms Tumor

Abdominal swelling or mass:	Manifestations resulting from
■ Firm	compression of tumor mass
■ Nontender	Secondary metabolic alterations
■ Confined to one side	from tumor or metastasis
Hematuria (less than one fourth	If metastasis, symptoms of lung
of cases)	involvement:
Fatigue and malaise	■ Dyspnea
Hypertension (occasionally)	■ Cough
Weight loss	■ Shortness of breath
Fever	■ Chest pain (sometimes)

tion) followed by the sudden onset of hemolysis and renal failure.

Pathophysiology

The primary site of injury appears to be the endothelial lining of the small glomerular arterioles, which become swollen and occluded with deposits of platelets and fibrin clots (intravascular coagulation). Red blood cells are damaged as they attempt to move through the partially occluded blood vessels. These damaged cells are removed by the spleen, causing acute hemolytic anemia. The platelet aggregation within the damaged blood vessels or the damage and removal of platelets produce the characteristic thrombocytopenia.

Diagnostic Evaluation

The triad of anemia, thrombocytopenia, and renal failure is sufficient for diagnosis (Box 27-4). Renal involvement is evidenced by proteinuria, hematuria, and urinary casts; BUN and serum creatinine levels are elevated. A low hemoglobin and hematocrit and a high reticulocyte count confirm the hemolytic nature of the anemia.

Therapeutic Management

The goals of therapy are early diagnosis and aggressive, supportive care of the ARF and hemolytic anemia. The most consistently effective treatment of HUS is hemodialysis or peritoneal dialysis, which is instituted in any child who has been anuric for 24 hours or who demonstrates oliguria with uremia or hypertension and seizures. Other treatments include use of pharmacologic agents, fresh-frozen plasma, and plasmapheresis. Blood transfusions with fresh, washed packed cells are administered for severe anemia but are used with caution to prevent circulatory overload from added volume.

Prognosis. With prompt treatment the recovery rate is about 95%, but residual renal impairment ranges from 10% to 50%. Long-term complications include chronic renal failure, hypertension, and central nervous system disorders. Death is usually caused by residual renal impairment or central nervous system injury.

Nursing Care Management

Nursing care is the same as that provided in ARF and, for children with continued impairment, includes management of chronic disease. Because of the sudden and life-threatening nature of the disorder in a previously well child, parents are often ill prepared for the impact of hospitalization and treat-

ment. Therefore support and understanding are especially important aspects of care.

WILMS TUMOR

Wilms tumor, or nephroblastoma, is the most common malignant renal and intraabdominal tumor of childhood. Its frequency is estimated to be 7.6 cases per million in Caucasian children less than 15 years of age (Dome, Perlman, Ritchey, and others, 2006). Wilms tumor occurs about three times more often in African-Americans than in East Asians in the United States. The peak age at diagnosis is approximately 3 years, and occurrence is slightly more frequent in boys than in girls. The majority of patients with Wilms tumor are diagnosed at younger than 5 years of age, with 1% to 2.5% having a familial origin. Unfortunately, there is no method of identifying gene carriers at this time.

Etiology

Wilms tumor probably arises from a malignant, undifferentiated cluster of primordial cells capable of initiating the regeneration of an abnormal structure. Its occurrence slightly favors the left kidney, which is advantageous because surgically this kidney is easier to manipulate and remove. In about 10% of cases both kidneys are involved. Studies have shown that development of Wilms tumor is frequently associated with aniridia, hemihypertrophy, Beckwith-Wiedemann syndrome, or genitourinary anomalies (Kline and Sevier, 2003; Dome, Perlman, Ritchey, and others, 2006).

Diagnostic Evaluation

In a child suspected of having Wilms tumor, special emphasis is placed on the history and physical examination for the presence of congenital anomalies, a family history of cancer, and signs of malignancy (e.g., weight loss, size of liver and spleen, indications of anemia, lymphadenopathy). Most children with Wilms tumor are brought to the practitioner because of abdominal swelling or an abdominal mass (Box 27-5). Specific tests include radiographic studies, including abdominal ultrasound and abdominal and chest computed tomography scan; hematologic studies; biochemical studies; and urinalysis. Studies to demonstrate the relationship of the tumor to the ipsilateral kidney and the presence of a normal functioning kidney on the contralateral side are essential. If a large tumor is present, an inferior venacavogram is necessary to demonstrate possible tumor involvement adjacent to the vena cava. A bone marrow aspiration may be performed to rule out metastasis, which is rare in children with Wilms tumor.

BOX 27-6

Staging of Wilms Tumor

Stage I—Tumor is limited to kidney and completely resected.
Stage II—Tumor extends beyond kidney but is completely resected.
Stage III—Residual nonhematogenous tumor is confined to abdomen.
Stage IV—Hematogenous metastases; deposits are beyond stage III, namely, to lung, liver, bone, and brain.
Stage V—Bilateral renal involvement is present at diagnosis.

NURSINGALERT

To reinforce the need for caution, it may be necessary to post a sign on the bed that reads "DO NOT PALPATE ABDOMEN." Careful bathing and handling are also important in preventing trauma to the tumor site.

Therapeutic Management

Combined treatment with surgery and chemotherapy with or without radiation is based on the histologic pattern and clinical stage (Box 27-6).

Surgery is scheduled as soon as possible after confirmation of a renal mass, usually within 24 to 48 hours of admission. A large transabdominal incision is performed for optimal visualization of the abdominal cavity. The tumor, affected kidney, and adjacent adrenal gland are removed. Great care is taken to keep the encapsulated tumor intact, since rupture can seed cancer cells throughout the abdomen, lymph channel, and bloodstream. The contralateral kidney is carefully inspected for evidence of disease or dysfunction. Regional lymph nodes are inspected, and a biopsy is performed when indicated. Any involved structures, such as part of the colon, diaphragm, or vena cava, are removed. Metal clips are placed around the tumor site for exact marking during radiotherapy.

If both kidneys are involved, the child may be treated with radiotherapy or chemotherapy before surgery to decrease the size of the tumor, allowing more conservative surgery. It may be possible to perform a partial nephrectomy on the less affected kidney, with a total nephrectomy on the opposite side. When a transplant is feasible, such as from a twin, sibling, or parent, bilateral nephrectomy is considered as a last resort.

Postoperative radiotherapy is indicated for children with large tumors, metastasis, residual postoperative disease, unfavorable histologic characteristics, or recurrence. Chemotherapy is indicated for all stages. The most effective agents for treating Wilms tumor are actinomycin D (dactinomycin), vincristine, and adriamycin, with the addition of cyclophosphamide for unfavorable histology or advanced disease (Dome, Perlman, Ritchey, and others, 2006). The duration of therapy ranges from 6 to 15 months.

Prognosis. Survival rates for Wilms tumor are the highest among all childhood cancers. Children with localized tumor (stages I and II) have a 90% chance of cure with multimodal therapy. Factors that favorably affect the success of further therapy include initial treatment with only vincristine and dactinomycin, relapse to the lungs only, relapse in the abdomen of a patient who received no prior abdominal irradiation, and relapse more than 12 months after diagnosis. Wilms tumor may recur, especially in the lungs. Both chemotherapy and radiotherapy can induce second malignancies, usually in areas that have been irradiated (Dome, Perlman, Ritchey, and others, 2006).

Nursing Care Management

Nursing care of the child with Wilms tumor is similar to that of children with other cancers treated with surgery, irradiation, and chemotherapy. However, there are some significant differences; these are discussed for each phase of nursing intervention.

Preoperative Care. The preoperative period is one of swift diagnosis. The nurse faces the challenge of preparing the child and parents for all laboratory and operative procedures within 24 to 48 hours of admission. Because of the minimal preparatory time, explanations should be simple, repetitive, and focused on the child's actual experiences. In addition to the usual preoperative observations, blood pressure is monitored, since hypertension from excess renin production is a possibility.

There are several special preoperative concerns, the most important of which is that the *tumor is not palpated unless absolutely necessary* because manipulation of the mass may cause dissemination of cancer cells to adjacent and distant sites.

Because radiotherapy and chemotherapy are usually begun immediately after surgery, parents need an explanation of what to expect, such as major benefits and side effects. The timing of the information should be considered to avoid overwhelming the family. Ideally, the nurse should be present during physician-parent conferences to answer questions as they arise. It is usually better to postpone telling the child about these side effects until after surgery. Alopecia, usually of most concern to older children, does not occur until approximately 2 weeks after the initial treatment regimen. Therefore the child can be prepared for the hair loss postoperatively.

Postoperative Care. Despite the extensive surgical intervention necessary in many children with Wilms tumor, the recovery is usually rapid. The major nursing responsibilities are the same as those after any abdominal surgery (see Surgical Procedures, Chapter 22). Because these children are at risk for intestinal obstruction from vincristine-induced ileus, radiation-induced edema, and postsurgical adhesion formation, the nurse carefully monitors gastrointestinal activity, such as bowel movements, bowel sounds, distention, vomiting, and pain. The nurse also monitors blood pressure, urinary output, and signs of infection, as well as instituting pulmonary hygiene to prevent postoperative pulmonary complications.

Family Support. The postoperative period is frequently difficult for parents. The shock of seeing their child immediately after surgery may be the first realization of the seriousness of the diagnosis. It also marks the confirmation of the stage of the tumor. During this period, the nurse should be with the parents to assure them of the child's recovery after surgery and to assess the parent's understanding of the total experience. They need an opportunity to express their feelings and need to be provided the same emotional care discussed in Chapter 18 for families who have a child with a life-threatening disorder.

Older children need an opportunity to deal with their feelings concerning the many procedures to which they have been subjected in rapid succession. Play therapy with dolls or puppets or through drawing can be extremely beneficial in helping them adjust. It is not unusual for children to feel angry because of the extent of surgery, the need for additional therapy, or the seriousness of the disorder.

RENAL FAILURE

Renal failure is the inability of the kidneys to excrete waste material, concentrate urine, and conserve electrolytes. It can occur suddenly (**acute renal failure [ARF]**) in response to inadequate perfusion, kidney disease, or urinary tract obstruction, or it can develop slowly (**chronic renal failure [CRF]**) as a result of longstanding kidney disease or an anomaly.

Azotemia and *uremia* are terms often used in relation to renal failure. **Azotemia** is the accumulation of nitrogenous waste within the blood. **Uremia** is a more advanced condition in which retention of nitrogenous products produces toxic symptoms. Azotemia is not life threatening, whereas uremia is a serious condition that often involves other body systems.

ACUTE RENAL FAILURE

ARF is said to exist when the kidneys suddenly are unable to regulate the volume and composition of urine appropriately in response to food and fluid intake and the needs of the organism. The principal feature of ARF is oliguria* associated with azotemia, metabolic acidosis, and diverse electrolyte disturbances. ARF is not common in childhood, but the outcome depends on the cause, associated findings, and prompt recognition and treatment.

The pathologic conditions that produce ARF caused by glomerulonephritis and HUS are discussed in relation to those disorders. ARF can also develop as a result of a large number of related or unrelated clinical conditions: poor renal perfusion; urinary tract obstruction; acute renal injury; or the final expression of chronic, irreversible renal disease. The most common cause in children is transient renal failure resulting from severe dehydration or other causes of poor perfusion that may respond to restoration of fluid volume.

Pathophysiology

ARF is usually reversible, but the deviations of physiologic function can be extreme, and mortality in the pediatric age-group remains high. There is severe reduction in the glomerular filtration rate, an elevated BUN level, and a significant reduction in renal blood flow.

The clinical course is variable and depends on the cause. In reversible ARF there is a period of severe oliguria, or a low-output phase, followed by an abrupt onset of diuresis, or a high-output phase, and then a gradual return to (or toward) normal urine volumes.

Diagnostic Evaluation

In many instances of ARF the infant or child is already critically ill with the precipitating disorder, and the explanation for development of oliguria may or may not be readily apparent

---

*The definition of oliguria varies extensively in the literature, from 1.8 to 4 dl/m²/24 hr.

(Box 27-7). When a previously well child develops ARF without obvious cause, a careful history is taken to reveal symptoms that may be related to glomerulonephritis, obstructive uropathy, or exposure to nephrotoxic chemicals (e.g., ingestion of heavy metals, inhalation of carbon tetrachloride or other organic solvents, or medications such as nonsteroidal antiinflammatory drugs [Krause, Cleper, Eisenstein, and others, 2005] known to be toxic to the kidneys). Significant laboratory measurements during renal shutdown that serve as a guide for therapy are BUN, serum creatinine, pH, sodium, potassium, and calcium.

Therapeutic Management

Treatment of ARF is directed toward (1) treatment of the underlying cause, (2) management of the complications of renal failure, and (3) provision of supportive therapy within the constraints imposed by the renal failure.

Treatment of poor perfusion resulting from dehydration consists of volume restoration, as described in Chapter 24 in treatment of dehydration. If oliguria persists after restoration of fluid volume or if the renal failure is caused by intrinsic renal damage, the physiologic and biochemical abnormalities that have resulted from kidney dysfunction must be corrected or controlled. Initially a Foley catheter is inserted to rule out urine retention, to collect available urine for analysis, and to monitor results of diuretic administration. The catheter may or may not be removed during the oliguric phase.

The amount of exogenous water provided should not exceed the amount needed to maintain zero water balance. It is calculated on the basis of estimated endogenous water formation and losses from sensible (primarily gastrointestinal) and insensible sources. No allotment is calculated for urine as long as oliguria persists.

When the output begins to increase, either spontaneously or in response to diuretic therapy, the intake of fluid, potassium, and sodium must be monitored and adequate replacement provided to prevent depletion and its consequences. Some patients pass enormous amounts of electrolyte-rich urine.

Complications. The child with ARF has a tendency to develop water intoxication and hyponatremia, which makes it difficult to provide calories in sufficient amounts to meet the child's needs and reduce tissue catabolism, metabolic acidosis, hyperkalemia, and uremia. If the child is able to tolerate oral foods, food sources high in concentrated carbohydrate and fat but low in protein, potassium, and sodium may be provided. However, many children have functional disturbances of the gastrointestinal tract, such as nausea and vomiting; therefore the IV route is generally preferred and usually consists of essential amino acids or a combination of essential and nonessential amino acids administered by the central venous route.

Control of water balance in these patients requires careful monitoring of feedback information, such as accurate intake and output, body weight, and electrolyte measurements. In general, during the oliguric phase, no sodium, chloride, or potassium is given unless there are other large, ongoing losses. Regular measurement of plasma electrolyte, pH, BUN, and creatinine levels is required to assess the adequacy of fluid therapy and to anticipate complications that require specific treatment.

Hyperkalemia is the most immediate threat to the life of the child with ARF. Hyperkalemia can be minimized and sometimes avoided by eliminating potassium from all food and fluid, by reducing tissue catabolism, and by correcting acidosis. Measures employed for the reduction of serum potassium levels are oral or rectal administration of an ion-exchange resin such as sodium polystyrene sulfonate (Kayexalate) and peritoneal dialysis or hemodialysis (p. 970). The resin produces its effect by exchange of its sodium for the potassium, thus binding potassium for removal from the body. This increased sodium concentration may contribute to fluid overload, hypertension, and cardiac failure. Dialysis removes potassium and other waste products from the serum by diffusion through a semipermeable membrane.

Hypertension is a frequent and serious complication of ARF, and to detect it early, blood pressure measurements are made every 4 to 6 hours. The most common cause of hypertension in ARF is overexpansion of extracellular fluid and plasma volume together with activation of the renin-angiotensin system. Hypertension is controlled with antihypertensive drugs. Other measures that may be used include limiting fluids and salt.

Anemia is frequently associated with ARF, but transfusion is not recommended unless the hemoglobin drops below 6 g/dl. Transfusions, if used, consist of fresh, packed red blood cells given slowly to reduce the likelihood of increasing blood volume, hypertension, and hyperkalemia.

Seizures occur often when renal failure progresses to uremia and are also related to hypertension, hyponatremia, and hypocalcemia. Treatment is directed to the specific cause when known. More obscure causes are managed with antiepileptic drugs.

Cardiac failure with pulmonary edema is almost always associated with hypervolemia. Treatment is directed toward reduction of fluid volume, with water and sodium restriction and administration of diuretics.

Prognosis. The prognosis of ARF depends largely on the nature and severity of the causative factor or precipitating event and the promptness and competence of management. The outcome is least favorable in children with rapidly progressive nephritis and cortical necrosis. Children in whom ARF is a result of HUS or AGN may recover completely, but residual renal impairment or hypertension is more often the rule. Complete recovery is usually expected in children whose renal failure is a result of dehydration, nephrotoxins, or ischemia. ARF after cardiac surgery is less favorable. It is often impossible to assess the extent of recovery for several months.

Nursing Care Management

Meticulous attention to fluid intake and output is mandatory and includes all of the physical measurements discussed previously in relation to problems of fluid balance. Monitoring fluid balance and vital signs is a continuous process, and observers are constantly on the alert for signs of complications so that appropriate interventions can be implemented. Because these children require intensive observation and often specialized treatment, such as dialysis, they are usually admitted to an intensive care unit in which needed equipment and trained personnel are available (see Nursing Care Plan).

Limiting fluid intake requires ingenuity on the part of caregivers to cope with the child who is thirsty. Rationing the daily intake in small amounts of fluid served in containers that give the impression of larger volumes is one strategy. Older children who understand the rationale of fluid limits can help determine how their daily ration should be distributed.

Meeting nutritional needs is sometimes a problem; the child may be nauseated, and encouraging concentrated foods without fluids may be difficult. When nourishment is provided by the IV route, careful monitoring is essential to prevent fluid overload. In addition, nursing measures such as maintaining an optimal thermal environment, reducing any elevation of body temperature, and reducing restlessness and anxiety are employed to decrease the rate of tissue catabolism.

The nurse must be continually alert for changes in behavior that indicate the onset of complications. Infection from reduced resistance, anemia, and general morbidity is a constant threat. Fluid overload and electrolyte disturbances can precipitate cardiovascular complications such as hypertension and cardiac failure. Fluid and electrolyte imbalances, acidosis, and accumulation of nitrogenous waste products can produce neurologic involvement manifested by coma, seizures, or alterations in sensorium.

Although children with ARF are usually quite ill and voluntarily diminish their activity, infants may become restless and irritable, and children are often anxious and frightened. Frequent, painful, and stress-producing treatments and tests must be performed. A supportive, empathetic nurse can provide comfort and stability in a threatening and unnatural environment.

Family Support. Providing support and reassurance to parents is among the major nursing responsibilities. The seriousness of ARF and its emergency nature are stressful to parents, and most feel some degree of guilt regarding the child's condition, especially when the illness is a result of ingestion of a toxic substance, dehydration, or a genetic disease. They need reassurance and a sympathetic listener. They also need to be

nursingcareplan | The Child with Acute Renal Dysfunction

Nursing Diagnosis	Expected Patient Outcomes	Nursing Interventions	Rationale
Risk for Injury related to accumulated electrolytes and waste products **Child's/Family's Defining Characteristics** *(Subjective and Objective Data)* Excesses in potassium, sodium, and phosphorus Evidence of hyperkalemia, hyperphosphatemia, uremia Excess blood urea nitrogen	Child will exhibit no evidence of waste product accumulation. **The Following NOC Concept Applies to These Outcomes** Risk Control	Assist with renal dialysis. Administer sodium polystyrene sulfate (Kayexalate). Provide diet low in potassium, sodium, and phosphorus. Observe for evidence of accumulated waste products. Increase water intake. **The Following NIC Concepts Apply to These Interventions** Risk Identification Medication Administration Surveillance Teaching: Disease Process	To maintain renal excretory function To reduce serum potassium levels To reduce excretory demand on kidneys To ensure prompt treatment To increase waste excretion by kidneys
Imbalanced Nutrition: Less Than Body Requirements related to restricted diet **Child's/Family's Defining Characteristics** *(Subjective and Objective Data)* Weight loss Inadequate growth Poor nutritional intake	Child will consume an adequate amount of appropriate foods. Child will show no evidence of deficiencies or weight loss. **The Following NOC Concepts Apply to These Outcomes** Nutritional Status: Nutrient Intake Nutritional Status: Food & Fluid Intake Weight Control	Provide dietary instructions for foods that reduce excretory demands on kidney and provide sufficient calories and protein for growth. Limit phosphorus, salt, and potassium as prescribed. Encourage intake of carbohydrates and foods high in calcium. Arrange for renal dietitian to meet with family to review allowable foods and assist in dietary planning. Help hemodialysis patient to fill out menu requests for meals. **The Following NIC Concepts Apply to These Interventions** Teaching: Prescribed Diet Vital Signs Monitoring Fluid Management Nutrition Management Nutrition Therapy Nutritional Monitoring	To provide an appropriate diet that can reduce kidney demands To prevent mineral excess To provide calories for growth and calcium to prevent bone demineralization To promote understanding of the child's dietary needs To promote appropriate food choice decisions

kept informed of the child's progress and provided explanations regarding the therapeutic regimen. The equipment and the child's behavior are sometimes frightening and anxiety provoking. Nurses can do much to help parents comprehend and deal with the stresses of the situation.

CHRONIC RENAL FAILURE

The kidneys are able to maintain the chemical composition of fluids within normal limits until more than 50% of functional renal capacity is destroyed by disease or injury. Chronic renal insufficiency or failure begins when the diseased kidneys can no longer maintain the normal chemical structure of body fluids under normal conditions. Progressive deterioration over months or years produces a variety of clinical and biochemical disturbances that eventually culminate in the clinical syndrome known as **uremia.**

A variety of diseases and disorders can result in CRF. The most frequent causes are congenital renal and urinary tract malformations, vesicoureteral reflux associated with recurrent UTI, chronic pyelonephritis, hereditary disorders, chronic glomerulonephritis, and glomerulonephropathy associated with systemic diseases such as anaphylactoid purpura and lupus erythematosus.

Pathophysiology

Early in the course of progressive nephrotic destruction, the child remains asymptomatic with only minimal biochemical abnormalities. Unless the presence of CRF is detected in the process of routine assessment, signs and symptoms that indicate advanced renal damage frequently emerge only late in the course of the disease. Midway in the disease process, as increasing numbers of nephrons are totally destroyed and most others are damaged to varying degrees, the few that remain intact are hypertrophied but functional. These few normal nephrons are able to make sufficient adjustments to stresses to maintain reasonable degrees of fluid and electrolyte balance. Definitive biochemical examination at this time will reveal restricted tolerance to excesses or restrictions. As the disease progresses to the end stage, because of a severe reduction in the number of functioning nephrons, the kidneys are no longer able to maintain fluid and electrolyte balance, and the features of uremic syndrome appear.

The accumulation of various biochemical substances in the blood, those that result from diminished renal function, produces complications such as the following:

Retention of waste products, especially the BUN and creatinine
Water and sodium retention, which contributes to edema and vascular congestion
Hyperkalemia of dangerous levels
Metabolic acidosis of a sustained nature because of continual hydrogen ion retention and bicarbonate loss
Calcium and phosphorus disturbances, resulting in altered bone metabolism, which in turn causes growth arrest or retardation, bone pain, and deformities known as **renal osteodystrophy**
Anemia caused by hematologic dysfunction, including shortened life span of red blood cells, impaired red blood cell production related to decreased production of erythropoietin, prolonged bleeding time, and nutritional anemia
Growth disturbance, probably caused by such factors as renal osteodystrophy, poor nutrition associated with dietary restrictions and loss of appetite, and biochemical abnormalities

Children with CRF seem to be more susceptible to infection, especially pneumonia, UTI, and septicemia, although the reason for this is unclear. These children become extraordinarily sensitive to changes in vascular volume that may cause pulmonary overload, central nervous system symptoms, hypertension, and cardiac failure.

Diagnostic Evaluation

The diagnosis of CRF is usually suspected on the basis of any number of clinical manifestations, a history of prior renal disease, or biochemical findings. The onset is usually gradual, and the initial signs and symptoms are vague and nonspecific (Box 27-8).

Laboratory and other diagnostic tools and tests are of value in assessing the extent of renal damage, biochemical disturbances, and related physical dysfunction (see Tables 27-1 to 27-3). Often they can help establish the nature of the underlying disease and differentiate between other disease processes and the pathologic consequences of renal dysfunction.

Therapeutic Management

In irreversible renal failure the goals of medical management are to (1) promote maximum renal function, (2) maintain body fluid and electrolyte balance within safe biochemical limits, (3) treat systemic complications, and (4) promote as active and normal a life as possible for the child for as long as possible. The child is allowed unrestricted activity and is allowed to set his or her own limits regarding rest and extent of exertion. School attendance is encouraged as long as the child is able. When the effort is too great, home tutoring is arranged.

Diet regulation is the most effective means, short of dialysis, for reducing the quantity of materials that require renal excretion. The goal of diet management in renal failure is to

---

BOX 27-8

Clinical Manifestations of Chronic Renal Failure

Early signs:
- Loss of normal energy
- Increased fatigue on exertion
- Pallor, subtle (may not be noticed)
- Elevated blood pressure (sometimes)

As the disease progresses:
- Decreased appetite (especially at breakfast)
- Less interest in normal activities
- Increased or decreased urinary output with compensatory intake of fluid
- Pallor more evident
- Sallow, muddy appearance of skin

Child may complain of:
- Headache
- Muscle cramps
- Nausea

Other signs and symptoms:
- Weight loss
- Facial edema
- Malaise
- Bone or joint pain
- Growth retardation
- Dryness or itching of the skin
- Bruised skin
- Sensory or motor loss (sometimes)
- Amenorrhea (common in adolescent girls)

Uremic syndrome (untreated):
- Gastrointestinal symptoms
  —Anorexia
  —Nausea and vomiting
- Bleeding tendencies
  —Bruises
  —Bloody diarrheal stools
  —Stomatitis
  —Bleeding from lips and mouth
- Intractable itching
- Uremic frost (deposits of urea crystals on skin)
- Unpleasant "uremic" breath odor
- Deep respirations
- Hypertension
- Congestive heart failure
- Pulmonary edema
- Neurologic involvement
  —Progressive confusion
  —Dulled sensorium
  —Coma (ultimately)
  —Tremors
  —Muscular twitching
  —Seizures

---

provide sufficient calories and protein for growth while limiting the excretory demands made on the kidney, to minimize metabolic bone disease (**osteodystrophy**), and to minimize fluid and electrolyte disturbances. Dietary protein intake is limited only to the reference daily intake (RDA) for the child's age. Restriction of protein intake below the RDA is believed to negatively affect growth and neurodevelopment. Malnutrition may develop in patients with CRF even before they need dialysis (Nailescu, Kaskel, and Kaskel, 2004).

Sodium and water are not usually limited unless there is evidence of edema or hypertension, and potassium is not usually restricted. However, restrictions of any or all three may be imposed in later stages or at any time that abnormal serum concentrations are evident.

Dietary phosphorus is controlled through reduction of protein and milk intake to prevent or correct the calcium/phosphorus imbalance. Phosphorus levels can be further reduced by oral administration of calcium carbonate preparations or other phosphate-binding agents that combine with the phosphorus to decrease gastrointestinal absorption and thus the serum levels of phosphate. Treatment with 25-OH vitamin D is begun to increase calcium absorption and suppress elevated parathyroid hormone levels.

Metabolic acidosis is alleviated through administration of alkalizing agents such as sodium bicarbonate or a combination of sodium and potassium citrate.

Growth failure is one major consequence of CRF, especially in the preadolescent. These children grow poorly both before and after the initiation of hemodialysis. The use of recombinant human growth hormone to accelerate growth in children with growth retardation secondary to CRF has been successful (Mehls, Schaefer, Tönshoff, and others, 2002; Vimalachandra, Hodson, Willis, and others, 2006). **Osseous deformities** that result from renal osteodystrophy, especially those related to ambulation, are troublesome and require correction if they occur. **Dental defects** are common in children with CRF, and the earlier the onset of the disease, the more severe are the dental manifestations (including hypoplasia, hypomineralization, tooth discoloration, alteration in size and shape of teeth, malocclusion, and ulcerative stomatitis). Therefore regular dental care is especially important in these children.

Anemia in children with CRF is related to decreased production of erythropoietin. Recombinant human erythropoietin (rHuEPO) is being offered to these children as thrice-weekly or weekly subcutaneous injections and is replacing the need for frequent blood transfusions. The drug corrects the anemia and in turn increases appetite, activity, and general well-being in the children who receive it.

Hypertension of advanced renal disease may be managed initially by cautious use of a low-sodium diet, fluid restriction, and perhaps diuretics such as hydrochlorothiazide or furosemide. Severe hypertension requires the use of antihypertensive agents, singly or in combination.

Intercurrent infections are treated with appropriate antimicrobials at the first sign of infection; however, any drug eliminated through the kidneys is administered with caution. Other complications are treated symptomatically (e.g., central-acting antiemetics for **nausea,** antiepileptics for **seizures,** and diphenhydramine [Benadryl] for **pruritus**).

Once evidence of **end-stage renal disease (ESRD)** appears in a child, the disease runs its relentless course and results in death in a few weeks, unless waste products and toxins are removed from body fluids by dialysis or kidney transplantation. These techniques have been adapted for infants and small children and are implemented in most cases of renal failure after conservative management is no longer effective (see Technologic Management of Renal Failure, p. 970).

Prognosis. Dialysis and transplantation are the only treatments currently available for children with ESRD. Although children may survive on dialysis, it is not an ideal long-term modality. Complications include infection of access sites, growth failure, and disruption of normal socialization. Many pediatric centers encourage families of children with ESRD to consider kidney transplantation. The North American Renal Transplantation in Children Report of the North American Pediatric Renal Trials and Collaborative Studies reports a graft survival of 90% at 1 year and 74% at 6 years for living donor kidneys, and 80% at 1 year and 58% at 6 years for cadaver kidneys (Benfield, McDonald, Bartosh, and others, 2003).

Posttransplant complications include infection, hypertension, steroid toxicity, hyperlipidemia, aseptic necrosis, malignancy, and growth retardation (Benfield, 2003). Long-term graft survival is not guaranteed, and many children require a second or third transplant. Successful kidney transplantation does improve rehabilitation of children with CRF, both educationally and psychologically. Increasing use of primary or preemptive kidney transplants is becoming the optimal form of renal replacement therapy, leading to substantial improvement in quality of life (Goldstein, Graham, Burwinkle, and others, 2006).

Nursing Care Management

The multiple complications of ESRD are managed according to evidence-based clinical practice guidelines such as the ESRD Clinical Performance Measures Project (Fadrowski, Frankenfield, Amaral, and others, 2007). However, progressive disease places a number of stresses on the child and family, including those of a potentially fatal illness (see Chapter 18). There is a continuing need for repeated examinations that often entail painful procedures, side effects, and frequent hospitalizations. Diet therapy becomes progressively more restricted and intense, and the child is required to take a variety of medications. Ever present in all aspects of the treatment regimen is the agonizing realization that without treatment, death is inevitable.

Some specific stresses related to ESRD and its treatment are predictable. When it first becomes apparent that ESRD is inevitable, both parents and child experience depression and anxiety. Acceptance is particularly difficult if renal failure progresses rapidly after diagnosis. Denial and disbelief are usually pronounced, especially among the parents. After renal failure is established and symptoms become progressively more distressing, the initiation of dialysis is usually perceived as a positive experience, and after experiencing initial concerns regarding the treatment, the child begins to feel better and parental anxiety is relieved for a time.

Initiating a dialysis regimen is a traumatic and anxiety-provoking experience for most children because it involves surgery for implantation of a graft, fistula, or peritoneal catheter. The initial experience with the dialysis procedure is frightening to most children. They need reassurance about the nature of the preparations for dialysis and the conduct of the treatment.

Both the graft and the fistula require needle insertions at each dialysis. The goal is to perform pain-free venipuncture. Using buffered lidocaine with a small-gauge needle (30 gauge) to anesthetize the area before venipuncture of the graft or fistula is one method. Using an anesthetizing topical preparation such as EMLA (eutectic mixture of local anesthetics [lidocaine and prilocaine]) 1 hour before venipuncture is another approach (see Pain Management, Chapter 7). External dual-lumen venous access devices eliminate the need for needles but are more prone to infection and other central line complications.

Adolescents, with their increased need for independence and their urge for rebellion, usually adapt less well than younger children. They resent the control and enforced dependence imposed by the rigorous and unrelenting therapy program. They resent being dependent on hemodialysis technology, their parents, and the professional staff. Depression or hostility is common in adolescents undergoing hemodialysis.

The availability of home peritoneal dialysis has offered a greater degree of freedom for persons undergoing long-term dialysis. The nurse is responsible for teaching the family about (1) the disease, its implications, and the therapeutic plan; (2) the possible psychologic effects of the disease and the treatment; and (3) the technical aspects of the procedure. The family learns to manage the various aspects of the dialysis procedure, how to maintain accurate records, and how to observe for signs of complications that need to be reported to the proper persons.

Body changes related to the disease process, such as pale or ashen skin color, growth retardation, and lack of sexual maturation, are stress provoking. Dietary restrictions are particularly burdensome for both children and parents. Children feel deprived when they are unable to eat foods previously enjoyed and that are unrestricted for other family members. Consequently, they may fail to cooperate. Diet restrictions may be interpreted as punishment. Some children, unable to understand fully the purpose of restrictions, will sneak forbidden food items at every opportunity. Allowing children, especially adolescents, maximum participation in and responsibility for their own treatment program is helpful.

After months or years of dialysis, the parents and child feel anxiety associated with the prognosis and continued pressures of the treatment. The relentless need for treatment interferes with family plans. The time spent in transportation to and from the dialysis unit and the time spent undergoing dialysis treatments cut into time for outside activities, including

school. Graft and fistula problems, as well as peritoneal catheter exit site infections, may develop and present a common source of aggravation (see Family Focus box).

The possibility of kidney transplantation often provides hope for relief from the rigors of hemodialysis and peritoneal dialysis. Most children and families respond well to a kidney transplant, and most children can be successfully rehabilitated.

The National Kidney Foundation* and other agencies provide a number of services and information for families of children with renal disease.

TECHNOLOGIC MANAGEMENT OF RENAL FAILURE

DIALYSIS

Dialysis is the process of separating colloids and crystalline substances in solution by the difference in their rate of diffusion through a semipermeable membrane. Methods of dialysis currently available for clinical management of renal failure are **peritoneal dialysis,** wherein the abdominal cavity acts as a semipermeable membrane through which water and solutes of small molecular size move by osmosis and diffusion according to their respective concentrations on either side of the membrane, and **hemodialysis,** in which blood is circulated outside the body through artificial membranes that permit a similar passage of water and solutes. A third type of dialysis is **hemofiltration,** in which blood filtrate is circulated outside the body by hydrostatic pressure exerted across a semipermeable membrane with simultaneous infusion of a replacement solution. Types of hemofiltration include **continuous venovenous hemofiltration, continuous venovenous hemodialysis,** and **continuous venovenous hemodiafiltration.** These continuous renal replacement therapies are used in ARF, severe fluid overload, and inborn errors of metabolism or after bone marrow transplant (Goldstein, 2003).

Peritoneal dialysis is the preferred form of dialysis for infants, for children and parents who wish to remain independent, for families who live a long distance from the medical center, and for children who prefer fewer dietary restrictions and a gentler form of dialysis. Chronic peritoneal dialysis is most often performed at home. The two types of peritoneal dialysis are **continuous ambulatory peritoneal dialysis** and **continuous cycling peritoneal dialysis.** In both methods, commercially available sterile dialysis solution is instilled into the peritoneal cavity through a surgically implanted indwelling catheter tunneled subcutaneously and sutured into place. The warmed solution is allowed to enter the peritoneal cavity by gravity and remains a variable length of time according to the rate of solute removal and glucose absorption in individual patients. The care and management of the procedure are the responsibility of the parents of young children. Some centers have initiated use of home health nurses to give parents respite from care. Older children and adolescents can carry out the procedure themselves, which provides them with some control and less dependency. This is especially important for adolescents.

---

*30 E. 33rd St., New York, NY 10016; (212) 889-2210, (800) 622-9010; http://www.kidney.org. In Canada: Kidney Foundation of Canada, 300-5165 Sherbrooke St. West, Montreal QC H4A 1T6; (514) 369-4806, (800) 361-7494; http://www.kidney.ca.

Hemodialysis requires the creation of a vascular access and the use of special dialysis equipment—the hemodialyzer, or so-called artificial kidney. Vascular access may be one of three types: fistulas, grafts, or external vascular access devices. An **arteriovenous fistula** is an access in which a vein and artery are connected surgically. The preferred site is the radial artery and a forearm vein that produces dilation and thickening of the superficial vessels of the forearm to provide easy access for repeated venipuncture. An alternative is the creation of a subcutaneous (internal) **arteriovenous graft** by anastomosing artery and vein, with a synthetic prosthetic graft for circulatory access. The most commonly used material is expanded polytetrafluoroethylene (ePTFE). Both the graft and the fistula require needle insertions with each dialysis treatment.

For external vascular access devices, percutaneous catheters are inserted in the femoral, subclavian, or internal jugular veins, even in very small children. A more permanent form of external access is available via a central catheter inserted surgically into the internal jugular vein. This catheter has a dual lumen, which allows a larger volume of blood flow with minimum recirculation. Catheters eliminate the need for skin punctures but may require some home care.

Hemodialysis is best suited to children who do not have someone in the family who is able to perform home peritoneal dialysis and to those who live close to a dialysis center. The procedure is usually performed three times per week for 4 to 6 hours, depending on the child's size. Hemodialysis achieves rapid correction of fluid and electrolyte abnormalities but can cause problems in association with this rapid change, such as muscle cramping and hypotension. Disadvantages include school absence during dialysis and strict fluid and dietary restrictions between dialysis sessions. Boredom for the child and family is often a problem during dialysis, and planned activities should be introduced (Fig. 27-3).

Most children show rapid clinical improvement with the implementation of dialysis, although it is directly related to the duration of uremia before dialysis and good nutrition. Growth rate and skeletal maturation improve, but recovery of normal growth is infrequent. In many cases, sexual development, although delayed, progresses to completion.

TRANSPLANTATION

Kidney transplantation is now an acceptable and effective means of therapy in the pediatric age-group. Although peritoneal dialysis and hemodialysis are life preserving, both require major alterations in lifestyle. Transplantation offers the opportunity for a relatively normal life and is the preferred form of treatment for children with ESRD. Primary or preemptive transplants maintain the greatest amount of normalcy in the family's life.

FIG. 27-3 ■ Diversional activities help lessen the boredom children can experience during hemodialysis.

Kidneys for transplant are available from two sources: a **living related donor,** usually a parent or a sibling, or a **cadaver donor,** wherein the family of a dead or brain-dead patient consents to donation of a healthy kidney. Retransplantation occurs frequently.

The primary goal in transplantation is the long-term survival of grafted tissue by securing tissue that is antigenically similar to that of the recipient and by suppressing the recipient's immune mechanism. The immunosuppressant therapy of choice has been corticosteroids (prednisone) in conjunction with cyclosporine or tacrolimus and mycophenolate mofetil. Other therapies include antilymphoblast globulin or monoclonal antibodies. New immunosuppressant medications are rapidly coming into clinical trials and into use in large transplant centers. It is important for the nurse to learn about the medications used in the antirejection protocol(s) and their side effects. Because the immunosuppressant medications are taken indefinitely, transplant patients experience many side effects of the drugs, including hypertension, growth retardation, cataracts, risk of infection, obesity, characteristics of Cushing syndrome, and hirsutism (Smith, Nemeth, and McDonald, 2003).

Rejection of the transplanted kidney is the most common cause of transplant failure. Rejection is treated aggressively with immunosuppressant medications and can often be reversed. Some patients do not respond to treatment of acute rejection or develop chronic rejection and must eventually return to dialysis or undergo another kidney transplant.

KEY POINTS

- Common inflammatory disorders of the genitourinary tract include UTI, nephrotic syndrome, and AGN.
- Management of UTIs is directed at eliminating infection, detecting and correcting functional or anatomic abnormalities, preventing recurrences, and preserving renal function.
- Vesicoureteral reflux is the retrograde flow of bladder urine into the ureters.
- Obstructive uropathy is a result of structural or functional abnormalities of the urinary system that obstruct the normal flow of urine.
- The more common defects of the genitourinary tract include phimosis, cryptorchidism, inguinal hernia, hydrocele, and hypospadias.
- Body-image concerns and castration anxiety are particularly intense in children with defects in the genital area.
- Nephrotic syndrome is characterized by increased glomerular permeability to protein, with massive urinary loss of protein resulting in hypoproteinemia and edema.
- Management of nephrotic syndrome is aimed at reducing excretion of protein, reducing or preventing fluid retention by tissues, and preventing infection and other complications.
- Common features of AGN are oliguria, edema, hypertension, circulatory congestion, hematuria, and proteinuria.
- Therapeutic management of AGN involves maintenance of fluid balance, treatment of hypertension, and antibiotic therapy.
- Management of HUS is aimed at control of complications and hematologic manifestations of renal failure.
- Wilms tumor is the most common malignant neoplasm of the kidney in infants and children.
- In ARF, management is directed at determining treatment of the underlying cause, managing complications of renal failure, and providing supportive therapy.
- Abnormalities in CRF are waste product retention, water and sodium retention, hyperkalemia, acidosis, calcium and phosphorus disturbance, anemia, and growth disturbances.
- The types of dialysis used in ESRD are peritoneal dialysis and hemodialysis.
- When the child will need home dialysis, the nurse educates the family about the disease, its implications, the therapeutic plan, possible psychologic effects of the disease, and the treatment and technical aspects of the procedure.
- The major concerns in kidney transplantation are tissue matching and prevention of rejection; psychologic concerns involve self-image as related to possible body changes as a result of the effects of corticosteroid therapy.

answers to CRITICAL THINKING EXERCISE

URINARY TRACT INFECTION AND CONSTIPATION

1. Yes. Lisa's mother reports a history of constipation with large, hard-formed stools occurring only every 3 or 4 days. Lisa was diagnosed with a UTI severe enough to be admitted to the hospital.
2. a. The structure of the lower urinary tract is believed to account for the increased incidence of bacteriuria in females.
   b. A history of hard, large stools occurring every 3 or 4 days is not a normal elimination pattern for 4-year-old children.
   c. A large stool mass within the colon is likely to cause pressure on the bladder and urethra and not allow the bladder to empty completely. Stasis of the urine can lead to infection.
3. The first priority at this time is to begin treatment for the UTI. Lisa's diet and fluid intake should be evaluated and a plan developed to prevent constipation in the future.
4. Yes. Lisa's history reflects chronic problems with constipation that must be addressed.
5. Lisa might have other risk factors associated with UTIs in children, and these should be explored further. The single most important host factor influencing the occurrence of UTI is urinary stasis. Other possible causes of urinary stasis may need to be considered.

REFERENCES

American Academy of Pediatrics: Task Force on Circumcision, *Pediatrics* 103(3):686-693, 1999.

Bailey DT, Dalton C, Daugherty F, and others: Can a concentrated cranberry extract prevent recurrent urinary tract infections in women? A pilot study, *Phytomedicine* 14(4):237-241, 2007.

Benfield MR: Current status of kidney transplant: update 2003, *Pediatr Clin North Am* 50(6):1301-1334, 2003.

Benfield MR, McDonald RA, Bartosh S, and others: Changing trends in pediatric transplantation: 2001 annual report of the North American Pediatric Renal Transplant Cooperative Study, *Pediatr Transplant* 7(4):321-335, 2003.

Davis ID, Avner ED: Conditions particularly associated with hematuria. In Behrman RE, Kliegman RM, Jenson HB, editors: *Nelson textbook of pediatrics*, ed 17, Philadelphia, 2004, Saunders.

Dome JS, Perlman EJ, Ritchey ML, and others: Renal tumors. In Pizzo PA, Poplack DP, editors: *Principles and practices of pediatric oncology*, ed 5, Philadelphia, 2006, Lippincott.

Fadrowski JJ, Frankenfield D, Amaral S, and others: Children on long-term dialysis in the United States: findings from the 2005 ESRD clinical performance measures project, *Am J Kidney Dis* 50(6):958-966, 2007.

Goldstein SL: Overview of pediatric renal replacement therapy in acute renal failure, *Artif Organs* 27(9):781-785, 2003.

Goldstein SL, Graham N, Burwinkle T, and others: Health-related quality of life in pediatric patients with ESRD, *Pediatr Nephrol* 21(6):846-850, 2006.

Jepson RG, Mihaljevic L, Craig J: Cranberries for preventing urinary tract infections, *Cochrane Database Syst Rev* (2):CD001321, 2004.

Kanellopoulos TA, Salakos C, Spiliopoulou I, and others: First urinary tract infection in neonates, infants and young children: a comparative study, *Pediatr Nephrol* 21(8):1131-1137, 2006.

Kass E: Timing of elective surgery on the genitalia of male children with particular reference to the risks, benefits, and psychological effects of surgery and anesthesia, *Pediatrics* 97(4):590-594, 1996.

Kirsch AJ, Perez-Brayfield MR, Scherz HC: Minimally invasive treatment of vesicoureteral reflux with endoscopic injection of dextranomer/hyaluronic acid copolymer: the Children's Hospital of Atlanta experience, *J Urol* 170(1):211-215, 2003.

Kline NE, Sevier N: Solid tumors in children, *J Pediatr Nurs* 18(2):96-102, 2003.

Krause I, Cleper R, Eisenstein B, and others: Acute renal failure, associated with non-steroidal anti-inflammatory drugs in healthy children, *Pediatr Nephrol* 20(9):1295-1298, 2005.

Lavelle MT, Conlin MJ, Skoog SJ: Subureteral injection of Deflux for correction of reflux: analysis of factors predicting success, *Urology* 65(3):564-567, 2005.

Mehls O, Schaefer F, Tönshoff B, and others: Effectiveness of growth hormone treatment in short children with chronic renal failure, *J Pediatr* 141(1):147-148, 2002.

Nailescu C, Kaskel PJ, Kaskel FJ: Nutrition and metabolism. In Avner ED, Harmon WE, Niaudet P, editors: *Pediatric nephrology*, ed 5, Philadelphia, 2004, Lippincott Williams & Wilkins.

National Kidney Foundation: *The National Kidney Foundation kidney disease outcomes quality initiative (NKF KDOQI™)*, retrieved February 8, 2007, from http://www.kidney.org/professionals/kdoqi.

Rosenthal M: Current concept in managing UTIs in children, *Infect Dis Child* 17(3):30-31, 2004.

Schaefer F: Management of peritonitis in children receiving chronic peritoneal dialysis, *Paediatr Drugs* 5(5):315-325, 2003.

Shaikh N, Morone NE, Bost JE, and others: Prevalence of urinary tract infection in childhood: a meta-analysis, *Pediatr Infect Dis J* 27(4):302-308, 2008.

Smith JM, Nemeth TL, McDonald RA: Current immunosuppressive agents: efficacy, side effects, and utilization, *Pediatr Clin North Am* 50(6):1283-1300, 2003.

Vimalachandra D, Hodson EM, Willis NS, and others: Growth hormone for children with chronic kidney disease, *Cochrane Database Syst Rev* (3): CD003264, 2006.

The Child with Cerebral Dysfunction

MARILYN J. HOCKENBERRY

CHAPTER OUTLINE

CEREBRAL DYSFUNCTION, 975
General Aspects, 975
Increased Intracranial Pressure, 975
Altered States of Consciousness, 976
 Levels of Consciousness, 976
 Coma Assessment, 976
Neurologic Examination, 977
 Vital Signs, 977
 Skin, 977
 Eyes, 977
 Motor Function, 978
 Posturing, 979
 Reflexes, 979
Special Diagnostic Procedures, 979
**NURSING CARE OF THE UNCONSCIOUS
CHILD, 981**
Respiratory Management, 982
Intracranial Pressure Monitoring, 982
 Nursing Activities, 983
 Suctioning, 984

Nutrition and Hydration, 984
 Altered Pituitary Secretion, 984
Medications, 984
Thermoregulation, 984
Elimination, 984
Hygienic Care, 985
Positioning and Exercise, 985
Stimulation, 985
 Regaining Consciousness, 985
Family Support, 985
CEREBRAL TRAUMA, 986
Head Injury, 986
Near-Drowning, 993
NERVOUS SYSTEM TUMORS, 995
Brain Tumors, 995
Neuroblastoma, 997

INTRACRANIAL INFECTIONS, 998
Bacterial Meningitis, 998
Nonbacterial (Aseptic) Meningitis, 1002
Encephalitis, 1002
Rabies, 1003
Reye Syndrome, 1004
SEIZURE DISORDERS, 1005
Epilepsy, 1005
Nursing Care Plan: The Child with
 Seizure Disorder, 1011
Febrile Seizures, 1016
CEREBRAL MALFORMATIONS, 1016
Cranial Deformities, 1016
Hydrocephalus, 1017

LEARNING OBJECTIVES

On completion of this chapter the reader will be able to:

- Describe the various modalities for assessment of cerebral function.
- Differentiate between the stages of consciousness.
- Formulate a care plan for the unconscious child.

- Distinguish between the types of head injuries and the serious complications.
- Describe the nursing care of a child with a tumor of the central nervous system.
- Outline a care plan for the child with bacterial meningitis.
- Differentiate between the various types of seizure disorders.

- Demonstrate an understanding of the manifestations of a seizure disorder and the management of a child with such a disorder.
- Describe the preoperative and postoperative care of a child with hydrocephalus.

RELATED TOPICS and ADDITIONAL RESOURCES

IN TEXT

Administration of Medication, *Ch. 22*
Childhood Mortality, *Ch. 1*
Family-Centered Care of the Child During
   Illness and Hospitalization, *Ch. 21*
Family-Centered Home Care, *Ch. 20*
Immunizations, *Ch. 10*
Impact of Chronic Illness or Disability on the
   Child, *Ch. 18*
Infection Control, *Ch. 22*
Maintaining Healthy Skin, *Ch. 22*
Neurologic Assessment, *Ch. 6*
Pain Assessment; Pain Management, *Ch. 7*
Preparation for Diagnostic and Therapeutic
   Procedures, *Ch. 22*

 COMPANION CD

Animations—Brain Lobes; Cervical Nerve
   Examination; Seizure, Generalized;
   Subdural Hematoma; Ventriculoperitoneal
   Shunt
Case Studies—Meningitis; Hydrocephalus
   with Myelomeningocele
Critical Thinking Exercise—Seizures
NCLEX Review Questions

evolve

evolve.elsevier.com/Wong/essentials/

NCLEX Review Questions
Critical Thinking Case Studies—Brain Tumor;
   Head Injury

Nursing Care Plans—The Unconscious
   Child; The Child with a Seizure Disorder;
   The Child with Bacterial Meningitis
Skill—Implementing Seizure Precautions
WebLinks

 **WONG'S CLINICAL MANUAL
OF PEDIATRIC NURSING, 7th Ed**

Nursing Care Plans—The Unconscious
   Child, *p. 464;* The Child with Bacterial
   Meningitis, *p. 469*
Patient and Family Education—Caring for an
   Intermittent Infusion Device, *p. 531;*
   Giving Oral Medications, *p. 523;* Giving
   Rectal Medications—Suppositories, *p. 538*

CEREBRAL DYSFUNCTION

Most of the information about the status of the brain is obtained by indirect measurements. Some of these measurements are discussed elsewhere in relation to numerous aspects of childcare (e.g., as part of assessments of health [Chapter 6], newborn status [Chapter 8], intellectual disability [Chapter 19], hypoxic injury [cerebral palsy, Chapter 32], and attainment of developmental milestones at each stage of development). Since increased intracranial pressure (ICP) and altered states of consciousness have such prominent places in neurologic dysfunction, they are described here, followed by techniques for neurologic assessment and diagnostic tests.

GENERAL ASPECTS

Children younger than 2 years of age require special evaluation, since they are unable to respond to directions designed to elicit specific neurologic responses. Early neurologic responses in infants are primarily reflexive; these responses are gradually replaced by meaningful movement in the characteristic cephalocaudal direction of development. This evidence of progressive maturation reflects more extensive myelinization and changes in neurochemical and electrophysiologic properties.

Most information about infants and small children is gained by observing their spontaneous and elicited reflex responses as they develop increasingly complex locomotor and fine motor skills and by eliciting progressively sophisticated communicative and adaptive behaviors. Delay or deviation from expected milestones helps identify high-risk children. Persistence or reappearance of reflexes that normally disappear indicates a pathologic condition. In evaluating the infant or young child, it is also important to obtain the pregnancy and delivery history to determine the possible impact of intrauterine environmental influences known to affect the orderly maturation of the central nervous system (CNS). These influences include maternal infections, chemicals, trauma, and metabolic insults.

General aspects of assessment that provide clues to the etiology of dysfunction include:

Family history—Sometimes offers clues regarding possible genetic disorders with neurologic manifestations
Health history—May provide valuable clues regarding the cause of dysfunction (e.g., an injury, short febrile illness, encounter with an animal or insect, ingestion of neurotoxic substances, inhalation of chemicals, a past illness, or known diabetes mellitus)
Physical evaluation of infants—Includes observation of:
- Size and shape of the head
- Spontaneous activity and postural reflex activity
- Sensory responses
- Attitude—normal flexed posture, extreme extension, opisthotonos, hypotonia
- Symmetry in movement of extremities
- Excessive tremulousness or frequent twitching movements
- Altered expiratory cycle—prolonged apnea, ataxic breathing, paradoxic chest movement, and hyperventilation
- Skin and hair texture
- Distinctive facial features
- A high-pitched, piercing cry
- Abnormal eye movements
- Inability to suck or swallow
- Lip smacking
- Asymmetric contraction of facial muscles
- Yawning (may indicate cranial nerve involvement)
- Muscular activity and coordination
- Level of development

INCREASED INTRACRANIAL PRESSURE

The brain, tightly enclosed in the solid bony cranium, is well protected but highly vulnerable to pressure that may accumulate within the enclosure. The cranium's total volume—brain (80%), cerebrospinal fluid (CSF) (10%), and blood (10%)—must remain approximately the same at all times. A change in the proportional volume of one of these components (e.g., increase or decrease in intracranial blood) must be accompanied by a compensatory change in another. In this way the

BOX 28-1

Clinical Manifestations of Increased Intracranial Pressure in Infants and Children

INFANTS
Tense and/or bulging fontanel
Separated cranial sutures
Macewen sign (cracked-pot sound on percussion)
Irritability
High-pitched cry
Increased occipitofrontal circumference
Distended scalp veins
Changes in feeding
Crying when disturbed
Setting-sun sign

CHILDREN
Headache
Nausea
Vomiting
Diplopia, blurred vision
Seizures

PERSONALITY AND BEHAVIORAL SIGNS
Irritability, restlessness
Indifference, drowsiness
Decline in school performance
Diminished physical activity and motor performance
Increased sleeping
Memory loss
Inability to follow simple commands
Lethargy and drowsiness

LATE SIGNS
Bradycardia
Lowered level of consciousness
Decreased motor response to commands
Decreased sensory response to painful stimuli
Alterations in pupil size and reactivity
Flexion or extension posturing
Cheyne-Stokes respirations
Papilledema
Coma

BOX 28-2

Levels of Consciousness

Full consciousness—Awake and alert; oriented to time, place, and person; behavior appropriate for age
Confusion—Impaired decision making
Disorientation—Disorientation to time and place, decreased level of consciousness
Lethargy—Limited spontaneous movement, sluggish speech, drowsiness
Obtundation—Arousable with stimulation
Stupor—Remaining in a deep sleep, responsive only to vigorous and repeated stimulation
Coma—No motor or verbal response to noxious (painful) stimuli
Persistent vegetative state (PVS)—The permanently lost function of the cerebral cortex; eyes following objects only by reflex or when attracted to the direction of loud sounds, all four limbs spastic but can withdraw from painful stimuli, hands showing reflexive grasping and groping, face grimacing, some food may be swallowed, and the child may groan or cry but utters no words

Modified from Seidel HM, Ball JW, Dains JE, and others, editors: *Mosby's guide to physical examination,* ed 6, St Louis, 2006, Mosby.

ALTERED STATES OF CONSCIOUSNESS

Consciousness implies awareness—the ability to respond to sensory stimuli and have subjective experiences. There are two components of consciousness: **alertness,** an arousal-waking state, including the ability to respond to stimuli; and **cognitive power,** including the ability to process stimuli and produce verbal and motor responses.

An altered state of consciousness usually refers to varying states of unconsciousness that may be momentary or may extend for hours, for days, or indefinitely. **Unconsciousness** is depressed cerebral function—the inability to respond to sensory stimuli and have subjective experiences. **Coma** is defined as a state of unconsciousness from which the patient cannot be aroused even with powerful stimuli.

Levels of Consciousness

Assessment of LOC remains the earliest indicator of improvement or deterioration in neurologic status. LOC is determined by observations of the child's responses to the environment. Other diagnostic tests, such as motor activity, reflexes, and vital signs, are more variable and do not necessarily directly parallel the depth of the comatose state. The most consistently used terms are described in Box 28-2.

Coma Assessment

Several scales have been devised in an attempt to standardize the description and interpretation of the degree of depressed consciousness. The most popular of these is the **Glasgow Coma Scale (GCS),** which consists of a three-part assessment: eye opening, verbal response, and motor response (Fig. 28-1). When LOC is being assessed in young children, it is often useful to have a parent present to help elicit a desired response. An infant or child may not respond in an unfamiliar environment or to unfamiliar voices. Children older than 3 years of age should be able to give their name, although they may not be cognizant of place or time.

Numeric values of 1 through 5 are assigned to the levels of response in each category. The sum of these numeric values

volume and pressure normally remain constant. Examples of compensatory changes are reduction in blood volume, decrease in CSF production, increase in CSF absorption, or shrinkage of brain mass by displacement of intracellular and extracellular fluid. Children with open fontanels compensate by skull expansion and widened sutures. However, at any age the capacity for spatial compensation is limited. An increase in ICP may be caused by tumors or other space-occupying lesions, accumulation of fluid within the ventricular system, bleeding, or edema of cerebral tissues. Once compensation is exhausted, any further increase in volume will result in a rapid rise in ICP.

Early signs and symptoms of increased ICP are often subtle and assume many patterns (Box 28-1). As pressure increases, signs and symptoms become more pronounced and the level of consciousness (LOC) deteriorates.

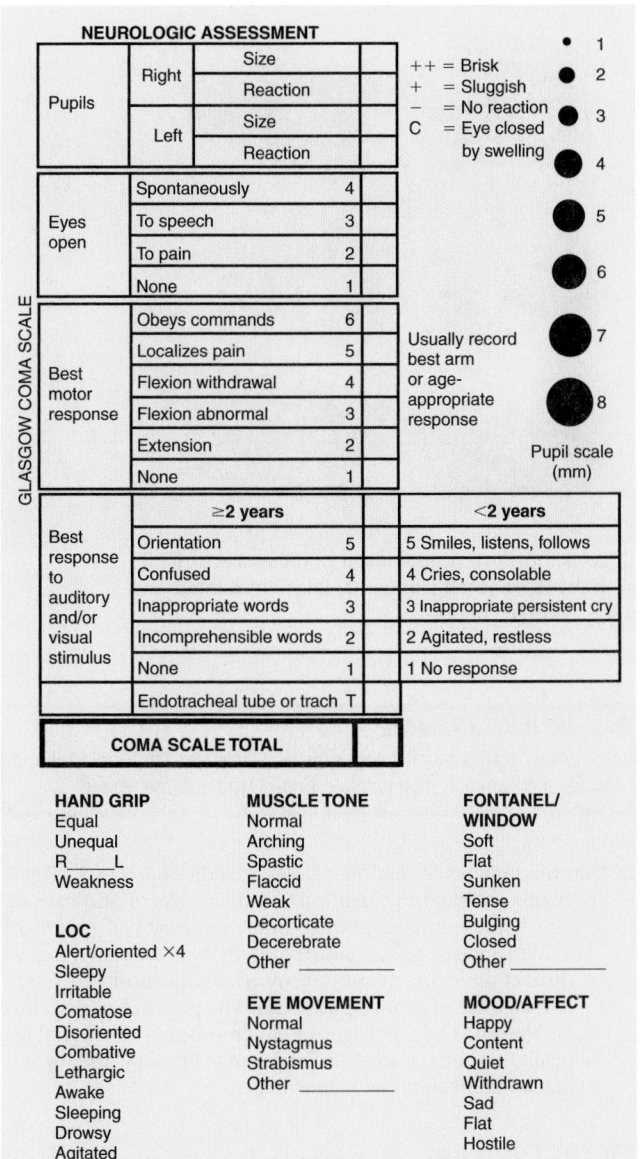

FIG. 28-1 ■ Pediatric coma scale.

provides an objective measure of the patient's LOC. The lower the score, the deeper the coma. A person with an unaltered LOC would score the highest, 15; a score of 8 or below is generally accepted as a definition of coma; the lowest score, 3, indicates deep coma. The Task Force for the Determination of Brain Death in Children has established physical examination criteria for cases of irreversible coma (1987).

NURSING ALERT

Lack of response to painful stimuli is abnormal and should be reported immediately.

NEUROLOGIC EXAMINATION

The purpose of the neurologic examination is to establish an accurate, objective baseline of neurologic information. It is essential that the neurologic examination be documented in a fashion that is able to be reproduced by others. This allows for

a comparison of the findings so the observer can detect subtle changes in the neurologic status that might not otherwise be evident. Descriptions of behaviors should be simple, objective, and easily interpreted: "Drowsy but awake and conversationally rational/oriented"; "Sleepy but arousable with vigorous physical stimuli. Pressure to nail base of right hand results in upper extremity flexion/lower extremity extension."

Vital Signs

Pulse, respiration, and blood pressure provide information regarding the adequacy of circulation and the possible underlying cause of altered consciousness. Autonomic activity is most intensively disturbed in cases of deep coma or brainstem lesions.

Body temperature is often elevated, and sometimes the elevation may be extreme. High temperature is most frequently a sign of an acute infectious process or heat stroke but may be caused by ingestion of some drugs (especially salicylates, alcohol, and barbiturates) or by intracranial bleeding, especially subarachnoid hemorrhage. Hypothalamic involvement may cause elevated or decreased temperature. Coma of a toxic origin may produce hypothermia.

The **pulse** is variable and may be rapid, slow and bounding, or feeble. **Blood pressure** may be normal, elevated, or at shock levels. The Cushing reflex, or pressor response, which causes a slowing of the pulse and an increase in blood pressure, is uncommon in children; when it occurs, it is a very late sign of ICP. Vital signs are also affected by medications. For assessment purposes, actual *changes* in pulse and blood pressure are more important than the direction of the change.

Respirations are often slow, deep, and irregular. Slow, deep breathing is often seen in the heavy sleep caused by sedatives, after seizures, or in cerebral infections. Slow, shallow breathing may result from sedatives or opioids (narcotics). Hyperventilation (deep and rapid respirations) is usually a result of metabolic acidosis or abnormal stimulation of the respiratory center in the medulla caused by salicylate poisoning, hepatic coma, or Reye syndrome (RS).

Breathing patterns have been described with a number of terms (e.g., apneustic, cluster, ataxic, Cheyne-Stokes). However, it is better to describe what is being observed rather than placing a label on it because the traditional terms are often used and interpreted incorrectly. Periodic or irregular breathing is an ominous sign of brainstem (especially medullary) dysfunction that often precedes complete apnea. The **odor** of the breath may provide additional clues (e.g., the fruity, acetone odor of ketosis; the foul odor of uremia; the fetid odor of hepatic failure; or the odor of alcohol).

Skin

The skin may offer clues to the cause of unconsciousness. The body surface should be examined for signs of injury, needle marks, petechiae, bites, and ticks. Evidence of toxic substances may be found on the hands, face, mouth, and clothing—especially in small children.

Eyes

Pupil size and reactivity are assessed (Fig. 28-2; see also Fig. 28-1). Pinpoint pupils are commonly observed in poisoning, such as opiate or barbiturate poisoning, or in brainstem dysfunction. Widely dilated and reactive pupils are often seen after seizures and may involve only one side. Dilated pupils may also be

FIG. 28-2 ■ Variations in pupil size with altered states of consciousness. **A,** Ipsilateral pupillary constriction with slight ptosis. **B,** Bilateral small pupils. **C,** Midposition, light fixed to all stimuli. **D,** Bilateral dilated and fixed pupils. **E,** Dilated pupils, left eye abducted with ptosis. **F,** Pinpoint pupils.

caused by eye trauma. Widely dilated and fixed pupils suggest paralysis of cranial nerve III secondary to pressure from herniation of the brain through the tentorium. A unilateral fixed pupil usually suggests a lesion on the same side. If pupils are fixed bilaterally for more than 5 minutes, brainstem damage is usually implied. Dilated and nonreactive pupils are also seen in hypothermia, anoxia, ischemia, poisoning with atropine-like substances, or prior instillation of mydriatic drugs.

> **NURSINGALERT**
> The sudden appearance of a fixed and dilated pupil(s) is a neurosurgical emergency.

The description of eye movements should indicate whether one or both eyes are involved and how the reaction was elicited. The parents should be asked about preexisting strabismus, which will cause the eyes to appear normal under compromise. Posttraumatic strabismus indicates cranial nerve VI damage.

Special tests, usually performed by qualified persons, include:

Doll's head maneuver—Elicited by rotating the child's head quickly to one side and then to the other. Conjugate (paired or working together) movement of the eyes in the direction opposite to the head rotation is normal. Absence of this response suggests dysfunction of the brainstem or oculomotor nerve (cranial nerve III).

> **NURSINGALERT**
> Any tests that require head movement are not attempted until after cervical spine injury has been ruled out.

Caloric test, or oculovestibular response—Elicited with the child's head up (head of bed is elevated 30 degrees) by irrigating the external auditory canal with 10 ml of ice water for 20 seconds, which normally causes conjugate movement of the eyes toward the side of stimulation. This movement is lost when the pontine centers are impaired, thus providing important information in assessment of the comatose patient.

> **NURSINGALERT**
> The caloric test is painful and is never performed on a child who is awake or on an individual with a ruptured tympanic membrane.

Funduscopic examination—Reveals additional clues. Papilledema will not be evident early in the course of unconsciousness because it takes 24 to 48 hours to develop, if it develops at all. Papilledema is characterized by optic disc swelling, indistinct optic disc margins, hemorrhage, tortuosity of vessels, and absence of venous pulsations. The presence of preretinal (subhyaloid) hemorrhages in children is almost invariably a result of acute trauma with intracranial bleeding, usually subarachnoid or subdural hemorrhage.

Motor Function

Observing spontaneous activity, posture, and response to painful stimuli provides clues to the location and extent of cerebral dysfunction. Even subtle movements (e.g., the outward rotation of a hip) should be noted and the child observed for other signs. Asymmetric movements of the limbs or absence of movement suggests paralysis. In hemiplegia the affected limb lies in external rotation and will fall uncontrollably when lifted and allowed to drop. These observations should be described rather than labeled.

In the deeper comatose states there is little or no spontaneous movement, and the musculature tends to be flaccid. There is considerable variability in the motor behavior in lesser degrees of coma. For example, the child may be relatively immobile or restless and hyperkinetic; muscle tone may be increased or decreased. Tremors, twitching, and spasms of muscles are common observations. The patient may display purposeless plucking or tossing movements. Combative or negativistic behavior is not uncommon. Hyperactivity is more common in acute febrile and toxic states than in cases of increased ICP. Seizures are common in children and may be present in coma from any cause. Any repetitive or seizure movements should be described.

FIG. 28-3 ■ **A,** Flexion posturing. **B,** Extension posturing.

Posturing

Primitive postural reflexes emerge as cortical control over motor function is lost in brain dysfunction. These reflexes are evident in posturing and motor movements directly related to the area of the brain involved. Posturing reflects a balance between the lower exciting and the higher inhibiting influences, and strong muscles overcome weaker ones. **Flexion posturing** (Fig. 28-3, *A*) is seen with severe dysfunction of the cerebral cortex or with lesions to corticospinal tracts above the brainstem. Typical flexion posturing includes rigid flexion, with arms held tightly to the body; flexed elbows, wrists, and fingers; plantar flexed feet; legs extended and internally rotated; and possibly presence of fine tremors or intense stiffness. **Extension posturing** (see Fig. 28-3, *B*) is a sign of dysfunction at the level of the midbrain or lesions to the brainstem. It is characterized by rigid extension and pronation of the arms and legs, flexed wrists and fingers, clenched jaw, extended neck, and possibly an arched back. Unilateral extension posturing is often caused by tentorial herniation.

Posturing may not be evident when the child is quiet but can usually be elicited by applying painful stimuli, such as a blunt object pressed on the base of the nail. Nurses should avoid applying thumb pressure to the supraorbital region of the frontal bone (risk of orbital damage). Noxious stimuli (e.g., suctioning) will elicit a response, as may turning or touching. When the nurse is describing posturing, the stimulus needed to provoke the response is as important as the reaction.

Reflexes

Testing of some reflexes may be of limited value. In general, the corneal, pupillary, muscle-stretch, superficial, and plantar reflexes tend to be absent in deep coma. The state of reflexes is variable in lighter grades of unconsciousness and depends on the underlying pathologic process and the location of the lesion. Absence of corneal reflexes and presence of a tonic neck reflex are associated with severe brain damage. The Babinski reflex (see Extremities, Chapter 6) may be of value if it is found to be present consistently in children older than 18 months. A positive Babinski reflex is significant in assessment

of pyramidal tract lesions when it is unilateral and associated with other pyramidal signs.

> **NURSING ALERT**
>
> Three key reflexes that demonstrate neurologic health in young infants are the Moro, tonic neck, and withdrawal reflexes.

SPECIAL DIAGNOSTIC PROCEDURES

Numerous diagnostic procedures are used for assessment of cerebral function. Laboratory tests that may help delineate the cause of unconsciousness include blood glucose, urea nitrogen, and electrolyte (pH, sodium, potassium, chloride, calcium, and bicarbonate) tests; clotting studies, hematocrit, and a complete blood count; liver function tests; blood cultures if there is fever; and sometimes studies to detect lead or other toxic substances, such as drugs.

An electroencephalogram (EEG) may provide important information. For example, generalized random, slow activity suggests suppressed cortical function, and localized slow activity suggests a space-occupying lesion. A flat tracing is one of the criteria used as evidence of brain death.

Examination of spinal fluid is carried out when toxic encephalopathy or infection is suspected. Lumbar puncture is ordinarily delayed if intracranial hemorrhage is suspected and is contraindicated in the presence of ICP because of the potential for tentorial herniation.

Auditory and visual evoked potentials are sometimes used in neurologic evaluation of very young children. Brainstem auditory evoked potentials are useful for evaluating the continuity of brainstem auditory tracts and are particularly useful for detecting demyelinating disease and neoplasms of the brainstem and distinguishing between brainstem and cortical lesions. For example, a normal evoked potential in a comatose patient suggests involvement of the cerebral hemispheres.

Highly sophisticated tests are carried out with specialized equipment. Two imaging techniques, computed tomography (CT) and magnetic resonance imaging (MRI), assist in diagnosis by scanning both soft tissues and solid matter. Most of these tests are outlined in Table 28-1. Because such tests can be threatening to children, the nurse needs to prepare patients for the tests and provide support and reassurance during the tests (see Preparation for Diagnostic and Therapeutic Procedures, Chapter 22). Children who are old enough to understand require careful explanation of the procedure, why it is being done, what they will experience, and how they can help. School-age children usually appreciate a more detailed description of why contrast material is injected. The importance of lying still for tests, particularly CT, needs to be stressed. Children unfamiliar with the machines can be shown a picture beforehand. Although radiographic examinations are not painful, the machinery is often so frightening in appearance that the child protests because of anxiety.

This is especially true of CT and MRI, both of which require that the child's head be placed within a special immobilizing device. Chin and cheek pads are sometimes used to prevent the slightest head movement, and straps are applied to the body to prevent a slight change in body position. The nurse can explain these events to a frightened child by comparing them to an astronaut's preparation for a space flight. It is important to emphasize to the child that at no time is the procedure painful.

TABLE 28-1

Neurologic Diagnostic Procedures

TEST	DESCRIPTION	PURPOSE	COMMENTS
Lumbar puncture (LP)	Spinal needle is inserted between L3-L4 or L4-L5 vertebral spaces into subarachnoid space; cerebrospinal fluid (CSF) pressure is measured, and sample is collected for examination.	Diagnostic—Measures spinal fluid pressure, obtains CSF for laboratory analysis Therapeutic—Injection of medication	Contraindicated in patients with increased intracranial pressure (ICP) or infected skin over puncture site.
Subdural tap	Needle is inserted into anterior fontanel or coronal suture (midline to pupil).	Helps rule out subdural effusions Removes CSF to relieve pressure	Place infant in semierect position after subdural tap to minimize leakage from site; prevent child from crying if possible. Check site frequently for evidence of leakage.
Ventricular puncture	Needle is inserted into lateral ventricle via coronal suture (midline to pupil).	Removes CSF to relieve pressure	Risk of intracerebral or ventricular hemorrhage.
Electroencephalography (EEG)	EEG records changes in electrical potential of brain. Electrodes are placed at various points to assess electrical function in a particular area. Impulses are recorded by electromagnetic pen or digitally.	Detects spikes, or bursts of electrical activity that indicate the potential for seizures Used to determine brain death	Patient should remain quiet during procedure; may require sedation. Minimize external stimuli during procedure.
Nuclear brain scan	Radioisotope is injected intravenously, then counted and recorded after fixed time intervals. Radioisotope accumulates in areas where blood-brain barrier is defective.	Identifies focal brain lesions (e.g., tumors, abscesses) Positive uptake of material with encephalitis and subdural hematoma Visualizes CSF pathways	Requires intravenous (IV) access; patient may require sedation. In normal children or noncommunicating hydrocephalus, no retrograde filling of ventricles occurs. Areas of concentrated uptake of material are termed *hot spots*.
Endocephalography	Pulses of ultrasonic waves are beamed through head; echoes from reflecting surfaces are recorded graphically.	Identifies shifts in midline structures from their normal positions as a result of intracranial lesions May show ventricular dilation	Simple, safe, rapid procedure. Fontanel must be patent.
Real-time ultrasonography (RTUS)	RTUS is similar to CT but uses ultrasound instead of ionizing radiation.	Allows high-resolution anatomic visualization in variety of imaging planes	Produces images similar to CT scan. Especially useful in neonatal central nervous system problems. Anterior fontanel must be patent.
Radiography	Skull films are taken from different views—lateral, posterolateral, axial (submentoventricular), half-axial.	Shows fractures, dislocations, spreading suture lines, craniosynostosis Shows degenerative changes, bone erosion, calcifications	Simple, noninvasive procedure.
Computed tomography (CT) scan	Pinpoint x-ray beam is directed on horizontal or vertical plane to provide series of images that are fed into computer and assembled in image displayed on video screen. CT uses ionizing radiation.	Visualizes horizontal and vertical cross section of brain in 3 planes (axial, coronal, sagittal) Distinguishes density of various intracranial tissues and structures—congenital abnormalities, hemorrhage, tumors, demyelinating and inflammatory processes, calcification	Requires IV access if contrast agent is used. Patient may require sedation. Rapid.
Magnetic resonance imaging (MRI)	MRI produces radiofrequency emissions from elements (e.g., hydrogen, phosphorus), which are converted to visual images by computer.	Permits visualization of morphologic feature of target structures Permits tissue discrimination unavailable with many techniques	MRI is noninvasive procedure except when IV contrast agent is used. No exposure to radiation occurs. Patient may require sedation. Parent or attendant can remain in room with child. MRI does not visualize bone detail or calcifications. No metal can be present in scanner.

TABLE 28-1
Neurologic Diagnostic Procedures—cont'd

TEST	DESCRIPTION	PURPOSE	COMMENTS
Positron emission tomography (PET)	PET involves IV injection of positron-emitting radionucleotide; local concentrations are detected and transformed into visual display by computer.	Detects and measures blood volume and flow in brain, metabolic activity, biochemical changes within tissue	Requires lengthy period of immobility. Minimum exposure to radiation occurs. Patient may require sedation.
Digital subtraction angiography (DSA)	Contrast dye is injected intravenously; computer "subtracts" all tissues without contrast medium, leaving clear image of contrast medium in vessels studied.	Visualizes vasculature of target tissue Visualizes finite vascular abnormalities	Safe alternative to angiography. Patient must remain still during procedure; may require sedation.
Single-photon emission computed tomography (SPECT)	SPECT involves IV injection of photon-emitting radionuclide; radionuclides are absorbed by healthy tissue at different rate than by diseased or necrotic tissue; data are transferred to computer that converts image to film.	Provides information regarding blood flow to tissues; analyzing blood flow to organ may help determine how well it is functioning	Requires lengthy period of immobility. Minimum exposure to radiation occurs. Patient may require sedation.

The nurse should not expect cooperation from a young child. Sedation may be required. Many different agents are currently used for sedation of children undergoing neurologic diagnostic procedures. Chloral hydrate or benzodiazepines have been used for decades as short-term sedative agents and remain safe methods of pediatric outpatient sedation (Kao, Adamson, Tatman, and others, 1999; Wetzell, 2007). Chloral hydrate is used alone for sedating children for procedures such as MRI. In recent years other sedative agents have been used safely, alone and in combination, for children in the outpatient setting. These include intravenous (IV) sodium pentobarbital (Nembutal), IV fentanyl (Sublimaze), IV midazolam (Versed) (Wetzell, 2007), and intranasal midazolam (Ljungman, Kreuger, Andreasson, and others, 2000; Lloyd, Alredy, and Lloyd, 2000). (See Pain Management, Chapter 7.)

Physical preparation for the diagnostic test may involve administration of a sedative. If so, children should be helped through the preparation and administration and assured that someone will remain with them (if possible). Children need continual support and reinforcement during procedures in which they remain conscious. Vital signs and physiologic responses to the procedure are monitored throughout. Many diagnostic procedures performed on an outpatient basis require sedation, and children need recovery time and observation. The nurse should review written instructions with parents if the child is discharged after a procedure. Children who have undergone a procedure with a general anesthetic require postanesthesia care, including positioning to prevent aspiration of secretions and frequent assessment of the vital signs and LOC. In addition, other neurologic functions such as pupillary responses, motor strength, and movement are tested at regular intervals. Any surgical wound resulting from the test is checked for bleeding, CSF leakage, and other complications. Children who undergo repeated subdural taps should have their hematocrit monitored to detect excessive blood loss from the procedure.

NURSING CARE OF THE UNCONSCIOUS CHILD

The unconscious child requires nursing attendance, with observation, recording, and evaluation of changes in objective signs. These observations provide valuable information regarding the patient's progress. Often they serve as a guide to diagnosis and treatment. Therefore careful and detailed observations are essential for the patient's welfare. In addition, vital functions must be maintained and complications prevented through conscientious and meticulous nursing care. The outcome of unconsciousness may be early and complete recovery, death within a few hours or days, persistent and permanent unconsciousness, or recovery with varying degrees of residual mental or physical disability. The outcome and recovery of the unconscious child may depend on the level of nursing care and observational skills.

Emergency measures are directed toward ensuring a patent airway, treatment of shock, and reduction of ICP (if it is increased). Delayed treatment often leads to increased damage. As soon as emergency measures have been implemented—and in many cases concurrently—therapies for specific causes are begun. Because nursing care is closely related to medical management, both are considered here.

Continual observation of LOC, pupillary reaction, and vital signs is essential to manage CNS disorders. Regular assessment of neurologic signs is a vital part of nursing comatose children. Vital signs are measured and recorded regularly. The frequency depends on the cause of coma, the status, and the progression of cerebral involvement. Intervals may be as short as every 15 minutes or as long as every 2 hours. Significant alterations are reported immediately. Temperature is taken every 2 to 4 hours, depending on the patient's condition.

An elevated temperature may occur in children with CNS dysfunction; therefore a light covering is sufficient. Vigorous efforts, such as tepid sponge baths or application of a hypothermia blanket, are needed to prevent brain damage if temperature exceeds 40° C (104° F) rectally.

The LOC is assessed periodically, including size, equality, and reaction of pupils to light. Signs of meningeal irritation such as nuchal rigidity are also assessed. Other aspects of LOC assessment include response to vocal commands, spontaneous behavior, resistance to care, and response to painful stimuli. Motions of any type, changes in muscle tone or strength, and body position are noted. Seizure activity is described according to the type and length of seizure and body areas involved. An antiepileptic drug such as phenytoin (Dilantin) or phenobarbital is ordered for control of seizure activity.

Pain management for the comatose child requires astute nursing observation and management. Signs of pain include changes in behavior (e.g., increased agitation and rigidity, alterations in physiologic parameters); increased heart rate, respiratory rate, and blood pressure; and decreased oxygen saturation. Since these findings are not specific for pain, the nurse should observe for their appearance during times of induced or suspected pain and their disappearance after the end of the inciting procedure or the administration of analgesia. A pain assessment record should be used to document indications of pain and the effectiveness of interventions (see Pain Assessment, Chapter 7).

The use of opioids, such as morphine, to relieve pain is controversial because they may mask signs of altered consciousness or depress respirations. However, unrelieved pain activates the stress response, which can elevate ICP. To block the stress response, some authorities advocate the use of analgesics, sedatives, and, in some cases such as head injury, paralyzing agents via continuous IV infusion. A frequently used combination is fentanyl, midazolam, and vecuronium (Norcuron). If there are concerns about assessing the LOC or respiratory depression, naloxone (Narcan) can be used to reverse the opioid effects. Acetaminophen and codeine may also be effective analgesics for mild to moderate pain. Regardless of which drugs are used, adequate dosage and regular administration are essential to provide optimal pain relief (see Pain Management, Chapter 7).

Other measures to relieve discomfort include providing a quiet, dimly lit environment; limiting visitors; preventing any sudden, jarring movement, such as banging into the bed; and preventing an increase in ICP. The last is most effectively achieved by proper positioning and prevention of straining, such as during coughing, vomiting, or defecating.

> **NURSINGALERT**
>
> When opioids are used, bowel elimination must be closely monitored because of the potential constipating effect. Stool softeners should be given with laxatives as needed to prevent constipation.

RESPIRATORY MANAGEMENT

Respiratory effectiveness is the primary concern in the care of the unconscious child, and establishment of an adequate airway is *always* the first priority. Carbon dioxide has a potent vasodilating effect and will increase cerebral blood flow (CBF) and ICP. Cerebral hypoxia that lasts longer than 4 minutes nearly always causes irreversible brain damage.

> **NURSINGALERT**
>
> Respiratory obstruction and subsequent compromise leads to cardiac arrest. Maintaining an adequate, patent airway is of the utmost importance.

Children in lighter states of coma may be able to cough and swallow, but those in deeper states are unable to handle secretions, which tend to pool in the throat and pharynx. Dysfunction of cranial nerves IX and X places the child at risk for aspiration and cardiac arrest; therefore the child is positioned to prevent aspiration of secretions, and the stomach is emptied to reduce the likelihood of vomiting. In infants, blockage of air passages from secretions can happen in seconds. In addition, upper airway obstruction from laryngospasm is a frequent complication in comatose children.

An oral airway can be used for the child who is suffering a temporary loss of consciousness, such as after a contusion, seizure, or anesthesia. For children who remain unconscious for a longer time, a nasotracheal or orotracheal tube is inserted to maintain the open airway and facilitate removal of secretions. A tracheostomy is performed in cases in which laryngoscopy for introduction of an endotracheal tube would be difficult or dangerous. Suctioning is used only as needed to clear the airway, exerting care to prevent increasing ICP. Respiratory status is observed and evaluated regularly. Signs of respiratory embarrassment may be an indication for ventilatory assistance.

When the respiratory center is involved, mechanical ventilation is usually indicated (see Chapter 22). Blood gas analysis is performed regularly, and oxygen is administered when indicated. Moderately severe hypoxia and respiratory acidosis are often present but are not always evident from clinical manifestations. Hyperventilation frequently accompanies unconsciousness and may lead to respiratory alkalosis, or it may represent the body's attempt to compensate for metabolic acidosis. Therefore blood gas and pH determinations are essential guides for electrolyte therapy. Chest physiotherapy is carried out on a regular basis, and the child's position is changed at least every 2 hours to prevent pulmonary complications.

INTRACRANIAL PRESSURE MONITORING

Management of the child with increased ICP is possibly the most formidable task and the most controversial subject in pediatric critical care. It appears that the outcome in pediatric neurologic injury may reflect the initial cerebral damage more than the subsequent intracranial hypertension. Of note, ICP gives little indication of the severity of the initial insult (Bayir, Kochanek, and Clark, 2003).

When increased ICP is a result of accumulation of CSF from obstruction of CSF flow, a ventricular tap will provide relief quickly and effectively. Evacuation of a hematoma reduces pressure from this source. Indications for inserting an ICP monitor are as follows:

■ GCS evaluation of 8
■ GCS evaluation of less than 8 with respiratory assistance
■ Deterioration of condition
■ Subjective judgment regarding clinical appearance and response

Four major types of ICP monitors are

1. Intraventricular catheter with fibroscopic sensors attached to a monitoring system
2. Subarachnoid bolt (Richmond screw)
3. Epidural sensor
4. Anterior fontanel pressure monitor.

Transducers for both ventricular and subarachnoid monitoring should be set up without the use of a flush device. Direct ventricular pressure measurement remains the gold standard of ICP monitoring.

The catheter method involves introduction of a catheter into the lateral ventricle on the nondominant side, if known, or placement in the subdural space. The catheter has the advantage of providing a means of extraventricular (or continuous) drainage to reduce pressure. A drainage bag attached to the system is kept at the level of the ventricles and can be lowered to decrease ICP (see Critical Thinking Exercise).

NURSINGALERT

If the external ventricular drain (EVD) is unclamped for CSF drainage, carefully monitor the level of the collection container. If the container is too low, improper CSF decompression could lower ICP too rapidly, causing bleeding and pain.

With the bolt method the end of the bolt is placed into the subarachnoid space. The bolt cannot be adequately secured in a small child's pliant skull, although special modifications have been developed for children younger than 6 years of age.

NURSINGALERT

The bolt is stabilized with dressings, but these are not changed or disturbed, even to check the site.

The placement of the bolt is not adjusted by anyone except the neurosurgeon who placed the device. The neurosurgeon is notified if a satisfactory waveform is not observed.

An epidural sensor can be placed between the dura and the skull through a burr hole and connected to a stopcock assembly and a transducer, which provides a readout of the pressure. Correlation of pressure readings is less invasive but may be inconsistent. In infants a fontanel transducer can be used to detect impulses from a pressure sensor and convert them to electrical energy. The electrical energy is then converted to visible waves or numeric readings on an oscilloscope. ICP measurement from the anterior fontanel is noninvasive but may prove to be inaccurate if the equipment is poorly placed or inconsistently recalibrated. The intraparenchymal pressure monitoring device (e.g., Camino) is a result of fiberoptic technology and performs reliably.

ICP can be increased by instillation of solutions; therefore antibiotics are administered systemically if a positive CSF culture is obtained. However, IV ICP monitoring rarely causes infection. Since CSF is a body fluid, standard precautions are implemented according to hospital policy (see Infection Control, Chapter 22).

Nurses caring for patients with intracranial monitoring devices must be acquainted with the system, assist with insertion, interpret the monitor readings, and be able to distinguish between danger signals and mechanical dysfunction.

??? CRITICAL THINKING EXERCISE

Hydrocephalus

Three-year-old Emma is 5 days postoperative for removal of a posterior fossa tumor. Although an external ventricular drain (EVD) was placed to treat her hydrocephalus, she continues to demonstrate signs of increased intracranial pressure (ICP), including holding the back of her head, anorexia, crying when moved or when strangers enter the room, and intermittent lethargy. On examination, fluid drainage is noted on the mother's clothes, and Emma is experiencing repetitive, rapid eyelid blinking.

QUESTIONS
1. Evidence—Is there sufficient evidence to draw conclusions about Emma's behavior, physical assessment findings, and ICP?
2. Assumptions—Describe any underlying assumption about each of the following:
   a. A preschool-age child who had a posterior fossa tumor removed 5 days ago
   b. A preschool-age child who has an EVD placed to treat the hydrocephalus
   c. A preschool-age child with an EVD who continues to demonstrate physical signs associated with increased ICP after recent surgery
3. What priorities for nursing care should be established?
4. Does the evidence support your nursing intervention?
5. What alternative perspectives might you have?

For increased ICP resulting from cerebral edema, several medical measures are available. Osmotic diuretics may provide rapid relief in emergency situations. Although their effect is transient, lasting only about 6 hours, they can be lifesaving in emergencies. These substances are rapidly excreted by the kidneys and carry with them large quantities of sodium and water. Mannitol (or sometimes urea) administered intravenously is the drug most frequently used for rapid reduction. The infusion is generally given slowly but may be pushed rapidly in cases of herniation or impending herniation. Because of the profound diuretic effect of the drug, an indwelling catheter is inserted to ensure bladder emptying. Adrenocorticosteroids are not recommended for cerebral edema secondary to head trauma. $Paco_2$ should be maintained at 25 to 30 mm Hg to produce vasoconstriction, which reduces CSF, thereby decreasing ICP.

Nursing Activities

In cases of high levels of increased ICP, nursing procedures tend to trigger reactive pressure waves in many patients. For example, increased intrathoracic or abdominal pressure will be transmitted to the cranium. Particular care should be taken in positioning these patients to avoid neck vein compression, which may further increase ICP by interfering with venous return.

The child can be propped to one side or the other, and the use of an alternating-pressure mattress reduces the chance of prolonged pressure to vulnerable areas. Frequent clinical assessment of the child cannot be replaced by an ICP monitoring device.

It is important to avoid activities that may increase ICP by causing pain or emotional stress. Gentle range-of-motion exercises can be carried out but should not be performed vigorously. Nontherapeutic touch can cause an increase in ICP. Any disturbing procedures to be performed should be scheduled to take advantage of therapies that reduce ICP, such as osmotherapy and sedation. Efforts are taken to minimize or eliminate environmental noise. Assessment and intervention to relieve pain are important nursing functions to decrease ICP. Individualizing nursing activities and minimizing environmental stimuli by decreasing noxious procedures help control ICP (El Bashir, Laundy, and Booy, 2003; Vernon-Levett, 1998).

Suctioning

Suctioning and percussion are poorly tolerated and are therefore contraindicated unless concurrent respiratory problems exist. Hypoxia and the Valsalva maneuver associated with cough both acutely elevate ICP. Vibration, which does not increase ICP, accomplishes excellent results and should be tried first if treatment is needed. If suctioning is necessary, it should be brief and preceded by hyperventilation with 100% oxygen, which can be monitored during suctioning with a pulse oxygen sensor reading to determine oxygen saturation.

NUTRITION AND HYDRATION

Fluids and calories are supplied initially by the IV route (see Chapter 22). An IV infusion is started early, and the type of fluid administered is determined by the patient's general condition. Fluid therapy requires careful monitoring and adjustment based on neurologic signs and electrolyte determinations. Often, comatose children are unable to cope with the same amounts of fluid they could tolerate at other times, and overhydration must be avoided to prevent fatal cerebral edema.

Hydration is maintained in the same manner (initially by IV and later by feeding tube). When cerebral edema is a threat, fluids may be restricted to reduce the chance of fluid overload. Skin and mucous membranes are examined for signs of dehydration. Observation for signs of altered fluid balance related to abnormal pituitary secretions is a part of nursing care.

Altered Pituitary Secretion

An altered ability to handle fluid loads is attributed in part to the syndrome of inappropriate antidiuretic hormone secretion (SIADH) and diabetes insipidus (DI) resulting from hypothalamic dysfunction (see Chapter 29). SIADH frequently accompanies CNS diseases such as head injury, meningitis, encephalitis, brain abscess, brain tumor, and subarachnoid hemorrhage. In the patient with SIADH, scant quantities of urine are excreted, electrolyte analysis reveals hyponatremia and hyposmolality, and manifestations of overhydration are evident. It is important to evaluate all parameters, since the reduced urinary output might be erroneously interpreted as a sign of dehydration.

The treatment of SIADH consists of restriction of fluids until serum electrolytes and osmolality return to normal levels. Since SIADH frequently occurs with meningitis in children, fluid restriction is often prescribed. Likewise, DI may occur after intracranial trauma. There is increased urine volume and the accompanying danger of dehydration. Adequate replacement of fluids is essential, and observation of electrolyte balance is necessary to detect signs of hypernatremia and hyperosmolality. Exogenous vasopressin may be administered.

MEDICATIONS

The cause of unconsciousness determines specific drug therapies. Children with infectious processes are given antibiotics appropriate to the disease and the infecting organism, and corticosteroids are prescribed for inflammatory conditions and edema. Cerebral edema is an indication for osmotherapy with osmotic diuretics. Sedatives or antiepileptics are prescribed for seizure activity (see p. 1008). Sedation in the combative child provides amnesic and anxiolytic properties in conjunction with a paralytic agent. The combination decreases ICP and allows treatment of cerebral edema. Usual drugs include morphine, midazolam, and pancuronium (Pavulon). Midazolam is attractive because of its short half-life.

Deep coma, induced by administration of barbiturates, is controversial in the management of ICP. Barbiturates are currently reserved for the reduction of increased ICP when all else has failed. Barbiturates decrease the cerebral metabolic rate for oxygen and protect the brain during times of reduced cerebral perfusion pressure. Barbiturate coma requires extensive monitoring, cardiovascular and respiratory support, and ICP monitoring to assess response to therapy. Paralyzing agents such as pancuronium also may be needed to aid in performing diagnostic tests, improving effectiveness of therapy, and reducing risks of secondary complications. Elevation of ICP and/or heart rate of patients who are being given paralyzing agents or are under sedation may indicate the need for another dose of either or both medications.

THERMOREGULATION

Hyperthermia often accompanies cerebral dysfunction; if it is present, measures are implemented to reduce the temperature to prevent brain damage and to reduce metabolic demands generated by the increased body temperature. Medically induced hypothermia assists in controlling ICP and may result in an improved outcome (Palmer, 2000). Antipyretics are the method of choice for fever reduction; cooling devices are used to induce hypothermia. Laboratory tests and other methods are used in an attempt to determine the cause, if any, of the hyperthermia.

ELIMINATION

A retention catheter is usually inserted in the acute phase, although diapers may be used and weighed to record urinary output. The child who formerly had bowel and bladder control is generally incontinent. If the child remains comatose for a long period, the indwelling catheter may be removed and periodic bladder emptying accomplished by intermittent catheterization. Stool softeners are usually sufficient to maintain bowel function, but suppositories or enemas may be needed occasionally for adequate elimination and to prevent an impaction. The passage of liquid stool after a period of no bowel activity is usually a sign of an impaction. To avoid this preventable problem, daily recording of bowel activity is essential.

HYGIENIC CARE

Routine measures for cleansing and maintaining skin integrity are an integral part of nursing care of the unconscious child (see Maintaining Healthy Skin, Chapter 22).

Mouth care is performed at least twice daily, since the mouth tends to become dry or coated with mucus. The teeth are carefully brushed with a soft toothbrush or cleaned with gauze saturated with saline. Commercially prepared cleansing devices, such as Toothettes, are convenient for cleansing the mouth and teeth. Lips are coated with ointment or other preparations to protect them from drying, cracking, or blistering.

The deeply comatose child is also prone to eye irritation. The corneal reflexes are absent; therefore the eyes are easily irritated or damaged by linen, dust, or other substances that may come in contact with them. There is excessive dryness as a result of incomplete closure of the eyes and/or decreased secretions, especially if the child is undergoing osmotherapy to reduce or prevent brain edema.

NURSINGALERT

The eyes should be examined regularly and carefully for early signs of irritation or inflammation. Artificial tears (methylcellulose) are placed in the eyes every 1 to 2 hours. Eye dressings may sometimes be needed to protect the eyes from possible damage.

POSITIONING AND EXERCISE

The unconscious child is positioned to prevent aspiration of saliva, nasogastric secretions, and vomitus and to minimize ICP. The head of the bed is elevated, and the child is placed in a side-lying or semiprone position. A small, firm pillow is placed under the head, and the uppermost limbs are flexed and supported with pillows. The weight of the body should not rest on the dependent arm. In the semiprone position the child lies with the dependent arm at the side behind the body, the opposite side supported on pillows, and the uppermost arm and leg flexed and resting on the pillows. This position prevents undue pressure on the dependent extremities. The dependent position of the face encourages drainage of secretions and prevents the flaccid tongue from obstructing the airway.

Normal range-of-motion exercises help maintain function and prevent contractures of joints. Exercises should be done gently and with full range of motion. A small rolled pad can be placed in the palms to help maintain proper position of fingers; footboards or boots can be used to help prevent footdrop; and splinting may be needed to prevent severe contractures of the wrist, knee, or ankle in decerebrate children.

STIMULATION

Sensory stimulation is important in the care of the unconscious child, just as it is in the care of the alert child. For the temporarily unconscious or semiconscious child, sensory stimulation helps arouse the child to the conscious state and orient the child in terms of time and place. Auditory and tactile stimulation are especially valuable. Tactile stimulation is not appropriate for the child in whom it may elicit an undesirable response. However, for other children tactile contact often has a relaxing and calming effect. When the child's condition permits, holding or rocking has a soothing effect and provides the body contact needed by young children.

The auditory sense is often present in a state of coma. Hearing is the last sense to be lost and the first one to be regained; therefore the child should be spoken to as any other child. Conversation around the child should not include thoughtless or derogatory remarks. A radio playing soft music or a music box or CD player is frequently used to provide auditory stimulation. Singing the child's favorite songs or reading a favorite story is a tactic used to maintain the child's contact with a familiar world. Playing songs or stories recorded in the parents' voices can provide a continuous source of familiar stimulation.

Regaining Consciousness

Awakening from a coma is a gradual process; however, sometimes children regain consciousness within a short time. Regaining orientation involves knowing person, place, and time, in that order.

Certain behaviors have been observed when children awaken from the unconscious state. The stress and anxiety they appear to feel in a strange and unfamiliar environment are consistently expressed in silent and withdrawn behavior. Children respond to basic questioning but usually do not display their prehospitalization personality and social behavior until they are transferred from the critical care area.

FAMILY SUPPORT

Helping parents of an unconscious child cope with the situation is especially difficult. They may demonstrate all the guilt, fear, hostility, and anxiety of any parent of a seriously ill child (see Chapter 18). In addition, these parents are faced with the uncertain outcome of the cerebral dysfunction. The fear of death, intellectual disability, or other permanent disability is present. Nursing intervention with parents depends on the nature of the pathologic condition, the parents' personality, and the parent-child relationship before the injury or illness.

If there is little or no residual effect, the child will be dismissed to home care fairly soon. The parents need the most intensive nursing intervention during the period of crisis and uncertainty. During the recovery phase they are given information, information is clarified, and they are encouraged to become involved in the child's care. Often the child's hospitalization is brief; however, some children require extended hospitalization for intensive therapy and rehabilitation.

Like parents who lose a child through death, the parents of the child lost to their world attempt to reconstitute a representation of the child. They bring items that belong to the child, such as favorite toys, music, and other objects cherished by the child. This is interpreted as an attempt to provide stimulation for the child in the hope of eliciting a response, to let the hospital staff know the child as the unique individual he or she was so that the parents' distress can be better appreciated, and to reconstitute an image of the child "lost" to them and for whom they mourn. An awareness of these behaviors and coping mechanisms provides nurses with the understanding that helps them support the parents in their grief process.

Superimposed on the process of grieving for the "lost" child, parents may be faced with difficult decisions. When the child's brain is so severely damaged that vital functions must be maintained by artificial means, the parents must make the final decision of whether to remove life-support systems. Since the decision is so difficult for parents, the practitioner is frequently placed in a position of making the decision indirectly. After providing the parents with all of the information, the practitioner will suggest that the child be removed from the life support to "see if the child can make it without help." The approach relieves the parents of the decision and can be effective, but it is based on an evaluation of the parents' intellectual level and emotional state. Sometimes parents may even choose to refuse treatment if they believe it to be best for the child and the family (informed dissent). At other times parents request that "everything possible" be done for the child.

When the child has survived the cerebral insult and is not comatose, but physical and/or mental capacity is limited, either minimally or severely, families must cope with the long and tedious rehabilitation process and the uncertain outcome. The drain on financial, emotional, and social resources can be enormous.

For parents who choose to care for their child at home, planning for home care begins early in the recovery process. The family should become involved with the child's care as soon as they indicate an interest and ability to do so. They need education and support in learning to care for the child, regular follow-up observation and assessment of the home management, and planning for some respite care of the child. Parents need to understand that it is important to plan for periodic relief from the continual care of the child (see Preparing for Discharge and Home Care, Chapter 21; and Family-Centered Home Care, Chapter 20).

CEREBRAL TRAUMA

HEAD INJURY

Head injury is a pathologic process involving the scalp, skull, meninges, or brain as a result of mechanical force. According to national statistics and Safe Kids Worldwide,* injuries are the number one health risk for children and the leading cause of death in children older than 1 year of age. Yearly, one in four children in the United States will suffer an injury serious enough to require medical attention. Tragically, 8000 children are killed every year by injuries. It has been estimated that 300 per 100,000 children per year have a traumatic brain injury and that 10 per 100,000 children per year die as a result of the brain injury. Studies indicate that as many as three fourths of the childhood deaths caused by mechanical trauma are the direct result of a brain injury. There is evidence to demonstrate that a previous head injury increases a child's risk of having a subsequent head injury (Swaine, Tremblay, Platt, and others, 2007).

Etiology

The three major causes of brain damage in childhood, in order of importance, are falls, motor vehicle injuries, and bicycle injuries. Neurologic injury accounts for the highest mortality rate, with boys affected twice as often as girls. In motor vehicle accidents children younger than 2 years of age are almost exclusively injured as passengers, whereas older children may also be injured as pedestrians or cyclists. The majority of deaths from brain trauma caused by bicycle injuries occur between the ages of 5 and 19 years. Bicycle helmet laws have been effective in reducing the risk of head injury by 85% and brain injury by 88% (Rivara and Grossman, 2007).

The exposed nature of the head renders it particularly vulnerable to external violence, and many of the physical characteristics of children predispose them to craniocerebral trauma. For example, infants are frequently left unattended on beds, in high chairs, and in other places from which they can fall. Because the head of an infant or toddler is proportionately larger and heavier in relation to other body parts, it is the most likely to be injured. Incomplete motor development contributes to falls at young ages, and the natural curiosity and exuberance of children also increase their risk of injury.

Pathophysiology

The pathology of brain injury is directly related to the force of impact. Intracranial contents (brain, blood, CSF) are damaged because the force is too great to be absorbed by the skull and musculoligamentous support of the head. The elastic, pliable skull of the infant and young child absorbs much of the direct energy of physical impact to the head and affords some protection to intracranial structures. Although nervous tissue is delicate, it usually requires a severe blow to cause significant damage.

A child's response to head injury is different from that of an adult. The larger head size and insufficient musculoskeletal support render the very young child particularly vulnerable to acceleration-deceleration injuries.

Primary head injuries are those that occur at the time of trauma and include skull fracture, contusions, intracranial hematoma, and diffuse injury. Subsequent complications include hypoxic brain damage, increased ICP, infection, and cerebral edema. The predominant feature of a child's brain injury is the amount of diffuse swelling that occurs. Hypoxia and hypercapnia threaten the energy requirements of the brain and increase CBF. The added volume across the blood-brain barrier, along with the loss of autoregulation, exacerbates cerebral edema. Pressure inside the skull that is greater than arterial pressure results in inadequate perfusion.

Cerebral hyperemia occurs more often in children than adults, and this volume expansion may account for their tendency to develop intracranial hypertension. However, because the cranium of very young children has the ability to expand and the thin skull is more compliant, they may tolerate increases in ICP better than older children and adults do. Children have a significantly higher percentage of good outcomes, a lower mortality rate, and a lower incidence of surgical mass lesions after severe head trauma. However, their thinner, softer skull may sustain greater long-term damage than previously suggested.

Physical forces act on the head through **acceleration, deceleration,** or **deformation.** Acceleration or deceleration is more descriptive of the circumstances responsible for most head injuries. When the stationary head receives a blow, the sudden acceleration causes deformation of the skull and mass movement of the brain. Continued movement of the intracranial contents allows the brain to strike parts of the skull (e.g., the sharp edges of the sphenoid or the irregular surface of the anterior fossa) or the edges of the tentorium.

Although the brain volume remains unchanged, significant distortion takes place as the brain changes shape in response to the force of impact to the skull. This movement can cause bruising at the point of impact (**coup**) and/or at a distance as

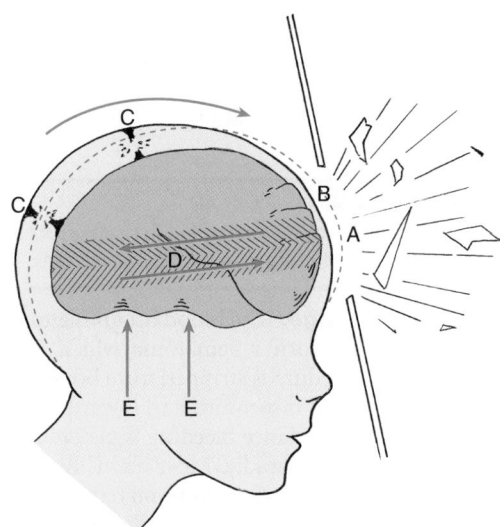

FIG. 28-4 ■ Mechanical distortion of cranium during closed head injury. *A,* Preinjury contour of skull. *B,* Immediate postinjury contour of skull. *C,* Torn subdural vessels. *D,* Shearing forces. *E,* Trauma from contact with floor of cranium. (Redrawn from Grubb RL, Coxe WS: Central nervous system trauma: cranial. In Eliasson SG, Presky AL, Hardin Jr WB, editors: *Neurological pathophysiology,* New York, 1974, Oxford University Press.)

FIG. 28-5 ■ **A,** Epidural (extradural) hematoma and compression of temporal lobe through tentorial hiatus. **B,** Subdural hematoma.

the brain collides with the unyielding surfaces far removed from the point of impact (**contrecoup**) (Fig. 28-4). Thus a blow to the occipital region can cause severe injury to the frontal and temporal areas of the brain. Sudden deceleration, such as takes place during a fall, causes the greatest cerebral injury at the point of impact. Children with an acceleration-deceleration injury demonstrate diffuse generalized cerebral swelling produced by increased blood volume or a redistribution of cerebral blood volume (cerebral hyperemia) rather than by increased water content (edema), as seen in adults.

Another effect of brain movement is shearing stresses, which may tear small arteries and cause subdural hemorrhages. Damage can also occur when severe compression of the skull causes the brain to be forced through the tentorial opening. This can produce irreparable damage to the brainstem (Fig. 28-5).

Concussion. The most common head injury is **concussion,** a transient and reversible neuronal dysfunction, with instantaneous loss of awareness and responsiveness, that results from trauma to the head and persists for a relatively short time, usually minutes or hours. It is generally followed by amnesia for the moment of the injury and a variable period after the injury. The common misconception that loss of consciousness is the hallmark of concussion is not true, especially for children. Concussion is correctly defined as a traumatically induced alteration in mental status. Confusion and amnesia following head injury are the hallmarks of concussion.

The pathogenesis of concussion is still unclear but may be a result of shearing forces that cause stretching, compression, and tearing of nerve fibers, particularly in the area of the central brainstem, the seat of the reticular activating system. It has also been suggested that the anatomic alterations of nerve fibers cause the release of large quantities of acetylcholine into the CSF and a reduction in oxygen consumption with increased lactate production.

Contusion and Laceration. The terms **contusion** and **laceration** are used to describe visible bruising and tearing of cerebral tissue. Contusions represent petechial hemorrhages along the superficial aspects of the brain at the site of impact (coup injury) or a lesion remote from the site of direct trauma (contrecoup injury). In serious accidents there may be multiple sites of injury.

The major areas of the brain susceptible to contusion or laceration are the occipital, frontal, and temporal lobes. Also, the irregular surfaces of the anterior and middle fossae at the base of the skull are capable of producing bruises or lacerations on forceful impact. Contusions may cause focal disturbances in strength, sensation, or visual awareness. The degree of brain damage in the contused areas varies according to the extent of vascular injury. Signs will vary from mild, transient weakness of a limb to prolonged unconsciousness and paralysis. However, the signs and symptoms may be clinically indistinguishable from those of concussion.

The lower incidence of cerebral contusion in infancy has been attributed to the infant's pliable skull with less convolutional markings of the inner space between brain tissue and bone. In addition, the infant's brain tissue has a softer consistency, which also reduces surface injury. However, infants who are roughly shaken (shaken baby syndrome) can sustain profound neurologic impairment, seizures, retinal hemorrhages, and intracranial subarachnoid or subdural hemorrhages. In addition to these classic injuries, high cervical spinal cord hemorrhages and contusions can occur.

Cerebral lacerations are generally associated with penetrating or depressed skull fractures. However, they may occur without fracture in small children. When brain tissue is actually torn, with bleeding into and around the tear, usually more severe and prolonged unconsciousness and paralysis occur, leaving permanent scarring and some degree of disability.

Fractures. Because of its flexibility, the immature skull is able to sustain a greater degree of deformation than the adult skull before it incurs a fracture. A great deal of force is required to produce a fracture in an infant's skull. However, the undersurface of the skull contains grooves in which the meningeal arteries lie. A fracture that runs through one of these grooves may tear the artery and produce severe and damaging hemorrhage. Hypovolemic hypotension can occur in infants with skull fractures.

The types of fractures that occur are as follows:

Linear fractures are those in which the lines of the fracture are predetermined by the site and velocity of the impact, as well as by the strength of the bone. These are uncommon before 2 to 3 years of age but constitute the majority of childhood skull fractures. Most linear skull fractures are associated with an overlying hematoma or soft-tissue swelling (Schutzman and Greenes, 2001).

Depressed fractures are those in which the bone is locally broken, usually into several irregular fragments that are pushed inward, causing pressure on the brain. The inner portion of the bone is more extensively fragmented than the outer portion, which almost invariably produces tears in the dura. These are uncommon before 2 to 3 years of age. In infants and very young children, the soft, malleable bone may become dented in a peculiar rounded or "Ping-Pong ball" depression, without laceration of either skin or dura.

Comminuted fractures consist of multiple associated linear fractures. They usually result from intense impact. These types of fractures often result from repeated blows against an object and may suggest child abuse.

Basilar fractures involve the basilar portion of the frontal, ethmoid, sphenoid, temporal, or occipital bones. Because of the proximity of the fracture line to structures surrounding the brainstem, this is a serious head injury. Approximately 80% of the cases may include clinical features such as subcutaneous bleeding in the posterior neck area and over the mastoid process (battle sign). Bleeding around the eyes (raccoon eyes) or bleeding behind the tympanic membrane (hemotympanum) may occur.

Open fractures cause communication between the skull and the scalp or the surfaces of the upper respiratory tract. Open fractures increase the risk of CNS infection. They may have an overlying laceration called a *compound fracture.* Open fractures can also create an opening in the paranasal sinuses or middle ear that can lead to CSF rhinorrhea or otorrhea. Facial paralysis, vertigo, tinnitus, or hearing loss may develop.

Diastatic fractures are traumatic separations of the cranial sutures. These most frequently affect the lambdoid suture and are rarely seen beyond the first 3 years of life. They require no specific treatment but should be observed for "growing fractures." Growing fractures are skull fractures associated with an underlying dural tear that may be caused by a leptomeningeal cyst, dilated ventricles, or a herniated brain. Neurologic symptoms include headache, seizures, and asymmetric cranial growth (Schutzman and Greenes, 2001). Infants and young children who have isolated skull fractures should be evaluated for growing skull fractures from 1 to 2 months after the injury (Schutzman and Greenes, 2001).

Complications

The major complications of trauma to the head are hemorrhage, infection, edema, and herniation through the tentorium. Infection is always a hazard in open injuries, and edema is related to tissue trauma. Vascular rupture may occur even in minor head injuries, causing hemorrhage between the skull and cerebral surfaces. Compression of the underlying brain produces effects that can be rapidly fatal or insidiously progressive.

> **NURSINGALERT**
>
> Posttraumatic meningitis should be suspected in children with increasing drowsiness and fever who also have basilar skull fractures.

Epidural Hemorrhage. The blood accumulates between the dura and the skull to form a hematoma, which, because of the difficulty with which dura is stripped from bone, forces the underlying brain contents downward and inward as the brain expands (see Fig. 28-5, *A*). Since bleeding is generally arterial, brain compression occurs rapidly. Most often the expanding hematoma is located in the parietotemporal region, forcing the medial portion of the temporal lobe under the edge of the tentorium, where it causes pressure on nerves and blood vessels. The lower incidence of epidural hematoma in childhood has been attributed to the fact that the middle meningeal artery is not embedded in the bone surface of the skull until approximately 2 years of age. Therefore a fracture of the temporal bone is less likely to lacerate the artery. Second, the dura closely adheres to the inner table of the skull, especially at the level of the sutures, making separation from bleeding less likely. However, a child's skull can be indented with sufficient force to tear the middle meningeal artery and rebound intact without causing a fracture. Hemorrhage can also derive from dural veins or the dural sinuses, especially in infants and small children, in whom fracture is less likely to occur. In 20% to 40% of children a skull fracture is not detectable. The classic clinical picture of epidural hemorrhage (momentary unconsciousness followed by a normal period, then lethargy or coma) is seldom evident in children (see Box 28-3 for clinical manifestations). The period of impaired consciousness is frequently lacking, and the symptom-free period is atypical because of nonspecific complaints such as irritability, headache, and vomiting. When it does occur, the symptom-free period frequently lasts longer than 48 hours.

Clinically significant epidural hematomas are uncommon in children younger than 4 years of age. These differences may be caused by the decreased tendency of the resilient skull to fracture; the ability of blood to escape through widened sutures, an open fontanel, or a fracture; bleeding from smaller vessels with less rapid and massive bleeding; lower systolic blood pressure in children; and possibly the decreased susceptibility of the child's brain to pressure changes.

Subdural Hemorrhage. A subdural hemorrhage is bleeding between the dura and the cerebrum, usually as a result of rupture of cortical veins that bridge the subdural space (see Fig. 28-5, *B*). Subdural hematomas are 10 times more frequent than epidural hematomas, occurring most often in infancy, with a peak incidence at 6 months.

Unlike epidural hemorrhage, which develops inwardly against the less resistant brain tissue, subdural hemorrhage tends to develop more slowly and spreads thinly and widely until it is limited by the dural barriers—the falx and tentorium. Subdural hematoma is fairly common in infants, frequently as a result of birth trauma, falls, assaults, or violent shaking. The small subdural space and dura firmly attached to the skull in this area are highly vulnerable to increased ICP.

BOX 28-3
Clinical Manifestations of Acute Head Injury

MINOR INJURY
May or may not lose consciousness
Transient period of confusion
Somnolence
Listlessness
Irritability
Pallor
Vomiting

SIGNS OF PROGRESSION
Altered mental status (e.g., difficulty rousing child)
Mounting agitation
Development of focal lateral neurologic signs (p. 990)
Marked changes in vital signs

SEVERE INJURY
Signs of increased intracranial pressure (see Box 28-1)
Increased head size (infant)
Bulging or full fontanel (infant)
Retinal hemorrhage
Extraocular palsies (especially cranial nerve VI)
Hemiparesis
Quadriplegia
Elevated temperature
Unsteady gait (older child)
Papilledema (older child)
Retinal hemorrhages

ASSOCIATED SIGNS
Scalp trauma
Other injuries (e.g., to extremities)

NURSINGALERT
Children with a subdural hematoma and retinal hemorrhages should be evaluated for the possibility of child abuse, especially shaken baby syndrome.

Repeated subdural taps often provide relief in the infant, as revealed by follow-up CT scans, improved neurologic status, and a flat anterior fontanel. Surgical evacuation of the hematoma is the treatment of choice in the older child and is frequently required in infants.

Cerebral Edema. Some degree of brain edema is expected, especially 24 to 72 hours after craniocerebral trauma. Cerebral edema caused by direct cellular injury or vascular injury induces vascular stasis, anoxia, and further vasodilation. If the progression continues unchecked, ICP exceeds arterial pressure and fatal anoxia ensues, and/or the pressure causes herniation of a portion of the brain over the edge of the tentorium, compressing the brainstem and occluding the posterior cerebral arteries. Diffuse cerebral swelling and changes in CBF are common patterns after head injury in children.

NURSINGALERT
If a child loses consciousness or vomits more than three times, medical attention should be sought.

Diagnostic Evaluation

A detailed history, especially a health history, both past and present, is essential in evaluating the child with a craniocerebral trauma. Certain disorders, such as drug allergies, hemophilia, diabetes mellitus, or epilepsy, may produce similar symptoms. Furthermore, even minor traumatic injury can aggravate a preexisting disease process. Events surrounding the injury often supply significant data. It must be determined whether the infant or child exhibited alterations in consciousness; any other signs and behaviors exhibited by the child must be noted. Since head injuries are frequently accompanied by injuries in other areas, the examination is performed with care to avoid further damage.

NURSINGALERT
Stabilize a child's spine after head injury until a spinal cord injury is ruled out.

Initial Assessment. Priorities in the initial stabilization phase of a child with a head injury include assessment of the ABCs (airway, breathing, circulation); evaluation for shock; a neurologic examination, especially LOC; assessment of pupillary symmetry and response to light; and observation for seizures (Bayir, Kochanek, and Clark, 2003). The assessment is carried out quickly in relation to vital signs (see Emergency Treatment box). Excited and irritable children may have a rapid pulse, hyperventilate, appear pale, and feel clammy shortly after an injury.

NURSINGALERT
Deep, rapid, periodic, or intermittent and gasping respirations; wide fluctuations or noticeable slowing of the pulse; and widening pulse pressure or extreme fluctuations in blood pressure are signs of brainstem involvement. Note that marked hypotension may represent internal injuries.

Ocular signs such as fixed and dilated pupils, fixed and constricted pupils, and pupils that are poorly reactive or nonreactive to light and accommodation indicate increased ICP or brainstem involvement. It is important to remain with the child who demonstrates fixed and dilated pupils, since these are ominous signs, with the probability of respiratory arrest. Dilated, nonpulsating blood vessels indicate increased ICP before the appearance of papilledema. Retinal hemorrhages are seen in acute head injuries.

NURSINGALERT
Observation of asymmetric pupils or one dilated, nonreactive pupil in a comatose child is a neurosurgical emergency.

Less urgent but important additional assessments include examination of the scalp for lacerations and palpation for other abnormalities. A significant amount of blood loss can occur from scalp lacerations.

NURSINGALERT
Bleeding from the nose or ears needs further evaluation, and a watery discharge from the nose (rhinorrhea) that is positive for glucose (as tested with Dextrostix) suggests leaking of CSF from a skull fracture.

An accurate assessment of clinical signs provides baseline information. Serial evaluations, preferably by a single ob-

Head Injury

Assess child:

    A—Airway (with cervical-spine immobilization)

        Use jaw thrust to open airway

    B—Bleeding

    C—Circulation

Clean any abrasions with soap and water.

- Apply clean dressing.
- If bleeding, apply ice to relieve pain and swelling.

Keep NPO (nothing by mouth) until instructed otherwise.

Assess pain, but do not give analgesics or sedatives.

Check pupil reaction every 4 hours (including twice during night) for 48 hours.

Awaken twice during the night to check level of consciousness.

Seek medical attention if any of the following apply:

- Injury sustained:
  - —At high speed (e.g., automobile)
  - —Fall from a significant distance (e.g., roof, tree, or height greater than that of the child)
  - —From great force (e.g., baseball bat)
  - —Under suspicious circumstances
- Loss of consciousness
- Amnesia
- Discomfort (crying) more than 10 minutes after injury
- Headache that is severe, worsening, interferes with sleep
- Fluid leak from ears or nose
- Vomiting three or more times
- Swelling in front of or above earlobe or increased swelling
- Confusion or not behaving normally
- Difficult to arouse from sleep
- Difficulty speaking
- Blurred vision or seeing double
- Unsteady gait
- Difficulty using extremities
- Neck pain
- Pupils dilated, unequal, or fixed
- Infant with full or bulging fontanel
- Bruising below the eyes

server, help to detect changes in the neurologic status. Alterations in mental status, evidenced by increased difficulty in rousing the child, mounting agitation, development of focal lateral neurologic signs, or marked changes in vital signs, usually indicate extension or progression of the basic pathologic process.

Special Tests. After a thorough clinical examination, a variety of diagnostic tests are helpful in providing a more definitive diagnosis of the type and extent of the trauma. The severity of a head injury may not be apparent on clinical examination of a child, but it will be detectable on a CT scan. Whenever the child has a history consistent with a serious head injury (unrestrained occupant in a severe motor vehicle accident or a fall from a significant height), it is important that a scan be performed even if the child initially appears alert and oriented. All children with head injuries who have any alteration of consciousness, headache, vomiting, skull fracture, seizure, or a predisposing medical condition should also undergo CT scanning.

MRI and neurobehavioral assessment following early head injury may be useful in documenting cognitive impairment in relation to structural alterations in the young brain. MRI provides details of soft tissues better than any other noninvasive device. Electroencephalography is not particularly helpful for early diagnosis but is useful for defining seizure activity or focal destructive lesions after the acute phase of illness. Lumbar puncture is rarely used in craniocerebral trauma and is contraindicated in the presence of increased ICP because of the possibility of herniation. In some centers monitoring ICP is part of the assessment.

Posttraumatic Syndromes. Posttraumatic syndromes can be clinically manifested because of structural complications resulting from a head injury and through the signs and symptoms demonstrated by the child. Structural complications can include hydrocephalus and focal deficits such as optic atrophy, cranial nerve palsies, motor deficits, DI, aphasia, and seizures. Behavioral disturbances include sleep disturbances, phobias, emotional lability, altered school performance, and changes related to aggressiveness or withdrawal. **Postconcussion syndrome** is a common sequela to brain injury and can occur within minutes to an hour after a head injury. The manifestations vary with the child's age. The syndrome occurs frequently in children younger than 1 year of age. The syndrome in adolescents is similar to that in adults. The duration of manifestations can vary from several days to several months. Death from concussion is preventable unless overwhelming secondary brain injury has occurred (Durkin, Olsen, Barlow, and others, 1998; Gennarelli, 1999).

Posttraumatic seizures occur in a number of children who survive a head injury and are more common in children than in adults. Seizures are more likely to occur within the first few days of the head injury (Chiaretti, De Benedictis, Polidori, and others, 2000). **Structural complications** (e.g., hydrocephalus) may occur after a head injury. The type of residual effect depends on the location and nature of the disorder. True intellectual disability occurs only after severe injuries.

Therapeutic Management

The majority of children with mild to moderate concussion who have not lost consciousness can be cared for and observed at home after careful examination reveals no serious intracranial injury. Nurses should provide parents with clear explanations and instructions and should encourage them to ask questions both before and after leaving the medical facility if clarification is needed (see Family Focus box).

The parents are instructed to check the child every 2 hours to determine any changes in responsiveness. The sleeping child should be wakened to see if he or she can be roused normally. Parents are advised to maintain contact with the health professional, who usually wishes to examine the child again in 1 or 2 days. The manifestations of epidural hematoma in children do not generally appear until 24 hours or more after injury.

Children with severe injuries, those who have lost consciousness for more than a few minutes, and those with prolonged and continued seizures or other focal or diffuse neurologic signs must be hospitalized until their condition is stable and their neurologic signs have diminished.

The child is maintained on nothing by mouth (NPO) or restricted to clear liquids, if able to take fluids by mouth, until it is determined that vomiting will not occur. IV fluids are

FAMILY FOCUS

Maintaining Contact

Maintaining contact with parents for continued observation and reevaluation of the child, when indicated, facilitates early diagnosis and treatment of possible complications from head injury, such as hematoma, hydrocephalus, cysts, and posttraumatic seizures. Children are generally hospitalized for 24 to 48 hours' observation if their family lives far from medical facilities or lacks transportation or a telephone that would provide access to immediate help. Other circumstances such as language or other communication barriers, or even emotional trauma, may hinder learning and make it difficult for families to feel confident in caring for their child at home.

indicated in the child who is comatose or displays dulled sensorium and in the child with persistent vomiting. Fluid balance is closely monitored by daily weights; accurate intake and output measurements; and serum osmolality to detect early signs of water retention, excessive dehydration, and states of hypertonicity or hypotonicity.

The volume of IV fluid is carefully monitored to avoid aggravating any cerebral edema and to minimize the possibility of overhydration in case of SIADH. However, damage to the hypothalamus or pituitary gland may produce DI with its accompanying hypertonicity and dehydration.

Restlessness can be satisfactorily managed, if necessary, with mild sedation, and headache is usually controlled with acetaminophen (Tylenol). Antiepileptics are used for seizure control and frequently in cases of suspected contusion or laceration. Antibiotics may be administered if lacerations, CSF leakage, or excessive cerebral tissue damage is present. Prophylactic tetanus toxoid is given as appropriate. Cerebral edema is managed as described for the unconscious child. Hyperthermia is controlled with tepid sponges or a hypothermia blanket.

Surgical Therapy. Scalp lacerations are sutured after the underlying bone is carefully examined. Depressed fractures require surgical reduction and removal of bone fragments. Torn dura is sutured. Ping-Pong ball skull fractures in very young infants ordinarily correct themselves within a few weeks and do not require specific treatment, although they can be reduced by pressure against the bone.

Prognosis. The outcome of craniocerebral trauma depends on the extent of injury and complications. However, the outlook is generally more favorable for children than for adults (Faillace, 2002; Masson, Thicoipe, Mokni, and others, 2003). More than 90% of children with concussions or simple linear fractures recover without symptoms after the initial period. The incidence of fatalities and neurologic sequelae is lower in children than in adults, even in those with severe head injuries. The prognosis for recovery is primarily related to the duration of coma and the degree of injury. The combination of impaired consciousness and skull fracture carries the highest risk of complication.

The concern regarding outcome is increasingly focused on cognitive, emotional, and mental problems. Children experience a higher frequency of psychologic disturbances after head injury, whereas adults are more prone to physical complaints. Children may be more vulnerable than adults to long-term cognitive and behavioral dysfunction after diffuse brain injury. Even with recovery, the effects of brain injury on a child's potential can never be known.

True coma (not obeying commands, eyes closed, and not speaking) usually does not last more than 2 weeks. A child's eventual outcome can range from brain death to a persistent vegetative state to complete recovery. However, even the best recovery may be associated with personality changes, including mood lability and loss of confidence; impaired short-term memory; headaches; and subtle cognitive impairments. Many children are left with significant disabilities after head injury that appear months later as learning difficulties, behavioral changes, or emotional disturbances (Faillace, 2002). Generally, within 6 months to 1 year after the injury, 90% of the long-term neurologic outcome has been achieved.

Nursing Care Management

The hospitalized child requires careful neurologic assessment and evaluation (including vital signs) repeated at frequent intervals to provide information needed to establish a correct diagnosis, reveal signs and symptoms of increased ICP, determine clinical management, prevent many complications, and provide support to the child and family during the recovery phases.

The child is placed on bed rest, usually with the head of the bed elevated slightly. Appropriate safety measures, such as side rails kept up and seizure precautions for children of all ages, are implemented. For the extremely restless child, hard surfaces may have to be padded and restraint used to prevent the possibility of further injury. Care is individualized according to the child's specific needs. The unconscious child is managed as described in the previous section, but most childhood head injuries are those causing momentary stunning or temporary unconsciousness. Children may be restless and irritable, but more often their reaction is to fall asleep when left undisturbed. A quiet environment helps reduce restlessness and irritability. Shining bright lights directly into the child's face is irritating and often aggravates the child, making assessment of ocular responses difficult.

Frequent examinations of vital signs, neurologic signs, and LOC are extremely important nursing observations. When possible, they should be performed by a single observer to better detect subtle changes that may indicate worsening neurologic status. Pupils are checked for size, equality, reaction to light, and accommodation. After the initial elevations usually seen following injury, the vital signs generally return to normal unless there is brainstem involvement. An axillary measurement of temperature is the safest method, since seizures are not uncommon and vomiting is a frequent response in children, especially when the child is disturbed.

The most important nursing observation is assessment of the child's LOC. Alterations in consciousness appear earlier in the progression of an injury than alterations of vital signs or focal neurologic signs. Some expected responses may be misinterpreted as deviations from the normal. Frequent examinations of alertness are fatiguing to the child; therefore the child often desires to fall asleep, which may be confused with depressed consciousness. When left alone, the child goes to sleep. It is not uncommon to observe ocular divergence through the partially closed eyelids.

A key nursing role is to provide sedation and analgesia for the child. The conflict between the need to promote comfort and relieve anxiety in the child vs the need to assess for neurologic changes presents a dilemma. However, both goals can be achieved with close observation of the child's LOC and response to analgesics, use of a pain assessment record, and effective communication with the practitioner. To differentiate between sedation from an opioid and sedation from the injury, naloxone can be given *slowly* to reverse the opioid's sedative effect. Decreasing restlessness after administration of an analgesic most likely reflects pain control rather than a declining LOC.

Observations of position and movement provide additional information. Any abnormal posturing is noted, as well as whether it occurs continuously or intermittently. Are the child's handgrips strong and equal in strength? Are there any signs of flexion or extension posturing? What is the child's response to stimulation? Is movement purposeful, random, or absent? Are movement and sensation equal on both sides or restricted to one side only?

The child may complain of headache or other discomfort. The child who is too young to describe a headache will be fussy and resist being handled. The child who suffers from vertigo will often assume a position of comfort and vigorously resist efforts to be moved. Forcible movement causes the child to vomit and display spontaneous nystagmus. Seizures, relatively common in children with craniocerebral trauma, may be of any type but are more often generalized, regardless of the type of injury. Any seizure activity should be carefully observed and described in detail. Children in postictal (postseizure) states are lethargic, with sluggish pupils.

Drainage from any orifice is noted. Bleeding from the ear suggests the possibility of a basal skull fracture. The amount and characteristics of the drainage are observed, and since the auditory canal may be a source of infection, dry, sterile cotton can be placed loosely at the orifice and changed when soiled.

NURSING ALERT

Suctioning through the nares is contraindicated because of the risk of the catheter entering the brain parenchyma through a fracture in the skull.

Head trauma is frequently accompanied by other undetected injuries; therefore any bruises, lacerations, or evidence of internal injuries or fractures of the extremities are noted and reported. Associated injuries are evaluated and treated appropriately.

The child with normal LOC is usually allowed clear liquids unless fluid is restricted. If the child has an IV infusion, it is maintained as prescribed. The diet is advanced to that appropriate for the child's age as soon as the condition permits. Intake and output are measured and recorded, and any incontinence of bowel or bladder is noted in the child who has been toilet trained.

The child should be observed for any unusual behavior, but behavior should be interpreted in relation to the child's normal behavior. For example, urinary incontinence during sleep would be of no consequence in a child who routinely wets the bed but would be highly significant for one who is always dry. In addition, a child who is subject to nightmares might cry out and demonstrate agitated behavior at night. There would be less concern about a child who falls asleep several times during the day if this were consistent with the child's usual behavior. Parents are valuable resources. Information obtained from parents at or shortly after admission is helpful in evaluating the child's behavior (e.g., the ease with which the child is roused normally, the usual sleeping position, how much the child sleeps during the day, motor activity the child is capable of [rolling over, sitting up, climbing], hearing and visual acuity, appetite, and manner of eating [spoon, bottle, cup]).

Family Support. The emotional and educational support of the family of children who have suffered head injury presents a formidable, challenging aspect to nursing care. Witnessing the parents' ordeal of grief and helplessness on seeing their child in an altered state, connected to monitoring equipment in an intensive care unit, evokes empathy. The nurse can encourage the family to be involved in the child's care, to bring in familiar belongings, or to make a tape recording of familiar voices and sounds. Parents may need a demonstration on how to touch or cuddle their child and may want to talk about their grief. The nurse can listen attentively, reinforce what is being done to assist the child, and direct parents toward signs and symptoms of recovery to instill hope without promises. A common phenomenon is for families to seek information from all health care providers, asking, "What will she be like? What do you know?" as they search for some clue that the child is recovering. Honesty and kindness, along with competent care, distinguish excellent nursing abilities.

When the child is discharged, the parents are advised of probable posttraumatic symptoms that may be expected, such as behavioral changes, sleep disturbances, phobias, and seizures. They should understand observations they need to make and how to contact the physician, nurse, or health facility in case the child develops any unusual signs or symptoms. The importance of follow-up evaluation should be emphasized. It is often advisable to refer the family to a public health agency for home follow-through to be certain that the child receives posthospital evaluation.

Rehabilitation. The rehabilitation and management of the child with permanent brain injury are essential aspects of care. Rehabilitation of brain-injured children is begun as soon as feasible and usually involves the family and a rehabilitation team. Careful assessment of the child's capabilities, limitations, and probable potential is made as early as possible, and appropriate interventions are implemented to maximize the residual capacities. The Brain Injury Association of America* provides information and listings of rehabilitation services and support groups throughout the country.

Pediatric trauma rehabilitation is a national concern. Coordinating care and services for early rehabilitation involves identifying the child's and family's response to the traumatic injury and disability, securing available resources, and recognizing the parental role in the process.

The child with a disability resulting from head trauma requires assessment on a physical, cognitive, emotional, and social level. The child has experienced separation, pain, sensory deprivation and overload, changes in circadian cycle, and fear of the unknown. Recovery and transition require new coping strategies at the same time that regressive and acting-out behavior may start. Parents and children need honest communication for decision making. A rehabilitation facility or home rehabilitation is advocated when the child has progressed beyond what can be provided in a hospital setting.

---

*1608 Spring Hill Road, Suite 110, Vienna, VA 22182; (703) 761-0750; fax: (703) 761-0755; http://www.biausa.org.

The Rancho Los Amigos Scale provides a systematic assessment of the possible progress a child may achieve following a severe head injury.

Prevention. Tremendous strides have been taken in the prevention of cerebral damage after head injury in children. New developments requiring research point to the prevention of cellular injury or the primary insult. However, the greatest benefit lies in prevention of head injuries. Nurses can exert a valuable influence on behalf of children through education. The reason injuries remain preventable is that unnecessary risks go unchecked. Inadequate supervision combined with a child's natural sense of indestructibility and exploration can lead to lethal results. Nurses are in the unique position of influencing caregivers in terms of growth and development. Banning the use of infant walkers is an example. This equipment does not help develop motor skills and places infants at risk for head and neck injuries from falls, especially down steps. Public education, coupled with legislative support, can prevent childhood injuries. (For extensive discussions of childhood injuries and prevention, see Chapters 10, 12, 13, 15, and 16. See also Childhood Mortality, Chapter 1.)

NEAR-DROWNING

Drowning is a major cause of accidental death in children over 1 year of age. Most cases of drowning are accidental, usually involving the following individuals:

- Children who are helpless in water, such as inadequately attended children in or near swimming pools or infants in bathtubs
- Small children who fall into ponds, streams, and flooded excavations, usually near home
- Occupants of pleasure boats who fail to wear life preservers
- Children who have diving accidents
- Children who are able to swim but overestimate their endurance

Accidental drowning occurs five times more often in boys than in girls; almost 40% of children are younger than age 5, and 90% of cases occur in private swimming pools (Kallas, 2004). Drowning can take place in any body of water, including such unlikely ones as a pail of water. Top-heavy toddlers fall head first into a pail of water, their arms become trapped, and they are unable to free themselves. Hot tubs and whirlpool spas have been implicated in childhood drowning injury. The suction created at the outlet is strong enough to trap even larger children underwater. Drowning as a form of fatal child abuse has also been recognized as a problem. Homicidal drownings are unwitnessed, they usually occur in the home, and the victims are either infants or toddlers. With expeditious treatment many children are being saved.

For purposes of this discussion, two terms need clarification:

Drowning—Death from asphyxia while submerged, regardless of whether fluid has entered the lungs
Near-drowning—Survival at least 24 hours after submersion in a fluid medium

Pathophysiology

The major pulmonary changes that occur in drowning are directly related to the length of submersion (regardless of the type and amount of fluid aspirated), the victim's physiologic response, and the development and degree of immersion hypothermia. In addition, cerebral recovery depends on the effectiveness of initial resuscitation and subsequent critical care measures to support cerebral salvage.

Physiologic factors that influence the extent of damage from immersion include resistance to asphyxia and anoxia, which shows some individual variation. There is greater resistance with diminishing age; young children can withstand longer periods of submersion. More important is the drowning, or diving, reflex. This neurologic response is triggered by immersion of the face in cold water. Blood is shunted away from the periphery, and the flow is concentrated in the brain and heart predominantly.

The problems created by near-drowning are (1) hypoxia and asphyxiation, (2) aspiration, and (3) hypothermia (except near-drowning in hot tubs). Cardiopulmonary arrest is secondary to asphyxiation.

Hypoxia is the primary problem because it results in global cell damage, and different cells tolerate variable lengths of anoxia. Neurons, especially cerebral cells, sustain irreversible damage after 4 to 6 minutes of submersion. The heart and lungs can survive up to 30 minutes. Regardless of the amount of water aspirated, there is arterial hypoxemia (resulting from atelectasis with shunting of blood through the nonventilated alveoli) and a combined respiratory acidosis (resulting from retained carbon dioxide) and metabolic acidosis (caused by buildup of acid metabolites from anaerobic metabolism). The pathologic events are directly related to the duration of submersion. The major difficulty is acute ventilatory insufficiency. Approximately 10% of drowning victims die without aspirating fluid but succumb from acute asphyxia as a result of prolonged reflex laryngospasm.

Aspiration of fluid occurs in the majority of drownings. The aspirated fluid results in pulmonary edema, atelectasis, airway spasm, and pneumonitis, which aggravates the hypoxia. It was previously thought that submersion in salt water vs fresh water altered the physiologic response to near-drowning. However, there is no clinically significant difference in the response of human survivors, and the type of water does not alter the therapy or outcome.

Hypothermia occurs rapidly in infants and children, partly because of their large surface area relative to body mass and partly as a result of the cold water itself. Water is an excellent heat conductor, and contact with the skin is increased by struggling. Hypothermia may make resumption or maintenance of cardiac function possible if body temperature is less than 30° C (86° F). Profound hypothermia is usually evidence of lengthy submersion.

Therapeutic Management

Resuscitative measures should begin at the scene of a drowning, and the victim should be transported to the hospital with maximal ventilatory and circulatory support. Many victims need care for some time after aspiration of fluid. In the hospital, intensive pulmonary care is implemented and continued according to the patient's needs.

In general, the management of the near-drowning victim is based on the degree of cerebral insult (Box 28-4). The first priority is to restore oxygen delivery to the cells and prevent further hypoxic damage. A spontaneously breathing child will do well in an oxygen-enriched atmosphere; the more severely affected child will require endotracheal intubation and mechanical ventilation. Blood gases and pH are monitored frequently as a guide to oxygen, fluid, and electrolyte therapies.

BOX 28-4
Clinical Manifestations of Near-Drowning

CATEGORY A
Awake, minimal injury
Fully conscious; may have mild hypothermia, mild chest radiograph changes, mild arterial blood gas abnormalities

CATEGORY B
Blunted sensorium, moderate injury
Obtund, stuporous, purposeful response to painful stimuli, mild to moderate hypothermia, frequent respiratory distress, abnormal chest radiographs, arterial blood gas abnormalities

CATEGORY C
Comatose, severe anoxia
Unarousable, abnormal response to pain, abnormal respiratory pattern, seizures, shock, marked arterial blood gas abnormalities, abnormal chest radiographs, arrhythmias, metabolic acidosis, hyperkalemia, hyperglycemia, disseminated intravascular coagulation
C1—Flexion posturing, Cheyne-Stokes respirations
C2—Extension posturing, central hyperventilation
C3—Flaccid, apneic, or cluster breathing
C4—Flaccid, apneic, no detectable circulation

NURSINGALERT

All children who have a near-drowning experience should be admitted to the hospital for observation. Although many patients do not appear to have suffered adverse effects from the event, complications (e.g., respiratory compromise, cerebral edema) may occur 24 hours after the incident.

nursingcareguidelines

Establishing Brain Death in Children

1. Coma and apnea must coexist. Child must exhibit complete loss of consciousness, vocalization, and volitional activity.
2. Brainstem function must be absent, as defined by:
   a. Midposition or fully dilated pupils that do not respond to light. Drugs may influence and invalidate pupillary assessment.
   b. Absence of spontaneous eye movements and those induced by oculocephalic and caloric (oculovestibular) testing.
   c. Absence of movement of bulbar musculature, including facial and oropharyngeal muscles. The corneal, gag, cough, sucking, and rooting reflexes are absent.
   d. Absence of respiratory movements when child is removed from respirator. Apnea testing using standardized methods can be performed but is done after other criteria are met.
3. Child must not be significantly hypothermic or hypotensive for age.
4. Flaccid tone and absence of spontaneous or induced movements, including spinal cord events such as reflex withdrawal or spinal myoclonus, should exist.
5. Examination should remain consistent with brain death throughout the observation and testing period.
6. Observation periods according to age:
   Seven days to 2 months—Two separate examinations and two electroencephalograms (EEGs), separated by at least 48 hours
   Two months to 1 year—Two separate examinations and two EEGs, separated by at least 24 hours
   Over 1 year—Two separate examinations separated by at least 12 hours; if irreversible cause exists, no laboratory testing needed; if difficult to assess extent of reversibility of brain damage, observation indicated for at least 24 hours

Modified from Task Force for the Determination of Brain Death in Children: Guidelines for the determination of brain death in children, *Ann Neurol* 21:616, 1987; Janakiraman N: Brain death, *Indian J Pediatr* 65:525-527, 1998; and Lutz-Dettinger N, de Jaeger A, Kerremanas I: Care of the potential pediatric organ donor, *Pediatr Clin North Am* 48:715-749, 2001.

Aspiration pneumonia is a frequent complication that occurs about 48 to 72 hours after the episode. Bronchospasm, alveolocapillary membrane damage, atelectasis, abscess formation, and acute respiratory distress syndrome are other complications that occur after aspiration of fluid.

Prognosis. Studies report that the best predictors of a good outcome were length of submersion in nonicy water (>5° C [41° F]) for less than 5 minutes and the presence of sinus rhythm, reactive pupils, and neurologic responsiveness at the scene. The worst prognoses—for death or severe neurologic impairment—were in children submerged for more than 10 minutes and not responding to advanced life support within 25 minutes. All children without spontaneous, purposeful movement and normal brainstem function 24 hours after near-drowning suffered severe neurologic deficits or death (Zuckerman, Gregory, and Santos-Damiani, 1998; Kallas, 2004). (See Nursing Care Guidelines box.)

Nursing Care Management

Nursing care depends on the child's condition. A child who survives may need intensive respiratory nursing care with attention to vital signs, mechanical ventilation and/or tracheostomy, blood gas determination, chest therapy, and IV infusion. Frequently the child is comatose for an indefinite period and requires the same care as an unconscious child. A difficult aspect in the care of the child victim of near-drowning is helping the parents cope with severe guilt reactions. The magni-

tude of the event is so great that efforts to provide comfort and support are of only limited success. Parents need to hear that everything possible is being done to treat the child, and this message needs to be repeated often.

The parents of the child who is saved from death are also faced with the anxiety of not knowing what the outcome will be. The situation generates such intense feelings of loneliness, it is important for families to know that they are not alone. They need to be reminded frequently that there are caring people to assist them both during the crisis and later. Additional sources of support that can be recommended are psychiatric and social work consultants, community services, and religious support. Self-help groups are excellent if these are available in the community.

Nurses often have difficulty relating to the parents if obvious neglect has precipitated the accident and subsequent problems; therefore it is important for those who care for these children and their families to assess their own feelings about the situation, as well as the family's coping abilities and resources. Caring for near-drowning victims and their families requires nurses to be sensitive to the needs of the child and family and to recognize their own reactions and emotions.

Prevention. Most drownings, particularly of infants or small children, can be prevented with adequate supervision. Water safety and survival training should be required for all school-age children, and nurses can be active advocates in their communities. Nurses are also in a position to emphasize the importance of adequate adult supervision when children are in the water. Aquatic programs for infants and toddlers do not decrease the risk of drowning; young children should never be left unattended when in or near the water (American Academy of Pediatrics, 2000b; Kallas, 2004). Parents with pools should know cardiopulmonary resuscitation techniques. (See also Injury Prevention, Chapters 10, 12, 13, 15, and 16.)

NERVOUS SYSTEM TUMORS

Brain tumor and neuroblastoma are two major forms of childhood cancer derived from neural tissue. CNS tumors account for approximately 20% of all childhood cancers, and approximately 3.3 cases per 100,000 occur in children under 15 years of age (Blaney, Kun, Hunter, and others, 2006). Both of these tumors are difficult to treat and have not demonstrated the dramatic improvements in survival seen in other forms of childhood cancer.

BRAIN TUMORS

Brain tumors are the most common solid tumors in children and are the second most common childhood cancer. The majority of tumors (about 60%) are **infratentorial** (below the tentorium cerebelli), which means that they occur in the posterior third of the brain, primarily in the cerebellum or brainstem. This anatomic distribution accounts for the frequency of symptoms resulting from increased ICP. The other tumors are **supratentorial,** or within the anterior two thirds of the brain, mainly the cerebrum.

Brain tumors, whether benign or malignant, can arise from any cell within the cranium. Consequently, the cranial cells' origin provides a histologic classification for major tumors. For instance, astrocytes (cells that form the supportive tissue for neurons) may form a common glial tumor called an astrocytoma. The major infratentorial tumors are medulloblastomas, cerebellar astrocytomas, brainstem gliomas, and ependymomas, and the major supratentorial tumors are astrocytomas, hypothalamic tumors, optic pathway tumors, and craniopharyngiomas.

Diagnostic Evaluation

The signs and symptoms of brain tumors are directly related to their anatomic location and size and, to some extent, the child's age. In infants, whose cranial sutures are still open, virtually no early detectable symptoms develop. It is not until spinal fluid obstruction causes markedly increased head size that a lesion may be suspected. Even in older children, clinical manifestations are nonspecific. However, the most common symptoms are headache, especially on awakening, and vomiting that is not related to feeding. Vomiting occurs from increased ICP that compresses the brainstem, directly stimulating the vomiting center in the medulla (Blaney, Kun, Hunter, and others, 2006).

Diagnosis of a brain tumor is based subjectively on presenting clinical signs and objectively on neurologic tests and histologic diagnosis via surgery. Because the signs and symptoms are vague and easily overlooked, early diagnosis relies on a high index of suspicion during history taking. A number of tests may be used in the neurologic evaluation, but the most common diagnostic procedure is MRI, which determines the location and extent of the tumor. Other tests that may be used include CT, angiography, electroencephalography, and lumbar puncture. Lumbar puncture is dangerous in the presence of increased ICP because of the possibility of brainstem herniation following a sudden release of pressure. The definitive diagnosis is based on brain tissue specimens obtained during surgery.

Therapeutic Management

Treatment may involve the use of surgery, radiotherapy, and chemotherapy. All three may be used, depending on the type of tumor. The treatment of choice is total removal of the tumor without residual neurologic damage. Patients with the most complete tumor removal have the greatest chance of survival. Radiotherapy is used to treat most tumors and to shrink the size of the tumor before attempting surgical removal. Chemotherapy has emerged in the past decade to delay radiation in children younger than 3 years of age because of the rapid brain development occurring in the first 3 years of life (Blaney, Kun, Hunter, and others, 2006; Murray-Ryan and Petriccione, 2002). Chemotherapy is also used as adjunct therapy for residual tumor, nonresectable tumor, or recurrent tumor. Water-soluble agents are able to penetrate the disrupted blood-brain barrier and attack brain tumor cells (Blaney, Kun, Hunter, and others, 2006; Murray-Ryan and Petriccione, 2002). Typically, the most commonly used chemotherapy agents are cisplatin, carboplatin, vincristine, cyclophosphamide, lomustine, carmustine, etoposide, ifosfamide, and topotecan. Surgery (biopsy, resection, laser, or stereotactic), radiotherapy (hyperfractionated, fractionated, or stereotactic), and multiagent chemotherapy are all instrumental in the treatment of brain tumors.

Prognosis. The prognosis for the child with a brain tumor depends on the type of brain tumor, the tumor's size, the extent of the disease, and the child's age. Problems associated with treatment and a relatively poor prognosis, primarily in infants and young children, are compounded by serious late effects of therapy. A decline in incidence of children with medulloblastoma has been significantly linked with a protective effect of maternal folate, iron, and multivitamin supplementation. Along with the recent advances in surgical instrumentation allowing aggressive surgical intervention (e.g., stereotactic surgery, radiosurgery), modifications in radiation (e.g., hyperfractionation, brain mapping) and use of chemotherapy (e.g., intrathecal, intratumoral) have increased the long-term survival rates for many children with brain tumors (Blaney, Kun, Hunter, and others, 2006; Alston, Newton, Kelsey, and others, 2003; Gupta and Berger, 2003; Murray-Ryan and Petriccione, 2002).

Nursing Care Management

A brain tumor is often suspected in a child admitted to the hospital with neurologic dysfunction, although the actual diagnosis may not yet be confirmed. Establishing a baseline of data with which to compare preoperative and postoperative changes is an essential step toward planning physical care and preventing complications. It also allows the nurse to assess the degree of physical incapacity and the family's emotional reaction to the diagnosis.

Vital signs, including blood pressure and pulse pressure (the difference between systolic and diastolic pressures), are taken routinely and more often when any change is noted. Any sudden variations are reported immediately. It is especially important to note a change in vital signs during or after diagnostic procedures. A routine neurologic assessment is also performed at the same time as vital signs, and head circumference is measured on infants and very young children.

The child is observed for evidence of headache, vomiting, and any seizure activity. The location, severity, and duration of the headache are noted, as well as its relationship to activity and time of day. Behaviors such as lying flat and facing away from light or refusing to engage in play are clues to discomfort in the nonverbal child. The child's gait is observed at least once daily. Head tilt and other changes in posturing are always noted.

Prevent Postoperative Complications. Usually the surgeon will prescribe specific orders for vital signs, neurologic checks, positioning, fluid regulation, and medication. These vary somewhat, depending on the location of the craniotomy. The following are general principles of care for infratentorial or supratentorial surgery. Additional aspects of care that are discussed elsewhere may include care of the child with seizures and neurologic assessment of the unconscious child.

Vital signs are taken as frequently as every 15 to 30 minutes until the child is stable. Temperature measurement is particularly important because of hyperthermia resulting from surgical intervention in the hypothalamus or brainstem and from some types of general anesthesia. To prepare for this reaction, a cooling blanket should be placed on the bed *before* the child returns to the unit so that it is ready for use when needed. The temperature is monitored carefully when any cooling measures are taken because hypothermia can occur suddenly. Recognizing signs of other complications such as increased ICP, meningitis, and respiratory tract infection is imperative.

> **NURSINGALERT**
>
> When temperature is elevated, an infectious process must always be suspected, particularly if the febrile state occurs 1 to 2 days after surgery.

Neurologic checks are an essential aspect of care and include pupillary reaction to light, LOC, sleep patterns, and response to stimuli. Although children may be comatose for a few days, once they regain consciousness, there should be a steady increase in alertness. Regression to a lethargic, irritable state indicates increasing pressure, possibly caused by meningitis or cerebral edema.

> **NURSINGALERT**
>
> Sluggish, dilated, or unequal pupils are reported immediately because they may indicate increased ICP and potential brainstem herniation, a medical emergency.

Observations for function are not instituted until the child regains consciousness. However, as soon as possible the nurse should begin testing reflexes, handgrip, and functioning of the cranial nerves. Muscle strength is usually diminished as a result of general weakness after surgery but should improve daily. Ataxia may be significantly worse with cerebellar intervention, but it will slowly improve. Edema near the cranial nerves may depress important functions such as the gag, blink, or swallowing reflex.

Dressings are observed for evidence of drainage. If soiled, the dressing is not removed but is reinforced with dry sterile gauze. The approximate amount of drainage is estimated and recorded. A drain may be placed in the operative site.

> **NURSINGALERT**
>
> To keep an accurate account of drainage, the soiled area is circled with a pen every hour or so. In this way, continuous bleeding is easily recognized. The presence of colorless drainage is reported immediately, since it most likely is CSF from the incisional area. A foul odor from the dressing may indicate an infection. Such a finding is reported, and a culture is taken.

Correct positioning after surgery is critical to prevent pressure against the operative site, reduce ICP, and avoid the danger of aspiration. If a large tumor was removed, the child is not placed on the operative side, since the brain may suddenly shift to that cavity, causing trauma to the blood vessels, linings, and the brain itself. The nurse confers with the surgeon to be certain of the correct position, including degree of neck flexion. The first 24 to 48 hours after brain surgery are critical. If the child's position is restricted, notice of this is posted above the head of the bed. When the child is turned, every precaution is used to prevent jarring or malalignment to prevent undue strain on the sutures. Two nurses are needed—one supporting the head and the other supporting the body. The use of a turning sheet may facilitate turning a heavy child.

The child with an infratentorial procedure is usually positioned on either side with the bed flat. When a supratentorial craniotomy is performed, the head of bed is elevated 20 to 30 degrees with the child on either side or on the back. In a supratentorial craniotomy the head elevation facilitates CSF drainage and decreases excessive blood flow to the brain to prevent hemorrhage. Pillows should be placed against the child's back, not head, to maintain the desired position. Ordinarily the head and neck are kept in midline with the body and the neck should not be flexed (Curley and Moloney-Harmon, 2001).

> **NURSINGALERT**
>
> The Trendelenburg position is contraindicated in both infratentorial and supratentorial surgeries because it increases ICP and the risk of hemorrhage. If shock is impending, the practitioner is notified immediately, before the head is lowered.

With an infratentorial craniotomy the child is allowed nothing by mouth for at least 24 hours, or longer if the gag and swallowing reflexes are depressed or the child is comatose. With a supratentorial operation, clear fluids may be resumed soon after the child is alert, sometimes within 24 hours. If the child vomits, oral liquids are stopped. Vomiting not only predisposes the child to aspiration, but also increases ICP and the potential for incisional rupture.

The child should be fed to conserve energy and minimize movement. If there is any sign of facial paralysis, the child is fed slowly to prevent choking or aspiration. Sometimes gavage feeding is necessary when body functions are too depressed to permit safe oral feedings or when the child refuses to eat or drink. IV fluids are continued until oral fluids are well tolerated. Because of the postoperative cerebral edema and danger of increased ICP, fluids are carefully monitored.

Headache may be severe and is largely a result of cerebral edema. Measures to relieve some of the discomfort include providing a quiet, dimly lit environment; restricting visitors; preventing any sudden jarring movement, such as banging into the bed; and preventing an increase in ICP. Avoiding increased ICP is most effectively achieved by proper positioning and prevention of straining, such as during coughing, vomiting, or defecating. The use of opioids, such as morphine, to relieve pain is controversial because it is thought that they may mask signs of altered consciousness or depress respirations. However, they can be given safely, since naloxone can be used to reverse opioid effects, such as sedation or respiratory depression. Acetaminophen and codeine are also effective analgesics for mild to moderate pain. Regardless of the drugs used, adequate dosage and regular administration are essential to providing optimal pain relief (see also Pain Assessment; Pain Management, Chapter 7). Placing an ice bag on the forehead may also provide some headache relief, especially if facial edema is severe.

Support Child and Family. The family's emotional needs are immense when the diagnosis is a brain tumor, and feelings are influenced by the extent of surgery, any neurologic deficits, the expected prognosis, and additional therapy.* Since few definitive answers can be given before surgery, the surgeon's report is a significant finding that can vary from a completely benign, resected neoplasm to a highly malignant, invasive, and only partially removed tumor. Although parents try to prepare themselves for a potentially fatal diagnosis, it is a shock for them.

Parents should be encouraged to verbalize their feelings about the diagnosis. Often they express tremendous guilt for viewing the insidious onset of symptoms, such as ataxia, visual difficulty, or headache, as "minor complaints" by the child. Any comments that insinuate that the parents should have sought medical advice sooner are avoided, since such remarks only add to the parents' guilt feelings.

During this period the nurse should also discuss with parents what they plan to tell the child. If the child was prepared honestly, the diagnosis can be expressed in a similar manner. During recovery the child will need additional explanation about the treatment and the reason for any residual neurologic effects, such as ataxia or blindness.

NEUROBLASTOMA

Neuroblastomas are the most common malignant extracranial solid tumors in children, accounting for 8% to 10% of all childhood cancers (Brodeur and Maris, 2006). They occur in about 1 per 10,000 live births, with a slightly higher incidence in boys. The majority of children with neuroblastoma manifest the disease before 10 years of age, with the median age of occurrence at 22 months (Brodeur and Maris, 2006). These tumors originate from embryonic neural crest cells that normally give rise to the adrenal medulla and the sympathetic ganglia. Consequently, the majority of tumors develop in the adrenal gland or the retroperitoneal sympathetic chain. Other sites may be in the head, neck, chest, or pelvis.

Neuroblastoma is a "silent" tumor. In more than 70% of cases, diagnosis is made after metastasis occurs, with the first signs caused by involvement in the nonprimary site, usually the lymph nodes, bone marrow, skeletal system, skin, or liver.

Diagnostic Evaluation

The objective of diagnosis is to locate the primary site and areas of metastasis. The signs and symptoms of neuroblastoma depend on the location and stage of the disease. Most presenting signs are caused by compression of adjacent structures. Skeletal survey; skull, neck, chest, abdominal, and bone CT scans; and bilateral bone marrow aspirations and biopsies are used to locate a tumor mass and metastasis. A metaiodobenzylguanidine (MIBG) scan is used to determine involvement of bone or tissue; however, it is only available at certain centers.

Urinary excretion of catecholamines is detected in approximately 95% of children with adrenal or sympathetic tumors. Analyzing the breakdown products excreted in the urine, namely vanillylmandelic acid (VMA), homovanillic acid (HVA), dopamine, and norepinephrine, permits detection of suspected tumor before and after medical-surgical intervention (Kline and Sevier, 2003; Brodeur and Maris, 2006). Amplification of proto-oncogene, known as the *N-myc* gene, and chromosomal abnormalities correlates strongly with advanced-stage disease, rapid tumor progression, and a poor prognosis (Brodeur and Maris, 2006).

Therapeutic Management

Accurate clinical staging is important for establishing initial treatment. Therefore surgery is used both to remove as much of the tumor as possible and to obtain biopsies. In early stages, complete surgical removal of the tumor is the treatment of choice. If the tumor is large, partial resection is attempted, with a course of irradiation postoperatively to shrink the tumor in the hope of complete removal at a later date. Surgery is usually limited to biopsy in stages III and IV because of the extensive metastasis, although the use of additional surgery to assess tumor regression or remove a regressed tumor is not unlikely.

Radiotherapy provides emergency management of a massive neuroblastoma that is causing spinal cord compression (Kline and Sevier, 2003; Nguyen, Sallah, Ludin, and others, 2000). Radiotherapy also offers palliation for metastatic lesions in the bones, lung, liver, or brain.

Chemotherapy is the mainstay of therapy for extensive local or disseminated disease. Agents used in various combinations include cyclophosphamide, doxorubicin, cisplatin, etoposide, vincristine, ifosfamide, carboplatin, topotecan, and teniposide. In children with high-risk disease or recurrent disease, retinoic acid, radiotherapy, and myeloablative chemotherapy with peripheral stem cell rescue may be used to obtain a longer remission, even though a poor overall survival rate is seen (Kline and Sevier, 2003; Brodeur and Maris, 2006).

Prognosis. If all stages are grouped together, the 5-year disease-free survival rates range from 88% to 90% for children in the low-risk stage, and from 22% to 30% in children in the high-risk stage (Brodeur and Maris, 2006). Generally, the younger the child at diagnosis (especially younger than 1 year of age), the better the survival rate. Neuroblastoma is one of the few tumors that demonstrate spontaneous regression (especially stage IV-S), possibly as a result of maturity of

---

*Excellent publications are available from the National Brain Tumor Foundation, 22 Battery St., Suite 612, San Francisco, CA 94111-5520; (800) 934-CURE (patient line); (415) 834-2873; http://www.braintumor.org. The pamphlet *When Your Child Is Ready to Return to School* is available from the American Brain Tumor Association, 2720 River Road, Des Plaines, IL 60018; (847) 827-9910; fax: (847) 827-9918; http://www.abta.org.

the embryonic cell or the development of an active immune system.

Nursing Care Management

Nursing considerations are similar to those discussed for leukemia and brain tumors, including psychologic and physical preparation for diagnostic and operative procedures; prevention of postoperative complications for abdominal, thoracic, or cranial surgery; and explanation of chemotherapy, radiotherapy, and their side effects.

Since this tumor carries a poor prognosis for many children, every consideration must be given the family in terms of coping with a life-threatening illness (see Chapter 18). Because of the high degree of metastasis at the time of diagnosis, many parents suffer substantial guilt for not having recognized signs earlier. Parents need much support in dealing with these feelings and expressing them to the appropriate people.

INTRACRANIAL INFECTIONS

The nervous system is subject to infection by the same organisms that affect other organs of the body. However, the nervous system is limited in the ways in which it responds to injury. Laboratory studies are needed to identify the causative agent. The inflammatory process can affect the meninges (meningitis) or brain (encephalitis).

Meningitis can be caused by a variety of organisms, but the three main types are (1) bacterial, or pyogenic, caused by pus-forming bacteria, especially meningococci, pneumococci, and *Haemophilus* organisms; (2) viral, or aseptic, caused by a wide variety of viral agents; and (3) tuberculous, caused by the tuberculin bacillus. The majority of children with acute febrile encephalopathy have either bacterial meningitis or viral meningitis as the underlying cause.

BACTERIAL MENINGITIS

Bacterial meningitis is an acute inflammation of the meninges and CSF. The advent of antimicrobial therapy has had a marked effect on the course and prognosis, although the introduction of conjugate vaccines against *Haemophilus influenzae* type b (Hib vaccine) in 1990 has led to the most dramatic change in the epidemiology of bacterial meningitis (Centers for Disease Control and Prevention, 2002; Prober, 2007; Scheifele, Halperin, Law, and others, 2005) (see Evidence-Based Practice box). In 1993 the incidence of *H. influenzae* was two cases per 100,000 children younger than 5 years, whereas in 1987 the incidence was 41 per 100,000 (Centers for Disease Control and Prevention, 2002). Today, *H. influenzae* type b infection has been virtually eradicated among young children in areas in the world where the Hib vaccine is administered routinely (Centers for Disease Control and Prevention, 2002; Yogev and Guzman-Cottrill, 2005). Routine use of the conjugated pneumococcal vaccine introduced in 2000 may lead to world trends in young children similar to those experienced with the Hib vaccine (Yogev and Guzman-Cottrill, 2005). Practitioners are optimistic that the use of the new pneumococcal conjugate vaccine will produce a rapid and adequate antibody response in young children. Bacterial meningitis from *Streptococcus pneumoniae* will soon be on the decline (Prober, 2007).

Bacterial meningitis remains a significant cause of illness in the pediatric age-groups because of the residual damage caused by undiagnosed and untreated or inadequately treated cases.

The majority of reported cases occur in children between 1 month and 5 years of age, with an increased mortality risk in the adolescent and young adult (Saez-Llorens and McCracken, 2003; Sotir, Ahrabi-Fard, Croft, and others, 2005).

Bacterial meningitis can be caused by a variety of bacterial agents. Currently *H. influenzae* type b, *S. pneumoniae*, and *Neisseria meningitidis* (meningococcus) are responsible for bacterial meningitis in 95% of children older than 2 months.

Other organisms are β-hemolytic streptococci, *Staphylococcus aureus*, and *Escherichia coli*. The leading causes of neonatal meningitis are group B streptococci, *E. coli*, and *Listeria monocytogenes*. *E. coli* infection is seldom seen beyond infancy. Meningococcal meningitis occurs in epidemic form and is the only type readily transmitted by droplet infection from nasopharyngeal secretions. Although this condition may develop at any age, the risk of meningococcal infection increases with the number of contacts; therefore it occurs predominantly in school-age children and adolescents.

There appear to be some seasonal variations. Meningitis caused by *H. influenzae* primarily occurs in autumn or early winter. Pneumococcal and meningococcal infections can occur at any time but are more common in later winter or early spring.

Pathophysiology

The most common route of infection is vascular dissemination from a focus of infection elsewhere. For example, organisms from the nasopharynx invade the underlying blood vessels and enter the cerebral blood supply or form local thromboemboli that release septic emboli into the bloodstream. Invasion by direct extension from infections in the paranasal and mastoid sinuses is less common. Organisms also gain entry by direct implantation after penetrating wounds, skull fractures that provide an opening into the skin or sinuses, lumbar puncture or surgical procedures, anatomic abnormalities such as spina bifida, or foreign bodies such as an internal ventricular shunt or an external ventricular device. Once implanted, the organisms spread into the CSF, by which the infection spreads throughout the subarachnoid space.

The infective process is like that seen in any bacterial infection: inflammation, exudation, white blood cell accumulation, and varying degrees of tissue damage. The brain becomes hyperemic and edematous, and the entire surface of the brain is covered by a layer of purulent exudate that varies with the type of organism. For example, meningococcal exudate is most marked over the parietal, occipital, and cerebellar regions; the thick, fibrinous exudate of pneumococcal infection is confined chiefly to the surface of the brain, particularly the anterior lobes; and the exudate of streptococcal infections is similar to that of pneumococcal infections, but thinner.

As infection extends to the ventricles, thick pus, fibrin, or adhesions may occlude the narrow passages and obstruct the flow of CSF.

Clinical Manifestations

The clinical manifestations of acute bacterial meningitis depend to a large extent on the child's age. The picture is also influenced to some degree by the type of organism, the effectiveness of therapy for antecedent illness, and whether it occurs as an isolated entity or as a complication of another illness or injury. The onset of illness is likely to be abrupt, with fever, chills, headache, and vomiting that are associated with

BOX 27-4
Clinical Manifestations of Hemolytic Uremic Syndrome

Vomiting	Oliguria or anuria
Irritability	Central nervous system
Lethargy	involvement:
Marked pallor	▪ Seizures
Hemorrhagic manifestations:	▪ Stupor or coma
▪ Bruising	Signs of acute heart failure
▪ Petechiae	(sometimes)
▪ Jaundice	
▪ Bloody diarrhea	

BOX 27-5
Clinical Manifestations of Wilms Tumor

Abdominal swelling or mass:	Manifestations resulting from
▪ Firm	compression of tumor mass
▪ Nontender	Secondary metabolic alterations
▪ Confined to one side	from tumor or metastasis
Hematuria (less than one fourth	If metastasis, symptoms of lung
of cases)	involvement:
Fatigue and malaise	▪ Dyspnea
Hypertension (occasionally)	▪ Cough
Weight loss	▪ Shortness of breath
Fever	▪ Chest pain (sometimes)

tion) followed by the sudden onset of hemolysis and renal failure.

Pathophysiology

The primary site of injury appears to be the endothelial lining of the small glomerular arterioles, which become swollen and occluded with deposits of platelets and fibrin clots (intravascular coagulation). Red blood cells are damaged as they attempt to move through the partially occluded blood vessels. These damaged cells are removed by the spleen, causing acute hemolytic anemia. The platelet aggregation within the damaged blood vessels or the damage and removal of platelets produce the characteristic thrombocytopenia.

Diagnostic Evaluation

The triad of anemia, thrombocytopenia, and renal failure is sufficient for diagnosis (Box 27-4). Renal involvement is evidenced by proteinuria, hematuria, and urinary casts; BUN and serum creatinine levels are elevated. A low hemoglobin and hematocrit and a high reticulocyte count confirm the hemolytic nature of the anemia.

Therapeutic Management

The goals of therapy are early diagnosis and aggressive, supportive care of the ARF and hemolytic anemia. The most consistently effective treatment of HUS is hemodialysis or peritoneal dialysis, which is instituted in any child who has been anuric for 24 hours or who demonstrates oliguria with uremia or hypertension and seizures. Other treatments include use of pharmacologic agents, fresh-frozen plasma, and plasmapheresis. Blood transfusions with fresh, washed packed cells are administered for severe anemia but are used with caution to prevent circulatory overload from added volume.

Prognosis. With prompt treatment the recovery rate is about 95%, but residual renal impairment ranges from 10% to 50%. Long-term complications include chronic renal failure, hypertension, and central nervous system disorders. Death is usually caused by residual renal impairment or central nervous system injury.

Nursing Care Management

Nursing care is the same as that provided in ARF and, for children with continued impairment, includes management of chronic disease. Because of the sudden and life-threatening nature of the disorder in a previously well child, parents are often ill prepared for the impact of hospitalization and treat-ment. Therefore support and understanding are especially important aspects of care.

WILMS TUMOR

Wilms tumor, or nephroblastoma, is the most common malignant renal and intraabdominal tumor of childhood. Its frequency is estimated to be 7.6 cases per million in Caucasian children less than 15 years of age (Dome, Perlman, Ritchey, and others, 2006). Wilms tumor occurs about three times more often in African-Americans than in East Asians in the United States. The peak age at diagnosis is approximately 3 years, and occurrence is slightly more frequent in boys than in girls. The majority of patients with Wilms tumor are diagnosed at younger than 5 years of age, with 1% to 2.5% having a familial origin. Unfortunately, there is no method of identifying gene carriers at this time.

Etiology

Wilms tumor probably arises from a malignant, undifferentiated cluster of primordial cells capable of initiating the regeneration of an abnormal structure. Its occurrence slightly favors the left kidney, which is advantageous because surgically this kidney is easier to manipulate and remove. In about 10% of cases both kidneys are involved. Studies have shown that development of Wilms tumor is frequently associated with aniridia, hemihypertrophy, Beckwith-Wiedemann syndrome, or genitourinary anomalies (Kline and Sevier, 2003; Dome, Perlman, Ritchey, and others, 2006).

Diagnostic Evaluation

In a child suspected of having Wilms tumor, special emphasis is placed on the history and physical examination for the presence of congenital anomalies, a family history of cancer, and signs of malignancy (e.g., weight loss, size of liver and spleen, indications of anemia, lymphadenopathy). Most children with Wilms tumor are brought to the practitioner because of abdominal swelling or an abdominal mass (Box 27-5). Specific tests include radiographic studies, including abdominal ultrasound and abdominal and chest computed tomography scan; hematologic studies; biochemical studies; and urinalysis. Studies to demonstrate the relationship of the tumor to the ipsilateral kidney and the presence of a normal functioning kidney on the contralateral side are essential. If a large tumor is present, an inferior venacavogram is necessary to demonstrate possible tumor involvement adjacent to the vena cava. A bone marrow aspiration may be performed to rule out metastasis, which is rare in children with Wilms tumor.

es

tration of *Haemophilus influenzae* type b (Hib), pneu-
ce and mortality associated with bacterial meningitis?

years, research-based articles (level 3 or lower), children

est Africa will be difficult unless long-lasting
ningococcal vaccines are incorporated into routine
zation schedules (Woods, Armstrong, Sackey, and

randomized trial in Gambia was conducted to assess
an Hib conjugate vaccine for the prevention of
neumonia, and other invasive diseases caused by *H.*
m March 1993 to October 1995, 42,848 infants were
inistered the conjugate vaccine Hib polysaccharide
n (PRP-T) mixed with diphtheria-tetanus-pertussis
or DTP alone at age 2 months, 3 months, and 4
doses of the vaccine were 95% effective in the
meningitis and pneumonia caused by *H. influenzae* in
nfants receiving the Hib vaccine (Mulholland, Hilton,
others, 1997).

DENCE: NURSING IMPLICATIONS

ic studies strongly suggest that all children should be
st the most common organisms responsible for bacterial
I. influenzae type b, *S. pneumoniae*, and *N. meningitidis*)
ccines to decrease the incidence of bacterial meningitis.
l stress to the parents, children, adolescents, and young
rtance of adhering to the immunization schedule to
against serious childhood diseases.

nacko CE, and others: Comparison of incidence in invasive *Strepto-*
e disease among children before and after introduction of conju-
cal vaccine, *Pediatr Infect Dis J* 24(4):320-330, 2005.
C, de Andrade JG, and others: Progress towards meningitis preven-
ate vaccines era, *Braz J Infect Dis* 7(5):315-324, 2003.
S, Adegbola R, and others: Randomised trial of *Haemophilus influ-*
us protein conjugate for prevention of pneumonia and meningitis
s, *Lancet* 349(9060):1191-1197, 1997.
R: Bacterial meningitis in childhood at the Children's Hospital of
1998, *Clin Pediatr (Phila)* 40(11):595-600, 2001.
MM, Hadler J, and others: Decline in invasive pneumococcal disease
tion of protein–polysaccharide conjugate vaccine, *N Engl J Med*
6, 2003.
ng G, Sackey SO, and others: Emergency vaccination against epi-
in Ghana: implications for the control of meningococcal disease in
et 355(9197):30-33, 2000.

: Evaluation

ncture is the definitive diagnostic test. The fluid
easured, and samples are obtained for culture,
blood cell count, and determination of glucose
ontent. The findings are usually diagnostic. Cul-
itivity testing are needed to identify the causative
inal fluid pressure is usually elevated, but inter-
 often difficult when the child is crying. Sedation

BOX 28-5
Clinical Manifestations of Bacterial Meningitis

CHILDREN AND ADOLESCENTS
Usually abrupt onset
Fever
Chills
Headache
Vomiting
Alterations in sensorium
Seizures (often the initial sign)
Irritability
Agitation
May develop:
- Photophobia
- Delirium
- Hallucinations
- Aggressive behavior
- Drowsiness
- Stupor
- Coma
Nuchal rigidity
- May progress to opisthotonos
Positive Kernig and Brudzinski signs
Hyperactive but variable reflex responses
Signs and symptoms peculiar to individual organisms:
- Petechial or purpuric rashes (meningococcal infection), especially when associated with a shocklike state
- Joint involvement (meningococcal and *Haemophilus influenzae* infection)
- Chronically draining ear (pneumococcal meningitis)

INFANTS AND YOUNG CHILDREN
Classic picture (above) rarely seen in children between 3 months and 2 years of age
Fever

Poor feeding
Vomiting
Marked irritability
Frequent seizures (often accompanied by a high-pitched cry)
Bulging fontanel
Nuchal rigidity (may or may not be present)
Brudzinski and Kernig signs not helpful in diagnosis
Difficult to elicit and evaluate in this age-group
Subdural empyema (*H. influenzae* infection)

NEONATES: SPECIFIC SIGNS
Extremely difficult to diagnose
Manifestations vague and nonspecific
Well at birth but within a few days begins to look and behave poorly
Refuses feedings
Poor sucking ability
Vomiting or diarrhea
Poor tone
Lack of movement
Weak cry
Full, tense, and bulging fontanel sometimes appearing late in course of illness
Neck usually supple

NEONATES: NONSPECIFIC SIGNS THAT MAY BE PRESENT
Hypothermia or fever (depending on the infant's maturity)
Jaundice
Irritability
Drowsiness
Seizures
Respiratory irregularities or apnea
Cyanosis
Weight loss

---

with fentanyl and midazolam can alleviate the child's pain and fear associated with this procedure. If there is evidence or suspicion of increased ICP (papilledema, focal neurologic deficits, bulging fontanel), a CT scan of the head may be warranted before the procedure.

The patient generally has an elevated white blood cell count, often predominantly polymorphonuclear leukocytes. The glucose level is reduced, generally in proportion to the duration and severity of the infection. The relationship between the CSF glucose and serum glucose levels is important in evaluating the glucose content of CSF; therefore a serum glucose sample is drawn approximately one half hour before the lumbar puncture. Protein concentration is usually increased.

A blood culture is advisable for all children suspected of having meningitis and occasionally will be positive when CSF culture is negative. Nose and throat cultures may provide helpful information in some cases.

Therapeutic Management
Acute bacterial meningitis is a medical emergency that requires early recognition and immediate institution of therapy to prevent death or residual disabilities. The initial therapeutic management includes:

- Isolation precautions
- Initiation of antimicrobial therapy
- Maintenance of hydration
- Maintenance of ventilation
- Reduction of increased ICP
- Management of systemic shock
- Control of seizures
- Control of temperature
- Treatment of complications

The child is isolated from other children, usually in an intensive care unit for close observation. An IV infusion is started to facilitate the administration of antimicrobial agents, fluids, antiepileptic drugs, and blood, if needed. The child is placed on a cardiac monitor and in respiratory isolation.

Drugs. Until the causative organism is identified, the choice of antibiotic is based on the known sensitivity of the organism most likely to be the infective agent. After identification of the organism, antimicrobial agents are adjusted accordingly.

Dexamethasone may play a role in the initial management of increased ICP and cerebral herniation, but its ability to reduce long-term complications of bacterial meningitis remains controversial. There is evidence that dexamethasone therapy

---

areas that have been irradiated (Dome, Perlman, and others, 2006).

Care Management

are of the child with Wilms tumor is similar to that n with other cancers treated with surgery, irradia-chemotherapy. However, there are some significant es; these are discussed for each phase of nursing ion.

erative Care. The preoperative period is one of nosis. The nurse faces the challenge of preparing the parents for all laboratory and operative procedures to 48 hours of admission. Because of the minimal ry time, explanations should be simple, repetitive, sed on the child's actual experiences. In addition to preoperative observations, blood pressure is moni-ce hypertension from excess renin production is a y.

are several special preoperative concerns, the most t of which is that the *tumor is not palpated unless necessary* because manipulation of the mass may semination of cancer cells to adjacent and distant

se radiotherapy and chemotherapy are usually begun tely after surgery, parents need an explanation of expect, such as major benefits and side effects. The the information should be considered to avoid over-g the family. Ideally, the nurse should be present dur-cian-parent conferences to answer questions as they s usually better to postpone telling the child about e effects until after surgery. Alopecia, usually of most to older children, does not occur until approximately after the initial treatment regimen. Therefore the be prepared for the hair loss postoperatively.

operative Care. Despite the extensive surgical in-n necessary in many children with Wilms tumor, the is usually rapid. The major nursing responsibilities ame as those after any abdominal surgery (see Surgi-dures, Chapter 22). Because these children are at risk stinal obstruction from vincristine-induced ileus, n-induced edema, and postsurgical adhesion forma-nurse carefully monitors gastrointestinal activity, such movements, bowel sounds, distention, vomiting, and e nurse also monitors blood pressure, urinary output, s of infection, as well as instituting pulmonary hygiene nt postoperative pulmonary complications.

ly Support. The postoperative period is frequently for parents. The shock of seeing their child immedi-er surgery may be the first realization of the serious-the diagnosis. It also marks the confirmation of the the tumor. During this period, the nurse should be parents to assure them of the child's recovery after and to assess the parent's understanding of the total ce. They need an opportunity to express their feel-need to be provided the same emotional care dis-n Chapter 18 for families who have a child with a atening disorder.

r children need an opportunity to deal with their feel-cerning the many procedures to which they have been d in rapid succession. Play therapy with dolls or pup-through drawing can be extremely beneficial in help-n adjust. It is not unusual for children to feel angry decreases the risk of neurologic sequelae in children with *H. influenzae* type b meningitis and should be considered for use in other bacterial types of meningitis (American Academy of Pediatrics, 2006; Prober, 2007). It should not be used if aseptic or nonbacterial meningitis is suspected (Bonthius and Karacay, 2002).

Signs of gastrointestinal hemorrhage or secondary infection may complicate steroid administration. Antibiotic treatment with cephalosporins demonstrates superiority for promptly sterilizing the CSF and reducing the incidence of severe hearing impairment.

Nonspecific Measures. Maintaining hydration is a prime concern, and IV fluids and the type and amount of fluid are determined by the patient's condition. The optimum hydration involves correction of any fluid deficits followed by fluid restriction as ordered to prevent cerebral edema. Cerebral edema and electrolyte disturbances are associated with poor neurologic outcome following bacterial meningitis (Bonthius and Karacay, 2002). Children with bacterial meningitis must be monitored for signs of increased ICP. If needed, measures to decrease ICP are implemented (see p. 982).

Complications are treated appropriately, such as aspiration of subdural effusion in infants and treatment for disseminated intravascular coagulation syndrome. Shock is managed by restoration of circulating blood volume and maintenance of electrolyte balance. Seizures can occur during the first few days of treatment. These are controlled with the appropriate antiepileptic drug. Hearing loss is not uncommon. The patient should undergo auditory evaluation 6 months after the illness has resolved.

Lumbar puncture is carried out as needed to determine the effectiveness of therapy. The patient is evaluated neurologically during the convalescent period.

Prognosis. Ten percent to 15% of cases of bacterial meningitis are fatal (Centers for Disease Control and Prevention, 2000). The child's age, duration of illness before antibiotic therapy, rapidity of diagnosis after onset, type of organism, and adequacy of therapy are important in the prognosis for bacterial meningitis. Bacterial meningitis can result in brain damage, hearing loss, or learning disability (Centers for Disease Control and Prevention, 2000; Prober, 2007).

Neonatal meningitis carries the highest mortality. However, with the development of new antibiotics and the advent of aggressive supportive care measures, the mortality rate for bacterial meningitis in children caused by *H. influenzae* type b, *S. pneumoniae*, and *N. meningitidis* is less than 10% in most studies (Prober, 2007).

The sequelae of bacterial meningitis are seen most often when the disease occurs in the first 2 months of life and least often in children with meningococcal meningitis. The residual deficits in infants are primarily a result of communicating hydrocephalus and the greater effects of cerebritis on the immature brain. In older children the residual effects are related to the inflammatory process itself or result from vasculitis associated with the disease. Bacterial meningitis continues to cause substantial morbidity in infants and children. The mortality rate and incidence of poor neurologic outcome are highest in patients with pneumococcal meningitis (Saez-Llorens and McCracken, 2003; Prober, 2007).

Hearing impairment is the most common sequela of this disease. Evaluation of cranial nerve VIII is needed for at least a 6-month follow-up period to assess for possible hearing loss.

Prevention. Vaccines are available for types A, C, Y, and W-135 meningococci and *H. influenzae* type b. Routine meningococcal polysaccharide vaccination of children is licensed for use only in children 2 years and older (Pichichero, 2005). The new quadrivalent meningococcal conjugate vaccine (Menactra) was licensed by the U.S. Food and Drug Administration (FDA) in January 2005 for children and adults from 11 to 55 years (Pichichero, 2005). However, routine vaccinations for *H. influenzae* type b are recommended for all children beginning at 2 months of age (see Immunizations, Chapter 12). Pneumococcal conjugate vaccine is now recommended for all children beginning at 2 months of age (American Academy of Pediatrics, 2000a).

> **NURSINGALERT**
>
> Nurses should take the necessary precautions to protect themselves and others from possible infection. Parents are taught the proper procedures and supervised in their application.

> **NURSINGALERT**
>
> A major priority of nursing care of a child suspected of having meningitis is to administer antibiotics as soon as they are ordered. The child is placed on respiratory isolation for at least 24 hours after initiation of antimicrobial therapy.

Nursing Care Management

The room is kept as quiet as possible, and environmental stimuli are kept to a minimum because most children with meningitis are sensitive to noise, bright lights, and other external stimuli. Most children are more comfortable without a pillow and with the head of the bed slightly elevated. A side-lying position is more often assumed because of nuchal rigidity. The nurse should avoid actions that cause pain or increase discomfort, such as lifting the child's head. Evaluating the child for pain and implementing appropriate relief measures are important during the initial 24 to 72 hours. Acetaminophen with codeine is often used. Measures are used to ensure safety because the child is often restless and subject to seizures.

The nursing care of the child with meningitis is determined by the child's symptoms and treatment. Observation of vital signs, neurologic signs, LOC, urinary output, and other pertinent data is carried out at frequent intervals. The child who is unconscious is managed as described previously (see p. 981), and all children are observed carefully for signs of the complications just described, especially increased ICP, shock, or respiratory distress. Frequent assessment of the open fontanels is needed in the infant because subdural effusions and obstructive hydrocephalus can develop as a complication of meningitis.

Fluids and nourishment are determined by the child's status. The child with dulled sensorium is usually given nothing by mouth. Other children are allowed clear liquids initially and, if these are tolerated, progress to a diet suitable for their age. Careful monitoring and recording of intake and output are needed to determine deviations that might indicate impending shock or increasing fluid accumulation, such as cerebral edema or subdural effusion.

One of the most difficult problems in the nursing care of children with meningitis is maintaining IV infusion for the length of time needed to provide adequate antimicrobial therapy (usually 10 days). Because continuous IV fluids are usually not necessary, an intermittent infusion device is used. In some cases children who are recovering uneventfully are sent home with the device, and the parents are taught IV drug administration.

Family Support. The sudden nature of the illness makes emotional support of the child and parents extremely important. Parents are upset and concerned about their child's condition and often feel guilty for not having suspected the seriousness of the illness sooner. They need much reassurance that the natural onset of meningitis is sudden and that they acted responsibly in seeking medical assistance when they did. The nurse encourages the parents to openly discuss their feelings to minimize blame and guilt. They also are kept informed of the child's progress and of all procedures, results, and treatments. In the event that the child's condition worsens, they need the same psychologic care as parents who face the possible death of their child (see Chapter 18).

NONBACTERIAL (ASEPTIC) MENINGITIS

Aseptic meningitis is caused by many different viruses. The onset may be abrupt or gradual. The initial manifestations are headache, fever, malaise, and gastrointestinal symptoms. Signs of meningeal irritation develop 1 or 2 days after the onset of illness. Onset is more insidious in infants and toddlers. Signs and symptoms are vague and are often thought to be associated with a minor illness.

Diagnosis is based on clinical features and CSF findings. Variations in CSF values in bacterial and viral meningitis are listed in Table 28-2. It is important to differentiate this self-limiting disorder from the more serious forms of meningitis.

Treatment is primarily symptomatic, such as acetaminophen for headache and muscle pain, maintenance of hydration, and positioning for comfort. Until a definitive diagnosis is made, antimicrobial agents may be administered and isolation enforced as a precaution against the possibility that the disease might be of bacterial origin. Nursing care is similar to the care of the child with bacterial meningitis.

ENCEPHALITIS

Encephalitis is an inflammatory process of the CNS that is caused by a variety of organisms, including bacteria, spirochetes, fungi, protozoa, helminths, and viruses. Most infections are associated with viruses, and this discussion is limited to those agents.

Etiology

Encephalitis can occur as a result of (1) direct invasion of the CNS by a virus or (2) postinfectious involvement of the CNS after a viral disease. Often the specific type of encephalitis may not be identified. The cause of more than half the cases reported in the United States is unknown. The majority of cases of known etiology are associated with the childhood diseases of measles, mumps, varicella, and rubella and, less often, with the enteroviruses, herpesviruses, and West Nile virus.

Herpes simplex encephalitis is an uncommon disease, but 30% of cases involve children. The initial clinical findings are nonspecific (fever, altered mental status), but most cases

TABLE 28-2

Variation of Cerebrospinal Fluid Analysis in Bacterial and Viral Meningitis

MANIFESTATIONS	BACTERIAL*	VIRAL
White blood cell count	Elevated; increased polys	Slightly elevated; increased lymphs
Protein content	Elevated	Normal or slightly increased
Glucose content	Decreased	Normal
Gram stain; bacteria culture	Positive	Turbid or cloudy
Color	Cloudy	Clear

*Results may vary in the neonate.

evolve to demonstrate focal neurologic signs and symptoms. Children may experience focal seizures. The CSF is abnormal in most cases. Because of a rise in the number of children with herpes simplex encephalitis, suspected cases require prompt attention, especially because the diagnosis can be difficult. The clinical diagnosis can be confirmed by the rapid appearance of immunoglobulin M antibody to herpes simplex virus type 1 in CSF and serum. The early use of IV acyclovir reduces mortality and morbidity. Empiric therapy with acyclovir is given before precise virologic diagnosis has been established. CSF should be sent for viral titers.

The multiplicity of causes of viral encephalitis makes diagnosis difficult. Most are those involved with arthropod vectors (togaviruses and bunyaviruses) and those associated with hemorrhagic fevers (arenaviruses, filoviruses, and hantaviruses). In the United States the vector reservoir for most agents pathogenic for humans is the mosquito (St. Louis or West Nile encephalitis); therefore most cases of encephalitis appear during the hot summer months and subside during the autumn.

The clinical features of encephalitis are similar regardless of the agent involved. Manifestations can range from a mild benign form that resembles aseptic meningitis, lasts a few days, and is followed by rapid and complete recovery, to a fulminating encephalitis with severe CNS involvement. The onset may be sudden or may be gradual with malaise, fever, headache, dizziness, apathy, nuchal rigidity, nausea and vomiting, ataxia, tremors, hyperactivity, and speech difficulties (Box 28-6). In severe cases the patient has high fever, stupor, seizures, disorientation, spasticity, and coma that may proceed to death. Ocular palsies and paralysis also may occur.

Diagnostic Evaluation

The diagnosis is made on the basis of clinical findings and, where possible, identification of the specific virus. Early in the course of encephalitis, CT scan results may be normal. Later, hemorrhagic areas in the frontotemporal region may be seen. Togaviruses (some of which were formerly labeled arboviruses) are rarely detected in the blood or spinal fluid, but viruses of herpes, mumps, measles, and enteroviruses may be found in the CSF. Serologic testing may be required. The first blood sample should be drawn as soon as possible after onset, with the second sample drawn 2 or 3 weeks later.

BOX 28-6
Clinical Manifestations of Encephalitis

ONSET: SUDDEN OR GRADUAL	SEVERE CASES
Malaise	High fever
Fever	Stupor
Headache	Seizures
Dizziness	Disorientation
Apathy	Spasticity
Lethargy	Coma (may proceed to death)
Neck stiffness	Ocular palsies
Nausea and vomiting	Paralysis
Ataxia	
Tremors	
Hyperactivity	
Speech difficulties: mutism	
Altered mental status	

BOX 28-7
Clinical Manifestations of Rabies

INITIAL SIGNS
General malaise
Fever
Sore throat

EXCITEMENT PHASE
Hypersensitivity
Increased reaction to external stimuli
Seizures
Maniacal behavior
Choking

SEVERE SPASM OF RESPIRATORY MUSCLES*
Apnea
Cyanosis
Anoxia

*From attempts at swallowing (characteristics from which the term *hydrophobia* was derived).

Therapeutic Management

Patients suspected of having encephalitis are hospitalized promptly for observation. Treatment is primarily supportive and includes conscientious nursing care, control of cerebral manifestations, and adequate nutrition and hydration, with observation and management as for other cerebral disorders. Viral encephalitis can cause devastating neurologic injury. Cerebral hyperemia occurs in severe viral encephalitis, and ICP monitoring to reduce the pressure may be needed (Prober, 2007). Follow-up care with periodic reevaluation and rehabilitation is important for patients who develop residual effects of the disease.

The prognosis for the child with encephalitis depends on the child's age, the type of organism, and residual neurologic damage. Very young children (younger than 2 years of age) may exhibit increased neurologic disability, including learning difficulties and seizure disorders.

Nursing Care Management

Nursing care of the child with encephalitis is the same as for any unconscious child and for the child with meningitis. Additional nursing interventions include observation for deterioration in consciousness. Isolation of the child is not necessary; however, good hand-washing technique must be followed. A main focus of nursing management is the control of rapidly rising ICP. Neurologic monitoring, administration of medications, and support of the child and parents are the major aspects of care.

RABIES

Rabies is an acute infection of the nervous system caused by a virus that is almost invariably fatal if left untreated. It is transmitted to humans by the saliva of an infected mammal and is introduced through a bite or skin abrasion. After entry into a new host, the virus multiplies in muscle cells and is spread through neural pathways without stimulating a protective host immune response.

Approximately 88% of rabies cases come from wild animals and 12% from domestic animals. Carnivorous wild animals (skunks, raccoons, and bats) are the animals most often infected with rabies and the cause of most indigenous cases of human rabies in the United States (Centers for Disease Control and Prevention, 2001; Toltzis, 2007). The likelihood of human exposure to a rabid domestic animal has decreased greatly.

The circumstances of a biting incident are important. An unprovoked attack is more likely than a provoked attack to indicate a rabid animal. Bites inflicted on a child attempting to feed or handle an apparently healthy animal can generally be regarded as provoked. Any child bitten by a wild animal is assumed to be exposed to rabies.

NURSING ALERT

Unusual behavior in an animal is cause for suspicion; children should be warned to beware of wild animals that appear to be friendly.

Although rabies is common among wildlife species, human rabies is rarely acquired. Modern-day prophylaxis is nearly 100% successful. The highest incidence occurs in children under age 15 years. The incubation period usually ranges from 1 to 3 months but may be as short as 10 days or as long as 8 months. Only 10% to 15% of persons bitten develop the disease, but once symptoms are present, rabies progresses to a fatal outcome. In the United States, human fatalities associated with rabies occur in people who fail to seek medical attention, usually because they are unaware of their exposure.

The disease is characterized by a period of general malaise, fever, and sore throat followed by a phase of excitement that features hypersensitivity and increased reaction to external stimuli, convulsions, maniacal behavior, and choking (Box 28-7). Attempts at swallowing may cause such severe spasm of respiratory muscles that apnea, cyanosis, and anoxia are produced—the characteristics from which the term *hydrophobia* was derived.

Diagnosis is made on the basis of history and clinical features. Treatment is of little avail once symptoms appear, but the long incubation period allows time for the induction of active and passive immunity before the onset of illness.

Therapeutic Management

Two types of immunizing products are available for use in humans: (1) the inactivated rabies vaccines, which induce an active immune response; and (2) the globulins, which contain preformed antibodies. The two types of products should be used concurrently for rabies postexposure treatment when prophylaxis is indicated.

The current therapy for a rabid animal bite consists of thorough cleansing of the wound and passive immunization with human rabies immunoglobulin as soon as possible after exposure to provide rapid, short-term passive immunity (Centers for Disease Control and Prevention, 1999; Toltzis, 2007).

Postexposure active immunity is conferred by administration of the human diploid cell rabies vaccine. The first intramuscular injection of the vaccine is given at the same time as the immunoglobulin (day 0) and is followed by injections at 3, 7, 14, and 28 days after the first dose (Centers for Disease Control and Prevention, 1999; Toltzis, 2007). Before antirabies prophylaxis is initiated, the local or state health department should be consulted.

Nursing Care Management

Parents and children are frightened by the urgency and seriousness of the situation. They need anticipatory guidance for the therapy and support and reassurance regarding the efficacy of the preventive measures for this dreaded disease. The vaccine is well tolerated by children, although they need preparation for the series of injections. Mass immunization is unnecessary and unlikely to be implemented. In areas in which rabies is rare, the schedule given is sufficient. However, certain circumstances may warrant preexposure vaccination, such as when a child is being taken to an area of the world where rabies in stray dogs is still a problem.

REYE SYNDROME

RS is a disorder defined as toxic encephalopathy associated with other characteristic organ involvement (Kamienski, 2003). It is characterized by fever, profoundly impaired consciousness, and disordered hepatic function.

The etiology of RS is not well understood, but most cases follow a common viral illness, most commonly influenza or varicella. RS is a condition characterized pathologically by cerebral edema and fatty changes of the liver. The onset of RS is notable for profuse vomiting and varying degrees of neurologic impairment, including personality changes and deterioration in consciousness (Carey and Balistreri, 2007). The cause of RS is a mitochondrial insult induced by different viruses, drugs, exogenous toxins, and genetic factors. Elevated serum ammonia levels tend to correlate with the clinical manifestations and prognosis.

Definitive diagnosis is established by liver biopsy. The staging criteria for RS are based on liver dysfunction and on neurologic signs that range from lethargy to coma (Box 28-8). As a result of improved diagnostic techniques, children who in the past would have been diagnosed with RS are now diagnosed with other illnesses such as viral or metabolic diseases. Cases of unrecognized, drug-induced encephalopathy by antiemetics given to children during viral illnesses have symptoms similar to those of RS.

The potential association between aspirin therapy for the treatment of fever in children with varicella or influenza and

---

BOX 28-8
Staging Criteria for Reye Syndrome

Stage I—Vomiting, lethargy, and drowsiness; liver dysfunction; type I electroencephalogram (EEG); follows commands; pupillary reaction brisk

Stage II—Disorientation, combativeness, delirium, hyperventilation, hyperactive reflexes, appropriate responses to painful stimuli; evidence of liver dysfunction; type I EEG; pupillary reaction sluggish

Stage III—Obtunded, coma, hyperventilation, flexion rigidity, preservation of pupillary light reaction and oculovestibular reflexes (although sluggish); type II EEG

Stage IV—Deepening coma, extension rigidity, loss of oculocephalic reflexes, large and fixed pupils, loss of doll's eye reflex, loss of corneal reflexes; minimal liver dysfunction; type III or IV EEG; evidence of brainstem dysfunction

Stage V—Seizures, loss of deep tendon reflexes, respiratory arrest, flaccidity; type IV EEG; usually no evidence of liver dysfunction

---

the development of RS precludes its use in these patients. However, by the time the FDA required aspirin product labeling in 1986, most of the decline in RS incidence had already occurred.

Therapeutic Management

The most important aspect of successful management of the child with RS is early diagnosis and aggressive therapy. Rapid progression through coma stages and high peak ammonia concentrations are associated with a more serious prognosis. Cerebral edema with increased ICP represents the most immediate threat to life. Recovery from RS is rapid and usually without sequelae if diagnosis is determined early and therapy is initiated promptly.

Prognosis. Although the incidence of RS has markedly decreased, health professionals must remind parents and caregivers to avoid using both aspirin and non-aspirin–containing salicylates during febrile illnesses in children (Bhutta, Van Savell, and Schexnayder, 2003; Kamienski, 2003). Survivors may have subtle neuropsychologic deficits. Generally, recovery is good given the gravity of the disease (Bhutta, Van Savell, and Schexnayder, 2003; Kamienski, 2003).

Nursing Care Management

The most important aspect of successful management of the child with RS is early diagnosis and aggressive therapy (Bhutta, Van Savell, and Schexnayder, 2003). Cerebral edema with increased ICP represents the most immediate threat to life. Recovery from RS is rapid and usually without sequelae if there has been early diagnosis and implementation of therapy. In about one third of patients, RS causes death or long-term neurologic sequelae.

Care and observations are implemented as for any child with an altered state of consciousness (see p. 976) and increasing ICP. Accurate and frequent monitoring of intake and output is essential for adjusting fluid volumes to prevent both dehydration and cerebral edema. Because of related liver dysfunction, laboratory studies to determine impaired coagulation, such as prolonged bleeding time, should be monitored.

Parents of children with RS need to be kept informed of the child's progress, to have diagnostic procedures and therapeutic management explained, and to be given concerned and sympathetic support.* Families need to be aware that salicylate, the alleged offending ingredient in aspirin, is contained in other products (e.g., Pepto-Bismol). They should refrain from administering any product for influenza-like symptoms without first checking the label for "hidden" salicylates.

SEIZURE DISORDERS†

Seizures are caused by excessive and disorderly neuronal discharges in the brain. The manifestation of seizures depends on the region of the brain in which they originate and may include unconsciousness or altered consciousness; involuntary movements; and changes in perception, behaviors, sensations, and posture. Seizures are the most common treatable neurologic disorder in children and can occur with a wide variety of conditions involving the CNS.

EPILEPSY

Epilepsy is a condition characterized by two or more unprovoked seizures and can be caused by a variety of pathologic processes in the brain. Seizures are a symptom of an underlying disease process. A single seizure event should not be classified as epilepsy and is generally not treated with long-term antiepileptic drugs. Some seizures may result from an acute medical or neurologic illness and cease once the illness is treated. In other cases, children may have a single seizure without the cause ever being known. Once it is determined that the child has had a seizure, it is important to classify the seizure, according to the International Classification of Epileptic Seizures, and assign it to the appropriate epilepsy syndrome, according to the International Classification of Epilepsies and Epileptic Syndromes. Optimum treatment and prognosis require an accurate diagnosis and a determination of the cause whenever possible.

Etiology

Seizures in children have many different causes. Seizures are classified not only according to type, but also according to etiology. Acute symptomatic seizures are associated with an acute insult such as head trauma or meningitis. Remote symptomatic seizures are those without an immediate cause but with an identifiable prior brain injury such as major head trauma, meningitis or encephalitis, hypoxia, stroke, or a static encephalopathy such as intellectual disability or cerebral palsy. Cryptogenic seizures are those occurring with no clear cause. Idiopathic seizures are genetic in origin. A partial list of causative factors is presented in Box 28-9.

Pathophysiology

Regardless of the etiologic factor or type of seizure, the basic mechanism is the same. Abnormal electrical discharges (1) may arise from central areas in the brain that affect consciousness; (2) may be restricted to one area of the cerebral cortex, producing manifestations characteristic of that particular anatomic focus; or (3) may begin in a localized area of the cortex

---

*National Reye's Syndrome Foundation, (800) 233-7393 (United States only) or (419) 924-9000; fax: (419) 924-9999; e-mail: nrsf@reyessyndrome.org; http://www.reyessyndrome.org.
†Rebecca J. Schultz, MSN, RN, CPNP, contributed this section.

BOX 28-9
Etiology of Seizures in Children

NONRECURRENT (ACUTE)	RECURRENT (CHRONIC)
Febrile episodes	Idiopathic epilepsy
Intracranial infection	Epilepsy secondary to:
Intracranial hemorrhage	■ Trauma
Space-occupying lesions (cyst, tumor)	■ Hemorrhage
	■ Anoxia
Acute cerebral edema	■ Infections
Anoxia	■ Toxins
Toxins	■ Degenerative phenomena
Drugs	■ Congenital defects
Tetanus	■ Parasitic brain disease
Lead encephalopathy	■ Hypoglycemia injury
Shigella, Salmonella organisms	Epilepsy—sensory stimulus
Metabolic alterations	Epilepsy-stimulating states
■ Hypocalcemia	■ Narcolepsy and catalepsy
■ Hypoglycemia	■ Psychogenic
■ Hyponatremia or hypernatremia	■ Tetany from hypocalcemia, alkalosis
■ Hypomagnesemia	Hypoglycemic states
■ Alkalosis	■ Hyperinsulinism
■ Disorders of amino acid metabolism	■ Hypopituitarism
■ Deficiency states	■ Adrenocortical insufficiency
■ Hyperbilirubinemia	■ Hepatic disorders
	Uremia
	Allergy
	Cardiovascular dysfunction or syncopal episodes
	Migraine

---

and spread to other portions of the brain and, if sufficiently extensive, produce generalized seizure activity.

In response to physiologic stimuli, such as cellular dehydration, severe hypoglycemia, electrolyte imbalance, sleep deprivation, emotional stress, and endocrine changes, these hyperexcitable cells activate normal cells in surrounding areas and in distant, synaptically related cells. A generalized seizure develops when the neuronal excitation from the epileptogenic focus spreads to the brainstem, particularly the midbrain and reticular formation. These centers within the brainstem, known as the **centrencephalic system,** are responsible for the spread of the epileptic potentials. The discharges can originate spontaneously in the centrencephalic system or be triggered by a focal area in the cortex. On the basis of these characteristic neuronal discharges (as recorded by the EEG), seizures are designated as partial, generalized, and unclassified epileptic seizures (Menkes and Sankar, 2000). In a large proportion of children focal seizures spread to other areas, ultimately becoming generalized with loss of consciousness.

Seizure Classification and Clinical Manifestations

There are many different types of seizures, and each has unique clinical manifestations. Seizures are classified into three major categories:

Partial seizures, which have a local onset and involve a relatively small location in the brain
Generalized seizures, which involve both hemispheres of the brain and are without local onset
Unclassified epileptic seizures

Descriptions of the different types of seizures are found in Box 28-10 and Table 28-3.

Diagnostic Evaluation

Establishing a diagnosis is critical for establishing a prognosis and planning the proper treatment. The process of diagnosis in a child suspected of having epilepsy includes (1) determining whether epilepsy or seizures exist and not an alternative diagnosis, and (2) defining the underlying cause, if possible. The assessment and diagnosis rely heavily on a thorough history, skilled observation, and several diagnostic tests.

It is especially important to differentiate epilepsy from other brief alterations in consciousness or behavior. Clinical entities that mimic seizures include migraine headaches, toxic effects of drugs, syncope (fainting), breath-holding spells in infants and young children, movement disorders (tics, tremor, chorea), prolonged QT syndrome, sleep disturbances (sleepwalking, night terrors), psychogenic seizures, rage attacks, and transient ischemic attacks (rare in children) (Browne and Holmes, 2004). Cocaine intoxication should be considered in the differential diagnosis of new-onset seizure activity in newborn infants.

The history of the seizure should be equally detailed, including the type of seizure or description of the child's behavior during the event, the age at onset, and the time at which the seizure occurs (e.g., early morning, before meals, while

---

BOX 28-10

Classification and Clinical Manifestations of Seizures

PARTIAL SEIZURES

Simple Partial Seizures with Motor Signs
Characterized by:
- Localized motor symptoms
- Somatosensory, psychic, autonomic symptoms
- Combination of these
- Abnormal discharges remaining unilateral

Manifestations:
- Aversive seizure (most common motor seizure in children)—Eye or eyes and head turn away from the side of the focus; awareness of movement or loss of consciousness
- Rolandic (Sylvan) seizure—Tonic-clonic movements involving the face, salivation, arrested speech; most common during sleep
- Jacksonian march (rare in children)—Orderly, sequential progression of clonic movements beginning in a foot, hand, or face and moving, or "marching," to adjacent body parts

Simple Partial Seizures with Sensory Signs
Characterized by various sensations, including:
- Numbness, tingling, prickling, paresthesia, or pain originating in one area (e.g., face or extremities) and spreading to other parts of the body
- Visual sensations or formed images
- Motor phenomena such as posturing or hypertonia

Uncommon in children younger than 8 years of age

Complex Partial Seizures (Psychomotor Seizures)
Observed more often in children from 3 years through adolescence
Characterized by:
- Period of altered behavior
- Amnesia for event (no recollection of behavior)
- Inability to respond to environment
- Impaired consciousness during event
- Drowsiness or sleep usually following seizure
- Confusion and amnesia possibly prolonged
- Complex sensory phenomena (aura)—Most frequent sensation is a strange feeling in the pit of the stomach that rises toward the throat; often accompanied by:
  —Odd or unpleasant odors or tastes
  —Complex auditory or visual hallucinations
  —Ill-defined feelings of elation or strangeness (e.g., déjà vu, a feeling of familiarity in a strange environment)
  —Strong feelings of fear and anxiety; distorted sense of time and self
  —In small children, emission of a cry or attempt to run for help

Patterns of motor behavior:
- Stereotypic
- Similar with each subsequent seizure
- May suddenly cease activity, appear dazed, stare into space, become confused and apathetic, and become limp or stiff or display some form of posturing
- May be confused
- May perform purposeless, complicated activities in a repetitive manner (automatisms), such as walking, running, kicking, laughing, or speaking incoherently, most often followed by postictal confusion or sleep
- May exhibit oropharyngeal activities, such as smacking, chewing, drooling, swallowing, and nausea or abdominal pain followed by stiffness, a fall, and postictal sleep
- Rarely manifests actions such as rage or temper tantrums; aggressive acts uncommon during seizure

GENERALIZED SEIZURES

Tonic-Clonic Seizures (Formerly Known as Grand Mal)
Most common and most dramatic of all seizure manifestations
Occur without warning

Tonic Phase
Lasts approximately 10 to 20 seconds
Manifestations:
- Eyes roll upward
- Immediate loss of consciousness
- If standing, falls to floor or ground
- Stiffens in generalized, symmetric tonic contraction of entire body musculature
- Arms usually flexed
- Legs, head, and neck extended
- May utter a peculiar piercing cry
- Apneic; may become cyanotic
- Increased salivation and loss of swallowing reflex

Clonic Phase
Lasts about 30 seconds but can vary from only a few seconds to a half hour or longer
Manifestations:
- Violent jerking movements as the trunk and extremities undergo rhythmic contraction and relaxation
- May foam at the mouth
- May be incontinent of urine and feces

As event ends, movements less intense, occurring at longer intervals, then ceasing entirely

BOX 28-10

Classification and Clinical Manifestations of Seizures—cont'd

GENERALIZED SEIZURES—cont'd
Tonic-Clonic Seizures (Formerly Known as Grand Mal)—cont'd
Status Epilepticus

Series of seizures at intervals too brief to allow the child to regain consciousness between the time one event ends and the next begins
- Requires emergency intervention
- Can lead to exhaustion, respiratory failure, and death

Postictal State

Manifestations:
- Appears to relax
- May remain semiconscious and difficult to arouse
- May awaken in a few minutes
- Remains confused for several hours
- Poor coordination
- Mild impairment of fine motor movements
- May have visual and speech difficulties
- May vomit or complain of severe headache
- When left alone, usually sleeps for several hours
- On awakening is fully conscious
- Usually feels tired and complains of sore muscles and headache
- No recollection of entire event

Absence Seizures (Formerly Called Petit Mal or Lapses)

Characterized by:
- Onset usually between 4 and 12 years of age
- More common in girls than in boys
- Usually cease at puberty
- Brief loss of consciousness
- Minimum or no alteration in muscle tone
- May go unrecognized because of little change in child's behavior
- Abrupt onset; suddenly develops 20 or more attacks daily
- Event often mistaken for inattentiveness or daydreaming
- Events possibly precipitated by hyperventilation, hypoglycemia, stresses (emotional and physiologic), fatigue, or sleeplessness

Manifestations:
- Brief loss of consciousness
- Appear without warning or aura
- Usually last about 5 to 10 seconds
- Slight loss of muscle tone may cause child to drop objects
- Ability to maintain postural control; seldom falls
- Minor movements such as lip smacking, twitching of eyelids or face, or slight hand movements
- Not accompanied by incontinence
- Amnesia for episode
- May need to reorient self to previous activity

Atonic and Akinetic Seizures (Also Known as Drop Attacks)

Characterized by:
- Onset usually between 2 and 5 years of age
- Sudden, momentary loss of muscle tone and postural control
- Events recurring frequently during the day, particularly in the morning hours and shortly after awakening

Manifestations:
- Loss of tone causing child to fall to the floor violently; unable to break fall by putting out hand; may incur a serious injury to the face, head, or shoulder
- Loss of consciousness only momentary

Myoclonic Seizures

A variety of seizure episodes
May be isolated as benign essential myoclonus
May occur in association with other seizure forms
Characterized by:
- Sudden, brief contractures of a muscle or group of muscles
- Occur singly or repetitively
- No postictal state
- May or may not be symmetric
- May or may not include loss of consciousness

Infantile Spasms

Also called infantile myoclonus, massive spasms, hypsarrhythmia, salaam episodes, or infantile myoclonic spasms
Most commonly occur during the first 6 to 8 months of life
Twice as common in boys as in girls
Numerous seizures during the day without postictal drowsiness or sleep
Poor outlook for normal intelligence
Manifestations:
- Possible series of sudden, brief, symmetric, muscular contractions
- Head flexed, arms extended, and legs drawn up
- Eyes sometimes rolling upward or inward
- May be preceded or followed by a cry or giggling
- May or may not include loss of consciousness
- Sometimes flushing, pallor, or cyanosis

Infants who are able to sit but not stand:
- Sudden dropping forward of the head and neck with trunk flexed forward and knees drawn up—the *salaam* or *jackknife* seizure

Less often: alternate clinical forms
- Extensor spasms rather than flexion of arms, legs, and trunk, and head nodding
- Lightning events involving a single, momentary, shocklike contraction of the entire body

---

TABLE 28-3

Comparison of Simple Partial, Complex Partial, and Absence Seizures

CLINICAL MANIFESTATIONS	SIMPLE PARTIAL	COMPLEX PARTIAL	ABSENCE
Age of onset	Any age	Uncommon before age 3 years	Uncommon before age 3 years
Frequency (per day)	Variable	Rarely over 1-2 times	Multiple
Duration	Usually <30 seconds	Usually >60 seconds, rarely <10 seconds	Usually <10 seconds, rarely >30 seconds
Aura	May be sole manifestation of seizure	Frequent	Never
Impaired consciousness	Never	Always	Always; brief loss of consciousness
Automatisms	Never	Frequent	Frequent
Clonic movements	Frequent	Occasional	Occasional
Postictal impairment	Rare	Frequent	Never
Mental disorientation	Rare	Common	Unusual

awake, or during sleep). Any factors that may have precipitated the seizure are important, including fever, infection, head trauma, anxiety, fatigue, sleep deprivation, menstrual cycle, alcohol, and activity (e.g., hyperventilation or exposure to strong stimuli such as bright flashing light or loud noises). If the child can describe any sensory phenomena, these are recorded. The duration and progression of the seizure (if any) and the postictal feelings and behavior (e.g., confusion, inability to speak, amnesia, headache, and sleep) are recorded. It is important to determine whether more than one seizure type exists. It is often more informative to ask parents to mime the seizure rather than relying on their oral description. Miming often reveals features, such as head turning, that would otherwise go unrecognized. Some seizures are overlooked by parents. For example, some parents may not identify brief head nods or brief single jerks as seizures unless specifically asked whether their child has these symptoms. The family history should include whether other family members have had a seizure, intellectual disability, cerebral palsy, or other neurologic disorders. A family history can offer clues to paroxysmal disorders such as migraine headaches, breath-holding spells, febrile seizures, or neurologic diseases.

A complete physical and neurologic examination, including developmental assessment of language, learning, behavior, and motor abilities, may provide clues to the cause of the seizures. A number of laboratory and neuroimaging tests may be ordered depending on the child's age, whether this is a new onset seizure, characteristics of the seizure, and the history. Laboratory studies that may prove to be of value include a venous lead level if the history warrants or white blood cell count (for signs of infection). Blood glucose may give evidence of hypoglycemic episodes, and serum electrolytes, blood urea nitrogen, calcium, serum amino acids, lactate, ammonia, and urine organic acids may indicate metabolic disturbances. Blood for chromosomal analysis may also be tested if a genetic etiology is suspected. A toxic screen may be done if alcohol or drug abuse or withdrawal is suspected. Lumbar puncture can confirm a suspected diagnosis of meningitis. CT may be done to detect a cerebral hemorrhage, infarctions, and gross malformations. MRI provides greater anatomic detail and is used to detect developmental malformations, tumors, and cortical dysplasias (Kuzniecky, 2001).

The EEG is obtained for all children with seizures and is the most useful tool for evaluating a seizure disorder. The EEG confirms the presence of abnormal electrical discharges and provides information on the seizure type and the focus. The EEG is carried out under varying conditions—with the child asleep, awake, awake with provocative stimulation (flashing lights, noise), and hyperventilating. Stimulation may elicit abnormal electrical activity, which is recorded on the EEG. Various seizure types produce characteristic EEG patterns: high-voltage spike discharges are seen in tonic-clonic seizures, with abnormal patterns in the intervals between seizures; a three-per-second spike and wave pattern is observed in an absence seizure; and absence of electrical activity in an area suggests a large lesion, such as an abscess or subdural collection of fluid.

A normal EEG does not rule out seizures because the EEG is only a surface recording and only represents approximately 1 hour of time and therefore may show normal interictal activity. If there is concern about whether a child has seizures or

the seizure type cannot be determined, then a long-term video EEG may be done to record the child during wakefulness and sleep. The full body image is recorded on video, with selected EEG channels displayed on the same screen for simultaneous recording and viewing. EEG monitoring is also available in digital EEG and digital video imaging, which allows for greater selection of EEG channels and is available in both routine and long-term EEGs. Polygraph equipment may also be used to monitor physiologic data such as respiratory effort, eye movements, heart rate, and systemic blood pressure. These techniques can be used concurrently and are especially valuable in differentiating epileptic activity from paroxysmal behavior or nonepileptic motor events.

Therapeutic Management

The goal of treatment of seizure disorders is to control the seizures or to reduce their frequency and severity, discover and correct the cause when possible, and help the child live as normal a life as possible. If the seizure activity is a manifestation of an infectious, traumatic, or metabolic process, the seizure therapy is instituted as part of the general therapeutic regimen. Management of epilepsy has four treatment options: drug therapy, the ketogenic diet, vagus nerve stimulation, and epilepsy surgery.

Drug Therapy. It is known that persons predisposed to epilepsy have seizures when their basal level of neuronal excitability exceeds a critical point; no event occurs if the excitability is maintained below this threshold. The administration of antiepileptic drugs serves to raise this threshold and prevent seizures. Consequently, the primary therapy for seizure disorders is the administration of the appropriate antiepileptic drug or combination of drugs in a dosage that provides the desired effect without causing undesirable side effects or toxic reactions. Antiepileptic drugs are believed to exert their effect primarily by reducing the responsiveness of normal neurons to the sudden, high-frequency nerve impulses that arise in the epileptogenic focus. Thus the seizure is effectively suppressed; however, the abnormal brain waves may or may not be altered. Complete control can be achieved in 75% of children with epilepsy; good control can be achieved in another 15% (Shafer, 1999).

Therapy is begun with a single drug known to be effective and have the lowest toxicity, that is, the safest side effect profile for the child's particular type of seizure. The dosage is gradually increased until the seizures are controlled or the child develops side effects. If the drug is effective but does not sufficiently control the seizures, a second drug is added in gradually increasing doses. Once seizures are controlled, the first drug may be tapered to reduce the potential adverse effects of polytherapy. However, this decision is individualized for each child (Browne and Holmes, 2004). Monotherapy remains the treatment method of choice for epilepsy, but polypharmacy may be a viable alternative for children who cannot attain seizure control with only one agent (Leppik, 2000).

Measurement of blood levels of the drug is important if the seizures continue once the child is on a therapeutic dose of medication, to adjust the dosage, and to assist in determining which medication may be causing the side effects if the child is on multiple antiepileptic medications. Some possible causes of low serum blood concentrations are noncompliance, poor absorption, and drug interactions. The dosage needs to be increased as the child grows. Blood cell counts, urinalysis, and liver function tests are obtained at frequent intervals in children receiving particular antiepileptic medications that can affect organ function.

If complete seizure control is maintained on an anticonvulsant drug for 2 years, it is safe to discontinue the drug for patients with no risk factors. Risk factors include children over 12 years of age at onset, history of neonatal seizures, numerous seizures before control is achieved, and the presence of a neurologic dysfunction (e.g., motor handicap or intellectual disability). Up to 25% of children whose medications are discontinued will experience seizure recurrence. Recurrence occurs most frequently within 6 months of discontinuation (Johnston, 2007).

When seizure medications are discontinued, the dosage is decreased gradually over several weeks. Sudden withdrawal of a drug is not recommended because it can cause an increase in the number and severity of seizures.

> ### NURSING ALERT
>
> Fosphenytoin is often used to treat seizures instead of IV phenytoin because of possible complications and drug interactions associated with IV phenytoin. If IV phenytoin is used, it should be administered via slow IV push at a rate that does not exceed 50 mg/min. Because phenytoin precipitates when mixed with glucose, only normal saline is used to flush the tubing or catheter. Fosphenytoin may be given in saline or glucose solutions at a rate of up to 150 mg PE (phenytoin equivalent)/min, and it may be given intramuscularly if necessary.

Ketogenic Diet. The ketogenic diet is a high-fat, low-carbohydrate, and adequate protein diet (Lefevre and Aronson, 2000). Consumption of such a diet forces the body to shift from using glucose as the primary energy source to using fat, and the individual develops a state of ketosis. The diet is rigorous. All foods and liquids the child consumes must be carefully weighed and measured. The diet is deficient in vitamins and minerals; therefore vitamin supplements are necessary. Potential side effects of the diet are constipation, weight loss, lethargy, and kidney stones. It is unknown whether long-term effects such as increased blood lipids will occur (Levy and Cooper, 2003).

The ketogenic diet has been shown to be an efficacious and tolerable treatment for difficult-to-control seizures (Freeman, Kossoff, and Hartman, 2007). Outcomes of 150 children with uncontrollable seizures revealed that 7% of the children were seizure free and another 20% had a 90% decrease in seizures 1 year after instituting the ketogenic diet (Freeman, Vining, Pillas, and others, 1998). Three to six years later, 27% of these children had few or no seizures while on the ketogenic diet (Hemingway, Freeman, Pillas, and others, 2001).

Vagus Nerve Stimulation. Vagus nerve stimulation uses an implantable device that reduces seizures in individuals who have not had effective control with drug therapy. It is currently indicated as adjunct therapy in patients 12 years and older with partial onset seizures (with or without secondary generalization). A programmable signal generator is implanted subcutaneously in the chest. Electrodes tunneled underneath the skin deliver electrical impulses to the left vagus nerve (cranial nerve X). The device is programmed noninvasively to deliver a precise pattern of stimulation to the left vagus nerve. The patient or caregiver can activate the device using a magnet at the onset of a seizure. Studies show that about one third of patients have a 50% or greater reduction in seizures after 1 year of therapy (Morris, Mueller, and Vagus Nerve Stimulation Study Group, 1999).

Surgical Therapy. When seizures are determined to be caused by a hematoma, tumor, or other cerebral lesion, surgical removal is the treatment. In children with epilepsy, surgery is reserved for those who suffer from incapacitating, refractory seizures. Refractory seizures are usually defined as the persistence of seizures despite adequate trials of three antiepileptic medications, alone or in combination (Browne and Holmes, 2004). The epileptogenic area should be in a surgically removable and functionally silent region of the brain. Early removal of the symptomatic area is associated with seizure control and decreased use of antiepileptic drugs (Mathern, Giza, Yudovin, and others, 1999). An extensive medical (e.g., invasive EEG monitoring), psychosocial, and psychoneurologic evaluation is required.

Status Epilepticus. Status epilepticus is a continuous seizure that lasts more than 30 minutes or a series of seizures from which the child does not regain a premorbid LOC (Shorvon and Walker, 2005; Treiman and Walker, 2006). The duration required for seizures to be considered status epilepticus continues to be debated (Chen and Wasterlain, 2006). The initial treatment is directed toward support and maintenance of vital functions, that is, attending to the ABCs of life support, administering oxygen, and gaining IV access, immediately followed by IV administration of antiepileptic agents.

Rectal diazepam is a simple, effective, and safe treatment for home or prehospital management (Pellock and Shinnar, 2005). It is available in a prefilled rectal gel syringe (Diastat) for easy administration. Rectal diazepam is not associated with respiratory depression when used as recommended (Pellock and Shinnar, 2005). Midazolam has been given successfully by intranasal route for treatment of acute epileptic seizures (Fisgin, Gurer, Senbil, and others, 2000; Kutlu, Yakinci, Dogrul, and others, 2000). Intranasal midazolam not only is safe and effective for stopping seizures, but is easier to administer than rectal diazepam (Harbord, Kyrkou, Kyrkou, and others, 2004).

For in-hospital management of status epilepticus, IV diazepam or lorazepam (Ativan) is the first-line drug of choice (Browne and Holmes, 2004). Lorazepam may be replacing IV diazepam as the drug of choice. It has a longer duration of action and causes less respiratory depression in children over 2 years of age. Concurrent IV loading with fosphenytoin is usually necessary for sustained control of seizures. Valproic acid has also been reported to be effective in status epilepticus when given rectally or intravenously (Yamamoto and Yim, 2000). The child must be closely monitored during administration to detect early alterations in vital signs that may indicate impending respiratory depression. When diazepam is ineffective, fosphenytoin or phenobarbital is given intravenously as the next line of treatment. This combination of therapy places the child at high risk for apnea, and therefore respiratory support is generally necessary. Children who continue to have seizures despite the above drug treatment may be given anesthetizing doses of midazolam, propofol, or pentobarbital. In this situation, continuous EEG monitoring is typically done to monitor for and treat electrographic seizures.

> **NURSINGALERT**
>
> Diazepam is incompatible with many drugs. To give intravenously, inject slowly and directly into the vein or through tubing as close as possible to the vein insertion site.

Nursing care of a child with status epilepticus includes, in addition to the ABCs of life support, monitoring blood pressure and body temperature. During the first 30 to 45 minutes of the seizure the blood pressure may be elevated. Thereafter the blood pressure typically returns to normal but may be decreased depending on the medications being administered for seizure control. Hyperthermia requiring treatment may occur as a result of increased motor activity.

Prognosis

Most children who experience a second seizure will experience additional seizures. Therefore a history of two seizures is sufficient to diagnose epilepsy (Shinnar, Berg, O'Dell, and others, 2000). Epidemiologic studies using population- or community-based cohorts show that the etiology and specific epilepsy syndromes are the most important factors affecting prognosis.

Children who have intellectual disability or cerebral palsy are at the highest risk for developing epilepsy. Seizures will remit in more than two thirds of children with childhood onset of seizure. Mortality is increased in children with epilepsy; those with neurologic abnormalities or seizures that are refractory to treatment are at the highest risk (Browne and Holmes, 2004).

Nursing Care Management

An important nursing responsibility is to observe the seizure episode and accurately document the events. Any alterations in behavior preceding the seizure and the characteristics of the episode, such as sensory-hallucinatory phenomena (e.g., an aura), motor effects (e.g., eye movements, muscular contractions), alterations in consciousness, and postictal state, are noted and recorded (Box 28-11). The nurse should describe only what is observed, rather than trying to label a seizure type. He or she notes the time that the seizure began and the duration of the seizure.

Based on a thorough assessment, several nursing diagnoses are identified. The more common diagnoses for the child with a seizure disorder are included in the Nursing Process box and Nursing Care Plan.

Text continued on p. 1015

BOX 28-11

General Observations: The Child During a Seizure

OBSERVATIONS DURING SEIZURE

General Description
Order of events (before, during, and after)
Duration of seizure
- Tonic-clonic—from first signs of event until jerking stops
- Absence—from loss of consciousness until consciousness is regained
- Complex partial—from first sign of unresponsiveness, motor activity, automatisms until there are signs of responsiveness to environment

Onset
Time of onset
Significant precipitating events—missed medication dosage, illness, stress, sleep deprivation, menses

Behavior
Change in facial expression
Cry or other sound
Stereotypic or automatous movements
Random activity (wandering)
Position of eyes, head, body, extremities
Unilateral or bilateral posturing of one or more extremities

Movement
Change of position, if any
Site of commencement—hand, thumb, mouth, generalized
Tonic phase—length, parts of body involved
Clonic phase—twitching or jerking movements, parts of body involved, sequence of parts involved, generalized, change in character of movements
Lack of movement or muscle tone of body part or entire body

Face
Color change—pallor, cyanosis, flushing
Perspiration
Mouth—position, deviation to one side, teeth clenched, tongue bitten, frothing at mouth, flecks of blood or bleeding
Lack of expression
Asymmetric expression

Eyes
Position—straight ahead, deviation upward or outward, conjugate or divergent gaze
Pupils—change in size, equality, reaction to light

Respiratory Effort
Presence and length of apnea

Other
Incontinence

POSTICTAL OBSERVATIONS
Duration of postictal period
State of consciousness
Orientation
Arousability
Motor ability
- Any change in motor function
- Ability to move all extremities
- Paresis or weakness
Speech
Sensations
- Complaint of discomfort or pain
- Any sensory impairment
Recollection of preseizure sensations (aura)

nursingprocess | The Child with Seizures

ASSESSMENT

Assess for signs and symptoms of seizures in children; observe any alterations in behavior preceding the seizure and the characteristics of the episode, motor effects, alterations in consciousness, and postictal state. A complete description of the general observations of a child experiencing a seizure is found in the Nursing Care Plan.

DIAGNOSIS (PROBLEM IDENTIFICATION)

After a thorough assessment, several nursing diagnoses are evident (see Nursing Care Plan below). Other nursing diagnoses include:

- Anxiety
- Ineffective Tissue Perfusion
- Interrupted Family Processes
- Self-Esteem Disturbance

PLANNING

Expected patient outcomes include:

- Child will be protected during a seizure.
- Influencing or triggering factors will be determined and adjustments made to lessen seizure events.
- Child will experience as few seizures as possible.
- Child and family will cope with the challenges associated with the disorder.
- Child will develop a positive self-image.

INTERVENTIONS

Numerous intervention strategies are discussed on pp. 1010-1016.

EVALUATION

The effectiveness of nursing interventions for the family and child with epilepsy is determined by continual assessment and evaluation of care based on the following guidelines:

- Observe child's behavior for evidence of seizure activity, and assess the environment for situations that could cause injury to child in the event of a seizure; interview family regarding management of child during a seizure.
- Interview child and family regarding adherence to the medication regimen and identification of triggering factors.
- Observe and interview family regarding their feelings and concerns and their understanding of child's condition.
- Observe child's interactions with others, and interview child about any feelings or concerns regarding health.

nursingcareplan | The Child with Seizure Disorder

Nursing Diagnosis	Expected Patient Outcomes	Nursing Interventions	Rationale
Risk for Injury related to central nervous system (CNS) dysfunction and inability to control self (motor) secondary to type of seizure	Child will not experience physical injury as a result of seizure activity.	Administer antiepileptic medication (AED).	To prevent seizure activity
	The Following NOC Concepts Apply to These Outcomes	Teach family and child, as appropriate, the purpose of AED medication, action, potential side effects, and administration of medications.	To prevent seizure activity and encourage self-care
Child's/Family's Defining Characteristics *(Subjective and Objective Data)*	Risk Control Personal Safety Behavior Safe Home Environment Falls Occurrence	Monitor for side effects of AED and therapeutic levels according to child's growth, illness factors that affect metabolism, and effects of drug.	To prevent secondary effects of AED and prevent seizure from subtherapeutic drug levels
Change in level of consciousness (LOC) Disorientation Clonic movements Automatisms Aura		Stress importance of compliance with medication regimen even if child has no evidence of seizure activity.	To prevent seizure activity
Postictal impairment (dependent on the type of seizure)		Advise family and child to avoid situations that are known to precipitate a seizure (e.g., blinking lights, fatigue, excess activity or exercise, physical factors).	To prevent exposure to situations that may cause a seizure
		Assess home care environment for risk factors that may produce childhood physical injury: loose rugs; unprotected stairway; access to water buckets, pool, or standing water.	To prevent physical harm
		Teach parents by anticipatory guidance risk factors for injury in environment based on child's developmental age and type of seizure (e.g., not leaving child in bathtub without adult supervision).	

Continued

Nursing Diagnosis	Expected Patient Outcomes	Nursing Interventions	Rationale
Risk for Injury related to central nervous system (CNS) dysfunction and inability to control self (motor) secondary to type of seizure—cont'd		Counsel female patients of childbearing age taking AEDs about contraception and birth defects associated with AEDs.	To prevent birth defects in offspring of women taking AEDs
		In the event of a tonic-clonic seizure: Place child on side. Time seizure.	To prevent injury and trauma To prevent aspiration and maintain a patent airway
		Protect child during seizure. Do not attempt to restrain child or use force. If child is standing or sitting in wheelchair at beginning of episode, ease child to floor. Do not put anything in child's mouth. Place small cushion or blanket under child's head. Remove eyeglasses. Loosen clothing. Prevent child from hitting head on objects. Remove hazards. Pad objects such as crib, side rails, or wheelchair. Keep side rails raised when child is sleeping, resting, or having a seizure. Allow seizure to end without interference.	
		Teach parents or caregiver how to care for child during seizure and in postictal state.	To protect child and caregiver from injury
		Protect child after seizure (postictal period). Time the period. Maintain child in a side-lying or recovery position. Call emergency medical services as necessary or ensure child receives medical evaluation after seizure.	To prevent trauma and implement therapeutic intervention
		The Following NIC Concepts Apply to These Interventions	
		Surveillance: Safety Environmental Management: Safety Medication Administration Teaching: Disease Process Neurologic Monitoring Seizure Precautions	

Nursing Diagnosis	Expected Patient Outcomes	Nursing Interventions	Rationale
Risk for Aspiration and Ineffective Breathing Pattern related to impaired motor activity, loss of consciousness, and loss of airway protection (tonic-clonic seizure)	Child's airway will remain patent. Child will have effective ventilations.	In the event of a seizure, place child in a side-lying position on a flat surface such as floor or bed.	To prevent aspiration and protect airway
	The Following NOC Concepts Apply to These Outcomes	Remain with child.	To determine need for emergency care
Child's/Family's Defining Characteristics *(Subjective and Objective Data)*	Aspiration Prevention Respiratory Status: Airway Patency Respiratory Status: Ventilation	Remove secretions, food, and liquids from mouth when seizure subsides.	To prevent choking, aspiration
Reduced LOC		If child has emesis, place on side.	To prevent choking, aspiration
Depressed cough reflex		In postictal state monitor oxygenation status.	To determine need for oxygen
Apnea Decreased inspiratory pressure		Administer oxygen as necessary to maintain pulse oximeter over 89%.	To prevent hypoxia

nursingcareplan | The Child with Seizure Disorder—cont'd

Nursing Diagnosis	Expected Patient Outcomes	Nursing Interventions	Rationale
Risk for Aspiration and Ineffective Breathing Pattern related to impaired motor activity, loss of consciousness, and loss of airway protection (tonic-clonic seizure)—cont'd		Suction oropharynx once seizure subsides as necessary to clear mucus or food. Administer medications intended to stop seizure (rectal diazepam [Diastat], rectal phenytoin, IV phenytoin). **The Following NIC Concepts Apply to These Interventions** Risk Identification Aspiration Precautions Oxygen Therapy Medication Administration	To prevent aspiration To prevent continued seizure activity

Nursing Diagnosis	Expected Patient Outcomes	Nursing Interventions	Rationale
Risk for Injury related to impaired consciousness and automatisms **Child's/Family's Defining Characteristics** *(Subjective and Objective Data)* Immediate loss of consciousness Tonic rigidity replaced by intense jerking movements May become incontinent of urine and feces Postictal impairment Change in vital signs, respiratory status, color Vomiting	Child will not experience physical injury and will remain calm. **The Following NOC Concepts Apply to These Outcomes** Risk Control Safe Home Environment Personal Safety Behavior Physical Injury Severity Falls Occurrence	Time seizure. Protect child during seizure. Do not attempt to restrain child or use force. Remove hazards in immediate environment. Redirect child to safe area, especially away from windows, stairs, heating elements, or sources of water. Talk in calm voice and reassuring manner. Watch to see whether seizure generalizes into a tonic-clinic seizure. Protect child after seizure (postictal period). Time the period. Stay with child until fully alert. **The Following NIC Concepts Apply to These Interventions** Risk Identification Environmental Management: Safety Surveillance Seizure Precautions	To establish duration and possible need for emergency care To prevent injury to child or self To prevent injury To prevent injury from falls, burns, and drowning To prevent further agitation To determine type of seizure To provide support, because child may be confused and frightened

Nursing Diagnosis	Expected Patient Outcomes	Nursing Interventions	Rationale
Anxiety/Fear (Parent), related to child having life-threatening and incapacitating seizure activity* **Child's/Family's Defining Characteristics** *(Subjective and Objective Data)* Anguish Fright Feelings of inadequacy and hopelessness Worry, apprehension Panic Excitement	Parent will cope with child's condition and receive adequate support. **The Following NOC Concepts Apply to These Outcomes** Anxiety Self-Control Coping Fear Self-Control	Allow parent(s) to remain with child during seizure. Instruct parent on proper protection interventions during child's seizure activity: positioning, safety, airway maintenance, reassurance techniques, emergency medication administration. Provide information regarding nature (type) of seizure, therapeutic interventions, and lifestyle modifications.	To decrease fear of unknown and allow parent to see measures taken to protect child To promote parent participation and to promote sense of control over situation To promote knowledge of condition, parental intervention, sense of control

*Nursing diagnosis may also apply to child in the postictal phase, depending on type of seizure and child's understanding and cognitive level.

Continued

nursingcareplan   The Child with Seizure Disorder—cont'd

Nursing Diagnosis	Expected Patient Outcomes	Nursing Interventions	Rationale
Anxiety/Fear (Parent), related to child having life-threatening and incapacitating seizure activity—cont'd		Encourage family involvement in daily care of child, with goal of normalization and promotion of optimal growth and development of child.	To provide hope and promote family functioning and coping
		Involve parents in discussion of fears and anxieties; discuss resource and support options available to family.	To promote family integrity and functioning

The Following NIC Concepts Apply to These Interventions

Support Group
Coping Enhancement
Anxiety Reduction
Family Process Maintenance
Active Listening
Counseling
Decision-Making Support
Family Involvement Promotion

emergencytreatment

Seizures

TONIC-CLONIC SEIZURE

During the Seizure

Remain calm.

Time seizure episode.

If child is standing or seated, ease child down to the floor.

Place pillow or folded blanket under child's head.

Loosen restrictive clothing.

Remove eyeglasses.

Clear area of any hazards or hard objects.

Allow seizure to end without interference.

If vomiting occurs, turn child to one side.

Do not:

- Attempt to restrain child or use force
- Put anything in child's mouth
- Give any food or liquids

After the Seizure

Time postictal period.

Check for breathing. Check position of head and tongue.

Reposition if head is hyperextended. If child is not breathing, give rescue breathing and call emergency medical services (EMS).

Keep child on side.

Remain with child.

Do not give food or liquids until child is fully alert and swallowing reflex has returned.

Call EMS when necessary.

Look for medical identification, and determine what factors occurred before onset of seizure that may have been triggering factors.

Check head and body for possible injuries.

Check inside of mouth to see if tongue or lips have been bitten.

COMPLEX PARTIAL SEIZURE

During the Seizure

Do not restrain.

Remove harmful objects from area.

Redirect to safe area.

Do not agitate; instead, talk in calm, reassuring manner.

Do not expect child to follow instructions.

Watch to see if seizure generalizes.

After the Seizure

Stay with child and reassure until fully conscious.

CALL EMERGENCY MEDICAL SERVICES IF

Child stops breathing.

There is evidence of injury or child is diabetic or pregnant.

Seizure lasts for more than 5 minutes (unless duration of seizure is typically longer than 5 minutes) and written medical order is present.

Status epilepticus occurs.

Pupils are not equal after seizure.

Child vomits continuously 30 minutes after seizure has ended (sign of possible acute problem).

Child cannot be awakened and is unresponsive to pain after seizure has ended.

Seizure occurs in water.

This is child's first seizure.

Modified from *Seizure recognition and first aid*, 2001, Epilepsy Foundation, retrieved March 5, 2007, from http://www.epilepsyfoundation.org.

The child must be protected from injury during the seizure; nursing observations made during the event provide valuable information for diagnosis and management of the disorder (see Emergency Treatment box).

It is impossible to halt a seizure once it has begun, and no attempt should be made to do so. The nurse must remain calm, stay with the child, and prevent the child from sustaining any harm during the seizure. If possible, the child should be isolated from the view of others by closing a door or pulling screens. A seizure can be upsetting to the child, other visitors, and their families. If other persons are present, they should be assured that everything is being done for the child. After the seizure, they can be given a simple explanation about the event as needed.

If the nurse is able to reach the child in time, a child who is standing or seated in a chair (including a wheelchair) is eased to the floor immediately. During (and sometimes after) the tonic-clonic seizure, the swallowing reflex is lost, salivation increases, and the tongue is hypotonic. Therefore the child is at risk for aspiration and airway occlusion. Placing the child on the side facilitates drainage and helps maintain a patent airway. Suctioning the oral cavity and posterior oropharynx may be necessary. Vital signs should be taken. The child is allowed to rest if at school or away from home. When feasible, the child is integrated into the environment as soon as possible. Sending a child with a chronic seizure disorder home from school is not necessary unless requested by the parents.

Seizure precautions are required for children who are known to have seizures or who are under observation for seizures. The extent of these measures depends on the type and frequency of the seizure (Box 28-12).

> **NURSINGALERT**
>
> Do not move or forcefully restrain the child during a tonic-clonic seizure, and do not place a solid object between the teeth.

Long-Term Care. Care of the child with a recurrent seizure disorder involves physical care and instruction regarding the importance of the drug therapy and, probably more significant, the problems related to the emotional aspects of the disorder. Few diseases generate as much anxiety among relatives as epilepsy. Fears and misconceptions about the disease and its treatment abound in the layperson's mind. For many, it represents the archetype of severe hereditary affliction. Nursing care is directed toward educating the child and family about epilepsy and helping them develop strategies to cope with the psychologic and sociologic problems related to epilepsy.

Children with epilepsy are prescribed antiepileptic medications. These medications are administered at regular intervals to maintain adequate levels in the blood. The most convenient times for administration seem to be with meals or at bedtime. It is important to impress on the family the necessity of giving the antiepileptic medication regularly and for as long as required. In general, antiepileptic medications are continued until the child has been seizure free for 2 years (Johnston, 2007). The medication is then slowly tapered over a period of weeks to avoid the possibility of precipitating a seizure. It is sometimes easy to skip doses or omit them for a variety of reasons, especially when the child is free of seizures most of the time. This is particularly so when the child is older and assumes responsibility for his or her medication. The seizure threshold may be lowered during any illness, but particularly with fever. Therefore parents should be aware that if their

> **BOX 28-12**
>
> ## Seizure Precautions
>
> The extent of precautions depends on type, severity, and frequency of seizures. They may include:
> - Side rails raised when child is sleeping or resting
> - Side rails and other hard objects padded
> - Waterproof mattress or pad on bed or crib
>
> Appropriate precautions during potentially hazardous activities may include:
> - Swimming with a companion
> - Showers preferred; bathing only with close supervision
> - Use of protective helmet and padding during bicycle riding, skateboarding, in-line skating
> - Supervision during use of hazardous machinery or equipment
>
> Have child carry or wear medical identification.
> Alert other caregivers to need for any special precautions.
> Child may not drive or operate hazardous machinery or equipment unless seizure free for designated period (varies by state).

child has an illness, he or she is at increased risk for seizures. Parents should contact their health professional if their child misses medications during an illness because of vomiting.

Rectal preparations of some antiepileptic medications are highly effective when a child is unable to take oral medications because of repeated vomiting, gastrointestinal surgery, or status epilepticus. Parents can learn to administer rectal antiepileptic medication for home treatment. Rectal diazepam is a useful adjunctive home treatment for children at risk for prolonged seizures or clusters of seizures. Hospitalization is minimized, and parental confidence is enhanced.

> **NURSINGALERT**
>
> Children taking phenobarbital or phenytoin should receive adequate vitamin D and folic acid, since deficiencies of both have been associated with these drugs. Phenytoin should not be taken with milk.

Nurses should educate the child and parents about the possible adverse reactions to the medications used to treat seizures. Parents should understand the common side effects and be encouraged to report their observations to their health care provider. Parents should understand that the child needs periodic physical assessment and laboratory studies. Possible adverse effects on the hematopoietic system, liver, and kidneys may be reflected in symptoms such as fever, sore throat, enlarged lymph nodes, jaundice, and bleeding (e.g., easy bruising, petechiae, ecchymoses, epistaxis). A common factor in status epilepticus is inadequate blood levels of antiepileptic drugs.

Although children with epilepsy are at increased risk for injury, limitations on activities should be relatively few. The degree to which activities are restricted is individualized for each child and depends on the type, frequency, and severity of the seizures; the child's response to therapy; and the length of time the seizures have been controlled. To prevent head injuries, children should always wear appropriate safety devices, such as helmets, and should avoid activities involving heights. Although bike riding is safe for most children, children with frequent seizures and impairment of consciousness should avoid it. Skating, in-line skating, and skateboarding should be restricted only in children with frequent seizures. Helmets must be worn while participating in these activities.

Children with epilepsy are at higher risk for drowning than children without epilepsy. Young children should never be left alone in the bathtub, even for a few seconds. Older children and adolescents should be encouraged to use a shower and reminded not to lock the bathroom door when showering. They should never swim unsupervised.

Because the child is encouraged to attend school, camp, and other normal activities, the school nurse and teachers should be made aware of the child's condition and therapy. They can help ensure regularity of medication administration and provision of any special care the child might need. Teachers, child care providers, camp counselors, youth organization leaders, coaches, and other adults who assume responsibility for children should be instructed regarding care of the child during a seizure so that they can act calmly for the child's welfare and influence the attitude of the child's peers.

Triggering Factors. Careful and detailed documentation of seizures over time may indicate a pattern. When this occurs, the nurse or responsible adult may intervene to identify the triggering factors and make changes in the environment that may prevent seizures or decrease their frequency. Often the necessary changes are simple but can make an enormous difference in the lives of the child and family.

The most common factors that may trigger seizures in children include emotional stress, sleep deprivation, fatigue, fever, and illness (Frucht, Quigg, Schwaner, and others, 2000; Nakken, Solaas, Kjeldsen, and others, 2005). Other precipitating factors include sleep, flickering lights, menstrual cycle, alcohol, heat, hyperventilation, and fasting (Frucht, Quigg, Schwaner, and others, 2000). Some individuals have pattern-sensitive epilepsy, that is, seizures precipitated by changes in dark-light patterns, such as those that occur with a flash on a camera, automobile headlights, reflections of light on snow or water, or rotating blades on a fan. A study by Radhakrishnan, Johnson, McClelland, and others (2005) showed that most of these individuals had absence, myoclonic, or generalized tonic-clonic seizures. Some children have seizures while playing video games. These children are sensitive to intermittent photic stimulation that can trigger an epileptic episode (Fylan, Harding, Edson, and others, 1999; Ricci and Vigevano, 1999). However, the overwhelming majority of children with epilepsy can play video or computer games and watch television without the risk of seizures.

FEBRILE SEIZURES

The International League Against Epilepsy defines a febrile seizure as "a seizure in association with a febrile illness in the absence of a central nervous system infection or acute electrolyte imbalance in children older than 1 month of age without prior afebrile seizures" (Baram and Shinnar, 2002). Febrile seizures are one of the most common neurologic conditions of childhood, affecting approximately 3% to 8% of children (Sadleir and Scheffer, 2007). Most febrile seizures occur between 6 months and 3 years of age, with the average age of onset between 12 and 30 months. They are unusual after 5 years of age. Boys are affected about twice as often as girls, and there appears to be an increased familial susceptibility.

The cause of febrile seizures is still uncertain. Both animal and human studies demonstrate an age-specific susceptibility to seizures induced by fever and that it is the peak temperature that is important, not the rapidity of the temperature elevation (Baram and Shinnar, 2002). The temperature usually exceeds 38.8° C (101.8° F), and the seizure occurs during the temperature rise rather than after a prolonged elevation. Sometimes it constitutes the dramatic beginning of an illness, often an upper respiratory tract or gastrointestinal infection.

Most febrile seizures have stopped by the time the child is taken to a medical facility. However, if the seizure continues, treatment consists of controlling the seizure with IV or rectal diazepam and reducing the temperature with acetaminophen. Antiepileptic prophylaxis is not indicated. Parental education and emotional support are important interventions. Parents need reassurance regarding the benign nature of febrile seizures. Several large studies show no difference in intelligence, behavior, or academic performance in children with febrile seizures compared with either population or sibling controls (Verity, Greenword, and Golding, 1998). Parents also need education on how to protect the child from harm and observe exactly what happens to the child during the event. Attempts to lower the temperature will not prevent a seizure. Tepid sponge baths are not recommended for several reasons: they are ineffective in significantly lowering the temperature, the shivering effect further increases metabolic output, and cooling causes discomfort to the child.

Long-term antiepileptic therapy is usually not required for children with simple febrile seizures. Antipyretic therapy during febrile illness offers symptomatic relief for fever-associated symptoms but appears to be ineffective in preventing a seizure (Sadleir and Scheffer, 2007).

> ### NURSINGALERT
> If a febrile seizure lasts more than 5 minutes, parents should seek medical attention right away. Instruct them to call for emergency assistance (911) and not to place the child who is actively having a seizure in the car.

CEREBRAL MALFORMATIONS
CRANIAL DEFORMITIES

In the normal newborn the cranial sutures are separated by membranous seams several millimeters wide. For the first few hours to 1 to 2 days after birth, the cranial bones are highly mobile, which allows them to mold and slide over one another, adjusting the circumference of the head to accommodate to the changing shape and character of the birth canal. The principal sutures in the infant's skull are the sagittal, coronal, and lambdoidal sutures, and the major soft areas at the juncture of these sutures are the anterior and posterior fontanels (see Fig. 8-6).

After birth, growth of the skull bones occurs in a direction **perpendicular** to the line of the suture, and normal closure occurs in a regular and predictable order. Although there are wide variations in the age at which closure takes place in individual children, normally all sutures and fontanels are ossified by the following ages:

Eight weeks—Posterior fontanel closed
Six months—Fibrous union of suture lines and interlocking of serrated edges
Eighteen months—Anterior fontanel closed
After 12 years—Sutures unable to be separated by increased ICP

Solid union of all sutures is not completed until late childhood. Closure of a suture before the expected time inhibits the perpendicular growth. Since normal increase in brain volume requires expansion, the skull is forced to grow in a direction *parallel* to the fused suture. This alteration in skull growth always produces a distortion of the head shape when the underlying brain growth is normal. The small head with closed and normal shape is a result of deficient brain growth; the suture closure is secondary to this brain growth failure. Failure of brain growth is not secondary to suture closure.

Various types of cranial deformities are encountered in early infancy. These include the enlarged head with frontal protrusion (**bossing**; characteristic of hydrocephalus), the parietal bossing that is seen in chronic subdural hematoma, the small head, and a variety of skull deformities. Some occur during prenatal development; in others, head circumference is usually within normal limits at birth, and the deviation from normal development becomes apparent with advancing age.

Prognosis. The majority of infants with craniosynostosis have normal brain development. The exceptions are those with genetic disorders that involve brain pathologic conditions.

Nursing Care Management

Nursing care of families in which there is a child with a cranial defect involves identifying children with deformities and referring them for evaluation. Since no therapy is available for children with microcephaly, nursing care is directed toward helping parents adjust to rearing a child with brain damage (see Chapter 19).

Caring for infants who benefit from surgery requires special emphasis on observation for signs of decreased hematocrit and hemoglobin because of the large blood loss during surgery (see Family Focus box). A cardiac monitor may demonstrate a resting heart rate of 200 beats/min. Nursing care includes observation for signs of hemorrhage, infection, pain, and swelling, as well as parental education for suture care and

FAMILY FOCUS

Blood Donation

Parents may wish to provide a compatible blood donor for their infant undergoing a planned surgical correction for craniosynostosis. Nurses need to inform and guide parents through this blood bank procedure.

safety. Surgical sutures should remain dry and intact. Parents need to observe for any signs of redness, drainage, or swelling and report any temperature greater than 38.4° C (101° F).

Early surgical management of craniosynostosis allows proper expansion of the brain and the creation of an acceptable appearance. Parents require special support and education during this time, especially from the health care team (Stal, Chebret, and McElroy, 1998).

HYDROCEPHALUS

Hydrocephalus is a condition caused by an imbalance in the production and absorption of CSF in the ventricular system. When production is greater than absorption, CSF accumulates within the ventricular system, usually under increased pressure, producing passive dilation of the ventricles.

Pathophysiology

The causes of hydrocephalus are varied, but the result is either (1) impaired absorption of CSF fluid within the subarachnoid space, obliteration of the subarachnoid cisterns, or malfunction of the arachnoid villi (**nonobstructive** or **communicating hydrocephalus**); or (2) obstruction to the flow of CSF through the ventricular system (**obstructive** or **noncommunicating hydrocephalus**) (Kinsman and Johnston, 2007). The terms *communicating* and *noncommunicating hydrocephalus* traditionally referred to obstructive and nonobstructive types of hydrocephalus when pneumoencephalography was used to establish the diagnosis; because other diagnostic methods are now used, the terms may be used only as a reference point in the diagnosis. Other authorities suggest that hydrocephalus be classified according to the cause and therefore refer to either congenital or acquired hydrocephalus (Rudy, 2005). Rarely, a tumor of the choroid plexus causes increased CSF secretion. Any imbalance of secretion and absorption causes an increased accumulation of CSF in the ventricles, which become dilated (ventriculomegaly) and compress the brain substance against the surrounding rigid bony cranium. When this occurs before fusion of the cranial sutures, it causes enlargement of the skull and dilation of the ventricles (Fig. 28-6). In children younger than 10 to 12 years of age, partially closed suture lines, especially the sagittal suture, may become diastatic or opened. After 12 years of age the sutures are fused and will not open.

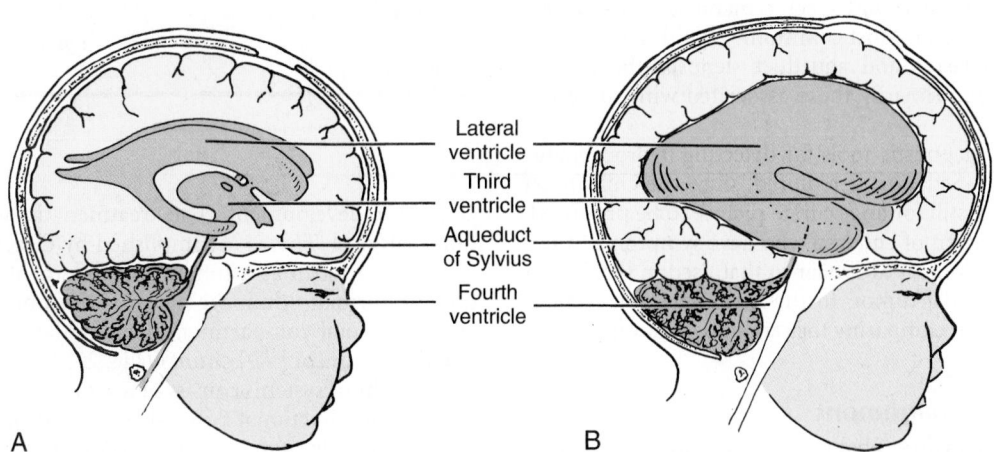

Lateral ventricle
Third ventricle
Aqueduct of Sylvius
Fourth ventricle

FIG. 28-6 ■ Hydrocephalus: a block in flow of cerebrospinal fluid. **A,** Patent cerebrospinal fluid circulation. **B,** Enlarged lateral and third ventricles caused by obstruction of circulation—stenosis of aqueduct of Sylvius.

Most cases of noncommunicating hydrocephalus are a result of developmental malformations. Although the defect usually is apparent in early infancy, it may become evident at any time from the prenatal period to late childhood or early adulthood. Other causes include neoplasms, infections, and trauma. An obstruction to the normal flow can occur at any point in the CSF pathway to produce increased pressure and dilation of the pathways proximal to the site of obstruction.

Developmental defects (e.g., Arnold-Chiari malformations, aqueduct stenosis, aqueduct gliosis, and atresia of the foramina of Luschka and Magendie [Dandy-Walker syndrome]) account for most cases of hydrocephalus from birth to 2 years of age. Hydrocephalus is so often associated with myelomeningocele that all infants with this condition should be observed for its development. In the remainder of cases there is a history of intrauterine infection, perinatal hemorrhage, and neonatal meningoencephalitis. In older children hydrocephalus is most often a result of space-occupying lesions, intracranial infections, hemorrhage, or preexisting developmental defects, such as aqueduct stenosis or the **Arnold-Chiari malformation** (a congenital anomaly in which the cerebellum and medulla oblongata extend down through the foramen magnum).

Diagnostic Evaluation

The two factors that influence the clinical picture in hydrocephalus are the time of onset and preexisting structural lesions. In infancy, before closure of the cranial sutures, head enlargement is the predominant sign, whereas in older infants and children the lesions responsible for hydrocephalus produce other neurologic signs through pressure on adjacent structures before causing CSF obstruction (Box 28-13).

In infancy the diagnosis of hydrocephalus is based on head circumference that crosses one or more grid lines on the measurement chart within a period of 2 to 4 weeks and on associated neurologic signs that are present and progressive. However, other diagnostic studies are needed to localize the site of CSF obstruction. Routine daily head circumference measurements are carried out in infants with myelomeningocele and intracranial infections. In evaluation of a preterm infant, specially adapted head circumference charts are consulted to distinguish abnormal head growth from rapid head growth that takes place normally.

The signs and symptoms in early to late childhood are caused by increased ICP, and specific manifestations are related to the focal lesion. Most commonly resulting from posterior fossa neoplasms and aqueduct stenosis, the clinical manifestations are primarily those associated with space-occupying lesions.

The primary diagnostic tools for detecting hydrocephalus are CT and MRI. Sedation is required, since the child must remain absolutely still for an accurate picture to be produced. Diagnostic evaluation of children who have symptoms of hydrocephalus after infancy is similar to that used in those with suspected intracranial tumor. In the neonate, echoencephalography is useful in comparing the ratio of lateral ventricle to cortex.

Therapeutic Management

The treatment of hydrocephalus is directed toward relief of the hydrocephalus, treatment of complications, and management of problems related to the effect of the disorder on psy-

BOX 28-13
Clinical Manifestations of Hydrocephalus

INFANCY (EARLY)
Abnormally rapid head growth
Bulging fontanels (especially anterior) sometimes without head enlargement:
- Tense
- Nonpulsatile
Dilated scalp veins
Separated sutures
Macewen sign (cracked-pot sound on percussion)
Thinning of skull bones

INFANCY (LATER)
Frontal enlargement, or bossing
Depressed eyes
Setting-sun sign (sclera visible above the iris)
Pupils sluggish, with unequal response to light

INFANCY (GENERAL)
Irritability
Lethargy
Infant cries when picked up or rocked and quiets when allowed to lie still
Early infantile reflex acts may persist
Normally expected responses fail to appear
May display:
- Change in level of consciousness
- Opisthotonos (often extreme)
- Lower extremity spasticity
- Vomiting
Advanced cases:
- Difficulty in sucking and feeding
- Shrill, brief, high-pitched cry
- Cardiopulmonary embarrassment

CHILDHOOD
Headache on awakening; improvement following emesis or upright posture
Papilledema
Strabismus
Extrapyramidal tract signs (e.g., ataxia)
Irritability
Lethargy
Apathy
Confusion
Incoherence
Vomiting

chomotor development. The treatment is, with few exceptions, surgical. This is accomplished by direct removal of an obstruction (such as a tumor) or placement of a shunt that provides primary drainage of the CSF from the ventricles to an extracranial compartment, usually the peritoneum (**ventriculoperitoneal [VP] shunt**) (Fig. 28-7).

Most shunt systems consist of a ventricular catheter, a flush pump, a unidirectional flow valve, and a distal catheter. In all models the valves are designed to open at a predetermined intraventricular pressure and close when the pressure falls below that level, thus preventing backflow of secretions.

FIG. 28-7 ■ Ventriculoperitoneal shunt. Catheter is threaded beneath the skin.

The initial shunt is placed when necessary to relieve CSF obstruction, and revisions are needed when signs of malfunction appear. In all mechanisms the initial success rate is relatively high; however, shunts are associated with complications that interfere with continued shunt function or threaten the child's life.

The major complications of VP shunts are infection and malfunction. All shunts are subject to mechanical difficulties, such as kinking, plugging, or separation or migration of the tubing. Malfunction is most often caused by mechanical obstruction either within the ventricles from particulate matter (tissue or exudate) or at the distal end from thrombosis or displacement as a result of growth. The child with a shunt obstruction is often first seen in an emergency department with clinical manifestations of increased ICP, frequently accompanied by worsening neurologic status.

The most serious complication, shunt infection, can occur at any time, but the period of greatest risk is 1 to 2 months after placement. The infection is generally a result of intercurrent infections at the time of shunt placement. Infections include septicemia, bacterial endocarditis, wound infection, shunt nephritis, meningitis, and ventriculitis. Meningitis and ventriculitis are of greatest concern, since any complicating CNS infection is a significant predictor of poor intellectual outcome. Infection is treated with massive doses of antibiotics administered by the IV route. A persistent infection requires removal of the shunt until the infection is controlled. External ventricular drainage (EVD) is used until CSF is sterile. The EVD allows for removal of CSF through a tube that is placed in the child's ventricle and flows by gravity into a collection device.

An alternative to shunt placement is the endoscopic third ventriculostomy in children with noncommunicating hydrocephalus. In this procedure, an endoscope is used to make a small opening in the floor of the third ventricle that allows the CSF to flow freely through the previously blocked ventricle. Aldana, Kestle, Brockmeyer, and others (2003) have shown that endoscopic septal fenestration has an overall patency rate of 81%, which may eliminate the need for a CSF shunt. The complication rate of the endoscopic septal fenestration procedure was 9.3% and included intraventricular hemorrhage,

sterile meningitis, and septostomy failure (Aldana, Kestle, Brockmeyer, and others, 2003).

Prognosis. The prognosis for children with treated hydrocephalus depends largely on the rate at which hydrocephalus develops, the duration of increased ICP, the frequency of complications, and the cause of the hydrocephalus. For example, malignant tumors may have a high mortality rate regardless of other complicating factors.

Surgically treated hydrocephalus with continued neurosurgical and medical management has a survival rate of about 80%, with the highest incidence of mortality occurring within the first year of treatment. Of the surviving children, approximately one third are both intellectually and neurologically normal, and one half have neurologic disabilities.

Nursing Care Management

Preoperatively the infant with diagnosed or suspected hydrocephalus is observed carefully for signs of increasing ICP. In infants the head is measured daily at the largest point, the occipitofrontal circumference (see Head Circumference, Chapter 6, for technique). Fontanels and suture lines are gently palpated for size, signs of bulging, tenseness, and separation. An infant with normal ICP will display bulging under certain circumstances such as straining or crying; therefore such accompanying behavior should be noted. Irritability, lethargy, or seizure activity, as well as altered vital signs and feeding behavior, may indicate an advancing pathologic condition.

In older children, who are usually admitted to the hospital for elective or emergency shunt revision, the most valuable indicator of increasing ICP is an alteration in the child's LOC and the way in which the child interacts with the environment. Changes are identified by observation and by comparison of present behavior with customary behavior, sleep patterns, developmental capabilities, and habits, all obtained through a detailed history and a baseline assessment. This baseline information serves as a guide for postoperative assessment and evaluation of shunt function.

General nursing care of the infant with hydrocephalus may present special problems. Maintaining adequate nutrition often requires flexible feeding schedules to accommodate diagnostic procedures, since feeding before or after handling can precipitate an episode of vomiting. Small feedings at more frequent intervals are often better tolerated than larger ones spaced farther apart. These infants are often difficult to feed and require extra time and innovation.

The nurse is responsible for preparing the child for diagnostic tests such as tomography and for assisting the practitioner with procedures such as a ventricular tap, which is often performed to relieve excessive pressure during the preoperative period and for CSF examination. Sedation is required, since the child must remain absolutely still during diagnostic testing. IV pentobarbital or oral chloral hydrate is commonly used for these procedures (see Preparation for Diagnostic and Therapeutic Procedures, Chapter 22).

NURSING ALERT

If surgery is anticipated, IV lines should not be placed in a scalp vein on a child with hydrocephalus.

Postoperative Care. Routine postoperative care and observation are instituted. In addition, the infant or child is positioned carefully on the unoperated side to prevent pressure on the shunt valve and pressure areas. The child is kept flat to avoid complications resulting from too-rapid reduction of intracranial fluid. When the ventricular size is reduced too rapidly, the cerebral cortex may pull away from the dura and tear the small interlacing veins, producing a subdural hematoma. This is not a problem in children with elective shunt revision, since their intraventricular size and pressure have been normal. The surgeon indicates the position to be maintained and the extent of activity allowed. If there is increased ICP, the surgeon will prescribe elevation of the head of the bed and allow the child to sit up to enhance gravity flow through the shunt. Pain management can usually be achieved with acetaminophen with or without codeine for mild to moderate pain and opioids for severe pain (see Pain Management, Chapter 7).

Observation is continued for signs of increased ICP, which indicates obstruction of the shunt. Neurologic assessment includes evaluation of pupillary dilation (pressure causes compression or stretching of the oculomotor nerve, producing dilation on the same side as the pressure) and blood pressure (hypoxia to the brainstem causes variability in these vital signs).

> **NURSINGALERT**
>
> Arbitrary pumping of the shunt may cause obstruction or other problems and should not be performed unless indicated by the neurosurgeon.

The child is also observed for abdominal distention, since CSF may cause peritonitis or a postoperative ileus as a complication of distal catheter placement. In addition, intake and output are carefully monitored. Children may be placed on fluid restriction with nothing by mouth for 24 hours. The IV infusion is closely monitored to prevent fluid overload. Routine feeding is resumed after the prescribed NPO period, but the presence of bowel sounds is determined before feeding a child with a VP shunt.

Since infection is the greatest hazard of the postoperative period, nurses are continually on the alert for the usual manifestations of CSF infection, such as elevated vital signs, poor feeding, vomiting, decreased responsiveness, and seizure activity. There may be signs of local inflammation at the operative sites and along the shunt tract. The child's diaper should be kept off the peritoneal dressing site or suture line. Antibiotics are administered by the IV route as ordered, and the nurse may also need to assist the practitioner with intraventricular instillation. The incision site is inspected for leakage, and any suspected drainage is tested for glucose, an indication of CSF.

Meticulous skin care is continued postoperatively, with extra care taken to prevent tissue damage from pressure. A pressure-reducing mattress or overlay pad underneath the child helps prevent pressure on prominent areas. Skin is inspected regularly for any signs of pressure, irritation, or infection.

Family Support. Specific needs and concerns of parents during periods of hospitalization are related to the reason for the child's hospitalization (shunt revision, infection, diagnosis) and the diagnostic and surgical procedures to which the child is subjected. Often parents have little understanding of anatomy; therefore they need further exploration and reinforcement of information that was given to them by the physician and neurosurgeon, as well as information about what they can expect. They are especially frightened of any procedure that involves the brain, and the fear of intellectual disability or brain damage is real and pervasive. Nurses can do much to allay their anxiety by explaining the rationale underlying the various nursing and medical activities, such as positioning or testing, and by simply being available and willing to listen to their concerns.

To prepare for the child's discharge and home care, the parents are instructed on how to recognize signs that indicate shunt malfunction or infection and how to pump the shunt, if necessary. Active children may have accidents, such as a fall, that can damage the shunt, and the tubing may pull out of the distal insertion site or become disconnected during normal growth.

Safe transportation is an essential issue to discuss with parents. The tendency for the enlarged head to fall forward and to turn to the side, combined with poor head control, influences the type of child restraint system needed. Small infants can be restrained reclining in an approved car-restraint bed.

The management of hydrocephalus in a child is a demanding task for both family and health professionals, and helping a family cope with the child is an important nursing responsibility. It is important to emphasize that hydrocephalus is a lifelong problem and that the child will require evaluation on a regular basis. The overall aim is to establish realistic goals and an appropriate educational program that will help the child to achieve his or her optimal potential.

Families can be referred to community agencies for support and guidance. The National Hydrocephalus Foundation* and the Hydrocephalus Association† provide information on the condition for families and assist interested groups in establishing local organizations. Helpful booklets are available from these and other sources.

---

*12413 Centralia Road, Lakewood, CA 90715-1653; (562) 924-6666, (888) 857-3434; http://www.nhfonline.org.
†870 Market St., Suite 705, San Francisco, CA 94102; (415) 732-7040, (800) 598-3789; http://www.hydroassoc.org. A booklet titled *About Hydrocephalus: A Book for Parents* is available in English or Spanish.

KEY POINTS

- LOC is the most important indicator of neurologic health; altered levels include full consciousness, confusion, disorientation, lethargy, obtundation, stupor, coma, and persistent vegetative state.
- Complete neurologic examination includes LOC; posture; motor, sensory, cranial nerve, and reflex testing; and vital signs.
- Nursing care of the unconscious child focuses on ensuring respiratory management; performing neurologic assessment; monitoring ICP; supplying adequate nutrition and hydration; providing drug therapy; promoting elimination, hygienic care, proper positioning, exercise, and stimulation; and providing family support.
- Fractures resulting from head injuries may be classified as depressed, compound, basilar, and diastatic.
- Primary head injury involves features that occur at the time of trauma, including fractured skull, contusions, intracranial hematoma, and diffuse injury. Secondary complications include hypoxic brain damage, increased ICP, infection, cerebral edema, and posttraumatic syndromes.

- The young child's response to head injury is different because of the following features: larger head size; expandable skull; larger blood volume to the brain; small subdural spaces; and thinner, softer brain tissue.
- Problems resulting from near-drowning include hypoxia and asphyxiation, aspiration, and hypothermia.
- Nursing care of the child with a brain tumor includes observing for signs and symptoms related to the tumor, preparing the child and family for diagnostic tests and operative procedures, preventing postoperative complications, planning for discharge, and promoting a return to optimal health.
- Nursing care of the child with meningitis includes administering antibiotics, taking isolation precautions, removing environmental stimuli, ensuring correct positioning, monitoring vital signs, administering IV therapy, promoting adequate fluid and nutritional status, and providing supportive care to the family.
- Routine immunization of infants with *H. influenzae* type b and pneumococcal conjugate vaccines has reduced the incidence of bacterial meningitis.
- Encephalitis may result from direct invasion of the CNS by a virus or from involvement of the CNS after viral disease.
- A seizure is a symptom of an underlying pathologic condition and may be manifested by sensory-hallucinatory phenomena, motor effects, sensorimotor effects, or loss of consciousness.
- Partial seizures are categorized as simple (without associated impairment of consciousness) or complex (with impaired consciousness); both types may become generalized.
- Generalized seizures are categorized as tonic-clonic convulsive absence, atonic and akinetic, myoclonic, and infantile spasms.
- Long-term care of the child with recurrent seizure disorders includes physical care and education regarding the importance of drug therapy and problems related to emotional aspects of the disorder.
- Febrile seizures are the most common type of childhood seizure.
- Many cranial deformities are amenable to surgical correction.
- Hydrocephalus is a symptom of underlying brain pathologic condition demonstrated by impaired absorption of CSF or obstruction to the flow of CSF within the ventricles.
- Therapy for hydrocephalus involves relief of the hydrocephalus, treatment of the underlying brain disorder if possible, prevention or treatment of complications, and management of problems related to psychomotor development.

answers to
CRITICAL THINKING EXERCISE

HYDROCEPHALUS

1. Yes. Emma's fussiness, holding the back of her head, intermittent periods of lethargy, and repetitive, rapid eye blinking are signs of increased ICP.
2. a. Emma's posterior fossa tumor removal places her at risk for cerebral edema with associated increased ICP.
   b. Emma's EVD may be occluded and should be assessed. Positioning of the EVD is important to evaluate, since the cerebrospinal fluid (CSF) drains by gravity; repositioning may be necessary to promote adequate drainage and decrease ICP.
   c. The physical signs and behavior are indicative of increased ICP, which may occur if Emma's EVD is obstructed or is draining improperly. There is evidence that CSF is draining on the mother's clothing, which is an abnormal finding with an EVD; the EVD is a closed system, and breakage or malfunction may cause the child further harm if bacteria colonize the reservoir.
3. The nurse should inspect the EVD site, assess Emma's neurologic status, and notify the medical provider of the findings. A transparent dressing should be placed over the EVD site to observe for CSF drainage, an abnormal finding. The EVD should remain positioned so that gravity drainage of CSF is enhanced (at the level of the external auditory meatus with the head at a 20- to 30-degree elevation); rapid CSF drainage is undesirable, since it may result in subdural complications. A computed tomography scan may be useful in determining the status of the drainage device.
4. Yes. Emma's signs of increased ICP and CSF drainage on her mother's clothes support the nurse's actions.
5. Another consideration for some of Emma's fussiness in the postoperative period is discomfort and pain. However, pain management should be monitored closely to avoid masking the signs of increased ICP. Once it is evident that the ICP is elevated, pain management measures should be performed, including an assessment of what Emma has taken previously to relieve pain. In addition, the nurse should explain the signs of elevated ICP to the mother and convey that obstruction of CSF flow from the EVD can cause these clinical signs and behaviors. Reassurance that the increased ICP will subside with removal of the EVD obstruction is important.

REFERENCES

Aldana PR, Kestle JRW, Brockmeyer DL, and others: Results of endoscopic septal fenestration in the treatment of isolated ventricular hydrocephalus, *Pediatr Neurosurg* 38(6):286-294, 2003.

Alston RD, Newton R, Kelsey A, and others: Childhood medulloblastoma in northwest England, 1954 to 1977: incidence and survival, *Dev Med Child Neurol* 45(5):308-314, 2003.

American Academy of Pediatrics, Committee on Infectious Diseases, Pickering L, editor: *Red book: 2006 report of the Committee on Infectious Diseases*, ed 27, Elk Grove Village, Ill, 2006, The Academy.

American Academy of Pediatrics: Recommendations for the prevention of pneumococcal infections, including the use of pneumococcal conjugant vaccine, pneumococcal polysaccharide vaccine and antibiotic prophylaxis, *Pediatrics* 106(2):362-366, 2000a.

American Academy of Pediatrics, Committee on Sports Medicine and Fitness and Committee on Injury and Poison Prevention: Swimming programs for infants and toddlers, *Pediatrics* 105:868-870, 2000b.

Baram TZ, Shinnar S: *Febrile seizures*, San Diego, 2002, Academic Press.

Bayir H, Kochanek PM, Clark RS: Traumatic brain injury in infants and children: mechanisms of secondary damage and treatment in the intensive care unit, *Crit Care Clin* 19(3):529-549, 2003.

Bhutta AT, Van Savell H, Schexnayder SM: Reye's syndrome: down but not out, *South Med J* 96(1): 43-45, 2003.

Blaney SM, Kun LE, Hunter J, and others: Tumors of the central nervous system. In Pizzo PA, Pollack DG, editors: *Principles and practice of pediatric oncology*, ed 5, Philadelphia, 2006, Lippincott-Raven.

Bonthius DJ, Karacay B: Meningitis and encephalitis in children: an update, *Neurol Clin* 20(4):1013-1038, 2002.

Brodeur GM, Maris JM: Neuroblastoma. In Pizzo PA, Pollack DG, editors: *Principles and practice of pediatric oncology*, ed 5, Philadelphia, 2006, Lippincott-Raven.

Browne TR, Holmes GL: *Handbook of epilepsy*, ed 3, Philadelphia, 2004, Lippincott Williams & Wilkins.

Carey RG, Balistreri W: Mitochondrial hepatopathies. In Behrman RE, Kliegman RM, Jenson HTS, and others, editors: *Nelson textbook of pediatrics*, ed 18, Philadelphia, 2007, Saunders.

Centers for Disease Control and Prevention: Progress toward elimination of *Haemophilus influenzae* type b invasive disease among infants and children—United States, 1998-2000, *MMWR* 51:234-239, 2002.

Centers for Disease Control and Prevention: Compendium of animal rabies prevention and control, 2001, National Association of State Public Health Veterinarians, Inc., *MMWR* 50(RR-8):1-9, 2001.

Centers for Disease Control and Prevention: *Meningococcal disease*, 2000, retrieved March 5, 2007, from http://www.cdc.gov/ncidod/dbmd/diseaseinfo/meningococcal_t.htm.

Centers for Disease Control and Prevention: Human rabies prevention—United States, 1999, *MMWR* 48(RR-1):1-21, 1999.

Chen JWY, Wasterlain CG: Status epilepticus: pathophysiology and management in adults, *Lancet Neurol* 5:246-256, 2006.

Chiaretti A, De Benedictis R, Polidori G, and others: Early post-traumatic seizures in children with head injury, *Childs Nerv Syst* 16(12):862-866, 2000.

Curley MAQ, Moloney-Harmon PA: *Critical care nursing of infants and children*, ed 2, Philadelphia, 2001, Saunders.

Durkin MS, Olsen S, Barlow B, and others: The epidemiology of urban pediatric neurological trauma: evaluation of, and implications for, injury prevention programs, *Neurosurgery* 42(2):300-310, 1998.

El Bashir H, Laundy M, Booy R: Diagnosis and treatment of bacterial meningitis, *Arch Dis Child* 88(7):814-819, 2003.

Faillace WJ: Management of childhood neurotrauma, *Surg Clin North Am* 82(2):349-363, 2002.

Fisgin T, Gurer Y, Senbil N, and others: Nasal midazolam effects on childhood acute seizures, *J Child Neurol* 15(12):833-835, 2000.

Freeman JM, Kossoff ER, Hartman AL: The ketogenic diet: one decade later, *Pediatrics* 119(3):535-543, 2007.

Freeman JM, Vining EP, Pillas DJ, and others: The efficacy of the ketogenic diet: 1998—a prospective evaluation of intervention in 150 children, *Pediatrics* 102(6):1358-1363, 1998.

Frucht MM, Quigg M, Schwaner C, and others: Distribution of seizure precipitants among epilepsy syndromes, *Epilepsia* 41(12):1543-1549, 2000.

Fylan F, Harding GF, Edson AS, and others: Mechanisms of video game epilepsy, *Epilepsia* 40(Suppl 4):28-30, 1999.

Gennarelli TA: Trauma to the head: general considerations. In Schwartz GR, editor: *Principles and practices of emergency medicine*, ed 4, Philadelphia, 1999, Lippincott Williams & Wilkins.

Gupta N, Berger MS: Brain mapping for hemispheric tumors in children, *Pediatr Neurosurg* 38(6):302-306, 2003.

Harbord JG, Kyrkou NE, Kyrkou MR, and others: Use of intranasal midazolam to treat acute seizures in paediatric community settings, *J Pediatr Child Health* 40(9-10):556-558, 2004.

Hemingway C, Freeman JM, Pillas DJ, and others: The ketogenic diet: a 3-to-6-years follow up of 150 children enrolled prospectively, *Pediatrics* 108(4):898-905, 2001.

Johnston MV: Seizures in childhood. In Behrman RE, Kliegman RM, Jenson HTS, and others, editors: *Nelson textbook of pediatrics*, ed 18, Philadelphia, 2007, Saunders.

Kallas HJ: Drowning and near-drowning. In Behrman RE, Kliegman RM, Jenson HTS, editors: *Nelson textbook of pediatrics*, ed 17, Philadelphia, 2004, Saunders.

Kamienski MC: Reye syndrome, *Am J Nurs* 103(7):54-57, 2003.

Kao SC, Adamson SD, Tatman LH, and others: A survey of post-discharge side-effects of conscious sedation using chloral hydrate in pediatric CT or MR imaging, *Pediatr Radiol* 29(4):287-290, 1999.

Kline NE, Sevier N: Solid tumors in children, *J Pediatr Nurs* 18(2):96-102, 2003.

Kinsman SL, Johnston MV: Congenital anomalies of the central nervous system. In Behrman RE, Kliegman RM, Jenson HTS, and others, editors: *Nelson textbook of pediatrics*, ed 18, Philadelphia, 2007, Saunders.

Kutlu NO, Yakinci C, Dogrul M, and others: Intranasal midazolam for prolonged convulsive seizures, *Brain Dev* 22(6):359-361, 2000.

Kuzniecky RI: Neuroimaging in pediatric epilepsy. In Pellock JM, Dodson WE, Bourgeois BFD, editors: *Pediatric epilepsy: diagnosis and therapy*, New York, 2001, Demos Medical Publishing.

Lefevre F, Aronson N: Ketogenic diet for the treatment of refractory epilepsy in children: a systematic review of efficacy, *Pediatrics* 105(4):e46, 2000, retrieved March 5, 2007, from http://www.pediatrics.org/cgi/content/full/105/4/e46.

Leppik IE: Monotherapy and polypharmacy, *Neurology* 55(Suppl 3):525-529, 2000.

Levy R, Cooper P: Ketogenic diet for epilepsy, *Cochrane Database Syst Rev* (3):CD001903, DOI:10.1002/14651858.CD001903, 2003.

Ljungman G, Kreuger A, Andreasson S, and others: Midazolam nasal spray reduces procedural anxiety in children, *Pediatrics* 105(1 Pt 1):73-78, 2000.

Lloyd CJ, Alredy T, Lloyd JC: Intranasal midazolam as an alternative to general anaesthesia in the management of children with oral and maxillofacial trauma, *Br J Oral Maxillofac Surg* 38(6):593-595, 2000.

Masson F, Thicoipe M, Mokni T, and others: Epidemiology of traumatic comas: a prospective population-based study, *Brain Inj* 17(4):279-293, 2003.

Mathern GW, Giza CC, Yudovin S, and others: Postoperative seizure control and antiepileptic drug use in pediatric epilepsy surgery patients: the UCLA experience, 1986-1997, *Epilepsia* 40(12):1740-1749, 1999.

Menkes JH, Sankar R: Paroxysmal disorders. In Menkes JH, Sarnat HB, editors: *Child neurology*, Philadelphia, 2000, Lippincott Williams & Wilkins.

Morris GL, Mueller WM, and Vagus Nerve Stimulation Study Group E01-E05: Long term treatment with vagus nerve stimulation in patients with refractory epilepsy, *Neurology* 53:1731-1735, 1999.

Murray-Ryan J, Petriccione MM: Central nervous system tumors. In Baggott CR, Kelly KP, Fochtman D, and others, editors: *Nursing care of children and adolescents with cancer*, ed 3, Philadelphia, 2002, Saunders.

Nakken KO, Solaas MH, Kjeldsen MJ, and others: Which seizure-precipitating factors do patients with epilepsy most frequently report? *Epilepsy Behav* 6(1):85-89, 2005.

Nguyen NP, Sallah S, Ludin A, and others: Neuroblastoma producing spinal cord compression: rapid relief with low dose of radiation, *Anticancer Res* 20(6c):4687-4690, 2000.

Palmer J: Management of raised intracranial pressure in children, *Intens Crit Care Nurs* 16:319-327, 2000.

Pellock JM, Shinnar S: Respiratory adverse events associated with diazepam rectal gel, *Neurology* 64(10):1768-1770, 2005.

Pichichero M: Meningococcal conjugate vaccine in adolescents and children, *Clin Pediatr* 44(6):479-489, 2005.

Prober CG: Central nervous system infections. In Behrman RE, Kliegman RM, Jenson HTS, and others, editors: *Nelson textbook of pediatrics*, ed 18, Philadelphia, 2007, Saunders.

Radhakrishnan K, Johnson JA, McClelland RL, and others: Pattern-sensitive epilepsy: electroclinical characteristics, natural history, and delineation of the epileptic syndrome, *Epilepsia* 46(1):48-58, 2005.

Ricci S, Vigevano F: The effect of video-game software in video-game epilepsy, *Epilepsia* 40(Suppl 4):31-37, 1999.

Rivara FP, Grossman D: Injury control. In Behrman RE, Kliegman RM, Jenson HTS, and others, editors: *Nelson textbook of pediatrics*, ed 18, Philadelphia, 2007, Saunders.

Rudy C: Hydrocephalus, *J Pediatr Health Care* 19(2):111, 127-128, 2005.

Sadleir LG, Scheffer IE: Febrile seizures, *BMJ* 334:307-311, 2007.

Saez-Llorens X, McCracken Jr GH: Bacterial meningitis in children, *Lancet* 361(9375):2139-2148, 2003.

Scheifele D, Halperin S, Law B, and others: Invasive *Haemophilus influenzae* type b infections in vaccinated and unvaccinated children in Canada, 2001-2003, *CMAJ* 172(1):53-56, 2005.

Schutzman SA, Greenes DS: Pediatric minor head trauma, *Ann Emerg Med* 37(1):65-74, 2001.

Shafer PO: Epilepsy and seizures: advances in seizure assessment, treatment, and self-management, *Nurs Clin North Am* 34(3):743-759, 1999.

Shinnar S, Berg AT, O'Dell C, and others: Predictors of multiple seizures in a cohort of children prospectively followed from the time of their first unprovoked seizure, *Ann Neurol* 48(2):140-147, 2000.

Shorvon S, Walker M: Status epilepticus in idiopathic generalized epilepsy, *Epilepsia* 46(Suppl 9):73-79, 2005.

Sotir MJ, Ahrabi-Fard S, Croft DR, and others: Meningococcal disease incidence and mortality in Wisconsin, 1993-2002, *Wisc Med J* 104(3):38-44, 2005.

Stal S, Chebret L, McElroy C: The team approach in the management of congenital and acquired deformities, *Clin Plast Surg* 25(4):485-491, 1998.

Swaine BR, Tremblay C, Platt RW, and others: Previous head injury is a risk factor for subsequent head injury in children: a longitudinal cohort study, *Pediatrics* 119(4):749-758, 2007.

Task Force for the Determination of Brain Death in Children: Guidelines for the determination of brain death in children, *Arch Neurol* 44(6):587-588, 1987.

Toltzis P: Rabies. In Behrman RE, Kliegman RM, Jenson HTS, and others, editors: *Nelson textbook of pediatrics*, ed 18, Philadelphia, 2007, Saunders.

Treiman DM, Walker MC: Treatment of seizure emergencies: convulsive and non-convulsive status epilepticus, *Epilepsy Res* 68S:S77-S82, 2006.

Verity CM, Greenword R, Golding J: Longterm intellectual and behavioral outcomes of children with febrile convulsions, *N Engl J Med* 338(24): 1723-1728, 1998.

Vernon-Levett P: Neurologic system. In Slota MC, editor: *Core curriculum for pediatric critical care nursing*, Philadelphia, 1998, Saunders.

Weiner WJ, Goetz CG: *Neurology for non-neurologists*, ed 5, Philadelphia, 2004, Lippincott Williams & Wilkins.

Wetzell RC: Anesthesia and perioperative care. In Behrman RE, Kliegman RM, Jenson HTS, and others, editors: *Nelson textbook of pediatrics*, ed 18, Philadelphia, 2007, Saunders.

Yamamoto LG, Yim GK: The role of intravenous valproic acid in status epilepticus, *Pediatr Emerg Care* 16(4):296-298, 2000.

Yogev R, Guzman-Cottrill J: Bacterial meningitis in children: critical review of current concepts, *Drugs* 65(8):1097-1112, 2005.

Zuckerman GB, Gregory PM, Santos-Damiani SM: Predictors of death and neurologic impairment in pediatric submersion injuries: the pediatric risk of mortality score, *Arch Pediatr Adolesc Med* 152:134-140, 1998.

29

The Child with Endocrine Dysfunction

MARILYN J. HOCKENBERRY

CHAPTER OUTLINE

DISORDERS OF PITUITARY FUNCTION, 1024
Hypopituitarism, 1024
Pituitary Hyperfunction, 1029
Precocious Puberty, 1029
Diabetes Insipidus, 1030
Syndrome of Inappropriate Antidiuretic Hormone, 1031
DISORDERS OF THYROID FUNCTION, 1032
Juvenile Hypothyroidism, 1032

Goiter, 1033
Lymphocytic Thyroiditis, 1033
Hyperthyroidism, 1034
DISORDERS OF PARATHYROID FUNCTION, 1035
Hypoparathyroidism, 1035
Hyperparathyroidism, 1036
DISORDERS OF ADRENAL FUNCTION, 1037
Acute Adrenocortical Insufficiency, 1037

Chronic Adrenocortical Insufficiency (Addison Disease), 1038
Cushing Syndrome, 1039
Congenital Adrenal Hyperplasia, 1040
Pheochromocytoma, 1042
DISORDERS OF PANCREATIC HORMONE SECRETION: DIABETES MELLITUS, 1042
Nursing Care Plan: The Child with Diabetes Mellitus, 1052

LEARNING OBJECTIVES

On completion of this chapter the reader will be able to:
- Differentiate between the disorders caused by hypopituitary and hyperpituitary dysfunction.
- Describe the manifestations of thyroid hypofunction and hyperfunction and the management of children with the disorders.

- Distinguish between the manifestations of adrenal hypofunction and hyperfunction.
- Differentiate among the various categories of diabetes mellitus.
- Discuss the management and nursing care of the child with diabetes mellitus in the acute care setting.

- Distinguish between a hypoglycemic and a hyperglycemic reaction.
- Design a teaching plan for a child with diabetes mellitus.
- Formulate a teaching plan for instructing the parents of a child with diabetes mellitus.

RELATED TOPICS and ADDITIONAL RESOURCES

 IN TEXT

Administration of Medication, *Ch. 22*
Altered Growth and Maturation, *Ch. 17*
Biologic Development (Adolescence), *Ch. 16*
Chronic Renal Failure, *Ch. 27*
Compliance, *Ch. 22*
Congenital Hypothyroidism, *Ch. 9*
Genetic Evaluation and Counseling, *Ch. 9*
Impact of Chronic Illness, Disability, or
     Death on the Child and Family, *Ch. 18*
Metabolic Complications, *Ch. 9*
Surgical Procedures, *Ch. 22*

 COMPANION CD

Animation—Adrenal Function
Case Study—Diabetes Mellitus
Critical Thinking Exercise—Hypothyroidism
NCLEX Review Questions

evolve

evolve.elsevier.com/Wong/essentials/

NCLEX Review Questions
Critical Thinking Case Study—Diabetes
     Insipidus

Nursing Care Plans—The Child with
     Diabetes Mellitus; The Child with Diabetic
     Ketoacidosis
WebLinks

 **WONG'S CLINICAL MANUAL
OF PEDIATRIC NURSING, 7th Ed**

Nursing Care Plans—The Child with
     Diabetes Mellitus, *p. 475;* The Child with
     Diabetic Ketoacidosis (DKA), *p. 478*

The endocrine system consists of three components: (1) the cell, which sends a chemical message by means of a hormone; (2) the target cells, or end organs, which receive the chemical message; and (3) the environment through which the chemical is transported (blood, lymph, extracellular fluids) from the site of synthesis to the sites of cellular action. The endocrine system controls or regulates metabolic processes governing energy production, growth, fluid and electrolyte balance, response to stress, and sexual reproduction (Baxter and Ribeiro, 2001). The endocrine glands, which are distributed throughout the body, are listed in Table 29-1; also listed are several additional structures sometimes considered endocrine glands, although they are not usually included.

DISORDERS OF PITUITARY FUNCTION

Deficiencies of the anterior pituitary hormones may be due to organic defects or have an idiopathic etiology and may occur as a single hormonal problem or in combination with other hormonal deficiencies. The clinical manifestations depend on the hormones involved and the age of onset. If the tropic hormones are involved, the resulting disorder reflects the altered stimulus to the target gland. For example, if thyroid-stimulating hormone (TSH) is deficient, thyroid hormone (TH) is also deficient and the child displays the manifestations of hypothyroidism.

An overproduction of the anterior pituitary hormones can result in gigantism (caused by excess growth hormone [GH] production during childhood), hyperthyroidism, hypercortisolism (Cushing syndrome), and precocious puberty from excessive gonadotropins. Overproduction may be caused by hyperplasia of the pituitary cells—which may eventually progress to a tumor (adenoma)—or a primary hypothalamic defect that results in an excess of the hormone's releasing factor. Although the initial clinical manifestations are a result of pituitary oversecretion, eventually pituitary insufficiency occurs, and the signs of panhypopituitarism become evident.

> **NURSINGALERT**
>
> Children with panhypopituitarism should wear medical identification, such as a bracelet.

HYPOPITUITARISM

Hypopituitarism is diminished or deficient secretion of pituitary hormones. The consequences of the condition depend on the degree of dysfunction and lead to gonadotropin deficiency with absence or regression of secondary sex characteristics; GH deficiency, in which children display retarded somatic growth; TSH deficiency, which produces hypothyroidism; and corticotropin deficiency, which results in manifestations of adrenal hypofunction. Hypopituitarism can result from any of the conditions listed in Box 29-1. The most common organic cause of pituitary undersecretion is tumors in the pituitary or hypothalamic region, especially the craniopharyngiomas.

Constitutional growth delay refers to individuals (usually boys) with delayed linear growth, generally beginning as a toddler, and skeletal and sexual maturation that is behind that of age-mates (Miller and Zimmerman, 2004; Halac and Zimmerman, 2004). Typically these children will reach normal adult height. Often there is a history of a similar pattern of growth in one of the child's parents or other family members. The untreated child will proceed through normal

> **BOX 29-1**
>
> **Clinical Manifestations of Hypopituitarism**
>
> Presenting complaint—short stature
> - Usually normal growth first year
> - Growth during second year drops below established percentile
> - Growth measurements below 5th percentile
>
> Premature aging common in later life
> Height may be retarded more than weight
> Appear well nourished
> Skeletal proportions normal
> Tend to be relatively inactive
> Less likely to participate in aggressive, sporting-type activities
> Bone age nearly always retarded but closely related to height age
> Usually primary teeth appear at expected age; eruption of permanent teeth delayed
> Teeth are overcrowded and malpositioned (because of underdeveloped jaw)
> Sexual development usually delayed but normal

TABLE 29-1

Hormones and Their Function

HORMONE	EFFECT	HYPOFUNCTION	HYPERFUNCTION
ADENOHYPOPHYSIS (ANTERIOR PITUITARY)*			
Somatotropic hormone (STH) or growth hormone (GH) (somatotropin) *Target tissue*—Bones	Promotes growth of bone and soft tissues. Has main effect on linear growth. Maintains a normal rate of protein synthesis. Conserves carbohydrate utilization and promotes fat mobilization. Is essential for proliferation of cartilage cells at epiphyseal plate. Is ineffective for linear growth after epiphyseal closure. Has hyperglycemic effect (antiinsulin action)	Epiphyseal fusion with cessation of growth. Prepubertal dwarfism. Pituitary cachexia (Simmonds disease). Generalized growth retardation. Hypoglycemia	Prepubertal gigantism. Acromegaly (after full growth is attained). Diabetes mellitus. Postpubertal hypoproteinemia
Thyrotropin (thyroid-stimulating hormone [TSH]) *Target tissue*—Thyroid gland	Promotes and maintains growth and development of thyroid gland. Stimulates thyroid hormone secretion	Hypothyroidism. Marked delay of puberty. Juvenile myxedema	Hyperthyroidism. Thyrotoxicosis. Graves disease
Adrenocorticotropic hormone (ACTH) *Target tissue*—Adrenal cortex	Promotes and maintains growth and development of adrenal cortex. Stimulates adrenal cortex to secrete glucocorticoids and androgens	Acute adrenocortical insufficiency (Addison disease). Hypoglycemia. Increased skin pigmentation	Cushing syndrome
Gonadotropins *Target tissue*—Gonads	Stimulate gonads to mature and produce sex hormones and germ cells	Absent or incomplete spontaneous puberty	Precocious puberty
Follicle-stimulating hormone (FSH) *Target tissue*—Ovaries, testes	*Male*—Stimulates development of seminiferous tubules; initiates spermatogenesis. *Female*—Stimulates graafian follicles to mature and secrete estrogen	Hypogonadism. Sterility. Absence or loss of secondary sex characteristics. Amenorrhea	Early epiphyseal closure. Precocious puberty. Primary gonadal failure. Hirsutism. Polycystic ovary. Early epiphyseal closure
Luteinizing hormone (LH)† *Target tissue*—Ovaries, testes	*Male*—Stimulates differentiation of Leydig cells, which secrete androgens, principally testosterone. *Female*—Produces rupture of follicle with discharge of mature ovum; stimulates secretion of progesterone by corpus luteum	Hypogonadism. Sterility. Impotence. Absence or loss of secondary sex characteristics. Ovarian failure. Eunuchism	Precocious puberty. Primary gonadal failure. Hirsutism. Polycystic ovary. Early epiphyseal closure
Prolactin (luteotropic hormone) *Target tissue*—Ovaries, breasts	Stimulates milk secretion. Maintains corpus luteum and progesterone secretion during pregnancy	Inability to lactate. Amenorrhea	Galactorrhea. Functional hypogonadism
Melanocyte-stimulating hormone (MSH) *Target tissue*—Skin	Promotes pigmentation of skin	Diminished or absent skin pigmentation	Increased skin pigmentation
NEUROHYPOPHYSIS (POSTERIOR PITUITARY)			
Antidiuretic hormone (ADH) (vasopressin) *Target tissue*—Renal tubules	Acts on distal and collecting tubules, making them more permeable to water, thus increasing reabsorption and decreasing excretion of urine	Diabetes insipidus	Syndrome of inappropriate secretion of ADH. Fluid retention. Hyponatremia
Oxytocin *Target tissue*—Uterus, breasts	Stimulates powerful contractions of uterus. Causes ejection of milk from alveoli into breast ducts (letdown reflex)		

*For each anterior pituitary hormone there is a corresponding hypothalamic-releasing factor. A deficiency in these factors caused by inhibiting anterior pituitary hormone synthesis produces the same effects. (See text for more detailed information.)

†In the male, LH is sometimes known as interstitial cell–stimulating hormone (ICSH).

Continued

TABLE 29-1

Hormones and Their Function—cont'd

HORMONE	EFFECT	HYPOFUNCTION	HYPERFUNCTION
THYROID			
Thyroid hormones—Thyroxine (T$_4$) and triiodothyronine (T$_3$)	Regulate metabolic rate; control rate of growth of body cells Especially important for growth of bones, teeth, and brain Promote mobilization of fats and gluconeogenesis	Hypothyroidism Myxedema Hashimoto thyroiditis General growth greatly reduced; extent dependent on age at which deficiency occurs Intellectual disability in infant	Exophthalmic goiter (Graves disease) Accelerated linear growth Early epiphyseal closure
Thyrocalcitonin	Regulates calcium and phosphorus metabolism Influences ossification and development of bone		
PARATHYROID GLANDS			
Parathyroid hormone (PTH)	Promotes calcium reabsorption from blood, bone, and intestines Promotes excretion of phosphorus in kidney tubules	Hypocalcemia (tetany)	Hypercalcemia (bone demineralization) Hypophosphatemia
ADRENAL CORTEX			
Mineralocorticoids Aldosterone	Stimulate renal tubules to reabsorb sodium, thus promoting water retention but potassium loss	Adrenocortical insufficiency	Electrolyte imbalance Hyperaldosteronism
Sex hormones—Androgens, estrogens, progesterone	Influence development of bone, reproductive organs, and secondary sex characteristics	Male feminization	Adrenogenital syndrome
Glucocorticoids Cortisol (hydrocortisone and compound F) Corticosterone (compound B)	Promote normal fat, protein, and carbohydrate metabolism Mobilize body defenses during periods of stress Suppress inflammatory reaction	Addison disease Acute adrenocortical insufficiency Impaired growth and sexual function	Cushing syndrome Severe impairment of growth with slowing in skeletal maturation In excess, tend to accelerate gluconeogenesis and protein and fat catabolism
ADRENAL MEDULLA			
Epinephrine (adrenaline), norepinephrine (noradrenaline)	Produce vasoconstriction of heart and smooth muscles (raise blood pressure) Increase blood glucose via glycolysis Inhibit gastrointestinal activity Activate sweat glands		Hyperfunction caused by: Pheochromocytoma Neuroblastoma Ganglioneuroma
ISLETS OF LANGERHANS OF PANCREAS			
Insulin (β cells)	Promotes glucose transport into the cells Increases glucose utilization, glycogenesis, and glycolysis Promotes fatty acid transport into cells and lipogenesis Promotes amino acid transport into cells and protein synthesis	Diabetes mellitus	Hyperinsulinism
Glucagon (α cells)	Acts as antagonist to insulin, thereby increasing blood glucose concentration by accelerating glycogenolysis Able to inhibit secretion of both insulin and glycogen		Hyperglycemia May be instrumental in genesis of diabetic ketoacidosis (DKA) in diabetes mellitus
Somatostatin (δ cells)	Able to inhibit secretion of both insulin and glycogen		

TABLE 29-1

Hormones and Their Function—cont'd

HORMONE	EFFECT	HYPOFUNCTION	HYPERFUNCTION
OVARIES			
Estrogen	Accelerates growth of epithelial cells, especially in uterus following menses Promotes protein anabolism Promotes epiphyseal closure of bones Promotes breast development during puberty and pregnancy Plays role in sexual function Stimulates water and sodium reabsorption in renal tubules Stimulates ripening of ova	Lack of or repression of sexual development	Precocious puberty, early epiphyseal closure
Progesterone	Prepares uterus for nidation of fertilized ovum and aids in maintenance of pregnancy Aids in development of alveolar system of breasts during pregnancy Inhibits myometrial contractions Has effect on protein catabolism Promotes salt and water retention, especially in endometrium		
TESTES			
Testosterone	Accelerates protein anabolism for growth Promotes epiphyseal closure Promotes development of secondary sex characteristics Plays role in sexual function Stimulates testes to produce spermatozoa	Delayed sexual development or eunuchoidism	Precocious puberty, early epiphyseal closure

changes as expected on the basis of bone age. These changes, although occurring later than in the average child, will appear in normal sequence and manner, and treatment with GH is not usually indicated. However, its use has become controversial, especially in relation to parental and child requests for treatment to accelerate growth.

Diagnostic Evaluation

Only a small number of children with delayed growth or short stature have hypopituitary dwarfism. In the majority of instances the cause is constitutional delay. Diagnostic evaluation is aimed at isolating organic causes, which, in addition to GH deficiency, may include hypothyroidism, oversecretion of cortisol, gonadal aplasia, chronic illness, nutritional inadequacy, Russell-Silver dwarfism, or hypochondroplasia.

A complete diagnostic evaluation should include a family history, a history of the child's growth patterns and previous health status, physical examination, psychosocial evaluation, radiographic surveys, and endocrine studies. Accurate measurement of height (using a calibrated stadiometer) and weight and comparison with standard growth charts are essential. Multiple height measures reflect a more accurate assessment of abnormal growth patterns (Box 29-2) (Hall, 2000).

A skeletal survey in children less than 3 years of age and radiographic examination of the hand-wrist for centers of ossification (bone age) (Box 29-3) in older children are important in evaluating growth.

Definitive diagnosis is based on absent or subnormal reserves of pituitary GH. Because GH levels are normally so low in children that differentiation from abnormal concentrations is unreliable, GH secretion should be stimulated, followed by measurement of blood levels. Exercise is a natural and benign stimulus for GH release, and elevated levels can be detected after 20 minutes of strenuous exercise in normal children. Also, GH levels are elevated 45 to 90 minutes after the onset of sleep.

Initial assessment of the serum insulin-like growth factor-I (IGF-I) and IGF binding protein 3 (IGFBP3) indicates a need for further evaluation of GH dysfunction if levels are less than -1 SD below the mean for age. It is recommended that GH stimulation tests be reserved for children with low serum IGF-I and IGFBP3 levels and poor growth (Hochberg, 1999).

Recent studies have shown that traditional GH stimulation test results can be substantially lower than previously accepted (Hilczer, Smyczynska, and Lewinski, 2006; Guyda, 2000; Mauras, Walton, Nicar, and others, 2000). GH-dependent growth factors

BOX 29-2

Evaluating the Growth Curve

Ensure reliability of measurements. Accurately obtain and plot height and weight measurements.

Determine absolute height. The child's absolute height bears some relationship to the likelihood of a pathologic condition. However, the majority of children who have a height below the lowest percentile (either 3rd or 5th percentile on the height curve) do not have a pathologic growth problem.

Assess height velocity. The most important aspect of a growth evaluation is the observation of a child's height over time, or height velocity. Accurate determination of height velocity requires at least 4 and preferably 6 months of observation. A substantial deceleration in height velocity (crossing several percentiles) between 3 and 12 or 13 years of age indicates a pathologic condition until proven otherwise.

Determine weight-to-height relationship. Determination of the weight-to-height ratio has some diagnostic value in ascertaining the cause of growth retardation in a short child.

Project target height. The height of a child can be judged inappropriately short only in the context of his or her genetic potential. Determine the target height of the child with the formula:

[Father's height (cm) + Mother's height (cm) + 13]/2 for boys

or

[Father's height (cm) + Mother's height (cm) − 13]/2 for girls

Most children achieve an adult stature within approximately 10 cm (4 inches) of the target height.

Modified from Vogiatzi MG, Copeland KC: The short child, *Pediatr Rev* 19(3):92-99, 1998.

BOX 29-3

Bone Age for Evaluating Growth Disorders

Bone age refers to a method of assessing skeletal maturity by comparing the appearance of representative epiphyseal centers obtained on x-ray examination with age-appropriate published standards.

Most conditions that cause poor linear growth also cause a delay in skeletal maturation and a retarded bone age. Observation of even a profoundly delayed bone age is never diagnostic or even indicative of a specific diagnosis. A delayed bone age merely indicates that the associated short stature is to some extent "partially reversible," since linear growth will continue until epiphyseal fusion is complete. In comparison, a bone age that is not delayed in a short child is of much greater concern and may, in fact, be of some diagnostic value under certain circumstances.

Modified from Vogiatzi MG, Copeland KC: The short child, *Pediatr Rev* 19(3):92-99, 1998.

may be more sensitive indicators of GH deficiency than GH stimulation tests. Increasingly sensitive radioimmunoassays for GH levels have been developed.

Therapeutic Management

Treatment of GH deficiency caused by organic lesions is directed toward correction of the underlying disease process (e.g., surgical removal or irradiation of a tumor). The definitive treatment of GH deficiency is replacement of GH, which is successful in 80% of affected children. A Cochrane Review of nine randomized controlled trials confirmed that GH therapy can increase short-term grown and improve final height (Bryant, Cave, and Milne, 2003). Reiter, Price, Wilton,

and others (2006) found final height within the midparental height range in 1258 patients with idiopathic GH deficiency treated at an early age.

The decision to stop GH therapy is made jointly by the child, family, and health care team. Radiologic evidence of epiphyseal closure is a criterion for ending therapy. Dosage is increased as the time of epiphyseal closure nears to optimize use of the GH. Children with other hormone deficiencies require replacement therapy to correct the specific disorders. This may involve administration of thyroid extract, cortisone, testosterone, or estrogens and progesterone. Treatment with the sex hormones is usually begun during adolescence to promote normal sexual maturation.

Nursing Care Management

The principal nursing consideration is identifying children with growth problems. Despite the fact that the majority of growth problems are not a result of organic causes, any delay in normal growth and sexual development poses special emotional adjustments for these children.

The nurse may be a key person in helping establish a diagnosis. For example, if serial height and weight records are not available, the nurse can question parents about the child's growth compared with that of siblings, peers, or relatives. Investigating clothing sizes is often helpful in determining growth at different ages. Parents may comment that the child wears out clothes before growing out of them or that, if the clothing fits the body, it often is too long in the sleeves or legs.

Because the behavioral or physical changes that suggest a tumor are insidious, they are frequently overlooked. It is important to correlate the onset of any positive findings with the initial evidence of growth retardation. For example, visual problems and headache are not uncommon in school-age children and can coincidentally occur after a growth problem is recognized. In fact, headache may represent the emotional trauma caused by short stature rather than be a symptom of a tumor. This line of questioning should be pursued cautiously to avoid alarming parents unduly about the possibility of a brain tumor.

Part of a nurse's role in helping establish a diagnosis is assisting with diagnostic tests. Preparation of the child and family is especially important if a number of tests are being performed, and the child requires particular attention during provocative testing. Blood samples are usually taken every 30 minutes for a 3-hour period. Children also have difficulty overcoming hypoglycemia generated by tests with insulin, so they must be observed carefully for signs of hypoglycemia, whereas those receiving glucagon are at risk of nausea and vomiting.

Child and Family Support. Children undergoing hormone replacement require additional support. The nurse should provide education for patient self-management during the school-age years.* Nursing functions include family education concerning medication preparation and storage, injection sites, injection technique, and syringe disposal (see Chapter 22). Administration of GH is facilitated by family routines that include a specific time of day for the injection. Younger

---

*Home care instructions on giving subcutaneous injections are available in Wilson D, Hockenberry M: *Wong's clinical manual of pediatric nursing,* ed 7, St Louis, 2008, Mosby.

children may enjoy using a calendar and colorful stickers to designate received injections.

> **NURSING TIP**
>
> Optimum dosing is often achieved when GH is administered at bedtime. Physiologic release is more normally stimulated as a result of pituitary release of GH during the first 45 to 90 minutes after the onset of sleep.

Even when hormone replacement is successful, these children attain their eventual adult height at a slower rate than their peers; therefore they need assistance in setting realistic expectations regarding improvement. Both sexes need guidance toward appropriate vocational goals. Because these children appear younger than their chronologic age, others frequently relate to them in infantile or childish ways. Children having school problems need special counseling. Parents and teachers benefit from guidance directed toward setting realistic expectations for the child based on age and abilities. For example, in the home such children should have the same age-appropriate responsibilities as their siblings. As they approach adolescence, they should be encouraged to participate in group activities with peers. They should wear styles that accentuate their actual age, not their size. If abilities and strengths are emphasized rather than physical size, such children are more likely to develop a positive self-image.

Professionals and families can find resources for research, education, support, and advocacy from the Human Growth Foundation.* The treatment is expensive, but the cost is often partially covered by insurance if the child has a documented deficiency. Children with panhypopituitarism should be advised to wear medical identification at all times.

PITUITARY HYPERFUNCTION

Excess GH before closure of the epiphyseal shafts results in proportional overgrowth of the long bones until the individual reaches a height of 2.4 m (8 feet) or more. Vertical growth is accompanied by rapid and increased development of muscles and viscera. Weight is increased but is usually in proportion to height. Proportional enlargement of head circumference also occurs and may result in delayed closure of the fontanels in young children. Children with a pituitary-secreting tumor may also demonstrate signs of increasing intracranial pressure, especially headache.

If oversecretion of GH occurs after epiphyseal closure, growth is in the transverse direction, producing a condition known as **acromegaly**. Typical facial features include overgrowth of the head, lips, nose, tongue, jaw, and paranasal and mastoid sinuses; separation and malocclusion of the teeth in the enlarged jaw; disproportion of the face to the cerebral division of the skull; increased facial hair; thickened, deeply creased skin; and increased tendency toward hyperglycemia and diabetes mellitus (DM).

Diagnostic Evaluation

Diagnosis is based on a history of excessive growth during childhood and evidence of increased levels of GH. Radiographic studies may reveal a tumor in an enlarged sella turcica,

normal bone age, enlargement of bones (such as the paranasal sinuses), and evidence of joint changes. Endocrine studies to confirm excess of other hormones, specifically thyroid, cortisol, and sex hormones, should also be included in the differential diagnosis.

Therapeutic Management

If a lesion is present, surgical treatment by cryosurgery or hypophysectomy is performed to remove the tumor when feasible. Other therapies aimed at destroying pituitary tissue include external irradiation and radioactive implants. Depending on the extent of surgical extirpation and degree of pituitary insufficiency, hormone replacement with thyroid extract, cortisone, and sex hormones may be necessary.

Nursing Care Management

The primary nursing consideration is early identification of children with excessive growth rates. Although medical management is unable to reduce growth already attained, further growth can be retarded. The earlier the treatment, the more control there is in predetermining a normal adult height. Nurses in ambulatory settings who are frequently involved in growth screening should refer children who demonstrate excessive linear growth for a medical evaluation. They should also observe for signs of a tumor, especially headache, and evidence of concurrent hormonal excesses, particularly the gonadotropins, which cause sexual precocity.

Children with excessive growth rates require as much emotional support as those with short stature. Children and their parents need an opportunity to express their thoughts. A compassionate nurse can be supportive to these children, especially before adolescence when they are larger than their peers. The nurse can emphasize to a tall girl that as boys grow older, they become taller and she will not always be looking down at them.

PRECOCIOUS PUBERTY

Manifestations of sexual development before age 9 years in boys or age 8 years in girls have traditionally been considered precocious development, and these children were recommended for further evaluation (Midyett, Moore, and Jacobson, 2003; Kempers and Otten, 2002). Recent examination of the age limit for defining when puberty is precocious reveals that the onset of puberty in girls is occurring earlier than previous studies have documented (Slyper, 2006; Biro, Huang, Crawford, and others, 2006). Mean onset of puberty was 10.2 and 9.6 years in Caucasian and African-American girls, respectively. Based on these findings, precocious puberty evaluation for a pathologic cause should be performed for Caucasian girls younger than 7 years of age or for African-American girls younger than 6 years of age. No change in the guidelines for evaluation of precocious puberty in boys is recommended. However, recent data suggest that boys may be beginning maturation earlier as well (Slyper, 2006; Herman-Giddens, 2006).

Normally the hypothalamic-releasing factors stimulate secretion of the gonadotropic hormones from the anterior pituitary at the time of puberty. In the male, interstitial cell–stimulating hormone stimulates Leydig cells of the testes to secrete testosterone; in the female, follicle-stimulating hormone (FSH) and luteinizing hormone stimulate the ovarian follicles to

---

*997 Glen Cove Ave., Suite 5, Glen Head, NY 11545; (800) 451-6434; e-mail: hgf1@hgfound.org; http://www.hgfound.org.

BOX 29-4

Causes of Precocious Puberty

CENTRAL PRECOCIOUS PUBERTY

Idiopathic, with or without hypothalamic hamartoma

Secondary

- Congenital anomalies
- Postinflammatory—Encephalitis, meningitis, abscess, granulomatous disease
- Radiotherapy
- Trauma
- Neoplasms

After effective treatment of longstanding pseudoisosexual precocity

PERIPHERAL PRECOCIOUS PUBERTY

Familial male-limited precocious puberty

Albright syndrome

Gonadal or extragonadal tumors

Adrenal

- Congenital adrenal hyperplasia
- Adenoma, carcinoma
- Glucocorticoid resistance

Exogenous sex hormones

Primary hypothyroidism

INCOMPLETE PRECOCIOUS PUBERTY

Premature thelarche

Premature menarche

Premature pubarche or adrenarche

Modified from Root AW: Precocious puberty, *Pediatr Rev* 21(1):10-19, 2000.

---

secrete estrogens (Nebesio and Eugster, 2007). This sequence of events is known as the **hypothalamic-pituitary-gonadal axis.** If for some reason the cycle undergoes premature activation, the child will display evidence of advanced or precocious puberty. Causes of precocious puberty are found in Box 29-4.

Isosexual precocious puberty is more common among girls than boys. Approximately 80% of children with precocious puberty have **central precocious puberty (CPP),** in which pubertal development is activated by the hypothalamic gonadotropin-releasing hormone (GnRH) (Greiner and Kerrigan, 2006). This produces early maturation and development of the gonads with secretion of sex hormones, development of secondary sex characteristics, and sometimes production of mature sperm and ova (Lee, 1999; Root, 2000). CPP may be the result of congenital anomalies; infectious, neoplastic, or traumatic insults to the central nervous system (CNS); or treatment of longstanding sex hormone exposure (Trivin, Couto-Silva, Sainte-Rose, and others, 2006). CPP occurs more frequently in girls and is usually idiopathic, with 95% demonstrating no causative factor (Nebesio and Eugster, 2007; Greiner and Kerrigan, 2006; Root, 2000). A CNS insult or structural abnormality is found in more than 90% of boys with CPP (Root, 2000).

Peripheral precocious puberty (PPP) includes early puberty resulting from hormone stimulation other than the hypothalamic GnRH–stimulated pituitary gonadotropin release. Isolated manifestations that are usually associated with puberty may be seen as variations in normal sexual development (Greiner and Kerrigan, 2006). They appear without other

signs of pubescence and are probably caused by unusual end-organ sensitivity to prepubertal levels of estrogen or androgen. Included are premature thelarche (development of breasts in prepubertal girls), premature pubarche (premature adrenarche, early development of sexual hair), and premature menarche (isolated menses without other evidence of sexual development).

Therapeutic Management

Treatment of precocious puberty is directed toward the specific cause when known. Precocious puberty of central (hypothalamic-pituitary) origin is managed with monthly injections of a synthetic analog of **luteinizing hormone–releasing hormone,** which regulates pituitary secretions (Greiner and Kerrigan, 2006; Muir, 2006). The available preparation, leuprolide acetate (Lupron Depot), is given in a dosage of 0.2 to 0.3 mg/kg intramuscularly once every 4 weeks. Breast development regresses or does not advance, and growth returns to normal rates, enhancing predicted height. Studies suggest that not all patients attain adult targeted heights and the addition of GH therapy may be warranted (Walvoord and Pescovitz, 1999). Treatment is discontinued at a chronologically appropriate time, allowing pubertal changes to resume. Psychologic management of the patient and family is an important aspect of care. Both parents and the affected child should be taught the injection procedure.

Nursing Care Management

Psychologic support and guidance of the child and family are the most important aspects of management. Parents need anticipatory guidance, support and information resources, and reassurance of the benign nature of the condition (Greiner and Kerrigan, 2006; O'Sullivan and O'Sullivan, 2002). Dress and activities for the physically precocious child should be appropriate to the chronologic age. Sexual interest is not usually advanced beyond the child's chronologic age, and parents need to understand that the child's mental age is congruent with the chronologic age and that the child's normal, overt manifestations of affection are age-appropriate and do not represent sexual advances.

Although the child's heterosexual behavior is appropriate for the chronologic age, the nurse should emphasize to parents that the child is fertile. Usually no form of contraception is necessary unless the child is sexually active. In this situation proper counseling is important because hormonal forms of birth control, such as estrogen pills, will prematurely initiate epiphyseal closure, resulting in stunted linear growth.

DIABETES INSIPIDUS

The principal disorder of posterior pituitary hypofunction is diabetes insipidus (DI), also known as **neurogenic DI,** resulting from undersecretion of **antidiuretic hormone (ADH),** or **vasopressin** (Pitressin), and producing a state of uncontrolled diuresis (Wong and Verbalis, 2002). This disorder is not to be confused with nephrogenic DI, a rare hereditary disorder affecting primarily males and caused by unresponsiveness of the renal tubules to the hormone.

Neurogenic DI may result from a number of different causes. Primary causes are familial or idiopathic; of the total cases, approximately 45% to 50% are idiopathic. Secondary causes include trauma (accidental or surgical), tumors, granulomatous disease, infections (meningitis or encephalitis), and vascular anomalies (aneurysm). Certain drugs, such as alcohol or phenytoin (diphenylhydantoin), can cause a transient polyuria.

The cardinal signs of DI are polyuria and polydipsia. In the older child, signs such as excessive urination accompanied by a compensatory insatiable thirst may be so intense that the child does little more than go to the toilet and drink fluids (Cheetham and Baylis, 2002). Frequently the first sign is enuresis. In the infant the initial symptom is irritability that is relieved with feedings of water but not milk. The infant is also prone to dehydration, electrolyte imbalance, hyperthermia, azotemia, and potential circulatory collapse.

Dehydration is usually not a serious problem in older children, who are able to drink larger quantities of water. However, any period of unconsciousness, such as after trauma or anesthesia, may be life threatening because the voluntary demand for fluid is absent. During such instances careful monitoring of urine volumes, blood concentration, and intravenous (IV) fluid replacement is essential to prevent dehydration.

> **NURSINGALERT**
> The child with DI complicated by congenital absence of the thirst center must be encouraged to drink sufficient quantities of liquid to prevent electrolyte imbalance.

Diagnostic Evaluation

The simplest test used to diagnose this condition is restriction of oral fluids and observation of consequent changes in urine volume and concentration. Normally, reducing fluids results in concentrated urine and diminished volume. In DI, fluid restriction has little or no effect on urine formation but causes weight loss from dehydration. Accurate results from this procedure require strict monitoring of fluid intake and urinary output, measurement of urine concentration (specific gravity or osmolality), and frequent weight checks. A weight loss between 3% and 5% indicates significant dehydration and requires termination of the fluid restriction.

> **NURSINGALERT**
> Small children require close observation during fluid deprivation to prevent them from drinking, even from toilet bowls, flower vases, or other unlikely sources of fluid.

If this test is positive, the child should be given a test dose of injected **aqueous vasopressin,** which should alleviate the polyuria and polydipsia. Unresponsiveness to exogenous vasopressin usually indicates nephrogenic DI. An important diagnostic consideration is to differentiate DI from other causes of polyuria and polydipsia, especially DM. DI may be the early sign of an evolving cerebral process (De Buyst, Massa, Christophe, and others, 2007).

Therapeutic Management

The usual treatment is hormone replacement, either with an intramuscular or subcutaneous injection of vasopressin tannate in peanut oil or with a nasal spray of aqueous lysine vasopressin (Verbalis, 2003). The injectable form has the advantage of lasting 48 to 72 hours, which affords the child a full night's sleep. However, it has the disadvantage of requiring frequent injections and proper preparation of the drug.

> **NURSINGTIP**
> To be effective, vasopressin must be thoroughly resuspended in the oil by being held under warm running water for 10 to 15 minutes and shaken vigorously before being drawn into the syringe. If this is not done, the oil may be injected minus the ADH. Small brown particles, which indicate drug dispersion, must be seen in the suspension.

Nursing Care Management

The initial objective is identification of the disorder. Because an early sign may be sudden enuresis in a child who is toilet trained, excessive thirst with bed-wetting is an indication for further investigation. Another clue is persistent irritability and crying in an infant that is relieved only by bottle-feedings of water. After head trauma or certain neurosurgical procedures, the development of DI can be anticipated; therefore these patients must be closely monitored.

Assessment includes measurement of body weight, serum electrolytes, blood urea nitrogen, hematocrit, and urine specific gravity taken before surgery and every other day after the procedure. Fluid intake and output should be carefully measured and recorded. Alert patients are able to adjust intake to urine losses, but unconscious or very young patients require closer fluid observation. In children who are not toilet trained, collection of urine specimens may require application of a urine-collecting device.

After confirmation of the diagnosis, parents need a thorough explanation regarding the condition with specific clarification that DI is a different condition from DM. They must realize that treatment is lifelong. If children are to receive the injectable vasopressin, ideally two caregivers should be taught the correct procedure for preparation and administration of the drug. Once children are old enough, they should be encouraged to assume full responsibility for their care.

For emergency purposes, these children should wear medical alert identification. Older children should carry the nasal spray with them for temporary relief of symptoms. School personnel need to be aware of the problem so they can grant children unrestricted use of the lavatory. Failure to permit this may result in embarrassing accidents that often lead to a child's unwillingness to attend school.

SYNDROME OF INAPPROPRIATE ANTIDIURETIC HORMONE

The disorder that results from oversecretion of the posterior pituitary hormone, or ADH, is known as syndrome of inappropriate antidiuretic hormone (SIADH). It is observed with increased frequency in a variety of conditions, especially those involving infections, tumors, or other CNS disease or trauma (Lin, Liu, and Lim, 2005).

The manifestations are directly related to fluid retention and hypotonicity. Excess ADH causes most of the filtered water to be reabsorbed from the kidneys back into central circulation. Serum osmolality is low, and urine osmolality is inappropriately elevated. When serum sodium levels are diminished to 120 mEq/L, affected children display anorexia, nausea (and sometimes vomiting), stomach cramps, irritability, and personality changes. With progressive reduction in sodium, other neurologic signs, stupor, and convulsions may be evident. The symptoms usually disappear when the underlying disorder is corrected.

The immediate management consists of restricting fluids. Subsequent management depends on the cause and severity.

Fluids continue to be restricted to one-fourth to one-half maintenance. When there are no fluid abnormalities but SIADH can be anticipated, fluids are often restricted expectantly at two-thirds to three-fourths maintenance.

Nursing Care Management

The first goal of nursing management is recognizing the presence of SIADH from symptoms described in patients at risk, especially those in the pediatric intensive care unit.

NURSINGALERT

Nausea, vomiting, and malaise may precede the onset of more severe stages such as disorientation, confusion, coma, and seizures (Majzoub and Muglia, 2003).

Accurately measuring intake and output, noting daily weight, and observing for signs of fluid overload are primary nursing functions, especially in the child receiving IV fluids. Seizure precautions are implemented, and the child and family need education regarding the rationale for fluid restrictions. The rare child with chronic SIADH will be placed on long-term ADH-antagonizing medication, and the child and family will require instructions for its administration.

DISORDERS OF THYROID FUNCTION

The thyroid gland secretes two types of hormones: **TH,** which consists of the hormones **thyroxine (T_4)** and **triiodothyronine (T_3),** and **calcitonin.** The secretion of thyroid hormones is controlled by TSH from the anterior pituitary, which in turn is regulated by thyrotropin-releasing factor (TRF) from the hypothalamus as a negative feedback response. Consequently, hypothyroidism or hyperthyroidism may result from a defect in the target gland or from a disturbance in the secretion of TSH or TRF. Because the functions of T_3 and T_4 are qualitatively the same, the term *thyroid hormone* (TH) is used throughout the discussion.

The synthesis of TH depends on available sources of dietary iodine and tyrosine. The thyroid is the only endocrine gland capable of storing excess amounts of hormones for release as needed. During circulation in the bloodstream, T_4 and T_3 are bound to carrier proteins (thyroxine-binding globulin). They must be unbound before they are able to exert their metabolic effect.

The main physiologic action of TH is to regulate the basal metabolic rate and thereby control the processes of growth and tissue differentiation. Unlike GH, TH is involved in many more diverse activities that influence the growth and development of body tissues. Therefore a deficiency of TH exerts a more profound effect on growth than that seen in hypopituitarism.

Calcitonin helps maintain blood calcium levels by decreasing the calcium concentration. Its effect is the opposite of parathyroid hormone (PTH) in that it inhibits skeletal demineralization and promotes calcium deposition in the bone.

JUVENILE HYPOTHYROIDISM

Hypothyroidism is one of the most common endocrine problems of childhood. It may be either congenital (see Chapter 9) or acquired and represents a deficiency in secretion of TH (Foley, 2001). Hypothyroidism from dietary insufficiency of iodine is now rare in the United States, since iodized salt is a readily available source of the nutrient.

BOX 29-5

Clinical Manifestations of Juvenile Hypothyroidism

Decelerated growth
  ■ Less when acquired at later age
Myxedematous skin changes
  ■ Dry skin
  ■ Puffiness around eyes
  ■ Sparse hair
  ■ Constipation
  ■ Sleepiness
  ■ Mental decline

Beyond infancy, primary hypothyroidism may be caused by a number of defects. For example, a congenital hypoplastic thyroid gland may provide sufficient amounts of TH during the first year or two but be inadequate when rapid body growth increases demands on the gland. A partial or complete thyroidectomy for cancer or thyrotoxicosis can leave insufficient thyroid tissue to furnish hormones for body requirements. Radiotherapy for Hodgkin disease or other malignancies may lead to hypothyroidism (Pizzo and Poplack, 2006). Infectious processes may cause hypothyroidism. It can also occur when dietary iodine is deficient.

Clinical manifestations depend on the extent of dysfunction and the child's age at onset. Primary congenital hypothyroidism is characterized by low levels of circulating thyroid hormones and raised levels of TSH at birth (Macchia, 2000). The GnRH test and baseline measurement of gonadotropin and sex hormone serum concentrations at 3 months of age are promising options for assessment of hypothalamic-pituitary-gonadal function in infants with congenital hypothyroidism (van Tijn, Schroor, Delemarre-van de Waal, and others, 2007). The presenting symptoms are decelerated growth from chronic deprivation of TH or thyromegaly. Impaired growth and development are less severe when hypothyroidism is acquired at a later age, and, because brain growth is nearly complete by 2 to 3 years of age, intellectual disability and neurologic sequelae are not associated with juvenile hypothyroidism. Other manifestations are myxedematous skin changes (dry skin, puffiness around the eyes, sparse hair), constipation, sleepiness, and mental decline (Box 29-5).

Therapy is TH replacement, the same as for hypothyroidism in the infant, although the prompt treatment needed in the infant is not required in the child. In children with severe symptoms, the restoration of euthyroidism is achieved more gradually with administration of increasing amounts of L-thyroxine over a period of 4 to 8 weeks to avoid symptoms of hyperthyroidism, which can occur with treatment of chronic hypothyroidism. Researchers have found that children treated early continue to have mild delays in reading, comprehension, and arithmetic but catch up by grade six (Rovet and Ehrlich, 2000). However, adolescents may demonstrate problems with memory, attention, and visuospatial processing.

Nursing Care Management

The importance of early recognition in the infant is discussed in Chapter 9. Growth cessation or retardation in a child whose growth has previously been normal should alert the observer to the possibility of hypothyroidism. After diagnosis and implementation of thyroxine therapy, the importance of compliance and periodic monitoring of response to therapy should be stressed to parents. Children should learn to take responsibility for their own health as soon as they are old enough, at about 9 or 10 years of age.

GOITER

A goiter is an enlargement or hypertrophy of the thyroid gland. It may occur with deficient (hypothyroid), excessive (hyperthyroid), or normal (euthyroid) TH secretion. It can be congenital or acquired. Congenital disease usually occurs as a result of maternal administration of antithyroid drugs or iodides during pregnancy. Acquired disease can result from increased secretion of pituitary TSH in response to decreased circulating levels of TH or from infiltrative neoplastic or inflammatory processes. In areas where dietary iodine (essential for TH production) is deficient, goiter can be endemic.

Enlargement of the thyroid gland may be mild and noticeable only when there is an increased demand for TH (e.g., during periods of rapid growth). Where iodine deficiency is severe, a large percentage of the population displays goiters. Enlargement of the thyroid at birth can be sufficient to cause severe respiratory distress. Sporadic goiter is usually caused by lymphocytic thyroiditis, and intrinsic biochemical defects in synthesis of the hormones are associated with goiters. TH replacement is necessary to treat the hypothyroidism and reverse the TSH effect on the gland.

Nursing Care Management

Large goiters are identified by their obvious appearance. Smaller nodules may be evident only on palpation. Nurses in ambulatory settings need to be aware of the possibility of goiters and report such findings. Benign enlargement of the thyroid gland may occur during adolescence and should not be confused with pathologic states. Nodules rarely are caused by a cancerous tumor but always require evaluation. Questions regarding exposure to radiation should be included in the assessment.

NURSING ALERT

If an infant is born with a goiter, immediate precautions are instituted for emergency ventilation, such as supplemental oxygen and a tracheostomy set nearby. Hyperextension of the neck often facilitates breathing.

Immediate surgery to remove part of the gland may be lifesaving in infants born with a goiter. When thyroid replacement is necessary, parents have the same needs regarding its administration as discussed for the parents of children who have hypothyroidism (see Chapter 9).

LYMPHOCYTIC THYROIDITIS

Lymphocytic thyroiditis (**Hashimoto disease, juvenile autoimmune thyroiditis**) is the most common cause of thyroid disease in children and adolescents and accounts for the largest percentage of juvenile hypothyroidism (Szymborska and Staroszczyk, 2000). It accounts for many of the enlarged thyroid glands formerly designated *thyroid hyperplasia of adolescence* or *adolescent goiter*. Although it can occur during the first 3 years of life, it occurs more frequently after age 6. It reaches a peak incidence during adolescence, and there is

---

BOX 29-6

Clinical Manifestations of Lymphocytic Thyroiditis

ENLARGED THYROID GLAND
Usually symmetric
Firm
Freely movable
Nontender

TRACHEAL COMPRESSION
Sense of fullness
Hoarseness
Dysphagia

HYPERTHYROIDISM (POSSIBLE)
Nervousness
Irritability
Increased sweating
Hyperactivity

---

evidence that the disease is self-limiting. The presence of a goiter and elevated thyroglobulin antibody with progressive increase in both thyroid peroxidase antibody and TSH may be predictive factors for future development of hypothyroidism (Radetti, Gottardi, Bona, and others, 2006).

The presence of the enlarged thyroid gland is usually detected by the practitioner during a routine examination, although it may be noted by parents when the youngster swallows. In most children the entire gland is enlarged symmetrically (though it may be asymmetric) and is firm, freely movable, and nontender. There may be manifestations of moderate tracheal compression (sense of fullness, hoarseness, and dysphagia), but it is extremely rare for a nontoxic diffuse goiter to enlarge to the extent that it causes mechanical obstruction. Most children are euthyroid, but some display symptoms of hypothyroidism. Other signs suggestive of hyperthyroidism are found in Box 29-6.

Diagnostic Evaluation

Thyroid function tests are usually normal, although TSH levels may be slightly or moderately elevated. With progressive disease the T_4 decreases, followed by a decrease in T_3 levels and an increase in TSH. A variety of abnormalities in radioactive iodine uptake may be noted. The majority of children have serum antibody titers to thyroid antigens, but fewer children have a positive red blood cell hemagglutination test result. When both tests are used, almost all children with thyroid autoimmunity are detected. However, levels in children are lower than in adults; therefore repeated measurements may be needed in doubtful cases, since titers may increase later in the disease.

Therapeutic Management

In many cases the goiter is transient and asymptomatic and regresses spontaneously within a year or two. Therapy of a nontoxic diffuse goiter is usually simple, uncomplicated, and effective. Oral administration of TH decreases the size of the gland significantly and provides the feedback needed to suppress TSH stimulation, and the hyperplastic thyroid gland gradually regresses in size. Surgery is contraindicated in this disorder. Untreated patients should be evaluated periodically.

Nursing Care Management

Nursing care consists of identifying the youngster with thyroid enlargement, reassuring the child that the condition is probably only temporary, and reinforcing instructions for thyroid therapy.

HYPERTHYROIDISM

The largest percentage of hyperthyroidism in childhood is caused by **Graves disease,** which is usually associated with an enlarged thyroid gland and exophthalmos (Ma, Xie, Kuang, and others, 2006; Streetman and Khanderia, 2004; Thompson, 2002). Most cases of Graves disease in children occur between ages 6 and 15, with a peak incidence at 12 to 14 years of age, but the disease may be present at birth in children of thyrotoxic mothers. The incidence is five times higher in girls than in boys.

The hyperthyroidism of Graves disease is apparently caused by an autoimmune response to TSH receptors, but no specific etiology has been identified. There is definitive evidence for familial association, with a high concordance incidence in twins. Patients with Graves disease possess the histocompatibility antigens A1, B8, and DR3 (Dallas and Foley, 2003; Simmonds, Howson, Heward, and others, 2005).

The development of manifestations is highly variable. Signs and symptoms develop gradually, with an interval between onset and diagnosis of approximately 6 to 12 months. The principal clinical features are excessive motion—irritability, hyperactivity, short attention span, tremors, insomnia, and emotional lability. Clinical manifestations are presented in Box 29-7.

Exophthalmos (protruding eyeballs), observed in many children, is accompanied by a wide-eyed staring expression, increased blinking, lid lag, lack of convergence, and absence of wrinkling of the forehead when looking upward. As protrusion of the eyeball increases, the child may not be able to completely cover the cornea with the lid. Visual disturbances may include blurred vision and loss of visual acuity. Ophthalmopathy can develop long before or after the onset of hyperthyroidism. A consistent pathogenic link between them has not been identified. It is now thought that Graves ophthalmopathy is a disorder of autoimmune origin caused by a complex interplay of endogenous and environmental factors (Bartalena, Tanda, Piantanida, and others, 2003).

Diagnostic Evaluation

The presence of a thyroid mass in a child requires a thorough history, including inquiry into prior irradiation to the head and neck and exposure to a goitrogen. The diagnosis is established on the basis of increased levels of T_4 and T_3. TSH is suppressed to unmeasurable levels (Ma, Xie, Kuang, and others, 2006). Other tests are rarely indicated.

Therapeutic Management

Therapy for hyperthyroidism is controversial, but all methods are directed toward retarding the rate of hormone secretion. The three acceptable modes available are the antithyroid drugs, which interfere with the biosynthesis of TH, including propylthiouracil (PTU) and methimazole (MTZ,

---

BOX 29-7

Clinical Manifestations of Hyperthyroidism (Graves Disease)

CARDINAL SIGNS
Emotional lability
Physical restlessness, characteristically at rest
Decelerated school performance
Voracious appetite with weight loss in 50% of cases
Fatigue

PHYSICAL SIGNS
Tachycardia
Widened pulse pressure
Dyspnea on exertion
Exophthalmos (protruding eyeballs)
Wide-eyed, staring expression with lid lag
Tremor
Goiter (hypertrophy and hyperplasia)
Warm, moist skin
Accelerated linear growth
Heat intolerance (may be severe)
Hair fine and unable to hold a curl
Systolic murmurs

THYROID STORM
Acute onset:
- Severe irritability and restlessness
- Vomiting
- Diarrhea
- Hyperthermia
- Hypertension
- Severe tachycardia
- Prostration
May progress rapidly to:
- Delirium
- Coma
- Death

Tapazole); subtotal thyroidectomy; and ablation with radioiodine (^{131}I iodide) (Streetman and Khanderia, 2004; Rivkees and Cornelius, 2003). Each is effective, but each has advantages and disadvantages.

When affected children exhibit signs and symptoms of hyperthyroidism (e.g., increased weight loss, pulse, pulse pressure, and blood pressure), their activity should be limited to classwork only. Vigorous exercise is restricted until thyroid levels are decreased to normal or near-normal values.

Thyrotoxicosis (thyroid "crisis" or thyroid "storm") may occur from sudden release of the hormone. Although thyrotoxicosis is unusual in children, a crisis can be life threatening. These "storms" are evidenced by the acute onset of severe irritability and restlessness, vomiting, diarrhea, hyperthermia, hypertension, severe tachycardia, and prostration. There may be rapid progression to delirium, coma, and even death. A crisis may be precipitated by acute infection, surgical emergencies, or discontinuation of antithyroid therapy. Treatment, in addition to antithyroid drugs, is administration of β-adrenergic blocking agents (propranolol), which provide relief from the adrenergic hyperresponsiveness that produces the disturbing side effects of the reaction. Therapy is usually required for 2 to 3 weeks.

The American Thyroid Association* has an extensive website with information related to prevention, treatment, and cure of thyroid disease.

Nursing Care Management

The initial nursing objective is identification of children with hyperthyroidism. Because the clinical manifestations often appear gradually, the goiter and ophthalmic changes may not be noticed, and the excessive activity may be attributed to behavioral problems. Nurses in ambulatory settings, particularly schools, need to be alert to signs that suggest this disorder, especially weight loss despite an excellent appetite, academic difficulties resulting from a short attention span and inability to sit still, unexplained fatigue and sleeplessness, and difficulty with fine motor skills such as writing. Exophthalmos may develop long before the onset of signs and symptoms of hyperthyroidism and may be the only presenting sign (Thompson, 2002). Exophthalmos is less common in adults than children (Jospe, 2001).

Much of these children's care is related to treating physical symptoms before a response to drug therapy is achieved. These children need a quiet, unstimulating environment that is conducive to rest. Sometimes hospitalization is necessary during the immediate treatment phase to remove a child from a troubled home. A regular routine is beneficial in providing frequent rest periods, minimizing the stress of coping with unexpected demands, and meeting the children's needs promptly. Physical activity is restricted. For example, school physical education classes are discontinued.

Emotional lability is often manifested by sudden episodes of crying or elation. Such behavior, coupled with irritability, disrupts interpersonal relationships, creating difficulties within and outside the home. Parents need help in understanding the uncontrollable nature of these outbursts and ways of minimizing them through decreased environmental stimulation, stress, and frustration. The child should be encouraged to express feelings about behavior and its effect on others. The nurse can encourage the child to concentrate on friendship with one special peer rather than a group until the condition is stabilized.

Heat intolerance may produce considerable family conflict. Preferring a cooler environment than others, the child is likely to open windows, complain about the heat, wear minimum clothing, and remove blankets while sleeping. Although the child should dress in accordance with climatic conditions, the use of light cotton clothing in the home, good ventilation, air conditioning or fans, frequent baths, and adequate hydration is helpful in providing comfort. Hygiene should be stressed because of excessive sweating.

Dietary requirements should be adjusted to meet the child's increased metabolic rate. Although the need for calories is increased, these should be provided in wholesome foods rather than "junk" foods. The child may require vitamin supplements to meet daily requirement. Rather than three large meals, the child's appetite may be better satisfied by five or six moderate meals throughout the day. Family members should refrain from making remarks about the child's appetite be-

cause the child may voluntarily restrict his or her eating to avoid such attention.

Once therapy is instituted, the nurse explains the drug regimen, emphasizing the importance of observing for side effects of antithyroid drugs. Untoward effects of propylthiouracil and related compounds include urticarial rash, fever, arthritis, or arthralgia. There may be enlargement of the salivary and cervical lymph glands, a diminished sense of taste, hepatitis, and edema of the lower extremities. Parents should also be aware of the signs of hypothyroidism, which can occur from overdose of the drugs. The most common indications are lethargy and somnolence.

> **NURSINGALERT**
>
> Children being treated with propylthiouracil or methimazole must be carefully monitored for side effects of the drug. Because sore throat and fever accompany the grave complication of leukopenia, these children should be seen by a practitioner if such symptoms occur. Parents and children should be taught to recognize and report symptoms immediately.

> **NURSINGALERT**
>
> The earliest indication of hypoparathyroidism may be anxiety and mental depression, followed by paresthesia and evidence of heightened neuromuscular excitability, such as:
>
> **Chvostek sign**—Facial muscle spasm elicited by tapping the facial nerve in the region of the parotid gland
>
> **Trousseau sign**—Carpal spasm elicited by pressure applied to nerves of the upper arm
>
> **Tetany**—Carpopedal spasm (sharp flexion of wrist and ankle joints), muscle twitching, cramps, seizures, and stridor

DISORDERS OF PARATHYROID FUNCTION

The parathyroid glands secrete **PTH,** the main function of which, along with vitamin D and calcitonin, is homeostasis of serum calcium concentration (Perheentupa, 2003). The effect of PTH on calcium is opposite that of calcitonin. The net result of the integrated action of PTH and vitamin D is maintenance of serum calcium levels within a narrow normal range and the mineralization of bone. Secretion of PTH is controlled by a negative feedback system involving the serum calcium ion concentration. Low ionized calcium levels stimulate PTH secretion, causing absorption of calcium by the target tissues; high ionized calcium concentrations suppress PTH.

HYPOPARATHYROIDISM

Hypoparathyroidism is a spectrum of disorders that result in deficient PTH. **Congenital hypoparathyroidism** may be caused by a specific defect in the synthesis or cellular processing of PTH or by aplasia or hypoplasia of the gland (Perheentupa, 2003).

Hypoparathyroidism can also occur secondary to other causes. Postoperative hypoparathyroidism may follow thyroidectomy with acute or gradual onset and be transient or permanent. Two forms of transient hypoparathyroidism may be present in the newborn, both of which are the result of a relative PTH deficiency. One type is caused by maternal hyperparathyroidism or maternal DM. A more common, later form appears almost exclusively in infants fed a milk formula with a high phosphate-to-calcium ratio.

Clinical signs of hypoparathyroidism are found in Box 29-8. Muscle cramps are an early symptom, progressing to

---

*6066 Leesburg Pike, Suite 550, Falls Church, VA 22041; (800) THYROID; e-mail: thyroid@thyroid.org; http://www.thyroid.org.

Clinical Manifestations of Hypoparathyroidism

PSEUDOHYPOPARATHYROIDISM
Short stature
Round face
Short, thick neck
Short, stubby fingers and toes
Dimpling of skin over knuckles
Subcutaneous soft tissue calcifications
Intellectual disability a prominent feature

IDIOPATHIC HYPOPARATHYROIDISM
None of the above physical characteristics observed
May include papilledema
May have intellectual disability

BOTH TYPES
Dry, scaly, coarse skin with eruptions
Hair often brittle
Nails thin and brittle with characteristic transverse grooves
Dental and enamel hypoplasia
Muscle contractions:
- Tetany
- Carpopedal spasm
- Laryngospasm (laryngeal stridor)
- Muscle cramps and twitching
- Positive Chvostek sign or Trousseau sign (see Nursing Alert on p. 1035)
- Paresthesias, tingling
Neurologic:
- Headache
- Seizures (generalized, absence, or focal)
- Swings of emotion
- Loss of memory
- Depression
- Confusion possible
Gastrointestinal:
- Muscle cramps
- Diarrhea
- Vomiting
Retarded skeletal growth

numbness, stiffness, and tingling in the hands and feet. A positive Chvostek or Trousseau sign or laryngeal spasms may be present. Convulsions with loss of consciousness may occur. These episodes may be preceded by abdominal discomfort, tonic rigidity, head retraction, and cyanosis. Headaches and vomiting with increased intracranial pressure and papilledema may occur and may suggest a brain tumor (Behrman, Kliegman, and Jenson, 2004).

Diagnostic Evaluation

The diagnosis of hypoparathyroidism is made on the basis of clinical manifestations associated with **decreased serum calcium** and **increased serum phosphorus.** Levels of plasma PTH are low in idiopathic hypoparathyroidism but high in pseudohypoparathyroidism. End-organ responsiveness is tested by the administration of PTH with measurement of urinary cyclic adenosine monophosphate (cAMP). Kidney function tests are included in the differential diagnosis to rule out renal insufficiency. Although bone radiographs are usually

normal, they may demonstrate increased bone density and suppressed growth.

Therapeutic Management

The objective of treatment is to maintain normal serum calcium and phosphate levels with minimum complications. Acute or severe tetany is corrected immediately by IV and oral administration of calcium gluconate and follow-up daily doses to achieve normal levels. Twice-daily serum calcium measurements are taken to monitor the efficacy of therapy and prevent hypercalcemia. When diagnosis is confirmed, **vitamin D therapy** is begun. Vitamin D therapy is somewhat difficult to regulate because the drug has a prolonged onset and a long half-life. Some authorities advocate beginning with a lower dose with stepwise increases and careful monitoring of serum calcium until stable levels are achieved. Others prefer rapid induction with higher doses and rapid reduction to lower maintenance levels (Behrman, Kliegman, and Jenson, 2004).

Long-term management consists of administration of massive doses of vitamin D, and oral calcium supplementation may be useful in maintaining adequate serum calcium levels, although it is not essential. Blood calcium and phosphorus are monitored frequently until the levels have stabilized; they are then monitored monthly and less often until the child is seen at 6-month intervals. Renal function, blood pressure, and serum vitamin D levels are measured every 6 months. Serum magnesium levels are measured every 3 to 6 months to permit detection of hypomagnesemia, which may raise the requirement for vitamin D.

Nursing Care Management

The initial objective is recognition of hypocalcemia. Unexplained convulsions, irritability (especially to external stimuli), gastrointestinal symptoms (diarrhea, vomiting, cramping), and positive signs of tetany should lead the nurse to suspect this disorder. Much of the initial nursing care is related to the physical manifestations and includes institution of seizure and safety precautions; reduction of environmental stimuli (e.g., avoiding sudden or loud noise, bright lights, stimulating activities); and observation for signs of laryngospasm such as stridor, hoarseness, and a feeling of tightness in the throat. A tracheostomy set and injectable calcium gluconate should be located near the bedside for emergency use. The administration of calcium gluconate requires precautions against extravasation of the drug and tissue destruction.

After initiating treatment, the nurse discusses with the parents the need for continuous daily administration of calcium salts and vitamin D. Because vitamin D toxicity can be a serious consequence of therapy, parents are advised to watch for signs that include weakness, fatigue, lassitude, headache, nausea, vomiting, and diarrhea. Early renal impairment is manifested by polyuria, polydipsia, and nocturia.

HYPERPARATHYROIDISM

Hyperparathyroidism is rare in childhood but can be primary or secondary. The most common cause of primary hyperparathyroidism is adenoma of the gland (Behrman, Kliegman, and Jenson, 2004). The most common causes of secondary hyperparathyroidism are chronic renal disease, renal osteodystrophy, and congenital anomalies of the urinary tract. The common factor is hypercalcemia. The clinical signs of hyperparathyroidism are listed in Box 29-9.

BOX 29-9
Clinical Manifestations of Hyperparathyroidism

GASTROINTESTINAL
Nausea
Vomiting
Abdominal discomfort
Constipation

CENTRAL NERVOUS SYSTEM
Delusions
Confusion
Hallucinations
Impaired memory
Lack of interest and initiative
Depression
Varying levels of consciousness

NEUROMUSCULAR
Weakness
Easy fatigability
Muscle atrophy (especially proximal muscles of lower limbs)
Tongue twitching
Paresthesias in extremities

SKELETAL
Vague bone pain
Subperiosteal resorption of phalanges
Spontaneous fractures
Absence of lamina dura around teeth

RENAL
Polyuria
Polydipsia
Renal colic
Hypertension

Diagnostic Evaluation

Blood studies to identify **elevated calcium** and **decreased phosphorus levels** are routinely performed. Measurement of PTH, as well as several tests to isolate the cause of the hypercalcemia, such as renal function studies, should be included. Other procedures used to substantiate the physiologic consequences of the disorder include electrocardiography and radiographic bone surveys.

Therapeutic Management

Treatment depends on the cause of hyperparathyroidism. The treatment of primary hyperparathyroidism is surgical removal of the tumor or hyperplastic tissue. Treatment of secondary hyperparathyroidism is directed at the underlying contributing cause, which subsequently restores the serum calcium balance. However, in some instances such as in chronic renal failure the underlying disorder is irreversible. In this case treatment is aimed at raising serum calcium levels to inhibit the stimulatory effect of low levels on the parathyroids. This includes oral administration of calcium salts, high doses of vitamin D to enhance calcium absorption, a low-phosphorus diet, and administration of a phosphorus-mobilizing aluminum hydroxide to reduce phosphate absorption.

Nursing Care Management

The initial nursing objective is recognition of the disorder. Because secondary hyperparathyroidism is a consequence of chronic renal failure, the nurse is always alert to signs that suggest this complication, especially bone pain and fractures. Because urinary symptoms are the earliest indication, assessment of other body systems for evidence of high calcium levels is indicated when polyuria and polydipsia coexist. Clues to the possibility of hyperparathyroidism include change in behavior, especially inactivity; unexplained gastrointestinal symptoms; and cardiac irregularities.

DISORDERS OF ADRENAL FUNCTION

The **adrenal cortex** secretes three main groups of hormones collectively called **steroids** and classified according to their biologic activity: (1) **glucocorticoids** (cortisol, corticosterone), (2) **mineralocorticoids** (aldosterone), and (3) **sex steroids** (androgens, estrogens, and progestins). Alterations in the levels of these hormones produce significant dysfunction in a variety of body tissues and organs. Because the adrenocortical cells are capable of producing any of the steroids, pathologic conditions may result in a deficiency or an excess of more than one type of hormone. However, most are rare in children.

The **adrenal medulla** secretes the **catecholamines epinephrine** and **norepinephrine.** Both hormones have essentially the same effects on various organs as those caused by direct sympathetic stimulation, except that the hormonal effects last several times longer. Catecholamine-secreting tumors are the primary cause of adrenal medullary hyperfunction.

ACUTE ADRENOCORTICAL INSUFFICIENCY

The acute form of adrenocortical insufficiency (**adrenal crisis**) may have a number of causes during childhood. Although a rare disorder, some of the more common etiologic factors include hemorrhage into the gland from trauma, which may be caused by a prolonged, difficult labor; fulminating infections, such as meningococcemia, which result in hemorrhage and necrosis (Waterhouse-Friderichsen syndrome); abrupt withdrawal of exogenous sources of cortisone or failure to increase exogenous supplies during stress; or congenital adrenogenital hyperplasia of the salt-losing type.

Early symptoms of adrenocortical insufficiency include increased irritability, headache, diffuse abdominal pain, weakness, nausea and vomiting, and diarrhea. Other clinical signs are found in Box 29-10. In the newborn, adrenal crisis is accompanied by extreme hyperpyrexia (high temperature), tachypnea, cyanosis, and seizures. Usually there is no evidence of infection or purpura. However, hemorrhage into the adrenal gland may be evident as a palpable retroperitoneal mass.

Diagnostic Evaluation

There is no rapid, definitive test for confirmation of acute adrenocortical insufficiency. Routine procedures such as measurement of plasma cortisol levels are too time-consuming to be practical. Therefore diagnosis is usually made based on clinical presentation, especially when a fulminating sepsis is accompanied by hemorrhagic manifestations and signs of circulatory collapse despite adequate antibiotic therapy. Because there is no real danger in administering a cortisol preparation for a short period, treatment should be instituted immediately. Improvement with cortisol therapy confirms the diagnosis.

BOX 29-10

Clinical Manifestations of Acute Adrenocortical Insufficiency

EARLY SYMPTOMS
Increased irritability
Headache
Diffuse abdominal pain
Weakness
Nausea and vomiting
Diarrhea

GENERALIZED HEMORRHAGIC MANIFESTATIONS (WATERHOUSE-FRIDERICHSEN SYNDROME)
Fever (increases as condition worsens)
Central nervous system signs:
- Nuchal rigidity
- Seizures
- Stupor
- Coma

SHOCKLIKE STATE
Weak, rapid pulse
Decreased blood pressure
Shallow respirations
Cold, clammy skin
Cyanosis
Circulatory collapse (terminal event)

NEWBORN
Hyperpyrexia
Tachypnea
Cyanosis
Seizures
Gland evident as palpable retroperitoneal mass (hemorrhagic)

Therapeutic Management

Treatment involves replacement of cortisol, replacement of body fluids to combat dehydration and hypovolemia, administration of glucose solutions to correct hypoglycemia, and specific antibiotic therapy in the presence of infection. Initially IV hydrocortisone (Solu-Cortef) is administered. Normal saline containing 5% glucose is given parenterally to replace lost fluid, electrolytes, and glucose. If hemorrhage has been severe, whole blood may be replaced. In the event that these measures do not reverse the circulatory collapse, vasopressors are used for immediate vasoconstriction and elevation of blood pressure.

Once the child's condition is stabilized, oral doses of cortisone, fluids, and salt are given, similar to the regimen used for chronic adrenal insufficiency. To maintain sodium retention, aldosterone is replaced by synthetic salt-retaining steroids.

Nursing Care Management

Because of the abrupt onset and potentially fatal outcome of this condition, prompt recognition is essential. Vital signs and blood pressure are taken every 15 minutes to monitor the hyperpyrexia and shocklike state. Seizure precautions are instituted, since convulsions from the elevated temperature are not uncommon. As soon as therapy is instituted, the nurse

should monitor the child's response to fluid and cortisol replacement. Too rapid administration of fluids can precipitate cardiac failure, whereas overdosage with cortisol produces hypotension and a sudden fall in temperature.

Once the acute phase is over and the hypovolemia is corrected, the child is given oral fluids, such as small quantities of ginger ale, fruit juice, or salted broth. Too rapid ingestion of oral fluids may induce vomiting, which increases dehydration. Therefore the nurse should plan a gradual schedule for reintroducing liquids. For children who refuse to drink, the prospect of having the IV infusion removed once oral fluids are increased is often a motivating factor.

NURSINGALERT

Monitor serum electrolyte levels and observe for signs of hypokalemia or hyperkalemia (e.g., weakness, poor muscle control, paralysis, cardiac dysrhythmias, and apnea). The condition is rapidly corrected with IV or oral potassium replacement.

NURSINGTIP

When an oral potassium preparation is given, it should be mixed with a small amount of strongly flavored fruit juice to disguise its bitter taste.

The sudden, severe nature of this disorder necessitates a great deal of emotional support for the child and family. The child may be placed in an intensive care unit where the surroundings are strange and frightening. Despite the need for emergency intervention, the nurse must be sensitive to the family's psychologic needs and prepare them for each procedure, even if this is a brief statement such as "The intravenous infusion is necessary to replace fluid that the child is losing." Because recovery within 24 hours is often dramatic, the nurse should keep the parents apprised of the child's condition, emphasizing signs of improvement, such as a lowered temperature and elevated blood pressure. If paralysis occurs, the nurse should assure them that this condition is temporary and quickly reversed.

CHRONIC ADRENOCORTICAL INSUFFICIENCY (ADDISON DISEASE)

Chronic adrenocortical insufficiency is rare in children. When it does occur, it is usually caused by a destructive lesion of the adrenal gland or neoplasms, or the cause is idiopathic. At one time, generalized tuberculosis was the leading cause of adrenal gland destruction.

Evidence of this disorder is usually gradual in onset, since 90% of adrenal tissue must be nonfunctional before signs of insufficiency are manifested. However, during periods of stress, when demands for additional cortisol are increased, symptoms of acute insufficiency may appear in a previously well child (Box 29-11).

Definitive diagnosis is based on measurements of functional cortisol reserve. The cortisol and urinary 17-hydroxycorticosteroid levels are low and fail to rise while plasma **adrenocorticotropic hormone (ACTH)** levels are elevated with corticotropin (ACTH) stimulation, the definitive test for the disease.

Therapeutic Management

Treatment involves replacement of **glucocorticoids (cortisol)** and **mineralocorticoids (aldosterone).** Some children are able to be maintained solely on oral supplements of cortisol

BOX 29-11

Clinical Manifestations of Chronic Adrenocortical Insufficiency

NEUROLOGIC SYMPTOMS
Muscular weakness
Mental fatigue
Irritability, apathy, and negativism
Increased sleeping, listlessness

PIGMENTARY CHANGES
Previous scars
Palmar creases
Mucous membranes
Hair
Hyperpigmentation over pressure points (elbows, knees, or waist)
Less frequently, vitiligo (loss of pigmentation)

GASTROINTESTINAL SYMPTOMS
Dehydration
Anorexia
Weight loss

CIRCULATORY SYMPTOMS
Hypotension
Small heart size
Dizziness
Syncopal (fainting) attacks

HYPOGLYCEMIA
Headache
Hunger
Weakness
Trembling
Sweating

OTHER SIGNS (SEEN IN SOME CHILDREN)
Recurrent, unexplained seizures
Intense craving for salt
Acute abdominal pain
Electrolyte imbalances

BOX 29-12

Etiology of Cushing Syndrome

Pituitary—Cushing syndrome with adrenal hyperplasia, usually attributed to an excess of adrenocorticotropic hormone (ACTH)
Adrenal—Cushing syndrome with hypersecretion of glucocorticoids, generally a result of adrenocortical neoplasms
Ectopic—Cushing syndrome with autonomous secretion of ACTH, most often caused by extrapituitary neoplasms
Iatrogenic—Cushing syndrome, frequently a result of administration of large amounts of exogenous corticosteroids
Food dependent—Inappropriate sensitivity of adrenal glands to normal postprandial increases in secretion of gastric inhibitory polypeptide

Adapted from: Magiakou MA, Mastorakos G, Oldfield EH, and others: Cushing's syndrome in children and adolescents. Presentation, diagnosis, and therapy, *N Engl J Med* 331(10):629-636, 1994.

(cortisone or hydrocortisone preparations) with a liberal intake of salt. During stressful situations, such as fever, infection, emotional upset, or surgery, the dosage must be tripled to accommodate the body's increased need for glucocorticoids. Failure to meet this requirement will precipitate an acute crisis. Overdosage produces appearance of cushingoid signs.

Children with more severe states of chronic adrenal insufficiency require mineralocorticoid replacement to maintain fluid and electrolyte balance. Other forms of therapy include monthly injections of desoxycorticosterone acetate or implantation of desoxycorticosterone acetate pellets subcutaneously every 9 to 12 months.

Nursing Care Management

Once the disorder is diagnosed, parents need guidance concerning drug therapy. They must be aware of the continuous need for cortisol replacement. Sudden termination of the drug because of inadequate supplies or inability to ingest the oral form because of vomiting places the child in danger of an acute adrenal crisis. Therefore parents should always have a spare supply of the medication in the home. Ideally they will have a prefilled syringe of hydrocortisone and be instructed in proper technique for intramuscular administration of the drug in case of crisis. Unnecessary administration of cortisone will not harm the child, but if it is needed, it may be lifesaving. Any evidence of acute insufficiency should be reported to the practitioner immediately.

Parents also need to be aware of side effects of the drugs. Undesirable side effects of cortisone include gastric irritation, which is minimized by ingestion with food or the use of an antacid; increased excitability and sleeplessness; weight gain, which may require dietary management to prevent obesity; and, rarely, behavioral changes, including depression or euphoria. Parents should be aware of signs of overdose and report these to the practitioner. In addition, the drug has a bitter taste, which creates a challenge for nurses and parents in its administration.

Because the body cannot supply endogenous sources of cortical hormones during times of stress, the home environment should be stable and relatively unstressful. Parents need to be aware that during periods of emotional or physical crisis the child requires additional hormone replacement. The child should wear medical identification, such as a bracelet, to permit medical personnel to adjust requirements during emergency care.

CUSHING SYNDROME

Cushing syndrome is a characteristic group of manifestations caused by excessive circulating free cortisol. It can result from a variety of causes, which generally fall into one of five categories (Box 29-12). Cushing syndrome in young children may be due to an adrenal tumor (Moshang, 2003).

Cushing syndrome is uncommon in children. When seen, it is often caused by excessive or prolonged steroid therapy that produces a cushingoid appearance (Fig. 29-1). This condition is reversible once the steroids are gradually discontinued. Abrupt withdrawal will precipitate acute adrenal insufficiency. Gradual withdrawal of exogenous supplies is necessary to allow the anterior pituitary an opportunity to secrete increasing amounts of ACTH to stimulate the adrenals to produce cortisol.

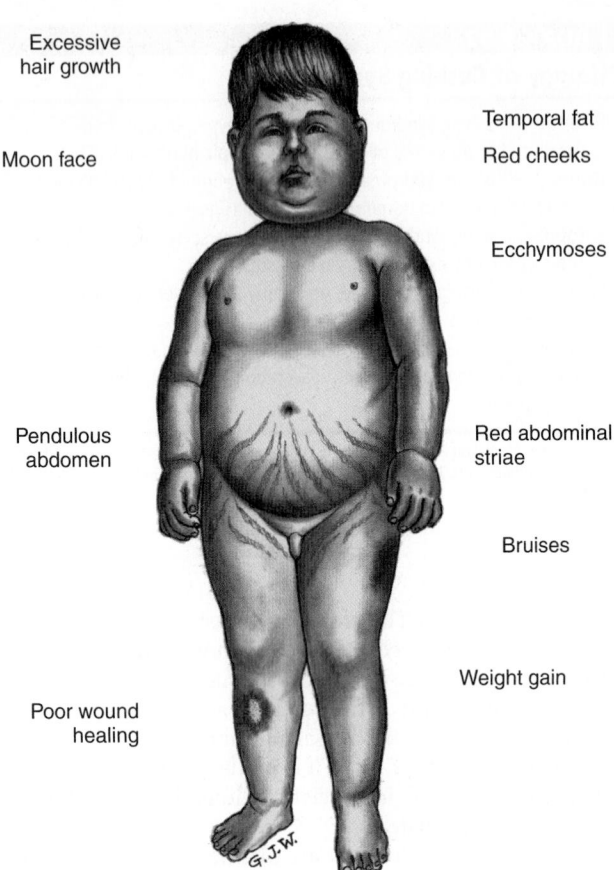

Excessive hair growth

Moon face

Temporal fat
Red cheeks

Ecchymoses

Pendulous abdomen

Red abdominal striae

Bruises

Weight gain

Poor wound healing

G.J.W.

FIG. 29-1 ■ Characteristics of Cushing syndrome.

Clinical Manifestations

Because the actions of cortisol are widespread, clinical manifestations are equally profound and diverse. Those symptoms that produce changes in physical appearance occur early in the disorder and are of considerable concern to school-age and older children. The physiologic disturbances, such as hyperglycemia, susceptibility to infection, hypertension, and hypokalemia, may have life-threatening consequences unless recognized early and treated successfully. Children with short stature may be responding to increased cortisol levels, resulting in Cushing syndrome. Cortisol inhibits the action of GH.

Diagnostic Evaluation

Several tests are helpful in confirming excess cortisol levels. They include fasting blood glucose levels for hyperglycemia, serum electrolyte levels for hypokalemia and alkalosis, 24-hour urinary levels of elevated 17-hydroxycorticoids and 17-ketosteroids, and radiographic studies of bone for evidence of osteoporosis and of the skull for enlargement of the sella turcica. Another procedure used to establish a more definitive diagnosis is the dexamethasone (cortisone) suppression test (Nieman and Ilias, 2005). Administration of an exogenous supply of cortisone normally suppresses ACTH production. However, in individuals with Cushing syndrome, cortisol levels remain elevated. This test is helpful in differentiating between children who are obese and those who appear to have cushingoid features.

Therapeutic Management

Treatment depends on the cause. In most cases surgical intervention involves bilateral adrenalectomy and postoperative replacement of the cortical hormones (the therapy for this is the same as that outlined for chronic adrenal insufficiency). If a pituitary tumor is found, surgical extirpation or irradiation may be chosen. In either of these instances, treatment of panhypopituitarism with replacement of GH, thyroid extract, ADH, gonadotropins, and steroids may be necessary for an indefinite period (Nieman and Ilias, 2005).

Nursing Care Management

Nursing care also depends on the cause. When cushingoid features are caused by steroid therapy, the effects may be lessened with administration of the drug early in the morning and on an alternate-day basis. Giving the drug early in the day maintains the normal diurnal pattern of cortisol secretion. If given during the evening, it is more likely to produce symptoms because endogenous cortisol levels are already low and the additional supply exerts more pronounced effects. An alternate-day schedule allows the anterior pituitary an opportunity to maintain more normal hypothalamic-pituitary-adrenal control mechanisms.

If an organic cause is found, nursing care is related to the treatment regimen. Although a bilateral adrenalectomy permanently solves one condition, it reciprocally produces another syndrome. Before surgery, parents need to be adequately informed of the operative benefits and disadvantages. Postoperative teaching regarding drug replacement is the same as discussed in the previous section.

> **NURSINGALERT**
> Postoperative complications of adrenalectomy are related to the sudden withdrawal of cortisol. Observe for shocklike symptoms (e.g., hypotension, hyperpyrexia).

Anorexia and nausea and vomiting are common and may be improved with the use of nasogastric decompression. Muscle and joint pain may be severe, requiring use of analgesics. The psychologic depression can be profound and may not improve for months. Parents should be aware of the physiologic reasons behind these symptoms in order to be supportive of the child.

CONGENITAL ADRENAL HYPERPLASIA

Congenital adrenal hyperplasia (CAH) is a family of disorders caused by decreased enzyme activity required for cortisol production in the adrenal cortex. The most common defect is **21-hydroxylase deficiency,** which constitutes more than 90% of all cases of CAH (American Academy of Pediatrics, 2000; Levine, 2000). This deficiency occurs in approximately 1 per 12,000 to 15,000 births and causes overproduction of the adrenal androgens, resulting in virilization of the female fetus.

Excessive androgens cause masculinization of the urogenital system at approximately the tenth week of fetal development. The most pronounced abnormalities occur in the girl, who is born with varying degrees of ambiguous genitalia. Masculinization of external genitalia causes the clitoris to enlarge so that it appears as a small phallus. Fusion of the labia produces a saclike structure resembling the scrotum without testes. However, no abnormal changes occur in the internal sexual organs, although the vaginal orifice is usually closed by the fused labia. The label *ambiguous genitalia* should be applied to any infant with hypospadias or micropenis and no palpable gonads, and a diagnostic evaluation for CAH should be contemplated. Males do not display genital abnormalities at birth (New and Ghizzoni, 2003).

Increased pigmentation of skin creases and genitalia caused by increased ACTH may be a subtle sign of adrenal insufficiency. A salt-wasting crisis frequently occurs, usually within the first few weeks of life (Behrman, Kliegman, and Jenson, 2004). Infants fail to gain weight, and hyponatremia and hyperkalemia may be significant. Cardiac arrest can occur.

Untreated CAH results in early sexual maturation, with enlargement of the external sexual organs; development of axillary, pubic, and facial hair; deepening of the voice; acne; and marked increase in musculature with changes toward an adult male physique. However, in contrast to precocious puberty, breasts do not develop in the female, and she remains amenorrheic and infertile. In the male the testes remain small, and spermatogenesis does not occur. In both sexes linear growth is accelerated, and epiphyseal closure is premature, resulting in short stature by the end of puberty.

Diagnostic Evaluation

Clinical diagnosis is initially based on congenital abnormalities that lead to difficulty in assigning sex to the newborn and on signs and symptoms of adrenal insufficiency or hypertension. Definitive diagnosis is confirmed by evidence of increased 17-ketosteroid levels in most types of CAH (Levine, 2000). Usually the level of 17-hydroxycorticoids is low or near normal. In complete 21-hydroxylase deficiency, blood electrolytes demonstrate loss of sodium and chloride and elevation of potassium. In older children bone age is advanced, and linear growth is increased. Chromosome typing for positive sex determination and to rule out any other genetic abnormality (e.g., Turner syndrome) is always done in any case of ambiguous genitalia.

Another test that can be used to visualize the presence of pelvic structures is ultrasonography, a noninvasive, painless imaging technique that does not require anesthesia or sedation. It is especially useful in CAH because it readily identifies the absence or presence of female reproductive organs in a newborn or child with ambiguous genitalia. Because ultrasonography yields immediate results, it has the advantage of determining the child's gender long before the more complex laboratory results for chromosome analysis or steroid levels are available.

Therapeutic Management

The initial medical objective is to confirm the diagnosis and assign a sex to the child, usually according to the genotype. In both sexes cortisone is administered to suppress the abnormally high secretions of ACTH. If cortisone is begun early enough, it is very effective. Cortisone depresses the secretion of ACTH by the adenohypophysis, which in turn inhibits the secretion of adrenocorticosteroids, which stems the progressive virilization. The signs and symptoms of masculinization in the female gradually disappear, and excessive early linear growth is slowed. Puberty occurs normally at the appropriate age.

The recommended oral dosage is divided to simulate the normal diurnal pattern of ACTH secretion. Because these children are unable to produce cortisol in response to stress, it is necessary to increase the dosage during episodes of infection, fever, or other stresses. Acute emergencies require immediate IV or intramuscular administration. Emergency situations include bacterial and viral infections, vomiting, surgery, fractures, major injuries, and sometimes insect stings.

Children with the salt-losing type of CAH require aldosterone replacement, as outlined under chronic adrenal insufficiency, and supplementary dietary salt. Frequent laboratory tests are conducted to assess the effects on electrolytes, hormonal profiles, and renin levels. The frequency of testing is individualized to the child.

Depending on the degree of masculinization in the female, reconstructive surgery may be required to reduce the size of the clitoris, separate the labia, and create a vaginal orifice (Miranda, Oliveira-Filho, Lemos-Marini, and others, 2004). Surgery is performed when the infant is physically able to withstand the procedure but before she is old enough to be aware of the abnormal genitalia. Plastic surgery is generally done in stages and yields excellent cosmetic results. Reports concerning sexual satisfaction after partial clitoridectomy indicate that the capacity for orgasm and sexual gratification is not necessarily impaired.

Unfortunately, not all children with CAH are diagnosed at birth and raised in accordance with their genetic sex. Particularly in the case of affected females, masculinization of the external genitalia may have led to sex assignment as a male. In males, diagnosis is usually delayed until early childhood, when signs of virilism appear. In these situations it is advisable to continue rearing the child as a male in accordance with assigned sex and phenotype. Hormone replacement may be required to permit linear growth and to initiate male pubertal changes. Surgery is usually indicated to remove the female organs and reconstruct the phallus for satisfactory sexual relations. These individuals are not fertile.

Nursing Care Management

Of major importance is recognition of ambiguous genitalia in newborns. If there is any question regarding assignment of sex, the parents need to be told immediately to prevent the embarrassing situation of informing family members of the child's sex and then having to change the announcement.

As soon as the sex is determined, parents should be informed of the findings and encouraged to choose an appropriate name, and the child should be identified as a male or female, with no reference to ambiguous sex. If the appearance of the enlarged genitalia in a girl concerns the parents, they should be encouraged to discuss their feelings. Suggesting ways to avoid questioning remarks from visitors, such as diapering the child in a separate room, is also helpful. If surgery is anticipated, showing parents before-and-after photographs of reconstruction helps to reinforce the expected cosmetic benefits.

In general, rearing the genetically female child as a girl is preferred because of the success of surgical intervention and the satisfactory results with hormones in reversing virilism and providing a prospect of normal puberty and the ability to conceive. This is in contrast to the choice of rearing the child as a boy, in which case the child is sterile and may never be able to function satisfactorily in heterosexual relationships. If the parents persist in their decision to assign a male sex to a genetically female child, a psychologic consultation should be requested to explore their motivations and ensure their understanding of the future consequences for the child.

Nursing care management regarding cortisol and aldosterone replacement are the same as those discussed for chronic adrenocortical insufficiency. Because infants are especially prone to dehydration and salt-losing crises, parents need to be aware of signs of dehydration and the urgency of immediate medical intervention to stabilize the child's condition. Parents should have injectable hydrocortisone available and know how to prepare and administer the intramuscular injection (see Chapter 22).

In the unfortunate situation in which the sex is erroneously assigned and the correct sex determined later, parents need a great deal of help in understanding the reason for the incorrect sex identification and the options for sex reassignment or medical-surgical intervention. Because children become aware of their sexual identity by 18 months to 2 years of age, it is believed that any reassignment after this period can cause tremendous psychologic conflicts in the child. Therefore sex rearing should be continued as previously established with medical-surgical intervention as required.

> **NURSINGALERT**
>
> The parents should be advised that there is no physical harm in treating for suspected adrenal insufficiency that is not present, whereas the consequence of not treating acute adrenal insufficiency can be fatal.

PHEOCHROMOCYTOMA

Pheochromocytoma is a rare tumor characterized by secretion of catecholamines. The tumor most commonly arises from the chromaffin cells of the adrenal medulla but may occur wherever these cells are found, such as along the paraganglia of the aorta or thoracolumbar sympathetic chain (Pacak, Eisenhofer, Ahlman, and others, 2007). Approximately 10% of these tumors are located in extraadrenal sites. In children they are frequently bilateral or multiple and are generally benign. Often there is a familial transmission of the condition as an autosomal dominant trait (Behrman, Kliegman, and Jenson, 2004).

The clinical manifestations of pheochromocytoma are caused by an increased production of catecholamines, producing hypertension, tachycardia, headache, decreased gastrointestinal activity with resultant constipation, increased metabolism with anorexia, weight loss, hyperglycemia, polyuria, polydipsia, hyperventilation, nervousness, heat intolerance, and diaphoresis. In severe cases, signs of congestive heart failure are evident.

Diagnostic Evaluation

The clinical manifestations mimic those of other disorders, such as hyperthyroidism or DM.

Therapeutic Management

Definitive treatment consists of surgical removal of the tumor. In children the tumors may be bilateral, requiring a bilateral adrenalectomy and lifelong glucocorticoid and mineralocorticoid therapy. The major complications that can occur during surgery are severe hypertension, tachyarrhythmias, and hypotension. The first two are caused by excessive release of catecholamines during manipulation of the tumor, and the latter results from catecholamine withdrawal and hypovolemic shock.

Preoperative medication to inhibit the effects of catecholamines is begun 1 to 3 weeks before surgery to prevent these complications. The major group of drugs used is the α-adrenergic blocking agents with or without β-adrenergic blocking agents. The most commonly used α-adrenergic blocker is phenoxybenzamine (Dibenzyline), a long-acting medication given orally every 12 hours. The shorter-acting phentolamine (Regitine) is equally effective but less satisfactory for long-term use, although it is useful for acute hypertension. To control catecholamine release when α-adrenergic blocking agents are inadequate, the child is given β-adrenergic blocking agents.

Success of therapy is judged by lowering of blood pressure to normal, absence of hypertensive attacks (flushing or blanching, fainting, headache, palpitations, tachycardia, nausea and vomiting, profuse sweating), heat tolerance, decrease in perspiration, and disappearance of hyperglycemia. A disadvantage of these drugs is their inability to block the effects of catecholamines on beta receptors.

Nursing Care Management

An initial nursing objective is identification of children with this disorder. Outstanding clues are hypertension and hypertensive attacks. Because of behavioral changes (nervousness, excitability, overactivity, even psychosis), increased cardiac and respiratory activity may appear to be related to an acute anxiety attack. Therefore a careful history of the onset of symptoms and association with stressful events is helpful in distinguishing between an organic and a psychologic cause for the symptoms.

Preoperative nursing care involves frequent monitoring of vital signs and observation for evidence of hypertensive attacks and congestive heart failure. Therapeutic effects are evidenced by normal vital signs and absence of glycosuria. Daily blood glucose levels, urine acetone, and any signs of hyperglycemia are noted and reported immediately.

> **NURSINGALERT**
>
> Do not palpate the mass. Preoperative palpation of the mass releases catecholamines, which can stimulate severe hypertension and tachyarrhythmias.

The environment is made conducive to rest and free of emotional stress. This requires adequate preparation during hospital admission and before surgery. Parents are encouraged to room-in with their child and to participate in care. Play activities need to be tailored to the child's energy level without being overly strenuous or challenging because these can increase metabolic rate and promote frustration and anxiety.

After surgery the child is observed for signs of shock from removal of excess catecholamines. If a bilateral adrenalectomy was performed, the nursing interventions are those discussed for chronic adrenocortical insufficiency.

DISORDERS OF PANCREATIC HORMONE SECRETION: DIABETES MELLITUS

DM is a chronic disorder of metabolism characterized by a partial or complete deficiency of the hormone **insulin.** It is the most common metabolic disease, resulting in metabolic adjustment or physiologic change in almost all areas of the

Acanthosis Nigricans

TABLE 29-2

Characteristics of Type 1 and Type 2 Diabetes Mellitus

CHARACTERISTIC	TYPE 1	TYPE 2
Age at onset	<20 years	Increasingly occurring in younger children
Type of onset	Abrupt	Gradual
Sex ratio	Affects males slightly more than females	Females outnumber males
Percentage of diabetic population	5%-8%	85%-90%
Heredity:		
Family history	Sometimes	Frequently
Human leukocyte antigen	Associations	No association
Twin concordance	25%-50%	90%-100%
Ethnic distribution	Primarily Caucasians	Increased incidence in Native Americans, Hispanics, African-Americans
Presenting symptoms	3 P's common: polyuria, polydipsia, polyphagia	May be related to long-term complications
Nutritional status	Underweight	Overweight
Insulin (natural):		
Pancreatic content	Usually none	>50% normal
Serum insulin	Low to absent	High or low
Primary resistance	Minimum	Marked
Islet cell antibodies	80%-85%	<5%
Therapy:		
Insulin	Always	20%-30% of patients
Oral agents	Ineffective	Often effective
Diet only	Ineffective	Often effective
Chronic complications	>80%	Variable
Ketoacidosis	Common	Infrequent

body. Approximately one in three children born in the United States will develop diabetes. The odds are higher for African-American and Hispanic children: nearly 50% of them will develop diabetes (Urrutia-Rojas and Menchaca, 2006). DM in children can occur at any age but has a peak incidence between ages 10 and 15 years, with 75% diagnosed before 18 years of age. The incidence in boys is slightly higher than in girls (1:1 to 1.2:1).

Traditionally DM had been classified according to the type of treatment needed. The old categories were insulin-dependent diabetes mellitus (IDDM), or type I; and non–insulin-dependent diabetes mellitus (NIDDM), or type II. In 1997 these terms were eliminated because treatment can vary (some people with NIDDM require insulin) and because the terms do not indicate the underlying problem. The new terms are *type 1* and *type 2,* using Arabic symbols to avoid confusion (e.g., type II could be read as type eleven) (American Diabetes Association, 2001). The characteristics of type 1 DM and type 2 DM are outlined in Table 29-2.

Type 1 DM is more prominent in Caucasians, with an incidence of 20 per 100,000; the incidence in African-Americans is 11 per 100,000; the incidence in Hispanics is 15.2 per 100,000; and the incidence in Cubans is 2.6 per 100,000. Native Americans tend to develop type 2 DM rather than type 1 DM even when diagnosed in childhood. The Pima Tribe reports a greater than 55% incidence of type 2 DM. Type 1 diabetes is characterized by destruction of the pancreatic β cells, which produce insulin; this usually leads to absolute insulin deficiency. Type 1 diabetes has two forms. Immune-mediated DM results from an autoimmune destruction of the β cells; it typically starts in children or young adults who are slim, but it

can arise in adults of any age. **Idiopathic type 1** refers to rare forms of the disease that have no known cause.

Type 2 diabetes usually arises because of insulin resistance, in which the body fails to use insulin properly, combined with relative (rather than absolute) insulin deficiency. People with type 2 can range from predominantly insulin resistant with relative insulin deficiency to predominantly deficient in insulin secretion with some insulin resistance. It typically occurs in those who are over 45, are overweight and sedentary, and have a family history of diabetes.

The symptomatology of diabetes is more readily recognizable in children than in adults, so it is surprising that the diagnosis may sometimes be missed or delayed. Diabetes is a great imitator; influenza, gastroenteritis, and appendicitis are the conditions most often diagnosed when it turns out that the disease is really diabetes (Box 29-13).

Pathophysiology

Insulin is needed to support the metabolism of carbohydrates, fats, and proteins, primarily by facilitating the entry of these substances into the cell. Insulin is needed for the entry of glucose into the muscle and fat cells, prevention of mobilization of fats from fat cells, and storage of glucose as glycogen in the cells of liver and muscle. Insulin is not needed for the entry of glucose into nerve cells or vascular tissue. The chemical composition and molecular structure of insulin are such that it fits into receptor sites on the cell membrane. Here it initiates a sequence of poorly defined chemical reactions that alter the cell membrane to facilitate the entry of glucose into the cell and stimulate enzymatic systems outside the cell that metabolize the glucose for energy production.

BOX 29-13
Clinical Manifestations of Type 1 Diabetes Mellitus

Polyphagia

Polyuria

Polydipsia

Weight loss

Enuresis or nocturia

Irritability; "not himself" or "herself"

Shortened attention span

Lowered frustration tolerance

Dry skin

Blurred vision

Poor wound healing

Fatigue

Flushed skin

Headache

Frequent infections

Hyperglycemia
- Elevated blood glucose levels
- Glucosuria

Diabetic ketosis
- Ketones and glucose in urine
- Dehydration in some cases

Diabetic ketoacidosis
- Dehydration
- Electrolyte imbalance
- Acidosis
- Deep, rapid breathing (Kussmaul)

With a deficiency of insulin, glucose is unable to enter the cell, and its concentration in the bloodstream increases. The increased concentration of glucose (**hyperglycemia**) produces an osmotic gradient that causes the movement of body fluid from the intracellular space to the interstitial space, then to the extracellular space and into the glomerular filtrate in order to "dilute" the hyperosmolar filtrate. Normally the renal tubular capacity to transport glucose is adequate to reabsorb all the glucose in the glomerular filtrate. When the glucose concentration in the glomerular filtrate exceeds the renal threshold (6180 mg/dl), glucose spills into the urine (**glycosuria**) along with an osmotic diversion of water (**polyuria**), a cardinal sign of diabetes. The urinary fluid losses cause the excessive thirst (**polydipsia**) observed in diabetes. This water "washout" results in a depletion of other essential chemicals, especially potassium.

Protein is also wasted during insulin deficiency. Because glucose is unable to enter the cells, protein is broken down and converted to glucose by the liver (**glucogenesis**); this glucose then contributes to the hyperglycemia. These mechanisms are similar to those seen in starvation when substrate (glucose) is absent. The body is actually in a state of starvation during insulin deficiency. Without the use of carbohydrates for energy, fat and protein stores are depleted as the body attempts to meet its energy needs. The hunger mechanism is triggered, but increased food intake (polyphagia) enhances the problem by further elevating blood glucose.

Ketoacidosis. When insulin is absent or insulin sensitivity is altered, glucose is unavailable for cellular metabolism, and the body chooses alternate sources of energy, principally fat. Consequently fats break down into fatty acids, and glycerol in the fat cells is converted by the liver to ketone bodies (β-hydroxybutyric acid, acetoacetic acid, acetone). Any excess is eliminated in the urine (**ketonuria**) or the lungs (**acetone breath**). The ketone bodies in the blood (ketonemia) are strong acids that lower serum pH, producing **ketoacidosis.**

Ketones are organic acids that readily produce excessive quantities of free hydrogen ions, causing a fall in plasma pH. Then chemical buffers in the plasma, principally bicarbonate, combine with the hydrogen ions to form carbonic acid, which readily dissociates into water and carbon dioxide. The respiratory system attempts to eliminate the excess carbon dioxide by increased depth and rate—**Kussmaul respirations,** or the hyperventilation characteristic of metabolic acidosis. The ketones are buffered by sodium and potassium in the plasma. The kidney attempts to compensate for the increased pH by increasing tubular secretion of hydrogen and ammonium ions in exchange for fixed base, thus depleting the base buffer concentration.

With cellular death, potassium is released from the cell (intracellular fluid) into the bloodstream (extracellular fluid) and excreted by the kidney, where the loss is accelerated by osmotic diuresis. The total body potassium is then decreased, even though the serum potassium level may be elevated as a result of the decreased fluid volume in which it circulates. Alteration in serum and tissue potassium can lead to cardiac arrest.

If these conditions are not reversed by insulin therapy in combination with correction of the fluid deficiency and electrolyte imbalance, progressive deterioration occurs, with dehydration, electrolyte imbalance, acidosis, coma, and death. **Diabetic ketoacidosis (DKA)** should be diagnosed promptly in a seriously ill patient and therapy instituted in an intensive care unit.

Long-Term Complications. Long-term complications of diabetes involve both the microvasculature and the macrovasculature. The principal microvascular complications are **nephropathy, retinopathy,** and **neuropathy.** Microvascular disease develops during the first 30 years of diabetes, beginning in the first 10 to 15 years after puberty, with renal involvement evidenced by proteinuria and clinically apparent retinopathy.

With poor diabetic control, vascular changes can appear as early as 2½ to 3 years after diagnosis; however, with good to excellent control, changes can be postponed for 20 or more years. Intensive insulin therapy appears to delay the onset and slow the progression of clinically important retinopathy, including vision-threatening lesions, nephropathy, and neuropathy. Hypertension and atherosclerotic cardiovascular disease are also major causes of morbidity and mortality in patients with DM (Karnik, Fields, and Shannon, 2007). The postpubertal duration, not the total duration, of type 1 DM is implicated as a risk factor for the development of microvascular disease (Schultz, Konopelska-Bahu, Dalton, and others, 1999). The process appears to be one of glycosylation, wherein proteins from the blood become deposited in the walls of small vessels (e.g., glomeruli), where they become trapped by "sticky" glucose compounds (glycosyl radicals). The buildup of these substances over time causes narrowing of the vessels, with subsequent interference with microcirculation to the affected areas (Beisswenger, Szwergold, and Yeo, 2001). Macrovascular disease develops after 25 years of diabetes and creates the predominant problems in patients with type 2 DM.

Other complications have been observed in children with type 1 DM. Hyperglycemia appears to influence thyroid function, and altered function is frequently observed at the time of diagnosis and in poorly controlled diabetes. Limited mobility of small joints of the hand occurs in 30% of 7- to 18-year-old children with type 1 DM and appears to be related to changes in the skin and soft tissues surrounding the joint as a result of glycosylation.

> **NURSINGALERT**
>
> Recurrent vaginal and urinary tract infections, especially with *Candida albicans,* are often an early sign of type 2 DM, especially in adolescents.

Diagnostic Evaluation

Three groups of children who should be considered as candidates for diabetes are (1) children who have glycosuria, polyuria, and a history of weight loss or failure to gain despite a voracious appetite; (2) those with transient or persistent glycosuria; and (3) those who display manifestations of metabolic acidosis, with or without stupor or coma. In every case diabetes must be considered if there is glycosuria, with or without ketonuria, and unexplained hyperglycemia.

Glycosuria by itself is not diagnostic of diabetes. Other sugars, such as galactose, can produce a positive result with certain test strips, and a mild degree of glycosuria can be caused by other conditions, such as infection, trauma, emotional or physical stress, hyperalimentation, and some renal or endocrine diseases.

An 8-hour fasting blood glucose level of 126 mg/dl or more, a random blood glucose value of 200 mg/dl or more accompanied by classic signs of diabetes, or an oral glucose tolerance test (OGTT) finding of 200 mg/dl or more in the 2-hour sample is almost certain to indicate diabetes (American Diabetes Association, 2005; Hoffman, 2003). Postprandial blood glucose determinations and the traditional OGTTs have yielded low detection rates in children and are not usually necessary for establishing a diagnosis. Serum insulin levels may be normal or moderately elevated at the onset of diabetes; delayed insulin response to glucose indicates impaired glucose tolerance.

Ketoacidosis must be differentiated from other causes of acidosis or coma, including hypoglycemia, uremia, gastroenteritis with metabolic acidosis, salicylate intoxication encephalitis, and other intracranial lesions. DKA is a state of relative insulin insufficiency and may include the presence of hyperglycemia (blood glucose level ≥330 mg/dl), ketonemia (strongly positive), acidosis (pH <7.30 and bicarbonate <15 mmol/L), glycosuria, and ketonuria (Magee and Bhatt, 2001). Tests used to determine glycosuria and ketonuria are the glucose oxidase tapes (Keto-Diastix).

Therapeutic Management

The management of the child with type 1 DM consists of a multidisciplinary approach involving the family; the child (when appropriate); and professionals, including a pediatric endocrinologist, diabetes nurse educator, nutritionist, and exercise physiologist. Often psychologic support from a mental health professional is also needed. Communication among the team members is essential and extends to other individuals in the child's life, such as teachers, school nurse, school guidance counselor, and coach.

The definitive treatment is replacement of insulin that the child is unable to produce. However, insulin needs are also affected by emotions, nutritional intake, activity, and other life events such as illnesses and puberty. The complexity of the disease and its management requires that the child and family incorporate diabetes needs into their lifestyle. Medical and nutritional guidance are primary, but management also includes continuing diabetes education, family guidance, and emotional support.

Insulin Therapy. Insulin replacement is the cornerstone of management of type 1 DM. Insulin dosage is tailored to each child based on home blood glucose monitoring. The goal of insulin therapy is maintaining near-normal blood glucose values while avoiding too frequent episodes of hypoglycemia. The goals of treatment are to maintain near-normal glucose levels of less than 126 mg/dl, and glycosylated hemoglobin (hemoglobin A_{1c}) of 7% or less (Hannon, Gungor, and Arslanian, 2006). Glycemic control decreases the likelihood of long-term complications in patients with DM (Petitti, Imperatore, Palla, and others, 2007). Insulin is administered as two or more injections per day or as continuous subcutaneous infusion using a portable insulin pump.

Healthy pancreatic cells secrete insulin at a low but steady basal rate with superimposed bursts of increased secretion that coincide with intake of nutrients. Consequently insulin levels in the blood increase and decrease coincidentally with rises and falls in blood glucose levels. In addition, insulin is secreted directly into the portal circulation; therefore the liver, which is the major site of glucose disposal, receives the largest concentration of insulin. No matter which method of insulin replacement is used, this normal pattern cannot be duplicated. Subcutaneous injection results in absorption of the drug into the general circulation, thus reducing the concentrations of insulin to which the liver is exposed.

Insulin Preparations. Insulin is available in highly purified pork preparations and in human insulin biosynthesized by and extracted from bacterial or yeast cultures. Most clinicians suggest human insulin as the treatment of choice. Insulin is available in rapid-, intermediate-, and long-acting preparations, and all are packaged in the strength of 100 units/ml. Some insulins are available as premixed insulins, such as 70/30 and 50/50 ratios, the first number indicating the percentage of intermediate-acting and the second number the percentage of rapid-acting insulin. The different types of insulin are found in Box 29-14.

> **NURSINGALERT**
>
> The human insulins from various manufacturers may be interchangeable, but human insulin and pork insulin or pure pork insulin should never be substituted for one another.

Dosage. Conventional management has consisted of a **twice-daily insulin** regimen of a combination of **rapid-acting** and **intermediate-acting** insulin drawn up into the same syringe and injected before breakfast and before the evening meal. The amount of morning regular insulin is determined by patterns in the late morning and lunchtime blood glucose values. The morning intermediate-acting dosage is determined by patterns in the late afternoon and supper blood glucose values. Fasting blood glucose patterns at breakfast help determine the evening dose of intermediate insulin, and the blood glucose patterns at bedtime help determine the evening dose of rapid-acting (regular) insulin. For some children, better morning glucose control is achieved by a later (bedtime) injection of intermediate-acting insulin.

Regular insulin is best administered at least 30 minutes before meals. This allows sufficient time for absorption and results in a significantly greater reduction in the postprandial rise in blood glucose than if the meal were eaten immediately after the insulin injection. Intensive therapy consists of mul-

Check insulin pump

Types of Insulin

There are four types of insulin, based on the following criteria:
- How soon the insulin starts working (onset)
- When the insulin works the hardest (peak time)
- How long the insulin lasts in the body (duration).

However, each person responds to insulin in his or her own way. That is why onset, peak time, and duration are given as ranges.

Rapid-acting insulin (e.g., NovoLog) reaches the blood within 15 minutes after injection. The insulin peaks 30 to 90 minutes later and may last as long as 5 hours.

Short-acting (regular) insulin (e.g., Novolin R) usually reaches the blood within 30 minutes after injection. The insulin peaks 2 to 4 hours later and stays in the blood for about 4 to 8 hours.

Intermediate-acting insulins (e.g., Novolin N) reach the blood 2 to 6 hours after injection. The insulins peak 4 to 14 hours later and stay in the blood for about 14 to 20 hours.

Long-acting insulin (e.g., Lantus) takes 6 to 14 hours to start working. It has no peak or a very small peak 10 to 16 hours after injection. The insulin stays in the blood between 20 and 24 hours.

Some insulins come mixed together (e.g., Novolin 70/30). For example, you can buy regular insulin and NPH insulins already mixed in one bottle, which makes it easier to inject two kinds of insulin at the same time. However, you cannot adjust the amount of one insulin without also changing how much you get of the other insulin.

Adapted from American Diabetes Association: *Resource guide 2005*, retrieved April 10, 2008, from http://www.diabetes.org/rg2005/insulin.jsp.

tiple injections throughout the day with a once- or twice-daily dose of long-acting (Ultralente) insulin to simulate the basal insulin secretion and injections of rapid-acting insulin before each meal. A multiple daily injection program reduces microvascular complications of diabetes in young, healthy patients who have type 1 DM.

The precise dose of insulin needed cannot be predicted. Therefore the total dosage and percentage of regular- to intermediate-acting insulin should be determined empirically for each child. Usually 60% to 75% of the total daily dose is given before breakfast, and the remainder before the evening meal. Furthermore insulin requirements do not remain constant but change continuously during growth and development; the need varies according to the child's activity level and pubertal status. For example, less insulin is required during spring and summer months, when the child is more active. Illness also alters insulin requirements. Some children require more frequent insulin administration. This includes children with difficult-to-control diabetes and children during the adolescent growth spurt.

Methods of Administration. Daily insulin is administered subcutaneously by twice-daily injections, by multiple-dose injections, or by means of an insulin infusion pump. The **insulin pump** is an electromechanical device designed to deliver fixed amounts of regular or lispro insulin continuously (basal rate), thereby more closely imitating the release of the hormone by the islet cells (Olohan and Zappitelli, 2003). Although the pump delivers a programmed amount of basal insulin, the child or parent must program a dose for the pump to deliver before each meal.

The system consists of a syringe to hold the insulin, a plunger, and a computerized mechanism to drive the plunger.

The insulin flows from the syringe through a catheter to a needle inserted into subcutaneous tissue (the abdomen or thigh), and the lightweight device is worn on a belt or a shoulder holster. The needle and catheter are changed every 48 to 72 hours by the child or parent, using aseptic technique, and then taped in place.

Although the pump provides more consistent insulin delivery, it has certain disadvantages. Pump therapy is expensive and requires commitment from the parent and child. A certain level of math skills is required to calculate infusion rates. It should also not be removed for more than 1 hour at a time, which may limit some activities. Skin infections are common; and, as with any other mechanical device, it is subject to malfunction. However, the pumps are equipped with alarms that signal problems, such as a depleted battery, an occluded needle or tubing, or a microprocessor malfunction.

Monitoring. Daily monitoring of blood glucose levels is an essential aspect of appropriate DM management. Plasma blood glucose and hemoglobin A_{1c} goal ranges are found in Table 29-3.

Blood Glucose. Self-monitoring of blood glucose (SMBG) has improved diabetes management and is used successfully by children from the onset of their diabetes. By testing their own blood, children are able to change their insulin regimen to maintain their glucose level in the euglycemic (normal) range of 80 to 120 mg/dl. Diabetes management depends to a great extent on SMBG. In general, children tolerate the testing well.

Glycosylated Hemoglobin. The measurement of glycosylated hemoglobin (hemoglobin A_{1c}) levels is a satisfactory method for assessing control of the diabetes. As red blood cells circulate in the bloodstream, glucose molecules gradually attach to the hemoglobin A molecules and remain there for the lifetime of the red blood cell, approximately 120 days. The attachment is not reversible; therefore this glycosylated hemoglobin reflects the average blood glucose levels over the previous 2 to 3 months. The test is a satisfactory method for assessing control, detecting incorrect testing, monitoring effectiveness of changes in treatment, defining patients' goals, and detecting nonadherence. Nondiabetic hemoglobin A_{1c} values are generally between 4% and 6% but can vary by laboratory. Diabetes control for children depends on age, with hemoglobin A_{1c} levels of 6.5% to 8% indicating a slightly elevated but acceptable range (American Diabetes Association, 2005). Hemoglobin A_{1c} levels of less than 7% are a well-established goal at most care centers.

Urine. Urine testing for glucose is no longer used for diabetes management; there is poor correlation between simultaneous glycosuria and blood glucose concentrations. However, urine testing can be carried out to detect evidence of ketonuria.

NURSINGALERT

It is recommended that urine be tested for ketones every 3 hours during an illness or whenever the blood glucose level is over 240 mg/dl when illness is not present.

Nutrition. Essentially the nutritional needs of children with diabetes are no different from those of healthy children. Children with diabetes need no special foods or supplements. They need sufficient calories to balance daily expenditure for energy and to satisfy the requirement for growth and development. Unlike the child without diabetes, whose insulin is se-

TABLE 29-3

Plasma Blood Glucose and Hemoglobin A₁c Goals for Type 1 Diabetes Mellitus by Age-Group

AGE	VALUE* BEFORE MEALS (mg/dl)	VALUE* AT BEDTIME/ OVERNIGHT (mg/dl)	HEMOGLOBIN A₁c (%)	IMPLICATIONS
Toddlers and preschoolers (<6 years)	100-180	110-200	≤8.5% (but ≥7.5%)	High risk and vulnerability to hypoglycemia
School age (6-12 years)	90-180	100-180	<8%	Risks of hypoglycemia and relatively low risk of complications before puberty
Adolescents (>12 years) and young adults	90-130	90-150	<7.5%	Risk of hypoglycemia Developmental and psychologic issues

Modified from American Diabetes Association: Standards of medical care in diabetes, *Diabetes Care* 28(Suppl):S4-36, 2005.
*Plasma blood glucose goal range.

Adult A1C is less than 7!!

creted in response to food intake, insulin injected subcutaneously has a relatively predictable time of onset, peak effect, duration of action, and absorption rate depending on the type of insulin used. Consequently the timing of food consumption must be regulated to correspond to the timing and action of the insulin prescribed.

Meals and snacks must be eaten according to peak insulin action, and the total number of calories and proportions of basic nutrients must be consistent from day to day. The constant release of insulin into the circulation makes the child prone to hypoglycemia between the three daily meals unless a snack is provided between meals and at bedtime. The distribution of calories should be calculated to fit the activity pattern of each child. For example, a child who is more active in the afternoon will need a larger snack at that time. This larger snack might also be split to allow some food at school and some food after school. Food intake should be altered to balance food, insulin, and exercise. Extra food is needed for increased activity.

Concentrated sweets are discouraged, and because of the increased risk for atherosclerosis in persons with DM, fat is reduced to 30% or less of the total caloric requirement. Dietary fiber has become increasingly important in dietary planning because of its influence on digestion, absorption, and metabolism of many nutrients. It has been found to diminish the rise in blood glucose after meals.

Correctly used, the diet allows for flexibility and the incorporation of preferred foods in most instances. For the growing child, food restriction should never be used for diabetes control, although caloric restrictions may be imposed for weight control if the child is overweight. In general, the child's appetite should be the guide for the amount of calories needed, with the total caloric intake adjusted to appetite and activity.

Exercise. Exercise is encouraged and never restricted unless indicated by other health conditions. Exercise lowers blood glucose levels, depending on the intensity and duration of the activity. Consequently exercise should be included as part of diabetes management, and the type and amount of exercise should be planned around the child's interests and capabilities. However, in most instances children's activities are unplanned, and the resulting decrease in blood glucose can be compensated for by providing extra snacks before (and, if the exercise is prolonged, during) the activity. In addition to a feeling of well-being, regular exercise aids in utilization of food and often results in a reduction of insulin requirements.

Hypoglycemia. Occasional episodes of hypoglycemia are an integral part of insulin therapy, and an objective of diabetes management is to achieve the best possible glycemic control while minimizing the frequency and severity of hypoglycemia. Even with good control, a child may frequently experience mild symptoms of hypoglycemia. If the signs and symptoms are recognized early and promptly relieved by appropriate therapy, the child's activity should be interrupted for no more than a few minutes

NURSINGALERT

Hypoglycemic episodes most commonly occur before meals, or when the insulin effect is peaking.

The signs and symptoms of hypoglycemia are caused by both increased adrenergic activity and impaired brain function. The increased adrenergic nervous system activity plus increased secretion of catecholamines produces nervousness, pallor, tremulousness, palpitations, sweating, and hunger. Weakness, dizziness, headache, drowsiness, irritability, loss of coordination, seizures, and coma are more severe responses and reflect CNS glucose deprivation and the body's attempts to elevate the serum glucose levels.

It is often difficult to distinguish between hyperglycemia and a hypoglycemic reaction (Table 29-4). Because the symptoms are similar and usually begin with changes in behavior, the simplest way to differentiate between the two is to test the blood glucose level. The blood glucose level is low in hypoglycemia, whereas in hyperglycemia the glucose level is significantly elevated. Urinary ketones may be present after hypoglycemia as a result of starvation ketone production. In doubtful situations it is safer to give the child some simple carbohydrate. This will help alleviate the symptoms in the case of hypoglycemia but will do little harm if the child is hyperglycemic.

Children are usually able to detect the onset of hypoglycemia, but some are too young to implement treatment. Parents should become adept at recognizing the onset of symptoms—for example, a change in a child's behavior, such as tearfulness or euphoria. In the majority of cases, 10 to 15 g of simple carbohydrate, such as 1 tablespoon of table sugar, will elevate the blood glucose level and alleviate the symptoms. The simpler the carbohydrate, the more rapidly it will be absorbed (8 ounces of milk equals 15 g of carbohydrate). The rapid-releasing sugar is followed by a complex carbohydrate such as a slice of bread or a cracker and by a protein such as peanut butter or milk.

TABLE 29-4

Comparison of Manifestations of Hypoglycemia and Hyperglycemia

VARIABLE	HYPOGLYCEMIA	HYPERGLYCEMIA
Onset	Rapid (minutes)	Gradual (days)
Mood	Labile, irritable, nervous, weepy	Lethargic
Mental status	Difficulty concentrating, speaking, focusing, coordinating	Dulled sensorium
	Nightmares	Confusion
Inward feeling	Shaky feeling	Thirst
	Hunger	Weakness
	Headache	Nausea and vomiting
	Dizziness	Abdominal pain
Skin	Pallor	Flushed
	Sweating	Signs of dehydration
Mucous membranes	Normal	Dry, crusty
Respirations	Shallow, normal	Deep, rapid (Kussmaul)
Pulse	Tachycardia, palpitations	Less rapid, weak
Breath odor	Normal	Fruity, acetone
Neurologic	Tremors	Diminished reflexes
		Paresthesia
Ominous signs	Late—Hyperreflexia, dilated pupils, seizure	Acidosis, coma
	Shock, coma	
Blood:		
Glucose	Low: <60 mg/dl	High: ≥250 mg/dl
Ketones	Negative	High, large
Osmolarity	Normal	High
pH	Normal	Low (≤7.25)
Hematocrit	Normal	High
Bicarbonate	Normal	<20 mEq/L
Urine:		
Output	Normal	Polyuria (early) to oliguria (late)
Glucose	Negative	Enuresis, nocturia
Ketones	Negative or trace	High
Visual	Diplopia	Blurred vision

For a mild reaction, milk or fruit juice is a good food to use in children. Milk supplies them with lactose or milk sugar, as well as a more prolonged action from the protein and fat (aids in decreased absorption). Other glucose sources include Insta-Glucose (cherry-flavored glucose), carbonated drinks (not sugarless), sherbet, gelatin, or cake icing. All children with diabetes should carry with them glucose tabs, Insta-Glucose, sugar cubes, or sugar-containing candy such as LifeSavers or Charms. A difficulty with candies or icing is that the child may learn to fake a reaction to get the sweets; therefore commercial treatment products such as Insta-Glucose or glucose tabs may be preferred.

Glucagon is sometimes prescribed for home treatment of hypoglycemia. It is available as an emergency kit that must be mixed at the time of use and is administered intramuscularly or subcutaneously. Glucagon functions by releasing stored glycogen from the liver and requires about 15 to 20 minutes to elevate the blood glucose level.

NURSINGALERT

Vomiting may occur after administration of glucagon; therefore precautions against aspiration must be taken (e.g., placing the child on the side), since the child often becomes unconscious.

Once the child is responsive, the lost glycogen stores are replaced by small amounts of sugar-containing fluid administered frequently until the child feels comfortable trying solid foods.

Morning Hyperglycemia. The management of elevated morning blood glucose levels depends on whether the increase is a true dawn phenomenon, insulin waning, or a rebound hyperglycemia (the **Somogyi effect**). **Insulin waning** is a progressive rise in blood glucose levels from bedtime to morning. It is treated by increasing the nocturnal insulin dose. The true dawn phenomenon shows a relatively normal blood glucose level until about 3 AM, when the level begins to rise. The Somogyi effect may occur at any time but often entails an elevated blood glucose level at bedtime and a drop at 2 AM with a rebound rise following. The treatment for this phenomenon is decreasing the nocturnal insulin dose to prevent the 2 AM hypoglycemia. The rebound rise in the blood glucose level is a result of counter-regulatory hormones (epinephrine, GH, and corticosteroids), which are stimulated by hypoglycemia. More frequent blood monitoring (especially at times of anticipated peak insulin action) will usually identify these conditions. Trace amounts of urinary ketones aid in identifying undetected hypoglycemia.

Illness Management. Illness alters diabetes management, and maintaining control is usually related to the seriousness of the illness. In the well-controlled child an illness will run its course as it does in the unaffected child. The goals during an illness are to restore euglycemia, treat urinary ketones, and maintain hydration. Blood glucose levels and urinary ketones should be monitored every 3 hours. Some hyperglycemia and ketonuria are expected in most illnesses, even with diminished food intake, and are an indication for increased insulin. Insulin should never be omitted during an illness, although dosage requirements may increase, decrease, or remain unchanged, depending on the severity of the illness and the child's appetite. Often the child will need supplemental insulin between usual dose times. If the child vomits more than once, if blood glucose levels remain above 240 mg/dl, or if urinary ketones remain high, the health care practitioner should be notified. Simple carbohydrates may be substituted for carbohydrate-containing exchanges in the meal plan. Although insulin and diet are important tools in sick-day care, fluids are the most important intervention. Fluids must be encouraged to prevent dehydration and to flush out ketones.

Therapeutic Management of Diabetic Ketoacidosis

DKA, the most complete state of insulin deficiency, is a life-threatening situation. Management consists of rapid assessment, adequate insulin to reduce the elevated blood glucose level, fluids to overcome dehydration, and electrolyte replacement (especially potassium).

Because DKA constitutes an emergency situation, the child should be admitted to an intensive care facility for management. The priority is to obtain a venous access for administration of fluids, electrolytes, and insulin. The child should be weighed, measured, and placed on a cardiac monitor. Blood glucose and ketone levels are determined at the bedside, and samples are obtained for laboratory measurement of glucose, electrolytes, blood urea nitrogen, arterial pH, Po_2, Pco_2, hemoglobin, hematocrit, white blood cell count and differential, calcium, and phosphorus.

Oxygen may be administered to patients who are cyanotic and in whom arterial oxygen is less than 80%. Gastric suction is applied to unconscious children to avoid the possibility of pulmonary aspiration. Antibiotics may be administered to febrile children after appropriate specimens are obtained for culture. A Foley catheter may or may not be inserted for urine samples and measurement. Unless the child is unconscious, a collection bag is usually sufficient for accurate assessments.

Fluid and Electrolyte Therapy. All patients with DKA suffer from dehydration (10% of total body weight in severe ketoacidosis) because of the osmotic diuresis, accompanied by depletion of electrolytes, sodium, potassium, chloride, phosphate, and magnesium. Serum pH and bicarbonate reflect the degree of acidosis. Prompt and adequate fluid therapy restores tissue perfusion and suppresses the elevated levels of stress hormones.

The initial hydrating solution is 0.9% saline solution. Traditionally deficits have been replaced at a rate of 50% over the first 8 to 12 hours and the remaining 50% over the next 16 to 24 hours. Current trends suggest more cautious fluid management to reduce the risk of cerebral edema. The fluid deficit is replaced evenly over a period of 24 to 48 hours.

> **NURSINGALERT**
>
> Potassium must never be given until the serum potassium level is known to be normal or low, and urinary voiding is observed. All maintenance IV fluids should include 20 to 40 mEq/L of potassium. Never give potassium as a rapid IV bolus, or cardiac arrest may result.

Serum potassium levels may be normal on admission, but after fluid and insulin administration the rapid return of potassium to the cells can seriously deplete serum levels, with the attendant risk of cardiac arrhythmias. As soon as the child has established renal function (is voiding at least 25 ml/hr) and insulin has been given, vigorous potassium replacement is implemented. The cardiac monitor is used as a guide to therapy, and configuration of T waves should be observed every 30 to 60 minutes to determine changes that might indicate alterations in potassium concentration (widening of the QT interval and the appearance of a U wave following a flattened T wave indicate hypokalemia; an elevated and spreading T wave and shortening of the QT interval indicate hyperkalemia).

Insulin should not be given until urinary ketones and a blood glucose level have been obtained. Continuous IV regular insulin is given at a dosage of 0.1 units/kg/hr. Insulin therapy should be started after the initial rehydration bolus, since serum glucose levels fall rapidly after volume expansion. Blood glucose levels should decrease by 50 to 100 mg/dl/hr. When blood glucose levels fall to 250 to 300 mg/dl, dextrose is added to the IV solution. The goal is to maintain blood glucose levels between 120 and 240 mg/dl by adding 5% to 10% dextrose. Sodium bicarbonate is used conservatively; it is used for pH less than 7.0, severe hyperkalemia, or cardiac instability. Because sodium bicarbonate has been associated with increased risk for cerebral edema, children receiving this substance must be carefully monitored for changes in level of consciousness (Glaser, Barnett, McCaslin, and others, 2001).

When the critical period is over, the task of regulating insulin dosage in relation to diet and activity is started. Children should be actively involved in their own care and are given responsibility according to their ability and the guidance of the nurse.

> **NURSINGALERT**
>
> Because insulin can chemically bind to plastic tubing and in-line filters, thereby reducing the amount of medication reaching the systemic circulation, an insulin mixture is run through the tubing to saturate the insulin-binding sites before the infusion is started.

Nursing Care Management

Children with DM may be admitted to the hospital at the time of their initial diagnosis; during illness or surgery; or for episodes of ketoacidosis, which may be precipitated by any of a variety of factors (see the Evidence-Based Practice box evaluating hospitalization compared to outpatient care for newly diagnosed children with type 1 DM). Many children are able to keep the disease under control with periodic assessment and adjustment of insulin, diet, and activity as needed under the supervision of a practitioner. Under most circumstances these children can be managed well at home and require hospitalization only for a serious illness or upset.

However, a small number of children with diabetes exhibit a degree of metabolic lability and have repeated episodes of DKA that require hospitalization, which interferes with education and social development. These children appear to display a characteristic personality structure. They tend to be unusually passive and nonassertive and to come from families that are inclined to smooth over conflicts without resolution. Children in this type of setting experience emotional arousal with little, if any, opportunity or ability to resolve it. Other children from psychosocially dysfunctional families display behavioral and personality problems. This emotional stress

EVIDENCE-BASED PRACTICE

Hospital Admission or Outpatient Care for Children Newly Diagnosed with Type 1 Diabetes Mellitus

ASK THE QUESTION   Is hospitalization necessary for children newly diagnosed with type 1 diabetes mellitus (DM) who are not acutely ill?

SEARCH FOR EVIDENCE
Search Strategies   Searched the literature to obtain clinical research studies related to this issue. Selection criteria included English; publications within past 10 years; research-based articles; infant, child, and adolescent populations.
Databases Used   PubMed, CINAHL, Cochrane Collaboration, AHRQ

CRITICALLY ANALYZE THE EVIDENCE

In a Cochrane Review, six studies were found evaluating routine hospital admission compared with outpatient or home care for children newly diagnosed with type 1 DM (Clar, Waugh, and Thomas, 2003). The overall quality of the six studies was low, making results of the review inconclusive. Overall it appears that outpatient home management of type 1 DM in children at diagnosis does not lead to any disadvantages in terms of metabolic control, acute diabetic complications and hospitalizations, adjustment to the disease, or total financial costs (Spaulding and Spaulding, 1976; Galatzer, Schoshana, Gil, and others, 1982; Chase, Crews, Garg, and others, 1992; Simell, Putto-Laurila, Nanto-Salonen, and others, 1995; Dougherty, Schiffrin, White, and others, 1998). However, high quality randomized controlled trials are needed.

One randomized controlled trial found that home-based management of children newly diagnosed with type 1 DM may lead to slight improvement in long-term metabolic control (Dougherty, Schiffrin, White, and others, 1998). No differences were found in any psychosocial or behavioral parameters evaluated or the rate of complications within 2 years of the diagnosis.

APPLY THE EVIDENCE: NURSING IMPLICATIONS

The main tasks after diagnosis of type 1 DM in children are to achieve metabolic stabilization and prevent complications, to provide support to the child and family, and to educate them on how to manage the disease. No definitive conclusion can be made from the research found on this issue. However, the few studies that exist suggest that there are no adverse effects associated with outpatient home management of a child newly diagnosed with type 1 DM.

References

Chase PH, Crews KR, Garg S, and others: Outpatient management vs in-hospital management of children with new-onset diabetes, *Clin Pediatr* 31(8):450-456, 1992.

Clar C, Waugh N, Thomas S: Routine hospital admission versus out-patient or home care in children at diagnosis of type 1 diabetes mellitus, *Cochrane Database Syst Rev* (3): CD004099, 2003.

Dougherty G, Schiffrin A, White D, and others: Home-based management can achieve intensification cost-effectively in type 1 diabetes, *Pediatrics* 103(1):122-128, 1998.

Galatzer A, Schoshana A, Gil R, and others: Crisis intervention programme in newly diagnosed diabetic children, *Diabetes Care* 5(4):414-419, 1982.

Simell T, Putto-Laurila A, Nanto-Salonen K, and others: Randomized prospective trial of ambulatory treatment and one-week hospitalisation of children with newly diagnosed IDDM, *Diabetes* 44(Suppl 1):162A, 1995.

Spaulding R, Spaulding W: The diabetic daycare unit: comparison of patients and costs of initiating insulin therapy in the unit and a hospital, *Can Med Assoc J* 114:780-783, 1976.

causes an increased production of endogenous catecholamines, which stimulate fat breakdown, leading to ketonemia and ketonuria.

Hospital Management. The child with DKA requires intensive nursing care. Vital signs should be observed and recorded frequently. Hypotension caused by the contracted blood volume of the dehydrated state may cause decreased peripheral blood flow, which can be particularly hazardous to the heart, lungs, and kidneys. An elevated temperature may indicate infection and should be reported so that treatment can be implemented immediately.

Careful and accurate records should be maintained, including vital signs (pulse, respiration, temperature, blood pressure), weight, IV fluids, electrolytes, insulin, blood glucose level, and intake and output. A urine collection device or retention catheter is used to obtain the urine measurements, which include volume, specific gravity, and glucose and ketone values. The volume relative to the glucose content is important because 5% glucose in a 300-ml sample is a significantly greater amount than a similar reading from a 75-ml sample. A diabetic flow sheet maintained at the bedside provides an ongoing record of the vital signs, urine and blood tests, amount of insulin given, and intake and output. The level of consciousness is assessed and recorded at frequent intervals. The comatose child generally regains consciousness

fairly soon after initiation of therapy but is managed like any unconscious child until then.

When the critical period is over, the task of regulating insulin dosage to diet and activity is begun. The same meticulous records of intake and output, urine glucose and acetone levels, and insulin administration are maintained. Capable children should be actively involved in their own care and are given responsibility for keeping the intake and output record, testing the blood and urine, and, when appropriate, administering their own insulin—all under the supervision and guidance of the nurse (see Nursing Process box and Nursing Care Plan).

Child and Family Education. Several organizations are prepared to assist with education and dissemination of knowledge about diabetes. The American Diabetes Association,* Canadian Diabetes Association,† Juvenile Diabetes Research Foundation International,‡ and American Association of Diabetes Educators§ are valuable resources for a wide variety of

---

*1701 N. Beauregard St., Alexandria, VA 22311; (800) 342-2383; http://www.diabetes.org.

†1400-522 University Ave., Toronto, ON M5G 2R5; (800) 226-8464; http://www.diabetes.ca.

‡120 Wall St., New York, NY 10005; (800) 533-CURE; http://www.jdrf.org.

§200 W. Madison St., Suite 800, Chicago, IL 60606; (800) 338-3633; e-mail: education@aadenet.org; http://www.diabeteseducator.org.

nursingprocess | The Child with Diabetes Mellitus

ASSESSMENT

Assess for signs and symptoms of type 1 diabetes mellitus (DM) in children (see Box 29-13). Common symptoms include polyphagia, polyuria, polydipsia, weight loss, and fatigue.

DIAGNOSIS (PROBLEM IDENTIFICATION)

After a thorough assessment, several nursing diagnoses are evident (see Nursing Care Plan, p. 1052). Other nursing diagnoses include:

- Risk for Infection related to reduced body defenses
- Altered Nutrition: Less Than Body Requirements
- Altered Family Processes related to a child with a life-threatening illness
- Activity Intolerance related to fatigue
- Body Image Disturbance
- Individual Coping: Ineffective

PLANNING

Expected patient outcomes include:

- Child and family will be educated about the disease, assessment techniques, and therapy.

- Child will experience minimum complications of diabetes.
- Child will develop a positive self-image.
- Child and family will receive adequate support.

IMPLEMENTATION

Numerous intervention strategies are discussed on pp. 1049-1057.

EVALUATION

The effectiveness of nursing interventions for the family and child with type 1 DM is determined by continual assessment and evaluation of care based on the following guidelines:

- Interview family to determine their understanding of the disease; have child and family demonstrate and discuss the needed assessment and therapeutic techniques.
- Interview family regarding their understanding of control; analyze and evaluate management records.
- Discuss the child's disease with him or her.
- Interview family and child regarding their feelings and concerns about the disease.

---

educational materials. The National Institute of Diabetes and Digestive and Kidney Diseases* publishes a number of comprehensive annotated bibliographies, including "Educational Materials for and About Young People with Diabetes," a compilation of resource materials for children, siblings, parents, teachers, and health professionals, and "Sports and Exercise for People with Diabetes."

Medical Identification. One of the first things the nurse should call to the parents' attention is the need for the child to wear some means of medical identification. Usually recommended is the MedicAlert identification, a stainless steel or silver- or gold-plated identification bracelet that is visible and immediately recognizable. It contains a collect telephone number that medical personnel can call around the clock for medical records and personal information.

Nature of Diabetes. The better the parents understand the pathophysiology of diabetes and the function and action of insulin and glucagon in relation to caloric intake and exercise, the better they will understand the disease and its effects on the child. Parents need answers to a number of questions (voiced or unvoiced) to increase their confidence in coping with the disease. For example, they may want to know about the various procedures performed on their child and treatment rationale, such as what is being put in the IV bottle and the expected effect.

Meal Planning. Normal nutrition is a major aspect of the family education program. Diet instruction is usually conducted by the nutritionist, with reinforcement and guidance from the nurse. The emphasis is on adequate intake for age, consistent menus, complex carbohydrates, and consistent eating times. The family is taught how the meal plan relates to the requirements of growth and development, the disease process, and the insulin regimen. Meals and snacks are modified based

on the child's preferences and current menu, preserving cultural patterns and preferences as much as possible. Extensive exchange lists are available that include foods compatible with most lifestyles.

Learning about foods within specific food groups helps in making choices. Weights and measures of foods are used as eye-training devices for defining serving sizes and should be practiced for about 3 months, with gradual progression to estimation of food portions. Even when the child and family become competent in estimating portion sizes, reassessment should take place weekly or monthly and when there is any change of brands.

Family members should also be guided in reading labels for the nutritional value of foods and food content. They need to become familiar with the carbohydrate content of food groups. Substitution with foods of equal carbohydrate content is the skill needed for successful carbohydrate counting. Substitution might be necessary if a food is not available in sufficient quantity or for the teenager who wishes to eat fast food with peers. The use of a multiple daily injection program lends flexibility to the timing of meals.

Lists of popular fast-food items and items served at the major fast-food chains can be obtained from the restaurants to help guide food selections. It is important that the child know the nutritional value of these items (the major chains are remarkably uniform), but the child should be cautioned to avoid high-fat and high-sugar/high-carbohydrate items; for example, the child could choose a plain hamburger instead of a double cheeseburger.

Children should use sugar substitutes in moderation in items such as soft drinks. Artificial sweeteners have been shown to be safe, but if there is any question about amounts, the physician, dietitian, or nurse specialist can provide guidelines based on body weight. Sugar-free chewing gum and candies made with sorbitol may be used in moderation by children with DM. Although sorbitol is less cariogenic than other varieties of sugar substitutes, it is an alcohol sugar that

---

*Office of Communications and Public Liaison, NIDDK, NIH, Building 31, Room 9A06, 31 Center Drive, MSC 2560, Bethesda, MD 20892-2560; (301) 496-3583; http://www.niddk.nih.gov.

nursingcareplan	The Child with Diabetes Mellitus

Nursing Diagnosis	Expected Patient Outcomes	Nursing Interventions	Rationale
Risk for Injury related to insulin deficiency	Child will demonstrate normal blood glucose levels.	Obtain blood glucose level.	To determine most appropriate dosage of insulin
Child's/Family's Defining Characteristics *(Subjective and Objective Data)*	**The Following NOC Concepts Apply to These Outcomes**	Administer insulin as prescribed.	To maintain normal blood glucose level
Polyphagia	Blood Glucose Control	Understand the action of insulin: differences in composition, time of onset, and duration of action for the various preparations.	To ensure accurate insulin administration
Polydipsia	Nutritional Status: Nutrient Intake		
Polyuria			
Weight loss		Employ aseptic techniques when preparing and administering insulin.	To prevent infection
Enuresis or nocturia		Rotate sites.	To enhance absorption of insulin
Abnormal blood profile—glucose, insulin			
Irritability		**The Following NIC Concepts Apply to These Interventions**	
Shortened attention span			
Fatigue		Health Education	
Dry skin		Hyperglycemia Management	
Blurred vision		Hypoglycemia Management	
Headache		Nutritional Management	
Frequent infections		Medication Administration	
Hyperglycemia			
Flushed skin			

Nursing Diagnosis	Expected Patient Outcomes	Nursing Interventions	Rationale
Risk for Injury related to hypoglycemia	Child will exhibit no evidence of hypoglycemia.	Recognize signs of hypoglycemia early. Be alert at times when blood glucose levels are lowest (before meals and snacks; 2-4 AM; after bursts of physical activity without additional food; or with delayed, omitted, or incompletely consumed meal or snack).	To prevent hypoglycemia
Child's/Family's Defining Characteristics *(Subjective and Objective Data)*	**The Following NOC Concept Applies to These Outcomes**		
Shaky feeling	Blood Glucose Control		
Hunger		Test blood glucose.	To evaluate glucose level
Headache		Offer 10-15 g of readily absorbed carbohydrates, such as orange juice, hard candy, or milk.	To elevate blood glucose level and alleviate symptoms of hypoglycemia
Dizziness			
Difficulty concentrating, speaking, or focusing		Follow with complex carbohydrate and protein, such as bread or cracker spread with peanut butter or cheese.	To maintain blood glucose level
Tremors			
Tachycardia		Administer glucagons to unconscious or combative child; position child to minimize risk of aspiration because vomiting may occur.	To elevate blood glucose level
Shallow respirations			
Can lead to convulsion, shock, and coma			
		The Following NIC Concepts Apply to These Interventions	
		Health Education	
		Hypoglycemia Management	

Nursing Diagnosis	Expected Patient Outcomes	Nursing Interventions	Rationale
Knowledge Deficit (Diabetes Management) related to care of a child with newly diagnosed diabetes mellitus	Child and family will have attitude conducive to learning.	Select methods, vocabulary, and content appropriate to learner's level.	To maximize learning
		Allow time for family and child to begin to adjust to initial impact of the diagnosis.	To allow child and family to set pace
Child's/Family's Defining Characteristics *(Subjective and Objective Data)*		Select an environment conducive to learning.	To promote learning
Lack of understanding		Involve all senses and employ a variety of teaching strategies, especially participation.	To promote effective learning
Inability to prepare and administer insulin			
Inability to follow meal planning guidelines		Provide pamphlets or other supplementary materials.	To promote learning
Difficulty describing treatment plan			

nursingcareplan | The Child with Diabetes Mellitus—cont'd

Nursing Diagnosis	Expected Patient Outcomes	Nursing Interventions	Rationale
Knowledge Deficit (Diabetes Management) related to care of a child with newly diagnosed diabetes mellitus—cont'd	Child and family will demonstrate understanding of meal planning	Emphasize relationship between normal nutritional needs and the disease.	To encourage sense of normalcy
		Become familiar with family's culture and food preferences.	To include culture preferences in meal planning
		Teach or reinforce learners' understanding of the basic food groups and the prescribed meal plan.	To reinforce existing knowledge base
		Help child and family estimate portion sizes by volume.	To provide a more practical method than weighing food
		Suggest low-carbohydrate snack items.	To promote appropriate food choices
		Guide family in assessing labels of food products for carbohydrate content.	To reinforce that consistency in carbohydrate portions is essential
	Child and family will demonstrate knowledge of and ability to administer insulin.	Teach child and family the characteristics of the insulins prescribed.	To increase understanding that there are several insulin preparations
		Teach proper mixing of insulins.	To prevent contaminating the vials
		Teach injection procedure.	To promote appropriate administration
		Teach basic techniques using an orange or similar item.	To build confidence
		Use demonstration and return demonstration techniques on another adult before injecting child.	To minimize stress for the child
		Help families and child work out a set rotational pattern.	To ensure maximum absorption of insulin and prevent hypertrophy at injection site
		Teach proper care of insulin and equipment.	To prevent contamination and minimize complications
	Child and family will demonstrate ability to test blood glucose level.	Teach family and child, if old enough, blood glucose monitoring or use of equipment, interpretation of results, and care and maintenance of equipment.	To ensure that child and family learn how to adjust insulin based on blood glucose level
	Child and family will demonstrate knowledge of management of hyperglycemia and hypoglycemia.	Instruct learners in how to recognize signs of hyperglycemia and hypoglycemia.	To prevent delay of treatment
		Explain relationship of insulin needs to illness, activity, and intense emotion.	To ensure appropriate treatment
		Teach how to adjust food, activity, and insulin at times of illness and during other situations that alter blood glucose levels.	To ensure appropriate treatment
		Suggest carrying source of carbohydrate, such as sugar cubes or hard candy, in pocket.	To prevent delay in treatment
		Instruct parents and child in how to treat hypoglycemia with food, simple sugars, or glucagons.	To establish health practices that last a lifetime
	Child and family will demonstrate understanding of proper hygiene.	Emphasize importance of personal hygiene.	To promote child's general health
		Encourage regular dental care and yearly ophthalmologic examinations.	To minimize risk of infection
		Teach proper care of cuts and scratches; teach proper foot care.	To prevent infection

The Following NOC Concepts Apply to These Outcomes

Blood Glucose Control
Knowledge: Medication
Knowledge: Treatment Regimen

The Following NIC Concepts Apply to These Interventions

Health Education
Hyperglycemia Management
Hypoglycemia Management

is metabolized to fructose and then to glucose. Furthermore, large amounts can cause osmotic diarrhea. Most dietetic foods contain sorbitol. They are more expensive than regular foods. Also, while a product may be sugar free, it is not necessarily carbohydrate free.

Traveling. Traveling requires planning, especially when a trip involves crossing time zones. A number of tips are included in pamphlets available free of charge. Suggestions for traveling encompass what will be needed from the practitioner before leaving, what and how much to take along, needs in transit, what to consider at the destination, and planning for when the child returns home. Planning is needed no matter what type of travel is considered—automobile, plane, bus, or train.

Insulin. Families need to understand the treatment method and the insulin prescribed, including the effective duration, onset, and peak action. They also need to know the characteristics of the various types of insulins, the proper mixing and dilution of insulins, and how to substitute another type when their usual brand is not available (insulin is a nonprescription drug). Insulin need not be refrigerated but should be maintained at a temperature between 15° and 29.4° C (59° and 85° F). Freezing renders insulin inactive.

Insulin bottles that have been "opened" (i.e., the stopper has been punctured) should be stored at room temperature or refrigerated for up to 28 to 30 days. After 1 month these vials should be discarded. Unopened vials should be refrigerated and are good until the expiration date on the label. Diabetic supplies should not be left in a hot environment.

Injection Procedure. Learning to give insulin injections is a source of anxiety for both parents and children. It is helpful for the learner to know that this important aspect of care will become as routine as brushing the teeth. First, the basic injection technique is taught, using an orange or similar item and sterile normal saline for practice. To gain children's confidence, the nurse can demonstrate the technique by giving a skillful injection to the parent and then having the parent return the demonstration by giving the nurse an injection. With practice and confidence, the parents will soon be able to give the insulin injection to their children, and their children will trust them. Another effective strategy is to instruct the children and then have them teach the technique to the parents while the nurse observes. Both parents should participate, and as little time as possible should elapse between instruction and the actual injection, especially with parents and teenage learners.

Insulin can be injected into any area in which there is adipose (fat) tissue over muscle; the drug is injected at a 90-degree angle. Newly diagnosed children may have lost adipose tissue, and care should be exerted not to inject intramuscularly. The pinch technique is the most effective method for tenting the skin to allow easy entrance of the needle to subcutaneous tissues in children. The site selected will sometimes depend on whether children or parents administer the insulin. The arms, thighs, hips, and abdomen are usual injection sites for insulin. The children can reach the thighs, abdomen, and part of the hip and arm easily but may require help to inject other sites. For example, a parent can pinch a loose fold of skin of the arm while the child injects the insulin.

The parents and child are helped to work out a rotation pattern to various areas of the body to enhance absorption, since insulin absorption is slowed by fat pads that develop in

FIG. 29-2 ■ School-age children are able to administer their own insulin.

TABLE 29-5

Onset and Duration of Action Related to Injection Site

	SITE OF INJECTION			
	ABDOMEN	**ARM**	**LEG**	**BUTTOCK**
Rate	Very fast	Fast	Slow	Very slow
Duration	Very short	Short	Long	Very long

From Albisser AM, Sperlich M: Adjusting insulins, *Diabetes Educ* 18(3):211-218, 1992.

overused injection areas. The most efficient rotation plan involves giving about four to six injections in one area (each injection about 2.5 cm [1 inch] apart, or the diameter of the insulin vial from the previous injection) and then moving to another area.

It is important to remember that the absorption rate varies in different parts of the body (Table 29-5). The methodical use of one anatomic area and then movement to another (as described in the previous paragraph) minimizes variations in absorption rates. However, absorption is also altered by vigorous exercise, which enhances absorption from exercised muscles; therefore it is recommended that a site be chosen other than the exercising extremity (e.g., avoiding legs and arms when playing in a tennis tournament).

Injection sites for an entire month can be determined in advance on a simple chart. For example, the "paper doll" (body outline) can be constructed and insulin sites marked by the child. After injection, the child places the date on the appropriate site. To keep in practice, it is a good idea for the parent to give two or three injections a week in areas that are difficult for the child to reach. The same basic methodology is used when teaching children to give their own insulin injections (Fig. 29-2). They should practice first on an orange or a doll, building courage gradually. Other devices are available for insulin injection and may offer advantages to some children. Children who do not wish to give themselves injections can be taught to use a syringe-loaded injector (Inject-Ease). With the device, puncture is always automatic. Adolescents respond well to a self-contained and compact device resembling a fountain pen (NovoPen), which eliminates conventional vials and syringes. Preloaded pens may also cause less pain, since the needle is not blunted by piercing the rubber top of the insulin vial (Lteif and Schwenk, 1999).

Continuous Subcutaneous Insulin Infusion. Some children are considered candidates for use of a portable insulin pump, and even some young children with unsatisfactory metabolic control can benefit from its use. The child and the parents are taught to operate the device, including the mechanics of the pump, battery changes, and alarm systems. A number of devices are on the market that vary in the basal rates they are able to deliver and in the cost of the equipment. Families can investigate the various devices and select the model that best suits their needs. Product information is available from pump manufacturers and distributors.*

Parents and children learn (1) the technical aspects of the pump and self-monitoring of blood glucose; (2) prevention and treatment for hyperglycemia, sick-day management, and meal planning; (3) the effects of exercise, stress, and diet on blood glucose levels; and (4) decision-making strategies to evaluate blood glucose patterns and make adjustments in all aspects of the regimen.

Numerous blood glucose measurements (at least four times per day) are an essential part of infusion pump use. Intensive education and supervision are critical to obtaining maximum efficiency and control. This is particularly important if the family has been accustomed to a conventional insulin regimen. They must realize that simply wearing the pump will not normalize blood glucose. The pump is merely an insulin delivery device, and frequent, routine blood glucose determinations are necessary to adjust the insulin delivery rate.

The major problem with use of the insulin pump is inflammation from irritation or infection at the insertion site. The site should be cleaned thoroughly before the needle is inserted and then covered with a transparent dressing. The site is changed and rotated every 48 to 72 hours (this may vary) or at the first sign of inflammation. Nurses working where pumps are part of the therapeutic regimen should become familiar with the operation of the specific device being used and the protocol of disease management. Others should be aware of this management technique and be prepared to assist patients using the pump.

Monitoring. Nurses should also be prepared to teach and supervise blood glucose monitoring. SMBG is associated with few complications, and although it does not necessarily lead to improved metabolic control, it provides a more accurate assessment of blood glucose levels than can be obtained with the historical urine testing. Blood glucose monitoring has the added advantage that it can be performed anywhere (see Atraumatic Care box).

Blood for testing can be obtained by two different methods: manually or with a mechanical bloodletting device. A mechanical device is recommended for children, although the child and family should learn to use both methods in the event of mechanical failure. Several lancet devices are avail-

FIG. 29-3 ■ Child using finger-stick device to obtain blood sample.

ATRAUMATIC CARE

Minimizing Pain of Blood Glucose Monitoring

- To enhance blood flow to the finger, hold it under warm water for a few seconds before the puncture.
- When obtaining blood samples, use the ring finger or thumb (blood flows more easily to these areas), and puncture the finger just to the side of the finger pad (more blood vessels and fewer nerve endings).
- To prevent a deep puncture, press the platform of the lancet device lightly against the skin and avoid steadying the finger against a hard surface.
- Use lancet devices with adjustable-depth tips. Begin with the shallowest setting.
- Use glucose monitors that require small blood samples (e.g., Ascensia Elite) to avoid repeated punctures.

---

able, and each provides a means for obtaining a large drop of blood for testing (Fig. 29-3).

NURSING ALERT

Caution children not to allow anyone else to use their lancet because of the risk of contracting hepatitis B virus or human immunodeficiency virus infection.

The blood sample may be obtained from fingertips or alternate sites such as the forearm. Alternate site testing requires a meter that can test a small volume of blood. Not all meters are capable of this.

Signs of redness and soreness at the site of finger puncture should be examined by the practitioner. It may be evidence of poor technique, poor hygiene, or poor skin healing relative to poor control. Many types of blood-testing meters are available for home use. Newer technology has brought about improvements in meter size and ease of use. The family should be shown features of several meters, including advantages and disadvantages, and allowed to choose equipment that best meets their needs.

---

*Medtronic MiniMed, http://www.minimed.com; Disetronic, http://www.disetronic-usa.com; Animas, http://www.animascorp.com.

FIG. 29-4 ■ Child using blood glucose monitor and reagent strips to test blood for glucose.

The least expensive testing method uses a reagent strip to which blood is applied (Fig. 29-4). After blotting, the color change is compared against a color scale for an estimation of the blood glucose level. The strips can be cut in half (although not all professionals recommend this) to obtain two readings per strip. This method is not accepted practice but may be necessary for some families or situations.

Urine Testing. Testing for urinary ketones is recommended during times of illness or when blood glucose values are elevated. Information on a specific ketone-testing product should include correct procedure, storage, and product expiration. Families need a clear understanding of home management of ketones: fluids and additional insulin as directed by the health care team.

Signs of Hyperglycemia. Severe hyperglycemia is most often caused by illness, growth, emotional upset, or missed insulin doses. Emotional stress from school finals or examinations or physical response to immunizations are examples of causes of hyperglycemia. With careful glucose monitoring, any elevation can be managed by adjustment of insulin or food intake. Parents should understand how to adjust food, activity, and insulin at the time of illness or when the child is treated for an illness with a medication known to raise the blood glucose level (e.g., steroids). The hyperglycemia is managed by increasing insulin soon after the increased glucose level is noted. Health care professionals should be aware that adolescent girls often become hyperglycemic around the time of their menses and should be advised to increase insulin dosages if necessary.

Signs of Hypoglycemia. Hypoglycemia is caused by imbalances of food intake, insulin, and activity. Ideally hypoglycemia should be prevented, and parents need to be prepared to prevent, recognize, and treat the problem. They should be familiar with the signs of hypoglycemia and instructed in treatment, including care of the child with seizures. Early signs are adrenergic, including sweating and trembling, which help raise the blood glucose level, much like the reaction when an individual is startled or anxious. The second set of symptoms that follow an untreated adrenergic

reaction is neuroglycopenic (also called brain hypoglycemia). These symptoms typically include difficulty with balance, memory, attention, or concentration; dizziness or lightheadedness; and slurred speech. Severe and prolonged hypoglycemia leads to seizures, coma, and possible death (Cryer, 2000). Hypoglycemia can be managed effectively as outlined in the Emergency Treatment box.

It is advisable for parents to plan for anticipated excitement or exercise. In addition, gastroenteritis may decrease insulin needs slightly as a result of poor appetite, vomiting, or diarrhea. If the blood glucose level is low but urinary ketones are present, the family should be aware of the increased need for simple carbohydrates and liquids.

Hygiene. All aspects of personal hygiene should be emphasized for the child with diabetes. The child should be cautioned against wearing shoes without socks, wearing sandals, or walking barefoot. Correct nail and extremity care tailored to the individual child (with the guidance of a podiatrist) can begin health practices that last a lifetime. Eyes should be checked once a year unless the child wears glasses, and then as directed by the ophthalmologist. Regular dental care is emphasized, and cuts and scratches should be treated with plain soap and water unless otherwise indicated. Diaper rash in infants and candidal infections in teens may indicate poor diabetes control.

Exercise. Exercise is an important component of the treatment plan. If the child is more active at one time of the day than at another time, food or insulin can be altered to meet that activity pattern. Food should be increased in the summer, when children tend to be more active. Decreased activity on return to school may require a decrease in food intake or increase in insulin dosage. The child who is active in team sports will need a snack about a half hour before the anticipated activity. Races or other competition may call for a slightly higher food intake than at practice times.

Food intake will usually need to be repeated for prolonged activity periods, often as frequently as every 45 minutes to 1 hour. Families should be informed that if increased food is not tolerated, decreased insulin is the next course of action. If the timing of the exercise is changed so that the supper meal is delayed, the insulin in the second or third dose of the day may be moved back to precede the mealtime. Sugar may sometimes be needed during exercise periods for quick response. Elevated blood glucose levels after extreme activity may represent the body's adrenergic response to exercise. If the blood glucose level is elevated ($\geq$240 mg/dl) before planned exercise, urinary ketones should be checked and the activity may need be postponed until the blood glucose is controlled.

> **NURSINGALERT**
>
> Ketonuria in the presence of hyperglycemia is an early sign of ketoacidosis and a contraindication to exercise.

Record Keeping. Home records are an invaluable aid to diabetes self-management. The nurse and family devise a method to chart insulin administered, blood glucose values, urine ketone results, and other factors and events that affect diabetes control. The child and family are encouraged to observe for patterns of blood glucose responses to events such as exercise. If lapses in management occur (such as eating a candy bar), the child should be encouraged to note this and not be criticized for the transgression.

Self-Management. Self-management is the key to close control. Being able to make changes when they are needed rather than waiting until the next contact with health care professionals is important for self-management and gives the individual and family the feeling they have control over the disease. Psychologically this helps family members feel they are useful and participating members of the team. Allowing the child to learn to look at records objectively promotes independence in self-management support. As children grow and assume more responsibility for self-management, they develop confidence in their ability to manage their disease and confidence in themselves as persons. They learn to respond to the disease and to make more accurate interpretations and changes in treatment when they become adults.

Puberty is associated with decreased sensitivity to insulin that normally would be compensated for by an increased insulin secretion. Health care professionals should anticipate that pubertal patients will have more difficulty maintaining glycemic control. Insulin doses commonly need to be increased, often dramatically (McConnell, Harper, Campbell, and others, 2001). Patients should be taught to give themselves additional doses of rapid-acting insulin (5% to 10% of their daily dose) when their blood glucose levels are increased. The use of supplemental rapid-acting insulin is preferred to withholding food in the adolescent.

Child or Adolescent and Family Support. Just as the physiologic responses affect the child, the parents and other family members of the child with newly diagnosed DM experience various emotional responses to the crisis. Care in the acute setting is short but may create fears and frustrations. The prospect of a chronic illness in their child engenders all the feelings and concerns that are faced by parents of children with other chronic illnesses (see Chapter 18). The threat of complications and death is always present, as well as the continuing drain on emotional and financial resources.

Certain fears may develop as a result of past experiences with the disease. A severe insulin reaction with seizures can contribute to fear of repetition. Once parents observe a seizure or the adolescent has one in a public place, the desire to maintain better control is reinforced. They must understand how to prevent problems and how to handle problems calmly and coolly if they occur, and they must understand the complexities of the body, the disease, and its complications. Young children usually adjust well to problems related to the disease. With toddlers and preschoolers, insulin injections and glucose testing may be difficult at first. However, they usually accept the procedures when the parents use a matter-of-fact approach, without calling attention to a "hurt," and treat the procedure like any other routine part of the child's life. After the injection, time with some special and positive attention, such as reading or talking, or another pleasant activity, is one way to convert children who initially refuse injections to those who accept them.

In the years before adolescence children probably accept their condition most easily. They are able to understand the basic concepts related to their disease and its treatment. They are able to test blood glucose and urine, recognize food groups, give injections, keep records, and distinguish fear or excitement from hypoglycemia. They understand how to recognize, prevent, and treat hypoglycemia. However, they still need considerable parental involvement.

> **NURSINGTIP**
>
> Ongoing motivation to adhere to a regimen is difficult. An older child and parent (or another caregiver) may enjoy negotiating a day off when the responsibility for testing and recording blood glucose is delegated from the child to the caregiver (or vice versa).

Adolescents appear to have the most difficulty adjusting. Adolescence is a time of stress in trying to be perfect and like one's peers, and no matter what others say, having diabetes is being different. Some adolescents are more upset about not being able to have a candy bar than about injections, diet, and other aspects of management. If children can accept the difference as a part of life—in other words, that each person is different in some way—then, with adequate parental support, they should be able to adjust well (see Critical Thinking Exercise).

Camping and other special group activities are useful. At diabetes camp, children learn that they are not alone. As a result, they become more independent and resourceful in other settings. Useful information about such camps and organizations can be obtained from the American Diabetes Association. A list of accredited camps specifically for children and teenagers with diabetes is also available from the American Camping Association.*

---

*5000 State Road 67 N., Martinsville, IN 46151; (765) 342-8456; http://www.acacamps.org.

??? CRITICAL THINKING EXERCISE

Type 1 Diabetes Mellitus

Rebecca, a 15-year-old with a 3-year history of type 1 diabetes mellitus (DM), has been admitted to the pediatric intensive care unit for treatment of diabetic ketoacidosis (DKA). This is her fifth hospital admission for DKA in the past year. Rebecca's parents are divorced, and she has four younger siblings, none of whom has diabetes. Rebecca's mother has maintained two jobs for the past 5 years and frequently leaves Rebecca in charge of the household. In anticipation of her discharge, you are planning a patient education program for Rebecca and her mother. What important issues regarding Rebecca's unstable diabetes management must you consider to plan the education program?

QUESTIONS

1. Evidence—Is there sufficient evidence to draw conclusions about Rebecca's recurrent episodes of DKA?
2. Assumptions—Describe an underlying assumption about each of the following:
   a. Type 1 DM in adolescence
   b. Type 1 DM and menses
   c. Emotional stress and elevated blood glucose levels
   d. Blood glucose monitoring for insulin management
3. What priorities for nursing care should be established for Rebecca?
4. Does the evidence support your nursing intervention?
5. What alternative perspectives might you have?

KEY POINTS

- The endocrine system has three components: the cell, which sends a chemical message via a hormone; target cells, which receive the message; and the environment through which the chemical is transported from the site of synthesis to the sites of cellular action.
- Pituitary dysfunction is manifested primarily by growth disturbance.
- The main physiologic action of TH is to regulate the basal metabolic rate and control the processes of growth and tissue differentiation.
- Disorders of thyroid function include hypothyroidism, autoimmune thyroiditis, goiter, and hyperthyroidism.
- Therapy for hyperthyroidism is directed at retarding the rate of hormone secretion and may include drug therapy, thyroidectomy, or radioiodine therapy.
- Classic forms of hypoparathyroidism in childhood are idiopathic (deficient production of PTH) and pseudohypoparathyroidism (increased PTH production with end-organ unresponsiveness to PTH).

- The adrenal cortex secretes three important groups of hormones: glucocorticoids, mineralocorticoids, and sex steroids.
- Disorders of adrenal function include acute adrenocortical insufficiency, chronic adrenocortical insufficiency, Cushing syndrome, and CAH.
- Five categories of Cushing syndrome are pituitary, adrenal, ectopic, iatrogenic, and food dependent.
- Management of CAH includes assignment of a sex according to genotype, administration of cortisone, and, possibly, reconstructive surgery.
- DM is categorized as type 1 diabetes and type 2 diabetes.
- The focus of type 1 DM is insulin replacement, diet, and exercise.
- Education of families includes explanation of diabetes, meal planning, administering insulin injections, monitoring general hygienic practices, promoting exercise, record keeping, and observing for complications.

??? answers to CRITICAL THINKING EXERCISE

TYPE 1 DIABETES MELLITUS

1. Yes. Rebecca has had five hospital admissions for DKA in the past year. Numerous factors must be involved with her unstable disease.
2. a. The normal tasks of adolescence can play a significant role in blood glucose instability.
   b. Adolescent girls with diabetes have frequent fluctuations of blood glucose levels immediately before, during, or after their menses.
   c. Rebecca's personal loss from the divorce, her mother's absence because of a heavy work schedule, and the added responsibilities of the household may cause significant stress, resulting in elevated blood glucose levels.
   d. Careful, frequent, consistent monitoring of blood glucose levels is essential for effective insulin management during adolescence.
3. The first priority would be to focus directly on the issues of hyperglycemia. Determination of Rebecca's practice of monitoring and managing her diabetes at home is essential. Areas of diabetes management that should be emphasized include careful dietary management, an appropriate exercise program, conscientious self-testing of blood glucose, appropriate administration of daily insulin, and adherence to sliding-scaling insulin therapy. Discussion of the emotional stressors she identifies at this time is appropriate.
4. Yes, Rebecca's history of DKA over the past year supports her inability to monitor and manage her diabetes.
5. It would be appropriate to make a referral for special support services for counseling and possible home care follow-up to assess her diabetes management skills at home.

REFERENCES

American Academy of Pediatrics, Section on Endocrinology and Committee on Genetics: Technical report: congenital adrenal hyperplasia, *Pediatrics* 106(6):1511-1518, 2000.

American Diabetes Association: Care of children and adolescents with type 1 diabetes, *Diabetes Care* 28:186-212, 2005.

American Diabetes Association: Report of the Expert Committee on the Diagnosis and Classification of Diabetes Mellitus, *Diabetes Care* 24(Suppl 1):S5-S20, 2001.

Bartalena L, Tanda ML, Piantanida E, and others: Oxidative stress and Graves' ophthalmopathy: in vitro studies and therapeutic implications, *Biofactors* 19(3-4):155-163, 2003.

Baxter JD, Ribeiro RCJ: Introduction to endocrinology. In Greenspan FS, Gardner DG, editors: *Basic and clinical endocrinology*, ed 6, New York, 2001, Lange Medical Books/McGraw-Hill.

Behrman RE, Kliegman RM, Jenson HB: *Nelson textbook of pediatrics*, ed 17, Philadelphia, 2004, Saunders.

Beisswenger P, Szwergold B, Yeo K: Glycated proteins in diabetes, *Clin Lab Med* 21(10):53-78, 2001.

Biro FM, Huang B, Crawford PB, and others: Pubertal correlates in black and white girls, *J Pediatr* 148(2):234-240, 2006.

Bryant J, Cave C, Milne R: Recombinant growth hormone for idiopathic short stature in children and adolescents, *Cochrane Database Syst Rev* (2): CD004440, DOI:10.1002/14651858.CD004440, 2003.

Cheetham T, Baylis PH: Diabetes insipidus in children: pathophysiology, diagnoses and management, *Paediatr Drugs* 4(12):785-796, 2002.

Cryer P: Glucose counterregulatory hormones: physiology, pathophysiology, and relevance to clinical hypoglycemia. In Le Roith D, Taylor S, Olefsky J, editors: *Diabetes mellitus: a fundamental and clinical text,* ed 5, Philadelphia, 2000, Lippincott Williams & Wilkins.

Dallas JS, Foley TP: Hyperthyroidism. In Lifshitz F, editor: *Pediatric endocrinology,* ed 4, New York, 2003, Marcel Dekker.

De Buyst J, Massa G, Christophe C, and others: Clinical, hormonal and imaging findings in 27 children with central diabetes insipidus, *Eur J Pediatr* 166(1):43-49, 2007.

Foley TP: Hypothyroidism. In Hoekelman RA, Adam HM, Nelson NM, and others, editors: *Primary pediatric care,* ed 4, St Louis, 2001, Mosby.

Glaser N, Barnett P, McCaslin I, and others: Risk factors for cerebral edema in children with diabetic ketoacidosis: the Pediatric Emergency Medicine Collaborative Research Committee of the American Academy of Pediatrics, *N Engl J Med* 344(4):264-269, 2001.

Greiner MV, Kerrigan JR: Puberty: timing is everything, *Pediatr Ann* 35(12):916-922, 2006.

Guyda HJ: Growth hormone testing and the short child, *Pediatr Res* 48(5):579-580, 2000.

Halac I, Zimmerman D: Evaluating short stature in children, *Pediatr Ann* 33(3):171-176, 2004.

Hall DMB: Growth monitoring, *Arch Dis Child* 82(1):10-15, 2000.

Hannon TS, Gungor N, Arslanian SA: Type 2 diabetes in children and adolescents: a review for the primary care provider, *Pediatr Ann* 35(12):880-887, 2006.

Herman-Giddens ME: Recent data on pubertal milestones in United States children: the secular trend toward earlier development, *Int J Androl* 29(1):241-246, 2006.

Hilczer M, Smyczynska J, Lewinski A: Limitations of clinical utility of growth hormone stimulating tests in diagnosing children with short stature, *Endocrinol Regul* 40(3):69-75, 2006.

Hochberg Z: *Practical algorithms in pediatric endocrinology,* Basel, Switzerland, 1999, Karger.

Hoffman RP: Juvenile diabetes: avoiding problems during therapy, *Clin Advisor* May 2003, pp 70-75.

Hoffman RP: Eating disorders in adolescents with type 1 diabetes: a closer look at a complicated condition, *Postgrad Med* 109(4):67-69, 73-74, 2001.

Jospe N: Hyperthyroidism. In Hoekelman RA, Adam HM, Nelson NM, and others, editors: *Primary pediatric care,* ed 4, St Louis, 2001, Mosby.

Karnik AA, Fields AV, Shannon RP: Diabetic cardiomyopathy, *Curr Hypertens Rep* 9(6):467-473, 2007.

Kempers MJ, Otten BJ: Idiopathic precocious puberty versus puberty in adopted children: auxological response to gonadotrophin-releasing hormone agonist treatment and final height, *Eur J Endocrinol* 147(5):609-616, 2002.

Lee PA: Central precocious puberty: an overview of diagnosis, treatment, and outcome, *Endocrinol Metab Clin North Am* 28(4):901-918, 1999.

Levine LS: Congenital adrenal hyperplasia, *Pediatr Rev* 21(5):159-170, 2000.

Lin M, Liu SJ, Lim IT: Disorders of water imbalance, *Emerg Med Clin North Am* 23(3):749-770, 2005.

Lteif AN, Schwenk WF: Accuracy of pen injectors versus insulin syringes in children with type 1 diabetes, *Diabetes Care* 22(10):137-140, 1999.

Ma C, Xie JW, Kuang AR, and others: Radioiodine treatment for pediatric Grave's disease (protocol), *Cochrane Database Syst Rev* (4):CD006294, DOI:10.1002/14651858, 2006.

Macchia PE: Recent advances in understanding the molecular basis of primary congenital hypothyroidism, *Mol Med Today* 6(1):36-42, 2000.

Magee MF, Bhatt BA: Management of decompensated diabetes: diabetic ketoacidosis and hyperglycemic hyperosmolar syndrome, *Crit Care Clin* 17(1):75-106, 2001.

Majzoub JA, Muglia LJ: Disorders of water homeostasis. In Lifshitz F, editor: *Pediatric endocrinology,* ed 4, New York, 2003, Marcel Dekker.

Mauras N, Walton P, Nicar M, and others: Growth hormone stimulation testing in both short and normal statured children: use of an immunofunctional assay, *Pediatr Res* 48(5):614-618, 2000.

McConnell EM, Harper R, Campbell M, and others: Achieving optimal diabetic control in adolescence: the continuing enigma, *Diabetes Metab Res Rev* 17(10):67-74, 2001.

Midyett LK, Moore WV, Jacobson JD: Are pubertal changes in girls before age 8 benign? *Pediatrics* 111(1):47-51, 2003.

Miller BS, Zimmerman D: Idiopathic short stature in children, *Pediatr Ann* 33(3):177-181, 2004.

Miranda ML, Oliveira-Filho AG, Lemos-Marini SH, and others: Labioscrotal island flap in feminizing genitoplasty, *J Pediatr Surg* 39(7):1030-1033, 2004.

Moshang T: Cushing's disease, 70 years later . . . and the beat goes on (editorial), *J Clin Endocrinol Metab* 88(1):31-33, 2003.

Muir A: Precocious puberty, *Pediatr Rev* 27(10):373-381, 2006.

Nebesio TD, Eugster EA: Current concepts in normal and abnormal puberty, *Curr Prob Pediatr Adolesc Health Care* 37(2):50-72, 2007.

Nieman LK, Ilias I: Evaluation and treatment of Cushing's syndrome, *Am J Med* 118(12):1340-1346, 2005.

New MI, Ghizzoni L: Update on congenital adrenal hyperplasia. In Lifshitz F, editor: *Pediatric endocrinology,* ed 4, New York, 2003, Marcel Dekker.

Olohan K, Zappitelli D: The insulin pump, *Am J Nurs* 103(4):48-56, 2003.

O'Sullivan E, O'Sullivan M: Precocious puberty: a parent's perspective, *Arch Dis Childhood* 86:320-321, 2002.

Pacak K, Eisenhofer G, Ahlman H, and others: Pheochromocytoma: recommendations for clinical practice from the First International Symposium, *Nat Clin Pract Endocrinol Metab* 3(2):92-102, 2007.

Perheentupa J: Hypoparathyroidism and mineral homeostasis. In Lifshitz F, editor: *Pediatric endocrinology,* ed 4, New York, 2003, Marcel Dekker.

Petitti BD, Imperatore G, Palla SL, and others: Serum lipids and glucose control: the SEARCH for Diabetes in Youth study, *Arch Pediatr Adolesc Med* 161(2):159-165, 2007.

Pizzo PA, Poplack DG: *Principles and theories of pediatric oncology,* Philadelphia, 2006, Lippincott Williams & Wilkins.

Radetti G, Gottardi E, Bona G, and others: The natural history of euthyroid Hashimoto's thyroiditis in children, *J Pediatr* 149(6):827-832, 2006.

Reiter EO, Price DA, Wilton P, and others: Effect of growth hormone (GH) treatment on the near-final height of 1258 patients with idiopathic GH deficiency: analysis of a large international database, *J Clin Endocrinol Metab* 91(6):2047-2054, 2006.

Rivkees SA, Cornelius EA: Influence of iodine-131 dose on the outcome of hyperthyroidism in children, *Pediatrics* 111(4):745-748, 2003.

Root AW: Precocious puberty, *Pediatr Rev* 21(1):10-19, 2000.

Rovet JF, Ehrlich R: Psychoeducational outcome in children with early-treated congenital hypothyroidism, *Pediatrics* 105(3):515-522, 2000.

Schultz CJ, Konopelska-Bahu T, Dalton RN, and others: Microalbuminuria prevalence varies with age, sex, and puberty in children with type 1 diabetes followed from diagnosis in a longitudinal study, *Diabetes Care* 22(3):495-502, 1999.

Simmonds MJ, Howson JM, Heward JM, and others: Regression mapping of association between the human leukocyte antigen region and Graves disease, *Am J Human Genet* 76(1):157-163, 2005.

Slyper AH: The pubertal timing controversy in the USA, and a review of possible causative factors for the advance in timing of onset of puberty, *Clin Endocrinol (Oxf)* 65(1):1-8, 2006.

Streetman DD, Khanderia U: Diagnosis and treatment of Graves disease, *Am J Nurse Pract* 8(1):27-36, 2004.

Szymborska M, Staroszczyk B: Thyroiditis in children, *Med Wieku Rozwoj* IV(4):383-391, 2000.

Thompson GB: Surgical management in Graves' disease, *Panminerva Med* 44(4):287-293, 2002.

Trivin C, Couto-Silva AC, Sainte-Rose Z, and others: Presentation and evolution of organic central precocious puberty according to the type of CNS lesion, *Clin Endocrinol (Oxford)* 65(2):239-245, 2006.

Urrutia-Rojas X, Menchaca J: Prevalence of risk for type 2 diabetes in school children, *J Sch Health* 76(5):189-194, 2006.

Van Tijn DA, Schroor EJ, Delemarre-van de Waal HA, and others: Early assessment of hypothalamic-pituitary-gonadal function in patients with congenital hypothyroidism of central origin, *J Clin Endocrinol Metab* 92(1):104-109, 2007.

Verbalis JG: Diabetes insipidus, *Rev Endocr Metab Disord* 4(2):177-185, 2003.

Walvoord EC, Pescovitz OH: Combined use of growth hormone and gonadotropin-releasing hormone analogues in precocious puberty: theoretic and practical considerations, *Pediatrics* 104(4 Pt 2):1010-1014, 1999.

Wong LL, Verbalis JG: Systemic diseases associated with disorders of water homeostasis, *Endocrinol Metab Clin North Am* 31(1):121-140, 2002.

30

The Child with Integumentary Dysfunction

SHANNON STONE McCORD, ROSE U. BAKER, AND MARY A. MONDOZZI

CHAPTER OUTLINE

INTEGUMENTARY DYSFUNCTION, 1061
Skin Lesions, 1061
  Skin of Younger Children, 1061
Wounds, 1062
  Epidermal Injuries, 1062
  Injury to Deeper Tissues, 1062
  Process of Wound Healing, 1062
  Factors That Influence Healing, 1065
General Therapeutic Management, 1065
  Dressings, 1067
  Topical Therapy, 1067
  Systemic Therapy, 1067
Nursing Care Management, 1067
  Wound Care, 1068
  Relief of Symptoms, 1068
  Topical Therapy, 1068
Home Care and Family Support, 1069

INFECTIONS OF THE SKIN, 1069
Bacterial Infections, 1069
Viral Infections, 1071
Dermatophytoses (Fungal Infections), 1071
Systemic Mycotic (Fungal) Infections, 1072
SKIN DISORDERS RELATED TO CHEMICAL OR PHYSICAL CONTACTS, 1074
Contact Dermatitis, 1074
Poison Ivy, Oak, and Sumac, 1075
Drug Reactions, 1076
Foreign Bodies, 1076
SKIN DISORDERS RELATED TO ANIMAL CONTACTS, 1076
Arthropod Bites and Stings, 1076
Scabies, 1079
Pediculosis Capitis, 1079

Rickettsial Diseases, 1082
Lyme Disease, 1082
Mammal Bites and Scratches, 1083
Pet and Wild Animal Bites, 1083
Human Bites, 1083
Cat Scratch Disease, 1083
MISCELLANEOUS SKIN DISORDERS, 1084
SKIN DISORDERS ASSOCIATED WITH SPECIFIC AGE-GROUPS, 1084
Diaper Dermatitis, 1084
Atopic Dermatitis (Eczema), 1086
Seborrheic Dermatitis, 1089
Acne, 1089
THERMAL INJURY, 1091
Burns, 1091
Sunburn, 1103
Cold Injury, 1103

LEARNING OBJECTIVES

On completion of this chapter the reader will be able to:
- Describe the distribution and configuration of various skin lesions.
- List the benefits of a moist environment for wound healing.
- Discuss the nursing care related to therapies for skin disorders.
- Contrast the manifestations of and therapies for bacterial, viral, and fungal infections of the skin.
- Compare the skin manifestations related to age in children.
- Outline a care plan to prevent and treat diaper dermatitis.
- Outline a care plan for a child with atopic dermatitis.
- Formulate a teaching plan for an adolescent with acne.
- Describe the methods for assessing a burn wound.
- Discuss the physical and emotional care of a child with a severe burn wound.

RELATED TOPICS and ADDITIONAL RESOURCES

 IN TEXT

Birthmarks, *Ch. 9*
Candidiasis, *Ch. 9*
Communicable Diseases, *Ch. 14*
Erythema Toxicum Neonatorum, *Ch. 9*
Immunizations, *Ch. 10*
Injury Prevention (Burns): Infant, *Ch. 10;*
   Toddler, *Ch. 12;* School-Age Child,
   Ch. 15; Adolescent, *Ch. 16*
Ostomies, *Ch. 22*
Pain Assessment; Pain Management, *Ch. 7*

Physical Examination: Skin, *Ch. 6;* Newborn,
   Ch. 8
Preparation for Diagnostic and Therapeutic
   Procedures, *Ch. 22*
Tanning, *Ch. 16*

 COMPANION CD

Animation—Burns in Children
Case Studies—Poison Ivy; Acne Vulgaris;
   Impetigo; Burns
NCLEX Review Questions

 evolve

evolve.elsevier.com/Wong/essentials/

Critical Thinking Case Study—Tinea Capitis
NCLEX Review Questions
Nursing Care Plan—The Child with Burns
WebLinks

**WONG'S CLINICAL MANUAL
OF PEDIATRIC NURSING, 7th Ed**

Nursing Care Plan—The Child with Burns,
   p. 489

INTEGUMENTARY DYSFUNCTION

SKIN LESIONS

Lesions of the skin result from a variety of etiologic factors. Skin lesions originate from (1) contact with injurious agents (infective organisms, toxic chemicals, and physical trauma), (2) hereditary factors, (3) external factors (e.g., allergens), or (4) systemic diseases (e.g., measles, lupus erythematosus, nutritional deficiency diseases). Responses to these agents or factors are highly individualized. An agent that is harmless to one individual may be damaging to another, and a single agent may produce varying degrees of response.

An important factor in the etiology of skin manifestations is the child's age. Infants are subject to "birthmark" malformations and atopic dermatitis (AD) that appear early in life; the school-age child is susceptible to ringworm of the scalp; and acne is a characteristic skin disorder of puberty. Contact dermatitis, such as poison ivy, is seen only when the noxious agent is found in the environment. Tension and anxiety may produce, modify, or prolong skin conditions.

Skin of Younger Children

The major skin layers arise from different embryologic origins. Early in the embryonic period, a single layer of epithelium forms from the ectoderm, while simultaneously the corium develops from the mesenchyme. In the infant and small child the epidermis is loosely bound to the dermis. This poor adherence causes the layers to separate easily during an inflammatory process to form blisters. This is especially true in preterm infants, who have a propensity to blister formation and separation of the skin with minor trauma such as the removal of adhesive tape. In contrast, the skin of the older child is thinner, and the cells of all the strata are more compressed.

Pathophysiology of Dermatitis

More than half of the dermatologic problems in children are forms of dermatitis. This implies a sequence of inflammatory changes in the skin that are grossly and microscopically similar but diverse in course and causation. Acute responses produce intercellular and intracellular edema, the formation of intradermal vesicles, and an initial infiltration of inflammatory cells into the epidermis. In the dermis there is edema, vascular dilation, and early perivascular cellular infiltration. The location and manner of these reactions produce the le-

sions characteristic of each disorder. The changes are usually reversible, and the skin ordinarily recovers without blemish unless complicating factors such as ulceration from the primary irritant, scratching, and infection are introduced or underlying vascular disease develops. In chronic conditions permanent effects are seen that vary according to the disorder, the general condition of the affected individual, and the available therapy.

Diagnostic Evaluation

Although the history and subjective symptoms of skin lesions are explored first, the obvious objective characteristics of the lesions are often noted simultaneously. Many skin lesions are easily diagnosed after careful inspection.

History and Subjective Symptoms. Many cutaneous lesions are associated with local symptoms. The most common local symptom is itching (**pruritus**), which varies in intensity. Pain or tenderness often accompanies some skin lesions. Other skin sensations such as burning, prickling, stinging, or crawling are also described. Alterations in local feeling include absence of sensation (**anesthesia**); excessive sensitiveness (**hyperesthesia**); diminished sensation (**hypesthesia** or **hypoesthesia**); or abnormal sensation, such as burning or prickling (**paresthesia**). These symptoms may remain localized or migrate; may be constant or intermittent; and may be aggravated by a specific activity, such as exposure to sunlight.

It is important to determine whether the child has an allergic condition such as asthma or hay fever or history of a previous skin disease. AD, often associated with allergies, frequently begins in infancy. Important questions for the parent include when the lesion or symptom first appeared; whether it occurred with ingestion of a food or other substance, including any medication; and whether the condition was related to activity such as contact with plants, insects, or chemicals.

Objective Findings. The distribution, size, morphology, and arrangement of skin lesions provide significant information. Extrinsic causes usually result from physical, chemical, or allergic irritants or from an infectious agent such as bacteria, fungi, viruses, or animal parasites. Skin manifestations are also produced by intrinsic causes such as an infection (measles or chickenpox), drug sensitization, or other allergic phenomena.

Types of Lesions. Skin lesions assume distinct characteristics that are related to the pathologic process. Nurses should become familiar with the common terms that are applied to skin lesions because these terms are used in the processes of record keeping and communication. These terms include:

Erythema—A reddened area caused by increased amounts of oxygenated blood in the dermal vasculature

Ecchymoses (bruises)—Localized red or purple discolorations caused by extravasation of blood into dermis and subcutaneous tissues

Petechiae—Pinpoint, tiny, and sharp circumscribed spots in the superficial layers of the epidermis

Primary lesions—Skin changes produced by a causative factor; common primary lesions in pediatric skin disorders are macules, papules, and vesicles (Fig. 30-1)

Secondary lesions—Changes that result from alteration in the primary lesions, such as those caused by rubbing, scratching, medication, or involution and healing (Fig. 30-2)

Distribution pattern—The pattern in which lesions are distributed over the body, whether local or generalized, and the specific areas associated with the lesions

Configuration and arrangement—The size, shape, and arrangement of a lesion or groups of lesions (e.g., discrete, clustered, diffuse, or confluent)

Laboratory Studies. If a skin problem is related to a systemic disease (e.g., collagen or immunodeficiency disease), laboratory studies are performed to identify these conditions. Diagnostic techniques include microscopic examination, cultures, skin scrapings or biopsy, cytodiagnosis, patch testing, Wood light examination, allergic skin testing, and other laboratory tests such as blood count and sedimentation rate.

WOUNDS

Wounds are structural or physiologic disruptions of the skin that activate normal or abnormal tissue repair responses. Wounds are classified as acute or chronic. **Acute wounds** are those that heal uneventfully within 2 to 3 weeks. **Chronic wounds** are those that do not heal in the expected time frame or are associated with complications. Cofactors that disrupt or delay wound healing include compromised perfusion, malnutrition, and infection. In children, most wounds are acute and can be prevented from becoming chronic wounds through appropriate nursing care. Wounds are also classified as surgical and nonsurgical and then further classified in the same manner as burns: superficial, partial thickness, or full thickness (complex wounds that include muscle or bone).

Epidermal Injuries

Abrasions are the most common epidermal wounds in children, usually in the form of a skinned knee or elbow. In most injuries the margins of the abraded area are superficial, involving only the outer layers of epidermis, although the central portion may extend into the dermis. Epithelial tissue is composed of labile cells, which are constantly destroyed and replaced throughout the life span. Therefore epidermal injuries usually result in rapid, uneventful healing and recovery.

Injury to Deeper Tissues

Tissues composed of **permanent cells** such as muscle and nerve cells are unable to regenerate. These tissues repair themselves by substituting fibrous connective tissue for the injured tissue. This fibrous tissue, or **scar,** serves as a patch to preserve or restore the continuity of the tissue. Wounds involving permanent cells include surgical incisions, lacerations, ulcers, evulsions, and full-thickness burns.

Process of Wound Healing

When the skin is injured, its normal protective barrier function is broken. In the healthy immunocompetent individual, acute traumatic abrasions, lacerations, and superficial skin and soft-tissue injuries heal spontaneously without complications. The process of tissue healing involves complex cellular interactions and biochemical reactions. The healing process is segregated into four phases that are characterized by the particular cells involved and the chemicals produced. The four stages of wound healing are hemostasis, inflammation, proliferation, and remodeling (Krasner, Rodeheaver, and Sibbald, 2001). Some authorities combine the first two phases.

In the **hemostasis** phase, platelets act to seal off the damaged blood vessels and to form a stable clot. Hemostasis occurs within minutes of the initial injury to the skin unless there is an underlying clotting disorder.

Inflammation, the second stage of wound healing, presents a clinical picture that involves erythema, swelling, and warmth, often associated with pain at the wound site. This stage usually lasts up to 4 days after injury. The inflammation phase involves white blood cells such as the neutrophils, monocytes, and macrophages. These cells mount an initial defense against microbial invasion and secrete proteolytic enzymes that destroy nonviable tissue and microorganisms in the wound area.

The **proliferative** phase, which includes **granulation** and **contracture,** is the third stage of healing. This phase lasts from 4 to 21 days in acute wounds, depending on the size of the wound. The phase involves the replacement of dermal tissues and subdermal tissues in deep wounds, as well as the contraction of the wound. The phase is characterized clinically by the presence of granulation tissue, the "beefy," pebbled red tissue in the wound base. Fibroblasts, or immature connective tissue cells, secrete collagen, which provides the foundation for dermal regeneration. Angiocytes regenerate the outer layers of capillaries, and endothelial cells produce the lining in a process called *angiogenesis*. The formation of granulation tissue, which provides the foundation for the wound, depends on angiogenesis. The keratinocytes are responsible for epithelialization. In the final stage of epithelialization, contracture occurs as the keratinocytes differentiate and form the protective outer layer, or stratum corneum, of the skin.

Remodeling, or **maturation,** is the final phase of the healing process. This phase occurs in the dermis as fibroblasts increase the tissue tensile strength and gradually replace type 3 collagen in the scar tissue with type 1 collagen, thicken the collagen fibers, and reorient the collagen fibers along the lines of tissue tension. Fibroblasts disappear as the wound becomes stronger. The wound edges are brought closer together, and a mature scar is formed. Children heal aggressively with abundant scar tissue, especially during growth spurts. The highly elastic quality of children's skin pulls on the wound, and the wound defends against this pull by forming scar tissue. Remodeling and maturation occur over several months and can take up to 2 years. Thus some wounds that appear to be completely healed can break down suddenly if attention is not paid to the initial causative factors.

The phases of wound healing are complex and may be interrupted by disease conditions, medications, and other sys-

Macule—flat; nonpalpable; circumscribed; less than 1 cm in diameter; brown, red, purple, white, or tan in color
Examples: Freckles; flat moles; rubella; rubeola

Plaque—elevated; flat topped; firm; rough; superficial papule greater than 1 cm in diameter; may be coalesced papules
Examples: Psoriasis; seborrheic and actinic keratoses

Patch—flat; nonpalpable; irregular in shape; macule that is greater than 1 cm in diameter
Examples: Vitiligo; port-wine marks

Wheal—elevated, irregularly shaped area of cutaneous edema; solid, transient, changing, variable diameter; pale pink with lighter center
Examples: Urticaria; insect bites

Papule—elevated; palpable; firm; circumscribed; less than 1 cm in diameter; brown, red, pink, tan, or bluish red in color
Examples: Warts; drug-related eruptions; pigmented nevi

Nodule—elevated; firm; circumscribed; palpable; deeper in dermis than papule; 1 to 2 cm in diameter
Examples: Erythema nodosum; lipomas

Vesicle—elevated; circumscribed; superficial; filled with serous fluid; less than 1 cm in diameter
Examples: Blister; varicella

Pustule—elevated; superficial; similar to vesicle but filled with purulent fluid
Examples: Impetigo; acne; variola

Bulla—vesicle greater than 1 cm in diameter
Examples: Blister; pemphigus vulgaris

Cyst—elevated; circumscribed; palpable; encapsulated; filled with liquid or semisolid material
Example: Sebaceous cyst

FIG. 30-1 ■ Primary skin lesions. (From Seidel HM, Ball JW, Dains JE, and others: *Mosby's guide to physical examination,* ed 6, St Louis, 2006, Mosby.)

Scale—heaped-up keratinized cells; flaky exfoliation; irregular; thick or thin; dry or oily; varied size; silver, white, or tan in color
Examples: Psoriasis; exfoliative dermatitis

Crust—dried serum, blood, or purulent exudate; slightly elevated; size varies; brown, red, black, tan, or straw in color
Examples: Scab on abrasion; eczema

Lichenification—rough, thickened epidermis; accentuated skin markings caused by rubbing or irritation; often involves flexor aspect of extremity
Example: Chronic dermatitis

Scar—thin to thick fibrous tissue replacing injured dermis; irregular; pink, red, or white in color; may be atrophic or hypertrophic
Example: Healed wound or surgical incision

Keloid—irregularly shaped, elevated, progressively enlarging scar; grows beyond boundaries of wound; caused by excessive collagen formation during healing
Example: Keloid from ear piercing or burn scar

Excoriation—loss of epidermis; linear or hollowed-out crusted area; dermis exposed
Examples: Abrasion; scratch

Fissure—linear crack or break from epidermis to dermis; small; deep; red
Examples: Athlete's foot; cheilosis

Erosion—loss of all or part of epidermis; depressed; moist; glistening; follows rupture of vesicle or bulla; larger than fissure
Examples: Varicella; variola following rupture

Ulcer—loss of epidermis and dermis; concave; varies in size; exudative; red or reddish blue
Examples: Decubiti; stasis ulcers

FIG. 30-2 ■ Secondary skin lesions. (From Seidel HM Ball JW, Dains JE, and others: *Mosby's guide to physical examination,* ed 6, St Louis, 2006, Mosby.)

TABLE 30-1

Factors That Delay Wound Healing

FACTOR	EFFECT ON HEALING
Dry wound environment	Allows epithelial cells to dry out and die; impairs migration of epithelial cells across wound surface
Nutritional deficiencies	
Vitamin A	Results in inadequate inflammatory response
Vitamin B$_1$	Results in decreased collagen formation
Vitamin C	Inhibits formation of collagen fibers and capillary development
Protein	Reduces supply of amino acids for tissue repair
Zinc	Impairs epithelialization
Immunocompromise	Results in inadequate or delayed inflammatory response
Impaired circulation	Inhibits inflammatory response and removal of debris from wound area
	Reduces supply of nutrients to wound area
Stress (pain, poor sleep)	Releases catecholamines that cause vasoconstriction
Antiseptics	
Hydrogen peroxide	Toxic to fibroblasts; can cause subcutaneous gas formation (mimics gas-forming infection)
Povidone-iodine	Toxic to white and red blood cells and fibroblasts
Chlorhexidine	Toxic to white blood cells
Medications	
Corticosteroids	Impair phagocytosis
	Inhibit fibroblast proliferation
	Depress formation of granulation tissue
	Inhibit wound contraction
Chemotherapy	Interrupts the cell cycle; damages DNA or prevents DNA repair
Antiinflammatory drugs	Decrease the inflammatory phase
Foreign bodies	Increase inflammatory response
	Inhibit wound closure
Infection	Increases inflammatory response
	Increases tissue destruction
Mechanical friction	Damages or destroys granulation tissue
Fluid accumulation	Accumulation in area inhibits tissues from approximating
Radiation	Inhibits fibroblastic activity and capillary formation
	May cause tissue necrosis
Diseases	
Diabetes mellitus	Inhibits collagen synthesis
	Impairs circulation and capillary growth
	Hyperglycemia impairs phagocytosis
Anemia	Reduces oxygen supply to tissues
Peripheral vascular disease	Reduces oxygen supply to wounds
Uremia	Decreases collagen and granulation tissue

DNA, Deoxyribonucleic acid.

temic and local factors that influence the healing process. When a wound does not follow the **"normal wound healing trajectory,"** it may become stuck in one of the stages and become a chronic wound. It is important that health care providers understand and address the factors that influence wound healing and prevent the development of chronic wounds.

Factors That Influence Healing

Wound care management has shifted from interventions aimed at maintaining a dry environment to those that promote a moist, crust-free environment that enhances the migration of epithelial cells across the wound and facilitates remodeling. An acute full-thickness wound kept in a moist environment usually reepithelializes in 12 to 15 days, whereas the same wound when kept open to the air heals in about 25 to 30 days.

Numerous factors can delay healing (Table 30-1). For example, traditional practices, such as the use of antiseptics (hydrogen peroxide and povidone-iodine [Betadine] solutions), which were once thought to prevent infection, are now known to have a cytotoxic effect on healthy cells and minimal effect on controlling infections. Povidone-iodine may also be absorbed through the skin in neonates and young children.

GENERAL THERAPEUTIC MANAGEMENT

Some skin disorders demand aggressive therapy, but by and large the major aim of treatment is to prevent further damage, eliminate the cause, prevent complications, and provide relief from discomfort while tissues undergo healing (McCord and Levy, 2006). Factors that contribute to the development of dermatitis and that prolong the course of the disease should be eliminated when possible. The most common causative agents of dermatitis in infants, children, and adolescents are environmental factors (soaps, bubble baths, shampoos, rough or tight clothing, wet diapers, blankets, and toys) and the natural elements (such as dirt, sand, heat, cold, moisture, and

TABLE 30-2

Common Wound Care Products

TYPE OF PRODUCT	INDICATIONS	FUNCTION	DRESSING CHANGE FREQUENCY	COMMENTS
Transparent film (e.g., Tegaderm)	Skin tears, IV and tube sites, partial-thickness wounds, primary and secondary dressings	Provides moist wound healing, impermeable to fluid and bacteria, promotes autolytic débridement, nonabsorptive	Daily, up to 7 days	Seals wound from contaminants
Hydrocolloid (e.g., DuoDERM)	Pressure ulcers, partial- and full-thickness wounds, skin tears, tape anchor	Occlusive, impermeable to bacteria and contaminants, promotes autolytic débridement, minimal absorption	Up to 7 days	Do not place over infected or heavily draining wounds
Alginates/hydrofibers—calcium, collagen, and silver (e.g., Aquacel, Fibracal)	Moderate to large drainage, partial- and full-thickness wounds, dehiscence, infection, bleeding	Absorptive	Daily, but depends on amount of drainage; silver impregnated, 3-7 days	Excellent for packing, tunneling, and undermining; trauma-free removal
Barrier dressings (e.g., Stomahesive wafer, Coloplast wafer)	Protect periwound, tube and tape anchor	Protect skin from drainage or adhesive stripping	Up to once weekly	Excellent around G tube sites; apply around wounds or on skin to attach tape
Barrier cream or ointment (e.g., Sensi-Care, Critic-Aid, Laniseptic)	Perineal and diaper areas	Protects skin from moisture	With each diaper change	Some impregnated with antifungals; choose those formulated to stick to moist lesions
Foam (e.g., Lyofoam, Mepilex, Allevyn, PolyMem)	Moderate to heavy drainage, partial- and full-thickness wounds	More absorptive than gauze	Depends on drainage; up to 7 days	Excellent around leaking tubes and tracheostomies, available with fenestration, comfortable, nonadherent, trauma-free removal
Silver (e.g., SilvaSorb dressing and gel, Arglaes powder)	Infected or colonized partial- and full-thickness wounds	Depends on dressing type; available in foam, hydrocolloid, hydrofiber, alginate, and powder	Depends on dressing type; usually 3-7 days	Consider in wounds recalcitrant to previous treatments; controls odor
Wound gels (e.g., Flaminal)	Dry, partial- and full-thickness wounds and burns	Adds moisture, promotes epithelialization, fills up dead space	Once or twice daily	Easy to use; base frequency on wound moisture
Hydrogel dressing (CarraGauze, CarraDres)	Burns, partial- and full-thickness wounds, painful wounds	Adds moisture, aids autolytic débridement, minimal to moderate absorption	Daily	Nonadherent, trauma- and pain-free removal
Becaplermin gel (Regranex)	Ulcers	Promotes granulation	Daily	Contraindicated in infected and necrotic wounds, refrigerate, expensive
Enzymatic débrider (Accuzyme)	Necrotic wounds in patients who are not surgical candidates	Selectively dissolves necrotic tissue	Once or twice daily	Cross-hatch eschar with a scalpel for enzyme penetration, cover with moist N/S gauze to activate, avoid use with silver or mercury
Gauze	All wound types	Minor absorption, mild débridement	3-4 times per day	Dries out, poor absorbency, can macerate periwound, increased labor costs and supplies secondary to dressing change frequency

From McCord SS, Moise L: Practical guide to pediatric wound care, *Semin Plast Surg* 20(3):192-199, 2006.
G tube, Gastrostomy tube; *IV,* intravenous; *N/S,* normal saline.

wind). Dermatitis may also result from home remedies and medications.

Dressings

No one dressing meets the needs of all wounds. The traditional **dry** gauze dressing should not be used on open wounds, since it allows the wound surface to dry, does little to prevent bacterial invasion, and adheres to the dried scab so that removal disturbs the newly regenerating epithelial cells. In most instances, traditional gauze dressings have been replaced by dressings that promote moist wound healing (Table 30-2). Moist wound healing increases the rate of collagen synthesis and reepithelialization and decreases pain and inflammation. It also creates an environment for autolytic débridement of necrotic tissue, which creates a clean wound bed and enhances granulation. However, a balance must be achieved between creating a moist wound bed and maintaining a dry periwound area that protects the skin and wound from maceration. The dressing type and frequency of dressing changes help to achieve this balance. The frequency of dressing changes is based on the presence of infection, the type of dressing, the location of the wound, and the amount of drainage. Dressings should always be changed when they are loose or soiled. They should be changed more frequently in areas where contamination is likely (e.g., the sacral area, the buttocks, the tracheal area) or when wound infection is suspected or present.

Topical Therapy

Several agents and methods are available for treatment. In selecting a therapeutic regimen, the practitioner considers (1) the choice of active ingredient, (2) the proper vehicle or base, (3) the cosmetic effect, (4) the cost, and (5) instructions for use. Several basic concepts must also be considered. Overtreatment is avoided. For example, when the dermatitis is acute, topical applications should be mild and bland to avoid further irritation. Broken or inflamed skin, especially in children, is more absorbent than intact skin, and chemicals that are nonirritating to intact skin may be quite irritating to inflamed skin.

Topical applications may be applied to treat the disorder, reduce itching, decrease external stimuli, or apply external heat or cold. The emollient action of soaks, baths, and lotions provides a soothing film over the skin surface that reduces external stimuli. Ordinarily, lukewarm, tepid, or cool applications offer the greatest relief.

> **NURSING ALERT**
>
> Application of heat tends to aggravate most conditions, and its use is usually reserved for reducing specific inflammatory processes, such as folliculitis and cellulitis.

Ointments in a petrolatum base provide protection from moisture. Therefore this type of ointment is indicated around gastrostomy tubes, in skinfolds, and in the diaper area. Creams are absorbed by the skin and are used for areas where a nongreasy "feel" is desired (e.g., face, hands).

Topical Corticosteroid Therapy. Glucocorticoids are the therapeutic agents used most frequently for skin disorders. Their local antiinflammatory effects are merely palliative, so the medication must be applied until the condition undergoes a remission or the causative agent is eliminated. Corticosteroids are applied directly to the affected area, are essentially nonsensitizing, and have only minor side effects. As with the

use of any steroids, their use in large amounts may mask signs of infection, and symptoms may be exacerbated after termination of the drug. Families are cautioned that the medication cannot be used for all skin disorders. The concentrations available without prescription are not adequate for stubborn skin conditions (e.g., psoriasis) and may further aggravate inflammation caused by fungus or bacteria. Most parents and children apply too much topical hydrocortisone; therefore they should be counseled that it is both effective and economical to apply only a thin film and to massage it into the skin. Parents and children should also be advised to use the application for no more than 5 to 7 days because these agents may cause depigmentation and other changes in the skin.

Other Topical Therapies. Other topical treatments include chemical cautery (especially useful for warts), cryosurgery, electrodesiccation (chiefly used for warts, granulomas, and nevi), ultraviolet (UV) therapy (primarily used in psoriasis and acne), laser therapy (especially for birthmarks), and acne therapies such as dermabrasion and chemical peels. New drugs called **topical immunomodulators** are effective in reducing the itching of AD (eczema) and preventing the recurrence of "flares."

Systemic Therapy

Systemic drugs may be used as an adjunct to topical therapy in some dermatologic disorders. The drugs most frequently used are corticosteroids, antibiotics, and antifungal agents. Corticosteroids are valuable because of their capacity to inhibit inflammatory and allergic reactions. Dosage is carefully adjusted and gradually tapered to the minimum dosage that is effective and tolerated. In infants and children, the dosage is larger than is usually calculated from body weight ratios. However, prolonged use may temporarily suppress growth.

Antibiotics are used in severe or widespread skin infections. However, because these drugs tend to produce hypersensitivity in some patients, they are used with caution. Antifungal agents are the only means for treating systemic fungal infections.

NURSING CARE MANAGEMENT

The child's subjective symptoms and the parent's history provide valuable information to help establish a diagnosis. Older children often describe the condition as painful, itching, or tingling or in other descriptive terms. However, much can be determined by also observing the younger child's behavior. Does the child scratch? Is the child restless or irritable? Does the child favor or avoid using a body part? A careful history provides important clues. Has the child had access to chemicals or been in the woods or around a woodpile? Has the child eaten a new food? Is the child taking medication? Has the child any known allergy? Do siblings or playmates have similar lesions? What soap or bubble bath is used for bathing?

It is important for nurses to not only describe but also assess skin lesions and wounds. The color, shape, and distribution of lesions and wounds are important. Individual lesions are described according to standard terminology. Sometimes two descriptors are used for a particular characteristic (e.g., maculopapular rash). To confirm or amplify the findings made by inspection, the nurse may gently palpate the skin to detect characteristics such as temperature, moisture, texture, elasticity, and edema. Wounds are assessed for depth of tissue damage, evidence of healing, and signs of infection.

The frequency of wound assessment depends on the severity and complexity of the wound. For example, simple or chronic wounds are assessed weekly; infected or complex wounds are assessed daily. Wounds are measured at least weekly (height, width, and depth). The wound bed is assessed for color, drainage, odor, necrosis, granulation tissue, fibrin slough, undermining and condition of the wound edges, and the color and condition of the surrounding skin.

Therapeutic programs are designed to include general measures such as rest, protection, and relief of discomfort and specific treatments such as medication and physical techniques. Only a few skin diseases are contagious; therefore it is usually not necessary to isolate the affected child, except from persons in danger of acquiring a secondary infection (e.g., a child receiving large doses of corticosteroids or other immunosuppressant drugs or a child with an immunologic deficiency disorder). However, if the skin manifestation is caused by a viral exanthema, such as measles or chickenpox, the child is prevented from exposing other susceptible children.

Wound Care

Parents can generally manage small skin lesions or wounds at home. The parents are instructed to wash their hands and then wash the wound gently with mild soap and water or normal saline. They are cautioned to avoid povidone-iodine, alcohol, and hydrogen peroxide because these products are toxic to wounds.

Open wounds are covered with a dressing, such as a commercial adhesive bandage, although larger wounds may benefit from the use of occlusive dressings (see Table 30-2). If occlusive dressings are applied, parents should learn how to apply and remove the dressings correctly. For example, hydrocolloid dressings adhere best if a wide margin is left around the wound and the dressing is pressed against intact skin until it adheres. If a dressing needs to be secured, a nonalcohol skin barrier can be applied to protect the skin, or the wound can be "picture framed" with hydrocolloid dressing and dressing tape can be secured to the hydrocolloid. This method of securing the dressing protects the skin when the tape is removed. Montgomery straps or stretch netting can also be used to secure dressings and to avoid the use of tape.

Dressings are removed carefully to protect intact skin and the epithelial surface of the wound. When removing transparent or hydrocolloid dressings, the nurse or parent should raise one edge of the dressing and pull *parallel* to the skin to loosen the adhesive. The longer the dressings are left on, the easier they are to remove. Less frequent dressing changes decrease wound contamination.

Lacerations present a special challenge. The injured child and family are usually distressed by the bleeding. In particular, scalp lacerations tend to bleed profusely. Parental guilt and shock usually accompany the injury. The initial nursing intervention is to apply pressure to the area and to attempt to calm the child before further examination. Unless there is bleeding from a severed artery, the wound is cleansed with a forced jet of sterile tepid water or saline (via syringe) and examined for extent; depth; and presence of foreign material such as dirt, glass, or fabric fragments.

The location of the wound facilitates assessment. Wounds over bony areas may contain bone chips, and clear fluid seeping from severe head wounds may indicate cerebrospinal fluid. A pressure dressing is applied for transfer to medical care. After the child is in a medical facility, he or she is prepared for suturing.

Puncture wounds that do not require a tetanus booster are soaked in warm water and soap for several minutes. Causing the wound to rebleed may be helpful. An adhesive bandage can be applied if desired. Puncture wounds of the head, chest, or abdomen or those that could still contain a portion of the puncturing object must be evaluated carefully.

Parents are cautioned against opening blisters or kissing a wound "to make it better." The wound can easily become contaminated from germs in the human mouth. If scabs form, they are allowed to slough off without assistance; picking or early removal may cause scarring and secondary infection. Parents are advised to seek medical help if there is evidence of infection.

Relief of Symptoms

Most therapeutic regimens for skin lesions are directed toward relief of pruritus, the most common subjective complaint. Cooling the affected area and increasing the skin pH with cool baths or compresses and alkaline applications (e.g., baking soda baths) are helpful in reducing the itching. Clothing and bed linen should be soft and lightweight to decrease the irritation from friction and stimulation.

During treatment, both the affected and unaffected skin is protected from damage and secondary infection. Preventing scratching is important. Older children can cooperate, although they may need to be reminded to stop scratching or rubbing. However, small or uncooperative children may require the use of devices such as mittens (especially during sleep) or special coverings. Keeping fingernails clean, short, and trimmed reduces the risk of secondary infection.

Antipruritic medications, such as diphenhydramine (Benadryl) or hydroxyzine (Atarax), may be prescribed for severe itching, especially if it disturbs the child's rest. Pain and discomfort are usually managed with nonpharmacologic measures and mild analgesia. Severe pain requires more potent medication. Occlusive dressings over wounds reduce pain. For suturing wounds a topical anesthetic or intradermal buffered lidocaine should be used (see Pain Management, Chapter 7).

Topical Therapy

The specific type of topical therapy and the mode of application depend on the nature and location of the lesion. It is especially important to wash the hands before and after application of any topical therapy. The skin is assessed before the application and reassessed after treatment. Any observed changes are noted and described.

Wet compresses or **dressings** cool the skin by evaporation, relieve itching and inflammation, and cleanse the area by loosening and removing crusts and debris. A variety of ingredients, such as plain water or Burow solution (available without a prescription), can be applied on Kerlix gauze; plain gauze; or (preferably) soft cotton cloths such as freshly laundered handkerchiefs or strips from diaper, sheeting, or pillowcase material.

Dressings immersed in the desired solution are wrung out slightly and applied to the affected area wet but not dripping. They are applied flat and smooth in such a way that motion is not totally restricted—fingers are wrapped separately, and arms and legs are wrapped so that elbows and knees can bend. Dressings are held in place by Kerlix or other cotton wrap, tubular stockinette, mittens, and socks (two pairs—one to hold the dressings in place, the other to protect from movement). When evaporation begins to dry them, the dressings are removed, rewet in the solution, and reapplied using aseptic technique. The solution is *not* poured or applied with a syringe directly over the dressings. As fluid evaporates, the solution becomes more concentrated, and this could damage sensitive lesions.

Fresh solution at room temperature is applied at 2-, 3-, or 4-hour intervals and allowed to remain on the lesion from 20 to 90 minutes. Wet dressings are seldom continued after about 48 hours. The child is protected against chilling during treatment, and no more than 20% of the body is covered with a dressing at one time to avoid the risk of hypothermia. After treatment, the skin is dried thoroughly by patting with a towel. Lotion or other medication (if prescribed) is applied at this time.

When children are uncooperative in the use of wet dressings, **soaks** are often used for removal of crusts and for their mild astringent action. The same solutions are used as for wet compresses. Gaining young children's cooperation for hand or foot soaks is difficult unless the procedure is accompanied by play. Older infants and toddlers delight in playing with brightly colored objects or poker chips scattered over the bottom of the receptacle, and preschoolers can be challenged to hold a floating item beneath the water's surface. However, these activities require supervision; infants and small children place items in their mouths, and children easily lose control with water play. Washing dishes, cars, dolls, or doll clothes will also occupy time during soaks.

Although older children can cooperate, they, too, need something to do during the procedure, such as listening to music or a story or watching television. Placing the solution and the extremity in a plastic sealable bag is an effective method to soak a hand or foot.

Baths are useful in the treatment of widespread dermatitis by evenly distributing the soothing antipruritic and antiinflammatory effects of the solution, usually oatmeal or mineral oil preparations. The solution is added to a tub of lukewarm water. The temperature of the bath is tepid, and the treatment usually lasts 15 to 30 minutes. Therapeutic baths are more interesting when toy boats or other items for water play accompany the procedure.

Topical applications are applied to skin lesions to ease discomfort, prevent further injury, and facilitate healing. A thin application of the ointment or cream may be covered with a plastic film and anchored with adhesive, covered with a commercial transparent dressing, or wrapped in Kerlix gauze and held in place by a stretchy net dressing. Topical preparations are applied systematically with the contour of the body surface (not simply up and down). Children love to be "painted," and lotion applications can be fun when an ordinary paintbrush is used. Regardless of the type of preparation used, parents need detailed information on how to apply it and how long the preparation should remain on the skin.

> **NURSINGALERT**
> Provide written instructions and demonstrate to parents the correct amount of topical medication to apply (e.g., size of a pea; thin film to cover). If more than one preparation is applied, mark the containers with numbers so the parents remember the correct order of application. Stress that more is not necessarily better with some medications, such as steroids.

HOME CARE AND FAMILY SUPPORT

Dermatologic conditions always involve the family, but few situations require hospitalization and most care is delivered at home. Because the family members must carry out the treatment plan, their cooperation is essential. Regimens that are simple to accomplish in the clinic, hospital, or primary care provider's office may be frustrating and baffling at home. The family may also need assistance in adapting equipment available for home therapy.

It is important that the child and family be given as detailed explanations as possible about both the expected and unexpected results of treatment, including any ill effects that might occur. If unexplained reactions develop, the family is directed to discontinue treatment and report the reactions to the appropriate person. The use of over-the-counter medicines is discouraged unless the preparations have been discussed with the health care provider and have received approval.

Because the skin is the most visible portion of the body, defects in its surface alter its appearance and cause distress for the child. Skin problems may also result in rejection by others. Parents of other children may fear that their children will "catch" the disorder. Occasionally the affected child's own family members reduce their interaction or physical contact with the child. This is seldom a problem with dermatitis of short duration, but chronic conditions can frequently create problems and affect the child's self-esteem.

INFECTIONS OF THE SKIN
BACTERIAL INFECTIONS

Normally, the skin harbors a variety of bacterial flora, including the major pathogenic varieties of staphylococci and streptococci. The degree of pathogenicity of the organism depends on its invasiveness and toxicity, the integrity of the skin, and the immune and cellular defenses of the host. Children with congenital or acquired immunodeficiency disorders (such as acquired immunodeficiency syndrome [AIDS]), those in a debilitated condition, those receiving immunosuppressant therapy, and those with a generalized malignancy such as leukemia or lymphoma are at risk for developing bacterial infections.

Because of the characteristic "walling-off" process of the inflammatory reaction (abscess formation), staphylococci are more difficult to treat, and the local infected area is associated

TABLE 30-3

Bacterial Infections

DISORDER AND ORGANISM	MANIFESTATIONS	MANAGEMENT	COMMENTS
Impetigo contagiosa (Fig. 30-3)—*Staphylococcus*	Begins as a reddish macule Becomes vesicular Ruptures easily, leaving superficial, moist erosion Tends to spread peripherally in sharply marginated irregular outlines Exudate dries to form heavy, honey-colored crusts Pruritus common *Systemic effects*—Minimal or asymptomatic	Careful removal of undermined skin, crusts, and debris by softening with 1:20 Burow solution compresses Topical application of bactericidal ointment Systemic administration of oral or parenteral antibiotics (penicillin) in severe or extensive lesions	Tends to heal without scarring unless secondary infection Autoinoculable and contagious Common in toddler, preschooler May be superimposed on eczema
Pyoderma—*Staphylococcus, Streptococcus*	Deeper extension of infection into dermis Tissue reaction more severe *Systemic effects*—Fever, lymphangitis	Soap and water cleansing Wet compresses Bathing with antibacterial soap as prescribed Do not share washcloths or towels Mupirocin to nares and lesions as prescribed Systemic antibiotics	Autoinoculable and contagious May heal with or without scarring
Folliculitis (pimple), furuncle (boil), carbuncle (multiple boils)—*Staphylococcus aureus*	Folliculitis—Infection of hair follicle Furuncle—Larger lesion with more redness and swelling at a single follicle Carbuncle—More extensive lesion with widespread inflammation and "pointing" at several follicular orifices *Systemic effects*—Malaise, if severe	Skin cleanliness Local warm, moist compresses Topical application of antibiotic agents Systemic antibiotics in severe cases Incision and drainage of severe lesions, followed by wound irrigations with antibiotics or suitable drain implantation	Autoinoculable and contagious Furuncle and carbuncle tend to heal with scar formation Never squeeze a lesion
Cellulitis—*Streptococcus, Staphylococcus, Haemophilus influenzae* (Fig. 30-4)	Inflammation of skin and subcutaneous tissues with intense redness, swelling, and firm infiltration Lymphangitis "streaking" frequently seen Involvement of regional lymph nodes common May progress to abscess formation *Systemic effects*—Fever, malaise	Oral or parenteral antibiotics Rest and immobilization of both affected area and child Hot, moist compresses to area	Hospitalization may be necessary for child with systemic symptoms Otitis media may be associated with facial cellulitis
Staphylococcal scalded skin syndrome—*S. aureus*	Macular erythema with "sandpaper" texture of involved skin Epidermis becoming wrinkled (in 2 days or less), and large bullae appearing	Systemic administration of antibiotics Gentle cleansing with saline, Burow solution, or 0.25% silver nitrate compresses	Infant subject to fluid loss, impaired body temperature regulation, and secondary infection, such as pneumonia, cellulitis, and septicemia Heals without scarring

with an increase in bacteria all over the skin surface that serves as a source of continuing infection. In previous years, methicillin-resistant *Staphylococcus aureus* (MRSA) infections were primarily seen in nursing homes and hospitals. In recent years, the number of MRSA community-acquired infections has risen (Kaplan, 2006). All these factors underline the importance of careful hand washing and cleanliness when caring for infected children and their lesions to prevent the spread of infection and as an essential prophylactic measure when caring for infants and small children. Common bacterial skin disorders are outlined in Table 30-3.

Nursing Care Management

The major nursing interventions related to bacterial skin infections are to prevent the spread of infection and to prevent complications. Impetigo contagiosa and MRSA infection can

easily spread by self-inoculation; therefore the child must be cautioned against touching the involved area. Hand washing is mandatory before and after contact with an affected child, and this practice is emphasized to all those who care for the child. Many children with AD are colonized with MRSA in the nares and under the fingernails. For many bacterial infections, and for MRSA infection in particular, the child should be provided with washcloths and towels separate from those of other family members. Pajamas, underwear, and other clothes should be changed daily and washed in hot water. Razors used for shaving should be discarded after each use and not shared. To prevent recurrence, some infectious disease specialists recommend bathing in a chlorine bath twice weekly with 1 tsp of chlorine per gallon of water.

Children and parents are often tempted to squeeze follicular lesions. They must be warned that squeezing will not has-

FIG. 30-3 ■ Impetigo contagiosa. (From Weston WL, Lane AT, Morelli JG: *Color textbook of pediatric dermatology,* ed 3, St Louis, 2002, Mosby.)

FIG. 30-4 ■ Cellulitis of cheek from puncture wound. (From Weston WL, Lane AT, Morelli JG: *Color textbook of pediatric dermatology,* ed 4, St Louis, 2007, Mosby.)

ten the resolution of the infection and that there is a risk of making the lesion worse or spreading the infection. No attempt should be made to puncture the surface of the pustule with a needle or sharp instrument. A child with a sty may waken with the eyelids of the affected eye sealed shut with exudate. The child or the parents are instructed to gently wipe the lid from the inner to the outer edge with warm water and a clean washcloth until the exudate is removed.

The child with limited cellulitis of an extremity is usually managed at home on a regimen of oral antibiotics and warm compresses. The parents are taught the procedures and instructed in administration of the medication. Children with more extensive cellulitis, especially around a joint with lymphadenitis or on the face, are usually admitted to the hospital for parenteral antibiotics with continued treatment at home. Nurses are responsible for teaching the family to administer the medication and apply compresses.

VIRAL INFECTIONS

Viruses are intracellular parasites that produce their effect by using the intracellular substances of the host cells. Composed of only a deoxyribonucleic acid (DNA) or ribonucleic acid

(RNA) core enclosed in an antigenic protein shell, viruses are unable to provide for their own metabolic needs or to reproduce themselves. After a virus penetrates a cell of the host organism, it sheds the outer shell and disappears within the cell, where the nucleic acid core stimulates the host cell to form more virus material from its intracellular substance. In a viral infection the epidermal cells react with inflammation and vesiculation (as in herpes simplex) or by proliferating to form growths (warts).

Many of the communicable viral diseases of childhood are associated with rashes, and each rash is characteristic. The type of lesion and the configuration of rubeola, rubella, and chickenpox are described in Table 14-1. Other common viral disorders of the skin are outlined in Table 30-4.

DERMATOPHYTOSES (FUNGAL INFECTIONS)

The dermatophytoses (ringworm) are infections caused by a group of closely related filamentous fungi that invade primarily the stratum corneum, hair, and nails. These are superficial infections that live on, not in, the skin. They are confined to the dead keratin layers and are unable to survive in the deeper layers. Because the keratin is desquamated constantly, the fungus must multiply at a rate that equals the rate of keratin production to maintain itself; otherwise the infection would be shed with the discarded skin cells. Common dermatophytoses are outlined in Table 30-5.

Dermatophytoses are designated by the Latin word *tinea,* with further designation related to the area of the body where they are found (e.g., tinea capitis [ringworm of the scalp]). Dermatophyte infections are most often transmitted from one person to another or from infected animals to humans. Diagnosis is made from microscopic examination of scrapings taken from the advancing periphery of the lesion, which almost always produces a scale.

Nursing Care Management

When teaching families how to care for ringworm, the nurse should emphasize good health and hygiene. Because of the infectious nature of the disease, affected children should not exchange grooming items, headgear, scarves, or other articles of apparel that have been in proximity to the infected area with other children. Affected children are provided with their own towels and directed to wear a protective cap at night to avoid transmitting the fungus to bedding, especially if they sleep with another person. Because the infection can be acquired by animal-to-human transmission, all household pets should be examined for the disorder. Other sources of infection are seats with headrests (theater seats), seats in public transportation vehicles, helmets, and gymnasium mats.

Both 2% ketoconazole and 1% selenium sulfide shampoos may reduce colony counts of dermatophytes. These shampoos can be used in combination with oral therapy to reduce the transmission of disease to others. The shampoo should be applied to the scalp for 5 to 10 minutes at least three times per week. The child may return to school once the therapy is initiated.

Alternately, if the child is treated with the drug griseofulvin, the therapy frequently continues for weeks or months, and because subjective symptoms subside, children or parents may be tempted to decrease or discontinue the drug. The nurse should emphasize to family members the importance of maintaining the prescribed dosage schedule and of taking the

TABLE 30-4

Viral Infections

INFECTION	MANIFESTATIONS	MANAGEMENT	COMMENTS
Verruca (warts) *Cause*—Human papillomavirus (various types)	Usually well-circumscribed, gray or brown, elevated, firm papules with a roughened, finely papillomatous texture Occur anywhere, but usually appear on exposed areas such as fingers, hands, face, and soles May be single or multiple Asymptomatic	Not uniformly successful Local destructive therapy, individualized according to location, type, and number—surgical removal, electrocautery, curettage, cryotherapy (liquid nitrogen), caustic solutions (lactic acid and salicylic acid in flexible collodion, retinoic acid, salicylic acid plasters), x-ray treatment, laser	Common in children Tend to disappear spontaneously Course unpredictable Most destructive techniques tend to leave scars Autoinoculable Repeated irritation will cause to enlarge Apply topical anesthetic EMLA
Verruca plantaris (plantar wart)	Located on plantar surface of feet and, because of pressure, are practically flat; may be surrounded by a collar of hyperkeratosis	Apply caustic solution to wart, wear foam insole with hole cut to relieve pressure on wart; soak 20 minutes after 2-3 days; repeat until wart comes out	Destructive techniques tend to leave scars, which may cause problems with walking Apply topical anesthetic EMLA
Herpes simplex virus Type I (cold sore, fever blister) Type II (genital)	Grouped, burning, and itching vesicles on inflammatory base, usually on or near mucocutaneous junctions (lips, nose, genitalia, buttocks) Vesicles dry, forming a crust, followed by exfoliation and spontaneous healing in 8-10 days May be accompanied by regional lymphadenopathy	Avoidance of secondary infection Burow solution compresses during weeping stages Topical therapy (penciclovir) to shorten duration of cold sores Oral antiviral (acyclovir) for initial infection or to reduce severity in recurrence Valacyclovir (Valtrex), an oral antiviral, used for episodic treatment of recurrent genital herpes; reduces pain, stops viral shedding, and has a more convenient administration schedule than acyclovir	Heal without scarring unless secondary infection Type I cold sores prevented by using sunscreens protecting against ultraviolet A (UVA) and ultraviolet B (UVB) light to prevent lip blisters Aggravated by corticosteroids Positive psychologic effect from treatment May be fatal in children with depressed immunity
Varicella-zoster virus (herpes zoster; shingles)	Caused by same virus that causes varicella (chickenpox) Virus has affinity for posterior root ganglia, posterior horn of spinal cord, and skin; crops of vesicles usually confined to dermatome following along course of affected nerve Usually preceded by neuralgic pain, hyperesthesias, or itching May be accompanied by constitutional symptoms	Symptomatic Analgesics for pain Mild sedation sometimes helpful Local moist compresses Drying lotions sometimes helpful Ophthalmic variety: use systemic corticotropin (adrenocorticotropic hormone [ACTH]) or corticosteroids Acyclovir Lidocaine (Lidoderm) topical anesthetic	Pain in children usually minimal Postherpetic pain does not occur in children Chickenpox may follow exposure; isolate affected child from other children in a hospital or school May occur in children with depressed immunity; can be fatal
Molluscum contagiosum *Cause*—Pox virus Small, benign tumors	Flesh-colored papules with a central caseous plug (umbilicated) Usually asymptomatic	Cases in well children resolve spontaneously in about 18 months Treatment reserved for troublesome cases Apply topical anesthetic EMLA and remove with curette Use tretinoin gel 0.01% or cantharidin (Cantharone) liquid* Curettage or cryotherapy	Common in school-age children Spread by skin-to-skin contact, including autoinoculation and fomite-to-skin contact

EMLA, Eutectic mix of lidocaine and prilocaine.
*Not available in the United States, but can be purchased in Canada.

medication with high-fat foods for best absorption. They are also instructed regarding possible drug side effects, such as headache, gastrointestinal upset, fatigue, insomnia, and photosensitivity. For children who take the drug over many months, periodic testing is required to monitor leukopenia and assess liver and renal function. Newer antifungal medications such as terbinafine, itraconazole, and fluconazole may be used when there are adverse reactions to griseofulvin. Currently, these drugs are being studied to determine their efficacy and safety in treating tinea capitis in children but are not approved by the U.S. Food and Drug Administration (FDA) for this indication at this time.

SYSTEMIC MYCOTIC (FUNGAL) INFECTIONS

Mycotic (systemic or deep fungal) infections have the capacity to invade the viscera, as well as the skin. The most common infections are the lung diseases, which are usually acquired by inhalation of fungal spores. These fungi produce a variable spectrum of disease, and some are common in certain geographic areas. They are not transmitted from person to person

TABLE 30-5

Dermatophytoses (Fungal Infections)

DISEASE/ORGANISM	MANIFESTATIONS	MANAGEMENT	COMMENTS
Tinea capitis—*Trichophyton tonsurans, Microsporum audouinii, Microsporum canis* (Fig. 30-5, *A*)	Lesions in scalp but may extend to hairline or neck Characteristic configuration of scaly, circumscribed patches or patchy, scaling areas of alopecia Generally asymptomatic, but severe, deep inflammatory reaction may occur that manifests as boggy, encrusted lesions (kerions) Pruritic Microscopic examination of scales is diagnostic	Oral griseofulvin Oral ketoconazole for difficult cases Selenium sulfide shampoos Topical antifungal agents (e.g., clotrimazole, haloprogin, miconazole)	Person-to-person transmission Animal-to-person transmission Rarely, permanent loss of hair *M. audouinii* transmitted from one human being to another directly or from personal items; *M. canis* usually contracted from household pets, especially cats Atopic individuals more susceptible
Tinea corporis—*Trichophyton rubrum, Trichophyton mentagrophytes, M. canis, Epidermophyton* (see Fig. 30-5, *B*)	Generally round or oval, erythematous scaling patch that spreads peripherally and clears centrally; may involve nails (tinea unguium) *Diagnosis*—Direct microscopic examination of scales Usually unilateral	Oral griseofulvin Local application of antifungal preparation such as tolnaftate, haloprogin, miconazole, clotrimazole; apply 1 inch beyond periphery of lesion; continual application 1-2 weeks after no sign of lesion	Usually of animal origin from infected pets Majority of infections in children caused by *M. canis* and *M. audouinii*
Tinea cruris ("jock itch")—*Epidermophyton floccosum, T. rubrum, T. mentagrophytes*	Skin response similar to tinea corporis Localized to medial proximal aspect of thigh and crural fold; may involve scrotum in males Pruritic *Diagnosis*—Same as for tinea corporis	Local application of tolnaftate liquid Wet compresses or sitz baths may be soothing	Rare in preadolescent children Health education regarding personal hygiene
Tinea pedis ("athlete's foot")—*T. rubrum, Trichophyton interdigitale, E. floccosum*	On intertriginous areas between toes or on plantar surface of feet Lesions vary: 　Maceration and fissuring between toes 　Patches with pinhead-sized vesicles on plantar surface Pruritic *Diagnosis*—Direct microscopic examination of scrapings	Oral griseofulvin Local applications of tolnaftate liquid and antifungal powder containing tolnaftate *Acute infections*—Compresses or soaks followed by application of glucocorticoid cream Elimination of conditions of heat and perspiration by clean, light socks and well-ventilated shoes; avoidance of occlusive shoes	Most frequent in adolescents and adults; rare in children, but occurrence increases with wearing of plastic shoes Transmission to other individuals rare despite general opinion to contrary Ointments not successful
Candidiasis (moniliasis)—*Candida albicans*	Grows in chronically moist areas Inflamed areas with white exudate, peeling, and easy bleeding Pruritic *Diagnosis*—Characteristic appearance	Amphotericin B, nystatin ointment, or other antifungal preparations to affected areas	Common form of diaper dermatitis (see Fig. 30-11) Oral form common in infants (see Chapter 9) Vaginal form in older females May be disseminated in immunosuppressed children

FIG. 30-5 ■ **A,** Tinea capitis. **B,** Tinea corporis. Both infections are caused by *Microsporum canis,* the "kitten" or "puppy" fungus. (From Habif TP: *Clinical dermatology: a color guide to diagnosis and therapy,* ed 4, St Louis, 2004, Mosby.)

TABLE 30-6

Systemic Mycoses

DISORDER/ORGANISM	SKIN MANIFESTATIONS	SYSTEMIC MANIFESTATIONS	MANAGEMENT	COMMENTS
North American blastomycosis— *Blastomyces dermatitidis*	Chronic granulomatous lesions and microabscesses in any part of body Initial lesion is a papule; undergoes ulceration and peripheral spread	Pulmonary symptoms, such as cough, chest pain, weakness, and weight loss May have skeletal involvement, with bone destruction and formation of cutaneous abscesses	Intravenous (IV) administration of amphotericin B	Usual portal of entry is lungs Source of infection unknown Noninfectious Pulmonary infections may be mild and self-limiting and require no treatment Progressive disease often fatal
Cryptococcosis— *Cryptococcus neoformans (Torula histolytica)*	Usually on face; acneiform, firm, nodular, painless eruption	*Central nervous system (CNS) manifestations*—Headache, dizziness, stiff neck, and signs of increased intracranial pressure Low-grade fever, mild cough, lung infiltration	IV amphotericin B; may be administered intrathecally for CNS involvement 5-Fluorocytosine for meningitis Excision and drainage of local lesions	Acquired by inhalation of dust but may enter through skin Prognosis serious Noninfectious Increased incidence in persons receiving corticosteroids with lymphoreticular malignancies, or type 2 diabetes
Histoplasmosis— *Histoplasma capsulatum*	Not distinctive or uniform, but most appear as punched-out or granulomatous ulcers	General systemic symptoms may include pallor, diarrhea, vomiting, irregular spiking temperature, hepatosplenomegaly, and pulmonary symptoms Any tissue of body may be involved with related symptoms	IV amphotericin B for severe cases Oral ketoconazole	Organism cultured from soil, especially where contaminated with fowl droppings Fungus enters through skin or mucous membranes of mouth and respiratory tract Endemic in Mississippi and Ohio River valleys Disseminated diseases most common in infants and children
Coccidioidomycosis (valley fever)— *Coccidioides immitis*	Erythema nodosum Erythema multiforme Erythematous maculopapular rash	Primary lung disease usually asymptomatic May be sign of acute febrile illness Disseminated disease is serious	IV amphotericin B IV miconazole (synthetic imidazole) Intraventricular miconazole plus oral ketoconazole for CNS involvement Surgical resection of persistent pulmonary cavities	Inhalation of aerospores from soil Endemic in southwestern United States Usually resolves spontaneously Increased incidence in dark-skinned races (Filipino, African-American, Mexican, Asian)

but appear to reside in the soil, from which their spores are airborne. The cutaneous lesions caused by deep fungal infections are granulomatous and appear as ulcers, plaques, nodules, fungating masses, and abscesses. The course of deep fungal diseases is chronic with slow progression that favors sensitization (Table 30-6).

SKIN DISORDERS RELATED TO CHEMICAL OR PHYSICAL CONTACTS

CONTACT DERMATITIS

Contact dermatitis is an inflammatory reaction of the skin to chemical substances, natural or synthetic, that evoke a hypersensitivity response or direct irritation. The initial reaction occurs in an exposed region, most commonly the face and neck, backs of the hands, forearms, male genitalia, and lower legs. Early in the reaction, there is usually a sharp delineation between inflamed and normal skin that ranges from a faint, transient erythema to massive bullae on an erythematous swollen base. Itching is a constant symptom.

The cause may be a primary irritant or a sensitizing agent. A **primary irritant** is one that irritates any skin. A **sensitizing agent** produces an irritation on those individuals who have met the irritant or something chemically related to it, have undergone an immunologic change, and have become sensitized. Prior exposure is not necessarily a factor in the reaction. A sensitizer irritates in relatively low concentrations only persons who are allergic to it.

In infants, contact dermatitis occurs on the convex surfaces of the diaper area (see Diaper Dermatitis, p. 1084). Other agents that produce contact dermatitis include plants (poison ivy, oak, or sumac), animal irritants (wool, feathers, and furs), metal (nickel found in jewelry and the snaps on sleepers and denim), vegetable irritants (oleoresins, oils, and turpentine), synthetic fabrics (e.g., shoe components), dyes, cosmetics, perfumes, and soaps (including bubble baths). The list is endless.

The major goal in treatment is to prevent further exposure of the skin to the offending substance. Provided there is no further irritation, the skin's normal recuperative powers will often produce healing without treatment. Otherwise, treatment of contact dermatitis is based on severity. Mild cases are treated with topical steroids. Mild to moderately severe cases may require a 2-week course of strong topical corticosteroids. Very severe cases require systemic corticosteroids (Kronemyer, 2003).

Nursing Care Management

Nurses frequently detect evidence of contact dermatitis during routine physical assessments. Skin manifestations in specific areas suggest limited contact, such as around the eyes (mascara), areas of the body covered by clothing but not protected by undergarments (wool), or areas of the body not covered by clothing (UV injury). Generalized involvement is more likely to be caused by bubble bath or soap. Often nurses can determine the offending agent and counsel families regarding management. However, if the lesions persist, are extensive, or show evidence of infection, medical evaluation is indicated.

POISON IVY, OAK, AND SUMAC

Contact with the dry or succulent portions of any of three poisonous plants (ivy, oak, and sumac) produces localized, streaked or spotty, oozing, and painful impetiginous lesions. The offending substance in these plants is an oil, **urushiol,** that is extremely potent. Sensitivity to urushiol is not inborn but is developed after one or two exposures and may change over a lifetime. All parts of the plants contain the oil, including dried leaves and stems (Fig. 30-6). Even smoke from burning brush piles can produce a reaction.

Animals do not seem to be affected by the oil; however, dogs or other animals that have run or played in the plants may carry the sap on their fur, and animals that eat the plants can transfer the oil in their saliva. Shoes, tools, and toys can transfer the oil. Golf balls that have been in the rough are another source of contact.

Urushiol takes effect as soon as it touches the skin. It penetrates through the epidermis and bonds with the dermal layer, where it initiates an immune response. The full-blown reaction is evident after about 2 days, with redness, swelling, and itching at the site of contact. Several days later, streaked or spotty blisters oozing serum from damaged cells produce the characteristic impetiginous lesions (Fig. 30-7). The lesions dry and heal spontaneously, and itching stops by 10 to 14 days.

Therapeutic Management

As soon as an exposure is realized, there is no time to waste. The earlier the skin is cleansed, the greater the chance of removing the urushiol before it attaches to the skin. The exposed skin can be cleansed with isopropyl alcohol followed by water. A shower with soap and warm water should follow. Clothes, tools, shoes and any other objects that had contact with the plants should be cleaned with alcohol and then water.

Treatment of the lesions includes calamine lotion, soothing Burow solution compresses, or Aveeno baths to relieve discomfort. Topical corticosteroid gel is effective for prevention or relief of inflammation, especially when applied before blisters form. Oral corticosteroids may be needed for severe reactions, and a sedative such as diphenhydramine may be ordered.

Nursing Care Management

When it is known that the child has made contact with the plant, the area is immediately flushed (preferably within 15 minutes) with *cold* running water to neutralize the urushiol

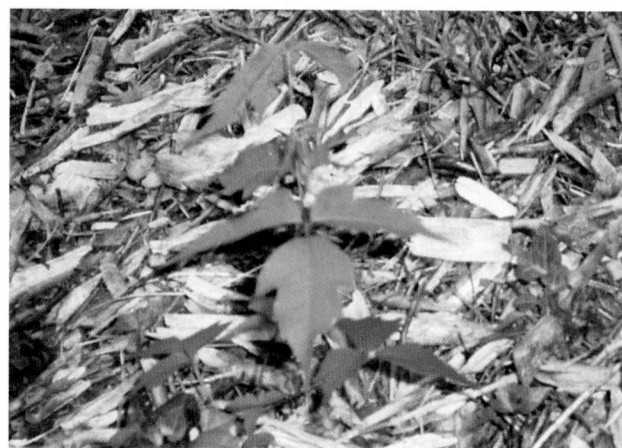

FIG. 30-6 ■ Poison ivy.

FIG. 30-7 ■ Poison ivy lesions. Note "streaked" blisters surrounding one large blister. (From Habif TP: *Clinical dermatology: a color guide to diagnosis and therapy,* ed 4, St Louis, 2004, Mosby.)

not yet bonded to the skin. If there is a stream nearby, an effective method is to have the child enter the water (clothes and all) and allow the water to rinse the oil from both skin and clothing. Harsh soap is contraindicated because it removes protective skin oils and dilutes the urushiol, allowing it to spread; hard scrubbing irritates the skin. All clothing that has come in contact with the plant is removed with care and thoroughly laundered in hot water and detergent. Every effort is made to prevent the child from scratching the lesions. Although the lesions do not spread by contact with the blister serum or from scratching, they can become secondarily infected (see Critical Thinking Exercise).

Prevention. Prevention is best accomplished by avoiding contact and removing the plant from the environment. All children, especially those known to be sensitive, should be taught to recognize the plant. Information regarding means for destroying plants can be obtained from the U.S. Department of Agriculture or U.S. Forestry Service. If poisonous plants are growing in public community area, the local authorities should be contacted to remove the plants. A cream that protects exposed skin from poison oak and ivy is Ivy Block.

??? CRITICAL THINKING EXERCISE

Poison Ivy

While at an overnight camp near a stream, Billy, age 9, runs up to the campfire and shows the nurse some leaves he has picked in the woods. The nurse recognizes the leaves as poison ivy. One of the adolescent assistants wants to throw the leaves on the campfire and scrub Billy's hands vigorously with soap. Billy's cabin mates ask the nurse: "Is poison ivy catching? Are we going to get it too?" What nursing actions should the camp nurse implement?

QUESTIONS

1. Evidence—Is there sufficient evidence to draw any conclusions at this time?
2. Assumptions—Describe some underlying assumptions about the following:
   a. The agent that causes poison ivy
   b. Effects of poison ivy on the skin
   c. Immediate treatment for poison ivy
   d. Contraindicated treatments for poison ivy
3. What implications and priorities for nursing care can be drawn at this time?
4. Does the evidence support this conclusion?
5. Are there alternative perspectives to your arguments?

DRUG REACTIONS

Adverse reactions to drugs are seen more often in the skin than in any other organ, although any organ of the body can be affected. The reaction may be a result of toxicity related to drug concentration, individual intolerance to the average dosage of the drug, or an allergic or idiosyncratic response. The manifestations may be associated with side effects or secondary effects of a drug, either of which are unrelated to its primary pharmacologic actions.

Although any drug is capable of producing a reaction in the susceptible individual, some drugs have a tendency to produce a particular reaction consistently, and others are more likely to produce an untoward effect. Many are allergenic responses that occur after a previous administration of the drug, even a topical application. Other factors influence a drug response in a particular individual. For example, the incidence increases with the amount and number of drugs given.

> **NURSING ALERT**
>
> Intravenous (IV) drugs are more likely to cause a reaction than oral drugs. Stop the drug, but maintain the infusion with normal saline.

Manifestations of drug reactions may be delayed or immediate. A period of 7 days is usually required for a child to develop sensitivity to a drug that has never been administered previously. With prior sensitivity the manifestations appear almost immediately. Rashes are the most common manifestation of adverse drug reactions in children. However, individual drug reactions may vary from a single lesion to extensive, generalized epidermal necrosis such as that seen in Stevens-Johnson syndrome (see Table 30-9). Cutaneous manifestations can resemble almost any skin disease and can be seen in almost any degree of severity. With few exceptions, the distribution of a drug eruption is widespread because it results from a circulating agent; appears as an inflammatory response with itching; is sudden in onset; and may be associated with constitutional symptoms such as fever, malaise, gastrointestinal upsets, anemia, or liver and kidney damage.

In most cases treatment for simple cutaneous reactions consists of discontinuing the drug. Sometimes a decision is made to continue the drug (such as an antibiotic in an infant or small child) until the cause of the rash is clearly indicated. In urticarial-type eruptions antihistamines may be ordered, and for widespread and severe lesions corticosteroids are beneficial. Severe anaphylactic reactions are a medical emergency (see Anaphylaxis, Chapter 25).

Nursing Care Management

The most effective means of management is prevention. Parents always remember a severe reaction. A careful history will elicit evidence of a previous drug reaction. The history should include the name of the drug, nature of the reaction, drug dosage, and how soon after administration the reaction occurred (see Chapter 6).

Nurses who suspect that a rash is caused by a medication should withhold any further dose and report the eruption to the practitioner. Frequent offenders in drug reactions are penicillin and sulfonamides, and nurses must be alert to this possibility. However, even commonplace drugs, including aspirin, barbiturates, chemical agents in some foods, flavoring agents, and preservatives, are capable of producing an undesired response. Persons who have severe reactions should wear a medical identification bracelet or necklace in case of emergency or inadvertent administration of the offending drug.

FOREIGN BODIES

Parents can remove small wooden splinters with a needle and tweezers that have been sterilized with alcohol or a flame. The area around the sliver is washed with soap and water before removal is attempted. The sliver is exposed with the needle, then grasped firmly by the tweezers and pulled out. Some foreign bodies, such as a fishhook, pieces of glass, a difficult-to-see object, or a deeply embedded object (such as a needle in a foot or near a joint), require medical evaluation.

Small cactus prickles or spines are troublesome to remove, but the following methods may prove helpful:

- Apply a thin layer of water-soluble household glue and cover with gauze; when the glue dries, peel off the gauze.
- Apply hair removal wax or body sugar, let dry, and remove.
- Place cellophane tape, sticky side down, over the spines and lift off.

SKIN DISORDERS RELATED TO ANIMAL CONTACTS

Arthropod Bites and Stings

Bites and stings account for a significant amount of mild to moderate discomfort in children. Most bites and stings are managed by simple symptomatic measures, such as compresses, calamine lotion, and prevention of secondary infection. **Arthropods** include insects and arachnids, such as mites, ticks, spiders, and scorpions. Most arthropods in the United States, including tarantulas, are relatively harmless. Although all spiders produce venom that is injected via fangs, some are unable to pierce the skin and others produce venom that is insufficiently toxic to be harmful. Only scorpions and two spiders—the brown recluse and the black widow—inject venom deadly enough to require immediate attention. Children bitten by these arachnids must receive medical attention as soon as possible. Major offending creatures, their manifestations, and management are outlined in Table 30-7.

When a hymenopteran (bees in particular) stings, its barbed stinger penetrates the skin. As long as the stinger remains in the skin, the muscles push the stinger deeper and the venom is pumped into the wound. The best approach is to remove the stinger as quickly as possible and to get away from the vicinity of other insects to prevent further injury. Children

TABLE 30-7

Skin Lesions Caused by Arthropods

MECHANISM AND CHARACTERISTIC	MANIFESTATIONS	MANAGEMENT
INSECT BITES—FLIES, GNATS, MOSQUITOES, FLEAS		
Mechanism—Foreign protein in insects' saliva introduced when skin is penetrated for a blood-sucking meal *Distribution:* Almost everywhere—Fleas, mosquitoes, ants Suburbs and rural areas—Bees Urban areas—Hornets, wasps, yellow jackets	Hypersensitivity reaction Papular urticaria Firm papules; may be capped by vesicles or excoriated Little or no reaction in nonsensitized person	*Treatment:* Use antipruritic agents and baths. Administer antihistamines. Prevent secondary infection. *Prevention:* Avoid contact. Remove focus, such as treating furniture, mattresses, carpets, and pets, where insects may live. Apply insect repellent when exposure is anticipated.
CHIGGERS—HARVEST MITES		
Mechanism—Attach with claws and secrete a digestive substance that liquefies the host's epidermis *Manifestations:* Erythematous papules Intense itching	Same as insect bites Favor warm areas of body, especially intertriginous areas and areas covered with clothing	Avoid contact, especially in areas of tall grass and underbrush. Apply insect repellant when exposure is anticipated. Administer systemic steroids for extensive bites.
HYMENOPTERANS—BEES, WASPS, HORNETS, YELLOW JACKETS, FIRE ANTS		
Mechanism: Injection of venom through stinging apparatus Venom contains histamine, allergenic proteins, and often a spreading factor, hyaluronidase Severe reactions caused by hypersensitivity or multiple stings	*Local reaction*—Small red area, wheal, itching, and heat *Systemic reactions*—May be mild to severe, including generalized edema, pain, nausea and vomiting, confusion, respiratory embarrassment, and shock	*Treatment:* Carefully scrape off stinger or pull out stinger as quickly as possible. Cleanse with soap and water. Apply cool compresses. Apply common household product (e.g., lemon juice, paste made with aspirin or baking soda). Administer antihistamines. *Severe reactions*—Administer epinephrine, corticosteroids; treat for shock. *Prevention:* Teach child to wear shoes; to avoid wearing bright clothing, flowery prints, shiny jewelry, or perfumed grooming products (cologne, scented hairspray), which might attract the insect; and to avoid places where the insect may be contacted. Hypersensitive children should wear medical identification to indicate allergy and therapy needed; family should keep emergency medication and be taught its administration.
BLACK WIDOW SPIDER		
Mechanism—Venom injected through a clawlike appendage; has neurotoxic action *Characteristics:* Shiny black spider, with a body about 1.25 cm (0.5 inch) long and a red or orange hourglass-shaped marking on underside Avoids light and bites in self-defense	Mild sting at time of bite Area becomes swollen, painful, and erythematous Dizziness, weakness, and abdominal pain May produce delirium, paralysis, seizures, and (if large amount of venom absorbed) death	*Treatment:* Cleanse wound with antiseptic. Apply cool compresses. Administer antivenin. Administer muscle relaxant, such as calcium gluconate; analgesics or sedatives; hydrocortisone or diazepam intravenously. *Prevention*—Teach children to avoid places that harbor the spider (e.g., woodpiles).

Continued

TABLE 30-7

Skin Lesions Caused by Arthropods—cont'd

MECHANISM AND CHARACTERISTIC	MANIFESTATIONS	MANAGEMENT
BROWN RECLUSE SPIDER *Mechanism:* Venom injected via fangs Venom contains powerful necrotoxin *Characteristics:* Slender spider, with long legs and body length of 1-2 cm; color is fawn to dark brown; recognized by fiddle-shaped mark on head Shy; bites only when annoyed or surprised Prefers dark areas where seldom disturbed	Mild sting at time of bite Transient erythema followed by bleb or blister; mild to severe pain in 2-8 hours; purple, star-shaped area in 3-4 days; necrotic ulceration in 7-14 days (Fig. 30-8) Systemic reactions may include fever, malaise, restlessness, nausea, vomiting, and joint pain Generalized petechial eruption Wounds heal with scar formation	*Treatment:* Apply cool compresses locally. Administer antibiotics, corticosteroids. Relieve pain. Wound may require skin graft. *Prevention*—Teach children to avoid possible nesting sites.
SCORPIONS *Mechanism:* Sting by means of a hooked caudal stinger that discharges venom Venom of more venomous species contains hemolysins, endotheliolysins, and neurotoxins *Characteristics*—Usual habitat southwestern United States	Intense local pain, erythema, numbness, burning, restlessness, vomiting Ascending motor paralysis with seizures, weakness, rapid pulse, excessive salivation, thirst, dysuria, pulmonary edema, coma, and death Some species produce only local tissue reaction with swelling at puncture site (distinctive) Symptoms subside in a few hours Deaths occur among children <4 years of age, usually in first 24 hours	*Treatment:* Delay absorption of venom by keeping child quiet; place involved area in dependent position. Administer antivenin. Relieve pain. Admit to pediatric intensive care unit for surveillance. *Prevention*—Teach children to avoid possible nesting sites.
TICKS *Mechanism*—In process of sucking blood, head and mouth parts are buried in skin *Characteristics:* Feed on blood of mammals Significant in humans because of pathologic organism carried May be vectors of various infectious diseases, such as Rocky Mountain spotted fever, Q fever, tularemia, relapsing fever, Lyme disease, tick paralysis Must attach and feed for 1-2 hours to transmit disease Usual habitat is wooded area	Tick usually attached to skin, head embedded Produce firm, discrete, intensely pruritic nodules at site of attachment May cause urticaria or persistent localized edema	*Treatment:* Grasp tick with tweezers (forceps) as close as possible to point of attachment. Pull straight up with steady, even pressure; if bare hands, use a tissue to touch tick during removal; wash hands thoroughly with soap and water. Remove any remaining part (e.g., head) with sterile needle. Cleanse wounds with soap and disinfectant. *Prevention*—Teach children to avoid areas where prevalent. Inspect skin (especially scalp) after being in wooded areas. (See discussion on p. 1082.)

FIG. 30-8 ■ Brown recluse spider bite. Note central necrosis surrounded by purplish area and blisters. (From Weston WL, Lane AT: *Color textbook of pediatric dermatology,* ed 4, St Louis, 2007, Mosby.)

who have become sensitized to hymenopteran bites may demonstrate a severe systemic response that can be life threatening. One sting can produce generalized urticaria, respiratory difficulty (from laryngeal edema), hypotension, and death. Intramuscular administration of epinephrine provides immediate relief and must be available for emergency use.

Hypersensitive children should wear a medical identification bracelet. They should also have a kit that contains epinephrine and a hypodermic syringe. Families are reminded to check the expiration date on the kit and to replace an outdated one. They should determine whether a nurse is available at the school and the school policy regarding administration of drugs. If a school nurse is not present, someone at the school should be designated to inject the epinephrine in case of an emergency.

SCABIES

Scabies is an endemic infestation caused by the scabies mite, *Sarcoptes scabiei.* Lesions are created as the impregnated female burrows into the stratum corneum of the epidermis (never into living tissue) to deposit her eggs and feces. The inflammatory response and intense itching occur after the host becomes sensitized to the mite, approximately 30 to 60 days after initial contact. If the person has been previously sensitized to the mite, the response occurs within 48 hours after exposure. After this time, the areas over which the mite has traveled will begin to itch and develop the characteristic eruption (Box 30-1). Consequently, mites will not necessarily be located at all sites of eruption.

There is great variability in the type of lesions. Infants often develop an eczematous eruption; therefore the observer must look for discrete papules, burrows, or vesicles.

Nursing Care Management

The treatment of scabies is the application of a scabicide. Currently, permethrin 5% cream (Elimite) is the drug of choice. Alternative drugs are 1% lindane cream or lotion and 10% crotamiton. Permethrin is preferred because it is safer, it avoids the risk of neurotoxicity, and it is more effective than lindane. Nurses instructing families in the use of scabicides should emphasize the importance of following directions carefully. Lindane should not be used immediately after a bath or shower. Permethrin is applied to all skin surfaces from the neck down to the toes (not just areas with rash, but also areas between the fingers and toes, the umbilicus, and the cleft of the buttocks). The cream should remain on the skin for 8 to 14 hours and then be removed by bathing. Lindane is removed by bathing after 8 to 12 hours. A second treatment with the same lotion may be required 7 to 10 days later. Lindane should not be used for preterm infants, young infants, people with known seizure disorders, people with hypersensitivity to the product, patients with crusted scabies, or patients with extensive dermatitis. Pregnant women and younger children are often treated with milder scabies medications. Crotamiton is applied once a day for 2 days, followed by a cleansing bath 48 hours after the last application. All clothes, bedding, and towels used by the infested person 3 days before treatment should be washed in hot water and dried in a hot dryer (Centers for Disease Control and Prevention, 2008).

Another prescription drug used to treat scabies is ivermectin (Frankowski and Weiner, 2002). Ivermectin is administered orally in a single dose for treatment of severe or crusted scabies. It should be considered for patients whose infestation is refractory or those who cannot tolerate topical scabicides. However, the safety and efficacy of ivermectin for pediatric patients younger than 5 years of age or children weighing less than 15 kg (33 pounds) is not established. This drug is not currently licensed for treatment of scabies by the FDA (American Academy of Pediatrics, 2006). Families need to know that although the mite that causes scabies will be killed with these treatments, the rash and the itch will not be eliminated until the stratum corneum is replaced in approximately 2 to 3 weeks. Soothing ointments or lotions can be applied for itching. Antibiotics may be given for secondary infection.

PEDICULOSIS CAPITIS

Pediculosis capitis (head lice) is an infestation of the scalp by *Pediculus humanus capitis,* a common parasite in school-age children. The adult louse lives only about 48 hours when away from a human host, and the life span of the average female is 1 month. The female lays her eggs at night at the junction of a hair shaft and close to the skin because the eggs need a warm environment. The **nits,** or eggs, hatch in approximately 7 to 10 days. Itching is usually the only symptom. Common areas involved are the occipital area, behind the ears, and the nape of the neck (Box 30-2).

Diagnostic Evaluation

Diagnosis is made by observation of the white eggs (nits) firmly attached to the hair shafts (Fig. 30-9). Because of their brief life span and mobility, adult lice are more difficult to locate. Nits must be differentiated from dandruff, lint, hair spray, and other items of similar size and shape. Scratch marks or inflammatory papules, caused by secondary infection, may also be found on the scalp in the vulnerable areas.

▌BOX 30-1

Clinical Manifestations of Scabies

LESION
Children—Minute grayish brown, threadlike (mite burrows), pruritic
- Black dot at end of burrow (mite)
Infants—Eczematous eruption, pruritic

DISTRIBUTION
Generally in intertriginous areas—Interdigital, axillary-cubital, popliteal, inguinal
Children older than 2 years of age—Primarily hands and wrists
Children younger than 2 years—Primarily feet and ankles

▌BOX 30-2

Clinical Manifestations of Pediculosis

Pruritus (caused by crawling insects and insect saliva on skin)
Nits observable on hair shaft (see Fig. 30-9)

DISTRIBUTION
Occipital area
Behind ears
Nape of neck
Eyebrows and eyelashes (occasionally) (caused by pubic lice)

FIG. 30-9 ■ **A,** Empty nit case. **B,** Viable nits. (From *The contemporary approach to the control of head lice in schools and communities,* Pittsburgh, 1991, SmithKline Beecham.)

Therapeutic Management

Treatment consists of the application of pediculicides and manual removal of nit cases. The drug of choice for infants and children is permethrin 1% cream rinse (Nix), which kills adult lice and nits. This product and preparations of pyrethrin with piperonyl butoxide (RID or A-200 Pyrinate) can be obtained without a prescription and are more effective and safer than lindane (Strong and Johnstone, 2008). The FDA has issued a warning regarding the use of lindane because of the potential for neurotoxicity (US Food and Drug Administration, 2003). Although the FDA believes that the benefits of lindane outweigh the risks when used as directed, patients should be treated with these medications when other treatments are not tolerable or have failed. Another product approved for treatment of head lice, malathion 0.5% (Ovide), is available only by prescription. However, malathion contains flammable alcohol, must remain on the hair for 8 to 12 hours, and is not recommended for children younger than 6 years of age.

Because of concerns that head lice may be developing resistance to chemical shampoos and that repeated exposure of children to strong chemicals on the scalp may be unwise, effective nonchemical control measures are essential. Daily removal of nits from the child's hair with a metal nit comb at least every 2 or 3 days is a control measure following treatment with a pediculicide (Mumcuoglu, Barker, Burgess, and others, 2007).

Nursing Care Management

An important nursing role is educating the parents about pediculosis. Nurses should emphasize that *anyone* can get pediculosis; it has no respect for age, socioeconomic level, or cleanliness. The louse does not jump or fly, but it can be transmitted from one person to another on personal items. Lice are more likely to infest Caucasian children, those with straight hair, and girls. Children are cautioned against sharing combs, hair ornaments, hats, caps, scarves, coats, and other items used on or near the hair. Children who share lockers are more likely to become infested, and slumber parties place children at risk. Lice are not carried or transmitted by pets.

Nurses or parents should carefully inspect children who scratch their head more than usual for bite marks, redness, and nits. The hair is systematically spread with two flat-sided sticks or tongue depressors, and the scalp is observed for any movement that indicates a louse. Nurses should wear gloves when examining the hair. Lice are small and grayish tan, have no wings, and are visible to the naked eye. The nits, or eggs, appear as tiny whitish oval specks adhering to the hair shaft about 6 mm (0.25 inch) from the scalp. The adherent nature of the nits distinguishes them from dandruff, which falls off readily. **Empty nit cases,** indicating hatched lice, are translucent rather than white and are located more than 6 mm from the scalp (see Fig. 30-9).

If evidence of infestation is found, it is important to treat the child according to the directions on the label of the pediculicide. Parents are advised to read the directions carefully before beginning treatment. The child is made as comfortable as possible during the application process because the pediculicide must remain on the scalp and hair for several minutes. Playing "beauty parlor" during the shampoo is a useful strategy. The child lies supine, with the head over a sink or basin, and covers the eyes with a dry towel or washcloth. This prevents medication, which can cause chemical conjunctivitis, from splashing into the eyes. If eye irritation occurs, the eyes must be flushed well with tepid water. It is not necessary to remove the nits after treatment because only live lice cause infestation. However, because none of the pediculicides is 100% effective in killing all the eggs, the makers of some pediculicides recommend manual removal of the nits after treatment (Centers for Disease Control and Prevention, 2005). An extra-fine-tooth comb that is included in many commercial pediculicides or is available at community pharmacies facilitates manual removal. If the comb is ineffective in removing the nit cases, the examiner should remove them by scraping them off the strands of hair with his or her fingernails.

Live lice survive for up to 48 hours away from the host, but nits are shed into the environment and are capable of hatching in 7 to 10 days; retreatment may be required (Centers for Disease Control and Prevention, 2005). Therefore measures must be taken to prevent further infestation (see Community Focus box). Spraying with insecticide is not recommended because of the danger to children and animals. Families should also be advised that the pediculicide is relatively expensive, especially when several members of the household require treatment. Families may be inclined to try home remedies to treat the lice. A recent study by Lee, Rios, Aten, and others (2004) showed that home remedies such as petroleum jelly, oils, vinegar, butter, alcohol, and mayonnaise did little to kill louse eggs but increased the risk for skin infection with *Staphylococcus aureus.* Another study by Pearlman (2004) showed that dry-on pediculicide lotions may effectively treat lice without the use of current shampoos with neurotoxins, nit removal, or extensive housecleaning. Another study (Goates, Atkin, Wilding, and others, 2006) demonstrated that one 3-minute application of hot air has the potential to eliminate lice infestations.

Prevention. The increasing incidence of pediculosis in schoolchildren is a serious concern for school nurses, parents, and community health agencies. However, school head lice screening programs have not proven to have a significant effect on the incidence of head lice in the school setting; parent education programs may be more helpful in the management of head lice. Children with head lice should be allowed to return to school after proper treatment. Both the American Academy of Pediatrics and the National Association of School Nurses discourage a "no nit" policy for schools (Frankowski and Weiner, 2002) (see Evidence-Based Practice box).

COMMUNITY FOCUS

Preventing the Spread and Recurrence of Pediculosis

- Machine wash all washable clothing, towels, and bed linens in hot water, and dry in a hot dryer for at least 20 minutes. Dry clean nonwashable items.
- Thoroughly vacuum carpets, car seats, pillows, stuffed animals, rugs, mattresses, and upholstered furniture.
- Seal nonwashable items in plastic bags for 14 days if unable to dry clean or vacuum.
- Soak combs, brushes, and hair accessories in lice-killing products for 1 hour or in boiling water for 10 minutes.

- In daycare centers, store children's clothing items such as hats and scarves and other headgear in separate cubicles.
- Discourage the sharing of items such as hats, scarves, hair accessories, combs, and brushes among children in group settings such as daycare centers.
- Avoid physical contact with infested individuals and their belongings, especially clothing and bedding.
- Inspect children in a group setting regularly for head lice.
- Provide educational programs on the transmission of pediculosis, its detection, and treatment.

Modified from Chin J, editor: *Control of communicable diseases manual,* Washington, DC, 2000, American Public Health Association.

EVIDENCE-BASED PRACTICE

No-Nit School Policies

ASK THE QUESTION   In schoolchildren, are pediculosis policies ("no-nit" policies) effective methods to decrease lice infestation?

SEARCH FOR EVIDENCE

Search Strategies   Databases were searched for the following key terms: head lice in children, pediculosis, head lice and school-age children, policies for head lice.

Databases Used   MEDLINE, PubMed, Ovid, and CINAHL

CRITICALLY ANALYZE THE EVIDENCE

To determine how often children were excluded from school inappropriately, health care providers and nonspecialists were invited to submit to the Harvard School of Public Health specimens that they found in children's hair when they suspected head lice (Pollack, Kiszewski, and Spielman, 2000). Analysis of 614 specimens revealed that lice and eggs were present in fewer than two thirds of these specimens, and only 53% of the specimens contained a live louse or viable eggs. Health professionals and nonspecialists both overdiagnosed pediculosis capitis and failed to distinguish active from extinct infestations. Eighty-two percent of the schools involved in this study had a no-nits policy, and noninfested children were excluded as often as children with active infestations.

In a study evaluating the presence of head lice in 1729 school-age children, a total of 28 children (1.6%) were found to have lice and 63 (3.6%) had nits with no lice (Williams, Reichert, MacKenzie, and others, 2001). Repeat assessment 2 weeks later revealed that only 18% of the children with nits alone developed lice. These researchers stated that having five or more nits within 6 mm (0.25 inch) of the head increased the risk of nit conversion, but most children with nits had no lice. The researchers concluded that school policies that excluded children with nits alone from school were not warranted.

The American Academy of Pediatrics (Frankowski and Weiner, 2002) have established guidelines for diagnosis and treatment of pediculosis. These guidelines state that no-nit policies in schools are detrimental, causing lost time in the classroom and inappropriate allocation of the school nurse's time, and that such a response is not warranted because pediculosis is not a serious medical condition (Frankowski, 2004).

No-nit policies state that when a school nurse finds head lice in a child's hair, that child is promptly sent home from school with directions for the parents to shampoo the child's hair and remove the lice. Parents

comply with these directions and send the child back to school after shampooing and meticulously combing the child's hair. If the school nurse finds a single egg or nit remaining in the child's hair, the school's no-nit policy demands that the nurse exclude the child from school until the eggs or nits are completely removed. The problem is that all nits are often not eliminated by treatment, but the nits left after treatment are inactive or dead, and harmless. Remnants of dead nits may remain attached to the hair for months or years. If the eggs are dead, there is no reason for a child to miss school.

APPLY THE EVIDENCE: NURSING IMPLICATIONS

A no-nit policy inflates the risks associated with lice infestations, increases the probability of overusing pediculicides, and may hinder academic performance by excluding children from school. Several practice implications can be derived from the studies: (1) school nurses should receive training and a microscope or magnifying glass to help them identify head lice correctly; (2) a diagnosis of head lice should be based on observation of live lice rather than dead eggs, dandruff, or other suspicious material in a child's hair; (3) a no-nit policy should be invoked only as a last resort; and (4) repeated failure of parents to rid a child's hair of nits is not a sound basis for suspecting neglect or abuse or instituting legal action against the parents.

References

Frankowski BL: American Academy of Pediatrics guidelines for the prevention and treatment of head lice infestation, *Am J Manage Care* 10(9):S269-S272, 2004.
Frankowski BL, Weiner LB: Head lice, *Pediatrics* 110(3):638-643, 2002.
Pollack RJ, Kiszewski AE, Spielman A: Overdiagnosis and consequent management of head louse infestations in North America, *Pediatr Infect Dis J* 19(8):689-693, 2000.
Williams LK, Reichert A, MacKenzie WR, and others: Lice, nits, and school policy, *Pediatrics* 107:1011-1015, 2001.

TABLE 30-8

Eruptions Caused by Rickettsiae

DISORDER, ORGANISM, AND HOST	MANIFESTATIONS	MANAGEMENT	COMMENTS
Rocky Mountain spotted fever—*R. rickettsii* *Arthropod*—Tick *Transmission*—Tick *Mammal source*—Wild rodents, dogs	*Gradual onset*—Fever, malaise, anorexia, myalgia *Abrupt onset*—Rapid temperature elevation, chills, vomiting, myalgia, severe headache Maculopapular or petechial rash primarily on extremities (ankles and wrists) but may spread to other areas, characteristically on palms and soles	*Control*—Protection from tick bite by wearing proper apparel, tick repellent Tetracycline or chloramphenicol Vigorous supportive therapy	Usually self-limiting in children Onset in children may resemble any infectious disease Severe disease rare in children Inspect children and dogs regularly if they play in wooded areas See Table 30-7 for management of ticks
Epidemic typhus— *R. prowazekii* *Arthropod*—Body louse *Transmission*—Infected feces into broken skin *Mammal source*—Humans	Abrupt onset of chills, fever, diffuse myalgia, headache, malaise Maculopapular rash becoming petechial 4-7 days later, spreading from trunk outward	*Control*—Immediate destruction of vectors Tetracycline or chloramphenicol Supportive treatment	Patient should be isolated until deloused See discussion on p. 1079 for management of pediculosis Excreta from infected lice also in dust; disinfect patient's clothing, bedding, and possessions and wash in hot water
Endemic typhus—*R. typhi* *Arthropod*—Rat fleas or lice *Transmission*—Flea bite; inhaling or ingesting flea excreta *Mammal source*—Rats	Headache, arthralgia, backache followed by fever; may last 9-14 days Maculopapular rash after 1-8 days of fever; begins in trunk and spreads to periphery; rarely involves face, palms, soles	*Control*—Eliminate rat reservoir, insect vectors, or both Tetracycline or chloramphenicol Supportive treatment	Fairly common in United States Shorter duration than epidemic typhus Mild, seldom fatal illness Difficult to distinguish from epidemic typhus
Rickettsialpox—*R. akari* *Arthropod*—Mouse mite *Transmission*—Mite *Mammal source*—House mouse	Maculopapular rash following primary lesion; eschar at site of bite; fever, chills, headache	*Control*—Eradication of rodent reservoir and mite vector Tetracycline or chloramphenicol Supportive treatment	Self-limiting nonfatal disease Endemic in New York City Found in many cities in United States

RICKETTSIAL DISEASES

The organisms responsible for a number of disorders are transmitted to human beings via arthropods (Table 30-8). Mammals become infected only through the bites of infected lice, fleas, ticks, and mites, all of which serve as both infectors and reservoirs. Rickettsiae are intracellular parasites, similar in size to bacteria that inhabit the alimentary tract of a wide range of natural hosts. Rickettsial diseases are more common in temperate and tropical climates where humans live in association with arthropods. Infection in humans is incidental (except epidemic typhus) and not necessary for the survival of the rickettsial species. However, after the organism invades a human, it causes a disease that varies in intensity from a benign, self-limiting illness to a disease that is fulminating and fatal.

LYME DISEASE

Lyme disease is the most common tick-borne disorder in the United States. It is caused by the spirochete *Borrelia burgdorferi*, which enters the skin and bloodstream through the saliva and feces of ticks, especially the deer tick. Most cases of Lyme disease are reported in the Northeast from southern Maine to northern Virginia. The disease may initially appear in any of three stages:

Stage 1 consists of the tick bite at the time of inoculation, followed in 3 to 31 days by the development of **erythema migrans** at the site of the bite (Fig. 30-10).

Stage 2, the most serious stage of the disease, is characterized by systemic involvement of neurologic, cardiac, and musculoskeletal systems that appears several weeks after the cutaneous phase is completed.

Stage 3, or the late stage, includes musculoskeletal pain that involves the tendons, bursae, muscles, and synovia. Arthritis may occur, and late neurologic problems include deafness and chronic encephalopathy.

Diagnostic Evaluation

Diagnosis is best made clinically during the early stages by recognizing the characteristic rash, erythema migrans. Serologic testing may be used to establish the diagnosis in later stages of the disease.

Therapeutic Management

Early and appropriate treatment is essential to prevent complications. Children older than 8 years of age are treated with oral doxycycline; amoxicillin is recommended for children younger than 8 years of age (American Academy of Pediatrics, 2006). For patients allergic to penicillin, alternative drugs include cefuroxime or erythromycin (Wade, 2000). Most experts treat individuals with early Lyme disease for 14 to 21 days. Persons who have removed ticks from themselves should be monitored closely for signs and symptoms of tickborne diseases for 30 days; in particular they should be monitored for erythema migrans, a red expanding skin lesion at the site of the tick bite that may suggest Lyme disease. People who de-

FIG. 30-10 ■ Lyme disease. Note annular red rings in erythema chronicum migrans. (From Weston WL, Lane AT: *Color textbook of pediatric dermatology,* ed 4, St Louis, 2007, Mosby.)

velop a skin lesion or viral infection–like illness within 1 month of an attached tick should seek prompt medical attention (Wormser, Dattwyler, Shapiro, and others, 2006). Treatment of erythema migrans most often prevents development of later stages of Lyme disease.

Nursing Care Management

The major thrust of nursing care should be educating parents to protect their children from exposure to ticks. Children should avoid tick-infested areas or wear light-colored clothing so that ticks can be spotted easily, tuck pant legs into socks, and wear a long-sleeved shirt tucked into pants when in wooded areas. Parents and children need to perform regular tick checks when they are in infested areas (with special attention to the scalp, neck, armpits, and groin areas). Parents should also be alert for signs of the skin lesion, especially if their children have been in tick-infested areas. Insect repellents containing diethyltoluamide (DEET) and permethrin can protect against ticks, but parents should use these chemicals cautiously. Although there have been reports of serious neurologic complications in children resulting from frequent and excessive application of DEET repellants, the risk is low when they are used properly. Products with DEET should be applied sparingly according to label instructions and not applied to a child's face, hands, or any areas of irritated skin. After the child returns indoors, treated skin should be washed with soap and water. Information about Lyme disease can be obtained from the American Lyme Disease Foundation, Inc.*

Mammal Bites and Scratches

PET AND WILD ANIMAL BITES

Animal bites are common in childhood. However, children are bitten more often by animals belonging to the family or to neighbors than by stray animals. The majority of victims of dog bites are boys between the ages of 5 and 9 years (Centers for Disease Control and Prevention, 2003; Bernardo, Gardner, O'Connor, and others, 2000). Most dog or cat injuries are to the upper extremities. Small children are likely to be bitten or scratched on the head, face, and neck because they tend to put their heads near the animal's head and flail their arms rather than protecting their heads. Animal bites are potentially serious

*PO Box 466, Lyme, CT 06371; e-mail: inquire@aldf.com; http://www.aldf.com.

because of the likelihood of significant infection. Injuries vary in intensity from small puncture wounds to complete evulsion of tissue that is associated with significant crush injury.

Therapeutic Management

General wound care consists of rinsing the wound with copious amounts of saline or Ringer's lactate under pressure via a large syringe and of washing the surrounding skin with mild soap. A clean pressure dressing is applied, and the extremity is elevated if the wound is bleeding. Medical evaluation is advised because of the danger of tetanus and rabies, although dogs in most urban areas must be immunized against rabies. Bites from wild animals, such as squirrels, bats, raccoons, foxes, and skunks, are also dangerous.

Prophylactic antibiotics are indicated for puncture wounds and wounds in areas that may prove to be cosmetically or functionally impaired if infected. Extensive lacerations are débrided and loosely sutured to allow drainage in the event of infection. Tetanus toxoid is administered according to standard guidelines (see Immunizations, Chapter 10), and rabies protocol is followed (see Rabies, Chapter 28). Injuries to poorly vascularized areas, such as the hands, are more likely to become infected than those in more vascularized areas, such as the face; puncture wounds are more likely to become infected than lacerations.

Nursing Care Management

The most important aspect related to animal bites is prevention. Children should understand animal behavior and develop respect for animals (see Community Focus box). Parents should monitor their children's behavior with a dog and instruct them not to tease or surprise a dog, invade its territory, interfere with its feeding or sleeping, take its toy, or interact with a sick or injured dog or a dog with pups. Parents who are considering getting a pet, especially a dog, for themselves or their children should select a dog that has a high level of sociability with, and is unlikely to be a danger to, children.

HUMAN BITES

Children often acquire lacerations from the teeth of other humans in rough play, during fights, or as victims of child abuse. Many preschool children bite others out of frustration or anger. Because human dental plaque and gingiva harbor pathogenic organisms, all human bites should receive attention. Delayed treatment increases the risk of infection.

If the laceration is less than 6 mm (0.25 inch) in length, the wound can be treated at home. The wound is washed vigorously with soap and water, and a pressure dressing is applied to stop bleeding. Ice applications minimize discomfort and swelling. Increased pain or redness at the wound site is an indication that the child should receive medical attention for antibiotic therapy. Tetanus toxoid is needed if the child is insufficiently immunized. Wounds larger than 6 mm should receive medical attention.

CAT SCRATCH DISEASE

Cat scratch disease is the most common cause of regional lymphadenitis in children and adolescents. It usually follows the scratch or bite of an animal (a cat or kitten in 99% of cases). The disease is usually a benign, self-limiting illness that resolves spontaneously in about 2 to 4 months. Diagnosis is made on the basis of (1) history of contact with a cat or kitten,

COMMUNITY FOCUS

Animal Safety

- Teach children to avoid all strange animals, especially wild, sick, or injured ones, who may be carriers of rabies (use the same techniques employed in teaching children not to talk to strangers).
- Teach children to avoid dangerous and nervous animals in the neighborhood.
- Vaccinate your own dog against rabies.
- Never permit children to break up an animal fight, even when their own pet is involved. Use a rake, broom, or garden hose to separate animals.
- Teach children the danger of mistreating or teasing pets (animals will bite if mauled, annoyed, or frightened).
- Spay or neuter your pets (spaying or neutering reduces aggression, not protectiveness).
- Avoid direct eye contact with a threatening dog, and remain motionless until a threatening dog leaves the area.
- Never hold your face close to an animal.
- Teach children not to disturb an animal that is eating; sleeping; or caring for young puppies, kittens, etc.
- Never tease; pull the tail; or take away food, a bone, or a toy with which an animal is playing.
- Never approach a strange dog that is confined or restrained; do not keep animals confined with short ropes or chains (this can make them aggressive or vicious, especially when teased).
- Do not run, ride a bicycle, or skate in front of a dog (it will startle the dog); teach children the importance of avoiding bike routes where dogs are known to chase vehicles.
- Do not allow an inexperienced child or adult to feed a dog (if the person pulls back when the animal moves to take the food, this can frighten and startle the animal).
- If a dog is asleep or unaware of your presence, or has not seen you approach, speak to the animal to make it aware of your presence to avoid startling the animal.
- Allow a dog to see and sniff a child before the child attempts to pet the animal.
- Do not permit a child to lead a large dog.
- Train or socialize a dog for appropriate behavior; avoid aggressive play with pets.
- Do not adopt pets for children until children demonstrate their maturity and ability to handle and care for pets.

From Humane Society of the United States: *Preventing and avoiding dog bites*, Washington, DC, 1998, The Society.

(2) the presence of regional lymphadenopathy for several days, and (3) serologic identification of the causative organism by indirect fluorescent antibody assay or polymerase chain reaction test. The disease may persist for several months before gradual resolution. In some children, especially those who are immunocompromised, the adenitis may progress to suppuration and serious complications. Treatment is primarily supportive, but antibiotic therapy may hasten the resolution of adenopathy in the disease (Centers for Disease Control and Prevention, 2002).

MISCELLANEOUS SKIN DISORDERS

A number of miscellaneous skin lesions occur in children. Some occur as a result of congenital disorders and are inherited as an autosomal dominant trait (Table 30-9). **Ichthyoses** are a heterogeneous group of disorders characterized by scal-

ing that create challenging problems in treatment. These disorders are not discussed in detail here because of their wide variability.

SKIN DISORDERS ASSOCIATED WITH SPECIFIC AGE-GROUPS

Several common dermatologic conditions are confined to children in specific age-groups. These conditions include diaper, atopic, and seborrheic dermatitis, which occurs predominantly in infants, and acne, which is most common in adolescence.

DIAPER DERMATITIS

Diaper dermatitis is common in infants and one of several acute inflammatory skin disorders caused either directly or indirectly by wearing diapers. The peak age of occurrence is 9 to 12 months of age, and the incidence is greater in bottle-fed infants than in breast-fed infants.

Pathophysiology and Clinical Manifestations

Diaper dermatitis is caused by prolonged and repetitive contact with an irritant (e.g., urine, feces, soaps, detergents, ointments, friction). Although the irritant in the majority of cases is urine and feces, a combination of factors contribute to irritation.

Prolonged contact of the skin with diaper wetness produces higher friction, greater abrasion damage, increased transepidermal permeability, and increased microbial counts. Healthy skin is less resistant to potential irritants.

Although ammonia was once thought to cause diaper rash because of the association between the strong odor on diapers and dermatitis, ammonia alone is not sufficient. The irritant quality of urine is related to an increase in pH from the breakdown of urea in the presence of fecal urease. The increased pH promotes the activity of fecal enzymes, principally the proteases and lipases, which act as irritants. Fecal enzymes also increase the permeability of skin to bile salts, another potential irritant in feces.

The eruption of diaper dermatitis is manifested primarily on convex surfaces or in folds. The lesions represent a variety of types and configurations. Eruptions involving the skin in most intimate contact with the diaper (e.g., the convex surfaces of buttocks, inner thighs, mons pubis, scrotum) but sparing the folds are likely to be caused by chemical irritants, especially from urine and feces (Fig. 30-11). Other causes are detergents or soaps from inadequately rinsed cloth diapers or the chemicals in disposable wipes. Perianal involvement is usually the result of chemical irritation from feces, especially diarrheal stools. *Candida albicans* infection produces perianal inflammation and a maculopapular rash with satellite lesions that may cross the inguinal fold (Fig. 30-12). It is seen in up to 90% of infants with chronic diaper dermatitis and should be considered in diaper rashes that are recalcitrant to treatment.

Nursing Care Management

Nursing interventions are aimed at altering the three factors that produce dermatitis: wetness, pH, and fecal irritants. The most significant factor amenable to intervention is the moist environment created in the diaper area. Changing the diaper as soon as it becomes wet eliminates a large part of the problem, and removing the diaper to expose healthy skin to air facilitates drying. The use of a hair dryer or heat lamp is not recommended because these devices can cause burns.

TABLE 30-9

Miscellaneous Skin Disorders

DISEASE AND CAUSATIVE AGENT	LOCAL MANIFESTATIONS	MANAGEMENT	COMMENTS
Urticaria—Usually allergic response to drugs or infection	Development of wheals Vary in size and configuration and tend to appear quickly, spread irregularly, and fade within a few hours May be constant or intermittent, sparse or profuse, small or large, discrete or confluent May be acute, chronic, or recurrent in acute attacks	Local soothing and antipruritic applications Antihistamines Epinephrine or ephedrine Cortisone in severe cases Severe upper respiratory tract involvement may require tracheostomy	Known etiologic agents should be avoided May be accompanied by malaise, fever, lymphadenopathy Severe cases may involve mucous membranes, internal organs, and joints Obstruction to air passages constitutes medical emergency (see Chapter 25)
Intertrigo—Mechanical trauma and aggravating factors of excessive heat, moisture, and sweat retention	Red, inflamed, moist, partially denuded, marginated areas, the shape of which is determined by location Appears where opposing skin surfaces rub together, such as intergluteal folds, groin, neck, and axilla Excessive moisture and obesity are often factors	Affected areas kept clean and dry Skinfolds kept separated with a generous supply of nonmedicated powder Expose to air and light Remove excess clothing	A form of diaper irritation Prevent recurrence by keeping susceptible areas clean and dry Frequently associated with overheating from too much clothing; common in tracheostomy patients with short necks and copious secretions
Psoriasis—Unknown; hereditary predisposition; may be triggered by stress	Round, thick, dry, reddish patches covered with coarse, silvery scales over trunk and extremities; first lesions commonly appear in scalp; facial lesions more common in children than in adults Affected cells proliferate at a much more rapid rate than normal cells	Tar preparations in combination with ultraviolet B (UVB) light or natural sunlight Topical corticosteroids Topical vitamin D analog calcipotriene Phenol and saline solutions followed by a tar shampoo to remove scales Keratolytic agents (salicylic acid) Acitretin Emollients may provide relief	Uncommon in children <6 years old Patients are otherwise healthy Coal tar acts synergistically with UVB light Keratolytic agents enhance absorption of corticosteroids Humidifiers may help in winter
Alopecia* Alopecia areata	Sudden onset of asymptomatic, noninflammatory, round, bald patches in hairy parts of body	Psychologic support Inducement of allergic contact dermatitis to stimulate growth of hair Minoxidil (peripheral vasodilator)	Family history in 10%-26% of cases Some concern regarding drug therapy safety Refer to support groups*
Traumatic alopecia	Traction alopecia around scalp margins from tight hair styles (e.g., braids, pony tails, corn rows)	Counseling regarding hair styling, use of hair cosmetics, hot combs, rollers	More prevalent in African-American children and adolescents Prolonged traction can produce fibrosis of hair root and permanent loss
Trichotillomania	Compulsive hair pulling	Determine and treat cause	Chronic hair pulling may require psychologic therapy
Tinea capitis	See Table 30-5	See Table 30-5	See Table 30-5
Erythema multiforme (Stevens-Johnson syndrome)—Unknown; associated with ingestion of some drugs; often follows upper respiratory tract infection	Erythematous papular rash Lesions enlarge by peripheral expansion, develop central vesicle Involves most skin surfaces except scalp May extend to mucous membranes, especially oral, ocular, and urethral	Symptomatic and supportive Maintain adequate intake of fluids (oral or intravenous), calories, and protein Moist wound care, hydrogels such as CarraGauze, Vaseline, or Aquaphor Appropriate treatment of complications Diligent monitoring of urine volume and specific gravity, hemoglobin and hematocrit, serum electrolyte levels, total body weight	Rash often preceded by fever and malaise Complications include renal failure and severe eye disease Respiratory involvement in a number of cases Self-limiting, but recovery may extend for weeks; skin lesions may subside without scarring; mucous membrane lesions may persist for months Recurrence rate 20%; mortality as high as 10% High mutation rate

TABLE 30-9
Miscellaneous Skin Disorders—cont'd

DISEASE AND CAUSATIVE AGENT	LOCAL MANIFESTATIONS	MANAGEMENT	COMMENTS
Neurofibromatosis—Inherited disorder; autosomal dominant inheritance pattern	Café-au-lait spots, pigmented nevi, axillary freckling Slow-growing cutaneous and subcutaneous neurofibromas	Symptomatic treatment of associated manifestations (e.g., speech defects, seizures, skeletal defects [scoliosis, kyphosis], learning disabilities) Surgical removal of troublesome tumors	Refer to support groups† Family needs to know about genetic implications

†Children's Tumor Foundation, 95 Pine St., 16th Floor, New York, NY 10005; (800) 323-7938 or (212) 344-6633; fax: (212) 747-0004; e-mail: info@ctf.org; http://www.ctf.org.

FIG. 30-11 ■ Irritant diaper dermatitis. Note sharply demarcated edges. (From Habif TP: *Clinical dermatology: a color guide to diagnosis and therapy*, ed 4, St Louis, 2003, Mosby.)

FIG. 30-12 ■ Candidiasis of diaper area. Note beefy red central erythema with satellite pustules. (From Weston WL, Lane AT, Morelli JG: *Color textbook of pediatric dermatology*, ed 4, St Louis, 2007, Mosby.)

Diaper construction has a significant impact on the incidence and severity of diaper dermatitis. Superabsorbent disposable paper diapers reduce diaper dermatitis. They contain an absorbent gelling material that binds water tightly to decrease skin wetness, maintains pH control by providing a buffering capacity, and decreases skin irritation by preventing mixing of urine and feces in the diaper. Another advance in diapers is the addition of an inner layer or top sheet that is impregnated with petrolatum (as in Pampers Swaddler with Absorb Away Liner).

FAMILY-CENTERED CARE

Controlling Diaper Rash
Keep skin dry.*
- Use superabsorbent disposable diapers to reduce skin wetness.
- If using cloth diapers, use only overwraps that allow air to circulate; avoid rubber pants.
- Change diapers as soon as soiled—especially with stool—whenever possible, preferably once during the night.
- Expose healthy or only slightly irritated skin to air, not heat, to dry completely.

Apply ointment, such as zinc oxide or petrolatum, to protect skin, especially if skin is very red or has moist, open areas.
- Avoid removing skin barrier cream with each diaper change; remove waste material and reapply skin barrier cream.
- To completely remove ointment, especially zinc oxide, use mineral oil; do not wash vigorously.

Avoid overwashing the skin, especially with perfumed soaps or commercial wipes, which may be irritating.
- May use a moisturizer or nonsoap cleanser, such as cold cream or Cetaphil, to wipe urine from skin.
- Gently wipe stool from skin using water and mild soap, such as Dove.
- When traveling, fill an old baby wipe container with soft paper towels and warm water.

*Powder helps keep the skin dry, but talc is dangerous if breathed into the lungs. Plain cornstarch or cornstarch-based powder is safer. When using any powder product, first shake it into your hand, then apply it to the diaper area. Store the container away from the infant's reach; keep the container closed when not in use.

Guidelines for controlling diaper rash are presented in the Family-Centered Care box. A common misconception about using cornstarch on skin is that it promotes the growth of *C. albicans*. Neither cornstarch nor talc promotes the growth of fungi under conditions normally found in the diaper area. Cornstarch is more effective in reducing friction and tends to cake less than talc when the skin is wet. On the basis of these properties and its safety in terms of inhalation injury, cornstarch is the preferred product. Talc should not be used.

ATOPIC DERMATITIS (ECZEMA)
Eczema or eczematous inflammation of the skin refers to a descriptive category of dermatologic diseases and not to a specific etiology. AD is a type of pruritic eczema that usually begins during infancy and is associated with allergy with a

---

BOX 30-3
Clinical Manifestations of Atopic Dermatitis

DISTRIBUTION OF LESIONS

Infantile form—Generalized, especially cheeks, scalp, trunk, and extensor surfaces of extremities (Fig. 30-13)

Childhood form—Flexural areas (antecubital and popliteal fossae, neck), wrists, ankles, and feet

Preadolescent and adolescent form—Face, sides of neck, hands, feet, face, and antecubital and popliteal fossae (to a lesser extent)

APPEARANCE OF LESIONS

Infantile Form

Erythema
Vesicles
Papules
Weeping
Oozing
Crusting
Scaling
Often symmetric

Childhood Form

Symmetric involvement
Clusters of small erythematous or flesh-colored papules or minimally scaling patches
Dry and may be hyperpigmented
Lichenification (thickened skin with accentuation of creases)
Keratosis pilaris (follicular hyperkeratosis) common

Adolescent or Adult Form

Same as childhood manifestations
Dry, thick lesions (lichenified plaques) common
Confluent papules

OTHER PHYSICAL MANIFESTATIONS

Intense itching
Unaffected skin dry and rough
African-American children likely to exhibit more papular or follicular lesions than are Caucasian children
May exhibit one or more of the following:
- Lymphadenopathy, especially near affected sites
- Increased palmar creases (many cases)
- Atopic pleats (extra line or groove of lower eyelid)
- Prone to cold hands
- Pityriasis alba (small, poorly defined areas of hypopigmentation)
- Facial pallor (especially around nose, mouth, and ears)
- Bluish discoloration beneath eyes ("allergic shiners")
- Increased susceptibility to unusual cutaneous infections (especially viral)

FIG. 30-13 ■ Infantile atopic dermatitis with oozing and crusting of lesions. (From Weston WL, Lane AT, Morelli JG: *Color textbook of pediatric dermatology,* ed 4, St Louis, 2002, Mosby.)

The diagnosis of AD is based on a combination of history and morphologic findings (Box 30-3). Children with AD have a lower threshold for cutaneous itching than do other children, and many authorities believe the dermatologic manifestations appear subsequent to scratching from the intense pruritus. For example, infants rub their faces against bed linen, and their crawling (a form of scratching) results in irritation of knees and elbows. Lesions disappear if the scratching is stopped.

The majority of children with infantile AD have a family history of eczema, asthma, food allergies, or allergic rhinitis, which strongly supports a genetic predisposition. The cause is unknown but appears to be related to abnormal function of the skin, including alterations in perspiration, peripheral vascular function, and heat tolerance. Manifestations of the chronic disease improve in humid climates and get worse in the fall and winter, when homes are heated and environmental humidity is lower. The disorder can be controlled but not cured.

Therapeutic Management

The major goals of management are to (1) hydrate the skin, (2) relieve pruritus, (3) reduce flare-ups or inflammation, and (4) prevent and control secondary infection. The general measures for managing AD focus on reducing pruritus and other aspects of the disease. Management strategies include avoiding exposure to skin irritants or allergens; avoiding overheating; and administrating medications such as antihistamines, topical immunomodulators, topical steroids, and (sometimes) mild sedatives as indicated.

Enhancing skin hydration and preventing dry, flaky skin are accomplished in a number of ways, depending on the child's skin characteristics and individual needs. A tepid bath with a mild soap (Dove or Neutrogena), no soap, or an emulsifying oil, followed immediately by application of an emollient (within 3 minutes), assists in trapping moisture and preventing its loss. Bubble baths and harsh soaps should be avoided. The bath may need to be repeated once or twice daily, depending on the child's status; excessive bathing without emollient application only dries out the skin. Some lotions are not effective, and emollients should be chosen carefully to prevent excessive skin drying. Aquaphor, Cetaphil, and Eucerin are acceptable lotions for skin hydration. A nighttime bath, followed by emollient application and dressing in soft cotton pajamas, may help alleviate most nighttime pruritus.

hereditary tendency (**atopy**). AD manifests in three forms based on the child's age and the distribution of lesions:

1. **Infantile (infantile eczema)**—Usually begins at 2 to 6 months of age; generally undergoes spontaneous remission by 3 years of age.
2. **Childhood**—May follow the infantile form; occurs at 2 to 3 years of age; 90% of children have manifestations by age 5 years.
3. **Preadolescent and adolescent**—Begins at about 12 years of age; may continue into the early adult years or indefinitely.

Sometimes colloid baths, such as the addition of 2 cups of cornstarch to a tub of warm water, provide temporary relief of itching and may help the child sleep if given before bedtime. Cool wet compresses are soothing to the skin and provide antiseptic protection.

Oral antihistamine drugs such as hydroxyzine or diphenhydramine usually relieve moderate or severe pruritus. Nonsedating antihistamines such as loratadine (Claritin) or fexofenadine (Allegra) may be preferred for daytime pruritus relief. Because pruritus increases at night, a mildly sedating antihistamine may be needed.

Occasional flare-ups require the use of topical steroids to diminish inflammation. Low-, moderate-, or high-potency topical corticosteroids are prescribed, depending on the degree of involvement, the area of the body to be treated, the child's age, the potential for local side effects (striae, skin atrophy, and pigment changes), and the type of vehicle to be used (e.g., cream, lotion, ointment). Patients receiving topical corticosteroid therapy for chronic conditions should be evaluated for risk factors for suboptimal linear growth and reduced bone density (American Academy of Dermatology, 2003). Topical immunomodulators, a new nonsteroidal treatment for AD, are best used at the beginning of a "flare up" just as the skin becomes red and itches. Two new immunomodulator medications used in children with AD are tacrolimus and pimecrolimus (Kronemyer, 2003). Tacrolimus is available in two ointment strengths (0.03% and 0.1%); the 0.03% concentration has been approved for use in children 2 years of age and older. Tacrolimus is recommended for intermittent therapy in patients who are not adequately responsive to, or are intolerant of, conventional therapy (Yetman and Parks, 2002). Pimecrolimus is available in a 1% cream that has no systemic accumulation or effects. This drug is approved for use in children with mild to moderate AD. Both drugs can be used freely on the face without worrying about steroid side effects.

If secondary skin infections occur in children with AD, these infections are managed with appropriate systemic antibiotics.

Nursing Care Management

Assessment of the child with AD includes a family history for evidence of atopy, a history of previous involvement, and any environmental or dietary factors associated with the present and previous exacerbations. The skin lesions are examined for type, distribution, and evidence of secondary infection. Parents are interviewed regarding the child's behavior, especially in relation to scratching, irritability, and sleeping patterns. Exploration of the family's feelings and methods of coping is also important.

The nursing care of the child with AD is challenging. Controlling the intense pruritus is imperative if the disorder is to be successfully managed, since scratching leads to new lesions and may cause secondary infection. In addition to the medical regimen, other measures can be taken to prevent or minimize the scratching. Fingernails and toenails are cut short, kept clean, and filed frequently to prevent sharp edges. Gloves or cotton stockings can be placed over the hands and pinned to shirtsleeves. One-piece outfits with long sleeves and long pants also decrease direct contact with the skin. If gloves or socks are used, the child needs time to be free from such restrictions. An excellent time to remove gloves, socks, or other

protective devices is during the bath or after receiving sedative or antipruritic medication.

Conditions that increase itching are eliminated when possible. Woolen clothes or blankets, rough fabrics, and furry stuffed animals are removed from the child's environment. Because heat and humidity cause perspiration (which intensifies itching), proper dress for climatic conditions is essential. Pruritus is often precipitated by exposure to the irritant effects of certain components of common products such as soaps, detergents, fabric softeners, perfumes, and powders. Most children experience less itching when soft cotton fabrics are worn next to the skin. During cold months, synthetic fabrics (not wool) should be used for overcoats, hats, gloves, and snowsuits. Exposure to latex products, such as gloves and balloons, should also be avoided.

Clothes and sheets are laundered in a mild detergent and rinsed thoroughly in clear water (without fabric softeners or antistatic chemicals). Putting the clothes through a second complete wash cycle without using detergent reduces the amount of residue remaining in the fabric.

Preventing infection is usually accomplished by preventing scratching. Baths are given as prescribed, the water is kept tepid, and soaps (except as indicated) and bubble baths are avoided, as are oils or powders. Skinfolds and diaper areas need frequent cleansing with plain water. A room humidifier or vaporizer may benefit children with extremely dry skin. The skin lesions are examined for signs of infection—usually honey-colored crusts or pustules with surrounding erythema. Any signs of infection are reported to the practitioner.

> **NURSINGALERT**
>
> If the child is being treated with baths for hydration, it is imperative that the emollient preparation be applied immediately after bathing (while the skin is still slightly moist) to prevent drying.

Wet soaks and compresses are applied and medications for pruritus or infection are administered as directed. The family is given explicit instructions on the preparation and use of soaks, special baths, and topical medications, including the order of application if more than one is prescribed. It is important to emphasize that one thick application of topical medication is *not* equivalent to several thin applications, and that excessive use of an agent (particularly steroids) can be hazardous. If children have difficulty remaining still for a 10- or 15-minute soak, bath, or dressing application, these can be carried out at naptime or when the child is engrossed in watching television, listening to a story, or playing with tub toys.

Diet modification is another source of frustration to parents. When a hypoallergenic diet is prescribed, parents need help to understand the reason for the diet and the guidelines for avoiding hyperallergenic foods (see Nursing Care Guidelines box). Because hypoallergenic diets take time before visible effects are apparent, parents need reassurance that results may not be seen immediately. If airborne allergens make eczema worse, the family is counseled about "allergy proofing" the home (see Asthma, Chapter 23).

Family Support. Parents are assured that the lesions will not produce scarring (unless secondarily infected) and that the disease is not contagious. However, the child may have repeated exacerbations and remissions. Spontaneous and per-

nursingcareguidelines

Preventing Atopy in Children

IDENTIFY CHILDREN AT RISK
Family history of allergy
Increased immunoglobulin E in cord blood and postnatal serum
Dry, flaky skin

PRENATAL PRECAUTIONS (LAST TRIMESTER)
Avoid any known food allergens
Avoid milk and other dairy products, peanuts, and eggs
Minimize ingestion of other hyperallergenic foods

POSTNATAL PRECAUTIONS
Breast milk or casein-whey hydrolysate formula (e.g., Nutramigen, Pregestimil, Alimentum) exclusively for at least 6 months
No solid food for first 6 months
No cow's milk or soy formula for 12 months
No eggs, fish, corn, citrus, peanuts, nuts, or chocolate for 12 to 18 months
One new food added at 5- to 7-day intervals to identify possible reaction

ENVIRONMENTAL CONTROL
Limited exposure to dust, molds, furry animals, and cigarette smoke

Data from Johnstone D: Strategy for intervention of food allergy in infants, *Int Pediatr* 4(4):319-325, 1989; Zeiger R, Heller S, Mellon M, and others: Effectiveness of dietary manipulation in the prevention of food allergy in infants, part II, *J Allergy Clin Immunol* 78(1 Pt 2):224-238, 1986; Wood RA: Prospects for the prevention of allergy in children, *Curr Opin Pediatr* 8(6):601-605, 1995.

manent remission takes place at approximately 2 to 3 years of age in most children with the infantile disorder.

During acute phases, emotional stress can become intense for the family. They need time to discuss negative feelings and to be reassured that these feelings are normal. Stress tends to aggravate the severity of the condition. Therefore efforts to relieve as much anxiety as possible in both the parents and the child have a beneficial emotional and physical effect.

SEBORRHEIC DERMATITIS

Seborrheic dermatitis is a chronic, recurrent, inflammatory reaction of the skin. It occurs most commonly on the scalp (cradle cap) but may involve the eyelids (blepharitis), external ear canal (otitis externa), nasolabial folds, and inguinal region. The cause is unknown, although it is more common in early infancy, when sebum production is increased. The lesions are characteristically thick, adherent, yellowish, scaly, oily patches that may or may not be mildly pruritic. Unlike AD, seborrheic dermatitis is not associated with a positive family history for allergy and is common in infants shortly after birth and in adolescents after puberty. Diagnosis is made primarily on the basis of the appearance and the location of the crusts or scales.

Nursing Care Management

Cradle cap may be prevented with adequate scalp hygiene. Not infrequently, parents omit shampooing the infant's hair for fear of damaging the "soft spots," or fontanels. The nurse

should discuss how to shampoo the infant's hair and emphasize that the fontanel is like skin anywhere else on the body—it does not puncture or tear with mild pressure.

When seborrheic lesions are present, the treatment is directed at removing the crusts. Parents are taught the appropriate procedure to clean the scalp. Education may need to include a demonstration. Shampooing should be done daily with a mild soap or commercial baby shampoo; medicated shampoos are not necessary, but an antiseborrheic shampoo containing sulfur and salicylic acid may be used. Shampoo is applied to the scalp and allowed to remain on the scalp until the crusts soften. Then the scalp is thoroughly rinsed. A fine-tooth comb or a soft facial brush helps remove the loosened crusts from the strands of hair after shampooing.

ACNE   *most severe causes scarring*

Acne vulgaris is the most common skin problem treated by physicians during patients' adolescence. Acne is not caused by dirt but by testosterone, a hormone present in males and females that increases during puberty. It stimulates the sebaceous glands of the skin to enlarge, or produce oil, and plug the pores. Whiteheads, blackheads, and pimples are present in teenage acne (American Academy of Dermatology, 2006).

One half of the adolescent population experiences acne by the end of the teenage years. Although the disorder can appear before the age of 10 years, the peak incidence occurs in middle to late adolescence (at age 16 to 17 years in girls and 17 to 18 years in boys). It is more common in boys than in girls. The degree to which an individual is affected may range from nothing more than a few isolated comedones to a severe inflammatory reaction. Although the disease is self-limiting and not life threatening, it has great significance to the adolescent. Health professionals should not underestimate the impact that acne has on teens.

Numerous factors affect the development and course of acne. Its distribution in families and a high degree of concordance in identical twins suggest hereditary factors. Premenstrual flares of acne occur in nearly 70% of adolescent girls, suggesting a hormonal cause. Studies do not indicate a clear association between stress and acne, but adolescents commonly cite stress as a cause for acne outbreaks. Cosmetics containing lanolin, petrolatum, vegetable oils, lauryl alcohol, butyl stearate, and oleic acid can increase comedone production. Exposure to oils in cooking grease can be a precursor in adolescents who work over fast-food restaurant hot oils. There is no known link between dietary intake and the development or worsening of acne.

Pathophysiology

Acne is a disease that involves the **pilosebaceous follicles** (the hair follicle and sebaceous gland complex) of the face, neck, chest, and upper back. Three pathophysiologic factors are involved in the development of acne: excessive sebum production, comedogenesis, and the overgrowth of *Propionibacterium acnes* (Mancini, 2000).

Comedogenesis (formation of comedones) results in a noninflammatory lesion that may be either an **open comedone** ("blackhead") or a **closed comedone** ("whitehead"). Inflammation occurs with the proliferation of *P. acnes,* which draws in neutrophils, causing inflammatory papules, pustules, nodules, and cysts (Fig. 30-14).

FIG. 30-14 ■ Acne vulgaris. **A,** Comedones with a few inflammatory pustules. **B,** Papulopustular acne. (From Weston WL, Lane AT: *Color textbook of pediatric dermatology,* ed 4, St Louis, 2007, Mosby.)

Therapeutic Management

Successful management of acne depends on a cooperative effort between the health care provider, the adolescent, and the parents. Unlike many other dermatologic conditions, acne lesions resolve slowly, and improvement may not be apparent for at least 6 weeks. Individual comedones can take several weeks to months to resolve, and papules and pustules usually resolve in about 1 week. The multifactorial causes of acne necessitate a combined approach for successful treatment. Treatment consists of general measures of care and specific treatments determined by the type of lesions involved.

General Measures. Improvement of the adolescent's overall health status is part of the general management. Adequate rest, moderate exercise, a well-balanced diet, reduction of emotional stress, and elimination of any foci of infection are all part of general health promotion.

Cleansing. Dirt or oil on the surface of the skin does not cause acne. Gentle cleansing with a mild cleanser once or twice daily is usually sufficient. Antibacterial soaps are ineffective and may be too drying when used in combination with topical acne medications. For some adolescents hygiene of the hair and scalp appears to be related to the clinical activity of the acne. Acne on the forehead may improve with brushing the hair away from the forehead and more frequent shampooing.

Medications. Treatment success depends on commitment from the adolescent. Before prescribing treatment, the practitioner should determine the adolescent's level of comfort and readiness to begin treatment.

Tretinoin (Retin-A) is the only drug that effectively interrupts the abnormal follicular keratinization that produces microcomedones, the invisible precursors of the visible comedones. Tretinoin alone is usually sufficient for management of comedonal acne (Russell, 2000). Tretinoin is available as a cream, gel, or liquid. This drug can be extremely irritating to the skin and requires careful patient education for optimal usage. The patient should be instructed to begin with a pea-sized dot of medication, which is divided into the three main areas of the face and then gently rubbed into each area. The medication should not be applied for at least 20 to 30 minutes after washing to decrease the burning sensation. The avoidance of sun and the daily use of sunscreen must be emphasized, since sun exposure can result in severe sunburn. Adolescents should be advised to apply the medication at night and to use a sunscreen with a sun protection factor (SPF) of at least 15 in the daytime.

Topical **benzoyl peroxide** is an antibacterial agent that inhibits the growth of *P. acnes* organisms. It is effective against both inflammatory and noninflammatory acne and is an effective first-line agent. This medication is available as a cream, lotion, gel, or wash. The patient should be informed that the medication may have a bleaching effect on sheets, bedclothes, and towels. The adolescent can be reassured that skin bleaching will not occur. Accommodation to the medication can be gained with a gradual increase in the strength and frequency of application.

When inflammatory lesions accompany the comedones, a **topical antibacterial agent** may be prescribed. These agents are used to prevent new lesions and to treat preexisting acne. Clindamycin, erythromycin, metronidazole, azelaic acid, and the combination of either benzoyl peroxide and erythromycin (Benzamycin) or benzoyl peroxide and glycolic acid are all choices for topical antibacterial therapy. The combination of 5% benzoyl peroxide and 3% erythromycin is especially beneficial, although the exact mechanism of action is not understood (Burkhart, Specht, and Neckers, 2000). Tretinoin improves the penetration of other topical agents, and combination therapy with tretinoin and an antibacterial treatment is the only way to address three of the pathogenic causes of acne: keratinization, *P. acnes,* and inflammation (Laude, 2000).

Systemic antibiotic therapy is used when moderate to severe acne does not respond to topical treatments. Oral antibiotics such as tetracycline, erythromycin, minocycline, and doxycycline are considered safe to use (American Academy of Dermatology, 2006).

Females with mild to moderate acne may respond well to topical treatment and the addition of an **oral contraceptive pill (OCP).** OCPs reduce the endogenous androgen production and decrease the bioavailability of the woman's circulating androgens. Both of these actions result in decreased acne.

Isotretinoin, 13-*cis*-retinoic acid (Accutane), is a potent and effective oral agent that is reserved for severe cystic acne that has not responded to other treatments. Isotretinoin is the only agent available that affects factors involved in the development of acne. However, treatment with isotretinoin should be managed *only* by a dermatologist. Adolescents with multiple, active, deep dermal or subcutaneous cystic and nodular acne lesions are treated for 20 weeks. Multiple side effects can occur, including dry skin and mucous membranes, nasal irritation, dry eyes, decreased night vision, photosensitivity, arthralgia, headaches, mood changes, aggressive or violent behaviors, depression, and suicidal ideation. Adolescents on this drug should be monitored for depression, depressive symptoms, and suicidal ideation (Jacobs, Deutsch, and Brewer, 2001). The drug should be given only at the recommended doses for no longer than the recommended duration. The most significant side effects of this drug are the teratogenic effects. Isotretinoin is absolutely contraindicated in pregnant women. Sexually active young women must be using an effective contraceptive method during treatment and for 1 month after treatment. Patients receiving isotretinoin should also be monitored for elevated cholesterol and triglyceride levels. Significant elevation may require discontinuation of the medication.

Nursing Care Management

Because acne is so common and its appearance may seem so mild, the health care provider may underestimate the relative importance of the disease to the adolescent. The nurse should assess the individual adolescent's level of distress, current management, and perceived success of any regimen before initiating a referral. If adolescents do not perceive the acne to be a problem, they may lack motivation to follow the treatment plan.

The nurse can provide ongoing support for the adolescent when a treatment plan is initiated. The family is also encouraged to support the adolescent in his or her efforts. Use of medications and basic skin care information should be discussed in detail with the adolescent. Written instructions should accompany the verbal discussion. Information to dispel myths regarding the use of abrasive cleansing products can prevent unnecessary costs and trauma to the skin.

Teenagers need education about the factors that aggravate and damage the skin, such as too vigorous scrubbing. In addition, picking, squeezing, and manual expression with fingernails break down the ductal walls of lesions and cause the acne to worsen. Mechanical irritation, such as vinyl helmet straps that rub areas predisposed to acne, can also cause the development of lesions.

THERMAL INJURY

BURNS

Burn injuries are usually attributed to extreme heat sources but may also result from exposure to cold, chemicals, electricity, or radiation. Most burns are relatively minor and do not require definitive medical treatment. However, burns involving a large body surface area, critical body parts, or the geriatric or pediatric population often benefit from treatment in specialized burn centers. The American Burn Association has established criteria to guide decisions regarding the severity of injury and the need for transfer for specialized care.* Burn prevention is also discussed in Chapters 10, 12, 15, and 16.

When burns are characterized by patients' age and type of injury, the following patterns become apparent: (1) hot-water scalds are most frequent in toddlers, (2) flame-related burns are more common in older children, (3) 10% to 20% of documented cases of child abuse include burn injuries (Herndon, 2007), and (4) children playing with matches or lighters account for 1 in 10 house fires.

The extent of tissue destruction is determined by the intensity of the heat source, the duration of contact or exposure, the conductivity of the tissue involved, and the rate at which the heat energy is dissipated by the skin. A brief exposure to high-intensity heat from a flame can produce burn injuries similar to those induced by long exposure to less intense heat in hot water.

Characteristics of Burn Injury

The physiologic responses, therapy, prognosis, and disposition of the injured child are all directly related to the *amount of tissue destroyed.* Therefore the severity of the burn injury is assessed on the basis of the percentage of **total body surface area (TBSA)** burned and depth of the burn. Among children in the school age–group or younger age-groups, a burn that is

*The American Burn Association offers an Advanced Burn Life Support Program; http://www.ameriburn.org/ablsnow.php.

10% TBSA can be life threatening if not treated correctly. Other important factors in determining the seriousness of the injury are the location of the wounds, the child's age and general health, the causative agent, the presence of respiratory involvement, and any associated injury or condition.

Type of Injury. The majority of burns result from contact with thermal agents such as a flame, hot surfaces, or hot liquids. Electrical injuries caused by household current have the greatest incidence in young children, who insert conductive objects into electrical outlets and bite or suck on connected electrical cords (Herndon, 2007). These burns occur most commonly during the spring and summer months and are also associated with risk-taking behaviors in boys. Direct contact with high- or low-voltage current, as well as lightning strikes, is the most frequent mechanism of injury. The resistance of the tissue and the path of the electric current are responsible for the damage incurred. Electric current travels through the body following the path of least resistance, which involves the tissues, fluid, blood vessels, and nerves. A more localized burn is produced if skin resistance is high at the area of contact, and a more systemic pattern of injury is produced if skin resistance is low. Often compared with a crush injury, serious electrical trauma results from current passing through vital organs, muscle compartments, and nerve or vascular pathways. Loss of limbs, cardiac fibrillation, respiratory collapse, and burns are common occurrences after exposure to electrical energy. Criteria for admission, as derived from evidence-based practice for electrical burn injuries, includes a history of loss of consciousness, electrocardiographic (ECG) changes, 10% TBSA affected, or the need for monitoring an affected extremity. Cardiac monitoring is therefore included in standard burn care when ECG changes are identified on admission (Arnoldo, Klein, and Gibran, 2006).

Chemical burns are seen in the pediatric population and can cause extensive injury. The severity of injury is related to the chemical agent (acid, alkali, or organic compound) and the duration of contact. The mechanism of injury differs from that in other burns in that there is a chemical disruption and alteration of the physical properties of the exposed body area. Noxious agents exist in many cleaning products commonly found in the home. In addition to concern for localized damage, the potential for systemic toxicity must be addressed. Of particular concern is the exposure of the eyes to chemical agents, the ingestion of caustic substances, and inhalation of toxic gases produced from chemicals.

Extent of Injury. The extent of a burn is expressed as a percentage of the TBSA. This is most accurately estimated by using specially designed age-related charts (Fig. 30-15). It is more efficient to use a chart designed to assign body proportions to children of different ages.

Depth of Injury. A thermal injury is a three-dimensional wound that is also assessed in relation to depth of injury. Traditionally the terms *first-, second-,* and *third-degree* have been used to describe the depth of tissue injury. However, with the current emphasis on wound healing, these have been replaced by more descriptive terms based on the extent of destruction to the epithelializing elements of the skin (Fig. 30-16).

Superficial (first-degree) burns are usually of minor significance. With these burns, there is often a latent period followed by erythema. Tissue damage is minimal, the protective functions of the skin remain intact, and systemic effects are rare. Pain is the predominant symptom, and the burn heals in

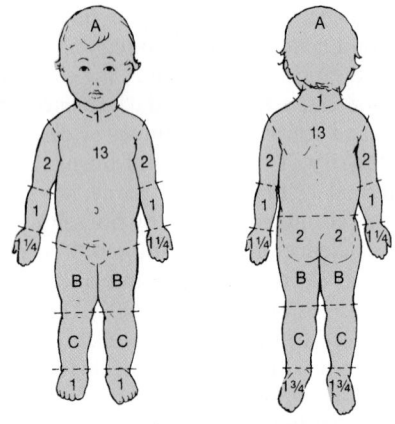

RELATIVE PERCENTAGES OF AREAS AFFECTED BY GROWTH

AREA	BIRTH	AGE 1 YR	AGE 5 YR
A = ½ of head	9½	8½	6½
B = ½ of one thigh	2¾	3¼	4
C = ½ of one leg	2½	2½	2¾

A

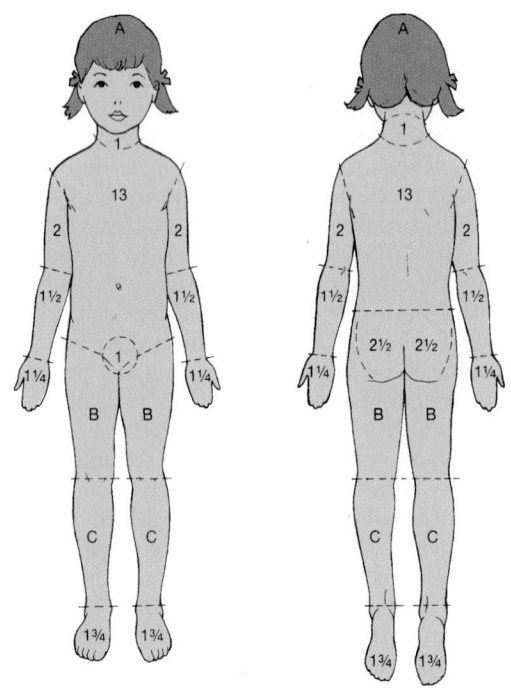

RELATIVE PERCENTAGES OF AREAS AFFECTED BY GROWTH

AREA	AGE 10 YR	AGE 15 YR	ADULT
A = ½ of head	5½	4½	3½
B = ½ of one thigh	4½	4½	4¾
C = ½ of one leg	3	3¼	3½

B

FIG. 30-15 ■ Estimation of distribution of burns in children. **A,** Children from birth to age 5 years. **B,** Older children.

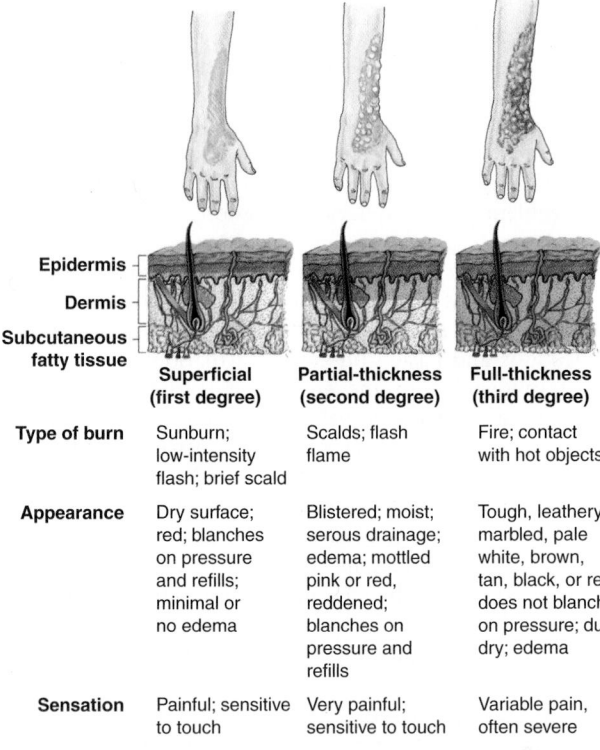

	Superficial (first degree)	Partial-thickness (second degree)	Full-thickness (third degree)
Type of burn	Sunburn; low-intensity flash; brief scald	Scalds; flash flame	Fire; contact with hot objects
Appearance	Dry surface; red; blanches on pressure and refills; minimal or no edema	Blistered; moist; serous drainage; edema; mottled pink or red, reddened; blanches on pressure and refills	Tough, leathery; marbled, pale white, brown, tan, black, or red; does not blanch on pressure; dull, dry; edema
Sensation	Painful; sensitive to touch	Very painful; sensitive to touch	Variable pain, often severe

FIG. 30-16 ■ Classification of burn depth. (Redrawn from Grant HD, Murray RH: *Emergency care,* ed 7, Upper Saddle River, NJ, 1995, Prentice-Hall.)

(Fig. 30-17). The wound is extremely sensitive to temperature changes, exposure to air, and light touch. Although classified as second-degree or partial-thickness burns, deep dermal burns resemble full-thickness injuries in many respects. Sweat glands and hair follicles remain intact. The burn may appear mottled, with pink, red, or waxy white areas exhibiting blisters and edema formation. Systemic effects are similar to those encountered with full-thickness burns. Although many of these wounds heal spontaneously, healing time may be extended beyond 14 days. These burn wounds often heal with extensive scarring.

Full-thickness (third-degree) burns are serious injuries that involve the entire epidermis and dermis and extend into subcutaneous tissue (see Fig. 30-16). Nerve endings, sweat glands, and hair follicles are destroyed. The burn varies in color from red to tan, waxy white, brown, or black and is distinguished by a dry, leathery appearance (Fig. 30-18). Normally, full-thickness burns lack sensation in the area of injury because of the destruction of nerve endings. However, most full-thickness burns have superficial and partial-thickness burned areas at the periphery of the burn, where nerve endings are intact and exposed. Excised eschar and donor sites also cause exposed nerve fibers. As the peripheral fibers regenerate, painful sensations return. Consequently, children often experience severe pain related to the size and depth of the burn. Full-thickness wounds are not capable of reepithelialization and require surgical excision and grafting to close the wound.

Fourth-degree burns are full-thickness injuries that involve underlying structures such as muscle, fascia, and bone. The wound appears dull and dry, and ligaments, tendons, and bone may be exposed (Fig. 30-19).

5 to 10 days without scarring. Mild sunburn is an example of a superficial burn.

Partial-thickness (second-degree) injuries involve the epidermis and varying degrees of the dermis. These wounds are painful, moist, red, and blistered. Superficial partial-thickness burns involve the epidermis and part of the dermis. Dermal elements are intact, and the wound should heal in approximately 14 days with variable amounts of scarring

FIG. 30-17 ■ Superficial partial-thickness burns on an African-American child. **A,** Blisters intact. **B,** Blisters removed. (Courtesy Hillcrest Medical Center, Tulsa, Oklahoma.)

FIG. 30-18 ■ *Bottom to top:* Deep partial-thickness burn *(red area)*; full-thickness burn *(white area)*; full-thickness burn with eschar *(brown area)*. (Courtesy Hillcrest Medical Center, Tulsa, Oklahoma.)

FIG. 30-19 ■ Full-thickness burn with muscle and fascia involved. (Courtesy Hillcrest Medical Center, Tulsa, Oklahoma.)

Severity of Injury. Burns are classified as minor, moderate, or major, which is useful in determining the disposition of the patient for treatment. Burn patients are categorized as (1) those with a **major burn injury,** who require the services and facilities of a specialized burn center; (2) those with a **moderate burn,** who may be treated in a hospital with expertise in burn care; and (3) those with **minor injuries,** who may be treated on an outpatient basis. The extent and depth of the burn (Table 30-10), the causative agent, the body area involved, the patient's age, and concomitant injuries and illnesses determine the severity of the injury.

Because the skin of infants is so thin, it is likely to sustain deeper injuries compared with older children. Children younger than 2 years of age, especially 6 months or younger, have a significantly higher mortality rate than older children with burns of similar magnitude. Acute or chronic illnesses or superimposed injuries also complicate burn care and response to treatment.

Inhalation Injury. Trauma to the tracheobronchial tree often follows inhalation of the heated gases and toxic chemicals produced during combustion. Although direct thermal injury to the upper airway may occur, heat damage below the vocal cords is rare. Inspired heated air is cooled in the upper airway before reaching the trachea. Reflex closure of the cords and laryngospasm also prevent full inhalation. However, evidence of direct thermal injury to the upper airway includes burns of the face and lips, singed nasal hairs, and laryngeal edema. Clinical manifestations may be delayed as long as 24 to

48 hours. Wheezing, increasing secretions, hoarseness, wet rales, and carbonaceous secretions are signs of respiratory tract involvement. Upper airway obstruction is often associated with burn shock and fluid resuscitation. In such situations, endotracheal intubation may also be necessary to preserve a patent airway.

Inhalation of carbon monoxide is suspected when the injury has occurred in an enclosed space. Mucosal erythema and edema followed by sloughing of the mucosa are manifestations of respiratory tract injury. A mucopurulent membrane replaces the mucosal lining and seriously compromises respiration and ventilation.

Early in the postburn period most pulmonary infections result from nosocomial exposure, immobility, and abdominal distention. The hematogenous variety occurs later and is related to the septic burn wound or other foci, such as phlebitis at the site of an invasive IV line. A significant increase in mortality has been observed when inhalation injury and pneumonia are both present.

Deep burns, especially those circling the thorax, may cause restriction of chest excursion as a result of edema and inelastic eschar formation. Young children are particularly at risk be-

TABLE 30-10			
Severity Grading System Adopted by the American Burn Association			
	MINOR*	MODERATE	MAJOR
Partial-thickness burns	<10% of total body surface area (TBSA)	>10%-20% TBSA	>20% TBSA
Full-thickness burns			All
Treatment	Usually outpatient; may require 1- to 2-day admission	Admission to hospital, preferably one with expertise in burn care	Admission to a burn center

From Vaccaro P, Trofino RB: Care of the patient with minor to moderate burns. In Trofino RB, editor: *Nursing care of the burn-injured patient*, Philadelphia, 1991, Davis.
*Minor burns exclude any burn involving the face, hands, feet, perineum, or crossing joints; electrical burns; any injury complicated by the presence of inhalation injury or concomitant trauma; children with psychosocial factors affecting the injury.

cause of the pliability of the skeletal structure. Restriction of the chest is relieved by an escharotomy incision, which allows expansion of the chest wall to facilitate ventilation.

Pathophysiology

Thermal injuries produce both local and systemic effects that are related to the extent of tissue destruction. In superficial burns the tissue damage is minimal. In partial-thickness burns there is considerable edema and more severe capillary damage. With a major burn greater than 30% TBSA, there is a systemic response involving an increase in capillary permeability, allowing plasma proteins, fluids, and electrolytes to be lost. Maximum edema formation in a small wound occurs about 8 to 12 hours after injury. After a larger injury, hypovolemia, associated with this phenomenon, will slow the rate of edema formation, with maximum effect at 18 to 24 hours.

Another systemic response is anemia, caused by direct heat destruction of red blood cells, hemolysis of injured red blood cells, and trapping of red blood cells in the microvascular thrombi of damaged cells. A long-term decrease in the number of red blood cells may occur as a result of increased red blood cell fragility. Initially there is an increased blood flow to the heart, brain, and kidneys, with decreased blood flow to the gastrointestinal tract. There is an increase in metabolism to maintain body heat, providing for the increased energy needs of the body.

Complications. Thermally injured children are subject to a number of serious complications, both from the wound and from systemic alterations resulting from the injury. The immediate threat to life is related to airway compromise and profound shock. During healing, infection—both local and systemic sepsis—is the primary complication. Mortality associated with thermal trauma in children increases with the severity of injury and decreases as age advances. In children older than 3 years, the mortality rate is similar to that of adults. Below this age, the survival rate with burns and their associated complications lessens considerably.

A less apparent respiratory tract injury is inhalation of carbon monoxide. Carbon monoxide has a greater affinity for hemoglobin than does oxygen, thereby depriving peripheral tissues and oxygen-dependent organs (such as the heart and brain) of the oxygen needed for survival. Treatment for either of these two problems is 100% oxygen, which reverses the situation rapidly.

Pulmonary problems are a major cause of fatality in children with either thermal burns or complications in the respiratory tract. Respiratory problems include inhalation injuries, aspiration in unconscious patients, bacterial pneumonia, pul-

monary edema, pulmonary embolus, posttraumatic pulmonary insufficiency, and atelectasis. The most common cause of respiratory failure in the pediatric age-group is bacterial pneumonia, which requires prolonged intubation and sometimes a tracheostomy. Tracheostomies increase the incidence of serious complications and are performed only in extreme cases.

A less common complication is pulmonary edema resulting from fluid overload or acute respiratory distress syndrome (ARDS) in association with gram-negative sepsis. ARDS results from pulmonary capillary damage and leakage of fluid into the interstitial spaces of the lung. A loss of compliance and interference with oxygenation are the consequences of pulmonary insufficiency in conjunction with systemic sepsis.

Wound Sepsis. Sepsis is a critical problem in the treatment of burns and an ever-present threat following the shock phase. Initially, burn wounds are relatively pathogen free unless they are contaminated with potentially infectious material, such as dirt or polluted water. However, dead tissue and exudate provide a fertile field for bacterial growth. On approximately the third postburn day, early colonization of the wound surface by a preponderance of gram-positive organisms (primarily staphylococci) changes to predominantly gram-negative opportunistic organisms, particularly *Pseudomonas aeruginosa*. By the fifth postburn day, bacterial invasion is well under way beneath the surface of the burn wound. Early surgical excision of eschar together with placement of autograft reduces the incidence of sepsis.

Therapeutic Management

Emergency Care. The initial management of the burn patient begins at the scene of injury. The first priority is to stop the burning process (see Emergency Treatment box). The child should then be transported immediately to the nearest medical facility for treatment and evaluation. The child and the family are usually extremely frightened and anxious; sensitivity to their emotional state and reassurance should be provided during the transport process.

Stop the Burning Process. The chief aim of rescue in flame burns is to smother the fire, not fan it. Children tend to panic and run, which spreads the flames and makes assistance more difficult. The injured child should be placed in a horizontal position and rolled in a blanket, rug, or similar article, with care taken not to cover the head and face because of the danger of inhalation of toxic fumes. If nothing is available, the victim should lie down and roll over slowly to extinguish the flames. Remaining in the vertical position may cause the hair to ignite or the inhalation of flames, heat, or smoke.

emergencytreatment

Burns

MINOR BURNS

Stop the burning process:

- Apply cool water to the burn or hold the burned area under cool running water.
- Do not use ice.

Do not disturb any blisters that form, unless the injury is from a chemical substance.

Do not apply anything to the wound.

Cover with a clean cloth if risk of damage or contamination.

Remove burned clothing and jewelry.

MAJOR BURNS

Stop the burning process:

- Flame burns—smother the fire.
- Place victim in the horizontal position.
- Roll victim in a blanket or similar object; avoid covering the head.

Assess for an adequate airway and breathing.

If child is not breathing, begin mouth-to-mouth resuscitation.

Remove burned clothing and jewelry.

Cover wound with a clean cloth.

Keep victim warm.

Transport to medical aid.

Begin intravenous and oxygen therapy as prescribed.

Major burns with large amounts of denuded skin should not be cooled. Heat is rapidly lost from burned areas, and additional cooling leads to a drop in core body temperature and potential circulatory collapse. Wet dressings also promote vasoconstriction because of cooling, resulting in impaired circulation to the burned area and increased tissue damage. Chemical burns require continuous flushing with large amounts of water before transport to a medical facility. The use of neutralizing agents on the skin is contraindicated, since a chemical reaction is initiated and further injury may result. If the chemical is in powder form, the addition of water may spread the caustic agent. The powder should be brushed off if possible.

Burned clothing is removed to prevent further damage from smoldering fabric and hot beads of melted synthetic materials. Jewelry is removed to eliminate the transfer of heat from the metal and constriction resulting from edema formation. This also provides access to the wound and prevents painful removal later.

Assess the Victim's Condition. As soon as the flames are extinguished, the child is assessed. Airway, breathing, and circulation are the primary concerns. Cardiopulmonary complications may result from exposure to electric current, inhalation of toxic fumes and smoke, hypovolemia, and shock. Emergency measures are instituted as appropriate.

Cover the Burn. The burn wound should be covered with a clean cloth to prevent contamination, decrease pain by eliminating air contact, and prevent hypothermia. No attempt should be made to treat the burn. Application of topical ointments, oils, or other home remedies is contraindicated.

Transport the Child to Medical Aid. The child with an extensive burn is not given anything by mouth to avoid aspiration in the presence of paralytic ileus and upper airway edema and to prevent water intoxication. The child is transported to the nearest medical facility. If this cannot be accomplished within a relatively short period, IV access should be established, if possible, with a large-bore catheter. Oxygen is administered, if available, at 100%. A report of the initial assessment and any interventions implemented is given to the medical facility assuming care of the child.

Provide Reassurance. Providing reassurance and psychologic support to both the family and the child helps immeasurably during the period of postinjury crisis. Reducing anxiety conserves energy the family and child will need to cope with the physiologic and emotional stress of injury.

Minor Burns. Treatment of burns classified as minor can usually be managed adequately on an outpatient basis when it is determined that the parent can be relied on to carry out instructions for care and observation. Patients with less than optimum circumstances may require close follow-up to ensure adherence with treatment.

The wound is cleansed with a mild soap and tepid water. Débridement of the wound includes removal of any embedded debris, chemicals, and devitalized tissue. Removal of intact blisters remains controversial. Some authorities argue that blisters provide a barrier against infection; others maintain that blister fluid is an effective medium for the growth of microorganisms. However, blisters should be broken if the injury is due to a chemical agent to control absorption. Most practitioners favor covering the wound with an antimicrobial ointment to reduce the risk of infection and to provide some form of pain relief. The dressing consists of nonadherent fine-mesh gauze placed over the ointment and a light wrap of gauze dressing that avoids interference with movement. This helps keep the wound clean and protect it from trauma. The caregiver is instructed to wash the wound, reapply the dressing, and return the child to the office or clinic as directed for wound observation. The frequency of dressing changes may vary from every other day to once a day.

Some practitioners prefer an occlusive dressing, such as a hydrocolloid, which is placed over the wound after cleansing. Hydrogel dressings, which are soothing and nonadherent, may also be used. The dressing is changed when leakage occurs—at regular intervals or at least weekly. This method eliminates the discomfort associated with frequent dressing changes but impairs visualization of the wound surface.

If there is a high probability of infection or other complications or if there is doubt about the ability to carry out instructions, the caregiver may be directed to bring the patient in daily for dressing changes and inspection. Another option is have a nurse make a home visit to inspect the wound and perform the dressing change. Frequent removal of the dressing is an effective mode of débridement. Soaking the dressing in tepid water or normal saline before removal helps loosen the dressing and debris and reduce discomfort. Burns of the face are usually treated by an open method. The wound is washed and débrided in the same manner, and a thin film of antimicrobial ointment is applied.

A tetanus history is obtained on admission. If there is no history of immunization, or if more than 5 years have passed since the last immunization, tetanus prophylaxis is administered. There is no evidence that systemic antibiotic prophylaxis decreases the incidence of infection in small burn wounds (Herndon, 2007). Therefore antibiotics should be used only when there is evidence of infection. A mild analgesic such as acetaminophen is usually sufficient to relieve discomfort; the antipyretic effect of the drug also alleviates the sensation of heat.

Most minor burns heal without difficulty, but if the wound margin becomes erythematous, gross purulence is noted, or the child develops evidence of systemic reaction, such as fever or tachycardia, hospitalization is indicated. The child should also be evaluated for functional impairment, and the caregiver should be instructed in the exercise and ambulation program. After wound healing, an evaluation of scar maturation and range of motion will indicate any need for further therapy.

Major Burns. The first priority is airway maintenance. The inhalation of noxious agents or respiratory burns is suggested when there is a history of injury in an enclosed space; edema of the oral and nasal membranes; thermal injury to the face, nares, and upper torso; hyperemia; and blisters or evidence of trauma to the upper respiratory passages. When respiratory involvement is suspected or evident, 100% oxygen is administered and blood gas values, including carbon monoxide levels, are determined.

If the child exhibits changes in sensorium, air hunger, or other signs of respiratory distress, an endotracheal tube is inserted to maintain the airway. When severe edema of the face and neck is anticipated, intubation is performed before swelling makes intubation difficult or impossible. Controlled intubation is preferred to an emergency procedure. Intubation allows for the delivery of humidified oxygen, the removal of secretions from respiratory passages, and the provision of ventilatory support.

When full-thickness burns encircle the chest, constricting eschar may limit chest wall excursion, and ventilation of the child becomes more difficult. Escharotomy of the chest relieves this constriction and improves ventilation.

Fluid Replacement Therapy. The objectives of fluid therapy are to (1) compensate for water and sodium lost to traumatized areas and interstitial spaces, (2) reestablish sodium balance, (3) restore circulating volume, (4) provide adequate perfusion, (5) correct acidosis, and (6) improve renal function.

Fluid replacement is required during the first 24 hours because of fluid shifts that occur after the injury. Various formulas are used to calculate fluid needs, and the one adopted depends on practitioner preference. Crystalloid solutions are used during this initial phase of therapy. Parameters such as vital signs (especially heart rate), urinary output volume, adequacy of capillary filling, and state of sensorium determine adequacy of fluid resuscitation.

After the initial 24-hour period, theoretically there is a capillary seal, and capillary permeability is restored. Colloid solutions such as albumin, Plasma-Lyte, or fresh frozen plasma are useful in maintaining plasma volume. However, children with burn injuries usually require fluids in excess of their calculated maintenance and replacement volume. Reasons for this may include underestimation of burn size (particularly in pediatric patients), pulmonary injury that sequesters resuscitation fluid in the lung, electrical injury with greater tissue destruction than that which is visible, and a delay in the initiation of fluid resuscitation. Irreversible burn shock that persists despite aggressive fluid resuscitation remains a significant cause of death in the immediate postburn period. Fluid balance may continue to be a problem throughout the course of treatment, especially during periods in which there may be considerable evaporative loss from the wound.

Nutrition. The enhanced metabolic requirements and catabolism in severe burns make nutritional needs of paramount importance and often difficult to satisfy. The diet must provide sufficient calories to meet the increased metabolic needs and enough protein to avoid protein breakdown. Hypoglycemia can result from the stress of the burn injury because the liver glycogen stores are rapidly depleted.

A high-protein, high-calorie diet is encouraged. Many children have poor appetites and are unable to meet energy requirements solely by oral feeding. Most children with burns in excess of 25% TBSA require supplementation with tube feeding. Early and continued nutritional support is an important part of therapy for seriously burned patients. Enteral feeding provides direct nourishment to the gastrointestinal tract and helps reverse the defective gut barrier that accompanies burn shock (Purdue, 2007).

If nutritional requirements cannot be met entirely by the enteral route, parenteral hyperalimentation is used to supplement intake. However, enteral feeding increases blood flow in the intestinal tract, preserves gastrointestinal function, and minimizes bacterial translocation by decreasing mucosal atrophy of the intestines. These factors make enteral feeding the preferred route of nutritional support (Herndon, 2007).

To facilitate growth and proliferation of epithelial cells, administration of vitamins A and C is begun early in the postburn period. Zinc is also supplemented because of its important role in wound healing and epithelialization.

Medication. Antibiotics are usually not administered prophylactically. The administration of systemic antibiotics to control wound colonization is not indicated, since decreased circulation to the injured area prevents delivery of the medication to areas of deepest injury. Surveillance cultures and monitoring of the clinical course provide the most reliable indicators of developing infection. Appropriate antibiotics are instituted to treat the specific identified organism. Otitis media should not be overlooked as a source of fever in the pediatric population.

Some form of sedation and analgesia is required in the care of burned children. Morphine sulfate is the drug of choice for severe burn injuries. Morphine has extensive distribution but is metabolized rapidly; continuous infusion or frequent administration is needed for pain management in burns. Morphine is administered intravenously and titrated to individual need. The unstable circulatory status and edema formation preclude intramuscular or subcutaneous administration. When combined, midazolam (Versed) and fentanyl (Sublimaze) also provide excellent IV sedation and analgesia to control procedural pain in children with burns (Herndon, 2007). The oral form of fentanyl, Oralet, provides effective analgesia in a convenient form that the child can suck. Dosage monitoring is important because tolerance to opioids may develop. IV analgesics are most effective when they are administered just before the onset of procedural pain.

The use of short-acting anesthetic agents, such as propofol (Diprivan) and nitrous oxide, has proved beneficial in eliminating procedural pain. Pharyngeal reflexes remain intact, thus ensuring a patent airway. Propofol is an IV sedative hypnotic agent that produces sedation in less than 1 minute and lasts only a few minutes. Nitrous oxide is a useful short-term analgesic when given in a mixture of gases on a fixed ratio of 50% nitrous oxide and 50% oxygen (Annequin, Carbajal, Chauvin, and others, 2000). Initiation of action is approximately 1 minute, with peak effect reached in 3 to 5 minutes. Nitrous oxide is useful to alleviate anxiety and raise the threshold of pain during procedures. The child may self-administer the nitrous oxide mixture with assistance. For any conscious or unconscious sedation, the child must be monitored continuously during the procedure (see Preoperative Care, Chapter 22; and Pain Assessment and Pain Management, Chapter 7).

Management of the Burn Wound. After the initial period of shock and the restoration of fluid balance, the primary concern is the burn wound. The objectives of wound management include prevention of infection, removal of devitalized tissue, and closure of the wound. The application of dressings and topical antimicrobial therapy reduce pain by minimizing the exposure to air.

Primary Excision. In children with large, full-thickness burn wounds, excision is performed as soon as the patient is hemodynamically stable after initial resuscitation. Because the burn wound precipitates an exaggerated physiologic response, many complications do not resolve until the eschar is excised and the wound is closed. Early excision of deep partial- and full-thickness burns reduces the incidence of infection and the threat of sepsis.

Débridement. Partial-thickness wounds require débridement of devitalized tissue to promote healing. Débridement is painful and requires analgesia and a sedative before the procedure. Medications given for pain need to be readily available during this procedure and may need to be titrated up during the procedure. Hydroxyzine and diphenhydramine are often needed for itching that occurs after whirlpool and débridement. The itching becomes particularly bothersome as the burns heal.

Hydrotherapy is employed to cleanse the wound and involves soaking in a tub or showering at least once a day for no more than 20 minutes. The water acts to loosen and remove sloughing tissue, exudate, and topical medications. Hydrotherapy helps to cleanse not only the wound but the entire body and aids in maintenance of range of motion. Mesh gauze serves to entrap the exudative slough and is readily removed during hydrotherapy. Any loose tissue is carefully trimmed away before the wound is redressed.

Topical Antimicrobial Agents. Methods used for managing the burn wound include:

Exposure—Wounds are left open to air; crust forms on partial-thickness wounds, and eschar forms on full-thickness burns.
Open—Topical antimicrobial agent is applied directly to the wound surface and the wound is left uncovered.
Modified—Antimicrobial agent is applied directly or impregnated into thin gauze and applied to the wound; gauze or net secures the area.
Occlusive—Antimicrobial agent is impregnated in gauze or applied directly to the wound; multiple layers of bulky gauze are placed over the primary layer and secured with gauze or net.

All these methods provide wound coverage and employ some type of topical agent. Topical agents do not eliminate organisms from the wound but can effectively inhibit bacterial growth. To be effective, a topical application must be non-toxic, capable of diffusing through eschar, harmless to viable tissue, inexpensive, and easy to apply. A topical ointment should not encourage the development of resistant strains of bacteria and should produce minimal electrolyte derangement. A comparison of commonly used agents is summarized in Table 30-11.

Biologic Skin Coverings. Permanent coverage of extensive burns is a prolonged process that requires repeated operative procedures using general anesthesia for atraumatic care in débridement and grafting. Early closure shortens the period of metabolic stress and decreases the likelihood of burn wound sepsis. In the acute phase, biologic dressings cover and protect the wound from contamination, reduce fluid and protein loss, increase the rate of epithelialization, reduce pain, and facilitate movement of joints to retain range of motion.

Allograft (homograft) skin is obtained from human cadavers that are screened for communicable diseases. Allograft is particularly useful in the coverage of surgically excised deep partial- and full-thickness wounds in extensive burns when available donor sites are limited. Severe immunosuppression occurs in massively burned children, and the allograft becomes adherent. The allograft can remain in place until suitable donor sites become available. Typically, rejection is seen approximately 3 to 4 weeks after application (Herndon, 2007). The availability of tissue banks and a supply of suitable donors limit the use of allografts.

Xenograft from a variety of species, most notably pigs, is commercially available. In large burns, the porcine xenograft is commonly applied when extensive early débridement is indicated to cover a partial-thickness burn; this provides a temporary covering for the wound until an available autograft can be applied to the full-thickness areas (Herndon, 2007). Pig-skin dressings are replaced every 1 to 3 days. They are particularly effective in children with partial-thickness scald burns of the hands and face because they allow relatively pain-free movement, which reduces contracture formation and has the added benefit of improving appetite and morale.

When applied early to a superficial partial-thickness injury, biologic dressings stimulate epithelial growth and faster wound healing. However, biologic dressings must be applied to clean wounds. If the dressing covers areas of heavy microbial contamination, infection occurs beneath the dressing. In the case of partial-thickness burns, such infection may convert the wound to a full-thickness injury.

Synthetic skin coverings are available for the management of partial-thickness burn wounds. Ideally, the dressing should provide the properties of human skin: adherence, elasticity, durability, and hemostasis. Synthetic skin substitutes are readily available, have an indefinite shelf life, and are relatively inexpensive.

Synthetic dressings are composed of a variety of materials and can be used successfully in the management of superficial partial-thickness burns and donor sites. Examples include adherent elastic films; hydroactive materials; or colloidal suspensions that are usually permeable to air, vapor, and fluids.

Biobrane is a flexible silicone-nylon membrane bonded to collagenous peptides of porcine skin. Calcium alginate is another treatment for donor sites. As with biologic dressings, it is important that the wound be free of debris before the dressing is applied. Body temperature elevation or evidence of purulence, erythema, or cellulitis around the wound edges may indicate that the wound has become infected beneath the

TABLE 30-11

Comparison of Common Topical Preparations

AGENT	DRESSINGS	ADVANTAGES	DISADVANTAGES
Silver nitrate 0.5% (AgNO$_3$)	Open, modified or occlusive; impedes joint movement; dressings changed twice daily; keep dressing moist, rewet at least every 2 hours	Greatly reduces evaporative losses; does not interfere with wound healing; bacteriostatic action against major burn flora, including *Pseudomonas* and *Staphylococcus* organisms; inexpensive	Does not penetrate eschar; ineffective on established burn wound infections; little effect on *Klebsiella* and *Aerobacter* groups; stains skin, clothing, linens; makes assessment of the wound difficult because of staining; hypotonicity pulls electrolytes from the wound, depleting sodium, potassium, chloride, and magnesium; stings on application
Silver sulfadiazine 1% (AgSD)	Occlusive; motion of joints maintained; applied twice daily; do not use with a history of allergy to sulfa	Little pain on application; bactericidal by altering DNA and cell metabolism; effective against gram-positive and gram-negative bacteria; easy to apply; nontoxic	Transient neutropenia; does not penetrate eschar; forms proteinaceous gel on wound surface that is painful to remove; occasional rashes and pruritus; decreases granulocyte formation
Mafenide acetate 10% (Sulfamylon)	*Cream*—Usually open; do not apply to face; apply twice daily *Solution*—Occlusive; keep dressing moist (rewet at least every 2 hours); protect solution from light	Penetrates eschar and diffuses rapidly into burn wound and underlying tissues; effective in deep flame, electrical, and infected wounds; biostatic against many gram-positive and gram-negative organisms, including *Pseudomonas* and *Clostridium*	Difficult and painful to remove cream; pain on application; metabolic acidosis, hypercapnia, and carbonic anhydrase inhibition; inhibits wound healing; hypersensitivity in some patients
Bacitracin	Open, modified; motion of joints maintained; change dressing twice daily	Bactericidal and bacteriostatic against gram-positive organisms; low toxicity; painless application; easy to apply	Limited activity against gram-negative organisms; allergic reaction in sensitive individuals

dressing. If this occurs, prompt discontinuance of the synthetic dressing is indicated. All synthetic dressings are reputed to hasten wound healing and reduce discomfort.

Permanent Skin Coverings. Permanent coverage of deep partial- and full-thickness burns is usually accomplished with a split-thickness skin graft. This graft consists of the epidermis and a portion of the dermis removed from an intact area of skin by a special instrument, the **dermatome** (Fig. 30-20). With extensive burns it is often difficult to find enough viable skin to cover the wounds; therefore available donor sites and special techniques are used. Split-thickness skin grafts may be sheet graft or mesh graft.

Sheet Graft. A sheet of skin, removed from the donor site, is placed intact over the recipient site and sutured in place; this is used in areas where cosmetic results are most visible (Fig. 30-21).

Mesh Graft. A sheet of skin is removed from the donor site and passed through a mesher, which produces tiny slits in the skin that allow the skin to cover 1.5 to 9 times the area of the sheet graft; this results in a less desirable cosmetic and functional outcome (Fig. 30-22).

The donor site is dressed with synthetic wound coverings or fine-mesh gauze until the dressing separates at 10 to 14 days, when the wound is healed. Dressings are not changed on donor sites to avoid damage to newly healed, delicate epithelium. Healed donor sites are available for reharvesting in patients with extensive burns and limited undamaged skin, but the quality of skin is decreased when multiple grafts are taken.

Artificial Skin. The development of Integra, a product that allows the dermis to regenerate, has produced significant im-

FIG. 30-20 ■ Removal of split-thickness skin graft with a dermatome.

provement in burn wound healing and decreased scar formation. It is applied to partial- and full-thickness burns. The two-layer membrane is made of collagen (a fibrous protein from animal tendons and cartilage) and silicone rubber (i.e., Silastic). The Silastic layer is peeled off after the dermis is formed. The application of artificial skin does not replace the grafting procedure, but it prepares the burn wound to accept an ultrathin autograft. Advantages include faster healing of the burn wound when integrity of the dermis is restored,

FIG. 30-21 ■ Sheet graft.

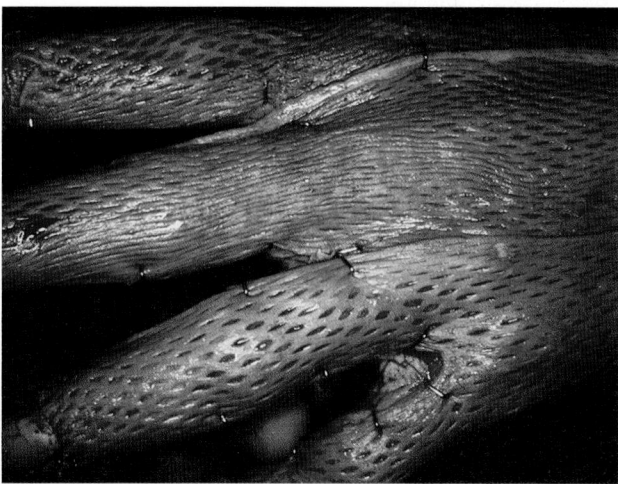

FIG. 30-22 ■ Mesh graft.

faster healing of donor sites with the use of ultrathin grafts, and restoration of sweat glands and hair follicles. A disadvantage is its high cost.

Cultured Epithelium. When burns are extensive and donor sites for split-thickness skin grafting are limited, it is possible to culture cells from a full-thickness skin biopsy and produce coherent sheets that can be applied to clean, excised full-thickness wounds. Epithelial cell culture grafts offer the possibility of an unlimited source of autografts in patients with extensive burns. Cultured epithelial autografts are effective in early wound closure. The child's own skin is fractionated and cultured in a porcine media to form a thin epithelial layer that is applied to the burn wound. This technique offers an improved rate of survival in patients with extensive burns and limited donor sites.

Prognosis. Children differ from adults in their responses to thermal injury, and the mortality rates in young children are significantly higher than those in older children and adults. Mortality is greatest for children younger than 48 months of age. Many children who do survive have long-term functional and cosmetic impairments.

Nursing Care Management

Because the care of burned children encompasses a broad range of skills, nursing care has been divided into segments that correspond with the major phases of burn treatment. The **acute phase,** also referred to as the *emergent* or *resuscitative* phase, involves the first 24 to 48 hours. The **management phase** extends from the completion of adequate resuscitation through wound coverage. The **rehabilitative phase** begins once the majority of the wounds have healed and rehabilitation has become the predominant focus of the care plan. This phase continues until all reconstructive procedures and corrective measures are accomplished (often a period of months or years).

Acute Phase. The primary emphasis during the emergent phase is the treatment of burn shock and the management of pulmonary status. Monitoring vital signs, output, fluid infusion, and respiratory parameters are ongoing activities in the hours immediately after injury. IV infusion is begun immediately and is regulated to maintain a urinary output of at least 1 to 2 ml/kg in children weighing less than 30 kg (66 pounds); an output of 30 to 50 ml/hr is expected in children weighing more than 30 kg. Urinary output and specific gravity, vital signs, laboratory data, and objective signs of adequate hydration guide the rate of fluid administration.

Children who are hospitalized with burns require constant observation and assessment for complications. Alterations in electrolyte balance produce clinical symptoms of confusion, weakness, cardiac irregularities, and seizures. Changes in respiratory function and gas exchange are reflected clinically by restlessness, irritability, increased work of breathing, and alterations in blood gas values. The loss of protective function of the skin exposes burned children to increased risk of hypothermia. Edema formation and circulatory impairment result in the loss of sensation and deep throbbing pain.

NURSINGALERT

Evaluate the burned extremity and check the pulse every hour. If unable to palpate, use Doppler to ascertain loss of circulation and pulse. If the pulse is lost, escharotomy may be necessary to relieve the edema causing pressure on blood vessels, to restore adequate circulation.

Burn units maintain a pictorial record of the wound to record progress and for legal purposes (if child abuse is suspected). The burn wound is treated according to the protocol of the specific burn facility. The burn team monitors infection control procedures and ensures that staff and visitors comply with established protocols to prevent cross-contamination in the burn unit.

Throughout the acute phase of care, the psychosocial needs of the children and their families should not be overlooked. The child is frightened, uncomfortable, and often confused. Children may be isolated from familiar persons and surroundings; the overwhelming physical needs at this time are the primary focus of the staff and parents. In addition to feeling concern for their child, the family experiences guilt, which may be related to the fact that the parents did not or could not protect their child from injury. Consistency in the information presented and in the attitude of the staff creates a sense of familiarity and stability during the acute phase of care. Consistent caregivers can also help decrease the patient's and family's anxiety and provide coordination of care. For example, when many teams of consultants and specialists are involved in the child's care, appointing one "spokesperson" decreases the confusion and enhances communication regarding the child's care.

Management and Rehabilitative Phases. After the patient's condition is stabilized, the management phase begins. The multidisciplinary team concentrates on preventing wound infections, closing the wound as quickly as possible, and managing the numerous complications. Although the rehabilitative phase begins when permanent wound closure has been achieved, rehabilitation issues are identified on admission and are included in the care plan throughout the hospital course.

> ### NURSINGALERT
> Disorientation in the burned patient is one of the first signs of overwhelming sepsis and may indicate inadequate hydration. Assessment of the sensorium is another important indicator of the adequacy of hydration. With inadequate hydration, a spiking fever and diminished bowel sounds accompanied by paralytic ileus are noted and progressively increase over 48 to 72 hours, after which the temperature falls to subnormal limits. At this time the wound deteriorates, the white blood cell count is depressed, and septic shock becomes manifest.

Comfort Management. The severe pain of the wound and resultant therapies, the anxiety generated by these experiences, sleep deprivation, itching related to wound healing, and the conscious and unconscious interpretations of traumatic events contribute to the psychologic behaviors commonly observed in children with burns. It is always difficult to deal with a child in pain, and inflicting pain on a helpless child is contrary to the empathic nature of nursing. Interventions to promote comfort may include medications (including IV morphine or midazolam and short-term anesthetics such as propofol), relaxation techniques, distraction therapy, behavioral techniques, operant conditioning (e.g., tokens, star chart), and family participation.

Children need age-appropriate explanations before all procedures. When children appear to accept pain with little or no response, psychologic consultation may be needed. Consistency in caregivers is important. If this is not possible, a carefully developed, multidisciplinary care plan is necessary to provide consistency.

Care of the Burn Wound. The nurse has a major responsibility for cleansing, débriding, and applying topical medications and dressings to the burn wound. Pain medication should be administered so that the peak effect of the drug coincides with the procedure. Children who have an understanding of the procedure to be performed and some perceived control demonstrate less maladaptive behavior. Children also respond well to participating in decisions (see Atraumatic Care box).

Outer dressings are removed. Any dressings that have adhered to the wound can be more easily removed by applying tepid water or normal saline. Loose or easily detached tissue is débrided during the cleansing process. In dressing the wound, it is important that all areas be clean, that medication be amply applied, and that no two burned surfaces touch each other (e.g., fingers or toes; ears touching the side of the head). If they are touching, the burned surfaces will heal together, causing deformity or dysfunction.

ATRAUMATIC CARE

Reducing the Stress of Burn Care Procedures
- Have all materials ready before beginning.
- Administer appropriate analgesics and sedatives.
- Remind the child of the impending procedure to allow sufficient time to prepare.
- Allow the child to test and approve the temperature of the water.
- Allow the child to select the area of the body on which to begin.
- Allow the child to request a short rest period during the procedure.
- Allow the child to remove the dressings if desired.
- Provide something constructive for the child to do during the procedure (e.g., holding a package of dressings or a roll of gauze).
- Inform the child when the procedure is near completion.
- Praise the child for cooperation.

Topical medications may be applied directly to the wound with a tongue blade or gloved hand or impregnated into fine-mesh gauze before application. Dressings are then applied to assist in exudate absorption, wound débridement, and increased patient comfort. All dressings applied circumferentially should be wrapped in a distal-to-proximal manner. The dressing is applied with sufficient tension to remain in place but not so tightly as to impair circulation or limit motion. Elastic bandages are applied over dressings to prevent epithelial breakdown, decrease edema, stimulate circulation, and improve mobility. A stable dressing is especially important when the child is ambulatory.

Standard precautions, including the use of protective garb and barrier techniques, should be followed when caring for patients with thermal injuries. Frequent hand and forearm washing is the single most important element of the infection control program. Strict policies for cleaning the environment and patient care equipment should be implemented to minimize the risk of cross-contamination. All visitors and members of other departments should be oriented to the infection control policies, including the importance of hand and forearm washing and use of protective garb. Visitors should be screened for infection and contagious diseases before patient contact.

Nutrition. Oral feedings are encouraged unless the child is intubated or paralytic ileus persists. Because children with burns often lack an appetite, the child needs encouragement, help, and patience. Consultation between the caregiver and the dietitian helps determine food preferences. Children who are old enough to participate should be included in meal planning. In addition, many children prefer an atmosphere more nearly like that provided at home. Therefore, when possible, many children enjoy sitting at a table and interacting with other children at mealtimes. Painful procedures should not be scheduled near mealtimes, since most children will be too physically exhausted and emotionally upset to eat.

Children who require enteral supplementation must be monitored for feeding intolerance and tube malposition. The nurse should also monitor and report any abdominal distention, diarrhea, or electrolyte and metabolic deviations.

Prevention of Complications

Acute Care. The maintenance of body temperature is important to the child with burns. Core body temperature is supported when energy is conserved with an environmental temperature of 28° to 33° C (82.4° to 91.4° F). Large areas of the body should not be exposed simultaneously during dressing changes. Warmed solutions, linens, occlusive dressings, heat shields, a radiant warmer, and warming blankets assist in preventing hypothermia.

The chief danger during acute care is infection—wound infection, generalized sepsis, or bacterial pneumonia. Accurate and ongoing assessments of all parameters that provide clues to the early diagnosis and treatment of infection are essential. Symptoms of sepsis include a change in the level of consciousness, a rising or falling white blood cell count, hypothermia or hyperthermia, a loss of the progression of wound healing, increasing fluid requirements, hypoactive or absent bowel sounds, a rising or falling blood glucose level, tachycardia, tachypnea, and thrombocytopenia.

Children are reluctant to move if movement causes pain, and they are likely to assume a position of comfort. Unfortunately, the most comfortable position often encourages the formation of contractures and loss of function. Ongoing efforts to prevent contractures include maintaining proper body alignment, positioning and splinting involved extremities in extension, providing active and passive physical therapy, and encouraging spontaneous movement when feasible. Frequent position changes are important to promote adequate bronchopulmonary hygiene and capillary perfusion to common pressure areas. Low–air loss beds are beneficial for the morbidly obese or children with posterior grafts. Special attention should be given to areas at risk for increased pressure, such as the posterior scalp, heels, sacrum, and areas exposed to mechanical irritation from splints and dressings.

Long-Term Care. The rehabilitative phase of care begins once wound coverage is achieved. Scar formation becomes a major problem as burn wounds heal (Fig. 30-23). Contractile properties of the scar tissue can result in disabling contractures, deformity, and disfigurement.

Uniform pressure applied to the scar decreases the blood supply. When pressure is removed, blood supply to the scar is immediately increased; therefore periods without pressure should be brief to avoid nourishment of the hypertrophic tissue. Continuous pressure to areas of scarring can be achieved by elastic bandages or commercially available pressure garments. Because these custom-made garments are often worn for months, revisions may be required as the child grows. It is much easier to prevent scarring and contracture of the wound than to resolve an existing problem. Splints and appliances may also be needed until wound maturation is achieved (Fig. 30-24).

Scar tissue has certain significant properties, particularly for growing children. Intense itching occurs in healing burn wounds and scar tissue until the scar is no longer active. Itching is usually treated with a combination of H_1 and H_2 antagonists such as cetirizine (Zyrtec) and cimetidine (Tagamet) (Baker, Zeller, Klein, and others, 2001); an H_1 antagonist alone; and frequent applications of a moisturizer, such as Vaseline, Cetaphil, Aquaphor, Eucerin, cocoa butter, or Nivea. Petrolatum-based ointments (Vaseline, Aquaphor) seem to spread more easily on friable skin than thick creams do. Massage therapy during the

FIG. 30-23 ▪ Extensive scars from flame burn. (Courtesy The Paul and Carol David Foundation Burn Institute, Akron, Ohio.)

FIG. 30-24 ▪ Child in elasticized (Jobst) garment and "airplane" splints.

application of moisturizers is also beneficial to stretch scar tissue and aid in contracture prevention. Scar tissue has no sweat glands, and children with extensive scarring may experience difficulty during hot weather. Caregivers should be alerted to this possibility and be prepared to institute alternate methods of cooling when necessary.

Scar tissue does not grow and expand, as does normal tissue, which may create difficulties, especially in functional areas such as on the hands and over joints. Additional surgery is sometimes required to allow independent functioning in daily activities, to improve cosmetic appearance, or to restore anatomic integrity.

The nursing activities in the rehabilitative phase of treatment focus on the child's and family's adaptation to the burn injury and their ability to reintegrate into the community. The psychologic pain and sequelae of severe burn injury are as intense as the physical trauma. The impact of severe burns taxes the coping mechanisms at all ages. Very young children, who suffer acutely from separation anxiety, and adolescents, who are developing an identity, are probably the most affected psychologically. Toddlers cannot understand why the parents they love and who have protected them can leave them in such a frightening and unfamiliar place. Adolescents, in the process of achieving independence from the family, find themselves in a dependent role with a damaged body. Being different from others at a time when conformity with peers is so important is difficult to accept.

Anticipation of the return to school can be overwhelming and frightening. It is essential that health care professionals recognize the importance of preparing teachers and classmates for the child's return. Teachers need to be provided with information to assist the child and family and to promote the child's optimal adjustment. Hospital-sponsored school reentry programs use a variety of methods to provide education and information about the implications of the injury, the garments and appliances, and the need for support and acceptance. Telephone calls, videotapes, information packets, and visits by members of the health care team offer opportunities to help with reintegration into the school environment—a focal point of the child's life.

Psychosocial Support of the Child. Children should begin early to do as much for themselves as possible and to be active participants in their care. Loss of control and perceived helplessness may result in acting-out behaviors. During illness, children regress to a previous developmental level that allows them to deal with stress. As children begin to participate in their care, they gain confidence and self-esteem. Fears and anxieties diminish with accomplishment and self-confidence. If the child demonstrates nonadherence in the rehabilitative phase, a behavior modification program can be initiated to promote or reward the child's accomplishment in care.

Children need to know that their injury and the treatments are not punishment for real or imagined transgressions and that the nurse understands their fear, anger, and discomfort. They also need body contact. This is often difficult to arrange for the child with massive burns. Stroking areas of unburned skin is comforting. Even older children enjoy sitting on the parent's lap and being cuddled and hugged. This can be a reward or a comfort in times of stress, but most of all it should be kept in mind that it is a natural part of childhood.

Psychosocial Support of the Family. Recognizing and respecting each family's strengths, differences, and methods of coping allow the nurse to respond to their unique needs by implementing a family-centered approach to care. In the acute phase, all attention is focused on the child, and the parents feel powerless and ineffectual. Most parents feel overwhelming guilt, whether or not the guilt is justified. They feel responsible for the injury. These feelings may impede the child's rehabilitation. Parents may indulge the child and allow nonadherent behaviors that affect physical and emotional recovery. Parents need to be informed of the child's progress and helped to cope with their feelings while providing support to their child. The nurse can help them understand that it is not selfish to look after themselves and their own needs to meet their child's needs. It is important to recognize the parents' need to grieve the change in their child's normal appearance as part of the

grieving process. Definitive professional help may be needed for parents whose response to the injury is severe or whose response to stress is manifested in destructive behavior.

The parents are members of the multidisciplinary team and participate in the development of the care plan. It is important to facilitate their input; to consider all aspects of the physical, emotional, social, and cultural factors affecting the child and family; and to establish a realistic home therapy program. The family's willingness to assume responsibility for care and their ability to implement the therapeutic regimen are assessed. Home, school, and other environmental factors are explored; financial concerns and available community resources are discussed; and a specific care plan for the child, with an anticipated follow-up program, is developed.

Prevention of Burn Injury. The best intervention is to prevent burns from occurring. Hot liquids in the kitchen and bathroom most commonly injure infants and toddlers. Hot liquids should be kept out of reach; tablecloths and dangling appliance cords are often pulled by toddlers, who spill hot grease and liquids on themselves. Electrical cords and outlets represent a potential risk to small children, who may chew on accessible cords and insert objects into outlets.

The Consumer Product Safety Commission recommends a reduction of water heater thermostats to a maximum of 48.9° C (120° F). The "dial-down" recommendation has been suggested by utility companies, burn treatment centers, medical personnel, and others interested in public safety. However, many water heaters continue to remain set at levels well above the safe level. Small children are especially at risk for scald injuries from hot tap water because of their decreased reaction time and agility, their curiosity, and the thermal sensitivity of their skin. Caregivers should never leave a child unattended in a bath and without adult supervision. Water should always be tested before a child is placed in the tub or shower.

The increased use of microwave ovens has resulted in burn injuries from the extremely hot internal temperatures generated in heated items. Baby formula, jelly-filled pastries, and hot liquids and dishes may result in cutaneous scalds or the ingestion of overheated liquids. Parents should use caution when removing items from the microwave oven and should always test the food before giving it to children.

As children mature, risk-taking behaviors increase. Matches and lighters are dangerous in the hands of the young. Adults must remember to keep potentially hazardous items out of the reach of children; a lighter, like a match, is a tool for adult use.

Education related to fire safety and survival should begin with the very young. They can practice "stop, drop, and roll" to extinguish a fire. The fire escape route, including a safe meeting place away from the home in case of fire, also should be practiced.

Community activities are also helpful in supporting burn survivors and preventing burns. The Aluminum Cans for Burned Children (ACBC) is an exemplary effort based at the Paul and Carol David Foundation Burn Institute, Akron, Ohio.* Activities funded by ACBC include Burn Survivors Support Group, Burn Camp, and meetings of Juvenile Firestoppers (for children with fire-setting behavior). Adult week-

*Akron Children's Hospital, One Perkins Square, Akron, OH 44308-1062; (330) 543-1000; fax: (330) 543-9998; http://www.akronchildrens.org.

end retreats and school and family education sessions are a part of this program. The burn center and fire department provide the personnel to present programs.

Additional information on burn care and prevention can be obtained from the American Burn Association* and the National Safety Council.† The Alisa Ann Ruch Burn Foundation‡ provides assistance to burn victims and burn centers. The Shriners Burn Institutes are staffed to treat pediatric patients after acute burn injuries and those requiring rehabilitative and reconstructive services as a result of scarring and functional impairment. Information can be obtained from local Shrine Temples and Shrine Clubs, from Shriners Hospitals, or by contacting the International Shrine Headquarters.§ The Alisa Ann Ruch Foundation and Shriners Hospitals for Crippled Children support research to improve burn care and treatment and promote public education in burn prevention.

SUNBURN

Sunburn is a common skin injury caused by overexposure to UV light waves. The sun emits a continuous spectrum of visible and nonvisible light rays that range in length from very short to very long. The shorter, higher-frequency waves are more damaging than longer wavelengths, but much of the light is filtered out as it travels through the atmosphere. Of the light that does filter through, **ultraviolet A (UVA) waves** are the longest and cause only minimum burning, but play a significant role in photosensitive and photoallergic reactions. They are also responsible for premature aging of the skin and potentiate the effects of **ultraviolet B (UVB)** waves. UVB waves are shorter and are responsible for tanning, burning, and most of the harmful effects attributed to sunlight, especially skin cancer.

Numerous factors influence the amount of UVB exposure. Maximum exposure occurs at midday (10 AM to 3 PM), when the distance from the sun to a given spot on the earth is shortest. There is more exposure at higher altitudes and near the equator, and less when the sky is hazy (although the amount of UV radiation that does penetrate is easily underestimated). Window glass effectively screens out UVB but not UVA rays. Fresh snow, water, and sand reflect UV rays, especially when the sun is directly overhead.

Sunburn is usually an epidermal burn, although severe sunburn can be a partial-thickness burn with blister formation. Treatment of sunburn involves stopping the burning process, decreasing the inflammatory response, and rehydrating the skin. Local application of cool tap water soaks, or immersion in a tepid-water bath (temperature slightly below 36.7° C [98° F]) for 20 minutes or until the skin is cool, limits tissue destruction and relieves the discomfort. After the cool applications, a bland oil-in-water moisturizing lotion can be applied. Partial-thickness burns are treated the same as those from any heat source (see earlier discussion on burns).

---

*625 North Michigan Ave., Suite 2550, Chicago, IL 60611; (312) 642-9260; fax: (312) 642-9130; e-mail: info@ameriburn.org; http://www.ameriburn.org.
†1121 Spring Lake Drive, Itasca, IL 60143-3201; (630) 285-1121, e-mail: info@nsc.org; http://www.nsc.org.
‡2501 W. Burbank Blvd., Suite 201, Burbank, CA 91505; (800) 242-BURN; http://www.aarbf.org.
§2900 Rocky Point Drive, Tampa, FL 33607; Shriners International Headquarters website: http://www.shrinershq.org; Shriners Hospitals for Children website: http://www.shriners.com/Hospitals/_Hospitals_for_Children.

Nursing Care Management

Protection from sunburn is the major goal of management, and the harmful effects of the sun on the delicate skin of infants and children are currently receiving increased attention. To protect skin exposed to the sun for extended periods, skin should be covered with clothing, and FDA-approved sun protection agents should be applied.

Two types of products are available for sun protection: **topical sunscreens,** which partially absorb UV light, and **sun blockers,** which block out UV rays by reflecting sunlight. The most frequently recommended sun blockers are zinc oxide and titanium dioxide ointments. Sunscreens are products containing an **SPF** based on evaluation of effectiveness against UV rays. The SPF is a number, such as 15, which indicates that if individuals normally burn in 10 minutes without a sunscreen, use of a sunscreen with SPF 15 allows them to remain in the sun 15 times 10, or 150 minutes (2½ hours) before acquiring the same degree of burns. The most effective sunscreens against UVB are **p-aminobenzoic acid (PABA)** and **PABA-esters.** However, many individuals are allergic to PABA, and sunscreens without PABA are encouraged to prevent these reactions in children.

Sunscreens are applied evenly to all exposed areas, with special attention to skinfolds and areas that might become exposed as clothing shifts. Parents are directed to read labels of sunscreen products carefully for the SPF and follow the manufacturer's directions for application.

> **NURSINGALERT**
>
> Sunscreens are not recommended for infants younger than 6 months of age. However, infants younger than 6 months of age may have sunscreen applied over small areas of skin such as the back of hands that may not be adequately covered by clothing when they are in the sun (American Academy of Pediatrics, 1999). Infants should be kept out of the sun or physically shaded from it. Fabric with a tight weave, such as cotton, offers good protection.

Individuals who work in the community, such as teachers, daycare workers, coaches, and youth-group leaders, and relatives, should all be made aware of sun safety for children. Sunscreens must be applied *liberally*.

COLD INJURY

Cold injuries are most commonly seen in very cold regions. The nature of the heat-regulating mechanisms of the body are such that the inner portion of the body, or core, produces heat, and the periphery, or outer area, conserves or dissipates heat. When the body attempts to conserve heat, the outer tissues are subjected to low temperatures, and local trauma may result.

Chilblain, redness and swelling of the skin, occurs when extremities, usually the hands, are exposed intermittently to temperatures of −1.1° to 15.5° C (30° to 60° F). The response may vary but is characterized by intense vasodilation that increases the temperature of involved tissues above that of unaffected tissue and produces edematous, reddish blue patches that itch and burn. As warming takes place, the sensations become more intense, but ordinarily they subside in a few days.

Frostbite is the term used to describe tissue damage caused when excessive heat loss to local tissues allows ice crystals to form in tissues. The frostbitten part appears white or blanched, feels solid, and is without sensation. Rapid rewarming is associated with less tissue necrosis than slow thawing. It restores blood flow and shortens the period of cellular damage. Rewarming produces a flush (sometimes deep purple) and a return of sensation, which is extremely painful. Large blisters may appear in 24 to 48 hours after rewarming and begin to reabsorb within 5 to 10 days, followed by the formation of a hard black eschar. Superficial injury often heals without incident. Rewarming is accomplished by immersing the part in well-agitated water at 37.8° to 42.2° C (100° to 108° F). Discomfort is managed with analgesics and sedatives. Care of blistered skin is similar to that described for burns. It is seldom possible to estimate the extent of tissue loss until new skin layers are revealed after the eschar layer separates.

KEY POINTS

- A variety of factors can produce lesions of the skin.
- It is important for nurses to be able to describe skin lesions accurately.
- The process of wound healing consists of hemostasis, inflammation, proliferation, and remodeling.
- A moist environment promotes wound healing.
- Bacterial, viral, and fungal infections are common in childhood.
- Some skin diseases are transmitted by arthropod vectors, especially ticks.
- The most common skin infestations of childhood—scabies and pediculosis capitis—affect children of any age and from any social class.
- Contact dermatitis may involve a primary irritant or a sensitizing agent.
- Adverse reactions to drugs are manifested more often in the skin than in any other body organ.
- The most common skin disorders of infancy are diaper dermatitis, seborrheic dermatitis, and AD.
- Acne, a disorder affecting many adolescents, is related to hormonal fluctuation, stimulation of the sebaceous glands, excessive sebum production, the formation of comedones, and the overgrowth of the *P. acnes* organism.
- Medication and gentle facial cleansing are the treatments of choice for acne.
- Burns are caused by thermal, chemical, electric, or radioactive agents.
- Burns are assessed on the extent, depth, and severity of the wound.

- Essentials of emergency care of burn injury include stopping the burning process, covering the burn, transporting the injured child to medical aid, and providing reassurance to the child and family.
- Management of minor burns consists of facilitating wound healing, relieving discomfort, and preventing complications.
- Management of major burns consists of facilitating wound healing, relieving discomfort, replacing destroyed skin, preventing or treating complications, and providing rehabilitation.
- Sunscreen is recommended for use when the skin is exposed to the damaging effects of the sun's rays.
- Thermal injuries to the skin can result from exposure to extreme cold.

answers to CRITICAL THINKING EXERCISE

POISON IVY

1. Yes, there are sufficient data to determine an effective intervention.
2. a. The leaves and stems of the poison ivy plant contain urushiol, an oil, that produces an immune reaction in the skin.
   b. When urushiol comes in contact with the skin, it penetrates the epidermis and bonds with the dermal layer. After about 2 days, localized, oozing, and painful impetiginous lesions are produced in the skin.
   c. When a child has contact with any part of the poison ivy plant, the skin areas should be immediately flushed with cold running water to neutralize the urushiol, and calamine lotion should be applied. Clothing that has come in contact with the plant should be removed and thoroughly laundered in hot water and detergent.
   d. Harsh soap is contraindicated because it removes the protective skin oils and dilutes the urushiol, allowing it to spread; hard scrubbing irritates the skin.
3. The most important immediate intervention is to rinse Billy's hands in cool water and apply calamine lotion. Because Billy's camp is near a stream, he can enter the water where it is shallow, and allow the water to rinse the oil of the poison ivy from his hands and clothes. The leaves should not be burned because contact with the smoke can cause a skin reaction and is also dangerous to the lungs if it is inhaled. Billy's clothes should be washed in hot water with detergent. Poison ivy lesions are not contagious, so the camp nurse should tell Billy's cabin mates that they will not "catch" his poison ivy.
4. Yes, the evidence supports these interventions.
5. The camp nurse should have realized she should have taught young campers and the adolescent assistants to recognize common hazardous plants, insects, and ticks found in the outdoor environment; strategies to prevent contact with these agents; and first aid measures to implement if contact does occur.

REFERENCES

American Academy of Pediatrics, Committee on Infectious Diseases, Pickering L, editor: *Red book: 2006 report of the Committee on Infectious Diseases,* ed 27, Elk Grove Village, Ill, 2006, The Academy.

American Academy of Pediatrics, Committee on Environmental Health: Ultraviolet light: a hazard to children, *Pediatrics* 104(2):328-333, 1999.

American Academy of Dermatology: *Acne,* 2006, retrieved Feb 1, 2007, from http://www.aad.org/public/Publications/pamphlets/Acne.htm.

American Academy of Dermatology: *Guidelines for the care of atopic dermatitis,* 2003, retrieved Feb 2, 2007, from http://www.aad.org/professionals/guidelines/AtopicDermatitis.htm.

Annequin D, Carbajal R, Chauvin P, and others: Fixed 50% nitrous oxide oxygen mixture for painful procedures: a French survey, *Pediatrics* 105(4):E47, 2000.

Arnoldo B, Klein M, Gibran NS: Practice guidelines for the management of electrical injuries, *J Burn Care Res* 27(4):439-447, 2006.

Baker RAU, Zeller RA, Klein RL, and others: Burn wound itch control using H_1 and H_2 antagonists, *J Burn Care Rehabil* 22(4):263-268, 2001.

Bernardo LM, Gardner MJ, O'Connor J, and others: Dog bites in children treated in a pediatric emergency department, *J Spect Pediatr Nurs* 5(2):87-95, 2000.

Burkhart CN, Specht K, Neckers D: Synergistic activity of benzoyl peroxide and erythromycin, *Skin Pharmacol Appl Skin Physiol* 13(5):292-296, 2000.

Centers for Disease Control and Prevention, Division of Parasitic Diseases: *Scabies,* Feb 4, 2008, retrieved April 22, 2008, from http://www.cdc.gov/ncidod/dpd/parasites/scabies/factsht_scabies.htm.

Centers for Disease Control and Prevention, Division of Parasitic Diseases: *Treating head lice infestation,* Aug 19, 2005, retrieved April 22, 2008, from http://www.cdc.gov/ncidod/dpd/parasites/lice/factsht_head_lice_treating.htm.

Centers for Disease Control and Prevention: Nonfatal dog bite–related injuries treated in hospital emergency departments—United States, 2001, *MMWR* 52(26):605-610, 2003.

Centers for Disease Control and Prevention: Cat-scratch disease in children—Texas, September 2000–August 2001, *MMWR* 51(10):212-214, 2002.

Food and Drug Administration: FDA issues health advisory regarding labeling changes for lindane products, April 2003, *HealthInfo Tx Rep,* retrieved March 4, 2007, from http://www.fda.gov/bbs/topics/ANSWERS/2003/ANS01205.html.

Goates BM, Atkin JS, Wilding KG, and others: An effective nonchemical treatment for head lice: a lot of hot air, *Pediatrics* 188(5):1962-1970, 2006.

Frankowski BL, Weiner LB: Head lice, *Pediatrics* 110(3):638-643, 2002.

Herndon DN, editor: *Total burn care,* ed 3, London, 2007, Saunders.

Jacobs DG, Deutsch NL, Brewer M: Suicide, depression, and isotretinoin: is there a causal link? *J Am Acad Dermatol* 45(5):S168-S175, 2001.

Kaplan SL: Community-acquired methicillin-resistant *Staphylococcus aureus* infections in children, *Semin Pediatr Infect Dis* 17(3):113-119, 2006.

Krasner DL, Rodeheaver GT, Sibbald RG: *Chronic wound care: a clinical source book for healthcare professionals,* ed 3, Wayne, Penn, 2001, HMP Communications.

Kronemyer B: Scratching the surface of atopic and contact dermatitis, *Infect Dis Child* 16(3):40, 2003.

Laude TA: Acne in childhood and adolescence: update on treatment choices, *Consultant* 3:457-465, 2000.

Lee MC, Rios Am, Aten MF, and others: Management and outcome of children with skin and soft tissue abscesses caused by community-acquired methicillin-resistant *Staphylococcus aureus, Pediatr Infect Dis J* 23(2):123-127, 2004.

Mancini AJ: Acne vulgaris: a treatment update, *Contemp Pediatr* 17(12):122-133, 2000.

McCord SS, Levy ML: Practical guide to pediatric wound care, *Semin Plast Surg* 20(3):92-199, 2006.

Mumcuoglu KY, Barker SC, Burgess IE, and others: International guidelines for effective control of head louse infestations, *J Drugs Dermatol* 6(4):409-414, 2007.

Pearlman DL: A simple treatment for head lice: dry on, suffocation based pediculicide, *Pediatrics* 114(3):e275-e279, 2004.

Purdue GF: American Burn Association presidential address 2006 on nutrition: yesterday, today, and tomorrow, *J Burn Care Res* 28(1):1-5, 2007.

Russell JJ: Topical therapy for acne, *Am Fam Physician* 61(2):357-366, 2000.

Strong M, Johnstone PW: Interventions for treating scabies, *Cochrane Database Syst Rev* 18(3):CD 000320, 2008.

Wade CF: Keeping Lyme disease at bay: an integrated approach to prevention, *Am J Nurs* 100(7):26-31, 2000.

Wormser GP, Dattwyler RJ, Shapiro ED, and others: The clinical assessment, treatment, and prevention of Lyme disease, human granulocytic anaplasmosis, and babesiosis: clinical practice guidelines by the Infections Diseases Society of America, *Clin Infect Dis* 43:1089-1134, 2006.

Yetman RJ, Parks D: Diagnosis and management of atopic dermatitis, *J Pediatr Health Care* 16(3):143-145, 2002.

The Child with Musculoskeletal or Articular Dysfunction

DAVID WILSON, MARTHA R. CURRY, AND MARILYN J. HOCKENBERRY

CHAPTER OUTLINE

THE IMMOBILIZED CHILD, 1107
Immobilization, 1107
  Physiologic Effects of Immobilization, 1107
  Psychologic Effects of Immobilization, 1108
  Effect on Families, 1109
TRAUMATIC INJURY, 1110
Soft-Tissue Injury, 1110
  Contusions, 1110
  Dislocations, 1111
  Sprains, 1111
  Strains, 1112
Fractures, 1112
  Epiphyseal (or Physeal) Injuries, 1112
  Types of Fractures, 1112
  Bone Healing and Remodeling, 1113
The Child in a Cast, 1115
  The Cast, 1115

The Child in Traction, 1117
  Purposes of Traction, 1117
  Types of Traction (General), 1118
  Upper Extremity Traction, 1118
  Lower Extremity Traction, 1118
  Cervical Traction, 1119
Distraction, 1121
  External Fixation, 1121
Amputation, 1121
CONGENITAL DEFECTS, 1122
Developmental Dysplasia
  of the Hip, 1122
Congenital Clubfoot, 1125
Metatarsus Adductus (Varus), 1126
Skeletal Limb Deficiency, 1127
Osteogenesis Imperfecta, 1127
ACQUIRED DEFECTS, 1128
Legg-Calvé-Perthes Disease, 1128

Slipped Capital Femoral Epiphysis, 1130
Kyphosis and Lordosis, 1130
Idiopathic Scoliosis, 1130
**INFECTIONS OF BONES
AND JOINTS, 1134**
Osteomyelitis, 1134
Septic Arthritis, 1135
Skeletal Tuberculosis, 1135
BONE AND SOFT-TISSUE TUMORS, 1136
General Concepts: Bone Tumors, 1136
Osteosarcoma, 1136
Ewing Sarcoma (Primitive
  Neuroectodermal Tumor), 1137
Rhabdomyosarcoma, 1138
DISORDERS OF JOINTS, 1139
Juvenile Idiopathic Arthritis (Juvenile
  Rheumatoid Arthritis), 1139
Systemic Lupus Erythematosus, 1142

LEARNING OBJECTIVES

On completion of this chapter the reader will be able to:

- Outline a care plan for a child immobilized with an injury or a degenerative disease.
- Develop a teaching plan for the parents of a child in a cast.
- Explain the functions of the various types of traction.

- Devise a nursing care plan for a child in traction.
- Differentiate among the various congenital skeletal defects.
- Design a teaching plan for the parents of a child with a congenital skeletal deformity.
- Describe the therapies and nursing care of a child with scoliosis.

- Outline a care plan for a child with osteomyelitis.
- Differentiate between osteosarcoma and Ewing sarcoma.
- Describe the nursing care of a child with juvenile idiopathic arthritis.
- Demonstrate an understanding of the management of a child with systemic lupus erythematosus.

RELATED TOPICS and ADDITIONAL RESOURCES

 IN TEXT

Childhood Morbidity, *Ch. 1*
Compliance, *Ch. 22*
Family-Centered Care of the Child During
    Illness and Hospitalization, *Ch. 21*
Injury Prevention: Infant, *Ch. 10;* Toddler,
    Ch. 12; Preschooler, *Ch. 13;* School-Age
    Child, *Ch. 15;* Adolescent, *Ch. 16*
Pain Assessment; Pain Management, *Ch. 7*
Physical Examination: Back and Extremities,
    Ch. 6
Preparation for Diagnostic and Therapeutic
    Procedures, *Ch. 22*
Surgical Procedures, *Ch. 22*

 COMPANION CD

Animations—Bone Fractures; Spine
    Structure
Case Studies—Fractures; Osteomyelitis;
    Developmental Dysplasia of the Hip
Critical Thinking Exercise—Osteogenic
    Sarcoma
NCLEX Review Questions
Pediatric Assessment Video Clip

 evolve

evolve.elsevier.com/Wong/essentials/

Critical Thinking Case Studies—Legg-Calvé-
    Perthes Disease; Scoliosis
NCLEX Review Questions
Pediatric Assessment Video Clip
Skill—Monitoring Neurovascular Status
WebLinks

**WONG'S CLINICAL MANUAL
OF PEDIATRIC NURSING, 7th Ed**

Patient and Family Education—Giving
    Nasogastric Tube Feedings, *p. 549;* Giving
    Gastrostomy Feedings, *p. 551;* Caring for
    the Child in a Cast, *p. 517;* Caring for an
    Intermittent Infusion Device, *p. 531*
Nursing Care Plan—The Child with Cancer,
    p. 480

THE IMMOBILIZED CHILD

IMMOBILIZATION

One of the most difficult aspects of illness in children is the immobility it imposes. Children by nature are usually active, and immobility, however temporary, may have lasting effects on the child's developmental progress. The most frequent reasons for immobility are congenital defects (e.g., spina bifida, arthrogryposis [a generalized immobility of the joints]); degenerative disorders (e.g., muscular dystrophy); and infections or injuries that impair the integumentary system (e.g., severe burns), the musculoskeletal system (e.g., multiple fractures, osteomyelitis), or the neurologic system (e.g., spinal cord injury, polyneuritis, head injury). At times therapies such as traction and spinal fusion are responsible for prolonged immobilization, although the increasing trends in health care are early mobilization and discharge and outpatient treatment.

Physiologic Effects of Immobilization

Many clinical studies, including space program research, have documented predictable consequences that occur after immobilization and the absence of gravitational force. Functional and metabolic responses to restricted movement can be noted in most of the body systems. Each has a direct influence on the child's growth and development because homeostatic mechanisms thrive on normal use and need feedback to maintain dynamic equilibrium. Inactivity leads to a decrease in the functional capabilities of the whole body as dramatically as the lack of physical exercise leads to muscle weakness.

Disuse from illness, injury, or a sedentary lifestyle can limit function and potentially delay age-appropriate milestones. Most of the pathologic changes that occur during immobilization arise from decreased muscle strength and mass, decreased metabolism, and bone demineralization, which are closely interrelated, with one change leading to or affecting the others. Some results of immobilization are primary and produce a direct effect; other pathophysiologic consequences occur frequently but seem to be more indirect and are therefore secondary effects. Many pathophysiologic changes affect more than one body system, with the primary or secondary effect being demonstrated in both systems.

The major effects of immobilization are outlined briefly in Table 31-1 and are related directly or indirectly to decreased muscle activity, which produces numerous primary changes in the musculoskeletal system with secondary alterations in the cardiovascular, respiratory, metabolic, and renal systems. The musculoskeletal changes that occur during disuse are a result of alterations in the effect of gravity and stress on the muscles, joints, and bones. Muscle disuse leads to tissue breakdown and loss of muscle mass (**atrophy**). Muscle atrophy causes decreased strength and endurance, which may take weeks or months to restore.

During immobilization a **joint contracture** begins when the arrangement of collagen, the main structural protein of connective tissues, is altered, resulting in a denser tissue that does not glide as easily. Eventually muscles, tendons, and ligaments can shorten and reduce joint movement, ultimately producing contractures that restrict function. The daily stresses on bone created by motion and weight bearing maintain the balance between bone formation (osteoblastic activity) and bone resorption (osteoclastic activity). During immobilization, increased calcium leaves the bone, causing osteopenia (demineralization of the bones), which may predispose bone to pathologic fractures.

The major musculoskeletal consequences of immobilization are:

▪ Significant decrease in muscle size, strength, and endurance
▪ Bone demineralization leading to osteoporosis
▪ Contractures and decreased joint mobility.

The larger the portion of the body immobilized and the longer the immobilization, the greater the hazards of immobility.

BOX 31-2
Clinical Manifestations of a Fracture

Signs of injury:
- Generalized swelling
- Pain or tenderness
- Deformity
- Diminished functional use of affected limb or digit

May also demonstrate:
- Bruising
- Severe muscular rigidity
- Crepitus (grating sensation at fracture site)

emergencytreatment

Fracture

Assess the extent of injury—5 *P*'s:
1. Pain and point of tenderness
2. Pulse—Pulse distal to the fracture site
3. Pallor
4. Paresthesia—Sensation distal to the fracture site
5. Paralysis—Movement distal to the fracture site

Determine the mechanism of injury.

Move the injured part as little as possible.

Cover open wounds with a sterile or clean dressing.

Immobilize the limb, including joints above and below the fracture site; do not attempt to reduce the fracture or push protruding bone under the skin.

Use a soft splint (pillow or folded towel) or rigid splint (rolled newspaper or magazine).

Uninjured leg can serve as a splint for a leg fracture if no splint is available.

Reassess neurovascular status.

Apply traction if circulatory compromise is present.

Elevate the injured limb if possible.

Apply cold to the injured area.

Call emergency medical services or transport to medical facility.

Therapeutic Management

The majority of children's fractures heal well, and nonunion is rare. Most fractures are readily reduced by simple traction and immobilization until healing takes place. However, the position of the bone fragments in relation to one another influences the rapidity of healing and the residual deformity. Healing is prompt and complete with end-to-end apposition, but a gap between fragments delays (or prevents) healing. The goals of fracture management are the following:

- To regain alignment and length of the bony fragments (reduction)
- To retain alignment and length (immobilization)
- To restore function to the injured parts
- To prevent further injury

Children with displaced fractures may have immediate reduction and internal fixation with intramedullary nails rather than being immobilized by traction. This practice is more common and holds true for all types of fractures, including femur fractures. The use of traction for fractures in children does vary by institution. The child's natural tendency to be active is usually sufficient to restore normal mobility, and physical therapy is rarely needed.

Children are most frequently hospitalized for fractures of the femur and the supracondylar area of the distal humerus, which may require internal fixation and pinning; displaced supracondylar fractures in children should be treated surgically (Do and Herrera-Soto, 2003). Fractures of the humerus, which usually result from a fall with the arm in extension, frequently involve the supracondylar portion. These fractures especially place the patient at risk for nerve damage and angulation deformities; therefore most children with a fractured humerus are taken to surgery for either a closed or open reduction with a percutaneous pinning of the fractured bone segments. Preoperatively the fracture is reduced with adequate analgesia and a temporary splint for immobilization.

If simple reductions cannot be achieved or if a neurovascular problem is detected after injury, observation in a hospital is indicated. Severe contusions with profound swelling cannot be treated with a cast, which would act as a tourniquet on the extremity. A badly malaligned fracture may require traction for a period before a cast is applied.

Wrist buckle fractures are common in a child who falls and extends the arm forward to break the fall. There are reports of radius and/or ulna buckle fractures in children treated with a removable splint for 3 to 4 weeks instead of a short arm cast (Plint, Perry, Correll, and others, 2006). The children treated with removable splints had better wrist function, had adequate bone healing, and experienced less inconvenience for bathing compared with the group of children placed in a short arm cast.

The major methods for immobilizing a fracture, casting and traction, are described later.

Nursing Care Management

Nurses are frequently the persons who make the initial assessment of a child with a suspected fracture (see Emergency Treatment box). The child and parents may be frightened and upset, and the child is often in pain. Therefore, if the child is alert and there is no evidence of hemorrhage, the initial nursing interventions are directed toward calming and reassuring the child and parents so that a more extensive assessment can be more easily accomplished.

While remaining calm and speaking in a quiet voice, the nurse can ask the parents and older child to describe what happened. The child may arrive with the limb supported in some manner; if not, careful support or immobilization may be provided to the affected site. In the event that the limb is supported or immobilized, it may be best not to touch the child but to ask him or her to point to the painful area and to wiggle the fingers or toes. By this time the child may feel relatively safe and will allow someone to gently touch the area just enough to feel the pulses and test for sensation. A child's anxiety is greatly influenced by previous experiences with injury and with health personnel. However, he or she needs to be told what will happen and what to do to help. The affected limb need not be palpated, and it should not be moved unless properly splinted. If the child is at home or if the practitioner is not present to examine the child, some type of splint is applied carefully for transport to the medical facility. Parental anxiety may be heightened by the child's pain reaction and fear, and possibly by other events surrounding the accident; thus it is important to communicate to the parent that the child will receive the necessary care, including pain management.

> **NURSINGALERT**
>
> The five P's of ischemia from a vascular injury should be included in an assessment of the injury:
> 1. Pain
> 2. Pallor
> 3. Pulselessness
> 4. Paresthesia
> 5. Paralysis

THE CHILD IN A CAST

The completeness of the fracture, the type of bone involved, and the amount of weight bearing influence how much of the extremity must be included in the cast to immobilize the fracture site completely. In most cases the joints above and below the fracture are immobilized to eliminate the possibility of movement that might cause displacement at the fracture site. Four major categories of casts are used for fractures: **upper extremity** to immobilize the wrist or elbow, **lower extremity** to immobilize the ankle or knee, **spinal** and **cervical** to immobilize the spine, and **spica casts** to immobilize the hip and knee.

The Cast

Casts are constructed from gauze strips and bandages impregnated with plaster of paris or, more commonly, from synthetic lighter weight and water-resistant materials (e.g., fiberglass and polyurethane resin).

Both types of casting produce heat from chemical reaction activated by water immediately after application. Plaster casts mold closely to the body part, take 10 to 72 hours to dry, have a smooth exterior, and are inexpensive. The newer synthetic casting material is lighter, dries in 5 to 30 minutes, permits earlier weight bearing, and is water resistant. The disadvantage of synthetic casting is its inability to mold closely to body parts; its rough exterior, which may scratch surfaces; and increased cost.

Synthetic casts have special advantages for children. They come in different colors and with designs (e.g., cartoons, stripes); and they are lightweight, durable, easy to clean, and relatively water resistant, depending on the type of inner lining used; only those with a Gore-Tex inner lining may be immersed in water without affecting the cast integrity. Bathing with a synthetic cast may be accomplished by covering the cast with a plastic bag; if the synthetic cast gets wet, it should be dried thoroughly. One drawback to immersion is the time necessary to completely dry the cast and padding. Synthetic casts are difficult to write on; a waterproof marker or color markers may be used.

Cast Application. The child's developmental age should be considered before the cast is applied. For preschoolers who fear bodily harm and fantasize the loss of an extremity, it may be helpful to use a plastic doll or stuffed animal to explain the procedure beforehand. Toddlers and preschoolers do not have easily defined body boundaries; if an extremity is wrapped in a bandage, cast, or splint, to the young child the extremity ceases to exist. It is also helpful to explain that some synthetic cast material will become warm but will not burn. During the application of the cast, various distraction methods can be used, including discussing favorite pets or activities at school, blowing bubbles, and so forth. In this age-group explanations such as "This will help your arm get better" are futile because the child has no concept of causality.

Before the cast is applied, the extremities are checked for any abrasions, cuts, or other alterations in the skin surface and for the presence of rings or other items that might cause constriction from swelling; such objects are removed. A tube of cloth stockinette or Gore-Tex liner is stretched over the area to be casted, and bony prominences are padded with soft cotton sheeting. Dry rolls of casting material are immersed in a pail of water. The wet rolls are put on in a bandage fashion and molded to the extremity. During application of the plaster cast, the underlying stockinette is pulled over the rough edges of the cast and secured with a layer of wet plaster 1.25 to 2.5 cm (0.5 to 1 inch) below the rim to form a smooth, padded edge to protect the skin.

If the practitioner does not form such a protective edge with stockinette, the rough edges of the plaster cast can be protected by a "petaled" edge. Small pieces approximately 5 to 7.5 cm (2 to 3 inches) long are cut from 2.5- or 3.8-cm (1- or 1.5-inch) wide adhesive tape or moleskin. The edges are rounded with scissors, and these "petals" are placed over the edge of the cast, with each petal slightly overlapping the previous petal to form a smooth, neat edge. It is easier to apply the petal to the underside of the cast first and then bring the loose edge to the front, pressing firmly so that the edges remain securely attached. Synthetic casts usually do not require additional padding on the edges, since they do not crack like plaster material might. However, the padding minimizes irritation and abrasions from the rough edges of the cast.

Nursing Care Management

The complete evaporation of the water from a hip spica cast can take 24 to 48 hours when older types of plaster materials are used. Drying occurs within minutes with fiberglass cast material. The cast must remain uncovered to allow it to dry from the inside out. Turning the child in a plaster cast at least every 2 hours will help to dry a body cast evenly and prevent complications related to immobility. A regular fan or cool-air hair dryer to circulate air may be helpful when the humidity is high.

> **NURSINGALERT**
>
> Heated fans or dryers are not used because they cause the cast to dry on the outside and remain wet beneath or cause burns from heat conduction by way of the cast to the underlying tissue.

A wet plaster cast should be supported by a pillow that is covered with plastic and handled by the palms of the hands to prevent indenting the cast, which can create pressure areas. A dry plaster-of-paris cast produces a hollow sound when it is tapped with the finger. If "hot spots" are felt on the cast surface (usually indicating infection beneath the area), this should be reported so that a window can be made in the cast to observe the site.

During the first few hours after a cast is applied, the chief concern is that the extremity may continue to swell to the extent that the cast becomes a tourniquet, shutting off circulation and producing neurovascular complications. To reduce the likelihood of this potential problem, the body part can be elevated, thereby increasing venous return. If edema is excessive, casts are bivalved (i.e., cut to make anterior and posterior halves that are held together with an elastic bandage). The cast and the involved extremity are observed frequently for neurovascular integrity and any signs of compromise. Permanent muscle and tissue damage can occur within 6 to 8 hours.

> **NURSING ALERT**
>
> Observations such as pain (unrelieved by pain medication 1 hour after administration), swelling, discoloration (pallor or cyanosis) of the exposed portions, decreased pulses, decreased temperature, or the inability to move the distal exposed part(s) should be reported immediately.

When an extremity that has sustained an open fracture is casted, a window is often left over the wound area to allow for observation and dressing of the wound. A surgical reduction is usually casted as a closed fracture. For the first few hours after surgery, substantial bleeding may soak through the cast. Periodically the circumscribed bloodstained area should be outlined with a waterproof marker and the time indicated to provide a guide for assessing the amount of bleeding.

Usually the child is discharged to home care after a cast is applied in the emergency department or clinic. Parents need instructions on drying and caring for the plaster cast because it takes longer to dry. Instructions are also given for checking for signs and symptoms that indicate the cast is too tight (see

> ![Family-Centered Care icon] **FAMILY-CENTERED CARE**
>
> ### Cast Care
>
> Keep the casted extremity elevated on pillows or similar support for the first day, or as directed by the health professional.
> Avoid denting the plaster cast with fingertips (use palms of hand to handle) while it is still wet to avoid creating pressure points.
> Observe the extremities (fingers or toes) for any evidence of swelling or discoloration (darker or lighter than a comparable extremity), and contact the health professional if noted.
> Check movement and sensation of the visible extremities frequently.
> Follow health professional's orders regarding any restriction of activities.
> Restrict strenuous activities for the first few days.
> - Engage in quiet activities but encourage use of muscles.
> - Move the joints above and below the cast on the affected extremity.
>
> Encourage frequent rest for a few days, keeping the injured extremity elevated while resting.
> Avoid allowing the affected limb to hang in a dependent position for any length of time.
> - Keep an injured upper extremity elevated (e.g., in a sling) while upright.
> - Elevate a lower limb when sitting and avoid standing for too long.
>
> Do not allow the child to put anything inside the cast. Keep small items that might be placed inside the cast away from small children.
> Keep a clear path for ambulation. Remove toys, hazardous floor rugs, pets, or other items over which the child might stumble.
> Use crutches appropriately if lower limb fracture requires non–weight bearing on affected extremity.
> The crutches should fit properly, have a soft rubber tip to prevent slipping, and be well padded at the axilla.
> With crutch walking the child's body weight is supported on the hand grips, not the axilla.

Family-Centered Care box). Parents should also be told to take the child to the health professional for attention if the cast becomes too loose, since a loose cast no longer serves its purpose.

Nurses can help families adapt the child's home environment to meet the temporary encumbrance of a large cast or one that restricts the child's mobility (e.g., long leg cast). Home care creates problems of varying magnitudes, especially for children in large casts (e.g., a hip spica [Fig. 31-3]). Commonplace situations become problematic (e.g., transporting a child safely and comfortably in a car). Standard seat belts and car seats may not be readily adapted for use by children in some casts. Specially designed car seats and restraints are available that meet safety requirements.* Alterations to standard car seats to accommodate the cast are not recommended, since the structure may be adversely altered and fail to properly restrain the child.

Parents are taught the proper care of the cast (or orthotic device) and are helped to devise means for maintaining cleanliness. A superabsorbent disposable diaper is tucked beneath the entire perineal opening of the cast. A larger diaper can be applied and fastened over the small diaper and cast to hold the smaller diaper in place. In the event that the larger diaper becomes wet or soiled, it is likely the cast is as well.

For tightly fitting casts, transparent film dressings can be cut into strips as for petaling, and one edge applied to the cast edge and the other directly to the perineum; this forms a continuous, waterproof bridge between the perineum and the cast to prevent leakage. An additional advantage to the

---

*For information on specially adapted molded-plastic chairs for children who have spica casts, contact Britax Hippo by SnugSeat, (800) 336-7684, http://www.snugseat.com. The E-Z-On vest is a special safety harness for larger children with poor trunk control. Additional safety restraints and a listing of distributors are available from SafetyBeltSafe U.S.A., http://www.carseat.org; (800) 745-SAFE; Spanish: (800) 747-SANO.

FIG. 31-3 ■ Spica cast with hip abductor. Note casts on doll as well.

use of this transparent dressing is that it keeps both the skin and the cast dry while allowing for observation of skin beneath the dressing.

Older infants and small children may stuff bits of food, small toys, or other items under the cast; parents should be alerted to this possibility so that they can initiate suitable preventive measures.

Feeding the infant in a hip spica cast offers problems in positioning. Very young infants can be fed in the supine position with the head elevated. With the infant's hips and legs supported on a pillow at the side, the parent can cuddle the infant in his or her arms during feeding. A somewhat similar position can be used for breastfeeding (i.e., with the infant supported on pillows or held in a "football" hold facing the mother with the legs behind her). An alternate position is to hold the infant upright on the caregiver's lap with the legs of the infant astride the adult's leg.

Children in spica casts usually find the prone position easier for self-feeding from a small table placed next to the dining table; alternatively, they may manage a semisitting position in bed or in a wheelchair (see Fig. 31-3). The use of a conventional toilet is almost impossible. A bedside toilet can be adapted for use. Small bedpans or other containers offer alternatives for elimination. The nurse may suggest waterproofing methods, by devising plastic wraps, for elimination and showers. Baths are possible only if the plaster cast is kept out of the water and covered to prevent it from becoming wet.

Cast Removal. Cutting the cast to remove it or to relieve tightness is frequently a frightening experience for children. They fear the sound of the cast cutter and are terrified that their flesh, as well as the cast, will be cut. The oscillating blade vibrates rapidly back and forth and will not cut when placed *lightly* on the skin. Children have described it as producing a

FIG. 31-4 ■ Young children usually adapt well to a cast but often fear the removal.

"tickly" sensation. The vibration also generates heat that may be felt by the child. Both these feelings should be explained.

Preparation for the procedure will help reduce anxiety, especially if a trusting relationship has been established between the child and the nurse. Many young children come to regard the cast as part of themselves, which intensifies their fear of removal (Fig. 31-4). They need continual reassurance that all is going well and that their behavior is accepted. After the cast is removed, the parents and child should be given the option of keeping the cast; it may be placed in a plastic bag because of the usual odor. If the cast has been in place for a lengthy period, decreased muscle mass will be noted. The child should be reassured that resuming exercise and routine activities will return function and appearance (provided there was no significant trauma beforehand).

After the cast is removed, the skin surface will be caked with desquamated skin and sebaceous secretions. Simple soaking in a bathtub is usually sufficient for their removal, but it may take several days to eliminate the accumulation completely. Application of oil or lotion may provide comfort. The parents and child should be instructed not to pull or forcibly remove this material with vigorous scrubbing, since it may cause excoriation and bleeding.

THE CHILD IN TRACTION

The ever-changing health care arena has witnessed the demise of many long-term treatments involving lengthy hospitalization; one such change is in the area of traction. Most balanced skeletal traction is applied in children after a severe or complex injury to allow physiologic stability, align bone fragments, and permit closer evaluation of the injured site. Newer technology has produced orthopedic fixation devices that allow partial or full mobility, thus preventing long-term immobilization and its consequences. In many situations, surgical intervention may be carried out within a matter of days; therefore skeletal traction devices described herein may be used infrequently in pediatrics.

Purposes of Traction

The six primary purposes of traction for reduction of fractures are:

1. To fatigue the involved muscles and reduce muscle spasm so that bones can be realigned
2. To position the distal and proximal bone ends in desired realignment to promote satisfactory bone healing
3. To immobilize the fracture site until realignment has been achieved and sufficient healing has taken place to permit casting or splinting
4. To help prevent or improve contracture deformity
5. To provide immobilization of specific areas of the body
6. To reduce muscle spasms (rare in children)

The three essential components of traction management are traction, countertraction, and friction (Fig. 31-5). To reduce or realign a fracture site, **traction** (forward force) is produced by attaching weight to the distal bone fragment; body weight provides **countertraction** (backward force); and the patient's contact with the bed constitutes the **frictional** force. These forces are used to align the distal and proximal bone fragments by adjusting the line of pull upward or downward and adducting or abducting the extremity.

To attain equilibrium, the amount of forward force is adjusted by adding weight to or subtracting weight from the traction, or countertraction can be increased by elevating the

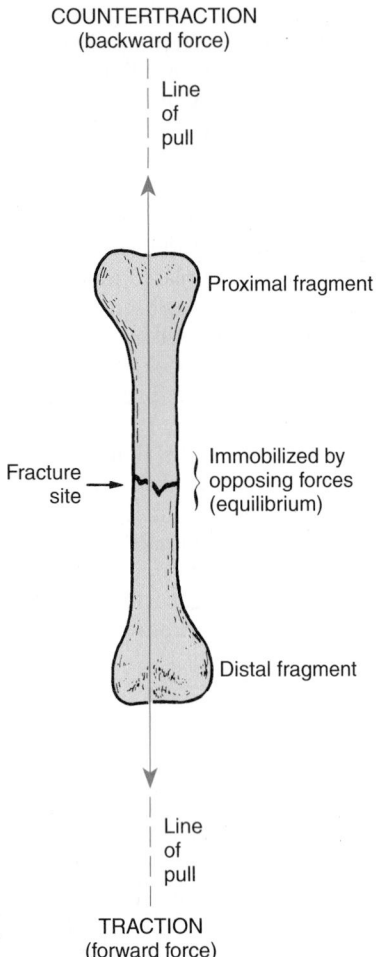

COUNTERTRACTION
(backward force)

Line
of
pull

Proximal fragment

Fracture
site

Immobilized by
opposing forces
(equilibrium)

Distal fragment

Line
of
pull

TRACTION
(forward force)

FIG. 31-5 ■ Application of traction to maintain bone alignment.

foot of the bed to create a greater gravitational pull to the backward force.

The **all-or-none law,** characteristic of muscle contractibility, influences the complete relaxation. When muscles are stretched, muscle spasm ceases, which permits the realignment of the bone ends. The continuous maintenance of traction is important during this phase because releasing the traction allows the muscle's normal contracting ability to again cause a malpositioning of the bone ends.

The realignment of the fragments is a gradual process that is achieved more rapidly in infants, who have limited muscle tone, than in muscular teenagers. The desired line of pull and callus formation are checked periodically by radiographic examination. The traction pull to some degree immobilizes the fracture site; however, adjunctive immobilizing devices such as splints or casts are sometimes used with skeletal traction. Immobilization with traction will be maintained until the bone ends are in satisfactory realignment, after which a less confining type of immobilization—a cast, pins, or external stabilization device—will be applied.

Types of Traction (General)

The pull needed for traction can be applied to the distal bone fragment in several ways (Box 31-3). The type of traction applied is determined primarily by the child's age, the condition

of the soft tissues, and the type and degree of displacement of the fracture. Fractures most commonly treated by application of traction are those involving the femur and vertebrae. The major types of traction for specific fractures are briefly discussed in the following sections.

Upper Extremity Traction

The use of upper extremity traction in children is uncommon. Newer surgical techniques allow for early mobilization and optimal results without traction. Nursing care of the child with upper extremity traction is the same as that for lower extremity traction, which is discussed below.

Lower Extremity Traction

The frequent site for a femoral fracture is in the middle third of the shaft. With this fracture there may be significant overriding but minimal displacement. In a fracture in the lower third of the shaft, the pull of the gastrocnemius muscle causes the distal fragment to become downwardly displaced.

Fractures of the femur can often be reduced with immediate application of a hip spica cast in young children. When traction is required, several types may be used, based on the initial assessment.

Bryant traction is a type of running traction in which the pull is in only one direction. Skin traction is applied to the legs, which are flexed at a 90-degree angle at the hips. The child's trunk (with buttocks raised slightly off the bed) provides countertraction.

Buck extension (Fig. 31-6) is a type of traction with the legs in an extended position. Except for fracture cases, turning from side to side with care is permitted to maintain the involved leg in alignment. Buck extension is used primarily for short-term immobilization, preoperatively with dislocated hips, for correcting contractures, or for bone deformities such as Legg-Calvé-Perthes disease. Buck traction may be accomplished with either skin straps or a special foam boot designed for traction.

Russell traction uses skin traction on the lower leg and a padded sling under the knee. Two lines of pull, one along the longitudinal line of the lower leg and one perpendicular to the leg, are produced. This combination of pulls allows realignment of the lower extremity and immobilizes the hip and knee in a flexed position. The hip flexion must be kept at the prescribed angle to prevent fracture malalignment, since there is no direct support under the fracture and the skin traction may

FIG. 31-6 ■ Buck extension traction. (Redrawn from Hilt NE, Schmitt EW: *Pediatric orthopedic nursing*, St Louis, 1975, Mosby.)

FIG. 31-7 ■ Ninety-ninety traction. (Redrawn from Hilt NE, Schmitt EW: *Pediatric orthopedic nursing*, St Louis, 1975, Mosby.)

FIG. 31-8 ■ **A,** Halo vest. **B,** Crutchfield tong traction. (**B,** Redrawn from Hilt NE, Schmitt EW: *Pediatric orthopedic nursing*, St Louis, 1975, Mosby.)

slip. Special nursing measures include carefully checking the position of the traction so that the amount of desired hip flexion is maintained and damage to the common peroneal nerve under the knee does not produce footdrop.

A common skeletal traction is 90-degree–90-degree traction (90-90 traction). The lower leg is supported by a boot cast or a calf sling, and a skeletal Steinmann pin or Kirschner wire is placed in the distal fragment of the femur, resulting in a 90-degree angle at both the hip and the knee (Fig. 31-7). From a nursing standpoint, this traction facilitates position changes, toileting, and prevention of complications related to traction.

Balanced suspension traction may be used with or without skin or skeletal traction. Unless used with another traction, the balanced suspension merely suspends the leg in a desired flexed position to relax the hip and hamstring muscles and does not exert any traction directly on a body part. A **Thomas splint** extends from the groin to midair above the foot, and a **Pearson attachment** supports the lower leg. Towels or pieces of felt covered with stockinette are clipped or pinned to the splints for leg support. When the child is lifted off the bed, the traction lifts with the child without loss of alignment. This traction requires careful checking of splints and ropes to make certain that no slippage or fraying has occurred. The traction is of great value in an older and heavier child when it is essential to lift the patient for care.

Cervical Traction

The cervical area is a vulnerable site for flexion or extension injuries to muscle, vertebrae, or the spinal cord. Cervical muscle trauma without other complications is treated with a cervical hard collar to relieve the weight of the head from the fracture site. When a child displaces or fractures a cervical vertebra, it may be necessary to reduce and immobilize the site with cervical skeletal traction. The spinal cord runs through the intravertebral canal, and dislocation or fracture of the ver-

tebrae can also cause spinal cord injury. Nursing assessment of neurologic function is essential to prevent further injury during the application and use of cervical skeletal traction.

Most cervical traction is accomplished with the use of a **halo brace** or **halo vest** (Fig. 31-8, *A*). This device consists of a steel halo attached to the head by four screws inserted into the outer skull; several rigid bars connect the halo to a vest that is worn around the chest, thus providing greater mobility of the rest of the body while avoiding cervical spinal motion altogether. If the injury has been limited to a vertebral fracture without neurologic deficit, a halo brace can be applied to permit earlier ambulation.

Cervical traction may also be accomplished by the insertion of **Crutchfield, Barton,** or **Gardner-Wells tongs** through burr holes in the skull, with weights attached to the hyperextended head (Fig. 31-8, *B*). As the neck muscles fatigue with constant traction pull, the vertebral bodies gradually separate so that the cord is no longer pinched between the vertebrae. Immobilization until fracture healing or surgical fixation can occur is an essential goal of cervical traction.

Nursing Care Management

To assess the child in traction, it is essential to know the purpose for which the traction is applied and to understand the basic principles of traction. Regular assessment of both the child and the traction apparatus is required (see Nursing Care Guidelines box). Many of the nursing problems associated with a child in traction are related to immobility. Modifying the child's diet, encouraging fluids, and offering a mild laxative may be necessary to prevent constipation.

When indicated by the attending practitioner, the nurse may remove nonadhesive skin traction. In these cases intermittent traction is periodically released and reapplied as ordered. A child may have several types of traction at one time, and each one must be assessed separately to avoid problems.

> **NURSING ALERT**
>
> Skeletal traction is never released by the nurse (except under direct supervision by the practitioner). This precaution includes not lifting the weights that are applying traction (e.g., for moving the child in bed, for repositioning).

In addition to routine skin observation and care, the child in skeletal traction will need special skin care at the pin site

nursingcareguidelines

Traction Care

UNDERSTAND THERAPY

Understand purpose of traction.

Understand function of traction in each specific situation.

MAINTAIN TRACTION

Check desired line of pull and relationship of distal fragment to proximal fragment. Check whether fragment is being directed upward, adducted, or abducted.

Check function of each component:

- Position of bandages, frames, splints, specialized boot
- Ropes—In center track of pulley, taut, no fraying, knots tied securely
- Pulleys—In original position on attachment bar; have not slid from original site; wheels freely movable
- Weights—Correct amount of weight, hanging freely, in safe location

Check bed position—Head or foot elevated as directed for desired amount of pull and countertraction.

Do not remove skeletal traction or adhesive traction straps on skin traction.

MAINTAIN ALIGNMENT

Observe for correct body alignment with emphasis on alignment of shoulder, hip, and leg.

Check after child has moved.

Maintain correct angles at joints.

SKIN TRACTION

Replace nonadhesive straps or elastic bandage on skin traction *when permitted* or absolutely necessary, but make certain that traction on limb is maintained by someone during procedure.

Assess straps or bandages to ascertain if they are correctly applied (diagonal or spiral) and not too loose or too tight, which could cause slippage and malalignment of traction.

Assess traction boot to ensure it has not slipped and is not causing compression of the foot, thus impairing the circulation.

SKELETAL TRACTION

Check pin sites frequently for signs of bleeding, inflammation, or infection.

Cleanse and dress pin sites per institution protocol or as ordered.

Apply topical antiseptic or antibiotic to pin sites daily as ordered.

Cover ends of pins with protective rubber or padding to prevent child's being scratched by pin.

Note pull of traction on pin; pull should be even.

Check pin screws to be certain that screws are tight in metal clamp that attaches traction apparatus to pin.

PREVENT SKIN BREAKDOWN

Provide alternating-pressure mattress underneath hips and back.

Make total-body skin checks for redness or breakdown, especially over areas that receive greatest pressure.

Wash and dry skin at least daily.

Inspect pressure points daily or more often if risk for breakdown is observed.

Use a skin breakdown assessment scale such as Modified Braden Q.

Stimulate circulation with gentle massage over pressure areas.

Change position at least every 2 hours to relieve pressure.

Encourage increase in intake of oral fluids.

Provide and encourage patient to eat a balanced diet, including vegetables and fruits.

PREVENT COMPLICATIONS

Check pulses in affected area and compare with pulses in contralateral site.

Assess circular dressings for excessive tightness.

Assess restrictive bandages or devices used to maintain traction on affected limb.

- Make certain that they are not too loose or too tight.
- Remove periodically and check for skin breakdown or pressure areas.

Encourage deep breathing or use of incentive spirometer.

Note any neurovascular changes, such as:

- Changes in color in skin and nail beds
- Alterations in sensation; increased pain
- Alterations in motor ability

Take immediate action to correct problem or report to practitioner if neurovascular changes are found.

Record findings of neurovascular changes.

Carry out passive, active, or active-with-resistance exercises of uninvolved joints.

Note if any tightness, weakness, edema, or contractures are developing in uninvolved joints and muscles.

Take measures to correct or prevent further development of weakness, such as applying footboard or foot orthoses to prevent footdrop.

---

according to hospital policy or practitioner preference. Pin sites should be frequently assessed and cleaned to prevent infection; after the first 48 to 72 hours pin site care may be performed once daily or weekly for mechanically stable pins (Holmes, Brown, and Pin Site Care Expert Panel, 2005). Use of a 2 mg/ml chlorhexidine solution has been proposed as best-practice care for skeletal pin sites by the National Association of Orthopaedic Nurses (Holmes, Brown, and Pin Site Care Expert Panel, 2005). Before the child's discharge, the family is taught pin site care, including how to observe for infection or pin instability, using a return demonstration method. A pressure reduction device, such as a special air mattress, decreases the chance of skin breakdown.

> **NURSINGTIP**
>
> A small hand mirror facilitates visualization of inaccessible skin areas.

When the child is first placed in traction, increased discomfort is common as a result of the traction pull fatiguing the muscle. It has been determined that orthopedic conditions are associated with a higher-than-average number of painful events and a higher percentage of bodily symptoms than other common conditions. IV opioids, including analgesics and muscle relaxants, help during this phase of care and should be administered liberally.

For skeletal traction to be effective, ensure that the weights are hanging freely at all times.

The specific nursing responsibilities for the patient in traction are outlined in the Nursing Care Guidelines box (p. 1120).

DISTRACTION

Unlike traction, which helps bones realign and fuse properly, **distraction** is the process of separating opposing bone to encourage regeneration of new bone in the created space. Distraction can also be used when limbs are of unequal lengths and new bone is needed to elongate the shorter limb.

External Fixation

The **Ilizarov external fixator (IEF)** is a common external fixation device. The IEF uses a system of wires, rings, and telescoping rods that permits limb lengthening to occur by manual distraction (Fig. 31-9). In addition to lengthening bones, the device can be used to correct angular or rotational defects or to immobilize fractures. The device is attached surgically by securing a series of external full or half rings to the bone with wires. External telescoping rods connect the rings to each other. Manual distraction is accomplished by manipulating the rods to increase the distance between the rings. A percutaneous osteotomy is performed when the device is applied to create a "false" growth plate. A special osteotomy or corticotomy involves cutting only the cortex of the bone while preserving its blood supply, bone marrow, endosteum, and periosteum. Capillary blood flow to the transected area is essential for proper bone growth. Cut bone ends typically grow at a rate of 1 cm (0.4 inches) per month. The IEF can result in up to a 15-cm (6-inch) gain in length.

Nursing Care Management

Success of the IEF depends on the child's and family's cooperation; therefore before surgery they must be fully informed of the appearance of the device, how it accomplishes bone growth and limits bone mobility, alterations in activities, and home and follow-up care. Children are involved in learning to adjust the device to accomplish distraction. Children and parents should be instructed in pin care, including observation for infection and loosening of the pins. Cleaning routines for the pin sites vary among practitioners but should not traumatize the skin.

Children who participate actively in their care report less discomfort. Because the device is external, the child and family need to be prepared for the reactions of others and assisted in camouflaging the device with appropriate apparel, such as wide-legged pants that close with self-adhering fasteners around the device. A loose sock or stockinette may also be used over the device to decrease public awareness. Partial weight bearing is allowed, and the child learns to walk with crutches. Alterations in activity include modifications at school and in physical education. Full weight bearing is not allowed until the distraction is completed and bone consolidation has occurred. Follow-up care is essential to maintain appropriate distraction until the desired limb length is achieved. The device is removed surgically after the bone has consolidated, and the child may need to use crutches or have a cast for 4 to 6 weeks after removal.

FIG. 31-9 ■ Child with Ilizarov external fixator during physical therapy on parallel bars.

AMPUTATION

A child may be born with the congenital absence of an extremity, have a traumatic loss of an extremity, or need a surgical amputation for a pathologic condition such as **osteosarcoma** (see p. 1136). With today's surgical technology and the quick thinking of bystanders who save a traumatically amputated body part, some children have had fingers and arms sewn back on with variable degrees of functional use regained.

For an amputated limb or body part that may be reattached, do the following:
1. Rinse limb gently with normal saline.
2. Loosely wrap limb in sterile gauze.
3. Place wrapped limb in a watertight bag.
4. Cool (without freezing) bag in ice water (do not pack in ice because this may harm tissue).
5. Label with child's name, date, and time, and transport with the child to the hospital.

Surgical amputation or the surgical repair of a permanently severed limb focuses on constructing an adequately nourished stump. A smooth, healthy, padded stump, free of nerve endings, is important in prosthesis fitting and subsequent ambulation. In some situations in which there is no vascular or neurologic deficit, a cast is applied to the stump immediately after the procedure, and a pylon, metal extension, and artificial foot are attached so that the patient can walk on the temporary prosthesis within a few hours.

Nursing Care Management

Stump shaping is done postoperatively with special elastic bandaging using a figure-eight bandage, which applies pressure in a cone-shaped fashion. This technique decreases stump edema, controls hemorrhage, and aids in developing desired contours so that the child will bear weight on the posterior aspect of the skin flap rather than on the end of the stump.

Stump elevation may be used during the first 24 hours, but after this time the extremity should not be left in this position, since contractures in the proximal joint will develop and seriously hamper ambulation. Monitoring proper body alignment will further decrease the risk of flexion contractures.

For older children and adolescents, arm exercises, bed pushups, and prosthesis-training programs using parallel bars help build up the arm muscles necessary for walking with crutches. Full range-of-motion exercises of joints above the amputation must be performed several times daily, using active and isotonic exercises. Young children are spontaneously active and require little encouragement.

Depending on the child's age, children or their parents will need to learn stump hygiene, including carefully washing with soap and water every day and checking for skin irritation, breakdown, or infection. A tube of stockinette or powder is used to slide the prosthesis on more easily. Skin must be checked carefully every time the prosthesis is removed, and prosthesis tolerance time must be adjusted to prevent skin breakdown.

For children who have had an amputation, **phantom limb sensation** is an expected experience because the nerve-brain connections are still present. Gradually these sensations fade, although in many amputees they persist for years. Preoperative discussion of this phenomenon will aid a child in understanding these "unusual feelings" and not hiding the experiences from others. Limb pain, especially pain that increases with ambulation, should be evaluated for the possibility of a neuroma at the free nerve endings in the stump, or other problems such as a poorly fitting prosthesis or joint instability.

CONGENITAL DEFECTS

Some skeletal defects may be diagnosed at birth or within days, weeks, or months after birth. In other cases the deviation may be difficult to detect without careful inspection. Therefore it is imperative that nurses become acquainted with signs of these defects and understand the principles of therapy in order to direct others in the care and management of these children.

DEVELOPMENTAL DYSPLASIA OF THE HIP

The broad term **developmental dysplasia of the hip (DDH)** describes a spectrum of disorders related to abnormal development of the hip that may occur at any time during fetal life, infancy, or childhood. A change in terminology from *congenital hip dysplasia* and *congenital dislocation of the hip* to DDH more properly reflects a variety of hip abnormalities in which there is a shallow acetabulum, subluxation, or dislocation.

The incidence of hip instability of some kind is approximately 10 per 1000 live births. The incidence of frank dislocation or a dislocatable hip is 1 per 1000 live births (Wall, 2000), and approximately 16% to 25% of infants with DDH are born breech (Hosalkar, Horn, Friedman and others, 2007). The left hip is involved in 60% of cases, the right hip in 20%, and both hips in 20%. Sixty percent of the patients are girls. Caucasian children have a higher incidence of developmental dysplasia than other groups (Maher, Salmond, and Pellino, 2002).

Pathophysiology

The cause of DDH is unknown, but certain factors such as gender, birth order, family history, intrauterine position, delivery type, joint laxity, and postnatal positioning are believed to affect the risk of DDH. Predisposing factors associated with

DDH may be divided into three broad categories: (1) physiologic factors, which include maternal hormone secretion and intrauterine positioning; (2) mechanical factors, which involve breech presentation, multiple fetus, oligohydramnios, and large infant size (other mechanical factors may include continued maintenance of the hips in adduction and extension that will in time cause a dislocation); and (3) genetic factors, which entail a higher incidence (6%) of DDH in siblings of affected infants and an even greater incidence (36%) of recurrence if a sibling and one parent were affected.

Some experts categorize DDH into two major groups: (1) **typical,** in which the infant is neurologically intact; and (2) **teratologic,** which involves a neuromuscular defect such as arthrogryposis or myelodysplasia. The teratologic forms usually occur in utero and are much less common.

Three degrees of DDH are illustrated in Fig. 31-10:

1. **Acetabular dysplasia** (or **preluxation**)—This is the mildest form of DDH, in which there is neither subluxation nor dislocation. There is a delay in acetabular development evidenced by osseous hypoplasia of the acetabular roof that is oblique and shallow, although the cartilaginous roof is comparatively intact. The femoral head remains in the acetabulum.
2. **Subluxation**—The largest percentage of DDH, subluxation, implies incomplete dislocation of the hip and is sometimes regarded as an intermediate state in the development from primary dysplasia to complete dislocation. The femoral head remains in contact with the acetabulum, but a stretched capsule and ligamentum teres cause the head of the femur to be partially displaced. Pressure on the cartilaginous roof inhibits ossification and produces a flattening of the socket.
3. **Dislocation**—The femoral head loses contact with the acetabulum and is displaced posteriorly and superiorly over the fibrocartilaginous rim. The ligamentum teres is elongated and taut.

Factors related to infant handling are indicated in the Cultural Awareness box.

Diagnostic Evaluation

DDH is often not detected at the initial examination after birth; thus all infants should be carefully monitored for hip dysplasia at follow-up visits throughout the first year of life. In the newborn period dysplasia usually appears as hip joint laxity rather than as outright dislocation (Fig. 31-11). Subluxation and the tendency to dislocate can be demonstrated by the Ortolani or Barlow tests (see Fig. 31-11, *B, C,* and *D*). The Ortolani and Barlow tests are most reliable from birth to 2 or 3 months of age. With the Barlow test the thighs are adducted, whereas the Ortolani test involves abducting the thighs to test for hip subluxation or dislocation (Seidel, Ball, Dains, and

---

🌐 **CULTURAL AWARENESS**

Developmental Dysplasia of the Hip

A striking relationship exists between the development of hip dislocation and methods of handling infants. Among the cultures with the highest incidence of dislocation, newly born infants are tightly wrapped in blankets or other swaddling material or are strapped to cradle boards. In cultures such as the Far East, where mothers traditionally carry infants on their backs or hips in the widely abducted straddle position, the disorder is virtually unknown.

Normal   Dysplasia   Subluxation   Dislocation

FIG. 31-10 ■ Configuration and relationship of structures in developmental dysplasia of the hip.

FIG. 31-11 ■ Signs of developmental dysplasia of the hip. **A,** Asymmetry of gluteal and thigh folds with shortening of the thigh (Galeazzi sign). **B,** Limited hip abduction, as seen in flexion (Ortolani test). **C,** Apparent shortening of the femur, as indicated by the level of the knees in flexion (Allis sign). **D,** Ortolani test with femoral head moving in and out of acetabulum (in infants 1 to 2 months old). **E,** Positive Trendelenburg sign with lordosis (if child is weight bearing).

BOX 31-4

Clinical Manifestations of Developmental Dysplasia of the Hip

INFANT
Shortening of limb on affected side
Restricted abduction of hip on affected side
Unequal gluteal folds (infant prone)
Positive Ortolani test
Positive Barlow test

OLDER INFANT AND CHILD
Affected leg shorter than the other
Telescoping or piston mobility of joint—Head of femur felt to move up and down in buttock when extended thigh is pushed first toward child's head and then pulled distally
Trendelenburg sign—When child stands first on one foot and then on the other (holding onto a chair, rail, or someone's hands) bearing weight on affected hip, pelvis tilts downward on normal side instead of upward, as it would with normal stability
Greater trochanter prominent and appearing above a line from anterosuperior iliac spine to tuberosity of ischium
Marked lordosis (bilateral dislocations)
Waddling gait (bilateral dislocations)

Front   Back

FIG. 31-12 ■ Child in Pavlik harness. (From Ball JW: *Mosby's pediatric patient teaching guides*, St Louis, 1998, Mosby.)

others, 2006). Other signs of DDH are shortening of the limb on the affected side (see Fig. 31-11, *C*), asymmetric thigh and gluteal folds (see Fig 31-11, *A*), and broadening of the perineum (in bilateral dislocation) (Box 31-4).

NURSING ALERT

These tests must be performed by an experienced clinician to prevent fracture or other damage to the hip. If these tests are performed too vigorously in the first 2 days of life, when the hip subluxates freely, persistent dislocation may occur.

Radiographic examination in early infancy is not reliable, since ossification of the femoral head does not normally take place until the third to sixth month of life. However, the cartilaginous head can be visualized directly by ultrasonography. Widespread newborn screening with ultrasound has been proposed; however, numerous studies reveal this approach has a high rate of false positives and subsequent overtreatment. Therefore ultrasound is recommended as an adjunct to other diagnostic procedures (American Academy of Pediatrics, 2000a). In infants older than age 4 months and in children, radiographic examination is useful in confirming the diagnosis. An upward slope in the roof of the acetabulum (the acetabular angle) greater than 40 degrees with upward and outward displacement of the femoral head is a frequent finding in older children. Computed tomography (CT) scan may be useful to assess the position of the femoral head relative to the acetabulum after closed reduction and casting. The American Academy of Pediatrics (2000a) has published extensive clinical guidelines for the early detection of DDH.

Therapeutic Management

Treatment is begun as soon as the condition is recognized, since early intervention is more favorable to the restoration of normal bony architecture and function. The longer treatment

is delayed, the more severe the deformity, the more difficult the treatment, and the less favorable the prognosis. The treatment varies with the child's age and the extent of the dysplasia. The goal of treatment is to obtain and maintain a safe, congruent position of the hip joint to promote normal hip joint development.

Newborn to Age 6 Months. The hip joint is maintained by dynamic splinting in a safe position with the proximal femur centered in the acetabulum in an attitude of flexion. Of the numerous devices available, the **Pavlik harness** is the most widely used, and with time, motion, and gravity, the hip works into a more abducted, reduced position (Fig. 31-12). The harness is worn continuously until the hip is proved stable on clinical and radiographic examination, usually in about 3 to 5 months.

When adduction contracture is present, other devices (such as skin traction) are used to slowly and gently stretch the hip to full abduction, after which wide abduction is maintained until stability is attained. When there is difficulty in maintaining stable reduction, a hip spica cast is applied and changed periodically to accommodate the child's growth. After 3 to 6 months, sufficient stability is acquired to allow transfer to a removable protective abduction brace. The duration of treatment depends on development of the acetabulum but is usually accomplished within the first year.

Ages 6 to 18 Months. In this age-group the dislocation is not recognized until the child begins to stand and walk, when attendant shortening of the limb and contractures of hip adductor and flexor muscles become apparent. Gradual reduction by traction is used for approximately 3 weeks. An individualized home traction program may be developed for the child preoperatively to decrease the length of hospitalization and maintain the home environment. The child then undergoes an attempted closed reduction of the hip using general anesthesia; if the hip is not reducible, an open reduction is performed. After reduction, the child is placed in a hip spica cast for 2 to 4 months until the hip is stable, at which time a flexion-abduction brace is applied.

Older Child. Correction of the hip deformity in older children is inherently more difficult than in the preceding age-groups, since secondary adaptive changes and other etiologic factors (such as juvenile arthritis or nonambulatory cerebral palsy) complicate the condition. Operative reduction, which may involve preoperative traction, tenotomy of contracted muscles, and any one of several innominate osteotomy procedures designed to construct an acetabular roof, is usually required. After cast removal and before weight bearing is permitted, range-of-motion exercises help restore movement. Successful reduction and reconstruction become increasingly difficult after the age of 4 years and are usually impossible or inadvisable in children older than 6 years of age because of severe shortening and contracture of muscles and deformity of the femoral and acetabular structures.

Nursing Care Management

Nurses are in a unique position to detect DDH in early infancy. During the infant assessment process and routine nurturing activities, the hips and extremities are inspected for any deviations from normal. These observations are reported to the attending practitioner, and the ambulatory child who displays a limp or an unusual gait should be referred for evaluation. This may indicate an orthopedic or neurologic problem. Nonambulatory children with cerebral palsy should also be assessed for evidence of dislocation.

The major nursing problems in the care of an infant or child in a cast or other device are related to maintenance of the device and adaptation of nurturing activities to meet the patient's needs. Generally, treatment and follow-up care of these children are carried out in a clinic, practitioner's office, or outpatient unit.

> **NURSING ALERT**
>
> The former practice of double- or triple-diapering for DDH is not recommended because it promotes hip extension, thus worsening proper hip development.

The primary nursing goal is teaching parents to apply and maintain the reduction device. The Pavlik harness allows for easy handling of the infant and usually produces less apprehension in the parent than heavy braces and casts. Because of the infant's rapid growth, the straps should be checked in the beginning of therapy every week for possible adjustments (Hart, Albright, Rebello, and others, 2006). It is important that parents understand the correct use of the appliance, which may or may not allow for its removal during bathing. Unbuckling or removing the harness is determined individually on the basis of the family's level of understanding and the degree of hip deformity. Parents are instructed not to adjust the harness without medical supervision. The child should be examined by the practitioner before any adjustment is attempted to make certain the hips are in correct placement before the harness is resecured.

Skin care is an important aspect of the care of an infant in a harness. The following instructions for preventing skin breakdown are stressed:

- Always put an undershirt (or a shirt with extensions that close at the crotch) under the chest straps, and put knee socks under the foot and leg pieces to prevent the straps from rubbing the skin.
- Check frequently (at least two or three times a day) for red areas under the straps and the clothing.

- Gently massage healthy skin under the straps once a day to stimulate circulation. In general, avoid lotions and powders because they can cake and irritate the skin.
- Always place the diaper under the straps.

Parents are encouraged to hold the infant with a harness and continue care and nurturing activities. The nurse can assist by being available for parents' questions about the necessary adaptations to daily care to decrease the parent's anxiety and possible feelings about the child being hurt by routine caring.

Casts and orthotic devices (braces) offer more challenging nursing and caregiver problems, since they cannot be removed for routine care, although sometimes a brace may be removed for bathing. Care of an infant or small child with a cast requires nursing innovation to reduce irritation and to maintain cleanliness of both the child and the cast, particularly in the diaper area. (See p. 1115 for care of the child in a cast.)

It is important for nurses, parents, and other caregivers to understand that children in corrective devices need to be involved in all the activities of any child in the same age-group. Confinement in a cast or appliance should not exclude children from family (or unit) activities. They can be held astride the lap for comfort and transported to areas of activity. The child may be allowed to walk in a cast or orthotic device. An adapted wheelchair, stroller, or scooter can offer mobility to the older infant or child.

CONGENITAL CLUBFOOT

Congenital **clubfoot** is a complex deformity of the ankle and foot that includes forefoot adduction, midfoot supination, hindfoot varus, and ankle equinus. Deformities of the foot and ankle are described according to the position of the ankle and foot. The more common positions involve the following variations:

Talipes varus—An inversion, or bending inward
Talipes valgus—An eversion, or bending outward
Talipes equinus—Plantar flexion, in which the toes are lower than the heel
Talipes calcaneus—Dorsiflexion, in which the toes are higher than the heel

Most cases of clubfoot are a combination of these positions, and the most frequently occurring type of clubfoot (approximately 95% of cases) is the composite deformity **talipes equinovarus (TEV),** in which the foot is pointed downward and inward in varying degrees of severity (Fig. 31-13). Unilateral clubfoot may occur as an isolated defect or in association with other disorders or syndromes, such as chromosomal aberrations, arthrogryposis, cerebral palsy, or spina bifida.

The incidence of clubfoot in the general population is 1 to 2 per 1000 live births, with boys affected twice as often as girls. Bilateral clubfeet occur in 50% of the cases (Gilmore and Thompson, 2003). The precise cause of clubfoot is unknown. Some authorities attribute the defect to abnormal positioning and restricted movement in utero, although the evidence is not conclusive. Other experts implicate arrested or abnormal embryonic development. Arrested development during this early stage tends to result in a rigid deformity, whereas mechanical pressures from intrauterine positioning are likely causes of more flexible deformities.

FIG. 31-13 ■ Bilateral congenital talipes equinovarus (congenital clubfoot) in 2-month-old infant. (From Zitelli BJ, Davis HW: *Atlas of pediatric physical diagnosis*, ed 4, St Louis, 2002, Mosby.)

FIG. 31-14 ■ Feet casted for correction of bilateral talipes equinovarus.

Classification

Clubfoot may be further divided into three categories: (1) positional clubfoot (also called transitional, mild, or postural clubfoot), which is believed to occur primarily from intrauterine crowding and responds to simple stretching and casting; (2) syndromic (or teratologic) clubfoot, which is associated with other congenital anomalies such as myelomeningocele or arthrogryposis and is a more severe form of clubfoot that is often resistant to treatment; and (3) congenital clubfoot, also referred to as idiopathic, which may occur in an otherwise normal child and has a wide range of rigidity and prognosis.

The mild, or postural, clubfoot may correct spontaneously or may require passive exercise or serial casting. There is no bony abnormality, but there may be tightness and shortening of the soft tissues medially and posteriorly. The teratologic clubfoot usually requires surgical correction and has a high incidence of recurrence. The congenital idiopathic clubfoot, or "true clubfoot," almost always requires surgical intervention because there is bony abnormality.

Diagnostic Evaluation

The deformity is readily apparent and easily detected prenatally through ultrasonography or at birth. However, it must be differentiated from some positional deformities that can be passively corrected or overcorrected. Paralytic changes in the lower extremity of children with neuromuscular involvement often produce equinovarus deformity. An increased risk of hip dysplasia is associated with clubfoot deformities.

Therapeutic Management

The goal of treatment for clubfoot is to achieve a painless, plantigrade, and stable foot. Treatment of clubfoot involves three stages: (1) correction of the deformity, (2) maintenance of the correction until normal muscle balance is regained, and (3) follow-up observation to avert possible recurrence of the deformity. Some feet respond to treatment readily; some respond only to prolonged, vigorous, and sustained efforts; and the improvement in others remains disappointing even with maximal effort on the part of all concerned.

Serial casting is begun shortly after birth, before discharge from the nursery. Successive casts allow for gradual stretching of skin and tight structures on the medial side of the foot (Fig. 31-14). Manipulation and casting are repeated frequently (ev-

ery week) to accommodate the rapid growth of early infancy. The extremity or extremities are casted until maximum correction is achieved, usually within 8 to 12 weeks. A Denis Browne splint may be used to manage feet that correct with casting and manipulation. A radiograph or ultrasound is then evaluated to see the relationship of the bones to each other. Failure to achieve normal alignment by 3 months indicates the need for surgical intervention. Current practice involves a percutaneous heel cord release at approximately 2 to 3 months of age followed by serial casting. This has decreased the number of children requiring more extensive surgery between 6 and 12 months of age. The foot (or feet) is immobilized postoperatively for approximately 6 to 12 weeks, and the child is allowed to walk after the cast is removed (Gilmore and Thompson, 2003).

Nursing Care Management

Nursing care of the child with clubfoot is the same as for any child who has a cast (see p. 1115). Because the child will spend considerable time in a corrective device, nursing care plans include both long-term and short-term goals. Conscientious observation of the skin and circulation is particularly important in young infants because of their rapid growth rate. Because treatment and follow-up care are handled in the orthopedist's office, clinic, or outpatient department, parent education and support are important in nursing care of these children.

Parents need to understand the overall treatment program, the importance of regular cast changes, and the role they play in the long-term effectiveness of the therapy. Reinforcing and clarifying the orthopedist's explanations and instructions, teaching parents about care of the cast or appliance (including vigilant observation for potential problems), and encouraging parents to facilitate normal development within the limitations imposed by the deformity or therapy are all part of nursing responsibilities.

METATARSUS ADDUCTUS (VARUS)

Metatarsus adductus, or metatarsus varus, is probably the most common congenital foot deformity. In most instances it is a result of abnormal intrauterine positioning, particularly in the firstborn child, and is usually detected at birth. The deformity is characterized by medial adduction of the toes and forefoot, frequently in association with inversion, and by convexity of the lateral border of the foot. Metatarsus adductus may be divided into three categories: type I, in which the forefoot is flexible and corrects easily with manipulation; type II, in which there is only partial flexibility in the forefoot and it corrects passively past neutral position but only to neutral position with active manipulation; and type III, in which the forefoot is rigid and will not stretch to neutral position with manipulation (Gilmore and Thompson, 2003). Unlike TEV, with which it is often confused, the angulation occurs at the tarsometatarsal joint, whereas the heel and ankle remain in a neutral position. Ankle range of motion is normal. This deformity often causes a pigeon-toed gait in the child.

Management depends on the rigidity and type of the deformity. With types I and II, correction can usually be accomplished by gentle manipulation and passive stretching of the foot, which the parent is taught to perform. Repeated and consistent stretching is continued for the first 6 weeks, after which the treatment is based on the flexibility of the foot. With type III, the child will usually require serial manipulation and casting to correct the defect. Casting is performed every 1 to 2 weeks for 6 to 8 weeks, after which a corrective shoe or orthosis may be used. Surgical correction is rarely required for the condition (Gilmore and Thompson, 2003).

Nursing Care Management

The nursing role primarily involves identifying the defect, so that early therapy and instruction of the parents can be initiated. The nurse teaches the parents how to hold the heel firmly and to stretch only the forefoot; otherwise, undue force on the heel may produce a valgus deformity. If casting or orthosis is required, the nurse instructs the parents in cast care and observation of the corrective device (see p. 1115).

SKELETAL LIMB DEFICIENCY

Congenital limb deficiencies, or reduction malformations, are manifested by a variety of degrees of loss of functional capacity. They are characterized by underdevelopment of skeletal elements of the extremities. The range of malformation can extend from minor defects of the digits to serious abnormalities, such as **amelia,** absence of an entire extremity; or **meromelia,** partial absence of an extremity, which includes **phocomelia** (seal limbs), the interposed deficiency of long bones with relatively good development of hands and feet attached at or near the shoulder or the hips. Most reduction defects are primary defects of development of the limb, but prenatal destruction of the limb can occur, such as full or partial amputation of a limb in utero from constriction of an amniotic band (**amniotic band syndrome**).

Pathophysiology

Limb deficiencies can be attributed to both heredity and environment and can originate at any stage of limb development. Formation of limbs may be suppressed at the time of limb bud formation, or there may be interference in later stages of differentiation and growth. Heredity appears to play a prominent role, and prenatal environmental insults have been implicated in a number of cases, such as the well-publicized **thalidomide** tragedy of the 1950s and early 1960s, which demonstrated a clear relationship between the time of exposure of the pregnant woman to the antiemetic drug and the presence and type

of limb deformity in the newborn. There still are many drugs that may have similar **teratogenic** effects in the first trimester of pregnancy; therefore medication administration during this period should be carefully evaluated by the practitioner. Unfortunately, during this period, the woman may not realize her pregnant condition unless the event is highly anticipated, and inadvertent consumption of harmful medications may occur. Deletion or shortening of digits or limbs may also be associated with **chorionic villus sampling,** especially before 10 to 12 weeks of gestation; however, the incidence and relationship remain uncertain.

Therapeutic Management

Children with congenital limb deficiencies should be fitted with prosthetic devices whenever possible, and the devices should be applied at the earliest possible stage of development in an attempt to match the infant's motor readiness. This favors natural progression of prosthetic use. For example, an infant with an upper extremity deficiency is fitted with a simple passive device, such as a mitten prosthesis, to encourage limb exploration, sitting (with the extremities needed for support), and bilateral hand activities.

Lower limb prostheses are applied when the infant begins sitting up and can maintain balance. In preparation for prosthetic devices, surgical modification may be necessary to ensure the most favorable use of the device, since severe deformity can interfere with its effective use. Phocomelic digits are preserved for controlling switches of externally powered appliances in upper extremities. Digits (in both upper and lower extremities) provide the child with surfaces for tactile exploration and stimulation. Prostheses are replaced to accommodate the child's growth and increasing capabilities.

Nursing Care Management

Prosthetic application training and habilitation are most successfully carried out in a center that specializes in meeting the special needs of these children, especially very young children and those with amputations or missing limbs. Management involves a **prosthetist,** who specializes in the development, fitting, and maintenance of prosthetic limbs, and other health care workers such as physical and occupational therapists. Parents need special attention and support and are encouraged to assist the child in making age-commensurate adjustments to the environment. Although these children need assistance, overprotection may produce overdependence, with later maladjustment to school and other situations.

OSTEOGENESIS IMPERFECTA

Osteogenesis imperfecta (OI) is the most common osteoporosis syndrome in childhood. OI is a heterogeneous, autosomal dominant disorder characterized by fractures and bone deformity. There are at least five types of OI, which accounts for significant disease variability. Clinical features may include varying degrees of bone fragility, deformity, and fracture; blue sclerae; hearing loss; and dentinogenesis imperfecta (hypoplastic discolored teeth). Although inheritance follows an autosomal dominant pattern in most cases, rare autosomal recessive inheritance exists (Box 31-5).

Most types of OI have defects in the *COL1A1* or *COL1A2* genes, which code for polypeptide chains in type 1 procollagen, a precursor of type 1 collagen, a major structural component of bone. The error results in faulty bone mineralization,

BOX 31-5
Classification of Osteogenesis Imperfecta

Type I*
A—Mild bone fragility; blue sclerae; normal teeth; hearing loss (occurs between ages 20 and 30 years); autosomal dominant inheritance
B—Same as A except dentinogenesis imperfecta instead of normal teeth
C—Same as B but no bone fragility
Type II—Lethal; stillborn or die in early infancy; severe bone fragility, multiple fractures at birth; 10% of cases of osteogenesis imperfecta (OI); autosomal recessive inheritance
Type III—Severe bone fragility leading to severe progressive deformities; normal sclerae; marked growth failure; most autosomal recessive inheritance; few autosomal dominant inheritance
Type IV
A—Mild to moderate bone fragility; normal sclerae; normal teeth; short stature; variable deformity; autosomal dominant inheritance
B—Same as A except dentinogenesis imperfecta instead of normal teeth; approximately 6% of cases of OI
Type V—Clinically similar to IV; hyperplastic callus; collagen mutation is negative
Type VI—Sclerae and dentition normal; moderate to severe bone fragility; diagnosis by bone biopsy because of similarities to other types; only identified in eight persons to date (Land, Rauch, Travers, and others, 2007)

*Two thirds of cases are type I.

abnormal bone architecture, and increased susceptibility to fracture.

OI has several classifications based on clinical features and patterns of inheritance (see Box 31-5). Clinically, type I is the most common, with wide variability of bone fragility; some affected family members have significant deformity and disability, whereas others lead agile, active lives. Type II variants are the most severe and are considered lethal in infancy. Type III OI is characterized by multiple fractures, bone deformity, and severe disability; affected individuals rarely live to 30 years of age. Type IV is similar to type I with blue or white sclerae. Another variant, or type V, has been described in which those affected have a hyperplastic callus, a radiodense metaphyseal band, and calcification of the interosseous membrane of the forearm; no collagen mutations are noted in this group (Marini, 2007). A type VI has been described with a characteristic mineralization defect, which does not respond to pamidronate therapy as do types I to V (Land, Rauch, Travers, and others, 2007). Children affected with this type have no dental involvement and normal sclerae; a bone biopsy is the only way to establish a diagnosis because of the similarities to other types.

Therapeutic Management

The treatment for OI is primarily supportive, although patients and families are optimistic about new research advances. Bone marrow transplant for severe OI was first reported in 1999 with positive results; however, this is still considered an experimental treatment. The use of bisphosphonate therapy with IV pamidronate to promote increased bone density and prevent fractures has become standard therapy for many children with OI.

The goals of a rehabilitative approach to management are directed to preventing (1) positional contractures and deformities, (2) muscle weakness and osteoporosis, and (3) malalignment of lower extremity joints prohibiting weight bearing.

Lightweight braces and splints help support limbs, prevent fractures, and aid in ambulation. Physical therapy helps prevent disuse osteoporosis and strengthens muscles, which in turn improves bone density.

Surgery is sometimes used to help treat the manifestations of the disease. Surgical techniques are used to correct deformities that interfere with bracing, standing, or walking. For the child with recurrent fractures, inserting an intramedullary rod provides stability to bones.

Nursing Care Management

Infants and children with this disorder require careful handling to prevent fractures. They must be supported when they are being turned, positioned, moved, and held. Even changing a diaper may cause a fracture in severely affected infants. These children should never be held by the ankles when being diapered but should be gently lifted by the buttocks or supported with pillows.

Both parents and the affected child need education regarding the child's limitations and guidelines in planning suitable activities that promote optimal development and protect the child from harm. Realistic occupational planning and genetic counseling are part of the long-term goals of care. Educational materials and information can be obtained from the Osteogenesis Imperfecta Foundation,* which also has a network that can put a family in contact with other families with a similar problem.

OI is a differential diagnosis that must be ruled out in the event of multiple fractures that could be attributed to nonaccidental injury. A detailed history, no evidence of associated soft-tissue injury, and the presence of other symptoms related to OI help to determine the diagnosis.

NURSINGALERT

Children with current fractures or healing fractures should be screened for OI. The assumption that abuse or neglect is the cause of fractures in children must be carefully evaluated by a multidisciplinary team.

ACQUIRED DEFECTS
LEGG-CALVÉ-PERTHES DISEASE

Legg-Calvé-Perthes disease, sometimes called *coxa plana* or *osteochondritis deformans juvenilis,* is a self-limiting disorder in which there is aseptic necrosis of the femoral head. The disease affects children ages 2 to 12 years, but most cases occur in boys between 4 and 8 years of age as an isolated event. In approximately 10% of cases the involvement is bilateral; most of the affected children have a skeletal age significantly below their chronologic age (Hosalkar, Horn, Friedman and others, 2007). The male/female ratio is 4:1 or 5:1. Caucasian children are affected 10 times more frequently than African-American children.

Pathophysiology

The cause of the disease is unknown, but there is a disturbance of circulation to the femoral capital epiphysis that produces an ischemic aseptic necrosis of the femoral head. During middle

*804 W. Diamond Ave., Suite 210, Gaithersburg, MD 20878; (800) 981-2663; http://www.oif.org.

BOX 31-6
Radiographic Stages of Legg-Calvé-Perthes Disease

Stage I: initial, or **avascular, stage**—Aseptic necrosis or infarction of the femoral capital epiphysis with degenerative changes producing flattening of the upper surface of the femoral head

Stage II: fragmentation, or **revascularization, stage**—Capital bone resorption and revascularization with fragmentation (vascular resorption of the epiphysis) that gives a mottled appearance on radiographs

Stage III: reossification, or **reparative, stage**—New bone formation, which is represented on radiographs as calcification and ossification or increased density in the areas of radiolucency; this filling-in process appears to take place from the periphery of the head centrally

Stage IV: residual, or **regenerative, stage**—Gradual reformation of the head of the femur without radiolucency and, it is hoped, to a spherical form

FAMILY FOCUS

Legg-Calvé-Perthes Disease

A family with five healthy children was one day startled to learn that their 2-year-old son could no longer walk. He was diagnosed with Legg-Calvé-Perthes disease. Through several years of prosthetic devices and numerous physician visits, hospitalizations, and surgeries, this family turned a potentially devastating experience into one with cherished memories.

Today, the parents reflect on how their family coped with the reality of a debilitating disease. It was difficult for the parents to observe an eager, energetic child watch other children riding bicycles, running, or playing outdoor games. They are warmed by memories of watching their other children make the difference for their sibling. They all developed a strong bond through caring and sharing with one another. Coping as a family was an easy adjustment and, most of all, therapeutic. Today, more than 20 years later, the parents believe that each family member has grown with feelings of faith and trust. The experience proved to them that life will go on, and that life is what you make it!

Shona Swenson Lenss, MS, RN, FNP
Cheyenne, Wyoming

childhood, circulation to the femoral epiphysis is more tenuous than at other ages and can become obstructed by trauma, inflammation, coagulation defects, and a variety of other causes. The pathologic events seem to take place in four stages (Box 31-6). The entire process may encompass as little as 18 months or continue for several years. The reformed femoral head may be severely altered or appear entirely normal.

Clinical Manifestations and Diagnostic Evaluation

The onset of Legg-Calvé-Perthes disease is usually insidious, and the history may reveal only intermittent appearance of a limp on the affected side or a symptom complex, including hip soreness, ache, or stiffness, which can be constant or intermittent. The parents may report seeing the child limping, and the limp becomes more pronounced with increased activity. The pain may be experienced in the hip, along the entire thigh, or in the vicinity of the knee joint. The pain and limp are usually most evident on arising and at the end of a long day of activities. The pain is usually accompanied by joint dysfunction and limited range of motion. There may be a vague history of trauma. The diagnosis is established by radiographic examination, with the definitive diagnosis being magnetic resonance imaging (MRI), which demonstrates osteonecrosis.

Therapeutic Management

Because deformity occurs early in the disease process, the aims of treatment are to eliminate hip irritability; restore and maintain adequate range of hip motion; prevent capital femoral epiphyseal collapse, extrusion, or subluxation; and ensure a well-rounded femoral head at the time of healing. Treatment varies according to the child's age at the time of diagnosis and the appearance of the femoral head vasculature and position within the acetabulum. Nonsurgical containment of the femoral head may be accomplished with abduction casts, whereas a pelvic or femoral osteotomy may be used to contain the femoral head. Activity causes microfractures of the soft ischemic epiphysis, which tend to induce synovitis, stiffness, and adductor contracture. The initial therapy is rest and non–weight bearing, which helps reduce inflammation and restore motion. Later, active motion is encouraged. In some cases traction is applied to stretch tight adductor muscles.

Containment can be accomplished in several ways. One is the use of non–weight-bearing devices, such as an abduction brace, leg casts, or a leather harness sling, which prevent weight bearing on the affected limb. Another includes the use of various weight-bearing appliances, such as abduction-ambulation braces or casts after a period of bed rest and traction. A third option consists of surgical reconstruction and containment procedures. Conservative therapy must be continued for 2 to 4 years, although braces constructed from lightweight materials allow the child to maintain a nearly normal activity level. Surgical correction, although subjecting the child to additional risks (e.g., from anesthesia, infection, blood transfusion), returns the child to normal activities in 3 to 4 months. The use of home traction has also been explored.

The disease is self-limiting, but the ultimate outcome of therapy depends on early and efficient treatment and the child's age at the onset of the disorder. Younger children (5 years and under), whose epiphyses are more cartilaginous, have the best prognosis for complete recovery. Children 10 years and older have a significant risk for degenerative arthritis, especially with femoral head deformity at the time of diagnosis. The later the diagnosis is made, the more femoral damage will have occurred before treatment is implemented. In most cases, with good patient compliance with the prescribed regimen, the prognosis is excellent.

Nursing Care Management

Nurses may be the first health professionals to identify affected children and to refer them for medical evaluation. They are also persons on whom the child and the family can rely to help them understand and adjust to the therapeutic measures. Because most of the child's care is conducted on an outpatient basis, the major emphasis of nursing care is teaching the family the care and management of the corrective appliance selected for therapy. The family needs to learn the purpose, function, application, and care of the corrective device and the importance of compliance to achieve the desired outcome (see Family Focus box).

One of the most difficult aspects associated with the disorder is coping with a normally active child who feels well but must remain relatively inactive during periods where non–weight bearing is required. Suitable activities must be devised to meet the needs of a child in the process of developing a sense of initiative or industry. Activities that meet the creative urges are well received.

SLIPPED CAPITAL FEMORAL EPIPHYSIS

Slipped capital femoral epiphysis (SCFE), or coxa vara, refers to the spontaneous displacement of the proximal femoral epiphysis in a posterior and inferior direction. It develops most frequently shortly before or during accelerated growth and the onset of puberty (children between the ages of 10 and 16 years; median age 13 for boys, 12 for girls) and is most frequently observed in males and obese children. Bilateral involvement occurs in up to 40% to 50% of cases (Greene, 2001).

Pathophysiology

Most cases of SCFE are idiopathic, although it can be associated with endocrine disorders, growth hormone therapy, renal osteodystrophy, and radiotherapy. The cause of idiopathic SCFE is multifactorial and includes obesity, physeal architecture and orientation, and pubertal hormone changes that affect physeal strength. Although obesity stresses the physeal plate, SCFE can also occur in children who are not obese. Radiographs show medial displacement of the epiphysis and uncovered upper portion of the femoral neck adjacent to the physis. There is a widened growth plate and irregular metaphysis. The capital femoral epiphysis remains in the acetabulum, but the femoral neck slips, deforming the femoral head and stretching blood vessels to the epiphysis.

Diagnostic Evaluation

The disorder is suspected when an adolescent or preadolescent youngster displays clinical signs or complains of hip, thigh, or knee pain (Box 31-7). The diagnosis is confirmed by anteroposterior and frog-leg radiographic examination.

Therapeutic Management

Treatment goals are to prevent further slippage and restore function (Perron, Miller, and Brady, 2002). Once the diagnosis is established, the child should be made completely non–weight bearing to prevent further slippage. Surgical treatment varies with the degree of displacement. Traditional methods included presurgery bed rest and traction followed by surgi-

---

BOX 31-7

Clinical Manifestations of Slipped Capital Femoral Epiphysis

Possible obesity
Limp on affected side
Pain in hip
- Continuous or intermittent
- Frequently referred to groin, anteromedial aspect of thigh, or knee
Restricted internal rotation on adduction with external rotation deformity
Loss of abduction and internal rotation as severity increases
Shortening of lower extremity

---

cal pinning; surgical pinning involves the placement of a single pin or multiple pins and screws, or osteotomy for deformity correction if needed. Postsurgical care includes non–weight bearing with crutch ambulation until acceptable, painless range of motion is achieved. SCFE is an emergency and requires early diagnosis and treatment to increase the likelihood of a satisfactory cure.

Nursing Care Management

Nursing care is the same as that for a child in a cast or in traction, as discussed earlier in this chapter. Postoperative care involves hemodynamic stabilization and assessment for complications.

KYPHOSIS AND LORDOSIS

The spine, consisting of numerous segments, can acquire deformity curves of three types: kyphosis, lordosis, and scoliosis (Fig. 31-15). **Kyphosis** is an abnormally increased convex angulation in the curvature of the thoracic spine (see Fig. 31-15, B). It can occur secondary to disease processes such as tuberculosis, chronic arthritis, osteodystrophy, or compression fractures of the thoracic spine. The most common form of kyphosis is postural. Children, especially during the time when skeletal growth outpaces growth of muscle, are prone to exaggeration of a normal kyphosis. They assume abnormal sitting and standing positions. **Scheuermann kyphosis** is a thoracic curve greater than 45 degrees with wedging greater than 5 degrees of at least three adjacent vertebral bodies and vertebral irregularity.

Postural kyphosis is almost always accompanied by a compensatory postural lordosis, an abnormally exaggerated concave lumbar curvature. Treatment of kyphosis consists of exercises to strengthen shoulder and abdominal muscles and bracing for more marked deformity. With adolescents, who are self-conscious about their appearance, the best approach is to emphasize the cosmetic value of corrective therapy and to place the responsibility on the adolescent for carrying out an exercise program at home with regular visits to and assessments by a therapist. Treatment with a brace may be indicated until skeletal maturity, and surgical fusion may be considered for severe, painful, or progressive thoracic curves such as Scheuermann kyphosis.

Lordosis is an accentuation of the cervical or lumbar curvature beyond physiologic limits (see Fig. 31-15, C). It may be a secondary complication of a disease process, a result of trauma, or idiopathic. It is often seen in association with flexion contractures of the hip, scoliosis, obesity, DDH, and SCFE. During the pubertal growth spurt, lordosis of varying degrees is observed in teenagers, especially girls. In obese children the weight of the abdominal fat alters the center of gravity, causing a compensatory lordosis. Unlike kyphosis, severe lordosis is usually accompanied by pain.

Treatment involves management of the predisposing cause when possible, such as weight loss and correction of deformities. Postural exercises or support garments are helpful in relieving symptoms in some cases; however, these do not usually effect a permanent cure.

IDIOPATHIC SCOLIOSIS

Idiopathic scoliosis is a complex spinal deformity in three planes, usually involving lateral curvature, spinal rotation causing rib asymmetry, and thoracic hypokyphosis. It is the most common spinal deformity and can be further classified according to age of onset: **infantile,** at birth or up to 3 years of age; **juvenile,** which develops during childhood; or, most commonly, **adolescent,** which develops during the growth spurt of early adolescence.

Idiopathic scoliosis can be caused by a number of conditions and may occur alone or in association with other diseases, particularly neuromuscular conditions. In most cases, however, there is no apparent cause, hence the name *idiopathic scoliosis.* There appears to be a genetic component to the etiology of idiopathic scoliosis; however, the exact relationship has yet to be established. The following section is limited to a discussion of adolescent idiopathic scoliosis.

Idiopathic scoliosis is most noticeable during the preadolescent growth spurt. Parents frequently bring a child for follow-up on an abnormal school scoliosis screening or because of ill-fitting clothes, such as poorly fitting slacks. School screening is somewhat controversial, since there are no controlled studies to demonstrate improved outcomes and a reported number of false positives lead to referrals (Bunnell, 2005); however, many experts suggest that school screening has increased public and professional awareness of scoliosis and has decreased the number of significant cases of serious deformity (Newton and Wenger, 2001). The American Academy of Pediatrics (2000b) recommends scoliosis screening at the time of primary practitioner visits in all preadolescent and adolescent children.

Diagnostic Evaluation

Observation is performed behind an undressed (in undergarments), standing child, noting asymmetry of shoulder height, scapular or flank shape, or hip height and alignment. When the child bends forward at the waist (the Adams test) with hanging arms, asymmetry of the ribs and flanks may be noted. A scoliometer is also used in the initial screening to measure truncal rotation (also measured by the Adams test). Often a primary curve and a compensatory curve will place the head in alignment with the gluteal cleft. However, in the uncompensated curve the head and hips are not aligned (see Fig.

31-15, *E* and *F*). (See Spine, Chapter 6, for additional information.) Definitive diagnosis is made by radiographs of the child in the standing position and use of the Cobb technique (standard measurement of angle curvature), which establishes the degree of curvature. The Risser scale is used to evaluate skeletal maturity on the radiographs; the scale assists in making a determination of the likely progression of the spinal angulature as the child's bones mature. Not all spinal curvatures are scoliosis. A curve of less than 10 degrees is considered a postural variation. Curves of less than 20 degrees are mild and, if nonprogressive, do not require treatment.

> **NURSING ALERT**
>
> Intraspinal conditions or other disease processes that can cause scoliosis must be ruled out. The presence of pain, sacral dimpling or hairy patches, cutaneous vascular changes, absent or abnormal reflexes, bowel or bladder incontinence, or left thoracic curve may indicate an intraspinal abnormality such as syringomyelia, diastematomyelia, or tethered cord syndrome. An MRI scan should be obtained for evaluation.

Therapeutic Management

Current management options include observation with regular clinical and radiographic evaluation, orthotic intervention (bracing), and surgical spinal fusion. Treatment decisions are based on the magnitude, location, and type of curve; the child's age and skeletal maturity; and any underlying or contributing disease process.

Bracing and Exercise. For many curves in the growing child and adolescent, bracing may be the treatment of choice. It is important to realize that *bracing is not curative,* but that it may slow the progression of the curvature to allow skeletal growth and maturity. The two most common types of bracing are (1) the **Boston** and **Wilmington braces,** which are underarm orthoses customized from prefabricated plastic shells, with corrective forces for each patient using lateral pads and decreasing lumbar lordosis, and (2) a **TLSO (thoracolumbosacral orthosis),** which is an underarm orthosis made of plastic that is custom molded to the body and then shaped to

FIG. 31-15 ■ Defects of spinal column. **A,** Normal spine. **B,** Kyphosis. **C,** Lordosis. **D,** Normal spine in balance. **E,** Mild scoliosis in balance. **F,** Severe scoliosis not in balance. **G,** Rib hump and flank asymmetry seen in flexion caused by rotary component. (Redrawn from Hilt NE, Schmitt EW: *Pediatric orthopedic nursing*, St Louis, 1975, Mosby.)

FIG. 31-16 ■ **A,** Standard thoracolumbosacral orthotic (TLSO) brace for idiopathic scoliosis. Brace may be decorated to make it more acceptable to adolescents. **B,** Variation of a standard TLSO brace that fastens in the back to provide needed support. **C,** Posterior view of same brace.

correct or hold the deformity (Fig. 31-16). The **Milwaukee brace,** which is an individually adapted brace that includes a neck ring, is rarely used in scoliosis but is sometimes used in the treatment of kyphosis. The **Charleston nighttime bending brace** is worn only when the child is in bed because it prevents walking because of the severity of the trunk bend. Bracing, although used as the gold standard treatment for mild to moderate curvatures, has not proved to be entirely effective in the treatment of scoliosis (Newton and Wenger, 2001), and some retrospective studies show only slight variation in outcomes in relation to the type of brace used. Compliance in wearing the brace is difficult because of the child's age and preoccupation with body image and appearance.

Exercises alone and chiropractic treatment are rarely of value for managing scoliosis; transcutaneous electrical nerve stimulation has also proved to be an ineffective treatment for this condition. Exercises are of benefit when used in conjunction with bracing to maintain and strengthen spinal and abdominal muscles during treatment.

Surgical Management. Surgical intervention may be required for correction of severe curves (usually 40 degrees or more). The degree of curvature and the cause inform the decision for surgery. Bracing and exercise have been universally disappointing in curves greater than 40 degrees, and paralytic and congenital curves, which will eventually progress, are best treated with early surgical stabilization if the child's health status will allow major surgery. The child's age and location of the curvature influence the decision for surgery, and any progressive or severe curve that does not respond to more conservative orthotic measures requires surgical correction. Difficulties with balance or seating, respiratory excursion, or pain are also considered.

The surgical technique consists of realignment and straightening with internal fixation and instrumentation combined with bony fusion (**arthrodesis**) of the realigned spine. The goals of surgical intervention are to correct the curvatures on the sagittal and coronal planes and to have a solid, pain-free fusion in a well-balanced torso, with maximum mobility of the remaining spinal segments.

Many instrumentation systems are available, including Harrington, Dwyer, Zielke, Luque, Cotrel-Dubousset, Isola, TSRH (Texas Scottish Rite Hospital), and Moss Miami. Selection of the system is individualized according to the patient's needs and surgeon's preference. Posterior or anterior approaches can be used.

The Harrington system, the first internal spinal instrumentation device, consists of distraction and compression rods, hooks, and nuts. The posterior elements are decorticated, and bone from the iliac crest or donor bone is placed across the vertebrae to provide fusion. Postoperatively the child is logrolled to prevent spinal motion and a molded plastic jacket is used to stabilize the spine until the fusion is solid.

The Luque-rod segmental spinal instrumentation provides segmental stability with the use of wires and L-shaped rods. By way of a posterior approach, the wires are threaded beneath the lamina of each vertebra and tightened around the rods resting along the transverse processes to stabilize the spine. Bone from the iliac crest or donor bone is used to fuse the spine. The advantage of this method is that the patient can be mobile within a few days and requires no postoperative immobilization. The disadvantage is the risk of nerve damage.

The Cotrel-Dubousset instrumentation combines the Harrington and L-rod approaches by using bilateral rods and hooks at many sites. Anterior approaches using the Dwyer or Zielke instrumentation involve screws into the vertebral bodies connected by a cable or rod. These systems require postoperative immobilization with a custom-fitted plastic jacket.

Nursing Care Management

Treatment for scoliosis extends over a significant portion of the affected child's period of growth. In adolescents this period is the one in which their identity, both physical and psychologic, is formed. The identification of scoliosis as a "deformity," in combination with unattractive appliances and a significant surgical procedure, can have a negative effect on the already fragile adolescent body image. The adolescent and family require excellent nursing care not only for physical needs to be met, but also for psychologic needs associated with the diagnosis, surgery, postoperative recovery, and eventual rehabilitation (Slote, 2002). Although adolescents with scoliosis are encouraged to participate in most peer activities, necessary therapeutic modifications are likely to make them feel different and apart. Nursing care of the adolescent who is facing scoliosis surgery, potential social isolation, pain, and uncertainty, not to mention misunderstood emotions and body image issues, must be evaluated from the adolescent's perspective to be successful in meeting the individual's needs (Napierkowski, 2007).

When a child or adolescent first faces the prospect of a prolonged period in a brace, jacket, or other device, the therapy program and the nature of the device must be explained thoroughly to both the child and the parents so that they will understand the anticipated results, how the appliance corrects the defect, the freedoms and constraints imposed by the device, and what they can do to help achieve the desired goal. Management involves the skills and services of a team of specialists, including the orthopedist, physical therapist, orthotist (a specialist in fitting orthopedic braces), nurse, social worker, and sometimes a thoracic or pulmonary specialist.

It is difficult for a child or adolescent to be restricted at any phase of development, but the adolescent needs continual positive reinforcement, encouragement, and as much independence as can be safely assumed during this time. Adolescents appreciate guidance and assistance regarding anticipated problems, such as selection of clothing and participation in social activities. Socialization with peers is strongly encouraged, and every effort is expended to help the adolescent feel attractive and worthwhile.

Preoperative Care. The preoperative workup usually involves a radiographic series, including bending and traction films, pulmonary function studies, and a number of routine laboratory studies (including prothrombin, partial thromboplastin, and bleeding times; blood count; electrolyte levels; urinalysis and urine culture; and blood levels of any medications). Because spinal surgery usually involves considerable blood loss, several options are considered preoperatively to maintain or replace blood volume. These options include autologous blood donations obtained from the patient before the surgery; intraoperative blood salvage; intraoperative hemodilution; erythropoietin administration; and controlled induced hypotension, which must be carefully monitored at all times to prevent physiologic instability (Newton and Wenger, 2001).

Surgery for spinal fusion is complex, and often adolescents who require the procedure because of idiopathic scoliosis are not familiar with medical terms, procedures, or experiences. Preoperative teaching is critical for the adolescent to be able to cooperate and participate in his or her treatment and recovery. Because the surgery is extensive, the patient is taught how to manage his or her own patient-controlled analgesia (PCA) pump; how to log-roll; and the use and function of other equipment, such as a chest tube (for anterior repair) and Foley catheter. It is recommended that the child or adolescent bring a favorite toy (age dependent) or personal items such as a favorite stuffed animal, laptop computer (for web surfing and e-mails), movie player, MP3 player, or portable compact disc player for postoperative use. Meeting with a peer who has undergone a similar surgery is also valuable (Slote, 2002).

Postoperative Care. After surgery, patients are monitored in an acute care setting and log-rolled when changing position to prevent damage to the fusion and instrumentation. Skin care is important, and pressure-relieving mattresses or beds may be needed to prevent pressure wounds (see Maintaining Healthy Skin, Chapter 22).

In addition to the usual postoperative assessments—of wound, circulation, and vital signs—the neurologic status of the patient's extremities requires special attention. Prompt recognition of any neurologic impairment is imperative because delayed paralysis may develop that requires surgical intervention. The most common postoperative problems after spinal fusion include neurologic injury or spinal cord injury, hypotension from acute blood loss, wound infection, delayed neurologic injury, and implanted hardware complications (Newton and Wenger, 2001). The child usually has considerable pain for the first few days after surgery and requires frequent administration of pain medication, preferably IV opioids administered on a regular schedule. For children able to understand the concept, PCA is recommended (see Pain Assessment; Pain Management, Chapter 7).

In most cases the patient begins ambulation as soon as possible, depending on the instrumentation used—generally by the second or third postoperative day. They are discharged by 1 week, depending on the surgical approach. In addition to pain management, the patient is evaluated for skin integrity, adequate urinary output, fluid and electrolyte balance, and ileus (Slote, 2002). The latter may be particularly distressful for the adolescent who is self-conscious. Discharge planning should include a timetable for follow-up with the practitioner and resumption of regular activities.

The patient may start physical therapy as soon as he or she is able, beginning with range-of-motion exercises on the first postoperative day and many of the activities of daily living in the following days. Self-care, such as washing and eating, is always encouraged. Throughout the hospitalization age-appropriate activities and contact with family and friends are important parts of nursing care and planning (see Immobilization, p. 1107).

The family is encouraged to become involved in the patient's care to facilitate the transition from hospital to home management. An organization that provides education and services to both families and professionals is the National Scoliosis Foundation.* The American Academy of Orthopaedic Surgeons† and Scoliosis Research Society,‡ an organization of physicians and scientists, have published an excellent

---

*Five Cabot Place, Stoughton, MA 02072; (800) 673-6922; http://www.scoliosis.org.

†6300 N. River Road, Rosemont, IL 60018-4262; (847) 823-7186; http://www.aaos.org.

‡611 E. Wells St., Suite 1100, Milwaukee, WI 53202; (414) 289-9107; http://www.srs.org.

book, *Scoliosis,* and the Scoliosis Research Society has educational information available on its website.

INFECTIONS OF BONES AND JOINTS

OSTEOMYELITIS

Osteomyelitis, an infectious process in the bone, can occur at any age but most frequently is seen in children 10 years of age or younger. *Staphylococcus aureus* is the most common causative organism. **Acute hematogenous osteomyelitis** results when a bloodborne bacterium causes an infection in the bone. Common foci include infected lesions, upper respiratory tract infections, otitis media, tonsillitis, abscessed teeth, pyelonephritis, and infected burns. **Exogenous osteomyelitis** is acquired from direct inoculation of the bone from a puncture wound, open fracture, surgical contamination, or adjacent tissue infection. **Subacute osteomyelitis** has a longer course and may be caused by less virulent microbes with a walled-off abscess or Brodie abscess, typically in the proximal or distal tibia. **Chronic osteomyelitis** is a progression of acute osteomyelitis and is characterized by dead bone, bone loss, and drainage and sinus tracts.

Generally, healthy bone is not likely to become infected. Factors that contribute to infection include inoculation with a large number of organisms, presence of a foreign body, bone injury, high virulence of an organism, immunosuppression, and malnutrition; certain types and locations of bone are also more vulnerable to infection.

Typically children with acute hematogenous osteomyelitis are seen with a 2- to 7-day history of pain, warmth, tenderness, and decreased range of motion in the affected limb, along with systemic symptoms of fever, irritability, and lethargy (Box 31-8). Symptoms often resemble those observed in other diseases involving bones such as arthritis or leukemia.

Pathophysiology

Osteomyelitis can be acquired exogenously by direct inoculation of bone during trauma or surgery; the hand and foot are commons sites. Hematogenous osteomyelitis is seeded by organisms from a preexisting infection such as tonsillitis or impetigo or from a contiguous source such as an adjacent infected bone or joint. Hematogenous osteomyelitis usually occurs in the metaphyses of long bones such as the femur or tibia. The infecting organism travels from the site of infection to the small end-artery capillary loops in the bone metaphyses, causing obstruction and initiating infection, with complications of bone destruction and abscess formation. In infants the diagnosis is challenging because of difficulty localizing symptoms and the increased likelihood of multiple bone involvement.

Diagnostic Evaluation

Organism identification and antibiotic susceptibility testing are essential for effective therapy. Cultures of aspirated subperiosteal pus along with cultures of blood, joint fluid, and infected skin samples should be obtained. Bone biopsy is indicated if blood culture results and radiographic findings are not consistent with osteomyelitis. Supporting evidence for osteomyelitis includes leukocytosis and elevated erythrocyte sedimentation rate. Radiographic signs, except for soft-tissue swelling, are evident only after 2 to 3 weeks. A three-phase technetium bone scan can show areas of increased blood flow, such as occurs in early stages in infected bone, and is useful in

---

BOX 31-8

Clinical Manifestations of Acute Osteomyelitis

GENERAL MANIFESTATIONS
History of trauma to affected bone (frequent)
Child appearing very ill
Irritability
Restlessness
Elevated temperature
Rapid pulse
Dehydration

LOCAL MANIFESTATIONS
Tenderness
Increased warmth
Diffuse swelling over involved bone
Involved extremity painful, especially on movement
Involved extremity held in semiflexion
Surrounding muscles tense and resistant to passive movement

---

locating multiple sites; however, it is not a diagnostic test. CT can detect bone destruction, and MRI provides anatomic details useful in delineating the area of involvement, especially if surgical intervention is planned. Sometimes the osteomyelitis may be unrecognized if it occurs as a complication of a severe toxic and debilitating disease.

Therapeutic Management

After culture specimens are obtained, empiric therapy is started with IV antibiotics covering the mostly likely organisms. For *S. aureus,* nafcillin or clindamycin is generally used; methicillin-resistant *S. aureus* may require vancomycin. When the infective agent is identified, administration of the appropriate antibiotic is initiated and continued for at least 4 weeks, but the length of therapy is determined by the duration of the symptoms, the response to treatment, and the sensitivity of the organism. In selected cases oral antibiotic therapy may follow a shorter IV course. Because of the prolonged duration of high-dose antibiotic therapy, it is important to monitor for hematologic, renal, hepatic, ototoxic, and other potential side effects.

Surgery may be indicated if there is no response to specific antibiotic therapy, persistent soft-tissue abscess is seen, or the infection spreads to the joint. Opinions differ regarding surgical intervention, but many advocate sequestrectomy and surgical drainage to decompress the metaphyseal space before pus erupts and spreads to the subperiosteal space, forming abscesses that strip the periosteum from bone or form draining sinuses. When these complications occur, a chronic infection usually persists. When surgical drainage is carried out, polyethylene tubes are placed in the wound; one tube instills an antibiotic solution directly into the infected area by gravity, and the other, connected to a suction apparatus, provides drainage.

Nursing Care Management

During the acute phase of illness any movement of the affected limb will cause discomfort; therefore the child is positioned comfortably with the affected limb supported. Moving and turning are carried out carefully and gently to minimize pain. The child may require pain medication or sedation. Vital signs are taken and recorded frequently, and measures are implemented to reduce a significant temperature elevation.

Antibiotic therapy requires careful observation and monitoring of the IV equipment and site. Because more than one antibiotic is usually administered, the compatibility of the drugs is determined and care is taken to avoid mixing incompatible drugs. For long-term antibiotic therapy, an intermittent infusion device or peripherally inserted central catheter is used. Antibiotic therapy is often continued at home.

Standard precautions are put in effect for children with open wounds, depending on the institution's policies. The wound is managed according to the practitioner's directions. Administration of antibiotic solution directly into the wound is most efficiently accomplished using a regular infusion setup that is prepared and regulated in the same manner as for any IV infusion. Intake and output are measured and recorded, and the character of both the wound and drainage is noted. The amount and character of drainage on the wound dressing are also noted.

Casts are sometimes used for immobilization, and, if so, routine cast care is carried out. The extremity is examined for sensation, circulation, and pain, and the area over the inflammation is usually left open for observation. The affected area, casted or uncasted, is assessed for color, swelling, heat, and tenderness.

The child usually has a poor appetite and may be prone to vomiting. The appetite returns as the acute symptoms recede. During convalescence, adequate nutrition must be maintained to aid healing and formation of new bone.

When the acute stage subsides, children begin to feel better, appetite improves, and they become interested in their surroundings and relationships. They wish to move about in bed and are allowed to do so. However, weight bearing on the affected limb is not permitted until healing is well under way in order to avoid pathologic fractures. Provision of diversional and constructive activities becomes an important nursing intervention. Children are usually confined to bed for some time after the acute phase but may be allowed to move about on a stretcher or in a wheelchair when isolation and bed rest are no longer necessary. At this stage the continuous IV infusion may be replaced by a heparin lock system to allow greater freedom.

As the infection subsides, physical therapy is instituted to ensure restoration of optimum function. The child is usually discharged on a regimen of oral antibiotics, and progress is followed closely for some time.

SEPTIC ARTHRITIS

Septic arthritis is a bacterial infection in the joint. It usually results from hematogenous spread or from direct extension of an adjacent cellulitis or osteomyelitis. Direct inoculation from trauma accounts for 15% to 20% of septic arthritis cases. The most common causative organism is *S. aureus*. Community-acquired methicillin-resistant *S. aureus* is commonly a cause of septic arthritis (Gutierrez, 2005). In addition to *S. aureus,* pathogens seen in neonates include group B streptococci, *Escherichia coli,* and *Candida albicans.* In children 2 months to 5 years of age, *S. aureus, Streptococcus pyogenes, Streptococcus pneumoniae,* and *Kingella kingae* are the primary organisms causing infection, whereas children older than 5 years are more likely to be infected by *S. aureus* and *S. pyogenes*; sexually active adolescents may be infected by *Neisseria gonorrhoeae* (Gutierrez, 2005).

Knees, hips, ankles, and elbows are the most common joints affected. Clinical manifestations include severe joint pain, swelling, warmth of overlying tissue, and occasionally erythema. The child is resistant to any joint movement. Features of systemic illness such as fever, malaise, headache, nausea, vomiting, and irritability may also be present.

Therapeutic Management and Nursing Care Management

The affected joint is aspirated and the specimen evaluated by Gram stain; culturing (including separate cultures for *Haemophilus influenzae* and *N. gonorrhoeae*); and determination of leukocyte count and glucose, lactate, and protein levels. An infection involving the hip, however, is considered a surgical emergency to prevent compromised blood supply to the head of the femur (Lampe, 2007). In addition, blood culture should be performed, and complete blood count with differential and erythrocyte sedimentation rate or C-reactive protein level should be obtained. Early radiographic findings are limited to soft-tissue swelling but may reveal a foreign body, and such films always provide a baseline for comparison. Technetium scans reveal areas of increased blood flow but will not differentiate between sites. MRI and CT scans provide more detailed images of cartilage loss, joint narrowing, erosions, and ankylosis of progressive disease.

Surgical intervention may also be required if there was a penetrating wound or a possible involvement of a foreign object. Physical therapy may be initiated for the child who is immobilized in a cast or traction to prevent flexion contractures.

Treatment is IV antibiotic therapy based on Gram stain results and the clinical presentation. The benefits of serial aspirations to demonstrate sterility of synovial fluid and reduce pressure or pain are controversial. Pain management is an important aspect of nursing care, particularly with involvement of a large joint such as the hip. Additional nursing care is the same as for osteomyelitis.

SKELETAL TUBERCULOSIS

In children tubercular infection of the bones and joints is acquired by lymphohematogenous spread at the time of primary infection. Occasionally it is from chronic pulmonary tuberculosis. Skeletal tubercular infection is not common in the United States but should be considered in communities with high tuberculosis case rates. The infection is most likely to involve the vertebrae, causing tubercular spondylitis. If the infection is progressive, it causes Pott disease with destruction of the vertebral bodies and results in kyphosis. Symptoms are insidious. The child may report persistent or intermittent pain. Other findings include joint swelling and stiffness; fever and weight loss are not common. Tubercular arthritis can also affect single joints such as a knee or hip and tends to cause severe destruction of adjacent bone. Infection in the fingers causes spina ventosa, a tuberculous dactylitis.

As with pulmonary tuberculosis, the index case should be located. A family and environmental history needs to be obtained and tuberculin skin tests (TSTs) performed. Results of TSTs are positive for the majority of children with tuberculous arthritis; however, the results are not diagnostic, and the clinical and laboratory features do not differentiate tubercular arthritis from a nontubercular septic arthritis. Diagnosis requires isolation of *Mycobacterium tuberculosis* from the site. Patients with the susceptible organism start treatment with combined antituberculosis chemotherapy (isoniazid, rifampin, and pyrazinamide); directly observed therapy (DOT) is preferred. (See also Chapter 23.)

Nursing Care Management

Nursing care depends on the site and extent of infection. Tuberculous spondylitis and hip infection may require immobilization, casting, and fusion. Nursing care is the same as for osteomyelitis and septic arthritis.

BONE AND SOFT-TISSUE TUMORS
GENERAL CONCEPTS: BONE TUMORS

Malignant bone tumors represent less than 5% of all malignant neoplasms, but 85% of all primary malignant bone tumors in children are either osteogenic sarcoma or Ewing sarcoma. The peak ages during childhood are 15 to 19 years. The sexes are affected equally until puberty, at which time the ratio approaches 2:1 in favor of males. This propensity for males with a peak incidence during adolescence is thought to result from the accelerated growth rate of osseous tissue.

Neoplastic disease can arise from any tissues involved in bone growth, such as osteoid matrix, bone marrow elements, fat, blood and lymph vessels, nerve sheath, and cartilage. They have several characteristics in common, which are discussed in the following sections. Specific information about each tumor is then presented.

Most malignant bone tumors produce localized pain in the affected site, which may be severe or dull and may be attributed to trauma or the vague complaint of "growing pains." The pain is often relieved by a flexed position, which relaxes the muscles overlying the stretched periosteum. Frequently it draws attention when the child limps, curtails physical activity, or is unable to hold heavy objects (Box 31-9).

Diagnostic Evaluation

Diagnosis begins with a thorough history and physical examination. A primary objective is to rule out causes such as trauma or infection. Careful questioning regarding pain is essential in determining the duration and rate of tumor growth. Physical assessment focuses on functional status of the affected area; signs of inflammation; size of the mass; involvement of regional lymph nodes; and any systemic indication of generalized malignancy, such as anemia, weight loss, and frequent infection.

Definitive diagnosis is based on radiologic studies, such as CT to determine the extent of the lesion; MRI to assess soft tissue, tumor boundaries, and nerve and vessel involvement; radioisotope bone scans to evaluate metastasis; and either needle or surgical bone biopsy to determine the histologic pattern. Radiologic findings are characteristic for each type of tumor. In osteogenic sarcoma, needlelike new bone formation growing at right angles to the diaphysis (shaft) produces a "sunburst" appearance. In Ewing sarcoma the deposits of new bone in layers under the periosteum produce an "onion skin" appearance. In both types of bone tumors, soft-tissue infiltration may be apparent.

At present there is no reliable biochemical test for bone cancers. Elevated alkaline phosphatase levels may occur in osteoid tumors. Several tests may be done for differential diagnosis in terms of secondary bone metastasis from Wilms tumor,

---

BOX 31-9
Clinical Manifestations of Bone Tumors

Pain localized at affected site
- May be severe or dull
- Often relieved by position of flexion

Frequently brought to attention when child:
- Limps
- Curtails own physical activity
- Is unable to hold heavy objects

---

neuroblastoma, retinoblastoma, rhabdomyosarcoma, lymphoma, or leukemia. Lung computerized tomography is usually a standard procedure, since pulmonary metastasis is the most common complication of primary bone tumors. Bone marrow aspiration is helpful in diagnosing Ewing sarcoma in the rare event that the child has bone marrow metastasis.

OSTEOSARCOMA

Osteosarcoma (osteogenic sarcoma) is the most common bone cancer in children. Its peak incidence is between 10 and 25 years of age (Link, Gebhardt, and Myers, 2006). It presumably arises from bone-forming mesenchyme, which gives rise to malignant osteoid tissue. Most primary tumor sites are in the metaphysis (wider part of the shaft, adjacent to the epiphyseal growth plate) of long bones, especially in the lower extremities. More than half occur in the femur, particularly the distal portion, with the rest involving the humerus, tibia, pelvis, jaw, and phalanges.

Therapeutic Management

Optimum treatment of osteosarcoma is surgery and chemotherapy. The surgical approach consists of surgical biopsy followed by either limb salvage or amputation. Depending on the tumor site, surgery includes amputation of the affected extremity at least 7.5 cm (3 inches) above the proximal tumor margin or above the joint proximal to the involved bone. With tumors of the distal femur, preservation of the hip joint may be possible. Other procedures include an above-the-knee amputation for tumors of the tibia or fibula, a hemipelvectomy for tumors of the innominate (hip) bone, and a forequarter amputation (removal of arm, scapula, and portion of the clavicle on the affected side) for tumors of the upper humerus.

The other surgical approach for selected patients is the **limb salvage procedure,** which involves en bloc resection of the primary tumor with prosthetic replacement of the involved bone. For example, with osteosarcoma of the distal femur, a total femur and joint replacement is performed. Frequently children undergoing a limb salvage procedure will receive preoperative chemotherapy in an attempt to decrease the tumor size and make surgery more manageable (Link, Gebhardt, and Myers, 2006).

Chemotherapy plays a vital role in treatment of osteosarcoma. Antineoplastic drugs, such as high-dose methotrexate with citrovorum factor rescue, doxorubicin, bleomycin, actinomycin D, cyclophosphamide, ifosfamide, and cisplatin, may be administered singly or in combination and may be employed both before and after surgery. When pulmonary metastasis is found, thoracotomy and chemotherapy have resulted in prolonged survival and potential cure. These combined-modality approaches have significantly improved the prognosis in osteosarcoma to approximately 85% in non-metastatic patients (Lanzkowsky, 2000). New trials have recently been completed using muramyl tripeptide phosphatidylethanolamine to eradicate micrometastases by stimulating macrophages to kill tumor cells not eliminated by chemotherapy (Link, Gebhardt, and Myers, 2006).

Nursing Care Management

Nursing care depends on the type of surgical approach. Obviously the family may have more difficulty adjusting to an amputation than a limb salvage procedure. In either instance, preparation of the child and family is critical. Straightforward honesty is essential in gaining the child's cooperation and trust. The diagnosis of cancer should not be disguised with false-hoods such as "infection." To accept the need for radical surgery, the child must be aware of the lack of alternatives for treatment. Although the responsibility of telling the child is generally left to the physician, the nurse should be present at the discussion or be aware of exactly what is said. The child should be told a few days before surgery to allow him or her time to think about the diagnosis and consequent treatment and to ask questions.

Sometimes children have many questions about the prosthesis, limitations on physical ability, and prognosis in terms of cure. At other times they react with silence or with a calm manner that belies their concern and fear. Either response must be accepted, since it is part of the grieving process of a loss. For those who desire information, it may be helpful to introduce them to another amputee before surgery or to show them pictures of the prosthesis.* However, the nurse must be careful not to overwhelm children with information. A sound approach is to answer questions without offering additional information. For those who do not pursue additional information, the nurse expresses a willingness to talk.

The child is also informed of the need for chemotherapy and its side effects before surgery. Caution must be exercised about offering too much information at one time. It is wise to discuss hair loss with an emphasis on positive aspects, such as wearing a wig. Because bone tumors affect adolescents and young adults, it is not unusual for them to become angry over all the radical body alterations.

If an amputation is performed, the child is usually fitted with a temporary prosthesis immediately after surgery, which permits early functioning and fosters psychologic adjustment. If this is not done, the child requires stump care, which is the same as for any amputee. A permanent prosthesis is usually fitted within 6 to 8 weeks. During hospitalization the child begins physical therapy to become proficient in the use and care of the device.

Phantom limb pain may develop after amputation. This symptom is characterized by sensations such as tingling, itching, and, more frequently, pain felt in the amputated limb. The child and family need to know that the sensations are real, not imagined. Amitriptyline (Elavil) has been used successfully in children to decrease the pain (Olsson, 1999).

Discharge planning must begin early in the postoperative period. Once the child has begun physical therapy, the nurse should consult with the therapist and practitioner to evaluate the child's physical and emotional readiness to reenter school. It is an opportune time to involve a community nurse in the child's home care. Every effort is made to promote normalcy and gradual resumption of realistic preamputation activities.* Role-playing in anticipation of such experiences is beneficial in preparing the child for the inevitable confrontation by others. Environmental barriers, such as stairs, are assessed in terms of the accessibility in the school and home, especially because the child may need to use crutches or a wheelchair before complete healing and prosthetic competency are achieved.

The nurse encourages the child to select clothing that best camouflages the prosthesis, such as pants or long-sleeved shirts. Well-fitted prostheses are so natural looking that girls can usually wear sheer stockings without revealing the device. Emphasizing feminine or masculine apparel helps the child regain a feeling of self-identity. Even during the postoperative period, encouraging the child to wear blue jeans and a T-shirt may distract attention from the deformity and focus it on familiar aspects of appearance.

The family and child need much support in adjusting not only to a life-threatening diagnosis but also to alteration in body form and function. Because loss of a limb entails a grieving process, those caring for the child need to recognize that the reactions of anger and depression are normal and necessary. Often parents view the anger as a direct affront to them for allowing the amputation to occur, or they see the depression as rejection. These are not personal attacks but the child's attempts to cope with a loss.

EWING SARCOMA (PRIMITIVE NEUROECTODERMAL TUMOR)

Ewing sarcoma, classified as a primitive neuroectodermal tumor (PNET), is the second most common malignant bone tumor (after osteosarcoma) in childhood. Ewing sarcoma arises in the marrow spaces of the bone rather than from osseous tissue. The tumor originates in the shaft of long and trunk bones, most often affecting the femur, tibia, fibula, humerus, ulna, vertebrae, scapula, ribs, pelvic bones, and skull (Link, Gebhardt, and Myers, 2006). It occurs almost exclusively in individuals under age 30, with the majority being between 4 and 25 years of age.

Therapeutic Management

Surgical amputation is not routinely recommended but may be considered when the results of radiotherapy render the extremity useless or deformed (e.g., from restricted growth in young children). The treatment of choice is intensive irradiation of the involved bone combined with chemotherapy. A widely used drug regimen includes vincristine, actinomycin D, cyclophosphamide or ifosfamide, etoposide, and doxorubicin. The addition of ifosfamide and etoposide has increased the 3-year survival to 80% (Lanzkowsky, 2000).

Nursing Care Management

The psychologic adjustment to Ewing sarcoma is typically less traumatic than it is to osteosarcoma because of the preservation of the affected limb. Many families accept the diagnosis

---

*Information about prostheses can be obtained from the National Amputation Foundation, 40 Church St., Malverne, NY 11565; (516) 887-3600; http://www.nationalamputation.org.

---

*Information about special programs for children with amputations is available from the Candlelighters Childhood Cancer Foundation, PO Box 498, Kensington, MD 20895; (800) 366-2223, (301) 962-3520; fax: (301) 962-3521; http://www.candlelighters.org.

with relief in knowing that this type of bone cancer does not necessitate amputation, and initially they may not be aware of the damaging effects on the irradiated site. Consequently they need preparation for the various diagnostic tests, including bone marrow aspiration and surgical biopsy, and adequate explanation of the treatment regimen. High-dose radiotherapy often causes a skin reaction of dry or moist desquamation followed by hyperpigmentation. The child should wear loose-fitting clothes over the irradiated area to minimize additional skin irritation. Because of increased sensitivity, the area is protected from sunlight and sudden changes in temperature, such as from heating pads or ice packs. The child is encouraged to use the extremity as tolerated. Occasionally the physical therapist may plan an active exercise program to preserve maximum function.

The child needs the same considerations for adjusting to the effects of chemotherapy as any other patient with cancer. The drug regimen usually results in hair loss, severe nausea and vomiting, peripheral neuropathy, and possibly cardiotoxicity. Every effort should be made to outline a treatment plan that allows the child maximum resumption of a normal lifestyle and activities (Kline and Sevier, 2003). (See also Nursing Care Plan: The Child with Cancer, Chapter 26.)

RHABDOMYOSARCOMA

Soft-tissue sarcomas are the fourth most common type of solid tumors in children. These malignant neoplasms originate from undifferentiated mesenchymal cells in muscles, tendons, bursae, and fascia, or in fibrous, connective, lymphatic, or vascular tissue. They derive their name from the specific tissue(s) of origin, such as myosarcoma (*myo*, muscle). Rhabdomyosarcoma (*rhabdo*, striated) is the most common soft-tissue sarcoma in children. Striated (skeletal) muscle is found almost anywhere in the body, so these tumors occur in many sites, the most common of which are the head and neck, especially the orbit. The disease occurs in children in all age-groups but is most common in children younger than 5 years of age. Its incidence is approximately 8.5 per 1 million for Caucasian children but only 4.0 per 1 million for African-American children in the age-group, from 2 to 19 years (Lanzkowsky, 2000). Rhabdomyosarcoma arises from embryonic mesenchyme.

The initial signs and symptoms are related to the site of the tumor and compression of adjacent organs (Box 31-10). Some tumor locations, particularly the orbit, produce symptoms early in the course of the illness and contribute to rapid diagnosis and an improved prognosis. Other tumors, such as those of the retroperitoneal area, produce no symptoms until they are large, invasive, and widely metastasized. Unfortunately, many of the signs and symptoms attributable to rhabdomyosarcoma are vague and frequently suggest a common childhood illness, such as "earache" or "runny nose." In some instances a primary tumor site is never identified.

Diagnostic Evaluation

Diagnosis begins with a careful examination of the head and neck area, particularly palpation of a nontender, hard mass. The nasopharynx and oropharynx are inspected for any evidence of a visible mass. Radiographic studies to isolate a tumor site are performed, accompanied by chest x-ray examinations, CT, MRI, bone surveys, and bone marrow aspiration to rule out metastasis. A lumbar puncture is indicated for head and neck tumors to examine the cerebrospinal fluid for malignant cells. An excisional biopsy is done to confirm the histologic type.

BOX 31-10

Clinical Manifestations of Rhabdomyosarcoma According to Tumor Site

CENTRAL NERVOUS SYSTEM
Headaches
Morning vomiting
Diplopia

ORBIT
Rapidly developing unilateral proptosis or exophthalmos
Ecchymosis of conjunctiva
Loss of extraocular movements (strabismus)
Orbital cellulitis

NASOPHARYNX
Stuffy nose (earliest sign)
Nasal obstruction—Dysphagia, nasal voice (obstruction of posterior nasal conchae)
Pain (sore throat and ear)
Epistaxis
Palpable neck nodes
Visible mass in oropharynx (late sign)

PARANASAL SINUSES
Nasal obstruction
Local pain, swelling
Discharge (may be unilateral)
Sinusitis

MIDDLE EAR
Signs of chronic serous otitis media
Pain, swelling
Mass in external canal
Sanguinopurulent drainage
Facial nerve palsy
Conductive hearing loss

RETROPERITONEAL AREA (USUALLY A "SILENT" TUMOR)
Abdominal mass
Pain
Signs of intestinal or genitourinary obstruction

PERINEUM
Visible superficial mass (scrotum, vaginal or cervical areas)
Bowel or bladder dysfunction (from tumor compression)
Vaginal bleeding or mucosanguineous discharge

EXTREMITY
Pain
Palpable fixed mass
Regional lymph node enlargement

Careful staging is extremely important for planning treatment and determining the prognosis. The Intergroup Rhabdomyosarcoma Study has established clinical staging (Wexler, Meyer, and Helman, 2006).

With the change in treatment from radical surgery or radiotherapy to a multimodal approach, survival rates for all stages have increased considerably. Five-year survival rates are approximately 65% (Lanzkowsky, 2000; Wexler, Meyer, and Helman, 2006). Data suggest that children who remain disease free for 2 years are probably cured; however, if relapse occurs, the prognosis for long-term survival is extremely poor.

Therapeutic Management

Because this tumor is highly malignant, with metastasis frequently occurring at the time of diagnosis, aggressive multimodal therapy is recommended. In the past, radical surgical removal of the tumor was the treatment of choice, but with improved survival from combined chemotherapy and irradiation, surgery plays a lesser role. Complete removal of the primary tumor is advocated whenever possible. However, only biopsy is required in certain tumor locations, such as those of the orbit, when followed by irradiation and chemotherapy. This is a fortunate change, since it avoids the devastating effects of enucleation, amputation, or pelvic exenteration.

High-dose irradiation to the primary tumor is recommended, except in group I tumors. Chemotherapy plays a major role in treatment of all groups. Drugs that are cytotoxic for rhabdomyosarcoma are vincristine, actinomycin D, ifosfamide, cisplatin, carboplatin, etoposide, cyclophosphamide, topotecan, melphalan, and doxorubicin, which are administered for 1 to 2 years, depending on the stage of the disease (Lanzkowsky, 2000).

Nursing Care Management

The nursing responsibilities are similar to those for other types of cancer, especially the solid tumors when surgery is employed. Specific objectives include (1) careful assessment for signs of the tumor, especially during well-child examinations; (2) preparation of the child and family for the multiple diagnostic tests, and (3) supportive care during each stage of multimodal therapy (Kline and Sevier, 2003).

DISORDERS OF JOINTS
JUVENILE IDIOPATHIC ARTHRITIS (JUVENILE RHEUMATOID ARTHRITIS)

Juvenile idiopathic arthritis (JIA) is a new name replacing *juvenile rheumatoid arthritis (JRA)* in the research literature and more slowly in clinical practice. The JRA nomenclature revision to JIA was due in part to the minimally applicable reference to "rheumatoid" in JRA. Only a small percentage of children have a positive rheumatoid factor, yet the name burdens the family with images of adult disfiguring rheumatoid arthritis. Furthermore, the JRA classification system focused more on disease at onset vs disease progression, which is more important (Warren, Perez, Curry, and others, 2001).

Semantics aside, JIA is a chronic autoimmune inflammatory disease causing inflammation of joints and other tissue with an unknown cause. JIA starts before age 16 years with peak onset between 1 and 3 years of age. Twice as many girls as boys are affected. The incidence is reported to be approximately 13.9 per 100,000 children per year among Caucasian children, with an overall prevalence of approximately 113 per 100,000 children (Miller and Cassidy, 2007). The cause is unknown, but two factors are hypothesized: immunogenic susceptibility and an environmental or external trigger such as a virus (e.g., rubella, Epstein-Barr virus, parvovirus B19) (Miller and Cassidy, 2007).

Pathophysiology

The disease process is characterized by chronic inflammation of the synovium with joint effusion and eventual erosion, destruction, and fibrosis of the articular cartilage. Adhesions between joint surfaces and ankylosis of joints occur if the inflammatory process persists.

Clinical Manifestations

The outcome of JIA is variable and unpredictable. The disease, even in severe forms, is rarely life threatening but can cause significant disability. The arthritis tends to wax and wane and eventually becomes inactive in approximately 70% of the cases; however, these children may have severe or minimal joint damage remaining when active arthritis abates. Approximately 30% of the children will have progressive arthritis into adulthood. Their arthritis can cause significant joint deformity and functional disability, requiring medication, physical therapy, and perhaps future joint replacement. Chronic and acute uveitis can cause permanent vision loss if undiagnosed and not aggressively treated.

Classification of Juvenile Idiopathic Arthritis

JIA is not a single disease, but a heterogeneous group of diseases. The universal Durban classification of JIA, revised and published in 1998, lists several disease categories, each with its own set of criteria and exclusions, which continue to be revised (Petty, Southwood, Manners, and others, 2004; Petty, Southwood, Baum, and others, 1998):

Systemic arthritis is arthritis in one or more joints associated with at least 2 weeks of fever, rash, lymphadenopathy, hepatosplenomegaly, and serositis.

Oligoarthritis is arthritis in one to four joints for the first 6 months of disease. It is subdivided to *persistent oligoarthritis* if it remains in four joints or less or becomes *extended oligoarthritis* if it involves more than four joints after 6 months.

Polyarthritis rheumatoid factor negative affects five or more joints in the first 6 months with a negative rheumatoid factor.

Polyarthritis rheumatoid factor positive also affects five or more joints in first 6 months, but these children have a positive rheumatoid factor.

Psoriatic arthritis is arthritis with psoriasis or an associated dactylitis, nail pitting, or onycholysis or psoriasis in a first-degree relative.

Enthesitis-related arthritis is arthritis and/or enthesitis (inflammation at the tendon insertion site) associated with at least two of the following: sacroiliac or lumbosacral pain, HLA-B27 antigen, arthritis in male older than 6 years, acute anterior uveitis, inflammatory bowel disease, Reiter syndrome, or acute anterior uveitis in a first-degree relative.

The JIA classification is replacing the JRA classification, which had three subtypes: pauciarticular, polyarticular, and systemic JRA.

Diagnostic Evaluation

JIA is a diagnosis of exclusion; there are no definitive tests. Classifications are based on the clinical criteria of age of onset before 16 years, arthritis in one or more joints for 6 weeks or longer, and exclusion of other causes. Laboratory tests may provide supporting evidence of disease. Sedimentation rate may or may not be elevated. Leukocytosis is frequently present during exacerbations of systemic JIA. Antinuclear antibodies are common in JIA but are not specific for arthritis; however, they help identify children who are at greater risk for uveitis. Plain radiographs are the best initial imaging studies and may show soft-tissue swelling and joint space widening from increased synovial fluid in the joint. Later films can reveal osteoporosis, narrow joint space, erosions, subluxation, and ankylosis. A slit lamp eye examination is necessary to diagnosis uveitis, inflammation in the anterior chamber of the eye, which is most common in antinuclear antibody–positive young girls with oligoarthritis. Routine examinations are necessary for early diagnosis and treatment to avoid sight-threatening disease (Kump, Castañeda, Androudi, and others, 2006).

Therapeutic Management

There is no cure for JIA. The major goals of therapy are to control pain, preserve joint range of motion and function, minimize effects of inflammation such as joint deformity, and promote normal growth and development. Outpatient care is the mainstay of therapy; lengthy hospitalizations are infrequent in this era of managed care. The treatment plan can be exhaustive and intrusive for the child and family, including medications, physical and occupational therapy, ophthalmologic slit lamp examinations, splints, comfort measures, dietary management, school modifications, and psychosocial support.

Medications. Many arthritis medications are available, and most are effective in suppressing the inflammatory process and relieving pain. These drugs may be given alone or in combination and are prescribed in a stepwise manner dependent on disease response to each level.

Nonsteroidal antiinflammatory drugs (NSAIDs) are the first drugs used. Naproxen, ibuprofen, and tolmetin are approved for use in children. They are effective with few common side effects other than gastrointestinal irritation and bruising; with naproxen, skin fragility is a possible side effect. NSAIDs must be taken with food. Aspirin, once the drug of choice, has been replaced by NSAIDs because they have fewer side effects and easier administration schedules.

Methotrexate is the second-line medication used in children who have failed with NSAIDs alone. It is started in combination with an NSAID. It is effective, with acceptable toxicity, which requires monitoring of complete blood cell counts and liver functions. Patient education about possible side effects, including discussions with teens about birth defects and avoiding alcohol, is essential.

Corticosteroids are potent immunosuppressives used for life-threatening complications, incapacitating arthritis, and uveitis. They are administered at the lowest effective dosage for the briefest period and discontinued on a tapering schedule. They may be administered orally, as intraarticular joint injections, as IV infusions, or in eye drop form for uveitis. A single intraarticular injection may provide effective relief for children with pauciarticular disease unresponsive to NSAIDs (Padeh and Passwell, 1998). Prolonged use of systemic steroids is associated with significant side effects, including Cushing syndrome, osteoporosis, increased infection risk, glucose intolerance, cataracts, and growth suppression.

Tumor Necrosis Factor Inhibition. **Etanercept** is a tumor necrosis factor-α receptor blocker and an effective drug for children with JIA unresponsive to methotrexate (Lovell, Giannini, Reiff, and others, 2003). It is given once or twice a week via subcutaneous injections. Possible side effects include transient allergic reaction at the injection site, increased infection risk, and rare reports of demyelinating disease and pancytopenia. The risk of malignancy is unknown. Parents and patients should be informed that biologic drugs are new therapies and more will be learned about potential side effects in the postmarketing period.

Slow-acting antirheumatic drugs (SAARDs) may require months to be effective and typically work in combination with NSAIDs. SAARDs include sulfasalazine, hydroxychloroquine, gold, and D-penicillamine. SAARDs are used less often because methotrexate has been recognized as second-line therapy.

Physical and Occupational Therapy. Programs of physical management are individualized for each child and designed to reach the ultimate goal: preserving function or preventing deformity. Physical therapy is directed toward specific joints, focusing on strengthening muscles, mobilizing restricted joint motion, and preventing or correcting deformities. Occupational therapy assumes responsibility for generalized mobility and performance of activities of daily living.

General treatment or maintenance programs vary; physical therapists may be involved several times weekly to monthly in management of a home program, or their visits may be limited to infrequent review of the home program for compliance, effectiveness, and need. Normal activities of daily living and the child's natural tendency to be active are usually sufficient to maintain muscle strength and joint mobility.

Exercising in a pool is excellent therapy, since it allows freedom of movement with support and minimal gravitational pull. If there is pain on motion, a hot pack or warm bath before therapy may help.

Practitioners may recommend nighttime splinting to help minimize pain and reduce flexion deformity. Joints most frequently splinted are the knees, wrists, and hands. Positioning during rest is also important. The child rests on a firm mattress with no pillow or a very low one and has no support under the knee. Loss of extension in the knee, hip, and wrist causes special problems and requires vigilance to detect the earliest signs of involvement and vigorous attention to prevent deformity with specialized passive stretching, positioning, and resting splints.

Nursing Care Management

Nursing the child with JIA involves assessment of the child's general health, the status of involved joints, and the child's emotional response to all ramifications of the disease—discomfort, physical restrictions, therapies, and self-concept.

The effects of JIA are manifest in every aspect of the child's life, including physical activities, social experiences, and personality development. Although children with severe disease may have more physical barriers to overcome, studies show that emotional and behavioral functioning is most closely linked with maternal depression and parental distress, not with physical disability (Frank, Hagglund, Schopp, and others, 1998). Nursing interventions to support the parents may foster successful adaptation for the entire family. Parental concerns about the disease prognosis, financial and insurance issues, spouse and sibling relationships, and job and schedule conflicts must all be addressed. Referral to social workers, counselors, or support groups may be needed.

Relieve Pain. The pain of JIA is related to several aspects of the disease: disease severity, functional status, individual pain threshold, family variables, and psychologic adjustment. The aim is to provide as much relief as possible with medication and other therapies to help children tolerate the pain and cope as effectively as possible. Opioid administration is not a routine therapy for the chronic pain of JIA. Nonpharmacologic modalities such as behavioral therapy and relaxation techniques have proved effective in modifying pain perception (see Pain Management, Chapter 7) and activities that aggravate pain. Opioid analgesics are typically avoided in juvenile arthritis; however, for children immobilized with refractory pain, short-term opioid analgesics can be part of a comprehensive plan that uses multiple pain relief techniques (Connelly and Schanberg, 2006).

Promote General Health. The child's general health must be considered. A well-balanced diet with sufficient calories to maintain growth is essential. If the child is relatively inactive, caloric intake needs to match energy needs to avoid excessive weight gain, which places additional stress on affected joints. Sleep and rest are essential for children with JIA. Some children will require rest during the day; however, daytime napping that interferes with nighttime sleepiness should be avoided. A bedtime routine that involves comfort measures can help induce sleep. A firm mattress, heated water bed, electric blanket, or sleeping bag helps provide warmth, comfort, and rest. Nighttime splints needed to maintain range of motion might initially be a source of bedtime conflict. The family needs to be instructed on how to use the splint appropriately; the splint should not be painful or impede sleep. Behavior modification programs that reward splint and exercise compliance may be helpful in reducing compliance barriers. Well-child care to assess growth, development, and immunization requirements needs to be coordinated between the primary care provider and the rheumatologist. Common childhood illnesses, such as upper respiratory tract infections, may cause arthritis to worsen; consequently, medical attention must be sought quickly for relatively minor illness to prevent arthritis flares. Effective communication between the family, the primary care provider, and the rheumatology team is essential for care coordination.

Children are encouraged to attend school, even on days when there may be some pain or discomfort. The school nurse's aid is enlisted so that a child is permitted to take the prescribed medication at school and to arrange for rest in the nurse's office during the day. Split days or half days may help a child remain involved in school. Permitting the child to come to school late allows time to gain joint movement and reduces the time at school to avoid exhaustion. It is important that the child attend school to learn skills and engage in social interaction, especially if the JIA continues to limit physical skills. Arranging for two sets of textbooks eliminates the need to carry books to and from school, thus reducing discomfort and difficulty walking. A formal school hearing may be necessary to obtain an individualized education plan, ensured by public law, which includes intensive school modifications.

Facilitate Compliance. The child and family are involved in the therapeutic plan. They need to know the pur-

pose and correct use of any splints and appliances and the medication regimen. The family is instructed regarding administration of medications and the value of a regular schedule of administration to maintain a satisfactory drug level in the body. They need to know that NSAIDs should not be given on an empty stomach and to be alert for signs of medication toxicity. If evidence of drug toxicity is noted, the family is instructed to notify the health professional and follow that person's instructions.

Encourage Heat and Exercise. Heat has been shown to be beneficial to children with arthritis. Moist heat is best for relieving pain and stiffness, and the most efficient and practical method is in the bathtub with warm water. In some cases a daily whirlpool bath, paraffin bath, or hot packs may be used as needed for temporary relief of acute swelling and pain. Hot packs are easily applied using a bath towel wrung out after being immersed in hot water or heated in a microwave oven, applied to the area, and covered with plastic for 20 minutes. Commercial pads that warm in only a few minutes in the microwave are also available. Painful hands or feet can be immersed in a pan of warm water for 10 minutes two or three times daily in addition to tub baths.

Pool therapy is the easiest method for exercising a large number of joints. Swimming activities strengthen muscles and maintain mobility in larger joints. Very small children who are frightened of the water can carry out their exercises in the bathtub. Small children love to splash, kick, and throw things in the water. Remember, adult supervision is necessary for all water activities.

Activities of daily living provide satisfactory exercise for older children to maintain maximal mobility with minimal pain. These children are encouraged in their efforts to be independent and patiently allowed to dress and groom themselves, to assume daily tasks, and to care for their belongings. It is often difficult for children to manipulate buttons, comb or brush hair, and turn faucets, but unless there is an acute flare, parents and other caregivers should not offer assistance. In addition, children should learn and understand why others do not help them. Many helpful devices, such as self-adhering fasteners, tongs for manipulating difficult items, and grab bars installed in bathrooms for safety, can be used to facilitate tasks. A raised (higher) toilet seat often makes the difference between dependent and independent toileting, since weak quadriceps muscles and sore knees inhibit the ability to raise the body from a low sitting position.

A child's natural affinity for play offers many opportunities for incorporating therapeutic exercises. Throwing or kicking a ball and riding a tricycle (with the seat raised to achieve maximum leg extension) are excellent moving and stretching exercises for a very young child whose daily living activities are physically limited.

An effective approach to beginning the day's activities is to awaken children early to give them their medication and then to allow them to sleep for an hour. On arising, children take a hot bath (or shower) and perform a simple ritual of limbering-up exercises, after which they commence the activities of the day, such as going to school. Exercise, heat, and rest are spaced throughout the remainder of the day according to the child's individual needs and schedules. Parents are instructed in exercises that meet the child's needs.

NURSINGTIP

Another method of supplying warmth before the child arises is to plug an electric blanket into an appliance timer. Set the blanket to medium or high and adjust the timer to turn on the blanket 1 hour before the child awakens (McIlvain-Simpson and Singsen, 1997).

The Arthritis Foundation* and the American Juvenile Arthritis Organization* provide services for both parents and professionals. Nurses should refer families to these agencies as an added resource.

Support Child and Family. JIA affects every aspect of life for the child and family. Physical limitations may interfere with self-care, school participation, and recreational activities. The intensive treatment plan, including multiple medications, physical therapy, comfort measures, and medical appointments, is intrusive and disruptive to the parents' work schedule and the family routine. To prevent isolation and foster independence, the family is encouraged to pursue their normal activities. Unfortunately, the adaptations necessary to make that occur take resourcefulness and commitment from all family members. At diagnosis and throughout the span of JIA, it is essential to recognize signs of stress and counterproductive coping and provide the necessary support to maximize adaptation. The problems and needs of these families are discussed in Chapter 18, and the reader is directed to that chapter for guidance in planning care.

SYSTEMIC LUPUS ERYTHEMATOSUS

Systemic lupus erythematosus (SLE) is a chronic, multisystem, autoimmune disease of the connective tissues and blood vessels characterized by inflammation in potentially any body tissue. Its course and symptoms are variable and unpredictable, with mild to life-threatening complications. In addition to SLE, there are other forms of lupus, such as neonatal lupus, which occurs when maternal autoantibodies cross the placenta and cause transient lupuslike symptoms in the newborn, with the potential serious complication of heart block. The remaining discussion focuses on SLE.

Recent reports suggest that survival rates in children with SLE have significantly improved; 5-year survival rates are said to be almost 100%, and 10-year survival rates are close to 90% (Ravelli, Ruperto, and Martini, 2005). SLE is more common in girls, with an approximate 5:1 female-to-male ratio, and typically occurs between the ages of 10 and 19 years. There is a familial tendency, although many newly diagnosed patients are unaware of other affected family members. SLE has been reported in all cultures, but within the United States there has been a disproportionately higher incidence in African-American, Asian, and Hispanic children.

The cause of SLE is not known. It appears to result from a complex interaction of genetics with an unidentified trigger that activates the disease. Suspected triggers include exposure to ultraviolet light, estrogen, pregnancy, infections, and drugs. Genetic predisposition to SLE is evidenced in an increased concordance rate in twins (tenfold), increased incidence within family members (10% to 16%), and increased frequency of certain gene alleles in population-based studies.

---

*PO Box 7669, Atlanta, GA 30357-0669; (800) 283-7800; http://www.arthritis.org. In Canada, the Arthritis Society may be contacted for locations of all local Canadian province offices: http://www.arthritis.ca.

BOX 31-11

Clinical Manifestations of Systemic Lupus Erythematosus Related to Tissues Involved

Constitutional—Fever, fatigue, weight loss, anorexia
Cutaneous—Erythematous butterfly rash over bridge of nose and across cheeks, discoid rash, photosensitivity, mucocutaneous ulceration, alopecia, periungual telangiectasias
Musculoskeletal—Arthritis, arthralgia, myositis, myalgia, tenosynovitis
Neurologic—Headache, seizure, forgetfulness, behavior change, change in school performance, psychosis, chorea, stroke, cranial and peripheral neuropathy, pseudotumor cerebri
Pulmonary and cardiac—Pleuritis, basilar pneumonitis, atelectasis, pericarditis, myocarditis, endocarditis
Renal—Glomerulonephritis, nephrotic syndrome, hypertension
Gastrointestinal—Abdominal pain, nausea, vomiting, blood in stool, abdominal crisis, esophageal dysfunction, colitis
Hepatic, splenic, and nodal—Hepatomegaly, splenomegaly, lymphadenopathy
Hematologic—Anemia, cytopenia
Ophthalmologic—Cotton wool spots, papilledema, retinopathy
Vascular—Raynaud phenomenon, thrombophlebitis, livedo reticularis

---

BOX 31-12

Diagnostic Criteria for Systemic Lupus Erythematosus

Four criteria must be met for diagnosis:
1. Malar rash—fixed malar erythema
2. Discoid rash—patchy erythematous lesions
3. Photosensitivity—rash with sun exposure
4. Oronasal ulcers—painless ulcers in mouth, nose
5. Arthritis—swelling, tenderness, or effusion in two or more peripheral joints (nonerosive)
6. Serositis—pleuritis, pericarditis
7. Renal disorder—proteinuria, casts
8. Neurologic disorder—psychosis, seizures
9. Hematologic disorder—hemolytic anemia, thrombocytopenia, leukopenia, lymphopenia
10. Immunologic disorder—anti–double-stranded deoxyribonucleic acid (DNA), anti-SM, antiphospholipid antibodies; lupus anticoagulant; false-positive syphilis test (rapid plasma reagin [RPR])
11. Antinuclear antibodies

Clinical Manifestations and Diagnostic Evaluation

The child with SLE may have any clinical manifestation with mild to life-threatening severity (Box 31-11). The diagnosis is established when 4 of the 11 diagnostic criteria are met (Box 31-12). Kidney involvement heralds progressive disease and the need for rigorous therapeutic management.

Therapeutic Management

The goal of treatment is to ensure the child's health by balancing the medications necessary to avoid exacerbation and complications while preventing or minimizing treatment-associated morbidity. Therapy involves the use of specific medications and general supportive care. The drugs used to control inflammation are corticosteroids administered in doses sufficient to control inflammation, then tapered to the lowest suppressive dose. Other drugs include antimalarial preparations, which are useful for rash and arthritis; NSAIDs, which relieve muscle and joint inflammation; and immunosuppressive agents, such as cyclophosphamide, for renal and central nervous system disease. Antihypertensives, aspirin, and antibiotics are just a few of the additional drugs that may be necessary to treat or avoid complications.

General supportive care includes sufficient nutrition, sleep and rest, and exercise. Exposure to the sun and ultraviolet B (UVB) light is limited because of its association with SLE exacerbation.

Nursing Care Management

The principal nursing goal is to help the child and family positively adjust to the disease and therapy. The child and family must learn to recognize subtle signs of disease exacerbation and potential complications of medication therapy and to communicate these concerns to their care provider. Consequently, patient and family education is an ongoing process initiated at diagnosis and tailored to the patient's individual needs. Referral to a social worker, psychologist, or support group may help the child and family make a successful adjustment. Support groups are associated with the Lupus Foundation of America* and the Arthritis Foundation.†

Key issues include therapy compliance; body-image problems associated with rash, hair loss, and steroid therapy; school attendance; vocational activities; social relationships; sexual activity; and pregnancy. (See Chapter 18 for a discussion on adjusting to a chronic illness.) Specific instructions for avoiding exposure to the sun and UVB light, such as using sunscreens, wearing sun-resistant clothing, and altering outdoor activities, must be provided with great sensitivity to ensure compliance while minimizing the associated feeling of being different from peers (see Sunburn, Chapter 30). Patients need to be instructed to maintain regular medical supervision and seek attention quickly during illness or before elective surgical procedures, such as dental extraction, because of potential needs for increased steroids or prophylactic antibiotics. People with SLE should carry medical identification for their disease and steroid dependence.

---

*2000 L St. NW, Suite 710, Washington, DC 20036; (202) 349-1155, (800) 558-0121; http://www.lupus.org.
†See footnote on facing page.

KEY POINTS

- Immobility has a profound effect on all aspects of growth and development.
- The major physical consequences of immobilization are loss of muscle strength, endurance, and muscle mass; bone demineralization; loss of joint mobility; and contractures.
- Features of children's fractures not observed in the adult include presence of growth plate, thicker and stronger periosteum, bone porosity, more rapid healing, and less joint stiffness.
- The goals of fracture management are to regain alignment and length of bony fragments, retain alignment and length, and restore function to injured parts.
- The method of fracture reduction is determined by the child's age, degree of displacement, amount of overriding, amount of edema, condition of the skin and soft tissues, sensation, and circulation distal to the fracture.
- The primary purposes of traction are to fatigue involved muscles and reduce muscle spasm, position bone ends in desired realignment, and immobilize the fracture site until realignment has been achieved to permit casting or splinting.
- The development of DDH appears to be related to intrauterine, genetic, and postnatal factors.
- Treatment of clubfoot consists of manipulation and casting to correct the deformity, maintenance of the correction, surgical heel cord release, and prevention of possible recurrence of the deformity.
- Acquired hip deformities are managed with non–weight-bearing devices (Legg-Calvé-Perthes disease) or surgical stabilization (SCFE).
- Observation for scoliosis is an important part of a routine physical assessment.
- Scoliosis is managed by bracing or surgical correction.
- Bone infections are managed with vigorous antibiotic therapy, immobilization of the affected part, and (sometimes) surgical drainage.
- Osteosarcoma is a neoplasm of bone-forming tissues; Ewing sarcoma is a neoplasm that arises from bone marrow spaces.
- Rhabdomyosarcoma may occur almost anywhere in the body, but the most common sites are the head and neck.
- Nursing care of the child with arthritis consists of promoting general health, relieving discomfort, preventing deformity, and preserving function.
- SLE is a chronic autoimmune disorder that affects the collagen tissues of the body.

REFERENCES

American Academy of Pediatrics: Clinical practice guideline: early detection of developmental dysplasia of the hip, *Pediatrics* 105(4):896-905, 2000a.
American Academy of Pediatrics: School health assessments, *Pediatrics* 105(4):875-877, 2000b; reaffirmed 2006, *Pediatrics* 118(3):1266-1267, 2006.
Bunnell WP: Selective screening for scoliosis, *Clin Orthop Relat Res* 434:40-45, 2005.
Connelly M, Schanberg L: Opioid therapy for the treatment of refractory pain in children with juvenile rheumatoid arthritis, *Natl Clin Pract Rheumatol* 2(12):636-637, 2006.

Curley MA, Razmus IS, Roberts KE, and others: Predicting pressure ulcer risk in pediatric patients: the Braden Q Scale, *Nurs Res* 52(1):22-33, 2003.
Do T, Herrera-Soto J: Elbow injuries in children, *Curr Opin Pediatr* 15(1):68-73, 2003.
Frank RG, Hagglund KJ, Schopp LH, and others: Disease and family contributors to adaptation in juvenile rheumatoid arthritis and juvenile diabetes, *Arthritis Care Res* 11(3):166-176, 1998.
Gilmore A, Thompson GH: Common childhood foot deformities, *Consult Pediatr* 2(2):63-71, 2003.

Greene WB, editor: *Essentials of musculoskeletal care*, ed 2, Rosemont, Ill, 2001, American Academy of Orthopaedic Surgeons.
Gutierrez K: Bone and joint infections in children, *Pediatr Clin North Am* 52(3):779-794, 2005.
Hart ES, Albright MB, Rebello GN, and others: Developmental dysplasia of the hip: nursing implications and anticipatory guidance for parents, *Orthop Nurs* 25(2):100-109, 2006.
Holmes SB, Brown SJ, Pin Site Care Expert Panel: Skeletal pin site care: National Association of Orthopaedic Nurses guidelines for orthopaedic nursing, *Orthop Nurs* 24(2):99-107, 2005.

Hosalkar HS, Horn D, Friedman JE, and others: The hip. In Kliegman RM, Behrman RE, Jenson HB, and others, editors: *Nelson textbook of pediatrics,* ed 18, Philadelphia, 2007, Saunders.

Kline NE, Sevier N: Solid tumors in children, *J Pediatr Nurs* 18(2):96-102, 2003.

Kump LI, Castañeda RA, Androudi SN, and others: Visual outcomes in children with juvenile idiopathic arthritis–associated uveitis, *Ophthalmology* 113(10):1874-1877, 2006.

Lampe RM: Osteomyelitis and suppurative arthritis. In Kliegman RM, Behrman RE, Jenson HB, and others, editors: *Nelson textbook of pediatrics,* ed 18, Philadelphia, 2007, Saunders.

Land C, Rauch F, Travers R, and others: Osteogenesis imperfecta type VI in childhood and adolescence: effects of cyclical intravenous pamidronate treatment, *Bone* 40(3):638-644, 2007.

Lanzkowsky P: *Manual of pediatric hematology and oncology,* San Diego, 2000, Academic Press.

Link MP, Gebhardt MC, Myers PA: Osteosarcoma. In Pizzo PA, Poplack DG, editors: *Principles and practices of pediatric oncology,* ed 5, Philadelphia, 2006, Lippincott.

Lovell DJ, Giannini EH, Reiff A, and others: Long-term efficacy and safety of etanercept in children with polyarticular-course juvenile rheumatoid arthritis: interim results from an ongoing multicenter, open-label, extended-treatment trial, *Arthritis Rheum* 48(1):218-226, 2003.

Maher AB, Salmond SW, Pellino TA: *Orthopaedic nursing,* ed 3, Philadelphia, 2002, Saunders.

Marini JC: Osteogenesis imperfect. In Kliegman RM, Behrman RE, Jenson HB, and others, editors: *Nelson textbook of pediatrics,* ed 18, Philadelphia, 2007, Saunders.

McIlvain-Simpson G, Singsen B: Decreasing morning stiffness, *Small* Talk 3(6):8, 1997.

Miller ML, Cassidy JT: Juvenile rheumatoid arthritis. In Kliegman RM, Behrman RE, Jenson HB, and others, editors: *Nelson textbook of pediatrics,* ed 18, Philadelphia, 2007, Saunders.

Napierkowski DB: Scoliosis: a case study in an adolescent boy, *Orthop Nurs* 26(3):147-153, 2007.

Newton PO, Wenger DR: Idiopathic and congenital scoliosis. In Morrissy RT, Weinstein SL, editors: *Lovell and Winter's pediatric orthopaedics,* Philadelphia, 2001, Williams & Wilkins.

Olsson GL: Neuropathic pain in children. In McGrath PJ, Finley GA, editors: *Chronic and recurrent pain in children and adolescents,* Seattle, 1999, IASP Press.

Padeh S, Passwell P: Intraarticular corticosteroid injection in the management of children with chronic arthritis, *Arthritis Rheum* 41(7):1210-1214, 1998.

Perron AD, Miller MD, Brady WJ: Orthopedic pitfalls in the ED: slipped capital femoral epiphysis, *Am J Emerg Med* 20(5):484-487, 2002.

Petty RE, Southwood TR, Baum J, and others: Revision of the proposed classification criteria for juvenile idiopathic arthritis: Durban, 1997, *J Rheumatol* 25(10):1991-1994, 1998.

Petty RE, Southwood TR, Manners P, and others: International League of Associations for Rheumatology classification of juvenile idiopathic arthritis, second revision, Edmonton, 2001, *J Rheumatol* 31(2):390-392, 2004.

Plint AC, Perry JJ, Correll R, and others: A randomized, controlled trial of removable splinting versus casting for wrist buckle fractures in children, *Pediatrics* 117(3):691-697, 2006.

Ravelli A, Ruperto N, Martini A: Outcome in juvenile onset lupus erythematosus, *Curr Opin Rheumatol* 17(5):568-573, 2005.

Samaniego IA: A sore spot in pediatrics: risk factors for pressure ulcers, *Pediatr Nurs* 29(4):278-283, 2003.

Seidel HM, Ball JW, Dains JE, and others: *Mosby's guide to physical examination,* ed 5, St Louis, 2006, Mosby.

Slote RJ: Psychological effects of caring for the adolescent undergoing spinal fusion for scoliosis, *Orthop Nurs* 21(6):19-28, 2002.

Wall EJ: Practical primary pediatric orthopaedics, *Nurs Clin North Am* 35(1):95-113, 2000.

Warren RW, Perez MD, Curry MR, and others: Juvenile idiopathic arthritis (juvenile rheumatoid arthritis). In Koopman WJ, editor: *Arthritis and allied conditions,* Philadelphia, 2001, Lippincott Williams & Wilkins.

Wexler LH, Meyer WH, Helman LJ: Rhabdomyosarcoma and the undifferentiated sarcomas. In Pizzo PA, Poplack DG, editors: *Principles and practices of pediatric oncology,* ed 5, Philadelphia, 2006, Lippincott.

32

The Child with Neuromuscular or Muscular Dysfunction

DAVID WILSON

CHAPTER OUTLINE

CONGENITAL NEUROMUSCULAR OR MUSCULAR DISORDERS, 1146
Cerebral Palsy, 1146
Nursing Care Plan: The Child with Cerebral Palsy, 1151
Spina Bifida (Myelomeningocele), 1154
    Latex Allergy, 1159

Spinal Muscular Atrophy, Type 1 (Werdnig-Hoffmann Disease), 1161
Spinal Muscular Atrophy, Type 3 (Kugelberg-Welander Disease), 1162
Muscular Dystrophies, 1162
Duchenne (Pseudohypertrophic) Muscular Dystrophy, 1162

ACQUIRED NEUROMUSCULAR DISORDERS, 1165
Guillain-Barré Syndrome (Infectious Polyneuritis), 1165
Tetanus, 1167
Botulism, 1168
    Infant Botulism, 1169
Spinal Cord Injuries, 1170

LEARNING OBJECTIVES

On completion of this chapter the reader will be able to:

- Discuss the nursing role in helping parents care for the child who has cerebral palsy.
- Formulate a nursing care plan for the preoperative and postoperative care of a child with myelomeningocele.

- Outline a care plan for a child with Guillain-Barré syndrome.
- Discuss the home care management of the child with a neuromuscular disease such as spinal muscular atrophy.
- Discuss the prevention and treatment of tetanus.

- Identify the causes of botulism in infants and children.
- List three causes of spinal cord injury in children.

RELATED TOPICS and ADDITIONAL RESOURCES

 IN TEXT

The Child with Cerebral Dysfunction, *Ch. 28*
Genetic Evaluation and Counseling, *Ch. 9*
The Immobilized Child, *Ch. 31*
Impact of the Child's Chronic Illness or Disability, *Ch. 18*
Neurologic Assessment, *Ch. 6*
Nursing Care of the High-Risk Newborn and Family, *Ch. 9*
Recommendations for Routine Immunizations: Tetanus, *Ch. 10*

 COMPANION CD

Animation—Guillain-Barré Syndrome
Critical Thinking Exercises—Myelomeningocele; Guillain-Barré Syndrome
NCLEX Review Questions

evolve
Critical Thinking Case Study—Cerebral Palsy
NCLEX Review Questions
Nursing Care Plan—The Child with Cerebral Palsy
WebLinks

 WONG'S CLINICAL MANUAL OF PEDIATRIC NURSING, 7th Ed

Patient and Family Education—Performing Clean Intermittent Bladder Catheterization, *p. 554*
Nursing Care Plans—The Child with Cerebral Palsy, *p. 471;* The Child with Myelomeningocele, *p. 473;* The Child with Respiratory Failure, *p. 423*

CONGENITAL NEUROMUSCULAR OR MUSCULAR DISORDERS

CEREBRAL PALSY

A new definition proposed in 2006 describes cerebral palsy (CP) as a "group of permanent disorders of the development of movement and posture, causing activity limitation, that are attributed to nonprogressive disturbances that occurred in the developing fetal or infant brain" (Rosenbaum, Paneth, Leviton, and others, 2007). In addition to motor disorders, the condition often involves disturbances of sensation, perception, communication, cognition, and behavior; secondary musculoskeletal problems; and epilepsy (Rosenbaum, Paneth, Leviton, and others, 2007). The etiology, clinical features, and course are variable and are characterized by abnormal muscle tone and coordination as the primary disturbances. CP is the most common permanent physical disability of childhood, and the incidence is reported to be between 1.5 and 3 in every 1000 live births in the United States (Ashwal, Russman, Blasco, and others, 2004; Dabney, Lipton, and Miller, 1997; Winter, Autry, Boyle, and others, 2002). Since the 1960s the prevalence of CP has risen approximately 20%, which most likely reflects the improved survival of extremely low–birth-weight and very low–birth-weight infants.

Although the prevalent traditional hypothesis has been that CP results from perinatal problems, especially birth asphyxia, it is now believed that CP results more often from existing **prenatal** brain abnormalities; however, the exact cause of these abnormalities remains elusive. It has been estimated that as many as 80% of CP cases are caused by unknown prenatal factors (Krigger, 2006). Intrauterine exposure to maternal chorioamnionitis is associated with an increased risk of CP in infants of normal birth weight and preterm infants (Gibson, MacLennan, Goldwater, and others, 2003; Volpe, 2001); however, not all term infants exposed to chorioamnionitis develop CP (Grether, Nelson, Walsh, and others, 2003; Wu, Escobar, Grether, and others, 2003). The prevalence of CP in infants born before 36 weeks of gestation and weighing less than 2000 g (4.4 pounds) has been reported to be 12%; the strongest independent risk factor for development of CP was periventricular leukomalacia (Han, Bang, Lim, and others, 2002). Damage occurring as a result of shaken baby syndrome may also result in CP in survivors. Additional factors that may contribute to the development of CP postnatally include bacterial meningitis, viral encephalitis, motor vehicle accidents (MVAs), and child abuse (Krigger, 2006). A significant percentage (15% to 60%) of children with CP will also have epilepsy, thus compromising issues of self-care and progression to normalization.

Pathophysiology

It is difficult to establish a precise location of neurologic lesions based on etiology or clinical signs because no characteristic pathologic pattern exists. Some patients have gross malformations of the brain; others may have evidence of vascular occlusion, atrophy, loss of neurons, and degeneration. A few exceptions occur and are related to anatomic areas such as spastic diplegia (associated with preterm birth), caused by hypoxic infarction or hemorrhage in the area adjacent to the lateral ventricles. Ataxic CP may occur in relation to cerebral hypoplasia and, in some cases, severe hypoglycemia (Volpe, 2001). The American College of Obstetricians and Gynecolo-

---

BOX 32-1

Clinical Classification of Cerebral Palsy

SPASTIC (PYRAMIDAL)

Characterized by persistent primitive reflexes, positive Babinski, ankle clonus, exaggerated stretch reflexes, eventual development of contractures

- 70% to 80% of all cases of cerebral palsy
- Diplegia—All extremities affected; lower more than upper (30% to 40% of spastic cerebral palsy [CP])
- Quadriplegia—All four extremities involved: legs and trunk, mouth, pharynx, and tongue (10% to 15% of spastic CP)
- Triplegia—Three limbs involved
- Monoplegia—Only one limb involved
- Hemiplegia—Motor dysfunction on one side of the body; upper extremity more affected than lower (20% to 30% of spastic CP)

Other features:

- Hypertonicity with poor control of posture, balance, and coordinated motion
- Impairment of fine and gross motor skills

DYSKINETIC (NONSPASTIC, EXTRAPYRAMIDAL)

Athetoid—Chorea (involuntary, irregular, jerking movements); characterized by slow, wormlike, writhing movements that usually involve the extremities, trunk, neck, facial muscles, and tongue

Dystonic—Slow, twisting movements of the trunk or extremities; abnormal posture

Involvement of the pharyngeal, laryngeal, and oral muscles causing drooling and dysarthria (imperfect speech articulation)

ATAXIC (NONSPASTIC, EXTRAPYRAMIDAL)

Wide-based gait

Rapid, repetitive movements performed poorly

Disintegration of movements of the upper extremities when the child reaches for objects

MIXED TYPE

Combination of spastic CP and dyskinetic CP

May be labeled mixed when no specific motor pattern is dominant; however, this term is losing favor to more precise descriptions of motor function and affected area of brain involved (see Rosenbaum, Paneth, Leviton, and others, 2007)

Data from Nehring W: Cerebral palsy. In Allen PJ, Vessey JA, editors: *Primary care of the child with a chronic condition*, St Louis, 2004, Mosby; Jones MW, Morgan E, Shelton JE, and others: Cerebral palsy: introduction and diagnosis, part 1, *J Pediatr Health Care* 21(3):146-152, 2007; and National Institute of Neurologic Disorders and Stroke: *Cerebral palsy: hope through research*, 2006, retrieved July 9, 2007, from http://www.ninds.nih.gov/disorders/cerebral_palsy/detail_cerebral_palsy.htm.

---

gists, in conjunction with the American Academy of Pediatrics (2003), published a report that defines neonatal encephalopathy. The report affirms that approximately 70% of cases of neonatal encephalopathy occur as a result of events before the onset of labor; it establishes criteria to define events sufficiently capable of causing intrapartum asphyxia and CP. Evidence indicates that events that cause the majority of CP cases occur not as a result of intrapartum asphyxia, but as a result of other causes that have been discussed previously (American Academy of Pediatrics and American College of Obstetricians and Gynecologists, 2003).

CP has been classified in several ways. A functional classification is based on the nature and distribution of neuromuscu-

BOX 32-2

Clinical Signs and Symptoms of Cerebral Palsy

SPASTIC TYPE

Increased muscle tone (hypertonicity)

Increased deep tendon reflexes and **clonus** (sudden dorsiflexion of the ankle or rapid distal movement of the patella resulting in alternating spasm and relaxation of the muscles being stretched)

Flexor, adductor, and internal rotator muscles more involved than extensor, abductor, and external rotator muscles

Difficulty with fine and gross motor skills

Most common contracture: that of the heelcord

Hip adductor contractures leading to progressive subluxation and dislocation

Knee contractures

Scoliosis common

Typical gait crouched, intoeing, scissoring

Elbow, wrist, and fingers in flexed position with thumb adducted

Motor weakness of antagonist muscle groups

DYSKINETIC TYPE

Purposeless, involuntary, uncontrollable movements of face and extremities

Increased movements with stress and voluntary movements, absent during sleep

Contractures rare

Normal deep tendon reflexes

ATAXIC TYPE

Disturbed coordination

Lack of equilibrium

Unsteady gait

Few orthopedic problems

Hyporeflexia

Loss of ability to gauge distance, speed, power of movement

Muscles hypotonic

Speech slurred, jerky, explosive

Nystagmus common

OTHER MANIFESTATIONS

Visual deficits (most common in spastic type)

Hearing impairment (most common in dyskinetic type)

Oral motor involvement resulting in drooling and feeding problems

Developmental delay (40% to 60%; most common in spastic quadriplegia)

Sensory impairment

Seizures (approximately 40% of those with spastic hemiplegia affected)

From Maher AB, Salmond SW, Pellino TA: *Orthopaedic nursing*, ed 3, Philadelphia, 2002, Saunders.

BOX 32-3

Early Signs of Cerebral Palsy

- Failure to meet any developmental milestones such as rolling over, raising head, sitting up, crawling
- Persistent primitive reflexes such as Moro, atonic neck
- Poor head control (head lag) and clenched fists after 3 months of age
- Stiff or rigid arms or legs; scissoring legs
- Pushing away or arching back; stiff posture
- Floppy or limp body posture, especially while sleeping
- Inability to sit up without support by 8 months
- Using only one side of the body, or only the arms to crawl
- Feeding difficulties
- Persistent gagging or choking when fed
- After 6 months of age, tongue pushing soft food out of the mouth
- Extreme irritability or crying
- Failure to smile by 3 months
- Lack of interest in surroundings

Data from Pathways Awareness Foundation: *Parents . . . if you see any of these warning signs . . . don't delay*, Chicago, 1991, The Foundation; Nehring W: Cerebral palsy. In Allen PJ, Vessey JA, editors: *Primary care of the child with a chronic condition*, St Louis, 2004, Mosby; and Jones MW, Morgan E, Shelton JE, and others: Cerebral palsy: introduction and diagnosis, part 1, *J Pediatr Health Care* 21(3):146-152, 2007.

pected brain abnormality and CP is now recommended for diagnostic assessment, with magnetic resonance imaging (MRI) preferred to computed tomography (CT) scan. Metabolic and genetic testing is recommended if no structural abnormality is identified by neuroimaging; laboratory tests are no longer recommended in the diagnostic process for CP (Ashwal, Russman, Blasco, and others, 2004).

Early recognition is made more difficult by the lack of reliable neonatal neurologic signs. However, infants with known etiologic risk factors should be monitored and evaluated closely in the first 2 years of life. The alert observer may be suspicious when a child demonstrates some of the manifestations outlined in Boxes 32-2 and 32-3. Because cortical control of movement does not occur until later in infancy, motor impairment associated with voluntary control is usually not apparent until after 2 to 4 months of age at the earliest. More often the diagnosis cannot be confirmed until the age of 2 years because motor tone abnormalities may be indicative of another neuromuscular illness.

The persistence of primitive reflexes may be of value in establishing the diagnosis: (1) either the asymmetric tonic neck reflex or persistent Moro reflex (beyond 4 months of age), and (2) the crossed extensor reflex. The tonic neck reflex normally disappears between 4 and 6 months of age. An "obligatory" response is considered abnormal. The crossed extensor reflex, which normally disappears by 4 months, is elicited by applying a noxious stimulus to the sole of one foot with the knee extended. Normally the contralateral foot responds with extensor, abduction, and then adduction movements. The possibility of CP is suggested if these reflexes are found after the age at which they should have disappeared.

Therapeutic Management

The goals of therapy for children with CP are early recognition and promotion of optimal development to enable affected children to attain normalization and their potential

lar dysfunction (Box 32-1). Additional classifications describe the area of the brain involved, the degree of motor involvement, accompanying impairments, anatomic distribution, and cause of CP (Rosenbaum, Paneth, Leviton, and others, 2007).

Diagnostic Evaluation

Infants at risk according to known etiologic factors associated with CP warrant careful assessment during early infancy to identify the signs of muscular dysfunction as early as possible. The neurologic examination and history are the primary modalities for diagnosis. Neuroimaging of the child with suswithin the limits of their existing health problems. The disorder is permanent, and therapy is primarily preventive and symptomatic.

Therapy has five broad aims:

1. To establish locomotion, communication, and self-help skills
2. To gain optimal appearance and integration of motor functions
3. To correct associated defects as effectively as possible
4. To provide educational opportunities adapted to the child's needs and capabilities
5. To promote socialization experiences with other affected and unaffected children

Each child is evaluated and managed on an individual basis. The scope of the child's needs requires multidisciplinary planning and care coordination among professionals and the child's family. The outcome for the child and family with CP is normalization and promotion of self-care activities that empower the child and family to achieve maximum potential.

Ankle-foot orthoses (AFOs, braces) are worn by many of these children and are used to help prevent or reduce deformity, increase the energy efficiency of gait, and control alignment. Other mobilization devices include wheeled scooter boards that allow children to propel themselves while on the abdomen, wheeled go-carts that provide sitting balance and serve as early "wheelchair" experience for young children, bicycle walkers, and special devices that leave the upper extremities free (Figs. 32-1 and 32-2). Strollers can be equipped with custom seats for dependent mobilization.

Orthopedic surgery may be required to correct contracture or spastic deformities, to provide stability for an uncontrollable joint, and to provide balanced muscle power. This includes tendon-lengthening procedures (especially heel-cord lengthening), release of spastic wrist flexor muscles, and correction of hip and adductor muscle spasticity or contracture to improve locomotion. Selective dorsal rhizotomy has provided marked improvement in some children with CP. The procedure involves selectively cutting dorsal column sensory rootlets that have an abnormal response to electrical stimulation. Achieving the benefits from the surgery requires intensive physical therapy and family commitment. Because the procedure results in flaccid muscles, the child must be retaught to sit, stand, and walk.

Surgical intervention is usually reserved for the child who does not respond to the more conservative measures, but it is also indicated for the child whose spasticity causes progressive deformities. Surgery is primarily used to improve function rather than for cosmetic purposes and is followed by physical therapy.

Intense pain may occur with muscle spasms in patients with CP. Pharmacologic agents given orally (dantrolene sodium, baclofen [Lioresal], and diazepam [Valium]) have had little effectiveness in improving muscle coordination in children with CP; however, they are effective in decreasing overall spasticity. The most common side effects of these agents include hepatotoxicity (dantrolene), drowsiness, fatigue, and muscle weakness; less commonly, diaphoresis and constipation may be seen with baclofen. Diazepam is used frequently but should be restricted to older children and adolescents.

Botulinum toxin A (Botox) is also used to reduce spasticity in targeted muscles. Botulinum toxin A is injected into a selected muscle (commonly the quadriceps, gastrocnemius, or medial hamstrings) after a topical anesthetic is applied. The drug acts to inhibit the release of acetylcholine into a specific muscle group, thereby preventing muscle movement. When it is administered early in the course of the illness, affected muscle contractures may be prevented, particularly in lower extremities, thus avoiding surgical procedures with possible adverse effects. The goal is to allow stretching of the muscle as it relaxes and permit ambulation with an AFO. The major reported adverse effect of botulinum toxin A injection is pain at the injection site (Roscigno, 2002). Prime candidates for botulinum toxin A injections are children with spasticity confined

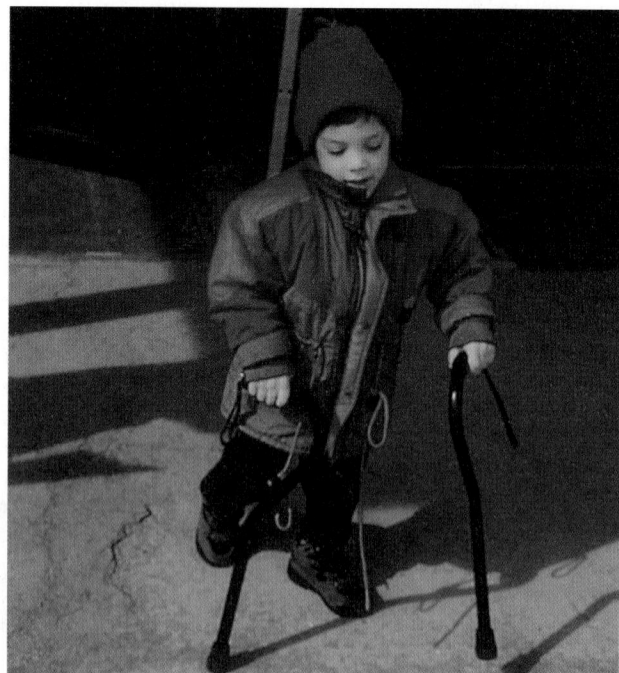

FIG. 32-1 ■ Mobilization device for child.

FIG. 32-2 ■ Bike walker used to provide mobility and to enhance leg muscle strength. (Courtesy Texas Children's Hospital, Houston.)

to the lower extremities; the drug weakens spasticity so the muscles can be stretched and the child may ambulate with or without orthoses. The onset of action occurs within 24 to 72 hours, with a peak effect observed at 2 weeks and a duration of action of 3 to 6 months (Green, Greenberg, and Hurwitz, 2003).

Children with CP may also experience pain as a result of surgical procedures intended to reduce contracture deformities, position and gastroesophageal reflux, and physical therapy (McKearnan, Kieckhefer, Engel, and others, 2004). Therefore pain management is an important aspect of care of the child with CP.

Neurosurgical and pharmacologic approach to managing the spasticity associated with CP involves the implantation of a pump to infuse baclofen directly into the intrathecal space surrounding the spinal cord to provide relief of spasticity. Intrathecal baclofen therapy is best suited for children with severe spasticity that interferes with activities of daily living (ADLs) and ambulation. Patients are screened before pump placement by the infusion of a "test dose" of intrathecal baclofen delivered via a lumbar puncture. Close monitoring for side effects (hypotonia, somnolence, seizures, nausea, vomiting, headache, and catheter- or pump-related problems [Albright, Gilmartin, Swift, and others, 2003]) and relief of spasticity occurs for several hours after the infusion. If a positive effect is noted, the patient is considered a candidate for pump placement. The implantation procedure is done in the operating room by a neurosurgeon. The pump, which is approximately the size of a hockey puck, is placed in the subcutaneous space of the midabdomen. An intrathecal catheter is tunneled from the lumbar area to the abdomen and connected to the pump. The pump is filled with baclofen and programmed to provide a set dose using a telemetry wand and a computer. Benefits of intrathecal baclofen include fewer systemic side effects than oral baclofen, dosage titration for maximizing effects, and reversibility of therapy with removal of the pump if so desired (Jacobs, 2001). The patient may remain hospitalized for 3 to 7 days to adjust the dosage and ensure proper healing. Outpatient visits to refill the pump and make dosage adjustments occur about every 4 to 6 weeks, depending on the patient's response to the treatment. This procedure is most suited for a multidisciplinary setting where rehabilitation specialists are readily available and consistently involved in the patient's ongoing care. Abrupt withdrawal of intrathecal baclofen, especially at high doses, may result in adverse effects such as rebound spasticity, pruritus, hyperthermia, rhabdomyolysis, disseminated intravascular coagulation, multiorgan failure, and death; in some cases intrathecal baclofen withdrawal may mimic sepsis.

Antiepileptic drugs (AEDs) such as carbamazepine (Tegretol) and divalproex (valproate sodium and valproic acid; Depakote) are prescribed routinely for children who have seizures. Gabapentin (Neurontin) has been used in adults with spinal cord injury (SCI) to decrease spasticity with success; no studies are available on the effectiveness of the drug in children. The α_2-adrenergic agonists clonidine (Catapres) and tizanidine (Zanaflex) have been used to decrease spasticity in adults with SCI and multiple sclerosis, but use in children with CP has yet to be reported (Krach, 2001). All medications should be monitored for maintenance of therapeutic levels and avoidance of subtherapeutic or toxic levels.

Dental hygiene is especially important. Regular visits to the dentist and prophylaxis, including brushing, fluoride, and flossing, should be instituted as soon as the teeth erupt. Dental care is especially important for children being given phenytoin, since they often develop gum hyperplasia. Additional problems common among children with CP include constipation caused by neurologic deficits and lack of exercise; poor bladder control and urinary retention; chronic respiratory tract infections and aspiration pneumonia, which occur as a result of gastroesophageal reflux, abnormal muscle tone, immobility, and altered positioning; and skin problems as a result of altered positioning, poor nutrition, and immobility.

A wide variety of technical aids is available to improve the functioning of children with CP. These include electromechanical toys that employ the concept of biofeedback and operate from a head unit. The toy is manipulated only when the head and trunk are in correct alignment. Eye-hand coordination can also be enhanced by computerized toys and games. Microcomputers combined with voice synthesizers aid children with speech difficulties to "speak." These and other devices print messages onto screen monitors and paper.

Many other electronic devices allow independent functioning. Sensors can be activated and deactivated by using a headstick or tongue, or other voluntary muscle movement over which the child has control. Voice-activated computer technology may also allow increased mobility and ambulation with specially designed devices such as wheelchairs. The application of this technology makes it possible for persons with CP to function eventually in their own residences and can be extended into the workplace.

Physical therapy is one of the most frequently used conservative treatment modalities. It requires the specialized skills of a qualified therapist with an extensive repertoire of exercise methods who can design a program to stimulate each child to achieve his or her functional goals.

An active therapy program involves the family; the physical therapist; and often other members of the health team, including the nurse. The most common approach uses traditional types of therapeutic exercises that consist of stretching, passive, active, and resistive movements applied to specific muscle groups or joints to maintain or increase range of motion, strength, or endurance.

Prognosis. In general, the more severe the functional disability, the worse the prognosis. Children with a severe physical disability, mental retardation, tube feedings, and severe seizures are known to have a shortened life expectancy. According to available data, approximately 30% to 50% of individuals with CP are mentally retarded, and an even higher percentage have mild cognitive and learning deficits (Green, Greenberg, and Hurwitz, 2003); however, many children with severe spastic quadriplegic CP have normal intelligence. Growth is affected in children with spastic quadriplegia, and many children remain below the 5th percentile for age and gender. As children with CP transition to adulthood, about 30% remain in the home and are cared for by a parent or caregiver; 50% of individuals with spastic quadriplegia live in independent settings and function at appropriate social levels considering their disability (Green, Greenberg, and Hurwitz, 2003). Vocational rehabilitation and higher education are possible for adults with CP, and one study found that 53% of all persons with CP were able to work outside the home in regular jobs; one third of the severely disabled adults with CP worked outside the home (Murphy, Molnar, and Lankasky, 2000).

NURSINGALERT

The use of mobile infant walkers is discouraged in children with CP. They pose a risk of injury to normal children and are especially hazardous for children with CP. Also, jumping seats, such as those that hang in doorways, should not be used.

Nursing Care Management

The nursing process in the care of the child with CP is outlined in the Nursing Process box.

Because children with CP are being identified and treated at an earlier age, parents are participating earlier in treatment programs for their disabled child. They are taught the proper handling and home care of young children with CP and need a carefully planned program so that their change of role from parent to caregiver can be melded into the already established relationship. Close work with other multidisciplinary team members is essential. Nurses reinforce the therapeutic plan and assist the family in devising and modifying equipment and activities to continue the therapy program in the home (see Nursing Care Plan).

Because children with CP expend so much energy in their efforts to accomplish ADLs, more frequent rest periods should be arranged to avoid the fatigue that may tax their limited capabilities. The diet should be tailored to the child's activity and metabolic needs. Gastrostomy feedings may be necessary to supplement regular feedings and ensure adequate weight gain, particularly in the child who is at risk for growth failure and chronic malnutrition. In children with severe CP and subsequent oral feeding difficulties, a feeding gastrostomy should be considered (Rogers, 2004). Gastrostomy feeding as a supplement to oral feeding is often recommended, especially when illness and decreased fluid or medication intake affect the child's well-being (Rogers, 2004). Oral feedings may be continued to maintain oral motor skills. Weight gain is perceived as an important measure of adequate oral feeding efficiency.

Parents may need assistance and advice with medication administration through a gastrostomy tube to prevent clotting. A skin-level gastrostomy is particularly suited for the child with CP. Because jaw control is often compromised, more normal control can be achieved if the feeder provides stability of the oral mechanism from the side or front of the face. When directed from the front, the middle finger of the nonfeeding hand is placed posterior to the body portion of the chin, the thumb is placed below the bottom lip, and the index finger is placed parallel to the child's mandible (Fig. 32-3). Manual jaw control from the side assists with head control, correction of neck and trunk hyperextension, and jaw stabilization. The middle finger of the nonfeeding hand is placed posterior to the bony portion of the chin, the index finger is placed on the chin below the lower lip, and the thumb is placed obliquely across the cheek to provide lateral jaw stability (Fig. 32-4).

Safety precautions are implemented, such as having children wear protective helmets if they are subject to falls or capable of injuring their heads on hard objects. Because the child with CP is at risk for altered proprioception and subsequent falls, the home and play environment should be adapted to the child's needs to prevent bodily harm. Appropriate immunizations should be administered to prevent childhood illnesses and protect against respiratory tract infections such

---

nursingprocess | The Child with Cerebral Palsy

ASSESSMENT

Nursing assessment includes risk identification of infants with etiologic factors that are associated with cerebral palsy (CP). Early recognition of CP is important so early interventions may be implemented (see Box 32-3). Ongoing assessment of infants for abnormal muscle tone, inability to achieve developmental milestones, and persistence of neonatal reflexes alert the nurse to investigate further.

DIAGNOSIS (PROBLEM IDENTIFICATION)

After a thorough assessment a number of nursing diagnoses are evident (see Nursing Care Plan, p. 1151). Other nursing diagnoses include:

- Imbalanced Nutrition: Less Than Body Requirements
- Delayed Growth and Development
- Interrupted Family Processes
- Risk for Aspiration

PLANNING

Expected outcomes for the child with CP include:

- Child will receive adequate nutrient intake for body growth (weight gain).
- Child will achieve developmental milestones to maximum potential.
- Family will cope with child's illness and functions to maximum potential.
- Child's airway will remain patent.

IMPLEMENTATION

Numerous intervention strategies for the child with CP are found on pp. 1150-1154.

EVALUATION

The effectiveness of nursing interventions for the family and child with CP is determined by continual reassessment and evaluation of care based on the following observational guidelines:

- Child's movements and use of mobilization devices
- Child's speech and ability to use communication devices
- Child's activities, especially those related to self-care
- Family perception regarding child's activities and school attendance
- Child's interactions with others and choice of activities; child's feelings and concerns
- Family feelings, concerns, and interaction with the child
- Child's behavior and responses during hospitalization

as influenza. Depending on the level of involvement, dental problems may be more common in children with CP, which creates a need for meticulous attention to all aspects of dental care.

The involvement of physical therapy, speech therapy, and occupational therapy is particularly important in establish-ment and maintenance of muscle function, development of adequate speech and phonation, and identification of modifi-cations necessary for the child's environment so that ADLs can be performed to the child's satisfaction.

As in all aspects of care, educational requirements are deter-mined by the child's needs and potential. Children with mild

nursingcareplan | The Child with Cerebral Palsy

Nursing Diagnosis	Patient Outcomes	Nursing Interventions	Rationale
Impaired Physical Mobility related to neuromuscular impairment	The infant or toddler will demonstrate active joint movement.	Carry out and teach family to perform stretching exercises on affected joints.	To prevent muscle contractures
Child's/Family's Defining Characteristics (Subjective and Objective Data)	The child will have adequate mobility to perform activities of daily living to maximum potential.	Use assistive devices such as wheelchair, ankle-foot orthoses (AFOs), and wrist splints.	To increase mobility
Postural instability during performance of routine activities of daily living	**The Following NOC Concepts Apply to These Outcomes**	Administer medications intended to decrease muscle spasticity.	To minimize pain and decrease spasticity
Limited ability to perform gross motor skills	Body Mechanics Performance Ambulation: Wheelchair	Encourage and teach parent(s) to use jaw control during feedings.	To facilitate eating
Limited range of motion	Joint Movement: Elbow, wrist, neck, knee, hip, ankle	Position child semiupright during feedings.	To decrease chance of aspiration and facilitate mobilization of food and fluids through esophagus
Limited ability to perform fine motor skills	Mobility		
Gait changes		Encourage play exercises that involve joint movement and promote fine and gross motor skill acquisition and repetition.	To promote joint movement To promote achievement of developmental milestones
Movement-induced tremor			
Persistence of primitive reflexes		**The Following NIC Concepts Apply to These Interventions**	
		Exercise Therapy: Joint Mobility Exercise Promotion: Stretching Self-Care Assistance	

Nursing Diagnosis	Patient Outcomes	Nursing Interventions	Rationale
Risk for Injury related to mobility limitation, neuromuscular impairment, and perception and cognition impairment	Child will remain injury free. Home physical environment will be safe.	Educate family regarding child's physical limitations that place him or her at greater risk for injury.	To prevent accidental injury during mobilization
Child's/Family's Defining Characteristics (Subjective and Objective Data)	**The Following NOC Concepts Apply to These Outcomes**	Instruct family in steps to avoid injury: padded furniture, lowered bed or side rails as appropriate, gates on stairs, avoidance of throw rugs, thick carpeting.	To promote family involvement in injury prevention
Physical factors: altered mobility Neuromuscular factors:	Personal Safety Behavior Falls Occurrence	Position child in semiupright position after feedings.	To prevent aspiration
■ Limited perception of danger		Use jaw support as needed during feedings.	To prevent choking
■ Uncontrollable muscular movements		Use appropriate mobilization devices and ensure they are safe for child's age.	To prevent muscle contractures
		Encourage mobilization and play activities that stretch muscles.	To promote personal safety
		Teach child which activities of daily living are safe and appropriate to perform without assistance of another person.	To promote self-care
		The Following NIC Concepts Apply to These Interventions	
		Risk Identification Environmental Management: Safety Surveillance: Safety Physical Restraint Parent Education: Childrearing Family	

Continued

primary caregiver. This respite may be crucial to the parent's well-being.

SPINA BIFIDA (MYELOMENINGOCELE)

Abnormalities that derive from the embryonic neural tube (**neural tube defects [NTDs]**) constitute the largest group of congenital anomalies that are consistent with multifactorial inheritance. Normally the spinal cord and cauda equina are encased in a protective sheath of bone and meninges (Fig. 32-5, *A*). Failure of neural tube closure produces defects of varying degrees (Box 32-4). They may involve the entire length of the neural tube or may be restricted to a small area.

In the United States, rates of NTDs have declined from 1.3 per 1000 births in 1970, to 0.3 per 1000 births after the introduction of mandatory food fortification with folic acid in 1998 (Honein, 2001). Further data indicate that the incidence of NTDs showed a 23% decline from 1996 to 2001 (Matthews, Honein, and Erickson, 2002). Increased use of prenatal diagnostic techniques and termination of pregnancies have also affected the overall incidence of NTDs (see also Prevention, p. 1157).

Myelodysplasia refers broadly to any malformation of the spinal canal and cord. Midline defects involving failure of the osseous (bony) spine to close are called **spina bifida (SB)**, the most common defect of the central nervous system. SB is categorized into two types: spina bifida occulta and spina bifida cystica.

Spina bifida occulta refers to a defect that is not visible externally. It occurs most frequently in the lumbosacral area (L5 and S1) (see Fig. 32-5, *B*). SB occulta may not be apparent unless there are associated cutaneous manifestations or neuromuscular disturbances.

Spina bifida cystica refers to a visible defect with an external saclike protrusion. The two major forms of SB cystica are **meningocele,** which encases meninges and spinal fluid but no neural elements (see Fig. 32-5, *C*), and **myelomeningocele** (or **meningomyelocele**), which contains meninges, spinal fluid, and nerves (see Fig. 32-5, *D*). Meningocele is not associated with neurologic deficit, which occurs in varying, often serious, degrees in myelomeningocele. Clinically the term *spina bifida* is used to refer to myelomeningocele.

Pathophysiology

Most authorities believe that the primary defect in NTDs is a failure of neural tube closure during the embryo's early development (the first 3 to 5 weeks). However, evidence also implicates a multifactorial etiology, including drugs, radiation, maternal malnutrition, chemicals, and possibly a genetic mutation in folate pathways in some cases, which may result in abnormal development. There is also evidence of a genetic component in the development of SB; myelomeningocele may occur in association with syndromes such as trisomy 18, PHAVER syndrome, and Meckel-Gruber syndrome (Shaer, Chescheir, and Schulkin, 2007). Additional factors predisposing children to an increased risk of NTDs include prepregnancy maternal obesity, maternal diabetes mellitus, previous NTD pregnancy, low maternal vitamin B_{12} status, maternal hyperthermia, and the use of AEDs in pregnancy.

The degree of neurologic dysfunction depends on where the sac protrudes through the vertebrae, the anatomic level of the defect, and the amount of nerve tissue involved. Most myelomeningoceles involve the lumbar or lumbosacral area

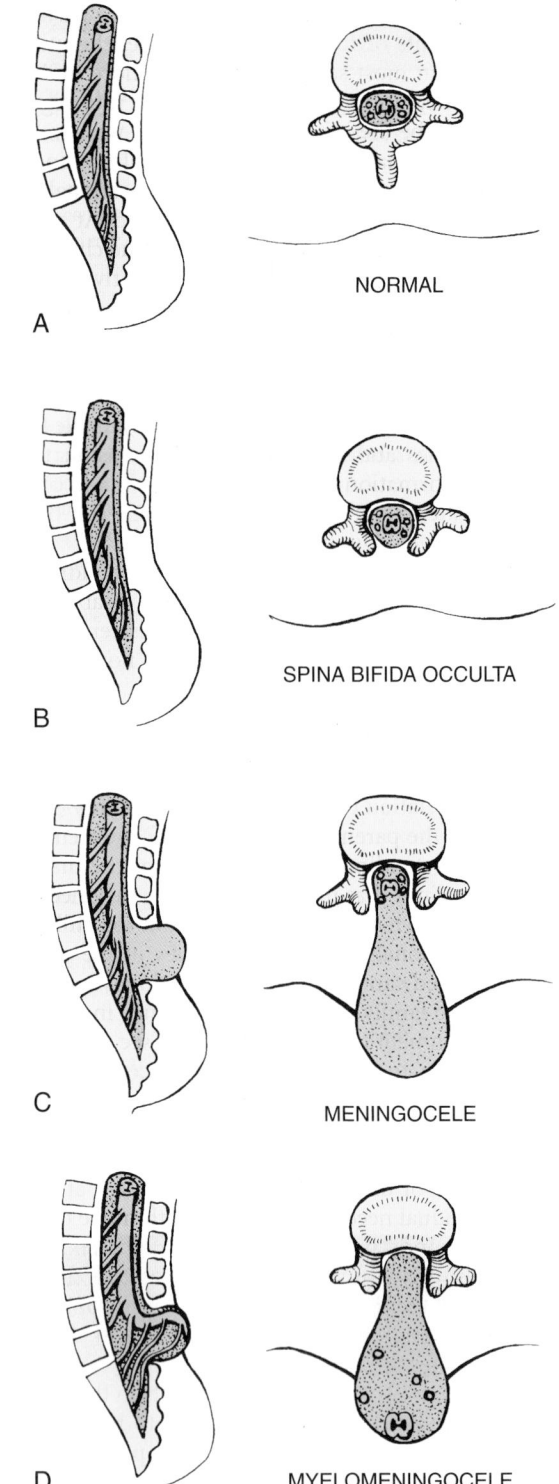

FIG. 32-5 ■ Midline defects of osseous spine with varying degrees of neural herniations.

(Fig. 32-6). Hydrocephalus is a frequently associated anomaly in 80% to 90% of the children.

Diagnostic Evaluation

The diagnosis of SB is made on the basis of clinical manifestations (Box 32-5) and examination of the meningeal sac. Diagnostic measures used to evaluate the brain and spinal cord

FIG. 32-6 ■ **A,** Myelomeningocele with intact sac. **B,** Myelomeningocele with ruptured sac. (Courtesy Dr. Robert C. Dauser, Neurosurgery, Baylor College of Medicine, Houston.)

BOX 32-4

Significant Neural Tube Defects

Cranioschisis—A skull defect through which various tissues protrude
Exencephaly—Brain totally exposed or extruded through an associated skull defect; fetus usually aborted
Anencephaly—If fetus with exencephaly survives, degeneration of the brain to a spongiform mass with no bony covering; incompatible with life usually beyond a few days
Encephalocele—Herniation of brain and meninges through a defect in the skull producing a fluid-filled sac; can be frontal or posterior
Rachischisis or **spina bifida**—Fissure in the spinal column that leaves the meninges and spinal cord exposed
Meningocele—Hernial protrusion of a saclike cyst of meninges filled with spinal fluid (see Fig. 32-5, *C*)
Myelomeningocele (meningomyelocele)—Hernial protrusion of a saclike cyst containing meninges, spinal fluid, and a portion of the spinal cord with its nerves (see Fig. 32-5, *D*)

BOX 32-5

Clinical Manifestations of Spina Bifida

SPINA BIFIDA CYSTICA
Sensory disturbances usually parallel to motor dysfunction
  ■ Below second lumbar vertebra:
    —Flaccid, partial paralysis of lower extremities
    —Varying degrees of sensory deficit
    —Overflow incontinence with constant dribbling of urine
    —Lack of bowel control
    —Rectal prolapse (sometimes)
  ■ Below third sacral vertebra:
    —No motor impairment
    —May have saddle anesthesia with bladder and anal sphincter paralysis
Joint deformities (sometimes produced in utero):
  ■ Talipes valgus or varus contractures
  ■ Kyphosis
  ■ Lumbosacral scoliosis
  ■ Hip dislocation or subluxation

SPINA BIFIDA OCCULTA
Frequently no observable manifestations
May be associated with one or more cutaneous manifestations:
  ■ Skin depression or dimple
  ■ Port-wine angiomatous nevi
  ■ Dark tufts of hair
  ■ Soft, subcutaneous lipomas
May have neuromuscular disturbances:
  ■ Progressive disturbance of gait with foot weakness
  ■ Bowel and bladder sphincter disturbances

include MRI, ultrasound, CT, and myelography. Laboratory examinations are used primarily to determine causative organisms for common complications associated with myelomeningocele: meningitis and urinary tract infections.

Prenatal Detection. It is possible to determine the presence of some major open NTDs prenatally. Ultrasonographic scanning of the uterus and elevated maternal concentrations of α-fetoprotein (AFP, or MS-AFP), a fetal-specific γ$_1$-globulin, in amniotic fluid may indicate anencephaly or myelomeningocele. The optimum time for performing these diagnostic tests is between 16 and 18 weeks of gestation, before AFP concentrations normally diminish and in sufficient time to permit a therapeutic abortion. It is recommended that such diagnostic procedures and genetic counseling be considered for all mothers who have borne an affected child, and testing is offered to all pregnant women (Kirkham, Harris, and Grzybowski, 2005). In addition, elective prelabor cesarean birth may result in less motor dysfunction. Chorionic villus sampling is also a method for prenatal diagnosis of NTDs; however, it carries certain risks (skeletal limb depletion) and is not recommended before 10 weeks of gestation.

Therapeutic Management

Early surgical closure of the myelomeningocele sac through fetal surgery has been evaluated in relation to prevention of injury to the exposed spinal cord tissue and improvement of neurologic and urologic outcomes in the affected child. Initial fetal surgical success and survival rates appear to be positive; however, reports vary in relation to the success of fetal surgery in the actual reduction of urologic problems, improvement of lower leg function, and prevention of hydrocephalus in the postnatal period. The overall mortality rate from fetal surgery is 4%, and complications include oligohydramnios, preterm delivery, and a smaller birth weight (Kaufman, 2004). The Management of Myelomeningocele Study, a clinical trial supported by the National Institutes of Health, is currently investigating the outcome of fetal surgery.

Management of the child who has a myelomeningocele requires a multidisciplinary approach involving the specialties of neurology, neurosurgery, pediatrics, urology, orthopedics, rehabilitation, physical therapy, and social services, along with intensive nursing care in a variety of specialty areas. The collaborative efforts of these specialists are focused on (1) the myelomeningocele and the problems associated with the defect—hydrocephalus, paralysis, orthopedic deformities, and genitourinary abnormalities; (2) possible acquired problems that may or may not be associated, such as meningitis, hypoxia, and hemorrhage; and (3) other conditions, such as cardiac or gastrointestinal malformations.

Infancy. Initial care of the newborn involves preventing infection; performing a neurologic assessment, including observing for associated anomalies; and dealing with the impact of the anomaly on the family. Although meningoceles are repaired early, especially if there is danger of rupture of the sac, the philosophy regarding skin closure of myelomeningocele varies. Most authorities believe that early closure, within the first 24 to 72 hours, offers the most favorable outcome. Early closure, preferably in the first 12 to 18 hours, not only prevents local infection and trauma to the exposed tissues, but also avoids stretching of other nerve roots (which may occur as the meningeal sac expands during the first hours after birth), thus preventing further motor impairment. Broad-spectrum antibiotics are initiated, and neurotoxic substances such as povidone-iodine are avoided at the malformation.

Associated problems are assessed and managed by appropriate surgical and supportive measures. Shunt procedures provide relief from imminent or progressive hydrocephalus (see Chapter 28). Meningitis, urinary tract infection, and ventriculitis are treated with vigorous antibiotic therapy and supportive measures. Surgical intervention for Chiari malformation (a downward herniation of the brain into the brainstem)

or for tethered cord (scar tissue binding the spinal cord) is indicated only when the child is symptomatic.

Improved surgical techniques do not alter the major physical disability, spinal defect, or chronic urinary tract infections that affect the quality of life for these children. Superimposed on the physical problems are the effects that the disorder has on family life and finances, including the need for long-term specialized school and health care services.

Orthopedic Considerations. According to most orthopedists, musculoskeletal problems that will affect later locomotion should be evaluated early, and treatment, where indicated, should be instituted without delay. Neurologic assessment will determine the neurosegmental level of the lesion and enable recognition of spasticity and progressive paralysis, potential for deformity, and functional expectations. Orthopedic management includes prevention of joint contractures, correction of the existing deformity, prevention or minimization of the effects of motor and sensory deficits, prevention of skin breakdown, and acquisition of the best possible function of affected lower extremities. Common orthopedic problems requiring attention in SB include deformities of the knees, hips, feet, and spine; fractures and insensate skin further complicate orthopedic care. Other problems that may occur later include kyphosis and scoliosis (Brown, 2001). Because children with this condition often have decreased sensitivity in lower extremities, preventive skin care is important. A high percentage (60%) of children seen in a wound clinic for skin breakdown had myelomeningocele (Samaniego, 2003). The status of the neurologic deficit remains the most important factor in determining the child's ultimate functional abilities.

With technologic advances, a variety of lightweight orthoses, including braces, special "walking" devices, and custom-built wheelchairs, are available to provide mobility to children with spinal cord lesions (see also Chapter 19). Early in infancy, intervention with passive range-of-motion exercises, positioning, and stretching exercises may help decrease the incidence of muscle contractures (Brown, 2001). Corrective surgical procedures, when indicated, are best initiated at an early age so that the child will not lag significantly behind agemates in developmental progress. Where there is little hope for lower extremity functioning, surgery is seldom recommended unless it will improve sitting position in a wheelchair and function for ADLs and mobility.

Management of Genitourinary Function. Myelomeningocele is one of the most common causes of **neuropathic (neurogenic) bladder dysfunction** among children. In infants the goal of treatment is to preserve renal function. In older children the goal is to preserve renal function and achieve optimal urinary continence. Urinary incontinence is a chronic, often debilitating problem for the child. In addition, the neuropathic bladder may produce **urinary system distress,** characterized by symptomatic urinary tract infections, ureterohydronephrosis, and vesicoureteral reflux or renal insufficiency. The characteristics of bladder dysfunction in children vary according to the level of the neurologic lesion and the influence of bony growth and development on the spine. Therefore ongoing urologic monitoring is essential. Evidence is growing that early intervention, based on evaluation during the neonatal period and before complications occur, serves to improve bladder function, reduces the risk of subsequent urinary system distress, and decreases the need for reconstructive surgery of the lower urinary tract (Snodgrass and Adams, 2004; Tarcan, Onol, Ilker, and others, 2006).

Treatment of renal problems includes (1) regular urologic care with prompt and vigorous treatment of infections; (2) a method of regular emptying of the bladder, such as **clean intermittent catheterization (CIC)** taught to and performed by parents and self-catheterization taught to children; (3) medications to improve bladder storage and continence, such as oxybutynin chloride (Ditropan) and tolterodine (Detrol); and (4) surgical procedures such as **vesicostomy** (bladder surgically brought out to the abdominal wall, allowing continuous urinary drainage) and **augmentation enterocystoplasty** (using a segment of bowel or stomach to increase bladder capacity, thereby reducing high bladder pressures).

However, despite the combined efforts of CIC, medication, and surgical intervention, some children with myelodysplasia may continue to experience debilitating urinary incontinence. Many of these children are able to attain social continence with a continent **urinary diversion** commonly referred to as a Mitrofanoff procedure. In this procedure, a catheterizable channel is surgically created from appendix, ureter, or tapered bowel. The proximal end of the channel is connected to the bladder with the distal end brought out as a small stoma on the abdominal wall, usually near the umbilicus. The bladder neck may be sutured to prevent urinary leakage from the urethra. CIC through the easily accessible abdominal route fosters greater independence in children, especially in those unable to transfer from wheelchair to toilet to perform CIC.

Bowel Control. Some degree of fecal continence can be achieved in most children with myelomeningocele with diet modification, regular toilet habits, and prevention of constipation and impaction. It is frequently a lengthy process. Dietary fiber supplements (recommended 10 g/day), laxatives, suppositories, or enemas aid in producing regular evacuation. Older children and adolescents seeking more independence may attain bowel continence and higher quality of life after undergoing an antegrade continence enema (ACE) procedure (Doolin, 2006). In a procedure similar to the Mitrofanoff, the appendix or ileum is used to create a catheterizable channel with attachment of the proximal end to the colon. The distal end of the channel exits through a small abdominal stoma. Every 1 or 2 days, a catheter is passed through the stoma, allowing enema solution to be instilled directly into the colon. After administration of the enema solution, the child sits on the toilet for 30 to 60 minutes as stool is flushed out through the rectum. Frequency of enemas and volume of solution used to completely evacuate the bowel vary among individuals.

Prognosis. The early prognosis for the child with myelomeningocele depends on the neurologic deficit present at birth, including motor ability, bladder innervation, and associated neurologic anomalies. Early surgical repair of the spinal defect, antibiotic therapy to reduce the incidence of meningitis and ventriculitis, prevention of urinary system dysfunction, and early detection and correction of hydrocephalus have significantly increased the survival rate and quality of life in such children. Many children with SB achieve partial independent living and gainful employment. Reports of survival rates vary, and many include adults who were born before medical advances and surgical techniques seen in the past 25 years. Researchers have noted that as adolescents with SB tran-

sition to young adulthood, they have increased difficulty obtaining centralized health care for the different health problems associated with SB (Lazzaretti and Pearson, 2004). This chronic condition has an array of associated complications, including hydrocephalus and shunt malfunctions, scoliosis, bowel and bladder management issues, latex allergy, and epilepsy. However, based on current medical knowledge and ethical considerations, aggressive, early management is favored for the child with myelomeningocele.

Prevention. The widespread use of folic acid among women of childbearing age is expected to significantly decrease the incidence of SB. It has been estimated that a daily intake of 0.4 mg of folic acid in women of childbearing age will prevent 50% to 70% of all cases of NTDs (Centers for Disease Control and Prevention, 2004). Preliminary data show a 24% decrease in cases of SB between 1996 and 2001 (Matthews, Honein, and Erickson, 2002). Although folic acid intake increased in 1999 to 2000 (compared with intake from 1988 to 1994), recent data indicate that serum folate concentrations among women of childbearing age decreased 16% from 2003 to 2004 in all ethnic groups studied. Lowest serum folate levels were seen in non-Hispanic whites in 2003 to 2004; however, overall serum folate levels remained below recommended levels in non-Hispanic blacks during all three periods studied (Centers for Disease Control and Prevention, 2007). These results indicate that nurses and other health care workers have an important task in disseminating information that may decrease the incidence of birth defects in children by promoting maternal consumption of folic acid.*

For women who have had a previous pregnancy affected by NTDs, folic acid intake is increased to 4 mg/day under supervision of a practitioner beginning 1 month before a planned pregnancy and continuing during the first trimester. Supplementation of 4 mg of folate should not be given in multivitamin preparations because of the risk of overdose of other vitamins.

To ensure adequate daily intake of the recommended amount of folic acid, women must take a folic acid supplement, eat a fortified breakfast cereal containing 100% of the recommended dietary allowance (RDA) of folic acid (e.g., Kellogg's Product 19, General Mills Total, Multigrain Cheerios Plus), or increase their consumption of other fortified foods (cereal, bread, rice, grits, pasta) and foods naturally rich in folate (green leafy vegetables and citrus fruits). The only population in which folic acid has *not proved* to be effective in decreasing the incidence of NTDs is epileptic women taking antiepileptic medications during pregnancy.

NURSING ALERT

Because approximately half of all pregnancies in the United States are unplanned (Henshaw, 1998), adolescent girls and women of childbearing age need to be educated about the necessity of folic acid to prevent NTDs. The daily dose of 0.4 mg (400 mcg) is most easily obtained from a multivitamin supplement.

---

*Information is available from Division of Birth Defects and Pediatric Genetics, NCBDDD, CDC, 1600 Clifton Road NE, Mailstop E-86, Atlanta, GA 30333; (404) 498-3800; e-mail: flo@cdc.gov; http://www.cdc.gov/ncbddd/folicacid. And from March of Dimes Resource Center, 1275 Mamaroneck Ave., White Plains, NY 10605; http://www.marchofdimes.com.

Nursing Care Management

At birth an examination is performed to assess the intactness of the membranous cyst. During transport to the nursery, every effort is made to prevent trauma to this protective covering. In addition to the routine assessment of the newborn (see Chapter 8), the infant is assessed for the level of neurologic involvement. Movement of extremities or skin response, especially an anal reflex, that might provide clues to the degree of motor or sensory impairment is noted. It is important to observe the infant's behavior in conjunction with the stimulus, since limb movements can be induced in response to spinal cord reflex activity that has no connection with the higher centers. Observation of urinary output, especially if a diaper remains dry, may indicate urinary retention. Abdominal assessment revealing bladder distention, even with a wet diaper, may indicate urinary overflow in a retentive bladder. The head circumference is measured daily (see Chapter 6), and the fontanels are examined for signs of tension or bulging.

Care of the Myelomeningocele Sac. The infant is usually placed in an incubator or warmer so that temperature can be maintained without clothing or covers that might irritate the spinal lesion. When an overhead warmer is used, the dressings over the defect require more frequent moistening because of the dehydrating effect of the radiant heat.

Before surgical closure the myelomeningocele is prevented from drying by the application of a sterile, moist, nonadherent dressing over the defect. The moistening solution is usually sterile normal saline. Dressings are changed frequently (every 2 to 4 hours), and the sac is closely inspected for leaks, abrasions, irritation, or any signs of infection. The sac must be carefully cleansed if it becomes soiled or contaminated. Sometimes the sac ruptures during delivery or transport, and any opening in the sac greatly increases the risk of infection to the central nervous system.

> **NURSINGTIP**
>
> To prevent stool contamination of the SB defect preoperatively, obtain a surgical drape (e.g., Steri-Drape). Cut a portion of the drape to fit the infant's sacrum, and secure the drape using nonlatex tape. Place the rest of the drape loosely over the dressing, covering the defect and thus preventing exposure to stool.

> **NURSINGALERT**
>
> Observe for early signs of infection, such as temperature instability (axillary), irritability, and lethargy, and for signs of increased intracranial pressure, which might indicate developing hydrocephalus.

> **NURSINGALERT**
>
> Avoid measuring rectal temperatures in infants with SB. Because bowel sphincter function is frequently affected, the thermometer can cause irritation and rectal prolapse.

One of the most important and challenging aspects in the early care of the infant with myelomeningocele is positioning. Before surgery the infant is kept in the prone position to minimize tension on the sac and the risk of trauma. The prone position allows for optimal positioning of the legs, especially in cases of associated hip dysplasia. The infant is placed prone with the hips slightly flexed and supported to reduce tension on the defect. The legs are maintained in abduction with a pad between the knees to counteract hip subluxation, and a small roll is placed under the ankles to maintain a neutral foot position. A variety of aids, including diaper rolls, pads, small foam pads, or specially designed frames and appliances, can be used to maintain the desired position.

Prevent Complications. The prone position affects other aspects of the infant's care. For example, in this position the infant is more difficult to keep clean, pressure areas are a constant threat, and feeding becomes a problem. The infant's head is turned to one side for feeding. Fortunately, most defects are repaired early, and the infant can be held for feeding soon after surgery. Special care must be taken to avoid pressure on the operative site.

Diapering the infant may be contraindicated until the defect has been repaired and healing is well advanced or epithelialization has taken place. The padding beneath the diaper area is changed as needed to keep the skin dry and free of irritation. When urinary retention is detected, CIC is employed. Because the bowel sphincter is frequently affected, there is continual passage of stool, often misinterpreted as diarrhea, which is a constant irritant to the skin and a source of infection to the spinal lesion.

Areas of sensory and motor impairment are subject to skin breakdown and therefore require meticulous care. Placing the infant on a special mattress or mattress overlay reduces pressure on the knees and ankles. Periodic cleansing, application of lotion, and gentle massage aid circulation.

Gentle range-of-motion exercises are carried out to prevent contractures, and stretching of contractures is performed when indicated. However, these exercises may be restricted to the foot, ankle, and knee joint. When the hip joints are unstable, stretching against tight hip flexors or adductor muscles, which act much like bowstrings, may aggravate a tendency toward subluxation. Consultation with a physical therapist is an important aspect of the short- and long-term management of infants with myelomeningocele.

Infants with unrepaired myelomeningocele may be held in the arms and cuddled as unaffected infants are, so their need for tactile stimulation is met by caressing, stroking, and other comfort measures. Individualized developmental care with age-appropriate stimulation is provided (see Developmental Outcome, Chapter 9).

Provide Postoperative Care. Postoperative care of the infant with myelomeningocele involves the same basic care as that of any postsurgical infant: monitoring vital signs, monitoring intake and output, providing nourishment, observing for signs of infection, and managing pain as needed. Care of the operative site is carried out under the direction of the surgeon and includes close observation for signs of leakage of cerebrospinal fluid (CSF). General care is continued as preoperatively.

The prone position is maintained after surgical closure, although many neurosurgeons allow a side-lying or partial side-lying position unless it aggravates a coexisting hip dysplasia or permits undesirable hip flexion. This offers an opportunity for position changes, which reduces the risk of pressure sores and facilitates feeding. If permitted, the infant can be held upright against the body, with care taken to avoid pressure on the operative site. After the effects of anesthesia have subsided and the infant is alert, feedings may be resumed unless there are other anomalies or associated complications.

Support Family and Educate About Home Care. As soon as the parents are able to cope with the infant's condition, they are encouraged to become involved in care. They need to learn how to continue at home the care that has been initiated in the hospital—positioning, feeding, skin care, and range-of-motion exercises when appropriate. They are taught CIC technique when it is prescribed. Parents also need to know the signs of complications (urinary, neurologic, orthopedic) and how to obtain assistance when needed.

The mother who wishes to breastfeed the infant is encouraged to do so, since this will be beneficial. Shortly after delivery the mother is started on a program of pumping to initiate and maintain milk supply until the infant is stable enough to begin breastfeeding (Hurtekant and Spatz, 2007). This process may require considerable support from nurses, physicians, and family members because of separation from the infant for surgical care and recovery.

The long-range planning with and support of the parents and newborn begin in the hospital and continue throughout childhood and even into young adulthood. The life expectancy of children with SB extends well into adulthood; therefore planning should involve long-term goals and plans for optimum function as an adult. Discussion about aspects of adulthood such as receiving educational or vocational training and education, living independently, having a mate, having sexual relationships, and bearing and rearing children is important and should not be overlooked. The unique service needs of adolescents with SB as they attempt to gain independence from family and establish a life of their own have not been adequately addressed in the literature (Buran, McDaniel, and Brei, 2002). Nurses assume an important role as a central member of the health team. As a care manager and coordinator, the nurse reviews information with the family, takes responsibility for family teaching, and acts as a liaison between inpatient and outpatient services. The child will need numerous hospitalizations over the years, and each one will be a source of stress to which the younger child is especially vulnerable (see Chapter 18 for a discussion of care of the child with a disability).

Habilitation involves not only solving problems of self-help and locomotion, but also solving the most distressing problem of urinary or bowel incontinence, which threatens the child's social acceptability. Assistance in preparing the child and the school regarding the child's special needs helps provide a better initial adjustment to this broader social experience. The Spina Bifida Association of America* is organized to provide services and support for families of children with spinal lesions.

Latex Allergy

Latex allergy was identified as a serious health hazard when a report linked intraoperative anaphylaxis with latex in children with SB. The high prevalence of latex allergy (up to 80%) in children with SB has been attributed to the repeated exposure to latex products during surgery and numerous bladder catheterizations and possible disease-associated factors. Some evidence suggests that children with SB are at increased risk for latex allergy as a result of the disease itself rather than repeated latex exposures (Eiwegger, Dehlink, Schwindt, and

*4590 MacArthur Blvd. NW, Suite 250, Washington, DC 20007-4226; (202) 944-3285, (800) 621-3141; http://www.spinabifidaassociation.org.

BOX 32-6

Medical Conditions Associated with Risk of Latex Allergy

- Spina bifida
- Urogenital anomalies
- Imperforate anus
- Tracheoesophageal fistula
- VATER association (*V*ertebral defects, imperforate *A*nus, Tracheo*E*sophageal fistula, and *R*adial and renal dysplasia)
- Preterm infants
- Ventriculoperitoneal shunt
- Mental retardation
- Cerebral palsy
- Spinal cord injuries
- Multiple surgeries
- Atopy

---

nursingcareguidelines

Identifying Latex Allergy

- Does your child have any symptoms, such as sneezing, coughing, rashes, or wheezing, when handling rubber products (e.g., balloons, tennis or Koosh balls, adhesive bandage strips) or when in contact with rubber hospital products (e.g., gloves, catheters)?
- Has your child ever had an allergic reaction during surgery?
- Does your child have a history of rashes; asthma; or allergic reactions to medication or foods, especially milk, kiwi, bananas, or chestnuts?
- How would you identify or recognize an allergic reaction in your child?
- What would you do if an allergic reaction occurred?
- Has anyone ever discussed latex or rubber allergy or sensitivity with you?
- Has your child had any allergy testing?
- When did your child last come in contact with any type of rubber product? Were you present?

Modified from Romanczuk A: Latex use with infants and children: it can cause problems, *MCN* 18(4):208-212, 1993.

---

others, 2006). Allergic reactions range from urticaria, wheezing, watery eyes, and rashes to anaphylactic shock. More severe reactions tend to occur when latex comes in contact with mucous membranes, wet skin, the bloodstream, or an airway. There also can be cross-reactions to a number of foods (e.g., banana, avocado, kiwi, chestnut). Latex allergy has been diagnosed in infants; symptoms manifested include wheezing, facial swelling, facial rash, and anaphylaxis (Kimata, 2004). In addition to patients with SB, high-risk populations include patients with urogenital anomalies or multiple surgeries and health care workers (see Box 32-6 for medical conditions associated with SB).

The most important goals are prevention of latex allergy and identification of children with a known hypersensitivity (see Nursing Care Guidelines box). High-risk and latex-allergic individuals must be managed in a **latex-free** environment. Care must be taken so that they do not come in direct or secondary contact with products or equipment containing latex *at any time* during medical treatment. Allergy testing has been used to identify latex allergy with varying success. Skin prick testing and provocation testing carry the risk of allergic reaction or anaphylaxis. The radioallergosorbent test (RAST) has been used to measure the serum level of latex-specific immunoglobulin E. The RAST has been shown to be 90% to 95% sensitive (Kellett, 1997). Pretreatment with an antihistamine and steroids (dexamethasone) before and after surgery to reduce the possibility of a serious reaction remains controversial, since it may interfere with healing.

Because children who have SB are prone to develop an allergy to latex, reducing exposure, from birth on, may decrease the chance of allergy development. Many health care facilities are establishing latex-safe environments when patients and health care workers are at risk. In the health care arena it is important to use products with the lowest potential risk of sensitizing patients and staff members.

Lists have been published of products, such as vinyl gloves, that may be substituted for latex (see footnote to Box 32-7). The U.S. Food and Drug Administration has proposed user labeling for latex-containing devices that come into contact, directly or indirectly, with live human tissue.*

---

*Additional information regarding latex allergy may be found at http://www.latex-allergy.org and http://latexallergylinks.tripod.com. For a list of latex products and alternative products, see Latex List on the Spina Bifida Association home page, http://www.spinabifidaassociation.org.

NURSING ALERT
Ask all patients, not only those at risk, about allergic reactions to latex during the health interview with the parent or child. Be certain that this is a routine part of all preoperative and preprocedural histories. Stress the importance of the allergy history to all personnel (e.g., phlebotomists).

The identification of those sensitive to latex is best accomplished through careful screening of *all* patients (see Nursing Care Guidelines box for questions related to latex allergy). Children with latex allergy should carry or wear some form of medical identification; those who have had serious reactions should also carry an injectable epinephrine pen and a pair of latex-free gloves for emergencies. Education programs regarding latex hypersensitivity are aimed at those who care for high-risk groups, such as children with SB, and may include relatives, school nurses, teachers, childcare workers, and baby-sitters. In addition to educating caregivers about the child's exposure to medical products that contain latex, nurses need to inform them of common nonmedical latex objects (Box 32-7). Parents should also be given literature explaining signs

---

BOX 32-7

Selected Items Possibly Containing Latex*

MEDICAL ITEMS

Adhesive bandage strips
Airways, masks (oxygen)
Anesthesia vent circuits, bags
Blood pressure cuffs and tubing
Bulb syringe
Catheters (indwelling, condom)
Chux (washable rubber pads)
Crutches (axillary, hand pads)
Dressings and wraps (various)
Elastic bandages
Electrode pads, bulbs
Endotracheal tubes
Finger cots
Gloves (sterile and examining, surgical and medical)
Heparin lock adapter
Intravenous tubing, injection ports, bags, burets
Medication vials
Nasogastric tubes
Ostomy supplies
Penrose drains
Pulse oximeters
Spacer (metered dose inhaler)
Stethoscope tubing
Suction tubing
Syringes (disposable)
Tape (cloth adhesive, paper)
Tourniquet
Urodynamics rectal pressure catheters
Vascular or compression stockings
Wheelchair cushions, tires

HOME AND COMMUNITY ITEMS

Art supplies (paint, markers, glue)
Balloons (not Mylar)
Balls (Koosh, tennis, bowling)
Cardiopulmonary resuscitation manikins
Carpet backing, gym floor, gym mats (Broadloom carpets contain no natural rubber latex. For other products, provide barrier cloth or mat.)
Chewing gum
Cleaning or kitchen gloves
Condoms, contraceptive sponges, diaphragms
Dental dams and equipment
Disposable diapers
Elastic exercisers
Elastic on legs, waist of clothing, some disposable diapers
Feeding nipples
Foam rubber lining on splints, braces
Electric toothbrush or massager (for chest physiotherapy)
Latex paints, sealants, stains (There is no natural rubber in latex paint, although it may be present in some waterproof paints and sealants.)
Pacifier
Playpits, playground surfaces with natural rubber latex
Racquet handles
Rubber bands
Water toys, swim, scuba equipment
Wheelchair cushions, tires
Zippered plastic storage bags

Modified from Spina Bifida Association of America Fact Sheet: *Latex in the hospital environment items and home and community items,* Washington, DC, 2003, The Association.
*It is difficult to obtain full and accurate information on the latex content of certain products, which may vary among companies and product series. Double-checking with suppliers before use with latex-allergic individuals is strongly recommended. For an updated list of latex-free items and alternative items, contact the Spina Bifida Association of America, 4590 MacArthur Blvd. NW, Suite 250, Washington, DC 20007-4226; Resource Center (800) 621-3141; http://www.spinabifidaassociation.org.

and symptoms of latex hypersensitivity and appropriate emergency treatment (see Anaphylaxis, Chapter 25).

SPINAL MUSCULAR ATROPHY, TYPE 1 (WERDNIG-HOFFMANN DISEASE)

Spinal muscular atrophy (SMA) type 1 (Werdnig-Hoffmann disease) is a disorder characterized by progressive weakness and wasting of skeletal muscles caused by degeneration of anterior horn cells. It is inherited as an autosomal recessive trait and is the most common paralytic form of the **floppy infant syndrome (congenital hypotonia)**. The sites of the pathologic condition are the anterior horn cells of the spinal cord and the motor nuclei of the brainstem, but the primary effect is atrophy of skeletal muscles. The age of onset is variable, but the earlier the onset, the more disseminated and severe the motor weakness. The disorder may be manifested early—often at birth—and almost always before 2 years of age; death may occur as a result of respiratory failure by age 2 years (Iannaccone and Burghes, 2002). The manifestations (Box 32-8) and prognosis are categorized according to the age of onset, severity of weakness, and clinical course; some children may fluctuate between exhibiting symptoms of types 1 and 2, or types 2 and 3, in regard to clinical function (Sarnat, 2007). A severe rare fetal form of SMA, classified as type 0, is reported to be quite lethal in the perinatal period (Sarnat, 2007).

Diagnostic Evaluation and Therapeutic Management

The diagnosis is based on the molecular genetic marker for the *SMN* (survival motor neuron) gene, which is located on chromosome 5q13. Prenatal diagnosis may be made by genetic analysis of circulating fetal cells in maternal blood (Beroud, Karliova, Bonnefont, and others, 2003) or circulating fetal cells in amniotic fluid. The risk of subsequent affected offspring in carriers of the mutant gene or in families with known cases of SMA may also be evaluated genetically. Further diagnostic studies include muscle electromyography (EMG), which demonstrates a denervation pattern, and muscle biopsy; however, the genetic analysis has become the gold standard for diagnosis of the condition.

There is no cure for the disease, and treatment is symptomatic and preventive, primarily preventing joint contractures and treating orthopedic problems, the most serious of which is scoliosis. Hip subluxation and dislocation may also occur. Many children benefit from powered chairs, lifts, special pressure-adjustable mattresses, and accessible environmental controls. Muscle and joint contractures require careful attention and care to prevent further complications. Nutritional growth failure may occur in infants and toddlers as a result of poor feeding; supplemental gastrostomy feedings may be required to maintain adequate nutritional status and maintain weight gain. The use of lower extremity orthoses may assist with ambulation, but eventually the child may be confined to a wheelchair as muscle atrophy progresses. Sleep-disordered breathing is common in children with SMA and often requires nocturnal mechanical ventilation. Noninvasive ventilation methods such as bilevel positive airway pressure (BiPAP) have decreased the morbidity and increased the survival rate of children with SMA types 1 and 2. Upper respiratory tract infections may occur and are treated with antibiotic therapy.

Prognosis. Prognosis varies according to age of onset or group as described in Box 32-8. Individuals with SMA type 1

BOX 32-8

Clinical Manifestations of Spinal Muscular Atrophy (SMA)

TYPE 1 (WERDNIG-HOFFMANN DISEASE)

Clinical manifestations within first few weeks or months of life

Onset within 6 months of life

Inactivity the most prominent feature

Infant lying in a frog-leg position with legs externally rotated, abducted, and flexed at knees

Generalized weakness

Absent deep tendon reflexes

Limited movements of shoulder and arm muscles

Active movement usually limited to fingers and toes

Diaphragmatic breathing with sternal retractions (diaphragmatic paralysis may occur)

Abnormal tongue movements (at rest)

Weak cry and cough

Poor suck reflex

Tiring quickly during feedings (if breastfed, may lose weight before noticeable)

Growth failure (nutritional)

Alert facies

Normal sensation and intellect

Affected infants not able to sit alone, roll over, or walk

Early death possible from respiratory failure or infection

TYPE 2 (INTERMEDIATE SMA)

Onset before age 18 months

Early—Weakness confined to arms and legs

Later—Becomes generalized

Legs usually involved to greater extent than arms

Prominent pectus excavatum

Movements absent during complete relaxation or sleep

Some infants able to sit if placed in position, but few can ambulate

Life span from 7 months to 7 years, although many have normal life expectancy

TYPE 3 (KUGELBERG-WELANDER SYNDROME; MILD SMA)

Onset of symptoms after 18 months of age

Normal head control and ability to sit unassisted by 6 to 8 months of age

Thigh and hip muscles weak

Scoliosis common

Failure to walk a common presentation

In those who manage to walk:

- Waddling gait
- Genu recurvatum
- Protuberant abdomen
- Ambulation becoming increasingly difficult
- Confinement to a wheelchair by second decade

Deep tendon reflexes possibly present early but disappear

NOTE: These classifications are general, but some research suggests there may be variations in life span and other characteristics (Iannaccone and Burghes, 2002; Russman, Iannaccone, Buncher, and others, 1992; Russman, 1996).

may succumb to respiratory infections or failure between 1 and 24 months of age (Iannaccone and Burghes, 2002); however, some may live into their third or fourth decade of life. A significant number of infants with SMA require a tracheotomy, and associated medical conditions in survivors include gastroesophageal reflux, scoliosis, early onset puberty, hip dysplasia, and recurrent oral candidiasis (Bach, 2007).

Nursing Care Management

The infant or small child with progressive muscle weakness requires nursing care similar to that of the immobilized patient (see Chapter 31). However, the underlying goal of treatment should be to assist the child and family in dealing with the illness while progressing toward a life of normalization within the child's capabilities. Special attention should be directed to preventing muscle and joint contractures, promoting independence in performance of ADLs, and becoming incorporated into the mainstream of school when possible. In addition, parents need support and resources to be able to provide for the child and remain an intact family. Because children with neuromuscular disease have abnormal breathing patterns that often contribute to early death, it is important to assess adequate oxygenation, especially during the sleep phase when shallow breathing occurs and hypoxemia may develop. Home pulse oximetry may be used to assess the child during sleep and provide noninvasive ventilation as necessary (Young, Lowe, Fitzgerald, and others, 2007; Bush, Fraser, Jardine, and others, 2005) (see Duchenne [Pseudohypertrophic] Muscular Dystrophy, below, for respiratory management). Supportive care also includes management of orthoses and other orthopedic equipment as required. Because children with SMA are intellectually normal, verbal, tactile, and auditory stimulation are important aspects of developmental care. Supporting them so that they can see the activities around them and transporting them in appropriate conveyances (e.g., wagon, power wheelchair) for a change of environment provide stimulation and a broader scope of contacts.

Children who are able to sit require proper support and attention to alignment to prevent deformities and other complications. Children who survive beyond infancy will need attention to educational needs and opportunities for social interaction with other children. The parents of a child who is chronically ill require much support and encouragement* (see Chapter 18). Parents who have not sought genetic counseling should be encouraged to do so to evaluate further risk potential.

SPINAL MUSCULAR ATROPHY, TYPE 3 (KUGELBERG-WELANDER DISEASE)

SMA type 3 (Kugelberg-Welander disease) is a result of anterior horn cell and motor nerve degeneration. The disease is characterized by a pattern of muscular weakness similar to that of infantile SMA (see Box 32-8). Several modes of inheritance have been reported for the disease: autosomal recessive, autosomal dominant, and X-linked recessive.

The onset occurs from younger than 1 year of age into adulthood, with symptoms resembling group 3 infantile SMA. Proximal muscle weakness (especially of the lower limbs) and muscular atrophy are the predominant features. The disease runs a slowly progressive course. Some children lose the ability to walk 8 to 9 years after the onset of symptoms, but many can still walk after 30 years or more. Many affected persons have a normal life expectancy (Iannaccone, 1998).

Therapeutic Management and Nursing Care Management

The management is primarily symptomatic and supportive and is related to maintaining mobility as long as possible, preventing complications such as skin breakdown, optimizing and maintaining respiratory function, and providing support to the child and family.

MUSCULAR DYSTROPHIES

Muscular dystrophies (MDs) constitute the largest and most important single group of muscle diseases of childhood. The MDs have a genetic origin in which there is gradual degeneration of muscle fibers, and they are characterized by progressive weakness and wasting of symmetric groups of skeletal muscles, with increasing disability and deformity. In all forms of MD there is insidious loss of strength, but each type differs in regard to muscle groups affected (Fig. 32-7), age of onset, rate of progression, and inheritance pattern. The most common form, **Duchenne muscular dystrophy (DMD)**, is considered separately in the next section.

Facioscapulohumeral (Landouzy-Dejerine) muscular dystrophy is inherited as an autosomal dominant disorder with onset in early adolescence. It is characterized by difficulty in raising the arms over the head, lack of facial mobility, and a forward slope of the shoulders. The progression is slow, and the life span is usually unaffected.

Limb-girdle muscular dystrophy is an autosomal recessive disease of later childhood, adolescence, or early adulthood with variable but usually slow progression. It is characterized by weakness of proximal muscles of the pelvic and shoulder girdles.

Treatment of the MDs consists mainly of supportive measures, including physical therapy, orthopedic procedures to minimize deformity, ventilation support, and assistance for the affected child in meeting the demands of daily living.

DUCHENNE (PSEUDOHYPERTROPHIC) MUSCULAR DYSTROPHY

DMD is the most severe and the most common MD of childhood. It is inherited as an X-linked recessive trait, and the single-gene defect is located on the short arm of the X chromosome. DMD has a reportedly high mutation rate, with a positive family history in 65% of all cases (Thompson and Berenson, 2001); therefore genetic counseling is an important aspect of the care of the family.

As in all X-linked disorders, males are affected almost exclusively. At the genetic level, both DMD and Becker MD (a milder variant) result from mutations of the gene that encodes dystrophin, a protein product in skeletal muscle. Dystrophin is absent from the muscle of children with DMD and is reduced or abnormal in children with Becker MD. Children with Becker MD have a later onset of symptoms, which are usually not as severe as those seen in DMD. The incidence is

---

*Family resources for SMA include Families of Spinal Muscular Atrophy, PO Box 196, Libertyville, IL 60048; (800) 886-1762; http://www.fsma.org; and Muscular Dystrophy Association–USA, 3300 E. Sunrise Drive, Tucson, AZ 85718; (800) 572-1717; http://www.mda.org. In Canada: Families of Spinal Muscular Atrophy Canada, PO Box 97, Rivers, MB R0K 1X0; (800) 866-0016; http://www.curesma.ca.

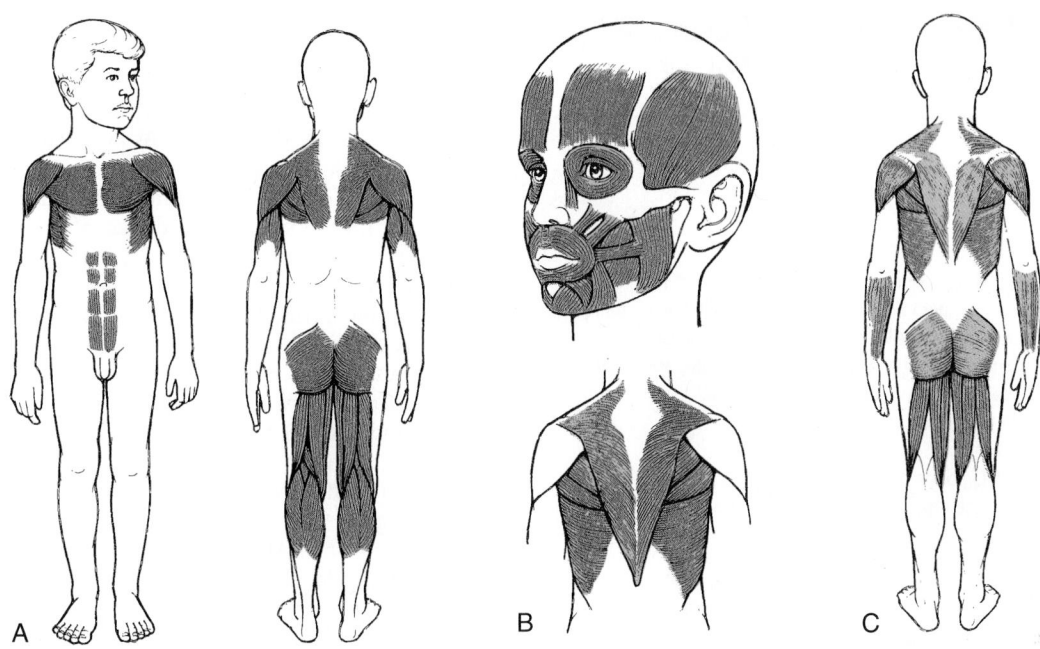

FIG. 32-7 ■ Initial muscle groups involved in muscular dystrophies. **A,** Pseudohypertrophic. **B,** Fascioscapulo-humeral. **C,** Limb girdle.

G.J.Wassilchenko

FIG. 32-8 ■ Child with Duchenne muscular dystrophy attains standing posture by kneeling, then gradually pushing his torso upright (with knees straight) by "walking" his hands up his legs (Gower sign). Note marked lordosis in upright position.

approximately 1 in 3600 male births for the Duchenne form and approximately 1 in 30,000 live births for the Becker type (Sarnat, 2007; Thompson and Berenson, 2001). Box 32-9 describes the characteristics of DMD.

Most children with DMD reach the appropriate developmental milestones early in life, although they may have mild, subtle delays. Evidence of muscle weakness usually appears during the third to seventh year, although there may have been a history of delay in motor development, particularly walking. Difficulties in running, riding a bicycle, and climbing stairs are usually the first symptoms noted. Later, abnormal gait on a level surface becomes apparent. In the early years, rapid developmental gains may mask the progression of the disease. Questioning the parents may reveal that the child has difficulty in rising from a sitting or supine position. Typically, affected boys have a waddling gait and lordosis, fall frequently,

---

BOX 32-9

Characteristics of Duchenne Muscular Dystrophy

- Early onset, usually between 3 and 7 years of age
- Progressive muscular weakness, wasting, and contractures
- Calf muscle hypertrophy in most patients
- Loss of independent ambulation by 9 to 12 years of age
- Slowly progressive, generalized weakness during teenage years

---

and develop a characteristic manner of rising from a squatting or sitting position on the floor (Gower sign; Fig 32-8). Parents may also notice the child has enlarged calves (Box 32-10).

Pseudohypertrophy is a term applied to muscular enlargement caused by fatty infiltration. Profound muscular atrophy

Clinical Manifestations of Duchenne Muscular Dystrophy

Relentless progression of muscle weakness; possible death from respiratory or cardiac failure
Waddling gait
Lordosis
Frequent falls
Gower sign (child turns onto side or abdomen, flexes knees to assume a kneeling position, then with knees extended gradually pushes torso to an upright position by "walking" the hands up the legs)
Enlarged (hypertrophied) muscles (especially calves, thighs, and upper arms); feel unusually firm or woody on palpation
Later stages—profound muscular atrophy
Mental deficiency (common)
- Mild (about 20 IQ points below normal)
- Mental deficit present in 25% to 30% of patients

Complications:
- Contracture deformities of hips, knees, and ankles
- Disuse atrophy
- Cardiomyopathy
- Obesity and at times undernutrition
- Respiratory compromise and cardiac failure

occurs in later stages, and as the disease progresses, contractures and deformities involving large and small joints are common complications. Ambulation usually becomes impossible by 12 years of age. Facial, oropharyngeal, and respiratory muscles are often spared until the terminal stages of the disease. Ultimately the disease process involves the diaphragm and auxiliary muscles of respiration, and cardiovascular involvement (cardiomyopathy, dysrhythmias, and heart failure) is common. Mild mental delay is common in roughly 30% of all individuals with MD, and many will have permanent learning disabilities; however, children with DMD should be transitioned into early learning programs and eventually into regular classrooms as much as possible. The eventual cause of death is usually respiratory tract infection or cardiac failure; however, much progress has been made in providing ventilatory methods to prolong and maintain quality of life.

Diagnostic Evaluation

The diagnosis of DMD is primarily established by blood polymerase chain reaction (PCR) for the dystrophin gene mutation (Sarnat, 2007). Prenatal diagnosis is also possible as early as 12 weeks of gestation. Serum enzyme measurement, muscle biopsy, and EMG may also be used in establishing the diagnosis. Serum creatine kinase levels are extremely high in the first 2 years of life, before the onset of clinical weakness. If the child demonstrates the usual characteristics, has a positive family history for DMD, and the PCR is positive, the muscle biopsy may be deferred.

Therapeutic Management

No effective treatment exists for childhood MD. The use of the corticosteroids prednisone and deflazacort has been evaluated as a treatment for DMD. Several clinical trials demonstrated increased muscle strength and improved performance and

pulmonary function, with significant decrease in the progression of weakness, when prednisone was administered for 6 months. The American Academy of Neurology has published a practice parameter for the administration of corticosteroids in the treatment of DMD (Moxley, Ashwal, Pandya, and others, 2005). Major side effects in these studies included weight gain and a cushingoid facial appearance. Deflazacort caused less weight gain than prednisone and was effective in decreasing muscle wasting in some children (Angelini, 2007). Deflazacort is not available in the United States but is in Canada.

Maintaining optimal function in all muscles for as long as possible is the primary goal; secondary is the prevention of contractures. Children with DMD who remain as active as possible are able to avoid wheelchair confinement for a longer time. Maintenance of function often involves stretching exercises, strength and muscle training, breathing exercises to increase and maintain vital lung capacity, range-of-motion exercises, surgery to release contracture deformities, bracing, and performance of ADLs.

Parents should always be involved in making decisions about the child's care, and teaching regarding home safety and prevention of falls is important as well. Parents should also be encouraged to have the child keep follow-up appointments for medical care and physical and occupational therapy. Because respiratory tract infections are most troublesome in these children, influenza and pneumococcal vaccines are encouraged, and contact with persons with respiratory tract infections should be avoided.

Eventually respiratory and cardiac problems become the central focus of the debilitating illness. Children with neuromuscular disease have abnormal breathing patterns, particularly during rapid-eye-movement sleep, and hypoxia may occur as a result of inadequate oxygenation (Birnkrant, 2002). The child and parents should be involved in a discussion of long-term ventilation options. Cardiac and respiratory assessment during wake-sleep cycles is imperative. Respiratory care for children with neuromuscular conditions such as SMA and DMD may involve the use of noninvasive ventilation with BiPAP on a temporary or full-time basis, mechanically assisted coughing (MAC), or tracheotomy and relief of airway obstruction with coughing and suctioning devices; the tracheotomy, however, is associated with more complications (Simonds, 2006; Young, Lowe, Fitzgerald, and others, 2007). Home pulse oximetry may be used to monitor oxygenation during sleep or to aid in decision making regarding the use of MAC to clear the airways.

Several devices are available for children with neuromuscular disease to assist in clearing the airway when the cough reflex is ineffective or diminished. The mechanical cough in-exsufflator (MIE) has been evaluated and found to be safe and effective in the daily management of respiratory function (Miske, Hickey, Kolb, and others, 2004). The MIE delivers positive inspiratory pressures at a set rate, followed by negative pressure exsufflation coordinated with the patient's own breathing rhythm; the exsufflation is designed to mimic a cough reflex so mucus can be effectively cleared. Airway suctioning after exsufflation is accomplished as necessary to clear the airways. In children the MIE may be connected directly to a tracheostomy or used with a mouthpiece or face mask.

Survival in individuals with DMD may be prolonged several years with the use of noninvasive ventilation and MAC as alternatives to tracheotomy and airway suctioning (Simonds, 2006). The American Thoracic Society (2004) has published extensive guidelines for respiratory monitoring and care of children and adults with DMD.

The American Academy of Pediatrics (2005) recommends an extensive cardiac evaluation of the child diagnosed with either DMD or Becker MD. Patients with neuromuscular conditions may not be seen with the typical signs and symptoms of cardiac dysfunction. Therefore symptoms such as weight loss, nausea and vomiting, cough, increased fatigue on performance of ADLs, and orthopnea should be carefully evaluated to detect early signs of cardiomyopathy.

Genetic counseling is also recommended for parents, female siblings, and maternal aunts and their female offspring. Long-term care, end-of-life directives, and palliative care options are issues that must be discussed with the child and family affected by MD. Professional counseling may be required to allow frank discussion of these issues in some cases, and referrals should be made as appropriate.

Research evaluating a number of treatments for DMD is in progress. These include clinical trials with glutamine and creatine monohydrate to preserve muscle strength; utrophin, a protein that is similar to dystrophin and in large quantities may counteract the effects of the deficiency of dystrophin (Chakkalakal, Thompson, Parks, and others, 2005); and the enzyme CT GalNAc transferase, which blocks muscle wasting in mice (Metules, 2002).

Nursing Care Management

The major emphasis of nursing care is to help the child and family cope with a chronic, progressive, incapacitating disease; to help design a program that will afford maximal independence and reduce the predictable and preventable disabilities associated with the disorder; and to help the child and family deal constructively with the limitations the disease imposes on their daily lives. Because of advances in technology, children with MD may live into early adulthood; therefore the goals of care should also involve decisions regarding quality of life, achievement of independence, and transition to adulthood.

Working closely with other team members, nurses assist the family in developing the child's self-help skills to give the child the satisfaction of being as independent as possible for as long as possible. This requires continual evaluation of the child's capabilities, which are often difficult to assess. Fortunately, most children with MD instinctively recognize the need to become as independent as possible and strive to do so.

Practical difficulties faced by families are physical limitations of housing and mobility. Some families live in houses or apartments that are unsuited to wheelchairs. Transportation may also be a barrier for families of children with MD. Assisting with these challenges requires team problem solving. Diet, nutritional needs, and nutrition modification are discussed according to the needs of the individual child and family.

The parents' social activities are also restricted, and the family's activities must be continually modified to accommodate the needs of the affected child. When the child becomes increasingly incapacitated, the family may consider home-based care, an assisted living facility, or respite care. Unless the child is severely incapacitated, he should also be involved in the decisions regarding such care. Nurses can assist with decision making by exploring all available options and resources

and support the child and family in the decision. Older boys with MD may also need psychiatric or psychologic counseling to deal with issues such as depression, anger, and quality of life. Parents also need to be encouraged to become involved in support groups because there is evidence that adequate social support from family, community, and other parents is crucial to appropriate coping in families with children with chronic illness.

Regardless of how successful the program or how well the family adapts to the disorder, superimposed on the physical and emotional problems associated with a child with a long-term disability is the constant knowledge of the ultimate outcome of the disease. All the manifestations seen in the child with a chronic fatal illness are encountered in these families (see Chapter 18).

Nurses are especially valuable health professionals as they come to know the family and the family's problems. Nurses can be alert to the family's problems and needs and make necessary referrals when supplementary services are indicated. The Muscular Dystrophy Association–USA* has branches in most communities to assist families in which there is a member with MD.

ACQUIRED NEUROMUSCULAR DISORDERS
GUILLAIN-BARRÉ SYNDROME (INFECTIOUS POLYNEURITIS)

Guillain-Barré syndrome (GBS), also known as infectious polyneuritis, is an uncommon acute demyelinating polyneuropathy with a progressive, usually ascending flaccid paralysis. Children are less often affected than adults; among children, those between ages 4 and 10 years have higher susceptibility. The male/female ratio is reported to be 1.5:1. Two peak time periods have been identified with an increased incidence of GBS: late adolescence and young adulthood. The incidence is also increased in pregnant and postpartum women (Newswanger and Warren, 2004).

Congenital GBS is rare yet may be seen in the neonatal period and consists of hypotonia, weakness, and decreased or absent reflexes; maternal neuromuscular disease may or may not be present. Diagnosis is established by the same criteria as in older children, but the symptoms gradually subside over the first few months of life and disappear by 12 months (Sarnat, 2007).

Pathophysiology

GBS is an immune-mediated disease often associated with a number of viral or bacterial infections or the administration of certain vaccines. It has been associated with infectious mononucleosis, measles, mumps, *Campylobacter jejuni* (gastroenteritis), cytomegalovirus, *Borrelia burgdorferi* (Lyme disease), Epstein-Barr virus, *Helicobacter pylori,* and *Mycoplasma* and *Pneumocystis* infections. Onset of GBS symptoms usually occurs within 10 days of the primary infection. Pathologic changes in spinal and cranial nerves consist of inflammation and edema with rapid, segmented demyelination and compression of nerve roots within the dural sheath. Nerve con-

---

*3300 E. Sunrise Drive, Tucson, AZ 85718; (800) 572-1717; http://www.mda.org. In Canada: Muscular Dystrophy Canada, 2345 Yonge St., Suite 900, Toronto, ON M4P 2E5; [0](866) MUSCLE-8; fax: (416) 488-7523; http://www.muscle.ca.

duction is impaired, producing ascending partial or complete paralysis of muscles innervated by the involved nerves. GBS has three phases:

1. **Acute**—Phase starts when symptoms begin and continues until new symptoms stop appearing or deterioration ceases; it may last as long as 4 weeks.
2. **Plateau**—Symptoms remain constant without further deterioration; it may last from days to weeks.
3. **Recovery**—Patient begins to improve and progress to optimal recovery; it usually lasts a few weeks to months depending on the deficits incurred by the illness.

Diagnostic Evaluation

Diagnosis of GBS is based on clinical manifestations (Box 32-11), CSF analysis, and EMG findings. CSF analysis reveals an increased protein concentration, and EMG shows evidence of acute muscle denervation; other laboratory studies are usually noncontributory. The symmetric nature of the paralysis helps differentiate this disorder from spinal paralytic poliomyelitis, which usually affects sporadic muscles.

Therapeutic Management

Treatment of GBS is primarily supportive. In the acute phase patients are hospitalized because respiratory and pharyngeal involvement may require assisted ventilation, sometimes with a temporary tracheotomy. Treatment modalities include aggressive ventilatory support, intravenous administration of immunoglobulin (IVIG), and steroids; plasmapheresis and immunosuppressive drugs may also be used. Plasmapheresis has been shown to decrease the length of recovery in patients with severe GBS yet is expensive, and side effects include hypotension, fever, bleeding disorders, chills, urticaria, and bradycardia. Further evidence reports equal benefits to treatment of GBS with IVIG administration or plasmapheresis; both sped up recovery time in studies reviewed (Hughes and Cornblath, 2005). Corticosteroids alone did not decrease the symptoms or shorten the duration of the disease. CSF filtration has been used in patients with GBS with some success;

CSF is removed, filtered, and replaced into the patient. This process presumably removes toxins and bacteria; however, further studies are needed to evaluate this treatment modality (Atkinson, Carr, Maybee, and others, 2006).

Medications that may be administered during the acute phase include a low-molecular-weight heparin to prevent deep vein thrombosis, a mild laxative or stool softener to prevent constipation, pain medication such as acetaminophen, and a histamine-antagonist to prevent stress ulcer formation. Chronic neuropathic pain following GBS may be treated with gabapentin, which is reported to be more effective than carbamazepine (Sarnat, 2007).

Course and Prognosis. Better outcomes are associated with younger age, no requirement for mechanical respiratory assistance, slower progression of disease, normal peripheral nerve function on EMG, and treatment with either IVIG or plasmapheresis. Recovery usually begins within 2 to 3 weeks, and most patients regain full muscle strength. The recovery of muscle strength progresses in the reverse order of onset of paralysis, with lower extremity strength being the last to recover. Poor prognosis with subsequent residual effects in children is reportedly associated with cranial nerve involvement, extensive disability at time of presentation, and intubation.

Most deaths associated with GBS are caused by respiratory failure; therefore early diagnosis and access to respiratory support are especially important. The rate of recovery is usually related to the degree of involvement and may extend from a few weeks to months. The greater the degree of paralysis, the longer the recovery phase.

Nursing Care Management

Nursing care is essentially supportive and is the same as that required for the child with immobilization and respiratory depression. The emphasis of care is on close observation to assess the extent of paralysis and on prevention of complications, including autonomic dysfunction (hypertension, orthostatic hypotension, syndrome of inappropriate antidiuretic hormone secretion, life-threatening dysrhythmias), respiratory dysfunction, fear and anxiety, and pain management.

During the acute phase of GBS the child's condition should be carefully observed for possible difficulty in swallowing and respiratory involvement. The child's respiratory function is closely monitored, and oxygen source, appropriate-sized resuscitation bag and mask, endotracheal intubation and suctioning equipment, tracheotomy tray, and vasoconstrictor drugs are kept available. Vital signs, including neurologic signs and level of consciousness, are monitored frequently. For the child who develops respiratory impairment, the care is the same as that for any child with respiratory distress requiring mechanical ventilation.

Throughout the recovery phase, special emphasis is placed on prevention of complications, including proper postural alignment, frequent change of position, assessment of skin at pressure points, and passive range-of-motion exercises. Respiratory care, should intubation be required, requires close monitoring of oxygenation status, usually by pulse oximetry and arterial blood gases; maintenance of an open airway with suctioning; and postural changes to prevent pneumonia. Children with oral and pharyngeal involvement may be fed via a nasogastric tube to ensure adequate feeding. Immobilization, which occurs with GBS, decreases gastrointestinal function; therefore attention to problems such as decreased gastric

---

BOX 32-11

Clinical Manifestations of Guillain-Barré Syndrome

INITIAL SYMPTOMS
Muscle tenderness
Paresthesia and cramps (sometimes)
Proximal symmetric muscle weakness
Ascending paralysis from lower extremities
Frequently involves muscles of trunk and upper extremities and those supplied by cranial nerves (especially facial)
Flaccid paralysis with loss of reflexes
May involve facial, extraocular, labial, lingual, pharyngeal, and laryngeal muscles
Intercostal and phrenic nerves:
  ■ Breathlessness in vocalizations
  ■ Shallow, irregular respirations

OTHER MANIFESTATIONS
Tendon reflexes depressed or absent
Variable degrees of sensory impairment
Muscle tenderness or sensitivity to slight pressure
Urinary incontinence or retention and constipation

emptying and constipation requires nursing assessment and appropriate collaborative interventions.

Prevention of deep vein thrombosis is accomplished with antiembolism devices, administration of a low-molecular-weight heparin, and early mobilization and ambulation. Temporary urinary catheterization may be required; urinary retention is not uncommon, and appropriate assessment of urinary output is vital. Sensory impairment and paralysis in the lower extremities makes the child susceptible to skin breakdown; therefore attention should be given to meticulous skin care. Although the child may have a generalized paralysis, cognitive function remains intact; therefore it is important for nursing care to involve communication with the child regarding procedures and treatments that may be frightening, especially if mechanical ventilation is required. Parents are encouraged to talk to the child and make eye and physical contact as much as possible to reassure the child during the illness. Psychosocial care of the child with GBS focuses on dealing with the child's anxiety and fear related to the disease itself and the unknown prognosis. In addition, the child's parents are allowed to express feelings and are encouraged to be involved in the child's daily care.

Pain management is crucial in the care of children with GBS. Although neuromuscular impairment may make pain perception more difficult to accurately evaluate, objective pain scales should be used.

Physical therapy is limited to passive range-of-motion exercises during the evolving phase of the disease. Later, as the disease stabilizes and recovery begins, an active physical therapy program is implemented to prevent contracture deformities and facilitate muscle recovery. This may include active exercise, gait training, and bracing.

Throughout the course of the illness, support of the child and parents is paramount. The usual rapidity of the paralysis and the long period of recovery greatly tax the emotional reserves of all family members. The parents and child benefit from repeated reassurance that recovery is occurring and from realistic information regarding the possibility of permanent disability. In the event of a residual disability, the family needs assistance in accepting and adjusting to the loss of function (see Chapter 18). The GBS/CIDP Foundation International* is a nonprofit organization devoted to support, education, and research. It provides support to families from recovered persons, publishes informational literature and a newsletter, and maintains a list of practitioners experienced with the disease.

TETANUS

Tetanus, or lockjaw, is an acute, preventable, but often fatal disease caused by an exotoxin produced by the anaerobic spore-forming, gram-positive bacillus *Clostridium tetani*. It is characterized by painful muscular rigidity primarily involving the masseter and neck muscles. There are four requirements for the development of tetanus: (1) presence of tetanus spores or vegetative forms of the bacillus, (2) injury to the tissues, (3) wound conditions that encourage multiplication of the organism, and (4) a susceptible host.

Tetanus spores are found in soil, dust, and the intestinal tracts of humans and animals, especially herbivorous animals.

The organisms are more prevalent in rural areas but are readily carried to urban areas by the wind. The organisms are not invasive but enter the body by way of wounds, particularly a puncture wound, burn, or crushed area. They may enter through a minor, unnoticed break in the skin, such as a thorn or needle prick, bee sting, or scratch. In the newborn, infection may occur through the umbilical cord, usually in situations in which infants are delivered in severely contaminated surroundings or the mother is not adequately immunized. The disease has the greatest incidence in months when persons are more involved in outdoor activities.

Pathophysiology

When prevention efforts are not effective and conditions are favorable, the organisms proliferate and form potent exotoxins, one of which is tetanospasmin. Tetanospasmin affects the central nervous system to produce the clinical manifestations of the disease. The ideal conditions for the organisms' growth are devitalized tissues without access to air, such as wounds that have not been washed or kept clean and those that have crusted over, trapping pus beneath. The exotoxin appears to reach the central nervous system by way of either the neuron axons or the vascular system. The toxin becomes fixed on nerve cells of the anterior horn of the spinal cord and the brainstem. The toxin acts at the myoneural junction to produce muscular stiffness and lower the threshold for reflex excitability.

The incubation period for tetanus varies from 2 days to months and averages 8 days; most cases occur within 14 days. In neonates it is usually 5 to 14 days. Shorter incubation periods have been associated with more heavily contaminated wounds, more severe disease, and a worse prognosis (American Academy of Pediatrics, 2006).

The manner of onset varies, but the initial symptoms are usually a progressive stiffness and tenderness of the muscles in the neck and jaw. Eventually all voluntary muscles are affected (Box 32-12). As the child recovers from the disease, the paroxysms become less frequent and gradually subside. Survival beyond 4 days usually indicates recovery, but complete recovery may require weeks.

Therapeutic Management

Preventive measures are based on the child's immune status and the nature of the injury. Specific prophylactic therapy after trauma is administration of **tetanus toxoid** (tetanus antitoxin is not available in the United States) (see Immunizations, Chapter 10, for age-specific recommendations).

The unprotected or inadequately immunized child who sustains a "tetanus-prone" wound (including wounds contaminated with dirt, feces, soil, and saliva; puncture wounds; avulsions; and wounds resulting from missiles, crushing, burns, and frostbite) should receive **tetanus immunoglobulin (TIG)**. Concurrent administration of both TIG and tetanus toxoid at separate sites is recommended both to provide protection and to initiate the active immune process. Once the individual has received primary tetanus immunization, antitoxin is believed to provide protection for at least 10 years and for a longer period after booster immunization (American Academy of Pediatrics, 2006). Completion of active immunization is carried out according to the usual pattern. Antibiotic treatment with oral or intravenous metronidazole (Flagyl) (alternatively parenteral penicillin G) is important in the

*The Holly Building, 104½ Forrest Ave., Narberth, PA 19072; (610) 667-0131, (866) 224-3301; http://gbs-cidp.org.

BOX 32-12
Clinical Manifestations of Tetanus

INITIAL SYMPTOMS
Progressive stiffness and tenderness of muscles in neck and jaw
Characteristic difficulty in opening the mouth (**trismus**)
Risus sardonicus (sardonic smile) caused by facial muscle spasm

PROGRESSIVE INVOLVEMENT
Opisthotonic positioning
Boardlike rigidity of abdominal and limb muscles
Difficulty swallowing
Extreme sensitivity to external stimuli (slight noise, gentle touch, or bright light):
  - Trigger paroxysmal muscle contractions that last seconds to minutes
  - Contractions recur with increased frequency until almost continuous (sustained, tetanic)
Laryngospasm and tetany of respiratory muscles:
  - Accumulated secretions
  - Respiratory arrest
  - Atelectasis
  - Pneumonia

OTHER ASPECTS
Mentation unaffected; patient alert
Pain, anxiety, and distress reflected in:
  - Rapid pulse
  - Sweating
  - Anxious facial expression
Fever usually absent or only mild

management of tetanus as an adjunct against vegetative forms of clostridia (American Academy of Pediatrics, 2006).

Aggressive supportive care is necessary to treat tetanus in the acute phase. The acutely ill child is best treated in an intensive care facility where close and constant observation and equipment for monitoring and respiratory support are readily available. A quiet environment is preferred to reduce external stimuli.

General supportive care is indicated, including maintaining adequate airway and fluid and electrolyte balance, managing pain, and ensuring adequate caloric intake. Indwelling oral or nasogastric feedings may be required to maintain adequate fluid and caloric intake; continued laryngospasm may necessitate total parenteral nutrition or gastrostomy feeding. Severe or recurrent laryngospasm or excessive secretions may require advanced airway management such as endotracheal intubation.

TIG therapy to neutralize toxins is the most specific therapy for tetanus. Antibiotics are administered to control the proliferation of the vegetative forms of the organism at the site of infection. Local care of the wound by surgical débridement and cleansing helps reduce the numbers of proliferating organisms at the site of injury. The cleansing should be repeated several times during the first 48 hours, and deep, infected lacerations are usually exposed and débrided.

Diazepam is the drug of choice for seizure control and muscle relaxation (Arnon, 2007b), but lorazepam (Ativan) may be used in some cases. Other AEDs may be administered as well. Intrathecal baclofen, magnesium sulfate, dantrolene sodium, and midazolam may also be used in the management of tetanus. Patients with severe tetanus and those who do not respond to other muscle relaxants may require the administration of a neuromuscular blocking agent, such as rocuronium or vecuronium; intrathecal baclofen may be used as a muscle relaxant but only in the intensive care unit because it often induces apnea. Because of their paralytic effect on respiratory muscles, use of these drugs requires mechanical ventilation with endotracheal intubation or tracheotomy and constant cardiopulmonary monitoring. Endotracheal tube insertion or tracheostomy is often indicated and should be performed before severe respiratory distress develops. Despite the absence of pain manifestation with these drugs, it is important to administer adequate analgesia. The administration of corticosteroids has met with success in some cases.

Nursing Care Management

The care of the child with tetanus requires supportive management with particular attention to airway and breathing. Respiratory status is carefully evaluated for any signs of distress, and appropriate emergency equipment is kept available at all times. The location, extent, and severity of muscle spasms are important nursing observations. Muscle relaxants, opioids, and sedatives that may be prescribed can also cause respiratory depression; therefore the child must be assessed for excessive central nervous system depression. Attention to hydration and nutrition involve monitoring an intravenous infusion, monitoring nasogastric or gastrostomy feedings, and suctioning oropharyngeal secretions when indicated.

In caring for the child with tetanus during the acute phase, the nurse makes every effort to control or eliminate stimulation from sound, light, and touch. Although a darkened room is ideal, sufficient light is essential so that the child can be carefully observed; light appears to be less irritating than vibratory or auditory stimuli. The infant or child is handled as little as possible, and extra effort is expended to avoid any sudden or loud noise to prevent seizures.

If a potent muscle relaxant such as vecuronium is used, the total paralysis makes oral communication impossible. The drug is not a sedative, however, and anxiety should be considered in children who are intubated. Therefore all the child's needs must be anticipated and procedures carefully explained beforehand.

Because their mental status is clear, children are aware of what is happening to them and are often extremely anxious. They should not be left alone, and all efforts should be made to reduce anxiety, which can contribute to muscle spasms. Parents are encouraged to stay with the child to offer security and support. They also need support, information and reassurance from the nurse.

BOTULISM

Botulism is an acute flaccid paralysis caused by the preformed toxin produced by the anaerobic bacillus *Clostridium botulinum*. In classic, or foodborne, botulism the most common source of the toxin is a contaminated food source. In addition to foodborne botulism, other forms include wound botulism; infant botulism; and man-made botulism, usually a result of bioterrorism (Arnon, 2007a). In foodborne illness, central nervous system symptoms appear abruptly within a few hours or gradually over several days after ingestion of contaminated

BOX 32-13

Clinical Manifestations of Botulism

GENERAL SIGNS

Weakness

Dizziness

Headache

Difficulty talking and speaking

Diplopia

Vomiting

Progressive, life-threatening respiratory paralysis

INFANT BOTULISM*

Constipation (a common symptom)

Generalized weakness

Decrease in spontaneous movements

Diminished or absent deep tendon reflexes

Loss of head control

Poor feeding

Weak cry

Reduced gag reflex

Progressive respiratory paralysis

*Most commonly diagnosed as "rule out sepsis" in the acute phase because of clinical presentation. Sometimes may be misdiagnosed as spinal muscular atrophy or metabolic disease.

food and may not be preceded by acute digestive disturbance (Box 32-13).

Treatment consists of intravenous administration of botulism antitoxin and general supportive measures, primarily respiratory and nutritional. Toxins vary in protein-binding capacity. Some have a relatively short half-life and do not bind to tissues firmly; therefore therapy is continued until paralysis abates. Other toxins appear to bind irreversibly to nerve endings and are therefore not amenable to neutralization.

Infant Botulism

Infant botulism, unlike the disease in older persons, is caused by ingestion of spores or vegetative cells of *C. botulinum* and the subsequent release of the toxin from organisms colonizing the gastrointestinal tract. *C. botulinum* types A and B are the most common causative strains of infant botulism. This form of botulism has become more prevalent than any other form. Many cases of infant botulism occur in breastfed infants who are being introduced to nonhuman milk substances (American Academy of Pediatrics, 2006). There appears to be no common food or drug source of the organisms; however, the *C. botulinum* organisms have been found in honey. Botulism may occur in infants as young as 1 week of age up to 12 months of age with peak incidence between 2 and 4 months of age.

The severity of the disease varies widely, from mild constipation to progressive sequential loss of neurologic function and respiratory failure (see Box 32-13). The affected infant is usually well before the onset of symptoms. Constipation is a common presenting symptom, and almost all infants exhibit generalized weakness and a decrease in spontaneous movements. Deep tendon reflexes are usually diminished or absent. Cranial nerve deficits are common, as evidenced by loss of head control, difficulty in feeding, weak cry, and reduced gag reflex. SMA type 1 and metabolic disorders are often mistaken

for infant botulism in the initial diagnostic phase because of the similarities in clinical manifestations of hypotonia, lethargy, and poor feeding (Francisco and Arnon, 2007). Presenting clinical signs also often mimic those of sepsis in young infants. Botulism toxin exerts its effect by inhibiting the release of acetylcholine at the myoneural junction, thereby impairing motor activity of muscles innervated by affected nerves.

Diagnosis is made on the basis of the clinical history, physical examination, and laboratory detection of the organism in the patient's stool and, less commonly, blood. However, isolation of the organism may take several days; therefore suspicion of botulism by clinical presentation should require emergent treatment (Arnon, 2007a). EMG may be helpful in establishing the diagnosis; however, results may be normal early in the course of the illness.

Treatment consists of immediate administration of botulism immune globulin intravenously (BIG-IV [BabyBIG]) (Francisco and Arnon, 2007), without delaying for laboratory diagnosis. Early administration of BIG-IV neutralizes the toxin and stops the progression of the disease. The human-derived botulism antitoxin (BIG-IV) has been evaluated and is now available nationwide for use only in infant botulism. In one study, infants treated with BIG-IV experienced a mean length of hospitalization decrease from 5.7 to 2.6 weeks and also had decreased time spent in intensive care, decreased mean duration of mechanical ventilation, and decreased mean duration of tube or intravenous feeding. In addition, the infants did not experience any adverse events related to BIG-IV; most infants received BIG-IV treatment within 3 to 18 days of hospitalization for botulism (Arnon, Schechter, Maslanka, and others, 2006). Approximately 50% of affected infants will require intubation and mechanical ventilation; therefore respiratory support is crucial, as is nutritional support since the infant is unable to feed. Trivalent equine botulinum antitoxin and bivalent antitoxin, used in adults and older children, is not administered to infants. Antibiotic therapy is not part of the management because the botulinum toxin is an intracellular molecule and antibiotics would not be effective; aminoglycosides in particular should not be administered because they may potentiate the blocking effects of the neurotoxin (Arnon, 2007a).

The prognosis is generally good if the patient is adequately treated, although recovery may be slow, requiring a few weeks after severe illness; the average length of stay for infant botulism is 44 days, and the fatality rate is reported to be less than 2%. Untreated patients may require a longer hospitalization.

NURSING ALERT

Although the precise source of *C. botulinum* spores has not been identified as originating from honey in many cases of infant botulism, it is still recommended that honey not be given to infants less than 12 months of age because the spores have been found in honey (Centers for Disease Control and Prevention, 2008).

Nursing Care Management

Nursing responsibilities include observing for and reporting signs of neuromuscular weakness or impairment and providing intensive nursing care when the infant is hospitalized (see Nursing Care of the High-Risk Newborn and Family, Chapter 9). Parental support and reassurance are important. Most infants recover when the disorder is recognized and therapy is implemented. Parents should be aware that, during recovery, patients tire easily when muscular action is sustained. This has important implications for timing the resumption of feedings because of the risk of aspiration. Parents should also be advised that normal bowel action may not return for several weeks; therefore a stool softener can be beneficial.

SPINAL CORD INJURIES

SCIs with major neurologic involvement traditionally have not been a common cause of physical disability in children. However, a sufficient number of children with these injuries are admitted to major medical centers, and because of the increased survival rate as a result of improved management, nurses are often involved in the care and rehabilitation of children with SCI.

Mechanisms of Injury

The most common cause of serious spinal cord damage in children is trauma involving MVCs (including automobile-bicycle, all-terrain vehicles, and snowmobiles), sports injuries (especially from diving, trampoline activities, gymnastics, and football), birth trauma, and nonaccidental trauma. The increased use of recreational activities involving motorized vehicles such as jet water skis, all-terrain vehicles, and motorcycles has also increased the incidence of SCIs in children. Congenital defects of the spine such as myelomeningocele also may in some cases produce the effects of SCI.

Transverse myelitis (inflammation of the spinal cord) has also been reported to develop from inadvertent intraarterial administration of long-acting penicillin injected into the buttocks. Damage can be extensive enough to result in paraplegia or even lower limb amputation.

In MVCs most SCIs in children are a result of indirect trauma caused by sudden hyperflexion or hyperextension of the neck, often combined with a rotational force. Trauma to the spinal cord without evidence of vertebral fracture or dislocation (SCIWORA) is particularly likely to occur in an MVC when proper safety restraints are not used. An unrestrained child becomes a projectile during sudden deceleration and is subject to injury from contact with a variety of objects inside and outside the vehicle. Individuals who use only a lap seat belt restraint are at greater risk of SCI than those who use a combination lap and shoulder restraint. High cervical spine injuries have been reported in children younger than 2 years of age who are improperly restrained in forward-facing car seats. Infants who are improperly restrained in an infant car seat may experience cervical trauma in a car crash. Small children may also be severely injured by deploying front seat air bags.

Falling from heights occurs less often in children than in adults, but vertebral compression from blows to the head or buttocks can occur in water sports (diving and surfing), falls from horses, or other athletic activities. Birth injuries may occur in breech deliveries from traction force on the spinal cord during delivery of the head and shoulders. When shaken, infants commonly sustain cervical cord damage, as well as subdural hematoma and retinal hemorrhage; mental retardation and death may occur subsequent to the traumatic event. Infants have weak neck muscles, and during vigorous shaking their large and heavy heads rapidly wobble back and forth. A significant number of adolescents receive SCIs secondary to gunshot wounds, stabbings, or other violent inflicted injury.

The injury sustained can affect any of the spinal nerves, and the higher the injury, the more extensive the damage. The child can be left with complete or partial paralysis of the lower extremities (**paraplegia**) or with damage at a higher level and without functional use of any of the four extremities (**quadriplegia**). A high cervical cord injury that affects the phrenic nerve paralyzes the diaphragm and leaves the child dependent on mechanical ventilation.

A mild but equally frightening form of cord trauma is **spinal cord compression,** a temporary neural dysfunction without visible damage to the cord. Complete quadriplegia can result but initially may not be differentiated from serious cord injury.

Therapeutic Management

The management of the child with SCI has changed dramatically in the past two decades as a result of improved technology, surgical procedures, and research into the complexity of the spinal cord and its neurologic components. Initial care begins at the scene of the accident; therefore education and training of first responder personnel in spinal immobilization, stabilization, and transfer techniques to prevent or reduce the severity of injury are critically important. Because of the complexity of these injuries, it is usually recommended that those with injuries be transported to a spinal injury center for care by specially trained health care personnel as soon as possible after the injury for appropriate diagnostic evaluation and intervention.

A number of special pediatric immobilization devices are now available that are physiologically appropriate for children's unique characteristics. A large head (proportionately), weak neck musculature, and weak tracheal cartilage predispose small children to airway compromise if placed supine; hence a spinal board with a built-in head drop may serve to protect the child's spine and neck and provide better airway management than the traditional flat board (DeBoer and Seaver, 2004).

Treatment with **functional electrical stimulation** (an implantable electrical stimulator with leads attached to the paralyzed muscles or nerves) has allowed children with certain SCIs greater mobility and functional use of paralyzed muscles to sit, stand, and walk with the aid of crutches, a walker, or other orthoses. Administration of pharmacologic agents such as clonidine hydrochloride may improve ambulation in patients with partial SCI, and exercise therapy through interactive locomotor training has been beneficial in helping some individuals with SCI regain ambulatory function.

SCI management guidelines and standards of care have recently been published for adult and pediatric patients with spinal injuries by the American Association of Neurological Surgeons and the Congress of Neurological Surgeons. For information regarding these guidelines and a more in-depth review of SCI care, the reader is referred to the Barker and Saulino (2002) reference for a synopsis of the guidelines, or see "Guidelines for the Management of Acute Cervical Spine and Spinal Cord Injuries" by Hadley, Walters, Grabb, and others (2002).

Nursing Care Management

The nursing care of the paraplegic or quadriplegic child is complex and challenging. A multidisciplinary SCI team is equipped to manage the acute phase of the injury, and some members, including the nurse, may follow the patient to eventual recovery. Nursing management is concerned with ensuring adequate initial stabilization of the entire spinal column with a rigid cervical collar with supportive blocks on a rigid backboard. During the acute phase of the injury it is imperative that airway patency be maintained and respiratory function monitored. It is important to evaluate the extent of the neurologic damage early to establish a baseline for neurologic functioning; continual assessment of function should occur to prevent further deterioration of neurologic status as a result of spinal cord edema. The American Spinal Injury Association (ASIA) Impairment Scale may be used to assess neurologic function on a routine basis during the patient's recovery (Barker and Saulino, 2002). Once the patient is admitted, further evaluation of the patient's abilities to perform ADLs can be made with the Functional Independence Measure (FIM) scale; this scale measures the patient's abilities during recovery and need for assistance (Barker and Saulino, 2002).

NURSINGALERT

In any situation in which SCI is suspected or a possibility, the child should be calmed, reassured, and told not to move; no one should be allowed to move the child unless he or she is able to stabilize the entire spine. A rigid cervical collar is used to immobilize the cervical spine, and the child is placed supine on a rigid immobilization board. Infants and small children may be removed in their car seats; no attempt should be made to take them out of the seat.

The nursing care of the child with an SCI is, in most respects, the same as that of any immobilized child (see The Immobilized Child, Chapter 31). Additional aspects of care that should be addressed on an individual basis include hypercalcemia in adolescent males, deep vein thrombosis, latex sensitization, and sleep-disordered breathing (Vogel, Hickey, Klaas, and others, 2004).

Respiratory care often focuses on maintaining an adequate airway and effective ventilation. The child with a high-level cervical injury (C3 and above) requires continuous ventilatory assistance. In most instances a tracheostomy is the method of choice for greater ease in clearing secretions and for less trauma to tissues during long-term ventilatory dependence. In some children breathing pacemaker devices (phrenic nerve stimulators) are implanted to stimulate the phrenic nerve and produce diaphragmatic contractions and lung expansion without assisted ventilation. In the child who does not require mechanical ventilation, special attention to clearance of secretions is vital because of decreased pulmonary function. In addition to chest physiotherapy, the child may require a cough-assist device to clear secretions effectively (see Duchenne Muscular Dystrophy: Therapeutic Management).

Temperature is often poorly regulated in children with SCI; therefore body temperature must be monitored closely for fluctuations. Response to environmental temperature changes may be slow or absent, and the ability to dissipate heat through the process of shivering may be compromised.

Children with SCI have unique needs in relation to skin care. Because of decreased sensation and impaired mobility, they depend on others to assess and assist in the management of intact skin. Skin care practices are the same as those for any child who is immobilized. A skin score scale such as the Braden Q Scale should be used to objectively evaluate risks for skin breakdown and skin conditions (Curley, Razmus, Roberts, and

FIG. 32-9 ■ Wheelchair allows adolescent mobility and independence. (Courtesy Texas Children's Hospital, Houston.)

others, 2003). An alternating-pressure mattress or other pressure relief or reduction device is kept underneath the child, and the skin is thoroughly inspected at least once a day (or more often if there is increased risk) for signs of pressure and breakdown, especially over bony prominences.

Bowel and bladder function is often affected in the child with SCI. CIC may be required to regularly empty the neurogenic bladder and prevent urinary tract infections. A regular bowel management program is tailored to the child's needs.

All adaptive devices help children increase their mobility, function, and endurance. The child with some lower extremity function progresses to parallel bars and then to a walker; the child with quadriplegia learns to use a wheelchair—among the most valuable aids available to the child with an SCI (Fig. 32-9). The wheelchair should be selected carefully in relation to where it will be used, the architectural barriers, and the child's functional capacity. For children with severe upper extremity paralysis, a variety of motorized wheelchairs are used; however, the more complex they are, the greater their cost, weight, and tendency to break down. Wheelchair tolerance is gained over time and is accompanied by measures to prevent orthostatic hypotension and pressure ulcers.

A variety of orthoses and other appliances can be adapted for use by many children. The primary purpose of lower extremity bracing in the child with an SCI is for ambulation, although correction of deformities may be attempted.

During the recovery and rehabilitation phase, patients with SCI must be carefully monitored for complications of immobility such as deep vein thrombosis and pulmonary embolus.

The child and family with SCI are prepared for the eventual discharge from the acute care facility to a rehabilitation center. The major aims of physical rehabilitation are to prepare the child and family to achieve normalization and resume life at home and in the community. Additional goals of rehabilitation in children with SCI are to promote independence in mobility and self-care skills, academic achievement, independent living, and employment.

The nurse is a crucial member of the health care team in relation to helping the family cope with the magnitude of the injury and disability, understand the extent of the disability, verbalize expected outcomes, and move toward eventual rehabilitation and normalization within the child's capabilities. The goals of rehabilitation include preparing the child and family to live at home and function as independently as possible.

KEY POINTS

- Clinical manifestations of CP include delayed gross motor development, altered motor performance, alterations of muscle tone and subsequent muscle contractures, abnormal posture, and associated disabilities such as seizures and sensory impairment.
- Therapy for CP takes into account the nature of the physical disability, defects associated with the disorder, and interpersonal and social influences encountered by the affected child.
- Care of the infant and child with myelomeningocele is directed toward protecting the meningeal sac, preventing infection and skin breakdown, observing for signs of urologic and bowel complications, promoting early parent-infant interaction, and planning appropriate interventions to optimize the child's development.

- SMA type 1 (Werdnig-Hoffmann disease) is characterized by progressive weakness and wasting of skeletal muscles caused by degeneration of anterior horn cells of the spinal cord.
- MDs are the most prevalent cause of neuromuscular dysfunction of childhood.
- Children with neuromuscular disease require careful monitoring of respiratory function and prompt interventions to prevent hypoxia and hypercarbia.
- Major complications of DMD include joint contractures, disuse atrophy, obesity, cardiomyopathy, sleep-disordered breathing, and respiratory failure as the condition progresses.
- Nursing care of the child with GBS consists of maintaining a patent airway; monitoring vital signs and neurologic signs; ensuring proper body alignment and positioning; and providing physical therapy, reassurance, and support to the child and family.
- Tetanus occurs when tetanus spores or vegetative bacilli enter a wound and multiply in a susceptible host.
- Clinical manifestations of infant botulism include constipation, decreased activity, poor feeding, and lethargy.
- Therapeutic management of SCI is directed toward immobilizing the entire spinal column at the scene of the traumatic event, transporting safely by health care personnel trained to transport possible spinal trauma victims, evaluating neurologic damage, preventing further neurologic damage, and implementing an aggressive rehabilitation program designed to help achieve independence and movement.

REFERENCES

Albright AL, Gilmartin R, Swift D, and others: Long-term intrathecal baclofen therapy for severe spasticity of cerebral origin, *J Neurosurg* 98(2):291-295, 2003.

American Academy of Pediatrics, Committee on Infectious Diseases, Pickering L, editor: *Red book: 2006 report of the Committee on Infectious Diseases,* ed 27, Elk Grove Village, Ill, 2006, The Academy.

American Academy of Pediatrics: Cardiovascular health supervision for individuals affected by Duchenne or Becker muscular dystrophy, *Pediatrics* 116(6):1569-1573, 2005.

American Academy of Pediatrics, American College of Obstetricians and Gynecologists: *Neonatal encephalopathy and cerebral palsy: defining the pathogenesis and pathophysiology,* Washington, DC, 2003, The College.

American Thoracic Society: Respiratory care of the patient with Duchenne muscular dystrophy, *Am J Respir Crit Care Med* 170(4):456-465, 2004.

Angelini C: The role of corticosteroids in muscular dystrophy: a critical appraisal, *Muscle Nerve* 36(4):424-435, 2007.

Arnon SS: Anaerobic bacterial infections: botulism (*Clostridium botulinum*). In Kliegman RM, Behrman RE, Jenson HB, and others, editors: *Nelson textbook of pediatrics,* ed 18, Philadelphia, 2007a, Saunders.

Arnon SS: Tetanus (*Clostridium tetani*). In Kliegman RM, Behrman RE, Jenson HB, and others, editors: *Nelson textbook of pediatrics,* ed 18, Philadelphia, 2007b, Saunders.

Arnon SS, Schechter R, Maslanka SE, and others: Human botulism immune globulin for the treatment of infant botulism, *N Engl J Med* 354(5):462-471, 2006.

Ashwal S, Russman BS, Blasco PA, and others: Practice parameter: diagnostic assessment of the child with cerebral palsy: report of the Quality Standards Subcommittee of the American Academy of Neurology and the Practice Committee of the Child Neurology Society, *Neurology* 62(6):851-863, 2004.

Atkinson SB, Carr RL, Maybee P, and others: The challenge of managing and treating Guillain-Barré syndrome during the acute phase, *Dimensions Crit Care Nurs* 25(6):256-263, 2006.

Bach JR: Medical considerations of long-term survival of Werdnig-Hoffmann disease, *Am J Phys Med Rehabil* 86(5):349-355, 2007.

Barker E, Saulino MF: Special report: first-ever guidelines for spinal cord injuries, *RN* 65(10):32-37, 2002.

Beroud C, Karliova M, Bonnefont JP, and others: Prenatal diagnosis of spinal muscular atrophy by genetic analysis of circulating fetal cells, *Lancet* 361(9362):1013-1014, 2003.

Birnkrant DJ: The assessment and management of the respiratory complications of pediatric neuromuscular diseases, *Clin Pediatr* 41(5):301-308, 2002.

Brown JP: Orthopaedic care of children with spina bifida: you've come a long way, baby! *Orthop Nurs* 20(4):51-58, 2001.

Buran CF, McDaniel AM, Brei TJ: Needs assessment in a spina bifida program: a comparison of the perceptions by adolescents with spina bifida and their parents, *Clin Nurs Spec* 16(5):256-262, 2002.

Bush A, Fraser J, Jardine E, and others: Respiratory management of the infant with type 1 spinal muscular atrophy, *Arch Dis Child* 90(7):709-711, 2005.

Centers for Disease Control and Prevention: *Botulism,* 2008, retrieved July 18, 2007, from http://www.cdc.gov/nczved/dfbmd/disease_listing/botulism_gi.html.

Centers for Disease Control and Prevention: Folate status in women of childbearing age, by race/ethnicity—United States, 1999-2000, 2001-2002, and 2003-2004, *MMWR* 55(51):1377-1380, 2007.

Centers for Disease Control and Prevention: Spina bifida and anencephaly before and after folic acid mandate—United States, 1995-1996 and 1999-2000, *MMWR* 53(17):362-365, 2004.

Chakkalakal JV, Thompson J, Parks RJ, and others: Molecular, cellular, and pharmacological therapies for Duchenne/Becker muscular dystrophies, *FASEB J* 19(8):880-891, 2005.

Curley MAQ, Razmus IS, Roberts KE, and others: Predicting pressure ulcer risk in pediatric patients: the Braden Q Scale, *Nurs Res* 52(1):22-33, 2003.

Dabney KW, Lipton GE, Miller F: Cerebral palsy, *Curr Opin Pediatr* 9(1):81-88, 1997.

DeBoer SL, Seaver M: Pediatric spinal immobilization: C-spines, car seats, and color-coded collars, *J Emerg Nurs* 30(5):481-484, 2004.

Doolin E: Bowel management for patients with myelodysplasia, *Surg Clin North Am* 86(2):505-514, 2006.

Eiwegger T, Dehlink E, Schwindt J, and others: Early exposure to latex products mediates latex sensitization in spina bifida but not in other diseases with comparable latex exposure rates, *Clin Exp Allergy* 36(10):1242-1246, 2006.

Francisco AM, Arnon SS: Clinical mimics of infant botulism, *Pediatrics* 119(4):826-828, 2007.

Gibson CS, MacLennan AH, Goldwater PN, and others: Antenatal causes of cerebral palsy: associations between inherited thrombophilias, viral and bacterial infection, and inherited susceptibility to infection, *Obstet Gynecol Surv* 58(3):209-220, 2003.

Green L, Greenberg GM, Hurwitz E: Primary care of children with cerebral palsy, *Clin Fam Pract* 5(2):1-21, 2003.

Grether JK, Nelson KB, Walsh E, and others: Intrauterine exposure to infection and risk of cerebral palsy in very preterm infants, *Arch Pediatr Adolesc Med* 157(1):26-32, 2003.

Hadley MN, Walters BC, Grabb PA, and others: Guidelines for management of acute cervical spine and spinal cord injuries, *Neurosurgery* 50(3 Suppl):S21-S29, 2002.

Han TR, Bang MS, Lim JY, and others: Risk factors of cerebral palsy in preterm infants, *Am J Phys Med Rehabil* 81(4):297-303, 2002.

Henshaw SK: Unintended pregnancy in the United States, *Fam Plan Perspect* 30:24-29, 1998.

Honein MA: Impact of folic acid fortification of the US food supply and occurrence of neural tube defects, *JAMA* 285(23):2981-2986, 2001.

Hughes RA, Cornblath DR: Guillain-Barré syndrome, *Lancet* 366(9497):1653-1666, 2005.

Hurtekant KM, Spatz DL: Special considerations for breastfeeding the infant with spina bifida, *J Perinat Neonatal Nurs* 21(1):69-75, 2007.

Iannaccone ST: Spinal muscular atrophy, *Semin Neurol* 18(1):19-26, 1998.

Iannaccone ST, Burghes A: Spinal muscular atrophies, *Adv Neurol* 88:83-98, 2002.

Jacobs JM: Management options for the child with spastic cerebral palsy, *Orthop Nurs* 20(3):53-59, 2001.

Kaufman BA: Neural tube defects, *Pediatr Clin North Am* 51(2):389-419, 2004.

Kellett PB: Latex allergy: a review, *J Emerg Nurs* 23(1):27-36, 1997.

Kimata H: Latex allergy in infants younger than 1 year, *Clin Exp Allergy* 34(12):1910-1915, 2004.

Kirkham C, Harris S, Grzybowski S: Evidence-based prenatal care, part I, General prenatal care and counseling issues, *Am Fam Physician* 71(7):1307-1316, 2005.

Krach LE: Pharmacotherapy of spasticity: oral medications and intrathecal baclofen, *J Child Neurol* 16(1):31-36, 2001.

Krigger KW: Cerebral palsy: an overview, *Am Fam Physician* 73(1):91-100, 101-102, 2006.

Lazzaretti CC, Pearson C: Myelodysplasia. In Allen PJ, Vessey JA, editors: *Primary care of the child with a chronic condition,* ed 4, St Louis, 2004, Mosby.

Matthews TJ, Honein MA, Erickson JD: Spina bifida and anencephaly prevalence—United States, 1991-2001, *MMWR Recomm Rep* 51(RR-13):9-11, 2002.

McKearnan KA, Kieckhefer GM, Engel JM, and others: Pain in children with cerebral palsy: a review, *J Neurosci Nurs* 36(5):252-259, 2004.

Metules T: Duchenne muscular dystrophy, *RN* 65(10):39-47, 2002.

Miske LJ, Hickey EM, Kolb SM, and others: Use of the mechanical in-exsufflator in pediatric patients with neuromuscular disease and impaired cough, *Chest* 125(4):1406-1412, 2004.

Moxley RT, Ashwal S, Pandya S, and others: Practice parameter: corticosteroid treatment of Duchenne dystrophy, *Neurology* 64(1):13-20, 2005.

Murphy KP, Molnar GE, Lankasky K: Employment and social issues in adults with cerebral palsy, *Arch Phys Med Rehabil* 81:807-811, 2000.

Newswanger DI, Warren CR: Guillain-Barré syndrome, *Am Fam Physician* 69(10):2405-2410, 2004.

Rogers B: Feeding method and health outcomes of children with cerebral palsy, *J Pediatr* 145(2 Suppl):S28-S32, 2004.

Roscigno CI: Addressing spasticity-related pain in children with spastic cerebral palsy, *J Neurosci Nurs* 34(3):123-131, 2002.

Rosenbaum P, Paneth N, Leviton A, and others: A report: the definition and classification of cerebral palsy April 2006, *Dev Med Child Neurol* 49(S109):1-44, 2007.

Russman BS: Function changes in spinal muscular atrophy II and III: the DCN/SMA group, *Neurology* 47(4):973-976, 1996.

Russman BS, Iannaccone ST, Buncher CR, and others: Spinal muscular atrophy: new thoughts on the pathogenesis and classification schema, *J Child Neurol* 7(4):347-353, 1992.

Samaniego IA: A sore spot in pediatrics: risk factors for pressure ulcers, *Pediatr Nurs* 29(4):278-282, 2003.

Sarnat HB: Neuromuscular disorders. In Kliegman RM, Behrman RE, Jenson HB, and others, editors: *Nelson textbook of pediatrics,* ed 18, Philadelphia, 2007, Saunders.

Shaer CM, Chescheir N, Schulkin J: Myelomeningocele: a review of the epidemiology, genetics, risk factors for conception, prenatal diagnosis, and prognosis for affected individuals, *Obstet Gynecol Surv* 62(7):471-479, 2007.

Simonds AK: Recent advances in respiratory care for neuromuscular disease, *Chest* 130(6):1879-1886, 2006.

Snodgrass WT, Adams R: Initial urologic management of myelomeningocele, *Urol Clin North Am* 31(3):427-434, viii, 2004.

Tarcan T, Onol FF, Ilker Y, and others: The timing of primary neurosurgical repair significantly affects neurogenic bladder prognosis in children with myelomeningocele, *J Urol* 176(3):1161-1165, 2006.

Thompson GH, Berenson FR: Other neuromuscular disorders. In Morrissy RT, Weinstein SL, editors: *Lovell and Winter's pediatric orthopaedics,* ed 5, Philadelphia, 2001, Lippincott Williams & Wilkins.

Vogel LC, Hickey KJ, Klaas SJ, and others: Unique issues in pediatric spinal cord injury, *Orthop Nurs* 23(5):300-308, 2004.

Volpe JJ: *Neurology of the newborn,* ed 4, Philadelphia, 2001, Saunders.

Winter S, Autry A, Boyle C, and others: Trends in the prevalence of cerebral palsy in a population-based study, *Pediatrics* 110(6):1220-1225, 2002.

Wu YW, Escobar GJ, Grether JK, and others: Chorioamnionitis and cerebral palsy in term and near-term infants, *JAMA* 290(20):2677-2684, 2003.

Young HK, Lowe A, Fitzgerald DA, and others: Outcome of noninvasive ventilation in children with neuromuscular disease, *Neurology* 68(3):198-201, 2007.

Denver II

Examiner:
Date:

Name:
Birthdate:
ID No.:

FIG. A-1 ■ A, Denver II. (From WK Frankenburg and JB Dodds, 1990.)

© 1969, 1989, 1990 W.K. Frankenburg and J.B. Dodds ©1978 W.K. Frankenburg

DIRECTIONS FOR ADMINISTRATION

1. Try to get child to smile by smiling, talking or waving. Do not touch him/her.
2. Child must stare at hand several seconds.
3. Parent may help guide toothbrush and put toothpaste on brush.
4. Child does not have to be able to tie shoes or button/zip in the back.
5. Move yarn slowly in an arc from one side to the other, about 8" above child's face.
6. Pass if child grasps rattle when it is touched to the backs or tips of fingers.
7. Pass if child tries to see where yarn went. Yarn should be dropped quickly from sight from tester's hand without arm movement.
8. Child must transfer cube from hand to hand without help of body, mouth, or table.
9. Pass if child picks up raisin with any part of thumb and finger.
10. Line can vary only 30 degrees or less from tester's line. /
11. Make a fist with thumb pointing upward and wiggle only the thumb. Pass if child imitates and does not move any fingers other than the thumb.

12. Pass any enclosed form. Fail continuous round motions.
13. Which line is longer? (Not bigger.) Turn paper upside down and repeat. (pass 3 of 3 or 5 of 6)
14. Pass any lines crossing near midpoint.
15. Have child copy first. If failed, demonstrate.

When giving items 12, 14, and 15, do not name the forms. Do not demonstrate 12 and 14.

16. When scoring, each pair (2 arms, 2 legs, etc.) counts as one part.
17. Place one cube in cup and shake gently near child's ear, but out of sight. Repeat for other ear.
18. Point to picture and have child name it. (No credit is given for sounds only.)
    If less than 4 pictures are named correctly, have child point to picture as each is named by tester.

19. Using doll, tell child: Show me the nose, eyes, ears, mouth, hands, feet, tummy, hair. Pass 6 of 8.
20. Using pictures, ask child: Which one flies?... says meow?... talks?... barks?... gallops? Pass 2 of 5, 4 of 5.
21. Ask child: What do you do when you are cold?... tired?... hungry? Pass 2 of 3, 3 of 3.
22. Ask child: What do you do with a cup? What is a chair used for? What is a pencil used for? Action words must be included in answers.
23. Pass if child correctly places and says how many blocks are on paper. (1, 5).
24. Tell child: Put block on table; under table; in front of me, behind me. Pass 4 of 4. (Do not help child by pointing, moving head or eyes.)
25. Ask child: What is a ball?... lake?... desk?... house?... banana?... curtain?... fence?... ceiling? Pass if defined in terms of use, shape, what it is made of, or general category (such as banana is fruit, not just yellow). Pass 5 of 8, 7 of 8.
26. Ask child: If a horse is big, a mouse is __? If fire is hot, ice is __? If the sun shines during the day, the moon shines during the __? Pass 2 of 3.
27. Child may use wall or rail only, not person. May not crawl.
28. Child must throw ball overhand 3 feet to within arm's reach of tester.
29. Child must perform standing broad jump over width of test sheet (8 1/2 inches).
30. Tell child to walk forward, ∞∞∞→ heel within 1 inch of toe. Tester may demonstrate. Child must walk 4 consecutive steps.
31. In the second year, half of normal children are non-compliant.

B OBSERVATIONS:

FIG. A-1, cont'd ■ B, Directions for administration of numbered items on Denver II. (From WK Frankenburg and JB Dodds, 1990.)

```
┌─────────────────────────────────────────────┬──────────────────────┐
│         DENVER ARTICULATION SCREENING EXAM    │  Name:               │
│          for children 2½ to 6 years of age    │                      │
│                                               │  Hosp. No.:          │
│  Instructions: Have child repeat each word    │                      │
│  after you. Circle the underlined sounds that │  Address:_____ │
│  he pronounces correctly. Total correct       │                      │
│  sounds is the Raw Score. Use charts on       │  _____ │
│  reverse side to score results.               │                      │
└─────────────────────────────────────────────┴──────────────────────┘
```

Date: _____   Child's age: _____   Examiner: _____   Raw score: ____
Percentile:_____   Intelligibility:_____   Result: _____

1. table   6. zipper   11. sock   16. wagon   21. leaf
2. shirt   7. grapes   12. vacuum   17. gum   22. carrot
3. door   8. flag   13. yarn   18. house
4. trunk   9. thumb   14. mother   19. pencil
5. jumping   10. toothbrush   15. twinkle   20. fish

Intelligibility: (circle one)
   1. Easy to understand   3. Not understandable
   2. Understandable ½ the time   4. Can't evaluate

Comments:

Date: _____   Child's age: _____   Examiner: _____   Raw score: ____
Percentile:_____   Intelligibility:_____   Result: _____

1. table   6. zipper   11. sock   16. wagon   21. leaf
2. shirt   7. grapes   12. vacuum   17. gum   22. carrot
3. door   8. flag   13. yarn   18. house
4. trunk   9. thumb   14. mother   19. pencil
5. jumping   10. toothbrush   15. twinkle   20. fish

Intelligibility: (circle one)
   1. Easy to understand   3. Not understandable
   2. Understandable ½ the time   4. Can't evaluate

Comments:

Date: _____   Child's age: _____   Examiner: _____   Raw score ____
Percentile:_____   Intelligibility:_____   Result: _____

1. table   6. zipper   11. sock   16. wagon   21. leaf
2. shirt   7. grapes   12. vacuum   17. gum   22. carrot
3. door   8. flag   13. yarn   18. house
4. trunk   9. thumb   14. mother   19. pencil
5. jumping   10. toothbrush   15. twinkle   20. fish

Intelligibility: (circle one)
   1. Easy to understand   3. Not understandable
   2. Understandable ½ the time   4. Can't evaluate

A

FIG. A-2 ■ A, Denver Articulation Screening Examination (DASE) for children 2½ to 6 years of age. (From AF Drumwright, University of Colorado Medical Center, 1971.)

To score DASE words: Note raw score for child's performance. Match raw score line (extreme left of chart) with column representing child's age (to the closest previous age group). Where raw score line and age column meet number in that square denotes percentile rank of child's performance when compared to other children that age. Percentiles above heavy line are ABNORMAL percentiles, below heavy line are NORMAL.

PERCENTILE RANK

Raw Score	2.5 yr.	3.0	3.5	4.0	4.5	5.0	5.5	6 years
2	1							
3	2							
4	5							
5	9							
6	16							
7	23							
8	31	2						
9	37	4	1					
10	42	6	2					
11	48	7	4					
12	54	9	6	1	1			
13	58	12	9	2	3	1	1	
14	62	17	11	5	4	2	2	
15	68	23	15	9	5	3	2	
16	75	31	19	12	5	4	3	
17	79	38	25	15	6	6	4	
18	83	46	31	19	8	7	4	
19	86	51	38	24	10	9	5	1
20	89	58	45	30	12	11	7	3
21	92	65	52	36	15	15	9	4
22	94	72	58	43	18	19	12	5
23	96	77	63	50	22	24	15	7
24	97	82	70	58	29	29	20	15
25	99	87	78	66	36	34	26	17
26	99	91	84	75	46	43	34	24
27		94	89	82	57	54	44	34
28		96	94	88	70	68	59	47
29		98	98	94	84	84	77	68
30		100	100	100	100	100	100	100

To score intelligibility:

	NORMAL	ABNORMAL
2½ years	Understandable ½ the time, or, "easy"	Not understandable
3 years and older	Easy to understand	Understandable ½ time Not understandable

Test result: 1. NORMAL on DASE and Intelligibility = NORMAL

2. ABNORMAL on DASE and/or Intelligibility = ABNORMAL

*If abnormal on initial screening, rescreen within 2 weeks.
If abnormal again, child should be referred for complete speech evaluation.

B

FIG. A-2, cont'd ■ B, Percentile rank. (From AF Drumwright, University of Colorado Medical Center, 1971.)

DENVER EYE SCREENING TEST

Name:
Hospital No:
Ward:
Address:

Vision Tests	1ST SCREENING: DATE: — Right Eye Normal / Abnormal / Untestable	Left Eye Normal / Abnormal / Untestable	RESCREENING: DATE: — Right Eye Normal / Abnormal / Untestable	Left Eye Normal / Abnormal / Untestable
1. E (3 years and above—3 to 5 trials)	3P / 3F / U	3P / 3F / U	3P / 3F / U	3P / 3F / U
2. Picture card (2½ to 2 11/12 years—3 to 5 trials)	3P / 3F / U	3P / 3F / U	3P / 3F / U	3P / 3F / U
3. Fixation (6 months to 2 5/12 years)	P / F / U	P / F / U	P / F / U	P / F / U
4. Squinting	Yes	Yes	Yes	Yes

Tests for Nonstraight Eyes	1ST SCREENING — Normal / Abnormal / Untestable	RESCREENING — Normal / Abnormal / Untestable
1. Do your child's eyes turn in or out, or are they ever not straight?	No / Yes	No / Yes
2. Cover test	P / F	P / F
3. Pupillary light reflex	P / F	P / F

Total Test Rating (Both Eyes)		
Normal (passed vision test plus no squint, plus passed 2 of 3 tests for nonstraight eyes)	Normal	Normal
Abnormal (abnormal on any vision test, squinting on 2 of 3 procedures for nonstraight eyes)	Abnormal	Abnormal
Untestable (untestable on any vision test or untestable on 2 of 3 tests for nonstraight eyes)	Untestable	Untestable
Future Rescreening Appointment for Total Test Rating (Abnormal or Untestable)	Date:	Date:

FIG. A-3 ■ Denver Eye Screening Test. (From WK Frankenburg and JB Dodds, University of Colorado Medical Center, 1969.)

SNELLEN SCREENING*

Preparation

1. Hang the Snellen chart on a light-colored wall so that the 20- to 30-foot lines are at eye level when children 6 to 12 years old are tested in the standing position (FIG. A-4).
2. Secure the chart to the wall with double-stick tape on the back side of all four corners. If the chart must be reversed for use of letter or E chart, secure it at the top and bottom with tacks. Make certain that the chart does not swing when in place.
3. The illumination intensity on the chart should be 10 to 30 footcandles, without any glare from windows or light fixtures. The illumination should be checked with a light meter.
4. Mark an exact 20-foot distance from the chart. Mark the floor with a piece of tape or "footprints" positioned so that the heels touch the 20-foot line.

*Modified from recommendations of the National Society to Prevent Blindness: *Guide to testing distance visual acuity,* Schaumburg, Ill, 1988, The Society.

FIG. A-4 ■ Snellen chart. **A,** Letter (alphabet) chart. **B,** Symbol E chart. (From National Society to Prevent Blindness, Inc., Schaumburg, Illinois.)

PROCEDURE

1. Place the child at the 20-foot mark, with the heel edging the line if the child is standing or with the back of the chair placed at the marker if the child is seated.
2. If the E chart is used, accustom the child to identifying which direction the "legs of the E" are pointing. Use a demonstration E card for this purpose.
3. Teach the child to use the occluder to cover one eye. Instruct the child to keep both eyes open during the test. Provide a clean cover card for each child and then discard after use.
4. If the child wears glasses, test only with glasses on.
5. Test both eyes together, then the right eye, then the left eye.
6. Begin with the 40- or 30-foot line and proceed with the test to include the 20-foot line.
7. With a child suspected of low vision, begin with the 200-foot line, and proceed until child can no longer correctly read three out of four or four out of six symbols on a line.
8. Use covers on the Snellen chart to expose only one symbol or one line at a time. When screening kindergarten or older children, expose one line but use a pointer to point to one symbol at a time.

RECORDING AND REFERRAL

1. Record the last line the child read correctly (three out of four or four out of six symbols).
2. Record visual acuity as a fraction. The numerator represents the distance from the chart, and the denominator represents the last line read correctly. For example, 20/30 means that the child read the 30-foot line at a 20-foot distance.
3. Observe the child's eyes during testing and record any evidence of squinting, head tilting, thrusting the head forward, excessive blinking, tearing, or redness.
4. Only make referrals after a second screening has been made on children who are potential candidates for referral.
5. The following children should be referred for a complete eye examination:
   a. Three-year-old children with vision in either eye of 20/50 or less (inability to correctly identify one more than half the symbols on the 40-foot line) *or* a two-line difference in visual acuity between the eyes in the passing range (e.g., 20/20 in one eye and 20/40 in the other)
   b. All other ages and grades with vision in either eye of 20/40 or less (inability to correctly identify one more than half the symbols on the 30-foot line)
   c. All children who consistently show any of the signs of possible visual disturbances, regardless of visual acuity

Growth Measurements

Height and Weight Measurements for Boys

| | HEIGHT BY PERCENTILES | | | | | | WEIGHT BY PERCENTILES | | | | | |
| | 5 | | 50 | | 95 | | 5 | | 50 | | 95 | |
AGE*	cm	inches	cm	inches	cm	inches	kg	lb	kg	lb	kg	lb
Birth	46.4	18¼	50.5	20	54.4	21½	2.54	5½	3.27	7¼	4.15	9¼
3 months	56.7	22¼	61.1	24	65.4	25¾	4.43	9¾	5.98	13¼	7.37	16¼
6 months	63.4	25	67.8	26¾	72.3	28½	6.20	13¾	7.85	17¼	9.46	20¾
9 months	68.0	26¾	72.3	28½	77.1	30¼	7.52	16½	9.18	20¼	10.93	24
1	71.7	28¼	76.1	30	81.2	32	8.43	18½	10.15	22½	11.99	26½
1½	77.5	30½	82.4	32½	88.1	34¾	9.59	21¼	11.47	25¼	13.44	29½
2†	82.5	32½	86.8	34¼	94.4	37¼	10.49	23¼	12.34	27¼	15.50	34¼
2½†	85.4	33½	90.4	35½	97.8	38½	11.27	24¾	13.52	29¾	16.61	36½
3	89.0	35	94.9	37¼	102.0	40¼	12.05	26½	14.62	32¼	17.77	39¼
3½	92.5	36½	99.1	39	106.1	41¾	12.84	28¼	15.68	34½	18.98	41¾
4	95.8	37¾	102.9	40½	109.9	43¼	13.64	30	16.69	36¾	20.27	44¾
4½	98.9	39	106.6	42	113.5	44¾	14.45	31¾	17.69	39	21.63	47¾
5	102.0	40¼	109.9	43¼	117.0	46	15.27	33¾	18.67	41¼	23.09	51
6	107.7	42½	116.1	45¾	123.5	48½	16.93	37¼	20.69	45½	26.34	58
7	113.0	44½	121.7	48	129.7	51	18.64	41	22.85	50¼	30.12	66½
8	118.1	46½	127.0	50	135.7	53½	20.40	45	25.30	55¾	34.51	76
9	122.9	48½	132.2	52	141.8	55¾	22.25	49	28.13	62	39.58	87¼
10	127.7	50¼	137.5	54¼	148.1	58¼	24.33	53¾	31.44	69¼	45.27	99¾
11	132.6	52¼	143.3	56½	154.9	61	26.80	59	35.30	77¾	51.47	113½
12	137.6	54¼	149.7	59	162.3	64	29.85	65¾	39.78	87¾	58.09	128
13	142.9	56¼	156.5	61½	169.8	66¾	33.64	74¼	44.95	99	65.02	143¼
14	148.8	58½	163.1	64¼	176.7	69½	38.22	84¼	50.77	112	72.13	159
15	155.2	61	169.0	66½	181.9	71½	43.11	95	56.71	125	79.12	174½
16	161.1	63½	173.5	68¼	185.4	73	47.74	105¼	62.10	137	85.62	188¾
17	164.9	65	176.2	69¼	187.3	73¾	51.50	113½	66.31	146¼	91.31	201¼
18	165.7	65¼	176.8	69½	187.6	73¾	53.97	119	68.88	151¾	95.76	211

Modified from National Center for Health Statistics, Health Resources Administration, Department of Health, Education and Welfare, Hyattsville, Md.
Conversion of metric data to approximate inches and pounds by Ross Laboratories.
*Years unless otherwise indicated.
†Height data include some recumbent length measurements, which make values slightly higher than if all measurements had been of stature (standing height).

FIG. B-1 ■ Weight-for-age percentiles, boys, birth to 36 months, CDC growth charts: United States. (Developed by the National Center for Health Statistics in collaboration with the National Center for Chronic Disease Prevention and Health Promotion, 2000.)

FIG. B-2 ■ Length-for-age percentiles, boys, birth to 36 months, CDC growth charts: United States. (Developed by the National Center for Health Statistics in collaboration with the National Center for Chronic Disease Prevention and Health Promotion, 2000.)

FIG. B-3 ■ Weight-for-length percentiles, boys, birth to 36 months, CDC growth charts: United States. (Developed by the National Center for Health Statistics in collaboration with the National Center for Chronic Disease Prevention and Health Promotion, 2000.)

FIG. B-4 ■ Head circumference-for-age percentiles, boys, birth to 36 months, CDC growth charts: United States. (Developed by the National Center for Health Statistics in collaboration with the National Center for Chronic Disease Prevention and Health Promotion, 2000.)

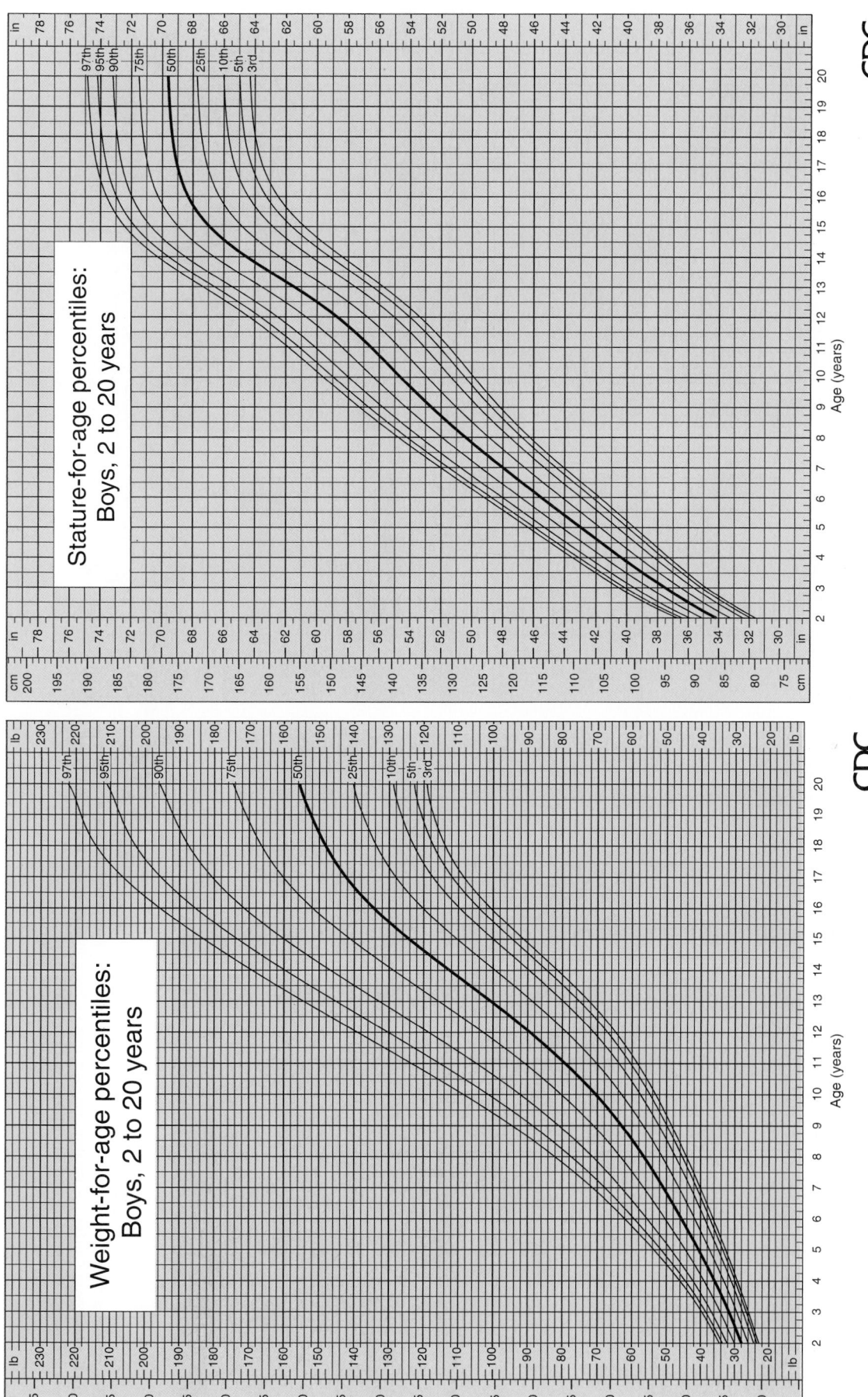

FIG. B-5 ■ Weight-for-age percentiles, boys, 2 to 20 years, CDC growth charts: United States. (Developed by the National Center for Health Statistics in collaboration with the National Center for Chronic Disease Prevention and Health Promotion, 2000.)

FIG. B-6 ■ Stature-for-age percentiles, boys, 2 to 20 years, CDC growth charts: United States. (Developed by the National Center for Health Statistics in collaboration with the National Center for Chronic Disease Prevention and Health Promotion, 2000.)

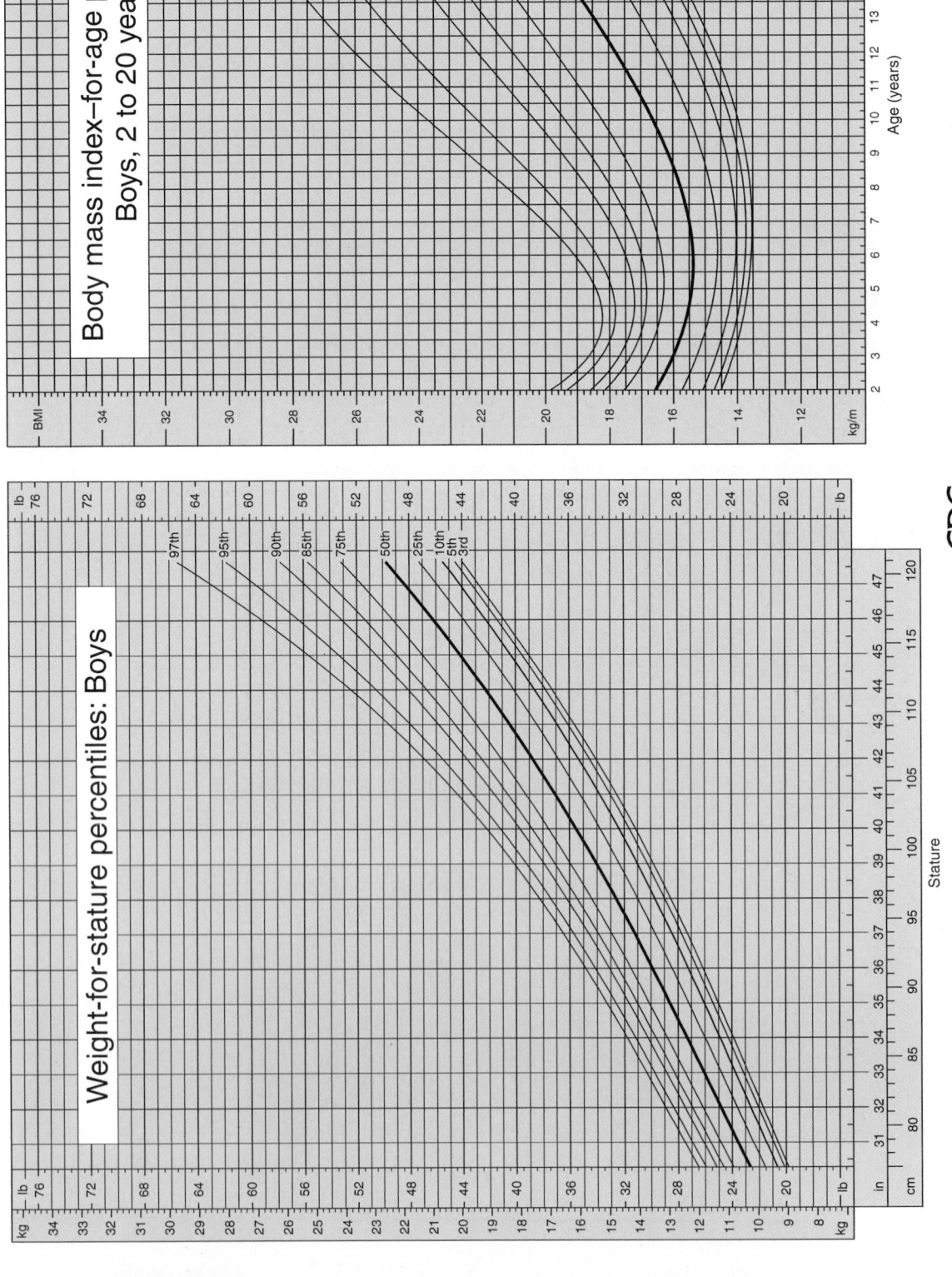

FIG. B-8 ■ Body mass index–for-age percentiles, boys, 2 to 20 years, CDC growth charts: United States. (Developed by the National Center for Health Statistics in collaboration with the National Center for Chronic Disease Prevention and Health Promotion, 2000.)

FIG. B-7 ■ Weight-for-stature percentiles, boys, CDC growth charts: United States. (Developed by the National Center for Health Statistics in collaboration with the National Center for Chronic Disease Prevention and Health Promotion, 2000.)

Height and Weight Measurements for Girls

	HEIGHT BY PERCENTILES						WEIGHT BY PERCENTILES					
	5		50		95		5		50		95	
AGE*	cm	inches	cm	inches	cm	inches	kg	lb	kg	lb	kg	lb
Birth	45.4	17¾	49.9	19¾	52.9	20¾	2.36	5¼	3.23	7	3.81	8½
3 months	55.4	21¾	59.5	23½	63.4	25	4.18	9¼	5.4	12	6.74	14¾
6 months	61.8	24¼	65.9	26	70.2	27¾	5.79	12¾	7.21	16	8.73	19¼
9 months	66.1	26	70.4	27¾	75.0	29½	7.0	15½	8.56	18¾	10.17	22½
1	69.8	27½	74.3	29¼	79.1	31¼	7.84	17¼	9.53	21	11.24	24¾
1½	76.0	30	80.9	31¾	86.1	34	8.92	19¾	10.82	23¾	12.76	28¼
2†	81.6	32¼	86.8	34¼	93.6	36¾	9.95	22	11.8	26	14.15	31¼
2½†	84.6	33¼	90.0	35½	96.6	38	10.8	23¾	13.03	28¾	15.76	34¾
3	88.3	34¾	94.1	37	100.6	39½	11.61	25½	14.1	31	17.22	38
3½	91.7	36	97.9	38½	104.5	41¼	12.37	27¼	15.07	33¼	18.59	41
4	95.0	37½	101.6	40	108.3	42¾	13.11	29	15.96	35¼	19.91	44
4½	98.1	38½	105.0	41¼	112.0	44	13.83	30½	16.81	37	21.24	46¾
5	101.1	39¾	108.4	42¾	115.6	45½	14.55	32	17.66	39	22.62	49¾
6	106.6	42	114.6	45	122.7	48¼	16.05	35½	19.52	43	25.75	56¾
7	111.8	44	120.6	47½	129.5	51	17.71	39	21.84	48¼	29.68	65½
8	116.9	46	126.4	49¾	136.2	53½	19.62	43¼	24.84	54¾	34.71	76½
9	122.1	48	132.2	52	142.9	56¼	21.82	48	28.46	62¾	40.64	89½
10	127.5	50¼	138.3	54½	149.5	58¾	24.36	53¾	32.55	71¾	47.17	104
11	133.5	52½	144.8	57	156.2	61½	27.24	60	36.95	81½	54.0	119
12	139.8	55	151.5	59¾	162.7	64	30.52	67¼	41.53	91½	60.81	134
13	145.2	57¼	157.1	61¾	168.1	66¼	34.14	75¼	46.1	101¾	67.3	148¼
14	148.7	58½	160.4	63¼	171.3	67½	37.76	83¼	50.28	110¾	73.08	161
15	150.5	59¼	161.8	63¾	172.8	68	40.99	90¼	53.68	118¼	77.78	171½
16	151.6	59¾	162.4	64	173.3	68¼	43.41	95¾	55.89	123¼	80.99	178½
17	152.7	60	163.1	64¼	173.5	68¼	44.74	98¾	56.69	125	82.46	181¾
18	153.6	60½	163.7	64½	173.6	68¼	45.26	99¾	56.62	124¾	82.47	181¾

Modified from National Center for Health Statistics, Health Resources Administration, Department of Health, Education and Welfare, Hyattsville, Md.
Conversion of metric data to approximate inches and pounds by Ross Laboratories.
*Years unless otherwise indicated.
†Height data include some recumbent length measurements, which make values slightly higher than if all measurements had been of stature.

FIG. B-9 ■ Weight-for-age percentiles, girls, birth to 36 months, CDC growth charts: United States. (Developed by the National Center for Health Statistics in collaboration with the National Center for Chronic Disease Prevention and Health Promotion, 2000.)

FIG. B-10 ■ Length-for-age percentiles, girls, birth to 36 months, CDC growth charts: United States. (Developed by the National Center for Health Statistics in collaboration with the National Center for Chronic Disease Prevention and Health Promotion, 2000.)

FIG. B-11 ▪ Weight-for-length percentiles, girls, birth to 36 months, CDC growth charts: United States. (Developed by the National Center for Health Statistics in collaboration with the National Center Fig Chronic Disease Prevention and Health Promotion, 2000.)

FIG. B-12 ▪ Head circumference-for-age percentiles, girls, birth to 36 months, CDC growth charts: United States. (Developed by the National Center for Health Statistics in collaboration with the National Center for Chronic Disease Prevention and Health Promotion, 2000.)

FIG. B-14 ■ Stature-for-age percentiles, girls, 2 to 20 years, CDC growth charts: United States. (Developed by the National Center for Health Statistics in collaboration with the National Center for Chronic Disease Prevention and Health Promotion, 2000.)

FIG. B-13 ■ Weight-for-age percentiles, girls, 2 to 20 years, CDC growth charts: United States. (Developed by the National Center for Health Statistics in collaboration with the National Center for Chronic Disease Prevention and Health Promotion, 2000.)

FIG. B-15 ■ Weight-for-stature percentiles, girls, CDC growth charts: United States. (Developed by the National Center for Health Statistics in collaboration with the National Center for Chronic Disease Prevention and Health Promotion, 2000.)

FIG. B-16 ■ Body mass index-for-age percentiles, girls, 2 to 20 years, CDC growth charts: United States. (Developed by the National Center for Health Statistics in collaboration with the National Center for Chronic Disease Prevention and Health Promotion, 2000.)

Growth Standards of Healthy Chinese Children

AGE	WEIGHT (kg)		HEIGHT (cm)		HEAD CIRCUMFERENCE (cm)	
	BOYS	GIRLS	BOYS	GIRLS	BOYS	GIRLS
Birth	3.27	3.17	50.6	50.0	34.3	33.7
1 month	4.97	4.64	56.5	55.5	38.1	37.3
2 months	5.95	5.49	59.6	58.4	39.7	38.7
3 months	6.73	6.23	62.3	60.9	41.0	40.0
4 months	7.32	6.69	64.4	62.9	42.0	41.0
5 months	7.70	7.19	65.9	64.5	42.9	41.9
6 months	8.22	7.62	68.1	66.7	43.9	42.8
8 months	8.71	8.14	70.6	69.0	44.9	43.7
10 months	9.14	8.57	72.9	71.4	45.7	44.5
12 months	9.56	9.04	75.6	74.1	46.3	45.2
15 months	10.15	9.54	78.3	76.9	46.8	45.6
18 months	10.67	10.08	80.7	79.4	47.3	46.2
21 months	11.18	10.56	83.0	81.7	47.8	46.7
24 months	11.95	11.37	86.5	85.3	48.2	47.1
2.5 years	12.84	12.28	90.4	89.3	48.8	47.7
3 years	13.63	13.16	93.8	92.8	49.1	48.1
3.5 years	14.45	14.00	97.2	96.3	49.4	48.5
4 years	15.26	14.89	100.8	100.1	49.7	48.9
4.5 years	16.07	15.63	103.9	103.1	50.0	49.1
5 years	16.88	16.46	107.2	106.5	50.2	49.4
5.5 years	17.65	17.18	110.1	109.2	50.5	49.6
6 years	19.25	18.67	114.7	113.9	50.8	50.0
7 years	21.01	20.35	120.6	119.3	51.1	50.2
8 years	23.08	22.43	125.3	124.6	51.4	50.6
9 years	25.33	24.57	130.6	129.5	51.7	50.9
10 years	27.15	27.05	134.4	134.8	51.9	51.3
11 years	30.13	30.51	139.2	140.6	52.3	51.7
12 years	33.05	34.74	144.2	146.6	52.7	52.3
13 years	36.90	38.52	149.8	150.7	53.0	52.8

Data from Bejing Children's Hospital, 1987, China.

Percentiles for Triceps Skinfold

| AGE-GROUP (years) | TRICEPS SKINFOLD PERCENTILES (mm) | | | | | | | | | |
| | MALES | | | | | FEMALES | | | | |
	5	25	50	75	95	5	25	50	75	95
1-1.9	6	8	10	12	16	6	8	10	12	16
2-2.9	6	8	10	12	15	6	9	10	12	16
3-3.9	6	8	10	11	15	7	9	11	12	15
4-4.9	6	8	9	11	14	7	8	10	12	16
5-5.9	6	8	9	11	15	6	8	10	12	18
6-6.9	5	7	8	10	16	6	8	10	12	16
7-7.9	5	7	9	12	17	6	9	11	13	18
8-8.9	5	7	8	10	16	6	9	12	15	24
9-9.9	6	7	10	13	18	8	10	13	16	22
10-10.9	6	8	10	14	21	7	10	12	17	27
11-11.9	6	8	11	16	24	7	10	13	18	28
12-12.9	6	8	11	14	28	8	11	14	18	27
13-13.9	5	7	10	14	26	8	12	15	21	30
14-14.9	4	7	9	14	24	9	13	16	21	28
15-15.9	4	6	8	11	24	8	12	17	21	32
16-16.9	4	6	8	12	22	10	15	18	22	31
17-17.9	5	6	8	12	19	10	13	19	24	37
18-18.9	4	6	9	13	24	10	15	18	22	30
19-24.9	4	7	10	15	22	10	14	18	24	34

From Frisancho A: New norms of upper limb fat and muscle areas for assessment of nutritional status, *Am J Clin Nutr* 34:2540-2545, 1981.

Percentiles of Upper Arm Circumference

| AGE-GROUP (years) | ARM CIRCUMFERENCE PERCENTILES (mm) | | | | | | | | | |
| | MALES | | | | | FEMALES | | | | |
	5	25	50	75	95	5	25	50	75	95
1-1.9	142	150	159	170	183	138	148	156	164	177
2-2.9	141	153	162	170	185	142	152	160	167	184
3-3.9	150	160	167	175	190	143	158	167	175	189
4-4.9	149	162	171	180	192	149	160	169	177	191
5-5.9	153	167	175	185	204	153	165	175	185	211
6-6.9	155	167	179	188	228	156	170	176	187	211
7-7.9	162	177	187	201	230	164	174	183	199	231
8-8.9	162	177	190	202	245	168	183	195	214	261
9-9.9	175	187	200	217	257	178	194	211	224	260
10-10.9	181	196	210	231	274	174	193	210	228	265
11-11.9	186	202	223	244	280	185	208	224	248	303
12-12.9	193	214	232	254	303	194	216	237	256	294
13-13.9	194	228	247	263	301	202	223	243	271	338
14-14.9	220	237	253	283	322	214	237	252	272	322
15-15.9	222	244	264	284	320	208	239	254	279	322
16-16.9	244	262	278	303	343	218	241	258	283	334
17-17.9	246	267	285	308	347	220	241	264	295	350
18-18.9	245	276	297	321	379	222	241	258	281	325
19-24.9	262	288	308	331	372	221	247	265	290	345

From Frisancho A: New norms of upper limb fat and muscle areas for assessment of nutritional status, *Am J Clin Nutr* 34:2540-2545, 1981.

Common Laboratory Tests

Common Laboratory Tests and Tests Results*

TEST/SPECIMEN	AGE/GENDER/REFERENCE	NORMAL RANGES			
		CONVENTIONAL UNITS		INTERNATIONAL UNITS (SI)	
Acetaminophen					
Serum or plasma	Therap. conc.	10-30 mcg/ml		66-200 μmol/L	
	Toxic conc.	>200 mcg/ml		>1300 μmol/L	
Ammonia nitrogen					
Plasma or serum	Newborn	90-150 mcg/dl		64-107 μmol/L	
	0-2 wk	79-129 mcg/dl		56-92 μmol/L	
	>1 mo	29-70 mcg/dl		21-50 μmol/L	
	Thereafter	0-50 mcg/dl		0-35.7 μmol/L	
Antistreptolysin O titer (ASO)					
Serum	2-4 yr	<160 Todd units			
	School-age children	170-330 Todd units			
Base excess					
Whole blood	Newborn	(−10)-(−2) mEq/L		(−10)-(−2) mmol/L	
	Infant	(−7)-(−1) mEq/L		(−7)-(−1) mmol/L	
	Child	(−4)-(+2) mEq/L		(−4)-(+2) mmol/L	
	Thereafter	(−3)-(+3) mEq/L		(−3)-(+3) mmol/L	
Bicarbonate (HCO₃)					
Serum	Arterial	21-28 mEq/L		21-28 mmol/L	
	Venous	22-29 mEq/L		22-29 mmol/L	
		Premature (mg/dl)	**Full term (mg/dl)**	**Premature (μmol/L)**	**Full term (μmol/L)**
Bilirubin, total					
Serum	Cord	<2.0	<2.0	<34	<34
	0-1 d	<8.0	<6.0	<137	<103
	1-2 d	<12.0	<8.0	<205	<137
	2-5 d	<16.0	<12.0	<274	<205
	Thereafter	<20.0	<10.0	<340	<171
Bilirubin, direct (conjugated)					
Serum		0.0-0.2 mg/dl		0-3.4 μmol/L	
Bleeding time					
Blood from skin puncture					
Ivy	Normal	2-7 min		2-7 min	
	Borderline	7-11 min		7-11 min	
Simplate (G-D)		2.75-8 min		2.75-8 min	
Blood volume					
Whole blood	Male	52-83 ml/kg		0.052-0.083 L/kg	
	Female	50-75 ml/kg		0.050-0.075 L/kg	
C-reactive protein (CRP)					
Serum	Cord	52-1330 ng/ml		52-1330 mcg/L	
	2-12 yr	67-1800 ng/ml		67-1800 mcg/L	
Calcium, ionized					
Serum, plasma, or whole blood	Cord	5.0-6.0 mg/dl		1.25-1.50 mmol/L	
	Newborn, 3-24 hr	4.3-5.1 mg/dl		1.07-1.27 mmol/L	
	24-48 hr	4.0-4.7 mg/dl		1.00-1.17 mmol/L	
	Thereafter	4.8-4.92 mg/dl or 2.24-2.46 mEq/L		1.12-1.23 mmol/L	

Modified from Kliegman RM, Behrman RE, Jenson HB, and others, editors: *Nelson textbook of pediatrics*, ed 18, Philadelphia, 2007, Saunders; McMillan JA, Deangelis CD, Feigin RD, and others, editors: *Oski's pediatrics: principles and practice*, ed 3, Philadelphia, 1999, Lippincott Williams & Wilkins; and Fischbach F: *A manual of laboratory and diagnostic tests*, ed 6, Philadelphia, 2000, Lippincott Williams & Wilkins.

*For a description of abbreviations, see p. 1200.

1192

Common Laboratory Tests and Tests Results—cont'd

TEST/SPECIMEN	AGE/GENDER/REFERENCE	NORMAL RANGES	
		CONVENTIONAL UNITS	INTERNATIONAL UNITS (SI)
Calcium, total			
Serum	Cord	9.0-11.5 mg/dl	2.25-2.88 mmol/L
	Newborn, 3-24 hr	9.0-10.6 mg/dl	2.3-2.65 mmol/L
	24-48 hr	7.0-12.0 mg/dl	1.75-3.0 mmol/L
	4-7 d	9.0-10.9 mg/dl	2.25-2.73 mmol/L
	Child	8.8-10.8 mg/dl	2.2-2.70 mmol/L
	Thereafter	8.4-10.2 mg/dl	2.1-2.55 mmol/L
Carbon dioxide, partial pressure (Pco_2)			
Whole blood, arterial	Newborn	27-40 mm Hg	3.6-5.3 kPa
	Infant	27-41 mm Hg	3.6-5.5 kPa
	Thereafter: Male	35-48 mm Hg	4.7-6.4 kPa
	Female	32-45 mm Hg	4.3-6.0 kPa
Carbon dioxide, total (tCO_2)			
Serum or plasma	Cord	14-22 mEq/L	14-22 mmol/L
	Premature (1 wk)	14-27 mEq/L	14-27 mmol/L
	Newborn	13-22 mEq/L	13-22 mmol/L
	Infant, child	20-28 mEq/L	20-28 mmol/L
	Thereafter	23-30 mEq/L	23-30 mmol/L
Cerebrospinal fluid (CSF)			
Pressure		70-180 mm H_2O	70-180 mm H_2O
Volume	Child	60-100 ml	0.06-0.10 L
	Adult	100-160 ml	0.10-0.16 L
Chloride			
Serum or plasma	Cord	96-104 mEq/L	96-104 mmol/L
	Newborn	97-110 mEq/L	97-110 mmol/L
	Thereafter	98-106 mEq/L	98-106 mmol/L
Sweat	Normal (homozygote)	<40 mEq/L	<40 mmol/L
	Marginal (e.g., asthma, Addison disease, malnutrition)	45-60 mEq/L	45-60 mmol/L
	Cystic fibrosis	>60 mEq/L	>60 mmol/L
Cholesterol, total			
Serum or plasma†	Acceptable	<170 mg/dl	<4.4 mmol/L
	Borderline	170-199 mg/dl	4.4-5.1 mmol/L
	High	≥200 mg/dl	≥5.2 mmol/L
Clotting time (Lee-White)			
Whole blood		5-8 min (glass tubes)	5-8 min
		5-15 min (room temp)	5-15 min
		30 min (silicone tube)	30 min
Creatine kinase (CK, CPK)			
Serum	Cord	70-380 U/L	70-380 U/L
	5-8 hr	214-1175 U/L	214-1175 U/L
	24-33 hr	130-1200 U/L	130-1200 U/L
	72-100 hr	87-725 U/L	87-725 U/L
	Adult	5-130 U/L	5-130 U/L
Creatinine			
Serum	Cord	0.6-1.2 mg/dl	53-106 μmol/L
	Newborn	0.3-1.0 mg/dl	27-88 μmol/L
	Infant	0.2-0.4 mg/d	18-35 μmol/L
	Child	0.3-0.7 mg/dl	27-62 μmol/L
	Adolescent	0.5-1.0 mg/dl	44-88 μmol/L
	Adult: Male	0.6-1.2 mg/dl	53-106 μmol/L
	Female	0.5-1.1 mg/dl	44-97 μmol/L
Urine, 24 hr	Premature	8.1-15.0 mg/kg/24 hr	72-133 μmol/kg/24 hr
	Full term	10.4-19.7 mg/kg/24 hr	92-174 μmol/kg/24 hr
	1.5-7 yr	10-15 mg/kg/24 hr	88-133 μmol/kg/24 hr
	7-15 yr	5.2-41 mg/kg/24 hr	46-362 μmol/kg/24 hr
Creatinine clearance (endogenous)			
Serum or plasma and urine	Newborn	40-65 ml/min/1.73 m^2	
	<40 yr: Male	97-137 ml/min/1.73 m^2	
	Female	88-128 ml/min/1.73 m^2	

†From National Cholesterol Education Program: Report of the expert panel on blood cholesterol levels in children and adolescents, *Pediatrics* 89(3 pt 2):527, 1992.

Continued

Common Laboratory Tests and Tests Results—cont'd

TEST/SPECIMEN	AGE/GENDER/REFERENCE	NORMAL RANGES	
		CONVENTIONAL UNITS	INTERNATIONAL UNITS (SI)
Digoxin			
Serum, plasma; collect at least 12 hr after dose	Therap. conc.		
	CHF	0.8-1.5 ng/ml	1.0-1.9 nmol/L
	Arrhythmias	1.5-2.0 ng/ml	1.9-2.6 nmol/L
	Toxic conc.		
	Child	>2.5 ng/ml	>3.2 nmol/L
	Adult	>3.0 ng/ml	>3.8 nmol/L
Eosinophil count			
Whole blood, capillary blood		50-250 cells/mm³ (μl)	50-250 × 10⁶ cells/L
Erythrocyte (RBC) count			
Whole blood	Cord	3.9-5.5 million/mm³	3.9-5.5 × 10¹² cells/L
	1-3 d	4.0-6.6 million/mm³	4.0-6.6 × 10¹² cells/L
	1 wk	3.9-6.3 million/mm³	3.9-6.3 × 10¹² cells/L
	2 wk	3.6-6.2 million/mm³	3.6-6.2 × 10¹² cells/L
	1 mo	3.0-5.4 million/mm³	3.0-5.4 × 10¹² cells/L
	2 mo	2.7-4.9 million/mm³	2.7-4.9 × 10¹² cells/L
	3-6 mo	3.1-4.5 million/mm³	3.1-4.5 × 10¹² cells/L
	0.5-2 yr	3.7-5.3 million/mm³	3.7-5.3 × 10¹² cells/L
	2-6 yr	3.9-5.3 million/mm³	3.9-5.3 × 10¹² cells/L
	6-12 yr	4.0-5.2 million/mm³	4.0-5.2 × 10¹² cells/L
	12-18 yr: Male	4.5-5.3 million/mm³	4.5-5.3 × 10¹² cells/L
	Female	4.1-5.1 million/mm³	4.1-5.1 × 10¹² cells/L
Erythrocyte sedimentation rate (ESR)			
Whole blood			
Westergren (modified)	Child	0-10 mm/hr	0-10 mm/hr
	<50 yr: Male	0-15 mm/hr	0-15 mm/hr
	Female	0-20 mm/hr	0-20 mm/hr
Wintrobe	Child	0-13 mm/hr	0-13 mm/hr
	Adult: Male	0-9 mm/hr	0-9 mm/hr
	Female	0-20 mm/hr	0-20 mm/hr
Fibrinogen			
Plasma	Newborn	125-300 mg/d	1.25-3.00 g/L
	Thereafter	200-400 mg/dl	2.00-4.00 g/L
Galactose			
Serum	Newborn	0-20 mg/dl	0-1.11 mmol/L
	Thereafter	<5 mg/dl	<0.28 mmol/L
Urine	Newborn	≤60 mg/dl	≤3.33 mmol/L
	Thereafter	<14 mg/24 hr	<0.08 mmol/d
Glucose			
Serum	Cord	45-96 mg/dl	2.5-5.3 mmol/L
	Newborn, 1 d	40-60 mg/dl	2.2-3.3 mmol/L
	Newborn, >1 d	50-90 mg/dl	2.8-5.0 mmol/L
	Child	60-100 mg/dl	3.3-5.5 mmol/L
	Thereafter	70-105 mg/dl	3.9-5.8 mmol/L
Whole blood	Adult	65-95 mg/dl	3.6-5.3 mmol/L
CSF	Adult	40-70 mg/dl	2.2-3.9 mmol/L
Urine (quantitative)		<0.5 g/d	<2.8 mmol/d
Urine (qualitative)		Negative	Negative

Glucose tolerance test (GTT), oral
Serum

Dosages		**Normal**	**Diabetic**	**Normal**	**Diabetic**
Adult: 75 g	Fasting	70-105 mg/dl	≥126 mg/dl	3.9-5.8 mmol/L	≥7.0 mmol/L
Child: 1.75 g/kg of ideal weight	60 min	120-170 mg/dl	≥200 mg/dl	6.7-9.4 mmol/L	≥11 mmol/L
up to maximum of 75 g	90 min	100-140 mg/dl	≥200 mg/dl	5.6-7.8 mmol/L	≥11 mmol/L
	120 min	70-120 mg/dl	≥200 mg/dl	3.9-6.7 mmol/L	≥11 mmol/L

Growth hormone (GH, somatotropin)

Plasma	1 d	5-53 ng/ml	5-53 mcg/L
	1 wk	5-27 ng/ml	5-27 mcg/L
	1-12 mo	2-10 ng/ml	2-10 mcg/L
	Fasting child/adult	<0.7-6.0 ng/ml	<0.7-6.0 mcg/L

Common Laboratory Tests and Tests Results—cont'd

TEST/SPECIMEN	AGE/GENDER/REFERENCE	NORMAL RANGES	
		CONVENTIONAL UNITS	INTERNATIONAL UNITS (SI)
Hematocrit (HCT, Hct)			
Whole blood	1 d (cap)	48%-69%	0.48-0.69 vol fraction
	2 d	48%-75%	0.48-0.75 vol fraction
	3 d	44%-72%	0.44-0.72 vol fraction
	2 mo	28%-42%	0.28-0.42 vol fraction
	6-12 yr	35%-45%	0.35-0.45 vol fraction
	12-18 yr: Male	37%-49%	0.37-0.49 vol fraction
	Female	36%-46%	0.36-0.46 vol fraction
Hemoglobin (Hb)			
Whole blood	1-3 d (cap)	14.5-22.5 g/dl	2.25-3.49 mmol/L
	2 mo	9.0-14.0 g/dl	1.40-2.17 mmol/L
	6-12 yr	11.5-15.5 g/dl	1.78-2.40 mmol/L
	12-18 yr: Male	13.0-16.0 g/dl	2.02-2.48 mmol/L
	Female	12.0-16.0 g/dl	1.86-2.48 mmol/L
Hemoglobin A			
Whole blood		>95% of total	>0.95 fraction of Hb
Hemoglobin F			
Whole blood	1 d	63%-92% HbF	0.63-0.92 mass fraction HbF
	5 d	65%-88% HbF	0.65-0.88 mass fraction HbF
	3 wk	55%-85% HbF	0.55-0.85 mass fraction HbF
	6-9 wk	31%-75% HbF	0.31-0.75 mass fraction HbF
	3-4 mo	<2%-59% HbF	<0.02-0.59 mass fraction HbF
	6 mo	<2%-9% HbF	<0.02-0.09 mass fraction HbF
	Adult	<2.0% HbF	<0.02 mass fraction HbF
Immunoglobulin A (IgA)			
Serum	Cord	1.4-3.6 mg/dl	14-36 mg/L
	1-3 mo	1.3-53 mg/dl	13-530 mg/L
	4-6 mo	4.4-84 mg/dl	44-840 mg/L
	7-12 mo	11-106 mg/dl	110-1060 mg/L
	2-5 yr	14-159 mg/dl	140-1590 mg/L
	6-10 yr	33-236 mg/dl	330-2360 mg/L
	Adult	70-312 mg/dl	700-3120 mg/L
Immunoglobulin D (IgD)			
Serum	Newborn	None detected	None detected
	Thereafter	0-8 mg/dl	0-80 mg/L
Immunoglobulin E (IgE)			
Serum	Male	0-230 IU/ml	0-230 kIU/L
	Female	0-170 IU/ml	0-170 kIU/L
Immunoglobulin G (IgG)			
Serum	Cord	636-1606 mg/dl	6.36-16.06 g/L
	1 mo	251-906 mg/dl	2.51-9.06 g/L
	2-4 mo	176-601 mg/dl	1.76-6.01 g/L
	5-12 mo	172-1069 mg/dl	1.72-10.69 g/L
	1-5 yr	345-1236 mg/dl	3.45-12.36 g/L
	6-10 yr	608-1572 mg/dl	6.08-15.72 g/L
	Adult	639-1349 mg/dl	6.39-13.49 g/L
Immunoglobulin M (IgM)			
Serum	Cord	6.3-25 mg/dl	63-250 mg/L
	1-4 mo	17-105 mg/dl	170-1050 mg/L
	5-9 mo	33-126 mg/dl	330-1260 mg/L
	10-12 mo	41-173 mg/dl	410-1730 mg/L
	2-8 yr	43-207 mg/dl	430-2070 mg/L
	9-10 yr	52-242 mg/dl	520-2420 mg/L
	Adult	56-352 mg/dl	560-3520 mg/L

Continued

Common Laboratory Tests and Tests Results—cont'd

TEST/SPECIMEN	AGE/GENDER/REFERENCE	NORMAL RANGES		
		CONVENTIONAL UNITS		INTERNATIONAL UNITS (SI)
Iron				
Serum	Newborn	100-250 mcg/dl		18-45 μmol/L
	Infant	40-100 mcg/dl		7-18 μmol/L
	Child	50-120 mcg/dl		9-22 μmol/L
	Thereafter: Male	65-170 mcg/dl		12-30 μmol/L
	Female	50-170 mcg/dl		9-30 μmol/L
	Intoxicated child	280-2550 mcg/dl		50.12-456.5 μmol/L
	Fatally poisoned child	>1800 mcg/dl		>322.2 μmol/L
Iron-binding capacity, total (TIBC)				
Serum	Infant	100-400 mcg/dl		17.90-71.60 μmol/L
	Thereafter	250-400 mcg/dl		44.75-71.60 μmol/L
Lead				
Whole blood	Child	<10 mcg/dl		<0.48 μmol/L
Urine, 24 hr		<80 mcg/L		<0.39 μmol/L
Leukocyte count (WBC count)		×1000 cells/mm³ (μl)		×10⁹ cells/L
Whole blood	Birth	9.0-30.0		9.0-30.0
	24 hr	9.4-34.0		9.4-34.0
	1 mo	5.0-19.5		5.0-19.5
	1-3 yr	6.0-17.5		6.0-17.5
	4-7 yr	5.5-15.5		5.5-15.5
	8-13 yr	4.5-13.5		4.5-13.5
	Adult	4.5-11.0		4.5-11.0
		×1000 cells/mm³ (μl)		×10⁶ cells/L
CSF (cell count)	Premature	0-25 mononuclear		0-25
		0-10 polymorphonuclear		0-10
		0-1000 RBC		0-1000
	Newborn	0-20 mononuclear		0-20
		0-10 polymorphonuclear		0-10
		0-800 RBC		0-800
	Neonate	0-5 mononuclear		0-5
		0-10 polymorphonuclear		0-10
		0-50 RBC		0-50
	Thereafter	0-5 mononuclear		0-5
Leukocyte differential count				
Whole blood	Myelocytes	0%	0 cells/mm³ (μl)	Number fraction 0
	Neutrophils—"bands"	3%-5%	150-400 cells/mm³ (μl)	Number fraction 0.03-0.05
	Neutrophils—"segs"	54%-62%	3000-5800 cells/mm³ (μl)	Number fraction 0.54-0.62
	Lymphocytes	25%-33%	1500-3000 cells/mm³ (μl)	Number fraction 0.25-0.33
	Monocytes	3%-7%	285-500 cells/mm³ (μl)	Number fraction 0.03-0.07
	Eosinophils	1%-3%	50-250 cells/mm³ (μl)	Number fraction 0.01-0.03
	Basophils	0%-0.75%	15-50 cells/mm³ (μl)	Number fraction 0-0.0075
Mean corpuscular hemoglobin (MCH)				
Whole blood	Birth	31-37 pg/cell		0.48-0.57 fmol/cell
	1-3 d (cap)	31-37 pg/cell		0.48-0.57 fmol/cell
	1 wk–1 mo	28-40 pg/cell		0.43-0.62 fmol/cell
	2 mo	26-34 pg/cell		0.40-0.53 fmol/cell
	3-6 mo	25-35 pg/cell		0.39-0.54 fmol/cell
	0.5-2 yr	23-31 pg/cell		0.36-0.48 fmol/cell
	2-6 yr	24-30 pg/cell		0.37-0.47 fmol/cell
	6-12 yr	25-33 pg/cell		0.39-0.51 fmol/cell
	12-18 yr	25-35 pg/cell		0.39-0.54 fmol/cell
	18-49 yr	26-34 pg/cell		0.40-0.53 fmol/cell

Common Laboratory Tests and Tests Results—cont'd

TEST/SPECIMEN	AGE/GENDER/REFERENCE	NORMAL RANGES	
		CONVENTIONAL UNITS	INTERNATIONAL UNITS (SI)
Mean corpuscular hemoglobin concentration (MCHC)			
Whole blood	Birth	30%-36% Hb/cell or g Hb/dl RBC	4.65-5.58 mmol Hb/L RBC
	1-3 d (cap)	29%-37% Hb/cell or g Hb/dl RBC	4.50-5.74 mmol Hb/L RBC
	1-2 wk	28%-38% Hb/cell or g Hb/dl RBC	4.34-5.89 mmol Hb/L RBC
	1-2 mo	29%-37% Hb/cell or g Hb/dl RBC	4.50-5.74 mmol Hb/L RBC
	3 mo–2 yr	30%-36% Hb/cell or g Hb/dl RBC	4.65-5.58 mmol Hb/L RBC
	2-18 yr	31%-37% Hb/cell or g Hb/dl RBC	4.81-5.74 mmol Hb/L RBC
	>18 yr	31%-37% Hb/cell or g Hb/dl RBC	4.81-5.74 mmol Hb/L RBC
Mean corpuscular volume (MCV)			
Whole blood	1-3 d (cap)	95-121 μm^3	95-121 fl
	0.5-2 yr	70-86 μm^3	70-86 fl
	6-12 yr	77-95 μm^3	77-95 fl
	12-18 yr: Male	78-98 μm^3	78-98 fl
	Female	78-102 μm^3	78-102 fl
Osmolality			
Serum	Child, adult	275-295 mOsm/kg H_2O	
Urine, random		50-1400 mOsm/kg H_2O, depending on fluid intake; after 12-hr fluid restriction: >850 mOsm/kg H_2O	
Urine, 24 hr		$\cong$300-900 mOsm/kg H_2O	
Oxygen, partial pressure (Po_2)			
Whole blood, arterial	Birth	8-24 mm Hg	1.1-3.2 kPa
	5-10 min	33-75 mm Hg	4.4-10.0 kPa
	30 min	31-85 mm Hg	4.1-11.3 kPa
	>1 hr	55-80 mm Hg	7.3-10.6 kPa
	1 d	54-95 mm Hg	7.2-12.6 kPa
	Thereafter (decreased with age)	83-108 mm Hg	11-14.4 kPa
Oxygen saturation (Sao_2)			
Whole blood, arterial	Newborn	85%-90%	Fraction saturated 0.85-0.90
	Thereafter	95%-99%	Fraction saturated 0.95-0.99
Partial thromboplastin time (PTT)			
Whole blood (Na citrate)			
Nonactivated		60-85 s (Platelin)	60-85 s
Activated		25-35 s (differs with method)	25-35 s
pH			H^+ concentration
Whole blood, arterial (must be corrected for body temperature)	Premature (48 hr)	7.35-7.50	31-44 nmol/L
	Birth, full term	7.11-7.36	43-77 nmol/L
	5-10 min	7.09-7.30	50-81 nmol/L
	30 min	7.21-7.38	41-61 nmol/L
	>1 hr	7.26-7.49	32-54 nmol/L
	1 d	7.29-7.45	35-51 nmol/L
	Thereafter	7.35-7.45	35-44 nmol/L
Urine, random	Newborn/neonate	5-7	0.1-10 μmol/L
	Thereafter	4.5-8 (average $\cong$6)	0.01-32 μmol/L (average $\cong$1.0 μmol/L)
Stool		7.0-7.5	31-100 nmol/L
Phenylalanine			
Serum	Premature	2.0-7.5 mg/dl	120-450 μmol/L
	Newborn	1.2-3.4 mg/dl	70-210 μmol/L
	Thereafter	0.8-1.8 mg/dl	50-110 μmol/L
Urine, 24 hr	10 d–2 wk	1-2 mg/d	6-12 μmol/d
	3-12 yr	4-18 mg/d	24-110 μmol/d
	Thereafter	Trace—17 mg/d	Trace—103 μmol/d
Plasma volume			
Plasma	Male	25-43 ml/kg	0.025-0.043 L/kg
	Female	28-45 ml/kg	0.028-0.045 L/kg
Platelet count (thrombocyte count)			
Whole blood (EDTA)	Newborn (after 1 wk, same as adult)	84-478 × 10^3/mm^3 (μl)	84-478 × 10^9/L
	Adult	150-400 × 10^3/mm^3 (μl)	150-400 × 10^9/L

Continued

Common Laboratory Tests and Tests Results—cont'd

TEST/SPECIMEN	AGE/GENDER/REFERENCE	NORMAL RANGES	
		CONVENTIONAL UNITS	INTERNATIONAL UNITS (SI)
Potassium			
Serum	Newborn	3.0-6.0 mEq/L	3.0-6.0 mmol/L
	Thereafter	3.5-5.0 mEq/L	3.5-5.0 mmol/L
Plasma (heparin)		3.4-4.5 mEq/L	3.4-4.5 mmol/L
Urine, 24 hr		2.5-125 mEq/d (varies with diet)	2.5-125 mmol/L
Protein			
Serum, total	Premature	4.3-7.6 g/dl	43-76 g/L
	Newborn	4.6-7.4 g/dl	46-74 g/L
	1-7 yr	6.1-7.9 g/dl	61-79 g/L
	8-12 yr	6.4-8.1 g/dl	64-81 g/L
	13-19 yr	6.6-8.2 g/dl	66-82 g/L
Total			
Urine, 24 hr		1-14 mg/dl	10-140 mg/L
		50-80 mg/d (at rest)	50-80 mg/d
		<250 mg/d (after intense exercise)	<250 mg/d (after intense exercise)
CSF		Lumbar: 8-32 mg/dl	80-320 mg/L
Prothrombin time (PT)			
One-stage (Quick)			
Whole blood (Na citrate)	In general	11-15 s (varies with type of thromboplastin)	11-15 s
	Newborn	Prolonged by 2-3 s	Prolonged by 2-3 s
Two-stage modified (Ware and Seegers)			
Whole blood (sodium citrate)		18-22 s	18-22 s
RBC count: see Erythrocyte (RBC) count			
Red blood cell volume			
Whole blood	Male	20-36 ml/kg	0.020-0.036 L/kg
	Female	19-31 ml/kg	0.019-0.031 L/kg
Reticulocyte count			
Whole blood	Adults	0.5%-1.5% of erythrocytes or 25,000-75,000/mm^3 (μl)	0.005-0.015 (number fraction) or 25,000-75,000 $\times$ 10^6/L
Capillary	1 d	0.4%-6.0%	0.004-0.060 (number fraction)
	7 d	<0.1%-1.3%	<0.001-0.013 (number fraction)
	1-4 wk	<0.1%-1.2%	<0.001-0.012 (number fraction)
	5-6 wk	<0.1%-2.4%	<0.001-0.024 (number fraction)
	7-8 wk	0.1%-2.9%	0.001-0.029 (number fraction)
	9-10 wk	<0.1%-2.6%	<0.001-0.026 (number fraction)
	11-12 wk	0.1%-1.3%	0.001-0.013 (number fraction)
Salicylates			
Serum, plasma	Therap. conc.	15-30 mg/dl	1.1-2.2 mmol/L
	Toxic conc.	>30 mg/dl	>18.5 mmol/L
Sedimentation rate: see Erythrocyte sedimentation rate (ESR)			
Sodium			
Serum or plasma	Newborn	134-146 mEq/L	134-146 mmol/L
	Infant	139-146 mEq/L	139-146 mmol/L
	Child	138-145 mEq/L	138-145 mmol/L
	Thereafter	136-146 mEq/L	136-146 mmol/L
Urine, 24 hr		40-220 mEq/L (diet dependent)	40-220 mmol/L
Sweat	Normal	<40 mEq/L	<40 mmol/L
	Indeterminate	45-60 mEq/L	45-60 mmol/L
	Cystic fibrosis	>60 mEq/L	>60 mmol/L
Specific gravity			
Urine, random	Adult	1.002-1.030	1.002-1.030
	After 12-hr fluid restriction	>1.025	>1.025
Urine, 24 hr		1.015-1.025	
Theophylline			
Serum, plasma	Therap. conc.		
Bronchodilator		10-20 mcg/ml	56-110 μmol/L
Premature apnea		5-10 mcg/ml	28-56 μmol/L
Toxic conc.		>20 mcg/ml	>110 μmol/L

Common Laboratory Tests and Tests Results—cont'd

TEST/SPECIMEN	AGE/GENDER/REFERENCE	NORMAL RANGES			
		CONVENTIONAL UNITS		INTERNATIONAL UNITS (SI)	
Thrombin time					
Whole blood (Na citrate)		Control time ±2 s when control is 9-13 s		Control time ±2 s when control is 9-13 s	
Thyroxine, total (T₄)					
Serum	Cord	8-13 mcg/dl		103-168 nmol/L	
	Newborn	11.5-24 mcg/dl (lower in low-birth-weight infants)		148-310 nmol/L	
	Neonate	9-18 mcg/dl		116-232 nmol/L	
	Infant	7-15 mcg/dl		90-194 nmol/L	
	1-5 yr	7.3-15 mcg/dl		94-194 nmol/L	
	5-10 yr	6.4-13.3 mcg/dl		83-172 nmol/L	
	Thereafter	5-12 mcg/dl		65-155 nmol/L	
	Newborn screen (filter paper)	6.2-22 mcg/dl		80-284 nmol/L	
Triglycerides (TG)		**Male** (mg/dl)	**Female** (mg/dl)	**Male** (g/L)	**Female** (g/L)
Serum, after ≥2-hr fast	Cord	10-98	10-98	0.10-0.98	0.10-0.98
	0-5 yr	30-86	32-99	0.30-0.86	0.32-0.99
	6-11 yr	31-108	35-114	0.31-1.08	0.35-1.14
	12-15 yr	36-138	41-138	0.36-1.38	0.41-1.38
	16-19 yr	40-163	40-128	0.40-1.63	0.40-1.28
Triiodothyronine (T₃), free					
Serum	Cord	20-240 pg/dl		0.3-3.7 pmol/L	
	1-3 d	200-610 pg/dl		3.1-9.4 pmol/L	
	6 wk	240-560 pg/dl		3.7-8.6 pmol/L	
	Adults (20-50 yr)	230-660 pg/dl		3.5-10.0 pmol/L	
Triiodothyronine, total (T₃-RIA)					
Serum	Cord	30-70 ng/dl		0.46-1.08 nmol/L	
	Newborn	72-260 ng/dl		1.16-4 nmol/L	
	1-5 yr	100-260 ng/dl		1.54-4 nmol/L	
	5-10 yr	90-240 ng/dl		1.39-3.70 nmol/L	
	10-15 yr	80-210 ng/dl		1.23-3.23 nmol/L	
	Thereafter	115-190 ng/dl		1.77-2.93 nmol/L	
Urea nitrogen					
Serum or plasma	Cord	21-40 mg/dl		7.5-14.3 mmol/L	
	Premature (1 wk)	3-25 mg/dl		1.1-9 mmol/L	
	Newborn	3-12 mg/dl		1.1-4.3 mmol/L	
	Infant/child	5-18 mg/dl		1.8-6.4 mmol/L	
	Thereafter	7-18 mg/dl		2.5-6.4 mmol/L	
Urine volume					
Urine, 24 hr	Newborn	50-300 ml/d		0.05-0.3 L/d	
	Infant	350-550 ml/d		0.35-0.5 L/d	
	Child	500-1000 ml/d		0.5-1 L/d	
	Adolescent	700-1400 ml/d		0.7-1.4 L/d	
	Thereafter: Male	800-1800 ml/d		0.8-1.8 L/d	
	Female	600-1600 ml/d (varies with intake and other factors)		0.6-1.6 L/d	
WBC: see Leukocyte count (WBC count)					

Abbreviations Used in Laboratory Tests

ABBREVIATION	TERM
cap	capillary
CHF	congestive heart failure
conc.	concentration
CSF	cerebrospinal fluid
d	day; diem
EDTA	ethylenediaminetetraacetate
g	gram
H^+	hydrogen ion
Hb	hemoglobin
hr	hour
IU	International unit
L	liter
m	meter
mEq	milliequivalent
min	minute
mm	millimeter
mm Hg	millimeters of mercury
mm H_2O	millimeters of water
mm^3	cubic millimeter
mo	month
mol	mole
mOsm	milliosmole
Na	sodium
Pa	pascal
RBC	red blood cells
s	second
temp	temperature
therap.	therapeutic
U	international unit of enzyme activity
vol	volume
WBC	white blood cells
wk	week
yr	year
>	greater than
≧	greater than or equal to
<	less than
≦	less than or equal to
±	plus/minus
≅	approximately equal to

Prefixes Denoting Decimal Factors

PREFIX	SYMBOL	AMOUNT
deci	d	one tenth (10^{-1})
centi	c	one hundredth (10^{-2})
milli	m	one thousandth (10^{-3})
micro	mc, μ	one millionth (10^{-6})
nano	n	one billionth (10^{-9})
pico	p	one trillionth (10^{-12})
femto	f	one quadrillionth (10^{-15})

Activity Intolerance
Activity Intolerance, Risk for
Airway Clearance, Ineffective
Allergy Response, Latex
Allergy Response, Risk for Latex
Anxiety
Anxiety, Death
Aspiration, Risk for
Attachment, Risk for Impaired Parent/Child
Autonomic Dysreflexia
Autonomic Dysreflexia, Risk for
Behavior, Risk Prone Health
Body Image, Disturbed
Body Temperature, Imbalanced, Risk for
Bowel Incontinence
Breastfeeding, Effective
Breastfeeding, Ineffective
Breastfeeding, Interrupted
Breathing Pattern, Ineffective
Cardiac Output, Decreased
Caregiver Role Strain
Caregiver Role Strain, Risk for
Comfort, Readiness for Enhanced
Communication, Impaired Verbal
Communication, Readiness for Enhanced
Conflict, Decisional
Conflict, Parental Role
Confusion, Acute
Confusion, Chronic
Confusion, Risk for Acute
Constipation
Constipation, Perceived
Constipation, Risk for
Contamination
Contamination, Risk for
Coping, Compromised Family
Coping, Defensive
Coping, Disabled Family
Coping, Ineffective
Coping, Ineffective Community
Coping, Readiness for Enhanced
Coping, Readiness for Enhanced Community
Coping, Readiness for Enhanced Family
Decision Making, Readiness for Enhanced
Denial, Ineffective
Dentition, Impaired
Development, Risk for Delayed
Diarrhea
Dignity, Risk for Compromised Human
Distress, Moral
Disuse Syndrome, Risk for
Diversional Activity, Deficient
Energy Field, Disturbed
Environmental Interpretation Syndrome, Impaired
Failure to Thrive, Adult
Falls, Risk for
Family Processes, Dysfunctional: Alcoholism
Family Processes, Interrupted
Family Processes, Readiness for Enhanced
Fatigue
Fear
Fluid Balance, Readiness for Enhanced
Fluid Volume, Deficient
Fluid Volume Excess

Fluid Volume, Risk for Deficient
Fluid Volume, Risk for Imbalanced
Gas Exchange, Impaired
Glucose, Risk for Unstable Blood
Grieving
Grieving, Complicated
Grieving, Risk for Complicated
Growth and Development, Delayed
Growth, Risk for Disproportionate
Health Maintenance, Ineffective
Health-Seeking Behaviors (specify)
Home Maintenance, Impaired
Hope, Readiness for Enhanced
Hopelessness
Hyperthermia
Hypothermia
Identity, Disturbed Personal
Immunization Status, Readiness for Enhanced
Incontinence, Functional Urinary
Incontinence, Overflow Urinary
Incontinence, Reflex Urinary
Incontinence, Stress Urinary
Incontinence, Total Urinary
Incontinence, Urge Urinary
Incontinence, Risk for Urge Urinary
Infant Behavior, Disorganized
Infant Behavior, Readiness for Enhanced Organized
Infant Behavior, Risk for Disorganized
Infant Feeding Pattern, Ineffective
Infection, Risk for
Injury, Risk for
Injury, Risk for Perioperative Positioning
Insomnia
Intracranial Adaptive Capacity, Decreased
Knowledge, Deficient (specify)
Knowledge, Readiness for Enhanced
Lifestyle, Sedentary
Liver Function, Risk for Impaired
Loneliness, Risk for
Memory, Impaired
Mobility, Impaired Bed
Mobility, Impaired Physical
Mobility, Impaired Wheelchair
Nausea
Neglect, Unilateral
Noncompliance
Nutrition, Imbalanced: Less Than Body Requirements
Nutrition, Imbalanced: More Than Body Requirements
Nutrition, Readiness for Enhanced
Nutrition, Risk for Imbalanced: More Than Body Requirements
Oral Mucous Membrane, Impaired
Pain, Acute
Pain, Chronic
Parenting, Impaired
Parenting, Readiness for Enhanced
Parenting, Risk for Impaired
Peripheral Neurovascular Dysfunction, Risk for
Poisoning, Risk for
Post-trauma Syndrome
Post-trauma Syndrome, Risk for
Power, Readiness for Enhanced

Powerlessness
Powerlessness, Risk for
Protection, Ineffective
Rape-Trauma Syndrome
Rape-Trauma Syndrome, Compound Reaction
Rape-Trauma Syndrome, Silent Reaction
Religiosity, Impaired
Religiosity, Readiness for Enhanced
Religiosity, Risk for Impaired
Relocation Stress Syndrome
Relocation Stress Syndrome, Risk for
Role Performance, Ineffective
Self-Care Deficit, Bathing/Hygiene
Self-Care Deficit, Dressing/Grooming
Self-Care Deficit, Feeding
Self-Care Deficit, Toileting
Self-Care, Readiness for Enhanced
Self-Concept, Readiness for Enhanced
Self-Esteem, Chronic Low
Self-Esteem, Situational Low
Self-Esteem, Risk for Situational Low
Self-Mutilation
Self-Mutilation, Risk for
Sensory Perception, Disturbed
Sexual Dysfunction
Sexuality Patterns, Ineffective
Skin Integrity, Impaired
Skin Integrity, Risk for Impaired
Sleep, Readiness for Enhanced
Sleep Deprivation
Social Interaction, Impaired
Social Isolation
Sorrow, Chronic
Spiritual Distress
Spiritual Distress, Risk for
Spiritual Well-Being, Readiness for Enhanced
Stress Overload
Sudden Infant Death Syndrome, Risk for
Suffocation, Risk for
Suicide, Risk for
Surgical Recovery, Delayed
Swallowing, Impaired
Therapeutic Regimen Management, Effective
Therapeutic Regimen Management, Ineffective
Therapeutic Regimen Management, Ineffective Community
Therapeutic Regimen Management, Ineffective Family
Therapeutic Regimen Management, Readiness for Enhanced
Thermoregulation, Ineffective
Thought Processes, Disturbed
Tissue Integrity, Impaired
Tissue Perfusion, Ineffective
Transfer Ability, Impaired
Trauma, Risk for
Urinary Elimination, Impaired
Urinary Elimination, Readiness for Enhanced
Urinary Retention
Ventilation, Impaired Spontaneous
Ventilatory Weaning Response, Dysfunction
Violence, Risk for Other-Directed
Violence, Risk for Self-Directed
Walking, Impaired
Wandering

North American Nursing Diagnosis Association–International: *Nursing diagnoses: definitions and classification 2007-2008,* Philadelphia, 2007, The Association.

		0	1	2	3	4	5
	0-5 coding	0	1	2	3	4	5
	0-10 coding	0	2	4	6	8	10
English		No Hurt	Hurts Little Bit	Hurts Little More	Hurts Even More	Hurts Whole Lot	Hurts Worst
Spanish		No duele	Duele un poco	Duele un poco más	Duele mucho	Duele mucho más	Duele el máximo
French		Pas mal	Un petit peu mal	Un peri plus mal	Encore plus mal	Très mal	Très mal
Italian		Non fa male	Fa male un poco	Fa male un po di piu	Fa male ancora di piu	Fa molto male	Fa maggior-mente male
Portuguese		Não doi	Doi um pouco	Doi um pouco mais	Doi muito	Doi muito mais	Doi o máximo
Bosnian		Ne boli	Boli samo malo	Boli malo više	Boli još više	Boli puno	Boli najviše
Vietnamese		Không dau	Hòi dau	Dau hòn chút	Dau nhiêu hòn	Dau thât nhiêu	Dau qúa dô
Chinese†		無痛	微痛	較痛	更痛	很痛	劇痛
Greek		Δεν Πονάϊ	Πονάϊ Λιγο	Πονάϊ Λιγο Πιο Πολν	Πονάϊ Πολν	Πονάϊ Πιο Πολν	Πονάϊ Παρα Πολν
Romanian		No doare	Doare puţin	Doare un pic mai mult	Doare şi mai mult	Doare foarte tare	Doare cel mai mult

Brief Word Instructions (Above)

Point to each face using the words to describe the pain intensity. Ask person to choose face that best describes own pain and record the appropriate number. Rating scale can be used with people 3 years and older.

NOTE: In a study of 148 children ages 4 to 5 years, there were no differences in pain scores when children used the original or brief word instructions. (In Wong D, Baker C: *Reference manual for the Wong-Baker FACES Pain Rating Scale,* Duarte, Calif, 1998, City of Hope Mayday Pain Resource Center; retrieved from http://evolve.elsevier.com/Wong/essentials).

Original Instructions

English. Explain to the person that each face is for a person who feels happy because he has no pain (hurt) or sad because he has some or a lot of pain. **Face 0** is very happy because he doesn't hurt at all. **Face 1** hurts just a little bit. **Face 2** hurts a little more. **Face 3** hurts even more. **Face 4** hurts a whole lot. **Face 5** hurts as much as you can imagine, although you don't have to be crying to feel this bad. Ask the person to choose the face that best describes how he or she is feeling.

Rating scale is recommended for persons ages 3 years and older.

Spanish. Expliquele a la persona que cada cara representa una persona que se siente feliz porque no tiene dolor o triste

---

*Wong-Baker FACES Pain Rating Scale:** Available at no charge from The Purdue Frederick Company, 100 Connecticut Ave., Norwalk, CT 06850-3590; http://www.partnersagainstpain.com. Spanish and Portuguese translations by Ellen Johnsen; French translation from Wong DL: *Soins infirmiers pediatrie,* Quebec, 2002, Editions Etudes Vivantes, Groupe Educalivres, Inc.; Italian translation by Madeline Mitchko; Bosnian translation by Barbara Bogomolov; Vietnamese translation by Yen B. Isle; Chinese translation by Hung-Shen Lin; Greek translation by Nicholas Mamalis; Romanian translation by Bogdan R. Dinu.

porque siente un poco o mucho dolor. **Cara 0** se siente muy feliz porque no tiene dolor. **Cara 1** tiene un poco de dolor. **Cara 2** tiene un poquito más de dolor. **Cara 3** tiene más dolor. **Cara 4** tiene mucho dolor. **Cara 5** tiene el dolor más fuerte que usted pueda imaginar, aunque usted no tiene que estar llorando para sentirse asi de mal. Pidale a la persona que escoja la cara que mejor describe su proprio dolor.

Esta escala se puede usar con personas de tres años de edad o más.

French. Expliquez à la personne que chaque visage représent une personne qui est heureux parce qu'elle n'a pas point du mal ou triste parce qu'elle a un peu ou beaucoup du mal. **Visage 0** est trés heureux parce qu'elle n'a pas point du mal. **Visage 1** a un petit peu de mal. **Visage 2** a plus du mal. **Visage 3** a encore plus du mal. **Visage 4** a beaucoup du mal. **Visage 5** a autant mal que vous pouvez imaginer, bien que ces mauvais sentiments ne finissent pas nécessairement a vous faire pleurer. Demandez à la personne de choisir le visage qui convient le mieux avec ses sentiments.

Ces evaluations sont recommendés pour des personnes de trois ans et davantage.

Italian. Spiegare a la persona che ogni facien è per una persona che si sente felice perchè non tiene dolore oppure triste perchè ha poco o molto dolore. **Faccia O** è molto felice perchè non tiene dolore. **Faccia 1** tiene poco dolore. **Faccia 2** tiene un po più di dolore. **Faccia 3** tiene più dolore. **Faccia 4** tiene molto dolore. **Faccia 5** tiene molto dolore che non puoi immaginare però non devi piangere per tenere dolore. Domandi ala persona di scegliere quale faccia meglio descrive come si sente.

Grado scale è raccomandata a la persona di tre anni in sù.

Portuguese. Explique a pessoa que cada face representa uma pessoa que está feliz porque não têm dor, ou triste por ter um pouco ou muita dor. **Face 0** está muito feliz porque não têm nenhuma dor. **Face 1** têm apenas um pouco de dor. **Face 2** têm um pouco mais de dor. **Face 3** têm ainda mais dor. **Face 4** têm muita dor. **Face 5** têm uma dor máxima, apesar de que nem sempre provoca o choro. Peça a pessoa que escolhe a face que melhor descreve como ele se sente.

Esta escala é aplicável a pessoas de tres anos de idade ou mais.

Romanian. Explicati copilului că fiecare desen (figură) corespunde unei persoane care este veselă, pentru ca nu are nici o durere, sau unei persoane care este tristă, pentru că are dureri. **Figura 0** este foarte fericită pentru că nu are nici o durere. **Figura 1** arată că doare doar un pic. **Figura 2** arată că doare ceva mai mult. **Figura 3** arată că doare şi mai mult. **Figura 4** arată că doare foarte tare. **Figura 5** arată că doare atât de tare cât se poate imagina, chiar dacă nu este însotita neapărat de lacrimi. Cereti copilului (persoanei) să indice figura care exprimă cel mai bine cum se simte el.

Scala de evaluare a durerii este recomandată pentru copiii în vârstùa de trei ani şi peste.

Bosnian. Objasnite osobi da je svako lice namjenjeno za osobu koja se osjeća sretnom jer ne osjeća bol ili tužnom jer osjeća malo ili puno boli. **Lice 0** je sretno jer ne osjeća nikakvu bol. **Lice 1** osjeća samo malu bol. **Lice 2** osjeća malo više boli. **Lice 3** osjeća još veću bol. **Lice 4** osjeća puno boli. **Lice 5** osjeća onoliku bol koju je moguće zamisliti, što ne znači da osoba koja osjeća tu bol mora plakati. Upitajte osobu da izabere lice koje najbolje opisuju kako se osjeća. Skala procijene bola se preporučuje za osobe starosti 3 godine ili više.

Upirati prstom na svako lice objašnjavajući riječima intensitet boli. Pitajte dijete da izabere lice koje najbolje opisuje njihovu bol i zabiljezue odgovarajući broj.

German. Erläutern Sie dem Kind, daβ jedes Gesicht zu einer Person gehört, die froh darüber ist, keine Schmerzen zu haben, oder die sehr traurig ist, weil sie mäβige bis starke Schmerzen hat. **Gesicht 0** ist sehr froh, weil es keine Schmerzen hat. **Gesicht 1** sagt, es tut ein biβchen weh. **Gesicht 2** hat ein biβchen mehr Schmerzen. **Gesicht 3** sagt, es tut noch mehr weh, und **Gesicht 4,** es tut ziemlich weh. **Gesicht 5** leidet unter so starken Schmerzen, wie Du Dir nur vorstellen kannst, auch wenn dabei nicht unbedingt Tränen flieβen müssen. Bitten Sie das Kind, das Gesicht auszuwählen, das seinem Empfinden am besten entspricht.

Empfohlen für Kinder ab drei Jahren.

Vietnamese

Xin cắt nghĩa cho mỗi người, từng khuôn mặt của một người căm thấy vui vẻ tại vì không có sự đau đớn hoặc, buồn vì có chút ít hay rất nhiều sự đau đớn.

Cái **mặt** với **số 0** thì rất là vui tại vì mặt ấy không có sự đau đớn. **Mặt số 1** chỉ đau một chút thôi. **Mặt số 2** hơi đau hơn một chút nữa. **Mặt số 3** đau hơn chút nữa. **Mặt số 4** đau thật nhiều. **Mặt số 5** đau không thể tưởng tượng, mặc dù người ta không cần phải khóc mới cảm thấy được sự buồn khổ như thế.

Bạn hỏi từng người tự chọn khuôn mặt nào diễn tả được sự đau đớn của chính mình.

Japanese

3歳以上の患者に望ましい。それぞれの顔は、患者の痛み (pain, hurt) がないのでご機嫌な感じ、または、ある程度の痛み・沢山の痛みがあるので悲しい感じを表現していることを説明して下さい。0＝痛みがまったくないから、とても幸せな顔をしている、1＝ほんの少し痛い、2＝もう少し痛い、3＝もっと痛い、4＝とっても痛い、5＝痛くて涙を流す必要はないけれども、これ以上の痛みは考えられないほど痛い。今、どのように感じているか最もよく表わしている顔を選ぶよう、患者に求めて下さい。

Chinese

解釋給人聽用每張臉譜來代表著一個人的感覺是因爲沒有疼痛〔傷痛〕而感快樂或是因爲些許疼痛或者是許多疼痛而感傷心。第零張臉是很快樂的因爲他一點也不覺得疼痛。第一張臉只痛一丁點兒。第二張臉又痛多了一些。第三張臉痛得更多了。第四張臉是非常痛了。第五張臉是爲人們所能想像到的劇痛既使感到這樣難過，卻不一定哭出來。請這人選擇出最能代表他現在感覺的一張臉譜。此量表適用於三歲以上的人。

ENGLISH PHRASE	SPANISH PHRASE	ENGLISH PHRASE	SPANISH PHRASE
PHYSICAL EXAMINATION		Up-to-date	Al día
Open your mouth	Abre la boca	Contagious	Contagioso
Breathe deeply	Respira profundo	Stool (various terms)	Excremento, heces, popo
Turn over	Voltéate	Has (she/he) had any chronic	¿Él (ella) ha tenido alguna
Hoarse	Ronco	illnesses?	enfermedad crónica?
Rash or skin lesion produced by	Rozadura o una lesión en la piel pro-	How many times did he/she	¿Cuántas veces vomitó hoy?
insect bite	ducida por una picadura de insecto	vomit today?	
Rash	Roncha, salpullido, rozadura	Wheezing or adventitious sounds	Pillido o ruidos en los pulmones
Ringworm	Tiña	(in lungs)	
To tighten (grip)	Apretar	Nasal secretions	Secreción nasal
To loosen	Relajar, aflojar	Stuffy nose	Bloqueo nasal
Bruise	Moretón	Breathing problems	Dificultad para respirar
Skin "spot" (like a blanching)	Mancha	Thick discharge	Flujo grueso
Snore, stertor	Roncar	Wound	Herida
Snoring sound	Ronquido	Blood pressure	Presión arterial
Swollen	Hinchado	Temperature	Temperatura
		Fever	Calentura, fiebre
SYMPTOMS		Pulse	Pulso
I would like to know if you have	Quisiera saber si tienes (o has tenido):	Heartbeat	Latido del corazón
(or have had):		Airway	Vía respiratoria
Cough	Tos	Vital signs	Signos vitals
Runny nose	Moquera		
Fever	Fiebre o calentura	**SPECIFIC CONDITIONS**	
Vomiting or nausea	Vómito o náusea	Flu	Gripa
Diarrhea	Diarrea	Croup	Crup
Constipation	Estreñimiento	Bronchitis	Bronquitis
Pain	Dolor	Burn	Quemadura
Allergic reaction	Reacción alérgica	Rash or dermatitis	Erupción o rozadura
Seizure	Convulsión	Pneumonia	Neumonía
Sore throat	Dolor de garganta	Pertussis	Tos ferina
Diaper dermatitis	Dermatitis por el pañal	Measles	Sarampión
Dizzy	Mareado(a)	Mumps	Paperas
		Chickenpox	Varicela
HISTORY		Rubella	Rubéola
Are you sleeping well?	¿Estás durmiendo bien?	Polio	Polio
Have you had any trauma?	¿Has tenido algún trastorno o algún	Tetanus	Tétano
	trauma?	Vomiting	Vómito
Have you had any hemorrhage or	¿Has tenido una hemorragia o pérdida	Diarrhea	Diarrea
loss of blood?	de sangre?	Asthma	Asma
Problems during pregnancy or	¿Problemas en el embarazo o parto?	Mucous	Moco
delivery?		Seizures	Convulsións
Born at term or premature?	¿Nació a tiempo o fue prematuro?	Drainage	Drenaje
Did he get better after the treat-	¿Mejoró después del tratamiento o	Immunization	Vacuna
ment or the medicine given?	después de haberle dado la medicina?	Poison ivy	Hiedra venenosa
How many times did (he/she)	¿Cuántas veces orinó hoy?	Bacterial infection	Infección bacterial
urinate today?		Viral infection	Infección viral
How many wet diapers has	¿Cuántos pañales ha mojado?	Diaper dermatitis	Dermatitis por causa del pañal
(he/she) had?		Rash or skin lesion produced by	Rozadura o lesión de la piel hecha por
How many dirty diapers?	¿Cuántos pañales sucios?	insect bite	una picadura de insecto
Where does it hurt?	¿Dónde te duele?	Ulcer (as in mouth ulcers or	Úlceras o llagas en la boca
When did it start?	¿Cuándo empezó?	chancre sores)	
Does (he/she) have any allergies	¿Él (ella) tiene alergia a alguna me-	Gastritis	Gastritis, agruras
to medicine or food?	dicina o comida?	Constipation	Estreñimiento

ENGLISH PHRASE	SPANISH PHRASE
SPECIFIC CONDITIONS—cont'd	
Home remedies	Tratamientos caseros
Fracture	Fractura
Intensive care	Cuidado intensivo
Immunizations	Vacunas
Animal bite	Mordida de animal
Menstrual period	Menstruación, período
Birth control	Anticonceptivo
EQUIPMENT	
Tube; can also mean nasogastric tube or urinary catheter, or any tube that has to be inserted into body (MicKey button, gastrostomy)	Sonda, catéter urinario, tubo que se introduce en el cuerpo
Gown	Bata
Suction	Succión
Sheet	Sábana
Diaper	Pañal
Bulb syringe	Saca mocos
Clothes, clothing	Ropa
Splint or cast	Férula o yeso
Dressing, bandage	Bendaje, gaza
Infusion pump	Máquina para infusion
Tape	Cinta
Teaspoon	Cucharadita
Cup (as in small medicine cup or drinking cup)	Taza
Syringe	Jeringa
Pill	Pastilla, píldora
Needle	Aguja
Antibiotic	Antibiótico
Cotton swab	Algodón
Pacifier	Chupón
Bottle, as in baby bottle or medicine bottle	Biberón
Juice	Jugo
Milk	Leche
BODY PARTS	
Bone	Hueso
Blood	Sangre
Tongue	Lengua
Head	Cabeza
Arm	Brazo
Finger	Dedo
Leg	Pierna
Neck	Cuello
Elbow	Codo
Foot	Pie
Ear	Oreja
Nose	Nariz
Mouth	Boca
Bladder	Vejiga
Back	Espalda
Chest	Pecho
Spleen	Bazo
Gallbladder	Vesícula
PAIN MANAGEMENT	
Do you have any pain in the . . .?	¿Tienes dolor . . .?
Headache	De cabeza
Stomachache	De estómago
Backache	De espalda

ENGLISH PHRASE	SPANISH PHRASE
Chest pain	En el pecho
In the arm	En el brazo
In the legs	En las piernas
In the mouth	En la boca
In the eyes	En los ojos
In the bladder	En la vejiga
How many hours, days, months, years have you had pain in the . . .?	¿Por cuántos (cuántas) horas, días, meses, años has tenido dolor en . . .?
Please show me where it hurts	Muéstreme dónde te duele, por favor.
What medicine are you taking for pain?	¿Qué medicina estás tomando para el dolor?
What medicine have you taken for pain?	¿Qué medicina has tomado para el dolor?
Calm down	Cálmate
This won't hurt	Esto no te va a doler
PROCEDURES	
Injection	Inyección
Lumbar puncture	Punción lumbar
Oral hydration solution (such as Pedialyte)	Suero oral o por la boca
Intravenous fluids	Suero intravenoso o por la vena
Start an intravenous line	Vamos a ponerle suero intravenoso o por la vena
Normal saline drops	Gotas de solución salina
Humidity	Humedad
Vaporizer	Vaporizador de aire
Breathing treatment	Tratamiento para la respiración
Humidity in the bathroom with a hot shower running	El vapor en el baño de la regadera o ducha de agua caliente
Stool sample	Muestra de heces (popo) excremento
We need to take some blood to see what exactly (illness) (he, she) has	Tenemos que tomar una muestra de sangre para saber con seguridad lo que el o ella tiene o padece
The results of your blood test show . . .	Los resultados de la sangre muestran . . .
The most important thing is to decrease the fever with Tylenol or Motrin	Lo más importante es reducir la fiebre con Tylenol o Motrin
We will have to catheterize (him/her)	Tendremos que ponerle una sonda en la vejiga
Topical treatment	Tratamiento tópico
To suture	Suturar
A suture	Sutura
To swab (as in "swab the mouth" or "to place a cream on . . .")	Untar
He/she should take lots of clear liquids	Debe tomar bastantes líquidos claros
To nurse, breastfeed	Amamantar
To burp	Eructar
X ray	Radiografía
Computed tomography scan	Tomografía
Nasal drops	Gotas nasales
Put ice on it	Póngale hielo
MISCELLANEOUS PHRASES	
He/she will need to be hospitalized for treatment (observation)	Tendrá que ser hospitalizado(a) para darle tratamiento (ser observado[a])
We need a urine specimen in this cup	Necesitamos su muestra de orina en esta taza
Take him/her to the primary doctor tomorrow	Llévelo mañana a su doctor principal o de cabecera
He/she's very sick	Está muy enfermo(a)

Dietary Reference Intakes

APPENDIX

Recommended Dietary Allowances (RDA) and Adequate Intake (AI)ᵃ of Major Nutrients

CATEGORY	AGE (yr) OR CONDITION	WEIGHT kg	WEIGHT lb	HEIGHT cm	HEIGHT in	PROTEIN RDA (g/kg)	FAT-SOLUBLE VITAMINS VITAMIN A RDA (mcg/d)ᵇ	VITAMIN D AI (mcg/d)ᶜ	VITAMIN E RDA (mg/d)ᵈ	VITAMIN K AI (mcg/d)
Infants	0.0-0.5	6	13	62	24		400	5	4	2
	0.5-1.0	9	20	71	28		500	5	5	2.5
Children	1-3	12	27	86	34	1.10	300	5	6	30
	4-8	20	44	115	45	0.95	400	5	7	55
Males	9-13	36	79	144	57	0.95	600	5	11	60
	14-18	61	134	174	68	0.85	900	5	15	75
	19-30	70	154	177	70	0.80	900	5	15	120
Females	9-13	37	81	144	57	0.95	600	5	11	60
	14-18	54	119	163	64	0.85	700	5	15	75
	19-30	57	126	163	64	0.80	700	5	15	90
Pregnant	≤18					+25 g/d	750	5	15	75
Lactating	≤18					+25 g/d	1200	5	19	75

Modified from the *Dietary Reference Intake* series, National Academy of Sciences, National Academies Press, 1997, 1998, 2000, 2001; and American Academy of Pediatrics: *Pediatric nutrition handbook* ed 5, Washington, DC, 2004, National Academies Press.

ᵃNOTE: For all nutrients, values for infants are AI.

ᵇRetinol equivalent (RAE). 1 RAE = 1 mcg retinol.

ᶜCholecalciferol. 1 mcg cholecalciferol = 40 IU vitamin D. Assumes an absence of adequate exposure to sunlight.

ᵈExpressed as α-tocopherol.

ᵉExpressed as niacin equivalents (NE); except for infants <6 months of age, expressed as preformed niacin. 1 mg niacin = 60 mg tryptophan.

ᶠExpressed as dietary folate equivalents (DFE); 1 DFE = 1 mcg food folate = 0.6 mcg folic acid from fortified food or as a supplement consumed with food = 5 mcg of a supplement taken on an empty stomach.

ᵍIn view of evidence linking folate intake with neural tube defects in the fetus, it is recommended that all women capable of becoming pregnant consume 400 mcg from supplements or fortified foods in addition to intake of food folate from the diet.

ʰIt is assumed all women will continue consuming 400 mcg from supplements or fortified food until their pregnancy is confirmed and they enter prenatal care, which ordinarily occurs after the end of the preconceptional period—the critical time for formation of the neural tube.

WATER-SOLUBLE VITAMINS							MINERALS						
VITAMIN C RDA (mg/d)	THIAMIN RDA (mg/d)	RIBOFLA-VIN RDA (mg/d)	NIACIN RDA (mg/d)[e]	VITAMIN B_6 RDA (mg/d)	FOLATE RDA (mcg/d)[f]	VITAMIN B_{12} RDA (mcg/d)	CALCIUM AI (mg/d)	PHOS-PHORUS RDA (mg/d)	MAGNE-SIUM RDA (mg/d)	IRON RDA (mg/d)	ZINC RDA (mg/d)	IODINE RDA (mg/d)	SELE-NIUM RDA (mg/d)
40	0.2	0.3	2	0.1	65	0.4	210	100	30	0.27	2	110	15
50	0.3	0.4	4	0.3	80	0.5	270	275	75	11	3	130	20
15	0.5	0.5	6	0.5	150	0.9	500	460	80	7	3	90	20
25	0.6	0.6	8	0.6	200	1.2	800	500	130	10	5	90	30
45	0.9	0.9	12	1	300	1.8	1300	1250	240	8	8	120	40
75	1.2	1.3	16	1.3	400	2.4	1300	1250	410	11	11	150	55
90	1.2	1.3	16	1.3	400	2.4	1000	700	400	8	11	150	55
45	0.9	0.9	12	1	300	1.8	1300	1250	240	8	8	120	40
65	1	1	14	1.2	400	2.4	1300	1250	360	15	9	150	55
75	1.1	1.1	14	1.3	400[g]	2.4	1000	700	310	18	8	150	55
80	1.4	1.4	18	1.9	600[h]	2.6	1300	1250	400	27	13	220	60
115	1.4	1.6	17	2	500	2.8	1300	1250	360	10	14	290	70

Estimated Safe and Adequate Daily Dietary Intakes of Selected Vitamins and Minerals*

| CATEGORY | AGE (yr) | VITAMINS | | TRACE ELEMENTS† | | | | |
		BIOTIN (mcg)	PANTOTHENIC ACID (mg)	COPPER (mg)	MANGANESE (mg)	FLUORIDE (mg)	CHROMIUM (mcg)	MOLYBDENUM (mcg)
Infants‡	0-0.5	10	2	0.4-0.6	0.3-0.6	0.1-0.5	10-40	15-30
	0.5-1	15	3	0.6-0.7	0.6-1.0	0.2-1.0	20-60	20-40
Children and adolescents	1-3	20	3	0.7-1.0	1.0-1.5	0.5-1.5	20-80	25-50
	4-6	25	3-4	1.0-1.5	1.5-2.0	1.0-2.5	30-120	30-75
	7-10	30	4-5	1.0-2.0	2.0-3.0	1.5-2.5	50-200	50-150
	11+	30-100	4-7	1.5-2.5	2.0-5.0	1.5-2.5	50-200	75-250
Adults		30-100	4-7	1.5-3.0	2.0-5.0	1.5-4.0	50-200	75-250

From Food and Nutrition Board, National Research Council: *Recommended dietary allowances,* ed 10, Washington, DC, 1989, National Academy of Sciences.
*Because there is less information on which to base allowances, these figures are not given in the main table of recommended dietary allowances and are provided here in the form of ranges of recommended intakes.
†Since the toxic levels for many trace elements may be only several times usual intakes, the upper levels for the trace elements given in this table should not be habitually exceeded.
‡For all nutrients, values for infants are adequate intake (AI).

Estimated Sodium, Chloride, and Potassium Minimum Requirements of Healthy Persons*

AGE	WEIGHT (kg)*	SODIUM (mg)*†	CHLORIDE (mg)*†	POTASSIUM (mg)‡
0-5 mo	4.5	120	180	500
6-11 mo	8.9	200	300	700
1 yr	11.0	225	350	1000
2-5 yr	16.0	300	500	1400
6-9 yr	25.0	400	600	1600
10-18 yr	50.0	500	750	2000
>18 yr§	70.0	500	750	2000

From Food and Nutrition Board, National Research Council: *Recommended dietary allowances,* ed 10, Washington, DC, 1989, National Academy of Sciences.
*No allowance has been included for large, prolonged losses from the skin through sweat.
†There is no evidence that higher intakes confer any health benefit.
‡Desirable intakes of potassium may considerably exceed these values (≈3500 mg for adults).
§No allowance included for growth. Values for those younger than 18 years of age assume a growth rate at the 50th percentile reported by the National Center for Health Statistics and averaged for males and females.

Median Heights and Weights and Estimated Energy Requirements (EERs)*

| CATEGORY | AGE (yr) OR CONDITION | WEIGHT | | HEIGHT | | ENERGY EER (kcal/day) (male/female) |
		kg	lb	cm	in	
Infants	0-0.5	6	13	60	24	570/520
	0.5-1	9	20	71	28	743/676
Children	1-3	12	27	86	34	1046/992
	4-8	20	44	115	45	1742/1642
Males	9-13	36	79	144	57	2279
	14-18	61	134	174	68	3152
	19-30	70	154	177	70	3067
Females	9-13	37	81	144	57	2071
	14-18	54	119	163	64	2368
	19-30	57	126	163	64	2403
Pregnant	1st trimester					2368
	2nd trimester					2708
	3rd trimester					2820
Lactating	1st 6 mo					2698
	2nd 6 mo					2768

Modified from the *Dietary reference intake series,* National Academy of Science, National Academies Press, 1997, 1998, 2000, 2001; and American Academy of Pediatrics: *Pediatric nutrition handbook,* ed 5, Washington, DC, 2004, National Academies Press.
The estimated energy requirement (EER) represents an average dietary energy intake that will maintain energy balance in a healthy individual based on gender, age, weight, and height. The values given are based on an "active" person at the reference height and weight and the midpoint age for each age-group until 19.

Index

A

Abbreviations, for laboratory tests, 1200
Abdominal circumference, of newborn, 205
Abdominal distention, in newborn, 205
Abdominal examination, 147-149
  in newborn, 205, 209, 210, 219t
Abdominal hernias, 849, 850t
Abdominal migraine, 829
Abdominal pain
  functional, 829
  in appendicitis, 829, 830
  in intussusception, 852
  paroxysmal, in infant, 395-396, 397, 397f
  recurrent (functional), 562-563
    management of, 192-193
Abdominal thrusts, 809-810, 810f
Abducens nerve, assessment of, 155t
Abduction, of newborns, prevention of, 221-222
ABO incompatibility, 281, 282, 282t, 944t, 945
Absence seizures, 1007b. See also Seizures.
Absolute neutrophil count (ANC), 913t
  calculation of, 935
Abstinence, sexual, 544t
Abstract thinking, 519
Abuse
  brain injury in, 987-988
  caregiver-child interaction and, 485
  child characteristics and, 481-482
  emotional, 480, 484b, 485, 486
  environment and, 482
  nursing care management in, 486-490
  nursing care plan for, 489
  parental characteristics and, 481
  physical, 480-482, 484b, 485, 486
  prevention of, 488
  recognition of, 483, 483b, 484b
  repeated, protection from, 486-487
  sexual, 482-483, 483b, 484b, 485, 486, 488, 490
  vs. folk remedies, 63, 64b
Acanthosis nigricans, 23, 24
Access to care, 2
Accessory nerve, assessment of, 155t
Accidents. See Safety concerns; Traumatic injuries.
Accommodation, pupillary, 135
Accomplishment, stage of, in school-age child, 494-495
Acculturation, 57
Accutane (isotretinoin), for acne, 1090
ACE inhibitors, for congestive heart failure, 878, 882
Acetaminophen (Tylenol)
  for circumcision pain, 227b
  for fever, 703
  for pain, 175, 176t, 180t
  poisoning with, 471b
Acetone breath, in diabetes mellitus, 1044
Achilles reflex, 154f
Achondroplastic dwarfism, 540
Acid mantle, of newborn skin, 225, 259
Acidosis, metabolic
  in acute renal failure, 966
  in chronic renal failure, 968, 969
  in diabetes mellitus, 1049

Acids, poisoning with, 471b
Acne, 1089-1091, 1090f
Acoustic feedback, 624
Acoustic nerve, assessment of, 155t
Acquaintance rape, 549-550, 549b
Acquired immunodeficiency syndrome. See HIV/AIDS.
Acrocyanosis, 217t
Acrodynia, in mercury poisoning, 475
Acromegaly, 1029
ACTH, 1025t
  hypersecretion of, 1038-1039
Actiq. See Fentanyl.
Activated charcoal, in poisoning treatment, 473
Activities of daily living, in chronic illness/disability, 590
Activity and exercise
  asthma and, 789
  in adolescent, 521, 522f, 528, 528f
  in anemia, 915
  in cognitive impairment, 616-617, 616f, 617f
  in congestive heart failure, 878
  in diabetes mellitus, 1047, 1056-1057
  in epilepsy, 1015-1016
  in hemophilia, 926, 927
  in juvenile idiopathic arthritis, 1140, 1141-1142
  in newborn, 214-215, 214t
  in preschooler, 448
  in school-age child, 505-506, 505f
  in toddler, 424
  obesity and, 552, 555-556
Acupressure, 6363
Acupuncture, 6363
Acute chest syndrome, in sickle cell anemia, 918, 922
Acute glomerulonephritis, 961-962
Acute illness, 10. See also Illness.
Acute leukemia, 930-937. See also Leukemia.
Acute lung injury, 781-782
Acute poststreptococcal glomerulonephritis, 961
Acute renal failure, 965-967
Acute respiratory distress syndrome (ARDS), 781-782, 903
Adams test, 1131
Adaptability, family, 31
Adaptive coping. See Coping mechanisms.
Addiction, 188, 189
Addison disease, 1038-1039, 1039b
Adenohypophysis, structure and function of, 1025t-1026t
Adenoidectomy, 764
Adenoids, 763, 763f
Adenosine
  for CPR, 807-809, 808t
  for supraventricular tachycardia, 897
Adenotonsillectomy, 764
  for sleep-disordered breathing, 803
Adequate intake, 113
Adherence, therapeutic, 698-700
Admission
  emergency, 680-681, 680b
  guidelines for, 668b
  preparation for, 665-668
  to intensive care unit, 681-683, 681b
Admission assessment, 665, 666b-667b

Adolescent
  acne in, 1089-1091, 1090f
  as emancipated minor, 689
  behavioral disorders in, 559-564
  biologic development of, 514-518, 515b, 516f, 517f, 525t
  body art and, 529
  body image of, self-concept and, 523-524
  chronic illness/disability in, 592t
  cognitive development of, 519, 525t
  communication with, 104-105
    about sexuality, 110-111, 110b
  confidentiality and, 689
  contraception for, 544-547
  cultural awareness of, 514
  definition of, 514, 525t
  dental health of, 528
  development of, 73t, 514-524, 525t. See also Development.
    stages of, 514, 525t
  diabetes mellitus in, 1057
  eating disorders in, 551-559
  family rules for, 533
  growth in, 515, 525t
  gynecologic examination in, 542
  health problems of, 536-571
  health promotion for, 524, 526-533
  hearing in, 529
  homosexual, suicide by, 569
  hospitalized, 673
  immunization of, 365, 526
  informed consent of, 689
  injury prevention in, 531-532, 531b
  interviewing, 526
  mental health issues in, 559-564
  moral development of, 520
  nutrition in, 526-528
  obesity in, 551-556
  personal care of, 528
  posture of, 529
  pregnant, 543-544
  privacy for, 544
  psychosocial development of, 518-519, 525t
  reproductive tract disorders in
    female, 540-542
    male, 542-543
  sex chromosome disorders in, 540-541, 541t
  sexual assault against, 549-550, 549b
  sexual development of, 515, 515b, 516f, 517f, 525t. See also Puberty.
    responses to, 524
  sexuality of, 522-523, 522f
    education and guidance for, 530-531
  sexually transmitted diseases in, 547
  sleep and activity in, 528, 528f
  social development of, 520-521, 525t
  spiritual development of, 520
  sports injuries in, 532, 538-540
  stress reduction for, 529, 530b, 530f
  substance abuse by, 564-568
  suicide by, 564
  tanning and, 529
  vaginitis in, 542
  vision in, 528
  vital signs in, 518
Adolescent Pediatric Pain Tool, 164-165, 165f
Adoption, 43-45

Page numbers followed by *f* indicate figures; *t*, tables; *b*, boxes.

Adrenal crisis, 1037
Adrenal disorders, 1037-1042
Adrenal hormones, 1026t, 1037
Adrenal hyperplasia, congenital, 1040-1042
Adrenal tumors, 1042
Adrenaline. *See* Epinephrine.
Adrenarche, 515
Adrenocortical insufficiency
    acute, 1037-1038, 1038b
    chronic, 1037-1039, 1038b, 1039b
    in congenital adrenal hyperplasia, 1041
Adrenocorticotropic hormone (ACTH), 1025t
    hypersecretion of, 1038-1039
Advance care planning, in home care, 654
Advanced life support, 805
Adventitious breath sounds, 145
Advil. *See* Ibuprofen (Advil, Motrin).
Aerosol therapy, 740-741
    for asthma, 788
Affect, in cognitive development, 330
Affinal relationships, 30
African Americans. *See also* Race/ethnicity.
    hair care for, 702
    health beliefs and practices of, 67t
    newborn, skin of, 207
    sickle-cell anemia in, 916-923
Agammaglobulinemia
    Swiss-type lymphopenic, 943
    X-linked lymphopenic, 943
Age
    bone, 1028b
    gestational, 202f-205f, 203-205, 204b
    of majority, 689
Agent, disease, 22
Aggression, in preschoolers, 447
Agnosia, 624
Agonal respiration, 145b
AIDS. *See* HIV/AIDS.
Air embolism, transfusion-related, 944t
Air enema, for intussusception, 853
Airway. *See also under* Pulmonary; Respiratory.
    patency of, in newborn, 215, 221
    suctioning of, 741-744, 743f
Airway burns, 782-783, 1093
Airway clearance, 809-810. *See also* Respiratory
        secretions.
Airway management. *See also* Ventilatory support.
    emergency, 809-810
    in anaphylaxis, 905
    in coma, 982
    in respiratory failure, 804-809
Airway obstruction
    by foreign body, 780-781
    emergency management of, 809-810
    in asthma, 785, 785f
Alae nasi, flaring of, 140-141
Albuterol, for asthma, 788-789
Alcohol use/abuse, 566-567
    birth defects due to, 311t
    in pregnancy, 303, 311t
Aldactone (spironolactone), for congestive heart
        failure, 879t
Aldosterone, 1026t
Alertness, 976
Alginate dressings, 1066t
Alkali poisoning, 471b
Allen card test, 137
Allen test, 715
Allergic conjunctivitis, 465b
Allergic reactions
    anaphylaxis in, 904-906
    asthma and, 784, 785b, 787-788
    atopic dermatitis and, 1086-1089
    environmental control in, 787-788
    history of, 109
    immunotherapy for, 789-790

Allergic reactions (*Continued*)
    skin testing in, 786, 788
    to animal dander, 787-788, 787b
    to drugs, 1076
        skin lesions in, 1076, 1085t
        Stevens-Johnson syndrome in, 1085t
    to food, 384-388, 385b
    to insect venom, 1079
    to latex, 1159-1161, 1159b, 1160b
    transfusion-related, 944t, 945t
Allis sign, 1123f, 1124
Allograft, for burns, 1097
Alloimmunization, transfusion-related, 945t
Alopecia, 1085t
    in chemotherapy, 937
Alternate cover test, 136, 136f
Alternate milk products, in infant formulas, 233
Alternative medicine. *See* Complementary and
        alternative therapies.
Amantadine (Symmetrel), for influenza, 765
Ambiguous genitalia, 958t
    in congenital adrenal hyperplasia, 1040-1041
Amblyopia, 135-136, 629t, 633
Ambulatory care, 679-680, 679b
Amelia, 1127
Amenorrhea, 541
    in athletes, 557
    in eating disorders, 557, 558
American Academy of Pediatrics
    breastfeeding and, 229-230
    circumcision and, 225-227
    formula feeding and, 232
    hearing screening and, 223
    HIV screening/prevention and, 223
American College of Obstetricians and Gynecolo-
        gists, on HIV transmission, 232
American Nurses Association Code of Ethics, 14,
        14b
American Sign Language, 626
Amethocaine gel, 184
Amino acid formulas, 232
5-Aminosalicylates, for ulcerative colitis, 834
Amiodarone, in CPR, 808t
Amitriptyline, for pain, 177t
Amniotic band syndrome, 1127
Amniotic fluid aspiration, 221
Amoxicillin, for otitis media, 766-767
Amphetamines, abuse of, 567
Ampules, glass, 720
Amputation, 1121-1122
    for bone cancer, 1137
    phantom limb sensation after, 1122, 1137
Amylase, 324
Anaclitic depression, 659
Anal examination, 151
    in newborn, 210, 220t
Anal patency, 210
Anal reflex, 151
Anal stage, 78
Anal stenosis, 854-855, 854t
Analgesia, 171-194. *See also* Pain management.
    addiction in, 188-189
    balanced, 191-192
    ceiling effect in, 178
    coanalgesics in, 178
    dosage in, 176t-178t, 178
    effectiveness of, 189-191
    epidural, 182t, 183-184
    equianalgesia in, 178, 180t
    first-pass effect in, 178
    for breakthrough pain, 183
    for dying child, 602-603
    for postoperative pain, 191-192
    for procedural pain, 191
    in evidence-based practice, 173-174, 185-187
    indications for, 177t

Analgesia (*Continued*)
    intradermal, 185
    multimodal, 191-192
    nonopioids in, 175, 176t-178t
    opioids in, 175-178, 176t-178t. *See also* Opioids.
    patient-controlled, 178-183, 181t, 183t, 191-192
    peak effect in, 187-188
    placebos in, 178
    preemptive, 191
    routes of administration for, 181t-182t, 183-185
    side effects in, 179t-180t, 188-189
    timing of, 187-188
    transmucosal, 181t, 184
Anaphylaxis, 904-906
Androgens, 515, 1026t
Anemia, 912-925
    aplastic, 924-925
    classification of, 912, 914f
    consequences of, 912
    Cooley, 923-924, 923b
    definition of, 912
    diagnosis of, 912, 913t, 914, 915
    Fanconi, 924-925
    hypoplastic, 924
    in acute renal failure, 966
    in chronic renal failure, 968
    in infant, 324
    in leukemia, 930, 935
    in newborn, 292t
    iron deficiency, 915-916
    nursing care for, 914-915
    physiologic, 324
    sickle-cell, 916-923
    treatment of, 914
Anencephaly, 1155b
Anesthesia
    complications of, 697
    induction of, 694-697
    malignant hyperthermia and, 697
    parental presence during, 694-696
    recovery after, 697
Anesthetic cream, 182t, 184
    for circumcision, 226, 227
    for venipuncture, 174, 224b, 717
Aneurysm, coronary, in Kawasaki disease, 902
Angel kiss, 249
Anger, in chronic illness/disability, 582
Angiography, renal, 952t
Angiotensin-converting enzyme inhibitors, for
        congestive heart failure, 878, 882
Angle of Louis, 143, 143f
Animal bites, 1083, 1084
Animism, 446
Anisometropia, 629t
Ankle clonus, 212t
Ankle clonus reflex, 212t
Ankle-foot orthoses, in cerebral palsy, 1148, 1148f
Ann Arbor staging system, 938
Anorectal malformations, 854-855, 854t
Anorexia, 702
    physiologic, in toddler, 422
Anorexia nervosa, 556-559, 557b
Antacids, for peptic ulcers, 837
Antegrade continence enema, 1157
Anterior fontanel, 207, 208f, 217t
Anthropometry, 115
    in physical examination, 121-124
Antianxiety agents, for pain, 178, 178t
Antiarrhythmics, 897
Antibiotics
    for acne, 1090
    for burns, 1096, 1097
    for cystic fibrosis, 798
    for inflammatory bowel disease, 834
    for Lyme disease, 1082-1083
    for osteomyelitis, 1134-1135

Antibiotics (Continued)
  for otitis media, 766-767
  for rickettsial disease, 1082-1083
  for tetanus, 1167-1168
  for urinary tract infections, 955, 956
  prophylactic
    for ophthalmia neonatorum, 222
    for sickle cell anemia, 919, 920
    for umbilicus, 225
Antibodies, in newborn, 200
Anticholinergics
  for asthma, 789
  for enuresis, 537
Anticipatory grief, 265, 605
Anticipatory guidance, 101
  in understanding adolescents, 532-533
  in understanding preschoolers, 450
  in understanding school-age children, 509, 511
  in understanding toddlers, 434
Anticonvulsants
  for bulimia nervosa, 558
  for pain, 178, 178t
  for seizures, 1008, 1015
    in cerebral palsy, 1149
    in status epilepticus, 1009
Anti-D antibody, for idiopathic thrombocytopenic
    purpura, 928b
Antidepressants
  for bulimia nervosa, 558
  for enuresis, 537
  for pain, 177t, 178, 178t, 193
Antidiuretic hormone, 1025t
  hypersecretion of, 1031-1032
    in coma, 984
  hyposecretion of, 1030-1031
  in newborn, 200
Antidiuretics, for enuresis, 537
Antidotes, for poisons, 473
Antiepileptics. See Anticonvulsants.
Antihemophilic factor deficiency, 925-927
Antihypertensives, 900, 901
Antilymphocyte globulin, for aplastic anemia, 925
Antipyretics, 703
Antiretroviral therapy, 940-941
Antiseizure agents. See Anticonvulsants.
Antispasmodics, for cerebral palsy, 1149
Antistreptolysin O titer, in rheumatic fever, 893
Antithymocyte globulin, for aplastic anemia,
    924-925
Anus. See also under Anal.
  examination of, 151
    in newborn, 210, 220t
  imperforate, 854
  of newborn, 210
Anxiety, separation
  in hospitalization, 659-661, 668-670
  in infant, 332, 335
Anxiolytics, for pain, 178, 178t
Aortic coarctation, 871b
Aortic stenosis, 871-872
Aortic valves, 146
Apgar score, 201-203, 202t
Aphasia, 624
Apheresis, 946
Aphthous stomatitis, 465
Apical impulse, 127, 146, 146f
Aplastic anemia, 924-925
Aplastic crisis, in sickle cell anemia, 918, 918b, 922
Apnea, 145b, 217t, 803-804
  obstructive sleep, 803
  of infancy, 404-406
  of prematurity, 291t
Apocrine glands, in newborn, 200
Apparent life-threatening event (ALTE), in infant,
    404-405
Appendicitis, 829-832

Appetite
  in toddler, 422
  loss of, 702
  regulation of, 552
Approach behaviors, 581, 581b
  in feeding, 234
  in newborn, 263, 263t
Appropriate-for-gestational-age (AGA) infant,
    204, 204f
Aqueous vasopressin, for syndrome of inappropri-
    ate antidiuretic hormone secretion, 1031
ARDS (acute respiratory distress syndrome), 781-
    782, 903
Arm circumference, 124, 1191
Arm recoil, 204b
Arm restraints, 709-710. See also Restraints.
Arnold-Chiari malformation, 1018
Arrhythmias, 219t, 324, 896-897
Art therapy, 107
Arterial blood sampling, 715
Arteriovenous fistula, in dialysis, 971
Arteriovenous graft, in dialysis, 971
Arthritis
  juvenile idiopathic, 1139-1142
  septic, 1135
Arthrodesis, for scoliosis, 1132
Arthropod bites and stings, 1076-1079, 1077t-
    1078t
Artificial skin, 1098-1099
Artificial tanning, 529
Artificial ventilation. See Ventilatory support.
Asafetida, 63
Ascariasis, 467t
Ascorbic acid, 390t-391t
Aseptic meningitis, 1002
Asian Americans. See also Race/ethnicity.
  epicanthal folds in, 136, 136f
  health beliefs and practices of, 67t, 68t, 69t
ASKED model, 66, 66b
ASO (ASLO) titer, in rheumatic fever, 893
Asphyxia, fetal, 198
Aspiration
  foreign body, 86, 87, 705-706, 780-781, 809-810,
    809f
    in infant, 365-369, 366b-367b
    in toddler, 428t, 433
  in near-drowning, 993
  in newborn, 221
  meconium, 291t
  pneumonia due to, 781
  prevention of, 696
  suprapubic, 954-955
    for specimen collection, 713, 714
  tracheoesophageal fistula and, 848
Aspiration biopsy, bone marrow, 711
Aspirin
  equianalgesic dose of, 180t
  for fever, 703
  for juvenile idiopathic arthritis, 1140
  for Kawasaki disease, 902
  poisoning with, 472b
  Reye syndrome and, 703, 1004-1005, 1004b
Assent, 688-689. See also Informed consent.
Assessment. See also Screening.
  admission, 665
  behavioral, 132
    in newborn, 213-215, 213b, 214t
  community needs, 24, 26
  developmental, 132
  family, 111, 112b-113b
  history in, 107-113
  nutritional, 113-118
  objective information in, 25
  of newborn, 201-215. See also Newborn, assess-
    ment of.
  physical, 118-156. See also Physical examination.

Assessment (Continued)
  review of systems in, 113, 114
  subjective information in, 24-25
Assimilation, 57
Assisted suicide, 596
Associative play, 84, 441
Asthma, 772t, 783-795
  age at onset of, 784
  allergens in, 784, 785b, 787-788, 791
  care plan for, 792
  classification of, 784, 784b
  diagnosis of, 785-786
  epidemiology of, 784
  etiology of, 784
  exercise-induced, 789
  family issues in, 794-795
  in adolescents, 794-795
  nursing care for, 791-795
  pathophysiology of, 785, 785f
  prognosis of, 790
  self-care in, 794
  severity of, 784, 784b
  status asthmaticus in, 790-791
  treatment of, 786-791
    acute care in, 794
    allergen control in, 787-788, 787b
    chest physical therapy in, 789
    drug therapy in, 788-789
    immunotherapy in, 789-790
    principles of, 787
  triggers in, 784, 785b
Astigmatism, 629t
Asymmetric tonic neck reflex, 212t, 213f
Asymmetry, of muscle tone, 211
Athlete's foot, 1073t
Athletics. See Sports participation.
Ativan. See Lorazepam (Ativan).
Atlantoaxial instability, in Down syndrome, 620
Atomoxetine (Strattera), for attention deficit
    hyperactivity disorder, 560
Atopic dermatitis, 1086-1089, 1087f, 1087t
Atraumatic care, 11
  immunizations and, 360
Atrial septal defect, 867, 868b
Atrioventricular block, 897
Atrioventricular canal defect, 869
Atrioventricular valves, 146
Atrophy, muscle, in immobilization, 1107, 1108t
Atropine, for CPR, 807-809, 808t
Attachment
  assessment of, 215, 215b
  development of, 331-332, 331f
  eye contact in, ophthalmia neonatorum pro-
    phylaxis and, 222
  high-risk newborn and, 265-267
  infant behavior and, 234, 234b
  maladaptive, in reactive attachment disorder,
    332
  maternal, 234-235, 234f
  multiple births/subsequent children and, 237,
    237f
  paternal, 235-236, 236f
  promotion of, 234-236, 234b, 234f, 236f
  sibling, 236, 236f
    high-risk newborn and, 267, 267f
Attachment behavior, in feeding, 234
Attention deficit hyperactivity disorder, 8,
    559-561
Auditory evoked potentials, 979
Auditory function. See Hearing.
Auditory nerve, assessment of, 155t
Auditory testing, 140, 141t
Augmentation enterocystoplasty, 1157
Aural temperature, 126t, 127b, 128
Auricle, 137-138

Auscultation
in blood pressure measurement, 129
of bowel sounds, 149
of breath sounds, 145, 145b, 740-741
in newborn, 209
of heart sounds, 146-147, 147f, 147t
in newborn, 209, 210
Authoritarian parent, 40
Authoritative parent, 41
Autism, 635-637
Autoimmune disorders
juvenile idiopathic arthritis, 1139-1142
systemic lupus erythematosus, 1142-1143
Autoimmune thyroiditis, 1033-1034
Automobile safety, 5, 591, 654
for adolescent, 531b, 532
for infant, 369-370, 369f
high-risk, 268
for newborn, 238-239, 268
at high risk, 268
for school-age child, 369-370, 369f, 510t
for toddler, 427t, 428-431, 429f, 430f
in chronic illness/disability, 591, 654
overheating during confinement in vehicle,
371-372, 431
Autonomic nervous system, of newborn, 201
Autonomy, 13
vs. shame and doubt, 79, 79t, 411-412, 412f
Avian influenza virus, 775-776
Avoidance behaviors, 581, 581b
Avulsed teeth, 507
Axillary hair, 132
Axillary nodes, 133, 134f
Axillary temperature, 126t, 127b, 128
in newborn, 205, 205f, 206
Azotemia, 965
Azotorrhea, in cystic fibrosis, 796

B

Babinski reflex, 152, 211, 211f, 212t, 979
Baby powder, aspiration of, 368
Baby-Friendly Hospital Initiative, 230
Bacille Calmette-Guérin vaccine, 779
Bacitracin, for burns, 1098t
Back. See also under Spinal.
examination of, 151-152
in newborn, 210, 220t
Back blows, for aspiration, 809, 809f
Baclofen, for cerebral palsy, 1149
Bacterial endocarditis, 891-893, 892b
Bacterial infections, of skin, 1069-1071, 1070t,
1071f
Bacterial meningitis, 998-1002
immunization for, 999, 1001
in sickle cell anemia, 919
Bacterial tracheitis, 769, 769t, 772
Bacteriuria, diagnosis of, 953t
Bag-mask ventilation, in CPR, 805
Balance, assessment of, 153
Ballard Scale, in gestational age assessment, 202f,
203
Balloons, in infant suffocation, 368
Balsalazide, for ulcerative colitis, 834
Bands, measurement of, 913t
Baptism, neonatal loss and, 270
Barbiturates
abuse of, 567
for status epilepticus, 1009
Barbiturate coma, 984
Bard Button, 747, 749f
Bariatric surgery, 554
Barlow test, 1122, 1123f
Barrel chest, 143
Barrier protection, 706, 707b
Bartholin glands, 151

Barton tongs, 1119
Basal metabolic rate (BMR), 76
fluid balance and, 815
obesity and, 552
Basophils, measurement of, 913t
Bathing, 701
in atopic dermatitis, 1088
in hyperthermia, 704
of newborn, 224-225, 225f
at high risk, 259
therapeutic, 1069
Bathing trunk nevus, 249
Batteries, ingestion of, 370-371
BCG vaccine, 779
Beds
infant suffocation and, 368
safety concerns for, 368, 705
sharing of
by family, 349, 402
by twins, 237, 237f, 262-263
Bed rest. See also Activity and exercise.
in congestive heart failure, 878, 882
Bed wetting, 537-538. See also Urinary incontinence.
in sickle cell anemia, 921-922
in syndrome of inappropriate antidiuretic
hormone secretion, 1031
Bee stings, 1076-1079, 1078t
Behavior
aggressive, in preschooler, 447
assessment of, 132
in newborn, 207, 213-215, 213b, 214t
feeding, 234
of abused/neglected child, 484b
of stressed/fatigued newborn, 263t
regression of, 422
Behavior modification, 42, 700
Behavioral contracts, 700
for eating disorders, 559
for pain management, 172
for suicidal behavior, 570
Behavioral measures, in pain assessment, 159-161,
159b, 160t-161t, 165-171
Behavioral Pain Score (BPS), 160t
Behavioral therapy
for attention deficit hyperactivity disorder, 560
for eating disorders, 558
for obesity, 555
Beneficence, 13
Benzoyl peroxide, for acne, 1090
Bereavement. See Grief.
Beta blockers, for congestive heart failure, 878
Beta-adrenergic agonists, for asthma, 788-789,
791-793
in status asthmaticus, 790
Bibliotherapy, 106b
Biceps reflex, 154f
Bicycle injuries, 5
prevention of, 508f, 509
Bidirectional shunt, 886f, 886t
Bile acid resins, 895
Biliary atresia, 842-843
Biliary cirrhosis, 841-842
Biliblanket, 278, 278f
Bilirubin, 275
Bilirubin encephalopathy, 277
Binge eating disorder, 556
Binocularity, development of, 325
Binuclear family, 34
Biobrane, 1097-1098
Biofeedback, 192
Biopsy
bone marrow, 711
renal, 952t
Biot respiration, 145b

Bird flu, 775-776
Birth defects. See Congenital anomalies and
specific defects.
Birth history, 109
Birth injuries, 244-247, 245f-247f
Birth order, 36-37, 37b
Birth practices, religious beliefs and, 65t-66t
Birth weight, 75, 206, 216t
blood pressure and, 252t
gestational age and, 203f, 204, 204f
hepatitis B vaccine and, 223
mortality and, 9
risk classification and, 250b. See also Newborn,
high-risk.
Birthmarks, 217t, 249-250, 249f
Bisacodyl, for opioid-related constipation, 179t
Bisexuality, 523
Bismuth, for peptic ulcers, 838
Bites
animal, 1083
arthropod, 1076-1079, 1077t-1078t, 1078f
rickettsial diseases due to, 1082-1083, 1082t
flea, 247-248, 1077t
human, 1083
Biting, by infant, 327
Biventricular pacing, for congestive heart failure, 878
Black eye, 630
Black widow spider bites, 1076-1079, 1077t
Bladder, neurogenic
in spina bifida, 1156, 1157
in spinal cord injuries, 1171
Bladder capacity, in school-age child, 494
Bladder catheterization
clean intermittent, 1157
in coma, 984
in specimen collection, 713-714
in spina bifida, 1157
Bladder exstrophy, 854, 958t
Bladder neck obstruction, 956-957, 957f
Blalock-Taussig shunt, 886f, 886t
Blanket, fiberoptic, for hyperbilirubinemia, 278,
278f
Blast cell leukemia, 930. See also Leukemia.
Blastomycosis, 1074t
Bleeding
in disseminated intravascular coagulation, 929
in hemophilia, 925-927
in hemostatic disorders, 925-930
in idiopathic thrombocytopenic purpura,
927-929
in leukemia, 930, 931t
intracranial
in head trauma, 987f, 988-989
in newborn, 293t
intraventricular, 293t
nasal, 929-930
subgaleal, 245-246, 245f
vitamin K deficiency, in newborn, 222, 292t
Bleeding disorders. See Hemostatic disorders.
Blended family, 33, 48
Blindisms, 631
Blindness. See Visual impairment.
Blinking reflex, in newborn, 212t
Blissymbols, 617-618
Blood, in stool, 914
Blood glucose testing, for diabetes mellitus
in diagnosis, 1045
in monitoring, 1045, 1046, 1055-1056
Blood group incompatibility, 944t, 945
hemolytic disease of newborn and, 281-282, 282f
Rh isoimmunization and, 282
Blood pressure. See also Hypertension;
Hypotension.
in newborn, 206, 206f, 217t
high-risk and, 252t

Blood pressure *(Continued)*
   in seizures, 1010
   measurement of, 129-132, 129t, 130f, 130t, 901
      by family member, 901
      in newborn, 206, 206f, 217t
      reference ranges for, 129t, 131, 900
Blood pressure tables, 131
Blood sampling, 710, 710f, 715-717. *See also*
      Venipuncture.
   arterial, 715
   capillary, 715
   central venous access device for, 725-730, 729f
   evidence based practice and, 717
   fear of blood loss and, 715-716
   from central venous catheter, 716
   heel lance for, 715, 716f, 717
   intermittent infusion devices for, 725, 729f
   positioning for, 710, 710f
   venous, 715-717
Blood tests
   in complete blood count, 912, 913t
   in genitourinary disorders, 954t
Blood transfusion. *See* Transfusion.
Blood urea nitrogen (BUN), 954t
Blood vessels, in newborn, 198-199
Blood volume, in newborn, 199
Blue spells, 884-886
Bodily injury fears, of hospitalized child, 672, 694
Body art, 529
Body fat. *See also* Obesity.
   measurement of, 124
Body image, 82
   development of
      in adolescent, 523-524
      in infant, 330-331, 331f
      in preschooler, 440
      in school-age child, 500
      in toddler, 414-415
   genital surgery and, 957-958
   in chronic illness/disability in, 590, 594
Body mass index (BMI), 121-122, 551, 553, 1189
   in adolescent girls vs. boys, 516, 518
Body surface area
   fluid balance and, 814-815
   in dosage calculation, 718
Body temperature. *See* Temperature.
Body water. *See under* Fluid.
Body weight. *See* Weight.
Boils, 1069-1071, 1070t
Bone
   cranial, in newborn, 207
   formation of, 75
   healing of, 1113
   immobilization effects on, 1108t
   infections of, 1134-1135
   ossification of, 76, 494
   structure of, 75
   tuberculosis of, 1135
Bone age, 75, 1028b
Bone disease, in chronic renal failure, 968, 969
Bone marrow aspiration biopsy, 711
Bone marrow transplantation. *See* Stem cell transplantation.
Bone remodeling, 1113
Bone tumors, 1136-1138
Booster seats, 429
Boston brace, 1131
Bottle feeding, 231-234. *See also* Formula feeding.
Bottle-mouth caries, 426
Botulinum toxin, for cerebral palsy, 1148-1149
Botulism, 1168-1170
Boundaries, family, 31-32

Bowel elimination. *See also* Constipation; Diarrhea; Fecal incontinence; Stool.
   in coma, 984-985
   in newborns and infants, 824
   in spina bifida, 1156
Bowel preparation, preoperative, 750
Bowlegs, 152, 152f
Braces
   for cerebral palsy, 1148, 1148f
   for developmental dysplasia of hip, 1124, 1124f, 1125
   for scoliosis, 1131-1133, 1132f
Brachial palsy, 211, 246-247, 247f
Brachial pulse, 146f
Bradycardia, 216t
Bradydysrhythmias, 896-897
Bradypnea, 145b
Braille, 631
Brain death, determination of, 994
Brain injury
   hypoxic-ischemic, in newborn, 293t
   in near-drowning, 993-995
   traumatic, 986-993. *See also* Head injury.
Brain tumors, 995-997
Brainstem evoked potentials, 979
Brazelton Neonatal Behavioral Assessment Scale (BNBAS), 213, 213b
Breakthrough pain, 183
Breast
   development of, 144, 515, 516f
   enlarged male, 144, 543
   examination of, 144
   of newborn, 200, 209
Breast milk jaundice, 275
Breastfeeding, 2, 229-231, 230b, 230f, 231f, 344
   contraindications to, 230
   donor milk for, 256-257
   expressed mother's milk for, 256
   growth patterns and, 122
   in cleft lip/cleft palate, 845
   jaundice associated with, 275
   newborn sense of smell and, 201
   nutritional value of human milk and, 228-229
   of high-risk newborn, 256-257
   of twins, 230-231, 230f
   promotion of, 231
   schedules for, 233
   stools and, in newborns, 200b
   suckling technique for, 231, 231f
   weaning from, 347
Breath odor, 977
   in diabetes mellitus, 1044
Breath sounds
   assessment of, 145, 145b, 740-741
   in newborn, 209
Breathing. *See also* Respiration.
   in neurologic examination, 977
   mouth-to-mouth/nose, 805, 806f
   periodic, in newborn, 209
   sleep-disordered, 803
British Sign Language, 626
Bronchial drainage, 741, 742f
Bronchiolitis, 772t, 773-774
Bronchitis, 772t, 773
Bronchodilators
   for asthma, 785, 785f, 788-789, 791-794
   for cystic fibrosis, 798, 798f
Bronchopneumonia, 774-777
Bronchoprovocation test, in asthma, 786
Bronchopulmonary dysplasia, 289, 291t
Bronchospasm
   exercise-induced, 789
   in asthma, 785, 785f, 791-794
Broviac catheter, 725-730, 727t
Brown adipose tissue, 199

Brown fat, 199
Brown recluse spider bites, 1076-1079, 1077t, 1078f
Bryant traction, 1118
Buck traction, 1118, 1119f
Buckle fractures, 1113f, 1114
Buddhism, 65t
Bulb syringe, for oropharyngeal suctioning, in newborn, 221
Bulimia nervosa, 556-559, 557b
Bullae, 1063f
Bullying, 498
Bupivacaine, for procedural pain, 191
Burial, 604
Burkitt lymphoma, 939
Burning, 64b
Burns, 5, 1091-1103
   age and, 1092f, 1093
   airway, 782-783, 1093
   analgesia for, 1096-1097
   carbon monoxide poisoning and, 783, 1093
   chemical, 1091
   comfort measures in, 1100
   complications of, 1094
      management of, 1101-1102
      prevention of, 1101-1102
   contractures in, prevention of, 1101, 1101f
   débridement of, 1095-1096, 1097
   depth of, 1091-1092, 1092f
   dressings for, 1095-1096
   drug therapy for, 1096-1097, 1098
   electrical, 1091
   emergency management of, 1094-1097
   extent of, 1091, 1092f
   family support in, 1102
   fluid management in, 1096
   fourth-degree, 1092, 1093f
   full-thickness (third-degree), 1092, 1092f, 1093f, 1094t
   grading of, 1093, 1094t
   hospitalization for, 1099
   in infant, 371-372
   in school-age child, 510t
   in sunburn, 1103
   in toddler, 427t, 431-432, 432f
   infection of, 1094, 1101
   inhalation injury and, 1093
   long-term care for, 1101-1102
   major, 1093, 1094t
      treatment of, 1096-1097
   minor, 1093, 1094t
      treatment of, 1095-1096
   moderate, 1093, 1094t
   nursing care for, 1099-1100
   nutritional support in, 1096, 1100
   of eye, 630
   partial-thickness (second-degree), 1092, 1092f, 1093f, 1094t
   pathophysiology of, 1094
   prevention of, 1102-1103
   psychosocial aspects of, 1101-1102
   rehabilitation in, 1099, 1100
   scald, 371, 432
   scarring in, 1101, 1101f
   sedation for, 1096-1097
   superficial (first-degree), 1091-1092, 1092f
   topical agents for, 1098
   total body surface area and, 1091, 1092f
   types of, 1091
   wound care for, 1095, 1096, 1097, 1100
Butorphanol, for opioid-related pruritus, 179t

C

Café-au-lait spots, 217t, 249
Caffeine, for opioid-related sedation, 179t

Calcitonin, 1026t, 1032
Calcium, 392t
Calcium chloride, for CPR, 807-809, 808t
Calcium imbalance
    in chronic renal failure, 969
    in hyperparathyroidism, 1037
Calendar method, 544
Callus, fracture, 1113
Caloric test, 978
Calories, daily requirements for, 76t
Campylobacter jejuni infection, 817-823, 819t. *See also* Diarrhea.
Cancer
    bone, 1136-1138
    brain, 995-997
    colon, in Crohn disease, 835
    leukemia, 930
    lymphoma, 937-939
    ocular, 633-635, 634f
    pain management in, 193-194
    renal, 963-965, 963b, 964b
    skin, prevention of, 89
    testicular, 542-543
Candida albicans, 248
Candidiasis, 1073t
    diaper area, 1084-1086, 1086f
    oral, in newborn, 218t, 248, 248f
Cannabis, 567
    intrauterine exposure to, 304-305
Capillary blood sampling, 715
Capillary hemangiomas, 249-250, 249f
Capillary refill time, 146
Caput succedaneum, 217t, 244, 245f
Car accidents, 5
Car seats/restraints
    for infant, 369-370, 369f
    for newborn, 238-239
        at high risk, 268
    for spica cast, 1116
    in chronic illness/disability, 591, 654
Car temperature, 371-372, 431
Carbamazepine, for pain, 177t
Carbon monoxide, end-tidal, hyperbilirubinemia and, 277
Carbon monoxide poisoning, 783, 1093m783
Carbuncles, 1069-1071, 1070t
Cardiac arrhythmias, 219t, 324, 896-897
Cardiac catheterization, 863-864, 864t
    for arrhythmias, 896
Cardiac examination, 145-147, 147f, 147t
    in newborn, 209-210, 219t
Cardiac glycosides, for congestive heart failure, 878
Cardiac pacing, 897
Cardiac surgery, for congenital heart disease, 867, 885, 886t, 888-891
Cardiac valves, 146
    abnormalities of, 871-872
Cardinal positions of gaze, 153, 154f
Cardiogenic shock, 902-904, 903t
Cardiomyopathy, 898-899
Cardiopulmonary resuscitation, 804-809
Cardiovascular dysfunction, 861-907. *See also* Heart disease.
    acquired, 891-899
    cardiac catheterization in, 863-864
    congenital, 862-891
    diagnosis of, 862-864
    echocardiography in, 863
    electrocardiography in, 863
    heart transplantation in, 899
    history in, 862
    in anaphylaxis, 904-906
    in cardiomyopathy, 898-899
    in dysrhythmias, 896-897
    in hyperlipidemia, 894-896

Cardiovascular dysfunction (*Continued*)
    in immobilization, 1108t
    in Kawasaki disease, 901-902
    in pulmonary artery hypertension, 897-898
    in shock, 902-907
    in systemic hypertension, 899-901
    nursing care in, 864-865
    physical examination in, 862
Cardioversion, 897
Care coordination, in home care, 646-647
Care plans
    for end-of-life care, 600-602
    in home care, 646-647
Caregivers, family, 641-655. *See also* Family; Home care.
Caries
    in school-age child, 506-507
    in toddler, 426, 426f
Caring, in therapeutic relationship, 12
Carotid pulse, 146f
Caruncles, 151
Carvedilol, for congestive heart failure, 878
Casanthranol/docusate sodium, for opioid-related constipation, 179t
Case management, in home care, 646-647, 647b
Casein-hydrolysate formulas, 232
Casts, 1115-1117, 1116f, 1117f
    application of, 1115
    care of, 1115-1117
    for clubfoot, 1126, 1126f
    for developmental dysplasia of hip, 1124, 1124f
    for fractures, 1115-1117, 1116f, 1117f
    for Legg-Calvé-Perthes disease, 1128-1130
    removal of, 1117
Casts, urinary, 953t
Cat bites, 1083, 1084
Cat scratch disease, 1083-1084
Catabolic state, 191
Cataracts, 629t
Catecholamines, 1037
Catheter toes, 255
Catheters/catheterization
    bladder, 713-714
        for neurogenic bladder, 1157
        for specimen collection, 713-714
        in coma, 984
    cardiac, 863-864, 864t
        for dysrhythmias, 896
    central venous, 725-730, 729f
        for blood sampling, 716
    for intravenous infusion, 733-738
    in dialysis, 971
    in intracranial pressure monitoring, 983
    intermittent infusion, 725, 729f
    tunneled, 725-730, 727t, 729f
Causal relationships, in cognitive development, 412, 439
Cavernous venous hemangiomas, 250
Cavopulmonary anastomosis, 886f, 886t
Ceiling effect, 178
Celiac disease, 855-856, 856t
Cellulitis, 1069-1071, 1070t, 1071f
Central auditory imperception, 624. *See also* Hearing impairment.
Central nervous system
    of infant, 323
    of newborn, 201
Central nervous system prophylaxis, in leukemia, 931
Central shunt, 886f, 886t
Central venous access device, 725-730, 728f
Central venous catheter, blood specimens from, 716
Centrencephalic system, 1005
Cephalhematoma, 217t, 244-245, 245f

Cephalocaudal growth, 72
Cephalopelvic disproportion, 244
Cerebellar function, assessment of, 153, 153b
Cerebral dysfunction, 974-1020
    assessment in, 975
        diagnostic procedures in, 979-981, 980t
        neurologic examination in, 977-979
    coma in, 976, 981-986
    in aseptic meningitis, 1002
    in bacterial meningitis, 998-1002
    in brain tumors, 995-997
    in encephalitis, 1002-1003
    in head trauma, 986-993
    in hydrocephalus, 1017-1020
    in near-drowning, 993-994
    in rabies, 1003-1004
    in Reye syndrome, 703, 1004-1005, 1004b
    in seizures, 1005-1016
    increased intracranial pressure in, 975-976, 976b. *See also* Increased intracranial pressure.
    nursing care in, 981-986
    overview of, 975
Cerebral edema. *See also* Increased intracranial pressure.
    drug therapy for, 984
    in chronic renal disease, 968
    in head trauma, 989
Cerebral hypoperfusion, 131
Cerebral palsy, 1146-1154
    care plan for, 1151-1152
    classification of, 1146-1147, 1146b
    definition of, 1146
    diagnosis of, 1147
    etiology of, 1146
    family support in, 1153
    hospitalization in, 1153-1154
    nursing care in, 1150-1154
    nursing process in, 1150
    pathophysiology of, 1146-1147
    prognosis of, 1149-1150
    signs and symptoms of, 1147b
    treatment of, 1147-1149
Cerebral trauma, 986-993. *See also* Head injury.
Cerebrospinal fluid
    collection and analysis of, 979, 980t
    analgesia for, 193
    in encephalitis, 1002
    in meningitis, 1000, 1002, 1002b
    positioning for, 710-711, 711f
    in hydrocephalus, 1017-1018, 1017f
Cerebrovascular accident, in sickle cell anemia, 918, 920-921, 922
Cerumen, 138
Cervical cap, 545t
Cervical esophagostomy, 848-849
Cervical nodes, 133, 134f
Cervical traction, 1119, 1119f
Changing table, fall from, 370
Charleston nighttime bending brace, 1132
Cheating, by school-age child, 501-502
Cheiloplasty, 846
Chelation therapy
    for heavy metal poisoning, 475
    for lead poisoning, 478-479, 480
Chemical burns, 1091. *See also* Burns.
Chemical conjunctivitis, 222b
Chemical dot thermometers, 127b
Chemotherapy
    extravasation in, 936
    for bone cancer, 1136-1137
    for brain tumors, 995
    for Ewing sarcoma, 1137-1138
    for Hodgkin disease, 938
    for leukemia, 931, 932, 935-936

Chemotherapy *(Continued)*
    for retinoblastoma, 634
    for Wilms tumor, 964
    late effects of, 932
    nursing care in, 935-937
    peripheral neuropathy in, 193
    safe handling of, 935-936
    side effects of, 935-937
Chest
    auscultation of
        for breath sounds, 145, 145b, 209, 740-741
        for heart sounds, 146-147, 147t, 209, 210
    barrel, 143
    examination of
        in cardiac assessment, 145-147, 147t
        in newborn, 209, 218t
        in respiratory assessment, 143-144, 143f
    movement of, 144, 144f
    percussion of, 741, 743f
    pigeon, 143
    shape of, 144
    size of, 143
        in newborn, 204, 216t
Chest circumference
    in newborn, 204, 216t
    in toddler, 410
Chest compression, in CPR, 807, 807f
Chest pain, in respiratory infections, 757b
Chest physical therapy, 741, 742f, 743f
    for asthma, 789
    for cystic fibrosis, 798, 801, 802
Chest thrusts, 809
Cheyne-Stokes respiration, 145b
Chickenpox, 454f, 454t-455t
    immunization against, 357
    maternal infection with, 305t
    Reye syndrome and, 703
Chief complaint, 107-108
Chigger bites, 1077t
Chilblain, 1103
Child abuse. *See* Abuse.
Child care facilities, for infants, 335, 340-341
Child center–based care, 340
Child health promotion, 2
Child pornography, 482
Childhood hysteria, 563
Childhood morbidity, 10
Childhood mortality, 9-10, 10t
Childrearing practices
    discipline/limit-setting and, 41-43
    infant temperament and, 335
Children's Hospital of Eastern Ontario Pain Scale
        (CHEOPS), 160t, 161
Chinese Americans. *See* Asian Americans.
Chlamydia, 547, 548t
    maternal infection with, 306t
    ophthalmia neonatorum due to, 222
Chloride, 392t
Chlorothiazide (Diuril), for congestive heart
        failure, 879t
Choking. *See* Aspiration, foreign body.
Cholecalciferol, 391t
Cholesterol, elevated serum, 894-896
Cholestyramine (Questran), 895
Choline magnesium trisalicylate (Trilisate), for
        pain, 175, 176t
Chordee, 220t, 958t
Chorea, in rheumatic fever, 894
Christian Scientists, 65t
Christmas disease, 925-927
Chromosome translocations, 619
Chronic active hepatitis, 840

Chronic illness/disability. *See also* Cognitive
        impairment; Hearing impairment; Visual
        impairment.
    activities of daily living in, 590
    assessment in, 585-586, 585b, 586t
    automobile safety and, 430-431
    coping mechanisms in
        of child, 584-585, 587-589
        of parents, 581, 586, 586b
        of siblings, 580-581, 590
    cultural aspects of, 577
    definition of, 576b
    developmental aspects of, 575-576, 583-584,
        591-594, 592t-593t
    early intervention in, 578
    end-of-life care in, 588b, 595-607. *See also*
        Death and dying.
    family support in, at time of diagnosis in,
        586-587
    family-centered care in, 576-578
    family–health provider communication in, 576,
        586-590
    family's adjustment to, 581-583
    family's emotional responses in, 581-583, 585,
        589
    functional burden in, 583, 583b
    health teaching in, 584-585
    home care in, 10, 11b, 577-578, 641-655
    managed care and, 578
    mobility in, 591
    normalization in, 577-578, 589-595, 642
    nursing care guidelines in, 588b, 589b
    nursing process in, 585
    overprotection in, 582, 583b
    overview of, 575
    pain assessment in, 171
    permanency planning in, 643
    primary health care in, 591
    realistic goals in, 594-595
    self-care in, 584-585
    shared decision making in, 577
    sibling needs and concerns in, 580-581, 580b,
        590
    support systems in, 583, 587-590
    terminology of, 576b
    therapeutic relationship in, 576
    type of, 585
Chronic leukemia, 930-937. *See also* Leukemia.
Chronic nonspecific diarrhea, 817
Chronic pain, 190
Chronic renal failure, 967-970
Church of Christ, Scientist, 65t
Church of Jesus Christ of Latter Day Saints, 65t
Cigarette smoking, 566
Ciliary muscles, 201
Circular reactions, in cognitive development, 330,
        412
Circulation
    enterohepatic, 275
    prenatal vs. postnatal, 866, 866f
Circulatory failure. *See* Shock.
Circulatory overload, transfusion-related, 944t
Circulatory system, of newborn, 198-199
Circumcision, 225-228
    analgesia for, 191, 226b-227b, 227-228
    cultural aspects of, 228
    female, 64b, 151, 228
    risks and benefits of, 225-227, 226b
    urinary tract infections and, 950
Circumstraint board, 227b, 228f
Cirrhosis, 841-842
Clarithromycin, for peptic ulcers, 838
Class, 54. *See also* Socioeconomic status.
Clavicle, fractures of, 1112
    during birth, 246

Clean intermittent catheterization, of neurogenic
        bladder, 1157
Clean-catch specimens, 712
Cleft lip/cleft palate, 209, 843-846, 844f, 847
Client/family teaching. *See* Health/family teaching.
Clinical care paths, in home care, 646-647
Clitoris, 151, 151f
    female genital mutilation and, 228
    of newborn, 210
Cloaca, 854
Clonidine
    for attention deficit hyperactivity disorder, 560
    for pain, 177t
Closed captioning, 626
Clostridial diarrhea, 817-823, 819t-820t. *See also*
        Diarrhea.
Clubbing, of fingers, 884, 884f
Clubfoot, 1125-1126, 1126f
Clubs, for school-age child, 497-498
Coagulation disorders. *See* Hemostatic disorders.
Coanalgesics, 178
Coarctation of aorta, 871b
Cobalamin, 390t
Cobedding, of twins, 237, 237f
    at high risk, 262-263
Cocaine, 567
    intrauterine exposure to, 303-304
Coccidioidomycosis, 1074t
Cochlear implants, 625
Cockroaches, allergy to, 787-788, 787b
Codeine, 175, 176t, 180t
Cognition, definition of, 80
Cognitive development, 79t, 80-81
    in adolescent, 519, 525t
    in infant, 327, 330, 330f
    in preschooler, 439, 445t
    in school-age child, 495, 496f, 502t
    in toddler, 412-413, 413f
    play in, 85, 330
Cognitive impairment, 611-623. *See also* Chronic
        illness/disability.
    behavioral signs of, 611b
    care plan for, 614-616
    child/family teaching in, 613
    classification of, 612, 612t
    communication in, 617-618
    definition of, 611
    developmental delay and, 611
    diagnosis of, 611-612, 611b
    dimensions of care for, 611b
    discipline in, 618
    education in, 613
    etiology of, 612
    hospitalization in, 618-619
    in autism, 635
    in cerebral palsy, 1149
    in Down syndrome, 619-622
    in fragile X syndrome, 622-623
    in hydrocephalus, 1019
    in Klinefelter syndrome, 541
    nursing care for, 612-619
    optimal development in, 616
    pain assessment in, 166-171
    placement in, 618
    play and exercise in, 616-617, 616f, 617f
    prevention of, 619
    self-care in, 613
    sexuality in, 618
    socialization in, 618
    treatment withholding in, 621
Cognitive power, 976
Cognitive-behavioral therapy, for abdominal pain,
        192-193
Coining, 63, 64b
Coitus interruptus, 544

Cold injury, 1103-1104
Cold sores, 465, 1072t
Colds, 759-762
Colectomy, for inflammatory bowel disease, 835, 836
Colestipol (Colestid), 895
Colic, 395-396, 397, 397f
Collarbone, fractures of, 1112
   during birth, 246
Colon cancer, in Crohn disease, 835
Colony-stimulating factor, for aplastic anemia, 925
Color tool, for pain assessment, 164, 164t
Color vision
   assessment of, 137
   in newborn, 201
Colostomies, 750-751
Coma, 976, 981-986
   assessment in, 976-977, 977f
   awakening from, 985
   barbiturate, 984
   drug therapy in, 984
   elimination in, 984-985
   exercises in, 985
   eye care in, 985
   family support in, 985-986
   home care in, 986
   hydration in, 984
   hygiene in, 985
   induced, 984
   nursing care in, 981-986
   nutrition in, 984
   oral care in, 985
   positioning in, 985
   respiratory management in, 982
   sensory stimulation in, 985
   suctioning in, 984
   syndrome of inappropriate antidiuretic hormone secretion in, 984
   thermoregulation in, 984
Comedones, 1089, 1090
Commitment, parent-infant attachment and, 235
Common cold, 759-762
Communal family, 34
Communication, 97-107. *See also* Interview.
   about sexuality, 110-111, 110b
   barriers in, 101, 102b
   cultural aspects of, 60-61, 62, 67t-69t, 100-101
   empathy in, 101
   guidelines for, 97-99
   illocutionary stage of, 103, 103b
   in autism, 635
   in chronic illness/disability, 576, 586-590
   in cognitive impairment, 617-618
   in hearing impairment, 626-627
   in home care, 649-650
   information overload in, 101
   listening skills in, 100-101
   locutionary stage of, 103, 103b
   nonverbal, 61, 107b
   play in, 105
   prelocutionary stage of, 103, 103b
   privacy and confidentiality in, 98-99
   setting for, 97
   silence in, 101
   with children, 102-107
      in adolescence, 104-105, 521
      in early childhood, 103-104
      in end-of-life care, 597
      in infancy, 103
      in school-age years, 104
      techniques of, 105, 106b-107b
   with deaf-blind, 633
   with non-English speakers, 60-61, 62, 101-102
   with parents, 99-102
   words to avoid in, 693

Community
   benefits of, 55-56
   definition of, 21
Community health diagnosis, 25
Community health nursing, 21
Community health programs, 25
Community needs assessment, 24, 26
Community planning, 25, 26
Community resources, for home care, 644-646, 644b
Community support, 55
Community-based nursing care, 20-27
   community concepts in, 21
   demography in, 22
   disease surveillance in, 21
   epidemiology in, 22-23
   health promotion in, 21
   nurse's roles and functions in, 21-22, 22b
   nursing process in, 24-27, 24b
   policy development in, 21
   populations served by, 21
Community-oriented care, 21
Complementary and alternative therapies, 63, 175
   classification of, 667b
   cultural aspects of, 63, 665
   for pain, 175
   hospitalization and, 665
   lead exposure from, 64
   types of, 667b
   vitamin imbalances due to, in infant, 379
Complete blood count (CBC), 912, 913t
Complete heart block, 897
Complex partial seizures, 1006b, 1014b. *See also* Seizures.
Compliance, 698-700
Complicated grief syndrome, 605
Compound nevi, 249
Computed tomography
   in cerebral dysfunction, 979, 980t
   in genitourinary disorders, 952t
Computers, privacy issues and, 99
Conceptual thinking, 495
Concrete operations stage, 79t, 80, 495
Concussions, 987. *See also* Head injury.
   postconcussion syndrome and, 990
Condoms, 544t-545t
Conductive hearing loss, 623, 624. *See also* Hearing impairment.
Confidentiality, 99
   for adolescents, 689
   parental notification and, 544
   suicide threats and, 570
Confusion, 976b
   opioid-related, 180t
Congenital adrenal hyperplasia, 1040-1042
Congenital aganglionic megacolon, 825-826, 825f
Congenital anomalies, 308-310. *See also* Chronic illness/disability *and specific anomalies*.
   assessment of, 308, 308b
   chemical agents causing, 309-310, 311t
   classification of, 308
   genetic etiology of, 309, 310t
   prenatal diagnosis of, 622
   psychologic considerations of, 317-318
Congenital heart disease, 862-891
   acyanotic, 866-867, 867f
   aortic coarctation in, 871b
   aortic stenosis in, 871b
   associated defects in, 865
   atrial septal defect in, 868b
   atrioventricular canal defect in, 870
   classification of, 866-870
   congestive heart failure in, 876-884
   cyanotic, 866-867, 867f, 884-886
   etiology of, 865

Congenital heart disease *(Continued)*
   family adjustment in, 886-887
   family teaching in, 887
   genetic factors in, 865
   hemodynamic defects in, 867-870, 870f
   home care in, 887-888
   hypoplastic left heart syndrome in, 876b
   hypoxemia in, 884-886
   in Down syndrome, 621
   incidence of, 865
   mixed defects in, 870
   neurologic complications in, 884
   nursing care in, 886-891
   obstructive, 867-870, 870f
   patent ductus arteriosus in, 869b-870b, 870
   pathophysiology of, 866
   perinatal circulatory changes and, 866, 866f
   pulmonary blood flow in, 867-870, 870f
   pulmonic stenosis in, 871b
   risk factors for, 865
   shunts in, 866, 866f
   stenotic, 867-870, 870f
   surgery for
      complications of, 889b
      discharge planning for, 891, 891b
      outcome in, 867
      patient/family preparation for, 888-889
      postoperative care in, 889-891
      preoperative care in, 888-889
      shunts in, 885, 886f, 886t
   tetralogy of Fallot in, 870, 873b
   total anomalous pulmonary venous connection in, 875b
   transposition of great arteries in, 874b
   tricuspid atresia in, 870, 873b-874b
   truncus arteriosus in, 870, 875b-876b
   ventricular septal defect in, 868b-869b
Congenital hypoparathyroidism, 1035-1036
Congenital hypothyroidism, 311-313, 312b
Congenital lactase deficiency, 387
Congenital limb deficiency, 1127
Congenital rubella, 307t
Congenital syphilis, 307t
Congestive heart failure, 876-884
   care plan for, 880-881
   clinical manifestations of, 877, 878b
   definition of, 876
   diagnosis of, 877
   etiology of, 876
   hypoxemia in, 884-886
   in acute renal failure, 966
   in cardiomyopathy, 898-899
   neurologic complications in, 884
   nursing care in, 879-884
   nursing process in, 880
   pathophysiology of, 877, 877f
   right- vs. left-sided, 877
   treatment of, 877-879
Conjugated bilirubin, 275
Conjunctiva
   bulbar, 135
   palpebral, 134
Conjunctivitis, 630
   chemical, 222b
   in newborn, 222, 248-249
   in toddler/preschooler, 464-465, 465b
Consanguineous relationships, 30
Conscience, 78, 439
Conscious mind, 78
Consciousness
   altered states of, 976-977
   assessment of, 976-977, 981
   levels of, 976, 976b
Consent. See Informed consent.

Conservation concept, in school-age children, 495, 496f
Constipation, 823-825
opioid-induced, 179t, 188
Constitutional delay, 540
in hypopituitarism, 1024-1027
Consummatory behavior, in feeding, 234
Consumption coagulopathy, 929
Contact dermatitis, 1074-1076
Contact precautions, 707, 707b
Contagious suicide, 570
Containment
for high-risk newborn, 262
in pain management, 173
Continuous ambulatory peritoneal dialysis, 970
Continuous cycling peritoneal dialysis, 970
Continuous venovenous hemodiafiltration, 970
Continuous venovenous hemodialysis, 970
Continuous venovenous hemofiltration, 970
Contraception, 544-547, 544t-546t
Contracts, behavioral, 172, 700
for suicidal behavior, 570
in eating disorders, 559
in pain management, 172
Contractures
in immobilization, 1107, 1108t
in wound healing, 1062
Contrecoup injury, 986-987, 987f
Control, loss of, in hospitalization, 661-663
Contusions
cerebral, 987, 987f
soft tissue, 1110-1111
Conversion disorder, 563
Cooley anemia, 923-924, 923b
Cooling measures, 703-704
Cooperative play, 85
Coordination, assessment of, 153
Coping mechanisms, 90
approach behaviors, 581, 581b
avoidance behaviors, 581, 581b
for pain, 171-173, 192-193
in chronic illness/disability
of child, 584-585, 589-590
of parents, 581, 587-589
of siblings, 580-581, 590
Coping styles, 90
Copper, 393t
Copycat suicides, 570
Cord blood stem cell transplantation, 946. See also
Stem cell transplantation.
Core temperature, 125, 127
Cornea, examination of, 135
in newborn, 208, 212t
Corneal light reflex, assessment of, 136, 136f, 208, 212t
Coronal suture, 208f
Coronary aneurysm, in Kawasaki disease, 902
Corporal punishment, 42-43
Corrosives, poisoning with, 471b
Corticosteroids
Cushing syndrome due to, 1039-1040
for asthma, 788, 794
for inflammatory bowel disease, 834
for juvenile idiopathic arthritis, 1140
for nephrotic syndrome, 960
for pain, 178t
for systemic lupus erythematosus, 1142-1143
mood changes due to, 937
moon face due to, 937
topical, 1067, 1068-1069
for atopic dermatitis, 1088
Corticosterone, 1026t
Cortisol, 1026t
deficiency of, 1038-1039
excess of, 1039-1040

Cortisone
for Addison disease, 1039
for congenital adrenal hyperplasia, 1041
Cosleeping, 349
SIDS and, 402
Costal angle, 143, 143f
Cotrel-Dubousset instrumentation, 1132
Cough
assessment of, 757b
for sputum collection, 717
in colds, 761
whooping, 458t-461t, 776
immunization for, 356
Cough reflex, 212t
Counseling, 13
genetic, 317-318
nutritional, toddler and, 422-423, 423b
telephone, 99, 100b
Coup injury, 986-987, 987f
Couplet care, 237
Cover test, 136, 136f
Cow's milk allergy, 386, 386b
Cow's milk-based formulas, 232
Coxa plana, 1128-1130
Coxa vara, 1130, 1130b
Coxsackieviruses, maternal infection with, 306t
Crackles, 145
in newborn, 209
Cradle cap, 1089
Cranial asymmetry, newborn sleeping position and, 221, 400-401, 401f
Cranial deformities, 1016-1017
Cranial nerves
assessment of, 155t
of newborn, 201
Cranial sutures, 207, 208f
closure of, 1016-1017
Cranioschisis, 1155b
Craniotabes, physiologic, 207, 217t, 246
Craniotomy, for congenital deformities, 1017
Crawl reflex, 212t, 213f
Crawling, 326, 329f
Creams, 1066t, 1067
Creatinine, reference ranges for, 954t
Creative activities, for hospitalized child, 674-675
Creeping, 326, 329f
Cremasteric reflex, 150, 150f
Crepitus, 246
Cribs, safety for, 705
infant suffocation and, 368
CRIES pain scale, 168t
Crime. See also Abuse; Violence.
newborn abduction, 221-222
Critical thinking, 14
Crohn disease, 833-836
Cromolyn sodium, for asthma, 788
Crotamiton, for scabies, 1079
Croup, 769, 769t, 770-771, 771b
spasmodic, 769, 769t, 771-772
Croup syndromes, 769-772, 769t
Crown-to-rump measurement, 204-205, 216t
Crusts, 1064f
Crying
in newborn, 215
nighttime, 348t
Cryptococcosis, 1074t
Cryptorchidism, 150, 958t
Cuban Americans. See Race/ethnicity.
Cued speech, 626
Cuff, blood pressure, 129-130, 130f
Cultural customs, 59-62
Cultural diversity, 56
Cultural factors
in adolescence, 514
in chronic illness/disability, 577

Cultural factors (Continued)
in circumcision, 228
in communication, 60, 61-62, 67t-69t, 100-101
in complementary and alternative therapy, 63, 665
in diet and nutrition, 58, 61-62, 63, 115b
in eye contact, 61
in family bed, 349
in health beliefs and practices, 60, 62-64, 67t-69t
in home care, 648-649
in lead poisoning, 476
in pain assessment, 171
in therapeutic relationship, 60-61
Cultural relativism, 57, 60
Cultural sensitivity, 57-58
Culturally competent care, 58
ASKED model for, 66, 66b
Culture, 52-69
acculturation and, 57
communities and, 55-56
definition of, 52
development and, 52
education and, 55
ethnicity and, 52. See also Race/ethnicity.
North American, 56
overview of, 52
peer, 56
religion and, 55, 64-67, 65t-66t. See also Religious beliefs.
self-esteem and, 53-54
standards and norms and, 52
subcultures and, 53
throat, 762, 763
values and, 52
Culture shock, 57
Cultured epithelium, for burns, 1099
Cupping, 64b
Curandero, 63
Cushing syndrome, 1039-1040, 1040f
Custody, 47
Customs, 59-62
Cyanosis
in anemia, 912
in congenital heart disease, 864-867, 867f
in congestive heart failure, 884-886
in respiratory disorders, 757b
race/ethnicity and, 133t
Cyclosporine, for aplastic anemia, 925
Cystic fibrosis, 795-803
clinical manifestations of, 797b
diagnosis of, 797
endocrine complications in, 796, 799-800
end-of-life care in, 802, 803
family support in, 801-803
gastrointestinal complications in, 796, 797b, 798
home care in, 801
hospital care in, 800-801
nursing care in, 800-803
pathophysiology of, 795-797, 796f
prognosis in, 800
reproductive complications in, 796, 803
respiratory complications in, 796, 797-799, 797b
transition to adulthood in, 803
treatment of, 797-800
Cystic fibrosis transmembrane regulator, 795
Cystitis, 950-956. See also Urinary tract infections.
hemorrhagic, cyclophosphamide-induced, 937
Cystoscopy, 952t
Cysts, 1063f
Cytomegalovirus, maternal infection with, 306t

D

Dance reflex, 212t
Date rape, 549-550, 549b
Date rape drugs, 549, 567

Dawn phenomenon, 1048
Daycare, 48, 49, 335, 340-341
    for HIV-infected children, 943
DDAVP, for hemophilia, 926
Dead space, 719-720
Deaf-blind, 633
Deafness, 623. *See also* Hearing impairment.
Death and dying. *See also* Mortality.
    at home, 603-604
    brain death in, 994
    communication with child in, 597
    decision making in
        by parents, 597
        by physician and health care team, 596-597
    ethical issues in, 595-596, 802
    family needs and concerns in, 603, 605-607
    fear of dying in, 603-604
    fear of suffering in, 602-603
    grief and, 605-607
    home care in, 599
    hospice care in, 599-600
    hospitalization in, 599, 604
    nurses' reactions to, 607
    nursing care plan for, 600-602
    of high-risk infant, 269-270
    organ donation and, 605
    pain management in, 193-194, 595, 596, 600-603
    palliative care in, 595
    postmortem care in, 604
    religious beliefs and practices in, 65t-66t
    signs of approaching death in, 604b
    sudden, of infant, 401-404
    symptom management in, 602-603
Death rattle, 604
Débridement
    enzymatic, 1066t
    of burns, 1095-1096, 1097
Decibels, 624, 624t
Decimal factor prefixes, 1200
Deep palpation, 149
Deep tendon reflexes, 153. *See also* Reflexes.
Defecation. *See* Bowel elimination.
Deferoxamine (Desferal), for thalassemia, 924
Deformational plagiocephaly, 400
Degree of fit, 78
Dehydration, 702, 814-817
    clinical manifestations of, 816t, 817
    diagnosis of, 816-817
    hypertonic, 816
    hypotonic, 816
    intake/output measurement in, 817
    isotonic, 816
    nursing care in, 817
    severity of, 816t
    types of, 815
Delayed gratification, 327
Deltoid, injection in, 720, 722, 722f
Demand feedings, 233
Demerol. *See* Meperidine (Demerol).
Democratic parent, 41
Demographic characteristics, 22
Demography, 22
Denial, in chronic illness/disability, 582
Dentition. *See* Teeth.
Denver Articulation Screening Examination, 447,
    1176-1177
Denver Developmental Screening Test, 93-94, 94b,
    1174-1175
Denver Eye Screening Test, 1178
Denver II, 93-94, 94b
Denver II Prescreening Developmental Question-
    naire, 94-95
Dependence
    in substance abuse, 188, 189, 564
    on opioids, 188, 189

Depo-Provera (medroxyprogesterone acetate),
    544, 546t
Depression, 563-564, 563b
    anaclitic, 659
    suicide and, 8, 564, 568-571
Deprivation dwarfism, 540
Depth perception, 325
Dermatitis, 1061-1062. *See also* Skin disorders.
    atopic, 1086-1089, 1087f, 1087t
    diaper, 248, 1084-1086, 1086f
    flea-bite, 247-248
    seborrheic, 1089
Dermatome, 1098, 1098f
Dermatophytoses, 1071-1072, 1073t
Desensitization, of preschoolers, 446
Desferal (deferoxamine), for thalassemia, 924
Desmopressin, for enuresis, 537
Dethronement, sibling rivalry and, 420
Detoxification, in substance abuse, 568
Deuteranomaly, 137
Development, 71-95
    biologic
        of adolescent, 514-518, 515b, 516f, 517f
        of infant, 323-327
        of preschooler, 438, 438f
        of school-age child, 493-494, 494f, 502t
        of toddler, 410-411
    cognitive, 79t, 80-81
        in adolescent, 519
        in infant, 327, 330, 330f
        in preschooler, 439
        in school-age child, 439, 502t
        in toddler, 412-413, 413f
    cultural influences in, 52
    definition of, 72
    differentiation in, 72-73
    emotional deprivation and, 88
    family, 32, 32b
    family influences on, 88
    general trends in, 74, 75t
    heredity and, 86
    home care and, 651-653, 653b
    in chronic illness/disability, 583-584, 591-594,
        592t-593t
    in first year, 336t-340t
    individual differences in, 74
    interpersonal relationships in, 88
    language, 81
        in infant, 332
        in preschooler, 439
        in toddler, 415-416
    mass media and, 90-93
    metabolism in, 76-77
    moral, 79t, 81, 439, 495-496, 519-520
        play in, 85-86
    motor, 132
    neglect and, 88
    neuroendocrine factors in, 86
    of body image
        in adolescent, 523-524
        in infant, 330-331, 331f
        in preschooler, 440
        in school-age child, 500
        in toddler, 414-415
    of self-concept, 82-83, 499-500, 523-524
    pace of, 73-74
    physical, 72, 75-77. *See also* Growth.
    physiologic changes in, 76-77
    play in, 83-86
        infant, 330, 331, 333, 333t-334t
        preschooler, 441-442, 441f, 442f
        toddler, 416-417, 416f
    preschooler, 438-442
    psychosexual, 78-79, 79t
    psychosocial, 79-80, 79t

Development *(Continued)*
    in adolescent, 518-519
    in infant, 327
    in preschooler, 438-439
    in school-age child, 494-495, 495f, 503t
    in toddler, 411
    sensitive periods in, 74
    sequence of, 73
    social, 331-333, 415, 416, 440-442, 497-499,
        520-521
    socioeconomic status and, 89
    spiritual, 79t, 81-82, 413-414, 439-440, 496-497
    stages of, 73t
    stress and, 89-90
    temperament and, 77-78
    toddler, 410-422, 418t-419t
Developmental assessment, 93-95, 132
Developmental delay, 611
Developmental history, 109-110
Developmental intervention, high-risk newborn
    and, 261-264
Developmental lactase deficiency, 387
Developmental tasks, 72, 79-80, 79t, 327, 411-412,
    438-439, 494-495
    in chronic illness/disability, 591-594, 592t-593t
Developmental theory, family, 32, 32b
Dexamethasone
    for bacterial meningitis, 1000-1001
    for pain, 177t
Dexamethasone suppression test, for Cushing
    syndrome, 1040
Dextroamphetamine (Dexedrine)
    for attention deficit hyperactivity disorder, 560
    for opioid-related sedation, 179t
Dextrocardia, 209, 219t
Diabetes insipidus, 1030-1031
Diabetes mellitus, 1042-1057
    activity and exercise in, 1047, 1056-1057
    care plan for, 1052-1053
    child/family support in, 1057
    child/family teaching in, 1050-1051
    clinical manifestations of, 1044t
    diagnosis of, 1045
    diet in, 1046-1047, 1051-1054
    exercise in, 1047
    family issues and concerns in, 1049-1050
    glucogenesis in, 1044
    glucose testing in
        in diagnosis, 1045
        in monitoring, 1045, 1046, 1047t, 1055-1056
    glycosuria in, 1044, 1045
    hospitalization in, 1049-1050
    hygiene in, 1056
    hyperglycemia in, 1044, 1048, 1048t, 1056
    hypoglycemia in, 1047-1048, 1048t, 1056, 1056b
    illness management in, 1048-1049
    in adolescents, 1057
    in cystic fibrosis, 796, 799
    insulin for, 1045-1046
        administration of, 1046, 1054-1055
        child/family teaching for, 1054
        dosage of, 1045-1046, 1048
        duration of action of, 1054
        for diabetic ketoacidosis, 1049
        in illness management, 1048-1049
        preparations of, 1045, 1046b
        pump for, 1055
        Somogyi effect and, 1046
        storage of, 1054
    ketoacidosis in, 1044, 1045, 1049
    long-term complications of, 1044
    maternal, 299-300, 299b
    MedicAlert identification in, 1051
    nursing care in, 1049-1058
    nursing process in, 1051

Diabetes mellitus (Continued)
  pathophysiology of, 1043-1044
  polydipsia in, 1044
  polyuria in, 1044
  psychological aspects of, 1049-1050
  record keeping in, 1057
  self-management in, 1057
  Somogyi effect in, 1048
  travel and, 1053
  treatment of, 1045-1049. See also Insulin,
      exogenous.
  type 1, 1043, 1043t
  type 2, 1043, 1043t
Diabetic ketoacidosis, 1044, 1045
  treatment of, 1049
Diabetic nephropathy, 1044
Diabetic neuropathy, 1044
Diabetic retinopathy, 1044
Diagnostic procedures. See Procedures.
Dialysis, 969-971
Diapers
  handling and disposal of, 707
  urine collection from, 712
Diaper dermatitis, 248, 1084
Diaphragm, contraceptive, 545t
Diaphragmatic hernia, 849, 850t
Diaphysis, 75
Diarrhea, 817-823
  acute, 817
  chronic, 817
    nonspecific, 817
  etiology of, 817-820, 818t-820t
  fluid management in, 702
  in celiac disease, 855, 856, 856b
  in inflammatory bowel disease, 833-834
  infectious, 817, 818t-820t
  intractable infantile, 817
  nursing care in, 822-823
  oral rehydration for, 821, 821b
  prevention of, 821-822, 823
  treatment of, 821
Diastasis recti, 148, 219t
Diazepam (Valium)
  for pain, 177t, 178
  for status epilepticus, 1009
  for tetanus, 1168
Dictatorial parent, 40
Diet, 702. See also Nutrition.
  caloric requirements in, 76t
  constipation and, 824, 825b
  cultural aspects of, 58, 61-62, 63, 115
  for adolescent, 527, 527f
  for hyperlipidemia, 894-895, 896
  for weight loss, 553, 555
  growth and, 88
  high-fiber, 824, 825b
  in acute renal failure, 965, 966
  in atopic dermatitis, 1088
  in celiac disease, 856
  in chronic renal failure, 968-969
  in cystic fibrosis, 799, 800-801
  in diabetes mellitus, 1046-1047, 1051-1054
  in diarrhea, 821-823
  in Down syndrome, 622
  in gastroesophageal reflux disease, 828
  in glomerulonephritis, 961
  in infant, 344-347
  in inflammatory bowel disease, 835-836
  in newborn, 228-234
  in toddler, 423-424
  iron sources in, 916
  ketogenic, 553, 1009
  low-cariogenic, 426
  protein requirements in, 76t
  race/ethnicity and, 58

Diet (Continued)
  religion and, 65t-66t
  vegetarian, in infant, 379-380, 380b
Dietary Guidelines for Americans, 553
Dietary history, 109, 114, 115b
Dietary reference intakes (DRIs), 113, 1206-1208
Diethylstilbestrol, 310
Differentiation, 72-73. See also Development.
Difficult temperament, 77-78
Digestion. See also under Gastrointestinal.
  in infant, 324
  in newborn, 199
  in toddler, 411
Digital subtraction angiography, in cerebral dys-
      function, 981t
Digital thermometers, 127b
  for newborns, 206
Digitalis, for congestive heart failure, 878
Digoxin (Lanoxin), for congestive heart failure,
      878, 879-882
Dilated cardiomyopathy, 898-899
Dilaudid. See Hydromorphone (Dilaudid).
Dinamap, 129, 206
Diphenhydramine, for opioid-related pruritus,
      179t
Diphtheria, 454-455
  immunization for, 351
Disability. See Chronic illness/disability.
Discharge planning, 644-646, 678-679
  for abused child, 488
  for newborn, 237-239, 238b
    after hyperbilirubinemia treatment, 280-281
    at high risk, 268-269
  in ambulatory care, 679-680
Discipline, 41-43
  for infant, 341-342
  for school-age child, 501
  in chronic illness/disability, 591
  in cognitive impairment, 618
Disease prevention. See Prevention.
Dishonesty, in school-age child, 501-504
Dislocations, 1111, 1111f
  congenital hip, 1122-1125, 1123f, 1124f
Disorientation, 976b
Disseminated intravascular coagulation, 929, 929b,
      929f
Distal intestinal obstruction syndrome, in cystic
      fibrosis, 796
Distraction, for pain, 172, 173
Distraction therapy
  for limb lengthening, 1121-1122, 1121f
  for scoliosis, 1132-1134
Distress behaviors, in pain, 159
Distributive shock, 902-904, 903t
Diuretics
  for congestive heart failure, 878, 879t, 883-884
  for increased intracranial pressure, 983
Diuril (chlorothiazide), for congestive heart
      failure, 879t
Diversity. See also under Cultural.
  in home care, 648-649
Diverticulum, Meckel, 831-833
Divided custody, 48
Divorce, 33-43, 45-48
  binuclear families and, 34
  blended families and, 33
  joint custody and, 34
  single-parent families and, 33-34
Dizygotic twins, 37, 38b
Dobutamine, in CPR, 808t
Documentation, of nursing process, 17-18, 18b
Docusate sodium, for opioid-related constipation,
      179t
Dog bites, 1083, 1084
Doll's eye reflex, in newborn, 212t

Doll's head maneuver, 978
Dolophine (methadone), 175, 176t
Domestic mimicry, 413
Dopamine, for CPR, 807-809, 808t
Doppler ultrasonography, in blood pressure mea-
      surement, 129
Dornase alfa (Pulmozyme), for cystic fibrosis, 798,
      798f
Dorsal penile nerve block, for circumcision, 227-
      228, 227b
Dorsalis pedis pulse, 146f
Double effect, 603
Down syndrome, 310t, 619-622. See also Cognitive
      impairment.
  palmar crease in, 133, 133f
Drainage, bronchial (postural), 741, 742f
  in cystic fibrosis, 798, 801, 802
Dramatic play, for hospitalized child, 675
Drawing, in communication, 107b
Dreams, sharing of, 106b
Dressings, 1065-1067, 1066t, 1068
  for burns, 1095-1096, 1100
  for intravenous line, 736
  for tracheostomy, 744-745, 745f
  wet, 1069
    for atopic dermatitis, 1069
Droperidol, for opioid-related nausea, 179t
Droplet precautions, 707, 707b
Drowning/near-drowning, 5, 993-995
  in infant, 372
  in toddler, 427t, 431
Drug abuse, 564-568. See also Substance abuse.
Drug reactions
  skin lesions in, 1076, 1085t
  Stevens-Johnson syndrome in, 1085t
Drug therapy. See also specific drugs.
  administration of, 718-732
    family teaching for, 731-732
    in home care, 731-732
    intradermal, 723, 724
    intramuscular, 719-723, 721f, 722f
    intravenous, 725-730
    nasal, 731, 731f
    nasogastric, 730
    optic, 730-731, 731f
    oral, 718-719, 720f
    orogastric, 730
    otic, 731
    rectal, 730
    subcutaneous, 723-724
    via gastrostomy, 730
  dosage in
    calculation of, 717-718
    checking of, 718
  for high-risk newborn, 261
  medication history in, 109
  patient identification for, 718
Drug withdrawal, signs of, in newborn, 302b
Dual-earner families, 48-49
Dubowitz scale, for gestational age assessment, 203
Duchenne muscular dystrophy, 1162-1165, 1163f
Ductus arteriosus, 866, 866f
  closure of, 198-199
  patent, 292t
Duodenal ulcers, 836-838
Duragesic. See Fentanyl.
Dust mite allergy, 787-788, 787b
Duvall's family life cycle stages, 32, 32b
Dwarfism
  hypopituitary, 1024-1027
  psychosocial, 540
Dwyer instrumentation, 1132
Dyad care, 237
Dysacusis, 624
Dysgraphia, 561

Dyslalia, 447
Dyslipidemia, 894-896
Dysmenorrhea, 542
Dysphoria, opioid-related, 180t
Dyspnea, 145b, 757b
Dysrhythmias, 219t, 324, 896-897
Dyssomnias, 347

E
Ear
  alignment of, 137-138, 138f
  examination of, 137-140, 138f-140f
    in newborn, 209, 218t
  foreign bodies in, 140
  in newborn, 272f
    examination of, 209, 218t
    hearing screening and, 223
  structure of, 137-138
Ear drops, administration of, 730, 731
Ear infections, 765-768
  hearing impairment and, 627-628
Ear wax, 138
Ear-based temperature, 126t, 127b, 128
  in newborn, 205-206
Eardrum. See Tympanic membrane.
Early intervention
  developmental, high-risk newborn and, 261-264
  educational, 578
Easy temperament, 77
Eating behavior, 702. See also Eating disorders;
        Feeding.
  in adolescents, 527, 527f
  in autism, 637
  psychologic factors in, 552-553
Eating disorders, 551-559
  anorexia nervosa, 556-559
  binge eating disorder, 556
  bulimia nervosa, 556-559
  not otherwise specified, 556
  obesity, 551-556. See also Obesity.
Ecchymosis, race/ethnicity and, 133t
Eccrine glands, in newborn, 200
Echocardiography, 863
Echovirus, maternal infection with, 306t
ECMO (extracorporeal membrane oxygenation),
        289, 294
Economics, health care, 23
Eczema, 1086-1089, 1087f, 1087t
Edema
  cerebral. See Cerebral edema; Increased intra-
        cranial pressure.
  laryngeal, in anaphylaxis, 905
Education. See also School.
  client/family. See Health/family teaching.
  early intervention in, 578
  early intervention programs in, 55, 578, 613
  home care and, 653
  in attention deficit hyperactivity disorder, 561
  in cerebral palsy, 1151-1152
  in cognitive impairment, 613
  in hearing impairment, 626-627
  in HIV infection, 943
  in hospitalization, 672-673
  in juvenile idiopathic arthritis, 1140
  in visual impairment, 631-632
  learning disabilities and, 559-561
  mainstreaming in, 578, 593-594
Edwards syndrome, 310t
Ego, 78, 412
Ego mastery, 499, 499f
Elbow
  dislocation of, 1111
  nursemaid's, 1111
Elbow restraints, 710
EleCare formula, 232

Electrical burns, 1091. See also Burns.
  prevention of, 371
Electrocardiography, 863
  for dysrhythmias, 896
Electroencephalography, 979, 980t
  for seizures, 1008
Electrolyte disturbances
  in acute renal failure, 966
  in diabetic ketoacidosis, 1049
  transfusion-related, 944t
Electronic pacemakers, 897
Electronic thermometers, 127, 127b
E-mail, privacy of, 99
Emancipated minors, 689
Embolism, air, transfusion-related, 944t
Emergency admission, 680-681, 680b
Emergency contraception, 546t
Emergency medical service (EMS), 805
EMLA cream, 182t, 184
  for circumcision, 226, 227
  for venipuncture, 174, 224b, 717
Emollients, 1066t, 1067
Emotional abuse/neglect, 480, 484b, 485, 486
  developmental effects of, 88
  psychosocial dwarfism due to, 540
Emotional bank, 89
Emotional instability, in adolescent, 519
Empathy, 101
Employment, work-family balance and, 48-49
Empowerment, 10
En face position, attachment and, 215, 234, 234f
Encephalitis, 1002-1003
Encephalocele, 1155b
Encephalopathy
  bilirubin, 277
  hypoxic-ischemic, 293t
Encopresis, 538, 823
Endemic typhus, 1082t
Endocarditis, bacterial, 891-893, 892b
Endocephalography, 980t
Endocrine disorders, 1023-1058
  adrenal, 1037-1042
  in cystic fibrosis, 796, 799-800
  pancreatic, 1042-1057. See also Diabetes
        mellitus.
    in cystic fibrosis, 796, 799
  parathyroid, 1035-1037
  pituitary, 1023-1032
  thyroid, 1032-1035
Endocrine system
  of newborn, 200-201
  structure and function of, 1025t-1027t
End-of-life care. See Death and dying.
Endoscopic third ventriculostomy, 1019
Endotracheal intubation, in CPR, 808t
End-stage liver disease, 841, 841b
End-stage renal disease, 969
End-tidal carbon monoxide, hyperbilirubinemia
        and, 277
Enemas, 750
  air, for intussusception, 853
  antegrade continence, 1157
  retention, for drug administration, 730
Energy needs, 76, 76t
  of high-risk newborn, 258-259
Enteral nutrition, 745-749. See also Nutritional
        support.
  drug administration in, 730
  for high-risk newborn, 256
  gastrostomy feeding in, 746-749
  gavage feeding in, 745-746, 747
  in congestive heart failure, 883
  in inflammatory bowel disease, 835, 836
  in necrotizing enterocolitis, 298
Enteric fever, 817-823, 818t. See also Diarrhea.

Enterobiasis, 468-469, 470b
Enterocolitis, 817-821, 818t-820t. See also
        Diarrhea.
  necrotizing, 297-298, 298b
Enterohepatic circulation, 275
Enterostomies, 750-751
Enterovirus, maternal infection with, 306t
Enucleation, 634-635
Enuresis, 537-538. See also Urinary incontinence.
  in sickle cell anemia, 921-922
  in syndrome of inappropriate antidiuretic
        hormone secretion, 1031
Environmental hazards, development and, 89
Enzymatic débridement, 1066t
Eosinophils, 200
  measurement of, 913t
Epicanthal fold, 136, 136f
Epidemic typhus, 1082t
Epidemiology, 22-23, 23f
Epidermal injuries, 1062. See also Wounds.
Epidermal stripping, 701
Epidural analgesia, 182t, 183-184
Epidural hematoma, 987f, 988
Epiglottitis, 769, 769t
Epilepsy, 1005-1016. See also Seizures.
Epinephrine, 1026t, 1037
  for anaphylaxis, 905
  for CPR, 807-809, 808t
Epiphyseal cartilage plate, 75
  injuries of, 1112
Epiphysis, 75
Epispadias, 220t, 958t
Epistaxis, 929-930
Epithelial pearls, 210, 220t
Epithelium, cultured, for burns, 1099
Epstein's pearls, 209, 218t
Equianalgesia, 178, 180t
Erb-Duchenne palsy, 211, 246-247, 247f
Ergocalciferol, 391t
Erikson's developmental tasks, 79-80, 79t, 327,
        411-412, 438-439, 494-495
Erosions, 1064f
Erythema, race/ethnicity and, 133t
Erythema infectiosum, 306t, 456-457, 456f
Erythema migrans, 1082-1083, 1083f
Erythema multiforme, 1085t
Erythema toxicum, 217t, 247-248
Erythroblastosis fetalis, 281-284, 282f, 282t
Erythrocytes. See Red blood cells.
Erythromycin, in ophthalmia neonatorum pro-
        phylaxis, 222
Escherichia coli infection
  gastrointestinal, 818t
  meningeal, 998-1002
Esophageal atresia, 846-849, 847f
Esotropia, 629t
Estimated average requirement, 113
Estrogen, 1026t, 1027t
  for dysmenorrhea, 542
  for Turner syndrome, 540, 541t
  in puberty, 514-515
Etanercept, for juvenile idiopathic arthritis, 1140
Ethical decision making, 13-14
  AMA Code of Ethics and, 14, 14b
  case study of, 621
  double effect in, 603
Ethical issues
  autonomy, 13
  beneficence, 13
  confidentiality, 99, 544
  in end-of-life care, 595-596
  in hospitalization, 669
  justice, 13
  nonmaleficence, 13
  parental notification, 544

Ethical issues *(Continued)*
  placebos, 178
  suicidal behavior, 570
  treatment withholding, 269, 621, 802
Ethnocentrism, 54
Euthanasia, 595-596. *See also* Treatment withholding.
Evaluation, in nursing process, 17
Evaporated milk formula, 233
Evaporative heat loss, 254
Evidence-based practice, 14-15, 15b, 15t
  nursing process and, 15, 15t
Evil eye, 62
Evoked potentials, 979
Ewing sarcoma, 1137-1138
Exanthem subitum, 456-457, 456f
Exchange transfusion. *See also* Transfusion.
  for hemolytic disease of newborn, 282-283
  for sickle cell anemia, 920-921
Excoriation, 1064f
Exencephaly, 1155b
Exercise. *See* Activity and exercise.
Exercise-induced asthma, 789
Exercises
  for scoliosis, 1132
  in coma, 985
Exhibitionism, 482
Exotropia, 629t
Exstrophy
  bladder, 958t
  cloacal, 854
Extended family, 33
Extension posturing, 979, 979f
External fixation, for distraction, 1121, 1121f
Extracellular fluid, 814
Extracorporeal membrane oxygenation, for newborn, 289, 294
Extravasation, in intravenous therapy, 738
Extremities. *See also under* Limb *and specific structures.*
  examination of, 152, 152f
    in newborn, 210-211, 211f, 220t
  prosthetics for, 1121-1122, 1127
Extremity venipuncture, positioning for, 710
Extrusion reflex, 212t
Eye
  "black," 630
  blood vessels of, 135, 135f
  cancer of, 633-635, 634f
  in newborn, 201, 208, 212t, 218t
  infections of, 630
  injuries of, 630, 633
  lazy, 135-136, 136f
  ophthalmia neonatorum prophylaxis and, 222
  prosthetic, 634-635, 634f
  structure of, 134f, 135f
  surgical removal of, 634-635
Eye care, in coma, 985
Eye contact
  cultural aspects of, 61
  in attachment, 222
Eye drops, administration of, 730-731, 731f
Eye examination, 134-137
  external structures in, 134-135, 134f
  funduscopic, 135, 135f
  in neurologic examination, 977-978, 978f
  in newborn, 208, 212t, 218t
  ocular alignment in, 135-136, 136f
  ophthalmoscopic, 135, 135f
  photoscreening, 136
  vision testing in, 135-137
Eyeglasses, 633
Eyelid, examination of, 134, 134f

F
Face, examination of, 132, 134
FACES Pain Rating Scale, 162t, 164
Facial nerve, assessment of, 155t
Facial paralysis, in newborn, 246, 246f
Facilitated communication, in hearing impairment, 626, 627
Facilitated tucking, 173, 262
Facilitative response, 106b
Facioscapulohumeral muscular dystrophy, 1162, 1163f
Factor VIII concentrate, for hemophilia, 926, 927
Factor VIII deficiency, 925-927
Factor IX deficiency, 925-927
Failure to thrive, 396-400. *See also* Growth failure.
  classification of, 397
  diagnosis of, 398
  factors in, 398
  feeding in, 399
  nursing care management of, 398-400, 399b, 399f
  prognosis of, 398
  treatment of, 398
Faith healing, 63-64
Falls, prevention of, 706
  in infants, 370
  in toddlers, 428t, 433
Family, 39-50
  abusive, 482
  affinal relationships in, 30
  blended (reconstituted), 33, 48
  communal, 34
  consanguineous relationships in, 30
  cultural values of, 67t-69t. *See also under* Cultural; Culture.
  definition of, 111
  developmental influence of, 88
  developmental stages of, 32, 32b
  dual-earner, 48-49
  extended, 33
  foster, 48
  functioning of, 34-35, 34b
  gay/lesbian, 34
  homeless, 54, 59
  immigrant, 54-55, 59
  North American, 56
  nuclear, 33
  nursing interventions for, 32-33, 33b
  of high-risk infant, 264-265, 265b
  of infant with SIDS, 403-404
  of special needs child, 579-583
  polyandric, 34
  polygamous, 34
  polygynous, 34
  roles and relationships in, 35-38. *See also* Parents; Siblings.
  single-parent, 33-34, 47-48
  size and configuration of, 35-36
  sororal/nonsororal, 34
  strengths of, 34-35, 34b
  stressors on, 32
  structure of, 33-34, 111, 112b
    newborn discharge and, 238
Family advocacy, 11-12
Family and Medical Leave Act, 49
Family assessment, 111, 112b-113b
  in home care, 650-651
Family bed, 349
  SIDS and, 402
Family boundaries, 31-32
Family caregivers, 641-655. *See also* Home care.
Family history, 111
Family life cycle, 32, 32b
Family of origin, 30
Family planning, 544-547, 544t-546t
Family stress theory, 31t, 32
Family systems theory, 30-32, 31t
Family teaching. *See* Health/family teaching.
Family theories, 30-32, 31t
Family-centered care, 10, 11b, 648-655. *See also* Home care.
  attachment process and, siblings in, 236, 236f, 267, 267f
  child safety home checklist and, 373
  cultural aspects of, 577
  guidance during adolescence and, 533
  guidance during school years and, 511
  guidelines for, 12
  helping children in school and, 501
  hyperbilirubinemia and, 280-281
  immunizations and, 360
  in chronic illness/disability, 576-578
  in hospitalization, 668-670
  infant feeding and, 346
  of high-risk newborn, 265-266
  sexual abuse and, 490
  shared decision making in, 577
  SIDS and, 403-404
Family-work balance, 48-49
Famotidine, for abdominal pain, 193
Fanconi syndrome, 924-925
Fasting, preoperative, 696, 696t, 732-733
  oral care in, 732
Fat
  body. *See also* Obesity.
    measurement of, 124
  brown, 199
  dietary, in hyperlipidemia, 894-895, 896
Father. *See also* Family; Parents.
  parent-infant attachment and, 235-236, 236f
  single, 47-48
Fatigue
  in newborn, 263t
  in radiation therapy, 938
Faucial tonsils, 763, 763f
Fears
  about surgery, 694-695
  in infants, 332, 335, 348t
  in preschoolers, 446
  in school-age children, 504
  in toddlers, 434
  of blood loss, 715-716
  of body alteration, 672, 694
  of dying child, 602-604
  of hospitalized child, 659-661, 668-670, 672
Febrile seizures, 704, 1016
Fecal incontinence, 538
  antegrade continence enema for, 1157
  in coma, 984-985
  in spina bifida, 1157
  in spinal cord injuries, 1171
Feces. *See* Stool.
Feedback, in family, 31
Feeding, 702, 745-746, 746f. *See also* Eating behavior.
  gavage, 745-746, 746f, 747. *See also* Enteral nutrition.
  in cerebral palsy, 1150, 1152f
  in cleft lip/cleft palate, 845
  in congestive heart failure, 883
  in Down syndrome, 622
  infant, 344-347. *See also* Breastfeeding; Formula feeding.
    difficulties with, 395-400
    failure to thrive and, 399
    growth patterns and, 122
    high-risk, 255-258, 298
  newborn, 228-234
  trophic, 256
    in necrotizing enterocolitis, 298

Feeding readiness, 257, 257f
Feeding resistance, 258
Feet. *See* Foot.
Female athlete triad, 557
Female condom, 545t
Female genital mutilation, 64b, 151, 228
Femoral head, aseptic necrosis of, 1128-1130
Femoral hernia, 148-149
Femoral pulse, 146f, 149, 149f
  in newborn, 210, 219t
Femoral venipuncture, positioning for, 710, 710f
Fentanyl, 175, 180t, 181t, 184
  abuse of, 567
  dosage of, 176t
  for burns, 1096
  for preoperative sedation, 696
  transdermal, 183
  transmucosal, 181t
Fetal alcohol syndrome, 303, 311t
Fetal asphyxia, 198
Fetal hemoglobin, in sickle cell anemia, 917, 921
Fetal shunts, closure of, 198
Fever, 702-705
  clinical definition of, 125b
  in coma, 984
  in Kawasaki disease, 901, 902
  in respiratory infections, 758
  seizures and, 704, 1016
  telephone triage for, 704
  temperature measurement in, 125-129, 125b, 125t-127t
  transfusion-related, 944t
Fever blisters, 465
Fiber, dietary, 824, 825b
Fiberoptic blanket, for hyperbilirubinemia, 278, 278f
Fibrinolysis, 925
Fifth disease, 456-457, 456f
Fine motor development, 325, 325f, 336t-340t, 438, 506
Finger spelling, 633
Fingernails
  assessment of, 132
  hematoma under, 1111
Fingers, clubbing of, 884, 884f
Finger-to-nose test, 153b
Fire ant stings, 1077t
Firearms, adolescents and, 532
First do no harm, 11
First-pass effect, 178
Fissures, 1064f
Fistulas
  arteriovenous, in dialysis, 971
  omphalomesenteric, 831
  tracheoesophageal, 846-849, 847f
FLACC Postoperative Pain Tool, 161, 161t
Flea bites, 247-248, 1077t
Fleet enema, 750
Flexion, in newborn, 207, 217t
Flexion creases, 133, 133f
Flexion posturing, 979, 979f
Flu, 764-765
  bird, 775-776
  Reye syndrome and, 703
Fluid
  extracellular, 814
  intracellular, 814
Fluid balance
  basal metabolic rate and, 815
  body surface area and, 814-815
  daily requirements for, 76, 815b
  determinants of, 814-815
  in infant, 325, 814-815
  in newborn, 199, 254
    hydration and, 255

Fluid balance (*Continued*)
  insensible losses and, 254, 814
  intake in, 76
  maintenance of, 732-738. *See also* Fluid management.
  renal function and, 815
Fluid management, 702, 732-738
  in acute renal failure, 966
  in adrenocortical insufficiency, 1038
  in burns, 1096
  in coma, 984
  in congestive heart failure, 878, 879t, 883-884, 885
  in diabetic ketoacidosis, 1049
  in diarrhea, 821, 821b
  in high-risk newborn, 255
  in hypoxemia, 885
  in respiratory infections, 758-759
  in resuscitation, 807-809, 904
  in shock, 904, 905
  in syndrome of inappropriate antidiuretic hormone secretion, 1031-1032
  intake and output measurement in, 732-733, 950
Fluid overload, transfusion-related, 944t
Fluid restriction, 732-733. *See also* Fluid management.
Fluid resuscitation, 807-809, 904, 905
  in near-drowning, 993-994
Fluid therapy, parenteral, 733-738. *See also* Intravenous administration, of fluids.
Flunitrazepam (Rohypnol), 549, 567
Fluoride, 393t
  dental health and, 349-350, 425, 426t
Fluoxetine, for bulimia nervosa, 558
Flush, 700
Flutter mucus clearance device, 798, 798f
Foam dressings, 1066t
Folic acid, 390t
  for spina bifida prevention, 1157
Folk medicine, 63. *See also* Complementary and alternative therapies.
Follicle-stimulating hormone, 1025t
Folliculitis, 1069-1071, 1070t
Follow-up formulas, 232-233
Fontanels, 207, 208f, 217t
Food. *See also* Diet; Feeding; Nutrition.
  aspiration of
    by infant, 367-368
    by toddler, 433
  "hot/cold," 63
  solid, for infants, 345-347
Food customs, 61-62, 63, 115
Food diary, 114
Food frequency questionnaire, 114
Food sensitivity, 384-388, 385b, 386b
Foot
  athlete's, 1073t
  catheter toes and, 255
  club, 1125-1126, 1126f
  congenital deformities of, 1125-1127
  examination of, 152
    in newborn, 211, 211f
  infant shoes and, 343
  of preterm infant, 272f
Foramen ovale, 198, 866, 866f
Foreign bodies
  aspiration of, 86, 87, 705-706, 780-781, 809-810
    by infant, 365-368, 366b-367b
    by toddler, 433
  in ear, 140
  in eye, 465b
  in skin, 1076
  ingestion of, by infant, 370-371
Foreign language speakers, communication with, 60-61, 62, 101-102

Foreskin, 210
  surgical removal of, 225-228. *See also* Circumcision.
Formal operations stage, 79t, 80
Formula feeding, 231-232, 344-345
  alternate milk products in, 233
  available formulas for, 232-233
  growth patterns and, 122
  iron deficiency anemia and, 915-916
  preparation of formula for, 233
  schedules for, 233
  stools and, in newborns, 200b
  weaning from, 347
Foster family, 48
Fovea centralis, 135, 135f, 201
Fowler's spiritual development theory, 79t, 81-82
Fractures, 1112-1121
  casts for, 1115-1117, 1116f, 1117f
  clinical manifestations of, 1113, 1114b
  diagnosis of, 1113
  during birth, 246
  emergency care for, 1114-1115
  epiphyseal injury in, 1112
  etiology of, 1112
  external fixation for, 1121, 1121f
  healing of, 1113
  in osteogenesis imperfecta, 1112, 1127-1128, 1128b
  nursing care for, 1114-1115
  of clavicle, 1112
  of skull, 988, 991. *See also* Head injury.
    during birth, 246
  reduction of, 1114
  stress, 539
  treatment of, 1114
  types of, 1112-1113, 1113b, 1113f
  vascular injury in, 1115
Fragile X syndrome, 622-623
Frenotomy, 209
Frenulum, 209
Freudian theory, psychosexual development in, 78-79, 79t
Friction, pressure ulcers and, 701
Friends, 55-56
  of adolescent, 521, 521f
  of school-age child, 497-498
Frontal bossing, 1017
Frontal suture, 208f
Frostbite, 1103-1104
Frustration, in preschoolers, 447
Fulminant hepatitis, 840
Functional abdominal pain, 562-563, 829
Functional asplenia, in sickle cell anemia, 921
Funduscopic examination, 135, 135f
  in neurologic examination, 978
Fungal infections
  of skin, 1071-1074, 1073f, 1073t, 1074t
  systemic, 1072-1074, 1074t
Furosemide (Lasix), for congestive heart failure, 879t
Furuncles, 1069-1071, 1070t

G

Gabapentin, for pain, 177t
Gag reflex, 141
  in newborn, 212t
Gait, assessment of, 152
Galactogogues, 230, 379
Galactosemia, 315-316
Galant reflex, 212t
Galeazzi sign, 1123f, 1124
Games, 84. *See also* Play.
  for hospitalized children, 673-674
  quiet, for school-age child, 499
Gamma globulin, for Kawasaki disease, 902

Gamma-hydroxybutyric acid (GHB), as date rape drug, 549
Gang violence, 498
Gardasil, 359
Gardner-Wells tongs, 1119
Gastric bypass surgery, 554
Gastric decontamination, for poisoning, 473
Gastric lavage, 473, 474
Gastric ulcers, 836-838
Gastric washing, for sputum collection, 780
Gastroenteritis, infectious, 817-823, 818t-820t. See also Diarrhea.
Gastroesophageal reflux disease, 823f, 827-829
Gastrointestinal disorders, 813-857
    abdominal migraine, 829
    appendicitis, 829-832
    celiac disease, 855-856, 856t
    cirrhosis, 841-842
    cleft lip/cleft palate, 843-846, 847
    clinical manifestations of, 815b
    constipation, 823-825
    Crohn disease, 833-836
    dehydration in, 814-817
    end-stage liver disease, 841, 841b
    esophageal atresia, 846-849, 847f
    functional abdominal pain, 829
    gastroesophageal reflux disease, 823f, 827-829
    hepatic, 838-843
    hepatitis, 839-841
    hernias, 849, 850f
    Hirschsprung disease, 825-826, 825f
    hypertrophic pyloric stenosis, 849-852
    in cystic fibrosis, 796, 797b, 799
    in immobilization, 1108t
    inflammatory, 829-843
    inflammatory bowel disease, 833-836
    intussusception, 852-853, 852f
    irritable bowel syndrome, 829
    malabsorption syndromes, 855-857
    malrotation, 853
    obstructive, 849-855
    short bowel syndrome, 856-857
    structural, 843-849
    tracheoesophageal fistula, 846-849, 847f
    ulcerative colitis, 833-836
    volvulus, 853
    vomiting, 826-827
Gastrointestinal hypersensitivity, immediate, 385
Gastrointestinal priming, of high-risk newborn, 256
    with necrotizing enterocolitis, 298
Gastrointestinal system
    of infant, 324
    of newborn, 199, 200b
        vitamin K and, 222, 292t
Gastroschisis, 219t, 849, 850t
Gastrostomy tube, for feeding, 746-749. See also Nutritional support.
    drug administration via, 730
Gauge, needle, 720
Gauze dressings, 1066t
Gavage feeding, 745-746, 746f, 747. See also Nutritional support.
    of high-risk newborn, 257-258
Gay and lesbian adolescents, suicide by, 569
Gay and lesbian family, 34
Gaze, cardinal positions of, 154f
Gel dressings, 1066t
Gender identity, development of, 415, 519
General systems theory, 30
Genetic counseling, 317-318
Genetic evaluation, 316-317, 317t
Genetic factors, in disease susceptibility, 58. See also specific diseases.
    newborn screening and, 223

Genitals
    ambiguous, 958t
        in congenital adrenal hyperplasia, 1040-1041
    anomalies of, 957, 958t
    cleansing of, 701
    examination of, 149-151, 150f, 151f, 542-543
        in newborn, 210, 219t-220t
        female, 150-151, 151f, 542
            in newborn, 200, 210, 219t, 272f
            mutilation of, 64b, 151, 228
        in newborn
            circumcision and, 225-228
            examination of, 210, 219t-220t
            female, 200-201, 210, 219t, 272f
            male, 210, 220t, 272f
        male, 149-150, 150f, 542-543
            disorders of, 542-543
            in newborn, 210, 220t, 272f
Genital herpes, 547, 548t, 1072t
Genital stage, 79
Genital surgery
    nursing care in, 958
    psychological aspects of, 957-958
Genital warts, 547, 548t
Genitourinary disorders, 949-971
    acute glomerulonephritis, 961-962
    acute renal failure, 965-967
    clinical manifestations of, 950, 955t
    congenital, 957, 958t
    glomerular, 958-962
    hemolytic uremic syndrome, 962-963, 963b, 965
    laboratory findings in, 950, 951t-954t
    nephrotic syndrome, 958-962, 960f
    nursing care in, 950, 958
    obstructive, 956-957
    surgery for
        nursing care in, 958
        psychologic aspects of, 957-958
    urinary tract infections, 950-956
    Wilms tumor, 963-965, 963b, 964b
Genu valgum, 152, 152f
Genu varum, 152, 152f
German measles. See Rubella.
Germinal matrix/intraventricular hemorrhage, 293t
Gestational age, 202f-205f, 203-205, 204b
    high-risk newborn and, 250b
GHB (g-hydroxybutyric acid), in date rape, 549
Giant pigmented nevus, 249
Giardiasis, 466-468, 468b, 468f
Gingiva, 142
Gingivitis, 507
Gingivostomatitis, herpetic, 465
Glabellar reflex, 212t
Glans, 150
Glasgow Coma Scale, 976-977, 977f
Glass ampules, 720
Glasses, 633
Glaucoma, 629t
Glenn shunt, 886f, 886t
Glomerular disease, 958-962
Glomerulonephritis, acute, 961-962
Glossopharyngeal nerve, assessment of, 155t
Gloves, 707-708
Glucagon, 1026t
    for diabetic hypoglycemia, 1048
Glucocorticoids
    endogenous, 1026t, 1037
    exogenous. See Corticosteroids.
Glucogenesis, in diabetes mellitus, 1044
Glucose, for venipuncture pain, 174, 224b
Glucose testing, in diabetes mellitus
    in diagnosis, 1045
    in monitoring, 1045, 1046, 1047t, 1055-1056
Glucosuria, 953t

Glucuronyl transferase, newborn liver function and, 199
Gluten-sensitive enteropathy, 855-856, 856t
Glycosuria, in diabetes mellitus, 1044, 1045
Glycosylated hemoglobin, in diabetes monitoring, 1046
Goals, definition of, 25
Goat's milk, 233
Goiter, 1033
Gomco technique, 228
Gonadotropins, 1025t
Gonorrhea, 547, 548t
    maternal, 306t
    ophthalmia neonatorum due to, 222
Gowns, 707-708
Graduated extinction method, for night crying, 348
Graft
    arteriovenous, in dialysis, 971
    organ. See Transplantation.
Graft versus host disease, 945-946
Granisetron, for opioid-related nausea, 179t
Granulation tissue
    at gastrostomy site, 747, 748f
    in wound healing, 1062
Granulocyte-macrophage colony-stimulating factor, for aplastic anemia, 925
Grasp
    palmar, 325
    pincer, 325, 325f
Grasp reflex, 152, 211, 211f
    in newborn, 212t
    in preterm infant, 273f
    psychosocial development and, 327
Gratification, delayed, 327
Graves disease, 1034-1035, 1034b
Grazing, as toddler nutritional approach, 423
Greenstick fractures, 1113f
Grief, 605-607
    anticipatory, 265, 605
    complicated, 605
    in children, 605
    in chronic illness/disability, 583
    parental, 606
    sibling, 606-607
Groshong catheter, 727t
Gross motor development, 325-327, 326f, 327f, 336t-340t, 438
Groups
    peer, 56
    primary, 53
    secondary, 53
Group A b-hemolytic streptococci, 755
    pharyngitis due to, 762-763
Group care, work-based, for infants, 340
Group identity, of adolescent, 518
Growth
    arm circumference and, 124
    assessment of, 121-124, 123f, 124f, 1028b
    biologic determinants of, 75
    body fat in, 122
    bone age and, 75, 1028b
    delayed, 540
    development and, 72. See also Development.
    directional, 72, 73f
    ethnic differences in, 122
    general trends in, 74, 75t
    head circumference and, 124
    height in, 75
    in acromegaly, 1029
    in adolescents, 514, 515-516, 518
    in health history, 109-110
    in infants, 323, 336t-340t
    in preschoolers, 438
    in school-age children, 493, 502t-503t

Growth (Continued)
  in toddlers, 410, 418t
  individual differences in, 74
  intrauterine, gestational age and, 203f, 204
  neuroendocrine factors in, 86
  normal variations in, 122, 123f
  nutrition and, 88
  of breast-fed vs. formula-fed infants, 122
  patterns of, 72-74, 73f
  proportional, 74
  rates of, 74, 74f
  reference ranges for, 1180-1191
  sensitive periods in, 74
  skeletal, 75-76
  skinfold thickness and, 124
  sleep and rest and, 77
  weight in, 75
Growth charts, 121-122, 1180-1191
Growth failure, 396-400, 540
  in chronic renal disease, 968
  in cystic fibrosis, 796-797, 800
  in hypopituitarism, 1024-1027
  psychosocial factors in, 540
Growth hormone, 1025t
  deficiency of, in hypopituitarism, 1024-1029
  excess of, in pituitary hyperfunction, 1029
Growth plate, 75
Growth spurt, 515
Guided imagery, for pain, 172
Guidelines for Adolescent Preventive Services
    (GAPS), 524-525
Guides, for visually impaired, 631
Guillain-Barré syndrome, 1165-1167, 1166b
Guilt
  in chronic illness/disability, 582
  in preschooler, 438
Gums, 142
Guns, adolescents and, 532
Guthrie blood test, 314
Gynecologic examination, 542
Gynecomastia, 144, 515, 543

H

H₂ receptor antagonists, for peptic ulcers, 837
Habits, in health history, 110, 110b
Habituation, neonatal, 213b
Haemophilus influenzae meningitis, 998-1002
Haemophilus influenzae type B vaccine, 357
Hair
  axillary, 132
  examination of, 132
  lanugo, 207
  nits in, 1079-1081
  pubic, 132
    in female, 151, 517f
    in male, 150, 517f
Hair care, 702
Hair follicles, in newborn, 200
Hair loss, 1085t
  in chemotherapy, 937
Hallucinations, opioid-related, 180t
Hallucinogens, 567
Halo vest, 1119, 1119f
Haloperidol, for opioid-related hallucinations,
    180t
Halotype, 945
Hand, flexion creases in, 133, 133f
Hard palate, 142, 142f
Hard-of-hearing, 623. See also Hearing
    impairment.
Hardy-Rand-Ritter test, 137
Harlequin color change, 217t
Harrington rods, 1132
Harvest mites, 1077t
Hashimoto disease, 1033-1034

Head. See also Skull.
  examination of, 133-134
    in newborn, 207, 208f, 217t
  growth of, 323
Head circumference, 124, 1187
  in newborn, 204, 216t
  in toddler, 410
Head control
  in infant, 325, 326f
  in newborn, 207, 208f
Head injury, 986-993
  cerebral edema in, 989
  cerebral lacerations in, 987-988
  complications of, 988-989
    long-term, 990
  concussions in, 987
  coup/contrecoup injury in, 986-987, 987f
  epidural hemorrhage in, 987f, 988
  etiology of, 986
  evaluation in, 989-990
  family support in, 992
  imaging studies in, 990
  in child abuse, 987-988
  increased intracranial pressure in, 898, 986, 988
  initial assessment in, 989-990
  pathophysiology of, 986-988, 987f
  prevention of, 993
  rehabilitation in, 992-993
  skull fractures in, 988
  subdural hemorrhage in, 987f, 988-989
  treatment of, 990-992
Head lag, 207, 208f
Head lice, 1079-1081
Head tilt–jaw thrust, 805, 806f
Head trauma, during birth, 244-246, 245f
Headache
  pain management for, 192
  postcraniotomy, 997
Headache diary, 192
Head-to-heel length, of newborn, 205, 205f, 216t
Head-to-tail growth, 72
Health beliefs and practices, 60, 62-64, 67t-69t
Health care
  access to, 2
  economic aspects of, 23
  in school, 508
Health care costs, home care and, 642
Health history. See History.
Health Insurance Portability and Accountability
    Act (HIPAA), 689
Health problems. See Illness.
Health promotion, 2. See also Pediatric nursing.
  dental care in, 3
  developmental influences on, 71-95. See also
    Development.
  disease prevention and, 12-13
  education in, 13. See also Health/family teaching.
  family in, 29-50. See also Family.
  immunizations in, 3
  in community-based nursing care, 21
  injury prevention in, 3-6
  nutrition in, 2-3
  substance abuse prevention in, 7-8
  violence prevention in, 6-7
Health/family teaching
  for compliance, 699-700
  for congenital heart disease, 888-889
  for drug administration, 731-732
  for HIV/AIDS, 941-942
  for newborn disease screening, 223
  for newborn home care, 237-238
    with high-risk infant, 264-265
  for nutritional support, 750
  for procedures, 692-693
    circumcision, 227

Health/family teaching (Continued)
  for stoma care, 751
  in chronic illness/disability, 584-585, 679
  in diabetes mellitus, 1050-1051
  in home care, 650, 678-679, 704-705
  in hospitalization, 675-676, 678-679
  in sickle cell anemia, 921-922
Healthy People 2010, 2, 2b
  breastfeeding and, 229
Hearing
  assessment of, 140, 141t
    in newborn, 209, 223
  in adolescent, 529
  in coma, 985
  in infant, 325
  in newborn, 201, 209, 223
  in toddler, 410
Hearing aids, 624, 625
Hearing impairment
  classification of, 624t
  communication in, 626-627
  conductive, 623
  definition of, 623
  diagnosis of, 140, 141t
    in newborn, 209, 223
  etiology of, 623
  family/child support in, 627
  hospitalization and, 627
  in bacterial meningitis, 1001
  noise-induced, 628
  nursing care for, 625-628
  pathology of, 623-624
  prevention of, 627-628
  sensorineural, 623-624
  severity of, 624, 624t
  treatment of, 624-625
  with visual impairment, 633
Hearing tests, 140, 141t
  in newborn, 209, 223
Hearing threshold, 624, 624t
Heart. See also under Cardiac; Cardiovascular.
  examination of, 145-147, 147f, 147t
    in newborn, 209-210, 219t
    in school-age child, 494
  position of, 145, 146f
Heart disease, 861-907
  acquired, 862, 891-899
    bacterial endocarditis, 891-893
    cardiomyopathy, 898-899
    dysrhythmias, 896-897
    rheumatic, 893-894
  cardiac catheterization in, 863-864
  congenital, 862-891. See also Congenital heart
    disease.
  diagnosis of, 862-864
  echocardiography in, 863
  electrocardiography in, 863
  history in, 862
  Kawasaki disease, 901
  nursing care in, 864-865
  physical examination in, 862
  transplantation for, 899
Heart failure. See Congestive heart failure.
Heart murmurs, 147, 148t
  in newborn, 210
Heart rate
  in infant, 324
  in newborn, 209
Heart sounds, 146-147, 147f, 147t
  in newborn, 209, 210
Heart transplantation, 899
Heart valves, 146
  abnormalities of, 871-872
Heat loss, in newborn, 221, 254, 254f
Heat regulation, in newborn, 199
Heat therapy, for juvenile idiopathic arthritis, 1141

Heavy metal poisoning, 475. *See also* Lead poisoning.
Heel lance, 715, 716f, 717
Heel sticks. *See* Venipuncture.
Heel-to-ear maneuver
    in newborn, 204b
    in preterm infant, 273f
Heel-to-shin test, 153b
Height. *See also* Growth.
    ethnic differences in, 122, 123f
    measurement of, 122-123, 123f
    normal increase in, 75, 75t, 323
    of adolescent, 515
    of preschooler, 438
    of toddler, 410
    reference ranges for, 1180-1191
    sitting, of newborn, 204-205, 216t
Heimlich maneuver, 809-810, 810f
Helicobacter pylori infection, in peptic ulcer disease, 836-838
Heliox, for status asthmaticus, 790-791
HELLP syndrome, 299
Helmet, for plagiocephaly, 400, 401f
Hemangiomas
    capillary (strawberry), 249-250, 249f
    cavernous venous, 250
Hemarthrosis, in hemophilia, 927
Hematologic disorders, 912-939
    anemia, 912-925
    complete blood count in, 912, 913t
    hemostatic, 925-930
    malignant, 930-939
Hematoma
    epidural, 987f, 988
    periorbital, 630
    subdural, 987f, 988-989
    subungual, 1111
Hematopoietic system, of newborn, 199
Hemimelia, 220t
Hemodialysis, 969-971
Hemofiltration, in chronic renal failure, 970
Hemoglobin
    fetal, in sickle cell anemia, 917, 921
    glycosylated, in diabetes monitoring, 1046
    measurement of, 913t
Hemoglobinopathies, 916
Hemolytic disease of the newborn, 281-284, 282f, 282t
Hemolytic transfusion reaction, 944t, 945
Hemolytic uremic syndrome, 962-963, 963b, 965
Hemophilia, 925-927
Hemopoietic system, development of, 324
Hemoptysis, in cystic fibrosis, 799
Hemorrhage. *See* Bleeding.
Hemorrhagic cystitis
    cyclophosphamide-induced, 937
    in chemotherapy, 937
Hemorrhagic disease of the newborn, 222, 292t
Hemorrhagic disorders. *See* Hemostatic disorders.
Hemostasis, 925
Hemostatic disorders, 925-930
    disseminated intravascular coagulation, 929, 929b, 929f
    epistaxis, 929-930
    hemophilia, 925-927
    idiopathic thrombocytopenic purpura, 927-929
Heparin, for catheter flushing, 726, 728t
Heparin lock, 725, 726
Hepatic disorders, 838-843
    biliary atresia, 842-843
    cirrhosis, 841-842
    end-stage liver disease, 841, 841b
    hepatitis, 839-841
    liver transplant for, 841-842, 843
Hepatic portoenterostomy, for biliary atresia, 842

Hepatic transplantation, 841-842, 843
Hepatitis
    chronic active, 840
    fulminant, 840
    subacute, 840
Hepatitis A, 838, 839t, 840-841
    immunization for, 351
Hepatitis B, 838-839, 839t, 840-841
    immunization for, 351
        in newborn, 222-223
    maternal transmission of, 306t
Hepatitis C, 839-841, 839t
Hepatitis D, 840
Hepatitis E, 840
Hepatitis G, 840
Hermaphroditism, 958t
Hernias, 849, 850f
    diaphragmatic, 849, 850t
    femoral, 148-149
    inguinal, 148, 150, 958t
        in newborn, 210
    umbilical, 148
Heroin, 567
Herpes genitalis, 547, 548t, 1072t
Herpes labialis, 1072t
    recurrent, 465
Herpes progenitalis, 547, 548t
Herpes simplex encephalitis, 1002-1003
Herpes simplex infection, in newborn, 222, 248-249
Herpes zoster, 463, 1072t
Herpetic gingivostomatitis, 465
Hiatal hernia, 849, 850t
Hickman catheter, 725-730, 727t
High chair, fall from, 370
High-density lipoproteins, in hyperlipidemia, 894-896
High-fiber diet, 824, 825b
High-risk newborn, 250-318. *See also under* Newborn.
Hinduism, 65t
Hip
    developmental dysplasia of, 1122-1125, 1123f, 1124f
    dislocation of, 1111
HIPAA (Health Insurance Portability and Accountability Act), 689
Hirschberg test, 136, 136f
Hirschsprung disease, 825-826, 825f
Hispanics. *See also* Race/ethnicity.
    health beliefs and practices of, 67t
    Spanish-English translation for, 1204
Histoplasmosis, 1074t
History, 107-113
    allergy, 109
    birth, 109
    chief complaint in, 107-108
    components of, 108b
    developmental, 109-110
    dietary, 109, 114, 115b
    direct vs. indirect, 107
    family, 111
    habits in, 110, 110b
    immunizations in, 109
    informant in, 107
    medication, 109
    nursing admission, 665, 666b-667b
    of present illness, 108, 108b
    of previous illnesses, 109
    psychosocial, 111-113
    review of systems in, 113, 114
    sexual, 110-111
HIV/AIDS, 547, 939-943
    in hemophilia, 927
    maternal infection with, 305t
    newborn screening for, 223

Hives, 1085t
HLA matching, 945, 946
Hodgkin disease, 937-939
Home care, 10, 11b, 577, 578, 641-655
    advance care planning in, 654
    benchmarking and, 648
    caregiver responsibilities in, 643, 644, 647
    caregiver support in, 644
    case management in, 646-647, 647b
    client diversity in, 648-649
    communication in, 649-650
    community resources for, 644-646, 644b, 654-655
    confidentiality and, 650
    cost of care and, 642
    cultural aspects of, 648-649
    death in, 603-604
    definition of, 641
    delegation in, 64
    developmental aspects of, 651-653, 653b
    dialysis in, 970
    discharge planning for, 644-646, 678-679
        after hyperbilirubinemia treatment, 280-281
        high-risk infant and, 268-269
        newborn and, 237-239, 238b, 268-269
    drug administration in, 731-732
    education and, 653
    evidence-based practice and, 648
    family assessment in, 650-651
    family support in, 654-655
    family teaching in, 650, 678-679, 704-705
    family-centered, 10, 11b, 648-655. *See also* Family-centered care.
    for infant, 335, 340
    house rules in, 651, 652b
    immobilization in, 1110
    in chronic illness/disability, 577-578
    in coma, 986
    in congestive heart failure, 884
    in skin disorders, 1069
    in terminal illness, 599
    individualized plan for, 645
    information resources for, 648b
    intermittent skilled nursing in, 644, 644b
    length of hospital stay and, 643
    medical equipment in, 654
    mobility in, 654
    nursing care standards for, 647-648
    nursing process in, 650-651
    nutritional support in, 750
    overview of, 641
    parent-professional collaboration in, 649-650, 650b
    permanency planning and, 643
    predischarge assessment for, 645, 645b
    private duty nursing in, 644, 644b
    quality improvement programs for, 648
    respite care and, 643
    safety concerns in, 653-654
    self-care in, 652-653
    services needed in, 644b
    stoma care in, 751
    technology in, 651
    telephone triage in, 651
    therapeutic boundaries in, 652
    training in, 647, 651, 653, 654
    transition to, 644-646, 677-678
    trends in, 642-643
    vs. hospice care, 641
    vulnerable child syndrome in, 654
Home care agencies
    certification of, 647
    selection of, 645b
Homelessness, 54, 59
Homograft, for burns, 1097

Homosexuality, 523
  suicide and, 569
Hookworm disease, 467t
Ho'oponopono, 63
Hopefulness, in chronic illness/disability, 584
Hormones. *See also* Endocrine system *and specific hormones.*
  in growth, 86
  sex, 1037
    in adolescent, 514-515
    in newborn, 200-201
Hornet stings, 1077t
Hospice care, 599-600
  vs. home care, 641
Hospitalization, 658-683
  activities in
    developmentally appropriate, 672-673
    diversional, 673-674
    expressive, 674-675
  admission in
    assessment for, 665, 666b-667b
    guidelines for, 668b
    preparation for, 665-668
  beneficial effects of, 663-664, 675-676
  child's response to, 659-664
  communication in, 677
  complementary and alternative therapies and, 665
  discharge planning in, 678-679
    for newborn, 237-239, 238b, 268-269
  ethical issues in, 669
  family issues and concerns in, 676-679
  family-centered care in, 668-670
  family's response to, 664
  fear of injury in, 672
  health teaching in, 675-676, 678-679
  hearing impairment and, 627
  in autism, 637
  in cognitive impairment, 618-619
  in intensive care unit, 681-683, 681b
  in terminal illness, 599, 604
  in visual impairment, 632
  isolation precautions in, 680
  length of stay in, 663-664
  long-term effects of, 663, 663b
  loss of control in, 661-663
    minimization of, 670-672
  newborn safety and, 221-222
  nurse's presence in, 668-670
  nursing interventions in, 668-676
  parent participation in, 677-678
  parental absence during, 669
  patient bill of rights for, 672, 672b
  play in, 673-675
  postvention in, 681
  preparation for, 664-668
  providing information in, 677
  room assignment in, 668
  routine in, 671, 671b
  self-care in, 671
  separation anxiety in, 659-661, 668-670
  sibling's response to, 664, 677
  stressors in, 659-664, 682b
  transition to home care after, 644-646, 678-679
  trends in, 663-664
Host factors, 22
Hot/cold classification, 63
HOTV test, 137
Huber needle, 727, 728f
Huffing, 567
Human bites, 1083
Human immunodeficiency virus infection. *See* HIV/AIDS.
Human milk. *See* Breastfeeding.
Human Milk Banking Association of North America, 256-257

Human papillomavirus infection, 547, 548t
  immunization for, 359
Humane care, 13
Humidification
  for respiratory infections, 756-758
  for tracheostomy, 745
Hyaline membrane disease, 284
Hydration. *See* Fluid management.
Hydrocarbons, poisoning with, 471b
Hydrocele, 210, 220t, 958
Hydrocephalus, 1017-1020, 1017f, 1018b, 1019f
Hydrocodone, 175, 176t, 178t
  abuse of, 567
Hydrocodone/acetaminophen (Lorcet, Lortab, Vicodin), 176t
Hydrocolloid dressings, 1066t, 1068
  for burns, 1095
Hydrocortisone, topical, 1067, 1068
Hydrofiber dressings, 1066t
Hydrogel dressings, 1066t
Hydromorphone (Dilaudid), 175, 176t, 180t, 183
  abuse of, 567
Hydronephrosis, 956-957
Hydrops fetalis, 282
Hydrotherapy, for burns, 1097
21-Hydroxylase deficiency, 1040-1042
Hydroxyzine, for opioid-related pruritus, 179t
Hygiene, 132, 700-702, 704-705
  in coma, 985
  oral. *See* Oral care.
  perineal, 701
Hymen, 151
Hymenal tag, 210
Hymenoptera stings, 1076-1079, 1078t
Hyperalbuminuria, 959
Hyperbilirubinemia, 274-281
  diagnosis of, 275-277, 276f
  nursing care management in, 279-281
  pathophysiology of, 275
  prognosis of, 279
  treatment of, 277-279, 278f
  types of, 274-275, 274t
Hypercalcemia, in hyperparathyroidism, 1037
Hypercyanotic spells, 884-886
Hyperglycemia, in diabetes mellitus, 1044, 1048, 1048t
Hyperhemolytic crisis, in sickle cell anemia, 918, 922
Hyperkalemia
  in acute renal failure, 966
  in chronic renal failure, 968
  transfusion-related, 944t
Hyperlipidemia, 894-896
Hyperopia, 628, 628t-629t
Hyperparathyroidism, 1036-1037, 1037b
Hyperphenylalaninemia, 313
Hyperpnea, 145b
Hypertension
  intracranial. *See* Increased intracranial pressure.
  persistent pulmonary, of newborn, 292t
  pulmonary artery, 897-898
  systemic, 899-901
    essential, 899
    in acute renal failure, 966
    in seizures, 1010
    pregnancy-induced, 299
    secondary, 899-900
Hyperthermia, 704. *See also* Fever.
  in coma, 984
  malignant, 697
Hyperthyroidism, 1034-1035, 1034b
Hypertonia, 220t
Hypertrophic cardiomyopathy, 898-899
Hypertrophic pyloric stenosis, 849-852
Hyperventilation, 145b

Hyperviscosity syndrome, 292t
Hypervolemia, transfusion-related, 944t
Hypoalbuminemia, 959
Hypocalcemia, in newborn, 284, 285t
Hypoglossal nerve, assessment of, 155t
Hypoglycemia
  in diabetes mellitus, 1047-1048, 1048t, 1056, 1056b
  in newborn, 284, 285t, 299
Hyponatremia, in acute renal failure, 966
Hypophosphatemia, in hyperparathyroidism, 1037
Hypopituitarism, 1024-1029
Hypoplastic anemia, 924
Hypoplastic left heart syndrome, 876b
Hyposensitization, for asthma, 789-790
Hypospadias, 220t, 958t
Hypotension, orthostatic, 131-132
Hypothalamic-pituitary-gonadal axis, 1030
Hypothermia
  in near-drowning, 993
  transfusion-related, 944t
Hypothyroidism, 1032-1033
  congenital, 311-313, 312b
Hypotonia, 211, 220t
  in Down syndrome, 620-622
Hypoventilation, 145b
Hypovolemic shock, 902-904, 903t
Hypoxemia, in congestive heart failure, 884-886
Hypoxia
  in congestive heart failure, 884-886
  in near-drowning, 993
  in sickle cell anemia, 918, 919b
Hypoxic-ischemic brain injury, in newborn, 293t
Hysteria, 563
Hysterical conversion reaction, 563

I

"I" messages, 106b
Ibuprofen (Advil, Motrin)
  for fever, 703
  for pain, 175, 176t
ICES therapy, 1112
Ichthyoses, 1084
Icterus, 274
Icterus neonatorum, 275
Id, 78, 412
Identical twins, 37, 38b
Identification
  of hospital personnel, 222
  of newborn, 221-222
Identity vs. role confusion, 79t, 80, 518-519
Idiopathic thrombocytopenic purpura, 927-929, 928b
IgA, 323-324
Ileocolic intussusception, 852-853, 852f
Ileostomy, 750-751
  for inflammatory bowel disease, 835, 836
Ileus
  meconium, 824
    in cystic fibrosis, 795-796, 797b, 799
  paralytic, 849
Ilizarov external fixator, 1121, 1121f
Illnesses
  acute, 10
  chronic. *See* Chronic illness/disability.
  common, 3-8
  development and, 89
  morbidity due to, 10
  susceptibility to, 58-59
Imaginary playmates, 442
Imaging studies
  in cerebral dysfunction, 980-981
  in genitourinary disorders, 951t-952t
  in head injury, 990

Imitation
    in cognitive development, 330, 413
    in play, 416
Immediate gastrointestinal hypersensitivity, 385
Immigrants. *See also* Race/ethnicity.
    children, 55
    families, 59
    migrant farmworkers, 54-55, 59
Immobilization, 1107-1110
    child's response to, 671
    family concerns and issues in, 1109
    in home care, 1110
    nursing care in, 1109-1110
    of fractures, 1115-1121. *See also* Casts; Traction.
    physiologic effects of, 1107, 1108t
    psychologic effects of, 1108
Immune globulin, botulism, 1169
Immune system
    development of, 324
    in infant, 324
    in newborn, 200
    in school-age child, 494
    in toddler, 411
Immunizations, 3, 350-365, 364t
    administration of, 359, 363-365
    adverse reactions to, 359
    autism and, 635, 636
    contraindications to, 359, 361t-363t
    current recommendations for, 350
    for adolescents, 365, 526
    for diphtheria, 351
    for *Haemophilus influenzae*, 357, 999, 1001
    for hepatitis A, 351, 839, 840t, 841
    for hepatitis B, 351, 839, 840t, 841
        for newborn, 222-223
    for human papillomavirus, 359
    for influenza, 358, 765
    for measles, 357
    for meningococcal disease, 358, 999, 1001
        in sickle cell anemia, 919
    for mumps, 357
    for newborn, 222-223
    for pertussis, 356
    for pneumococcal infection, 357-358, 776
        in sickle cell anemia, 919, 920
    for poliomyelitis, 356-357
    for rabies, 1004
    for rotavirus, 359
    for rubella, 357
    for tetanus, 351, 356, 356t, 1167
        in burns, 1095
    for tuberculosis, 779
    for varicella, 357
    improving rates of, 365
    in health history, 109
    in HIV/AIDS, 941
    precautions for, 359, 361t-363t
    schedule for, 121f, 350-351, 352f-354f, 355t
    with BCG vaccine, 779
Immunodeficiency disorders, 939-943
    HIV/AIDS, 939-943
    severe combined immunodeficiency disease, 943
    Wiskott-Aldrich syndrome, 943
Immunoglobulin, tetanus, 1167
Immunoglobulin A (IgA), 323-324
Immunologic disorders, 939-943
Immunomodulators, topical, 1067
Immunoreactive trypsinogen analysis, for cystic
    fibrosis, 797
Immunosuppression, after heart transplantation,
    899
Immunotherapy
    for aplastic anemia, 924-925
    for asthma, 789-790
    for inflammatory bowel disease, 834
Imperforate anus, 854

Impetigo, 1069-1071, 1070t, 1071f
    poststreptococcal glomerulonephritis and, 961
Implanon (levonorgestrel), 546t
Implanted ports, 725-730, 727t, 728f
    preslit, 734, 735f
Implementation, in nursing process, 17
Inactivity. *See also* Activity and exercise.
    obesity and, 552
Inborn errors of metabolism, 310-316
Incest, 482, 483
Incidence, 22
Incontinence
    fecal, 538
        in coma, 984-985
    urinary, 537-538. *See also* Enuresis.
        in coma, 984
Increased intracranial pressure, 975-976, 976b
    in head trauma, 986, 988, 989
    monitoring of, 982-983
    nursing care in, 983-984
    suctioning and, 984
Incubators, 254
Individual family service plan (IFSP), 653
Individuation, separation and, 331, 415
Industry vs. inferiority, 79t, 80, 494
Infant. *See also* Newborn.
    abduction of, from hospital, 221-222
    airway clearance in, 809, 809f
    apnea in, 404-406
    bathing of, 701
    biologic development of, 323-327
        fine motor skills in, 325, 325f, 336t-340t
        gross motor skills in, 325-327, 326f, 327f,
            336t-340t
        maturation of systems in, 323-325
        proportional changes in, 323
    biting by, 327
    bodily damage to, 372
    body image of, 330-331, 331f
    burns in, 371-372
    child care arrangements for, 335, 340-341
    chronic illness/disability in, 592t
    colic in, 395-396, 397, 397f
    communication with, 103
    dental health of, 349-350
    discipline for, 341-342
    drowning of, 372
    fluid balance in, 814-815
    food sensitivity in, 384-388
    health problems of, 378-407
    heel lance in, 715, 716f, 717
    immunizations for, 350-365. *See also*
        Immunizations.
    injury prevention in, 365-374
    kangaroo care for, 77
    limit setting for, 341-342
    nutrition in, 343-347
    play activities for, 333t-334t
    poisoning of, 370-371
    proper holding of, 708, 708f
    separation anxiety in, 332, 335
    shaken baby syndrome in, 481
    shoes for, 343
    sleep and activity in, 347-349, 348t
    sudden death of, 401-404
    suffocation of, 368-369
    teething in, 342-343, 343f
    temperament of, 334-335
    vegetarian diet in, 379-380, 380b
    weaning of, 347
Infant botulism, 1169-1170
Infant feeding. *See also* Breastfeeding; Formula
    feeding.
    growth patterns and, 122
    in cleft lip/cleft palate, 845
    in congestive heart failure, 883

Infant holds, 708, 708f
Infant mortality, 8-9, 8t, 9t
Infant seat, fall from, 370
Infant walkers, falls and, 370
Infection
    communicable, 453-469
    high-risk newborn and, 296-299
    maternal, neonatal complications of, 305-308,
        305t-307t
    musculoskeletal, 1134-1136
    newborn defenses against, 200
    transfusion-related, 945t
Infection control, 706-708
    for newborns, 221-228
        at high risk, 254-255
        bathing and, 224-225
        circumcision and, 225-227
        umbilicus and, 225
    for toddlers/preschoolers, 462-464
    handwashing in, 708
    isolation precautions in, 680, 707b
    sharps handling in, 708
    transmission-based precautions in, 706-707,
        707b
Infectious diarrhea. *See* Diarrhea.
Infectious mononucleosis, 768
Infective endocarditis, 891-893, 892b
Infertility
    in cystic fibrosis, 796, 803
    pelvic inflammatory disease and, 547-549
    radiation therapy and, 938-939
Infiltration, in intravenous therapy, 738
Inflammation, in wound healing, 1062
Inflammatory bowel disease, 833-836
Infliximab (Remicade), for inflammatory bowel
    disease, 834-835
Influenza, 764-765
    immunization for, 358
    Reye syndrome and, 703
Information overload, 101
Information technology
    in home care, 651
    nursing informatics and, 99
    privacy issues and, 99
Informed consent
    assent and, 688-689
    essential components of, 687
    evidence of, 689
    for procedures, 687-689
    of minors, 689
    of non-English speakers, 102
    of parents or guardians, 689
    requirements for, 687-689
    treatment in absence of, 689
Infrared thermometers, 127, 127b
    for newborns, 206
Infusion locks, 725, 726
Infusion pumps
    in baclofen administration, 1149
    in intravenous therapy, 735
    in patient-controlled analgesia, 178-183
Inguinal hernia, 148, 150, 958t
    in newborn, 210
Inguinal nodes, 133, 134f
Inhalant abuse, 567
Inhalation injury, 782-783, 1093
Inhalational poisoning, of infant, 371
Initiative, sense of, development of, 438-439
Initiative vs. guilt, 79-80, 79t
Injections
    insulin, 723-724
    intradermal, 723, 724
    intramuscular, 22f, 719-723, 721f
    needleless systems for, 723
    subcutaneous, 723-724

Injection therapy, for asthma, 789-790
Injuries. *See* Traumatic injuries.
In-line skate safety, 509
Insect bites and stings, 1076-1079, 1077t-1078t
Insulin, 1026t
　dosage errors for, 724
　endogenous, 1042, 1043
　　deficiency of. *See* Diabetes mellitus.
　　functions of, 1043-1044
　exogenous, 1045-1046. *See also* Diabetes mellitus, insulin for.
　injection of, 723-724
Insulin pump, 1055
Insulin waning, 1046
Intake and output measurement, 732-733
　in genitourinary disorders, 950
　urine collection for, 732, 960
Integumentary system. *See also under* Hair; Skin.
　of newborn, 200
Intelligence quotient, in cognitive impairment, 612, 612t
Intensive care unit, 681-683
Intercostal retractions, in newborn, 209
Intercostal spaces, 143, 143f
Intermittent infusion device, 725, 729f
Intermittent skilled nursing, in home care, 644, 644b
Internet
　developmental effects of, 93
　nursing informatics and, 99
Interpreters, 101-102
　children as, 102
Intersex, 958t
Interstitial pneumonia, 774-777
Intertrigo, 1085t
Interview
　history taking in, 107-113
　privacy and confidentiality for, 98-99
　setting for, 98-99
Intestinal malrotation, 853
Intestinal obstruction
　in anorectal malformations, 854-855, 854t
　in cystic fibrosis, 796, 797b
　in intussusception, 852-853, 852f
　in pyloric stenosis, 849-852
Intestinal transplantation, for short bowel syndrome, 857
Intestinal volvulus, 853
Intestine. *See also under* Gastrointestinal.
　of newborn, 199
Intracellular fluid, 814
Intracranial hemorrhage
　in head trauma, 987f, 988-989
　in newborn, 293t
Intracranial hypertension. *See* Increased intracranial pressure.
Intracranial infections, 998-1002
Intracranial pressure, increased, 975-976, 976b
Intramuscular drugs, 22f, 719-723, 721f. *See also* Drug therapy.
Intraosseous infusion, 733
Intrathecal analgesia, 182t
Intrauterine device, 546t
Intrauterine growth, gestational age and, 203f, 204
Intrauterine transfusion, Rh isoimmunization and, 282
Intravenous administration
　of drugs, 725-730
　　central venous access device for, 725-730, 728f
　　complications of, 729-730
　　heparin flush for, 726
　　peripheral intermittent infusion device for, 725, 729f
　　site care in, 729

Intravenous administration *(Continued)*
　of feeding solutions, 749-750
　of fluids
　　administration set change in, 737
　　complications of, 738
　　extravasation in, 738
　　for diarrhea, 822
　　infiltration in, 738
　　line removal in, 737-738
　　line securement in, 735-736, 735f
　　parenteral fluid, 733-738
　　site care in, 736
Intravenous pyelography, 951t
Intraventricular hemorrhage, 293t
Intussusception, 852-853, 852f
Invisible poverty, 54
Iodines, 393t
Iontocaine, 184, 185f
Iontophoresis, lidocaine, 184-187, 185f
Ipecac, 473
IQ, in cognitive impairment, 612, 612t
Iris, examination of, 134f, 135
　in newborn, 208
Iron, 393t
　for anemia, 916
　injection of, 916
Iron deficiency anemia, 915-916
Iron overload, transfusion-related, 924
Iron poisoning, 472b
Iron-rich diet, 916
Irritable bowel syndrome, 829
Irritant dermatitis, 1074-1076
Ishihara test, 137
Islam, 65t
Isoimmunization, Rh, 281, 282
Isolation precautions, 680
Isoniazid, for tuberculosis, 779
Isotretinoin (Accutane), for acne, 1090
Itching. *See* Pruritus.
Ivermectin, for scabies, 1079

J

Jacket restraint, 709
Jacob syndrome, 541t
Japanese Americans. *See also* Race/ethnicity.
　health beliefs and practices of, 67t
Jaundice, 274, 274t, 279, 281. *See also* Hyperbilirubinemia.
　breast milk, 275
　in biliary atresia, 842
　in cirrhosis, 841
　in hepatitis, 840
　physiologic, 275
　race/ethnicity and, 133t
Jaw thrust, in CPR, 805, 806f
Jehovah's witnesses, 66t
Jejunostomy feeding, 745
Jewish culture, circumcision in, 228
Jitteriness, in newborn, 294-295
Jobst garments, 1101, 1101f
Jock itch, 1073t
Joint Commission on Accreditation of Healthcare Organizations (JCAHO), 708
Joint contractures, in immobilization, 1107, 1108t
Joint custody, 34, 48
Joint disorders, 1139-1143
　in hemophilia, 927
　rheumatoid, 1139-1143
　traumatic, 1111-1112, 1111f
Joints, examination of, 152-153
Jones criteria, for rheumatic fever, 893, 893b
Judaism, 66t
Junctional nevi, 249
Justice, 13
Juvenile autoimmune thyroiditis, 1033-1034

Juvenile hypothyroidism, 1032-1033
Juvenile idiopathic arthritis, 1139-1142
Juvenile melanoma, 249

K

Kahunas, 63
Kangaroo care, 77, 173-175, 175f
　for high-risk newborn, 262
　in pain management, 173-175
　in thermoregulation, 254
Kasabach-Merritt syndrome, 250
Kasai procedure, for biliary atresia, 842
Kawasaki disease, 901
Keloids, 1064f
Kernicterus, 277
Ketamine
　for neuropathic pain, 194
　in date rape, 549
Ketoacidosis, diabetic, 1045
　treatment of, 1049
Ketogenic diet, 553, 1009
Ketonuria, 953t
　in diabetes mellitus, 1044
Kidnapping, of newborn, 221-222
Kidney. *See under* Renal.
Kindergarten, experience of, 442-443
Klinefelter syndrome, 310t, 540-541, 541t
Klippel-Trenaunay-Weber syndrome, 249
Klumpke palsy, 211, 247
Knee, ligament injuries of, 1112
Knee jerk reflex, 153, 154f
Knee-chest position, for hypercyanotic spells, 885, 885f
Knock-knee, 152, 152f
Kohlberg's moral development theory, 79t, 81, 439, 495-496, 519-520
Knock-knee, 152, 152f
Kugelberg-Welander disease, type 3, 1161b, 1162
Kussmaul respirations, 145b, 1044
Kwashiorkor, 381, 383
　marasmic, 383
Kyphosis, 1130, 1131f

L

Labia minora/majora, 151, 151f
　female genital mutilation and, 228
　of newborn, 200, 210
Laboratory tests
　abbreviations for, 1200
　reference ranges for, 1192-1199
Lacerations. *See also* Wounds.
　cerebral, 987-988
　nursing care for, 1068
　scalp, 991
Lacrimal punctum, 134-135
Lactase deficiency, 387
Lactation. *See* Breastfeeding.
Lacto-ovo vegetarians, 380
Lactose intolerance, 387-388
Lactovegetarians, 380
Lactulose, for opioid-related constipation, 179t
Laissez-faire parent, 40-41
LaLeche League International, 231
Lambdoid suture, 207, 208f
Language. *See also* Communication; Speech.
　foreign, communication and, 60-61, 62
　sign, 626
Language development, 81
　in infant, 332
　in preschooler, 439, 447
　in toddler, 415-416
Language disorders, in autism, 635
Lanoxin (digoxin), for congestive heart failure, 878, 879-882
Lanugo, 207
Large-for-gestational-age (LGA) infant, 204, 204f

Larva migrans, 467t
Laryngeal edema, in anaphylaxis, 905
Laryngitis, 769t, 770
Laryngotracheobronchitis, 769, 769t, 770-771, 771b
Lasix (furosemide), for congestive heart failure, 879t
LATCH system
    for infant car seat, 369
    for toddler car seat, 430, 430f
Latchkey children, 500-501
Latency period, 78, 494
Latex allergy, 1159-1161, 1159b, 1160b
Latinos. See also Race/ethnicity.
    health beliefs and practices of, 67t
    Spanish-English translation for, 1204
Lavage, gastric, for sputum collection, 780
Lavage solution, for bowel preparation, 750
Lazy eye, 135-136, 136f
Lead poisoning, 475-480
    anticipatory guidance in, 478
    causes of, 476, 476b
    clinical manifestations of, 476-477, 477f
    cultural aspects of, 476
    diagnosis of, 477-478
    from complementary and alternative therapies, 64
    nursing care management in, 479-480
    pathophysiology of, 476
    prognosis of, 479
    screening for, 478
    treatment of, 478-479, 480
Learning, in cognitive impairment, 613
Learning disabilities, 559-561. See also Cognitive impairment.
    attention deficit hyperactivity disorder and, 559-561
    definition of, 559
    school placement and, 561
Lea's shield, 545t
Left-to-right shunt, 866, 866f
Leg, examination of, 152, 152f
Leg restraints, 709-710
Legal blindness, 628
Legg-Calvé-Perthes disease, 1128-1130
Length. See also Growth; Height.
    crown-to-rump, 204-205, 216t
    head-to-heel, 205, 205f, 216t
    measurement of, 122, 123f
Lesbian adolescents, suicide by, 569
Lesbian family, 34
Lethargy, 976b
Leukemia, 930-937
    acute, 930
    blast cell, 930
    care plan for, 932-934
    chronic, 930
    classification of, 930
    clinical manifestations of, 931, 931t
    diagnosis of, 931
    pathophysiology of, 930-931, 931t
    prognosis of, 931-932, 937
    stem cell, 930
    treatment of, 931
        late effects of, 932
        nursing care for, 932-937
Leukocytes. See White blood cells.
Leukokoria, 633, 634f
Leukotrienes, for asthma, 789
Levalbuterol, for asthma, 788-789
Lever lock, 734, 735f
Levonorgestrel implant (Implanon), 546t
Levonorgestrel intrauterine system (Mirena), 546t
Levorphanol (Levo-Dromoran), 175, 176t

Lice, head, 1079-1081
Lichenification, 1064f
Lidocaine
    for circumcision pain, 226
    for CPR, 807-809, 808t
    iontophoretic, 184-187, 185f
Lidocaine lubricants, for bladder catheterization, 713-714
Ligament injuries, 1112
Light reflex
    corneal, 136, 136f
    otoscopic, 140
    pupillary, 135, 212t
Limb salvage procedure, 1136-1137
Limb-girdle muscular dystrophy, 1162, 1163f
Lindane
    for head lice, 1080
    for scabies, 1079
Lingual frenulum, 209
Lingual tonsils, 763, 763f
Lip
    cleft, 209, 843-846, 844f, 847
    herpes infection of, 1072t
        recurrent, 465
Lipase, 324
Lipid-lowering agents, 895-896
Lipids, elevated serum, 894-896
Lipreading, 626
Liquid crystal skin contact thermometers, 127, 127b
Listening skills, 100-101
Listerial meningitis, 998-1002
Listeriosis, maternal, 307t
Liver. See also under Hepatic.
    in infant, 324
    in newborn, 199, 210, 219t
    palpation of, 149
        in newborn, 210, 219t
LMX, 174, 182t, 184
Lobar pneumonia, 774-777
Locks, infusion, 725, 726, 734, 735f
Locomotion, 326-327, 329f
Lorazepam (Ativan)
    for pain, 177t
    for status epilepticus, 1009
Lorcet (hydrocodone/acetaminophen), 176t
Lordosis, 1130, 1131f
Lortab (hydrocodone/acetaminophen), 176t
Loss of control, feeding and, 702
Low birth weight, morbidity and mortality due to, 9, 9t
Low income status, 54
Low-density lipoproteins, in hyperlipidemia, 894-896
Lower limb prostheses, 1121-1122, 1127
Low-fat diet, in hyperlipidemia, 894-895, 896
LSD, 567
Lubricants, for bladder catheterization, 713-714
Luer connection, 727
Lumbar puncture, 979, 980t. See also Cerebrospinal fluid.
    analgesia for, 193
    positioning for, 710-711, 711f
Lumirubin, 277
Lung. See also under Pulmonary; Respiratory.
    examination of, 144-145, 144f, 145b
        in newborn, 209, 219t
    in newborn, 198, 209, 219t, 285, 288-289
    percussion of, 144-145
    structure of, 144, 144f
Luque rods, 1132
Luteinizing hormone, 1025t
Luteinizing hormone–releasing hormone, 1030
Lying, in school-age child, 501
Lyme disease, 1082-1083, 1083f

Lymph nodes
    examination of, 133, 134f
        in newborn, 210
    location of, 134f
Lymphangiography, 938
Lymphocytes, 200
    measurement of, 913t
Lymphocytic thyroiditis, 1033-1034
Lymphoid tissue, development of, 76
Lymphoma, 937-939
    Hodgkin disease, 937-939
    non-Hodgkin, 939
Lysergic acid diethylamide (LSD), 567

M

Macrobiotics, 380
Macrominerals, 379
Macula, examination of, 135, 135f
Macules, 1063f
Mafenide (Sulfamylon), for burns, 1098t
Magical thinking, 439
Magnesium, 394t
    for CPR, 807-809, 808t
Magnesium citrate, for opioid-related constipation, 179t
Magnesium sulfate, for status asthmaticus, 790, 791
Magnetic resonance imaging, in cerebral dysfunction, 979, 980t
Mainstreaming. See also Education; School.
    in chronic illness/disability, 578, 593-594
    in cognitive impairment, 613
Majority, age of, 689
Malathion, for head lice, 1080
Malignant hyperthermia, 697
Malnutrition, protein-energy, 381, 383-384
Malocclusion, 507
Malrotation, 853
Maltreatment, 480-490. See also Abuse; Neglect.
Managed care, in chronic illness/disability, 578
Manubrium
    auricular, 139f, 140
    sternal, 14f, 143
Marasmus, 381, 383
Marijuana, 567
    intrauterine exposure to, 304-305
Marriage, divorce and, 33-34, 45-48
Mask, oxygen, 738
Masked deprivation, 88
Mass spectrometry, tandem, 223
Masturbation, in preschooler, 446
Maternal diabetes, 299-300, 299b
Maternal infections, 305-308, 305t-307t
Maternal sensitive period, attachment and, 234
Maturation, 72. See also Development.
Maturity rating, for newborn, 202f, 203
McBurney point, 830
Mean arterial pressure, 129, 129t
Mean corpuscular hemoglobin (MCH), 913t
Mean corpuscular hemoglobin concentration (MCHC), 913t
Mean corpuscular volume (MCV), 913t
Measles, 458-459, 458f
    immunization for, 357
Meatus, nasal, 141, 141f
Mechanical ventilation
    in respiratory distress syndrome, 287, 287t
    tracheostomy for, 741-744, 743f
Meckel diverticulum, 831-833, 849
Meconium, 200b
    aspiration of, 291t
Meconium ileus, 824
    in cystic fibrosis, 795-796, 797b, 799
Meconium plug, 824

MedicAlert identification, in diabetes mellitus, 1051
Medication history, 109
Medicine cups, 719
Medroxyprogesterone acetate (Depo-Provera), 544, 546t
Megacolon, congenital aganglionic, 825-826, 825f
Meibomian glands, 134
Melanin, in newborn, 200
Melanocyte-stimulating hormone, 1025t
Melanoma, juvenile, 249
Menarche, 515, 541
Meningism, in pneumonia, 776
Meningitis
    aseptic, 1002
    bacterial, 998-1002
    immunization for, 358, 999, 1001
    in sickle cell anemia, 919
Meningocele, 1154-1161
Meningococcal disease, immunization for, 358, 999, 1001
    in sickle cell anemia, 919
Meningomyelocele, 1154-1161. *See also* Spina bifida.
Menstruation
    absence of, 541
        in athletes, 557
        in eating disorders, 557, 558
    pain in, 541-542
    tampon use in, toxic shock syndrome and, 907, 907t
Mental health, 3, 4
Mental health problems, 8
Mental representation, in cognitive development, 330
Mental retardation. *See* Chronic illness/disability; Cognitive impairment.
Meperidine (Demerol), 180t, 183
    abuse of, 567
Mercury poisoning, 475
Mercury thermometers, 206
Mercy killing, 596. *See also* Treatment withholding.
Meromelia, 1127
Mesalamine, for ulcerative colitis, 834
Mesh grafts, for burns, 1098, 1099f
Metabolic acidosis
    in acute renal failure, 966
    in chronic renal failure, 968, 969
    in diabetes mellitus, 1049
Metabolic disorders, in newborn, 284, 285t
Metabolic rate
    fluid balance and, 815
    in newborn, 199
Metabolism
    inborn errors of, 310-316
    rate of, 76
        obesity and, 552
Metalloporphyrins, for hyperbilirubinemia, 277
Metaphysis, 75
Metatarsus adductus (varus), 1126-1127
Metered-dose inhalers, 740
    for asthma, 788, 793
Metformin, for weight loss, 553
Methadone (Dolophine)
    for opioid dependence, 189
    for pain, 175, 176t, 180t
Methamphetamine, 567
    fetal/neonatal effects of, 304
Methicillin-resistant *Staphylococcus aureus* infection, cutaneous, 1069-1071, 1072
Methotrexate
    for inflammatory bowel disease, 834, 835
    for juvenile idiopathic arthritis, 1140
Methylphenidate
    for attention deficit hyperactivity disorder, 560
    for opioid-related sedation, 179t

Metronidazole, for peptic ulcers, 838
Mexican Americans. *See also* Race/ethnicity.
    health beliefs and practices of, 67t
Mexican-Americans, Spanish-English translation for, 1204
Mexiletine, for pain, 178t
MIC-KEY device, 747, 749f
Microminerals, 379
Midazolam (Versed)
    for burns, 1096
    for pain, 178
    for preoperative sedation, 696
    for status epilepticus, 1009
Middle-ear hearing loss, 623, 624. *See also* Hearing impairment.
Midstream specimen, 712
Migraine, abdominal, 829
Migrant farmworkers, 54-55, 59
Milia, 200, 217t
Miliaria, 217t
Milk
    breast. *See also* Breastfeeding.
        donor, 256
        expressed, 256
        newborn sense of smell and, 201
        nutrition and, 228-229
    evaporated, 233
    goat's, 233
    iron deficiency anemia and, 915
    witch's, 200, 209
Milk babies, 915
Milk of magnesia, for opioid-related constipation, 179t
Milk stool, 200b
Millard rotational advancement, for cleft lip/cleft palate, 844
Milwaukee brace, 1132
Mineral imbalances, in infant, 379, 392t, 395t
Mineral oil, for opioid-related constipation, 179t
Mineralocorticoids, 1037
Minimal change nephrotic syndrome, 958-961
Minimal enteral feedings, 256
    for necrotizing enterocolitis, 298
Minorities, 56-57. *See also* Culture; Race/ethnicity.
Minors. *See also* Adolescent.
    emancipated, 689
Mirena (levonorgestrel intrauterine system), 546t
Mixed conductive-sensorineural hearing loss, 624. *See also* Hearing impairment.
Mixed gonadal dysgenesis, 958
MMR vaccine, autism and, 635, 636
Mobility. *See also* Movement.
    in cerebral palsy, 1148, 1148f
    in chronic illness/disability, 591
    in Duchenne muscular dystrophy, 1164, 1165
    in hospitalization, 671
    in spina bifida, 1156, 1159
    in spinal cord injuries, 1171
    in visual impairment, 631
    range of motion and, in newborn, 211
Modeling, of aggression, 447
Modified Behavioral Pain Score (MBPS), 160t
Modified Blalock-Taussig shunt, 886f, 886t
Mohel, 228
Molestation, 482
Molluscum contagiosum, 1072t
Mongolian spots, 217t
Moniliasis. *See* Candidiasis.
Monocytes, 200
    measurement of, 913t
Mononucleosis, 768
Monospot test, 768
Monotropy, 237
Monozygotic twins, 37, 38b
Mons pubis, 151

Mood changes, steroid-related, 937
Moon face, steroid-related, 937
Moral development, 79t, 81, 439, 495-496, 519-520
    play in, 85-86
Morbidity, childhood, 10
Morbidity rates, 22, 23b
Morbidity statistics, 10
Mormons, 65t
Moro reflex, 212t, 213f
Morphine, 175, 176t, 180t, 183
    for neuropathic pain, 193, 194
Morphogenesis, 308
Mortality, 8-10. *See also* Death and dying.
    causes of, 3, 4t, 9, 9t
    childhood, 9-10, 10t
    high-risk newborn and, 250b
    infant, 8-9, 8t, 9t
Mortality rates, 22, 23b
Mosaicism, 619
Mosquito bites, 1077t
Mother. *See also* Family; Parents.
    working, 48
Mother-infant attachment. *See* Attachment.
Mother-infant (dyad) care, 237
Motivation, in learning, 613
Motor development
    assessment of, 132
    fine, 325, 325f, 336t-340t, 411, 438, 506
    gross, 325-327, 326f, 327f, 336t-340t, 411, 438
    in newborn, 211
    in preschooler, 438
    in school-age child, 506
    in toddler, 411
Motor examination, in neurologic examination, 978
Motor vehicle accidents. *See* Automobile safety.
Motrin. *See* Ibuprofen (Advil, Motrin).
Mourning. *See* Grief.
Mouth. *See also under* Oral.
Mouth-to-mouth/nose breathing, 805, 806f
Movement. *See also* Mobility.
    assessment of, 132
    in newborn, 211
Movies
    closed captioning for, 626
    violence in, 90-91
Moxibustion, 6363
Mucocutaneous lymph node system, 901-902
Mucositis
    in chemotherapy, 936-937
    oral, 465-466, 466f
Mucous membranes
    in newborn, 200
    nasal, 141
    oral, 142
Mucus, pulmonary. *See* Respiratory secretions.
Multicultural nursing. *See under* Cultural; Culture.
Multiple births. *See also* Twins.
    attachment process and, 237, 237f
Mummy restraint, 709, 710f
Mumps, 458-459
    immunization for, 357
Munchausen syndrome by proxy, 481
Murmurs, 147
    in newborn, 210
Muscle atrophy, in immobilization, 1107, 1108t
Muscle contusions, 1110-1111, 1111f
Muscle strains, 1112
Muscle tone, in newborn, 211, 220t
Muscular dystrophy, 1162-1165
    Duchenne, 1162-1165, 1163f
    facioscapulohumeral, 1162, 1163f
    limb-girdle, 1162, 1163f
Musculoskeletal disorders
    acquired, 1128-1134
    amputation for, 1121-1122

Musculoskeletal disorders *(Continued)*
  casts for, 1115-1117
  congenital, 1122-1128
  distraction therapy for, 1121
  infectious, 1134-1136
  neoplastic, 1136-1139
  traction for, 1117-1121
  traumatic, 76, 1110-1115
Musculoskeletal system
  of newborn, 200, 211
  of school-age child, 494
Music, in hospitalization, 674-675, 682
Muslims, 65t
Mutilation fears, 672
Mutual play, 442
Mutual storytelling, 106b
Mycotic infections, 1072-1074, 1074t
Myelin, 201
Myelination, 201
Myelodysplasia, 1154-1161. *See also* Spina bifida.
Myelomeningocele, 1154-1161, 1155f. *See also*
    Spina bifida.
Myelosuppression, in leukemia, 930-931, 935
Myopia, 628, 628t
Myositis ossificans, 1111
MyPyramid food guide, 553
MyPyramid for Kids, 381, 381b, 382f, 423b
Myringotomy, 767

N

Nails
  examination of, 132
  hematoma under, 1111
Naloxone
  for CPR, 807-809, 808t
  for respiratory depression, 179t
Naproxen (Naprosyn), 175, 176t
Narcissism, in infants, 327
Nasal anatomy, 140-141, 141f
Nasal bleeding, 929-930
Nasal cannula/prongs, 738
Nasal congestion, 757b, 758
  in Down syndrome, 622
Nasal decongestants, 758
Nasal discharge, in newborn, 218t
Nasal drug administration, 730, 731, 731f
Nasal examination, 140
  in newborn, 209, 218t
Nasal patency, in newborn, 209, 218t
Nasal polyps, in cystic fibrosis, 799
Nasal septum, 141, 141f
Nasal turbinates, 141, 141f
Nasal washings, 717
Nasoduodenal feeding, 749
Nasogastric feeding, 745-746, 746f, 747. *See also*
    Nutritional support.
Nasojejunal feeding, 749
Nasopharyngitis, 759-762, 761b
Natal rates, 22, 23b
Natal teeth, 209, 218t
National Center for Missing and Exploited Chil-
    dren (NCMEC), 221, 222
National Childhood Vaccine Injury Act, 365
National Children's Study, 2
Native Americans. *See also* Race/ethnicity.
  health beliefs and practices of, 67t
Nausea
  fluid management in, 702
  in chemotherapy, 936
  opioid-induced, 179t, 188
Near-drowning, 993-995
Near-to-far growth, 72
Nebulizers, 740
  for asthma, 793, 795f

Neck. *See also under* Cervical; Spinal.
  examination of, 133-134
    in newborn, 209, 218t
Necrotizing enterocolitis, 297-298, 298b
Nedocromil, for asthma, 788
Needles
  for intramuscular drugs, 719-720
  for intraosseous infusion, 733
  gauge of, 720
  handling of, 708
  Huber, 727, 728f
Needle sticks, prevention of, 708
Needleless systems, 734
  for intramuscular injections, 723
  for intravenous infusion, 734
Negativism, in toddlers, 412, 421-422
Neglect, 480, 484b, 485, 486
  development and, 88
  psychosocial dwarfism due to, 540
Neocate formula, 232
Neonatal Abstinence Scoring System, 302
Neonatal abstinence syndrome, 211, 300
Neonatal Infant Pain Scale (NIPS), 167t
Neonatal Intensive Care Unit Network Neurobe-
    havioral Scale, 302
Neonatal mortality, 8-9, 8t, 9t
Neonatal Pain, Agitation, and Sedation Scale
    (NPASS), 166, 168t
Neonatal teeth, 209
  vs. natal teeth, 209
Neonatal Withdrawal Inventory, 302
Neonate. *See* Newborn.
Nephroblastoma, 963-965, 963b, 964b
Nephropathy, diabetic, 1044
Nephrotic syndrome, 958-962, 959f, 960b
Nerves, cranial, 155t
  of newborn, 201
Nerve block, for circumcision, 227-228, 227b
Nerve deafness, 623-624. *See also* Hearing
    impairment.
Neural tube defects, 1154-1161. *See also* Spina
    bifida.
Neurofibromatosis, 1086t
Neurogenic bladder
  in spina bifida, 1156, 1157
  in spinal cord injuries, 1171
Neurogenic diabetes insipidus, 1030-1031
Neurohypophysis, structure and function of,
    1025t-1026t
Neurologic development, 76
Neurologic disorders, in newborn, 292t, 294
Neurologic examination, 153-155, 977-979
  of newborn, 211, 212t, 213f
Neurologic system
  of infant, 323
  of newborn, 201, 211
Neuromuscular disorders, 1145-1172
  acquired, 1165-1172
  cerebral palsy, 1146-1154
  congenital, 1146-1165
Neuropathy
  diabetic, 1044
  in chemotherapy, 937
  pain in, 193-194
Neutrophils, 200
  measurement of, 913t
Nevus
  bathing trunk, 249
  compound, 249
  giant pigmented, 249
  junctional, 249
  telangiectatic, 217t
Nevus flammeus, 217t, 249, 249f
New Ballard Scale (NBS), in gestational age assess-
    ment, 202f, 203

New morbidity, 3
Newborn. *See also* Infant; Neonatal.
  abdominal circumference of, 205
  abdominal examination in, 210, 219t
  adjustment of, to extrauterine life, 198-201,
    200b
  alcohol-exposed, 303
  anemia in, 292t
  assessment of, 201-215
    Apgar scoring in, 201-203, 202t
    attachment behaviors in, 215, 215b
    behavioral, 207, 213-215, 213b, 214t
    clinical, 202f-206f, 203-211, 204b, 208f, 211f,
      212t
    general appearance in, 207, 217t
    general measurements in, 204-207, 205f, 206f,
      216t
    gestational age in, 202f-205f, 203-205, 204b
    high-risk infant and, 251-252
    initial, 201-203, 202t
    physical examination in, 207-211, 208f, 211f,
      212t, 215, 215b, 216b, 217t-220t
    transitional, 211-213
  attachment behaviors in, 215, 215b
    ophthalmia neonatorum prophylaxis and,
      222
  auditory acuity in, 201
  bathing of, 224-225
  behavior of, 207, 213-215, 213b, 214t
  birth injuries in, 244-247, 245f-247f
  birthmarks in, 217t, 249-250, 249f
  blood pressure in, 206, 206f, 217t
  blood volume in, 199
  brachial palsy in, 246-247, 247f
  breasts of, 200, 209
  cardiovascular complications in, 292t, 294
  cerebral complications in, 292t, 294
  chest of, 209, 218t
  circulatory system of, 198-199
  cocaine-exposed, 303-304
  color preferences of, 201
  congenital anomalies in, 308-310
  conjunctivitis in, 222
  crying in, 215
  death of, 269-270
  discharge planning for, 237-239, 238b
    after hyperbilirubinemia treatment, 280-281
    high-risk infant and, 268-269
  drug-exposed, 300-305
    clinical manifestations of, 300, 302, 302b
    diagnosis of, 300-301
    nursing care management of, 302-303, 302b
    prognosis of, 302
    treatment of, 301-302
  ears of, 201, 209, 218t, 275f
    hearing screening and, 223
  endocrine system of, 200-201
  erythema toxicum neonatorum in, 247-248
  eyes of, 201, 208, 212t, 218t
    ophthalmia neonatorum prophylaxis and,
      222
  facial paralysis in, 246, 246f
  fatigue in, 263t
  feeding of, 228-234
    high-risk infant and, 255-258
  flexion in, 207, 217t
  fluid and electrolyte balance in, 199
  functional capacity in, 204
  gastrointestinal system of, 199, 200b
    vitamin K and, 222, 292t
  genitals of, 200, 210, 219t-220t, 272f
    circumcision and, 225-228
  gestational age of, 202f-205f, 203-205, 204b
  head circumference of, 204, 216t
  head evaluation in, 207, 208f

Newborn (*Continued*)
  hearing in, 201, 209
    screening of, 223
  heart rate in, 206, 209, 216t
  hemolytic disease of, 281-284, 282f, 282t
  hemorrhagic disease of, 222, 292t
  hepatitis in, 839-841
  herpes infection in, 248-249
  high-risk
    classification of, 250-251, 250b
    developmental outcome in, 261-264
    discharge planning for, 268-269
    drug-exposed, 300-305
    energy conservation in, 258-259
    ethical issues with, 269
    family support and, 264-265
    hydration in, 255
    hyperbilirubinemia in, 274-281
    identification of, 250
    inborn errors of metabolism in, 310-316
    infection prevention in, 254-255, 305-308
    loss of, 269-270
    maternal conditions and, 299-308
    medications for, 261
    metabolic complications in, 284, 285t
    nutrition in, 255-258
    parent-infant relationships and, 265-267
    physiologic monitoring of, 252, 252t
    positioning of, 259, 259f
    postterm, 273-274
    preterm, 271-273, 272f-273f
    respiratory distress in, 289-290
    respiratory support for, 252
    sepsis in, 296-297, 297b
    skin care in, 259-261
    systematic assessment of, 251-252
    thermoregulation in, 252-254, 254f
  HIV screening in, 223
  hypocalcemia in, 284, 285t
  hypoglycemia in, 284, 285t, 299
  identification of, 221-222
  immunization of, for hepatitis B, 222-223
  infection in. *See also specific type.*
    defenses against, 200
    maternal infections and, 305-308, 305t-307t
    prevention of, 221-228, 254-255
    sepsis, 296-297, 297b
  integumentary system of, 200
  kangaroo care for, 77, 173-175, 175f
  marijuana-exposed, 304-305
  maturity rating for, 202f, 203
  metabolic rate in, 199
  methamphetamine-exposed, 304
  mortality rates for, 8-9, 8t, 9t
  mucous membranes of, 200
  musculoskeletal system of, 200
  neurologic system of, 201, 211, 212t, 213f
  nose of, 209, 218t
  nutrition for, 228-234
    high-risk infant and, 255-258
  of diabetic mother, 299-300
  oral cavity of, 209, 218t
  pain assessment in, 159-161
  patent airway in, maintenance of, 215, 221
  periods of reactivity in, 211-213
  persistent pulmonary hypertension of, 292t
  posture of, 207, 217t, 272f
  pseudomenstruation in, 200, 210
  reflexes in, 212t. *See also specific reflexes.*
  renal system of, 200
  respiratory distress syndrome in, 284-288
  respiratory rate in, 206, 217t
  respiratory system of, 198, 209, 219t
    complications involving, 288-289, 291t, 294
    support for, 252

Newborn (*Continued*)
  salivary glands in, 199
  screening of, for disease, 223, 224b
  seizures in, 294-295, 294b, 295t
  sensory functions of, 201
  siblings of, 236, 236f
    high-risk infant and, 267, 267f
  sitting height of, 204-205, 216t
  skin of, 200, 207, 217t
    acid mantle of, 225, 259
    high-risk infants and, 259-261
  sleep/activity patterns in, 214-215, 214t
  smell in, 201
  stooling patterns in, 199, 200b
  stress in, 263t
  tactile sensation in, 201
  taste in, 201
  thermoregulation in, 199
    high-risk infant and, 252-254, 254f
    maintenance of stable temperature and, 221
  viability of, 250
  vision in, 201
  vital signs of, 205-207, 205f, 206f, 216t-217t
    high-risk infant and, 252, 252t
  vitamin K for, 222, 292t
  weight loss in, 205, 216t
  zinc deficiency in, 259-260
Niacin, 389t
Nicotinic acid, 389t
Nightmares, vs. sleep terrors, 449, 449t
Ninety-ninety traction, 1119, 1119f
Nipple
  examination of, 144
  supernumerary, 209
Nipple feeding, of high-risk newborn, 257, 257f
Nissen fundoplication, 828, 828f
Nitric oxide, for respiratory complications, in
    newborn, 289, 294
Nitrous oxide, 191
  for burns, 1096-1097
Nits, 1079-1081
Nodules, 1063f
No-harm contracts, 571
Noise-induced hearing impairment, 628
Non-communicating Children's Pain Checklist,
    166, 169f-170f
Non-English speakers, communication with,
    60-61, 62, 101-102
Nonmaleficence, 13
Nonnutritive sucking, 258, 342
  in pain management, 173
  pacifier aspiration in, 368
Nonshivering thermogenesis, 199
Nonsororal family, 34
Nonsteroidal antiinflammatory drugs (NSAIDs)
  for fever, 703
  for juvenile idiopathic arthritis, 1140
  for pain, 175, 176t-178t, 180t. *See also* Analgesia.
Nonsummativity, 31
Nonsynostotic plagiocephaly, 400
Nontherapeutic relationship, 11
Nonverbal communication, 61, 62
Normalization, in chronic illness/disability,
    577-578, 589-595, 642
Norms, 52
North American blastomycosis, 1074t
Nortriptyline, for pain, 177t
Norwalk virus infection, 817-823, 818t. *See also*
    Diarrhea.
Nose. *See also under* Nasal.
  examination of, 140
    in newborn, 209, 218t
  structure of, 140-141, 141f
Nose drops, administration of, 730, 731, 731f

Nosebleeds, 929-930
Nothing by mouth (NPO) status, 696, 696t,
    732-733
  oral care in, 732
NSAIDs. *See* Nonsteroidal antiinflammatory drugs
    (NSAIDs).
Nuclear brain scan, 980t
Nuclear family, 33
Numby Stuff, 184
Numeric pain scale, 163t, 164
Nursemaid's elbow, 1111
Nurses, cultural background of, 64-67
Nurses Assessment of Pain Inventory (NAPI), 160t
Nursing. *See also* Pediatric nursing.
  definition of, 10
Nursing admission history, 665, 666b-667b
Nursing care plans
  for end-of-life care, 600-602
  in home care, 646-647
Nursing caries, 426, 426f
Nursing diagnoses, 16-17, 16b, 1201
Nursing education, for home care, 647
Nursing informatics, 99
Nursing Interventions Classification, 16
Nursing Outcomes Classification, 16
Nursing practice, evidence-based practice in,
    14-15, 15b, 15t
Nursing process, 15-18, 16b
  assessment in, 16
  documentation of, 17-18, 18b
  evaluation in, 17
  evidence-based practice and, 15, 15t
  implementation in, 17
  in community-based nursing care, 24-27, 24b
  nursing diagnoses in, 16-17, 16b
  planning in, 17
Nursing research, 14
Nursing shortage, home care and, 644
Nutrition, 2-3. *See also* Diet; Eating; Feeding;
    Food.
  cultural aspects of, 58, 61-62, 63
  for adolescent, 526-528
  for infant, 343-347
  for newborn, 228-234
    at high risk, 255-258
  for preschooler, 447-448, 448f
  for school-age child, 504-505
  for toddler, 422-424, 423b
  growth and, 88
  parenteral. *See* Parenteral nutrition.
  race/ethnicity and, 58
Nutritional assessment, 113-118
  clinical examination in, 115-118, 116b-118b
  dietary intake in, 113-115, 115b
  evaluation of, 118
Nutritional counseling, for obesity, 555, 555b
Nutritional disorders. *See also specific disorders or*
    nutrients.
  in infants, 378-388
    nursing care management of, 380-381
Nutritional support
  drug administration in, 730
  enteral nutrition in, 745-749. *See also* Enteral
    nutrition.
  family teaching for, 750
  feeding techniques in, 745-750
  in anorexia nervosa, 558
  in burns, 1096, 1100
  in cerebral palsy, 1150
  in coma, 984
  in congestive heart failure, 883
  in gastroesophageal reflux disease, 828
  in inflammatory bowel disease, 834, 835-836
  in short bowel syndrome, 857

Nutritional support (Continued)
refeeding syndrome in, 558
total parenteral nutrition in, 749-750. See also Total parenteral nutrition.
NuvaRing, 546t
Nystagmus, in newborn, 208

O

OASIS (Outcome and Assessment Information Set), 648
Obedience, punishment and, moral development and, 439
Obesity, 3, 551-556
body mass index and, 121-122, 553
complications of, 551
diagnosis of, 553
etiology and pathophysiology of, 551-553
nursing care for, 554-556
nursing process in, 554
prevention of, 556
treatment of, 553-554
Object permanence
in infant, 330, 330f
in toddler, 412-413
Objective information, 25
Objective Pain Score, 160t
Objects, transitional, 415, 415f
Obstipation, 823
Obstructive sleep apnea syndrome, 803
Obstructive uropathy, 956-957, 957f
Obtundation, 976b
Occupational therapy, in juvenile idiopathic arthritis, 1140
Octreotide, for weight loss, 553-554
Oculomotor nerve, assessment of, 155t
Oculovestibular response, 978
Odors
breath, 977
in diabetes mellitus, 1044
newborn reactions to, 201
Ointments, 1066t, 1067
Olfaction
assessment of, 141, 155t
in newborn, 201
in toddler, 410
Olfactory nerve, assessment of, 155t
Olsalazine, for ulcerative colitis, 834
Omphalocele, 210, 219t, 849, 850t
Omphalomesenteric fistula, 831
Ondansetron, for opioid-related nausea, 179t
Onlooker play, 84
Only children, 37
Open fractures, 1113, 1113f
Ophthalmia neonatorum, prevention of, 222
Ophthalmoscopy, 135, 135f
Opioids, 175, 176t. See also Analgesia.
abuse of, 567
dependence on, 188-189
dosage of, 176t, 178, 180t
for dying child, 194
for neuropathic pain, 193
for postoperative pain, 697
in patient-controlled analgesia, 178-183, 181t, 183t
routes of administration for, 181t-182t
side effects of, 179t-180t, 188-189
weaning from, 188, 190t
Opisthotonic posturing, 220t
Optic disc, examination of, 135, 135f
Optic nerve, assessment of, 155t
Oral allergy syndrome, 385
Oral candidiasis, in newborn, 218t, 248, 248f
Oral care, 701-702
in cerebral palsy, 1149
in chemotherapy, 936-937

Oral care (Continued)
in coma, 985
in NPO status, 732-733
Oral contraceptives, 545t, 547
for dysmenorrhea, 542
Oral drugs, 718-719, 720f. See also Drug therapy.
Oral examination, 141-143, 142f
in newborn, 209, 218t
Oral rehydration therapy, 821
Oral stage, 78
Oral temperature, 126t, 127b, 128
Oral transmucosal fentanyl. See Fentanyl.
Oral ulcers, 465-466, 466f
in chemotherapy, 936-937
Oralet. See Fentanyl.
Organ donation, 605. See also Transplantation.
Orientation, neonatal, 213b
Orogastric feeding, 745-746, 746f
Oropharyngeal suctioning, in newborn, 221
Ortho Evra transdermal system, 546t
Orthodox Judaism, 66t
Orthophoric eyes, 136, 136f
Orthopnea, 757b
Orthoses
for cerebral palsy, 1148, 1148f
for developmental dysplasia of hip, 1124, 1124f, 1125
for juvenile idiopathic arthritis, 1140
for scoliosis, 1131-1133, 1132f
Orthostatic hypotension, 131-132
Ortolani test, 1122, 1123f
Oscillometry, in blood pressure measurement, 129, 130t
in newborn, 206, 206f, 217t
Oseltamivir (Tamiflu), 765
Osteochondritis, heel lance and, 715
Osteochondritis deformans juvenilis, 1128-1130, 1129b
Osteodystrophy, renal, 968, 969
Osteogenesis imperfecta, 1112, 1127-1128, 1128b
Osteomyelitis, 1134-1135
Osteoporosis
in anorexia nervosa, 557, 558
in cystic fibrosis, 799-800
in female athlete triad, 557
Osteosarcoma, 1135-1137
amputation for, 1121
Ostium primum defect, 868b
Ostium secundum defect, 868b
Ostomies, 750-751. See also specific types.
OTFC (oral transmucosal fentanyl). See Fentanyl.
Otitis media, 765-766
hearing impairment and, 627-628
Otoscopic examination, 138-140, 139f, 140f
Oucher Faces Pain Scale, 162t, 164, 171
Outcome and Assessment Information Set (OASIS), 648
Outcomes, 17
Outpatient care, 679-680, 679b
Ovarian hormones, 1027t
Overprotection, in chronic illness/disability, 582
Overuse syndromes, sports-related, 538-539
Overweight, 551. See also Obesity.
Oxybutynin, for opioid-related hallucinations, 180t
Oxycodone, 175, 176t, 180t
Oxygen therapy, 738-740, 739f, 740f
delivery devices for, 738-739, 739f
for carbon monoxide poisoning, 783
for congestive heart failure, 879t, 883
for cystic fibrosis, 798, 800
for sickle cell anemia, 919
for status asthmaticus, 790-791
monitoring in, 739-740
toxicity of, 739
Oxytocin, 1025t

P

Pacemakers, 897
Pacifiers, 258, 342
aspiration of, 368
in pain management, 173
Padded boards, for intravenous infusion, 737
Pain
abdominal. See Abdominal pain.
assessment of, 108
behavioral response to, 159-161, 159b, 159f
breakthrough, 183
chronic, 190
headache, 192
in cancer, 193-194
in cerebral palsy, 1148, 1149
in circumcision, 226b-227b, 227-228
in HIV/AIDS, 942
in juvenile idiopathic arthritis, 1140
in leukemia, 932-935
in menstruation, 541-542
in sickle cell anemia, 918, 918b, 921, 922
in terminal illness, 193-194, 595, 596, 600-603
neuropathic, 193-194
phantom limb, 1122, 1137
postoperative, 191-192, 697
procedural, 173-174, 184
in circumcision, 226b-227b, 227-228
stress response in, 189-190
Pain assessment
behavioral measures in, 159-161, 159b, 160t-161t, 165-171
cultural factors in, 171
in chronic illness, 171
in cognitive impairment, 166-171, 169f-170f
in complex pain, 171
in infants and neonates, 165-166, 167t-169t
multidimensional measures in, 164-165
physiologic measures in, 161-162
self-report measures in, 162-164, 162t-164t
tools for, 160t-161t
Pain Assessment Tool (PAT), 167t
Pain Indicator for Communicatively Impaired Children, 166-171
Pain management, 171-194. See also Analgesia.
cognitive-behavioral therapy in, 192-193
complementary and alternative therapies in, 175, 192
coping strategies in, 171-173, 192-193
effectiveness of, 189-191
for abdominal pain, 192-193
for burns, 1096-1097
for headache, 192
for postoperative pain, 191-192
for procedural pain, 137-174, 184, 191
in cancer, 193
in circumcision, 226b-227b, 227-228
for subcutaneous injections, 723-724
for venipuncture, 173-174, 184-185, 717
in end-of-life care, 193-194, 595, 596, 600-603
in evidence-based practice, 173-174, 185-187
nonpharmacologic, 171-175
pharmacologic, 175-194
postoperative, 697
Palate, 142, 142f
of newborn, 209
Palatine tonsils, 142-143, 142f, 763, 763f
Palatoplasty, 846
Palivizumab, for respiratory syncytial virus infection, 774
Palliative care, 595, 596-603. See also Death and dying.
Pallor, race/ethnicity and, 133t
Palmar flexion creases, 133, 133f
Palmar grasp, 325

Palpation
  deep, 149
  of abdomen, 149, 149f
    in newborn, 210, 219t
  of scrotum, 150, 150f
  of skull, 134
    in newborn, 207, 208f
  superficial, 149
Palpebral conjunctiva, 134, 134f
Palpebral fissure, 134, 134f
Pancreatic enzymes, for cystic fibrosis, 799
Pancreatic fibrosis, in cystic fibrosis, 796
Pancreatic hormones, 1026t
Pancreatic insufficiency, in cystic fibrosis, 796,
    799
Paper doll technique, 118, 119f
Papules, 1063f
Papulopustular acne, 1090
Parachute reflex, 325, 327f
Parallel play, 84, 416
Paralysis
  facial, in newborn, 246, 246f
  in Guillain-Barré syndrome, 1165-1167, 1166b
  in newborn, 246-247, 246f, 247f
  in spina bifida, 1154-1161
  in spinal cord disorders, 1170-1172
Paralytic ileus, 849
Paraplegia, 1170. *See also* Paralysis.
Parasitic diseases, intestinal, 465-469
Parasomnias, 347
Parasuicide, 568
Parathyroid disorders, 1035-1036
  hyperparathyroidism, 1036-1037, 1037b
  hypoparathyroidism, 1035-1036
Parathyroid hormones, 1026t
Parents, 38-45. *See also* Family; Father; Mother.
  abusive, child's interactions with, 485
  adolescent child's relationship with, 520, 525t
  adoptive, 43-45
  age of, 39
  anticipatory guidance for, 101
    understanding toddlers and, 434
  authoritarian, 40
  authoritative, 41
  communication with, 99-102. *See also*
    Communication.
  coping strategies of, 40
  democratic, 41
  dictatorial, 40
  discipline by, 41-43
  divorced, 33-34, 45-48
  grieving by, 606
  limit setting by, 41
  motivations for parenthood, 38-39
  of dying child, 603-607
  of hospitalized child, 664
  of special needs child, 579-581
  parenting styles of, 40-41
  preparation for parenthood, 39
  roles of, 35
  school programs and, 500
  single, 33-34, 47-48
  support for, 40
  transition to parenthood, 39-40
Parental notification, 544
Parenteral fluid therapy, 733-738
  administration set change in, 737
  complications of, 738
  equipment for, 733-735, 733f
  extravasation in, 738
  infiltration in, 738
  infusion sites in, 733, 733f
  line removal in, 737-738
  line securement in, 735-736, 735f
  site care in, 736

Parenteral nutrition. *See also* Nutritional support;
    Total parenteral nutrition.
  central venous catheter for, 725-730
Parent-infant attachment. *See* Attachment.
Parent's Postoperative Pain Rating Scale (PPPRS),
    161
Paroxysmal abdominal pain, in infant, 395-396,
    397, 397f
Partial seizures, 1006b. *See also* Seizures.
Parvovirus B19, 306t, 463
Patch, cutaneous, 1063f
Patch therapy, 633
Patellar reflex, 153
Patent ductus arteriosus, 292t, 869-870
Paternal engrossment, attachment and, 235-236,
    236f
Patient bill of rights, 672, 672b
Patient-controlled analgesia, 178-183, 181t, 183t
  for postoperative pain, 191-192
Pavlik harness, 1124, 1124f, 1125
Peak expiratory flow meter, in asthma, 786, 786b,
    791-794
Peak expiratory flow rate, 786, 786b
Pearson attachment, 1119f
Pedestrian injuries, 5
Pediatric nurse, roles of, 11-14
Pediatric nursing, 1-18. *See also* Nursing.
  access to, 2
  atraumatic care in, 11
  caring in, 12
  community-based, 20-27. *See also* Community-
    based nursing.
  coordination and collaboration in, 13
  ethical decision making in, 13-14. *See also under*
    Ethical.
  evidence-based practice in, 14-15, 15b, 15t
  family advocacy in, 11-12
  family-centered care in, 10, 11b
  goals of, 2, 2b
  humane care in, 13
  philosophy of care in, 10
  scope of, 11-14
  support and counseling in, 13
  therapeutic care in, 11
  therapeutic relationship in, 11
Pediatric Pain Questionnaire, 165
Pediatric social illness, 3
Pediculosis capitis, 1079-1081
Pedophilia, 482
Peer relations, 56
  of adolescent, 520-521, 525t
  of school-age child, 497-498
Pelvic examination, 542
Pelvic inflammatory disease, 547-549
Penicillin
  allergy to, 905
  prophylactic, for sickle cell anemia, 919, 920
Penile nerve block, for circumcision, 227-228,
    227b
Penis
  care for, after circumcision, 228
  disorders of, 542-543
  examination of, 150
    in newborn, 210, 220t
Peptic index score, 193
Peptic ulcer disease, 836-838
Perceptive deafness, 623-624. *See also* Hearing
    impairment.
Perceptual thinking, 495
Percocet, 175, 176t
Percodan, 175, 176t
Percussion
  of chest, 741, 743f
  of lung, 144-145
Perez reflex, 212t

Perineal care, 701
Periodic breathing, in newborn, 209
Periodontal disease, 507
Periodontitis, 507
Periorbital hematoma, 630
Peripheral blood smear, 913t
Peripheral blood stem cells
  removal of, 946
  transplantation of. *See* Stem cell
    transplantation.
Peripheral intermittent infusion device, 725, 729f
Peripheral intravenous lines, 733-738. *See also*
    Intravenous administration.
Peripheral neuropathy, 193
Peripheral vision, assessment of, 137
Peristalsis, 149
Peristaltic waves, 148
Peritoneal dialysis, 969-971
Peritonitis, in appendicitis, 829-830
Permanency planning, 643
Permethrin
  for head lice, 1080
  for scabies, 1079
Permissive parent, 40-41
PERRLA, 135
Persistent pulmonary hypertension of newborn,
    292t
Persistent vegetative state, 976b
Personal care, in adolescence, 528
Personnel
  identification of, 222
  in atraumatic care, 11
Pertussis, 458t-461t, 776
  immunization for, 356
Pet allergies, 787-788, 787b
Pet bites, 1083, 1084
Petechiae, race/ethnicity and, 133t
pH, urine, 953t
Phallic stage, 78
Phantom limb sensation, 1122, 1137
Pharyngeal tonsils, 763, 763f
Pharyngitis, 761b, 762-763, 762f
Phenylketonuria (PKU), 313-315, 313f
  newborn screening for, 223, 224b
Pheochromocytoma, 1042
Phimosis, 958t
Phobia, school, 562
Phocomelia, 220t, 1127
Phosphorus, 394t
  imbalance of
    in chronic renal failure, 969
    in hyperparathyroidism, 1037
Photoscreening, for amblyopia, 136
Phototherapy, for hyperbilirubinemia, 277-278,
    278f, 279-280
Phrenic nerve paralysis, 247
Physeal injury, 1112
Physical abuse, 480-482, 484b, 485, 486. *See also*
    Abuse.
Physical development, 72, 74-75. *See also*
    Growth.
Physical disabilities. *See* Chronic illness/disability.
Physical distress, 11
Physical examination, 118-156
  general appearance in, 132
  growth measurements in, 121-124, 123f, 124f
  guidelines for, 119
  in abused/neglected child, 486
  in newborn assessment, 207-211, 208f, 211f,
    215, 215b, 216b, 217t-220t
  in nutritional assessment, 115-118, 116b-118b
  of abdomen, 147-149
    in newborn, 209, 210, 219t
  of anus, 151
    in newborn, 210, 220t

Physical examination (*Continued*)
of chest, 143-144, 143f
in newborn, 209, 218t
of ear, 137-140
in newborn, 209, 218t
of extremities, 152
in newborn, 210-211, 211f, 220t
of eye, 134-137
in newborn, 208, 218t
of genitals, 149-151, 150f, 151f
in newborn, 210, 219t-220t
of head and neck, 133-134
in newborn, 207, 208f, 209, 217t, 218t
of heart, 145-147, 147f, 147t
in newborn, 209-210, 219t
of joints, 152-153
in newborn, 211
of lungs, 144-145, 144f, 145b
in newborn, 209, 219t
of lymph nodes, 133, 134f
in newborn, 210
of mouth and throat, 141-143, 142f
in newborn, 209, 218t
of nervous system, 153-155
of nose, 140
in newborn, 209, 218t
of skin, 132-133, 133f, 133t
in newborn, 207, 217t
of spine, 151-152
in newborn, 210, 220t
physiologic measurements in, 124-132. *See also*
Vital signs.
positioning for, 120t
preparation of child for, 118-121, 119f, 120t
Physical neglect, 480, 484b
Physical therapy
for cerebral palsy, 1149
for juvenile idiopathic arthritis, 1140
Physician-assisted suicide, 596. *See also* Treatment
withholding.
Physiologic anemia, 324
Physiologic anorexia, in toddler, 422
Physiologic craniotabes, 207, 217t, 246
Physiologic jaundice, 275
Physiologic splitting, of heart sounds, 146
Piaget's cognitive theory, 79t, 80-81, 327, 330,
412-413, 495, 519
Piercing, 529
Pigeon chest, 143
Pigeon toe, 152
Pigmentation, race/ethnicity and, 58
Pilonidal sinus, 210
Pincer grasp, 325, 325f
Pink eye, 465b
Pinna, 137-138
angle of, 138, 138f
in newborn, 209
Pinworms, 468-469, 470b
Pituitary
anterior, 1025t
posterior, 1025t-1026t
Pituitary disorders, 1023-1032
acromegaly, 1029
diabetes insipidus, 1030-1031
hyperfunction, 1029
hypopituitarism, 1024-1029
precocious puberty, 1029-1030, 1030t
syndrome of inappropriate antidiuretic hor-
mone secretion, 984, 1031-1032
Pituitary hormones, 1025t-1026t
Pizotifen, for abdominal pain, 193
Placebos, 178
Placing reflex, 212t
Plagiocephaly, 221, 400-401, 401f

Planning. *See also* Nursing care plans.
in nursing process, 17
Plantar reflex, 152
Plantar wart, 1072t
Plants, poisonous, 370, 470b, 472b
Plaque, cutaneous, 1063f
Plastibell procedure, 228
Plastic bags, infant suffocation in, 369
Plastic oxygen hood, 738, 739f
Platelet count, 913t
Platelet transfusion, apheresis in, 946
Play, 83-86
associative, 441
classification of, 84
content of, 83-84
for procedures, 694, 695b
functions of, 85-86
games in, 84
in autism, 635
in cognitive development, 330, 439
in cognitive impairment, 616-617, 616f, 617f
in communication, 105, 107b
in hospitalization, 673-675, 673b
in social development
of infant, 331, 333, 333t-334t
of preschooler, 441-442, 441f, 442f
of school-age child, 498-499, 499f
of toddler, 416-417, 416f
in visual impairment, 631
infant activities for, 333t-334t
mutual, 442
parallel, 416
preschooler activities for, 441-442, 441f, 442f
social character of, 84-85
solitary, 333
teams in, 499
therapeutic, 674
toddler activities for, 416-417, 416f
toys in, 86, 87
Play therapy, 674
Pneumatosis intestinalis, 298
Pneumococcal disease, 776
antibiotic prophylaxis for, in sickle cell anemia,
920
immunization for, 357-358
in sickle cell anemia, 919, 920
Pneumocystis carinii pneumonia, 940-941
Pneumonia, 774-777
aspiration, 781. *See also* Aspiration.
in near-drowning, 993
prevention of, 696
bacterial, 776
bronchopneumonia, 774
in avian influenza, 775-776
in cystic fibrosis, 796, 797-799
in SARs, 775
interstitial, 774
lobar, 774
Pneumocystis carinii, 940-941
primary atypical, 775
signs and symptoms of, 775b
viral, 775-776
Pneumonitis, 774-775
Pneumothorax, 289, 291t
Point of maximum intensity, 146, 146f
in newborn, 209
Poison control center, 470
Poison ivy/oak/sumac, 1075-1076, 1075f
Poisoning, 5-6
assessment of, 473
carbon monoxide, 783, 1093
emergency treatment for, 470, 473
gastric decontamination for, 473
heavy metal, 475-480
in infant, 370-371

Poisoning (*Continued*)
in preschooler, 469-480
in school-age child, 510t
in toddler, 427t, 432-433, 432f
lead, 475-480
recurrent, prevention of, 474-475
Poker chip tool, 163t, 164
Poliomyelitis, 460-461
immunization for, 356-357
Polyandry, 34
Polycythemia, 292t
in hypoxemia, 884
Polydactyly, 152, 210, 220t
Polydipsia
in diabetes mellitus, 1031
in syndrome of inappropriate antidiuretic
hormone secretion, 1031
Polyethylene glycol, for constipation, 824
Polygamy, 34
Polygyny, 34
Polyps, nasal, in cystic fibrosis, 799
Polys, measurement of, 913t
Polyuria
in diabetes mellitus, 1031
in syndrome of inappropriate antidiuretic
hormone secretion, 1031
Popliteal angle, 204b
Popliteal pulse, 146f
Populations, 21
Pornography, child sexual abuse and, 482
Ports, implanted, 725-730, 727t, 728f
preslit, 734, 735f
Port-wine stain, 217t, 249, 249f
Position. *See also* Posture.
knee-chest, for hypercyanotic spells, 885, 885f
recovery, 810, 810f
tripod, 769
Positional plagiocephaly, 215, 221, 400-401, 401f
Positioning
en face, attachment and, 215, 234, 234f
for breastfeeding, 231, 231f
for bronchial drainage, 741, 742f
for circumcision, 228, 228f
for coma, 985
for congestive heart failure, 883
for cranial surgery, 996
for ear examination, 138
for extremity venipuncture, 710
for femoral venipuncture, 710, 710f
for gavage feeding, 746, 746f
for genital examination, 150-151, 150f
for gynecologic examination, 542
for high-risk newborn, 259, 259f
for hypercyanotic spells, 885, 885f
for lumbar puncture, 710-711, 711f
for oral drug administration, 719, 720f
for oral examination, 141, 142f
for pain management, 173
for physical examination, 120t
for procedures, 710-711
for respiratory emergencies, 810, 810f
for sleep, in newborn, 215, 221
Positive self-talk, for pain, 172
Positron emission tomography, in cerebral dysfunction, 981t
Postanesthesia care, 694-697
Postcoital contraception, 546t
Postconcussion syndrome, 990
Posterior fontanel, 207, 208f, 217t
Posterior tibial pulse, 146f
Postmortem care, 604
Postneonatal mortality, 8-9, 8t, 9t
Postoperative care, 697-698
Postoperative pain management, 697. *See also*
Analgesia; Pain management.

Postoperative Pain Score, 167t
Postpubescence, 514
Poststreptococcal glomerulonephritis, 961
Postterm infants, 273-274
Posttraumatic seizures, 990
Posttraumatic stress disorder, 562
Postural drainage, 741, 742f
  in cystic fibrosis, 798, 801, 802
Postural hypotension, 131-132
Posture. *See also* Position.
  assessment of, 132
    gestational age and, 204b
    in newborn, 207, 217t, 272f
  of adolescent, 529
  opisthotonic, 220t
Posturing, in neurologic examination, 979, 979f
Postvention, 681
Potassium, 394t
Potassium imbalance
  in acute renal failure, 966
  in chronic renal failure, 968
  in diabetic ketoacidosis, 1049
  transfusion-related, 944t
Pouch, ostomy, 750-751
Poverty, 54
  development and, 89
  disease susceptibility and, 59
  homelessness and, 54
Povidone-iodine, in ophthalmia neonatorum
    prophylaxis, 222
Preadolescence, 494
Precautions
  airborne, 706-707, 707b
  contact, 707, 707b
  droplet, 707, 707b
  isolation, 680, 706, 707b
  standard, 706, 707b
    high-risk newborn and, 255
    newborn bathing and, 224
  transmission-based, 706-707, 707b
Precocious puberty, 1029-1030
Prefeeding behavior, 234
Pregnancy
  adolescent, 543-544
  drug use during, 300-305, 311t
  in cystic fibrosis, 796, 803
  infections in, 305-308, 305t-307t
  prenatal diagnosis in, 622
Pregnancy-induced hypertension, 299
Prehension, 325
Premature Infant Pain Profile (PIPP), 166, 168t
Prenatal diagnosis
  of Down syndrome, 622
  of spina bifida, 1155-1156
Preoperational stage, 79, 79t, 413, 414b, 439
Preoperative care, 694-697
  for circumcision, 228
Preoperative fasting, 696, 696t, 732-733
  oral care in, 732
Prepubescence, 494, 514
Prepuce, 210
Preschooler
  biologic development of, 438, 438f
  body image of, 440
  chronic illness/disability in, 592t
  cognitive development of, 439
  communication with, 103-104
  dental health of, 450
  fears of, 446
  imaginary playmates and, 442
  injury of, prevention of, 450
  masturbation in, 446
  nutrition in, 447-448, 448f
  personal-social behavior of, 440-441, 441f
  poisoning in, 469-480

Preschooler (*Continued*)
  preschool/kindergarten experience of, 442-443
  sex education for, 443-446
  sexual development of, 440
  sleep and activity in, 448-450, 449t
  social development of, 440-442, 441f, 442f
  speech problems in, 447
  spiritual development of, 439-440
  stress in, 446-447
Preslit injection ports, 734
Pressure garments, for burns, 1101
Pressure ulcers, 700-701
  prevention of, in coma, 985
Preterm infant, 271, 271b. *See also* Newborn,
    high-risk.
  apnea in, 291t
  car seat for, 268
  diagnostic evaluation of, 271-273, 272f-273f
  ethical considerations for, 269
  hepatitis B vaccine in, 223
  retinopathy in, 289, 293t
  therapeutic management of, 273
Prevalence, 22
Prevention, 12-13
  anticipatory guidance in, 13
  health teaching in, 13
  primary, 22-23
  secondary, 23
  tertiary, 23
  time line for, 121f
Priapism, in sickle cell anemia, 921
Primary groups, 53
Primitive neuroectodermal tumor, 1137-1138
Primitive reflexes, 201
Privacy, 98-99
  of Internet communications, 99
  parental notification and, 544
Private duty nursing, in home care, 644, 644b
Probiotics, lactose intolerance and, 387-388
Procedures, 686-751. *See also specific procedures.*
  compliance with, 698
  distraction for, 689-690, 693, 694, 695b
  for cardiovascular disorders, 864-865, 864b
  for drug administration, 717-732
  for elimination problems, 750-751
  for fluid management, 732-738
  for general hygiene and care, 700-705
  for respiratory disorders, 738-745
  for specimen collection, 710-717
  guidelines for, 690b
  health teaching for, 692-693
  informed consent for, 687-689
  pain management for, 173-174, 184. *See also*
      Analgesia; Pain management.
    in cancer, 193
  parental presence and support for, 690-692
  performance of, 693-694
  play for, 694, 695b
  positioning for, 710-711. *See also* Safety
      concerns.
  postprocedure care in, 694
  preparation for, 689-693
    developmental aspects of, 691t-692t
    physical, 693
    psychological, 689-693
  restraint for, 708-710
  surgical, 694-698. *See also* Surgery.
Progesterone, 1026t, 1027t
Prolactin, 1025t
Promethazine, for opioid-related nausea, 179t
Pros and cons technique, 107b
Prosthetic eye, 634-635, 634f
Prosthetic limbs, 1121-1122, 1127, 1137
Prostitution, of children, 482
Protanomaly, 137

Protein, daily requirements for, 76t
Protein-energy malnutrition (PEM), 381,
    383-384
Proteinuria, 953t
Proton pump inhibitors, for peptic ulcers, 837
Proximity, parent-infant attachment and, 235
Proximodistal growth, 72
Pruritus
  excoriation in, 1064f
  in atopic dermatitis, 1087
  in burns, 1101
  in pediculosis capitis, 1079-1080
  in scabies infestation, 1079
  in skin disorders, 1061
  opioid-induced, 179t, 188
  treatment of, 1067, 1068
Pseudohermaphroditism, 958t
Pseudohypertrophy, in Duchenne muscular dys-
    trophy, 1163-1164
Pseudomenstruation, in newborn, 200, 210, 219t
Pseudostrabismus, 136, 136f
Psoriasis, 1085f
Psychedelics, 567
Psychologic dependence, on opioids, 189
Psychologic distress, 11
Psychologic tasks, for parents of high-risk infant,
    265, 265b
Psychosexual development, 78-79, 79t
Psychosocial development, 79-80, 79t
  in adolescent, 518-519
  in infant, 327
  in preschooler, 438-439
  in school-age child, 494-495, 495f, 503t
  in toddler, 411
Psychosocial dwarfism, 540
Psychosocial history, 111-113
Psychotherapy
  for abdominal pain, 192-193
  for eating disorders, 558
  for obesity, 555
Ptyalin, 324
Puberty. *See also* Sexual development.
  breast development in, 144
  definition of, 514
  delayed, 515, 540
    radiation therapy and, 938-939
  hormonal changes of, 514-515
  menstruation in, 541
  precocious, 1029-1030
  responses to, 524
Pubic hair, 132
  in female, 151, 517f
  in male, 150, 517f
Pudendum, 151, 151f
Puerto Ricans. *See also* Race/ethnicity.
  health beliefs and practices of, 69t
Pulled elbow, 1111
Pulmonary artery hypertension, 897-898
Pulmonary aspiration. *See* Aspiration.
Pulmonary function tests, in asthma, 785-786
Pulmonary hypertension, persistent, of newborn,
    292t
Pulmonic stenosis, 872
Pulmonic valves, 146
Pulmozyme (dornase alfa), for cystic fibrosis, 798,
    798f
Pulses
  apical, 127, 146, 146f
  brachial, 146, 146f
  carotid, 146, 146f
  dorsalis pedis, 146, 146f
  femoral, 149, 149f
    in newborn, 210, 219t
  grading of, 129t
  location of, 146, 146f

Pulses *(Continued)*
  measurement of, 127-129
    in newborn, 206, 209, 216t
  popliteal, 146, 146f
  posterior tibial, 146, 146f
Pulse oximetry, 739-740, 740f
Pulsus paradoxus, 757b
Pumps, infusion
  in baclofen administration, 735
  in intravenous therapy, 735
  in patient-controlled analgesia, 178-183
Puncture wounds, 1068
Punishment, 41-43
  corporal, 42-43
  moral development and, 439
Pupil
  examination of, 134f, 135
    in newborn, 208, 212t
  of newborn, 201, 208, 212t
Pupillary light reflex, 135, 212t
Purpura
  definition of, 927-928
  idiopathic thrombocytopenic, 927-929
Pustules, 1063f
Pyelonephritis, 950. *See also* Urinary tract infections.
Pyloric stenosis, 849-852
Pyloromyotomy, 851-852, 851f
Pyoderma, 1069-1071, 1070t
Pyrazinamide, for tuberculosis, 779
Pyridoxine, 390t

Q
Quadriceps reflex, 153, 154f
Quadriplegia, 1170. *See also* Paralysis.
Questran (cholestyramine), 895
Quiet activities, of school-age child, 499, 499f

R
Rabies, 1003-1004
Race/ethnicity, 53-54, 56-57. *See also* Immigrants.
  adoption and, 44-45
  anemia and, 914
  childhood mortality and, 9-10
  culture and, 52, 53-54. *See also under* Cultural;
      Culture.
  diet and, 58, 61-62
  growth patterns and, 122
  hair characteristics and, 132
  infant mortality and, 9
  obesity and, 551
  of nurses, 64-67
  physical characteristics and, 58
  self-esteem and, 53
  skin color and, 58, 132, 133t, 207
Rachischisis. *See* Spina bifida.
Radial pulse, 146f
Radiant warmer, 254, 254f
Radiation therapy
  for brain tumors, 995
  for Ewing sarcoma, 1137-1138
  for Hodgkin disease, 938
  for leukemia, 931, 932
  for Wilms tumor, 964
  side effects of, 938-939
Radiofrequency ablation, for dysrhythmias, 896, 897
Radiography
  in cerebral dysfunction, 980t
  of bone tumors, 1136
  of fractures, 1113
Radionuclide cystogram, 951t
Range of motion, in newborn, 211
Range-of-motion exercises, in coma, 985
Rape, 549. *See also* Sexual abuse.
  date rape drugs and, 549, 567

Rape trauma syndrome, 550
Rapprochement, 415
Rash. *See also* Skin disorders.
  diaper, 1084-1086, 1086f
  in chickenpox, 454f
  in erythema infectiosum, 456, 456f
  in exanthem subitum, 456, 456f
  in measles, 458, 458f
  in rickettsial diseases, 1082
  in rubella, 460, 460f
  newborn, 247-248
Rating game, 106b
Reactive attachment disorder, 332
Reactive hyperemia, 700
Reactivity, periods of, in newborn, 211-213
Reading ability, in school-age child, 495, 499, 499f
Reading materials, developmental effects of, 90
Real-time ultrasonography, in cerebral dysfunction, 980t
Rebound effect, after phototherapy, 280
Recidivism, in substance abuse, 568
Reciprocity, parent-infant attachment and, 235
Recommended dietary allowance (RDA), 113, 380
Reconstituted family, 33, 48
Recovery position, 810, 810f
Rectal patency, 210, 220t
Rectal prolapse, in cystic fibrosis, 796, 799
Rectal suppositories, 730
  for anticonvulsants, 1015
Rectal temperature, 126t, 127b, 128
  vs. axillary temperature, in newborn, 205
Rectal ulcers, in chemotherapy, 937
Red blood cells
  in urine, 953t
  morphology of, 912, 914b
  sickled, 917-918, 917f
Red blood cell indices, 913t
Red reflex, 135
  in newborn, 208
Reduction deformities, 1127
Reed-Sternberg cells, 938
Refeeding syndrome, 558
Reflexes
  Achilles, 154f
  anal, 151
  ankle clonus, 212t
  assessment of, 153
    in newborn, 212t
  Babinski, 152, 211, 211f, 212t, 979
  biceps, 154f
  cognitive development and, 330
  corneal light, 136, 136f, 208, 212t
  cough, 212t
  crawl, 212t, 213f
  cremasteric, 150, 150f
  dance, 212t
  deep tendon, 153
  doll's eye, 212t
  examination of, 979
  extrusion, 212t
  gag, 141, 212t
  Galant, 212t
  glabellar, 212t
  grasp, 152, 211, 211f, 212t, 273f, 327
    in cerebral palsy, 1147b, 1148
  knee jerk, 153, 154f
  Moro, 212t, 213f
  otoscopic light, 140
  parachute, 325, 327f
  patellar, 153, 154f
  Perez, 212t
  placing, 212t
  plantar, 152
  primitive, 201
  pupillary light, 135, 212t

Reflexes *(Continued)*
  quadriceps, 153
  red, 135, 208
  rooting, 209, 212t
  sneeze, 212t
  startle, 209, 212t
  step, 212t
  sucking, 209, 212t, 218t
  tonic neck, 212t, 213f
  triceps, 154f
  trunk incurvation, 212t
  yawn, 212t
Reflux
  gastroesophageal, 823f, 827-829
  vesicoureteral, 954, 955
Refractive errors, 628, 628t-629t, 633
Refrigerant sprays, 184
Regression, in toddler behavior, 422
Regurgitation, 395
Rehabilitation
  in head injury, 992-993
  in substance abuse, 568
Rehydration. *See also* Fluid management.
  in diarrhea, 821, 821b
Relative poverty, 54
Relaxation techniques, for pain, 172
Religious beliefs, 55, 64, 65t-66t. *See also under*
      Spiritual.
  birth and death practices and, 65t-66t
  diet and, 65t-66t
  faith healing and, 63-64
  neonatal loss and, 270
  vs. spirituality, 64
Remicade (infliximab), for inflammatory bowel
      disease, 834-835
Renal angiography, 952t
Renal biopsy, 952t
Renal cancer, 963-965, 963b, 964b
Renal dialysis, 969-971
Renal disease, end-stage, 969
Renal failure
  acute, 965-967
  chronic, 967-970
Renal function
  assessment of, 950, 953t-954t
  fluid balance and, 815
Renal osteodystrophy, 968, 969
Renal palpation, in newborn, 210, 219t
Renal system
  of infant, 325
  of newborn, 200
Renal transplantation, 969, 971
Repetitive microtrauma, in athletes, 539
Reporting, of suicidal behavior, 570
Research, nursing, 14
Resiliency model of family stress, adjustment and
      adaptation, 32
Respiration. *See also* Breathing.
  assessment of, 144, 757
  chest movements in, 144, 144f
    in newborn, 209
  Cheyne-Stokes, 145b
  in neurologic examination, 977
  Kussmaul, 145b, 1044
  patterns of, 145b, 757b
Respiratory arrest, 803-804
Respiratory depression, opioid-induced, 179t, 188
Respiratory disorders
  acute lung injury, 781-782
  acute respiratory distress syndrome, 781-782, 903
  aerosol therapy for, 740-741
  asthma, 783-795
  bronchial (postural) drainage for, 741, 742f
  chest physical therapy for, 741, 742f

Respiratory disorders *(Continued)*
emergency management of, 803-810
foreign body aspiration, 780-781
in cystic fibrosis, 796, 797-799, 797b
in Down syndrome, 622
in immobilization, 1108t
infectious. *See* Respiratory infections.
noninfectious, 780-810
oxygen therapy for, 738-740
second-hand smoke and, 783, 784b
smoke inhalation injury, 782-783
Respiratory distress
in congestive heart failure, 883
in newborn, 221b, 284
Respiratory distress syndrome, 284-288
diagnosis of, 286, 286b, 286f
nursing care management in, 288
nursing care plan for, 289-290
pathophysiology of, 284-286
prevention of, 288
prognosis of, 288
treatment of, 286-287, 287t
Respiratory emergencies, 803-810
Respiratory failure, 803-804
cardiopulmonary resuscitation for, 804-809
in Duchenne muscular dystrophy, 1164-1165
Respiratory infections, 755-759. *See also specific*
infections.
age and, 755
avian influenza, 775-776
bacterial tracheitis, 769, 769t, 772
bronchiolitis, 773
bronchitis, 773
clinical manifestations of, 756, 756t, 757b
croup, 769, 769t, 770-771, 771b
croup syndromes, 769-770, 769t
epiglottitis, 769-770, 769t
etiology of, 755-756
fungal, 1072-1074
humidification for, 756
in cystic fibrosis, 796, 797-799
infectious mononucleosis, 768
influenza, 764-765
laryngitis, 769, 769t, 770
laryngotracheobronchitis, 769, 769t, 770-771,
771b
lower tract, 772-777
nasopharyngitis, 759-762
nursing care for, 756-759
nursing care plan for, 759-761
nursing process in, 757
pertussis, 776
pharyngitis, 761b, 762-763
pneumonia, 774-777
respiratory syncytial virus infection, 773-774
SARS, 775
spasmodic laryngitis, 769, 769t, 771-772
tonsillitis, 763-764, 763f
tuberculosis, 776-780
upper tract, 759-768
Respiratory movements, 144, 144f
in newborn, 209
Respiratory rate
maturation of, in infant, 323
measurement of, 129, 144
in newborn, 206, 217t
Respiratory secretions
clearance of
chest physical therapy in, 741, 742f, 743f
in cystic fibrosis, 798, 798f, 800, 801
sampling of, 717
Respiratory syncytial virus infection, 772t,
773-774
secretion sampling in, 717

Respiratory tract
in newborn, 198, 209
complications involving, 288-289, 291t, 294
in toddler, 410-411
reaction portion of, 772
Respite care, 643
Rest. *See also* Activity and exercise.
in congestive heart failure, 878, 882
Restraints, 708-710
automobile. *See* Car seats/restraints.
behavioral, 170f, 709-710
for gavage feeding, 746
medical-surgical, 708-709
Restrictive cardiomyopathy, 898-899
Resuscitation
cardiopulmonary, 804-809
fluid, 807-809, 904, 905. *See also* Fluid
management.
in near-drowning, 993-994
Resynchronization therapy, for congestive heart
failure, 878
Rete pegs, 200, 259
Retention enema, for drug administration, 730
Reticulocyte count, 913t
Retin-A (tretinoin), for acne, 1090
Retinoblastoma, 633-635, 634f
Retinoic acid (Acutane), for acne, 1090
Retinol, 388t
Retinopathy
diabetic, 1044
of prematurity, 289, 293t
Retrograde pyelography, 952t
Review of systems, 113, 114
Revised Infant Temperament Questionnaire,
334-335
Rewarming, for frostbite, 1104
Reye syndrome, 703, 1004-1005, 1004b
Rh incompatibility, 281-282, 282f
prevention of, 282
Rhabdomyosarcoma, 1138-1139, 1138b
Rheumatic fever, 893-894
Rheumatoid arthritis, juvenile, 1139-1142
Ribavirin, for respiratory syncytial virus infection,
774
Riboflavin, 389t
Ribs, 14f, 143
RICE therapy, 1112
in hemophilia, 927
Rickets, vitamin D–deficiency, 378
Rickettsial diseases, 1082-1083, 1082t
Rickettsialpox, 1082t
Rifampin, for tuberculosis, 779
Right-to-left shunt, 866, 866f
Riley Infant Pain Scale (RIPS), 160t
Rimantadine, for influenza, 765
Ring block, for circumcision anesthesia, 227-228,
227b
Ringworm, 1071-1072, 1073f, 1073t, 1085t
Risk factors, 16
demographic, 22
Ritalin (methylphenidate), for attention deficit
hyperactivity disorder, 560
Ritualism
in school-age children, 498-499
in toddlers, 412
Rocky Mountain spotted fever, 1082t
Rohypnol (flunitrazepam), 549, 567
Role continuity/discontinuity, 35
Roles
definition of, 52
family, 35
social, 52-53
Rolling over, 325
Roman Catholics, 66t
Romberg test, 153, 153b

Rooting reflex, 209, 212t
Roseola infantum, 456-457, 456f
Rotavirus infection, 817-823, 818t. *See also*
Diarrhea.
immunization for, 359
Roxicodone (oxycodone), 175, 176t
Rubella, 460-461, 460f
congenital, 307t
immunization for, 357
Rubeola, 458-459, 458f
Rules, in play, of school-age children, 498-499
Russell traction, 1118-1119, 1119f

S

S_1 heart sound, 146, 147t
S_2 heart sound, 146, 147t
S_3 heart sound, 146, 147t
S_4 heart sound, 146, 147t
Safety concerns, 3-6, 705-710. *See also* Traumatic
injuries.
developmental stage and, 4
for animals, 1084
for beds, 368, 705
for bicycle accidents, 5, 508f, 509
for burns, 5, 1102-1103
for chemotherapy, 936
for drowning, 5
for environmental hazards, 89, 705
for fires, 1102-1103
for guns, 5, 6
for insulin injections, 724
for motor vehicle accidents. *See* Automobile
safety.
for newborn, 221-228
for pedestrian accidents, 5
for poisoning, 5-6
for restraints, 709
for special needs children, 5, 591
for suffocation, 5
for toys, 86, 87, 367, 433, 705-706
for violence, 5, 6-7
for water safety, 995
gender and, 4t
home checklist for, 373
in epilepsy, 1015-1016
in home care, 653-654
Sagittal suture, 208f
Saline lock, 725, 726
Salivary glands, of newborn, 199
Salmeterol (Serevent), for asthma, 789
Salmon patch, 249
Salmonellosis, 817-823, 818t. *See also* Diarrhea.
Same sex family, 34
Sample collection. *See* Specimen collection.
Sandifer syndrome, 828
Sarcoma. *See also* Cancer.
Ewing, 1137-1138
osteogenic, 1136-1137
soft tissue, 1138-1139, 1138b
SARs, 775
Satiety behavior, in feeding, 234
Scabies, 1079
Scald burns. *See also* Burns.
in infant, 371
in toddler, 432
Scale, 1064f
Scale for Use in Newborns (SUN), 168t
Scales, for weighing, 124, 124f
Scalp
ringworm of, 1071-1072, 1073f, 1073t, 1085t
seborrheic dermatitis of, 1089
Scalp veins, for intravenous infusion, 733
Scarf sign, 204b, 272f
Scarlet fever, 462-463, 462f

Scars, 1062, 1064f
  burn, 1101, 1101f
  keloid, 1064f
Scheduled feedings, 233
Scheuermann kyphosis, 1130
School. *See also* Education.
  as cultural influence, 55
  cheating in, 501-502
  child's experience of, 500
  socialization in, 55, 626-627
School avoidance, 562
School phobia, 562
School refusal, 562
School vision, 628
School-age child
  attention deficit hyperactivity disorder in,
    559-561
  behavioral disorders in, 559-564
  bodily damage to, 510t
  burns in, 510t
  chronic illness/disability in, 592t
  cognitive development of, 495, 496f, 502t
  dental health of, 506-507, 506f
  discipline for, 501
  dishonest behavior in, 501-504
  elimination problems in, 537-538
  family-centered care for, 501
  fears in, 504
  fine motor skills of, 506
  health problems of, 536-571
  injury prevention in, 508-509, 508f, 510t
  latchkey, 500-501
  learning disabilities in, 559-561
  limit setting for, 501
  mental health issues in, 559-564
  moral development of, 495-496
  nutrition in, 504-505
  obesity in, 551-556
  poisoning of, 510t
  sex chromosome disorders in, 540-541, 541t
  sex education for, 507-508
  sleep in, 505
  social development of, 497-499, 497f, 499f
  spiritual development of, 496-497
  sports injuries in, 538-540
  stress in, 504
  suicide by, 564
Scintigraphy, in gastroesophageal reflux disease, 828
Sclera, 135
  of newborn, 208
Sclerema, 217t
Sclerosing agents, extravasation of, 738
Scolding, 42
Scoliosis, 1130-1134
  screening for, 151
Scorpion stings, 1076-1079, 1078t
Screening, 23. *See also* Assessment.
  developmental, 93-95, 132
  for cystic fibrosis, 797
  for hepatitis C, 840
  for hyperlipidemia, 895
  for hypertension, 901
  for lead poisoning, 478
  for PKU, 223, 224b
  for scoliosis, 151
  for sickle cell anemia, 918
  for vision problems, 136-137
  for visual impairment, 136-137, 1178-1179
  hearing, 223
  HIV, 223
  neonatal, 223, 224b
  schedule for, 121f
Scrotum, 150
  examination of, 150
    in newborn, 210

Sebaceous glands
  in newborn, 200
  of eyelid, 134
Seborrheic dermatitis, 1089
Secondary groups, 53
Second-hand smoke, 783, 784b
Secretin, for autism, 635
Securement devices, for intravenous line, 735,
    735f, 736
Sedation
  for burns, 1096-1097
  for dying child, 194
  in coma, 984
  opioid-induced, 179t, 188
  preoperative, 696-697
Seesaw respirations, 145b
Seizures, 1005-1016
  care plan for, 1011-1014
  classification of, 1005-1006, 1006b-1007b
  clinical manifestations of, 1010b
  diagnosis of, 1006-1008
  etiology of, 1005, 1005b
  febrile, 704, 1016
  in acute renal failure, 966
  in cerebral palsy, 1146, 1147b, 1149
  in coma, 984
  in status epilepticus, 1007, 1007b, 1009-1010
  meperidine-induced, 183
  neonatal, 294-295, 294b, 295t
  nursing process in, 1011
  pathophysiology of, 1005
  postictal state in, 1010b, 1014b
  posttraumatic, 990
  prognosis for, 1010
  treatment of, 1008-1010
    drug therapy in, 1008-1009
    emergency, 1014
    for status epilepticus, 1009-1010
    ketogenic diet in, 1009
    surgery in, 1009
    vagus nerve stimulation in, 1009
  triggering factors for, 1016
  types of, 1005-1006, 1006b-1007b
  vagus nerve stimulation for, 1009
Selective dorsal rhizotomy, for cerebral palsy, 1148
Selenium, 394t
Self-accusation, chronic illness/disability and, 582
Self-care
  hygiene in, 132, 700-702, 704-705
  in chronic illness/disability, 584-585
  in cognitive impairment, 584-585
  in home care, 652-653
  in hospitalization, 671
Self-concept, development of, 82-83, 499-500,
    523-524
Self-esteem, 82-83
  culture and, 53
Self-mastery, in hospitalization, 676
Semilunar valves, 146
Semi-vegetarians, 380
Senna, for opioid-related constipation, 179t
Sensorimotor stage, 79, 79t, 327, 330, 330f,
    412-413
  play in, 85
Sensorineural hearing loss, 623-624, 625. *See also*
    Hearing impairment.
Sensory function
  impaired, 623-635. *See also* Hearing impair-
    ment; Visual impairment.
  in infant, 325
  in newborn, 201
  in toddler, 410
Sensory stimulation, in coma, 985
Sentence completion, 106b
Separation, cognitive development and, 327

Separation anxiety
  in hospitalization, 659-661, 668-670
  in infant, 332, 335
Separation-individuation, 331, 415, 440
Sepsis, neonatal, 296-297, 297b
Septic arthritis, 1135
Septic shock, 906-907, 906b, 907t
Sequestration crisis, in sickle cell anemia, 918,
    918b, 922
Serevent (salmeterol), for asthma, 789
Severe acute respiratory syndrome (SARS), 775
Severe combined immunodeficiency disease
    (SCID), 943
Sex assignment, in congenital adrenal hyperplasia,
    1041-1042
Sex characteristics, pubertal development of, 514
Sex chromosome disorders, 540-541, 541t
Sex education
  for adolescents, 530-531
  for preschoolers, 443-446
  for school-age children, 507-508
Sex hormones, 1037
  in adolescent, 514-515
  in newborn, 200-201
Sex-role identity, in adolescent, 519
Sex-typing, 440
Sexual abuse, 482-483, 483b, 484b, 485, 486, 490.
    See also Abuse.
  prevention of, 488
Sexual assault, 549
  date rape drugs and, 549, 567
Sexual development. *See also* Puberty.
  in congenital adrenal hyperplasia, 1040-1041
  in females, 515, 515b, 516f, 517f
  in males, 515, 515b, 517f
  in precocious puberty, 1029-1030
  in preschooler, 440
Sexual history, 110-111
Sexual orientation, 523
  suicide and, 569
Sexuality
  adolescent, 522-523, 522f
    guidance and education for, 530-531
  communication about, 110-111, 110b
  in cognitive impairment, 618
  problems related to, 543-544
Sexually transmitted diseases, 547-549
Shaken baby syndrome, 481, 987. *See also* Abuse.
Shampooing, 702
Shampoos, for ringworm, 1071-1072, 1073t
Sharps, handling of, 708
Shear, pressure ulcers and, 701
Sheet grafts, for burns, 1098, 1099f
Shigellosis, 817-823, 819t. *See also* Diarrhea.
Shingles, 463, 1072t
Shivering, 324-325, 703-704
Shock
  anaphylactic, 904-906
  cardiogenic, 903t
  compensated, 903-904, 903t
  decompensated, 903-904, 903t
  distributive, 903t
  hypovolemic, 902-903, 903t
  in toxic shock syndrome, 907, 907t
  irreversible, 903t, 904
  septic, 906-907, 906b, 907t
Shoes, for infants, 343
Short bowel syndrome, 856-857
Shoulder, dislocation of, 1111
Showers, 701
Shunts
  fetal, closure of, 198
  intracardiac, 866
  surgical, 886, 886t
  ventriculoperitoneal, 1018-1020, 1019f

Siblings, 36-38
  attachment process and, 236, 236f
    high-risk newborn and, 267, 267f
  birth order of, 36-37, 37b
  developmental influence of, 88
  functions of, 36
  grieving by, 606-607
  of dying child, 603
  of hospitalized child, 664
  of special needs child, 580-581, 580b, 587, 590
  rivalry between, 420-421, 421f
  spacing of, 36
Sibutramine, for weight loss, 553-554
Sick-child care, 340
Sickle cell anemia, 916-923
  acute chest syndrome in, 918, 922
  clinical manifestations of, 918, 918b
  crises in, 918, 918b, 921, 922
  diagnosis of, 918
  emergency situations in, 922
  ethical decision-making in, 919
  evidence-based practice in, 920
  family teaching in, 921-922
  genetic factors in, 917
  nursing care in, 921-923
  pain in, 918, 918b, 921
  pathophysiology of, 917-918, 917f
  prognosis in, 921
  prophylactic penicillin for, 919, 920
  stroke in, 918, 920-921, 922
  treatment of, 918-921
  types of, 917
Sickle cell disease, 916-917
Sickle cell trait, 917
Sickle cell-C disease, 917
Sickle cell–hemoglobin E disease, 917
Sickle thalassemia disease, 917
Sickle-turbidity test (Sickledex), 918
Sign language, 626
Signs and symptoms, 17
Silence, in communication, 101
Silver dressings, 1066t
  for burns, 1098t
Silver nitrate
  for burns, 1098t
  in ophthalmia neonatorum prophylaxis, 222
Silver sulfadiazine, for burns, 1098t
Single-parent family, 33-34, 47-48
Single-photon emission computed tomography
    (SPECT), in cerebral dysfunction, 981t
Sinus arrhythmia, 219t, 324
Sinus tachycardia, 897
Sinus venosus defect, 868b
Site care. See Skin care.
Sitting ability, development of, 325-326, 328f
Skateboard safety, 509
Skeletal system. See also Musculoskeletal system.
  in adolescent, 516
  in newborn, 200
Skin
  artificial, 1098-1099
  examination of, 132-133, 133f, 133t
    in newborn, 207, 217t
  foreign bodies in, 1076
  iatrogenic injury of, 701
  in newborn, 200, 207, 217t
    at high risk, 259-261
    bathing and, 225, 259
    birthmarks and, 217t, 249-250, 249f
    in diaper dermatitis, 248
    in erythema toxicum neonatorum, 247-248
  structure of, 1061
Skin cancer, prevention of, 89
Skin care, 700-701
  for amputation stump, 1121-1122
  for enterostomy, 751

Skin care (Continued)
  for external fixation, 1121
  for gastrostomy, 747
  for Pavlik harness, 1125
  for peripheral intravenous lines, 729, 736
  for tracheostomy, 744
  for traction, 1120
  in diaper area, 1086
  in newborn, 225
  in spina bifida, 1158
  in spinal cord injuries, 1171
Skin color, 58, 132, 133t
  in newborn, 207, 217t
Skin disorders, 1060-1104. See also Dermatitis;
    Rash.
  animal-related, 1076-1084
  burns, 1091-1103
  cold injury, 1103-1104
  dermatitis, 1061-1062
  diagnosis of, 1061-1062
  family support in, 1069
  from chemical/physical irritants, 1074-1076
  home care for, 1069
  infectious, 1069-1074, 1070t, 1072t, 1073t
    bacterial, 1069-1071, 1070t, 1071f
    fungal, 1071-1074, 1073t, 1074t
    viral, 1071, 1072t
  lesions in, 1061-1062, 1063f-1064f
  miscellaneous, 1084-1091, 1085t-1086t
  nursing care in, 1067-1069
  pathophysiology of, 1061
  signs and symptoms of, 1061-1062
  terminology for, 1062
  topical therapy for, 1066t, 1067
  treatment of, 1065-1067
  wounds in, 1062-1065. See also Wounds.
Skin grafts, for burns, 1097, 1098-1099, 1098f,
    1099f
Skin substitutes, synthetic, 1097-1098
Skin tests
  for allergies, 786, 788
  for asthma, 786
  for tuberculosis, 778, 778b, 779b, 780
Skin texture, in newborn, 207
Skin turgor, 132
Skinfold thickness, 124
Skin-level device, for gastrostomy feeding, 747,
    749f
Skin-to-skin care, 77, 173-175, 175f
  for high-risk newborn, 262
  in thermoregulation, 254
Skull
  flattening of, positional plagiocephaly and,
    400-401
  fractures of, 988, 991. See also Head injury.
    during birth, 246
  malformations of, 1016-1017
  palpation of, 134
    in newborn, 207, 208f
Sleep
  age-related changes in, 77
  family bed and, 349
    SIDS and, 402
  in adolescent, 528, 528f
  in infant, 347-349, 348t
  in newborn, 214-215, 214t
    for patent airway maintenance, 215, 221
  in preschooler, 447-449, 448t
  in school-age child, 505
  in toddler, 424
  need for, 77
  positional plagiocephaly from, 215, 221,
    400-401, 401f
Sleep disorders
  in attention deficit hyperactivity disorder, 560
  obstructive sleep apnea, 803

Sleep terrors, vs. nightmares, 449, 449t
Slipped capital femoral epiphysis, 1130, 1130b
Slow-acting antirheumatic drugs, for juvenile
    idiopathic arthritis, 1140
Slow-to-warm-up temperament, 78
Small-for-gestational-age (SGA) infant, 204, 204f
Smegma, 210
Smell
  assessment of, 141, 155t
  in newborn, 201
  in toddler, 410
Smoke inhalation injury, 782-783
Smokeless tobacco, 566
Smoking, 565
  in pregnancy, fetal effects of, 311t
  second-hand smoke and, 783, 784b
Sneeze reflex, 212t
Snellen letter chart, 137, 1179
Sniffing, 567
Soaks, 1069
  for atopic dermatitis, 1088
Social development
  of adolescent, 520-521, 525t
  of infant, 331-333
  of preschooler, 440-442, 441f, 442f, 445t
  of school-age child, 497-499, 497f, 499f
  of toddler, 415, 416
Social roles, 52-53
Socialization, 52, 412. See also under Cultural;
    Culture.
  in autism, 635
  in chronic illness/disability, 618
  in hearing impairment, 626-627
  in home care, 654-655
  in hospitalization, 676
  in visual impairment, 631
Socioeconomic status
  class and, 54
  development and, 89
  disease susceptibility and, 58-59
  homelessness and, 54
  poverty and, 54
Sodium, 395t
Sodium bicarbonate
  for CPR, 807-809, 808t
  for diabetic ketoacidosis, 1049
Sodium imbalance
  in acute renal failure, 966
  in chronic renal failure, 968
Soft palate, 142, 142f
Soft spots, of newborn skull, 207
Soft tissue injuries, 1110-1112, 1111f
  birth-related, 244
Soft tissue sarcoma, 1138-1139, 1138b
Solid foods, for infants, 345-347
Solitary play, 333
Solutions
  dialysis, 970
  feeding, 749-750. See also Nutritional support.
  lavage, for bowel preparation, 750
Somatostatin, 1026t
Somatotropic hormone, 1025t
Somogyi effect, 1048
Sore throat, 761b, 762-763
  in infectious mononucleosis, 768
Sororal family, 34
Sound intensity, 624t
Soy-based formulas, 232
Spacer devices, 740
Spanish-English translations, 1204
Spanking, 42-43
Spasmodic laryngitis, 769, 769t, 771-772
Spasticity, in cerebral palsy, 1147b, 1148-1149
Special education. See Education.
Special needs children. See Chronic illness/
    disability; Cognitive impairment.

Specimen collection
    for blood. *See* Blood sampling; Venipuncture.
    for cerebrospinal fluid, 193, 710-711, 711f. *See also* Lumbar puncture.
    for respiratory secretions, 717
    for stool, 715
    for tissue. *See* Biopsy.
    for urine, 711-715
SPECT, in cerebral dysfunction, 981t
Speech. *See also* Communication; Language.
    cued, 626
    in hearing impairment, 626
Speech deficits, 626
    in autism, 635
    in cleft lip/cleft palate, 845
    in preschoolers, 447
Speech language therapy, 626
Spermicides, 545t
Spica casts, 1116, 1116f
    for developmental dysplasia of hip, 1124, 1124f
Spider bites, 1076-1079, 1077t-1078t, 1078f
Spina bifida, 210, 1154-1161
    bladder management in, 1156-1157
    bowel control in, 1157
    classification of, 1154, 1154f
    clinical manifestations of, 1155b, 1156-1157
    latex allergy in, 1159-1161
    mobility in, 1156
    nursing care in, 1158-1159
    pathophysiology of, 1154-1155
    prenatal diagnosis of, 1155-1156
    prevention of, 1157
    prognosis in, 1157
    spinal defects in, 1154, 1154f
    treatment of, 1156-1157
Spina bifida cystica, 1154, 1154f, 1155b
Spina bifida occulta, 1154, 1154f, 1155b
Spinal analgesia, 182t, 183-184, 184f
Spinal cord compression, 1170-1172
Spinal cord injuries, 1170-1172
Spinal curvature
    abnormal, 151, 1130-1134, 1131f
    screening for, 151
Spinal examination, 151-152
    in newborn, 210, 220t
Spinal fusion, for scoliosis, 1132-1133
Spinal muscular atrophy, 1161-1162, 1161b
Spiritual development, 79t, 81-82
    in adolescent, 520
    in preschooler, 439-440
    in school-age child, 496-497
    in toddler, 413-414
Spirituality
    definition of, 64
    faith healing and, 63-64
    neonatal loss and, 270
    vs. religion, 64. *See also* Religious beliefs.
Spironolactone (Aldactone), for congestive heart failure, 879t
Spitting up, 395
Spleen, palpation of, in newborn, 210, 219t
Splenectomy, for sickle cell anemia, 921
Splenic sequestration, in sickle cell anemia, 922
Splinters, 1076
Splints
    for burns, 1101, 1101f
    for intravenous infusion, 737
    for juvenile idiopathic arthritis, 1140
Split custody, 48
Sponge bath, cooling, 704
Sports participation, 505-506
    eating disorders in, 557
    injuries in, 532, 538-540
    refractive errors and, 633
Spot test, for infectious mononucleosis, 768

Sprains, 1111-1112
Sputum sample, collection of, 717, 757b, 780
Square window measurement, gestational age and, 204b
Stadiometer, 123, 123f
Stammering, 447
Standard precautions, 706, 707b
    high-risk newborn and, 255
    newborn bathing and, 224
Staphylococcal gastroenteritis, 817-823, 820t
Staphylococcal meningitis, 998-1002
Staphylococcal scalded skin syndrome, 1069-1071, 1070t, 1071f
Startle reflex, 209, 212t
Statin drugs, 895-896
Stature. *See* Height.
Status epilepticus, 1007, 1007b, 1009-1010
Statutory rape, 549-550, 549b
Stealing, in school-age child, 502-504
Steatorrhea, in cystic fibrosis, 796
Stem cell leukemia, 930. *See also* Leukemia.
Stem cell transplantation, 945-946
    apheresis in, 946
    for aplastic anemia, 925
    for leukemia, 931
    for severe combined immunodeficiency disease, 943
    for sickle cell anemia, 921
    graft versus host disease in, 945-946
    HLA matching in, 945-946
    nursing care in, 946
    types of, 946
Step reflex, 212t
Stereopsis, 325
Sternal angle, 143, 143f
Sternum, 143, 143f
Steroids. *See* Corticosteroids.
Stevens-Johnson syndrome, 1085t
Stimulants
    abuse of, 567
    for attention deficit hyperactivity disorder, 560
Stimulation, of newborn, 198
Stings, 1076-1079
    insect, 1076-1079, 1077t-1078t
Stoma care
    for enterostomy, 750-751
    for gastrostomy, 747
    for tracheostomy, 744-745, 745f
Stomatitis, 465-466, 466f
    in chemotherapy, 936-937
Stool. *See also under* Fecal.
    examination for occult blood, 914
    of newborn, 199, 200b
    specimen collection for, 715
Stool softeners, 824
Stork bites, 217t, 249
Storytelling, 106b
Strabismus, 135-136, 136f, 629t, 633
    amblyopia and, 629t, 633
    in newborn, 208
Strains, 1112
Stranger fear, in infants, 332, 335
Strangulation, infant, 368
Straterra (atomoxetine), for attention deficit hyperactivity disorder, 560
Strawberry hemangiomas, 249-250, 249f
Strep throat, 761b, 762-763
Streptococcal infection
    glomerulonephritis and, 961
    pharyngeal, 761b, 762-763
Streptococcal meningitis, 998-1002
Stress
    definition of, 89
    development and, 89-90
    family, 32

Stress *(Continued)*
    growth failure due to, 540
    in adolescent, 529, 530b, 530f
    in hospitalization
        child's response to, 659-664
        family's response to, 664, 664b
        in intensive care unit, 681-682, 681b
    in preschooler, 446-447
    in school-age child, 504
    newborn, 263t
    pain and, 189-190
Stress fractures, sports-related, 539
Stress management
    coping methods in, 90. *See also* Coping methods.
    emotional bank in, 89
    in Addison disease, 1039
Stroke, in sickle cell anemia, 918, 920-921, 922
Strongyloidiasis, 467t
Stump care, 1122
Stupor, 976b
Sturge-Weber syndrome, 249
Stuttering, 447
Subacute bacterial endocarditis, 891-893, 892b
Subcultures, 53. *See also* Race/ethnicity.
Subcutaneous injections, 723-724
Subdiaphragmatic abdominal thrusts, 809-810, 810f
Subdural hematoma, 987f, 988-989
Subdural tap, 980t
Subgaleal hemorrhage, 245-246, 245f
Subjective information, 24-25
Sublimaze (fentanyl), 175, 176t
Submandibular nodes, 133, 134f
Submental nodes, 133, 134f
Subpopulations, 21
Substance abuse, 7-8, 564-568
    addiction in, 188, 189, 564
    dependence in, 188, 189, 564
    in pregnancy, 300-305, 311t
    tolerance in, 188-189, 564
    withdrawal symptoms in, 188, 568
        newborn and, 302b
Subtotal colectomy, for inflammatory bowel disease, 835, 836
Subungual hematoma, 1111
Sucking, nonnutritive, 258, 342
    in pain management, 173
    pacifier aspiration in, 368
Sucking reflex, 209, 212t, 218t
Suckling technique, 231, 231f
Sucrose
    for circumcision pain, 227b
    for venipuncture pain, 174, 224b
Suctioning
    increased intracranial pressure and, 984
    oropharyngeal, in newborn, 221
Sudamina, 217t
Sudden infant death syndrome (SIDS), 401-404, 402t
Suffocation
    infant, 368-369
    toddler, 428t, 433
Suicide, 8, 564, 568-571
    assisted, 596
    attempted, 568
    physician-assisted. *See also* Treatment withholding.
    suicidal ideation and, 568, 570
Sulfamylon (mafenide), for burns, 1098t
Sunburn, 1103
    in infant, 371
    in toddler, 432
Sunscreen, 89
Superego, 78, 412, 439

Superficial palpation, 149
Supernumerary nipples, 209
Support groups
  for parents of high-risk newborns, 267
  for weight loss, 555
  in home care, 654-655
Suppositories, rectal, 730
  for anticonvulsants, 1015
Supraglottitis, 669t, 769-770
Suprapubic aspiration, 954-955
  for specimen collection, 713, 714
Suprasternal notch, 143, 143f
Supraventricular tachycardia, 896, 897
Surfactant
  for respiratory distress syndrome, 287
  in newborn, 198, 285
Surgery
  bariatric, 554
  body image and, 957-958
  bowel preparation for, 750
  cranial, 991
    for brain tumors, 995-996
  for amputation, 1121-1122
  for anorectal malformations, 854-855
  for appendicitis, 830-831
  for biliary atresia, 842
  for bladder exstrophy, 854-855
  for bone cancer, 1136-1137
  for cerebral palsy, 1148
  for cleft lip/cleft palate, 844-846
  for clubfoot, 1126
  for congenital heart disease, 867, 885, 886t,
    888-891. See also Congenital heart disease,
    surgery for.
  for cranial deformities, 1017
  for developmental dysplasia of hip, 1124-1125
  for esophageal atresia, 848-849
  for Ewing sarcoma, 1137-1138
  for gastroesophageal reflux disease, 828, 828f
  for Hirschsprung's disease, 826
  for hydrocephalus, 1018-1019, 1019f
  for inflammatory bowel disease, 835, 836
  for intussusception, 853
  for Meckel diverticulum, 832-833
  for obstructive uropathy, 957
  for osteomyelitis, 1134
  for peptic ulcers, 838
  for pyloric stenosis, 851-852, 851f
  for scoliosis, 1132-1134
  for seizures, 1009
  for short bowel syndrome, 857
  for sickle cell anemia, 921
  for sleep-disordered breathing, 803
  for spina bifida, 1156, 1158
  for tonsillitis/adenoiditis, 763-764
  for tracheoesophageal fistula, 848-849
  for weight loss, 554
  for Wilms tumor, 964
  genitourinary
    nursing care in, 958
    psychological aspects of, 957-958
  hospitalization for. See Hospitalization.
  outpatient, 679-680
  postoperative care in, 697-698
  postoperative pain in, 191-192
  preoperative care in, 694-697
  transplant. See Transplantation.
Sutures, cranial, 207, 208f
Swaddle restraint, 709, 710f
Swaddling
  for high-risk newborn, 262
  in pain management, 173
Sweat chloride test, 797
Swiss-type lymphopenic agammaglobulinemia, 943
Symbols, in cognitive development, 330

Symmetrel (amantadine), for influenza, 765
Sympathy, 101
Symptoms, 17
Syndactyly, 152, 210, 220t
Syndrome of inappropriate antidiuretic hormone
    secretion, 1031-1032
  in coma, 984
Synthetic skin, for burns, 1097-1098
Syphilis, 547, 548t
  congenital, 307t
Syringe. See also Needles.
  family teaching for, 731-732
  for intramuscular drugs, 719-720
  for needless intravenous systems, 734, 735f
  for oral medications, 719
Syrup of ipecac, 473
Systemic inflammatory response syndrome,
    906-907, 906b, 907t
Systemic lupus erythematosus, 1142-1143

T

T₃, 1026t, 1032
T₄, 1026t, 1032
Tachycardia, 216t
Tachydysrhythmias, 216t, 897
Tachypnea, 145b, 217t
Tactile sensation
  in newborn, 201
  in toddler, 410
Tactile stimulation, of newborn, 198
Talipes calcaneus, 1125
Talipes equinovarus, 1125-1126
Talipes equinus, 1125
Talipes valgus, 1125
Talipes varus, 1125
Tamiflu (oseltamivir), 765
Tampons, toxic shock syndrome and, 907, 907t
Tandem mass spectrometry, 223
Tanner scale, 515, 541
Tanning. See also Sunburn.
  by adolescents, 529
Tantrums, 421
Taping, 701
Tapping method, 631
Target populations, 21
Task analysis, 613
Taste
  in newborn, 201
  in toddler, 410
Tattooing, 529
Teachers, child's experience with, 500
Teaching. See Health/family teaching.
Team play, 499
Tear glands, 201
Teaspoons, for oral drugs, 719, 731
Teenager. See Adolescent.
Teeth. See also under Dental.
  avulsed, 507
  care of, 3, 701-702
    for adolescent, 528
    for infant, 349-350
    for preschooler, 450
    for school-age child, 506-507, 506f
    for toddler, 424-426, 425f, 426f, 426t
    in cerebral palsy, 1149
    in infant, 349-350
    in preschooler, 450
    in school-age child, 506-507, 506f
  deciduous, loss of, 493, 494f
  examination of, 142
  natal, vs. neonatal teeth, 209, 218t
Teething, 324, 342-343, 343f
Telangiectatic nevi, 217t
Telecommunication devices for the deaf (TDD),
    626

Telegraphic speech, 440
Telephone triage, 99, 100b
  for fever, 704
  in home care, 651
Teletypewriters, 626
Television
  closed captioning for, 626
  developmental effects of, 91-92
  obesity and, 552
Temper tantrums, 421
Temperament, 77-78, 77b, 334-335
  childrearing practices and, 335
Temperature, 77
  axillary, 126t, 127b, 128
    in newborn, 205, 205f, 216t
  core, 125, 127
  ear-based, 126t, 127b, 128
    in newborn, 205-206
  elevated. See Fever.
  inside parked car, 371-372, 431
  measurement of, 125-129, 125b, 125t-127t
  oral, 126t, 127b, 128
  rectal, 126t, 127b, 128
  regulation of, 77, 703
  stable, maintenance for newborns, 221
  temporal artery, 126t, 128
    in newborn, 206
  tympanic membrane, 205-206
Temperature regulation
  in infant, 324-325
  in newborn, 199
    at high risk, 252-254, 254f
  in toddler, 411
Temporal artery temperature, 126t, 128
  in newborn, 206
Tennison-Randall triangular flap, for cleft lip/cleft
    palate, 844
Tent, oxygen, 739
Teratogens, 308, 309-310, 311t
Terbutaline, for asthma, 788-789
Terminal care. See Death and dying.
Terrorism, toddler fears about, 434
Tertiary circular reactions, in cognitive develop-
    ment, 412
Testis
  cancer of, 542-543
  examination of, 150
    in newborn, 210
    self-examination, 543-544
  undescended, 150
Testosterone, 515, 1027t
Tet spells, 884-886
Tetanus, 1167-1168
  immunization for, 351, 356, 356t
  in burns, 1095
Tetracycline, in ophthalmia neonatorum prophy-
    laxis, 222
Tetralogy of Fallot, 870, 873b
  hypercyanotic spells in, 884-886
β-Thalassemia, 923-924, 923b
Thalidomide, limb deficiency and, 1127
Thelarche, 515
Therapeutic care, 11
Therapeutic holding, 709, 709f
Therapeutic play, 85, 674
Therapeutic procedures. See Procedures.
Therapeutic relationship, 11
  cultural aspects of, 60-61
  in family-centered care, 576-577
Thermal stimulus, in newborn, 198
Thermogenesis, 324-325
Thermometers, 127, 127b, 704-705
  for newborn, 205-206

Thermoregulation
  in coma, 984
  in infant, 324-325
  in newborn, 199, 221
Thiamine, 389t
Thimerosal, autism and, 635, 636
Third ventriculostomy, 1019
Third-person technique, 106b
Thirst
  in diabetes mellitus, 1044
  in syndrome of inappropriate antidiuretic
    hormone secretion, 1031
Thomas splint, 1119f
Thoracolumbosacral orthosis, 1131-1132, 1132f
Thorax. See Chest.
Thought stopping, for pain, 172
Three wishes technique, 106b
Throat, strep, 761b, 762-763
Throat culture, 762, 763
Thrush, in newborn, 218t, 248, 248f
Thumb sucking, 342
Thyrocalcitonin, 1026t, 1032
Thyroid, structure and function, 1026t
Thyroid crisis, 1034-1035
Thyroid disorders, 1032-1035
  goiter, 1033
  hyperthyroidism, 1034-1035, 1034b
  juvenile hypothyroidism, 1032-1033
  lymphocytic (Hashimoto) thyroiditis,
    1033-1034
Thyroid hormones, 1032
Thyroid storm, 1034-1035
Thyroiditis, lymphocytic (Hashimoto), 1033-1034
Thyroid-stimulating hormone, 1025t
Thyrotoxicosis, 1034-1035
Thyrotropin, 1025t
Thyroxine, 1026t, 1032
Tick bites, 1076-1079, 1077t
  rickettsial diseases due to, 1082-1083, 1082t
Time-out, 42, 43b
Tinea infections, 1071-1072, 1073f, 1073t, 1085t
Tissue turgor, 132
TLSO brace, 1131-1132, 1132f
Tobacco use, 565-566
  maternal, congenital effects of, 311t
Tocopherol, 391t
Toddler
  behavioral regression in, 422
  biologic development of, 410-411
  bodily damage to, 428t, 433-434
  body image of, 414-415
  burns in, 427t, 431-432, 432f
  chronic illness/disability in, 592t
  cognitive development of, 412-413, 413f
  communication with, 103-104
  dental health of, 424-426, 425f, 426f, 426t
  drowning of, 427t, 431
  gender identity of, 415
  injury of, prevention of, 426-434
  language development of, 415-416
  negativism in, 421-422
  personal-social behavior of, 416
  poisoning of, 427t, 432-433, 432f
  sensory functions of, 410
  sibling rivalry and, 420-421, 421f
  sleep and activity in, 424
  social development of, 415, 415f
  spiritual development of, 413-414
  suffocation of, 368-369, 428t
  temper tantrums in, 421
  terrorism and, 434
  toilet training of, 417-420, 420f
Toddler-Preschooler Postoperative Pain Scale
    (TPPPS), 161
Toeing in, 152

Toes
  catheter, 255
  clubbing of, 884
Toilet training, 417-420, 420f
Tolerable upper intake level, 114
Tolerance, 564
  to opioids, 188-189
Tolmetin (Tolectin), 175, 176t
Tongue
  examination of, 142
    in newborn, 209
  protruding, in Down syndrome, 622
Tongue-tie, 209
Tonic neck reflex, 212t, 213f
Tonic-clonic seizures, 1006b, 1014b. See also
    Seizures.
Tonsillar nodes, 133, 134f
Tonsillectomy, 763-764
  for sleep-disordered breathing, 803
Tonsillitis, 763-764, 763f
Tonsils, 142-143, 142f
Tooth. See Teeth.
Topical therapy, for skin lesions, 1067, 1068-1069
Topiramate, for bulimia nervosa, 558
TORCH complex, 305
Torticollis, 133, 218t
  positional plagiocephaly and, 400
Total anomalous pulmonary venous connection,
    875b
Total body surface area, in burns, 1091, 1092f
Total body water volume, in newborn, 199
Total parenteral nutrition, 749-750. See also Nutri-
    tional support.
  central venous catheter for, 725-730
  in inflammatory bowel disease, 835, 836
  in short bowel syndrome, 857
Touch
  for stimulation of newborn, 198
  in newborn, 201
  in toddler, 410
Touchpoints, for regression, in toddler develop-
    ment, 422
Toxic shock syndrome, 907, 907t
Toxocariasis, intestinal, 467t
Toxoplasmosis, maternal, 307t
Toys, 86, 617. See also Play.
  aspiration of, 367, 433
  for infants, 334t
  in hospitalization, 670, 673-674
  safety concerns for, 86, 87, 367, 433, 705-706
Trace elements, 379
Tracheal suctioning, increased intracranial pres-
    sure and, 984
Tracheitis, 769-770, 769t, 772
Tracheobronchitis, 772t, 773
Tracheoesophageal fistula, 846-849, 847f
Tracheomalacia, 848
Tracheostomy, 741-745
  emergency care of, 744-745, 745f
  routine care of, 744-745, 745f
  suctioning of, 741-744, 743f
Traction, 1117-1121, 1118f, 1119f
Transcutaneous bilirubinometry, 276-277
Transcutaneous oxygen monitoring, 740
Transesophageal electrocardiography, 896
Transfusion, 943-945, 944t
  administration of, 943-945
  apheresis in, 946
  complications of, 944t-945t
  for hemolytic disease of newborn, 282-283
  for hemophilia, 926, 927
  for sickle cell anemia, 920-921
  for thalassemia, 923-924
  HIV/AIDS transmission via, 927
  intrauterine, Rh isoimmunization and, 282

Transfusion (Continued)
  iron overload due to, 924
  platelet, 946
Transilluminators, 733, 733f, 734
Transitional objects, 415, 415f
Transitional stools, 200b
Translations
  for Wong-Baker FACES Pain Rating Scale,
    1202-1203
  Spanish-English, 1204
Translocations, chromosomal, 619
Transmission-based precautions, 706-707, 707b
Transparent film dressings, 1066t
Transplantation
  heart, 899
  intestinal, 857
  kidney, 969, 971
  liver, 841-842, 843
  organ donation for, 605
  stem cell
    for aplastic anemia, 925
    for sickle cell anemia, 921
Transport, of infants and children, 708
Transportation safety. See Automobile safety.
Transposition of great arteries, 874b
Traumatic alopecia, 1085t
Traumatic injuries, 3-6. See also Safety concerns.
  birth-related, 244-247, 245f-247f
  cerebral, 986-993. See also Head injury.
  dental, 507
  in infants, 365-374
  in preschoolers, 450
  intentional. See Abuse.
  mortality due to, 8t, 9-10, 9t
  musculoskeletal, 76, 1110-1117
  prevention of
    in adolescent, 531-532, 531b
    in school-age child, 508-509, 508f, 510t
  risk factors for, 5
  soft tissue, 1062-1065. See also Wounds.
  sports-related, 532, 538-540
  tetanus prophylaxis after, 356t
Travel. See also Automobile safety.
  diabetes mellitus and, 1053
Treatment. See also under Therapeutic.
Treatment compliance, 698-700
Treatment withholding
  in cystic fibrosis, 802
  in Down syndrome, 621
  in prematurity, 269
Tremor, in newborn, 295
Tretinoin (Retin-A), for acne, 1090
Triage, telephone, 99, 100b
Triceps reflex, 153f
Triceps skinfold, 1191
Trichomoniasis, 547, 548t
Trichotillomania, 1085t
Trichuriasis, 467t
Tricuspid atresia, 870, 873b-874b
Tricuspid valve, 146
Trigeminal nerve, assessment of, 155t
Triglycerides, elevated serum, 894-896
Triiodothyronine, 1026t, 1032
Trilisate (choline magnesium trisalicylate), for
    pain, 175, 176t
Triple drug therapy, for peptic ulcers, 838
Triple X superfemale, 541t
Tripod position, 769
Trisomy 13, 310t
Trisomy 18, 310t
Trisomy 21, 310t, 619-622
Trochlear nerve, assessment of, 155t
Trophic feedings, 256
  in necrotizing enterocolitis, 298
Truncus arteriosus, 865, 870, 875b-876b

Trunk incurvation reflex, 212t
Trust vs. mistrust, 79, 79t, 327
Trypsin, 324
Tubal tonsils, 763, 763f
Tuberculin skin test, 778, 778b, 779b, 780
Tuberculosis, 776-780
    skeletal, 1135-1136
Tumbling E test, 137
Tumors. See also Cancer.
    bone, 1136-1138
Tumor necrosis factor inhibitors, for juvenile
    idiopathic arthritis, 1140
Tunneled catheters, 725-730, 727t, 729f
Turgor, tissue, 132
Turner syndrome, 310t, 540, 541t
24-hour recall, 114
24-hour urine collection, 712-713
Twins, 37-38, 38b
    attachment process and, 237, 237f
    breastfeeding of, 230-231, 230f
    high-risk, developmental interventions for,
        262-263
Tylenol. See Acetaminophen (Tylenol).
Tylox, 175, 176t
Tympanic membrane
    examination of, 139-140, 139f, 140f
        in newborn, 209
    incision of, 767
    temperature measurement via, in newborn,
        205-206
Tympanostomy tubes, 767
Typewriter, Braille, 631-632
Typhoid fever, diarrhea in, 817-823, 818t
Typhus
    endemic, 1082t
    epidemic, 1082t
Tyrosine, PKU and, 313

U
Ugly duckling stage, 493
Ulcers
    cutaneous, 1064f
    oral, 465-466
        in chemotherapy, 936-937
    peptic, 836-838
    pressure, 700-701
        in coma, 985
    rectal, in chemotherapy, 937
Ulcerative colitis, 833-836
Ultrasonography
    in cerebral dysfunction, 980t
    in genitourinary disorders, 951t
Umbilical cord, examination of, 210, 219t
Umbilical cord blood stem cell transplantation,
        946. See also Stem cell transplantation.
Umbilical hernia, 148, 849, 850t
Umbilicus, 210
    abdominal circumference measurement and,
        205
    care of, infection control and, 225
    examination of, 148
Umbo, 139f, 140
Unconjugated bilirubin, 275
Unconscious mind, 78
Unconsciousness, 976. See also Coma.
    assessment in, 976-977, 977f
    nursing care in, 981-986
Undescended testis, 150
United Nations' Declaration of the Rights of the
        Child, 12, 13b
Upper respiratory infections, 759-768. See also
        Respiratory infections.
Uremia, 965, 967-970
Urethral meatus
    in female, 151, 151f
    in male, 150, 150f

Urethritis, 950-956. See also Urinary tract
        infections.
Uric acid, reference ranges for, 954t
Urinary catheterization, 713-714
    for neurogenic bladder, 1157
    for specimen collection, 713-714
    in coma, 984
Urinary diversion, 957
    for neurogenic bladder, 1157
Urinary elimination
    in coma, 984-985
    in diabetes mellitus, 1044
    in immobilization, 1108t
    in spina bifida, 1108t
    in spinal cord injuries, 1171
Urinary incontinence, 537-538. See also Enuresis.
    in coma, 984
    in sickle cell anemia, 921-922
    in spina bifida, 1156-1157
    in spinal cord injuries, 1171
Urinary retention, opioid-related, 180t
Urinary stasis, 954
Urinary system distress, in spina bifida, 1156-1157
Urinary tract infections, 950-956
    anatomic factors in, 950-954
    bacteriuria in, 950
    circumcision and, 950
    classification of, 950-954
    diagnosis of, 954-955
    etiology of, 950-954
    febrile, 950
    in obstructive uropathy, 957
    nursing care for, 955-956
    persistent, 950
    prevention of, 956
    prognosis of, 955
    recurrent, 950
    terminology for, 950
    treatment of, 955
Urinary tract obstruction, 956-957, 957f
Urine
    characteristics of, 953t
    volume of, in newborn, 200
Urine collection
    for intake and output measurement, 732, 960
    for urine testing, 711-715, 712f, 713f, 954, 956
Urine collection bag, 711-712, 712f
Urine specimens
    clean-catch, 712
    collection of, 711-715, 712f, 713f, 954, 956, 960
    midstream, 712
    twenty-four hour, 712-713
Urine tests, 951t
    for culture and sensitivity, 951t
    for glucose, in diabetes mellitus, 1046, 1056
    in renal assessment, 952t
Urobilinogen, 275
Urodynamic studies, 952t
Urostomy, 957
    for neurogenic bladder, 1157
Urticaria, 1085t
Urushiol, 1075
Uvula, 142, 142f
    of newborn, 209

V
Vaccines. See also Immunizations.
    autism and, 635, 636
    product brand names for, 364t
Vaccine Adverse Event Reporting System, 365
Vaccine Compensation Amendments, 365
Vaccine information statement, 365
VACTERL syndrome, 846, 854
Vagina, examination of, 151
    in newborn, 210
Vaginal discharge, in newborn, 200, 210, 219t

Vaginitis, 542
Vagus nerve, assessment of, 155t
Vagus nerve stimulation, for seizures, 1009
Valium. See Diazepam (Valium).
Valley fever, 1074t
Valproic acid, for status epilepticus, 1009
Values, culture and, 64-67
Varicella, 454f, 454t-455t
    immunization for, 357
    maternal infection with, 305t
    Reye syndrome and, 703
Varicella-zoster virus infection, 1072t
Vascular access, 725-730, 729f. See also Catheters/
        catheterization; Venipuncture.
    for intravenous infusion, 733-734
Vascular birthmarks, 249-250, 249f
Vasooclusive crisis, in sickle cell anemia, 918, 918b,
        921, 922
Vasopressin
    for hemophilia, 926
    for syndrome of inappropriate antidiuretic
        hormone secretion, 1031
    in newborn, 200
Vastus lateralis, injection in, 720, 721, 721f
VATER syndrome, 846, 854
Vegans, 380
Vegetarian diet, in infant, 379-380, 380b
Vehicular safety. See Automobile safety.
Venipuncture, 715-717
    extremity, positioning for, 710, 710f
    femoral, positioning for, 710
    for parenteral fluid therapy, 733, 733f
    pain management for, 173-174, 184-185, 224b,
        717
Venous hemangiomas, 250
Ventilation
    bag-mask, in CPR, 805
    in respiratory distress syndrome, 287, 287t
Ventilatory support. See also Airway management.
    in anaphylaxis, 905
    in Duchenne muscular dystrophy, 1164-1165
    in shock, 904
    in spinal cord injuries, 1171
    tracheostomy for, 741-744, 743f, 745f
Ventricular puncture, 980t
Ventricular septal defect, 867, 868b
Ventriculoperitoneal shunt, 1018-1020, 1019f
Ventriculostomy, endoscopic third, 1019
Ventrogluteal site, for injections, 720, 721, 721f
Vernix caseosa, 207, 324
Verruca, 1072t
Versed. See Midazolam (Versed).
Vesicants, extravasation of, 738
Vesicles, 1063f
Vesicostomy, for neurogenic bladder, 1157
Vesicoureteral reflux, 954, 955
Vestibulocochlear nerve, assessment of, 155t
Vibrio cholerae infection, 817-823, 819t. See also
        Diarrhea.
Vicodin (hydrocodone/acetaminophen), 176t
Video games, 92-93
    obesity and, 552
Vietnamese Americans. See also Race/ethnicity.
    health beliefs and practices of, 69t
Vinblastine, neurotoxicity of, 937
Vincristine, neurotoxicity of, 937
Violence, 5, 6-7. See also Abuse.
    bullying and, 498
    fears of, in toddlers, 434
    in mass media, 90-93
    mortality due to, 9-10, 9t-10t
Viral conjunctivitis, 465b
Viral encephalitis, 1002-1003
Viral infections, of skin, 1071, 1072t
Viral meningitis, 1002, 1002b
Viral pneumonia, 775-776

Virilization, in congenital adrenal hyperplasia, 1041
Virtual reality, in pain management, 173
Visceral larva migrans, 467t
Visible poverty, 54
Vision. *See also* Eye.
    color, 137
        in newborn, 201
    in adolescent, 528
    in infant, 325
    in newborn, 201
    peripheral, 137
Vision loss. *See* Visual impairment.
Vision testing, 135-137, 630
Visual acuity testing, 137
Visual aids, 632
Visual analog pain scale, 164, 164t
Visual evoked potentials, 979
Visual impairment, 628-635
    classification of, 628
    definition of, 628
    diagnosis of, 135-137, 630
    education in, 631-632
    etiology of, 628-630
    hospitalization in, 632
    independence in, 631
    mobility in, 631
    parent-child attachment in, 631
    play and socialization in, 631
    prevention of, 632-633
    rehabilitation in, 631
    screening for, 136-137, 1178-1179
    types of, 628t-629t
    with hearing impairment, 633
Visually evoked potentials, 137
Vital signs, 124-132
    in adolescent, 518
    in neurologic examination, 977
    in newborn, 205-207, 205f, 206f, 216t-217t
        at high risk, 252, 252t
    postoperative, 697, 698t
    pulse, 127-129
    respiratory rate, 129
    temperature, 124-127
Vitamin A, 388t
Vitamin B$_1$, 389t
Vitamin B$_2$, 389t
Vitamin B$_6$, 390t
Vitamin B$_{12}$, 390t
Vitamin C, 390t-391t
Vitamin D, 391t
Vitamin E, 391t
Vitamin imbalances, in infant, 378-379, 388t-392t
Vitamin K, 392t
    for newborn, 222, 292t
Voice, adolescent changes in, 516
Voiding. *See under* Urinary.
Voiding cystourethrography, 951t
Volvulus, intestinal, 853
Vomiting, 826-827
    fluid management in, 702
    in bulimia nervosa, 556-559

Vomiting *(Continued)*
    in chemotherapy, 936
    in pyloric stenosis, 849-850, 851t
Von Willebrand disease, 925-927
Voodoo, 63
Vulnerable child syndrome, 280, 654
Vulva, 151, 151f

W
Waldeyer tonsillar ring, 763, 763f
Walkers, infant, falls and, 370
Walking. *See also* Mobility.
    development of, 326-327, 329f
Warmer, radiant, 254, 254f
Warming techniques, in frostbite, 1104
Warts
    cutaneous, 1072t
    genital, 547, 548t
Wasp stings, 1077t
Water. *See also under* Fluid.
    daily requirements for, 76, 815, 815b
Water intoxication, in acute renal disease, 968
Waterhouse-Friderichsen syndrome, 1037
Weaning
    from opioids, 188, 190t
    of infant, 347
Weight. *See also* Growth.
    birth. *See* Birth weight.
    body mass index and, 121-122
    ethnic differences in, 122, 123f
    genetic factors in, 552
    measurement of, 123-124, 124f
        in newborn, 205, 216t
    reference ranges for, 1180-1191
    regulation of, 551-552
Weight gain. *See also* Obesity.
    in preschooler, 438
    in toddler, 410
    normal, 75, 75t
Weight loss
    in anorexia, 556-559
    in newborn, 205, 216t
    methods of, 553-556
Werdnig-Hoffmann disease, 1161-1162, 1161b
West nomogram, 718
Wet compresses, 1069
Wet dressings, 1069
    for atopic dermatitis, 1088
    for burns, 1095-1096
Wharton jelly, 219t
Wheals, 1063f
Wheelchairs, 591
Wheezes, 145, 757b
Whey-hydrolysate formulas, 232
Whitaker perfusion test, 952t
White blood cells
    in complete blood count, 913t
    in urine, 953t
Whooping cough, 458t-461t, 776
    immunization for, 356

Wilmington brace, 1131
Wilms tumor, 963-965, 963b, 964b
Wiskott-Aldrich syndrome, 943
Witchcraft, 63
Witch's milk, 200, 209
Withdrawal
    coital, 544
    in substance abuse, 568
        newborn and, 302b
    opioid, 188, 189, 568
Wong-Baker FACES Pain Rating Scale, 162t, 164
    translations for, 1202-1203
Word association game, 106b
Word-graphic rating scale, 163t, 164
Work-based group care, for infants, 340
Work-family balance, 48-49
Working mothers, 48
Wounds, 1062-1065. *See also* Skin disorders.
    acute, 1062
    assessment of, 1067-1068
    chronic, 1062
    healing of, 1062-1065, 1065t
    scars from, 1062, 1064f
Wound care, 1065-1067, 1066t
    dressings in, 1065-1067, 1066t, 1068. *See also* Dressings.
    enzymatic débridement in, 1066t
    for animal bites, 1083
    for burns, 1095, 1096, 1097, 1100
    for human bites, 1083
    nursing care in, 1068
    symptom relief in, 1068
    topical therapy in, 1067, 1068-1069
Wound sepsis, in burn patients, 1094
Wrist, fractures of, 1113f, 1114
Wryneck, 133, 218t

X
Xenograft, for burns, 1097
X-linked inheritance, dominant with reduced penetrance, 622
X-linked lymphopenic agammaglobulinemia, 943

Y
Yawn reflex, 212t
Yellow jacket stings, 1077t
Yersinia enterocolitis, 812-823, 819t. *See also* Diarrhea.
Yin and yang, 63
Yogurt, lactose intolerance and, 387-388

Z
Zanamivir, for influenza, 765
Zielke instrumentation, 1132
Zinc, 395t
    deficiency of, in newborn, 259-260
Zoster, 463, 1072t
Z-plasty, for cleft lip/cleft palate, 844

Blood Pressure (BP) Levels for Girls by Age and Height Percentile

AGE (yr)	BP PERCENTILE	SYSTOLIC BP (mm Hg) PERCENTILE OF HEIGHT							DIASTOLIC BP (mm Hg) PERCENTILE OF HEIGHT						
		5th	10th	25th	50th	75th	90th	95th	5th	10th	25th	50th	75th	90th	95th
1	50th	83	84	85	86	88	89	90	38	39	39	40	41	41	42
	90th	97	97	98	100	101	102	103	52	53	53	54	55	55	56
	95th	100	101	102	104	105	106	107	56	57	57	58	59	59	60
	99th	108	108	109	111	112	113	114	64	64	65	65	66	67	67
2	50th	85	85	87	88	89	91	91	43	44	44	45	46	46	47
	90th	98	99	100	101	103	104	105	57	58	58	59	60	61	61
	95th	102	103	104	105	107	108	109	61	62	62	63	64	65	65
	99th	109	110	111	112	114	115	116	69	69	70	70	71	72	72
3	50th	86	87	88	89	91	92	93	47	48	48	49	50	50	51
	90th	100	100	102	103	104	106	106	61	62	62	63	64	64	65
	95th	104	104	105	107	108	109	110	65	66	66	67	68	68	69
	99th	111	111	113	114	115	116	117	73	73	74	74	75	76	76
4	50th	88	88	90	91	92	94	94	50	50	51	52	52	53	54
	90th	101	102	103	104	106	107	108	64	64	65	66	67	67	68
	95th	105	106	107	108	110	111	112	68	68	69	70	71	71	72
	99th	112	113	114	115	117	118	119	76	76	76	77	78	79	79
5	50th	89	90	91	93	94	95	96	52	53	53	54	55	55	56
	90th	103	103	105	106	107	109	109	66	67	67	68	69	69	70
	95th	107	107	108	110	111	112	113	70	71	71	72	73	73	74
	99th	114	114	116	117	118	120	120	78	78	79	79	80	81	81
6	50th	91	92	93	94	96	97	98	54	54	55	56	56	57	58
	90th	104	105	106	108	109	110	111	68	68	69	70	70	71	72
	95th	108	109	110	111	113	114	115	72	72	73	74	74	75	76
	99th	115	116	117	119	120	121	122	80	80	80	81	82	83	83
7	50th	93	93	95	96	97	99	99	55	56	56	57	58	58	59
	90th	106	107	108	109	111	112	113	69	70	70	71	72	72	73
	95th	110	111	112	113	115	116	116	73	74	74	75	76	76	77
	99th	117	118	119	120	122	123	124	81	81	82	82	83	84	84
8	50th	95	95	96	98	99	100	101	57	57	57	58	59	60	60
	90th	108	109	110	111	113	114	114	71	71	71	72	73	74	74
	95th	112	112	114	115	116	118	118	75	75	75	76	77	78	78
	99th	119	120	121	122	123	125	125	82	82	83	83	84	85	86
9	50th	96	97	98	100	101	102	103	58	58	58	59	60	61	61
	90th	110	110	112	113	114	116	116	72	72	72	73	74	75	75
	95th	114	114	115	117	118	119	120	76	76	76	77	78	79	79
	99th	121	121	123	124	125	127	127	83	83	84	84	85	86	87
10	50th	98	99	100	102	103	104	105	59	59	59	60	61	62	62
	90th	112	112	114	115	116	118	118	73	73	73	74	75	76	76
	95th	116	116	117	119	120	121	122	77	77	77	78	79	80	80
	99th	123	123	125	126	127	129	129	84	84	85	86	86	87	88
11	50th	100	101	102	103	105	106	107	60	60	60	61	62	63	63
	90th	114	114	116	117	118	119	120	74	74	74	75	76	77	77
	95th	118	118	119	121	122	123	124	78	78	78	79	80	81	81
	99th	125	125	126	128	129	130	131	85	85	86	87	87	88	89
12	50th	102	103	104	105	107	108	109	61	61	61	62	63	64	64
	90th	116	116	117	119	120	121	122	75	75	75	76	77	78	78
	95th	119	120	121	123	124	125	126	79	79	79	80	81	82	82
	99th	127	127	128	130	131	132	133	86	86	87	88	88	89	90
13	50th	104	105	106	107	109	110	110	62	62	62	63	64	65	65
	90th	117	118	119	121	122	123	124	76	76	76	77	78	79	79
	95th	121	122	123	124	126	127	128	80	80	80	81	82	83	83
	99th	128	129	130	132	133	134	135	87	87	88	89	89	90	91
14	50th	106	106	107	109	110	111	112	63	63	63	64	65	66	66
	90th	119	120	121	122	124	125	125	77	77	77	78	79	80	80
	95th	123	123	125	126	127	129	129	81	81	81	82	83	84	84
	99th	130	131	132	133	135	136	136	88	88	89	90	90	91	92
15	50th	107	108	109	110	111	113	113	64	64	64	65	66	67	67
	90th	120	121	122	123	125	126	127	78	78	78	79	80	81	81
	95th	124	125	126	127	129	130	131	82	82	82	83	84	85	85
	99th	131	132	133	134	136	137	138	89	89	90	91	91	92	93
16	50th	108	108	110	111	112	114	114	64	64	65	66	66	67	68
	90th	121	122	123	124	126	127	128	78	78	79	80	81	81	82
	95th	125	126	127	128	130	131	132	82	82	83	84	85	85	86
	99th	132	133	134	135	137	138	139	90	90	90	91	92	93	93
17	50th	108	109	110	111	113	114	115	64	65	65	66	67	67	68
	90th	122	122	123	125	126	127	128	78	79	79	80	81	81	82
	95th	125	126	127	129	130	131	132	82	83	83	84	85	85	86
	99th	133	133	134	136	137	138	139	90	90	91	91	92	93	93

The 90th percentile is 1.28 SD, the 95th percentile is 1.645 SD, and the 99th percentile is 2.326 SD over the mean.